CASTLE CONNOLLY
TOP DOCTORS
New York Metro Area

16th Edition

Top Doctors Make A Difference

America's Trusted Source For Identifying Top Doctors

For more information, please contact:

Castle Connolly Medical Ltd., 42 West 24th St, New York, New York 10010
212-367-8400x110
E-mail: info@castleconnolly.com
Web site: http://www.castleconnolly.com.

Library of Congress Control Number: 2012939941
ISBN   1-883769-60-4   978-1-883769-60-4   (paperback)
ISBN   1-883769-58-2   978-1-883769-58-1   (hardcover)
Printed in the United States of America

Table of Contents

Table of Contents

Table of Contents

Table of Contents

Table of Contents

Table of Contents

Table of Contents

Hippocratic Oath

I swear by Apollo the physician, and Asklepios, and health, and All-Heal and all the gods and goddesses, that, according to my ability and judgement, I will keep this Oath and this stipulation — to reckon him who taught me this Art equally dear to me as my parents, to share my substance with him, and relieve his necessities if required; to look upon his offspring in the same footing as my own brothers, and to teach them this Art, if they should wish to learn it, without fee or stipulation; and that by precept, lecture and every other mode of instruction, I will impart a knowledge of the Art to my own sons, and those of my teachers, and to disciples bound by a stipulation and oath according to the law of medicine, but to none others.

I will follow that system of regimen which, according to my ability and judgement, I consider for the benefit of my patients, and abstain from whatever is deleterious and mischievous. I will give no deadly medicine to anyone if asked nor suggest any such counsel; and in like manner I will not give to a woman a pessary to produce abortion. With purity and wholeness I will pass my life and practice my Art.

I will not cut persons labouring under the stone, but will leave this to be done by men who are practitioners of this work. Into whatever houses I enter, I will go into them for the benefit of the sick, and will abstain from every voluntary act of mischief and corruption; and, further, from the seduction of females or males, of freemen and slaves. Whatever, in connection with my professional practice, or not in connection with it, I see or hear, in the life of men, which ought not to be spoken of abroad, I will not divulge, as reckoning that all such should be kept secret. While I continue to keep this Oath unviolated, may it be granted to me to enjoy life and the practice of the art, respected by all men, in all times! But should I trespass and violate this Oath, may the reverse be my lot!

From Dorland's Illustrated Medical Dictionary. 27th ed. (Philadelphia) W.B. Saunders Co., 1988. Hippocratic Oath. [Hippocrates. Greek physician, 460-377 B.C.]

About the Publishers

John K. Castle, the Chairman of Castle Connolly Medical Ltd., has spent much of the last three decades involved with healthcare institutions and issues. Mr. Castle served as Chairman of the Board of New York Medical College for eleven years, an institution where he served on the Board of Trustees for twenty-two years.

Mr. Castle has been extensively involved in other healthcare and voluntary activities as well. He served for five years as a commissioner and officer of the Joint Commission formerly known as (JCAHO), the body which accredits most public and private hospitals throughout the United States. Mr. Castle has also served as a trustee of five different hospitals in the metropolitan New York region, including NewYork Presbyterian Hospital, where he continues to serve.

Mr. Castle has also served as the Chairman of the Columbia Presbyterian Science Advisory Council and as a Director of the Whitehead Institute for Biomedical Research. He is a Fellow of New York Academy of Medicine and has served as a Trustee of the Academy. He was Chairman of the United Hospital Fund of New York's Capital Campaign and continues as Director Emeritus of the United Hospital Fund. He is a Life Member of the MIT Corporation, the governing body of the Massachusetts Institute of Technology.

Mr. Castle received his bachelor's degree from the Massachusetts Institute of Technology, his MBA as a Baker Scholar with High Distinction from Harvard, and two Honorary Doctorate degrees.

Mr. Castle's goal, as is the goal of Dr. John Connolly and all the Castle Connolly team, is to publish *America's Top Doctors®*, *America's Top Doctors® for Cancer*, *Top Doctors: New York Metro Area*, and other materials as well as build websites to help the public identify the very best in healthcare resources.

John J. Connolly, Ed.D., - the nation's foremost expert on identifying top physicians, is the President & CEO of Castle Connolly Medical Ltd. publisher of *America's Top Doctors*® and other consumer guides to help people find the best healthcare. He is also Vice-Chairman of Castle Connolly Graduate Medical Ltd., which publishes review manuals to assist resident physicians and fellows in preparing for their board exams.

Dr. Connolly served as President of New York Medical College, the nation's second largest private medical college, for more than ten years. He is a Fellow of the New York Academy of Medicine, a Fellow of the New York Academy of Sciences, a Director of the Northeast Business Group on Health, a member of the President's Council of the United Hospital Fund, and a member of the Board of the American Swiss Foundation.

Dr. Connolly has served as trustee of two hospitals and as Chairman of the Board of one. He is extensively involved in healthcare and community activities and has served on a number of voluntary and corporate boards including the Board of the American Lyme Disease Foundation, of which he is a founder and past chairman, and the Culinary Institute of America for over 20 years where he is now Chairman Emeritus. He also served as a director and Chairman of the Professional Examination Service and is presently on the board of the American Swiss Foundation. His current corporate board service includes: Baker and Taylor; Air Methods Corporation; Dearborn Risk Management and the Advisory Board of the Hudson Group. He holds a Bachelor of Science degree from Worcester State College, a Master's degree from the University of Connecticut, and a Doctor of Education degree in College and University Administration from Teacher's College, Columbia University, honorary doctorates (LHD) from Mercy College and Worcester State University.

Over the years, Dr. Connolly has served on the boards of, and as an officer of, numerous not-for-profit organizations including: President, Sullivan County Association for Retarded Children; Director and Chairman United Way of Dutchess County; Director and Founding Chairman Dutchess County Industrial Development Agency; Director and Founder Dutchess County Economic Development Association, President, Westchester County Historical Society.

Medical Advisory Board

Castle Connolly Medical Ltd. is pleased to be associated with a distinguished group of medical leaders who offer invaluable advice and wisdom in its efforts to assist consumers in making good healthcare choices. We thank each member of the Medical Advisory Board for their valuable contributions.

Foreword

Dear Reader:

Choosing a doctor is one of the most important choices in your life. However, most of us put little effort into this selection. We simply pick a name from a list or get a recommendation from a friend.

Most of us have very little information about our doctors, and/or don't know where to get it. With the publication of this Castle Connolly Guide—Top Doctors: New York Metro Area, you can learn about doctors' medical school education, residency, training, fellowships, board certifications, hospital appointments and much more. The Guide also describes in simple terms what information you should ascertain about each doctor and how to evaluate it. This information gathering is essential for anyone who wants to find a good doctor to truly meet his or her healthcare needs.

As an administrator and nurse who deals with the problems of health on a daily basis, I know well the importance of getting the best healthcare. Our center assists medical malpractice victims. The human tragedy we often encounter is heartbreaking.

In many cases, had the patient taken a few minutes to make a modest effort to learn more about his or her doctor's background, a serious incident may have been avoided.

That is why *Top Doctors: New York Metro Area* is so important to consumers. In this new and rapidly changing healthcare environment, patients must be well informed. Many do not trust the healthcare system. They are not confident that their health plan, their hospital, or even their doctor, is motivated to protect them and to ensure that they get excellent care.

The Castle Connolly Guide is a comprehensive guide chock full of valuable information. It is completely consumer-friendly, giving readers all that they need to know to make intelligent, informed choices.

Use it well and in good health!

Sincerely,

Sandra Gainer, R.N.
Associate Director
National Center for Patient Rights

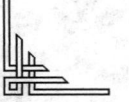
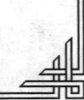

The Best in American Medicine
www.CastleConnolly.com

Introduction

A savvy consumer, searching for a car, restaurant, house or even a spouse, can easily find a guidebook to help. Yet, when it comes to choosing healthcare providers, the bookshelves are nearly bare.

Top Doctors: New York Metro Area has been written to fill that void. It will guide you in making critical —even lifesaving—choices.

This Guide Has Two Goals:

- To provide you with a base of information and a framework of understanding so that you can participate in the important healthcare choices that will maximize your own health, your family's health and the quality of your life.

- To provide detailed information on more than 6,000 well-trained, highly competent physicians from which you may confidently choose your personal best doctors for your own healthcare needs and those of your family.

Medicine is often described as a combination of art and science. This description holds true for the process of selecting the best medical care. This book describes the "science" of making that selection. It is not magical or even difficult. It is simply a matter of knowing what information you should have and where to find it.

The "art" is what you will bring to the selection process. It is based upon your feelings, your needs and the chemistry that develops between you and those who provide your healthcare. Castle Connolly's *Top Doctors: New York Metro Area* will help you prepare for that interaction and will guide you in getting the most from it.

Most importantly, Castle Connolly's *Top Doctors: New York Metro Area* will tell you how to combine the art and science so that you can make the best choices.

How to Use This Guide

This book has been written as a basic, "how to" guide for selecting the best healthcare. Section One provides important information on how to choose the best doctors. Doctors are the most important providers of healthcare and regardless of the type of medical insurance you have, you want the very best doctors to attend to your healthcare needs. Section Three contains listings of doctors as well as information on hospitals invited to participate in the Guide's Partnership for Excellence program. Section Four includes information on "Centers of Excellence"—special programs and services—offered by a number of the hospitals participating in the Partnership for Excellence program. Section Five contains seven appendices with important and interesting information.

Introduction

There Are Two Effective Ways to Use This Guide:

- Start at the beginning. This method will give you a broad understanding of the healthcare field and a clearer perspective of where you, the patient, fit in it. This method will arm you with necessary information for making informed choices and will help you find the best doctors.

- Study the doctor listings. While at least a brief reading of some or all of the introductory chapters is recommended so that, in the end, you will make well-informed choices, it is understandable that you may wish to go straight to the physician listings. The organization of these listings is outlined on pages 71 to 79. You will find guidelines for effectively using the listings on these pages.

Each chapter begins with explanations of terms that may be new to you. Reviewing these terms will help you read the section more easily.

In preparing this book, we've left little to chance or question. We hope to inspire you to assume a curious and insistent attitude as you make the healthcare choices that will take you and your family through life.

The Doctor of Choice

Primary Care Physicians

Quick Tips

- The time to establish a relationship with a doctor is while you are healthy. The top doctor to establish your relationship with is the one who is most likely to keep you healthy: A primary care doctor.

- Primary means first, so a primary care doctor is the first one you see for most health problems.

- It is difficult for any doctor, however skilled, to make judgements based on only one visit or a single test.

- Your primary care doctor can educate you about the "hows" and "whys" of health maintenance and disease prevention and follow up to help you stay faithful to the course the two of you have agreed upon.

- Any doctor with a license can practice in any specialty he/she chooses. Board certification is your assurance that the doctor has appropriate training in the specialty.

- When considering recommendations, use the old navigational technique of triangulation: focus on doctors whose names are mentioned by three or more people.

- Hospital telephone referral lines are not designed to distinguish among hundreds of doctors who may be more or less well regarded by other doctors, or who may be better suited to a particular caller when factors other than location, insurance coverage and office hours are taken into consideration.

- Many local medical societies publish directories, some of which are intended primarily for doctor-to-doctor referrals, while others are distributed to the public. They provide information but do not address quality.

- The internet provides many websites that provide lists of doctors: some are of questionable quality. Be careful that the information is from a trusted source.

Quick Take

... Primary care physician. That's a hot term in healthcare today. Who is this physician? How do you find one?...

Key Terms

Lupus Erythematosus - An autoimmune disorder, also referred to as SLE, or simply "lupus". It can cause inflammation and possible damage to a number of vital organs and is commonly marked by joint pain, facial and other rashes, abnormally high antibody levels, and diminished red blood cell levels.

Lyme Disease - An infectious disease, transmitted through the bite of a deer tick, which may or may not produce a distinctive bull's-eye rash at the site of the tick bite. First identified in Lyme, Connecticut, the infection may also produce other symptoms, including flu-like aches, arthritic joint pain, and, in complicated cases, cardiac abnormalities.

Managed Care - The process of integrating the finance and delivery of healthcare to control costs and improve quality. A managed care plan typically involves a group of practitioners who "manage" care for a specified population.

Osteopath - A healthcare professional who has earned a degree in osteopathic medicine, a D.O. Osteopathic medicine emphasizes massage and bone manipulation while traditional western allopathic medicine emphasizes treatment with drugs and surgery.

Preventive Medicine/Care - Health services that are aimed at maintaining good health and preventing illness. These services include routine physical examinations, immunizations, certain screening tests such as mammograms or Pap tests, as well as the practice of good health habits.

Primary Care Physician - The first doctor consulted for any health problem, a Primary Care Physician is a specialist who offers basic, including preventive, medical care. It is important to maintain an ongoing relationship with your primary care physician.

Specialist - A physician who practices in one or more of the 25 specialties defined by the American Board of Medical Specialties (ABMS). The term is also used to denote a physician's area of practice, such as pediatrics, geriatrics, surgery, etc.

Subspecialist - A specialist who obtains further training and certification in one or more of the 70 subspecialties approved by the American Board of Medical Specialties. The physician must first be certified in a specialty. For example, a board certified internist may become certified in cardiology or gastroenterology.

Primary Care Physicians

When it comes to choosing a doctor, too many people let the decision slide until they are sick or hurt and need immediate medical attention. That's unfortunate if an illness that could have been managed successfully develops to a stage where it becomes difficult to control or cure. It's even more unfortunate if the illness could have been prevented in the first place.

The time to establish a relationship with a doctor is while you are healthy, and the best one to establish your relationship with is the one who is most likely to keep you healthy: a primary care doctor.

Primary means first, so a primary care doctor is the first one you see for any health problem. Primary also means basic, so a primary care doctor offers the kind of fundamental care that can keep you healthy.

Yes, You Do Need a Doctor When You're Healthy.

Here are four good reasons why you should start your search for a primary care doctor now:

Reason One

A primary care doctor can put your current medical condition into a context that consists of your medical history, current condition as compared with past medical status, and changes in your body and environment over time. It is difficult for any doctor, however skilled, to make informed medical judgments based on only one visit or a single test. Conditions well out of normal range are easy to pick up, but extreme variations do not always occur and a serious illness may develop slowly with only a gradual increase in symptoms. The operative word is continuity: ideally, your medical care should not be interrupted by changes in providers.

Reason Two

A primary care doctor is better able to treat you as a whole person. Medicine has become very specialized and procedure-oriented, but the human body is not a loose collection of unrelated parts. It is a "whole" with strong interrelationships among all biological systems. Some of the poorest medical care results from people jumping from subspecialist to subspecialist. Despite talent, skill and training, no specialist knows the patient well enough, or for long enough, to be able to take the whole person into consideration and track the normal patterns of evolution and change. We end up with a specialist for every organ and system instead of a doctor who will care for the whole person.

Reason Three

A primary care doctor can establish preventive programs. Our healthcare system does not place enough emphasis on preventing illness; most healthcare dollars are spent on curative, rather than preventive, medicine. However, the status quo is slowly changing, and it is within primary care that the change is most evident. Your primary care doctor can educate you about the hows and whys of health maintenance and disease prevention and can follow up to help you stay faithful to the course the two of you have agreed upon. Only an ongoing relationship makes this possible.

Reason Four

A primary care doctor can save you money. Managed care advocates, among others, have long deplored the waste inherent in a system in which patients can simply call any specialist any time they have an ache or pain or are not feeling well. Primary care doctors can monitor referrals to specialists, following the patient closely to put together a variety of observations, opinions, and test results in order to treat each person on an individual basis. This improves the quality of care and also controls costs.

Patients who visit specialists without some guidance from a primary care doctor may choose the wrong specialist based on a general observation and self-diagnosis about the problem or illness they're experiencing. While in some cases the problem may be obvious (for example, an eye injury), in others it may be more subtle. Diseases such as lupus erythematosus and Lyme disease, for example, often have a myriad of symptoms that are easily misinterpreted by laypersons; in fact, they are often difficult even for doctors to diagnose accurately. While certain problems may require the collaboration of several specialists, it is important to have a primary care doctor navigating the course.

Finally, it is estimated that almost half of all emergency room visits in some areas are for non-emergencies; it's the most expensive place to receive primary care. When people have primary care doctors, they tend to turn to them rather than to hospital emergency departments.

If you are enrolled in any kind of managed care program, health maintenance organization (HMO) or other program, you will almost always be required to select a primary care doctor from its roster. Managed care executives recognize the necessity of a primary care doctor, not only for delivering quality healthcare, but also for controlling costs.

How to Find a Doctor

Unless you already have a primary care doctor you are satisfied with, you will have to find one. How? Here are five possible avenues to begin the process of finding the doctor that best suits your needs; each has limits, however.

Doctor Referrals

If you are moving and are leaving a trusted doctor behind, get a recommendation or two before you go. Furthermore, ask in what context and how well your doctor knows the new doctor—they may not have met since medical school.

Friends and Relatives

Always keep in mind that such recommendations are based largely on what may be "simpatico," or a personal affinity. Ask why your friend likes the doctor. It might be because the fees are low or the doctor makes house calls or is warm and sociable—all valid considerations, but certainly not principal determinants. So be wary of the generalized recommendation that "Dr. Jones is just wonderful." When considering recommendations, use the old navigational technique of triangulation: focus on doctors whose names are mentioned by three or more people.

Hospital Referral Services

Hospital telephone referral lines are not designed to distinguish among hundreds of doctors who may be more or less well regarded by other doctors, or who may be better suited to a particular caller when factors other than location, insurance coverage and office hours are taken into consideration. It would be impolitic for hospital referral services to rate their doctors. Their recommendations are based on specialty and geographic proximity, usually by way of a computer that rotates through the lists to "recommend" the next three names in line, and all members of the medical staff are eligible to participate.

Medical Society Directories

Many local medical societies publish directories, some of which are intended primarily for doctor-to-doctor referrals, while others are distributed to the public. These directories usually provide names, addresses, phone numbers and specialties and can be useful sources. However, they do not distinguish among doctors in any way. All members of the medical society, usually a countywide organization, are eligible for inclusion. This also applies to the referral lines offered by many medical societies.

The Internet

There are many websites that provide information on doctors. Some are directories or internet phone books. These can be helpful. Some claim to be based on quality measures. Many of these require physicians to pay, others are of questionable quality. Be sure the site sponsor or source is a trusted one.

Chapter 1

Many Ways to Say Doctor

In this guide, the term "doctor" is used to describe only medical doctors who have received a Doctor of Medicine degree (MD) and osteopaths who have received a Doctor of Osteopathic Medicine degree (DO). Doctors who have been trained in the British system may hold a degree of Bachelor of Medicine (MB), Bachelor of Surgery (BS), or Bachelor of Chirurgia (BCh), which is based on the ancient Greek term that refers to surgery.

The more formal term for any of these practitioners is "physician." However, most people use the more popular term "doctor," which is the one generally used in this book. Our discussions do not include other kinds of doctors such as dentists, podiatrists, psychologists or chiropractors, who also deliver healthcare.

Primary Care: The Fundamental Four

There is not complete agreement in medicine on which specialties are practiced by the group of doctors known as primary care specialists. For the purposes of this book, we have included the following specialties: Internal Medicine, Pediatrics, Family Practice and Obstetrics and Gynecology. Most adults choose general internists as their primary care doctors and select pediatricians for their children. There is also another type of specialist, the family practitioner, who cares for both children and adults. In addition to such generalists, many women also select an obstetrician/gynecologist as their primary care providers.

- A **general internist**, specializing in internal medicine, is trained to treat all internal organs and systems of the body. Many internists also are board certified in a subspecialty such as cardiology, gastroenterology or geriatric medicine. Therefore, if you have a history of heart disease, you may wish to select an internist who has additional training in cardiology, but who primarily practices general internal medicine. On the other hand, your primary care doctor may refer you to a cardiologist when necessary, and both may treat you over a period of years. In fact, it is not unusual for a patient with a serious or complex illness to be followed by two or three doctors, with the primary care doctor "quarterbacking" the team.

- A **family practitioner** is very broadly trained. Such doctors come closest to the general practitioner of the past. They are qualified to treat all family members, including children.

- A **pediatrician** is the doctor you would choose for the care of your children. As with doctors in internal medicine, pediatricians often have a subspecialty such as cardiology, rheumatology or endocrinology.

- **Obstetricians and Gynecologists** are the subject of significant debate in terms of their appropriateness as primary care doctors. The American Board of Obstetrics and Gynecology states that these doctors are specialists and are not generally trained for primary care. However, the reality is that many, particularly those who solely practice gynecology, often serve as a woman's primary care doctor. Gynecologists are divided on the issue. One recent study showed that 95 percent of visits to ob-gyns are self-referred and that about 60 percent of visits to these specialists are for diagnostic services and preventive services. Another study, by the American College of Obstetricians and Gynecologists, showed that 54 percent of women who see a gynecologist use these doctors for primary care. Reflecting the reality of current medical practice, we have included these specialists in the primary care category.

A businessman in his late fifties, a long-time competitive runner, had surgery in one of New York's top hospitals to repair a badly torn Achilles tendon. At his first follow-up visit to the orthopaedic surgeon, he was assured that "everything was healing perfectly," that he had nothing to be concerned about, and that he would soon be up and running again. Shortly thereafter, just before a summer camping trip, he decided to have his yearly physical examination. The primary care doctor examined the site of the surgery, probing up and down the whole length of the leg. Explaining that he was concerned about certain swelling and discoloration, the doctor arranged for a further examination with ultrasound imaging. This sophisticated test showed that a blood clot had formed in the upper part of the leg, which could have caused severe disability and even death had it gotten into the bloodstream and traveled to the heart or brain. It was the primary care doctor, who knew the patient well, who discovered the potentially fatal condition while carefully conducting a full physical exam.

What Makes A "Top" Doctor

Chapter 2

Quick Tips

- If in doubt about a doctor's training, ask the doctor if the residency completed was in the specialty of his/her practice. If not, ask why not.

- Board certification and recertification are the best ways to measure competence and training.

- The easiest way you can assess the quality of a doctor's residency program is to see if it took place in a large medical center with a name you recognize.

- If a doctor does not have admitting privileges or is not on the attending staff of a hospital, you might consider choosing another doctor.

- There are many excellent, well-trained doctors at community hospitals and they should be as carefully evaluated and considered in your search as a doctor at a teaching hospital.

- Doctors who are full-time academicians may be in the forefront of new techniques and research, but they are not necessarily better doctors.

- The best care is provided by a combination of primary care doctors and other specialists and subspecialists.

- Do not hesitate to ask how frequently your doctor has performed a procedure and with what degree of success. Practice may not lead to perfection, but it improves skills and enhances the probability of success.

- Check the date of graduation from medical school or completion of residency if you want to know precisely how long a doctor has been in practice.

Quick Take

... If a doctor does not have admitting privileges or is not on the attending staff of a hospital, you might consider choosing another doctor. ...

Key Terms

Academic Medical Center - A large medical complex that centers around a teaching hospital in which residency and fellowship programs are offered, where the medical school faculty practices full time and where major clinical research activities occur.

Board Certified - Term signifying that a doctor is qualified for specialization by one of the American Board of Medical Specialties (ABMS) boards. Qualification includes completing an approved residency and passing a rigid exam.

Board Eligible - Term signifying that a doctor has completed an approved residency but has not yet taken the exam given by one of the ABMS recognized boards. The term conveys no official status in the eyes of the ABMS.

Clinical - Medical care that involves direct contact with patients.

Credentialing - A process of screening conducted by hospitals wherein they review the training and licenses of doctors applying to practice on their medical staffs.

Indemnity - A form of health insurance coverage that pays for healthcare but permits the patients to select their provider. Until 1990, indemnity insurance covered most insured people in the United States.

Licensure - Official credentials by individual states that permit a doctor to practice medicine in that state. In some states, doctors may be licensed with no more than one year of post-graduate training.

Residency - A training period spent in a hospital by a graduate of a medical school before going into practice. Residents have earned a medical degree and, therefore, are doctors, but must complete an approved residency and pass an exam to become board certified.

Tertiary Care - Medical services provided by a hospital or medical center that include complex treatments and procedures such as open heart surgery, organ transplants and burn care.

What Makes A "Top" Doctor

Castle Connolly's Top Doctors™ selection process begins with surveys of physicians and healthcare professionals. Each year, Castle Connolly surveys thousands of physicians and other healthcare professionals and asks them to identify excellent doctors in every specialty in their region and throughout the nation. When we began the research for the first edition of America's Top Doctors®, we surveyed over 230,000 of the nation's leading medical specialists, department chairs, residency program directors, vice presidents of medical affairs and presidents of the nation's leading medical centers and specialty hospitals.

In addition to mail and online surveys, the Castle Connolly physician-led research team makes thousands of phone calls each year, talking with leading specialists, chairs of clinical departments and vice presidents of medical affairs, seeking to identify top specialists for most diseases and procedures.

The Castle Connolly physician-led research team carefully reviews the credentials of every physician being considered for inclusion in Castle Connolly Guides, magazine articles and website. The review includes, among other factors, scrutiny of medical education, training, hospital appointments, administrative posts, professional achievements, and malpractice and disciplinary history.

Information on outcomes, procedure volume and malpractice is becoming increasingly available, but the public disclosure varies from state to state. Castle Connolly uses its best efforts to gather the information that is available and use it effectively. Ultimately, however, it is the professional judgment of the Castle Connolly editors, the Chief Medical and Research Officer and the research staff, which determines Castle Connolly Top Doctor™ selection.

Physicians may also be removed from the Castle Connolly lists if, in the judgment of the selection team, that is warranted. Some of the reasons physicians are removed include retirement, change in practice (taking a full time administrative post, for example), unavailability to patients, malpractice or disciplinary issues, negative physician or patient feedback, professional demeanor or a change in the "mix" of specialists Castle Connolly will present for a given community. Being removed from a Castle Connolly list does not necessarily indicate something negative about the physician. At the same time, Castle Connolly does not claim to identify every excellent physician in the nation or a region. The physicians identified through the Castle Connolly research process are clearly among the very best, but there are always other very good physicians not identified by Castle Connolly and that is why our guides, websites and other distribution channels for this critical information describe a process whereby consumers can identify excellent physicians using their own efforts.

There are four basic criteria for selecting your own best doctor: professional preparation, professional reputation, office and practice arrangements and personal or bedside manner. The first three of these assessments can be made prior to your first visit, which is when you can make your fourth evaluation.

Professional Preparation

Education

Your review of your prospective doctor's education and training should begin with medical school. While you may feel that the institution where someone earned a bachelor's degree could be an indication of the quality of the doctor, most people in the medical field do not believe it plays a major role. A degree from a highly selective undergraduate college or university will help an aspiring doctor gain admission to a medical school, but once there, all students are peers. However, the information on undergraduate colleges, if important to you, is available in the American Board of Medical Specialties (ABMS) Compendium of Certified Medical Specialists and other medical directories.

American medical schools are highly standardized, at least in terms of minimum quality. All U.S. medical schools that grant medical degrees (MDs) and osteopathic degrees (DOs) are accredited by a group known as the LCME (Liaison Committee for Medical Education). Most are also accredited by the appropriate state agency, if one exists, and by regional accrediting agencies that accredit colleges and universities of all kinds.

Furthermore, U.S. medical schools have universally high standards for admission, including success on the undergraduate level and on the Medical College Admissions Tests (MCATs). Although frequently criticized for being slow to change and for training too many specialists, the system of medical education in the United States has insured high quality in medical practice. One recent positive change is a strong effort in most medical schools to diversify the composition of the student body. While these schools have been less successful in enrolling racial minorities, the number of women in U.S. medical schools has increased to the point where they now make up about 50 percent of most classes. In certain specialties preferred by female medical graduates (pediatrics, for example), it is possible that, in coming years, the majority of specialists will be female.

Most doctors practicing in the United States are graduates of U.S. medical schools. There are two other groups of doctors in practice who make up a substantial proportion of the total doctor population. They are: (1) foreign nationals who graduated from foreign schools; and (2) U.S. nationals who graduated from foreign schools (Canadian medical schools are not considered foreign). About one out of three physicians currently practicing in the U.S. represent these groups.

Foreign Medical Graduates

Foreign medical schools vary greatly in quality. Even some of the oldest and finest European schools have become virtually "open door institutions," with huge numbers of unscreened students who make teaching and learning difficult. Others are excellent and provided the model for our own system of medical education.

The fact that someone graduated from a foreign school does not mean that he or she is a poor doctor. Foreign schools, like U.S. schools, produce good doctors and poor doctors. Foreign medical graduates must pass the same exam taken by U.S. graduates for licensure, but the failure rate for foreign graduates is significantly higher. In the first year of using the new United States Medical Licensing Exam (USMLE), 93 percent of U.S. medical school graduates passed Step II, the clinical exam, as compared with 39 percent of foreign graduates. It is clear that the quality of foreign schools, if not individual doctors, is not the same as U.S. medical schools, at least as measured by our standards. Nonetheless, many communities and patients have been well served by foreign medical graduates practicing in this country—often in areas where it has been difficult to attract graduates of American schools.

Residency

Most doctors practicing today have at least three years of postgraduate training (following the MD or DO) in an approved residency program. This is not only an important step in the process of becoming a competent doctor, but it is also a requirement for board (specialty) certification. Most people assume that a prospective doctor needs to complete a three-year residency program to obtain a medical license. This is not true in some states. New York State, for example, requires only one postgraduate year. However, since all approved residencies last at least three years, and some, such as neurosurgery, general surgery, orthopaedic surgery and urology, may extend for five or more years, it is important to know the details of a doctor's training. Licensure alone is not enough of a basis on which to make a good choice.

Without undertaking extensive and detailed research on every residency program, the best assessment you can make of a doctor's residency program is to see if it took place in a large medical center whose name you recognize. The more prestigious institutions tend to attract the best medical students, sometimes regardless of the quality of the individual residency program. If in doubt about a doctor's training, ask the doctor if the residency completed was in the specialty of his/her practice. If not, ask why.

It is also important to be certain that a doctor completed a residency that has been approved by the appropriate governing board of the specialty such as the American Board of Surgery, the American Board of Radiology or the American Osteopathic Board of Pediatrics. These board groups are listed in Appendix A. If you are really concerned about a doctor's training, you should first call the hospital that offered the residency and ask if the residency was approved by the appropriate specialty group. If still in doubt, review the publication Directory of Graduate Medical Education Programs, often called the "green book," found in medical school or hospital libraries, which lists all approved residencies.

Board Certification

With an MD or DO degree and a license, an individual may practice any kind of medicine—with or without additional special training. For example, doctors with a license but no special training may call themselves cardiologists or pediatricians. This is why board certification is such an important factor. Twenty-five specialties are recognized by the American Board of Medical Specialties (ABMS). (Visit www.abms.org or call (312) 436-2600 for more information.) Eighteen boards certify in 106 specialties under the aegis of the American Osteopathic Association (AOA). (Visit www.osteopathic.org or call 800-621-1773 for more information.) Doctors who have qualified for such specialization are called board certified; they have completed an approved residency and passed the board's exam. (See Appendix A for an approved ABMS and AOA list; see pages 81-87 for a description of each specialty and subspecialty.) While many doctors who are not board certified do call themselves specialists, board certification is the best standard by which to measure competence and training.

You can be confident that doctors who are board certified have at a minimum the proper training in their specialty and have demonstrated their proficiency through supervision and testing. While there are many non-board certified doctors who are highly competent, it is more difficult to assess the level of their training. Board certification alone does not guarantee competence, but it is a standard that reflects successful completion of an appropriate training program.

Recertification

A relatively new focus of the specialty boards is the area of recertification. Until recently, board certification lasted for an unlimited time period. Now, almost all of the boards have put time limits on the certification period. For example, in internal medicine, it is ten years; in family practice seven years. In osteopathic medicine, some of the boards need to set a recertification period within 10 years. Many have done so already. These more stringent standards reflect an increasing emphasis, by both the medical boards and state agencies responsible for licensing doctors, on recertification.

Since the policies of the boards vary widely, it is good procedure to ask a doctor if certification was awarded and when. If the date was seven to ten years ago, ask if he/she has been recertified. Note: The most recent date of board certification or recertification is indicated in each physician's listing in this guide.

Unfortunately, many boards permit "grandfathering," whereby already certified doctors do not have to be recertified, and recertification demands apply only to newly certified doctors. Appendix A contains a list of the names and addresses of the boards and the certification period for each board specialty. Even if recertification is not required, it is good professional practice for doctors to undertake the process. It assures you, the patient, that they are attempting to stay current.

Many states have a continuing medical education (CME) requirement for doctors. These states typically require a minimum number of CME credits for a doctor to maintain a medical license. Seven states require 150 CME credits over a three-year period. Osteopathic doctors are required to take 120 hours of CME credits within three years to maintain certification.

Board Eligibility

Many doctors who have been recently trained are waiting to take the boards. They are sometimes described as "board eligible," a common term that the ABMS advocates abandoning because of its ambiguity. Board eligible means that the doctor has completed an approved residency and is qualified to sit for the related board's exam.

Each member board of the ABMS has its own policy regarding the use and recognition of the board eligible term. Therefore, the description "board eligible" should not be viewed as a genuine qualification, especially if a doctor has been out of medical school long enough to have taken the certification exam. To the boards, a doctor is either board certified or not. Furthermore, most of the specialty boards permit unlimited attempts to pass the exam and, in some cases, doctors who have failed the exam twice or even ten times continue to call themselves board eligible. In osteopathic medicine, the board eligible status is recognized only for the first six years after completion of a residency.

Self-Designated Medical Specialties

In addition to the ABMS and AOA-approved list of specialties and subspecialties, there is a wide variety of other doctors, and groups of doctors, who may call themselves "specialists". There are, at present, at least 100 such groups called self-designated medical specialties. They range from doctors who are working to create a recognized body of knowledge and subspecialty training to less formal groups interested in a particular approach to the practice of medicine. These groups may or may not have standards for membership. There is no way of determining the true extent of their members' training, and they are not recognized by the ABMS* or the AOA. While you should be cautious of doctors who claim they are specialists in these areas, many do have advanced training and the groups at least offer a listing of people interested in a particular approach to medical care. Rely on board certification to assure yourself of basic competence and use membership in one of these groups to indicate strong interest and possible additional training in a particular aspect of medicine. A list of these self-designated medical specialties may be found in Appendix B.

Fellowships

The purpose of a fellowship is to provide advanced training in the clinical techniques and research of a particular subspecialty. In the U.S. there are a variety of fellowship programs available to doctors, and they fall into two broad categories: approved and unapproved. Approved fellowships are those approved by the appropriate medical specialty board (e.g., the American Board of Radiology) and that lead to a subspecialty certificate. Fellowship programs that are not approved are often in the same areas of training as those that are, but they do not lead to a subspecialty

---

* One subspecialty, not yet recognized by the ABMS - Pediatric Neurosurgery - has been included because the retaining and certification process is rigorous and meaningful.

certificate. Unfortunately, all too often, unapproved fellowships exist only to provide relatively inexpensive labor for the research and/or patient care activities of a clinical department in a medical school or hospital. In such cases, the learning that takes place is secondary and may be a good deal less than in an approved fellowship. On the other hand, any fellowship is better than none at all and some unapproved fellowships have that status for a valid reason, which should not reflect negatively on the program. For example, the fellowship may have been recently created with approval being sought. To check that a fellowship is an approved one, call the hospital where the training took place or the medical board for that specialty.

Professional Reputation

There are doctors who meet every professional standard on paper, but who are simply not good doctors. In all probability, the medical community has ascertained that while the individual may still practice medicine, his or her reputation will reflect that collective assessment. There are also doctors who are outstanding leaders in their fields because of research or professional activities, but who are not particularly strong or perhaps even active in patient care. It is important to distinguish that kind of professional reputation from a reputation as a competent, caring doctor in delivering patient care. In a consumer survey conducted by the management consulting firm Towers Perrin, the chief criterion by which the respondents selected doctors was reputation. This was the most important factor for those enrolled in either managed care or indemnity plans.

Hospital Appointment

Most doctors are on the medical staff of one or more hospitals and are known as attendings. If a doctor does not have admitting privileges or is not on the attending staff of a hospital, you may wish to consider choosing another doctor. It can be very difficult to ascertain whether the lack of hospital appointment is for a good reason or not. For example, it is understandable that some doctors who are raising families or heading toward retirement choose not to meet the demands (meetings, committees, etc.) of being an attending. However, if you need care in a hospital, the lack of such an appointment means that another doctor will have to oversee that care. In some specialties such as dermatology and psychiatry, doctors may conduct their entire practices in the office, and a hospital appointment is not as essential, or as good a criterion for assessment, as in other specialties.

While mistakes are made, most hospitals are quite careful about admissions to their medical staffs. The best hospitals are highly selective, so a degree of screening (or "credentialing") has been done for you. In other words, the best doctors practice at the best hospitals. Since caring for a patient in the hospital is often a team effort involving a number of specialists, the reputation of the hospital where the doctor admits patients carries special weight. Hospital medical staffs also review their colleagues credentials before authorizing them to perform specific procedures. In addition, they typically reappoint their medical staffs—and review them—every two or three years. In effect, this is an additional screening to protect patients. It is especially true of hospitals that have what are known as closed staffs, where it is impossible to obtain admitting privileges unless there is a vacancy that the administration and medical staff deem necessary to fill. If you are having some type of surgical procedure and are concerned about the doctor's skill or experience with it, it may be worthwhile to call the Medical Affairs office at the doctor's hospital to see if he or she is authorized to perform that procedure in the hospital.

The reasons for a hospital's selectivity are easy to understand: every hospital wants to have the best reputation possible in order to attract patients, and no hospital, excellent or not, wishes to expose itself to liability. Obviously, the quality of the medical staff is immensely important in creating that reputation. Unfortunately, some hospitals are less diligent when a major group practice of doctors, all of whom have previously been affiliated with the institution, adds new members. In such cases, the hospital may almost automatically grant privileges without conducting the same intensive review given to individual doctors who are not members of a group practice. Also, some hospitals are less selective in granting privileges when beds are empty than when beds are full, since additional attendings provide additional patients.

A last and very important reason why a hospital appointment is an essential requirement in your choice of a doctor is that many states permit doctors to practice without malpractice insurance. If you are injured as a result of the doctor's poor care, you could be without recourse. However, few hospitals permit doctors to practice in them unless they carry malpractice insurance. This not only protects the hospital, but the patient as well.

Many people believe that they should choose a doctor with an appointment at a major medical center as opposed to a community hospital. This assumption is incorrect on two counts. For one thing, there are many excellent, well-trained doctors at community hospitals and they should be as carefully evaluated and considered in your search as a doctor at a large institution. What's more, the term "medical center" has less significance today than it did years ago when the term was used to describe only the major university hospitals of medical schools. A true medical center is a teaching hospital that offers multiple residency programs and at which the medical school faculty practices full-time, with fellowship programs and major clinical research activities an integral part of the teaching of medical students. These large centers also are involved in tertiary care, offering services such as organ transplants, burn care and cardiovascular surgery.

Today many community hospitals have added the term medical center to their name. They do this for two purposes: to indicate that they, too, offer advanced and sophisticated medical programs, and to compete for patients with the academic medical centers. With academic medical centers turning out many well-trained specialists and subspecialists who establish practices in nearby communities and then want to continue the highly specialized techniques they have learned, many community hospitals have initiated tertiary care programs of their own, further blurring the distinction between medical centers and hospitals.

In any case, most of our healthcare today is delivered outside of the hospital in ambulatory outpatient settings. Those who are hospitalized for acute illness (e.g., surgery, serious infection) will find that community hospitals and their staffs are well-suited to the task.

When extremely difficult and complex problems develop, or when tertiary care is needed, many communities have excellent academic medical centers. Of course, they offer primary care as well, especially to those who live nearby. This illustrates the point, once again, that medical care is a local issue.

Medical School Faculty Appointment

Many doctors have appointments on the faculties of medical schools. There is a range of categories from "straight" appointments—meaning full-time appointment as professor, associate professor, assistant professor or instructor—to clinical ranks that may reflect lesser degrees of involvement in teaching or research. If someone carries what is known as a straight academic rank (i.e., professor of surgery, without "clinical" in the title), this usually means that the individual is engaged full-time in medical school research and/or teaching activities. The title "professor of clinical surgery" usually describes a doctor who has a full-time appointment in a medical school, but who puts a greater emphasis on clinical practice (patient care) than on research or teaching. The title "clinical professor of surgery" usually specifies a part-time or adjunct appointment and less direct involvement in medical school activities.

Doctors who are full-time academicians may be in the forefront of new techniques and research, but they are not necessarily better doctors. Nonetheless, you can be assured that they have the support of other faculty, residents and medical students.

When you are seeking a subspecialist, a doctor's relationship to a medical school becomes more meaningful since medical school faculties tend to be made up of subspecialists. You are less likely to find large numbers of general or primary care practitioners engaged full-time on a medical school faculty. The newest approaches and techniques in medicine, for the most part, are explored and developed by medical school faculties in their laboratories and clinical practice settings. This is where they practice their subspecialties, as well as teach and perform research. Such leading specialists are not necessarily better doctors than community doctors—they are trained to provide a different kind of medical care. The best care is provided by a combination of primary care doctors and other specialists and subspecialists.

Medical Society Membership

Most medical society memberships sound very prestigious and some are; however, there are many societies that are not selective and which virtually any doctor can join. In addition, membership in many of the more prestigious societies is based on research and publication, or on leadership in the field, and may have little to do with direct patient care. While it is clearly an honor to be invited to join these groups, membership may be less than helpful in discerning whether a doctor can meet your needs.

Board certified doctors are referred to as Diplomates of the Board. Some of the colleges of medical specialties (e.g., the American College of Radiology and the American College of Surgeons) have multiple levels of recognition. The first is basic membership and the second, more prestigious and difficult to obtain, is status as a Fellow. Fellowship status in the colleges is meaningful and is based on experience, professional achievement and recognition by one's peers, including extensive experience in patient care. It should be viewed as a significant professional qualification.

Experience

Experience is difficult to assess. Obviously, in most cases, an older doctor has more experience; on the other hand, a younger doctor has been more recently immersed in residency, the challenge of medical school, or even a fellowship, and may be the most up-to-date. If a doctor is board certified, you may assume that assures at least a minimal amount of experience, but it could be as little as a year. In this guide the board certification date may reflect a doctor's most recent recertification, so check the date of graduation from medical school or completion of residency if you want to know precisely how long a doctor has been in practice.

There is a good deal of evidence that there is a positive relationship between quantity of experience and quality of care. That is, the more often a doctor performs a procedure, the better he/she becomes at it. That is why it is important to ask a doctor about his or her experience with the procedure that you need. Does the doctor see and treat similar cases every day, every week or only rarely? Of course, with some rare conditions, rarely is the only possible answer, but it is relative frequency that is critical. Major metropolitan areas, especially New York and San Francisco, became leaders in the treatment of AIDS because of the large number of patients seen in those metropolitan areas. Doctors in the suburbs of New York City (especially in New York's Westchester, Nassau and Suffolk counties) and in Fairfield County, Connecticut became leaders in the research and treatment of Lyme disease because that region is the epicenter of the disease.

In some states, data is available on volume or numbers of certain procedures performed at hospitals. Likewise, The Leapfrog Group (www.leapfroggroup.org) compares hospitals' performance on the national standards of safety, quality and efficiency - areas of healthcare that are most relevant to consumers and this information is later used to improve hospital quality, save healthcare spending and assist hospital employees with purchasing strategies. The federal government has posted outcome data for hospitals, but for a limited number of procedures, on a website www.hospitalcompare.hhs.gov/hospital-search.aspx. There is a good deal of controversy, however, on the validity and usefulness of such data. Opponents cite the fact that some of the data is produced from Medicare patient records only and, thus, is based solely on an elderly population that does not represent the total activity of a hospital or doctor. Proponents of the use of such volume data agree that it is not perfect, but suggest that it can be one useful criterion in selecting the best places to receive care for these specific problems. Recognizing the limitations of such data, the healthcare consumer may, nonetheless, find it of interest and use.

Office and Practice Arrangements

Although clearly not as important as training or reputation, office and practice arrangements are usually of great significance to patients. Practice arrangements include office hours, office location, billing procedures and office testing among the many factors that result in how well the office is run.

Many years ago most doctors practiced independently in private offices. They were called solo practitioners and usually had agreements with other doctors to respond to their patients' calls when they were unavailable. In recent decades, most doctors have entered group practices; indeed, this is becoming the most common way for young doctors to begin to practice. Two or more doctors in the same specialty, or in different specialties (a multi-specialty group), share offices and staff to lower their costs of operations. They also cover for each other on rotation for weekends, evenings and vacations. As a patient you may prefer one of the following: a solo practitioner who is covered occasionally; a group where you usually, but not always, see the same doctor; or a multi-specialty group where, if a consultation or referral is necessary, the specialist is at the same location. The choice is really one of personal preference.

There are other factors relating to practice arrangements that may or may not be important to an individual when choosing a doctor. One is the location of the office. A consumer poll conducted for the Robert Wood Johnson Foundation identified office location as one of the two most important factors in the selection of a doctor (the other was a recommendation by a relative or friend). Actually, the site of the office can be very important in choosing a doctor you may visit on a regular basis. If the location is inconvenient, you may be discouraged from making needed visits.

Another important factor concerns the use of nurse practitioners and physician's assistants in the office. Licensed nurse practitioners are advanced practice nurses in primary care. They have additional training beyond the basic requirements for nursing licensure, usually a master's degree or special certificate. They perform a broad range of nursing functions as well as functions that, historically, have been performed by doctors, including assessing and diagnosing, conducting physical examinations, ordering diagnostic tests, implementing treatment plans and monitoring patient status. Physician's assistants are licensed to provide medical care in many states. However, unlike nurses, they may practice only under a doctor's direction and supervision. According to an article in the professional journal Family Practice Management, these "midlevel providers," as they are called, "can handle 80 to 90 percent of the problems that occasion office visits." These providers have become more of a presence in healthcare in recent years, especially in medical groups and HMOs. If you don't think you will be satisfied having your office visit and examination conducted by anyone but the doctor, you should determine up front how many midlevel providers are on staff and how extensive their responsibilities are.

Narrowing the Choice

Here are 10 additional questions that will guide you in assessing if the practice patterns or arrangements of a doctor meet your needs. If there are other items not listed that are important to you, add them to the list before you make your initial appointment. You should try to obtain as much of the information as possible from the staff.

- Are you currently accepting new patients and, if so, is a referral required?
- On average, how long does a patient have to wait for an appointment?
- Are you open on weekends? In the evening?
- If lab work and X-rays are performed in the office what are the qualifications of the people doing the tests?
- Are full payment, deductibles or co-payments required at the time of the appointment?
- Do you accept my insurance plan? Medicare? Medicaid? Workers' compensation? No-fault insurance?
- Do you accept credit cards and, if so, which do you accept?
- Do you accept patient phone calls?
- Will you care for patients in their homes?
- Is your office handicapped-accessible?

If you have a chronic illness or disease, there may be certain additional aspects of a doctor's practice that could be particularly important to you. You should discuss any chronic problems when first establishing a relationship with a doctor. In fact, you may want to find a doctor with special interest or training in that problem.

House calls also continue to be important to some people. Yes, some doctors still do make house calls! In fact, a recent American Medical News article suggested that 43 percent of internal medicine specialists and 65 percent of family practice specialists made one or more house calls a year. However, it is important to point out that the number of doctors making house calls has declined because of technology, liability risks and time pressures. Important diagnostic equipment often cannot be carried around in a doctor's little black bag and is only available in the office or hospital. Also, the time required to visit one patient at home markedly reduces the time available to see other patients.

Personal or Bedside Manner

To many patients, once they have determined that a doctor is competent, the doctor's professional manner—also known as bedside manner—is the most important part of their choice. The Towers Perrin report cited earlier indicated that after reputation, skill in communicating was the most important factor sought in doctors. Patients prefer sensitive and caring doctors who listen carefully and demonstrate their concern. Studies show that such doctors are sued less often than others!

What characteristics make up a doctor's personal manner? The four described below may, when considered together, give you a clear idea of whether a particular doctor will be your personal "top" doctor.

- **Listening**. Professional manner includes the doctor's willingness to listen to patients, be supportive and understanding, explain procedures and exhibit concern and respect. These skills are expressed at the bedside, in the office, or in any setting where there is doctor/patient contact. Listening is also a valuable diagnostic tool. Unfortunately, these skills often have not been taught well in medical schools and the lack of them forms the primary basis for complaints from patients. However, there is growing emphasis on these vital interpersonal and communications skills in medical schools today and with good reason. They are critically important to most patients.

- **Cultural Sensitivity.** Some patients may prefer doctors who speak their language or are familiar with their cultural background. The term "culturally competent physician" is a relatively new one describing doctors who have the needed skills and attitudes to effectively treat patients from minority cultures.

- **Ethical, Religious and Philosophical Views.** Religion, or at least views on issues such as abortion, utilization of life-sustaining measures, natural childbirth, breast-feeding and other such matters can also be important. It is perfectly appropriate to ask doctors their views on sensitive issues.

- **Decision-making Procedures.** Years ago patients took the words of the doctor as law, not to be questioned or perhaps even discussed. That is not the case today. Consumers are better informed about health issues and may want to be actively involved in the decision making that affects their health. Some patients do not feel this way and are comfortable accepting a doctor's diagnosis or course of treatment without question. Some doctors—in diminishing numbers, thankfully—feel uncomfortable with patients who want everything explained to them or want to be involved in decision-making. Consider how you feel about this issue and discuss it with your doctor to be certain you are on compatible wavelengths.

Of course, what ultimately makes a "top" doctor are the results, the "outcomes," of care. Unfortunately, there is relatively little information available to consumers on the outcomes of physicians and hospitals. Some states, New York for example, have produced studies on outcomes for cardiac surgery. Also, some HMOs are talking about producing report cards for doctors. Generally, however, consumers will have difficulty finding outcome studies for individual doctors.

On the other hand, there is a growing movement to track and publish outcomes data on hospitals. The federal government has taken the lead by releasing outcomes data by hospitals for selected procedures. Visit www.hospitalcompare.hhs.gov.

One woman—a long-time City resident who moved to the suburbs to be near her children—found out the hard way about advice when she selected a doctor on the basis of her neighbor's glowing praise. During the initial visit, the patient's numerous questions about her chronic arthritis condition went unanswered while the doctor merely patted her on the shoulder and assured her that he would "take care of everything." While the paternalistic attitude might have suited the neighbor's needs, it fell far short for this senior patient, who was used to a good give-and-take with her former internist. She resumed her search for a doctor—this time with the assistance of the Castle Connolly guide, a more reliable source than a friend's recommendation.

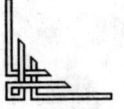
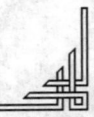

The Best in American Medicine
www.CastleConnolly.com

You And
Your Doctor:
A Team

Chapter 3

Quick Tips

- Always obtain copies of all medical records and tests for your files.

- When selecting a doctor, especially a primary care doctor, it is appropriate to request an interview to get acquainted.

- Good doctors listen, good patients talk.

- Always bring a pad and pencil with you to medical appointments. When the doctor gives you instructions, take notes.

- The Physician's Desk Reference, commonly known as the PDR, is available in most libraries and is an excellent resource for learning more about medications. (The PDR web page is at http://www.pdr.net)

- Do not hesitate to ask your pharmacist about side effects, generic substitutions and other questions related to your medications.

Quick Take

... The best doctor-patient relationship is based on a two-way dialogue. Be open and honest and seek a doctor who is the same. ...

Key Terms

American Medical Association - A membership organization of physicians and their professional associations dedicated to promoting the art and science of medicine and the betterment of public health through establishing and promoting ethical, educational, and clinical standards for the medical profession. It represents the interests of physicians on the national level.

Baseline Tests - A series of basic, routine medical tests—such as electrocardiogram, complete blood count, blood pressure measurement, weight measurement, and chest X-ray—that are usually completed by a physician upon a patient's initial visit in order to provide a standard for comparison during subsequent health examinations.

Generic Drugs - Prescription medications that have been marketed by one company under a proprietary or brand name and which may be sold, after the original exclusive patent expires, under a generic name or the name assigned to it during an early stage of development. Most generic drugs are less expensive than proprietary versions and are just as effective except in cases when, because of different manufacturing processes, they are not bioequivalent or handled by the body in an identical manner.

Third Party Payer - An organization such as indemnity insurance company or managed care organization that provides individual and group health insurance, or a governmental department which assumes responsibility for the payment of an individual's healthcare, either directly to the healthcare provider or by means of reimbursement to the individual (Medicare and Medicaid are such government programs).

You And Your Doctor: A Team

Trust and respect between doctors and patients have reached a low point in modern American society. A recent poll of consumers sponsored by the American Medical Association (AMA) concluded that approximately 70 percent of those who responded agreed with the statement that "people are beginning to lose faith in their doctors." (Despite concerns about doctors in general, much research has shown that patients tend to rate their own doctors well.)

Trust between doctors and patients has declined for many reasons, including unrealistic expectations on the part of some patients and the patronizing attitudes of some doctors, which clash with the higher education level and medical sophistication of many patients. This has been further complicated by changing financial arrangements, particularly those involving the government and third-party payers, and the perception that some doctors seem to be motivated not by the values of the Hippocratic Oath (See page xiii), but by those of the marketplace. The AMA poll cited earlier found that 69 percent of respondents agreed that doctors "are too interested in making money." Perhaps a significant factor in creating this atmosphere is that in many cases the relationship between doctor and patient now has another dimension, the managed care organization. Another significant contributor is the huge amount of paperwork required from doctors. Generated by quality-assurance efforts, regulation, complex billing and managed care procedures, this burden reduces the time doctors are able to spend with patients.

Given the formidable obstacles, it might seem impossible to find a primary care doctor who is well suited to your needs. If you have carefully read the preceding chapters, your work is half done. What remains is to find that special individual who fits the criteria.

The Initial Interview

When selecting a doctor, especially a primary care doctor, it is appropriate to request an exploratory interview. Frequently, doctors will engage in such brief interviews at no charge, at a reduced fee or by telephone. It is preferable to find out about a doctor's credentials, office hours and billing procedures from the staff beforehand so you don't waste time asking about basic facts. This leaves time to ask the doctor questions that will allow you to determine what kind of relationship could develop. It is interesting that many parents will insist on interviewing a pediatrician for their child but wouldn't think of interviewing a physician for themselves.

Ask the Right Questions

The most important aspect of this session is to see if you can develop a positive doctor/patient relationship. Are you comfortable with the doctor's manner, style and general personality? Do you feel a strong sense of trust in the doctor? Here are five questions to ask the doctor plus two questions to ask yourself that may lead you closer to a selection.

- What is your experience in treating _____ (if you are seeking care for a particular illness or condition)?

- Are you open to treatments and therapies that do not rely heavily on medication?

- What preventive programs do you suggest for someone of my age, sex and health status?

- How do you feel about involving patients in decision-making?

- What are your views on_____(ethical and moral issues of importance to you as a patient)?

Even when the doctor is responding to your questions, you should ask yourself:

- Is the doctor paying attention to me and really considering my questions or do the impersonal "stock" answers indicate that the doctor's thoughts are elsewhere?

- Does this doctor speak about good health and prevention with the personal knowledge of someone who seems to practice it?

If your prospective doctor seems to measure up to your standards, get the relationship off to a good start by making an appointment for a complete check-up. During this appointment, you will have an opportunity to share your medical and family history and baseline tests will be performed to serve as a standard in the years ahead.

Talking with Your Doctor

After you have selected your doctor, your first appointment should include an extensive review of your medical history. Your doctor should spend time with you, ask questions and listen to your responses carefully.

Medical students are often told, "Listen to your patients. They'll tell you what's wrong with them." This conveys an important lesson not only for doctors, but for patients: Good doctors listen; good patients talk.

Analysis of doctor/patient conversations has revealed that many patients wait until the end of a conversation, even until they are saying goodbye, to tell their doctors what is really bothering them. This is just a small example of the dynamics of doctor/patient relationships. It is also a good example of a waste of valuable time—the doctor's and the patient's. One reason doctors need to be trained to be good listeners is that they frequently must ascertain what is troubling the patient not by what is said directly, but by what is said indirectly, not at all or through body language and other signs. However, it is always easier, less time-consuming and certainly more effective if a patient can describe problems completely and accurately.

Before you even see a doctor, you should prepare thoroughly. You should have a complete record of your medical history, including a record of X-rays and any other diagnostic tests, as well as blood workups. You need information about childhood diseases, chronic conditions, hospitalizations, past and present medications, doses and drug reactions, if any, and, if possible, something about the health history of your parents and even their siblings. Except for the last item, these are available to patients from their previous doctors or hospitals. That is why it is useful to obtain copies of all medical records and tests for your own files. Not only will this save you time and effort, but may avoid additional testing and expense. Your doctor will also ask many seemingly personal questions about your work, education, sex life and even drug and alcohol use. These are all part of a complete medical history and will help your doctor better understand you and your state of health.

If you have a particular problem or concern, describe all your symptoms. Try not to minimize or exaggerate and, most of all, don't deny.

If you have questions to ask your doctor, make a list. Always bring a pad and pencil with you to medical appointments. When the doctor gives you instructions, take notes or ask the doctor to write them down for you. If a prescription is written, ask about doses, side effects, efficacy and alternative medications as well as generic substitutes. The Physician's Desk Reference, commonly known as the PDR, is available in most libraries and is an excellent resource for learning more about medications. There is also a PDR web page on the Internet at http://www.pdr.net. You can also get a great deal of information on medications from another health professional, your pharmacist. Do not hesitate to ask your pharmacist about side effects, generic substitutions and other questions related to your medications. However, if the information you receive conflicts with that given by your doctor, consult with the doctor and follow his or her directions.

A Matter of Time

Patients want and expect doctors who listen, express concern, explain conditions and procedures in a clear and understandable manner, discuss medications and their effects and side effects thoroughly, return calls, are available when needed and, perhaps most importantly, spend sufficient time with them. With increasing demands on their time, many doctors are left with an uneasy feeling of "running to stay in place." The end result may be a tendency, unintended for the most part, to rush through a patient visit. This situation contributes to the erosion of the doctor/patient relationship.

Also contributing to this problem is pervasive lateness on the part of doctors. Patients frequently complain that they spend hours in a doctor's waiting room, long past the appointed hour (research has shown the average wait is 20 minutes).

Unfortunately, the duration of a patient visit is not always predictable and unexpected delays may occur if the diagnosis is complicated or if a patient needs to discuss what is on his or her mind. The doctor who spends extra time with another patient is probably the doctor you want for yourself. If the lateness is excessive, persistent and without apparent good reason, discuss it with your doctor and, if it is interfering with your relationship, consider changing doctors.

Today many primary care physicians are changing their practices to a new model known as concierge or "private medicine." In this model, physicians reduce their practice patient load from, say, 2,200 patients to 600. Each patient who remains in, or enters, a concierge practice is required to pay an annual fee typically ranging from $1,500 to $5,000, or even more. As a function of the reduced patient load, the physicians have far greater time to spend with each patient and can offer faster appointments or better access sometimes even around the clock. The physician can also focus more on preventive medicine and other aspects of sound patient care, a luxury and benefit to the patient that many physicians in a primary care practice cannot enjoy.

After a delay of two hours in his doctor's office, one patient, a self-employed marketing consultant, made sure that it would never happen again. Did he have a showdown with the doctor? Did he decide never to return? Not at all. He simply made it a point to call the doctor's office two hours before his scheduled appointment to see how the schedule was running. He then adjusted his own schedule to coincide with the doctor's.

Strengthening
Your Team

Chapter 4

Quick Tips

- The more complex and difficult the problem, the more important reputation is. In fact, you might well narrow your focus to doctors on the staffs of certain medical centers noted for excellence with specific problems.

- Doctors typically refer patients to doctors on the staffs of the same hospitals where they practice.

- If the lateness of your doctor is excessive, persistent and without apparent good reason, discuss it with him or her.

- If you are not comfortable with your primary care doctor's referral, ask for a number of options. If necessary, you may consider going "out of network" even if you have to pay some or all of the fee.

- In many cases, insurance companies will pay for second opinions, but check ahead of time to make sure your insurance plan does cover them.

- One way HMOs control costs is by limiting second opinions.

- Doctors may have different solutions to the same problem — and any one or more could work.

Quick Take

... The old adage, two heads are better than one, often applies in healthcare, too. Expanded options include referrals, second opinions, alternative therapies and clinical trials. ...

Key Terms

Alternative Therapy - Non-traditional forms of healthcare — including acupuncture, homeopathy, naturopathy, massage, reflexology, biofeedback, hypnotherapy, herbology, therapeutic touc, and prayer — that are often based on ancient healing methods and have not been tested in a conventional scientific manner.

Clinical Trial - An experimental trial of a new drug or therapy in a selected group of human volunteers who suffer from the condition for which the experimental drug or treatment is to be used.

Double Blind Study - One form of a clinical trial in which two groups of volunteers — one group receiving the real drug or treatment and the other receiving a placebo or dummy — are followed for a specific period of time by researchers who do not know themselves who is receiving which therapy.

Protocol - A rigid set of rules set up for a clinical trial by the Food and Drug Administration (FDA) which must be followed strictly by all researchers and volunteers participating in the trial.

Strengthening Your Team

When You Need a Specialist

For the most part, selecting a specialist is similar to choosing a primary care doctor. There is one major difference, however; typically you will be referred to a specialist by your primary care doctor. Suggesting a consultation does not show a weakness on the part of the doctor. On the contrary, the real weakness lies in a doctor's reluctance to suggest consultations when advisable. Your primary care doctor will receive a written report from any consultation or referral. You should request a copy as well.

Ask your doctor why this particular specialist is being recommended. Find out about the specialist's training and experience. If your doctor has sent many patients to the same doctor for the same treatment, you should find out how successful the treatment was and if the patients were satisfied. You might also ask if the specialist would be the one selected for your doctor's own personal care. You should feel comfortable about seeing the specialist and, if you are not, ask for another recommendation or find a different one on your own.

Frequently, patients do seek out specialists on their own. If you are attempting to find a specialist or subspecialist without the guidance of your primary care doctor, use the various selection procedures described in Chapters One, Two and Three. When selecting a physician on your own, even greater emphasis should be placed on board certification in the relevant specialty. If you are trying to find someone to treat a very specific problem, make certain that the individual is well trained in that area. You may check to see if a doctor is board certified by calling the American Board of Medical Specialties at (312) 436-2600 or visiting their web site at www.abms.org.

You will also want to know if the specialist you select is well respected. The more complex and difficult the problem, the more important reputation is. In fact, you might narrow your focus to doctors on the staffs of certain medical centers noted for excellence in treating your specific problem. There are a number of books and magazine articles such as the annual U.S. News & World Report issue on America's best hospitals that offer views on the best medical centers for specific problems.

Finally, make certain your doctor and the specialist communicate easily about your case. If you should have a problem with a specialist, or if you are not pleased with the care given, let your primary care doctor know about it right away.

Doctors typically refer patients to doctors on the staffs of the same hospitals at which they practice. There are good and poor reasons for this, as explained below.

Why Doctors Usually Refer to Doctors in the Same Hospitals

Good Reasons:

- They know the doctors better.

- They continue to be involved in the case.

- Coordination of multiple specialists may be easier.

Poor Reasons:

- It is easier.

- They will get referrals back.

- It reduces the chance of losing the patient to another doctor.

- It may help build social or professional relationships.

- The hospital may pressure doctors to refer within the institution.

In today's managed care environment doctor referrals usually are restricted to other doctors in the managed care organization's network. Sometimes the referring doctor may not even be familiar with the other doctor's qualifications. If you are not comfortable with your primary care doctor's referral, ask for a number of options. If necessary, you may consider going "out of network" even if you have to pay some or all of the fee.

Second Opinions

Second opinions are a valuable medical tool, infrequently used in many instances, overused in others. Clearly, you do not want to get another doctor's opinion on every ailment or problem, but there are definitely times you should seek out a second opinion:

- Before major surgery.

- When the diagnosis is serious or life-threatening.

- If a rare disease is diagnosed.

- If the diagnosis is uncertain.

- If you think the number of tests or procedures recommended is excessive.

- If a test result has serious implications—a positive Pap smear for example—have the test re-done immediately before taking further action.

- If the treatment suggested is risky or expensive.

- If you are uncomfortable with the diagnosis and treatment recommended.
- If a course of treatment is not working.
- If you question your doctor's competence.
- If your insurance company requires it.

Most doctors will be supportive if you request a second opinion and many will even recommend it. In many cases, insurance companies will pay for second opinions, but check ahead of time to make sure your insurance plan does indeed cover them. In an HMO, you may have to be more assertive because one way that HMOs control costs is by limiting second opinions. This is especially true if you want an opinion outside the plan's network.

Often, the opinion of a second doctor will affirm the opinion of the first, but the reassurance may be worth the time and extra cost. On the other hand, if the second opinion differs from the first, you have two remaining alternatives: seek the opinion of a third doctor, or educate yourself as much as possible by talking with both doctors and reading up on the problem (trusting your instincts about which diagnosis is correct). If the diagnosis is the same but the recommended treatments differ, remember that doctors may have different solutions to the same problem—and any one or more could be efficient. For example, an orthopaedic surgeon may recommend surgery to correct a knee injury while a physiatrist (a doctor certified in physical medicine and rehabilitation) may recommend rehabilitation. One might work better than the other or they could both work equally well. The choice may be based on your preference. Remember, however, that surgical solutions can rarely be reversed. It usually is best to try a non-surgical solution first, if possible.

Complementary Medicine: Exploring Your Options

A recent study conducted by the University of Florida estimated that 86 percent of households in the U.S. use some type of complementary therapies (a term that implies that these therapies are used along with conventional medical treatment rather than in place of them). Total out-of-pocket expenditures for complementary/alternative medicine approach $30 billion annually, estimates David Eisenberg, MD and colleagues at the Harvard/Beth Israel Center for the Study of Alternative Medicine Research. They further point out that total visits to complementary/alternative providers numbered 629 million in 1997 as compared to 386 million visits to primary care physicians.

One of the reasons conventional medical therapies are conventional is that most have been proven to be effective in a rigorous scientific manner, while many complementary/alternative therapies have not been tested under accepted scientific conditions. You should always consider the possibility that some alternative therapies, since they are unproven, may do more harm than good. The alternative approaches in use today range from legitimate searches for new therapies to outright quackery and fraud. Without the guidance of the scientific and medical community, it is sometimes impossible for doctors, let alone consumers, to tell the difference.

Nonetheless, doctors are becoming more open to the use of complementary/alternative approaches. One study reported that about 30 percent of doctors questioned in the Los Angeles area said that they were open to complementary/alternative practices in one form or another and that acceptance is growing. Medical scientists are also indicating a new interest in studying approaches to health that may complement the strengths of Western medicine. Some of the therapies being explored include mind-body medicine, hypnotherapy, biofeedback, chiropractic, vital energy, metabolic therapy, naturopathy, homeopathy, therapeutic touch, acupuncture, prayer and the use of herbs.

Alternative healthcare often complements rather than replaces Western medicine. As such, the terms complementary or integrative, which accurately describe the relationship between Western and alternative healthcare, are used with increased frequency as this type of approach towards medicine becomes more commonplace.

In a New England Journal of Medicine study, 72 percent of the respondents who used unconventional therapies did not inform their medical doctor that they had done so. That is unfortunate, because such treatments could be greatly enhanced with the support and advice of a primary care doctor. More worrisome is the great danger that some people may use alternative treatments in lieu of, rather than as a supplement to, more conventional and proven medical therapies. A classic and tragic example of this was the surge of patients who traveled to Mexico to seek a "magic bullet" cure for cancer promised by the drug Laetrile (made from apricot pits). There was no magic; indeed, patients lost money, hope and, in some cases, the opportunity for timely use of proven treatment. If you do explore alternative therapies, be certain to let your doctor know about it. Some may be harmful, especially if you are undergoing another treatment under your doctor's direction.

To learn more about complementary/alternative medicine, contact the National Center for Complementary and Alternative Medicine Clearinghouse to locate a source of reliable information on the practice you are considering (see Appendix E).

How to Use Complementary/Alternative Medicine Wisely and Well

- Try to learn everything you can about the particular therapy that interests you. Your local library and the Internet both have substantial materials on complementary/alternative medicine.

- Discuss your plans with your doctor. You might gain some insight into the therapy in terms of its possible risks. Furthermore, if you are currently under medical treatment, you should make certain that the two approaches will not conflict in some way.

- If you start an alternative therapy and it does not appear to be providing relief, or seems to be worsening the condition, contact your doctor immediately.

Clinical Trials: Should You Participate?

Each year, more than half a million Americans, some of them sick, but even more of them healthy, volunteer to take part in experimental trials of new drugs and therapies. Before drugs, vaccines, biological agents and medical devices are made available for general use by doctors and their patients, they must go through extensive testing on animals and humans called "clinical trials." There is probably at least one clinical trial in process at some medical center for almost every serious disease.

On the plus side, a clinical trial offers the opportunity for prompt use of a drug or other treatment that seems promising, and comes with the bonus of regular and thorough medical examinations at no cost to you (some trials even make allowances for participants' travel and other expenses). Moreover, patients are encouraged to discuss all of their experiences regarding the trial. You will probably learn more about your condition and feel more in control, which can have a very positive effect. On the downside, you may be giving up standard treatment for something that may or may not be better. There is even the possibility that you will not get a drug at all, because most trials are conducted by the double-blind method, in which half of the participants get the drug and half get a placebo, or "dummy" medicine. Even the doctors conducting the trials do not know who is getting which drug.

What to Know Before You Get Involved

If you are considering participating in a clinical trial, you will want to know:

- Who is the sponsor? Look for a federal government, major health organization, drug company or university-sponsored trial.

- Do any impartial authorities monitor the trial? Every hospital conducting research has an institutional review board (IRB) consisting of medical professionals and community leaders who approve that hospital's participation. There are also data and safety monitoring boards that oversee trials.

- What is the financial relationship, if any, between the doctor, hospital and the company or agency sponsoring the trial?

- Will there be pain or discomfort? Will diagnostic tests be involved? Get detailed answers to these concerns before you sign any form.

- How often will I be examined? This depends on the guidelines of the trial (called the protocol). You should make every effort to keep your appointments.

- Does my own doctor get a record of my participation in the trial? Routine health information is sent to your doctor, but details relevant to a "blinded" trial are not disclosed until the trial is over.

- Is the drug in this trial approved for treatment of any other disorder? If the answer is yes, you then know that the drug has a prior safety record.

- After the study has ended, if I have responded well to the drug, will I be able to continue using it, even before it is approved?

- Can I drop out?

If you are interested in participating in a clinical trial, make your desire known to your doctor, who can track down openings in trials being conducted by medical centers, private foundations, drug companies, physician groups and the federal government. You can also access information on clinical trials by visiting the CenterWatch Clinical Trials Listing Service at www.centerwatch.com or the web site of the National Cancer Institute at www.cancer.gov/clinicaltrials.

*E*asy Access *to specialists and subspecialists, especially in large metropolitan areas, presents certain problems in coordination of care that a patient should be aware of. This difficulty is probably epitomized by one woman who was treated by a dermatologist, an ophthalmologist, a rheumatologist, a psychiatrist and an allergist, all of whom had office space in her very large apartment complex on Manhattan's upper west side-thus eliminating her need to even put on her coat. Fortunately, all were quite competent and had all the necessary qualifications. Unfortunately, each was affiliated with a different medical center, which made coordinating her care with her primary care doctor very complex.*

Changing Your Doctor

Quick Tips

- Surgical solutions can rarely be reversed. It usually is best to try a non-surgical solution first, if possible.

- You should always consider the possibility that alternative therapies - simply because they are unproven - may do more harm than good.

- If you do explore alternative therapies, be certain to let your doctor know about it. Some may be harmful, especially if you are undergoing another treatment under your doctor's direction.

- Before you decide to part company with your doctor, ask yourself if you've been a responsible patient.

- A doctor-patient relationship is like a marriage — both sides have to work to make it successful.

- Expressing your dissatisfaction may open the communication lines between you and your doctor; you might even end up in a better relationship with your present doctor

- Unless the situation is intolerable or the doctor is impaired, stay with your current doctor until you have found another one that you like

- When changing doctors, you may have to sign a release with your new doctor approving the transfer of all your medical records to the new office. These records cannot be withheld for any reason, even if you have not yet paid your last bill.

Quick Take

... There's a big difference between doctor-hopping and changing doctors for a good reason. Most failed doctor-patient relationships can be attributed to some common complaints but sometimes are a matter of self-defense...

Key Terms

National Practitioner Data Bank - A computerized listing, created by an Act of Congress, to track health professionals who are disciplined for unprofessional behavior and to deter them from simply moving their practicies from one state to another.

Public Citizen Health Research Group - A Washington, D.C. based consumer advocacy group that has been publicly critical of many medical practices that the group considers detrimental to public healthcare.

Changing Your Doctor

Obviously, at times there are good reasons for changing doctors. Some are very simple and straightforward, such as a doctor's retirement, illness or death, your own relocation or a change in your health plan. About 40 percent of people enrolling in managed care plans have to change their doctor to one who is affiliated with their plan.

The onset of a chronic condition may also prompt a change to a different medical specialist, such as a rheumatologist or cardiologist, if a condition needs to be managed by a specialist other than a primary care doctor.

If you have continuing symptoms that your doctor has been unable to diagnose or if, after a diagnosis, your problems continue to linger without improvement, you should at least consider getting a second opinion and, depending on that opinion, possibly change doctors. Doctors often have different approaches to the same problem. A different doctor may offer a different perspective and, perhaps, a solution.

You might also change doctors in order to find one who includes complementary/ alternative medicine in the treatment or to find one who can help you enroll in a clinical trial.

People who have hostile feelings toward organized medicine tend to change doctors frequently; their complaints then become a self-fulfilling prophecy. They don't get continuous, quality care because it's impossible for anyone to deliver it. On the other hand, negative feelings may be prompted by unfortunate encounters with incompetent doctors or by the patronizing or otherwise inappropriate attitudes expressed by some doctors toward patients. Patients on the receiving end of such a relationship should continue their search for a doctor who better meets their needs.

Eight Reasons to Say Goodbye

Here are the eight most common complaints about "doctors I don't go to anymore."

Poor Bedside Manner

Good medical care is more than diagnosis and treatment; it's also an attitude on the part of the doctor that sparks a sense of trust in the patient. Being under the care of a doctor who is impersonal, abrupt, bored, arrogant, condescending or sarcastic may, in the end, be counterproductive.

The doctor's aloofness could have a more serious explanation: substance abuse or psychological impairment, which, according to a recent American Medical Association report, affect 30,000 to 40,000 physicians. Mood swings and detachment are signs to watch for.

Too Vague and Evasive

A doctor who dismisses problems with "it's nothing to worry about" or "let me take care of it" or who uses medical jargon isn't interested in having you as a partner in your healthcare. The effect of this evasiveness can be anger, fear and confusion, leading to failure to follow directions and failure of treatment.

Never on Schedule

Medical emergencies can make appointment scheduling an inexact science, but when snafus become chronic, it's a sign of trouble. An explanation can ease the frustration, but make-up time should not be at your expense.

Couldn't Diagnose the Problem

Some conditions can't be diagnosed on-the-spot. Others aren't attributable to one specific cause. That doesn't excuse an incomplete workup, however, which may leave you with a condition that could have been treated earlier.

Ordered too Many Tests

Sophisticated technology is available and doctors tend to use it, although some testing may not be necessary. The number of tests performed for diagnosis seems to be reduced in patient-doctor relationships where communication is strong.

Discouraged Second Opinions

A doctor who dissuades you from talking to another doctor may perceive it as questioning his or her professional abilities.

Didn't Protect My Medical Privacy

No patient should have to discuss the reason for a visit, payment or payment problems within earshot of other patients or staff.

Under certain conditions, medical records can be requested by and turned over to insurance companies, lawyers, employers and certain others without your consent, but you can certainly see them, too, to make sure they contain the proper information. In all 50 states and the District of Columbia, federal law grants patients access to their medical records.

Unpleasant Office Staff

Repeated incidents such as rudeness over the telephone, a brusque physician's assistant or being kept waiting in an examining room for a long time before the doctor shows up are all annoying indications that a staff could do better.

The staff takes its cues from the chief. A doctor who doesn't demand the highest level of performance from a staff may be sending a message about his or her own laxity in diagnosis and treatment.

Should You Switch?

If these conditions exist in your doctor-patient relationship, it may be time to consider finding a new doctor. But before you decide to part company with your doctor, ask yourself if you've been a responsible patient. Often problems arise when patients don't reveal their full medical history or if they forget to alert their doctor about other drugs they are taking. A doctor-patient relationship is like a marriage—both sides have to work to make it successful.

If you're sure the problem isn't on your side, however, confront your doctor with your grievances. Or, if it's easier for you, you may want to write them in a letter. Expressing your dissatisfaction may open the communication lines between you and your doctor. You might even end up in a better relationship with your present doctor. Sometimes doctors aren't aware that they are in the midst of a deteriorating relationship until a patient wants to leave.

But if you are still unhappy with your doctor and you've decided a change is necessary, you can make a clean break by simply going to another doctor. Keep in mind, however, that your most important concern should be continuity of care. So, unless the situation is intolerable or the doctor is impaired, stay with your current doctor until you have found another one that you like.

Generally, medical records are kept by your doctor until you have found a new one. You will then have to sign a release with your new doctor approving the transfer of all your medical records to the new office. These records cannot be withheld for any reason, even if you have not yet paid your last bill.

Finally, don't feel embarrassed or guilty if you decide to change doctors. Remember, good quality medical care is your right!

Self Defense: Avoiding Questionable Doctors

In addition to finding good doctors, you also want to be able to identify and avoid doctors who have a history of professional problems. One way to do this is to make certain a doctor has not been disciplined by your state or, in fact, any state. You can call the appropriate state agency (listed in Appendix E) or check the web sites of those state agencies that make this information available. These sites list the names of doctors who have been disciplined by their state or by the federal government. The disciplinary actions were taken for a variety of reasons, including overprescribing or misprescribing medications, criminal convictions, alcohol or drug abuse and patient sexual abuse.

You also may visit the 'Vital Healthcare Info' section of the Castle Connolly Medical Ltd. web site (www.CastleConnolly.com) for links to those states with discipline information on their sites. You may also visit the American Medical Association (AMA) at www.ama-assn.org and American Board of Medical Specialities (ABMS) at www.abms.org. For the websites for biographical information about doctors, including board certification see Appendix D.

The Public Citizen Health Research Group, which publishes a report on the number of physicians disciplined in each state, believes that many states are not aggressive enough in monitoring doctors. They have been leading the call for public access to the National Practitioner Data Bank. The Data Bank was created in 1986 by an Act of Congress to track professionals who are disciplined for unprofessional behavior and to deter them from simply moving their practices from one state to another. The Data Bank became operational in 1990 and contains a record of adverse actions such as license removal, loss of clinical privileges and professional society membership actions taken against doctors and other licensed health professionals such as dentists. It contains the names of more than 170,000 health practitioners who have either a licensing action or malpractice judgment or settlement against them. There is strong pressure from some medical groups either to do away with the Data Bank or to place even stricter controls on access to it. They support their position with examples of errors in the handling of sensitive information. It is unlikely that Congress would permit the elimination of the Data Bank. In fact, it is possible that at some time in the future, access may be made more available to the public. However, at the present time there is no public general access to this information. After intense pressure a restricted data bank can now be accessed by research and journalism groups, provided they agree to newly imposed restrictions, which may be found unworkable.

A data service used by lawyers to check on a doctor's or hospital's malpractice history is LEXIS/NEXIS, the computerized legal information service. Some libraries will do a LEXIS/NEXIS search for a fee. Public access to the listing of malpractice payments is one issue on which doctors are very sensitive, and rightfully so. Many malpractice payments are made by insurance companies over the objections of doctors because the insurers feel it's cheaper to settle than to fight. Yet, doctors who feel they are blameless contend that these settlements reflect negatively on them. Also, since so many specialists, such as those in obstetrics and gynecology, are subject to more frequent lawsuits because of the nature of their practices, doctors are concerned about how patients will interpret a malpractice settlement. A few states, for example Massachussetts, make this information available on the State Health Department website. Check to see if it is available in your state. (See Vital Healthcare Information on the Castle Connolly Medical Ltd website (www.CastleConnolly.com.)

People who believe they have a problem with a doctor, whether in regard to fees, treatment or ethics, may contact the appropriate local medical society in the county in which the doctor practices or the state medical society. State health departments are also places consumers may turn to for assistance or information on disciplinary actions taken against doctors. The health department, typically, will only divulge that an action has been taken but will not give you any specific information about it (See Appendix E for phone numbers and addresses).

Changing your doctor should not be considered a setback in your search for the best doctor to meet your needs. As you may have come to understand throughout preceding chapters in this book, the personal and treatment styles doctors bring to their practices vary greatly. What is important for you, as a patient, to realize is that these subtle and immeasurable characteristics can be as important as clinical skills. There is, in fact, substantial empirical and anecdotal evidence demonstrating that confidence in the healer and the healing process plays a major role in many cures. Your main objective is to find the therapy—in combination with the professional who is providing the therapy—that works best for you.

In one case involving a woman in her mid-thirties, the doctor-patient relationship was severed over what was basically a conflict in personalities: the woman wished to have more control over her healthcare, and the doctor was reluctant to give it. The impasse was reached before the two could attempt any kind of a compromise, and the woman went off in search of a doctor who would better suit her personal needs. A year later, after a fruitless search for a doctor whose medical expertise she respected, she returned to her original doctor.

The Best in American Medicine
www.CastleConnolly.com

Choosing a Doctor in a Health Plan

Quick Tips

- A data service used by lawyers to check on a doctor's or hospital's malpractice history is Lexis/Nexis, the computerized legal information service. Lexis will do a search and issue a report on any malpractice awards or settlements ordered by a court.

- State health departments are also places consumers may turn to for assistance or information on disciplinary actions taken against doctors.

- There is substantial empirical and anecdotal evidence demonstrating that confidence in the healer and the healing process plays a major role in many cures.

- People who belive they have a problem with a doctor in regard to fees, treatment, or ethics, may contact the appropriate local medical society in the county in which the doctor practices, or the state medical society.

- When choosing a doctor in a health plan, use the same criteria you would apply to selecting a doctor in a fee-for-service practice.

- Typically, you will be sent a list with little information other than the doctor's name, specialty and address. Find out more about those doctors you may be considering.

- In some cases, a health plan will agree to pay at least a consultation fee if you feel strongly that you need to discuss your problem with another doctor outside of the health plan network

- If method of health plan payment to physicians is an issue of concern to you, it may be wise to ask your doctor about the method of compensation in the health plan in which you are enrolled.

Quick Take

... The rules are different but they are not difficult to play by. The first step is to sort out the alphabet soup of models. The model of health plan usually determines how your care will be delivered and often your satisfaction with it ...

Key Terms

Capitation - A method of payment to physicians and other healthcare providers whereby a fixed amount of money is allotted for each patient served.

EPO - An Exclusive Provider Organization is similar to a PPO except the patients must use only providers in the EPO.

Group Model HMO - A model of an HMO in which the HMO contracts with large multi-specialty groups of doctors to provide care, usually from a number of central locations.

Health Maintenance Organization (HMO) - One type of managed care organization that provides for a wide range of comprehensive healthcare services for its members in return for a fixed, predetermined fee. The care is provided by a network or group of physicians affiliated with the organization and possibly other healthcare professionals. The term "health plan" is a more common name in use today, which applies to all of the various health insurance organizations described in this list.

IPA - An Independent Practice Association is one model of health maintenance organization (HMO) in which the organization contracts with individual doctors, or groups of doctors, to provide care for the enrolled patients in the doctors' own offices.

PHO - A Physician Hospital Organization is an organization of a hospital and its physicians that may contract with managed care organizations (MCO) or may become licensed as an MCO itself.

PPO - A Preferred Provider Organization is a managed care model that offers healthcare provided by a group of doctors and/or hospitals that have negotiated discounted rates, either capitated or fee-for-service, for enrollees while continuing to provide care for other patients. Patients typically pay less if they use the PPO provider.

PSO - A Provider Service Organization, sometimes called a provider service network (PSN), is a group of doctors that are organized to provide care to a large number of patients, typically under contract to managed care organizations.

Staff Model HMO - A managed care model where the HMO employs the doctors, usally on salary. Care is provided out of a number of centralized locations.

Choosing a Doctor in a Health Plan

At one time only doctors looking for new patients joined HMOs. Today, there is a new reality. Although HMO's still exist, a more common name is health plan. Almost all doctors—more than 80 percent—participate in some kind of managed care arrangement. So it is likely that you will find the best for your own care if you know how to work the system.

When managed care achieves a significant market penetration and begins to control the flow of large numbers of patients, more doctors sign on. Also, many hospitals encourage their doctors to sign on with as many different plans as possible in order to ensure that the hospital does not lose any potential patients. Managed care now enrolls more than one out of every three people in the country, and more than 80 percent of workers who get health insurance through their employer are in some form of managed care. Today, more people are enrolled in PPOs (Preferred Provider Organization), which tend to be more flexible in choices of physicians, than are enrolled in HMOs. However, we will use health plan as "shorthand" for both.

The main factors to focus on in assessing a health plan or a PPO are its resources, primarily doctors and hospitals. First, is there an ample selection of primary care doctors near where you live and work? Second, are the doctors well qualified? This can be answered by following the approach outlined in this book for finding the best doctors. When choosing doctors, it is usually a good idea to call their offices to confirm they are still affiliated with the particular plan. Doctors frequently change affiliations with managed care plans. Also, it is a good idea to check on the procedure for using the doctor listed.

Health plans may list hundreds of doctors but not all of them are necessarily accessible to all members. A large health plan, for example, may restrict the number of specialists that primary care doctors can refer to for various reasons, including location, hospital capacity and general resource allocation. So although you may see the name of an ophthalmologist, gynecologist or other specialist you want to use, and indeed that doctor may be affiliated with the health plan, it does not necessarily follow that your primary care doctor is free to refer you to them. Those specialists may see health plan patients only on a certain basis—for specific procedures, for example, or in a certain geographic region—and then possibly only after a rigorous screening process. These possibilities illustrate the varying styles of operation you will find in managed care plans.

Doctors in health plans are bound by the same professional ethics that guide all doctors. However, there is a major difference; in a health plan, the plan is responsible for providing you with care as well as with a doctor. If your doctor leaves the plan, you don't follow him or her. The plan provides a new doctor for you.

Selecting Doctors in a Health Plan

Selecting a doctor in a health plan can be a greater challenge than selecting one when you have indemnity insurance that leaves you free to select a doctor without the restrictions of the plan. Obviously, in a health plan arrangement you need to select a doctor who belongs to that plan. Studies have shown that about 40 percent of enrollees in managed care plans have to choose a new doctor when they join. However, even in a plan of small size, you will usually have the option of choosing among a number of primary care doctors as well as other specialists and subspecialists. In doing so, utilize the same criteria you would apply to selecting a doctor in a fee-for-service practice.

The first doctor you select in a health plan is your primary care doctor. Typically, you will be sent a list with little information other than the doctor's name, specialty and address. Find out more about those doctors you may be considering. Use the process described earlier in this book. If you make a selection and are not satisfied, request a change. Ask about the procedure for changing doctors before you join the plan.

When you need a specialist, it is your primary care doctor who will refer you, as in traditional indemnity plans. But, unlike indemnity plans in which you can find a specialist on your own if you choose, in managed care plans you must be referred to see a specialist. Again, your choices will be limited in selecting specialists, but be assertive. Ask for a choice of doctors and ask why your primary care doctor recommends a particular specialist. One disadvantage to the IPA model and the network referral process is that primary care doctors can end up making referrals to specialists and/or subspecialists that they do not know. This may result in poor communication between the primary care doctor and the specialist, which is not in the patient's best interest. If you are not satisfied with the choices offered, ask to go outside the plan. Choice of providers outside a plan is built into certain managed care plans (PPOs or POS, Point of Service) and is permitted in many others under certain conditions.

However, if you do not have a choice, or if the choices are not ones with which you agree, consider going outside the health plan. Although you are likely to have to pay more, it may be worth it if you get a correct diagnosis and appropriate treatment for your problem. In some cases, the health plan will agree to pay at least a consultation fee if you feel strongly that you need to discuss your problem with another doctor outside the health plan network. After the consultation, if you still feel the need for a different doctor, at least your choice will be based on more complete information.

One of the most popular options offered by health plans permits going outside of the network of doctors and hospitals—but at an added cost. The point of service, or POS plan, one of the fastest growing offerings of many health plans, permits the health plan member to use doctors, hospitals, and other services that are not part of the health plan network. Typically, the member will pay an additional fee for this choice—for example, 20 percent or 30 percent of the cost—whereas if the member stays "in-network" the health plan will pay all or close to all of the cost.

When leaving the network of a POS, however, patients should find out exactly how much it will cost to do so. Some health plans will pay a percentage of "usual and customary fees" while others will pay a percentage of their own fee schedule, which is usually lower.

HMO Models

Although a large alphabet soup of health plan models has appeared since the big move toward managed care began in the late 1980s, and we now have PPOs, PSOs, and EPOs, two models are most important to the healthcare consumer. One is the staff or group model where patients visit their doctors in a single, or perhaps in a few, locations and where all the doctors and most, if not all, diagnostic and treatment facilities are located. The second is the independent practice association or IPA model where doctors see patients in their private offices. Organizations such as PPOs, EPOs and PSOs tend to be organized on the IPA model.

Whether a group/staff model or an IPA, all health plans require a primary care physician and all have certain protocols, usually involving referral by the primary care physician, to access a specialist.

Doctor Compensation

There is virtually no difference in the types of doctors who practice in the two plan models and each should be evaluated in terms of benefits to the individual patient. There is, however, a separate matter of how doctors in HMOs are compensated, and this issue has become a major concern to both patients and doctors.

Health plans compensate doctors in a number of ways. Doctors who are employed by staff model health plans are usually on salary, perhaps with a quality bonus based on patient satisfaction. In group model health plans, the physician group has a contract with the health plan and the doctors are employed by the group, usually on salary and, again, often with a quality bonus.

In the IPA model, or in PPOs, EPOs, PSOs and other types of managed care organizations the doctors are usually paid in one of two ways. In the past, the predominant payment method was a negotiated fee schedule, typically designed at some discount to the doctor's normal fee. Doctors simply traded the promise of higher volume for a reduced fee. Today, a major method of payment in an IPA is capitation. While this is fast becoming the most common method of payment in IPAs it is also the one generating the most controversy.

Under a capitated or capitation system doctors are paid a set amount per month or per year to provide care to a patient during that time period. So, for example, a primary care physician may be paid $25 per member per month.

Health plans have moved toward capitation as a method of payment because they found that discounted fee-for-service payment methods did not reduce costs as much as had been hoped, if at all. To make up for discounted fees of 20 percent, for instance, some doctors simply scheduled 20 percent more patient visits so that their incomes would not decrease. Doctors openly comment that discounted fees translate to discounted time with patients!

Capitation has helped to control costs. However, it also has introduced a number of important ethical issues for doctors, other healthcare providers, and for patients. Many are troubled by the notion that a doctor could be placed in a situation that appears to promise rewards for not providing care. It is generally recognized that under a fee-for-service system doctors have an incentive to provide more care, even if it is not necessary, because they are paid by the amount of care they deliver. But the reverse is not accepted in such a benign fashion: the concept of a doctor being rewarded to provide less care is of major concern to many people, including many doctors.

Another technique involved in payment systems utilized by managed care companies is called "withholds" or "set-asides." This method is also used to motivate doctors to control costs and, as in capitation, raises similar ethical concerns. Under this method, for example, a group of pediatricians is contracted to care for 1,000 children. That contract is based on a budget of $15,000 a month. A certain amount of that budget, say 20 percent, is reserved for referrals to subspecialists and another 20 percent is set aside or withheld. If the group of doctors uses fewer subspecialist referrals than budgeted they receive the 20 percent that was set aside. If they use more subspecialist referrals than were budgeted the extra amount comes out of the set-aside. The more set-aside that is used for referrals, the less doctors will be able to receive from it.

A great deal of controversy has ensued over these payment mechanisms. Some states, in fact, are legislating to prohibit or restrict these practices. Individual "horror stories" of patients who have been denied appropriate care, such as not being referred to a subspecialist in a timely manner, have been used to demonstrate the issue in human terms.

Some studies demonstrate that when physician-run health plans are paid by capitation and are in control they reduce costs more substantially than other plans. Some doctors strongly support capitation. They believe it makes them, rather than managers, responsible for allocating resources and making medical decisions.

And, despite the outcry, most of the studies of health plan patients versus non-plan patients demonstrate no differences in their health status.

In fact, there is a substantial body of research suggesting that health plan members receive more in the way of preventive services than do non-health plan populations.

If method of payment is an issue of concern to you, it may be wise to ask your doctor about the method of compensation in the health plan in which you are enrolled. If you believe the method would work against you as a patient you should discuss it with your doctor and ask if and how it influences the manner of care for patients. If you are not satisfied by the answer you may want to change doctors or, better yet, change health plans, if possible.

While the wisest course of action is to ask about this issue before joining a health plan, rather than after you have become a member, most plan members have not done this. If you believe you are not receiving appropriate care because of a health plan policy, you can contact your state health insurance department (see Appendix E).

In response to patient and physician concerns about payment policies, groups of doctors in various parts of the country have formed organizations to receive and investigate complaints against HMOs. You can contact them with any grievances you have about your plan (see Physicians Who Care, Appendix D).

How Doctors and Patients Feel about Managed Care

People enrolled in health plans tend to be satisfied by their plans. However, most doctors do not like managed care—and understandably so! Managed care organizations negotiate deep discounts in fees for doctors. There is no reason doctors should prefer this process, but when managed care controls so many patients there is little choice but to join managed care and negotiate.

Managed care organizations also require doctors to do a substantial amount of paperwork and to follow policies and procedures that control costs and monitor quality. All of this creates a level of business management most doctors resent.

At least a portion of these negative attitudes toward managed care can be ascribed to differences in the organization of medical practices in different parts of the country.

The northeast, south, and southwest regions have been the slowest to accept managed care because doctors generally resisted it more strongly than those in other parts of the country. Doctors in large group practices, which are more common in the far west and midwest than in the east, adapted to managed care more readily. In the northeast, where doctors practice solo or in small groups, the change has been greater and the adjustment more difficult.

Most doctors have adapted and learned to practice successfully in this new medical environment. According to a survey conducted by the American Medical Association, just over a third (210,811) of physicians in this country are now members of group practices. In 1995 group practices numbered 19,788, an increase of 361 percent since 1965. From 1991 to 1995, the number of groups increased by 16.4 percent and the number of group physicians by 14.3 percent.

The survey shows that, in an environment that is organizationally complex, medical groups have changed how they are organized legally, with partnerships declining to 13.8 percent and professional corporations increasing to 77.9 percent. In the latter group, control of decision making remains largely in the physician's hands. This ability to retain decision making power has dramatically altered physicians' attitudes towards managed care.

The view of patients and the public, however, is decidedly more positive about managed care.

A study sponsored by the Medstat Group, J.D. Power and Associates and the New England Medical Center reported that in 20 markets across the United States, health plans received more top scores than PPOs and fee-for-service plans.

The study asked plan members to assess their health plans on choice of providers, physician care, premiums and deductibles and access to care. Health plans topped fee-for-service and point-of-service plans in more than half of the markets.

One of the findings uncovered in a Louis Harris Associates poll of consumers was that of the majority surveyed, 59 percent, believed the trend toward managed care was a good thing as compared to 28 percent who viewed it as a bad thing. Also, 48 percent as compared to 39 percent believed managed care would improve quality, and 59 percent versus 30 percent believed it would help contain the costs of care. Of note was that the response of those people in communities with a high penetration by managed care tended to be the most positive!

There are many studies that have examined the quality of care and the satisfaction of patients in managed care settings. Most show that members of health plans and other managed care organizations are at least as satisfied or more satisfied with their care than people covered by indemnity insurance. Some studies have shown indemnity-covered people are more satisfied, particularly when it relates to choice of doctors. In fact, the issue of greatest concern to health plan enrollees is usually access, particularly to specialists. Advocates of either view can point to studies to support managed care or to criticize it. The key may lay in the studies that have demonstrated that when individuals have a choice, and select a managed care plan, they tend to be more satisfied than those who have no choice.

In terms of quality, the conclusion is similar. While critics may contend that the care delivered by managed care organizations is not adequate, and a study of Medicaid patients is frequently cited to support this view, the overwhelming majority of studies demonstrate no difference in the health status and quality of care of those people covered by managed care plans or by indemnity insurance.

The variability in the results of all of the studies on quality and satisfaction in managed care reinforces the important premise that, as there are good doctors and poor doctors, there are good health plans and poor health plans. It is important for consumers to know how to discern the difference and to put some effort, however modest, into finding the best.

Points to Remember

- To summarize, there is basically no difference in quality between doctors who participate in health plans and those who do not accept insurance. You can find excellent doctors if you're a member of a health plan and you can find poor ones, just as you can find excellent and poor doctors if you carry indemnity insurance. The key is making sure that you find the best available for your own needs and the needs of your family.

Some simple guidelines to remember:

- Review the credentials and training of any doctor who cares for you.

- Make certain that a doctor you select is taking new patients and the waiting period for an appointment is not unreasonable.

- Be sure the health plan has a sufficient number of specialists and subspecialists you may need to see and that they are of high quality. For example, if you have diabetes, you will want to make sure that the plan has endocrinologists on staff or as part of its network. If you have coronary heart disease, you will want to make sure that the plan has first rate cardiologists and an arrangement with an outstanding center where the doctors perform invasive and non-invasive diagnostic techniques and which has a good record for open heart surgery.

- Determine beforehand the health plan's policy for patient referral to subspecialists, especially whether or not you will have a choice and how it may be exercised.

- Inquire about the rules for changing doctors in the plan if you are not satisfied with your initial choice. You will want to know not only the procedure but how often such change is allowed.

- Ask about your options to go out of network and what your additional percentage of payment will be if you exercise this option. In determining what percentage the health plan pays, try to find out whether their payment is based on the health plan fee scale or "usual and customary" fees.

- Ask your doctor about the health plan's compensation system. You want to be sure that the system for paying your doctor will not have a negative influence on your care.

The Best in American Medicine
www.CastleConnolly.com

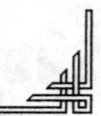

Directory of Doctors

Includes
Partnership for Excellence
Program

The Best in American Medicine
www.CastleConnolly.com

How to use the Directory of Doctors

Castle Connolly Medical Ltd. provides healthcare consumers with an invaluable source of information to identify leading physicians in their own community. This thirteenth edition of the Castle Connolly Guide, *Top Doctors: New York Metro Area*, contains vital information on more than 6,000 of the finest doctors in the region. Our guides are the result of a methodical process requiring a complete credential, licensing and disciplinary review of all doctors nominated for inclusion in the guide.

Why This Book Is Your Best Guide

Top Doctors: New York Metro Area is unique in a number of ways. The first edition of the Guide, published in 1994, was the first selective directory of doctors who practice in the New York metropolitan region. Castle Connolly recognizes that most healthcare is provided locally and people generally obtain their healthcare where they live or work. Therefore, by identifying excellent, caring physicians in every community and in every hospital, we apprise consumers of the best healthcare available to them within their own communities. Healthcare consumers in the New York metropolitan region are very fortunate with the abundance of doctors—approximately 55,000—who practice in the area. On the other hand, making a selection of one out of such a multitude can be a daunting task; it's hard even to know where to start. With *Top Doctors: New York Metro Area* in hand, you are already well on your way to finding the very best doctor for your individual needs and the needs of your family members.

With the profusion of outstanding academic medical centers, tertiary care teaching hospitals and fine regional hospitals in the New York metropolitan area, virtually any medical procedure or treatment can be found close to home. By virtue of this fact, it would be a simple matter to compile a book identifying the outstanding leaders in medical research and academic medicine in the region. Although many of these doctors are included in the listings, their names are to be found among the many excellent and caring doctors who deliver outstanding patient care in every community in the area. The goal—first and foremost—is to help you find the best doctors to meet your healthcare needs where you live and work. Again, a good reason why the Castle Connolly Guide is exceptional.

Further, the Castle Connolly Guide is different from most other listings of doctors in its selection process. Our selection is predicated on an extensive nomination procedure and a set of exacting standards which each nominated doctor was required to meet. To you, this means that the basis for inclusion of every one of the doctors in the listings was twofold: respect of their peers and medical excellence. Doctors do not pay to be listed. Our goal is to serve consumers, not doctors, hospitals or health plans.

How Castle Connolly Selects the Top Doctors

The basis of the Castle Connolly selection process is peer nomination. In some ways, this resembles an enhancement of the process in which a personal physician provides a patient with a referral to another physician for a particular problem. However, if the recommendation of one doctor is good, the recommendation of many doctors is even better. So, we ask thousands of randomly-selected physicians in the New York metropolitan area for their nominations.

How do we accomplish this enormous task? Over the years, the Castle Connolly physician-directed research team developed its extensive database of physicians through periodic mail, telephone and email surveys in the following counties:

New York State: New York, Bronx, Kings, Queens, Richmond, Nassau, Suffolk, Rockland, Westchester

New Jersey: Bergen, Essex, Hudson, Mercer, Middlesex, Monmouth, Morris, Passaic, Somerset, Union

Connecticut: Fairfield, New Haven

This cumulative database is systematically maintained and continuously updated. Surveyed physicians nominate top doctors in both their own and related specialties—especially those to whom they would refer their patients and their own family members. The database is also updated through further mail and telephone surveys. Each year we build on our prior research and supplement our database by inviting leading physicians at major medical centers in the metropolitan area, the thousands of top doctors included in earlier editions of our guide, and local leaders in the various medical specialties to offer their nominations for *Top Doctors: New York Metro Area*.

In addition to nominations obtained directly from practicing physicians, Castle Connolly solicits nominations from each area hospital's:

- President or Chief Executive Officer
- Vice President of Medical Affairs or the equivalent position
- Chief of Service in:
  - Anesthesiology
  - Medicine
  - Neurology
  - Obstetrics/Gynecology
  - Pathology
  - Pediatrics
  - Radiology
  - Surgery

Considerations for Inclusion Among the Top Doctors

Castle Connolly considers the following among the varied criteria used to determine physician eligibility for inclusion in our guides.

Professional Qualifications

- Education
- Residency
- Board certification
- Fellowships
- Professional reputation
- Hospital appointment
- Medical school faculty appointment
- Experience
- Disciplinary history

Personal Characteristics/Qualities

Not only do we seek nominations of physicians who excel in academic medicine and research, but most importantly, those who exhibit excellence in patient care. We ask physicians in our survey to consider not only the training and clinical skills of the physicians they nominate, but also interpersonal skills such as the following:

- Listening and communicating effectively
- Demonstrating empathy
- Educating and informing
- Instilling trust and confidence

Verification/Credential Review

The Castle Connolly research staff reviews and refines the pool of nominated physicians in a region, validates nominations and verifies credentials. This results in the development of a preliminary list of physicians. Each provisionally selected physician is then required to complete a comprehensive professional biographical form including their special practice interests (see the "SPECIALTY & SPECIAL EXPERTISE INDEX"). The information contained in the biographical form becomes an integral part of each selected physician's listing in the guide.

The last phase of the process refines the list of provisionally selected doctors by cross-referencing their names against a variety of databases providing confirmation of:

- Board certification and recertification
- Licensing
- Disciplinary history

In some regions, a small number of peer-nominated physicians who are not board-certified may be included in a guide. These are doctors recognized by their colleagues as having exceptional demonstrated clinical practice experience.

Physicians ultimately selected for inclusion in *Top Doctors: New York Metro Area* receive formal notification of their nomination for listing upon completion of the final confirmation of their professional credentials.

How You Can Select the Top Doctors

How can you begin to make a choice from such a compilation of names? There is, in fact, a basic step-by-step process which varies somewhat depending on your individual needs as you approach the list. Here are the possibilities:

ONE: **If You are Looking for a Doctor in a Particular County**

The key: Physicians listed in the following pages are organized under the county in which their office is located so that you can go directly to the section listing doctors in your county of residence.

Key fact: Like most healthcare consumers, you probably receive your healthcare locally. If you think about it, you usually have been treated by doctors close to where you live and in community hospitals. If necessary, you may be referred to regional specialists and nearby medical centers.

TWO: **If You are Looking for a Primary Care Physician — a Generalist**

The key: The doctors who practice predominantly primary care, in the specialties of internal medicine, family practice, pediatrics, and obstetrics/gynecology, are designated by the notation a in the listing.

Key fact: Every board certified physician is a specialist. The term "having boards" signifies that a physician has completed an approved residency in a given specialty and has passed a rigorous examination given by that particular board. Therefore, doctors who practice primary care—internists, family practitioners, pediatricians, and Ob/Gyns—are specialists in their respective fields, as are urologists, otolaryngologists and radiologists. These specialists are considered primary care physicians.

THREE: If You are Looking for a Physician in a Particular Specialty

The key: Each entry contains the specialty practiced by the doctor and, in most cases, the most recent year of board certification.

Key fact: Many physicians specialize in fields of medicine that are not primary care. These specialists have completed an approved residency in a given specialty and have passed a rigorous exam given by that specialty board. For example, some physicians are board certified in psychiatry, surgery, allergy and immunology or dermatology.

Many doctors choose to specialize further. They choose an additional training program called a fellowship and upon completion of the program, they are required to take another exam in order to be certified as a subspecialist. An example of such subspecialization is an internist (initially board certified in internal medicine) who subspecialize in nephrology or cardiology. This doctor would be termed "double boarded" and would very likely practice nephrology or cardiology rather than internal medicine as a primary care physician.

FOUR: If You are Looking for a Doctor with Expertise in a Particular Disease or Technique

The key: Particular skills and interests of the doctors are found under the heading "SPECIALTY & SPECIAL EXPERTISE INDEX."

Key fact: A physician may have a special expertise interest in a particular field of medicine without actually being board certified in that area. Special expertise interests should not be confused with a board certified medical specialty. For example, cosmetic surgery is not an American Board of Medical Specialties recognized specialty, but it may constitute a major practice activity for many plastic surgeons. Certain doctors may develop a reputation as "specialists" in AIDS, diabetes or arthroscopic surgery. None of these are recognized medical specialties, yet they are indications of a doctor's expertise in a disease or medical or surgical procedure which may be helpful if you have the disease or need the procedure.

Many doctors who have a strong interest in, or consider themselves "specializing in," a particular health problem or medical technique form special interest groups referred to as "self-designated medical specialties." These groups are often confused with recognized medical specialties, which they are not. Some of the groups would like to be recognized by the ABMS and may even work toward that goal. For example, adolescent medicine was a special interest and self-designated specialty that is now an ABMS recognized subspecialty.

Choosing a doctor with a special practice interest is an additional step to be considered after you have already narrowed your choices to particular specialists and/or subspecialists. The "SPECIALTY & SPECIAL EXPERTISE INDEX" lists the doctors' special area or areas of expertise and can be particularly useful in identifying physicians who embrace alternative or complementary practices. Self-designated medical specialties are listed in Appendix B.

FIVE: **If You are Looking for a Doctor by Name**

The key: The "ALPHABETICAL LISTING OF DOCTORS" indicates the page on which information on the doctor's credentials can be found. The listing is arranged in last name, first name order.

Key fact: Most people start their search for a doctor through recommendation by family and friends. As a savvy healthcare consumer you realize that such recommendations are often based on personal "chemistry" and may be made by someone who actually knows very little about doctors or healthcare. Therefore, you will want to check the credentials of any recommended doctor and follow the additional recommendations that we have outlined in Sections one and two.

SIX: **If You want Detailed Information on a Particular Doctor**

The key: Each doctor's listing includes a substantial amount of information about the doctor.

Key fact: Wise choices in healthcare are made by consumers who have gathered as much information as possible about a particular doctor. If a professional information form was not returned by a doctor in time for inclusion in the book, our research staff verified certain major points of information (name, address, telephone, hospital affiliation, and specialty) from public sources and we have included this limited information. Even if a doctor's full credentials are included in this book, it is possible that, since the time of publication, the doctor has moved his or her office(s), changed telephone number(s), joined new medical groups, resigned from or joined hospital staffs, and, especially, changed relationships with HMOs and PPOs. Nonetheless, you can, in most cases, track down the doctor by using the following sources:

- Doctor's office—call the office number listed in the directory and ask for a new number.

- Hospitals—call the hospital listed in the directory and ask for help in locating a particular doctor.

- State Health Department—all state health department numbers are listed in Appendix E.

- American Board of Medical Specialties—a complete listing of ABMS Specialty Boards is found in Appendix A.

- American Osteopathic Association—a complete listing of AOA Specialty Boards is found in Appendix A.

Conclusion

You are now ready to work with our directory of more than 5,000 of the finest doctors in the New York metropolitan area. Although you may be well-informed as a result of reading Sections one and two of this book, it is possible that choosing the doctor will seem to be a complex endeavor. The tendency might be to try to get the job done as quickly as possible by choosing a doctor based solely on the convenience of the office's location. To do so would be a big mistake. You want the best healthcare. You deserve it. A little effort will help you to get the best.

There are many excellent doctors in the region not listed in this book. You can identify them by using the process we have described in Sections one and two or, if a doctor in this book is unable to meet your needs, ask about other physicians highly regarded by that doctor.

We believe that this book will educate and enlighten you throughout its pages and that it will prove its value in the end—when you decide on the doctor with whom you plan to have a lasting relationship.

Obtaining Additional Doctor Information

You may wish to call a doctor's office to make an appointment or to help determine if the doctor is the one you want to care for you. Here are some questions you may want to ask:

1. Is a referral required?

2. Are you accepting new patients?

3. Which health plans/insurance do you accept?

4. Do you accept Medicare? Medicaid? Workers' compensation? No-fault insurance?

5. Are payments of deductible and co-payments required at the time of appointment?

6. Do you accept credit cards?

7. Do you see patients in the evening? On weekends?

8. Is the office handicapped-accessible?

9. Do you accept phone calls from patients?

10 Do you communicate with patients via the internet?

11. If you are not comfortable addressing the doctor in English, ask if your native language is spoken by the doctor or by someone else in the office.

Sample Listing

Smith, John MD [IM] *PCP - Spec Exp: Ulcers; Crohn's Disease;*

<u>   </u>   <u>   </u>

Name [specialty] &   Special Expertise(s)
Primary Care Physician indication

Hospital: NYU Med Ctr (page 130); **Address:** 100 Tenth St, FL 5 - Ste 3A, MC-1234, New York, NY 10010;

admitting hospital(s) &   Office address   Mail code   City, state zip
Hospital Information page(s)

Phone: (904) 296-0000; **Board Cert:** IM 70, GE 74; **Med School:** U Fla Coll Med 66;

Office phone   *Board certification(s) & date(s)   Medical school & year of degree

Resid: IM, NYU Med Ctr, 69; **Fellow:** GE, Lenox Hill Hosp, 72;

Residency(ies) & location(s)   Fellowship(s) & location(s)

Fac Appt: Assoc Clin Prof Med, NYU Sch Med

Faculty appointment & location

* Indicates the most recent date of board certification or recertification.

In our listings of the professional information on doctors, we have abbreviated hospitals and medical schools. The abbreviations are designed to be self-explanatory, but if you need assistance, refer to Appendix D: Hospitals Listings.

Note on Special Expertise(s):

These are not medical specialties as described on pages 81-87, but the areas of expertise or practice interests indicated by the doctor.

The information reported in each doctor's listing is, for the most part, provided by the doctor or his/her office staff. Castle Connolly attempts to verify the data through other sources but cannot guarantee that in all cases all data have been so verified or are accurate. All such information is subject to change from time to time due to changes in physician practices. Many doctors participate in several health plans and/or switch plans frequently. Therefore, you should verify with the doctor's office whether your health plan is currently accepted.

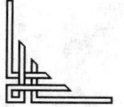
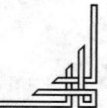

The Best in American Medicine
www.CastleConnolly.com

Medical Specialties
and Subspecialties

In the pages that follow, each list of doctors in a medical specialty or subspecialty is preceded by a brief description of that specialty (or subspecialty) and the training required for board certification.

Critical Care Medicine has been excluded because in emergency situations there is neither time nor opportunity for choice. A number of other specialities not relevant to most patients (e.g., Forensic Psychiatry) have not been included as well.

The following descriptions of medical specialties and subspecialties were provided by the American Board of Medical Specialties (ABMS), an organization comprised of the 24 medical specialty boards that provide certification in 25 medical specialties. A complete listing of all specialists certified by the ABMS can be found in The Official ABMS Directory of Board Certified Medical Specialists, is published by Marquis Who's Who. It is available (either in a multi-volume directory or on CD-ROM) in most public libraries, hospital libraries, university libraries and medical libraries. The ABMS also operates a toll-free phone line at 1-866-275-2267 and a website at www.abms.org to verify the certification status of individual doctors.

The following important policy statement, approved by the ABMS Assembly on March 19, 1987, remains valid.

The Purpose Of Certification

The intent of the certification process, as defined by the member boards of the American Board of Medical Specialties, is to provide assurance to the public that a certified medical specialist has successfully completed an approved educational program and an evaluation, including an examination process designed to assess the knowledge, experience and skills requisite to the provision of high quality patient care in that specialty.

Medical Specialties and Subspecialties

Medical Specialty and Subspecialty Descriptions and Abbreviations

The following medical specialties and subspecialties are indicated in the doctors' listings by their abbreviations. Specialties are indicated in bold, subspecialties in italics, and the four primary care specialties in bold capitals. To review the official American Board of Medical Specialties (ABMS) organization of specialties, refer to Appendix A.

Addiction Psychiatry   AdP
Deals with habitual psychological and physiological dependence on a substance or practice which is beyond voluntary control.

Adolescent Medicine   AM
Involves the primary care treatment of adolescents and young adults.

Allergy & Immunology   **A&I**
Diagnosis and treatment of allergies, asthma and skin problems such as hives and contact dermatitis.

Anesthesiology   **Anes**
Provides pain relief in maintenance or restoration of a stable condition during and following an operation. Anesthesiologists also diagnose and treat acute and long standing pain problems.

Cardiac Electrophysiology (Clinical)   CE
Involves complicated technical procedures to evaluate heart rhythms and determine appropriate treatment for them.

Cardiovascular Disease   Cv
Involves the diagnosis and treatment of disorders of the heart, lungs and blood vessels.

Child & Adolescent Psychiatry   ChAP
Deals with the diagnosis and treatment of mental diseases in children and adolescents.

Child Neurology   ChiN
Diagnosis and medical treatment of disorders of the brain, spinal cord and nervous system in children.

Clinical Genetics   **CG**
Deals with identifying the genetic causes of inherited diseases and ailments and preventing, when possible, their occurrence.

Colon and Rectal Surgery   **CRS**
Surgical treatment of diseases of the intestinal tract, colon and rectum, anal canal and perianal area.

Critical Care Medicine   CCM
Involves diagnosing and taking immediate action to prevent death or further injury of a patient. Examples of critical injuries include shock, heart attack, drug overdose and massive bleeding.

Dermatology   **D**

Diagnosis and treatment of benign and malignant disorders of the skin, mouth, external genitalia, hair and nails, as well as a number of sexually transmitted diseases.

Diagnostic Radiology   DR

Involves the study of all modalities of radiant energy in medical diagnoses and therapeutic procedures utilizing radiologic guidance.

Endocrinology, Diabetes & Metabolism   EDM

Involves the study and treatment of patients suffering from hormonal and chemical disorders.

FAMILY MEDICINE   **FP**

Deals with and oversees the total healthcare of individual patients and their family members. Family practitioners are more common in rural areas and may perform procedures more commonly performed by specialists (e.g., minor surgery).

Forensic Psychiatry   FPsy

Concerns the evaluation of certain diagnostic groups of patients that include those with sexual disorders, antisocial personality disorders, paranoid disorders and addictive disorders.

Gastroenterology   Ge

The study, diagnosis and treatment of diseases of the digestive organs including the stomach, bowels, liver and gallbladder.

Geriatric Medicine   Ger

Deals with diseases of the elderly and the problems associated with aging.

Geriatric Psychiatry   GerPsy

Involves the diagnosis, prevention and treatment of mental illness in the elderly.

Gynecologic Oncology   GO

Deals with cancers of the female genital tract and reproductive systems.

Hand Surgery   HS

Involves the treatment of injury to the hand through surgical techniques.

Hematology   Hem

Involves the diagnosis and treatment of diseases and disorders of the blood, bone marrow, spleen and lymph glands.

Hospice and Palliative Medicine   H&PM

Palliative care relieves the suffering and provides the best quality of life to people suffering from serious and severe chronic illness. Hospice care focuses on the palliation of a terminally ill patient's symptoms and also provides passionate support to both the patient and their surrounding loved ones.

Infectious Disease   Inf

The study and treatment of diseases caused by a bacterium, virus, fungus or animal parasite.

INTERNAL MEDICINE   **IM**

Diagnosis and nonsurgical treatment of diseases, especially those of adults. Internists may act as primary care specialists, highly trained family doctors or they may subspecialize in specialties such as cardiology or nephrology.

Maternal & Fetal Medicine MF

Involves the care of women with high-risk pregnancies and their unborn fetuses.

Medical Oncology Onc

Refers to the study and treatment of tumors and other cancers.

Neonatal-Perinatal Medicine NP

Involves the diagnosis and treatments of infants prior to, during and one month beyond birth.

Nephrology Nep

Concerned with disorders of the kidneys, high blood pressure, fluid and mineral balance, dialysis of body wastes when the kidneys do not function and consultation with surgeons about kidney transplantation.

Neurological Surgery **NS**

Involves surgery of the brain, spinal cord and nervous system.

Neurology **N**

Diagnosis and medical treatment of disorders of the brain, spinal cord and nervous system.

Neuroradiology NRad

Involves the utilization of imaging procedures during diagnosis as they relate to the brain, spine and spinal cord, head, neck and organs of special sense in adults and children.

Nuclear Medicine **NuM**

Evaluation of the functions of all the organs in the body and treatment of thyroid disease, benign and malignant tumors and radiation exposure through the use of radioactive substances.

Nuclear Radiology NR

Involves the use of radioactive substances to diagnose and treat certain functions and diseases of the body.

OBSTETRICS & GYNECOLOGY **ObG**

Deals with the medical aspects of and intervention in pregnancy and labor and the overall health of the female reproductive system.

Occupational Medicine OM

Concentrates on the effect of the work environment on the health of employees.

Ophthalmology **Oph**

Diagnosis and treatment of diseases of and injuries to the eye.

Orthopaedic Surgery **OrS**

Involves operations to correct injuries which interfere with the form and function of the extremities, spine and associated structures.

Otolaryngology   **Oto**

Explores and treats diseases in the interrelated areas of the ears, nose and throat.

Otology/Neurotology   ON

Concentrates on the management, prevention, cure and care of patients with diseases of the ear and temporal bone, including disorders of hearing and balance.

Pain Medicine   PM

Involves providing a high level of care for patients experiencing problems with acute or chronic pain in both hospital and ambulatory settings.

Pediatric Cardiology   PCd

Involves the diagnosis and treatment of heart disease in children.

Pediatric Critical Care Medicine   PCCM

Involves the care of children who are victims of life threatening disorders such as severe accidents, shock and diabetes acidosis.

Pediatric Dermatology   PD

Diagnosis and treatment of benign and malignant disorders of the skin, mouth, external genitalia, hair and nails in children.

Pediatric Endocrinology   PEn

Involves the study and treatment of children with hormonal and chemical disorders.

Pediatric Gastroenterology   PGe

The study, diagnosis and treatment of diseases of the digestive tract in children.

Pediatric Hematology-Oncology   PHO

The study and treatment of cancers of the blood and blood-forming parts of the body in children.

Pediatric Infectious Disease   PInf

The study and treatment of diseases caused by a virus, bacterium, fungus or animal parasite in children.

Pediatric Nephrology   PNep

Deals with the diagnosis and treatment of disorders of the kidneys in children.

Pediatric Otolaryngology   POto

Involves the diagnosis and treatment of disorders of the ear, nose and throat which affect children.

Pediatric Pulmonology   PPul

Involves the diagnosis and treatment of diseases of the chest, lungs, and chest tissue in children.

Pediatric Radiology   PR

Involves diagnostic imaging as it pertains to the newborn, infant, child and adolescent.

Pediatric Rheumatology   PRhu

Involves the treatment of diseases of the joints and connective tissues in children.

Pediatric Surgery   PS

Treatment of disease, injury or deformity in children through surgical techniques.

PEDIATRICS   **Ped**

Diagnosis and treatment of diseases of childhood and monitoring of the growth, development and well-being of preadolescent.

Physical Medicine & Rehabilitation   **PMR**

The use of physical therapy and physical agents such as water, heat, light electricity and mechanical manipulations in the diagnosis, treatment and prevention of disease and body disorders.

Plastic Surgery   **PlS**

Involves reconstructive and cosmetic surgery of the face and other body parts.

Preventive Medicine   **PrM**

A specialty focusing on the prevention of illness and on the health of groups rather than individuals.

Psychiatry   **Psyc**

Examination, treatment and prevention of mental illness through the use of psychoanalysis and/or drugs.

Public Health & General Preventive Medicine   PHGPM

Involves the investigation of the causes of epidemic disease and the prevention of a wide variety of acute and chronic illness.

Pulmonary Disease   Pul

Involves the diagnosis and treatment of diseases of the chest, lungs and airways.

Radiation Oncology   RadRo

Involves the use of radiant energy and isotopes in the study and treatment of disease, especially malignant cancer.

Reproductive Endocrinology   RE

Deals with the endocrine system (including the pituitary, thyroid, parathyroid, adrenal glands, placenta, ovaries and testes) and how its failure relates to infertility.

Rheumatology   Rhu

Involves the treatment of diseases of the joints, muscles, bones and associated structures.

Sleep Medicine   Sleep Med

Involves the investigation and of patients with sleep disorders.

Spinal Cord Injury Medicine   SpCdInj

Involves the prevention, diagnosis, treatment and management of traumatic spinal cord injuries.

Sports Medicine   SM

Refers to the practice of an orthopedist or other physician who specializes in injuries to the bone or other soft tissues (muscles, tendons, ligaments) caused by participation in athletic active.

Surgery   S

Treatment of disease, injury and deformity by surgical procedures.

Surgery of the Hand   SHd

Involves providing appropriate care for all structures in the upper extremity directly affecting the hand and wrist function.

Surgical Critical Care   SCC

Involves specialized care in the management of the critically ill patient, particularly the trauma victim and postoperative patient in the emergency department, intensive care unit, trauma unit, burn unit and other similar settings.

Thoracic & Cardiac Surgery   T&CS

Involves surgery on the heart, lungs and chest area.

Urology   U

Diagnosis and treatment of diseases of the genitals in men and disorders of the urinary tract and bladder in both men and women.

Vascular & Interventional Radiology   VIR

Involves diagnosing and treating diseases by percutaneous methods guided by various radiologic imaging modalities.

Vascular Surgery   VascS

Involves the operative treatment of disorders of the blood vessels excluding those to the heart, lungs or brain.

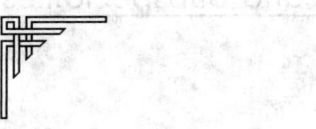

The Best in American Medicine
www.CastleConnolly.com

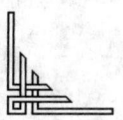

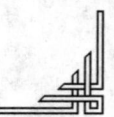

Partnership for Excellence
The Hospital Information Program

There are more than 200 acute care and specialty hospitals in the New York metropolitan area, many of which have extraordinary capabilities for superior patient care. Castle Connolly Medical Ltd. has received many requests from book buyers to provide information about hospitals. In response, we have invited a select group of outstanding hospitals to profile their services in this guide through the medium of paid advertorials. This program, called the Hospital Information Program is totally separate from the physician selection process, which is based upon a completely independent review system. Hospitals that sponsored pages in the Hospital Information Program are organized into three groups: Major Medical Centers, Specialty Hospitals and Regional Medical Centers.

Major Medical Centers begin on the next page and are followed by the Specialty Hospital pages. This section is followed by the listings of doctors. Regional Medical Centers and Hospitals are found at the beginning of each county section - within the doctor listings. The information gives you an overview of programs and services offered by these hospitals, as well as vital information related to their accreditation and sponsorship. Each hospital profile also contains a physician referral number, should you wish to ask the hospitals for recommendations of physicians not listed in the Castle Connolly Guide.

The "Centers of Excellence" section was also developed in response to requests from our readers who want to know which hospitals have special programs or services focusing on a particular illness or health need. The "Centers of Excellence" described here are also offered by hospitals participating in the Partnership for Excellence section of this guide. They reflect the depth of commitment of these hospitals, which provides the staff, resources and financial support necessary to develop these special programs. We believe you will find this information helpful in your search for the best healthcare — from both physicians and hospitals— for you and your family.

We are pleased to have these distinguished institutions as partners in our effort to help you meet your healthcare needs.

The following pages contain vital information on ten of the region's Major Medical Centers. A Major Medical Center is an acute care hospital with tertiary care services, residency programs, a major affiliation with a medical school and clinical research programs. A major medical center draws its patients from a broad geographic region, even nationally and internationally and, in many instances, is the center of a network or consortium of hospitals.

The New York metropolitan region is nationally and internationally known for its major medical centers and their excellent programs and services. Some of the nation's leading academic centers are in this region and, in addition to superior patient care and cutting edge patient research, they produce thousands of talented, well trained physicians and other health professionals each year. Castle Connolly Medical Ltd. has invited a number of major medical centers in the region to sponsor the profiles and information that follows.

Major Medical Centers

Atlantic Health System

Continuum Health Partners

Hackensack University Medical Center

Maimonides Medical Center

Montefiore Medical Center

Mount Sinai Medical Center

NewYork-Presbyterian Hospital

North Shore-LIJ Health System

NYU Langone Medical Center

SUNY Downstate Medical Center

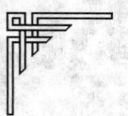

The Best in American Medicine
www.CastleConnolly.com

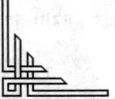
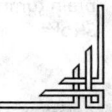

ATLANTIC HEALTH SYSTEM

Morristown Medical Center • Overlook Medical Center • Newton Medical Center • Goryeb Children's Hospital

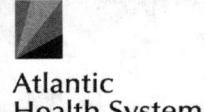

Atlantic Health System

Atlantic Neuroscience Institute • Carol G. Simon Cancer Center • Gagnon Cardiovascular Institute • Atlantic Rehabilitation Institute • Atlantic Sports Health

Atlantic Health System, 475 South Street, P.O. Box 1905, Morristown, NJ 07962
www.atlantichealth.org

To find a doctor, call 800-247-9580 or visit us online

Sponsorship: Voluntary Not–for–Profit • Beds: 1,310 • Accreditation: Joint Commission

Atlantic Health System is at the forefront of medicine, setting standards for quality health care in New Jersey and beyond. The nationally recognized physicians, experienced nurses and skilled staff provide outstanding and compassionate care. Atlantic Health System owns and operates Morristown Medical Center in Morristown, NJ; Overlook Medical Center in Summit, NJ; Newton Medical Center in Newton, NJ; and Goryeb Children's Hospital in Morristown, NJ. Official health care partner of the New York Jets, an official health care provider of the New Jersey Devils and official sports medicine and rehabilitation partner of the New Jersey Interscholastic Athletic Associations, the Atlantic Sports Health program has established itself as a leader in the field of sports medicine. Atlantic Health System is a clinical and academic affiliate of The Mount Sinai Hospital and Mount Sinai School of Medicine and a Major Clinical Research Affiliate of the Cancer Institute of New Jersey.

Morristown Medical Center – 100 Madison Avenue, Morristown, NJ 07960

Morristown Medical Center has been serving the Morris County community for more than 100 years, providing high-level patient care in first-rate facilities with a full range of medical specialties and services. Morristown Medical Center is named a Level 1 Regional Trauma Center by the American College of Surgeons and a Level II Trauma Center by the state. The cardiac surgery program is the largest in the state. Morristown Medical Center is designated a Regional Perinatal Center, which allows the hospital to treat the most complicated obstetrical cases and provide specialized care to sick or premature infants.

In 2012, U.S. News & World Report ranked Morristown Medical Center as a top hospital nationwide for cardiology, heart surgery and gynecology, in the publication's annual Best Hospitals list. Morristown Medical Center also ranked among the best hospitals in New Jersey and as a "Best Regional Hospital" for Cancer, Diabetes & Endocrinology, Neurology and Neurosurgery, Orthopedics as well as Gastroenterology, Geriatrics, Nephrology, Pulmonology and Urology.

Morristown Medical Center performs more joint replacements than any other New Jersey hospital. The surgical success rates are among the highest in the country, earning the hospital the Gold Seal from the Joint Commission. The Stroke Center at Morristown Medical Center is the only accredited stroke trauma center in Morris County and specializes in diagnosis and treatment of acute neurological trauma and stroke.

Morristown Medical Center was re-designated a Magnet Hospital for Excellence in Nursing Service, the highest level of recognition by American Nurses Credentialing Center for facilities that provide acute care services, a distinction awarded to less than 5 percent of U.S. hospitals. Morristown Medical Center is accredited by the Joint Commission.

Part of Morristown Medical Center, Urgent Care at Hackettstown offers board-certified physicians and skilled health care professionals who provide immediate medical services for all ages, including physicals, screenings, diagnostics and treatment, vaccinations, on-site lab and X-ray services.

Overlook Medical Center - 99 Beauvoir Avenue, Summit, NJ 07901

Overlook Medical Center is a pioneer in medical technology. Overlook has the state's first combined PET/CT scanner for functional brain imaging and stereotactic radiosurgery cancer treatment program, and was the first in the northeast U.S. to acquire magnetoencephalography (MEG) technology for functional brain mapping prior to brain surgery. The Brain Tumor Center is the only place in New Jersey to offer two brain tumor vaccine trials. Overlook's Neuroscience Institute is home to New Jersey's first Comprehensive Stroke Center and a comprehensive Level IV Epilepsy Center, as well as research and treatment programs in

Movement and Memory Disorders. The largest neuro-interventional radiology service in New Jersey also is housed at Overlook. The Minimally Invasive Surgery Program utilizes a wide range of robotics in the operating room, including the first robot, ViKY, in New Jersey to use voice recognition technology for surgeries in the gastrointestinal, urologic, thoracic and gynecologic regions.

Carol G. Simon Cancer Center offers the most advanced methods to diagnose, treat, and manage all types of cancers. Board-certified physicians and oncology-trained professionals provide multidisciplinary care in surgical, medical, and radiation oncology using state-of-the-art technology. Overlook is #5 in the world for the number of prostate cancer patients treated with CyberKnife® technology.

In 2012, U.S. News & World Report ranked Overlook Medical Center among the best hospitals in central New Jersey and as a "Best Regional Hospital" for Neurology and Neurosurgery as well as Gastroenterology, Geriatrics, Nephrology, Pulmonology and Urology.

Nationally recognized for Overlook's Emergency Department, the satellite ED in Union received the prestigious Lantern Award of the Emergency Nurses Association. Overlook is one of five NJ hospitals approved to provide emergency angioplasty in a community hospital setting. Overlook is one of only two hospitals to be certified for wound healing in NJ and is one of 17 hospitals in the country to receive this honor.

Newton Medical Center – 175 High Street, Newton, NJ 07860

Newton Medical Center, part of Atlantic Health System, is a fully accredited, 148-bed acute care, not-for-profit hospital serving more than 250,000 people in Sussex and Warren counties in New Jersey, Pike County in Pennsylvania, and southern Orange County in New York. Specialty service areas include cardiology, general and vascular surgery, orthopedics, gastroenterology, nephrology, oncology and neurology, mental health and sleep medicine. As the premier medical facility in the region, Newton Medical Center's expertise in these areas has earned multiple accolades, including an award for Clinical and Operational Excellence by the VHA, and three-year accreditations by both the Commission on Cancer for comprehensive treatment of cancer patients, and by the American College of Radiology for digital mammography services. The Charles L. Tice Heart Center for Diagnostic Services offers the latest diagnostic cardiac technology. Newton Medical Center's Echocardiography Laboratory is accredited by the Intersocietal Commission for Accreditation of Echocardiography Laboratories (ICAEL).

Newton Medical Center recently opened a state-of-the-art, wide-bore magnetic resonance imaging (MRI) scanner for outpatient appointments in addition to providing diagnostic scanning for hospital inpatients.

Newton Medical Center also operates Milford Health & Wellness Center, Sparta Health & Wellness Center, and in Home Health Services Inc., offering a variety of quality care services close to home. Newton also includes Urgent Care at Vernon which provides care for illnesses and injuries, including suture repairs and fracture care, and offers physicals, vaccines, routine screenings and access to the best private practice physicians in the region. In Pennsylvania, Newton's Urgent Care at Milford also provides care for illnesses and injuries.

Newton Medical Center is accredited by the Joint Commission.

Goryeb Children's Hospital

Upon opening its doors in 2002, Goryeb Children's Hospital quickly became the hospital of choice for families through the area. A decade later, physicians at Goryeb treat more than 50,000 pediatric patients annually across 20 different areas of medical and surgical care, including 750 patients annually in the Foley Pediatric Intensive Care Unit and more than 2,500 inpatients.

Goryeb Children's Hospital is a state-designated children's hospital. More than 100 board certified pediatric specialists at Goryeb provide care to patients at multiple locations throughout the state. In addition, Goryeb has more than 250 community pediatricians on staff.

The physicians and staff at Goryeb subscribe to a patient- and family-centered philosophy of care, partnering together with families to generate the best possible outcomes. Families and caregivers are educated, supported and empowered to make informed decisions about their child's care and to cope confidently with their child's condition or illness.

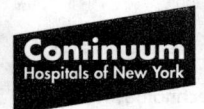

Continuum
Hospitals of New York

Beth Israel Medical Center
Beth Israel Brooklyn
Roosevelt Hospital
St. Luke's Hospital
NY Eye and Ear Infirmary

800.420.4004   www.chpnyc.org

Sponsorship: Voluntary Not-for-profit   **Beds:** 2,180 certified beds
Accreditation: Joint Commission of Accreditation of Healthcare Organizations (JCAHO),
Accreditation Council for Graduate Medical Education, Medical Society of New York,
in conjunction with the Accreditation Council for Continuing Medical Education

A STRONG PARTNERSHIP WITH A PROUD HERITAGE

Continuum Health Partners is a partnership of five venerable health care providers: Beth
Israel Medical Center-Milton and Carroll Petrie Division, Beth Israel Brooklyn,
St. Luke's Hospital, Roosevelt Hospital, and The New York Eye and Ear Infirmary. Each
of the five partner institutions was established more than a century ago by individuals
committed to improving health and health care in their communities. Today, the system
represents over 4,000 physicians and dentists and is superbly equipped to respond to the
health care needs of the populations we serve. Continuum providers also see patients in
group and private practice settings and in ambulatory centers in New York City and
Westchester County.

LOCATIONS

Continuum Health Partners has campuses in Manhattan and Brooklyn. Beth Israel Med-
ical Center has two divisions: the Milton and Caroll Petrie Division on the East Side, and
Beth Israel Brooklyn. The Phillips Ambulatory Care Center, a state-of-the-art outpatient
center, is located at Union Square. St. Luke's Hospital is in Morningside Heights and
Roosevelt Hospital is in the Columbus Circle and Lincoln Center neighborhoods on the
West Side. The New York Eye and Ear Infirmary is located on
Second Avenue and 14th Street.

ACADEMIC AFFILIATIONS

Beth Israel Medical Center is the University Hospital and Manhattan Campus for the
Albert Einstein College of Medicine. St. Luke's-Roosevelt Hospital Center is an Academic
Affiliate of Columbia University College of Physicians and Surgeons. The New York Eye
and Ear Infirmary is the primary teaching center of the New York Medical College and affiliated teaching hospitals in the areas of ophthalmology and otolaryngology.

For a referral to a great doctor in your neighborhood, call 800.420.4004.
Our Physician Referral Service can help you find a primary care
physician or specialist affiliated with
Beth Israel, St. Luke's, Roosevelt, or The New York Eye and Ear Infirmary.
Visit our Website at www.chpnyc.org

Cancer

The Continuum Cancer Centers of New York offer early detection, diagnosis, and treatment of a wide range of cancers. Our nationally recognized physicians offer innovative and highly successful programs coupled with superb support services. Our cancer services are state of the art, supported by sophisticated programs in medical oncology, surgical oncology, and radiation oncology.

Cardiac Services

The cardiology, cardiac surgery, and cardiac rehabilitation experts at Continuum offer a full range of diagnostic and treatment services. Some highlights of our cardiac programs are minimally invasive robotic cardiac surgery, arrhythmia services, 24-hour cardiac catheterization labs, and expertise in congestive heart failure.

Neurological Services

Continuum is home to many world leaders in neurology, neurosurgery and interventional neuroradiology. Our physicians are recognized authorities who establish innovative care protocols, chart new venues in therapy and develop the technologies that set the standards in the neuroscience fields.

Orthopedic Services

Continuum's orthopedic physicians are leading providers of general orthopedic, sports medicine, spine and rheumatologic care. Our specialists offer state-of-the-art care to patients throughout the New York metropolitan region. Many of our orthopedic surgeons are leaders in their field and are fellowship trained in their areas of sub-specialty.

Ear, Nose and Throat

Continuum offers eye, ear, nose and throat services throughout our system. The New York Center for Head and Neck combines the formidable medical and surgical capabilities of the five hospitals of Continuum. The center comprises 45 physicians across 14 specialties and subspecialties, including world-renowned surgeons and educators.

HIV/AIDS

We are one of the largest providers of HIV/AIDS care in New York City, with comprehensive-care clinics and facilities in multiple locations. Our facilities offer a complete range of health care services for individuals with HIV: diagnostic procedures, the latest treatments, and support services.

Pain Management

Our Department of Pain Medicine and Palliative Care offers a broad array of therapies for chronic pain of all types. The highly trained medical team includes pain specialists with backgrounds in neurology, rehabilitation medicine, anesthesiology and psychology.

Substance Abuse

Continuum offers extensive chemical dependency treatment services through The Addiction Institute of New York, the Stuyvesant Square Chemical Dependency Treatment Program, and the Department of Psychiatry and Behavioral Health. Our services include inpatient detoxification and outpatient programs, services for the mentally ill, family services, and after-care programs.

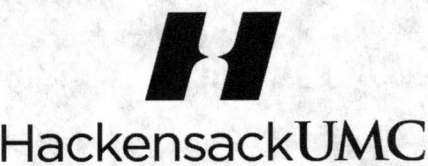

HackensackUMC

30 Prospect Avenue, Hackensack, NJ, 07601 • 551-996-2000
www.HackensackUMC.org

Number of beds: 775

Number of employees: 6,637

2011 Admissions: 39,900

Sponsorship: A not-for-profit, teaching and research hospital affiliated with the University of Medicine and Dentistry of New Jersey – New Jersey Medical School, St. George's University School of Medicine in Grenada, and Stevens Institute of Technology in Hoboken, NJ.

Beds: A 775-bed, Level II Trauma Center, providing tertiary and regional services for the New York/New Jersey metropolitan area.

Accreditation: Joint Commission

HackensackUMC is the recipient of 18 Gold Seals of Approval™ for healthcare quality from the Joint Commission, the only medical facility in the United States to achieve this record-number of the Joint Commission Disease-Specific Care Certifications.

The medical center holds the Joint Commission Disease-Specific Care Certifications in: Acute Myocardial Infarction; Asthma; Bone Marrow Transplantation; Breast Cancer; Chronic Obstructive Pulmonary Disease; Colorectal Cancer; Coronary Artery Disease; Depression Program; Geriatric Delirium; Heart Failure; Hip Replacement; Inpatient Diabetes Program; Knee Replacement; Pediatric Asthma; Pneumonia Disease; Primary Stroke Center; Trauma; and Uterine/Ovarian cancer.

BACKGROUND

Hackensack University Medical Center (HackensackUMC) is a 775-bed teaching and research hospital that provides the largest number of admissions in New Jersey. Founded in 1888 with 12 beds and as Bergen County's first hospital, HackensackUMC has demonstrated more than a century of growth and progress. At HackensackUMC, quality means pushing medicine further to prove that "impossible" is just an opinion – leading the pursuit of excellence in healthcare. HackensackUMC is a nationally recognized healthcare organization offering patients the most comprehensive services, state-of-the-art technologies, and facilities. Honors include being named one of America's 50 Best Hospitals™ by HealthGrades® for six years in a row. HackensackUMC is the only hospital in New Jersey, New York and New England to receive this honor for six consecutive years. *U.S. News & World Report* ranked HackensackUMC the number one hospital in New Jersey and one of the top four New York metro hospitals. The medical center also received nine national rankings and four New York metro area rankings. It was also named one of the 50 Best Hospitals in America by *Becker's Hospital Review*. HackensackUMC is a Magnet® recognized hospital for nursing excellence – the first in New Jersey and second in the nation – receiving its fourth designation in April 2009. It is the Hometown Hospital of the New York Football Giants as well as the New York Red Bulls soccer team.

MEDICAL AND DENTAL STAFF

Since HackensackUMC is one of the region's most comprehensive and progressive medical centers, it easily attracts many of the area's leading physicians – nearly 1,600 of them. These doctors, many of whom are on the cutting-edge in their fields and have received their training at our nation's most prominent institutions, have selected HackensackUMC as their place to practice their best medicine.

NURSING EXCELLENCE

Our medical staff is joined by a team of extraordinary nurses. As a Magnet® Hospital, HackensackUMC attracts and retains nurses who are tops in their fields. Making history in 1995 as the first official Magnet® Hospital in New Jersey, HackensackUMC is the only hospital in New Jersey with four designations from the American Nurses Credentialing Center.

WORLD-CLASS CARDIAC CARE

HackensackUMC is home to one of America's most comprehensive cardiac and vascular hospitals: its new Heart & Vascular Hospital – a "hospital within a hospital" – which integrates preventive, diagnostic and treatment services, with a special focus on cardiovascular disease management and breakthrough research. Inpatients and outpatients are treated for all types of cardiac and vascular diseases, including heart problems, such as: blocked arteries and irregular heartbeats; peripheral vascular disease; and neurovascular diseases, such as stroke and aneurysm. Housing all of these services within one specialized location allows for more efficient, effective patient care.

U.S. News & World Report ranked HackensackUMC #27 out of more than 700 hospitals in the nation for Cardiology & Heart Surgery. HackensackUMC is also one of HealthGrades® America's 100 Best Hospitals for Cardiac Care™ in 2012, and is five-star rated (out of a possible five-stars) in the following areas: Overall Cardiac Services; Cardiology Services; Coronary Bypass Surgery; Coronary Interventional Procedures; Treatment of Heart Attack; and Treatment of Heart Failure.

ONE OF THE NATION'S LARGEST AND MOST COMPREHENSIVE CANCER CENTERS

At John Theurer Cancer Center, we believe cancer is hard enough for patients and their loved ones. It is this belief that drives our passion to deliver extraordinary care every day, helping us to become one of the nation's top 50 cancer centers, ranked #31 out of more than 900 hospitals by U.S. News & World Report – the highest-ranked cancer center in New Jersey with this recognition.

In January 2011, we opened a new building that houses 14 specialty divisions, research and support services. This state-of-the-art facility offers a wide range of free resources to help patients become active participants in their treatment and support their fight against cancer. These resources include yoga, fitness, interactive nutrition classes in the Cooking Studio, art workshops, a patient resource librarian to help patients find credible health information online, and more.

Over the past 25 years we have become one of the largest cancer centers in the United States, but we have kept our focus on the unique needs of our patients. Prevention, treatment, and research advances have grown exponentially during this time. We are not only keeping up with the change of pace, we are at the forefront of providing tomorrow's treatment today by:

• Taking multi-disciplinary care to a new level with teams of disease-specific experts under one roof;
• Delivering personalized medicine focused on novel therapies, participatory treatment, predictive measures, and preventive care;
• Advancing research through biomarker-driven clinical trials and translational research;
• Providing holistic care that includes a wide range of complementary services important to the well-being of our patients that can be easily integrated into their care; and
• Creating a comforting environment in a new high-tech, high-touch building.

We believe our model is the next step towards the future of patient care, changing the cancer care experience one patient at a time. To receive information on John Theurer Cancer Center's services, call 551-996-5900 or visit jtcancercenter.org.

ONE OF THE NATION'S RENOWNED PEDIATRIC PROGRAMS

The Joseph M. Sanzari Children's Hospital at HackensackUMC is a state-designated children's hospital and an award-winning facility that has been recognized as one of the top-ranked children's hospitals in New Jersey and in the country. It ranked among the top 25 Best Children's Hospitals for neurology and neurosurgery in the 2012-13 Best Children's Hospitals rankings by U.S. News & World Report — the first hospital in New Jersey to be ranked in any Best Children's Hospitals specialty.

The Joseph M. Sanzari Children's Hospital was one of the first hospitals in New Jersey to have a separate, dedicated pediatric emergency room (PER) and is an American College of Surgeons designated Level II Trauma Center that cares for pediatric patients. The PER is staffed 24 hours a day, seven days a week with physicians and nurses who are specialized in the care of children requiring emergency medical services. It houses more than 30 specialties in a patient- and family-centered environment that includes children's play and family kitchen areas, and private inpatient rooms with computers, Internet access, and flat-screen plasma televisions.

The cutting-edge technologies facilities, expert staff, dedicated PER and specialty units that distinguish the Joseph M. Sanzari Children's Hospital are second to none.

For more information on any of the services offered at HackensackUMC, please call 551-996-2000, or visit www.HackensackUMC.org.

Maimonides Medical Center

4802 Tenth Avenue • Brooklyn, New York 11219
Phone: 718.283.6000
Physician Referral: 888.MMC.DOCS (662.3627)
www.maimonidesmed.org

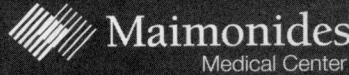
Maimonides
Medical Center

Sponsorship:	Voluntary, Not-for-Profit
Beds:	705 acute, 70 psychiatric
Accreditation:	The Joint Commission
	American College of Surgeons
	American Council of Graduate Medical Education (ACGME)

Maimonides Medical Center is among the largest independent teaching hospitals in the US, and trains more than 450 medical and surgical residents each year. Widely recognized for major achievements in medical technology and patient safety, Maimonides is a conductor of clinical trials for new treatments and therapies, and cited for overall clinical excellence by numerous health care evaluation services. The Cardiology, Stroke, Cancer and Critical Care divisions at Maimonides are rated among the best in the nation.

Significant Accomplishments

Excellence in cardiac care is historic: the first successful human heart transplant in the US was performed at Maimonides in 1967, and Maimonides is ranked by the Centers for Medicare & Medicaid Services among those hospitals that consistently achieve excellent ratings in heart attack, heart failure and pneumonia patient outcomes.

Physicians at Maimonides were among the first in the US to use computers to enter patient orders, thereby reducing the risk of errors, increasing efficiency, and speeding the healing process.

Maimonides has appeared on the American Hospital Association's "Most Wired" list more often than any other health care institution in the metropolitan area.

More babies are born at Maimonides than at any other single-campus hospital in the state of New York – due in no small part to its designation as a Regional Perinatal Center with Obstetric and Pediatric services which are unrivaled in this area.

Centers of Excellence

Cancer Center
The Maimonides Cancer Center offers a fully integrated approach that includes prevention, screening, diagnostics, treatment, palliative care and clinical research. Staffed by leading oncologists, radiologists, surgeons, nurses and social workers, the Center provides compassionate, patient-centered, state-of-the-art care. The newly built Breast Cancer Center is located just around the corner, and features a spa-like decor in which our dedicated team of breast cancer specialists treat patients.

Cardiac Institute

Renowned for its Catheterization Lab and pioneering new surgical procedures, the Maimonides Cardiac Institute includes an electrophysiology (EP) lab, hybrid OR, two ICUs, Chest Pain Observation Unit, Advanced Cardiac Care Unit, Congestive Heart Failure program and Atrial Fibrillation Center. The first successful heart transplant in America was performed at Maimonides in 1967. Today, its Cardiology division continues to innovate. Maimonides has been ranked by the Centers for Medicare & Medicaid Services among those hospitals achieving excellent ratings in both heart attack and heart failure patient outcomes. Its Left Ventricular Assist Device (LVAD) Program, the first and only one in Brooklyn, recently received advanced certification from the Joint Commission.

Stroke Center

The Jaffe Stroke Center at Maimonides is ranked among the best in the nation. It is currently the site of clinical trials for new stroke medications, medical devices and stroke protocols. The Center is one of the few that provides interventional neuroradiology techniques to remove stroke-causing blood clots from the brain – without surgery – significantly reducing the debilitating effects of stroke.

Infants & Children's Hospital

The Maimonides Infants & Children's Hospital, one of only five accredited children's hospitals in NYC, includes comprehensive inpatient services and over 30 pediatric subspecialties. With a Child Life & Creative Arts Therapies Program fully integrated with family-centered care, the Maimonides Infants & Children's Hospital also provides a Pediatric ICU, Neonatal ICU, Outpatient Services and Pediatric ER.

Vascular Institute

The Vascular Institute at Maimonides provides comprehensive diagnostic, clinical and vascular surgical services for patients with circulatory complications related to hypertension, diabetes, arteriosclerosis and other diseases. One of only five centers in New York certified to train vascular surgeons, the Institute includes a Diagnostic Lab, Vein Center, Vascular Surgery Center and Wound Center.

Stella & Joseph Payson Birthing Center

More babies are delivered at Maimonides than at any other single-campus hospital in New York State. The Payson Birthing Center offers a home-like setting with physicians, nurses, midwives and doulas, combined with advanced technology which includes a perinatal testing center with 3-D ultrasound and 24/7 neonatology.

Geriatrics Program

Maimonides serves one of the oldest inpatient populations in New York City, with one quarter of inpatients over the age of 75. The Geriatrics Program is fully equipped to meet the special needs of these seniors, including the assessment of memory loss and expertise in geriatric syndromes such as incontinence, falls and frailty. The Program encompasses inpatient and outpatient services, features the Acute Care for Elderly (ACE) Unit, the Safe at Home program and home-visiting service.

Montefiore
Inspired Medicine

111 East 210th Street
Bronx, New York 10467
1-800-MD-MONTE
www.montefiore.org

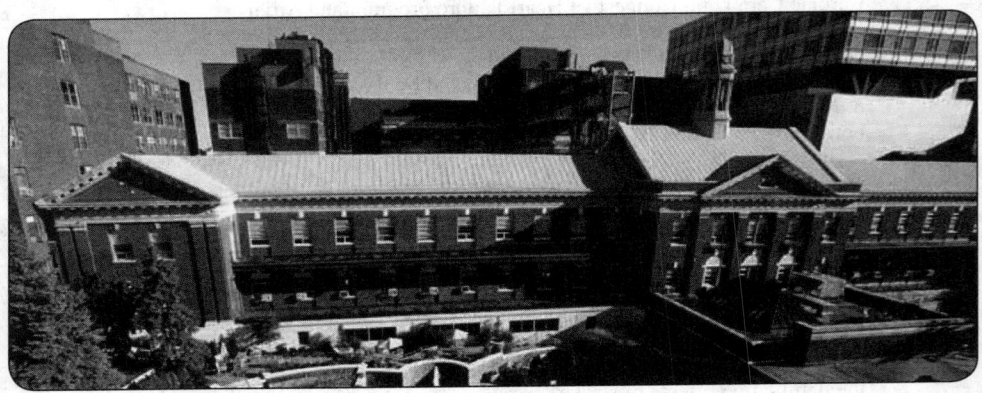

Montefiore Medical Center serves as a tertiary care referral center for patients from across the New York metropolitan area and beyond, and offers a full range of healthcare services to two million residents throughout the neighboring counties of Westchester and the Bronx, one of the most culturally and economically diverse urban communities in the United States. As the University Hospital and academic medical center for Albert Einstein College of Medicine, Montefiore is recognized by *U.S. News & World Report* as a national and regional leader in specialty and chronic care for both adults and children. The Children's Hospital at Montefiore (CHAM) was ranked among the best in the country by *U.S. News & World Report* for the fifth consecutive year.

Comprising four hospitals with 1,491 beds, Montefiore has more than 90,000 annual hospital admissions and provides more than 2.6 million ambulatory visits through a network of over 130 locations. Montefiore's emergency department is one of the busiest in the nation, with approximately 300,000 visits annually, and its nationally renowned home healthcare program provides more than 500,000 visits annually. In addition to having one of the largest school health programs in the country, Montefiore Medical Center includes a 23-site medical group practice integrated throughout the Bronx and Westchester and a care management organization providing services to nearly 200,000 health plan members.

Montefiore is a national leader in the research and treatment of acute and chronic diseases and is known and respected for its model of care emphasizing accountability and interdisciplinary programs. With notable centers of excellence in heart and vascular care, cancer care, transplantation, children's health, surgery, neurosciences, orthopaedics, ophthalmology and women's health, Montefiore defines clinical excellence and delivers premier care in a compassionate environment.

Montefiore Medical Center Hospitals

Montefiore Hospital	Wakefield Hospital	Weiler Hospital	The Children's Hospital
111 East 210th Street	600 East 233rd Street	1825 Eastchester Road	at Montefiore
Bronx, New York 10467	Bronx, New York 10466	Bronx, New York 10461	3415 Bainbridge Avenue
			Bronx, New York 10467

The Children's Hospital at Montefiore

Since opening in 2001, The Children's Hospital at Montefiore (CHAM) has quickly established itself as one of the most advanced hospitals for children in the nation. It is consistently recognized among the nation's top children's hospitals by *U.S. News & World Report*. CHAM's internationally renowned specialists combine clinical expertise, innovative research and leading-edge technology with an integrated, family-centric approach to achieve exceptional outcomes. As the pediatric hospital for Albert Einstein College of Medicine, CHAM is educating the next generation of healthcare professionals and transforming the future of children's health.

Montefiore Einstein Center for Cancer Care

Bringing together internationally known experts with the latest technologies and cutting-edge research, Montefiore Einstein Center for Cancer Care is known for its achievements in the prevention, diagnosis and treatment of rare and common cancers. Our multidisciplinary teams include medical, surgical and radiation oncologists, along with pathologists, radiologists and support specialists. They work together to provide each patient with the most effective, individualized treatment plan possible. Partnering with the National Cancer Institute–designated Albert Einstein Cancer Center, the Center for Cancer Care is the first facility in the Northeast to offer three types of "regional" chemotherapy treatments that deliver concentrated, targeted doses of anticancer drugs, avoiding the side effects of standard chemotherapy and improving effectiveness.

Montefiore Einstein Center for Heart & Vascular Care

A national leader in the prevention, diagnosis and treatment of cardiovascular disease, Montefiore Einstein Center for Heart & Vascular Care provides innovative therapies and clinical best practices for adult and pediatric patients. The Heart & Vascular Center's vast offerings include cardiac imaging, interventional cardiology, arrhythmia services and the most advanced surgical care for mitral valve repair, aneurysms and heart failure. Montefiore surgeons are also distinguished experts in the use of mechanical assist devices, as well as robotic and minimally invasive cardiac surgery. The Heart & Vascular Center is a three-year recipient of the Society of Thoracic Surgeons' three-star rating, placing it among the top 12 percent of the nation's cardiac surgery programs.

Montefiore Einstein Center for Transplantation

The Center for Transplantation is widely recognized for its excellent outcomes and holistic approach to care. Uniting Montefiore's clinical and surgical practices with the world-renowned faculty and researchers of Albert Einstein College of Medicine, the Transplantation Center treats adults and children with end-stage organ disease who receive all aspects of treatment and counseling in one convenient location. Additionally, the Transplantation Center's one-year survival rates exceed 90 percent in all areas (heart, liver, kidney and pancreas), surpassing the national average of 75 to 80 percent.

Neurosciences at Montefiore

Experience and expertise are the hallmarks of Montefiore's neuroscience programs. The Departments of Neurology and Neurosurgery treat adults and children with the full spectrum of neurological conditions. Notable services include intraoperative imaging, microneurosurgery, endovascular coiling, comprehensive programs in neurotoxicology, aging and dementia, gait disorders and frailty, stroke and neuro-oncology. Our pioneering Headache, Sleep-Wake Disorders, Cerebrovascular, and Comprehensive Epilepsy Centers offer world-renowned expertise. Our clinical programs are bolstered by a robust research enterprise that includes NIH- and foundation-sponsored studies focusing on autism, neurodegenerative diseases and other neurologic disorders.

Surgery at Montefiore

Montefiore is a recognized leader in the development of innovative new surgical procedures. With a proven reputation for performing even the most complex surgeries, our renowned surgeons provide both adults and children with extensive expertise in every surgical discipline. Employing state-of-the-art diagnostic, minimally invasive and robotic technologies, Montefiore continues to enhance surgical precision, reduce patient discomfort and speed recovery. Through cutting-edge research, our surgeons offer the most advanced surgical procedures available anywhere today.

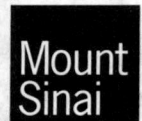
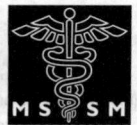

THE MOUNT SINAI MEDICAL CENTER

One Gustave L. Levy Place
Fifth Avenue and 100th Street
New York, NY 10029-6574
Physician Referral: 1-800-MD-SINAI (637-4624)
www.mountsinai.org

MOUNT SINAI
SCHOOL OF
MEDICINE

Sponsorship: Voluntary Not-for-Profit
Beds: 1,171
Accreditation: The Joint Commission;
Commission for Accreditation of Rehabilitation Facilities;
Magnet Award for Nursing Excellence

For 160 years, The Mount Sinai Medical Center has been a leader in patient care and translational research, with generations of patients benefitting from our teams of physicians and scientists working together to convert research into better medicine.

Located between the Upper East Side and East and Central Harlem—New York City's most and least affluent communities—Mount Sinai provides services to meet the needs of every patient. The Medical Center consists of The Mount Sinai Hospital and Mount Sinai School of Medicine, both of which continue to be ranked among the nation's best by *U.S. News & World Report*.

In 2012, Mount Sinai was again named among America's Best Hospitals, earning a spot on *U.S. News & World Report's* "Honor Roll" and ranking 14th out of 5,000 hospitals nationwide. We also ranked highly in 11 specialties: geriatric care; digestive disorders; cardiology and heart surgery; rehabilitation; diabetes and endocrinology; ear, nose and throat; psychiatry; neurology and neurosurgery; kidney disorders; gynecology; and urology. In addition, our School of Medicine was ranked 18th by the "Best Graduate Schools" edition.

Under the direction of Valentin Fuster, MD, PhD, **Mount Sinai Heart** incorporates world-class resources, innovative thinking and interdisciplinary programs to prevent and treat cardiovascular disease. In a statewide study, our Cardiac Catheterization Laboratory was deemed both the busiest and, with the lowest 30-day risk-adjusted mortality rate, the safest. Building on the expertise of our internationally renowned cardiologists, interventionalists and cardiac surgeon, we provide patients with the most advanced approach to care.

The Tisch Cancer Institute coordinates a full-service diagnostic and treatment program for cancer patients. Our programs include those in cancer of the liver, breast, prostate, and head and neck, as well as hematological malignancies, such as myeloproliferative disorders. In 2011, we opened the **Dubin Breast Center**, which provides advanced detection and treatment - and addresses every aspect of breast health – all in one centralized location. In October 2012, the **Derald H. Ruttenberg Treatment Center**, the Institute's outpatient cancer facility, will double in size upon its move one block north to the new **Leon and Norma Hess Center for Science and Medicine**. In addition, the Hess Center will house two full floors dedicated to cancer research.

Recognized as a national leader in organ transplantation, **The Recanati/Miller Transplantation Institute** is one of the few places in the country that provides multi-organ transplantation. Our surgeons were the first in New York State to perform many combined transplant procedures, including liver and kidney transplantation, pediatric liver transplantation, and living adult - and pediatric-donor liver transplantation.

The Department of Genetics and Genomic Sciences is one of the largest medical genetics centers in the nation, providing expert diagnostic, therapeutic, and counseling services for patients and families with or at risk for genetic disorders or birth defects. The department performs sophisticated diagnostic tests in its state-of-the-art molecular, biochemical, and cytogenetic laboratories, which are New York State and Clinical Laboratory Improvement Amendments (CLIA) licensed, and accredited by the College of American Pathologists (CAP).

balanced and integrated approach to improving the quality of life for New York's elderly. Ranked second in the country for geriatrics by *U.S. News & World Report* in 2012, we remain a national pioneer in geriatric medicine.

Our internationally recognized **Neurosurgery and Neurology** services rank as premier destinations for care. Our neurosurgeons have expertise in skull-base surgery, cerebrovascular disease, pituitary disorders, acoustic tumors, spinal reconstruction, epilepsy, radiosurgery, stereotactic and primary brain tumor surgery, and neuroendoscopy. Our neurologists lead internationally recognized centers for patient care, research and physician training that provide interdisciplinary expertise on brain and nervous system disorders including Parkinson's disease, dystonia, multiple sclerosis, epilepsy, headache, stroke, dementia, and neuromuscular disease.

Mount Sinai's **Gastrointestinal and Surgical** specialists have developed and advanced numerous techniques to help patients with Crohn's disease, ulcerative colitis, Barrett's esophagus and other digestive disorders lead healthier lives. They have led the way in caring for patients in need of advanced gastrointestinal endoscopy procedures and in developing innovative medical and surgical approaches for inflammatory bowel disease.

Rehabilitation Medicine offers comprehensive care for people with spinal cord injuries, brain injuries, major limb amputations and a variety of other neuromuscular, musculoskeletal, and chronic conditions. We are accredited by the Commission on Accreditation of Rehabilitation Facilities for the treatment of inpatient spinal cord and brain injury and amputations. We also offer comprehensive outpatient rehabilitation services, including physical, occupational, speech and neuropsychological therapies.

Dedicated to the preservation and restoration of the musculoskeletal system, members of our **Department of Orthopaedics** provide personalized treatments using the latest technology. They excel in total joint replacement, microvascular, cancer, and minimally invasive procedures, and surgeries of the foot and ankle, knee, hip, hand, elbow, shoulder, and spine. Our Joint Replacement Center offers easy access to care at all levels: pre-operative assessment, recovery, and therapy.

Mount Sinai's **Department of Urology** provides diagnosis and treatment for many conditions including prostate, bladder and kidney cancers. Our urologists are leaders in advancing emerging diagnostic techniques and treatments, and rank as experts in open, laparoscopic and robotic surgery. This combination of skills makes them uniquely qualified to determine the best approach for each patient. Consistently voted among the country's top doctors, our team has been recognized for the depth of its knowledge, experience and compassion.

A leader in diabetes treatment, management, and research, our **Division of Endocrinology, Diabetes, and Bone Disease** provides a full range of services to treat this epidemic. Patients with type 1 or type 2 diabetes are cared for by accomplished endocrinologists, nurse practitioners, and registered dietitians, who provide specialized, state-of-the-art treatment to help patients manage their condition safely.

Our **Department of Surgery** boasts highly skilled and talented clinicians and educators, who are pioneers in their respective fields. We are one of the oldest surgical departments in the country, and celebrate a rich history of offering unsurpassed patient care. We also train the next generation of surgeons, and have the highest caliber of surgical residents who graduate and go on to become leaders at institutions across the globe.

The Kravis Children's Hospital was named among the best children's hospitals in the country by *U.S. News & World Report*, and ranked in six specialties: gastroenterology, diabetes and endocrinology, urology, nephrology, cancer, and pulmonology. We offer advanced treatment, supported by research, community outreach, and advocacy programs. We treat heart, brain, and spine disorders; epilepsy; cancers and blood diseases; diabetes; gastrointestinal tract conditions; renal diseases; hypertension; asthma and other respiratory system illnesses; sleep problems; allergies; fetal and newborn conditions, and perform life-saving organ transplantations.

⌐ NewYork-Presbyterian
¬ The University Hospital of Columbia and Cornell

Affiliated with Columbia University College of Physicians and Surgeons and Weill Cornell Medical College

NewYork-Presbyterian Hospital	NewYork-Presbyterian Hospital
Columbia University Medical Center	Weill Cornell Medical Center
622 West 168th Street	525 East 68th Street
New York, NY 10032	New York, NY 10065

1-877-NYP-WELL (1-877-697-9355)   www.nyp.org

Sponsorship:	Voluntary Not-for-Profit
Beds:	2,409
Accreditation:	Joint Commission on Accreditation of Healthcare Organizations (JCAHO), Commission on Accreditation of Rehabilitation Facilities (CARF) and College of American Pathologists (CAP)

The #1 hospital in New York. 12 years running. Once again, we are proud to be named the top-ranked hospital in the New York metro area. NewYork-Presbyterian placed higher on the Honor Roll of 'America's Best Hospitals' than any other hospital in the region. This is the 12th consecutive year that we've been recognized to the Honor Roll by *U.S. News & World Report*™. NewYork-Presbyterian has the most physicians listed in *New York Magazine's* "Best Doctors" issue and is recognized for having more top doctors than any other hospital in the nation.

Overview

NewYork-Presbyterian Hospital, based in New York City, is the nation's largest not-for-profit, non-sectarian hospital, with 2,409 beds. The Hospital has nearly 2 million inpatient and outpatient visits in a year, including 12,797 deliveries and 195,294 visits to its emergency departments. NewYork-Presbyterian's 6,144 affiliated physicians and 19,376 staff provide state-of-the-art inpatient, ambulatory and preventive care in all areas of medicine. The Hospital enjoys a unique affiliation with two of the nation's leading Ivy League medical schools—Columbia University College of Physicians and Surgeons and the Joan and Sanford I. Weill Medical College of Cornell University.

NewYork-Presbyterian Hospital Features Renowned CENTERS OF EXCELLENCE Including:

Morgan Stanley Children's Hospital and the Komansky Center for Children's Health— One of the largest, most comprehensive children's hospitals in the world, providing highly sophisticated pediatric medical, surgical, and intensive care services—including a pediatric cardiovascular center and prenatal pediatric center—in a family-friendly, compassionate environment.

NewYork-Presbyterian Cancer Centers—Featuring two of the country's top cancer centers: Herbert Irving Comprehensive Cancer Center (one of only three comprehensive NCI-designated cancer centers in New York State) and the Weill Cornell Cancer Center. We treat more than 7,000 patients newly diagnosed with cancer each year. Through a multidisciplinary team approach, we combine the expertise and talents of all of the individuals responsible for a patient's care—surgical, medical, and radiation oncologists, specialized oncology nurses, social workers, and nutritionists—to deliver seamless care and conduct pioneering research.

NewYork-Presbyterian Digestive Disease Services—Our experts take a collaborative team approach to the care of patients with digestive cancers and nonmalignant digestive diseases, such as inflammatory bowel disease, pancreatic and biliary disorders. We have an exceptional track record performing routine and advanced procedures (particularly interventional endoscopy), prevention programs, and basic science and clinical research aimed at developing novel therapies.

NewYork-Presbyterian Heart—The optimal care of patients with heart disease is achieved by combining an experienced team of clinicians with the latest advances in technology. Basic science and clinical research efforts are aimed at developing more effective, less invasive ways to prevent, diagnose, and treat the full spectrum of cardiac disorders.

NewYork-Presbyterian Neuroscience Centers—Our team provides the most sophisticated diagnostic and treatment services for Alzheimer's disease, multiple sclerosis, Parkinson's disease, aneurysms, epilepsy, brain tumors, strokes, and other neurological disorders. Our scientific investigators are conducting research aimed at better understanding these diseases and further improving patient care.

NewYork-Presbyterian Psychiatry—NewYork-Presbyterian Hospital's behavioral health and psychiatric services for adults, children, and adolescents offer a full continuum of programs at all levels of care— including inpatient, outpatient, partial hospital, day treatment, and residential services. Specialized services are available in neuropsychiatry, chemical dependency, and eating disorders.

NewYork-Presbyterian Transplant Institute—NewYork-Presbyterian Hospital features the largest transplant program in the country. Our experts are internationally known for performing adult and pediatric heart, liver, kidney, pancreas, lung, bone marrow/stem cell, and intestinal and ex vivo transplantation.

NewYork-Presbyterian Vascular Care Center—We provide comprehensive, multidisciplinary preventive, diagnostic, and treatment services for aortic aneurysm, carotid artery disease, blood clots, peripheral vascular diseases, venous insufficiency, and venous ulcers. We take a minimally invasive approach to these diseases whenever possible.

William Randolph Hearst Burn Center—NewYork-Presbyterian Hospital is home to the largest and busiest burn center in the nation, caring for more than 900 inpatients and 4,000 outpatients annually. Our investigators also conduct research to improve survival and enhance the quality of life of burn victims.

In addition, the Hospital offers extraordinary expertise, comprehensive programs, and specialized resources in the fields of:

AIDS—The Center for Special Studies at NewYork-Presbyterian/Weill Cornell and the AIDS Care Program at NewYork-Presbyterian/Columbia provide comprehensive care for men, women, and children with HIV/AIDS. Both sites are designated as AIDS centers by New York State and by the National Institutes of Health.

Reproductive Medicine and Infertility—Our leading physicians and scientists in reproductive medicine use innovative technology for the comprehensive treatment of infertility in women and men. Our prestigious program is renowned for achieving success rates that are among the best in the world.

Trauma Center—Level 1 designations as an Adult Trauma Unit and a Pediatric Trauma Unit ensure the Hospital upholds the highest standards of 24-hour preparedness and treatment.

Women's Health Care—One of the first hospitals dedicated to women's health, NewYork-Presbyterian has established comprehensive programs which provide health care to women through all stages of their lives. The Hospital offers outstanding services in maternal-fetal health, gynecologic oncology, and a full range of preventive, primary, and specialty care.

NewYork-Presbyterian Healthcare System

NewYork-Presbyterian provides a comprehensive network of healthcare providers throughout the New York metropolitan area, including northern New Jersey, Westchester County, the Hudson Valley, and Fairfield, Connecticut. The full-service system includes 23 acute-care and community hospitals, 2 specialty institutions, 4 long-term facilities, and over 100 outpatient care centers.

Physician Referral: To find a NewYork-Presbyterian Hospital affiliated physician to meet your needs, call toll free **1-877-NYP-WELL** (1-877-697-9355) or visit our website at **www.nyp.org**

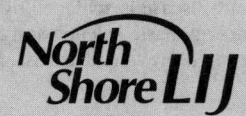

North Shore-LIJ Health System
Administration Offices
145 Community Drive
Great Neck, New York 11021
www.northshorelij.com
(516) 465-8000

A Network of Award Winning Hospitals and Programs.
Your Partner in Quality Care.

The nation's third-largest, non-profit, secular healthcare system, North Shore-LIJ delivers world-class clinical care throughout the New York metropolitan area. We are pioneering medical research at The Feinstein Institute for Medical Research, and highlighting a visionary approach to medical education through the Hofstra North Shore-LIJ School of Medicine. With nearly $7 billion in revenue and a workforce of more than 44,000, North Shore-LIJ is the largest employer on Long Island and the third-largest private employer in New York City.

North Shore-LIJ cares for people at every stage of life at 16 hospitals including a dedicated children's hospital, long-term care facilities and more than 270 ambulatory care centers throughout the region. North Shore-LIJ's owned hospitals and long-term care facilities house more than 6,000 beds, employ more than 10,000 nurses and have affiliations with more than 9,400 physicians. **In the most recent rankings by** *U.S. News and World Report*, **North Shore-LIJ hospitals were recognized with 57 national and regional designations, more than any other health system in New York.**

In addition to our network of hospitals, our health system delivers clinical care through the North Shore-LIJ Medical Group, the nation's sixth-largest physician group practice with more than 2,400 full-time physicians.

North Shore-LIJ Network of Hospitals

- **Five tertiary hospitals**
  - **Lenox Hill Hospital,** Manhattan
    - Manhattan Eye, Ear and Throat Hospital
  - **Long Island Jewish Medical Center,** New Hyde Park - Zuckerberg Pavilion
  - **North Shore University Hospital,** Manhasset
  - **Southside Hospital,** Bay Shore
  - **Staten Island University Hospital,** North

- **Three specialty care hospitals**
  - **South Oaks Hospital,** Amityville
  - **Steven & Alexandra Cohen Children's Medical Center of New York,** New Hyde Park
  - **The Zucker Hillside Hospital,** Glen Oaks

- **Seven community hospitals**
  - **Forest Hills Hospital**
  - **Franklin Hospital,** Valley Stream
  - **Glen Cove Hospital**
  - **Huntington Hospital**
  - **Plainview Hospital**
  - **Staten Island University Hospital,** South
  - **Syosset Hospital**

- **One affiliate hospital**
  - **Nassau University Medical Center,** East Meadow

To find a doctor: **1-888-321-DOCS** or visit **www.northshorelij.com**

A Home to Learning and Discovery

Beyond care delivery, North Shore-LIJ is home to the Feinstein Institute for Medical Research, which ranks among the nation's top five percent of all institutions that receive funding from the National Institutes of Health. At the Feinstein, scientists and investigators are conducting breakthrough research in oncology, immunology, psychiatry, neurology and many other specialties, and are leading more than 1,300 clinical trials involving 12,000 subjects.

As an academic medical center, North Shore-LIJ is also committed to educating the next generation of physicians. In 2011, the Hofstra North Shore-LIJ School of Medicine welcomed its inaugural class of 40 students. The School is the nation's 133rd medical school and New York State's first new allopathic medical school in 40 years.

Find the North Shore-LIJ Healthcare Provider That's Right for You

We make it easy to find the North Shore-LIJ specialist you need. Our knowledgeable staff will provide information on specialists, primary care physicians and special services. We're available to take your call 24 hours a day, 7 days a week.

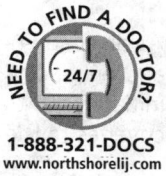

1-888-321-DOCS
www.northshorelij.com

North Shore-LIJ's Award Winning Programs and Services include:

- The Arthur Smith Institute for Urology
- Bariatric Surgery
- Behavioral Health
- Cohen Children's Medical Center of NY (Pediatrics)
- Cushing Neuroscience Institute
- The Feinstein Institute for Medical Research
- North Shore-LIJ Katz Institute for Women's Health
- North Shore-LIJ Cancer Institute
- North Shore-LIJ Cardiovascular Services
- North Shore-LIJ Center for Emergency Medical Services

- North Shore-LIJ Home Care Network
- North Shore-LIJ Imaging
- North Shore-LIJ Laboratories
- North Shore-LIJ Orthopaedic Institute
- North Shore-LIJ Rehabilitation Network
- Obstetrics & Gynecology
- Radiation Medicine
- Robotic Surgery
- North Shore-LIJ Medical Group Urgent Care Centers

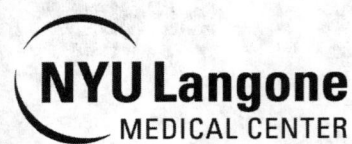

550 First Avenue *(at 31st Street)*
New York, NY 10016

www.NYULMC.org

Physician Referral: **888-7-NYU-MED** *(888-769-8633)*

NYU LANGONE MEDICAL CENTER

NYU Langone Medical Center is one of the nation's premier centers of excellence in health care, biomedical research, and medical education. For over 170 years, Medical Center physicians and researchers have made countless contributions to the practice and science of health care.

NYU Langone is comprised of Tisch Hospital, Rusk Institute of Rehabilitation Medicine, Hospital for Joint Diseases, Hassenfeld Pediatric Center, and NYU School of Medicine.

In a culture where treating the whole person and not simply the disease is the norm, NYU Langone Medical Center is renowned for clinical excellence across a wide array of specialties, including cardiology, cardiac and vascular surgery, cancer, musculoskeletal (including orthopaedics and rehabilitation), neurosurgery and children's services.

As an academic medical center, NYU Langone's clinical services are continually informed and enhanced by hundreds of basic and clinical research projects, as well as by major initiatives in translational research that promise to speed the transfer of laboratory discoveries to the patient's bedside.

Looking for information on our expert physicians? 1-888-769-8633

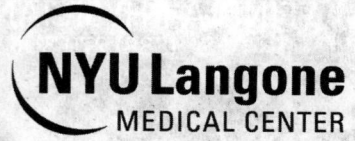

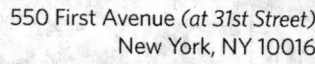

550 First Avenue *(at 31st Street)*
New York, NY 10016
www.NYULMC.org
Physician Referral: **888-7-NYU-MED** *(888-769-8633)*

Additional Areas of Expertise:

Adult Cardiovascular Services	Pediatric Cardiology
Internal Medicine	Pediatric Critical Care
Behavioral Health	Pediatric Gastroenterology
Cardiac Surgery	Pediatric Hematology/Oncology
Child and Adolescent Psychiatry	Pediatric Infectious Diseases
Clinical Genetics	Pediatric Pulmonology
Colon and Rectal Surgery	Pediatric Rheumatology
Dermatology	Pediatric Surgery
Gastroenterology	Program for IVF Reproductive
Geriatric Medicine	Psychiatry
Hand Surgery	Pulmonology
Hematology/Oncology	Radiology
Infectious Diseases	Radiation Oncology
Maternal Fetal Medicine	Reconstructive Plastic Surgery
Minimally Invasive Surgery	Rheumatology
Neonatal-Perinatal Medicine	Thoracic Surgery
Nuclear Medicine	Urology
Obstetrics and Gynecology	Vascular Surgery
Orthopaedic Services	Wound Care
Otolaryngology	Weight Management

Looking for information on our expert physicians? 1-888-769-8633

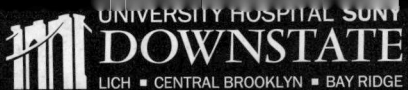

UNIVERSITY HOSPITAL SUNY
DOWNSTATE
LICH ■ CENTRAL BROOKLYN ■ BAY RIDGE

FIND A PHYSICIAN
(888) 270-SUNY
physicians.downstate.edu

SUNY Downstate Medical Center

SUNY Downstate Medical Center is Brooklyn's only academic medical center and one of the nation's leading urban medical centers, providing care to over 300,000 patients annually.

SUNY Downstate's University Hospital of Brooklyn at Central Brooklyn, in East Flatbush, is a full-service, comprehensive hospital comprised of 16 Departments providing over 150 specialty and subspecialty clincal services. Downstate also operates 3 community-based health centers in the Brooklyn neighborhoods of East New York, Bedford Stuyvesant and Midwood; a Dialysis Center; a Sleep Disorders Center; and the only Transplant and Pediatric Dialysis Centers in Brooklyn.

SUNY Downstate Long Island College Hospital is located in the Brooklyn Heights/ Cobble Hill neighborhood. LICH prides itself on combining the best features of a major medical center with the personal, caring approach of a community-centered hospital. Specialty centers include the Othmer Cancer Center, a Comprehensive Stroke Center, Sports Medicine Clinic, and pediatric and obstetric services.

SUNY Downstate Bay Ridge features a walk-in Urgent Care Center, as well as an Ambulatory Surgery Center, Advanced Endoscopy Center and Laser Vision Correction Center. Additionally, it includes onsite laboratory and diagnostic radiology facilities, and medical offices for doctors in many clinical specialties. Downstate Bay Ridge provides a wide range of options for patients in the Bay Ridge, Dyker Heights, Bensonhurst and Sunset Park communities.

Providing advanced care to the borough of Brooklyn at three major locations:

SUNY Downstate Central Brooklyn	SUNY Downstate Long Island College Hospital	SUNY Downstate Bay Ridge
450 Clarkson Avenue	339 Hicks Street	699 92nd Street
Brooklyn, NY 11203	Brooklyn, NY 11201	Brooklyn, NY 11228
Phone (718) 270-1000	Phone (718) 780-1000	Phone (718) 567-1234

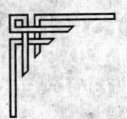

The Best in American Medicine
www.CastleConnolly.com

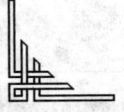
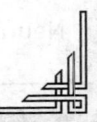

The New York metropolitan region is unique in its concentration of excellent Specialty Hospitals. Specialty Hospitals include those with a specific patient and disease focus such as cardiac care, psychiatric care and care of diseases and problems of eyes and ears. Many of these hospitals are nationally and internationally known for their outstanding care in these specialty areas and draw patients from the region and beyond who seek their excellent specialized care.

Castle Connolly Medical Ltd. has invited the following outstanding Specialty Hospitals to present important facts and information on their hospitals by sponsoring the profiles that follow.

Specialty Hospitals

Calvary Hospital

Hospital for Special Surgery

Memorial Sloan-Kettering Cancer Center

New York Eye & Ear Infirmary

NYU Hassenfeld Pediatric Center

NYU Hospital for Joint Diseases

NYU Rusk Institute of Rehabilitation

St Francis Hospital - The Heart Center

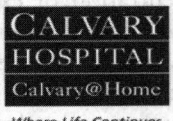

	1740 Eastchester Road	150 55th Street
	Bronx, NY 10461	Brooklyn, NY 11220
	Tel: (718) 518-2000	Tel: (718) 518-2000
	Fax: (718) 518-2674	Fax: (718) 518-2670

www.calvaryhospital.org

Beds:	225 (200 in Bronx, 25 at Brooklyn Satellite located at Lutheran Medical Center)
Accreditation:	The Joint Commission, College of American Pathologists (CAP)

SETTING THE STANDARD FOR PALLIATIVE CARE

Founded in 1899, Calvary Hospital is the nation's only fully accredited acute care specialty hospital dedicated to providing palliative care to adult advanced cancer patients. We care for patients at a 200-bed Bronx facility and a 25-bed satellite at Lutheran Medical Center in Brooklyn. Calvary's family-centric approach helps more than 6,000 patients and families each year with inpatient care, outpatient care, Calvary Home Care and Hospice, and the Center for Curative and Palliative Wound Care. The Joint Commission gave Calvary Hospital and our Home Care/Hospice program the Gold Seal of Approval™ in 2009. Press Ganey consistently ranks Calvary in the top one percent of its peers in patient satisfaction. Calvary received a 2012 Circle of Life Award® for innovative palliative and end-of-life care. To learn more or sign up for the e-newsletter, *Calvary Life*, please go to www.calvaryhospital.org.

Palliative Care Institute

Calvary's research and education arm, offers a curriculum for medical students, residents, postdoctoral fellows, and senior health practitioners, as well as health lectures for the community.

Acute Inpatient Care

One-page form expedites admissions process. Adults with advanced cancer are assigned a primary physician and a care team: nurse, social worker, dietitian, and case manager. Goal is to maximize physical, spiritual, and emotional comfort. Pastoral care and bereavement support are integral to care.

Outpatient and Wound Care

Outpatient clinic for cancer patients undergoing active treatment or who do not require acute inpatient care. The Center for Curative and Palliative Wound Care treats complex wounds related to cancer, diabetes, vascular disease, and other illnesses.

Calvary@Home: Home Care, Hospice, Nursing Home Hospice

Certified Home Health Agency

We provide a full range of home care services, not limited to patients with advanced cancer, in Bronx, Queens, northern Manhattan, and southern Westchester. Care is coordinated by patient's community physician or Calvary doctor. Nurse is available 24/7 for telephone consults.

Hospice & Nursing Home Hospice (NHH)

For people with all terminal diagnoses who are primarily cared for at home. Emphasis on quality of life, control of pain and symptoms, and support for family. Serves patients in Bronx, Brooklyn, Manhattan, Queens, Westchester, Nassau, and Rockland. Care may be coordinated by community physician or Calvary doctor. Nurse is available 24/7 by telephone. Bereavement support. Short-term hospitalization is available for acute symptom management. NHH is for nursing home residents suffering from all end-stage illnesses. Goal is to promote quality of life. Through a partnership with Mary Manning Walsh Home in Manhattan, Calvary provides an inpatient level of care for a select number of patients.

Family Care

Focuses on the impact of cancer on the family. Extensive bereavement support for adults, teens, and children, including bereavement camp for children and teens who participate in our support groups.

Pastoral Care

Calvary's Clinical Pastoral Education (CPE) program achieved certification by the Association for Clinical Pastoral Education – less than 2 years after the program was re-established. The 20-week, 400-hour program is the country's only CPE program exclusively focused on giving students hands-on experience solely with terminally ill patients in a hospital and home hospice setting.

Memorial Sloan-Kettering Cancer Center
The Best Cancer Care. Anywhere.

ESTABLISHED 1884

1275 York Avenue
New York, NY 10065
Make an Appointment: (800) 525-2225
www.mskcc.org

Beds: 470
Sponsorship/Network Affiliation: Private, Non-Profit
Make an Appointment: (800) 525-2225

THE MEMORIAL SLOAN-KETTERING ADVANTAGE: CANCER IS OUR ONLY FOCUS

At Memorial Sloan-Kettering Cancer Center, our only focus is cancer. Internationally recognized as one of the world's premier facilities for cancer care, we are consistently ranked as one of the nation's top cancer centers by *U.S. News & World Report*. We are proud to be a National Cancer Institute Comprehensive Cancer Center and a member of the National Comprehensive Cancer Network.

A TEAM APPROACH TO CANCER CARE

Our patients benefit from individualized treatment plans developed by a team of specialists with unsurpassed depth and breadth of experience. Teams include surgeons, medical and radiation oncologists, radiologists, pathologists, nurses, and others who are specialists in a specific type of cancer. They develop treatment plans that reflect their combined expertise, so patients who need several different types of therapy will receive the best combination for them.

GREATER PRECISION IN DIAGNOSIS

Getting the correct diagnosis right from the start is crucial. We use the most advanced imaging technologies, such as combined PET/CT and nuclear medicine scans, to accurately detect and precisely locate cancer. Our highly specialized pathologists analyze some 60,000 tumor samples annually to determine an exact diagnosis and the extent of disease. Increasingly, they use new technology to identify molecular differences among tumors, allowing even greater precision in diagnosis.

UNPARALLELED SURGICAL EXPERTISE

Recent studies have shown that, for many cancers, patients have fewer complications and better outcomes if they have surgery at a hospital where high volumes of these operations are performed by surgeons experienced in the procedure. Our surgeons are among the most experienced cancer surgeons in the world. They use the latest surgical technology, including robotic and minimally invasive techniques, as well as interventional radiology for embolization, thermal ablation, and chemical ablation of tumors. In their quest to spare or reconstruct organs and preserve function, they are renowned for not only saving lives, but preserving the quality of life.

ADVANCES IN CHEMOTHERAPY

Our medical oncologists are leaders in developing new chemotherapy drugs that are safer and more effective than standard therapies. They also help manage any side effects of chemotherapy, such as nausea and fatigue, so patients can continue their usual activities wherever possible. Increasingly, our medical oncologists use advanced technologies, such as immunotherapies or vaccines, often in combination with chemotherapy.

LEADERS IN RADIATION THERAPY

Our radiation oncologists are skilled in complex treatment planning and delivery techniques. Through their efforts, intensity-modulated radiation therapy was enhanced with image guidance (IGRT). IGRT enables our radiation oncologists to precisely sculpt multiple radiation beams to the contours of a tumor, sparing nearby normal tissue. The higher doses of radiation possible in IGRT also have a greater chance of killing tumors. Our doctors may use radiation combined with chemotherapy to make tumors more sensitive to the radiation, enhancing the chances of success.

RESEARCH EXPANDS TREATMENT OPTIONS

Through close collaboration between clinicians and research scientists, new therapies developed in the laboratory can be quickly translated into improved treatment options for patients.

INSURANCE

Memorial Sloan-Kettering Cancer Center is in-network with most New York–area insurance plans.

MAKE AN APPOINTMENT: (800) 525-2225

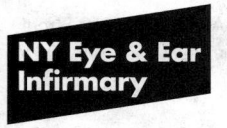

THE NEW YORK EYE AND EAR INFIRMARY

NY Eye & Ear Infirmary

Continuum Health Partners, Inc.

310 East 14th Street
New York, New York 10003
Tel. 212.979.4000   Fax. 212.228.0664
www.nyee.edu

BEDS:	69; Operating Rooms: 17; Surgical Cases: 27,000+ a year
Sponsorship:	Voluntary Not-for-Profit
Accreditation:	The Joint Commission
	College of American Pathologists

GENERAL OVERVIEW

The New York Eye and Ear Infirmary is one of the world's leading facilities for the diagnosis and treatment of diseases of the eyes, ears, nose, throat and related conditions. Founded in 1820, it is the first and most historic specialty hospital in the nation, as well as one of the busiest.

ACADEMIC AND CLINICAL AFFILIATIONS

A voluntary, not-for-profit institution, the Infirmary is a member of Continuum Health Partners, Inc. and an affiliated teaching hospital of New York Medical College. There are highly regarded residency programs in ophthalmology and otolaryngology, plus some two dozen post-graduate fellowship positions.

THE MEDICAL STAFF

The Medical Staff includes more than 600 board-certified attending physicians and surgeons throughout the metropolitan area. Many are renowned for their breakthrough research introducing widely practiced techniques.

SPECIALTIES

Ophthalmology: Within this area are subspecialties of cataract, glaucoma, retina, cornea and external disease, ocular plastic surgery, pediatric ophthalmology and strabismus, neuro-ophthalmology. ocular tumor and uveitis. Laser, photography, fluorescein angiography and electrophysiological testing are among the most advanced services available anywhere.

Otolaryngology: The department is in the forefront of treatment modalities using highly sophisticated endoscopic and laser equipment. Subspecialties include rhinology, laryngology, head & neck surgery, otology/neurotology, facial plastic surgery, pediatric otolaryngology, audiology, speech therapy and hearing aid dispensing.

Plastic & Reconstructive Surgery: Microsurgical capabilities and premium patient accommodations provide an optimum environment for facial plasty, liposuction, breast surgery and repair of defects from disease or trauma.

RELATED SERVICES

New York Eye Trauma Center: An advanced program for emergency treatment of eye injuries, it also is the Eye Injury Registry of New York State and leading collector of data which will help develop preventative strategies.

Ambulatory Surgery: A comprehensive Ambulatory Surgery Center is designed to expedite admission testing, pre-op preparation and post-op recovery in an efficient and comfortable setting.

Pediatric Specialty Care: Services of eye and ear, nose and throat specialists are coordinated with other professional and support staff especially sensitive to the youngest patients.

RESEARCH AND EDUCATION

The New York Eye and Ear Infirmary is a national and international leader in research in its specialties, achieving many "firsts" in successful surgical procedures and medical treatments. Laboratories include Cell Culture, Ocular Imaging, and Microsurgical Education. Over a hundred studies and clinical trials are currently being conducted.

Physician Referral: Call 1.800.449.HOPE (4673)

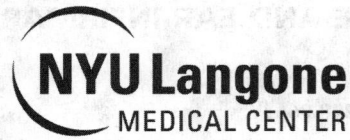

HASSENFELD PEDIATRIC CENTER

The new Hassenfeld Pediatric Center (HPC) is a full-service specialty children's hospital that works as a cohesive team across all children's health services at NYU Langone Medical Center. At HPC, newborns, children, adolescents and young adults receive the most comprehensive and advanced care possible from a team of pediatricians and pediatric specialists across more than 30 medical and surgical disciplines. With more than 150 full-time pediatric specialists, as well as pediatric nurses, child life specialists and social workers, the Hassenfeld Pediatric Center is uniquely equipped to provide innovative pediatric subspecialty care in a highly personalized manner.

About Children's Services at NYU Langone
NYU Langone Medical Center is nationally recognized in many pediatric specialty fields, including craniofacial anomalies, cardiac surgery, orthopaedic surgery, rehabilitation medicine, brain tumors, leukemia, sarcoma, and epilepsy. Our specialists work collaboratively to optimize care for each child, from the operating room and pediatric intensive care unit to the Emergency Department and pediatric inpatient unit.

A Family-Centered Approach
Integral to the care we provide is a myriad of support services for children and their families. We recognize that the best outcomes are achieved when the child's family is actively involved in every step of care. For that reason, our trained specialists address the needs of not just the patient, but of parents and siblings through ongoing education and communication.

The Future Shape of Pediatric Care at HPC
In 2017, a 160,000 square foot pediatric hospital, on the Medical Center's main campus, will become the inpatient centerpiece of the Hassenfeld Pediatric Center. This state-of-the-art facility will enhance the Center's ability to deliver world-class care through all private rooms, a feature that increases patient safety by decreasing exposure to infections, while providing a private, supportive environment for the patients and their families. HPC will be the only pediatric inpatient facility in Manhattan with this amenity, which will also include a "family zone" offering a sleep-in couch, storage, and Web access for each room.

The new pediatric hospital will also include a child-friendly pre-operative unit along with recovery bays where parents can be by the child's bedside during post-operation. Rounding out the new hospital will be a Family Center for orientation activities geared to patients, space for child-life activities and performances, as well as support, education and respite services for families.

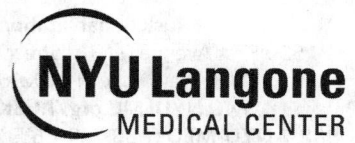

HOSPITAL FOR JOINT DISEASES

About the Hospital for Joint Diseases

The Hospital for Joint Diseases at NYU Langone Medical Center (HJD) is one of the nation's leading inpatient orthopaedic and rheumatologic specialty hospitals, and is ranked among the nation's top 10 for both orthopaedics and rheumatology in the 2012-2013 *U.S. News & World Report* annual survey of "Best Hospitals" in America. HJD is dedicated to the prevention and treatment of musculoskeletal diseases, providing some of the most advanced programs in the region for musculoskeletal disorders and the largest pediatric orthopaedic program in New York City. HJD also offers a number of unique and highly specialized services to provide tailored, world-class care to patients with specific musculoskeletal conditions and needs. We specialize in the following areas:

Orthopaedic Surgery

The clinical expertise of our internationally-renowned surgeons represents the full range of subspecialty areas of orthopaedic surgery, including Adult Reconstructive, Sports Medicine, Spine, Shoulder & Elbow, Foot & Ankle, Hand Surgery, Trauma & Fracture, Orthopaedic Oncology, and Pediatric Orthopaedics; additional areas of focus include minimally-invasive hip surgery and robotic-assisted joint replacement.

Rheumatology

HJD houses the Division of Rheumatology's Osteoporosis Center, offering a multidisciplinary approach to the evaluation and treatment of osteoporosis, including a range of advanced drug therapies.

Rehabilitation

Rehabilitation care at HJD is provided by the world-renowned Rusk Rehabilitation. Rusk's CARF-Accredited Brain Injury Rehabilitation Program is a center of innovation and excellence for the treatment of disabling neurological and neurocognitive disorders. HJD also houses Rusk's Orthopaedic Rehabilitation Unit, where an expert multidisciplinary rehabilitation team aids patients in their recovery after orthopaedic surgery or injury.

Neurology – Spine & Nerve

HJD provides a broad range of diagnostic and therapeutic services to patients with neurological disorders. Its outstanding clinical staff includes specialists in pain management, spine and nerve pain, and cerebral palsy.

Radiology

HJD provides complete diagnostic orthopaedic radiology services, including MRI, computed tomography, ultrasonography and conventional radiography, as well as a multitude of musculoskeletal interventional procedures. The medical team includes several internationally-known musculoskeletal radiologists with expertise in all aspects of osteoradiology.

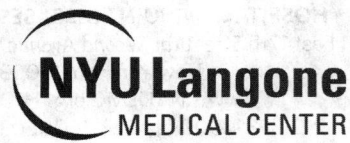

RUSK INSTITUTE OF REHABILITATION MEDICINE

Rusk Rehabilitation at NYU Langone Medical Center (Rusk) has been ranked the best rehabilitation hospital in New York and among the top ten in the country by *U.S. News & World Report* for 23 consecutive years. Rusk is internationally renowned for the treatment of adults and children with disabilities, providing the full continuum of inpatient and outpatient rehabilitation care at multiple, state-of-the-art NYU Langone facilities and across all specialties: physical, occupational, speech/swallowing and vocational therapy, psychology, music and recreational therapy, nutrition, nursing, and social work.

Rusk's CARF-Accredited Brain Injury Rehabilitation Program is tailored for patients who have medical, physical, cognitive, and behavioral changes as a result of a brain injury or neurological illness.

The Amputee Program provides specialized limb deficiency rehabilitation to patients who have undergone amputations.

The Joan and Joel Smilow Cardiac and Pulmonary Rehabilitation & Prevention Center offers a model of transitional care for patients with cardiac and lung conditions.

Orthopaedic/Musculoskeletal Rehabilitation is offered for patients with back, neck, hip, elbow and shoulder disorders, arthritis-related joint pain, conditions affecting the bones, tendon, ligaments and muscles, and for pre- and post-surgical patients.

The Spinal Cord Injury program offers a comprehensive, patient-centered array of specialized and innovative clinical and educational programs to optimize quality of life.

Sports Injury Rehabilitation addresses the needs of patients with sports-related conditions, including post-operative rehabilitation for patients who require orthopaedic surgery.

Rusk's CARF-Accredited Stroke Program offers an interdisciplinary team with specialized training in the medical, nursing or therapeutic care and treatment of stroke patients.

Vestibular Rehabilitation addresses the evaluation and treatment of patients suffering from dizziness and imbalance.

The Women's Health Program addresses issues that uniquely affect women, including pelvic floor muscle dysfunction/pain, urinary incontinence, cancer rehabilitation and lymphedema, and prenatal and postpartum musculoskeletal conditions.

Chest Physical Therapy cares for individuals with lung congestion, secretion retention or areas of lung collapse.

The Outpatient Rehabilitation Psychology Service provides care to patients with neurological and medical conditions on an outpatient basis.

Speech-Language Pathology & Swallowing is dedicated to patients with communication disorders due to neurological problems as well as diagnosis and management of swallowing and feeding disorders.

Vocational Services provides disabled individuals with the competencies needed to return to school or work and to lead a productive life.

St. Francis Hospital The Heart Center®

100 Port Washington Blvd.
Roslyn, New York 11576
www.stfrancisheartcenter.com
(516) 562-6000   1-888-HEARTNY

St. Francis Hospital, The Heart Center® is New York State's only specialty designated cardiac center and a nationally recognized leader in cardiac care. Founded in 1922 by the Franciscan Missionaries of Mary, the Hospital is an innovator in the delivery of specialized cardiovascular services in an environment where excellence and compassion are emphasized. St. Francis also offers an outstanding program in non-cardiac surgery, including some of the most advanced technology and minimally invasive techniques available for vascular, prostate, ear-nose-throat (ENT), abdominal, oncologic, gastrointestinal, and orthopedic surgery and procedures.

Cardiac Diagnostics and Treatment

St. Francis Hospital performs one of the highest volumes of cardiac surgical, interventional and arrhythmia procedures in the nation and has been consistently recognized for its outstanding quality of care. In 2012-13, St. Francis Hospital was ranked one of America's best hospitals by *U.S. News & World Report*.

Cardiac surgery: : In 2011, 1,477 open-heart surgeries were performed at St. Francis Hospital. The Hospital's cardiothoracic surgical staff has the combined experience of over 20,000 open-heart procedures in the last 10 years alone and are experts in all types of heart surgery, from conventional, open-heart bypass to off-pump coronary artery bypass (OPCAB) to the newest, minimally invasive valve procedures, including surgical techniques designed to treat certain cardiac arrhythmias or irregular heart rhythms.

Cardiac catheterization: In 2011, St. Francis interventional cardiologists performed 7,959 cardiac catheterizations and 3,046 percutaneous coronary interventions (angioplasty and insertion of stents). The Hospital is also recognized as one of the East Coast's highest volume centers for catheter-based techniques to close atrial septal defects (ASDs) and patent foramen ovale (PFO).

Arrhythmia and Pacemaker Center: St. Francis has a leading national program for pacemaker implantation and the diagnosis and treatment of cardiac rhythm abnormalities. The Center has unparalleled expertise in radiofrequency cardiac ablation, including treatment of atrial fibrillation.

Research and Technology: At the St. Francis Cardiac Research Institute, a team of world-renowned researchers is working with the latest noninvasive imaging technology, including advanced techniques and world-class expertise in cardiac CT angiography, cardiac magnetic resonance imaging (MRI), cardiac PET/CT and three-dimensional echocardiography. This multimodality approach to investigating the heart's function and disease processes is aimed at improving methods of diagnosing heart disease.

Prevention and Education

St. Francis Hospital's satellite campus, The DeMatteis Center for Cardiac Research and Education, in Greenvale, New York, is one of the few freestanding campuses in the U.S. dedicated to the prevention of heart disease. It is the site of community health lectures, as well as the largest medically staffed cardiac fitness and rehabilitation program on Long Island.

Physician referral: **1-888-HEARTNY**
Sponsorship: Voluntary not-for-profit
Beds: 306
Accreditation: Awarded accreditation from the Joint Commission.

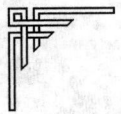

The Best in American Medicine
www.CastleConnolly.com

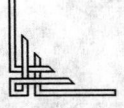
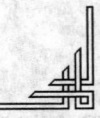

New York State Metropolitan Regional Medical Centers and Hospitals

The New York metropolitan region is fortunate to have a large number of truly excellent Regional Medical Centers and Hospitals. Many of these institutions offer sophisticated services that in years past were offered only at academic medical centers. However, with advancements in medical technology, Regional Medical Centers and Hospitals have access to the equipment, and by virtue of the medical schools and teaching hospitals in the region, the well-trained physicians and staff, to offer these programs.

Regional Medical Centers and Hospitals range in size from the small (100 beds) to the very large (800 beds) but they share a common theme: a primary focus on patient care.

We have invited a select number of excellent Regional Medical Centers and Hospitals to provide readers of the Castle Connolly Guide with information on their institutions and services by sponsoring profiles, which are included at the end of individual county sections in the physician listings that follow.

Regional Medical Centers and Hospitals

Children's & Women's Physicians of Westchester, LL

Greenwich Hospital

Hackensack University Health Network

Hackensack UMC at Pascack Valley

Hackensack UMC Mountainside

Holy Name Medical Center

New York Hospital Queens

New York Methodist Hospital

Northern Westchester Hospital

Phelps Memorial Hospital Center

Stamford Hospital

SUNY Downstate Medical Center (Univ Hosp of Brooklyn) - Central Brooklyn

SUNY Downstate Medical Center (Univ Hosp of Brooklyn) - LI College Hospital

Trinitas Regional Medical Center

Valley Hospital

White Plains Hospital Center

Winthrop-University Hospital

Yale Medical Group

SECTION THREE

Physician Listings

The State of New York

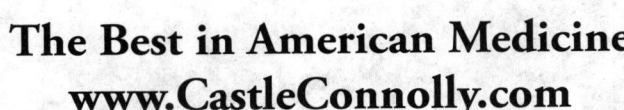

The Best in American Medicine
www.CastleConnolly.com

New York (Manhattan)

New York (Manhattan)

Addiction Psychiatry

Collins, Eric D MD (AdP) - **Spec Exp:** Addiction/Substance Abuse; Alcohol Abuse; **Hospital:** NY-Presby/Columbia Univ Med Ctr, NY (page 104); **Address:** 180 Ft Washington Ave, Box HP-260, New York, NY 10032; **Phone:** 212-305-8732; **Board Cert:** Psychiatry 2005; Addiction Psychiatry 2007; Psychosomatic Medicine 2008; **Med School:** Columbia P&S 1990; **Resid:** Psychiatry, NY State Psyc Inst 1994; **Fellow:** Psychosomatic Medicine, NY-Presby/Columbia Univ Med Ctr 1995; Substance Abuse, NY State Psyc Inst 1996; **Fac Appt:** Asst Prof Psyc, Columbia P&S

Frances, Richard J MD (AdP) - **Spec Exp:** Addiction/Substance Abuse; Anxiety & Mood Disorders; Forensic Psychiatry; **Hospital:** Silver Hill Hosp, NYU Langone Med Ctr (page 108); **Address:** 510 E 86th St, Ste 1D, New York, NY 10028; **Phone:** 212-861-0570; **Board Cert:** Psychiatry 1976; Addiction Psychiatry 2002; **Med School:** NYU Sch Med 1971; **Resid:** Psychiatry, Bronx Meml Hosp 1974; **Fellow:** Psychoanalysis, NY Psychoanalitic Inst 1984; **Fac Appt:** Clin Prof Psyc, NYU Sch Med

Galanter, I Marc MD (AdP) - **Spec Exp:** Alcohol Abuse; Drug Abuse; **Hospital:** NYU Langone Med Ctr (page 108), Bellevue Hosp Ctr; **Address:** 285 Central Park West, New York, NY 10024-3006; **Phone:** 212-877-4093; **Board Cert:** Psychiatry 1974; Addiction Psychiatry 2011; **Med School:** Albert Einstein Coll Med 1967; **Resid:** Psychiatry, Bronx Muni Hosp-Einstein 1971; **Fac Appt:** Prof Psyc, NYU Sch Med

Kleber, Herbert MD (AdP) - **Spec Exp:** Opiate Addiction; Cocaine Addiction; Marijuana Abuse; Drug Abuse; **Hospital:** NY-Presby/Columbia Univ Med Ctr, NY (page 104), NY State Psychiatric Inst; **Address:** 1051 Riverside Drive, Room 3713, Unit 66, New York, NY 10032-1007; **Phone:** 212-543-5570; **Med School:** Jefferson Med Coll 1960; **Resid:** Psychiatry, Yale-New Haven Hosp 1964; **Fac Appt:** Prof Psyc, Columbia P&S

Levin, Frances R MD (AdP) - **Spec Exp:** Addiction/Substance Abuse; Dual Diagnosis; Substance Abuse in ADHD Patients; **Hospital:** NY State Psychiatric Inst, NY-Presby/Columbia Univ Med Ctr, NY (page 104); **Address:** NYSPI, Dept Psychiatry-RFMH, 1051 Riverside Drive, Box 66, New York, NY 10032; **Phone:** 212-543-5896; **Board Cert:** Psychiatry 1990; Addiction Psychiatry 2002; **Med School:** Cornell Univ-Weill Med Coll 1985; **Resid:** Psychiatry, Payne Whitney Clin 1989; **Fellow:** Substance Abuse, Univ Maryland/NIDA 1990; **Fac Appt:** Assoc Prof Psyc, Columbia P&S

Paul, Edward MD (AdP) - **Spec Exp:** Opiate Addiction; Alcohol Abuse; Smoking Cessation; Cocaine Addiction; **Hospital:** NYU Langone Med Ctr (page 108); **Address:** 155 E 31st St, Ste 25J, New York, NY 10016; **Phone:** 212-447-5712; **Board Cert:** Psychiatry 1987; Addiction Psychiatry 2003; **Med School:** Columbia P&S 1982; **Resid:** Psychiatry, Payne Whitney Clinic 1987; Psychoanalysis, NYU Med Ctr 1993; **Fellow:** Substance Abuse, New York Hosp 1987; **Fac Appt:** Asst Clin Prof Psyc, NYU Sch Med

Rosenberg, Kenneth P MD (AdP) - **Spec Exp:** Addiction/Substance Abuse; Sexual Dysfunction; Physicians' Health-Psychiatric; **Hospital:** NY-Presby/Weill Cornell Med Ctr, NY (page 104); **Address:** 49 E 78th St, Ste 2A, New York, NY 10075; **Phone:** 212-861-8807; **Board Cert:** Psychiatry 1992; Addiction Psychiatry 2009; **Med School:** Albert Einstein Coll Med 1983; **Resid:** Psychiatry, NY Hosp-Cornell Med Ctr 1988; **Fellow:** Substance Abuse, NY Hosp-Cornell Med Ctr 1991; Public Health, NY Hosp-Cornell Med Ctr 1992; **Fac Appt:** Assoc Clin Prof Psyc, Cornell Univ-Weill Med Coll

Weiss, Carol J MD (AdP) - **Spec Exp:** Drug Abuse; Alcohol Abuse; **Hospital:** NY-Presby/Weill Cornell Med Ctr, NY (page 104); **Address:** 1044 Madison Ave, Ste PH1, New York, NY 10075; **Phone:** 212-988-1209; **Board Cert:** Psychiatry 1989; Addiction Psychiatry 2003; Addiction Medicine 2009; **Med School:** Johns Hopkins Univ 1983; **Resid:** Psychiatry, New York Hosp 1987; **Fellow:** Addiction Psychiatry, New York Hosp 1989; **Fac Appt:** Asst Clin Prof Psyc, Cornell Univ-Weill Med Coll

Adolescent Medicine

Diaz, Angela MD (AM) - **Spec Exp:** Adolescent Gynecology; Abuse/Neglect; **Hospital:** Mount Sinai Med Ctr (page 102); **Address:** 320 E 94th St Fl 2, New York, NY 10128-5604; **Phone:** 212-423-2900; **Board Cert:** Pediatrics 1987; **Med School:** Columbia P&S 1981; **Resid:** Pediatrics, Mt Sinai Med Ctr 1984; **Fellow:** Adolescent Medicine, Mt Sinai Med Ctr 1985; **Fac Appt:** Prof Ped, Mount Sinai Sch Med

Lopez, Ralph I MD (AM) - **Spec Exp:** Growth/Development Disorders; Eating Disorders; Learning Disorders; Parenting Issues; **Hospital:** NY-Presby/Weill Cornell Med Ctr, NY (page 104); **Address:** 418 E 71st St, New York, NY 10021-4894; **Phone:** 212-772-8989; **Board Cert:** Pediatrics 1972; **Med School:** NYU Sch Med 1967; **Resid:** Pediatrics, Bellevue Hosp 1969; Pediatrics, Chldns Hosp 1970; **Fellow:** Adolescent Medicine, Chldns Hosp 1971; **Fac Appt:** Clin Prof Ped, Cornell Univ-Weill Med Coll

Marks, Andrea M MD (AM) - **Spec Exp:** Eating Disorders; Adolescent Gynecology; Psychosomatic Disorders; Parenting Issues; **Hospital:** Mount Sinai Med Ctr (page 102); **Address:** 14 E 90th St, Ste 1-B, New York, NY 10128-0671; **Phone:** 212-987-1414; **Board Cert:** Pediatrics 1977; **Med School:** Univ Pennsylvania 1972; **Resid:** Pediatrics, Chldns Hosp 1974; **Fellow:** Adolescent Medicine, Chldns Hosp 1975; **Fac Appt:** Assoc Clin Prof Ped, Mount Sinai Sch Med

Nucci-Sack, Anne T MD (AM) - **Spec Exp:** Adolescent Gynecology; Vaccines; **Hospital:** Mount Sinai Med Ctr (page 102); **Address:** Mount Sinai Adolescent Health Center, 312 E 94th St, New York, NY 10128; **Phone:** 212-423-3000; **Board Cert:** Pediatrics 1986; Adolescent Medicine 2009; **Med School:** NY Med Coll 1981; **Resid:** Pediatrics, Bronx Municipal Hosp 1984; **Fellow:** Adolescent Medicine, Montefiore Hosp 1990; **Fac Appt:** Asst Prof Ped, Mount Sinai Sch Med

Pegler, Cynthia R MD (AM) - **Spec Exp:** Adolescent Gynecology; Eating Disorders; **Hospital:** NY-Presby/Weill Cornell Med Ctr, NY (page 104); **Address:** 992 5th Ave, New York, NY 10028; **Phone:** 212-517-5313; **Board Cert:** Pediatrics 2010; Adolescent Medicine 2009; **Med School:** Albany Med Coll 1984; **Resid:** Pediatrics, N Shore Univ Hosp 1987; **Fellow:** Adolescent Medicine, N Shore Univ Hosp 1990

Rudy, Bret J MD (AM) - **Spec Exp:** HIV in Adolescents; AIDS/HIV; **Hospital:** NYU Langone Med Ctr (page 108); **Address:** 227 E 30th St, rm 713, New York, NY 10016; **Phone:** 212-263-6425; **Board Cert:** Pediatrics 1998; Adolescent Medicine 2001; **Med School:** Univ Pittsburgh 1985; **Resid:** Pediatrics, Chldns Hosp of Philadelphia 1989; **Fellow:** Immunology, Chldns Hosp of Philadelphia 1991

Allergy & Immunology

Bassett, Clifford MD (A&I) - **Spec Exp:** Asthma & Sinusitis; Food Allergy; Pet Allergy; Skin Allergies; **Hospital:** NYU Langone Med Ctr (page 108), SUNY Downstate Med Ctr (Univ Hosp of Bklyn) - LICH (page 420); **Address:** 381 Park Ave S, Ste 1020, New York, NY 10016; **Phone:** 212-260-6078; **Board Cert:** Allergy & Immunology 2006; **Med School:** NY Med Coll 1985; **Resid:** Internal Medicine, Hackensack Med Ctr 1989; **Fellow:** Allergy & Immunology, LI College Hosp 1993; **Fac Appt:** Asst Clin Prof Med, NYU Sch Med

Buchbinder, Ellen MD (A&I) - **Spec Exp:** Asthma & Allergy; Rhinitis; Hives; Food & Drug Allergy; **Hospital:** Mount Sinai Med Ctr (page 102); **Address:** 111B E 88th St, New York, NY 10128; **Phone:** 212-410-3246; **Board Cert:** Internal Medicine 1981; Allergy & Immunology 1983; **Med School:** Tulane Univ 1978; **Resid:** Internal Medicine, New England Deaconess Hosp 1981; **Fellow:** Allergy & Immunology, Mass Genl Hosp 1983; **Fac Appt:** Asst Clin Prof Med, Mount Sinai Sch Med

Burton, Daniel A MD (A&I) - **Spec Exp:** Rhinitis; Asthma; Food & Drug Allergy; Urticaria; **Hospital:** NY-Presby/Weill Cornell Med Ctr, NY (page 104), Hosp For Special Surgery (page 115); **Address:** 235 E 67th St, Ste 203, New York, NY 10065; **Phone:** 212-288-9300; **Board Cert:** Internal Medicine 1989; Allergy & Immunology 1989; **Med School:** Wright State Univ 1984; **Resid:** Internal Medicine, St Lukes-Roosevelt Hosp Ctr 1987; **Fellow:** Allergy & Immunology, NY Hosp 1989; **Fac Appt:** Asst Prof Med, Cornell Univ-Weill Med Coll

Chandler, Michael MD (A&I) - **Spec Exp:** Asthma; Sinus Disorders; Airway Disorders; **Hospital:** Mount Sinai Med Ctr (page 102); **Address:** 115 E 61st St Fl 12, New York, NY 10065; **Phone:** 212-486-6715; **Board Cert:** Internal Medicine 1984; Allergy & Immunology 1987; **Med School:** Wayne State Univ 1981; **Resid:** Internal Medicine, Northwestern Meml Hosp 1984; **Fellow:** Allergy & Immunology, Northwestern Meml Hosp 1986; **Fac Appt:** Asst Clin Prof Med, Mount Sinai Sch Med

Corn, Beth E MD (A&I) - **Spec Exp:** Asthma; **Hospital:** Mount Sinai Med Ctr (page 102); **Address:** 5 E 98th St, Box 1089, New York, NY 10029; **Phone:** 212-241-0764; **Board Cert:** Allergy & Immunology 2005; **Med School:** Albert Einstein Coll Med 1989; **Resid:** Internal Medicine, St Lukes-Roosevelt Hosp 1992; **Fellow:** Clinical Immunology, Mt Sinai Med Ctr 1994; **Fac Appt:** Asst Prof Med, Mount Sinai Sch Med

Cunningham-Rundles, Charlotte MD/PhD (A&I) - **Spec Exp:** Immunotherapy; Immunodeficiency Disorders; **Hospital:** Mount Sinai Med Ctr (page 102); **Address:** 5 E 98th St Fl 11, New York, NY 10029; **Phone:** 212-659-9268; **Board Cert:** Internal Medicine 1972; **Med School:** Columbia P&S 1969; **Resid:** Internal Medicine, Bellevue Hosp Ctr 1972; **Fellow:** Allergy & Immunology, NYU Med Ctr 1974; **Fac Appt:** Prof Med, Mount Sinai Sch Med

Feldman, B Robert MD (A&I) - **Spec Exp:** Asthma; Allergic Rhinitis; Food Allergy; Eczema; **Hospital:** Morgan Stanley Children's Hosp of NY-Presby, NY (page 104); **Address:** Morgan Stanley Chlds Hosp NY-Presby, 3959 Broadway, New York, NY 10032; **Phone:** 212-305-2300; **Board Cert:** Pediatrics 1965; Allergy & Immunology 1972; **Med School:** Ros Franklin Univ/Chicago Med Sch 1959; **Resid:** Pediatrics, Michael Reese Hosp 1962; Allergy & Immunology, Michael Reese Hosp 1963; **Fellow:** Allergy & Immunology, Columbia-Presby Med Ctr 1964; **Fac Appt:** Clin Prof Ped, Columbia P&S

Frenkel, Renata MD (A&I) - **Spec Exp:** Asthma; Allergy; Sinus Disorders; Urticaria; **Hospital:** St. Luke's - Roosevelt Hosp Ctr - Roosevelt Div (page 94), Lenox Hill Hosp (page 106); **Address:** 30 W 60th St, Ste 1U, New York, NY 10023-7906; **Phone:** 212-265-1990; **Board Cert:** Allergy & Immunology 1979; **Med School:** Austria 1968; **Resid:** Allergy & Immunology, Roosevelt Hosp 1975; **Fac Appt:** Assoc Clin Prof Ped, Columbia P&S

Grubman, Samuel MD (A&I) - **Spec Exp:** Asthma & Allergy; Food Allergy; Immunodeficiency Disorders; Pediatric Allergy & Immunology; **Hospital:** NYU Langone Med Ctr (page 108); **Address:** 154 W 14th St, Fl 4, New York, NY 10011; **Phone:** 212-616-4122; **Board Cert:** Pediatrics 1987; Allergy & Immunology 2009; **Med School:** Mount Sinai Sch Med 1983; **Resid:** Pediatrics, NYU Med Ctr 1986; **Fellow:** Allergy & Immunology, Montefiore Med Ctr 1988; **Fac Appt:** Asst Prof Ped, NYU Sch Med

Lubitz, Arthur M MD (A&I) - **Spec Exp:** Allergy; Asthma; Immunotherapy; **Hospital:** Lenox Hill Hosp (page 106), NYU Langone Med Ctr (page 108); **Address:** 250 W 57th St, Ste 1231, New York, NY 10107; **Phone:** 212-247-7447; **Board Cert:** Internal Medicine 1984; Allergy & Immunology 2001; **Med School:** SUNY Downstate 1980; **Resid:** Internal Medicine, Coney Island Hosp 1983; **Fellow:** Allergy & Immunology, Long Island Coll Hosp 1985

Mazza, David S MD (A&I) - **Spec Exp:** Asthma; Sinus Disorders; Eczema; **Hospital:** St. Luke's - Roosevelt Hosp Ctr - Roosevelt Div (page 94); **Address:** 7 Lexington Ave, Ste P3, New York, NY 10010-5517; **Phone:** 212-677-7170; **Board Cert:** Pediatrics 1983; Allergy & Immunology 2008; **Med School:** Univ VT Coll Med 1977; **Resid:** Pediatrics, NYU-Bellevue Hosp 1980; **Fellow:** Pediatric Allergy & Immunology, Bellevue Hosp 1982; **Fac Appt:** Assoc Prof Ped, Columbia P&S

Rubin, James MD (A&I) - **Spec Exp:** Asthma; Rhinitis; Sinus Disorders; **Hospital:** Beth Israel Med Ctr - Petrie Division (page 94); **Address:** 35 E 35th St, Ste 202, New York, NY 10016-3823; **Phone:** 212-685-4225; **Board Cert:** Internal Medicine 1968; Allergy & Immunology 1972; **Med School:** NY Med Coll 1960; **Resid:** Internal Medicine, Beth Israel Hosp 1964; **Fellow:** Allergy & Immunology, Jewish Hosp 1965; **Fac Appt:** Assoc Clin Prof Med, Albert Einstein Coll Med

Shepherd, Gillian M MD (A&I) - **Spec Exp:** Food & Drug Allergy; Rhinosinusitis & Asthma; Urticaria; Insect Allergies; **Hospital:** NY-Presby/Weill Cornell Med Ctr, NY (page 104); **Address:** 235 E 67th St, Ste 203, New York, NY 10065; **Phone:** 212-288-9300; **Board Cert:** Internal Medicine 1979; Allergy & Immunology 1981; **Med School:** NY Med Coll 1976; **Resid:** Internal Medicine, Lenox Hill Hosp 1979; **Fellow:** Allergy & Immunology, New York Hosp-Cornell 1981; **Fac Appt:** Assoc Clin Prof Med, Cornell Univ-Weill Med Coll

Slankard, Marjorie MD (A&I) - **Spec Exp:** Sinus Disorders; Asthma; Food Allergy; Hereditary Angioedema; **Hospital:** NY-Presby/Columbia Univ Med Ctr, NY (page 104), Valley Hosp (page 689); **Address:** 16 E 60th St, Ste 321, New York, NY 10022-1002; **Phone:** 212-326-8410; **Board Cert:** Internal Medicine 1974; Allergy & Immunology 1977; **Med School:** Univ MO-Columbia Sch Med 1971; **Resid:** Internal Medicine, New York Hosp 1974; Internal Medicine, Rockefeller Univ Hosp 1974; **Fellow:** Immunology, New York Hosp-Cornell 1976; Immunology, Mount Sinai Med Ctr 1980; **Fac Appt:** Clin Prof Med, Columbia P&S

Tolston, Evelyn MD (A&I) - **Spec Exp:** Rhinitis; Asthma; Allergy; Sinusitis; **Hospital:** NYU Langone Med Ctr (page 108), Beth Israel Med Ctr - Petrie Division (page 94); **Address:** 161 Madison Ave, Ste 3A, New York, NY 10016; **Phone:** 646-424-0400; **Board Cert:** Allergy & Immunology 2005; **Med School:** Ukraine 1982; **Resid:** Internal Medicine, Cabrini Med Ctr 1993; Allergy & Immunology, Albert Einstein Coll Med 1995

Young, Stuart H MD (A&I) - **Spec Exp:** Asthma; Nasal & Sinus Disorders; Urticaria; Eczema; **Hospital:** Mount Sinai Med Ctr (page 102); **Address:** 121 E 60th St, New York, NY 10022-1102; **Phone:** 212-826-0815; **Board Cert:** Pediatrics 1968; Allergy & Immunology 1972; **Med School:** SUNY Downstate 1963; **Resid:** Pediatrics, Kings Co Hosp 1966; **Fellow:** Allergy & Immunology, Natl Jewish Hosp 1970; **Fac Appt:** Assoc Clin Prof Med, Mount Sinai Sch Med

Cardiac Electrophysiology

Biviano, Angelo MD (CE) - **Spec Exp:** Catheter Ablation; Defibrillators; Pacemakers; Atrial Fibrillation; **Hospital:** NY-Presby/Columbia Univ Med Ctr, NY (page 104); **Address:** 161 Fort Washington Ave, Ste 648, New York, NY 10032; **Phone:** 212-305-8559; **Board Cert:** Cardiovascular Disease 2004; Cardiac Electrophysiology 2006; **Med School:** Harvard Med Sch 1997; **Resid:** Internal Medicine, NewYork-Presby Hosp/Columbia Univ Med Ctr 2001; Cardiovascular Disease, NewYork-Presby Hosp/Columbia Univ Med Ctr 2004; **Fellow:** Cardiac Electrophysiology, NewYork-Presby Hosp/Columbia Univ Med Ctr 2005; **Fac Appt:** Asst Prof Med, Columbia P&S

Chinitz, Larry MD (CE) - **Spec Exp:** Arrhythmias; Pacemakers; Defibrillators; Atrial Fibrillation; **Hospital:** NYU Langone Med Ctr (page 108); **Address:** 403 E 34th St, Heart Rhythm Center, 4th Fl, New York, NY 10016-6402; **Phone:** 212-263-7149; **Board Cert:** Internal Medicine 1982; Cardiovascular Disease 1985; **Med School:** NYU Sch Med 1979; **Resid:** Internal Medicine, Bellevue Hosp Ctr 1983; **Fellow:** Cardiovascular Disease, NYU Med Ctr/Bellevue Hosp Ctr 1986; Cardiac Electrophysiology, Montefiore Hosp 1985; **Fac Appt:** Assoc Prof Med, NYU Sch Med

Evans, Steven J MD (CE) - **Spec Exp:** Arrhythmias; Electrophysiologic Testing; Defibrillators; Pacemakers; **Hospital:** Beth Israel Med Ctr - Petrie Division (page 94); **Address:** Beth Israel Med Ctr, 10 Union Square E, Ste 2A, New York, NY 10003; **Phone:** 212-844-8830; **Board Cert:** Internal Medicine 1987; Cardiovascular Disease 1989; Cardiac Electrophysiology 2002; **Med School:** NYU Sch Med 1984; **Resid:** Internal Medicine, Manhattan VA Med Ctr 1987; **Fellow:** Cardiovascular Disease, Cedars-Sinai Med Ctr 1990; Cardiac Electrophysiology, Cedars-Sinai Med Ctr 1990; **Fac Appt:** Asst Prof Med, Albert Einstein Coll Med

Garan, Hasan MD (CE) - **Spec Exp:** Arrhythmias; Cardiac Catheterization; Pacemakers/Defibrillators; **Hospital:** NY-Presby/Columbia Univ Med Ctr, NY (page 104); **Address:** 161 Fort Washington Ave, Ste 546, New York, NY 10032; **Phone:** 212-305-7646; **Board Cert:** Internal Medicine 1977; Cardiovascular Disease 1979; **Med School:** Harvard Med Sch 1974; **Resid:** Internal Medicine, Hosp Univ Penn 1976; **Fellow:** Cardiovascular Disease, Mass Genl Hosp 1978; Cardiac Electrophysiology, Mass Genl Hosp 1979; **Fac Appt:** Prof Med, Columbia P&S

Gomes, J Anthony MD (CE) - **Spec Exp:** Arrhythmias; Heart Attack; Atrial Fibrillation; Pacemakers; **Hospital:** Mount Sinai Med Ctr (page 102); **Address:** Mount Sinai Medical Ctr, One Gustave L Levy Pl, New York, NY 10029-6500; **Phone:** 212-241-7272; **Board Cert:** Internal Medicine 1974; Cardiovascular Disease 1977; **Med School:** India 1970; **Resid:** Internal Medicine, Mt Sinai Med Ctr 1973; **Fellow:** Cardiovascular Disease, Mt Sinai Med Ctr 1975; Cardiac Electrophysiology, USPHS Cardio-Pulmonary Lab 1976; **Fac Appt:** Prof Med, Mount Sinai Sch Med

Lerman, Bruce MD (CE) - **Spec Exp:** Catheter Ablation; Atrial Fibrillation; Defibrillators; Arrhythmias; **Hospital:** NY-Presby/Weill Cornell Med Ctr, NY (page 104); **Address:** NY Weill Cornell Med Ctr, 520 E 70th St, Starr 4, New York, NY 10021-9800; **Phone:** 212-746-2169; **Board Cert:** Internal Medicine 1980; Cardiovascular Disease 1985; Cardiac Electrophysiology 2012; **Med School:** Loyola Univ-Stritch Sch Med 1977; **Resid:** Internal Medicine, Northwestern Univ Hosp 1980; Internal Medicine, Univ Michigan Med Ctr 1981; **Fellow:** Cardiovascular Disease, Hosp Univ Penn 1982; Cardiovascular Disease, Johns Hopkins Hosp 1983; **Fac Appt:** Prof Med, Cornell Univ-Weill Med Coll

Markowitz, Steven M MD (CE) - **Spec Exp:** Arrhythmias; **Hospital:** NY-Presby/Weill Cornell Med Ctr, NY (page 104); **Address:** 520 E 70th St, Starr Bldg - Fl 4, New York, NY 10021; **Phone:** 212-746-2655; **Board Cert:** Cardiovascular Disease 2005; Cardiac Electrophysiology 2006; **Med School:** Harvard Med Sch 1988; **Resid:** Internal Medicine, New York Hosp 1991; **Fellow:** Cardiovascular Disease, NY Hosp-Cornell 1995; Cardiac Electrophysiology, NY Hosp-Cornell 1996; **Fac Appt:** Prof Med, Cornell Univ-Weill Med Coll

Matos, Jeffrey A MD (CE) - **Spec Exp:** Arrhythmias; Pacemakers; Defibrillators; **Hospital:** Lenox Hill Hosp (page 106); **Address:** Arrhythmia Associates, 1421 Third Ave Fl 5, New York, NY 10028; **Phone:** 212-772-6384; **Board Cert:** Internal Medicine 1980; Cardiovascular Disease 1983; **Med School:** Harvard Med Sch 1975; **Resid:** Internal Medicine, Beth Israel Hosp 1978; **Fellow:** Cardiovascular Disease, Peter Bent Brigham Hosp 1980; **Fac Appt:** Assoc Clin Prof Med, NYU Sch Med

Mehta, Davendra MD/PhD (CE) - **Spec Exp:** Arrhythmias; Congenital Heart Disease-Adult; Atrial Fibrillation; Heart Failure; **Hospital:** Mount Sinai Med Ctr (page 102); **Address:** One Gustave L Levy Pl, Box 1030, New York, NY 10029-6501; **Phone:** 212-241-7272; **Board Cert:** Cardiovascular Disease 2009; Cardiac Electrophysiology 2009; **Med School:** India 1979; **Resid:** Internal Medicine, Leicester Royal Infirmary 1983; **Fellow:** Cardiovascular Disease, Groby Road Hosp 1986; Electrocardiography, St George's Hosp 1989; **Fac Appt:** Prof Med, Mount Sinai Sch Med

Suri, Ranjit MD (CE) - **Spec Exp:** Arrhythmias; Atrial Fibrillation; Pacemakers; Heart Failure; **Hospital:** Lenox Hill Hosp (page 106), NY Hosp Queens (page 206); **Address:** Cardiac Arrythmia Ctr, Lenox Hill Hosp, 100 E 77th St, New York, NY 10075; **Phone:** 212-434-6500; **Board Cert:** Internal Medicine 2007; Cardiovascular Disease 2006; Cardiac Electrophysiology 2001; **Med School:** India 1982; **Resid:** Internal Medicine, Univ Conn Sch Med 1994; **Fellow:** Cardiovascular Disease, Univ Conn Sch Med 1993; Cardiac Electrophysiology, Mass Genl Hosp 2000; **Fac Appt:** Asst Clin Prof Med, Cornell Univ-Weill Med Coll

Whang, William MD (CE) - **Spec Exp:** Catheter Ablation; Arrhythmias; Atrial Fibrillation; Pacemakers/Defibrillators; **Hospital:** NY-Presby/Columbia Univ Med Ctr, NY (page 104); **Address:** 161 Fort Washington Ave, Fl 6, rm 648, New York, NY 10032; **Phone:** 212-305-8559; **Board Cert:** Cardiovascular Disease 2004; Cardiac Electrophysiology 2005; **Med School:** Columbia P&S 1998; **Resid:** Internal Medicine, NY-Presby Hosp/Columbia Univ Med Ctr 2001; **Fellow:** Cardiovascular Disease, Mass Genl Hosp 2004; Cardiac Electrophysiology, Mass Genl Hosp 2006; **Fac Appt:** Asst Clin Prof Med, Columbia P&S

Cardiovascular Disease

Andersen, Holly S MD (Cv) - **Spec Exp:** Preventive Cardiology; Women's Health; Mitral Valve Prolapse; **Hospital:** NY-Presby/Weill Cornell Med Ctr, NY (page 104); **Address:** 425 E 61st St Fl 6, New York, NY 10021; **Phone:** 212-628-6100; **Board Cert:** Internal Medicine 2002; Cardiovascular Disease 2005; **Med School:** Univ Rochester 1989; **Resid:** Internal Medicine, NY Presby-Cornell Med Ctr 1992; **Fellow:** Cardiovascular Disease, NY Presby-Cornell Med Ctr 1995; **Fac Appt:** Assoc Clin Prof Med, Cornell Univ-Weill Med Coll

Askanas, Aleksander MD (Cv) - **Spec Exp:** Arrhythmias; Angina; Congestive Heart Failure; **Hospital:** Beth Israel Med Ctr - Petrie Division (page 94), NYU Langone Med Ctr (page 108); **Address:** 242 E 19th St, Office #1, New York, NY 10003; **Phone:** 212-369-3080; **Board Cert:** Internal Medicine 1972; Cardiovascular Disease 1974; **Med School:** Poland 1960; **Resid:** Internal Medicine, VA Med Ctr 1971; **Fellow:** Cardiovascular Disease, VA Med Ctr 1972; **Fac Appt:** Asst Prof Med, Mount Sinai Sch Med

Berdoff, Russell L MD (Cv) - **Spec Exp:** Coronary Artery Disease; Heart Valve Disease; Preventive Cardiology; **Hospital:** Beth Israel Med Ctr - Petrie Division (page 94); **Address:** 67 Irving Pl, Fl 7, New York, NY 10003-2202; **Phone:** 212-979-9224; **Board Cert:** Internal Medicine 1978; Cardiovascular Disease 1981; **Med School:** NY Med Coll 1975; **Resid:** Internal Medicine, DC Genl Hosp 1978; **Fellow:** Cardiovascular Disease, Johns Hopkins Hosp 1980; **Fac Appt:** Assoc Clin Prof Med, Albert Einstein Coll Med

Berger, Marvin MD (Cv) - **Spec Exp:** Echocardiography; **Hospital:** Beth Israel Med Ctr - Petrie Division (page 94); **Address:** Heart Inst, 10 Union Square, Ste 2A, New York, NY 10003; **Phone:** 212-420-2068; **Board Cert:** Internal Medicine 1969; Cardiovascular Disease 1977; **Med School:** Ros Franklin Univ/Chicago Med Sch 1961; **Resid:** Internal Medicine, Beth Israel Hosp 1964; **Fellow:** Cardiovascular Disease, Mount Sinai Hosp 1965; **Fac Appt:** Clin Prof Med, Albert Einstein Coll Med

Bergmann, Steven R MD/PhD (Cv) - **Spec Exp:** Nuclear Cardiology; Cardiac Imaging; **Hospital:** Beth Israel Med Ctr - Petrie Division (page 94); **Address:** Beth Israel Med Ctr, Heart Institute, 1st Ave at 16th St, Baird Hall, 5th fl, New York, NY 10003; **Phone:** 212-420-4681; **Board Cert:** Internal Medicine 1998; Nuclear Cardiology 1999; **Med School:** Washington Univ, St Louis 1985; **Resid:** Internal Medicine, Barnes-Jewish Hosp 1988; **Fellow:** Cardiovascular Disease, Barnes-Jewish Hosp 1990; **Fac Appt:** Prof Med, Albert Einstein Coll Med

Blake, James A MD (Cv) - **Spec Exp:** Congestive Heart Failure; Nuclear Cardiology; Echocardiography; Hypertension; **Hospital:** NY-Presby/Weill Cornell Med Ctr, NY (page 104), Hosp For Special Surgery (page 115); **Address:** 133 E 58th St, Ste 301, New York, NY 10022; **Phone:** 212-755-8700; **Board Cert:** Internal Medicine 1984; Cardiovascular Disease 1987; Echocardiography 2009; Nuclear Cardiology 2009; **Med School:** Albert Einstein Coll Med 1981; **Resid:** Internal Medicine, NY Hosp 1984; **Fellow:** Cardiovascular Disease, NY Hosp 1987; **Fac Appt:** Assoc Clin Prof Med, Cornell Univ-Weill Med Coll

Blumenthal, David S MD (Cv) - **Spec Exp:** Heart Valve Disease; Preventive Cardiology; Coronary Artery Disease; **Hospital:** NY-Presby/Weill Cornell Med Ctr, NY (page 104); **Address:** 407 E 70th St, Fl 1, New York, NY 10021-5302; **Phone:** 212-861-3222; **Board Cert:** Internal Medicine 1978; Cardiovascular Disease 1981; **Med School:** Cornell Univ-Weill Med Coll 1975; **Resid:** Internal Medicine, NY Hosp 1978; Internal Medicine, NY Hosp 1981; **Fellow:** Cardiovascular Disease, Johns Hopkins Hosp 1980; **Fac Appt:** Clin Prof Med, Cornell Univ-Weill Med Coll

Cemaletin, Nevber S MD (Cv) - **Hospital:** Lenox Hill Hosp (page 106), Lenox Hill Hosp (Manh Eye, Ear & Throat Hosp) (page 106); **Address:** 110 E 59th St, Ste 9B, New York, NY 10022; **Phone:** 212-583-2899; **Board Cert:** Internal Medicine 1988; Cardiovascular Disease 1989; **Med School:** NY Med Coll 1984; **Resid:** Internal Medicine, Lenox Hill Hosp 1987; **Fellow:** Cardiovascular Disease, Lenox Hill Hosp 1989

Cohen, Howard A MD (Cv) - **Spec Exp:** Interventional Cardiology; Carotid Artery Stent Placement; **Hospital:** Lenox Hill Hosp (page 106); **Address:** Lenox Hill Hospital, Interventional Cardiology, 130 E 77th St Fl 9, New York, NY 10075; **Phone:** 212-434-2606; **Board Cert:** Internal Medicine 1974; Cardiovascular Disease 1977; **Med School:** NYU Sch Med 1970; **Resid:** Internal Medicine, Bellevue Hosp Ctr 1974; **Fellow:** Cardiovascular Disease, Johns Hopkins Hosp 1976

Cohen, Michael H MD (Cv) - **Spec Exp:** Congestive Heart Failure; Coronary Artery Disease; Hypertension; Cholesterol/Lipid Disorders; **Hospital:** NY-Presby/Columbia Univ Med Ctr, NY (page 104); **Address:** 161 Fort Washington Ave, rm 328, New York, NY 10032-3713; **Phone:** 212-305-5440; **Board Cert:** Internal Medicine 1971; **Med School:** Johns Hopkins Univ 1965; **Resid:** Internal Medicine, NY-Presby Hosp/Columbia Univ 1971; **Fellow:** Cardiovascular Disease, NY-Presby Hosp/Columbia Univ 1970; **Fac Appt:** Clin Prof Med, Johns Hopkins Univ

Cole, William J MD (Cv) - **Spec Exp:** Coronary Artery Disease; Hypertension; Cholesterol/Lipid Disorders; **Hospital:** NYU Langone Med Ctr (page 108); **Address:** 530 First Ave, Ste 3-D, New York, NY 10016; **Phone:** 212-263-7071; **Board Cert:** Internal Medicine 1983; Cardiovascular Disease 1987; **Med School:** NYU Sch Med 1980; **Resid:** Cardiovascular Disease, NYU Med Ctr 1984; **Fac Appt:** Asst Clin Prof Med, NYU Sch Med

Coppola, John T MD (Cv) - **Spec Exp:** Cardiac Catheterization; Angioplasty; **Hospital:** NYU Langone Med Ctr (page 108), Bellevue Hosp Ctr; **Address:** 275 7th Ave Fl 3, New York, NY 10001; **Phone:** 646-660-9999; **Board Cert:** Internal Medicine 1981; Cardiovascular Disease 1983; Interventional Cardiology 2009; **Med School:** NY Med Coll 1978; **Resid:** Internal Medicine, St Vincent Catholic Med Ctr 1981; **Fellow:** Cardiovascular Disease, St Vincent Catholic Med Ctr 1983

Dangas, George MD (Cv) - **Spec Exp:** Acute Coronary Syndromes; Angioplasty & Stent Placement; Hypertrophic Cardiomyopathy; Percutaneous Vascular Interventions; **Hospital:** Mount Sinai Med Ctr (page 102); **Address:** Cardiovascular Medicine Associates, Guggenheim Pavillion, 1190 5 Ave S, New York, NY 10029; **Phone:** 212-241-7014; **Board Cert:** Internal Medicine 1994; Cardiovascular Disease 2007; Interventional Cardiology 2009; **Med School:** Greece 1989; **Resid:** Internal Medicine, Miriam Hosp 1994; **Fellow:** Cardiovascular Disease, Mount Sinai Med Ctr 1997; Internal Medicine, Mount Sinai Med Ctr 1998; **Fac Appt:** Prof Med, Mount Sinai Sch Med

Deutsch, Adam MD (Cv) - **Spec Exp:** Hypertension; Cholesterol/Lipid Disorders; Echocardiography; Congestive Heart Failure; **Hospital:** NY-Presby/Weill Cornell Med Ctr, NY (page 104), Lenox Hill Hosp (page 106); **Address:** Park Avenue Cardiology, 1036 Park Ave, New York, NY 10028; **Phone:** 212-879-9000; **Board Cert:** Internal Medicine 2006; Cardiovascular Disease 2009; **Med School:** Albert Einstein Coll Med 1992; **Resid:** Internal Medicine, Columbia-Presby Med Ctr 1995; **Fellow:** Cardiovascular Disease, Columbia-Presby Med Ctr 1998

Devereux, Richard B MD (Cv) - **Spec Exp:** Marfan's Syndrome; **Hospital:** NY-Presby/Weill Cornell Med Ctr, NY (page 104); **Address:** 525 E 68th St, rm K-415, New York, NY 10065; **Phone:** 212-746-4655; **Board Cert:** Internal Medicine 1974; Cardiovascular Disease 1977; **Med School:** Univ Pennsylvania 1971; **Resid:** Internal Medicine, New York Hosp 1974; **Fellow:** Cardiovascular Disease, Hosp Univ Penn 1976; **Fac Appt:** Prof Med, Cornell Univ-Weill Med Coll

Drusin, Ronald MD (Cv) - **Spec Exp:** Heart Failure; Coronary Artery Disease; Heart Valve Disease; Transplant Medicine-Heart; **Hospital:** NY-Presby/Columbia Univ Med Ctr, NY (page 104); **Address:** Herbert Irving Pavillion, 161 Ft Washington Ave, Ste 647, New York, NY 10032; **Phone:** 212-305-5371; **Board Cert:** Internal Medicine 1973; Cardiovascular Disease 1975; **Med School:** Columbia P&S 1966; **Resid:** Internal Medicine, Presby Hosp 1969; **Fellow:** Cardiovascular Disease, Columbia-Presby Hosp 1973; **Fac Appt:** Clin Prof Med, Columbia P&S

Epstein, Stanley MD (Cv) - **Spec Exp:** Non-Invasive Cardiology; Preventive Cardiology; Hypertension; Cholesterol/Lipid Disorders; **Hospital:** NY-Presby/Columbia Univ Med Ctr, NY (page 104), Montefiore Med Ctr-Moses Campus, NY (page 100); **Address:** 15 W 72 St, Ste 22B, New York, NY 10023; **Phone:** 212-362-2079; **Board Cert:** Internal Medicine 1967; Cardiovascular Disease 1975; **Med School:** Ros Franklin Univ/Chicago Med Sch 1958; **Resid:** Internal Medicine, Jewish Hosp 1960; Internal Medicine, San Francisco Genl Hosp 1961; **Fellow:** Cardiovascular Disease, Montefiore Hosp Med Ctr 1967; **Fac Appt:** Clin Prof Med, Columbia P&S

Friedman, Howard S MD (Cv) - **Spec Exp:** Atrial Fibrillation; Coronary Artery Disease; Hypertension; **Hospital:** NYU Langone Med Ctr (page 108); **Address:** 650 First Ave, Fl 3, New York, NY 10016-3240; **Phone:** 212-889-9393; **Board Cert:** Internal Medicine 1971; Cardiovascular Disease 1974; Geriatric Medicine 2004; **Med School:** SUNY Buffalo 1966; **Resid:** Internal Medicine, Mt Sinai Med Ctr 1969; Cardiovascular Disease, Mt Sinai Med Ctr 1973; **Fac Appt:** Clin Prof Med, NYU Sch Med

Friedman, Sanford MD (Cv) - **Spec Exp:** Preventive Cardiology; **Hospital:** Mount Sinai Med Ctr (page 102); **Address:** 941 Park Ave, New York, NY 10028; **Phone:** 212-988-3772; **Board Cert:** Internal Medicine 1980; Cardiovascular Disease 1977; **Med School:** Tufts Univ 1971; **Resid:** Internal Medicine, Mt Sinai Med Ctr 1974; **Fellow:** Cardiovascular Disease, Mt Sinai Med Ctr 1976; **Fac Appt:** Assoc Clin Prof Med, Mount Sinai Sch Med

Fuchs, Richard MD (Cv) - **Spec Exp:** Coronary Artery Disease; Heart Valve Disease; Preventive Cardiology; **Hospital:** NY-Presby/Weill Cornell Med Ctr, NY (page 104); **Address:** 310 E 72nd St, New York, NY 10021; **Phone:** 212-717-2254; **Board Cert:** Internal Medicine 1979; Cardiovascular Disease 1981; **Med School:** Harvard Med Sch 1976; **Resid:** Internal Medicine, New York Hosp 1979; **Fellow:** Cardiovascular Disease, Johns Hopkins Hosp 1982; **Fac Appt:** Clin Prof Med, Cornell Univ-Weill Med Coll

Fuster, Valentin MD/PhD (Cv) - **Spec Exp:** Coronary Artery Disease; Heart Valve Disease; Congenital Heart Disease; Preventive Cardiology; **Hospital:** Mount Sinai Med Ctr (page 102); **Address:** One Gustave Levy Pl, Box 1030, MS 10029, New York, NY 10029-6500; **Phone:** 212-241-7911; **Board Cert:** Internal Medicine 1976; Cardiovascular Disease 1977; **Med School:** Spain 1967; **Resid:** Internal Medicine, Mayo Clin 1972; Cardiovascular Disease, Mayo Clin 1974; **Fellow:** Cardiovascular Disease, Univ Edinburgh 1971; **Fac Appt:** Prof Med, Mount Sinai Sch Med

Gliklich, Jerry MD (Cv) - **Spec Exp:** Heart Valve Disease; Arrhythmias; **Hospital:** NY-Presby/Columbia Univ Med Ctr, NY (page 104); **Address:** 173 Fort Washington Ave, Ste 606, New York, NY 10032; **Phone:** 212-305-5588; **Board Cert:** Internal Medicine 1978; Cardiovascular Disease 1981; **Med School:** Columbia P&S 1975; **Resid:** Internal Medicine, NY Hosp 1978; **Fellow:** Cardiovascular Disease, Columbia-Presby Med Ctr 1981; **Fac Appt:** Clin Prof Med, Columbia P&S

Goldberg, Harvey MD (Cv) - **Hospital:** NY-Presby/Weill Cornell Med Ctr, NY (page 104), Lenox Hill Hosp (page 106); **Address:** 425 E 61st St, Fl 6, New York, NY 10021-8795; **Phone:** 212-752-2000; **Board Cert:** Internal Medicine 1979; Cardiovascular Disease 1981; **Med School:** Cornell Univ-Weill Med Coll 1976; **Resid:** Internal Medicine, NY Hosp 1979; **Fellow:** Cardiovascular Disease, NY Hosp 1981; **Fac Appt:** Assoc Clin Prof Med, Cornell Univ-Weill Med Coll

Goldberg, Nieca MD (Cv) - **Spec Exp:** Heart Disease in Women; Preventive Cardiology; Echocardiography; Women's Health; **Hospital:** NYU Langone Med Ctr (page 108), Lenox Hill Hosp (page 106); **Address:** Joan H. Tisch Ctr for Women's Hlth, 207 E 84th St, New York, NY 10028; **Phone:** 212-289-2045; **Board Cert:** Internal Medicine 1987; Cardiovascular Disease 2005; **Med School:** SUNY Downstate 1984; **Resid:** Internal Medicine, St Lukes Roosevelt Hosp Ctr 1987; **Fellow:** Cardiovascular Disease, SUNY Hlth Sci Ctr 1990; **Fac Appt:** Assoc Clin Prof Med, NYU Sch Med

Goldman, Martin E MD (Cv) - **Spec Exp:** Heart Valve Disease; Echocardiography; Diagnostic Problems; **Hospital:** Mount Sinai Med Ctr (page 102); **Address:** 1190 5th Ave, New York, NY 10029-6504; **Phone:** 212-241-3078; **Board Cert:** Internal Medicine 1979; Cardiovascular Disease 1981; **Med School:** Albert Einstein Coll Med 1976; **Resid:** Internal Medicine, Peter Bent Brigham Hosp 1978; **Fellow:** Cardiovascular Disease, Mount Sinai Hosp 1980; **Fac Appt:** Prof Med, NYU Sch Med

Goodman, Dennis A MD (Cv) - **Spec Exp:** Preventive Cardiology; Cholesterol/Lipid Disorders; Complementary Medicine; **Hospital:** NYU Langone Med Ctr (page 108); **Address:** 635 Madison Ave Fl 3, New York, NY 10022; **Phone:** 212-439-6690; **Board Cert:** Internal Medicine 1984; Cardiovascular Disease 1989; Integrative Medicine 1995; **Med School:** South Africa 1979; **Resid:** Internal Medicine, Montefiore Med Ctr 1984; **Fellow:** Cardiovascular Disease, Baylor Coll Med 1987; **Fac Appt:** Clin Prof Med, NYU Sch Med

Gotto Jr, Antonio M MD (Cv) - **Spec Exp:** Cholesterol/Lipid Disorders; **Hospital:** NY-Presby/Weill Cornell Med Ctr, NY (page 104); **Address:** NY-Presby/Weill Cornell Med Ctr, Cardiac Disease Prevention Ctr, 1305 York Ave Fl 8, New York, NY 10021; **Phone:** 646-962-6004; **Board Cert:** Internal Medicine 1980; **Med School:** Vanderbilt Univ 1965; **Resid:** Internal Medicine, Mass Genl Hosp 1967; **Fac Appt:** Prof Med, Cornell Univ-Weill Med Coll

Halperin, Jonathan L MD (Cv) - **Spec Exp:** Peripheral Vascular Disease; Atrial Fibrillation; **Hospital:** Mount Sinai Med Ctr (page 102); **Address:** 1190 Fifth Ave, New York, NY 10029; **Phone:** 212-241-7243; **Board Cert:** Internal Medicine 1980; Cardiovascular Disease 1981; **Med School:** Boston Univ 1975; **Resid:** Internal Medicine, Mass Genl Hosp 1977; **Fellow:** Vascular Medicine, Boston Univ Med Ctr 1978; Cardiovascular Disease, Boston Univ Med Ctr 1980; **Fac Appt:** Prof Med, Mount Sinai Sch Med

Hecht, Alan MD (Cv) - **Spec Exp:** Heart Valve Disease; Coronary Artery Disease; Arrhythmias; **Hospital:** Mount Sinai Med Ctr (page 102); **Address:** 1075 Park Ave, New York, NY 10128; **Phone:** 212-876-0845; **Board Cert:** Internal Medicine 1984; Cardiovascular Disease 1987; **Med School:** Northwestern Univ 1981; **Resid:** Internal Medicine, Mt Sinai Hosp 1984; **Fellow:** Cardiovascular Disease, Mt Sinai Hosp 1986; **Fac Appt:** Assoc Clin Prof Med, Mount Sinai Sch Med

Horn, Evelyn M MD (Cv) - **Spec Exp:** Pulmonary Hypertension; Heart Failure; Ventricular Assist Device (LVAD); Heart Disease-Complex; **Hospital:** NY-Presby/Weill Cornell Med Ctr, NY (page 104); **Address:** 520 E 70th St Starr Bldg Fl 4 - Ste 443, New York, NY 10021; **Phone:** 212-746-2381; **Board Cert:** Internal Medicine 1983; Cardiovascular Disease 1985; Advanced Heart Failure & Transplant Cardiology 2010; **Med School:** Mount Sinai Sch Med 1980; **Resid:** Internal Medicine, Mt Sinai Hosp 1983; **Fellow:** Cardiovascular Disease, Cedars-Sinai Med Ctr 1985; **Fac Appt:** Clin Prof Med, Cornell Univ-Weill Med Coll

Inra, Lawrence A MD (Cv) - **Spec Exp:** Coronary Artery Disease; Preventive Cardiology; Cholesterol/Lipid Disorders; Hypertension; **Hospital:** NY-Presby/Weill Cornell Med Ctr, NY (page 104), Hosp For Special Surgery (page 115); **Address:** 407 E 70th St, New York, NY 10021; **Phone:** 212-249-1011; **Board Cert:** Internal Medicine 1979; Cardiovascular Disease 1981; **Med School:** Johns Hopkins Univ 1976; **Resid:** Internal Medicine, NY Hosp 1979; **Fellow:** Cardiovascular Disease, Mt Sinai Hosp 1981; **Fac Appt:** Assoc Clin Prof Med, Cornell Univ-Weill Med Coll

Kalman, Jill MD (Cv) - **Spec Exp:** Heart Failure; Cardiomyopathy; Heart Disease in Women; **Hospital:** Mount Sinai Med Ctr (page 102); **Address:** 1 Gustave L Levy Pl, Ste 178, GP Bldg Fl 6, Box 1030, MS 10029, New York, NY 10029-6501; **Phone:** 212-241-0511; **Board Cert:** Cardiovascular Disease 2005; **Med School:** Mount Sinai Sch Med 1987; **Resid:** Internal Medicine, Mt Sinai Med Ctr 1991; **Fellow:** Cardiovascular Disease, Mt Sinai Med Ctr 1995; **Fac Appt:** Assoc Prof Med, Mount Sinai Sch Med

Kamen, Mazen MD (Cv) - **Spec Exp:** Heart Valve Disease; Cholesterol/Lipid Disorders; Hypertension; Congenital Heart Disease; **Hospital:** NY-Presby/Weill Cornell Med Ctr, NY (page 104); **Address:** 1021 Park Ave, Ste 101, New York, NY 10028; **Phone:** 212-427-5800; **Board Cert:** Cardiovascular Disease 2006; **Med School:** NYU Sch Med 1983; **Resid:** Internal Medicine, NYU Med Ctr 1986; **Fellow:** Cardiovascular Disease, NY-Presby/Weill Cornell Med Ctr 1990; **Fac Appt:** Asst Prof Med, Cornell Univ-Weill Med Coll

Katz, Edward MD (Cv) - **Spec Exp:** Echocardiography; Cholesterol/Lipid Disorders; Coronary Artery Disease; **Hospital:** NYU Langone Med Ctr (page 108), NYU Hosp For Joint Diseases (page 119); **Address:** NYU Cardiology Associates, 530 1st Ave, Ste 9U, New York, NY 10016; **Phone:** 212-263-7751; **Board Cert:** Cardiovascular Disease 2009; Internal Medicine 1988; Echocardiography 2005; **Med School:** NYU Sch Med 1985; **Resid:** Internal Medicine, NYU Med Ctr 1988; **Fellow:** Cardiovascular Disease, NYU Med Ctr 1991; **Fac Appt:** Assoc Prof Med, NYU Sch Med

Katz, Stuart D MD (Cv) - **Spec Exp:** Heart Failure; Transplant Medicine-Heart; **Hospital:** NYU Langone Med Ctr (page 108); **Address:** NYU Cardiology Assocs, 530 First Ave, Ste 9U, New York, NY 10016; **Phone:** 212-263-7751; **Board Cert:** Internal Medicine 1986; Cardiovascular Disease 1989; Advanced Heart Failure & Transplant Cardiology 2010; **Med School:** SUNY Downstate 1983; **Resid:** Internal Medicine, Francis Scott Key Med Ctr 1986; **Fellow:** Cardiovascular Disease, Montefiore Med Ctr 1989; **Fac Appt:** Prof Med, NYU Sch Med

Kligfield, Paul MD (Cv) - **Hospital:** NY-Presby/Weill Cornell Med Ctr, NY (page 104); **Address:** 525 E 68th St, Ste L195, New York, NY 10021; **Phone:** 212-746-4686; **Board Cert:** Internal Medicine 1973; Cardiovascular Disease 1975; **Med School:** Harvard Med Sch 1970; **Resid:** Internal Medicine, Beth Israel Deaconess Med Ctr 1972; Cardiovascular Disease, St George's Hosp 1973; **Fellow:** Cardiovascular Disease, New York Hosp 1975; **Fac Appt:** Prof Med, Cornell Univ-Weill Med Coll

Kronzon, Itzhak MD (Cv) - **Spec Exp:** Heart Valve Disease; Echocardiography; Cardiac Imaging; Pericardial Diseases; **Hospital:** Lenox Hill Hosp (page 106); **Address:** 100 E 77th St, Unit 2 East, New York, NY 10075; **Phone:** 212-434-6119; **Board Cert:** Internal Medicine 1979; Cardiovascular Disease 1981; Echocardiography 2002; **Med School:** Israel 1964; **Resid:** Internal Medicine, Hadassah Hosp 1969; **Fellow:** Cardiovascular Disease, Montefiore Med Ctr 1973; Cardiovascular Disease, NYU Med Ctr 1974; **Fac Appt:** Prof Med, NYU Sch Med

Kutnick, Richard T MD (Cv) - **Spec Exp:** Echocardiography; **Hospital:** Lenox Hill Hosp (page 106); **Address:** 1421 3rd Ave Fl 6, New York, NY 10028; **Phone:** 212-879-2628; **Board Cert:** Internal Medicine 1979; Cardiovascular Disease 1981; **Med School:** Tufts Univ 1976; **Resid:** Internal Medicine, Lenox Hill Hosp 1979; **Fellow:** Cardiovascular Disease, Lenox Hill Hosp 1981; **Fac Appt:** Asst Prof Med, NYU Sch Med

Lazar, Eliot J MD (Cv) - **Spec Exp:** Hypertension; Coronary Artery Disease; **Hospital:** NY-Presby/Weill Cornell Med Ctr, NY (page 104); **Address:** NY-Presby/Weill Cornell Med Ctr, 525 E 68th St, Box 262, New York, NY 10065; **Phone:** 212-746-0386; **Board Cert:** Internal Medicine 1984; Cardiovascular Disease 1987; Geriatric Medicine 2006; **Med School:** SUNY Upstate Med Univ 1981; **Resid:** Internal Medicine, Bronx Muni Hosp 1984; **Fellow:** Cardiovascular Disease, Mount Sinai Med Ctr 1987; **Fac Appt:** Assoc Clin Prof Med, Cornell Univ-Weill Med Coll

Lewis, Benjamin H MD (Cv) - **Spec Exp:** Cardiac Stress Testing; Heart Disease & Gender; Echocardiography; Preventive Cardiology; **Hospital:** NY-Presby/Columbia Univ Med Ctr, NY (page 104), Lenox Hill Hosp (page 106); **Address:** 16 E 60th St Fl 3, New York, NY 10022; **Phone:** 212-326-8425; **Board Cert:** Internal Medicine 1980; Cardiovascular Disease 1983; **Med School:** UCSF 1977; **Resid:** Internal Medicine, Columbia-Presby Hosp 1980; **Fellow:** Cardiovascular Disease, Brigham Womens Hosp 1982; **Fac Appt:** Assoc Prof Med, Columbia P&S

Mancini, Donna M MD (Cv) - **Spec Exp:** Congestive Heart Failure; Transplant Medicine-Heart; **Hospital:** NY-Presby/Columbia Univ Med Ctr, NY (page 104); **Address:** 622 W 168 St Fl 12 West - rm 134, New York, NY 10032; **Phone:** 212-305-4600; **Board Cert:** Internal Medicine 1983; Cardiovascular Disease 1987; Advanced Heart Failure & Transplant Cardiology 2010; **Med School:** Albert Einstein Coll Med 1980; **Resid:** Internal Medicine, Bronx Municipal Hosp 1983; **Fellow:** Cardiovascular Disease, Montefiore Med Ctr 1986; **Fac Appt:** Prof Med, Columbia P&S

Masri, Bassem M MD (Cv) - **Spec Exp:** Cholesterol/Lipid Disorders; Coronary Artery Disease; Preventive Cardiology; Hypertension; **Hospital:** NY-Presby/Weill Cornell Med Ctr, NY (page 104); **Address:** NY-Presby/Weill Cornell Med Ctr, Cardiac Disease Prevention Ctr, 1305 York Ave Fl 8, New York, NY 10021; **Phone:** 646-962-6004; **Med School:** Lebanon 1988; **Resid:** Internal Medicine, American Univ of Beirut 1991; **Fellow:** Cardiovascular Disease, Baylor Coll Med; **Fac Appt:** Assoc Prof Med, Cornell Univ-Weill Med Coll

Matta, Raymond J MD (Cv) - **Hospital:** Mount Sinai Med Ctr (page 102); **Address:** 1120 Park Ave, Ste 1C, New York, NY 10128-1242; **Phone:** 212-410-5800; **Board Cert:** Internal Medicine 1973; Cardiovascular Disease 1975; **Med School:** Univ Pittsburgh 1969; **Resid:** Internal Medicine, Mass Genl Hosp 1971; **Fellow:** Cardiovascular Disease, Peter Bent Brigham Hosp 1975; **Fac Appt:** Assoc Clin Prof Med, Mount Sinai Sch Med

Mattes, Leonard MD (Cv) - **Hospital:** Mount Sinai Med Ctr (page 102); **Address:** 1199 Park Ave, Ste 1F, New York, NY 10128-1713; **Phone:** 212-876-7045; **Board Cert:** Internal Medicine 1972; Cardiovascular Disease 1975; **Med School:** Tulane Univ 1962; **Resid:** Internal Medicine, Mt Sinai Hosp 1967; Cardiovascular Disease, Mt Sinai Hosp 1969; **Fellow:** Cardiovascular Disease, Mt Sinai Hosp 1968; **Fac Appt:** Asst Clin Prof Med, Mount Sinai Sch Med

Meller, Jose MD (Cv) - **Hospital:** Mount Sinai Med Ctr (page 102); **Address:** 941 Park Ave, New York, NY 10028; **Phone:** 212-988-3772; **Board Cert:** Internal Medicine 1973; Cardiovascular Disease 1975; **Med School:** Chile 1969; **Resid:** Internal Medicine, Elmhurst Hosp 1971; Internal Medicine, Mt Sinai Med Ctr 1972; **Fellow:** Cardiovascular Disease, Mt Sinai Med Ctr 1974; **Fac Appt:** Clin Prof Med, Mount Sinai Sch Med

Messerli, Franz Hannes MD (Cv) - **Spec Exp:** Hypertension; Heart Failure; Coronary Artery Disease; **Hospital:** St. Luke's - Roosevelt Hosp Ctr - Roosevelt Div (page 94); **Address:** University Medical Practice Assocs, Div Cardiology, 425 W 59th St, Ste 9C, New York, NY 10019; **Phone:** 212-492-5550; **Board Cert:** Internal Medicine 1978; **Med School:** Switzerland 1970; **Resid:** Internal Medicine, Univ of Bern Inselspital 1970; **Fellow:** Cardiovascular Disease, Hotel Dieu Hospital 1973

Miller, David H MD (Cv) - **Spec Exp:** Hypertension; **Hospital:** NY-Presby/Weill Cornell Med Ctr, NY (page 104); **Address:** NY-Presby/Weill Cornell Med Ctr, 520 E 70th St, Ste 443, New York, NY 10021; **Phone:** 212-746-2144; **Board Cert:** Internal Medicine 1980; Cardiovascular Disease 1981; **Med School:** Univ VA Sch Med 1976; **Resid:** Internal Medicine, NY Hosp-Cornell Med Ctr 1979; **Fellow:** Cardiovascular Disease, NY Hosp-Cornell Med Ctr 1981; **Fac Appt:** Assoc Prof Med, Cornell Univ-Weill Med Coll

Mueller, Richard L MD (Cv) - **Spec Exp:** Vein Disorders; Stress Echocardiography; Hypertension; Echocardiography; **Hospital:** NY-Presby/Weill Cornell Med Ctr, NY (page 104), St. Luke's - Roosevelt Hosp Ctr - St Luke's Hosp (page 94); **Address:** Cardiovascular Diagnostics, Cosmetic Vein-Sutton Place Vein/Hair, 401 E 55th St, New York, NY 10022-6158; **Phone:** 212-593-9800; **Board Cert:** Internal Medicine 2010; Cardiovascular Disease 2000; Echocardiography 1999; Vascular Medicine 2006; **Med School:** UCSF 1987; **Resid:** Internal Medicine, North Shore Univ Hosp 1991; Internal Medicine, Meml Sloan Kettering Cancer Ctr 1990; **Fellow:** Cardiovascular Disease, New York Hosp 1994; **Fac Appt:** Asst Clin Prof Med, Cornell Univ-Weill Med Coll

Myerson, Merle MD (Cv) - **Spec Exp:** Preventive Cardiology; Cholesterol/Lipid Disorders; **Hospital:** St. Luke's - Roosevelt Hosp Ctr - Roosevelt Div (page 94), St. Luke's - Roosevelt Hosp Ctr - St Luke's Hosp (page 94); **Address:** 425 W 59th St, Ste 9C, Ctr for CV Disease Prevention, New York, NY 10019; **Phone:** 212-492-5550; **Board Cert:** Cardiovascular Disease 2003; **Med School:** SUNY Downstate 1993; **Resid:** Internal Medicine, Duke Univ Med Ctr 1996; **Fellow:** Cardiovascular Disease, Mary Imogene Basset Hosp 1997; Cardiovascular Disease, Columbia Univ Med Ctr 2001; **Fac Appt:** Asst Prof Med, Columbia P&S

O'Brien, Francis J MD (Cv) - **Spec Exp:** Preventive Cardiology; **Hospital:** NYU Langone Med Ctr (page 108), Bellevue Hosp Ctr; **Address:** 347 E 37th St Fl 2, New York, NY 10016; **Phone:** 212-726-7457; **Board Cert:** Internal Medicine 1985; Cardiovascular Disease 1989; **Med School:** Harvard Med Sch 1982; **Resid:** Internal Medicine, NYU Med Ctr 1983; **Fellow:** Cardiovascular Disease, Bellevue-NYU Hosp 1988; **Fac Appt:** Assoc Clin Prof Med, NYU Sch Med

Pinney, Sean MD (Cv) - **Spec Exp:** Transplant Medicine-Heart; Heart Failure; Pulmonary Hypertension; Congenital Heart Disease; **Hospital:** Mount Sinai Med Ctr (page 102); **Address:** Cardiovascular Medicine Associates, 5 E 98th St Fl 3, Box 30, New York, NY 10029; **Phone:** 212-241-7300; **Board Cert:** Cardiovascular Disease 2011; **Med School:** Georgetown Univ 1994; **Resid:** Internal Medicine, Bet Israel Deaconess Med Ctr 1999; **Fellow:** Cardiovascular Disease, Columbia Presby Hosp 2001; Transplant Medicine, Columbia Presby Hosp 2002; **Fac Appt:** Asst Prof Med, Mount Sinai Sch Med

Porder, Joseph B MD (Cv) - **Spec Exp:** Preventive Cardiology; Nutrition; Echocardiography; Preventive Medicine; **Hospital:** Mount Sinai Med Ctr (page 102); **Address:** 1160 5th Ave, Ste 102, New York, NY 10029; **Phone:** 212-860-5500; **Board Cert:** Internal Medicine 1985; Cardiovascular Disease 1987; **Med School:** Columbia P&S 1982; **Resid:** Internal Medicine, Mt Sinai Hosp 1985; **Fellow:** Cardiovascular Disease, Mt Sinai Hosp 1987

Post, Martin R MD (Cv) - **Spec Exp:** Coronary Artery Disease; Cholesterol/Lipid Disorders; **Hospital:** NY-Presby/Weill Cornell Med Ctr, NY (page 104); **Address:** 425 E 61st St, New York, NY 10021-8722; **Phone:** 212-752-2000; **Board Cert:** Internal Medicine 1974; Cardiovascular Disease 1974; **Med School:** SUNY Upstate Med Univ 1967; **Resid:** Internal Medicine, Ohio State Univ Hosp 1970; **Fellow:** Cardiovascular Disease, New York Hosp 1972; **Fac Appt:** Asst Prof Med, Cornell Univ-Weill Med Coll

Radwaner, Bradley A MD (Cv) - **Spec Exp:** Preventive Cardiology; Cholesterol/Lipid Disorders; Interventional Cardiology; **Hospital:** Lenox Hill Hosp (page 106); **Address:** 885 Park Ave, New York, NY 10075; **Phone:** 212-717-0666; **Board Cert:** Internal Medicine 1983; Cardiovascular Disease 1985; **Med School:** Cornell Univ-Weill Med Coll 1980; **Resid:** Internal Medicine, Lenox Hill Hosp 1983; **Fellow:** Cardiovascular Disease, St Lukes Hosp 1985; Interventional Cardiology, NYU Med Ctr 1986; **Fac Appt:** Asst Clin Prof Med, Cornell Univ-Weill Med Coll

Reichstein, Robert P MD (Cv) - **Spec Exp:** Preventive Cardiology; Cholesterol/Lipid Disorders; Aneurysm-Aortic; **Hospital:** Mount Sinai Med Ctr (page 102); **Address:** 1185 Park Ave, Ste 1L, New York, NY 10128; **Phone:** 212-996-2900; **Board Cert:** Internal Medicine 1980; Cardiovascular Disease 1983; **Med School:** Ros Franklin Univ/Chicago Med Sch 1977; **Resid:** Internal Medicine, Mt Sinai Hosp 1981; **Fellow:** Cardiovascular Disease, Mt Sinai Hosp 1984; **Fac Appt:** Asst Clin Prof Med, Mount Sinai Sch Med

Rentrop, K Peter MD (Cv) - **Hospital:** Lenox Hill Hosp (page 106), NYU Langone Med Ctr (page 108); **Address:** 920 Broadway, Ste 600, New York, NY 10010; **Phone:** 212-475-8066; **Board Cert:** Internal Medicine 1973; Nuclear Medicine 2002; **Med School:** Germany 1966; **Resid:** Internal Medicine, Detroit Med Ctr 1970; Internal Medicine, Cleveland Clinic 1971; **Fellow:** Cardiovascular Disease, Cleveland Clinic 1973; **Fac Appt:** Prof Med, NY Med Coll

Romanello, Paul P MD (Cv) - **Spec Exp:** Cholesterol/Lipid Disorders; Coronary Artery Disease; Hypertension; Nuclear Cardiology; **Hospital:** Lenox Hill Hosp (page 106); **Address:** 158 E 84th St, New York, NY 10028; **Phone:** 212-535-6340; **Board Cert:** Internal Medicine 1987; Cardiovascular Disease 1989; Nuclear Cardiology 2008; **Med School:** SUNY Upstate Med Univ 1983; **Resid:** Internal Medicine, Lenox Hill Hosp 1987; **Fellow:** Cardiovascular Disease, Lenox Hill Hosp 1989

Rosenbaum, Marlon S MD (Cv) - **Spec Exp:** Congenital Heart Disease-Adult; Heart Valve Disease; **Hospital:** NY-Presby/Columbia Univ Med Ctr, NY (page 104); **Address:** 161 Fort Washington Ave, Fl 6, rm 628, New York, NY 10032-3729; **Phone:** 212-305-6936; **Board Cert:** Internal Medicine 1983; Cardiovascular Disease 1985; **Med School:** NYU Sch Med 1980; **Resid:** Internal Medicine, Columbia-Presby Med Ctr 1983; **Fellow:** Cardiovascular Disease, Westchester Med Ctr 1985; Cardiovascular Disease, Mass Genl Hosp 1986; **Fac Appt:** Assoc Clin Prof Med, Columbia P&S

Rozanski, Alan MD (Cv) - **Spec Exp:** Nuclear Cardiology; Stress Management; **Hospital:** St. Luke's - Roosevelt Hosp Ctr - Roosevelt Div (page 94); **Address:** 1111 Amsterdam Ave, New York, NY 10025; **Phone:** 212-523-4011; **Board Cert:** Internal Medicine 1978; Cardiovascular Disease 1983; Nuclear Medicine 1983; **Med School:** Tufts Univ 1975; **Resid:** Internal Medicine, Mount Sinai 1977; **Fellow:** Cardiovascular Disease, Mount Sinai 1980; Nuclear Medicine, Cedars-Sinai Med Ctr 1982; **Fac Appt:** Prof Med, Columbia P&S

Schiffer, Mark B MD (Cv) - **Spec Exp:** Preventive Cardiology; Coronary Artery Disease; Cholesterol/Lipid Disorders; **Hospital:** Lenox Hill Hosp (page 106); **Address:** 158 E 84th St, New York, NY 10028-1802; **Phone:** 212-535-6340; **Board Cert:** Internal Medicine 1980; Cardiovascular Disease 1983; **Med School:** Northwestern Univ 1977; **Resid:** Internal Medicine, Lenox Hill Hosp 1981; **Fellow:** Cardiovascular Disease, Lenox Hill Hosp 1983

Schulman, Ira MD (Cv) - **Spec Exp:** Angina; Heart Failure; Cholesterol/Lipid Disorders; **Hospital:** NYU Langone Med Ctr (page 108), NY Downtown Hosp; **Address:** 111 Broadway, Fl 2, New York, NY 10006; **Phone:** 212-263-9700; **Board Cert:** Internal Medicine 1977; Cardiovascular Disease 1979; **Med School:** NYU Sch Med 1974; **Resid:** Internal Medicine, Bellevue Hosp 1977; **Fellow:** Cardiovascular Disease, Montefiore Med Ctr 1979; **Fac Appt:** Assoc Prof Med, NYU Sch Med

Schulze, Paul Christian MD/PhD (Cv) - **Spec Exp:** Heart Failure; Vascular Disease; Vasculitis; **Hospital:** NY-Presby/Columbia Univ Med Ctr, NY (page 104); **Address:** Columbia Presbyterian Hosp, 622 W 168th St, rm 1267, New York, NY 10032; **Phone:** 212-305-7912; **Board Cert:** Internal Medicine 2008; Cardiovascular Disease 2009; Echocardiography 2009; Nuclear Cardiology 2009; **Med School:** Germany 1998; **Resid:** Internal Medicine, Boston Univ Med Ctr 2007; **Fellow:** Cardiovascular Disease, NY Presby-Columbia Med Ctr 2009; **Fac Appt:** Asst Prof Med, Columbia P&S

Schwartz, Allan MD (Cv) - **Hospital:** NY-Presby/Columbia Univ Med Ctr, NY (page 104); **Address:** 173 Fort Washington Ave, Ste 4-600C, New York, NY 10032; **Phone:** 212-305-5367; **Board Cert:** Internal Medicine 1977; Cardiovascular Disease 1979; **Med School:** Columbia P&S 1974; **Resid:** Internal Medicine, Columbia-Presby Med Ctr 1976; **Fellow:** Cardiovascular Disease, Mass Genl Hosp 1978; **Fac Appt:** Clin Prof Med, Columbia P&S

Schwartz, William J MD (Cv) - **Spec Exp:** Coronary Artery Disease; Cardiac Catheterization; Congestive Heart Failure; **Hospital:** Mount Sinai Med Ctr (page 102); **Address:** Mt Sinai Multispecialty Physicians, 150 E 77th St, Ste 1E, New York, NY 10075; **Phone:** 212-439-6000; **Board Cert:** Internal Medicine 1978; Cardiovascular Disease 1981; **Med School:** Albert Einstein Coll Med 1975; **Resid:** Internal Medicine, Bronx Municipal Hosp 1978; **Fellow:** Cardiovascular Disease, Bronx Municipal Hosp 1979

Seinfeld, David MD (Cv) - **Spec Exp:** Preventive Cardiology; **Hospital:** Lenox Hill Hosp (page 106), Montefiore Med Ctr-Moses Campus, NY (page 100); **Address:** 20 E 68th St, Ste 214, New York, NY 10065-5841; **Phone:** 212-288-1538; **Board Cert:** Internal Medicine 1976; Cardiovascular Disease 1979; **Med School:** Albert Einstein Coll Med 1973; **Resid:** Internal Medicine, Montefiore Med Ctr 1976; **Fellow:** Cardiovascular Disease, Montefiore Med Ctr 1978; **Fac Appt:** Assoc Clin Prof Med, Albert Einstein Coll Med

Sherman, Warren MD (Cv) - **Spec Exp:** Angioplasty; Interventional Cardiology; **Hospital:** NY-Presby/Columbia Univ Med Ctr, NY (page 104); **Address:** 161 Ft Washington Ave Fl 6, New York, NY 10032; **Phone:** 212-305-7060; **Board Cert:** Internal Medicine 1980; Cardiovascular Disease 1983; Interventional Cardiology 2000; **Med School:** SUNY Upstate Med Univ 1977; **Resid:** Internal Medicine, Rochester Genl Hosp 1980; **Fellow:** Cardiovascular Disease, Oregon Hlth Sci Univ 1982; **Fac Appt:** Assoc Clin Prof Med, Columbia P&S

Shimony, Rony MD (Cv) - **Spec Exp:** Coronary Artery Disease; Arrhythmias; Heart Failure; Non-Invasive Cardiology; **Hospital:** Mount Sinai Med Ctr (page 102); **Address:** 485 Madison Ave Fl 17, New York, NY 10022; **Phone:** 212-752-2700; **Board Cert:** Internal Medicine 1987; Cardiovascular Disease 1989; **Med School:** SUNY Buffalo 1984; **Resid:** Internal Medicine, Lenox Hill Hosp 1987; **Fellow:** Cardiovascular Disease, Lenox Hill Hosp 1989; Cardiac Electrophysiology, Lenox Hill Hosp 1992

Siegal, Michael S MD (Cv) - **Spec Exp:** Coronary Artery Disease; **Hospital:** St. Luke's - Roosevelt Hosp Ctr - Roosevelt Div (page 94); **Address:** 30 Central Park S, Ste 13A, New York, NY 10019; **Phone:** 212-319-1700; **Board Cert:** Internal Medicine 1980; Cardiovascular Disease 1983; **Med School:** Columbia P&S 1977; **Resid:** Internal Medicine, Bellevue/NYU Med Ctr 1980; **Fellow:** Cardiovascular Disease, Mt Sinai Hosp 1982

Siegel, Stephen MD (Cv) - **Spec Exp:** Sports Medicine-Cardiology; Preventive Cardiology; Cholesterol/Lipid Disorders; Hypertension; **Hospital:** NYU Langone Med Ctr (page 108); **Address:** 245 E 35th St, New York, NY 10016; **Phone:** 212-684-1108; **Board Cert:** Internal Medicine 1981; Cardiovascular Disease 1983; **Med School:** Med Coll VA 1978; **Resid:** Internal Medicine, NYU Med Ctr/Bellevue Hosp Ctr 1981; **Fellow:** Cardiovascular Disease, NYU Med Ctr/Bellevue Hosp Ctr 1983; **Fac Appt:** Asst Clin Prof Med, NYU Sch Med

Sklaroff, Herschel J MD (Cv) - **Spec Exp:** Angina; Syncope; Hypertension; Diagnostic Problems; **Hospital:** Mount Sinai Med Ctr (page 102); **Address:** 1175 Park Ave, New York, NY 10128-1211; **Phone:** 212-289-6500 x2; **Board Cert:** Internal Medicine 1969; Cardiovascular Disease 1977; **Med School:** Univ Pennsylvania 1961; **Resid:** Internal Medicine, Mt Sinai Hosp 1965; Cardiovascular Disease, Mt Sinai Hosp 1966; **Fac Appt:** Clin Prof Med, Mount Sinai Sch Med

Slater, William R MD (Cv) - **Spec Exp:** Arrhythmias; Heart Valve Disease; Cardiac Electrophysiology; **Hospital:** NYU Langone Med Ctr (page 108); **Address:** NYU Medical Ctr, Div Cardiology, 530 First Ave, Ste 9U, New York, NY 10016; **Phone:** 212-263-7463; **Board Cert:** Internal Medicine 1981; Cardiovascular Disease 1985; Cardiac Electrophysiology 2002; **Med School:** Harvard Med Sch 1978; **Resid:** Internal Medicine, NYU-Bellevue Med Ctr 1981; **Fellow:** Cardiovascular Disease, Mt Sinai Hosp 1984; Cardiovascular Disease, Mass Genl Hosp/Brigham-Womens Hops 1986; **Fac Appt:** Assoc Prof Med, NYU Sch Med

Stein, Richard A MD (Cv) - **Spec Exp:** Preventive Cardiology; Coronary Artery Disease; Cardiac Rehabilitation; **Hospital:** NYU Langone Med Ctr (page 108); **Address:** NYU Cardiology Associates, 530 First Ave, Ste 9U, New York, NY 10016; **Phone:** 212-263-7751; **Board Cert:** Internal Medicine 1973; Cardiovascular Disease 1975; Sports Medicine 2007; **Med School:** NYU Sch Med 1967; **Resid:** Internal Medicine, Univ Hosp 1969; **Fellow:** Cardiovascular Disease, Univ Hosp 1974; **Fac Appt:** Prof Med, NYU Sch Med

Steingart, Richard M MD (Cv) - **Spec Exp:** Heart Failure; Nuclear Cardiology; Heart Disease in Cancer Patients; Cardiac Effects of Cancer/Cancer Therapy; **Hospital:** Meml Sloan-Kettering Cancer Ctr (page 116); **Address:** 1275 York Ave, New York, NY 10065; **Phone:** 212-639-8488; **Board Cert:** Internal Medicine 1977; Cardiovascular Disease 1979; **Med School:** Mount Sinai Sch Med 1974; **Resid:** Internal Medicine, Yale-New Haven Hosp 1977; **Fellow:** Cardiovascular Disease, Mt Sinai Med Ctr 1979; **Fac Appt:** Prof Med, Cornell Univ-Weill Med Coll

Tenenbaum, Joseph MD (Cv) - **Spec Exp:** Heart Valve Disease; Coronary Artery Disease; Atrial Fibrillation; **Hospital:** NY-Presby/Columbia Univ Med Ctr, NY (page 104); **Address:** 161 Ft Washington Ave, Ste 5-520, Irving Pavilion, New York, NY 10032; **Phone:** 212-305-5288; **Board Cert:** Internal Medicine 1977; Cardiovascular Disease 1979; **Med School:** Harvard Med Sch 1974; **Resid:** Internal Medicine, Columbia-Presby Med Ctr 1977; **Fellow:** Cardiovascular Disease, Mt Sinai Hosp 1979; **Fac Appt:** Prof Med, Columbia P&S

Tyberg, Theodore MD (Cv) - **Spec Exp:** Coronary Artery Disease; Cholesterol/Lipid Disorders; **Hospital:** NY-Presby/Weill Cornell Med Ctr, NY (page 104); **Address:** 425 E 61st St, Fl 6, New York, NY 10065; **Phone:** 212-752-2000; **Board Cert:** Internal Medicine 1978; Cardiovascular Disease 1981; **Med School:** Rush Med Coll 1975; **Resid:** Internal Medicine, New York Hosp 1978; **Fellow:** Cardiovascular Disease, Yale-New Haven Hosp 1980; **Fac Appt:** Assoc Clin Prof Med, Cornell Univ-Weill Med Coll

Unger, Allen MD (Cv) - **Spec Exp:** Cholesterol/Lipid Disorders; Hypertension; Preventive Cardiology; Coronary Artery Disease; **Hospital:** Mount Sinai Med Ctr (page 102); **Address:** 12 E 86th St, New York, NY 10028-0506; **Phone:** 212-734-6000; **Board Cert:** Internal Medicine 1968; Cardiovascular Disease 1977; **Med School:** SUNY Upstate Med Univ 1960; **Resid:** Internal Medicine, Mount Sinai Hosp 1967; **Fellow:** Cardiovascular Disease, Mount Sinai Hosp 1966; **Fac Appt:** Asst Clin Prof Med, Mount Sinai Sch Med

Varriale, Philip MD (Cv) - **Spec Exp:** Coronary Artery Disease; Arrhythmias; Congestive Heart Failure; Pacemakers; **Hospital:** Beth Israel Med Ctr - Petrie Division (page 94); **Address:** 222 E 19th St, Ste 2D, New York, NY 10003-2666; **Phone:** 212-777-3219; **Board Cert:** Internal Medicine 1966; Cardiovascular Disease 1970; **Med School:** SUNY Hlth Sci Ctr 1959; **Resid:** Internal Medicine, Brooklyn VA Hosp 1962; Internal Medicine, St Vincent's Med Ctr 1963; **Fellow:** Cardiovascular Disease, St Vincent's Med Ctr 1964; **Fac Appt:** Assoc Clin Prof Med, Mount Sinai Sch Med

Weintraub, Howard S MD (Cv) - **Spec Exp:** Hypertension; Echocardiography; Preventive Cardiology; Cholesterol/Lipid Disorders; **Hospital:** NYU Langone Med Ctr (page 108); **Address:** 345 E 37th St, Ste 308, New York, NY 10016-3217; **Phone:** 212-599-5030; **Board Cert:** Internal Medicine 1979; Cardiovascular Disease 1985; **Med School:** NYU Sch Med 1976; **Resid:** Internal Medicine, NYU Med Ctr 1979; **Fellow:** Pulmonary Disease, NYU Med Ctr 1980; Cardiovascular Disease, NYU Med Ctr 1982; **Fac Appt:** Assoc Clin Prof Med, NYU Sch Med

Weisenseel, Arthur C MD (Cv) - **Spec Exp:** Coronary Artery Disease; Cholesterol/Lipid Disorders; Congestive Heart Failure; Preventive Cardiology; **Hospital:** Mount Sinai Med Ctr (page 102); **Address:** 12 E 86th St, New York, NY 10028-0506; **Phone:** 212-734-6000; **Board Cert:** Internal Medicine 1969; Cardiovascular Disease 1973; **Med School:** Georgetown Univ 1963; **Resid:** Internal Medicine, Mount Sinai Hosp 1966; **Fellow:** Cardiovascular Disease, Mount Sinai 1967; **Fac Appt:** Assoc Clin Prof Med, Mount Sinai Sch Med

Wolk, Michael MD (Cv) - **Spec Exp:** Coronary Artery Disease; Heart Failure; Hypertension; **Hospital:** NY-Presby/Weill Cornell Med Ctr, NY (page 104); **Address:** 425 E 61st St, Fl 6, New York, NY 10021; **Phone:** 212-752-2000; **Board Cert:** Internal Medicine 1971; Cardiovascular Disease 1973; **Med School:** Columbia P&S 1964; **Resid:** Internal Medicine, Univ Hosp 1967; **Fellow:** Cardiovascular Disease, New England Med Ctr 1969; Cardiovascular Disease, New York Hosp-Cornell 1970; **Fac Appt:** Clin Prof Med, Cornell Univ-Weill Med Coll

Child & Adolescent Psychiatry

Abright, A Reese MD (ChAP) - **Spec Exp:** Mood Disorders; ADD/ADHD; Anxiety Disorders; **Hospital:** Elmhurst Hosp Ctr; **Address:** 140 E 40th St, Ste 1B, New York, NY 10016; **Phone:** 212-867-3131; **Board Cert:** Psychiatry 1978; Child & Adolescent Psychiatry 1981; **Med School:** Univ Tex SW, Dallas 1973; **Resid:** Psychiatry, St Vincent's Hosp 1974; Psychiatry, NY Hosp-Cornell Med Ctr 1977; **Fellow:** Child & Adolescent Psychiatry, NY Hosp-Cornell Med Ctr 1979; **Fac Appt:** Clin Prof Psyc, NY Med Coll

Bartell, Abraham MD (ChAP) - **Spec Exp:** Psychiatry in Cancer; Psychiatry in Physical Illness; **Hospital:** Meml Sloan-Kettering Cancer Ctr (page 116); **Address:** 1275 York Ave, New York, NY 10065; **Phone:** 646-888-0060; **Board Cert:** Psychiatry 2010; **Med School:** SUNY Downstate 1993; **Resid:** Psychiatry, Emma P Bradley Hosp 1986; **Fellow:** Child & Adolescent Psychiatry, Emma P Bradley Hosp 1998

Becker, Ina MD (ChAP) - ; **Address:** 262 Central Park W, Ste 1A, New York, NY 10024; **Phone:** 917-441-0880; **Board Cert:** Psychiatry 2005; Psychosomatic Medicine 2008; **Med School:** Germany 1087

Bird, Hector MD (ChAP) - **Spec Exp:** ADD/ADHD; Anxiety & Depression; Personality Disorders; **Address:** 300 W 72nd St, Ste 1F, New York, NY 10023-2004; **Phone:** 212-874-5311; **Board Cert:** Psychiatry 1975; Child & Adolescent Psychiatry 1977; **Med School:** Yale Univ 1965; **Resid:** Psychiatry, NY State Psych Inst 1971NY State Psych Inst 1972; **Fellow:** Psychoanalysis, WA White Institute 1977; **Fac Appt:** Prof Emeritus Psyc, Columbia P&S

Boorady, Roy J MD (ChAP) - **Spec Exp:** Psychopharmacology; Anxiety & Mood Disorders; ADD/ADHD; **Hospital:** NYU Langone Med Ctr (page 108); **Address:** Child Mind Institution, 445 Park Ave at 56th St, New York, NY 10022; **Phone:** 212-308-3118; **Board Cert:** Psychiatry 1993; Child & Adolescent Psychiatry 1994; **Med School:** SUNY Buffalo 1987; **Resid:** Psychiatry, Mass Mental Hlth Ctr 1991; **Fellow:** Child & Adolescent Psychiatry, Mass Genl Hosp 1993

Burkes, Lynn MD (ChAP) - **Spec Exp:** Diagnostic Problems; ADD/ADHD; Divorce/Family Issues; Developmental Disorders; **Hospital:** NYU Langone Med Ctr (page 108); **Address:** 185 West End Ave, Ste 1E, New York, NY 10023-5539; **Phone:** 212-362-5920; **Board Cert:** Psychiatry 1977; Child & Adolescent Psychiatry 1978; **Med School:** Drexel Univ Coll Med 1970; **Resid:** Psychiatry, Albert Einstein 1973; **Fellow:** Psychiatry, Bellevue Hosp 1975; **Fac Appt:** Assoc Clin Prof Psyc, NYU Sch Med

Coffey, Barbara J MD (ChAP) - **Spec Exp:** Tourette's Syndrome; ADD/ADHD; Obsessive-Compulsive Disorder; Psychopharmacology; **Hospital:** Mount Sinai Med Ctr (page 102); **Address:** Tics & Tourette's Clin & Rsch Program, 1240 Park Ave, New York, NY 10029; **Phone:** 212-659-1663; **Board Cert:** Psychiatry 1981; Child & Adolescent Psychiatry 1986; **Med School:** Tufts Univ 1975; **Resid:** Psychiatry, Boston Univ Med Ctr 1978; **Fellow:** Child & Adolescent Psychiatry, Tufts Univ 1980; **Fac Appt:** Prof Psyc, Mount Sinai Sch Med

Fox, Sarah J MD (ChAP) - **Spec Exp:** Anxiety & Mood Disorders; Eating Disorders; Psychoanalysis; **Hospital:** NY-Presby/Columbia Univ Med Ctr, NY (page 104); **Address:** 210 W 89th St, New York, NY 10024; **Phone:** 212-874-4558; **Board Cert:** Psychiatry 1991; Child & Adolescent Psychiatry 1994; **Med School:** Tufts Univ 1982; **Resid:** Pediatrics, Jacobi Med Ctr 1983; Psychiatry, Albert Einstein 1985; **Fellow:** Child & Adolescent Psychiatry, Columbia-Presby Med Ctr 1987

Gabbay, Vilma MD (ChAP) - **Spec Exp:** Depression; **Hospital:** NYU Langone Med Ctr (page 108), Bellevue Hosp Ctr; **Address:** NYU Child Study Ctr, 1 Park Ave Fl 7, New York, NY 10016; **Phone:** 646-754-4926; **Board Cert:** Psychiatry 2005; Child & Adolescent Psychiatry 2007; **Med School:** Israel 1994; **Resid:** Psychiatry, Montefiore Med Ctr 2001; **Fellow:** Child & Adolescent Psychiatry, NYU Med Ctr 2003; **Fac Appt:** Asst Prof ChAP, NYU Sch Med

Havens, Jennifer MD (ChAP) - **Spec Exp:** Bereavement/Traumatic Grief; **Hospital:** Bellevue Hosp Ctr, NYU Langone Med Ctr (page 108); **Address:** NYU Child Study Ctr, One Park Ave, Fl 7th, New York, NY 10016; **Phone:** 212-263-6622; **Board Cert:** Psychiatry 1991; Child & Adolescent Psychiatry 1993; **Med School:** Tufts Univ 1986; **Resid:** Psychiatry, Payne Witney Clinic/Cornell Med Ctr 1988; Child Psychiatry, NYS Psych Inst/CPMC 1991; **Fellow:** Child & Adolescent Psychiatry, Columbia Presby Med Ctr 1991; **Fac Appt:** Assoc Prof ChAP, NYU Sch Med

Hertzig, Margaret MD (ChAP) - **Spec Exp:** Developmental Disorders; ADD/ADHD; **Hospital:** NY-Presby/Weill Cornell Med Ctr, NY (page 104); **Address:** 525 E 68th St, Box 140, New York, NY 10021-4870; **Phone:** 212-746-5712; **Board Cert:** Psychiatry 1968; Child & Adolescent Psychiatry 1975; **Med School:** NYU Sch Med 1960; **Resid:** Pediatrics, Jewish Hosp 1962; Psychiatry, Bellevue Psych Hosp 1964; **Fellow:** Psychiatric Research, NYU Sch Med 1966; **Fac Appt:** Prof Psyc, Cornell Univ-Weill Med Coll

Hirsch, Glenn S MD (ChAP) - **Spec Exp:** Anxiety & Mood Disorders; Tourette's Syndrome; Bipolar/Mood Disorders; ADD/ADHD; **Hospital:** NYU Langone Med Ctr (page 108), Bellevue Hosp Ctr; **Address:** NYU Child Study Center, 1 Park Ave Fl 7, New York, NY 10016; **Phone:** 212-263-8704; **Board Cert:** Psychiatry 1984; Child & Adolescent Psychiatry 1985; **Med School:** Albert Einstein Coll Med 1979; **Resid:** Psychiatry, New York Hosp-Cornell 1982; **Fellow:** Child & Adolescent Psychiatry, Columbia-Presby Med Ctr 1984; **Fac Appt:** Asst Prof ChAP, NYU Sch Med

Koplewicz, Harold S MD (ChAP) - **Spec Exp:** Anxiety & Mood Disorders; Psychopharmacology; ADD/ADHD; **Address:** Child Mind Inst, 445 Park Ave at 56th St, New York, NY 10022; **Phone:** 212-308-3118; **Board Cert:** Psychiatry 1983; Child & Adolescent Psychiatry 1984; **Med School:** Albert Einstein Coll Med 1978; **Resid:** Psychiatry, NY Hosp-Westchester Div 1981; Psychiatry, NY State Psych Inst 1983; **Fellow:** Psychiatric Research, NY State Psych Inst 1985

Kron, Leo L MD (ChAP) - **Spec Exp:** Psychopharmacology; Psychotherapy; **Hospital:** St. Luke's - Roosevelt Hosp Ctr - Roosevelt Div (page 94); **Address:** 30 E 76th St, Ste 3A, New York, NY 10021; **Phone:** 212-861-7001; **Board Cert:** Psychiatry 1977; Child & Adolescent Psychiatry 1986; **Med School:** Univ British Columbia Fac Med 1971; **Resid:** Psychiatry, Albert Einstein Affil Hosp 1976; **Fellow:** Child & Adolescent Psychiatry, St Lukes Hosp 1978; **Fac Appt:** Asst Clin Prof Psyc, Columbia P&S

Leventhal, Bennett MD (ChAP) - **Spec Exp:** Autism; ADD/ADHD; Psychopharmacology; **Hospital:** NYU Langone Med Ctr (page 108); **Address:** 577 First Ave, New York, NY 10016; **Phone:** 212-263-8696; **Board Cert:** Psychiatry 1979; Child & Adolescent Psychiatry 1980; **Med School:** Louisiana State U, New Orleans 1974; **Resid:** Psychiatry, Duke Univ Med Ctr 1978; **Fellow:** Child & Adolescent Psychiatry, Duke Univ Med Ctr 1977; **Fac Appt:** Prof Psyc, NYU Sch Med

Lewis, Owen MD (ChAP) - **Spec Exp:** Psychotherapy; Psychopharmacology; **Hospital:** NY-Presby/Columbia Univ Med Ctr, NY (page 104); **Address:** 11 E 87th St, New York, NY 10128-0527; **Phone:** 212-996-8196; **Board Cert:** Psychiatry 1982; Child & Adolescent Psychiatry 1986; **Med School:** Mount Sinai Sch Med 1976; **Resid:** Psychiatry, NY Hosp 1980; **Fellow:** Child & Adolescent Psychiatry, NY Hosp 1982; **Fac Appt:** Clin Prof Psyc, Columbia P&S

Moreau, Donna L MD (ChAP) - **Spec Exp:** Psychotherapy & Psychopharmacology; Anxiety & Mood Disorders; **Hospital:** Morgan Stanley Children's Hosp of NY-Presby, NY (page 104); **Address:** 110 East End Ave, New York, NY 10028-7412; **Phone:** 212-772-9205; **Board Cert:** Psychiatry 1985; Child & Adolescent Psychiatry 1991; **Med School:** SUNY Hlth Sci Ctr 1980; **Resid:** Psychiatry, NY Hosp 1984; **Fellow:** Child & Adolescent Psychiatry, NY Hosp 1986; **Fac Appt:** Assoc Clin Prof Psyc, Columbia P&S

Newcorn, Jeffrey H MD (ChAP) - **Spec Exp:** Psychopharmacology; ADD/ADHD; Developmental Disorders; Behavioral Disorders; **Hospital:** Mount Sinai Med Ctr (page 102); **Address:** Mount Sinai Hosp, Dept Psychiatry, One Gustave L Levy Pl, Box 1230, New York, NY 10029; **Phone:** 212-659-8705; **Board Cert:** Psychiatry 1982; Child & Adolescent Psychiatry 1984; **Med School:** Univ Rochester 1977; **Resid:** Psychiatry, Tufts-New England Med Ctr 1980; **Fellow:** Child & Adolescent Psychiatry, Tufts-New England Med Ctr 1982; **Fac Appt:** Assoc Prof Psyc, Mount Sinai Sch Med

Perry, Richard MD (ChAP) - **Spec Exp:** Pervasive Development Disorders; Behavioral Disorders; Psychopharmacology; **Hospital:** Bellevue Hosp Ctr, NYU Langone Med Ctr (page 108); **Address:** 55 W 74th St, New York, NY 10023-2429; **Phone:** 212-595-0116; **Board Cert:** Psychiatry 1976; Child & Adolescent Psychiatry 1985; **Med School:** Belgium 1970; **Resid:** Psychiatry, Bellevue Hosp 1972; **Fellow:** Child & Adolescent Psychiatry, Bellevue Hosp 1974; **Fac Appt:** Clin Prof Psyc, NYU Sch Med

Shatkin, Jess P MD (ChAP) - **Spec Exp:** Behavioral Disorders; Anxiety & Mood Disorders; ADD/ADHD; Autism; **Hospital:** NYU Langone Med Ctr (page 108), Bellevue Hosp Ctr; **Address:** One Park Ave, Fl 7th, New York, NY 10016; **Phone:** 646-754-4900; **Board Cert:** Psychiatry 2001; Child & Adolescent Psychiatry 2003; **Med School:** SUNY Hlth Sci Ctr 1996; **Resid:** Psychiatry, UCLA NPI 1999; **Fellow:** Child & Adolescent Psychiatry, UCLA NPI 2001; **Fac Appt:** Assoc Clin Prof ChAP, NYU Sch Med

Spencer, Elizabeth Kay MD (ChAP) - **Hospital:** NYU Langone Med Ctr (page 108); **Address:** 121 E 31st St, Ste 1B, New York, NY 10016-6835; **Phone:** 212-684-3810; **Board Cert:** Psychiatry 1990; Child & Adolescent Psychiatry 1992; **Med School:** Geo Wash Univ 1979; **Resid:** Pediatrics, Univ Maryland Hosp 1982; Psychiatry, NYU Med Ctr 1986; **Fellow:** Behavioral Pediatrics, Univ Maryland Hosp 1984; Child & Adolescent Psychiatry, NYU Med Ctr 1988; **Fac Appt:** Asst Clin Prof Psyc, NYU Sch Med

Turecki, Stanley K MD (ChAP) - **Spec Exp:** Temperamentally Difficult Child; ADD/ADHD; Parenting Issues; **Hospital:** Lenox Hill Hosp (page 106); **Address:** 136 E 64th St, Ste 1B, New York, NY 10065; **Phone:** 212-355-2535; **Board Cert:** Psychiatry 1978; Child & Adolescent Psychiatry 1981; **Med School:** South Africa 1961; **Resid:** Psychiatry, Tara Hospital 1969; Psychiatry, Mt Sinai Hosp 1971

Walkup, John MD (ChAP) - **Spec Exp:** Anxiety Disorders; **Hospital:** NY-Presby/Weill Cornell Med Ctr, NY (page 104); **Address:** NY Presby Hosp-Weill Cornell, Dept Psych, 525 E 68th St, Box 140, New York, NY 10065; **Phone:** 212-746-1891; **Board Cert:** Psychiatry 1987; Child & Adolescent Psychiatry 1992; **Med School:** Univ Minn 1982; **Resid:** Psychiatry, Yale Univ Med Sch 1985; **Fellow:** Child Psychiatry, Yale Chld Study Ctr 1988; **Fac Appt:** Asst Prof Psyc, Johns Hopkins Univ

Walsh, Peter MD (ChAP) - **Hospital:** NY-Presby/Columbia Univ Med Ctr, NY (page 104); **Address:** 115 Central Park W, Ste 5, New York, NY 10023; **Phone:** 212-579-5552; **Med School:** Georgetown Univ 1991; **Resid:** Psychiatry, NY Presby-Columbia Med Ctr 1994; **Fellow:** Child & Adolescent Psychiatry, NY Presby-Columbia Med Ctr 1996

Child Neurology

Allen, Jeffrey MD (ChiN) - **Spec Exp:** Neuro-Oncology; Brain Tumors; Neurofibromatosis; **Hospital:** NYU Langone Med Ctr (page 108); **Address:** Hassenfeld Childrens Ctr, 160 E 32nd St Fl 2 - Ste L3, New York, NY 10016; **Phone:** 212-263-9907; **Board Cert:** Child Neurology 1977; **Med School:** Harvard Med Sch 1969; **Resid:** Pediatrics, Montreal Chldns Hosp 1973; Pediatric Neurology, Montreal Neur Inst/McGill 1976; **Fac Appt:** Prof Ped, NYU Sch Med

De Vivo, Darryl C MD (ChiN) - **Spec Exp:** Metabolic Disorders; Neuromuscular Disorders; Spinal Muscular Atrophy (SMA); **Hospital:** NY-Presby/Columbia Univ Med Ctr, NY (page 104); **Address:** Neurological Institute, 710 W 168th St, Ste NI 101, New York, NY 10032; **Phone:** 212-305-5244; **Board Cert:** Child Neurology 1972; **Med School:** Univ VA Sch Med 1964; **Resid:** Pediatrics, Mass Genl Hosp 1966; Neurology, Mass Genl Hosp 1967; **Fellow:** Neurology, Natl Inst Hlth 1969; Child Neurology, Children's Hosp 1970; **Fac Appt:** Prof N, Columbia P&S

Kaufman, David M MD (ChiN) - **Spec Exp:** Epilepsy/Seizure Disorders; Headache; Learning Disorders; Autism; **Hospital:** Mount Sinai Med Ctr (page 102), Lenox Hill Hosp (page 106); **Address:** 3 E 83rd St, New York, NY 10028-0459; **Phone:** 212-737-4911; **Board Cert:** Pediatrics 1980; **Med School:** Boston Univ 1975; **Resid:** Pediatrics, New York Hosp 1977; Neurology, Mount Sinai Hosp 1978; **Fellow:** Child Neurology, Mount Sinai Hosp 1980; **Fac Appt:** Assoc Clin Prof N, Mount Sinai Sch Med

Kosofsky, Barry MD/PhD (ChiN) - **Spec Exp:** Developmental Disorders; Autism; Stroke; **Hospital:** NY-Presby/Weill Cornell Med Ctr, NY (page 104); **Address:** NY-Cornell Med Ctr, Dept Pediatrics, 505 E 70th St, Helmsley Tower Fl 3, New York, NY 10021; **Phone:** 212-746-3321; **Board Cert:** Child Neurology 1993; **Med School:** Johns Hopkins Univ 1985; **Resid:** Pediatrics, Chldns Hosp 1987; Child Neurology, Mass Genl Hosp 1990; **Fellow:** Neurological Biology, Mass Genl Hosp 1992; **Fac Appt:** Prof Ped, Cornell Univ-Weill Med Coll

Miles, Daniel K MD (ChiN) - **Spec Exp:** Pediatric Neurology; Tuberous Sclerosis; Epilepsy; **Hospital:** NYU Langone Med Ctr (page 108); **Address:** New York Epilepsy & Neurology, 223 E 34th St Fl 1, New York, NY 10016; **Phone:** 646-558-0808; **Board Cert:** Child Neurology 1994; **Med School:** UMDNJ-NJ Med Sch, Newark 1983; **Resid:** Pediatrics, St Christopher's Hosp 1986; Pediatric Neurology, Chlds Meml Hosp 1989; **Fellow:** Epilepsy, Boston Chlds Hosp 1990

Molofsky, Walter J MD (ChiN) - **Spec Exp:** Seizure Disorders; Headache; ADD/ADHD; Stroke; **Hospital:** Beth Israel Med Ctr - Petrie Division (page 94), St. Luke's - Roosevelt Hosp Ctr - Roosevelt Div (page 94); **Address:** Beth Israel Medical Center, 10 Union Square East, Ste 5G, New York, NY 10003; **Phone:** 212-844-6910; **Board Cert:** Pediatrics 1982; Child Neurology 1986; **Med School:** NYU Sch Med 1976; **Resid:** Pediatrics, Columbia-Presby Med Ctr 1978; **Fellow:** Child Neurology, Columbia-Presby Med Ctr 1981; **Fac Appt:** Assoc Prof N, Albert Einstein Coll Med

Nass, Ruth D MD (ChiN) - **Spec Exp:** Autism; ADD/ADHD; Learning Disorders; Migraine; **Hospital:** NYU Langone Med Ctr (page 108); **Address:** 1 Park Ave Fl 7, New York, NY 10016; **Phone:** 212-263-6622; **Board Cert:** Pediatrics 1980; Child Neurology 1981; **Med School:** Albert Einstein Coll Med 1975; **Resid:** Pediatrics, NY Hosp 1977; Child Neurology, Columbia-Presby 1980; **Fellow:** Neurology, NY Hosp 1982; **Fac Appt:** Prof N, NYU Sch Med

Riviello Jr, James J MD (ChiN) - **Spec Exp:** Epilepsy/Seizure Disorders; Epilepsy in Tuberous Sclerosis; Electrical Status Epilepticus Of Sleep; **Hospital:** NYU Langone Med Ctr (page 108); **Address:** NYU Epilepsy and Neurology Center, 223 E 34th St Fl 1, New York, NY 10016; **Phone:** 646-558-0808; **Board Cert:** Pediatrics 1984; Child Neurology 1985; Clinical Neurophysiology 2006; **Med School:** Tufts Univ 1978; **Resid:** Pediatrics, St Christopher Hosp Chldn 1980; Neurology, Temple Univ Hosp 1983; **Fellow:** Pediatric Neurology, St Christopher Hosp Chldn 1983; **Fac Appt:** Prof N, NYU Sch Med

Wolf, Steven M MD (ChiN) - **Spec Exp:** Epilepsy; Headache; Migraine; **Hospital:** Beth Israel Med Ctr - Petrie Division (page 94), St. Luke's - Roosevelt Hosp Ctr - Roosevelt Div (page 94); **Address:** Beth Israel Med Ctr, Dept Ped Neurology, 10 Union Square East, Ste 5J, New York, NY 10003; **Phone:** 212-844-6944; **Board Cert:** Child Neurology 2006; Pediatrics 2011; Clinical Neurophysiology 2008; **Med School:** Albany Med Coll 1989; **Resid:** Pediatrics, Montefiore Med Ctr 1991; Child Neurology, Montefiore Med Ctr 1994; **Fellow:** Epilepsy, Montefiore Med Ctr 1995; **Fac Appt:** Asst Prof N, Albert Einstein Coll Med

Clinical Genetics

Anyane-Yeboa, Kwame MD (CG) - **Spec Exp:** Dysmorphology; Prenatal Diagnosis; **Hospital:** Morgan Stanley Children's Hosp of NY-Presby, NY (page 104); **Address:** Morgan Stanley Chldn's Hosp NY, 3959 Broadway, rm 601A, New York, NY 10032; **Phone:** 212-305-6731; **Board Cert:** Pediatrics 1979; Clinical Genetics 1982; **Med School:** Ghana 1972; **Resid:** Pediatrics, Harlem Hosp 1977; **Fellow:** Clinical Genetics, Babies Hosp-Columbia Presby 1980; **Fac Appt:** Assoc Prof Ped, Columbia P&S

Chung, Wendy Kay MD (CG) - **Spec Exp:** Cancer Genetics; Metabolic Genetic Disorders; Arrhythmias; **Hospital:** NY-Presby/Columbia Univ Med Ctr, NY (page 104); **Address:** 3959 Broadway Ave, New York, NY 10032; **Phone:** 212-305-6731; **Board Cert:** Clinical Genetics 2002; Clinical Molecular Genetics 2005; **Med School:** Cornell Univ 1998; **Resid:** Clinical Genetics, NY-Presby/Columbia Univ Med Ctr 2002; **Fellow:** Genetics, NY-Presby/Columbia Univ Med Ctr 2003; **Fac Appt:** Asst Prof Ped, Columbia P&S

Davis, Jessica G MD (CG) - **Spec Exp:** Marfan's Syndrome; Mental Retardation; Neurofibromatosis; Ehlers-Danlos Syndrome; **Hospital:** NY-Presby/Weill Cornell Med Ctr, NY (page 104), Hosp For Special Surgery (page 115); **Address:** 505 E 70th St, Box 128, New York, NY 10065; **Phone:** 646-962-2205; **Board Cert:** Clinical Genetics 1984; **Med School:** Columbia P&S 1959; **Resid:** Pediatrics, St Luke's Hosp 1962; Clinical Genetics, Albert Einstein Coll Med 1965; **Fellow:** Cytogenetics, Albert Einstein Coll Med 1966; Pediatrics, Albert Einstein Col Med 1968; **Fac Appt:** Assoc Clin Prof Ped, Cornell Univ-Weill Med Coll

Desnick, Robert John MD/PhD (CG) - **Spec Exp:** Inherited Metabolic Disorders; Lysosomal Disease; Gaucher Disease; Porphyria; **Hospital:** Mount Sinai Med Ctr (page 102); **Address:** Mount Sinai School of Medicine, Icahn Medical Institute, 1425 Madison Ave, Fl 14, rm 14-34, Box 1498, New York, NY 10029; **Phone:** 212-659-6700; **Board Cert:** Clinical Genetics 1982; Clinical Biochemical Genetics 1982; Clinical Molecular Genetics 2009; **Med School:** Univ Minn 1971; **Resid:** Pediatrics, Univ Minn Hosps 1973; **Fac Appt:** Prof Emeritus CG, Mount Sinai Sch Med

Colon & Rectal Surgery

Arnell, Tracey D MD (CRS) - **Spec Exp:** Laparoscopic Surgery; Diverticulitis; Inflammatory Bowel Disease; Anorectal Disorders; **Hospital:** NY-Presby/Columbia Univ Med Ctr, NY (page 104); **Address:** 161 Fort Washington Ave Fl 8, New York, NY 10032; **Phone:** 212-342-1734; **Board Cert:** Surgery 2009; Colon & Rectal Surgery 2010; **Med School:** Univ Wash 1992; **Resid:** Surgery, Harbor-UCLA Med Ctr 1998; **Fellow:** Colon & Rectal Surgery, Lahey Clinic 1999; **Fac Appt:** Asst Prof S, Columbia P&S

Brandeis, Steven MD (CRS) - **Spec Exp:** Hemorrhoids; Anal Disorders & Reconstruction; Colon & Rectal Cancer; Anorectal Disorders; **Hospital:** NY Downtown Hosp, NYU Langone Med Ctr (page 108); **Address:** 251 E 33rd St Fl 2 - Ste 2N, New York, NY 10016; **Phone:** 212-696-5411; **Board Cert:** Surgery 1981; Colon & Rectal Surgery 2001; **Med School:** NYU Sch Med 1975; **Resid:** Surgery, NYU Med Ctr-Bellevue Hosp 1980; **Fellow:** Colon & Rectal Surgery, RWJ Univ Hosp 1981; **Fac Appt:** Asst Prof S, NYU Sch Med

Chessin, David B MD (CRS) - **Spec Exp:** Laparoscopic Surgery; Colon & Rectal Cancer & Surgery; **Hospital:** Mount Sinai Med Ctr (page 102); **Address:** 25 E 69th St, New York, NY 10021; **Phone:** 212-517-8600; **Board Cert:** Surgery 2008; Colon & Rectal Surgery 2010; **Med School:** UMDNJ-RW Johnson Med Sch 2000; **Resid:** Surgery, Mt Sinai Med Ctr 2007; **Fellow:** Colon & Rectal Surgery, Mt Sinai Med Ctr 2008; **Fac Appt:** Asst Clin Prof S, Mount Sinai Sch Med

Gorfine, Stephen R MD (CRS) - **Spec Exp:** Anal Disorders & Reconstruction; Hemorrhoids; Rectal Cancer; Anal Cancer; **Hospital:** Mount Sinai Med Ctr (page 102), Lenox Hill Hosp (page 106); **Address:** 25 E 69th St, New York, NY 10021-4925; **Phone:** 212-517-8600; **Board Cert:** Internal Medicine 1981; Surgery 2007; Colon & Rectal Surgery 1988; **Med School:** Univ Mass Sch Med 1978; **Resid:** Internal Medicine, Mt Sinai Hosp 1981; Surgery, Mt Sinai Hosp 1985; **Fellow:** Colon & Rectal Surgery, Ferguson Hosp 1987; **Fac Appt:** Clin Prof S, Mount Sinai Sch Med

Guillem, Jose MD (CRS) - **Spec Exp:** Colon & Rectal Cancer; Rectal Cancer/Sphincter Preservation; Colon & Rectal Cancer-Hereditary; Peritoneal Mucinous Carcinomatosis; **Hospital:** Meml Sloan-Kettering Cancer Ctr (page 116); **Address:** 1275 York Ave, New York, NY 10065; **Phone:** 212-639-8278; **Board Cert:** Surgery 2004; Colon & Rectal Surgery 2005; **Med School:** Yale Univ 1983; **Resid:** Surgery, Columbia-Presby Med Ctr 1990; **Fellow:** Colon & Rectal Surgery, Lahey Clinic 1991; **Fac Appt:** Prof CRS, Cornell Univ-Weill Med Coll

Lee, Sang Won MD (CRS) - **Spec Exp:** Inflammatory Bowel Disease; Diverticulitis; Anorectal Disorders; Colon & Rectal Cancer & Surgery; **Hospital:** NY-Presby/Weill Cornell Med Ctr, NY (page 104); **Address:** NY-Presby/Weill Cornell Med Ctr, 525 E 68th St, Box 172, New York, NY 10021; **Phone:** 212-746-6030; **Board Cert:** Surgery 2003; Colon & Rectal Surgery 2004; **Med School:** NYU Sch Med 1993; **Resid:** Surgery, Beth Israel Deaconess Med Ctr 2001; **Fellow:** Laparoscopic Surgery, NY-Presby/Weill Cornell Med Ctr 2002; Colon & Rectal Surgery, NY-Presby/Weill Cornell Med Ctr 2003; **Fac Appt:** Asst Prof S, Cornell Univ-Weill Med Coll

Milsom, Jeffrey W MD (CRS) - **Spec Exp:** Inflammatory Bowel Disease; Laparoscopic Surgery; Colon & Rectal Cancer; Crohn's Disease; **Hospital:** NY-Presby/Weill Cornell Med Ctr, NY (page 104); **Address:** NY Cornell Med Ctr, Div Colorectal Surgery, 1315 York Ave Fl 2, New York, NY 10065-5304; **Phone:** 212-746-6030; **Board Cert:** Colon & Rectal Surgery 1986; **Med School:** Univ Pittsburgh 1979; **Resid:** Surgery, Roosevelt Hosp 1981; Surgery, Univ Virginia Med Ctr 1984; **Fellow:** Colon & Rectal Surgery, Ferguson Hosp 1985; **Fac Appt:** Prof S, Cornell Univ-Weill Med Coll

Penzer, Jason MD (CRS) - **Spec Exp:** Hemorrhoids; Colon & Rectal Cancer; Diverticulitis; Inflammatory Bowel Disease; **Hospital:** Lenox Hill Hosp (page 106), Beth Israel Med Ctr - Petrie Division (page 94); **Address:** 515 Madison Ave, Ste 705, New York, NY 10022; **Phone:** 212-675-2997; **Board Cert:** Surgery 2002; Colon & Rectal Surgery 2003; **Med School:** Yale Univ 1996; **Resid:** Surgery, St Vincent's Hosp 2001; **Fellow:** Colon & Rectal Surgery, UMDNJ Med Ctr 2002; **Fac Appt:** Asst Clin Prof S, NY Med Coll

Sonoda, Toyooki MD (CRS) - **Spec Exp:** Inflammatory Bowel Disease; Laparoscopic Surgery; Colon & Rectal Cancer & Surgery; Crohn's Disease; **Hospital:** NY-Presby/Weill Cornell Med Ctr, NY (page 104); **Address:** NY Presbyterian-Cornell Medical Ctr, 525 E 68th St, Box 172, New York, NY 10065; **Phone:** 212-746-6030; **Board Cert:** Surgery 2010; Colon & Rectal Surgery 2011; **Med School:** Yale Univ 1993; **Resid:** Surgery, UCSF Med Ctr 1995; Surgery, Cleveland Clinic 1998; **Fellow:** Laparoscopic Surgery, Mt Sinai Med Ctr 1999; Colon & Rectal Surgery, Cleveland Clinic 2000; **Fac Appt:** Asst Prof S, Cornell Univ-Weill Med Coll

Steinhagen, Randolph MD (CRS) - **Spec Exp:** Colostomy Avoidance; Colon & Rectal Cancer; Inflammatory Bowel Disease/Crohn's; Ulcerative Colitis; **Hospital:** Mount Sinai Med Ctr (page 102), St. John's Riverside Hosp-Andrus Pavil; **Address:** Div Colon & Rectal Surgery, 5 E 98th St Fl 14, Box 1259, New York, NY 10029-6501; **Phone:** 212-241-3547; **Board Cert:** Surgery 2002; Colon & Rectal Surgery 1985; **Med School:** Wayne State Univ 1977; **Resid:** Surgery, Mount Sinai Hosp 1982; **Fellow:** Colon & Rectal Surgery, Cleveland Clinic 1983; **Fac Appt:** Prof S, Mount Sinai Sch Med

Temple, Larissa MD (CRS) - **Spec Exp:** Colon & Rectal Cancer; Anal Cancer; Laparoscopic Surgery; **Hospital:** Meml Sloan-Kettering Cancer Ctr (page 116); **Address:** 1275 York Ave Fl 10, New York, NY 10065; **Phone:** 212-639-6081; **Board Cert:** Surgery 2011; Colon & Rectal Surgery 2005; **Med School:** Univ Calgary 1994; **Resid:** Surgery, Univ Toronto 2000; **Fellow:** Surgical Oncology, Meml Sloan Kettering Cancer Ctr 2002

Weiser, Martin R MD (CRS) - **Spec Exp:** Colon & Rectal Cancer; Laparoscopic Surgery; Cancer Surgery; **Hospital:** Meml Sloan-Kettering Cancer Ctr (page 116); **Address:** Meml Sloan Kettering Cancer Ctr, 1275 York Ave, Ste C1075, New York, NY 10065; **Phone:** 646-497-9065; **Board Cert:** Surgery 2009; Colon & Rectal Surgery 2012; **Med School:** Univ Chicago-Pritzker Sch Med 1991; **Resid:** Surgery, Brigham & Women's Hosp 1998; Colon & Rectal Surgery, Mount Sinai Med Ctr 2002; **Fellow:** Research, Harvard Med Sch 1995; Surgical Oncology, Meml Sloan Kettering Cancer Ctr 2000; **Fac Appt:** Assoc Prof S, Cornell Univ-Weill Med Coll

Whelan, Richard L MD (CRS) - **Spec Exp:** Laparoscopic Surgery; Colon & Rectal Cancer; **Hospital:** St. Luke's - Roosevelt Hosp Ctr - Roosevelt Div (page 94); **Address:** 425 W 59th St, Ste 7B, New York, NY 10019; **Phone:** 212-523-8172; **Board Cert:** Surgery 1997; Colon & Rectal Surgery 1989; **Med School:** Columbia P&S 1982; **Resid:** Surgery, Columbia Presby Hosp 1987; **Fellow:** Colon & Rectal Surgery, Univ Minn Med Ctr 1988; **Fac Appt:** Assoc Clin Prof S, Columbia P&S

Critical Care Medicine

Bahr, Gerald S MD (CCM) - **Spec Exp:** Ethics; Critical Care-Complex; **Hospital:** Lenox Hill Hosp (page 106); **Address:** Lenox Hill Hosp - Medicine, 110 E 59th St, Ste 9A, New York, NY 10022-1304; **Phone:** 212-583-2878; **Board Cert:** Internal Medicine 1976; Critical Care Medicine 2009; **Med School:** NY Med Coll 1972; **Resid:** Internal Medicine, Lenox Hill Hosp 1976; **Fellow:** Internal Medicine, Lenox Hill Hosp 1976; **Fac Appt:** Assoc Clin Prof Med, NYU Sch Med

Benjamin, Ernest MD (CCM) - **Spec Exp:** Respiratory Distress Syndrome; Sepsis; **Hospital:** Mount Sinai Med Ctr (page 102); **Address:** Mount Sinai Hosp, SICU, 1 Gustave Levy Pl, Box 1264, New York, NY 10029; **Phone:** 212-241-8867; **Board Cert:** Anesthesiology 1988; Critical Care Medicine 1989; **Med School:** France 1971; **Resid:** Critical Care Medicine, Univ Lyon Affil Hosps 1978; Internal Medicine, North Genl Hosp 1982; **Fellow:** Anesthesiology, Mount Sinai Hosp 1983; **Fac Appt:** Prof S, Mount Sinai Sch Med

Halpern, Neil A MD (CCM) - **Hospital:** Meml Sloan-Kettering Cancer Ctr (page 116), Mount Sinai Med Ctr (page 102); **Address:** 1275 York Ave, Ste C-1179H, New York, NY 10065; **Phone:** 212-639-6731; **Board Cert:** Internal Medicine 1984; Critical Care Medicine 2009; **Med School:** Mount Sinai Sch Med 1981; **Resid:** Internal Medicine, Mount Sinai Hosp 1984; **Fellow:** Critical Care Medicine, Univ Pittsburgh 1985; **Fac Appt:** Prof Med, Cornell Univ-Weill Med Coll

Dermatology

Albom, Michael J MD (D) - **Spec Exp:** Mohs' Surgery; Cosmetic Dermatology; Botox Therapy; Reconstructive Surgery; **Hospital:** NYU Langone Med Ctr (page 108), Lenox Hill Hosp (Manh Eye, Ear & Throat Hosp) (page 106); **Address:** 33 E 70th St, New York, NY 10021; **Phone:** 212-517-2121; **Board Cert:** Dermatology 1976; **Med School:** Boston Univ 1970; **Resid:** Dermatology, Boston Univ Med Ctr 1974; **Fellow:** Mohs Surgery, NYU Med Ctr 1975; **Fac Appt:** Clin Prof D, NYU Sch Med

Amin, Snehal P MD (D) - **Spec Exp:** Skin Laser Surgery; Mohs' Surgery; Skin Cancer; **Hospital:** NY-Presby/Weill Cornell Med Ctr, NY (page 104); **Address:** 800 Second Ave, Ste 200A, New York, NY 10017; **Phone:** 212-661-3376; **Board Cert:** Dermatology 2004; **Med School:** Albert Einstein Coll Med 2000; **Resid:** Dermatology, NY Presby-Weill Cornell Med Ctr 2004; **Fellow:** Mohs Surgery, Skin Laser Surgery Spec-NY/NJ 2005; **Fac Appt:** Asst Prof D, Cornell Univ-Weill Med Coll

Aranoff, Shera M MD (D) - **Spec Exp:** Skin Cancer; Cosmetic Dermatology; Acne; Dermatologic Surgery; **Hospital:** Lenox Hill Hosp (page 106); **Address:** 975 Park Ave, Ste 1-A, New York, NY 10028; **Phone:** 212-772-9305; **Board Cert:** Dermatology 1980; **Med School:** NY Med Coll 1973; **Resid:** Dermatology, Westchester Co Med Ctr 1980

Avram, Marc R MD (D) - **Spec Exp:** Hair Restoration/Transplant; Skin Laser Surgery; Cosmetic Dermatology; Botox Therapy; **Hospital:** NY-Presby/Weill Cornell Med Ctr, NY (page 104), SUNY Downstate Med Ctr (Univ Hosp of Bklyn) - LICH (page 420); **Address:** 905 5th Ave, MS 10021, New York, NY 10021-2650; **Phone:** 212-734-4007; **Board Cert:** Dermatology 2012; Hair Restoration Surgery 2007; **Med School:** SUNY Downstate 1989; **Resid:** Dermatology, Mass Genl Hosp 1994; **Fac Appt:** Clin Prof D, Cornell Univ-Weill Med Coll

Becker, David S MD (D) - **Spec Exp:** Mohs' Surgery; Dermatologic Surgery; Skin Cancer; Laser Surgery; **Hospital:** NY-Presby/Weill Cornell Med Ctr, NY (page 104); **Address:** The Dermatologic Society of Greater NY, 205 E 69th St, Ste 1C, New York, NY 10021; **Phone:** 212-772-3600; **Board Cert:** Dermatology 2001; **Med School:** UCSF 1989; **Resid:** Dermatology, UCSF Med Ctr 1993; **Fellow:** Dermatologic Surgery, Mass Genl Hosp 1994

Belsito, Donald V MD (D) - **Spec Exp:** Contact Dermatitis; Cutaneous Lymphoma; Psoriasis; Atopic Dermatitis; **Hospital:** NY-Presby/Columbia Univ Med Ctr, NY (page 104); **Address:** Columbia Doctors Eastside, 16 E 60th St Fl 3 - Ste 300, New York, NY 10022; **Phone:** 212-305-5293; **Board Cert:** Internal Medicine 1979; Dermatology 1983; Clinical & Laboratory Dematologic Immunology 1985; **Med School:** Cornell Univ-Weill Med Coll 1976; **Resid:** Internal Medicine, Case West Res Univ Hosps 1979; Dermatology, NYU Med Ctr 1982; **Fellow:** Dermatologic Research, NYU Med Ctr 1983; **Fac Appt:** Clin Prof D, Columbia P&S

Bernstein, Robert M MD (D) - **Spec Exp:** Hair Restoration/Transplant; Hair Loss in Women; **Hospital:** NY-Presby/Columbia Univ Med Ctr, NY (page 104); **Address:** 110 E 55th St, Fl 11, New York, NY 10022; **Phone:** 212-826-2400; **Board Cert:** Dermatology 1982; Hair Restoration Surgery 1998; **Med School:** UMDNJ-NJ Med Sch, Newark 1978; **Resid:** Dermatology, Montefiore Med Ctr 1982; **Fac Appt:** Clin Prof D, Columbia P&S

Berson, Diane S MD (D) - **Spec Exp:** Aging Skin; Acne; Skin Cancer; **Hospital:** NY-Presby/Weill Cornell Med Ctr, NY (page 104); **Address:** 211 E 53rd St, Ste 3, New York, NY 10022-4803; **Phone:** 212-355-3511; **Board Cert:** Dermatology 2009; **Med School:** NYU Sch Med 1984; **Resid:** Dermatology, SUNY Hlth Sci Ctr 1988; **Fac Appt:** Assoc Prof D, Cornell Univ-Weill Med Coll

Bickers, David R MD (D) - **Spec Exp:** Skin Cancer; Photodynamic Therapy; Psoriasis; Phototherapy; **Hospital:** NY-Presby/Columbia Univ Med Ctr, NY (page 104); **Address:** 16 E 60th St, Ste 300, New York, NY 10022-1002; **Phone:** 212-326-8465; **Board Cert:** Dermatology 1974; **Med School:** Univ VA Sch Med 1967; **Resid:** Dermatology, NYU Med Ctr 1973; **Fellow:** Pharmacology, Rockefeller Univ Hosp 1974; **Fac Appt:** Prof D, Columbia P&S

Brademas, Mary Ellen MD (D) - **Spec Exp:** Skin Diseases; Cosmetic Dermatology; Nail Diseases; **Hospital:** NYU Langone Med Ctr (page 108), Bellevue Hosp Ctr; **Address:** 11 5th Ave, Ste F, New York, NY 10003; **Phone:** 212-477-1515; **Board Cert:** Dermatology 1983; **Med School:** Georgetown Univ 1979; **Resid:** Dermatology, Johns Hopkins Hosp 1981; Dermatology, NYU Med Ctr 1983; **Fac Appt:** Assoc Clin Prof D, NYU Sch Med

Brandt, Fredric S MD (D) - **Spec Exp:** Botox Therapy; Cosmetic Dermatology; **Address:** Laser & Skin Surgery Ctr, 323 E 34th St Fl 2, New York, NY 10016; **Phone:** 212-889-7096; **Board Cert:** Internal Medicine 1978; Dermatology 1981; **Med School:** Hahnemann Univ 1975; **Resid:** Internal Medicine, VA Hosp 1981; Dermatology, Univ Miami Hosps 1983

Buchness, Mary Ruth MD (D) - **Spec Exp:** Skin Infections; Skin Cancer; Cosmetic Dermatology; Psoriasis; **Address:** 560 Broadway, Ste 406, New York, NY 10012; **Phone:** 212-822-3515; **Board Cert:** Dermatology 1986; **Med School:** Columbia P&S 1982; **Resid:** Dermatology, Columbia Univ Med Ctr 1986; **Fac Appt:** Assoc Prof Med, NY Med Coll

Burke, Karen E MD/PhD (D) - **Spec Exp:** Skin Cancer; Cosmetic Dermatology; Aging Skin; **Hospital:** Mount Sinai Med Ctr (page 102); **Address:** 429 E 52nd St, New York, NY 10022-6430; **Phone:** 212-754-1100; **Board Cert:** Dermatology 1985; **Med School:** NYU Sch Med 1978; **Resid:** Dermatology, NYU Med Ctr 1983; **Fac Appt:** Asst Clin Prof D, Mount Sinai Sch Med

Carucci, John A MD/PhD (D) - **Spec Exp:** Mohs' Surgery; **Hospital:** NYU Langone Med Ctr (page 108); **Address:** Dermatologic Surgery Assocs, 530 First Ave, Ste 7H, New York, NY 10016; **Phone:** 212-263-7019; **Board Cert:** Dermatology 2007; **Med School:** SUNY Downstate 1994; **Resid:** Dermatology, NYU Med Ctr 1998; **Fellow:** Mohs Surgery, Yale-New Haven Hosp 2000; **Fac Appt:** Asst Prof D, Cornell Univ-Weill Med Coll

Clark, Sheryl MD (D) - **Spec Exp:** Melanoma; Skin Cancer; Skin Laser Surgery; Cosmetic Dermatology; **Hospital:** NY-Presby/Weill Cornell Med Ctr, NY (page 104); **Address:** 109 E 61st St, New York, NY 10065; **Phone:** 212-750-2905; **Board Cert:** Dermatology 1988; **Med School:** Case West Res Univ 1982; **Resid:** Internal Medicine, Mount Sinai-Univ Hosp 1983; Dermatology, Barnes Hosp-Wash Univ 1988; **Fellow:** Dermatology, Barnes Hosp-Wash Univ 1988; **Fac Appt:** Asst Clin Prof D, Cornell Univ-Weill Med Coll

Cohen, David E MD (D) - **Spec Exp:** Occupational Dermatology; Contact Dermatitis; **Hospital:** NYU Langone Med Ctr (page 108); **Address:** NYU Dermatologic Assocs, 530 1st Ave, Ste 7R, New York, NY 10016; **Phone:** 212-263-5889; **Board Cert:** Dermatology 2003; Occupational Medicine 1996; **Med School:** SUNY Stony Brook 1989; **Resid:** Dermatology, NYU Med Ctr 1993; **Fellow:** Occupational Medicine, Columbia Univ Sch of Public Hlth 1994; **Fac Appt:** Assoc Prof D, NYU Sch Med

Davis, Joyce MD (D) - **Spec Exp:** Acne; Hair loss; Cosmetic Dermatology; **Hospital:** Beth Israel Med Ctr - Petrie Division (page 94), Mount Sinai Med Ctr (page 102); **Address:** 69 Fifth Avenue at 15th St, New York, NY 10003; **Phone:** 212-242-3066; **Board Cert:** Dermatology 1983; **Med School:** Albert Einstein Coll Med 1979; **Resid:** Dermatology, Mount Sinai Med Ctr 1983

DeLeo, Vincent A MD (D) - **Spec Exp:** Photosensitive Skin Diseases; Contact Dermatitis; Facial Rejuvenation; Eczema; **Hospital:** St. Luke's - Roosevelt Hosp Ctr - Roosevelt Div (page 94), Beth Israel Med Ctr - Petrie Division (page 94); **Address:** 1090 Amsterdam Ave, Fl 11, New York, NY 10025; **Phone:** 212-523-5898; **Board Cert:** Dermatology 2009; **Med School:** Louisiana State U, New Orleans 1969; **Resid:** Dermatology, Columbia-Presby Med Ctr 1976; **Fac Appt:** Clin Prof D, Columbia P&S

Demar, Leon K MD (D) - **Spec Exp:** Skin Cancer; Acne; Cosmetic Dermatology; Pediatric Dermatology; **Hospital:** Lenox Hill Hosp (page 106), NY-Presby/Columbia Univ Med Ctr, NY (page 104); **Address:** 985 5th Ave, New York, NY 10075; **Phone:** 212-988-9010; **Board Cert:** Dermatology 1977; **Med School:** NYU Sch Med 1973; **Resid:** Dermatology, Stanford Med Ctr 1975; Dermatology, Columbia-Presby Med Ctr 1977; **Fac Appt:** Asst Clin Prof D, Columbia P&S

Felderman, Lenora MD (D) - **Spec Exp:** Cosmetic Dermatology; Facial Rejuvenation; Acne & Rosacea; Skin Cancer; **Hospital:** NY-Presby/Weill Cornell Med Ctr, NY (page 104); **Address:** 1317 3rd Ave, Fl 8, New York, NY 10021-2995; **Phone:** 212-734-0091; **Board Cert:** Dermatology 2009; **Med School:** NY Med Coll 1981; **Resid:** Internal Medicine, Montefiore Med Ctr 1982; Dermatology, Montefiore Med Ctr 1985; **Fac Appt:** Asst Clin Prof D, Cornell Univ-Weill Med Coll

Franks Jr, Andrew G MD (D) - **Spec Exp:** Lupus/SLE; Raynaud's Disease; Scleroderma; Dermatomyositis; **Hospital:** NYU Langone Med Ctr (page 108); **Address:** NYU Dermatologic Assocs, Faculty Practice Tower, 530 First Ave Fl 7 - Ste 7R, New York, NY 10016; **Phone:** 212-263-5889; **Board Cert:** Internal Medicine 1975; Dermatology 1977; Rheumatology 1978; **Med School:** NY Med Coll 1971; **Resid:** Internal Medicine, Beth Israel Med Ctr 1974; Dermatology, Columbia-Presby Med Ctr 1975; **Fellow:** Rheumatology, Columbia-Presby Med Ctr 1977; **Fac Appt:** Prof D, NYU Sch Med

Garzon, Maria C MD (D) - **Spec Exp:** Pediatric Dermatology; Vascular Anomalies; Mycosis Fungoides; **Hospital:** NY-Presby/Columbia Univ Med Ctr, NY (page 104); **Address:** Columbia Univ, Dept Dermatology, 161 Ft Washington Ave Fl 12, New York, NY 10032; **Phone:** 212-305-5293; **Board Cert:** Dermatology 2004; Pediatric Dermatology 2004; **Med School:** Columbia P&S 1988; **Resid:** Pediatrics, Columbia Presby-Babies Hosp 1991; **Fellow:** Dermatology, Columbia Presby Med Ctr 1995; **Fac Appt:** Assoc Clin Prof D, Columbia P&S

Gendler, Ellen C MD (D) - **Spec Exp:** Cosmetic Dermatology; Contact Dermatitis; Botox Therapy; Facial Rejuvenation; **Hospital:** NYU Langone Med Ctr (page 108); **Address:** 1035 Fifth Ave, New York, NY 10028; **Phone:** 212-288-8222; **Board Cert:** Dermatology 1985; **Med School:** Columbia P&S 1981; **Resid:** Dermatology, NYU Med Ctr 1985; **Fac Appt:** Assoc Clin Prof D, NYU Sch Med

Geronemus, Roy G MD (D) - **Spec Exp:** Skin Laser Surgery; Cosmetic Dermatology; Mohs' Surgery; Skin Cancer; **Hospital:** New York Eye & Ear Infirm (page 117); **Address:** 317 E 34 St, Ste 11N, New York, NY 10016-4974; **Phone:** 212-686-7306; **Board Cert:** Dermatology 1983; **Med School:** Univ Miami Sch Med 1979; **Resid:** Dermatology, NYU-Skin Cancer Unit 1983; **Fellow:** Mohs Surgery, NYU-Skin Cancer Unit 1984; **Fac Appt:** Clin Prof D, NYU Sch Med

Goldberg, David J MD (D) - **Spec Exp:** Mohs' Surgery; Skin Cancer; Cosmetic Dermatology; Laser Surgery; **Hospital:** Mount Sinai Med Ctr (page 102), Hackensack Univ Med Ctr (page 96); **Address:** 115 E 57th St, Ste 710, New York, NY 10022; **Phone:** 212-750-8900; **Board Cert:** Dermatology 1984; Clinical & Laboratory Dematologic Immunology 1987; **Med School:** Yale Univ 1980; **Resid:** Dermatology, NYU Med Ctr 1984; **Fellow:** Mohs Surgery, NYU Med Ctr 1985; **Fac Appt:** Clin Prof D, Mount Sinai Sch Med

Gordon, Marsha MD (D) - **Spec Exp:** Cosmetic Dermatology; Botox Therapy; Facial Rejuvenation; **Hospital:** Mount Sinai Med Ctr (page 102); **Address:** 5 E 98th St Fl 5, New York, NY 10029-6574; **Phone:** 212-241-9728; **Board Cert:** Dermatology 1988; **Med School:** Univ Pennsylvania 1984; **Resid:** Dermatology, Mt Sinai Hosp 1988; **Fac Appt:** Clin Prof D, Mount Sinai Sch Med

Green, Michele S MD (D) - **Spec Exp:** Cosmetic Dermatology; Skin Laser Surgery; Facial Rejuvenation; Botox Therapy; **Hospital:** Lenox Hill Hosp (page 106); **Address:** 156 E 79th St, Ste 1B, New York, NY 10075; **Phone:** 212-535-3088; **Board Cert:** Dermatology 2004; **Med School:** Mount Sinai Sch Med 1991; **Resid:** Dermatology, Mt Sinai Hosp 1995

Greenberg, Robert MD (D) - **Spec Exp:** Skin Laser Surgery; Cosmetic Dermatology; Botox Therapy; **Hospital:** NYU Langone Med Ctr (page 108); **Address:** 117 E 72nd St, New York, NY 10021-4249; **Phone:** 212-861-2580; **Board Cert:** Dermatology 1977; **Med School:** Univ Mich Med Sch 1970; **Resid:** Dermatology, Univ of Miami Hosps 1975; Dermatology, New York Univ 1977; **Fellow:** Dermatology, Univ Miami Hosp 1974; **Fac Appt:** Asst Clin Prof D, NYU Sch Med

Greenspan, Alan H MD (D) - **Spec Exp:** Skin Cancer; Dermatologic Surgery; Phototherapy; **Hospital:** NYU Langone Med Ctr (page 108), NY Downtown Hosp; **Address:** 39 Broadway, Ste 3005, New York, NY 10006; **Phone:** 212-509-5200; **Board Cert:** Dermatology 2009; **Med School:** Northwestern Univ 1979; **Resid:** Internal Medicine, Northwestern Univ 1981; Dermatology, NYU Med Ctr 1984; **Fac Appt:** Asst Clin Prof D, NYU Sch Med

Gross, Dennis F MD (D) - **Hospital:** NYU Langone Med Ctr (page 108); **Address:** 105 E 37th St, Ground Fl, New York, NY 10016; **Phone:** 212-725-4555; **Board Cert:** Dermatology 1990; **Med School:** SUNY Stony Brook 1986; **Resid:** Dermatology, NYU Med Ctr 1990; **Fac Appt:** Asst Clin Prof D, NYU Sch Med

Grossman, Melanie MD (D) - **Spec Exp:** Skin Laser Surgery; Facial Rejuvenation; Body Contouring; Cosmetic Dermatology; **Hospital:** NY-Presby/Columbia Univ Med Ctr, NY (page 104); **Address:** 161 Madison Ave, Ste 4NW, New York, NY 10016-5405; **Phone:** 212-725-8600; **Board Cert:** Dermatology 2010; **Med School:** NYU Sch Med 1988; **Resid:** Internal Medicine, Yale-New Haven Hosp 1989; Dermatology, Columbia-Presby Med Ctr 1992; **Fellow:** Laser Surgery, Mass Genl Hosp 1995; **Fac Appt:** Asst Clin Prof D, Columbia P&S

Hale, Elizabeth K MD (D) - **Spec Exp:** Skin Cancer; Laser Surgery; Cosmetic Dermatology; **Hospital:** NYU Langone Med Ctr (page 108); **Address:** 317 E 34th St, Fl 11, New York, NY 10016; **Phone:** 212-686-7306; **Board Cert:** Dermatology 2002; **Med School:** NYU Sch Med 1998; **Resid:** Dermatology, NYU Med Ctr 2002; **Fellow:** Mohs Surgery, NYU Med Ctr 2003; **Fac Appt:** Assoc Clin Prof D, NYU Sch Med

Halpern, Allan C MD (D) - **Spec Exp:** Skin Cancer; Melanoma; Melanoma Early Detection/Prevention; **Hospital:** Meml Sloan-Kettering Cancer Ctr (page 116); **Address:** 160 E 53rd St Fl 2, New York, NY 10022; **Phone:** 212-610-0766; **Board Cert:** Internal Medicine 1984; Dermatology 1988; **Med School:** Albert Einstein Coll Med 1981; **Resid:** Internal Medicine, Montefiore Hosp 1985; Dermatology, Hosp Univ Penn 1989; **Fellow:** Epidemiology, Hosp Univ Penn 1989; **Fac Appt:** Assoc Prof Med, Cornell Univ-Weill Med Coll

Hatcher, Virgil MD (D) - **Spec Exp:** Cosmetic Dermatology; Psoriasis; Viral Infections; **Hospital:** NYU Langone Med Ctr (page 108); **Address:** 420 W 23rd St, Ste A-GF, New York, NY 10011-2172; **Phone:** 212-675-4244; **Board Cert:** Dermatology 2009; **Med School:** UCSF 1978; **Resid:** Dermatology, NYU Med Ctr 1982; **Fellow:** Virology, NYU Med Ctr 1983; **Fac Appt:** Asst Clin Prof D, NYU Sch Med

Hochman, Herbert A MD (D) - **Spec Exp:** Cosmetic Dermatology; Skin Laser Surgery; Skin Cancer; **Hospital:** Lenox Hill Hosp (page 106); **Address:** 1020 Park Ave, New York, NY 10028-0913; **Phone:** 212-861-1656; **Board Cert:** Dermatology 1977; **Med School:** Tulane Univ 1970; **Resid:** Dermatology, Montefiore Med Ctr 1976

Jacobs, Michael Ira MD (D) - **Spec Exp:** Skin Cancer; Melanoma; Cosmetic Dermatology; **Hospital:** NY-Presby/Weill Cornell Med Ctr, NY (page 104), Hosp For Special Surgery (page 115); **Address:** 407 E 70th St Fl 2, New York, NY 10021-5302; **Phone:** 212-772-7190; **Board Cert:** Dermatology 1981; **Med School:** Cornell Univ-Weill Med Coll 1977; **Resid:** Dermatology, New York Hosp 1981; **Fac Appt:** Assoc Clin Prof D, Cornell Univ-Weill Med Coll

Katz, Bruce MD (D) - **Spec Exp:** Laser Surgery; Cosmetic Surgery; Liposuction & Body Contouring; Cosmetic Dermatology; **Hospital:** Mount Sinai Med Ctr (page 102); **Address:** 60 E 56th St Fl 2, New York, NY 10022-3350; **Phone:** 212-688-5882; **Board Cert:** Dermatology 1983; **Med School:** McGill Univ 1977; **Resid:** Internal Medicine, Columbia Presby Med Ctr 1979; Dermatology, Columbia Presby Med Ctr 1982; **Fac Appt:** Clin Prof D, Mount Sinai Sch Med

Katz, Susan MD (D) - **Spec Exp:** Psoriasis; Skin Cancer & Moles; Cutaneous Lymphoma; Cosmetic Dermatology; **Hospital:** NYU Langone Med Ctr (page 108); **Address:** 111 Broadway Fl 2, New York, NY 10006; **Phone:** 212-263-9700; **Board Cert:** Dermatology 2009; **Med School:** NYU Sch Med 1977; **Resid:** Internal Medicine, Roosevelt Hosp 1979; Dermatology, Montefiore Med Ctr 1983; **Fac Appt:** Asst Clin Prof D, Albert Einstein Coll Med

Kauvar, Arielle B MD (D) - **Spec Exp:** Laser Surgery; Cosmetic Dermatology; Mohs' Surgery; Botox Therapy; **Hospital:** NYU Langone Med Ctr (page 108), New York Eye & Ear Infirm (page 117); **Address:** 1044 Fifth Ave, New York, NY 10028; **Phone:** 212-249-9440; **Board Cert:** Dermatology 2011; **Med School:** Harvard Med Sch 1989; **Resid:** Dermatology, NYU Med Ctr 1993; **Fellow:** Mohs Surgery, Laser & Skin Surgery Ctr 1994; **Fac Appt:** Assoc Clin Prof D, NYU Sch Med

Kenet, Barney J MD (D) - **Spec Exp:** Dermatologic Surgery; Cosmetic Dermatology; Liposuction; **Hospital:** NY-Presby/Weill Cornell Med Ctr, NY (page 104); **Address:** 25 E 86th St, Lobby A, New York, NY 10028; **Phone:** 212-535-9753; **Board Cert:** Dermatology 2012; **Med School:** Brown Univ 1988; **Resid:** Dermatology, New York Hosp 1992

Kline, Mitchell A MD (D) - **Spec Exp:** Melanoma; Skin Cancer; Mohs' Surgery; Cosmetic Dermatology; **Hospital:** NY-Presby/Weill Cornell Med Ctr, NY (page 104); **Address:** 700 Park Ave, New York, NY 10021; **Phone:** 212-517-6555; **Board Cert:** Dermatology 2009; **Med School:** Univ Pennsylvania 1985; **Resid:** Internal Medicine, Graduate Hosp 1987; Dermatology, New York Hosp 1990

Kriegel, David MD (D) - **Spec Exp:** Mohs' Surgery; Laser Surgery; Skin Cancer; Cosmetic Surgery; **Hospital:** Mount Sinai Med Ctr (page 102); **Address:** 250 W 57th St, Ste 825, New York, NY 10107-0809; **Phone:** 212-489-6669; **Board Cert:** Dermatology 2003; **Med School:** Boston Univ 1987; **Resid:** Dermatology, New England Med Ctr 1991; **Fellow:** Mohs Surgery, Stony Brook Univ Hosp 1993; **Fac Appt:** Assoc Prof D, Mount Sinai Sch Med

Lebwohl, Mark G MD (D) - **Spec Exp:** Skin Cancer; Psoriasis; Cutaneous Lymphoma; Pseudoxanthoma Elasticum; **Hospital:** Mount Sinai Med Ctr (page 102); **Address:** 5 E 98th St, Fl 5, New York, NY 10029-6501; **Phone:** 212-241-9728; **Board Cert:** Internal Medicine 1981; Dermatology 1983; **Med School:** Harvard Med Sch 1978; **Resid:** Internal Medicine, Mt Sinai Hosp 1981; Dermatology, Mt Sinai Hosp 1983; **Fellow:** Dermatology, Mt Sinai Hosp 1983; **Fac Appt:** Prof D, Mount Sinai Sch Med

Lombardo, Peter C MD (D) - **Spec Exp:** Skin Cancer; Cosmetic Dermatology; **Hospital:** St. Luke's - Roosevelt Hosp Ctr - Roosevelt Div (page 94), NY-Presby/Columbia Univ Med Ctr, NY (page 104); **Address:** Sutton Place Dermatology, 445 E 58th St, New York, NY 10022-2302; **Phone:** 212-838-0270; **Board Cert:** Dermatology 2009; **Med School:** Albany Med Coll 1959; **Resid:** Dermatology, Columbia-Presby 1965; Internal Medicine, St Luke's-Roosevelt Hosp Ctr 1966; **Fac Appt:** Assoc Clin Prof D, Columbia P&S

Marmur, Ellen S MD (D) - **Spec Exp:** Cosmetic Dermatology; Mohs' Surgery; Laser Surgery; **Hospital:** Mount Sinai Med Ctr (page 102); **Address:** 5 E 98th St, Fl 5, New York, NY 10029; **Phone:** 212-241-5778; **Board Cert:** Dermatology 2003; **Med School:** Albert Einstein Coll Med 1999; **Resid:** Dermatology, NY Hosp-Cornell Univ 2003; **Fellow:** Mohs Surgery, Hackensack Hosp 2004; Cosmetic Dermatology, Hackensack Hosp 2004; **Fac Appt:** Assoc Prof D, Mount Sinai Sch Med

Myskowski, Patricia L MD (D) - **Spec Exp:** AIDS-Kaposi's Sarcoma; Cutaneous Lymphoma; Skin Cancer; **Hospital:** Meml Sloan-Kettering Cancer Ctr (page 116); **Address:** 160 E 53 St, New York, NY 10022; **Phone:** 212-610-0768; **Board Cert:** Dermatology 1980; Clinical & Laboratory Dermatologic Immunology 1985; **Med School:** Brown Univ 1975; **Resid:** Internal Medicine, Bronx VA Hosp; Dermatology, NY Hosp-Cornell Med Ctr 1980; **Fellow:** Dermatology, Meml Sloan Kettering Cancer Ctr 1981; **Fac Appt:** Assoc Prof D, Cornell Univ-Weill Med Coll

Orbuch, Philip MD (D) - **Spec Exp:** Pediatric Dermatology; Skin Cancer; **Hospital:** NYU Langone Med Ctr (page 108), Bellevue Hosp Ctr; **Address:** 345 E 37th St, Ste 307, New York, NY 10016; **Phone:** 212-532-5355; **Board Cert:** Dermatology 2009; **Med School:** Israel 1981; **Resid:** Dermatology, NYU Med Ctr 1985; **Fellow:** Dermatology, NYU Med Ctr 1986; **Fac Appt:** Assoc Clin Prof D, NYU Sch Med

Orentreich, David S MD (D) - **Spec Exp:** Dermatologic Surgery; Liposuction; Hair Restoration/Transplant; Laser Surgery; **Hospital:** Mount Sinai Med Ctr (page 102); **Address:** 909 5th Ave, New York, NY 10021; **Phone:** 212-794-0800; **Board Cert:** Dermatology 1984; **Med School:** Columbia P&S 1980; **Resid:** Dermatology, Mt Sinai Med Ctr 1984; **Fac Appt:** Asst Clin Prof D, Mount Sinai Sch Med

Orlow, Seth J MD/PhD (D) - **Spec Exp:** Pediatric Dermatology; Birthmarks/Hemangiomas; Psoriasis/Eczema; **Hospital:** NYU Langone Med Ctr (page 108); **Address:** 530 1st Ave, Ste 7R, New York, NY 10016-6402; **Phone:** 212-263-5889; **Board Cert:** Dermatology 2009; Pediatric Dermatology 2004; **Med School:** Albert Einstein Coll Med 1986; **Resid:** Pediatrics, Mt Sinai Hosp 1987; Dermatology, Yale-New Haven Hosp 1989; **Fellow:** Pediatric Dermatology, Yale-New Haven Hosp 1990; **Fac Appt:** Prof D, NYU Sch Med

Ostad, Ariel MD (D) - **Spec Exp:** Skin Cancer; Mohs' Surgery; Skin Laser Surgery; Cosmetic Dermatology; **Hospital:** NYU Langone Med Ctr (page 108), Lenox Hill Hosp (page 106); **Address:** 897 Lexington Ave, New York, NY 10021; **Phone:** 212-517-7900; **Board Cert:** Dermatology 2004; **Med School:** NYU Sch Med 1991; **Resid:** Dermatology, NYU Med Ctr 1995; **Fellow:** Dermatologic Surgery, UCLA Med Ctr 1996; **Fac Appt:** Asst Prof D, NYU Sch Med

Podwal, Mark H MD (D) - **Spec Exp:** Skin Cancer; **Hospital:** NYU Langone Med Ctr (page 108); **Address:** 55 E 73rd St, New York, NY 10021; **Phone:** 212-288-7488; **Board Cert:** Dermatology 1975; **Med School:** NYU Sch Med 1970; **Resid:** Dermatology, Kings Co Hosp Ctr 1972; Dermatology, Bellevue Hosp 1974; **Fac Appt:** Assoc Clin Prof D, NYU Sch Med

Polis, Laurie MD (D) - **Spec Exp:** Cosmetic Dermatology; Skin Laser Surgery; Facial Rejuvenation; **Hospital:** Mount Sinai Med Ctr (page 102); **Address:** 62 Crosby St, New York, NY 10012; **Phone:** 212-431-1600 x227; **Board Cert:** Dermatology 1989; **Med School:** Mount Sinai Sch Med 1983; **Resid:** Dermatology, Montefiore Med Ctr 1989; **Fac Appt:** Asst Prof D, Mount Sinai Sch Med

Prioleau, Philip G MD (D) - **Spec Exp:** Melanoma; Skin Cancer; Mohs' Surgery; **Hospital:** NY-Presby/Weill Cornell Med Ctr, NY (page 104); **Address:** 1035 Fifth Ave, Ste C, New York, NY 10028; **Phone:** 212-794-3548; **Board Cert:** Surgery 1973; Anatomic Pathology 1979; Dermatopathology 1980; Dermatology 1983; **Med School:** Med Univ SC 1967; **Resid:** Surgery, Univ Va Hosp 1972; Plastic Surgery, Duke Univ Hosp 1975; **Fellow:** Pathology, Barnes Jewish Hosp 1980; Dermatopathology, NYU Med Ctr 1981; **Fac Appt:** Assoc Prof D, Cornell Univ-Weill Med Coll

Prystowsky, Janet MD (D) - **Spec Exp:** Mohs' Surgery; Cosmetic Dermatology; Skin Cancer; Laser Surgery; **Hospital:** St. Luke's - Roosevelt Hosp Ctr - Roosevelt Div (page 94); **Address:** 110 E 55th St Fl 7, New York, NY 10022; **Phone:** 212-230-1212; **Board Cert:** Dermatology 1987; **Med School:** Univ Chicago-Pritzker Sch Med 1983; **Resid:** Internal Medicine, Univ Chicago Hosps 1984; Dermatology, Hosp Univ Penn 1987; **Fellow:** Mohs Surgery, SUNY Stony Brook

Ramsay, David L MD (D) - **Spec Exp:** Cutaneous Lymphoma; Skin Cancer; **Hospital:** NYU Langone Med Ctr (page 108); **Address:** 530 1st Ave, Ste 7G, New York, NY 10016-6402; **Phone:** 212-683-6283; **Board Cert:** Dermatology 1974; **Med School:** Indiana Univ 1969; **Resid:** Dermatology, NYU Med Ctr 1973; **Fellow:** Dermatology, Univ Ill Hosp 1973; **Fac Appt:** Clin Prof D, NYU Sch Med

Ratner, Desiree MD (D) - Spec Exp: Mohs' Surgery; Skin Cancer; Dermatologic Surgery; **Hospital:** NY-Presby/Columbia Univ Med Ctr, NY (page 104); **Address:** Columbia Presbyterian Med Ctr, 161 Fort Washington Ave Fl 12, New York, NY 10032; **Phone:** 212-305-3625; **Board Cert:** Dermatology 2003; **Med School:** Johns Hopkins Univ 1989; **Resid:** Dermatology, Univ Michigan Med Ctr 1993; **Fellow:** Mohs Surgery, New England Med Ctr 1994; Mohs Surgery, Lahey Clinic 1995; **Fac Appt:** Prof D, Columbia P&S

Rigel, Darrell S MD (D) - Spec Exp: Melanoma; Skin Cancer; Cosmetic Dermatology; **Hospital:** NYU Langone Med Ctr (page 108), Mount Sinai Med Ctr (page 102); **Address:** 35 E 35th Street, Ste 208, New York, NY 10016-3823; **Phone:** 212-684-5964; **Board Cert:** Dermatology 1983; **Med School:** Geo Wash Univ 1978; **Resid:** Dermatology, NYU Med Ctr 1982; **Fellow:** Dermatologic Surgery, NYU Med Ctr 1983; **Fac Appt:** Clin Prof D, NYU Sch Med

Romano, John MD (D) - Spec Exp: Cosmetic Dermatology; **Hospital:** NY-Presby/Weill Cornell Med Ctr, NY (page 104); **Address:** 58 W 15th St, Grnd Fl, New York, NY 10011; **Phone:** 212-242-5815; **Board Cert:** Dermatology 1980; **Med School:** Cornell Univ-Weill Med Coll 1973; **Resid:** Internal Medicine, St. Vincents Hosp 1976; Dermatology, New York Hosp 1978; **Fac Appt:** Asst Clin Prof D, Cornell Univ-Weill Med Coll

Roth, Jeffrey S MD/PhD (D) - Spec Exp: Melanoma; Skin Cancer; HIV-Related Skin Disorders; Cosmetic Dermatology; **Hospital:** Mount Sinai Med Ctr (page 102); **Address:** Park Avenue Dermatology Assocs, 580 Park Ave, New York, NY 10065-7313; **Phone:** 212-752-3692; **Board Cert:** Dermatology 2001; **Med School:** Columbia P&S 1989; **Resid:** Dermatology, Columbia-Presby Hosp 1993; **Fac Appt:** Asst Clin Prof D, Mount Sinai Sch Med

Safai, Bijan MD (D) - Spec Exp: Dermatologic Surgery; Skin Cancer; Skin Laser Surgery; **Hospital:** Metropolitan Hosp Ctr - NY; **Address:** 625 Park Ave, New York, NY 10021-6545; **Phone:** 212-988-8918; **Board Cert:** Dermatology 1974; **Med School:** Iran 1965; **Resid:** Internal Medicine, VA Med Ctr 1970; Dermatology, NYU Med Ctr 1973; **Fellow:** Immunology, Meml Sloan-Kettering Cancer Ctr 1974; **Fac Appt:** Prof D, NY Med Coll

Schultz, Neal MD (D) - Spec Exp: Cosmetic Dermatology; Melanoma Early Detection/Prevention; Skin Laser Surgery; Tattoo Removal; **Hospital:** Mount Sinai Med Ctr (page 102); **Address:** 1130 Park Ave, New York, NY 10128; **Phone:** 212-369-9600; **Board Cert:** Dermatology 1978; **Med School:** Columbia P&S 1973; **Resid:** Internal Medicine, Mt Sinai Hosp 1975; Dermatology, Mt Sinai Hosp 1978; **Fac Appt:** Asst Clin Prof D, Mount Sinai Sch Med

Seidenberg, Roy Stern MD (D) - Spec Exp: Cosmetic Dermatology; Acne; **Hospital:** NYU Langone Med Ctr (page 108); **Address:** 317 E 34th St Fl 6, New York, NY 10016; **Phone:** 212-421-7546; **Board Cert:** Dermatology 2008; **Med School:** NY Med Coll 1991; **Resid:** Internal Medicine, Montefiore Med Ctr 1994; Dermatology, Cooper Hosp 1998; **Fellow:** Dermatologic Surgery, Boston Univ Med Ctr 1995; **Fac Appt:** Asst Clin Prof D, NYU Sch Med

Shelton, Ronald M MD (D) - Spec Exp: Cosmetic Dermatology; Mohs' Surgery; Skin Laser Surgery; **Hospital:** Mount Sinai Med Ctr (page 102); **Address:** 260 E 66 St, New York, NY 10065; **Phone:** 212-593-1818; **Board Cert:** Dermatology 1990; **Med School:** SUNY Upstate Med Univ 1984; **Resid:** Dermatology, Brooke Army Med Ctr 1990; **Fellow:** Mohs Surgery, UCSF Med Ctr 1993; **Fac Appt:** Assoc Clin Prof D, Mount Sinai Sch Med

Shim-Chang, Helen MD (D) - Spec Exp: Dermatopathology; **Hospital:** Mount Sinai Med Ctr (page 102); **Address:** Dermatology Assocs, 5 E 98th St Fl 5, New York, NY 10029; **Phone:** 212-241-9728; **Board Cert:** Anatomic Pathology 1997; Dermatopathology 1998; Dermatology 2008; **Med School:** Hahnemann Univ 1991; **Resid:** Internal Medicine, Mt Sinai Sch Med 1993; Dermatology, Mt Sinai Sch Med 1997; **Fellow:** Dermatopathology, Mt Sinai Hosp 1998

Shupack, Jerome L MD (D) - **Spec Exp:** Rare Skin Disorders; Psoriasis; Eczema; Blistering Diseases; **Hospital:** NYU Langone Med Ctr (page 108); **Address:** 530 1st Ave, HCC 7F, New York, NY 10016-6402; **Phone:** 212-263-7344; **Board Cert:** Dermatology 1970; **Med School:** Columbia P&S 1963; **Resid:** Internal Medicine, Mt Sinai Hosp 1965; Dermatology, NYU Med Ctr 1970; **Fac Appt:** Prof D, NYU Sch Med

Silverberg, Nanette B MD (D) - **Spec Exp:** Pediatric Dermatology; Vitiligo; Atopic Dermatitis; Viral Infections; **Hospital:** St. Luke's - Roosevelt Hosp Ctr - Roosevelt Div (page 94), Beth Israel Med Ctr - Petrie Division (page 94); **Address:** 425 W 59th St, Ste 5C, New York, NY 10019; **Phone:** 212-523-6003; **Board Cert:** Dermatology 2006; Pediatric Dermatology 2004; **Med School:** SUNY Downstate 1994; **Resid:** Dermatology, SUNY Downstate 1998; **Fellow:** Pediatric Dermatology, Chldn's Meml Hosp 1999; **Fac Appt:** Clin Prof D, Columbia P&S

Sobel, Howard MD (D) - **Spec Exp:** Cosmetic Dermatology; Botox Therapy; Liposuction; Laser Surgery; **Hospital:** Lenox Hill Hosp (page 106), Beth Israel Med Ctr - Petrie Division (page 94); **Address:** 960A Park Ave, New York, NY 10028-0325; **Phone:** 212-288-0060; **Med School:** Albert Einstein Coll Med 1975; **Resid:** Dermatology, Emory Univ Hosp 1979

Soter, Nicholas A MD (D) - **Spec Exp:** Urticaria; Psoriasis; Vasculitis; Phototherapy; **Hospital:** NYU Langone Med Ctr (page 108); **Address:** 240 E 38th St Fl 12, New York, NY 10016-6402; **Phone:** 212-263-5889; **Board Cert:** Dermatology 1970; Diagnostic Lab Immunology 1985; **Med School:** Univ Tex SW, Dallas 1965; **Resid:** Dermatology, Baylor Med Ctr 1968; Dermatology, Mass Genl Hosp 1969; **Fellow:** Immunology, Harvard Med Sch 1973; **Fac Appt:** Prof D, NYU Sch Med

Tanenbaum, Diane G MD (D) - **Spec Exp:** Skin Cancer; **Hospital:** Lenox Hill Hosp (page 106), NYU Langone Med Ctr (page 108); **Address:** 16 E 79th St, Ste 22, New York, NY 10075-0150; **Phone:** 212-249-6122; **Board Cert:** Dermatology 1971; **Med School:** SUNY Downstate 1964; **Resid:** Dermatology, NYU Med Ctr 1970; **Fac Appt:** Assoc Clin Prof D, NYU Sch Med

Tesser, Mark F MD (D) - **Spec Exp:** Cosmetic Dermatology; Skin Cancer; **Hospital:** Mount Sinai Med Ctr (page 102); **Address:** 1107 Park Ave, New York, NY 10128; **Phone:** 212-996-9600; **Board Cert:** Internal Medicine 1977; Dermatology 1980; **Med School:** Albert Einstein Coll Med 1974; **Resid:** Internal Medicine, Mount Sinai Hosp 1977; Dermatology, Mount Sinai Hosp 1979; **Fac Appt:** Asst Clin Prof D, Mount Sinai Sch Med

Unger, Walter P MD (D) - **Spec Exp:** Hair Restoration/Transplant; **Hospital:** Mount Sinai Med Ctr (page 102); **Address:** 710 Park Ave, New York, NY 10021-6591; **Phone:** 212-249-9393; **Board Cert:** Dermatology 1968; Hair Restoration Surgery 2008; **Med School:** Univ Toronto 1963; **Resid:** Dermatology, Philadelphia Skin-Cancer Hosp 1967; Internal Medicine, Sunny Brook Hosp 1968; **Fac Appt:** Clin Prof D, Mount Sinai Sch Med

Vogel, Louis N MD (D) - **Spec Exp:** Cosmetic Dermatology; Botox Therapy; Hair Removal-Laser; **Hospital:** NYU Langone Med Ctr (page 108); **Address:** 16 Park Ave, Ste 1D, New York, NY 10016-4329; **Phone:** 212-447-5443; **Board Cert:** Internal Medicine 1980; Dermatology 1983; **Med School:** Boston Univ 1977; **Resid:** Internal Medicine, NYU Med Ctr 1980; Dermatology, NYU Med Ctr 1983; **Fac Appt:** Asst Clin Prof D, NYU Sch Med

Walther, Robert MD (D) - **Spec Exp:** Acne; Skin Cancer; Psoriasis; **Hospital:** NY-Presby/Columbia Univ Med Ctr, NY (page 104); **Address:** 16 E 60th St, Ste 300, New York, NY 10022; **Phone:** 212-326-8465; **Board Cert:** Dermatology 2009; Internal Medicine 1977; **Med School:** Univ NC Sch Med 1973; **Resid:** Internal Medicine, Univ Miami Hosps 1975; Dermatology, Columbia-Presby Hosp 1978; **Fellow:** Dermatology, Rockefeller Univ Hosp 1980; **Fac Appt:** Clin Prof D, Columbia P&S

Warner, Robert MD (D) - **Spec Exp:** Laser Surgery; Laser Hair Removal; Cosmetic Dermatology; Botox Therapy; **Hospital:** Mount Sinai Med Ctr (page 102); **Address:** 580 Park Ave, New York, NY 10065; **Phone:** 212-752-3692; **Board Cert:** Dermatology 1981; **Med School:** SUNY Hlth Sci Ctr 1977; **Resid:** Dermatology, Mount Sinai Hosp 1981; **Fac Appt:** Asst Clin Prof D, Mount Sinai Sch Med

Wattenberg, Debra J MD (D) - **Spec Exp:** Cosmetic Dermatology; Botox Therapy; Skin Laser Surgery; Acne; **Hospital:** Mount Sinai Med Ctr (page 102); **Address:** 875 Fifth Ave, New York, NY 10065; **Phone:** 212-288-3200; **Board Cert:** Dermatology 2001; **Med School:** Mount Sinai Sch Med 1988; **Resid:** Internal Medicine, Beth Israel Med Ctr 1989; Dermatology, Mount Sinai Hosp 1992; **Fac Appt:** Assoc Clin Prof D, Mount Sinai Sch Med

Wechsler, Amy B MD (D) - **Spec Exp:** Cosmetic Dermatology; Acne; Skin Laser Surgery; **Address:** 3 E 69th St, New York, NY 10021; **Phone:** 212-396-2500; **Board Cert:** Psychiatry 2010; Dermatology 2005; **Med School:** Cornell Univ 1995; **Resid:** Psychiatry, Payne Whitney Clinic 1999; **Fellow:** Child & Adolescent Psychiatry, Payne Whitney Clinic 2001; Dermatology, SUNY Downstate 2004

Wexler, Patricia MD (D) - **Spec Exp:** Facial Rejuvenation; Liposuction; Botox Therapy; Acne; **Hospital:** Mount Sinai Med Ctr (page 102); **Address:** 145 E 32nd St Fl 7, New York, NY 10016; **Phone:** 212-684-2626; **Board Cert:** Internal Medicine 1983; Dermatology 1986; **Med School:** Belgium 1979; **Resid:** Internal Medicine, Beth Israel Med Ctr 1982; Dermatology, Mt Sinai Hosp 1986; **Fellow:** Infectious Disease, Beth Israel Med Ctr 1983; **Fac Appt:** Assoc Clin Prof D, Mount Sinai Sch Med

Diagnostic Radiology

Abramson, Sara J MD (DR) - **Spec Exp:** Pediatric Radiology; **Hospital:** Meml Sloan-Kettering Cancer Ctr (page 116); **Address:** 444 E 68th St, New York, NY 10065; **Phone:** 212-639-2184; **Board Cert:** Diagnostic Radiology 1976; **Med School:** Mount Sinai Sch Med 1971; **Resid:** Pediatrics, Mt Sinai Hosp 1973; Diagnostic Radiology, Chldns Mercy Hosp 1976; **Fellow:** Pediatric Radiology, Chldns Hosp 1981; **Fac Appt:** Prof Rad, Cornell Univ-Weill Med Coll

Adler, Ronald S MD/PhD (DR) - **Spec Exp:** Musculoskeletal Imaging; Ultrasound; Power Doppler Imaging; **Hospital:** NYU Langone Med Ctr (page 108), NYU Hosp For Joint Diseases (page 119); **Address:** Ctr for Musculoskeletal Care-Radiology Dept, 333 E 38th St Fl 6, New York, NY 10016; **Phone:** 646-501-7289; **Board Cert:** Diagnostic Radiology 1988; **Med School:** Wayne State Univ 1984; **Resid:** Diagnostic Radiology, Univ Mich Med Ctr 1988; **Fellow:** Ultrasound/CT/MRI, Univ Mich Med Ctr 1989; **Fac Appt:** Prof Rad, Cornell Univ-Weill Med Coll

Austin, John H M MD (DR) - **Spec Exp:** Lung Cancer; Thoracic Radiology; **Hospital:** NY-Presby/Columbia Univ Med Ctr, NY (page 104); **Address:** 177 Fort Washington Ave, Milstein Hosp Bldg 3-202C, New York, NY 10032-3784; **Phone:** 212-305-2639; **Board Cert:** Diagnostic Radiology 1970; **Med School:** Yale Univ 1965; **Resid:** Diagnostic Radiology, UCSF Med Ctr 1968; **Fellow:** Diagnostic Radiology, UCSF Med Ctr 1970; **Fac Appt:** Prof Emeritus Rad, Columbia P&S

Baer, Jeanne W MD (DR) - **Spec Exp:** Abdominal Imaging; **Hospital:** St. Luke's - Roosevelt Hosp Ctr - St Luke's Hosp (page 94); **Address:** St Luke's Hosp, Dept Radiology, 1111 Amsterdam Ave, New York, NY 10025; **Phone:** 212-523-4272; **Board Cert:** Diagnostic Radiology 1971; **Med School:** Columbia P&S 1964; **Resid:** Internal Medicine, Geo Wash Univ Med Ctr 1967; **Fellow:** Diagnostic Radiology, St Luke's-Roosevelt Hosp Ctr 1970; **Fac Appt:** Assoc Clin Prof Rad, Columbia P&S

Barone, Clement MD (DR) - **Spec Exp:** Women's Imaging; Mammography; Bone Densitometry; **Address:** 1440 York Ave, Ste P-1, New York, NY 10075; **Phone:** 212-988-1303; **Board Cert:** Diagnostic Radiology 1974; **Med School:** NY Med Coll 1968; **Resid:** Diagnostic Radiology, Mt Sinai Hosp 1970; Diagnostic Radiology, Mt Sinai Hosp 1974; **Fac Appt:** Asst Clin Prof, Mount Sinai Sch Med

Berson, Barry MD (DR) - **Spec Exp:** Mammography; Breast Imaging; Bone Densitometry; **Hospital:** Mount Sinai Med Ctr (page 102); **Address:** 165 E 84th St, New York, NY 10028-0302; **Phone:** 212-535-9770; **Board Cert:** Diagnostic Radiology 1990; **Med School:** Mount Sinai Sch Med 1984; **Resid:** Diagnostic Radiology, Mount Sinai Hosp 1990; **Fellow:** Neuroradiology, NYU Med Ctr 1992

Brill, Paula MD (DR) - **Spec Exp:** Pediatric Radiology; Bone Imaging; **Hospital:** NY-Presby/Weill Cornell Med Ctr, NY (page 104); **Address:** 525 E 68th St, New York, NY 10065; **Phone:** 212-746-2554; **Board Cert:** Pediatrics 1970; Diagnostic Radiology 1971; Pediatric Radiology 2005; **Med School:** Cornell Univ-Weill Med Coll 1962; **Resid:** Pediatrics, New York Hosp 1968; Diagnostic Radiology, New York Hosp 1971; **Fellow:** Diagnostic Radiology, Cornell Univ 1971; **Fac Appt:** Prof, Cornell Univ-Weill Med Coll

Cohen, Burton A MD (DR) - **Spec Exp:** CT Scan; MRI; PET Imaging; **Hospital:** Mount Sinai Med Ctr (page 102); **Address:** 165 E 84th St, New York, NY 10028; **Phone:** 212-535-9770; **Board Cert:** Diagnostic Radiology 1979; **Med School:** NY Med Coll 1975; **Resid:** Diagnostic Radiology, Mt Sinai Hosp 1979; **Fac Appt:** Assoc Clin Prof Rad, Mount Sinai Sch Med

Dershaw, D David MD (DR) - **Spec Exp:** Breast Imaging; Breast Cancer; Mammography; **Hospital:** Meml Sloan-Kettering Cancer Ctr (page 116); **Address:** 300 E 66th St, rm 727, New York, NY 10065; **Phone:** 646-888-4505; **Board Cert:** Diagnostic Radiology 1978; **Med School:** Jefferson Med Coll 1974; **Resid:** Diagnostic Radiology, New York Hosp 1978; **Fellow:** Ultrasound, Thos Jefferson Univ Hosp 1979; **Fac Appt:** Prof Rad, Cornell Univ-Weill Med Coll

Edelstein, Barbara A MD (DR) - **Spec Exp:** Breast Cancer; Women's Imaging; **Address:** 1045 Park Ave, New York, NY 10028; **Phone:** 212-860-7700; **Board Cert:** Diagnostic Radiology 1983; **Med School:** NY Med Coll 1977; **Resid:** Diagnostic Radiology, Montefiore Hosp 1982

Fefferman, Nancy R MD (DR) - **Spec Exp:** Pediatric Radiology; **Hospital:** NYU Langone Med Ctr (page 108); **Address:** 560 First Ave Fl 2 - Ste 234, New York, NY 10016; **Phone:** 212-263-5362; **Board Cert:** Radiology 1996; Pediatric Radiology 2009; **Med School:** NYU Sch Med 1991; **Resid:** Radiology, NYU Langone Med Ctr 1996; **Fellow:** Pediatric Radiology, NYU Langone Med Ctr 1997; **Fac Appt:** Asst Prof Rad, NYU Sch Med

Fried, Karen O MD (DR) - **Spec Exp:** Ultrasound; Thyroid Ultrasound; Vascular Ultrasound; **Address:** Lenox Hill Radiology, 61 E 77th St, New York, NY 10075; **Phone:** 212-772-3111; **Board Cert:** Diagnostic Radiology 1990; **Med School:** Albany Med Coll 1985; **Resid:** Diagnostic Radiology, LIJ Med Ctr 1990; **Fellow:** Cross Sectional Imaging, LIJ Med Ctr 1991

Genieser, Nancy B MD (DR) - **Spec Exp:** Neonatal Radiology; Pediatric Radiology; Child Abuse Imaging; **Hospital:** NYU Langone Med Ctr (page 108), Bellevue Hosp Ctr; **Address:** 462 1st Ave, NBV 3W33, New York, NY 10016-9196; **Phone:** 212-263-6373; **Board Cert:** Radiology 1967; Pediatric Radiology 2005; **Med School:** Med Coll PA Hahnemann 1962; **Resid:** Diagnostic Radiology, NYU Med Ctr 1966; **Fac Appt:** Prof Rad, NYU Sch Med

Ginsberg, Michelle S MD (DR) - **Spec Exp:** Lung Cancer; Thoracic Radiology; Pulmonary Embolism; Gastrointestinal Imaging; **Hospital:** Meml Sloan-Kettering Cancer Ctr (page 116); **Address:** Meml Sloan Kettering Cancer Ctr, 1275 York Ave, Dept Radiology, New York, NY 10021; **Phone:** 212-639-7292; **Board Cert:** Diagnostic Radiology 1995; **Med School:** Brown Univ 1990; **Resid:** Radiology, Montefiore Med Ctr- Weiler Div 1995; **Fellow:** Diagnostic Radiology, Meml Sloan Kettering Cancer Ctr 1996; **Fac Appt:** Assoc Prof Rad, Cornell Univ-Weill Med Coll

Henschke, Claudia L MD/PhD (DR) - **Spec Exp:** Lung Cancer; Lung Disease; Thoracic Radiology; **Hospital:** Mount Sinai Med Ctr (page 102); **Address:** Mt Sinai Med Ctr, Radiology Dept, 1 Gustave Levy Pl, Box 1234, New York, NY 10029; **Phone:** 212-241-2420; **Board Cert:** Diagnostic Radiology 1981; **Med School:** Howard Univ 1977; **Resid:** Diagnostic Radiology, Brigham & Womens Hosp 1983; **Fac Appt:** Prof Rad, Cornell Univ-Weill Med Coll

Herman, Zeva W MD (DR) - **Spec Exp:** Breast Imaging; Ultrasound; MRI; **Hospital:** Mount Sinai Med Ctr (page 102); **Address:** 525 Park Ave, New York, NY 10065; **Phone:** 212-888-1000 x1574; **Board Cert:** Diagnostic Radiology 1993; **Med School:** Mount Sinai Sch Med 1989; **Resid:** Diagnostic Radiology, Lenox Hill Hosp 1992; **Fellow:** Body Imaging, Meml Sloan Kettering Cancer Ctr 1993; **Fac Appt:** Rad, Mount Sinai Sch Med

Holliday, Roy MD (DR) - **Spec Exp:** Head & Neck Imaging; **Hospital:** New York Eye & Ear Infirm (page 117), Beth Israel Med Ctr - Petrie Division (page 94); **Address:** 310 E 14th St, New York, NY 10003; **Phone:** 212-979-4397; **Board Cert:** Diagnostic Radiology 1986; **Med School:** NYU Sch Med 1982; **Resid:** Diagnostic Radiology, NYU Med Ctr 1986; **Fellow:** Neurological Radiology, NYU Med Ctr 1987; **Fac Appt:** Clin Prof Rad, NYU Sch Med

Hricak, Hedvig MD/PhD (DR) - **Spec Exp:** Prostate Cancer-MR Spectroscopy (MRSI); Breast Imaging; Breast Cancer; **Hospital:** Meml Sloan-Kettering Cancer Ctr (page 116); **Address:** 1275 York Ave, Ste C278, New York, NY 10065; **Phone:** 800-525-2225; **Board Cert:** Diagnostic Radiology 1978; **Med School:** Yugoslavia 1970; **Resid:** Diagnostic Radiology, St Joseph Mercy Hosp 1977; **Fellow:** Ultrasound/CT, Henry Ford Hosp 1978; **Fac Appt:** Prof Rad, Cornell Univ-Weill Med Coll

Jacobs, Morton MD (DR) - **Spec Exp:** Neuroradiology; Head & Neck Imaging; Musculoskeletal Imaging; **Address:** Manhattan Diagnostic Radiology, 400 E 66th St, New York, NY 10065; **Phone:** 212-838-4243; **Board Cert:** Diagnostic Radiology 1976; Neuroradiology 1996; **Med School:** Univ Chicago-Pritzker Sch Med 1972; **Resid:** Diagnostic Radiology, New York Hosp 1976; **Fellow:** Neuroradiology, New York Hosp 1979

Levy, Miriam MD (DR) - **Spec Exp:** Breast Imaging; Mammography; Women's Imaging; **Address:** Medical Imaging of Manhattan, 635 Madison Ave Fl 16, New York, NY 10022; **Phone:** 212-794-2500; **Board Cert:** Diagnostic Radiology 1983; **Med School:** Albert Einstein Coll Med 1979; **Resid:** Diagnostic Radiology, Geo Wash Univ Hosp 1982; Diagnostic Radiology, St Vincents Hosp 1983; **Fellow:** Ultrasound/CT/MRI, New York Hosp 1984; **Fac Appt:** Asst Clin Prof Path, Mount Sinai Sch Med

Math, Kevin MD (DR) - **Spec Exp:** Musculoskeletal Imaging; **Hospital:** Beth Israel Med Ctr - Petrie Division (page 94); **Address:** East Manhattan Diagnostic Imaging, 604 2nd Ave, at 33rd St, New York, NY 10116; **Phone:** 212-683-6200; **Board Cert:** Diagnostic Radiology 1993; **Med School:** SUNY Upstate Med Univ 1988; **Resid:** Diagnostic Radiology, SUNY Hlth Sci Ctr 1993; **Fellow:** Musculoskeletal Imaging, Hosp Special Surgery/Weill Cornell Med Ctr 1994; **Fac Appt:** Assoc Prof Rad, Albert Einstein Coll Med

Megibow, Alec J MD (DR) - **Spec Exp:** Abdominal Imaging; Gastrointestinal Imaging; CT Body Scan; **Hospital:** NYU Langone Med Ctr (page 108), Bellevue Hosp Ctr; **Address:** 550 1st Ave, HHC 232, New York, NY 10016; **Phone:** 212-263-5222; **Board Cert:** Diagnostic Radiology 1978; **Med School:** SUNY Upstate Med Univ 1974; **Resid:** Diagnostic Radiology, Bellevue/NYU Med Ctr 1978; **Fellow:** Abdominal Imaging, NYU Med Ctr 1978; **Fac Appt:** Prof Rad, NYU Sch Med

Miller, Theodore MD (DR) - **Spec Exp:** Musculoskeletal Imaging; Ultrasound; **Hospital:** Hosp For Special Surgery (page 115); **Address:** Dept Radiology, 535 E 70th St, New York, NY 10021; **Phone:** 212-606-1127; **Board Cert:** Diagnostic Radiology 1993; **Med School:** Vanderbilt Univ 1987; **Resid:** Radiology, Mt Sinai Hosp 1992; **Fellow:** Radiology, Hosp for Spec Surg 1993; **Fac Appt:** Assoc Prof Rad, Cornell Univ-Weill Med Coll

Mitnick, Julie MD (DR) - **Spec Exp:** Mammography; Breast Cancer; **Address:** 650 1st Ave, New York, NY 10016; **Phone:** 212-686-4440; **Board Cert:** Diagnostic Radiology 1977; **Med School:** NYU Sch Med 1972; **Resid:** Diagnostic Radiology, NYU Med Ctr 1977; **Fellow:** Pediatric Radiology, NYU Med Ctr 1978; **Fac Appt:** Assoc Clin Prof Rad, NYU Sch Med

Morris, Elizabeth A MD (DR) - **Spec Exp:** Breast Imaging; Breast MRI; Breast Cancer; **Hospital:** Meml Sloan-Kettering Cancer Ctr (page 116); **Address:** 300 E 66th St Fl 7, New York, NY 10065; **Phone:** 646-888-4510; **Board Cert:** Diagnostic Radiology 1994; **Med School:** UCSF 1989; **Resid:** Diagnostic Radiology, NY-Cornell Med Ctr 1993; **Fellow:** Breast Imaging, Meml Sloan-Kettering Cancer Ctr 1994; **Fac Appt:** Assoc Prof Rad, Cornell Univ-Weill Med Coll

Naidich, David P MD (DR) - **Spec Exp:** Chest Radiology; Chronic Lung Disease; Lung Cancer; Pulmonary Embolism; **Hospital:** NYU Langone Med Ctr (page 108), Bellevue Hosp Ctr; **Address:** NYU Medical Center, Dept Radiology, 560 1st Ave, rm 236, New York, NY 10016; **Phone:** 212-263-5229; **Board Cert:** Diagnostic Radiology 1980; **Med School:** NYU Sch Med 1975; **Resid:** Diagnostic Radiology, Johns Hopkins Hosp 1979; **Fellow:** Cross Sectional Imaging, Johns Hopkins Hosp 1980; **Fac Appt:** Prof Rad, NYU Sch Med

Neistadt, L Daniel MD (DR) - **Spec Exp:** CT Body Scan; Gastrointestinal Imaging; Ultrasound; PET Imaging; **Address:** Manhattan Diagnostic Radiology, 400 E 66th St, New York, NY 10065; **Phone:** 212-838-4243; **Board Cert:** Internal Medicine 1975; Nuclear Medicine 1977; Diagnostic Radiology 1980; **Med School:** Stanford Univ 1972; **Resid:** Nuclear Medicine, New York Hosp 1977; Diagnostic Radiology, New York Hosp 1980; **Fellow:** Ultrasound/CT, New York Hosp 1981

Newhouse, Jeffrey MD (DR) - **Spec Exp:** Abdominal Imaging; Pelvic Imaging; **Hospital:** NY-Presby/Columbia Univ Med Ctr, NY (page 104); **Address:** 177 Fort Washington Ave, Millstein Bldg, 3rd Fl-Radiology, New York, NY 10032; **Phone:** 212-305-7898; **Board Cert:** Diagnostic Radiology 1972; **Med School:** Harvard Med Sch 1967; **Resid:** Diagnostic Radiology, Mass Genl Hosp 1972; **Fac Appt:** Prof, Columbia P&S

Novick, Mark D MD (DR) - **Spec Exp:** Breast Imaging; Mammography; MRI; **Address:** Lenox Hill Radiology, 61 E 77th St, New York, NY 10075; **Phone:** 212-772-3111; **Board Cert:** Diagnostic Radiology 1983; **Med School:** Univ Tenn Coll Med 1978; **Resid:** Diagnostic Radiology, Univ Tenn Med Ctr 1982; **Fellow:** Magnetic Resonance Imaging, UCSF Med Ctr

Panicek, David M MD (DR) - **Spec Exp:** Bone Cancer; Soft Tissue Tumors; Musculoskeletal Tumor Imaging; **Hospital:** Meml Sloan-Kettering Cancer Ctr (page 116); **Address:** 1275 York Ave, Ste C276G, Meml Sloan Kettering Cancer Ctr, New York, NY 10065; **Phone:** 800-525-2225; **Board Cert:** Diagnostic Radiology 1984; **Med School:** Cornell Univ-Weill Med Coll 1980; **Resid:** Diagnostic Radiology, NY Hosp-Cornell Med Ctr 1984; **Fac Appt:** Prof Rad, Cornell Univ-Weill Med Coll

Pavlov, Helene MD (DR) - **Spec Exp:** Sports Medicine Radiology; Musculoskeletal Imaging; Orthopaedic Imaging; **Hospital:** Hosp For Special Surgery (page 115), NY-Presby/Weill Cornell Med Ctr, NY (page 104); **Address:** Hosp for Special Surgery, 535 E 70th St, New York, NY 10021-4892; **Phone:** 212-606-1132; **Board Cert:** Diagnostic Radiology 1976; **Med School:** Temple Univ 1972; **Resid:** Diagnostic Radiology, Germantown Hosp 1976; **Fellow:** Musculoskeletal Imaging, Hosp For Special Surg 1977; **Fac Appt:** Prof Rad, Cornell Univ-Weill Med Coll

Pfaff, H Charles MD (DR) - **Spec Exp:** Musculoskeletal Imaging; Neuroradiology; **Hospital:** Beth Israel Med Ctr - Petrie Division (page 94), New York Eye & Ear Infirm (page 117); **Address:** New York Radiology Associates, 55 E 34th St, New York, NY 10016; **Phone:** 212-252-6071; **Board Cert:** Diagnostic Radiology 1992; **Med School:** Univ NC Sch Med 1987; **Resid:** Diagnostic Radiology, NY-Presby/Columbia Med Ctr 1992; **Fellow:** Nephrology, NY Presby/Columbia Med Ctr 1993; **Fac Appt:** Asst Prof Rad, Albert Einstein Coll Med

Potter, Hollis G MD (DR) - **Spec Exp:** Musculoskeletal Imaging; Cartilage Damage; Arthroplasty Imaging; **Hospital:** Hosp For Special Surgery (page 115); **Address:** Hosp for Special Surgery, MRI-basement, 535 E 70th St, Ste MRI, New York, NY 10021-4892; **Phone:** 212-606-1023; **Board Cert:** Diagnostic Radiology 1990; **Med School:** NY Med Coll 1985; **Resid:** Diagnostic Radiology, North Shore Univ Hosp 1990; **Fellow:** Diagnostic Radiology, Hosp Special Surgery 1991; **Fac Appt:** Prof Rad, Cornell Univ-Weill Med Coll

Prince, Martin R MD/PhD (DR) - **Spec Exp:** MRI Angiography; Abdominal Imaging; **Hospital:** NY-Presby/Weill Cornell Med Ctr, NY (page 104), NY-Presby/Columbia Univ Med Ctr, NY (page 104); **Address:** 416 E 55th St, New York, NY 10022; **Phone:** 212-746-6880; **Board Cert:** Diagnostic Radiology 1993; **Med School:** Harvard Med Sch 1985; **Resid:** Radiology, Mass Genl Hosp 1993; **Fellow:** Magnetic Resonance Imaging, Mass Genl Hosp 1993; Angiography, Mass Genl Hosp 1989; **Fac Appt:** Prof Rad, Cornell Univ-Weill Med Coll

Recht, Michael MD (DR) - **Spec Exp:** Musculoskeletal Imaging; **Hospital:** NYU Langone Med Ctr (page 108); **Address:** NYU Sch Med, Dept Radiology, rm IRM 229, New York, NY 10016; **Phone:** 212-263-9530; **Board Cert:** Diagnostic Radiology 1987; **Med School:** Univ Pennsylvania 1983; **Resid:** Radiology, Hosp Univ Penn 1987; **Fellow:** Interventional Radiology, Hosp Univ Penn 1987; Musculoskeletal Imaging, UCSD Med Ctr 1992

Rifkin, Matthew D MD (DR) - **Spec Exp:** CT Scan; MRI; Ultrasound; **Address:** Canal Street Radiology, 212 Canal St, Ste 203, New York, NY 10013; **Phone:** 212-349-5799; **Board Cert:** Diagnostic Radiology 1978; **Med School:** Albert Einstein Coll Med 1974; **Resid:** Diagnostic Radiology, Montefiore Hosp 1978; **Fellow:** Ultrasound/CT, Johns Hopkins Hosp 1979

Rosenberg, Zehava MD (DR) - **Spec Exp:** Musculoskeletal Imaging; **Hospital:** NYU Langone Med Ctr (page 108), NYU Hosp For Joint Diseases (page 119); **Address:** NYU Hosp for Joint Diseases, 301 E 17th St, rm 600, New York, NY 10003; **Phone:** 212-598-6373; **Board Cert:** Diagnostic Radiology 1985; **Med School:** Univ Conn 1980; **Resid:** Diagnostic Radiology, Einstein Affil Hosp 1984; **Fellow:** Musculoskeletal Imaging, NY Columbia-Presby Hosp 1986; **Fac Appt:** Prof Rad, NYU Sch Med

Rosenblatt, Ruth MD (DR) - **Spec Exp:** Breast Cancer; **Hospital:** NY-Presby/Weill Cornell Med Ctr, NY (page 104); **Address:** 425 E 61st St Fl 9, New York, NY 10065; **Phone:** 212-821-0600; **Board Cert:** Diagnostic Radiology 1969; **Med School:** Med Coll PA Hahnemann 1964; **Resid:** Diagnostic Radiology, Montefiore Med Ctr 1968; **Fac Appt:** Clin Prof, Cornell Univ-Weill Med Coll

Rosenfeld, Stanley MD (DR) - **Spec Exp:** Mammography; Ultrasound; Breast MRI; **Hospital:** Mount Sinai Med Ctr (page 102); **Address:** 1421 3rd Ave, Rosetta Radiology, New York, NY 10028; **Phone:** 212-744-5538; **Board Cert:** Diagnostic Radiology 1978; **Med School:** Albert Einstein Coll Med 1974; **Resid:** Diagnostic Radiology, Montefiore Hosp Med Ctr 1978; **Fac Appt:** Asst Prof Rad, Mount Sinai Sch Med

Ruzal-Shapiro, Carrie MD (DR) - **Spec Exp:** Pediatric Radiology; **Hospital:** NY-Presby/Columbia Univ Med Ctr, NY (page 104); **Address:** 3959 Broadway, Dept Radiology, Chony 3 North, New York, NY 10032; **Phone:** 212-305-9665; **Board Cert:** Diagnostic Radiology 1988; Pediatric Radiology 2004; **Med School:** Columbia P&S 1982; **Resid:** Radiology, Columbia-Presby Med Ctr 1988; **Fellow:** Pediatric Radiology, Columbia-Presby Med Ctr 1989; **Fac Appt:** Clin Prof Rad, Columbia P&S

Schwartz, Lawrence H MD (DR) - **Spec Exp:** Prostate Cancer; MRI; **Hospital:** NY-Presby/Columbia Univ Med Ctr, NY (page 104); **Address:** 180 Ft Washington Ave, Harkness Pav, rm 320, New York, NY 10032; **Phone:** 212-305-8994; **Board Cert:** Diagnostic Radiology 1991; **Med School:** Boston Univ 1986; **Resid:** Diagnostic Radiology, NY Hosp-Cornell Med Ctr 1991; **Fellow:** Ultrasound/CT/MRI, Brigham & Women's Hosp 1991; **Fac Appt:** Prof Rad, Cornell Univ-Weill Med Coll

Som, Peter MD (DR) - **Spec Exp:** Head & Neck Imaging; **Hospital:** Mount Sinai Med Ctr (page 102); **Address:** Mount Sinai Med Ctr, Dept Radiology, 1 Gustave Levy Pl, New York, NY 10029-6504; **Phone:** 212-241-7420; **Board Cert:** Diagnostic Radiology 1972; **Med School:** NYU Sch Med 1967; **Resid:** Diagnostic Radiology, Mt Sinai Hosp 1971; **Fac Appt:** Prof, Mount Sinai Sch Med

Sonnenblick, Emily B MD (DR) - **Spec Exp:** Women's Imaging; Breast MRI; **Hospital:** Mount Sinai Med Ctr (page 102); **Address:** Rosetta Radiology, 1421 Third Ave, New York, NY 10028; **Phone:** 212-744-5538; **Board Cert:** Diagnostic Radiology 1987; **Med School:** Cornell Univ-Weill Med Coll 1982; **Resid:** Diagnostic Radiology, Hosp U Penn 1984; Diagnostic Radiology, Columbia-Presby Med Ctr 1986; **Fellow:** Ultrasound, Mt Sinai Med Ctr 1987

Wolff, Steven D MD/PhD (DR) - **Spec Exp:** Cardiovascular Imaging; Cardiac MRI; **Hospital:** Lenox Hill Hosp (page 106), NY-Presby/Columbia Univ Med Ctr, NY (page 104); **Address:** 62 E 88th St, Lower Level, New York, NY 10128; **Phone:** 212-369-9200; **Board Cert:** Diagnostic Radiology 1994; **Med School:** Duke Univ 1989; **Resid:** Diagnostic Radiology, Johns Hopkins Hosp 1994

Yankelevitz, David MD (DR) - **Spec Exp:** Lung Cancer; Thoracic Radiology; **Hospital:** Mount Sinai Med Ctr (page 102); **Address:** Mt Sinai Med Ctr, Radiology Dept, 1 Gustave Levy Pl, Box 1234, New York, NY 10029; **Phone:** 212-241-2420; **Board Cert:** Diagnostic Radiology 1987; Nuclear Medicine 1987; **Med School:** SUNY Hlth Sci Ctr 1981; **Resid:** Diagnostic Radiology, Long Island Coll Hosp 1984; Nuclear Medicine, NY-Cornell Med Ctr 1987; **Fellow:** Diagnostic Radiology, NY-Cornell Med Ctr 1987; **Fac Appt:** Prof Rad, Cornell Univ-Weill Med Coll

Endocrinology, Diabetes & Metabolism

Bergman, Donald MD (EDM) - **Spec Exp:** Osteoporosis; Thyroid Disorders; Calcium Disorders; Paget's Disease of Bone; **Hospital:** Mount Sinai Med Ctr (page 102); **Address:** 1199 Park Ave, Ste 1F, New York, NY 10128; **Phone:** 212-876-7333; **Board Cert:** Internal Medicine 1975; Endocrinology, Diabetes & Metabolism 1977; **Med School:** Jefferson Med Coll 1971; **Resid:** Obstetrics & Gynecology, Mt Sinai Hosp 1972; Internal Medicine, Mt Sinai Hosp 1975; **Fellow:** Endocrinology, Diabetes & Metabolism, Mt Sinai Hosp 1977; **Fac Appt:** Clin Prof Med, Mount Sinai Sch Med

Bilezikian, John P MD (EDM) - **Spec Exp:** Osteoporosis; Bone Disorders-Metabolic; Parathyroid Disorders; **Hospital:** NY-Presby/Columbia Univ Med Ctr, NY (page 104); **Address:** Columbia Metabolic Bone Disease Program, Harkness Pavilion, 180 Ft Washington Ave Fl 9 - Ste 904, New York, NY 10032; **Phone:** 212-305-2663; **Board Cert:** Internal Medicine 1975; Endocrinology, Diabetes & Metabolism 1977; **Med School:** Columbia P&S 1969; **Resid:** Internal Medicine, Columbia-Presby Hosp 1975; **Fellow:** Endocrinology, Diabetes & Metabolism, Natl Inst Health 1977; **Fac Appt:** Prof Med, Columbia P&S

Bloomgarden, Zachary T MD (EDM) - **Spec Exp:** Diabetes; Diabetic Kidney Disease; Cholesterol/Lipid Disorders; **Hospital:** Mount Sinai Med Ctr (page 102); **Address:** 35 E 85th St, New York, NY 10028-0954; **Phone:** 212-879-5933; **Board Cert:** Internal Medicine 1977; Endocrinology, Diabetes & Metabolism 1979; **Med School:** Albert Einstein Coll Med 1974; **Resid:** Internal Medicine, Montefiore Med Ctr 1977; **Fellow:** Endocrinology, Diabetes & Metabolism, Vanderbilt Univ Med Ctr 1979; **Fac Appt:** Assoc Clin Prof Med, Mount Sinai Sch Med

Blum, Conrad B MD (EDM) - **Spec Exp:** Cholesterol/Lipid Disorders; Thyroid Disorders; Diabetes; **Hospital:** NY-Presby/Columbia Univ Med Ctr, NY (page 104); **Address:** 16 E 60th St, Ste 320, New York, NY 10022-1002; **Phone:** 212-326-8421; **Board Cert:** Internal Medicine 1976; Endocrinology, Diabetes & Metabolism 1977; **Med School:** Northwestern Univ 1971; **Resid:** Internal Medicine, Brigham Women & Chldn's Hosp 1976; **Fellow:** Endocrinology, Diabetes & Metabolism, Northwestern Univ Med Sch 1977; **Fac Appt:** Clin Prof Med, Columbia P&S

Bockman, Richard S MD/PhD (EDM) - **Spec Exp:** Bone Disorders-Metabolic; Osteoporosis; Parathyroid Disorders; Paget's Disease of Bone; **Hospital:** Hosp For Special Surgery (page 115), NY-Presby/Weill Cornell Med Ctr, NY (page 104); **Address:** 519 E 72nd St, Ste 206, New York, NY 10021; **Phone:** 212-606-1458; **Board Cert:** Internal Medicine 1975; **Med School:** Yale Univ 1968; **Resid:** Internal Medicine, NYU Med Ctr 1975; **Fellow:** Internal Medicine, NY-Cornell Med Ctr 1973; **Fac Appt:** Prof Med, Cornell Univ-Weill Med Coll

Brett, Elise M MD (EDM) - **Spec Exp:** Diabetes; Osteoporosis; **Hospital:** Mount Sinai Med Ctr (page 102); **Address:** 1192 Park Ave, New York, NY 10128; **Phone:** 212-831-2100; **Board Cert:** Internal Medicine 2007; Endocrinology, Diabetes & Metabolism 2009; **Med School:** Mount Sinai Sch Med 1994; **Resid:** Internal Medicine, Mt Sinai Hosp 1997; **Fellow:** Endocrinology, Diabetes & Metabolism, Mt Sinai Hosp 1999; **Fac Appt:** Assoc Clin Prof Med, Mount Sinai Sch Med

Brillon, David J MD (EDM) - **Spec Exp:** Diabetes; Thyroid Disorders; Clinical Trials; **Hospital:** NY-Presby/Weill Cornell Med Ctr, NY (page 104); **Address:** Cornell-Weill Physicians-Endocrinology, 525 E 68th St, Box 136, New York, NY 10065; **Phone:** 212-746-6290; **Board Cert:** Internal Medicine 1983; Endocrinology, Diabetes & Metabolism 1987; **Med School:** Brown Univ 1980; **Resid:** Internal Medicine, Rochester Genl Hosp 1983; **Fellow:** Endocrinology, Rochester Genl Hosp 1986; Endocrinology, Diabetes & Metabolism, UCSD Med Ctr 1988; **Fac Appt:** Clin Prof Med, Cornell Univ-Weill Med Coll

Bukberg, Phillip MD (EDM) - **Spec Exp:** Diabetes; Cholesterol/Lipid Disorders; **Hospital:** Beth Israel Med Ctr - Petrie Division (page 94); **Address:** 317 E 17th St Fl 7, Fierman Hall, New York, NY 10003; **Phone:** 212-420-2777; **Board Cert:** Internal Medicine 1977; Endocrinology, Diabetes & Metabolism 1979; **Med School:** SUNY Downstate 1973; **Resid:** Internal Medicine, St Vincent's Hosp & Med Ctr 1977; **Fellow:** Endocrinology, Meml Sloan Kettering Cancer Ctr 1979; Endocrinology, Mt Sinai Hosp 1982

Davies, Terry F MD (EDM) - **Spec Exp:** Thyroid Disorders in Pregnancy; Graves' Disease; Hashimoto's Disease; Thyroid Cancer; **Hospital:** Mount Sinai Med Ctr (page 102), VA Hudson Valley-FDR/Montrose; **Address:** 5 E 98th St, Box 1055, New York, NY 10029-6500; **Phone:** 212-241-7975; **Med School:** England, UK 1971; **Resid:** Internal Medicine, Univ Newcastle 1975; **Fellow:** Endocrinology, Diabetes & Metabolism, Univ Newcastle 1977; Endocrinology, Diabetes & Metabolism, Natl Inst Hlth 1979; **Fac Appt:** Prof Med, Mount Sinai Sch Med

Goland, Robin MD (EDM) - **Spec Exp:** Diabetes; **Hospital:** NY-Presby/Columbia Univ Med Ctr, NY (page 104); **Address:** 1150 St Nicholas Ave Fl 2, Naomi Berrie Diabetic Ctr, New York, NY 10032; **Phone:** 212-851-5494; **Board Cert:** Internal Medicine 1983; Endocrinology 1989; **Med School:** Columbia P&S 1980; **Resid:** Internal Medicine, Columbia-Presby Med Ctr 1984; **Fellow:** Endocrinology, Diabetes & Metabolism, Columbia-Presby Med Ctr 1987; **Fac Appt:** Assoc Prof Med, Columbia P&S

Greene, Loren Wissner MD (EDM) - **Spec Exp:** Thyroid Disorders; Osteoporosis; Pituitary Disorders; Diabetes; **Hospital:** NYU Langone Med Ctr (page 108), NY Downtown Hosp; **Address:** 650 First Ave, Fl 7th, New York, NY 10016-6402; **Phone:** 212-263-7449; **Board Cert:** Internal Medicine 1978; Endocrinology, Diabetes & Metabolism 1981; **Med School:** NYU Sch Med 1975; **Resid:** Internal Medicine, Bellevue Hosp Ctr-NYU 1978; **Fellow:** Endocrinology, Bellevue Hosp Ctr-NYU 1980; **Fac Appt:** Assoc Clin Prof Med, NYU Sch Med

Jacobs, Thomas MD (EDM) - **Spec Exp:** Adrenal Disorders; Pituitary Disorders; Calcium Disorders; Thyroid Disorders; **Hospital:** NY-Presby/Columbia Univ Med Ctr, NY (page 104); **Address:** 161 Fort Washington Ave, rm 210, MS 10032, New York, NY 10032-3713; **Phone:** 212-305-5578; **Board Cert:** Internal Medicine 1973; Endocrinology, Diabetes & Metabolism 1975; **Med School:** Johns Hopkins Univ 1968; **Resid:** Internal Medicine, Columbia Presby Hosp 1973; **Fellow:** Endocrinology, Diabetes & Metabolism, Univ Wash Med Ctr 1975; **Fac Appt:** Clin Prof Med, Columbia P&S

Kleinberg, David L MD (EDM) - **Spec Exp:** Pituitary Disorders; Neuroendocrinology; **Hospital:** NYU Langone Med Ctr (page 108); **Address:** 530 1st Ave, Ste 4C, New York, NY 10016; **Phone:** 212-263-6772; **Board Cert:** Internal Medicine 1972; Endocrinology 1975; **Med School:** Univ Miami Sch Med 1966; **Resid:** Internal Medicine, Maimonides Med Ctr 1968; Internal Medicine, Columbia-Presby Med Ctr 1971; **Fellow:** Endocrinology, Diabetes & Metabolism, Columbia-Presby Med Ctr 1970; **Fac Appt:** Prof Med, NYU Sch Med

Klyde, Barry J MD (EDM) - **Spec Exp:** Thyroid Disorders; Adrenal Disorders; Reproductive Endocrinology; Bone Disorders-Metabolic; **Hospital:** NY-Presby/Weill Cornell Med Ctr, NY (page 104); **Address:** 520 E 72nd St, Ste L0, New York, NY 10021-4840; **Phone:** 212-772-3333; **Board Cert:** Internal Medicine 1977; Endocrinology, Diabetes & Metabolism 1981; **Med School:** Stanford Univ 1974; **Resid:** Internal Medicine, New York Hosp 1977; **Fellow:** Endocrinology, Diabetes & Metabolism, New York Hosp & Rockefeller Univ 1979; **Fac Appt:** Asst Clin Prof Med, Cornell Univ-Weill Med Coll

Levine, Alice C MD (EDM) - **Spec Exp:** Adrenal Disorders; Pituitary Disorders; Reproductive Endocrinology; **Hospital:** Mount Sinai Med Ctr (page 102); **Address:** Mt Sinai School of Med, Dept of Medicine - Endocrinology, 5 E 98th St Fl 11, New York, NY 10029; **Phone:** 212-241-7975; **Board Cert:** Internal Medicine 1984; Endocrinology, Diabetes & Metabolism 1987; **Med School:** Columbia P&S 1981; **Resid:** Internal Medicine, NYU/Manhattan VA Hosp 1984; **Fellow:** Endocrinology, Diabetes & Metabolism, Mt Sinai Med Ctr 1986; **Fac Appt:** Assoc Prof Med, Mount Sinai Sch Med

McConnell, Robert J MD (EDM) - **Spec Exp:** Thyroid Disorders; Thyroid Ultrasound; **Hospital:** NY-Presby/Columbia Univ Med Ctr, NY (page 104); **Address:** 161 Fort Washington Ave, Ste 210, New York, NY 10032-3713; **Phone:** 212-305-5579; **Board Cert:** Internal Medicine 1978; Endocrinology, Diabetes & Metabolism 1981; **Med School:** Columbia P&S 1973; **Resid:** Internal Medicine, Barnes Hosp 1975; **Fellow:** Endocrinology, Diabetes & Metabolism, Columbia-Presby Hosp 1978; **Fac Appt:** Clin Prof Med, Columbia P&S

Mechanick, Jeffrey I MD (EDM) - **Spec Exp:** Nutrition; Thyroid Disorders; Thyroid Cancer; Bone Disorders-Metabolic; **Hospital:** Mount Sinai Med Ctr (page 102); **Address:** 1192 Park Ave, New York, NY 10128; **Phone:** 212-831-2100; **Board Cert:** Internal Medicine 1988; Endocrinology, Diabetes & Metabolism 2003; Clinical Nutrition 2001; **Med School:** Mount Sinai Sch Med 1985; **Resid:** Internal Medicine, Baylor Affil Hosp 1988; **Fellow:** Endocrinology, Diabetes & Metabolism, Mt Sinai Hosp 1990; **Fac Appt:** Clin Prof Med, Mount Sinai Sch Med

Peck, Valerie H MD (EDM) - **Spec Exp:** Osteoporosis; Thyroid Disorders; Obesity; Weight Management; **Hospital:** NYU Langone Med Ctr (page 108); **Address:** 135 E 37th St, New York, NY 10016; **Phone:** 212-213-3233; **Board Cert:** Internal Medicine 1977; Endocrinology, Diabetes & Metabolism 1979; **Med School:** NYU Sch Med 1974; **Resid:** Internal Medicine, Bellevue Hosp Ctr 1977; **Fellow:** Endocrinology, Bellevue Hosp Ctr 1978; **Fac Appt:** Assoc Clin Prof Med, NYU Sch Med

Poretsky, Leonid MD (EDM) - **Spec Exp:** Diabetes; Thyroid Disorders; **Hospital:** Beth Israel Med Ctr - Petrie Division (page 94); **Address:** 317 E 17th St Fl 7, New York, NY 10003; **Phone:** 212-420-2226; **Board Cert:** Internal Medicine 1983; Endocrinology, Diabetes & Metabolism 1985; **Med School:** Russia 1977; **Resid:** Internal Medicine, Coney Island Hosp 1983; **Fellow:** Endocrinology, Beth Israel Hosp 1985; **Fac Appt:** Prof Med, Albert Einstein Coll Med

Seltzer, Terry MD (EDM) - **Spec Exp:** Diabetes; Thyroid Disorders; Calcium Disorders; Pheochromocytoma; **Hospital:** NYU Langone Med Ctr (page 108); **Address:** 530 1st Ave, Ste 4D, New York, NY 10016-6402; **Phone:** 212-263-8717; **Board Cert:** Internal Medicine 1980; Endocrinology 1983; **Med School:** Harvard Med Sch 1977; **Resid:** Internal Medicine, NYU-Bellevue Hosp 1980; **Fellow:** Endocrinology, Diabetes & Metabolism, NYU-Bellevue Hosp 1982; **Fac Appt:** Asst Prof Med, NYU Sch Med

Seplowitz, Alan H MD (EDM) - **Spec Exp:** Thyroid Disorders; Cholesterol/Lipid Disorders; Diabetes; **Hospital:** NY-Presby/Columbia Univ Med Ctr, NY (page 104); **Address:** 161 Fort Washington Ave, Ste 4-422, New York, NY 10032-3729; **Phone:** 212-305-5503; **Board Cert:** Internal Medicine 1975; Endocrinology 1977; **Med School:** Columbia P&S 1972; **Resid:** Internal Medicine, Columbia-Presby Med Ctr 1974; **Fellow:** Lipid Metabolism, Natl Insts Hlth 1976; Endocrinology, Diabetes & Metabolism, Columbia-Presby Med Ctr 1978; **Fac Appt:** Assoc Clin Prof Med, Columbia P&S

Shane, Elizabeth MD (EDM) - **Spec Exp:** Bone Disorders-Metabolic; Osteoporosis; Parathyroid Disorders; **Hospital:** NY-Presby/Columbia Univ Med Ctr, NY (page 104); **Address:** 180 Ft Washington Ave, rm 904, New York, NY 10032; **Phone:** 212-305-2663; **Board Cert:** Internal Medicine 1978; Endocrinology 1981; **Med School:** Univ Toronto 1975; **Resid:** Internal Medicine, Columbia-Presby Hosp 1978; **Fellow:** Endocrinology, Columbia-Presby Hosp 1981; **Fac Appt:** Clin Prof Med, Columbia P&S

Silverberg, Shonni J MD (EDM) - **Spec Exp:** Osteoporosis; Parathyroid Disorders; Calcium Disorders; **Hospital:** NY-Presby/Columbia Univ Med Ctr, NY (page 104); **Address:** 180 Fort Washington Ave, Ste 920, New York, NY 10032; **Phone:** 212-305-2663; **Board Cert:** Internal Medicine 1983; Endocrinology, Diabetes & Metabolism 1985; **Med School:** Cornell Univ-Weill Med Coll 1980; **Resid:** Internal Medicine, NY Hosp 1983; **Fellow:** Endocrinology, Diabetes & Metabolism, Columbia-Presby Med Ctr 1986; **Fac Appt:** Prof Med, Columbia P&S

Siris, Ethel MD (EDM) - **Spec Exp:** Osteoporosis; Paget's Disease of Bone; Bone Disorders-Metabolic; **Hospital:** NY-Presby/Columbia Univ Med Ctr, NY (page 104); **Address:** 180 Ft Washington Ave, HP Bldg - Fl 9 - Ste 964, New York, NY 10032-3710; **Phone:** 212-305-9531; **Board Cert:** Internal Medicine 1974; Endocrinology, Diabetes & Metabolism 1977; **Med School:** Columbia P&S 1971; **Resid:** Internal Medicine, Columbia-Presby Med Ctr 1974; **Fellow:** Research, Natl Inst Hlth 1976; Endocrinology, Diabetes & Metabolism, Columbia-Presby Med Ctr 1977; **Fac Appt:** Prof Med, Columbia P&S

Tuttle, R Michael MD (EDM) - **Spec Exp:** Thyroid Cancer; **Hospital:** Meml Sloan-Kettering Cancer Ctr (page 116); **Address:** Meml Sloan Kettering Cancer Ctr, 1275 York Ave, New York, NY 10065; **Phone:** 646-888-2716; **Board Cert:** Endocrinology, Diabetes & Metabolism 2004; **Med School:** Univ Louisville Sch Med 1987; **Resid:** Internal Medicine, DD Eisenhower Army Med Ctr 1990; **Fellow:** Endocrinology, Diabetes & Metabolism, Madigan Army Med Ctr 1993; **Fac Appt:** Prof Med, Cornell Univ-Weill Med Coll

Wardlaw, Sharon MD (EDM) - **Spec Exp:** Pituitary Disorders; Neuroendocrinology; **Hospital:** NY-Presby/Columbia Univ Med Ctr, NY (page 104); **Address:** 180 Fort Washington Ave, rm 970, New York, NY 10032; **Phone:** 212-305-2254; **Board Cert:** Internal Medicine 1978; Endocrinology, Diabetes & Metabolism 1979; **Med School:** Cornell Univ-Weill Med Coll 1975; **Resid:** Internal Medicine, Case Western Univ Hosp 1977; **Fellow:** Endocrinology, Diabetes & Metabolism, Columbia-Presby 1980; **Fac Appt:** Prof Med, Columbia P&S

Young, Iven MD (EDM) - **Spec Exp:** Thyroid Disorders; Osteoporosis; Pituitary Disorders; Cushing's Syndrome; **Hospital:** NYU Langone Med Ctr (page 108); **Address:** 275 W Seventh Ave Fl 2, MS 10001, New York, NY 10001; **Phone:** 212-675-9332; **Board Cert:** Internal Medicine 1966; Endocrinology, Diabetes & Metabolism 1973; **Med School:** NYU Sch Med 1959; **Resid:** Internal Medicine, VA Med Ctr 1963; **Fellow:** Endocrinology, NYU Med Ctr 1966; **Fac Appt:** Assoc Clin Prof Med, NYU Sch Med

Zweig, Susan B MD (EDM) - **Spec Exp:** Thyroid Disorders; **Hospital:** NYU Langone Med Ctr (page 108), Bellevue Hosp Ctr; **Address:** 135 E 37th St, New York, NY 10016; **Phone:** 212-725-7841; **Board Cert:** Internal Medicine 2010; Endocrinology, Diabetes & Metabolism 2002; **Med School:** Israel 1997; **Resid:** Internal Medicine, St Lukes Roosevelt Hosp Ctr 2000; **Fellow:** Endocrinology, Beth Israel Med Ctr 2002; **Fac Appt:** Asst Clin Prof Med, NYU Sch Med

Family Medicine

Calman, Neil S MD (FMed) *PCP* - **Hospital:** Beth Israel Med Ctr - Petrie Division (page 94), Mount Sinai Med Ctr (page 102); **Address:** The Institute for Family Health, 16 E 16th St, New York, NY 10003-3105; **Phone:** 212-924-7744; **Board Cert:** Family Medicine 2003; **Med School:** Rush Med Coll 1975; **Resid:** Family Medicine, Montefiore Hosp Med Ctr 1978; **Fac Appt:** Prof FMed, Mount Sinai Sch Med

Kligler, Benjamin E MD (FMed) *PCP* - **Spec Exp:** Complementary Medicine; Acupuncture; **Hospital:** Beth Israel Med Ctr - Petrie Division (page 94); **Address:** Continuum Ctr for Health & Healing, 245 Fifth Ave Fl 2, New York, NY 10016; **Phone:** 646-935-2257; **Board Cert:** Family Medicine 2008; **Med School:** Boston Univ 1990; **Resid:** Family Medicine, Albert Einstein Affil Hosps 1994; **Fac Appt:** Asst Prof FMed, Albert Einstein Coll Med

Leeds, Gary E MD (FMed) *PCP* - **Spec Exp:** Asthma & Allergy; Hypertension; Cholesterol/Lipid Disorders; **Hospital:** Beth Israel Med Ctr - Petrie Division (page 94); **Address:** 22 W 15th St, New York, NY 10011-6842; **Phone:** 212-206-7717; **Board Cert:** Family Medicine 2002; **Med School:** Brown Univ 1978; **Resid:** Family Medicine, Georgetown Univ Hosp 1981

Levy, Albert MD (FMed) *PCP* - **Spec Exp:** Hypertension; Diabetes; Sexual Dysfunction; **Hospital:** Mount Sinai Med Ctr (page 102), Lenox Hill Hosp (page 106); **Address:** 911 Park Ave, New York, NY 10075; **Phone:** 212-288-7193; **Board Cert:** Family Medicine 2006; **Med School:** Brazil 1973; **Resid:** Surgery, Maimonides Hosp 1978; Family Medicine, Kings County Hosp 1980; **Fac Appt:** Asst Prof Med, Mount Sinai Sch Med

Lyon, Valerie K MD (FMed) *PCP* - **Spec Exp:** Preventive Medicine; **Hospital:** NYU Langone Med Ctr (page 108), Lenox Hill Hosp (page 106); **Address:** 59 E 54th St Fl 2, New York, NY 10022; **Phone:** 212-750-8330; **Board Cert:** Family Medicine 2006; **Med School:** Temple Univ 1986; **Resid:** Family Medicine, South Nassau Comm Hosp 1989

Schiller, Robert MD (FMed) *PCP* - **Spec Exp:** Complementary Medicine; **Hospital:** Beth Israel Med Ctr - Petrie Division (page 94), SUNY Downstate Med Ctr (Univ Hosp of Bklyn) - LICH (page 420); **Address:** Sidney Hillman Family Practice, 16 E 16th St Fl 3, New York, NY 10003-3105; **Phone:** 212-924-7744; **Board Cert:** Family Medicine 2006; **Med School:** NYU Sch Med 1982; **Resid:** Family Medicine, Montefiore Med Ctr 1985; **Fac Appt:** Asst Prof FMed, Albert Einstein Coll Med

Gastroenterology

Ackert, John MD (Ge) - **Spec Exp:** Endoscopy; Colonoscopy; Gastroesophageal Reflux Disease (GERD); **Hospital:** NYU Langone Med Ctr (page 108); **Address:** 232 E 30th St, Grnd Fl, New York, NY 10016; **Phone:** 212-889-5544; **Board Cert:** Internal Medicine 1975; Gastroenterology 1977; **Med School:** NYU Sch Med 1972; **Resid:** Internal Medicine, NYU Med Ctr 1975; **Fellow:** Gastroenterology, NYU Med Ctr 1977; **Fac Appt:** Asst Prof Med, NYU Sch Med

Adler, Howard MD (Ge) - **Spec Exp:** Colon Cancer; Colonoscopy; Endoscopy; **Hospital:** Lenox Hill Hosp (page 106), Beth Israel Med Ctr - Petrie Division (page 94); **Address:** 35 Sutton Pl, New York, NY 10022-2464; **Phone:** 212-421-3696; **Board Cert:** Internal Medicine 1967; Gastroenterology 1977; **Med School:** Albert Einstein Coll Med 1960; **Resid:** Internal Medicine, Herbert C Moffitt Hosp 1962; Internal Medicine, Bronx Municipal Hosp 1965; **Fellow:** Gastroenterology, Cornell U-Bellevue Hosp 1967; **Fac Appt:** Assoc Clin Prof Med, Albert Einstein Coll Med

Aisenberg, James MD (Ge) - **Spec Exp:** Colon Cancer Screening; Inflammatory Bowel Disease; Gastroesophageal Reflux Disease (GERD); Crohn's Disease; **Hospital:** Mount Sinai Med Ctr (page 102); **Address:** 311 E 79th St, Ste 2-A, New York, NY 10075; **Phone:** 212-996-6633; **Board Cert:** Gastroenterology 2000; **Med School:** Harvard Med Sch 1987; **Resid:** Internal Medicine, Columbia-Presby Med Ctr 1990; **Fellow:** Gastroenterology, Mt Sinai Hosp 1993; **Fac Appt:** Assoc Prof Med, Mount Sinai Sch Med

Baiocco, Peter J MD (Ge) - **Spec Exp:** Inflammatory Bowel Disease; Colon Cancer Screening; Gastroesophageal Reflux Disease (GERD); Endoscopy; **Hospital:** Lenox Hill Hosp (page 106); **Address:** 1317 3rd Ave Fl 5, New York, NY 10021-2995; **Phone:** 212-734-8811; **Board Cert:** Internal Medicine 1981; Gastroenterology 1983; **Med School:** Mount Sinai Sch Med 1978; **Resid:** Internal Medicine, Lenox Hill Hosp 1981; **Fellow:** Gastroenterology, Lenox Hill Hosp 1983; **Fac Appt:** Asst Clin Prof Med, NYU Sch Med

Basuk, Paul M MD (Ge) - **Spec Exp:** Gallbladder Disease; Pancreatic Disease; Esophageal Disorders; **Hospital:** NY-Presby/Weill Cornell Med Ctr, NY (page 104); **Address:** 210 E 86th St, Ste 201, New York, NY 10028; **Phone:** 212-861-9715; **Board Cert:** Internal Medicine 1983; Gastroenterology 1987; **Med School:** Northwestern Univ 1980; **Resid:** Internal Medicine, UCSF Med Ctr 1983; **Fellow:** Gastroenterology, UCSF Med Ctr 1987; **Fac Appt:** Asst Prof Med, Cornell Univ Weill Med Coll

Bednarek, Karl T MD (Ge) - **Spec Exp:** Colon & Rectal Cancer Detection; **Hospital:** Beth Israel Med Ctr - Petrie Division (page 94); **Address:** 10 Union Square E, Ste 2G, New York, NY 10003; **Phone:** 212-844-6335; **Board Cert:** Internal Medicine 1985; **Med School:** Mount Sinai Sch Med 1982; **Resid:** Internal Medicine, Beth Israel Med Ctr 1986; **Fellow:** Gastroenterology, Beth Israel Med Ctr 1988; **Fac Appt:** Asst Prof Med, Albert Einstein Coll Med

Ben-Zvi, Jeffrey MD (Ge) - **Spec Exp:** Inflammatory Bowel Disease/Crohn's; Gastroesophageal Reflux Disease (GERD); Swallowing Disorders; Colon Cancer Screening; **Hospital:** Lenox Hill Hosp (page 106), NY-Presby/Columbia Univ Med Ctr, NY (page 104); **Address:** 212 E 70th St, New York, NY 10075; **Phone:** 212-772-8730; **Board Cert:** Internal Medicine 2004; Gastroenterology 2004; Geriatric Medicine 2004; **Med School:** Columbia P&S 1983; **Resid:** Internal Medicine, St Lukes-Roosevelt Hosp 1986; **Fellow:** Gastroenterology, St Lukes-Roosevelt Hosp 1988; **Fac Appt:** Asst Clin Prof Med, Columbia P&S

Bernstein, Brett B MD (Ge) - **Spec Exp:** Gastroesophageal Reflux Disease (GERD); Capsule Endoscopy; Colon Cancer Screening; **Hospital:** Beth Israel Med Ctr - Petrie Division (page 94); **Address:** 10 Union Square East, Ste 2G, New York, NY 10003; **Phone:** 212-844-6330; **Board Cert:** Gastroenterology 2005; **Med School:** Mount Sinai Sch Med 1988; **Resid:** Internal Medicine, Beth Israel Med Ctr 1991; **Fellow:** Gastroenterology, Beth Israel Med Ctr 1994; **Fac Appt:** Asst Prof Med, Albert Einstein Coll Med

Borcich, Anthony S MD (Ge) - **Spec Exp:** Liver Disease; Hepatitis C; HIV & Hepatitis co-infection; **Hospital:** Mount Sinai Med Ctr (page 102), Lenox Hill Hosp (page 106); **Address:** 800A 5th Ave, New York, NY 10065; **Phone:** 212-722-8400; **Board Cert:** Internal Medicine 1987; Gastroenterology 1989; **Med School:** Northwestern Univ-Feinberg Sch Med 1984; **Resid:** Internal Medicine, St Lukes-Roosevelt Hosp 1987; **Fellow:** Gastroenterology, St Lukes-Roosevelt Hosp 1989; **Fac Appt:** Asst Clin Prof Med, Mount Sinai Sch Med

Brown Jr, Robert S MD (Ge) - **Spec Exp:** Hepatitis; Liver Disease; Transplant Medicine-Liver; Autoimmune Liver Disease; **Hospital:** NY-Presby/Columbia Univ Med Ctr, NY (page 104), NY-Presby/Weill Cornell Med Ctr, NY (page 104); **Address:** Ctr for Liver Disease & Transplantation, 622 W 168th St, PH Bldg - Fl 14, rm 105, New York, NY 10032; **Phone:** 212-305-1305; **Board Cert:** Internal Medicine 2002; Gastroenterology 2005; Transplant Hepatology 2010; **Med School:** NYU Sch Med 1989; **Resid:** Internal Medicine, Beth Israel Deaconess Med Ctr 1992; **Fellow:** Gastroenterology, UCSF Med Ctr 1994; Hepatology, UCSF Med Ctr 1995; **Fac Appt:** Prof Med, Columbia P&S

Cantor, Michael C MD (Ge) - **Spec Exp:** Colon Cancer; Hepatitis; Liver Disease; **Hospital:** NY-Presby/Weill Cornell Med Ctr, NY (page 104); **Address:** 310 E 72nd St Fl Level C, New York, NY 10021-4703; **Phone:** 212-472-3333; **Board Cert:** Internal Medicine 1985; Gastroenterology 1989; **Med School:** Columbia P&S 1982; **Resid:** Internal Medicine, New York Hosp 1985; **Fellow:** Gastroenterology, New York Hosp 1988; **Fac Appt:** Asst Clin Prof Med, Cornell Univ-Weill Med Coll

Carr-Locke, David L MD (Ge) - **Spec Exp:** Pancreatic/Biliary Endoscopy (ERCP); Pancreatic & Biliary Disease; Endoscopy; **Hospital:** Beth Israel Med Ctr - Petrie Division (page 94); **Address:** 1st & 16th St, New York, NY 10003; **Phone:** 212-420-4015; **Board Cert:** Internal Medicine 1974; **Med School:** England, UK 1972; **Resid:** Obstetrics & Gynecology, Orsett Hosp 1974; Internal Medicine, Leicester Hosp 1976; **Fellow:** Gastroenterology, Leicester Hosp 1978; Research, New Eng Baptist Hosp 1979; **Fac Appt:** Assoc Prof Med, Harvard Med Sch

Chapman, Mark L MD (Ge) - **Spec Exp:** Inflammatory Bowel Disease/Crohn's; Peptic Ulcer Disease; Gastrointestinal Motility Disorders; **Hospital:** Mount Sinai Med Ctr (page 102); **Address:** 12 E 86th St, New York, NY 10028-0506; **Phone:** 212-861-2000; **Board Cert:** Internal Medicine 1968; Gastroenterology 1970; **Med School:** SUNY Downstate 1961; **Resid:** Internal Medicine, Montefiore Med Ctr 1963; Internal Medicine, Mt Sinai Hosp 1964; **Fellow:** Gastroenterology, Mt Sinai Hosp 1966; **Fac Appt:** Assoc Clin Prof Med, Mount Sinai Sch Med

Cohen, Jonathan MD (Ge) - **Spec Exp:** Pancreatic/Biliary Endoscopy (ERCP); Colonoscopy; Barrett's Esophagus; Gastrointestinal Cancer; **Hospital:** NYU Langone Med Ctr (page 108); **Address:** 232 E 30th St, New York, NY 10016-8202; **Phone:** 212-889-5544; **Board Cert:** Gastroenterology 2005; **Med School:** Harvard Med Sch 1990; **Resid:** Internal Medicine, Beth Israel Hosp 1993; **Fellow:** Gastroenterology, UCLA Med Ctr 1995; Endoscopy, Wellesley Hosp 1995; **Fac Appt:** Clin Prof Med, NYU Sch Med

Cohen, Lawrence B MD (Ge) - **Spec Exp:** Gastroesophageal Reflux Disease (GERD); Esophageal Disorders; Colon & Rectal Cancer; Endoscopy; **Hospital:** Mount Sinai Med Ctr (page 102); **Address:** 311 E 79th St, Ste 2A, New York, NY 10075; **Phone:** 212-996-6633; **Board Cert:** Internal Medicine 1981; Gastroenterology 1983; **Med School:** Hahnemann Univ 1978; **Resid:** Internal Medicine, Mt Sinai Hosp 1981; **Fellow:** Gastroenterology, Mt Sinai Hosp 1983; **Fac Appt:** Assoc Clin Prof Med, Mount Sinai Sch Med

Cohen, Seth A MD (Ge) - **Spec Exp:** Pancreatic/Biliary Endoscopy (ERCP); Colonoscopy; Endoscopy; **Hospital:** Beth Israel Med Ctr - Petrie Division (page 94), Lenox Hill Hosp (page 106); **Address:** 305 Second Ave, Lower Level Suite #3, New York, NY 10003; **Phone:** 212-734-8874; **Board Cert:** Internal Medicine 1989; Gastroenterology 2004; **Med School:** Columbia P&S 1986; **Resid:** Internal Medicine, Mount Sinai Med Ctr 1989; **Fellow:** Gastroenterology, St Luke's-Roosevelt Hosp Ctr 1991; Gastroenterology, Beth Israel Hosp 1992

Connor, Bradley A MD (Ge) - **Spec Exp:** Travel Medicine; Parasitic Infections; Diarrheal Diseases; Tropical Diseases; **Hospital:** NY-Presby/Weill Cornell Med Ctr, NY (page 104); **Address:** 50 E 69th St, New York, NY 10021; **Phone:** 212-988-2800; **Board Cert:** Internal Medicine 1982; Gastroenterology 1985; **Med School:** Univ Tex SW, Dallas 1978; **Resid:** Internal Medicine, UT Hlth Sci Ctr-Bexar Co/A Murphy VA Hosps 1981; **Fellow:** Gastroenterology, NY Hosp 1984; **Fac Appt:** Assoc Clin Prof Med, Cornell Univ-Weill Med Coll

Cooper, Robert B MD (Ge) - **Spec Exp:** Colon Cancer Screening; Gastroesophageal Reflux Disease (GERD); Celiac Disease; Gallbladder Disease; **Hospital:** NY-Presby/Weill Cornell Med Ctr, NY (page 104); **Address:** 635 Madison Ave Fl 17, New York, NY 10022; **Phone:** 212-717-4967; **Board Cert:** Internal Medicine 1984; Gastroenterology 1989; **Med School:** Cornell Univ-Weill Med Coll 1981; **Resid:** Internal Medicine, NY Hosp/Weill Cornell Med Ctr 1984; **Fellow:** Gastroenterology, NY Hosp/Weill Cornell Med Ctr 1987; **Fac Appt:** Asst Prof Med, Cornell Univ-Weill Med Coll

Dieterich, Douglas T MD (Ge) - **Spec Exp:** Hepatitis; AIDS/HIV-Gastrointestinal Complications; Liver Disease; Endoscopy; **Hospital:** Mount Sinai Med Ctr (page 102); **Address:** 5 E 98th St Fl 11, New York, NY 10029; **Phone:** 212-241-7270; **Board Cert:** Internal Medicine 1981; Gastroenterology 1987; **Med School:** NYU Sch Med 1978; **Resid:** Internal Medicine, Bellevue Hosp Ctr-NYU 1981; **Fellow:** Gastroenterology, Bellevue Hosp Ctr-NYU 1983; **Fac Appt:** Prof Med, Mount Sinai Sch Med

Faust, Michael J MD (Ge) - **Spec Exp:** Gastrointestinal Disorders; **Hospital:** NYU Langone Med Ctr (page 108); **Address:** 345 E 37th St, Ste 207, New York, NY 10016-3256; **Phone:** 212-986-3330; **Board Cert:** Internal Medicine 1981; Gastroenterology 1983; **Med School:** NYU Sch Med 1978; **Resid:** Internal Medicine, Bellevue Hosp/NYU Med Ctr 1981; **Fellow:** Gastroenterology, Bellevue Hosp/NYU Med Ctr 1983; **Fac Appt:** Asst Prof Med, NYU Sch Med

Ferran, Elena Nascimbeni MD (Ge) - **Spec Exp:** Colonoscopy; Endoscopy; Irritable Bowel Syndrome; Liver Disease; **Hospital:** Lenox Hill Hosp (page 106); **Address:** 121 E 69th St, New York, NY 10021; **Phone:** 212-861-9268; **Board Cert:** Gastroenterology 2008; **Med School:** Italy 1989; **Resid:** Internal Medicine, St Vincent's Hosp 1994; **Fellow:** Gastroenterology, St Vincent's Hosp 1997; Hepatology, Mt Sinai Hosp 1998

Field, Steven P MD (Ge) - **Spec Exp:** Irritable Bowel Syndrome; **Hospital:** NYU Langone Med Ctr (page 108); **Address:** 245 E 35th St, New York, NY 10016; **Phone:** 212-686-9477; **Board Cert:** Internal Medicine 1980; Gastroenterology 1983; **Med School:** NYU Sch Med 1977; **Resid:** Internal Medicine, Bellevue Hosp 1981; **Fellow:** Gastroenterology, Mt Sinai Hosp 1983; **Fac Appt:** Asst Clin Prof Med, NYU Sch Med

Fochios, Steven E MD (Ge) - **Spec Exp:** Endoscopy; **Hospital:** Lenox Hill Hosp (page 106); **Address:** 117 E 65th St, New York, NY 10065; **Phone:** 212-861-4278; **Board Cert:** Internal Medicine 1980; Gastroenterology 1985; **Med School:** Geo Wash Univ 1976; **Resid:** Internal Medicine, Lenox Hill Hosp 1979; **Fellow:** Gastroenterology, Lenox Hill Hosp 1981

Foong, Anthony MD (Ge) - **Spec Exp:** Endoscopy; Colonoscopy; Gastrointestinal Disorders; Hemorrhoids; **Hospital:** Beth Israel Med Ctr - Petrie Division (page 94); **Address:** 210 Canal St, Ste 601, New York, NY 10013; **Phone:** 212-693-2100; **Board Cert:** Internal Medicine 1984; Gastroenterology 1987; **Med School:** Tufts Univ 1981; **Resid:** Internal Medicine, Univ Md Hosp 1984; **Fellow:** Gastroenterology, St Luke's-Roosevelt Hosp Ctr 1986

Frank, Michael MD (Ge) - **Spec Exp:** Inflammatory Bowel Disease/Crohn's; Colonoscopy; Endoscopy; **Hospital:** Lenox Hill Hosp (page 106); **Address:** 9 E 63rd St, New York, NY 10065; **Phone:** 212-593-7170; **Board Cert:** Internal Medicine 1977; Gastroenterology 1979; **Med School:** Albert Einstein Coll Med 1974; **Resid:** Internal Medicine, Bronx Municipal Hosps 1977; **Fellow:** Gastroenterology, Montefiore Med Ctr 1979; **Fac Appt:** Assoc Clin Prof Med, Albert Einstein Coll Med

Freiman, Hal MD (Ge) - **Spec Exp:** Gastroesophageal Reflux Disease (GERD); Biliary Disease; Pancreatic/Biliary Endoscopy (ERCP); Hepatitis; **Hospital:** Beth Israel Med Ctr - Petrie Division (page 94), NYU Langone Med Ctr (page 108); **Address:** 59 W 12th St, Ste 1D, New York, NY 10011-8520; **Phone:** 212-206-0074; **Board Cert:** Internal Medicine 1981; Gastroenterology 1983; **Med School:** Albany Med Coll 1978; **Resid:** Internal Medicine, St Vincent's Hosp 1981; **Fellow:** Gastroenterology, Westchester Co Med Ctr 1983

Friedlander, Charles N MD (Ge) - **Spec Exp:** Colonoscopy; Irritable Bowel Syndrome; **Hospital:** NYU Langone Med Ctr (page 108); **Address:** 232 E 30th St, New York, NY 10016-8202; **Phone:** 212-889-5544; **Board Cert:** Internal Medicine 1974; Gastroenterology 1977; **Med School:** SUNY Downstate 1968; **Resid:** Internal Medicine, Bellevue Hosp 1971; Internal Medicine, Bellevue Hosp 1974; **Fellow:** Gastroenterology, NYU Med Ctr 1976; **Fac Appt:** Assoc Prof Med, NYU Sch Med

Gerdes, Hans MD (Ge) - **Spec Exp:** Endoscopy; Endoscopic Ultrasound; Barrett's Esophagus; Gastrointestinal Cancer; **Hospital:** Meml Sloan-Kettering Cancer Ctr (page 116); **Address:** 1275 York Avenue, New York, NY 10065; **Phone:** 800-525-2225; **Board Cert:** Internal Medicine 1987; Gastroenterology 1989; **Med School:** Cornell Univ-Weill Med Coll 1983; **Resid:** Internal Medicine, New York Hosp 1986; **Fellow:** Gastroenterology, Meml Sloan Kettering Cancer Ctr 1989

Gerson, Charles MD (Ge) - **Spec Exp:** Irritable Bowel Syndrome; Diarrheal Diseases; **Hospital:** Mount Sinai Med Ctr (page 102); **Address:** 80 Central Park West, Ste B, New York, NY 10023-5204; **Phone:** 212-496-6161; **Board Cert:** Internal Medicine 1970; Gastroenterology 1972; **Med School:** SUNY Downstate 1962; **Resid:** Internal Medicine, Bellevue Hosp 1964; Internal Medicine, Mount Sinai Hosp 1965; **Fellow:** Gastroenterology, Bellevue Hosp 1968; Gastroenterology, Mount Sinai Hosp 1969; **Fac Appt:** Clin Prof Med, Mount Sinai Sch Med

Goldberg, Myron D MD (Ge) - **Spec Exp:** Colon Cancer Screening; Colonoscopy; Endoscopy; Hepatitis B & C; **Hospital:** Lenox Hill Hosp (page 106), NYU Langone Med Ctr (page 108); **Address:** 110 E 59th St, Ste 10D, New York, NY 10022-1304; **Phone:** 212-583-2900; **Board Cert:** Internal Medicine 1977; Gastroenterology 1979; **Med School:** Albert Einstein Coll Med 1971; **Resid:** Internal Medicine, Montefiore Med Ctr 1973; Internal Medicine, Lenox Hill Hosp 1974; **Fellow:** Gastroenterology, Columbia-Presby Hosp 1977; Gastroenterology, Lenox Hill Hosp 1978; **Fac Appt:** Asst Clin Prof Med, NYU Sch Med

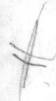

Goldin, Howard MD (Ge) - **Spec Exp:** Inflammatory Bowel Disease/Crohn's; Endoscopy; Liver Disease; **Hospital:** NY-Presby/Weill Cornell Med Ctr, NY (page 104), Rockefeller Univ; **Address:** 646 Park Ave, New York, NY 10065; **Phone:** 212-249-0404; **Board Cert:** Internal Medicine 1968; Gastroenterology 1973; **Med School:** Cornell Univ-Weill Med Coll 1961; **Resid:** Internal Medicine, New York Hosp 1964; **Fellow:** Gastroenterology, New York Hosp 1966; **Fac Appt:** Clin Prof Med, Cornell Univ-Weill Med Coll

Green, Peter H R MD (Ge) - **Spec Exp:** Celiac Disease; Endoscopy; Colonoscopy; Malabsorption Syndrome; **Hospital:** NY-Presby/Columbia Univ Med Ctr, NY (page 104); **Address:** Celiac Disease Ctr, Harkness Bldg, 180 Fort Washington Ave, Ste 936, New York, NY 10032-3713; **Phone:** 212-305-5590; **Med School:** Australia 1970; **Resid:** Internal Medicine, North Shore Med Ctr 1974; **Fellow:** Gastroenterology, North Shore Med Ctr 1976; Gastroenterology, Beth Israel Hosp 1977; **Fac Appt:** Clin Prof Med, Columbia P&S

Haber, Gregory B MD (Ge) - **Spec Exp:** Endoscopy; Pancreatic/Biliary Endoscopy (ERCP); Endoscopic Ultrasound; Barrett's Esophagus; **Hospital:** Lenox Hill Hosp (page 106); **Address:** 100 E 77th St Fl 2, New York, NY 10075; **Phone:** 212-434-6279; **Med School:** Univ Toronto 1970; **Resid:** Internal Medicine, Univ Toronto Med Ctr 1975; **Fellow:** Gastroenterology, Univ Toronto Med Ctr 1978

Hammerman, Hillel S MD (Ge) - **Spec Exp:** Swallowing Disorders; Liver Disease; Colonoscopy; **Hospital:** Lenox Hill Hosp (page 106); **Address:** 210 E 73rd St, Ste 1C, New York, NY 10021; **Phone:** 212-288-1030; **Board Cert:** Internal Medicine 1981; Gastroenterology 1983; **Med School:** Cornell Univ-Weill Med Coll 1978; **Resid:** Internal Medicine, Baltimore City Hosps 1981; **Fellow:** Gastroenterology, Lahey Clin 1983

Harary, Albert M MD (Ge) - **Spec Exp:** Endoscopy & Colonoscopy; Gastroesophageal Reflux Disease (GERD); Swallowing Disorders; **Hospital:** Lenox Hill Hosp (page 106), NYU Langone Med Ctr (page 108); **Address:** 110 E 55th St Fl 17, New York, NY 10022; **Phone:** 212-702-0123; **Board Cert:** Internal Medicine 1982; Gastroenterology 1985; **Med School:** Columbia P&S 1979; **Resid:** Internal Medicine, Univ Miami Affil Hosp 1982; **Fellow:** Gastroenterology, Univ Miami Affil Hosp 1984; **Fac Appt:** Asst Clin Prof Med, NYU Sch Med

Itzkowitz, Steven H MD (Ge) - **Spec Exp:** Colon & Rectal Cancer; Colon & Rectal Cancer Detection; Inflammatory Bowel Disease; Hereditary Cancer; **Hospital:** Mount Sinai Med Ctr (page 102); **Address:** 5 E 98th St, Box 1625, New York, NY 10029-6501; **Phone:** 212-241-4299; **Board Cert:** Internal Medicine 1982; Gastroenterology 1985; **Med School:** Mount Sinai Sch Med 1979; **Resid:** Internal Medicine, Bellevue Hosp/NYU Med Ctr 1982; **Fellow:** Gastroenterology, UCSF Med Ctr 1984; **Fac Appt:** Prof Med, Mount Sinai Sch Med

Jacobson, Ira M MD (Ge) - **Spec Exp:** Liver & Biliary Disease; Pancreatic Disease; Hepatitis; Hepatitis C; **Hospital:** NY-Presby/Weill Cornell Med Ctr, NY (page 104); **Address:** 1305 York Ave Fl 4, New York, NY 10021-5016; **Phone:** 646-962-4040; **Board Cert:** Internal Medicine 1982; Gastroenterology 2009; Transplant Hepatology 2006; **Med School:** Columbia P&S 1979; **Resid:** Internal Medicine, UCSF Med Ctr 1982; **Fellow:** Gastroenterology, Mass Genl Hosp 1984; **Fac Appt:** Prof Med, Cornell Univ-Weill Med Coll

Jaffin, Barry W MD (Ge) - **Spec Exp:** Gastrointestinal Motility Disorders; Inflammatory Bowel Disease; **Hospital:** Mount Sinai Med Ctr (page 102); **Address:** 620 Columbus Ave, New York, NY 10024; **Phone:** 212-721-2600; **Board Cert:** Internal Medicine 1984; Gastroenterology 1987; **Med School:** Mount Sinai Sch Med 1981; **Resid:** Internal Medicine, Med Ctr Hosp 1984; **Fellow:** Gastroenterology, Boston Univ Med Ctr 1986; **Fac Appt:** Asst Clin Prof Med, Mount Sinai Sch Med

Kahaleh, Michel MD (Ge) - **Spec Exp:** Pancreatic & Biliary Disease; Pancreatic/Biliary Endoscopy (ERCP); Endoscopy; **Hospital:** NY-Presby/Weill Cornell Med Ctr, NY (page 104); **Address:** 1305 York Ave Fl 4, New York, NY 10065; **Phone:** 646-962-4000; **Board Cert:** Internal Medicine 2009; Gastroenterology 2009; **Med School:** Belgium 1994; **Resid:** Internal Medicine, Univ Chicago Med Ctr 1999; **Fellow:** Gastroenterology, Esrasme Hosp/Univ Brussels; **Fac Appt:** Asst Prof Med, Cornell Univ-Weill Med Coll

Kairam, Indira R MD (Ge) - **Spec Exp:** Colon Cancer; Peptic Ulcer Disease; Hepatitis C; **Hospital:** St. Luke's - Roosevelt Hosp Ctr - St Luke's Hosp (page 94), St. Luke's - Roosevelt Hosp Ctr - Roosevelt Div (page 94); **Address:** 945 West End Ave, Ste 1D, New York, NY 10025-3573; **Phone:** 212-865-7355; **Board Cert:** Internal Medicine 1978; **Med School:** India 1973; **Resid:** Internal Medicine, St Clare's Hosp 1978; **Fellow:** Gastroenterology, Lahey Clinic 1980; **Fac Appt:** Asst Prof Med, NY Med Coll

Kim, Michelle K MD (Ge) - **Spec Exp:** Endscopic Ultrasound; Endoscopy; Gastrointestinal Cancer; **Hospital:** Mount Sinai Med Ctr (page 102); **Address:** Mt Sinai Faculty Practice, 5 E 98th St Fl 11, Box 1069, New York, NY 10029; **Phone:** 212-241-4299; **Board Cert:** Internal Medicine 2002; Gastroenterology 2005; **Med School:** Stanford Univ 1999; **Resid:** Internal Medicine, Weill Cornell Med Ctr 2002; **Fellow:** Gastroenterology, Weill Cornell Med Ctr 2007

Kim-Schluger, Hyung Leona MD (Ge) - **Spec Exp:** Transplant Medicine-Liver; Liver Disease; Hepatitis C; **Hospital:** Montefiore Med Ctr-Moses Campus, NY (page 100); **Address:** 5 E 98 St Fl 12, New York, NY 10029; **Phone:** 212-659-8031; **Board Cert:** Internal Medicine 2002; Gastroenterology 2003; Transplant Hepatology 2008; **Med School:** Columbia P&S 1988; **Resid:** Internal Medicine, NY-Presby/Columbia Univ Med Ctr 1991; **Fellow:** Gastroenterology, NY-Presby/Columbia Univ Med Ctr 1993; Transplant Hepatology, Mount Sinai Med Ctr 2008

Kimball, Annetta MD (Ge) - **Spec Exp:** Hepatitis; Inflammatory Bowel Disease/Crohn's; Irritable Bowel Syndrome; **Hospital:** St. Luke's - Roosevelt Hosp Ctr - Roosevelt Div (page 94); **Address:** 315 W 57th St, Ste 301, New York, NY 10019; **Phone:** 212-371-8900; **Board Cert:** Internal Medicine 1972; Gastroenterology 1973; **Med School:** Boston Univ 1968; **Resid:** Internal Medicine, Roosevelt Hosp 1970; Internal Medicine, Mount Sinai Hosp 1971; **Fellow:** Gastroenterology, Mount Sinai Hosp 1973; **Fac Appt:** Assoc Clin Prof Med, Columbia P&S

Knapp, Albert B MD (Ge) - **Spec Exp:** Colonoscopy/Polypectomy; Endoscopy; Liver Disease; Transplant Medicine-Liver; **Hospital:** NYU Langone Med Ctr (page 108), Lenox Hill Hosp (page 106); **Address:** 760 Park Ave, New York, NY 10021-4152; **Phone:** 212-737-3446; **Board Cert:** Internal Medicine 1982; Gastroenterology 1987; **Med School:** Columbia P&S 1979; **Resid:** Internal Medicine, Albert Einstein Med Ctr 1982; **Fellow:** Gastroenterology, Brigham & Women's Hosp 1985; Virology, Pasteur Inst 1975; **Fac Appt:** Clin Prof Med, NYU Sch Med

Kotler, Donald P MD (Ge) - **Spec Exp:** Esophageal Disorders; Nutrition & AIDS; Hepatitis; **Hospital:** St. Luke's - Roosevelt Hosp Ctr - St Luke's Hosp (page 94); **Address:** 1111 Amsterdam Ave, SR 12, New York, NY 10025; **Phone:** 212-523-3670; **Board Cert:** Internal Medicine 1976; Gastroenterology 1979; **Med School:** Albert Einstein Coll Med 1973; **Resid:** Internal Medicine, Jacobi Med Ctr 1976; **Fellow:** Gastroenterology, Hosp Univ Penn 1978; **Fac Appt:** Prof Med, Columbia P&S

Krumholz, Michael MD (Ge) - **Spec Exp:** Colonoscopy; Colon Cancer Screening; **Hospital:** Lenox Hill Hosp (page 106), Mount Sinai Med Ctr (page 102); **Address:** 111 E 80th St, Ste 1C, New York, NY 10021-0350; **Phone:** 212-734-5533; **Board Cert:** Internal Medicine 1983; Gastroenterology 1987; **Med School:** Mount Sinai Sch Med 1980; **Resid:** Internal Medicine, Beth Israel Hosp 1984; **Fellow:** Gastroenterology, Lenox Hill Hosp 1986; **Fac Appt:** Med, NYU Sch Med

Kummer, Bart A MD (Ge) - **Spec Exp:** Colonoscopy; Endoscopy; **Hospital:** NYU Langone Med Ctr (page 108), NY Downtown Hosp; **Address:** NYU Langone Trinity Ctr, 111 Broadway Fl 2, New York, NY 10006; **Phone:** 212-263-9700; **Board Cert:** Internal Medicine 1982; Gastroenterology 1985; **Med School:** Cornell Univ-Weill Med Coll 1979; **Resid:** Internal Medicine, Harlem Hosp 1982; **Fellow:** Gastroenterology, St Luke's-Roosevelt Hosp Ctr 1985; **Fac Appt:** Asst Prof Med, NYU Sch Med

Kurtz, Robert C MD (Ge) - **Spec Exp:** Pancreatic Cancer(Familial); Gastrointestinal Cancer; Endoscopy; Cancer Prevention; **Hospital:** Meml Sloan-Kettering Cancer Ctr (page 116); **Address:** 1275 York Ave, New York, NY 10065; **Phone:** 212-639-7620; **Board Cert:** Internal Medicine 1971; Gastroenterology 1977; **Med School:** Jefferson Med Coll 1968; **Resid:** Internal Medicine, NY Hosp/Meml Sloan Kettering Cancer Ctr 1971; **Fellow:** Gastroenterology, Meml Sloan Kettering Cancer Ctr 1973; **Fac Appt:** Prof Med, Cornell Univ-Weill Med Coll

Lambroza, Arnon MD (Ge) - **Spec Exp:** Swallowing Disorders; Gastroesophageal Reflux Disease (GERD); Barrett's Esophagus; Achalasia; **Hospital:** NY-Presby/Weill Cornell Med Ctr, NY (page 104), Lenox Hill Hosp (page 106); **Address:** 1085 Park Ave, New York, NY 10128-0320; **Phone:** 212-517-7570; **Board Cert:** Internal Medicine 1987; Gastroenterology 2011; **Med School:** Albert Einstein Coll Med 1984; **Resid:** Internal Medicine, Hosp Univ Penn 1987; **Fellow:** Gastroenterology, New York Hosp 1990; **Fac Appt:** Assoc Clin Prof Med, Cornell Univ-Weill Med Coll

Lax, James D MD (Ge) - **Spec Exp:** Liver Disease; Gastroesophageal Reflux Disease (GERD); Barrett's Esophagus; Eosinophilic Esophogitis; **Hospital:** St. Luke's - Roosevelt Hosp Ctr - Roosevelt Div (page 94), Lenox Hill Hosp (page 106); **Address:** 160 E 72nd St, New York, NY 10021-4364; **Phone:** 212-988-5740; **Board Cert:** Internal Medicine 1984; Gastroenterology 1987; **Med School:** NYU Sch Med 1981; **Resid:** Internal Medicine, St Luke's-Roosevelt Hosp Ctr 1984; **Fellow:** Gastroenterology, St Luke's-Roosevelt Hosp Ctr 1986; **Fac Appt:** Asst Clin Prof Med, Columbia P&S

Lebwohl, Oscar MD (Ge) - **Spec Exp:** Endoscopy; Inflammatory Bowel Disease/Crohn's; Ulcerative Colitis; Gastrointestinal Cancer; **Hospital:** NY-Presby/Columbia Univ Med Ctr, NY (page 104); **Address:** 161 Fort Washington Ave, rm 420, New York, NY 10032-3713; **Phone:** 212-305-5363; **Board Cert:** Internal Medicine 1975; Gastroenterology 1977; **Med School:** Harvard Med Sch 1972; **Resid:** Internal Medicine, Mt Sinai Med Ctr 1975; **Fellow:** Gastroenterology, Columbia-Presby Med Ctr 1976; Hepatology, Mt Sinai Med Ctr 1977; **Fac Appt:** Clin Prof Med, Columbia P&S

Lewis, Blair MD (Ge) - **Spec Exp:** Endoscopy; Capsule Endoscopy; **Hospital:** Mount Sinai Med Ctr (page 102); **Address:** 1067 5th Ave, New York, NY 10128-0101; **Phone:** 212-369-6600; **Board Cert:** Internal Medicine 1985; Gastroenterology 1987; **Med School:** Albert Einstein Coll Med 1982; **Resid:** Internal Medicine, Montefiore Med Ctr 1985; **Fellow:** Gastroenterology, Mt Sinai Med Ctr 1987; **Fac Appt:** Clin Prof Med, Mount Sinai Sch Med

Lightdale, Charles J MD (Ge) - **Spec Exp:** Barrett's Esophagus; Gastrointestinal Cancer; Endoscopic Ultrasound; **Hospital:** NY-Presby/Columbia Univ Med Ctr, NY (page 104); **Address:** Columbia-Presby Med Ctr, Irving Pavilion, 161 Fort Washington Ave, rm 812, New York, NY 10032-3713; **Phone:** 212-305-3423; **Board Cert:** Internal Medicine 1972; Gastroenterology 1973; **Med School:** Columbia P&S 1966; **Resid:** Internal Medicine, Yale-New Haven Hosp 1968; Internal Medicine, NY Hosp-Cornell 1969; **Fellow:** Gastroenterology, NY Hosp-Cornell 1973; **Fac Appt:** Clin Prof Med, Columbia P&S

Loria, Jeffrey Michael MD (Ge) - **Hospital:** Lenox Hill Hosp (page 106); **Address:** 178 E 85th St, Fl 4, New York, NY 10028; **Phone:** 212-288-2278; **Board Cert:** Internal Medicine 2012; Gastroenterology 2005; **Med School:** NY Med Coll 1987; **Resid:** Internal Medicine, Lenox Hill Hosp 1990; Internal Medicine, Lenox Hill Hosp 1991; **Fellow:** Gastroenterology, Elmhurst Hosp Ctr 1994

Lucak, Susan L MD (Ge) - **Spec Exp:** Irritable Bowel Syndrome; Liver Disease; **Hospital:** Lenox Hill Hosp (page 106), St. Luke's - Roosevelt Hosp Ctr - Roosevelt Div (page 94); **Address:** 121 E 69th St, New York, NY 10021; **Phone:** 212-861-0481; **Board Cert:** Internal Medicine 1984; Gastroenterology 2001; **Med School:** Albert Einstein Coll Med 1981; **Resid:** Internal Medicine, Montefiore Med Ctr 1985; **Fellow:** Gastroenterology, Montefiore Med Ctr 1987; Research, Columbia Presby Med Ctr 1991; **Fac Appt:** Asst Clin Prof Med, Columbia P&S

Lustbader, Ian J MD (Ge) - **Spec Exp:** Hepatitis C; Colonoscopy; Crohn's Disease; **Hospital:** NYU Langone Med Ctr (page 108); **Address:** 245 E 35th St Fl 1, New York, NY 10016-4283; **Phone:** 212-685-5252; **Board Cert:** Internal Medicine 1985; Gastroenterology 1987; **Med School:** Columbia P&S 1982; **Resid:** Internal Medicine, St Luke's-Roosevelt Hosp Ctr 1985; **Fellow:** Gastroenterology, Bellevue Hosp 1987; **Fac Appt:** Asst Clin Prof Med, NYU Sch Med

Magun, Arthur M MD (Ge) - **Spec Exp:** Hepatitis; Ulcerative Colitis; Endoscopy; Crohn's Disease; **Hospital:** NY-Presby/Columbia Univ Med Ctr, NY (page 104); **Address:** 161 Fort Washington Ave, Herbert Irving Pavillion Fl 3 - rm 338, New York, NY 10032-3713; **Phone:** 212-305-5287; **Board Cert:** Internal Medicine 1980; Gastroenterology 1983; **Med School:** Mount Sinai Sch Med 1977; **Resid:** Internal Medicine, Columbia-Presby Med Ctr 1980; **Fellow:** Gastroenterology, Columbia-Presby Med Ctr 1983; **Fac Appt:** Clin Prof Med, Columbia P&S

Marion, James MD (Ge) - **Spec Exp:** Colonoscopy; Colitis; Crohn's Disease; **Hospital:** Mount Sinai Med Ctr (page 102); **Address:** 12 E 86th St, New York, NY 10028; **Phone:** 212-861-2000; **Board Cert:** Internal Medicine 2003; Gastroenterology 2005; **Med School:** Columbia P&S 1989; **Resid:** Internal Medicine, Columbia Presby Hosp 1992; **Fellow:** Gastroenterology, Mt Sinai Hosp 1995; **Fac Appt:** Assoc Clin Prof Med, Mount Sinai Sch Med

Markowitz, Arnold J MD (Ge) - **Spec Exp:** Endoscopy; Gastrointestinal Cancer; **Hospital:** Meml Sloan-Kettering Cancer Ctr (page 116); **Address:** 1275 York Avenue, New York, NY 10065; **Phone:** 212-639-2901; **Board Cert:** Gastroenterology 2003; **Med School:** NYU Sch Med 1987; **Resid:** Internal Medicine, NYU Med Ctr 1990; **Fellow:** Gastroenterology, Univ Mich Med Ctr 1992; Gastroenterology, Univ Penn Med Ctr 1994; **Fac Appt:** Asst Prof Med, Cornell Univ-Weill Med Coll

Markowitz, David D MD (Ge) - **Spec Exp:** Gastroesophageal Reflux Disease (GERD); Esophageal Disorders; **Hospital:** NY-Presby/Columbia Univ Med Ctr, NY (page 104); **Address:** 161 Ft Washington Ave, Ste 853, New York, NY 10032; **Phone:** 212-305-1024; **Board Cert:** Internal Medicine 1988; Gastroenterology 2011; **Med School:** Columbia P&S 1985; **Resid:** Internal Medicine, Columbia-Presby Hosp 1988; **Fellow:** Gastroenterology, Columbia-Presby Hosp 1991; **Fac Appt:** Assoc Prof Med, Columbia P&S

Marsh Jr, Franklin MD (Ge) - **Spec Exp:** Colon Cancer; Liver Disease; Gastrointestinal Motility Disorders; **Hospital:** NY-Presby/Weill Cornell Med Ctr, NY (page 104); **Address:** 342 E 67th St, Ste 1D, New York, NY 10065-6238; **Phone:** 212-288-8820; **Board Cert:** Internal Medicine 1981; Gastroenterology 1985; **Med School:** SUNY Buffalo 1978; **Resid:** Internal Medicine, Harlem Hosp 1982; **Fellow:** Gastroenterology, New York Hosp 1984; **Fac Appt:** Asst Clin Prof Med, Cornell Univ-Weill Med Coll

Mayer, Lloyd MD (Ge) - **Spec Exp:** Inflammatory Bowel Disease/Crohn's; Ulcerative Colitis; **Hospital:** Mount Sinai Med Ctr (page 102); **Address:** 1425 Madison Ave, rm 11-20, New York, NY 10029; **Phone:** 212-659-9266; **Board Cert:** Internal Medicine 1979; Gastroenterology 1981; **Med School:** Mount Sinai Sch Med 1976; **Resid:** Internal Medicine, Bellevue Hosp 1979; **Fellow:** Gastroenterology, Mt Sinai Hosp 1981; **Fac Appt:** Prof Med, Mount Sinai Sch Med

Milano, Andrew MD (Ge) - **Spec Exp:** Endoscopy; Inflammatory Bowel Disease/Crohn's; Esophageal Disorders; **Hospital:** NYU Langone Med Ctr (page 108); **Address:** 530 1st Ave, Ste 4K, New York, NY 10016-6402; **Phone:** 212-263-7483; **Board Cert:** Internal Medicine 1977; Gastroenterology 1972; **Med School:** NYU Sch Med 1964; **Resid:** Internal Medicine, NYU-Bellevue Hosp 1967; **Fellow:** Gastroenterology, NYU-Bellevue Hosp 1968; **Fac Appt:** Clin Prof Med, NYU Sch Med

Min, Albert D MD (Ge) - **Spec Exp:** Hepatitis B & C; Liver Disease; **Hospital:** Beth Israel Med Ctr - Petrie Division (page 94); **Address:** Beth Israel Medical Ctr, 1st Ave at 16th St, New York, NY 10003; **Phone:** 212-420-4751; **Board Cert:** Internal Medicine 1988; Gastroenterology 2002; **Med School:** Univ Rochester 1985; **Resid:** Gastroenterology, SUNY Stony Brook 1988; **Fellow:** Hepatology, Montefiore Med Ctr 1991; **Fac Appt:** Assoc Clin Prof Med, Albert Einstein Coll Med

Miskovitz, Paul MD (Ge) - **Spec Exp:** Endoscopy; Liver Disease; Biliary Disease; **Hospital:** NY-Presby/Weill Cornell Med Ctr, NY (page 104); **Address:** 635 Madison Ave, Fl 17, New York, NY 10022; **Phone:** 212-717-4966; **Board Cert:** Internal Medicine 1978; Gastroenterology 1981; **Med School:** Cornell Univ-Weill Med Coll 1975; **Resid:** Internal Medicine, NY Hosp 1978; **Fellow:** Gastroenterology, NY Hosp 1980; **Fac Appt:** Clin Prof Med, Cornell Univ-Weill Med Coll

Nagler, Jerry MD (Ge) - **Spec Exp:** Inflammatory Bowel Disease; Irritable Bowel Syndrome; **Hospital:** NY-Presby/Weill Cornell Med Ctr, NY (page 104); **Address:** 407 E 70th St, FL 5, New York, NY 10021-5302; **Phone:** 212-628-7777; **Board Cert:** Internal Medicine 1976; Gastroenterology 1983; **Med School:** Yale Univ 1973; **Resid:** Internal Medicine, Columbia-Presby Hosp 1976; **Fellow:** Gastroenterology, NY Hosp/Cornell Med Ctr 1978; **Fac Appt:** Asst Clin Prof Med, Cornell Univ-Weill Med Coll

Ottaviano, Lawrence MD (Ge) - **Spec Exp:** Peptic Ulcer Disease; Colitis; **Address:** 60 Gramercy Park N, Ste 1B, New York, NY 10010; **Phone:** 212-254-1220; **Board Cert:** Internal Medicine 1988; Gastroenterology 2006; **Med School:** West Indies 1984; **Resid:** Internal Medicine, Cabrini Med Ctr 1987; **Fellow:** Gastroenterology, Cabrini Med Ctr 1989; **Fac Appt:** Asst Clin Prof Med, NY Med Coll

Pochapin, Mark B MD (Ge) - **Spec Exp:** Pancreatic Cancer; Endoscopic Ultrasound; Colon & Rectal Cancer Detection; Diarrheal Diseases; **Hospital:** NYU Langone Med Ctr (page 108); **Address:** 207 E 84th St Fl 4, 1315 York Ave Fl Ground, New York, NY 10028; **Phone:** 646-501-6760; **Board Cert:** Gastroenterology 2004; **Med School:** Cornell Univ-Weill Med Coll 1988; **Resid:** Internal Medicine, NY Hosp-Cornell Med Ctr 1991; **Fellow:** Gastroenterology, Montefiore Med Ctr 1993; **Fac Appt:** Assoc Clin Prof Med, Cornell Univ-Weill Med Coll

Poneros, John M MD (Ge) - **Spec Exp:** Endoscopy; Pancreatic Disease; Biliary Disease; Malabsorption; **Hospital:** NY-Presby/Columbia Univ Med Ctr, NY (page 104); **Address:** 161 Fort Washington Ave Fl 8 - Ste 862, New York, NY 10032; **Phone:** 212-305-1021; **Board Cert:** Gastroenterology 2011; Gastroenterology ; **Med School:** Columbia P&S 1995; **Resid:** Internal Medicine, NY Presby-Columbia Med Ctr 1998; **Fellow:** Gastroenterology, Mass General Hosp 2001; Advanced Endoscopy, Brigham & Women's Hosp 2002; **Fac Appt:** Asst Prof Med, Columbia P&S

Rieber, Jonathan M MD (Ge) - **Spec Exp:** Gastroesophageal Reflux Disease (GERD); Inflammatory Bowel Disease; Colonoscopy; **Hospital:** NY-Presby Hosp/The Allen Hosp (page 104), Lawrence Hosp Ctr; **Address:** 5030 Broadway, Ste 707, New York, NY 10034; **Phone:** 718-412-3445; **Board Cert:** Internal Medicine 2008; Gastroenterology 2010; **Med School:** NY Med Coll 1994; **Resid:** Internal Medicine, NY Presby-Columbia Med Ctr 1997; **Fellow:** Gastroenterology, NYU Med Ctr 2000; **Fac Appt:** Asst Clin Prof Med, Columbia P&S

Robilotti, James G MD (Ge) - **Spec Exp:** Irritable Bowel Syndrome; Peptic Ulcer Disease; Gastroesophageal Reflux Disease (GERD); Colon Cancer Screening; **Hospital:** Beth Israel Med Ctr - Petrie Division (page 94); **Address:** 29 Washington Sq West, New York, NY 10011-9180; **Phone:** 212-475-4030; **Board Cert:** Internal Medicine 1972; Gastroenterology 1981; **Med School:** UMDNJ-NJ Med Sch, Newark 1965; **Resid:** Internal Medicine, St Vincent's Hosp 1968; **Fellow:** Gastroenterology, St Vincent's Hosp 1970; **Fac Appt:** Assoc Clin Prof Med, NY Med Coll

Romeu, Jose MD (Ge) - **Spec Exp:** Colonoscopy/Polypectomy; Gastroscopy; Gastrointestinal Cancer; Gastroesophageal Reflux Disease (GERD); **Hospital:** Mount Sinai Med Ctr (page 102), Lenox Hill Hosp (page 106); **Address:** 1107 5th Ave, New York, NY 10128-0145; **Phone:** 212-534-6747; **Board Cert:** Internal Medicine 1973; Gastroenterology 1975; **Med School:** NYU Sch Med 1970; **Resid:** Internal Medicine, Mt Sinai Hosp 1973; **Fellow:** Gastroenterology, Mt Sinai Hosp 1976; **Fac Appt:** Asst Prof Med, Mount Sinai Sch Med

Rubin, Moshe MD (Ge) - **Spec Exp:** Enteroscopy-Small Bowel; Colonoscopy; Celiac Disease; Inflammatory Bowel Disease/Crohn's; **Hospital:** NY Hosp Queens (page 206); **Address:** 1020 Park Ave, Fl 1, New York, NY 10028; **Phone:** 212-772-1012; **Board Cert:** Internal Medicine 1986; Gastroenterology 1989; **Med School:** Yale Univ 1983; **Resid:** Internal Medicine, NY Hosp 1986; **Fellow:** Gastroenterology, Columbia-Presby Hosp 1988; **Fac Appt:** Assoc Prof Med, Cornell Univ-Weill Med Coll

Ruoff, Michael MD (Ge) - **Spec Exp:** Esophageal Disorders; Malabsorption; **Hospital:** NYU Langone Med Ctr (page 108); **Address:** 232 E 30 St Fl 1, New York, NY 10016-8202; **Phone:** 212-889-5544; **Board Cert:** Internal Medicine 1980; Gastroenterology 1972; **Med School:** NYU Sch Med 1963; **Resid:** Internal Medicine, Bellevue Hosp 1966; **Fellow:** Gastroenterology, NYU Med Ctr 1967; **Fac Appt:** Clin Prof Med, NYU Sch Med

Sachar, David B MD (Ge) - **Spec Exp:** Inflammatory Bowel Disease-Consult; **Hospital:** Mount Sinai Med Ctr (page 102); **Address:** One Gustave L Levy Pl, New York, NY 10029; **Phone:** 212-241-4514; **Board Cert:** Internal Medicine 1969; Gastroenterology 1972; **Med School:** Harvard Med Sch 1963; **Resid:** Internal Medicine, Beth Israel Hosp 1965; Internal Medicine, Beth Israel Hosp 1968; **Fellow:** Gastroenterology, Mount Sinai Hosp 1970; **Fac Appt:** Clin Prof Med, Mount Sinai Sch Med

Salik, James MD (Ge) - **Spec Exp:** Colonoscopy; Liver Disease; Inflammatory Bowel Disease; **Hospital:** NYU Langone Med Ctr (page 108); **Address:** 232 E 30th St, New York, NY 10016-8202; **Phone:** 212-889-5544; **Board Cert:** Internal Medicine 1983; Gastroenterology 1985; **Med School:** NYU Sch Med 1980; **Resid:** Internal Medicine, Bellevue Hosp 1983; **Fellow:** Gastroenterology, Bellevue Hosp 1985; **Fac Appt:** Asst Prof Med, NYU Sch Med

Scherl, Ellen MD (Ge) - **Spec Exp:** Inflammatory Bowel Disease; Crohn's Disease; Ulcerative Colitis; **Hospital:** NY-Presby/Weill Cornell Med Ctr, NY (page 104), Beth Israel Med Ctr - Petrie Division (page 94); **Address:** 1315 York Ave, Mezzanine Level, New York, NY 10021; **Phone:** 212-746-5077; **Board Cert:** Internal Medicine 1983; **Med School:** NY Med Coll 1977; **Resid:** Internal Medicine, Beth Israel Med Ctr 1981; **Fellow:** Gastroenterology, Mt Sinai Med Ctr 1983; **Fac Appt:** Asst Prof Med, Cornell Univ-Weill Med Coll

Schiano, Thomas D MD (Ge) - **Spec Exp:** Liver Disease; Transplant Medicine-Liver; Transplant Medicine-Bowel; Hepatitis; **Hospital:** Mount Sinai Med Ctr (page 102); **Address:** 5 E 98th St, Fl 12, Box 1104, MS 10029, New York, NY 10029; **Phone:** 212-241-8035; **Board Cert:** Internal Medicine 2000; Gastroenterology 2005; Transplant Hepatology 2006; **Med School:** Mexico 1987; **Resid:** Internal Medicine, Maimonides Med Ctr 1992; Gastroenterology, Temple Univ 1995; **Fellow:** Nutrition, Meml Sloan-Kettering Cancer Ctr 1993; Hepatology, Mt Sinai Med Ctr 1996; **Fac Appt:** Prof Med, Mount Sinai Sch Med

Schmerin, Michael J MD (Ge) - **Spec Exp:** Colonoscopy; Gastroscopy; Gastroesophageal Reflux Disease (GERD); **Hospital:** NY-Presby/Weill Cornell Med Ctr, NY (page 104), Lenox Hill Hosp (page 106); **Address:** 1060 Park Ave, Ste 1G, New York, NY 10128-1095; **Phone:** 212-348-3166; **Board Cert:** Internal Medicine 1976; Gastroenterology 1977; **Med School:** Jefferson Med Coll 1973; **Resid:** Internal Medicine, New York Hosp 1976; **Fellow:** Gastroenterology, New York Hosp-Cornell 1977; **Fac Appt:** Asst Prof Med, Cornell Univ-Weill Med Coll

Schneebaum, Cary MD (Ge) - **Spec Exp:** Colon Cancer Screening; **Hospital:** Beth Israel Med Ctr - Petrie Division (page 94); **Address:** 155 5th Ave, Fl 2, New York, NY 10010; **Phone:** 212-741-6100; **Board Cert:** Internal Medicine 1984; **Med School:** SUNY Hlth Sci Ctr 1981; **Resid:** Internal Medicine, Beth Israel Med Ctr 1984; **Fellow:** Gastroenterology, Beth Israel Med Ctr 1986

Schneider, Lewis P MD (Ge) - **Spec Exp:** Colon Cancer; Gastrointestinal Cancer; Esophageal Cancer; **Hospital:** NY-Presby/Columbia Univ Med Ctr, NY (page 104); **Address:** 16 E 60th St, rm 322, New York, NY 10022; **Phone:** 212-326-8426; **Board Cert:** Internal Medicine 1981; **Med School:** SUNY Downstate 1978; **Resid:** Internal Medicine, Columbia-Presby Hosp 1981; **Fellow:** Gastroenterology, Columbia-Presby Hosp 1983

Starpoli, Anthony A. MD (Ge) - **Spec Exp:** Gastroesophageal Reflux Disease (GERD); **Hospital:** Lenox Hill Hosp (page 106), NYU Langone Med Ctr (page 108); **Address:** 80 5th Ave, Ste 1605, New York, NY 10011; **Phone:** 212-673-2721; **Board Cert:** Internal Medicine 1989; Gastroenterology 2003; **Med School:** Univ IL Coll Med 1986; **Resid:** Internal Medicine, Sound Shore Med Ctr 1989; **Fellow:** Gastroenterology, St Vincents Hosp 1991; **Fac Appt:** Asst Clin Prof Med, NY Med Coll

Stein, Jeffrey A MD (Ge) - **Spec Exp:** Gallbladder Disease; Pancreatic Disease; **Hospital:** NY-Presby/Columbia Univ Med Ctr, NY (page 104); **Address:** 161 Ft Washington Ave, rm 328, New York, NY 10032; **Phone:** 212-305-5444; **Board Cert:** Internal Medicine 1971; Gastroenterology 1973; **Med School:** Harvard Med Sch 1965; **Resid:** Internal Medicine, Presbyterian Hosp 1970; **Fellow:** Gastroenterology, Presbyterian Hosp 1971; **Fac Appt:** Clin Prof Med, Columbia P&S

Tobias, Hillel MD (Ge) - **Spec Exp:** Liver Disease; Hepatitis B & C; Liver & Biliary Disease; **Hospital:** NYU Langone Med Ctr (page 108); **Address:** 232 E 30th St, New York, NY 10016-8202; **Phone:** 212-889-5544; **Board Cert:** Internal Medicine 1967; Gastroenterology 1979; Transplant Hepatology 2006; **Med School:** Washington Univ, St Louis 1960; **Resid:** Internal Medicine, Bellevue Hosp 1963; Hepatology, Royal Free Hosp 1965; **Fellow:** Hepatology, Mount Sinai Hosp 1967; **Fac Appt:** Prof Med, NYU Sch Med

Traube, Morris MD (Ge) - **Spec Exp:** Esophageal Disorders; Swallowing Disorders; Gastroesophageal Reflux Disease (GERD); **Hospital:** NYU Langone Med Ctr (page 108); **Address:** NYU Gastroenterology Associates, 530 First Ave, Ste 9N, New York, NY 10016; **Phone:** 212-263-3095; **Board Cert:** Internal Medicine 1981; Gastroenterology 1983; **Med School:** SUNY Downstate 1978; **Resid:** Internal Medicine, Maimonides Med Ctr 1981; **Fellow:** Gastroenterology, Yale-New Haven Hosp 1984; **Fac Appt:** Prof Med, NYU Sch Med

Ullman, Thomas A MD (Ge) - **Spec Exp:** Irritable Bowel Syndrome; Ulcerative Colitis; Inflammatory Bowel Disease/Crohn's; Colon & Rectal Cancer; **Hospital:** Mount Sinai Med Ctr (page 102); **Address:** 5 E 98th St Fl 11, New York, NY 10028; **Phone:** 212-241-4299; **Board Cert:** Gastroenterology 2009; **Med School:** Cornell Univ-Weill Med Coll 1992; **Resid:** Internal Medicine, New York Hosp 1995; **Fellow:** Gastroenterology, Yale-New Haven Hosp 1999; **Fac Appt:** Assoc Prof Med, Mount Sinai Sch Med

Wang, Timothy C MD (Ge) - **Hospital:** NY-Presby/Columbia Univ Med Ctr, NY (page 104); **Address:** 161 Fort Washington Ave, Ste 862, New York, NY 10032; **Phone:** 212-305-1021; **Board Cert:** Internal Medicine 1986; Gastroenterology 1989; **Med School:** Columbia P&S 1983; **Resid:** Internal Medicine, Barnes Jewish Hosp 1986; **Fellow:** Gastroenterology, Mass General Hosp 1989; **Fac Appt:** Prof Med, Columbia P&S

Waye, Jerome D MD (Ge) - **Spec Exp:** Endoscopy; Colon Cancer; Colonoscopy; **Hospital:** Mount Sinai Med Ctr (page 102), Lenox Hill Hosp (page 106); **Address:** 650 Park Ave, New York, NY 10065; **Phone:** 212-439-7779; **Board Cert:** Internal Medicine 1965; Gastroenterology 1970; **Med School:** Boston Univ 1958; **Resid:** Internal Medicine, Mt Sinai Hosp 1961; **Fellow:** Gastroenterology, Mt Sinai Hosp 1962; **Fac Appt:** Clin Prof Med, Mount Sinai Sch Med

Weiss, Robert A MD (Ge) - **Spec Exp:** Colon Cancer; Gastroesophageal Reflux Disease (GERD); Endoscopy; **Hospital:** Beth Israel Med Ctr - Petrie Division (page 94); **Address:** 380 2nd Ave, Ste 1004, New York, NY 10010; **Phone:** 212-473-4100; **Board Cert:** Internal Medicine 1987; Gastroenterology 1989; **Med School:** Mount Sinai Sch Med 1983; **Resid:** Internal Medicine, Beth Israel Med Ctr 1986; **Fellow:** Gastroenterology, Elmhurst Hosp Ctr-Mt Sinai 1988; **Fac Appt:** Asst Clin Prof Med, Albert Einstein Coll Med

Geriatric Medicine

Adelman, Ronald MD (Ger) - **Hospital:** NY-Presby/Weill Cornell Med Ctr, NY (page 104); **Address:** Irving Sherwood Wright Ctr on Aging, 1481 1st Ave, New York, NY 10075; **Phone:** 212-746-7000; **Board Cert:** Internal Medicine 1982; Geriatric Medicine 2009; **Med School:** Albert Einstein Coll Med 1978; **Resid:** Internal Medicine, Montefiore Med Ctr 1981

Bloom, Patricia A MD (Ger) - **Spec Exp:** Complementary Medicine; Dementia; Pain Management; **Hospital:** Mount Sinai Med Ctr (page 102); **Address:** 1440 Madison Ave, New York, NY 10029-6542; **Phone:** 212-659-8552; **Board Cert:** Internal Medicine 1978; Geriatric Medicine 2011; **Med School:** Univ Minn 1975; **Resid:** Internal Medicine, Montefiore Med Ctr 1978; **Fac Appt:** Assoc Prof Med, Mount Sinai Sch Med

Callahan, Eileen MD (Ger) - **Spec Exp:** Frail Elderly; Preventive Medicine; Dementia; **Hospital:** Mount Sinai Med Ctr (page 102); **Address:** Martha Stewart Ctr for Living, 1440 Madison Ave, New York, NY 10029; **Phone:** 212-659-8552; **Board Cert:** Internal Medicine 2004; Geriatric Medicine 2008; Hospice & Palliative Medicine 2005; **Med School:** UMDNJ-NJ Med Sch, Newark 1991; **Resid:** Internal Medicine, St Vincents Hosp Med Ctr 1994; **Fellow:** Geriatric Medicine, Mount Sinai Hosp 1996; **Fac Appt:** Assoc Prof Med, Mount Sinai Sch Med

Chang, Christine MD (Ger) - **Spec Exp:** Alzheimer's Disease; Dementia; **Hospital:** Mount Sinai Med Ctr (page 102); **Address:** 1440 Madison Ave, New York, NY 10029; **Phone:** 212-659-8552; **Board Cert:** Internal Medicine 2008; Geriatric Medicine 2010; **Med School:** Duke Univ 1995; **Resid:** Internal Medicine, Univ Pitt Hlth Sys 1998; **Fellow:** Geriatric Medicine, Johns Hopkins Hosp 2000; **Fac Appt:** Asst Prof Med, Mount Sinai Sch Med

Chun, Audrey K MD (Ger) - **Spec Exp:** Dementia; Depression; **Hospital:** Mount Sinai Med Ctr (page 102); **Address:** Martha Stewart Center for Living, 1440 Madison Ave, New York, NY 10029; **Phone:** 212-659-8552; **Board Cert:** Geriatric Medicine 2002; **Med School:** Baylor Coll Med 1998; **Resid:** Internal Medicine, Baylor Affil Hosp 2001; **Fellow:** Geriatric Medicine, Mt Sinai Hosp 2003; **Fac Appt:** Asst Prof Med, Mount Sinai Sch Med

Feher, Laszlo A DO (Ger) *PCP* - **Spec Exp:** Preventive Medicine; **Hospital:** NYU Langone Med Ctr (page 108), NYU Hosp For Joint Diseases (page 119); **Address:** 251 E 33rd St, Ste 2F, New York, NY 10016; **Phone:** 212-686-4212; **Board Cert:** Internal Medicine 2007; Geriatric Medicine 2008; **Med School:** NY Coll Osteo Med 1993; **Resid:** Internal Medicine, St Lukes Roosevelt Hosp 1996; **Fellow:** Geriatric Medicine, NYU Med Ctr 1998

Finkelstein, Martin S MD (Ger) - **Hospital:** NYU Langone Med Ctr (page 108); **Address:** 314 E 30th St, New York, NY 10016-6402; **Phone:** 646-370-2000; **Board Cert:** Internal Medicine 1970; **Med School:** NYU Sch Med 1964; **Resid:** Internal Medicine, Bellevue Hosp 1966; Internal Medicine, Stanford Univ Med Ctr 1967; **Fellow:** Infectious Disease, Stanford Univ Med Ctr 1968; **Fac Appt:** Assoc Clin Prof Med, NYU Sch Med

Fogel, Joyce MD (Ger) *PCP* - **Spec Exp:** Memory Disorders; Geriatric Functional Assessment; Preventive Medicine; **Hospital:** Beth Israel Med Ctr- Kings Hwy Div (page 94); **Address:** 275 8th Ave, New York, NY 10011-8305; **Phone:** 212-463-0101; **Board Cert:** Internal Medicine 1985; Geriatric Medicine 2011; **Med School:** SUNY Downstate 1982; **Resid:** Internal Medicine, Kings Co Hosp 1986; **Fellow:** Geriatric Medicine, Bellevue/NYU Med Ctr 1989; **Fac Appt:** Assoc Clin Prof Med, NY Med Coll

Karp, Adam H MD (Ger) *PCP* - **Spec Exp:** Falls in the Elderly; **Hospital:** NYU Hosp For Joint Diseases (page 119), NYU Langone Med Ctr (page 108); **Address:** 301 E 17th St, rm 208A, New York, NY 10003; **Phone:** 212-598-6738; **Board Cert:** Internal Medicine 2010; Geriatric Medicine 2012; **Med School:** Albert Einstein Coll Med 1987; **Resid:** Internal Medicine, Maimonides Med Ctr 1990; **Fellow:** Geriatric Medicine, Bellevue Hosp/NYU Med Ctr 1992; **Fac Appt:** Asst Prof Med, NYU Sch Med

Korc, Beatriz MD/PhD (Ger) - **Spec Exp:** Alzheimer's Disease; Diabetes; Preventive Medicine; **Hospital:** Meml Sloan-Kettering Cancer Ctr (page 116); **Address:** 1275 York Ave, New York, NY 10065; **Phone:** 646-888-3154; **Board Cert:** Internal Medicine 2007; Geriatric Medicine 2002; **Med School:** Uruguay 1983; **Resid:** Internal Medicine, Univ Rochester Med Ctr 1997; **Fellow:** Geriatric Medicine, Univ Rochester 2002; **Fac Appt:** Asst Prof Med, Mount Sinai Sch Med

Lachs, Mark S MD (Ger) - **Spec Exp:** Abuse/Neglect; **Hospital:** NY-Presby/Weill Cornell Med Ctr, NY (page 104); **Address:** Irving Sherwood Wright Med Ctr on Aging, 1484 First Ave, New York, NY 10075; **Phone:** 212-746-7000; **Board Cert:** Internal Medicine 1988; Geriatric Medicine 2002; **Med School:** NYU Sch Med 1985; **Resid:** Internal Medicine, Hosp Univ Penn 1988; **Fellow:** Geriatric Medicine, Yale-New Haven Hosp 1990; **Fac Appt:** Prof Med, Cornell Univ-Weill Med Coll

Leipzig, Rosanne M MD (Ger) *PCP* - **Spec Exp:** Medications in the Elderly; **Hospital:** Mount Sinai Med Ctr (page 102); **Address:** Martha Stewart Center for Living, 1440 Madison Ave, New York, NY 10029; **Phone:** 212-689-8552; **Board Cert:** Internal Medicine 1982; Geriatric Medicine 2008; **Med School:** Univ Mich Med Sch 1978; **Resid:** Internal Medicine, Strong Meml Hosp 1982; **Fellow:** Clinical Pharmacology, New York Hosp 1985; **Fac Appt:** Prof Med, Mount Sinai Sch Med

Morrison, R Sean MD (Ger) - **Spec Exp:** Palliative Care; **Hospital:** Mount Sinai Med Ctr (page 102); **Address:** Martha Stewart Center for Living, 1440 Madison Ave, New York, NY 10029; **Phone:** 212-659-8552; **Board Cert:** Internal Medicine 2003; Geriatric Medicine 2006; Hospice & Palliative Medicine 2008; **Med School:** Univ Chicago-Pritzker Sch Med 1990; **Resid:** Internal Medicine, NY Hosp/Cornell Med Ctr 1993; **Fellow:** Geriatric Medicine, Mt Sinai Med Ctr; **Fac Appt:** Prof Med, Mount Sinai Sch Med

Raman, Bharathi MD (Ger) - **Hospital:** NY-Presby/Weill Cornell Med Ctr, NY (page 104); **Address:** Irving Sherwood Wright Ctr on Aging, 1484 1st Ave, New York, NY 10075; **Phone:** 212-746-7000; **Board Cert:** Internal Medicine 1988; Geriatric Medicine 2011; **Med School:** India 1973; **Resid:** Internal Medicine, Woodhill Med Ctr 1988; **Fellow:** Geriatric Medicine, Mt Sinai Med Ctr 1990; **Fac Appt:** Asst Prof Med, Cornell Univ-Weill Med Coll

Sherman, Fredrick T MD (Ger) *PCP* - **Spec Exp:** Frail Elderly; Falls in the Elderly; Polypharmacology (Excess Medications); Memory Disorders; **Hospital:** Mount Sinai Med Ctr (page 102); **Address:** Archcare Senior Life, 1432 5th Ave, New York, NY 10035; **Phone:** 646-289-7700; **Board Cert:** Internal Medicine 1975; **Med School:** Temple Univ 1972; **Resid:** Internal Medicine, Med Coll Penn Hosp 1975; **Fac Appt:** Clin Prof Med, Mount Sinai Sch Med

Siegler, Eugenia L MD (Ger) *PCP* - **Spec Exp:** Dementia; **Hospital:** NY-Presby/Weill Cornell Med Ctr, NY (page 104); **Address:** Irving Sherwood Wright Ctr on Aging, 1484 First Ave, New York, NY 10021; **Phone:** 212-746-7000; **Board Cert:** Internal Medicine 1986; Geriatric Medicine 2010; **Med School:** Johns Hopkins Univ 1983; **Resid:** Internal Medicine, Bellevue Hosp 1987; **Fellow:** Geriatric Medicine, Hosp Univ Penn 1989; **Fac Appt:** Assoc Prof Med, Cornell Univ-Weill Med Coll

Geriatric Psychiatry

Devanand, Davangere MD (GerPsy) - **Spec Exp:** Memory Disorders; Alzheimer's Disease; Depression; Cognitive Loss in Aging; **Hospital:** NY State Psychiatric Inst; **Address:** NY State Psychiatric Inst, 1051 Riverside Dr, Unit 126, New York, NY 10032; **Phone:** 212-543-5612; **Board Cert:** Psychiatry 1985; Geriatric Psychiatry 2010; **Med School:** India 1979; **Resid:** Psychiatry, SUNY Upstate Med Ctr 1982; Psychiatry, Yale-New Haven Hosp 1984; **Fellow:** Biological Psychiatry, NY Presby-Columbia Med Ctr 1985; **Fac Appt:** Clin Prof Psyc, Columbia P&S

Reisberg, Barry MD (GerPsy) - **Spec Exp:** Alzheimer's Disease; Dementia; Cognitive Loss in Aging; Depression; **Hospital:** NYU Langone Med Ctr (page 108); **Address:** 145 E 32 St, Fl 5, Ste 508, rm 508, New York, NY 10016-6055; **Phone:** 212-263-8550; **Board Cert:** Psychiatry 1976; Geriatric Psychiatry 2012; **Med School:** NY Med Coll 1972; **Resid:** Psychiatry, Metropolitan Hosp 1975; **Fellow:** Psychiatric Research, Univ London 1975; **Fac Appt:** Prof Psyc, NYU Sch Med

Serby, Michael J MD (GerPsy) - **Spec Exp:** Alzheimer's Disease; Depression; Parkinson's Disease; **Hospital:** Beth Israel Med Ctr - Petrie Division (page 94); **Address:** 317 E 17th St, Fl 9, New York, NY 10003; **Phone:** 212-420-2421; **Board Cert:** Psychiatry 1979; Geriatric Psychiatry 2010; **Med School:** Emory Univ 1969; **Resid:** Psychiatry, Bellevue Hosp-NYU 1976; **Fac Appt:** Clin Prof Psyc, Albert Einstein Coll Med

Gynecologic Oncology

Abu-Rustum, Nadeem R MD (GO) - **Spec Exp:** Ovarian Cancer; Uterine Cancer; Cervical Cancer; Vulvar Disease/Cancer; **Hospital:** Meml Sloan-Kettering Cancer Ctr (page 116); **Address:** 1275 York Ave, New York, NY 10065; **Phone:** 212-639-7051; **Board Cert:** Obstetrics & Gynecology 2009; Gynecologic Oncology 2009; **Med School:** Lebanon 1990; **Resid:** Obstetrics & Gynecology, Greater Baltimore Med Ctr 1994; **Fellow:** Gynecologic Oncology, Meml Sloan-Kettering Cancer Ctr 1997; **Fac Appt:** Assoc Prof ObG, Cornell Univ-Weill Med Coll

Barakat, Richard R MD (GO) - **Spec Exp:** Laparoscopic Surgery; Ovarian Cancer; Uterine Cancer; Robotic Surgery; **Hospital:** Meml Sloan-Kettering Cancer Ctr (page 116); **Address:** 1275 York Ave, rm H1305, New York, NY 10065; **Phone:** 646-497-9055; **Board Cert:** Obstetrics & Gynecology 2012; Gynecologic Oncology 2012; **Med School:** SUNY Hlth Sci Ctr 1985; **Resid:** Obstetrics & Gynecology, Bellevue Hosp 1989; **Fellow:** Gynecologic Oncology, Meml Sloan Kettering Cancer Ctr 1991; **Fac Appt:** Assoc Prof ObG, Cornell Univ-Weill Med Coll

Brown, Carol MD (GO) - **Spec Exp:** Ovarian Cancer; Cervical Cancer; Uterine Cancer; Laparoscopic Surgery; **Hospital:** Meml Sloan-Kettering Cancer Ctr (page 116); **Address:** 1275 York Ave, rm H1311, New York, NY 10065; **Phone:** 212-639-7659; **Board Cert:** Obstetrics & Gynecology 2010; Gynecologic Oncology 2010; **Med School:** Columbia P&S 1986; **Resid:** Obstetrics & Gynecology, Hosp Univ Penn 1990; **Fellow:** Gynecologic Oncology, Meml Sloan Kettering Cancer Ctr 1992; Research, Meml Sloan Kettering Cancer Ctr 1994; **Fac Appt:** Asst Prof ObG, Cornell Univ-Weill Med Coll

Caputo, Thomas A MD (GO) - **Spec Exp:** Cervical Cancer; Ovarian Cancer; Uterine Cancer; Vulvar Disease/Cancer; **Hospital:** NY-Presby/Weill Cornell Med Ctr, NY (page 104); **Address:** NY Presby Hosp-Weill Cornell, 525 E 68th St, Ste J130, New York, NY 10021; **Phone:** 212-746-3179; **Board Cert:** Obstetrics & Gynecology 1993; Gynecologic Oncology 1977; **Med School:** UMDNJ-NJ Med Sch, Newark 1965; **Resid:** Obstetrics & Gynecology, Martland Hosp 1969; **Fellow:** Gynecologic Oncology, Emory Univ Hosp 1974; **Fac Appt:** Clin Prof ObG, Cornell Univ-Weill Med Coll

Chi, Dennis S MD (GO) - **Spec Exp:** Ovarian Cancer; Uterine Cancer; Cervical Cancer; Gynecologic Surgery-Complex; **Hospital:** Meml Sloan-Kettering Cancer Ctr (page 116); **Address:** 1275 York Ave, New York, NY 10065; **Phone:** 212-639-5016; **Board Cert:** Obstetrics & Gynecology 2011; Gynecologic Oncology 2011; **Med School:** NYU Sch Med 1990; **Resid:** Obstetrics & Gynecology, NYU Med Ctr 1994; **Fellow:** Gynecologic Oncology, Meml Sloan Kettering Cancer Ctr 1997; **Fac Appt:** Prof ObG, NYU Sch Med

Curtin, John P MD (GO) - **Spec Exp:** Uterine Cancer; Ovarian Cancer; Laparoscopic Surgery; Gestational Trophoblastic Disease; **Hospital:** NYU Langone Med Ctr (page 108); **Address:** NYU Clin Cancer Ctr, 160 E 34th St Fl 4, New York, NY 10016-6402; **Phone:** 212-731-5345; **Board Cert:** Obstetrics & Gynecology 2011; Gynecologic Oncology 2011; **Med School:** Creighton Univ 1979; **Resid:** Obstetrics & Gynecology, Univ Minn Med Ctr 1984; **Fellow:** Gynecologic Oncology, Meml Sloan-Kettering Cancer Ctr 1988; **Fac Appt:** Prof ObG, NYU Sch Med

Dottino, Peter R MD (GO) - **Spec Exp:** Laparoscopic Surgery; Gynecologic Cancer; **Hospital:** Mount Sinai Med Ctr (page 102); **Address:** 800-A 5th Ave, Ste 405, The Group for Women, New York, NY 10065; **Phone:** 212-888-8439; **Board Cert:** Obstetrics & Gynecology 2007; Gynecologic Oncology 2007; **Med School:** Georgetown Univ 1979; **Resid:** Obstetrics & Gynecology, SUNY Downstate Med Ctr 1983; **Fellow:** Gynecologic Oncology, Mt Sinai Hosp 1985

Fishman, David A MD (GO) - **Spec Exp:** Gynecologic Cancer; Ovarian Cancer-Early Detection; Minimally Invasive Surgery; Ultrasound; **Hospital:** Mount Sinai Med Ctr (page 102); **Address:** 5 E 98th St, Fl 2, New York, NY 10029; **Phone:** 212-427-9898; **Board Cert:** Obstetrics & Gynecology 2011; Gynecologic Oncology 2011; **Med School:** Texas Tech Univ 1988; **Resid:** Obstetrics & Gynecology, Yale-New Haven Hosp 1992; **Fellow:** Gynecologic Oncology, Yale-New Haven Hosp 1994; **Fac Appt:** Prof ObG, Mount Sinai Sch Med

Herzog, Thomas J MD (GO) - **Spec Exp:** Cervical Cancer; Gynecologic Cancer; Laparoscopic Surgery; Ovarian Cancer; **Hospital:** NY-Presby/Columbia Univ Med Ctr, NY (page 104); **Address:** Herbert Irving Pavilion, 161 Fort Washington Ave, 8-837, New York, NY 10032; **Phone:** 212-305-3410; **Board Cert:** Obstetrics & Gynecology 2008; Gynecologic Oncology 2008; **Med School:** Univ Cincinnati 1986; **Resid:** Obstetrics & Gynecology, Good Samaritan Hosp 1990; **Fellow:** Gynecologic Oncology, Barnes Jewish Hosp 1993; **Fac Appt:** Prof ObG, Columbia P&S

Holcomb, Kevin M MD (GO) - **Spec Exp:** Robotic Surgery; Laparoscopic Surgery; Ovarian Cancer; **Hospital:** NY-Presby/Weill Cornell Med Ctr, NY (page 104); **Address:** 525 E 68th St, Ste J 130, New York, NY 10021; **Phone:** 212-746-7553; **Board Cert:** Obstetrics & Gynecology 2011; Gynecologic Oncology 2011; **Med School:** NY Med Coll 1992; **Resid:** Obstetrics & Gynecology, NY Hosp-Cornell Med Ctr 1996; **Fellow:** Gynecologic Oncology, Downstate Med Ctr 1999; **Fac Appt:** Assoc Clin Prof ObG, Cornell Univ-Weill Med Coll

Koulos, John P MD (GO) - **Spec Exp:** Uterine Cancer; Ovarian Cancer; Cervical Cancer; **Hospital:** Beth Israel Med Ctr - Petrie Division (page 94); **Address:** Beth Israel Hosp Cancer Ctr, 10 Union Square E, Ste 4C, New York, NY 10003; **Phone:** 212-844-5729; **Board Cert:** Obstetrics & Gynecology 2010; Gynecologic Oncology 2010; **Med School:** Northwestern Univ 1978; **Resid:** Obstetrics & Gynecology, Northwestern Univ Med Sch 1982; **Fellow:** Gynecologic Oncology, Meml Sloan Kettering Cancer Ctr 1984; **Fac Appt:** Assoc Prof ObG, Albert Einstein Coll Med

Poynor, Elizabeth A MD/PhD (GO) - **Spec Exp:** Gynecologic Cancer; Gynecologic Surgery-Complex; Laparoscopic Surgery; Breast Cancer; **Hospital:** Lenox Hill Hosp (page 106); **Address:** 1050 5th Ave, New York, NY 10028; **Phone:** 212-426-2700; **Board Cert:** Obstetrics & Gynecology 2010; Gynecologic Oncology 2010; **Med School:** Columbia P&S 1988; **Resid:** Obstetrics & Gynecology, Hosp Univ Penn 1992; **Fellow:** Gynecologic Oncology, Meml Sloan-Kettering Cancer Ctr 1995

Rahaman, Jamal MD (GO) - **Spec Exp:** Minimally Invasive Surgery; Gynecologic Cancer; Robotic Surgery; Laparoscopic Surgery; **Hospital:** Mount Sinai Med Ctr (page 102); **Address:** 1136 Fifth Ave, New York, NY 10128-0122; **Phone:** 212-427-1415; **Board Cert:** Obstetrics & Gynecology 2011; Gynecologic Oncology 2011; **Med School:** Jamaica 1984; **Resid:** Obstetrics & Gynecology, Lincoln Med Ctr 1991; Obstetrics & Gynecology, Mt Sinai Med Ctr 1993; **Fellow:** Cardiovascular Surgery, Texas Heart Inst 1990; Gynecologic Oncology, Mt Sinai Med Ctr 1995; **Fac Appt:** Assoc Prof ObG, Mount Sinai Sch Med

Sonoda, Yukio MD (GO) *PCP* - **Spec Exp:** Laparoscopic Surgery; Fertility Preservation in Cancer; **Hospital:** Meml Sloan-Kettering Cancer Ctr (page 116); **Address:** 1275 York Ave, New York, NY 10065; **Phone:** 212-639-6450; **Board Cert:** Obstetrics & Gynecology 2006; Gynecologic Oncology 2006; **Med School:** Geo Wash Univ 1992; **Resid:** Obstetrics & Gynecology, SUNY Buffalo 1997

Wallach, Robert C MD (GO) - **Spec Exp:** Vulvar & Vaginal Cancer; Ovarian Cancer; Cervical Cancer; Peritoneal Carcinomatosis; **Hospital:** NYU Langone Med Ctr (page 108), Bellevue Hosp Ctr; **Address:** NYU Clinical Cancer Ctr, 160 E 34th St, New York, NY 10016; **Phone:** 212-731-5345; **Board Cert:** Obstetrics & Gynecology 1967; Gynecologic Oncology 1974; **Med School:** Yale Univ 1960; **Resid:** Obstetrics & Gynecology, Beth Israel Med Ctr 1965; **Fellow:** Gynecologic Oncology, SUNY Downstate Med Ctr 1966; **Fac Appt:** Prof ObG, NYU Sch Med

Zakashansky, Konstantin MD (GO) - **Spec Exp:** HPV-Human Papilloma Virus; Hysterectomy Alternatives; Robotic Surgery; **Hospital:** Mount Sinai Med Ctr (page 102), Lutheran Med Ctr - Brooklyn; **Address:** 1176 5th Ave, Box 1173, New York, NY 10029; **Phone:** 212-241-5034; **Board Cert:** Obstetrics & Gynecology 2007; Gynecologic Oncology 2010; **Med School:** SUNY Stony Brook 2000; **Resid:** Obstetrics & Gynecology, Beth Israel Med Ctr 2004; **Fellow:** Gynecologic Oncology, Mt Sinai 2007; **Fac Appt:** Asst Prof ObG, Mount Sinai Sch Med

Hand Surgery

Athanasian, Edward MD (HS) - **Spec Exp:** Bone & Soft Tissue Tumors; Hand & Upper Extremity Tumors; Hand & Upper Extremity Surgery; **Hospital:** Hosp For Special Surgery (page 115), Meml Sloan-Kettering Cancer Ctr (page 116); **Address:** Hospital for Special Surgery, 535 E 70th St, New York, NY 10021; **Phone:** 212-606-1962; **Board Cert:** Orthopaedic Surgery 2008; Hand Surgery 2008; **Med School:** Columbia P&S 1988; **Resid:** Surgery, Beth Israel Hosp 1989; Orthopaedic Surgery, Hosp Special Surgery 1993; **Fellow:** Hand Surgery, Mayo Clinic 1994; Orthopaedic Oncology, Meml Sloan Kettering Cancer Ctr 1995; **Fac Appt:** Asst Prof OrS, Cornell Univ-Weill Med Coll

Barron, O Alton MD (HS) - **Spec Exp:** Shoulder Arthroscopic Surgery; Elbow Surgery; Nerve & Tendon Reconstruction; Shoulder Reconstruction; **Hospital:** St. Luke's - Roosevelt Hosp Ctr - Roosevelt Div (page 94); **Address:** CV Starr Hand Surgery Ctr, 1000 10th Ave Fl 9, New York, NY 10019; **Phone:** 212-523-7590; **Board Cert:** Orthopaedic Surgery 2009; Hand Surgery 2009; **Med School:** Tulane Univ 1989; **Resid:** Surgery, Tulane Univ Affil Hosps 1994; **Fellow:** Shoulder Surgery, Columbia Presby Hosp 1995; Hand Surgery, St Lukes Roosevelt Hosp 1996; **Fac Appt:** Asst Clin Prof S, Columbia P&S

Beldner, Steven MD (HS) - **Spec Exp:** Elbow Surgery; Hand & Wrist Surgery; Scleroderma; **Hospital:** Beth Israel Med Ctr - Petrie Division (page 94), St. Luke's - Roosevelt Hosp Ctr - St Luke's Hosp (page 94); **Address:** 321 E 34th St, New York, NY 10016; **Phone:** 212-340-0000; **Board Cert:** Orthopaedic Surgery 1999; Hand Surgery 2001; **Med School:** UMDNJ-NJ Med Sch, Newark 1991; **Resid:** Orthopaedic Surgery, Bellevue Hosp 1996; **Fellow:** Hand Surgery, NYU Med Ctr 1997; **Fac Appt:** Asst Prof OrS, Albert Einstein Coll Med

Botwinick, Nelson MD (HS) - **Spec Exp:** Trauma; Carpal Tunnel Syndrome; Arthritis Hand Surgery; **Hospital:** NY Downtown Hosp; **Address:** 170 William St Fl 8, New York, NY 10038; **Phone:** 212-312-5598; **Board Cert:** Orthopaedic Surgery 2009; Hand Surgery 2009; **Med School:** NYU Sch Med 1980; **Resid:** Orthopaedic Surgery, NYU Med Ctr 1985; **Fellow:** Orthopaedic Surgery, NYU Med Ctr 1986; **Fac Appt:** Assoc Clin Prof OrS, NYU Sch Med

Carlson, Michelle Gerwin MD (HS) - **Spec Exp:** Sports Injuries; Hand & Upper Extremity Surgery; Pediatric Hand/Arm Surgery; Cerebral Palsy; **Hospital:** Hosp For Special Surgery (page 115); **Address:** 523 E 72nd St, Fl 4, rm 439, New York, NY 10021; **Phone:** 212-606-1546; **Board Cert:** Orthopaedic Surgery 2007; Hand Surgery 2007; **Med School:** Cornell Univ-Weill Med Coll 1987; **Resid:** Surgery, Hosp Special Surg 1992; **Fellow:** Hand Surgery, Hosp Special Surg 1993; **Fac Appt:** Assoc Prof OrS, Cornell Univ-Weill Med Coll

Catalano III, Louis W MD (HS) - **Spec Exp:** Hand & Upper Extremity Surgery; Wrist Surgery; Rotator Cuff Surgery; **Hospital:** St. Luke's - Roosevelt Hosp Ctr - Roosevelt Div (page 94); **Address:** 1000 10th Ave, Fl 3rd, New York, NY 10019; **Phone:** 212-523-7590; **Board Cert:** Orthopaedic Surgery 2003; Hand Surgery 2004; **Med School:** NYU Sch Med 1994; **Resid:** Surgery, Barnes Jewish Hosp 1995; Orthopaedic Surgery, Barnes Jewish Hosp 1999; **Fellow:** Hand Surgery, St. Lukes Roosevelt Hosp 2000; **Fac Appt:** Asst Clin Prof OrS, Columbia P&S

Glickel, Steven Z MD (HS) - **Spec Exp:** Hand & Wrist Surgery; Elbow Surgery; Peripheral Nerve Surgery; **Hospital:** St. Luke's - Roosevelt Hosp Ctr - Roosevelt Div (page 94); **Address:** 1000 10th Ave Fl 3, New York, NY 10019-1147; **Phone:** 212-523-7590; **Board Cert:** Orthopaedic Surgery 1985; Hand Surgery 2010; **Med School:** Harvard Med Sch 1976; **Resid:** Surgery, Columbia Presby Med Ctr 1978; Orthopaedic Surgery, Harvard Comb Ortho 1981; **Fellow:** Hand Surgery, St Luke's-Roosevelt Hosp Ctr 1983; Research, Columbia Presby Med Ctr 1982; **Fac Appt:** Clin Prof OrS, Columbia P&S

King, William MD (HS) - **Spec Exp:** Carpal Tunnel Syndrome; Hand Reconstruction; Microvascular Surgery; Fractures; **Hospital:** NYU Hosp For Joint Diseases (page 119), Lenox Hill Hosp (page 106); **Address:** 424 Madison Ave Fl 9, New York, NY 10017; **Phone:** 212-813-2104; **Board Cert:** Orthopaedic Surgery 2009; **Med School:** Columbia P&S 1974; **Resid:** Surgery, St Lukes-Roosevelt Hosp Ctr 1976; Orthopaedic Surgery, Columbia-Presby Med Ctr 1979; **Fellow:** Hand & Microvascular Surgery, Univ Colorado Hosp 1980; **Fac Appt:** Asst Prof OrS, NYU Sch Med

Lee, Steve K MD (HS) - **Spec Exp:** Peripheral Nerve Surgery; Tendon Surgery; Wrist/Hand Injuries; Ligament Reconstruction; **Hospital:** Hosp For Special Surgery (page 115); **Address:** 523 E 72nd St, Fl 4, New York, NY 10021; **Phone:** 212-606-1730; **Board Cert:** Orthopaedic Surgery 2010; Hand Surgery 2011; **Med School:** Duke Univ 1993; **Resid:** Orthopaedic Surgery, Yale-New Haven Hosp 1998; **Fellow:** Hand Surgery, NYU Hosp for Joint Diseases 2003; **Fac Appt:** Assoc Prof OrS, Cornell Univ-Weill Med Coll

Lenzo, Salvatore MD (HS) - **Spec Exp:** Carpal Tunnel Syndrome; Arthritis Hand Surgery; Hand & Wrist Injuries; Congenital Hand Deformities; **Hospital:** NYU Hosp For Joint Diseases (page 119), NYU Langone Med Ctr (page 108); **Address:** 955 5th Ave, New York, NY 10075; **Phone:** 212-734-9949; **Board Cert:** Orthopaedic Surgery 2010; Hand Surgery 2010; **Med School:** NYU Sch Med 1981; **Resid:** Orthopaedic Surgery, Bellevue Hosp 1986; **Fellow:** Hand Surgery, Bellevue Hosp 1987; **Fac Appt:** Assoc Prof OrS, NYU Sch Med

Melone Jr, Charles P MD (HS) - **Spec Exp:** Wrist Surgery; Fractures; **Hospital:** Beth Israel Med Ctr - Petrie Division (page 94); **Address:** 321 E 34th St, New York, NY 10016; **Phone:** 212-340-0000; **Board Cert:** Orthopaedic Surgery 1976; Hand Surgery 2004; **Med School:** Georgetown Univ 1969; **Resid:** Surgery, Nassau Co Med Ctr 1971; Orthopaedic Surgery, Nassau Co Med Ctr 1974; **Fellow:** Hand Surgery, NYU Langone Med Ctr 1975; **Fac Appt:** Prof OrS, Albert Einstein Coll Med

Polatsch, Daniel B MD (HS) - **Spec Exp:** Hand & Elbow Surgery; **Hospital:** Beth Israel Med Ctr - Petrie Division (page 94); **Address:** 321 E 34th St, New York, NY 10016; **Phone:** 212-340-0000; **Board Cert:** Orthopaedic Surgery 2005; Hand Surgery 2008; **Med School:** NYU Sch Med 1997; **Resid:** Orthopaedic Surgery, Hosp for Joint Dis 2002

Pruzansky, Mark E MD (HS) - **Spec Exp:** Arthritis Hand Surgery; Carpal Tunnel Syndrome; Sports Injuries; Wrist Surgery; **Hospital:** Mount Sinai Med Ctr (page 102), Lenox Hill Hosp (page 106); **Address:** 975 Park Ave, Ste 1B, MS 10028, New York, NY 10028; **Phone:** 212-249-8700; **Board Cert:** Orthopaedic Surgery 1980; Hand Surgery 2012; Orthopaedic Sports Medicine 2007; **Med School:** Mount Sinai Sch Med 1974; **Resid:** Orthopaedic Surgery, Mount Sinai Med Ctr 1978; **Fellow:** Hand Surgery, South Baptist Hosp 1978; Hand Surgery, Pacific Presby Hosp 1979; **Fac Appt:** Asst Prof OrS, Mount Sinai Sch Med

Raskin, Keith B MD (HS) - **Spec Exp:** Wrist/Hand Injuries; Arthritis; Carpal Tunnel Syndrome; Elbow Surgery; **Hospital:** NYU Langone Med Ctr (page 108), NYU Hosp For Joint Diseases (page 119); **Address:** 317 E 34th St, Fl 3, New York, NY 10016; **Phone:** 212-263-4263; **Board Cert:** Orthopaedic Surgery 2002; Hand Surgery 2002; **Med School:** Geo Wash Univ 1983; **Resid:** Orthopaedic Surgery, NYU Med Ctr 1988; **Fellow:** Hand Surgery, Union Mem Hosp 1989; **Fac Appt:** Assoc Clin Prof OrS, NYU Sch Med

Rettig, Michael MD (HS) - **Spec Exp:** Fractures; Arthritis; Nerve Disorders/Surgery; **Hospital:** NYU Langone Med Ctr (page 108), NYU Hosp For Joint Diseases (page 119); **Address:** 317 E 34th St Fl 3, New York, NY 10016-4974; **Phone:** 212-263-4263; **Board Cert:** Orthopaedic Surgery 2005; Hand Surgery 2005; **Med School:** SUNY Upstate Med Univ 1986; **Resid:** Orthopaedic Surgery, NYU Med Ctr 1991; **Fellow:** Hand Surgery, Mayo Clinic 1992; **Fac Appt:** Asst Prof OrS, NYU Sch Med

Rosenwasser, Melvin P MD (HS) - **Spec Exp:** Carpal Tunnel Syndrome; Sports Injuries; Elbow Surgery; Trauma; **Hospital:** NY-Presby/Columbia Univ Med Ctr, NY (page 104); **Address:** New York Orthopedic Hospital Associates, 622 W 168th St, PH 11, rm 1150, New York, NY 10032; **Phone:** 212-305-8036; **Board Cert:** Orthopaedic Surgery 1999; Hand Surgery 2011; **Med School:** Columbia P&S 1976; **Resid:** Surgery, Roosevelt Hosp 1979; Orthopaedic Surgery, Columbia Presby Hosp 1982; **Fellow:** Hand Surgery, Columbia Presby Hosp 1983; **Fac Appt:** Prof OrS, Columbia P&S

Strauch, Robert MD (HS) - **Spec Exp:** Hand Reconstruction; Hand & Elbow Nerve Disorders; Hand & Wrist Surgery; Elbow Surgery; **Hospital:** NY-Presby/Columbia Univ Med Ctr, NY (page 104); **Address:** 622 W 168th St, rm PH-11-1119, New York, NY 10032; **Phone:** 212-305-4272; **Board Cert:** Orthopaedic Surgery 2005; Hand Surgery 2005; **Med School:** Columbia P&S 1986; **Resid:** Orthopaedic Surgery, Columbia-Presby Hosp 1991; **Fellow:** Hand Surgery, Indiana Hand Center 1992; **Fac Appt:** Prof OrS, Columbia P&S

Weiland, Andrew J MD (HS) - **Spec Exp:** Wrist/Hand Injuries; Hand Reconstruction; **Hospital:** Hosp For Special Surgery (page 115), NY-Presby/Weill Cornell Med Ctr, NY (page 104); **Address:** Hospital for Special Surgery, 535 E 70th St, New York, NY 10021-4872; **Phone:** 212-606-1575; **Board Cert:** Orthopaedic Surgery 1977; **Med School:** Wake Forest Univ 1968; **Resid:** Surgery, Univ Michigan Med Ctr 1970; Orthopaedic Surgery, Johns Hopkins Hosp 1975; **Fellow:** Hand Surgery, Kleinert Hosp 1975; **Fac Appt:** Prof OrS, Cornell Univ-Weill Med Coll

Wolfe, Scott W MD (HS) - **Spec Exp:** Wrist Surgery; Nerve Disorders/Surgery; Fractures; **Hospital:** Hosp For Special Surgery (page 115); **Address:** Hospital for Special Surgery, 535 E 70 St, New York, NY 10021; **Phone:** 212-606-1529; **Board Cert:** Orthopaedic Surgery 2003; Hand Surgery 2003; **Med School:** Cornell Univ-Weill Med Coll 1984; **Resid:** Surgery, St Luke's Roosevelt Hosp Ctr 1986; Orthopaedic Surgery, Hosp Special Surg 1989; **Fellow:** Hand & Microvascular Surgery, Columbia Presby Med Ctr 1990; **Fac Appt:** Prof OrS, Cornell Univ-Weill Med Coll

Yang, S Steven MD (HS) - **Spec Exp:** Shoulder Surgery; Congenital Hand Deformities; **Hospital:** Lenox Hill Hosp (page 106), NYU Hosp For Joint Diseases (page 119); **Address:** 130 E 77th St Fl 7, New York, NY 10021; **Phone:** 212-744-8114; **Board Cert:** Orthopaedic Surgery 2009; Hand Surgery 2003; **Med School:** Duke Univ 1988; **Resid:** Orthopaedic Surgery, Lenox Hill Hosp 1994; **Fellow:** Hand Surgery, Hosp for Special Surgery 1995; **Fac Appt:** Asst Clin Prof OrS, NYU Sch Med

Hematology

Aledort, Louis M MD (Hem) - **Spec Exp:** Bleeding/Coagulation Disorders; Platelet Disorders; Paroxysmal Nocturnal Hemoglobinuria; **Hospital:** Mount Sinai Med Ctr (page 102); **Address:** 5 E 98 St, Fl 4, rm e, Box 1006, 1190 Fifth Ave, Box 1006, New York, NY 10029; **Phone:** 212-860-0205; **Board Cert:** Internal Medicine 1966; Hematology 1972; **Med School:** Albert Einstein Coll Med 1959; **Resid:** Internal Medicine, Univ Va Hlth Sci Ctr 1961; Hematology, Nat Inst Health 1963; **Fellow:** Internal Medicine, Strong Meml Hosp 1964; Hematology, Strong Meml Hosp 1966; **Fac Appt:** Prof Med, Mount Sinai Sch Med

Amorosi, Edward L MD (Hem) - **Hospital:** NYU Langone Med Ctr (page 108); **Address:** NYU Clinical Cancer Ctr, 160 E 34th St, New York, NY 10016; **Phone:** 212-731-5187; **Board Cert:** Internal Medicine 1966; Hematology 1972; Medical Oncology 1977; **Med School:** NYU Sch Med 1959; **Resid:** Internal Medicine, Bellevue Hosp Ctr- NYU 1962; Internal Medicine, Francis Delafield Hosp 1963; **Fellow:** Hematology, NYU Med Ctr 1965; **Fac Appt:** Prof Med, NYU Sch Med

Ansell, Jack Edward MD (Hem) - **Spec Exp:** Thrombotic Disorders; **Hospital:** Lenox Hill Hosp (page 106); **Address:** 100 E 77th St, New York, NY 10075; **Phone:** 212-434-2140; **Board Cert:** Internal Medicine 1975; Hematology 1976; **Med School:** Univ VA Sch Med 1972; **Resid:** Internal Medicine, Tufts- New England Med Ctr 1974; **Fellow:** Hematology, Boston Univ/Boston City Hosp 1975; Hematology, Boston VA Hosp 1977

Brower, Mark S MD (Hem) - **Spec Exp:** Bleeding/Coagulation Disorders; Hematologic Malignancies; Breast Cancer; **Hospital:** NY-Presby/Weill Cornell Med Ctr, NY (page 104); **Address:** 310 E 72nd St, New York, NY 10021-4703; **Phone:** 212-717-2995; **Board Cert:** Internal Medicine 1977; Hematology 1982; Medical Oncology 1979; **Med School:** Johns Hopkins Univ 1974; **Resid:** Internal Medicine, NY Hosp/Cornell Med Ctr 1977; **Fellow:** Hematology & Oncology, NY Hosp/Cornell Med Ctr 1980; **Fac Appt:** Clin Prof Med, Cornell Univ-Weill Med Coll

Castro-Malaspina, Hugo MD (Hem) - **Spec Exp:** Myelodysplastic Syndromes; Bone Marrow Failure Disorders; Bone Marrow Transplant; Anemia-Aplastic; **Hospital:** Meml Sloan-Kettering Cancer Ctr (page 116); **Address:** 1275 York Ave, New York, NY 10065; **Phone:** 800-525-2225; **Med School:** Peru 1971; **Resid:** Internal Medicine, St Louis Hosp; **Fellow:** Hematology & Oncology, Andean Biology Inst; Pediatric Hematology-Oncology, St Louis Hosp

Cook, Perry MD (Hem) - **Spec Exp:** Bone Marrow Transplant; Leukemia; Lymphoma; **Hospital:** NYU Langone Med Ctr (page 108); **Address:** 160 E 34th St Fl 7, New York, NY 10016; **Phone:** 212-731-5184; **Board Cert:** Internal Medicine 1980; Hematology 1982; Medical Oncology 1983; **Med School:** Univ Iowa Coll Med 1977; **Resid:** Internal Medicine, St Luke's-Roosevelt Hosp Ctr 1979; Internal Medicine, Columbia-Presby Med Ctr 1980; **Fellow:** Hematology & Oncology, Columbia-Presby Med Ctr 1983; **Fac Appt:** Assoc Clin Prof Med, NYU Sch Med

Diaz, Michael MD (Hem) - **Spec Exp:** Anemia; Bleeding/Coagulation Disorders; Lymphoma; **Hospital:** Mount Sinai Med Ctr (page 102); **Address:** 1112 Park Ave, New York, NY 10128; **Phone:** 212-876-4500; **Board Cert:** Internal Medicine 1979; Hematology 1986; **Med School:** St Louis Univ 1971; **Resid:** Internal Medicine, Lenox Hill Hosp 1974; **Fellow:** Hematology, Elmhurst Hosp 1976; **Fac Appt:** Asst Clin Prof Med, Mount Sinai Sch Med

Diuguid, David L MD (Hem) - **Spec Exp:** Bleeding/Coagulation Disorders; **Hospital:** NY-Presby/Columbia Univ Med Ctr, NY (page 104); **Address:** 161 Ft Washington Ave, Irving Bldg Fl 10, New York, NY 10032; **Phone:** 212-305-0527; **Board Cert:** Internal Medicine 1982; Hematology 1986; Medical Oncology 1985; **Med School:** Cornell Univ-Weill Med Coll 1979; **Resid:** Internal Medicine, Boston Univ Med Ctr 1983; **Fellow:** Hematology & Oncology, New England Med Ctr 1986; **Fac Appt:** Assoc Prof Med, Columbia P&S

Fruchtman, Steven M MD (Hem) - **Spec Exp:** Myeloproliferative Disorders; Polycythemia Rubra Vera; **Address:** 1150 Park Ave, Ste Medical, New York, NY 10128; **Phone:** 212-427-7700; **Board Cert:** Internal Medicine 1980; Hematology 1984; **Med School:** NY Med Coll 1977; **Resid:** Internal Medicine, Univ Hosp 1981; **Fellow:** Hematology, Mount Sinai Med Ctr 1984; Hematology, Meml Sloan Kettering Cancer Ctr 1985; **Fac Appt:** Assoc Prof Hem & Onc, NY Med Coll

Goldenberg, Alec MD (Hem) - **Spec Exp:** Breast Cancer; Lymphoma; Bleeding/Coagulation Disorders; **Hospital:** NYU Langone Med Ctr (page 108); **Address:** 157 E 32nd St Fl 2, New York, NY 10016; **Phone:** 212-689-6791; **Board Cert:** Internal Medicine 1986; Medical Oncology 1987; **Med School:** Johns Hopkins Univ 1980; **Resid:** Internal Medicine, Bellevue Hosp-NYU 1984; **Fellow:** Hematology & Oncology, Meml Sloan Kettering Canc Ctr 1988; **Fac Appt:** Assoc Clin Prof Med, NYU Sch Med

Gruenstein, Steven MD (Hem) - **Spec Exp:** Hematologic Malignancies; Breast Cancer; Gastrointestinal Cancer; Lung Cancer; **Hospital:** Mount Sinai Med Ctr (page 102), Lenox Hill Hosp (page 106); **Address:** 12 E 86th St, Central Park Hematology, New York, NY 10028-0506; **Phone:** 212-861-6660; **Board Cert:** Internal Medicine 1988; **Med School:** Italy 1984; **Resid:** Internal Medicine, Metropolitan Hosp Ctr 1987; **Fellow:** Hematology & Oncology, Beth Israel Med Ctr 1990; **Fac Appt:** Assoc Clin Prof Med, Mount Sinai Sch Med

Halperin, Ira MD (Hem) - **Spec Exp:** Leukemia; Myeloproliferative Disorders; **Hospital:** Beth Israel Med Ctr - Petrie Division (page 94); **Address:** 2 Fifth Ave, Ste 9, New York, NY 10011-8855; **Phone:** 212-254-5940; **Board Cert:** Internal Medicine 1970; Hematology 1976; Medical Oncology 1979; **Med School:** NYU Sch Med 1962; **Resid:** Internal Medicine, St Vincents Hosp 1966; **Fellow:** Hematology, Mt Sinai Hosp 1969

Hymes, Kenneth B MD (Hem) - **Spec Exp:** Bleeding/Coagulation Disorders; Leukemia & Lymphoma; Cutaneous Lymphoma, T-cell; Mycosis Fungoides; **Hospital:** NYU Langone Med Ctr (page 108); **Address:** NYU Clinical Cancer Center, 160 E 34th St, Fl 7, New York, NY 10016-6402; **Phone:** 212-731-5189; **Board Cert:** Internal Medicine 1978; Hematology 1980; Medical Oncology 1981; **Med School:** SUNY Upstate Med Univ 1975; **Resid:** Internal Medicine, Barnes Hosp 1978; **Fellow:** Hematology, NYU Med Ctr 1980; Medical Oncology, NYU Med Ctr 1981; **Fac Appt:** Assoc Prof Hem & Onc, NYU Sch Med

Isola, Luis M MD (Hem) - **Spec Exp:** Bone Marrow Transplant; Stem Cell Transplant; Myelodysplastic Syndromes; Anemia; **Hospital:** Mount Sinai Med Ctr (page 102); **Address:** 1190 Fifth Ave, New York, NY 10029; **Phone:** 212-241-6021; **Board Cert:** Internal Medicine 1986; Hematology 1988; **Med School:** Argentina 1979; **Resid:** Internal Medicine, Ctr for Med Education 1983; **Fellow:** Hematology, Mt Sinai Med Ctr 1985; **Fac Appt:** Assoc Prof Med, Mount Sinai Sch Med

Kempin, Sanford J MD (Hem) - **Spec Exp:** Bleeding/Coagulation Disorders; Leukemia; Lymphoma; Thrombotic Disorders; **Hospital:** Beth Israel Med Ctr - Petrie Division (page 94); **Address:** 325 W 15th St, New York, NY 10011; **Phone:** 212-604-6010; **Board Cert:** Internal Medicine 1976; Medical Oncology 1977; Hematology 1978; **Med School:** Belgium 1971; **Resid:** Internal Medicine, Lemuel Shattuck Hosp 1972; **Fellow:** Hematology, St Jude Chldns Rsch Hosp 1975; Medical Oncology, Meml Sloan Kettering Cancer Ctr 1976; **Fac Appt:** Asst Prof Hem & Onc, Albert Einstein Coll Med

Leonard, John P MD (Hem) - **Spec Exp:** Lymphoma; Multiple Myeloma; Hematologic Malignancies; Leukemia; **Hospital:** NY-Presby/Weill Cornell Med Ctr, NY (page 104); **Address:** NY Presby Hosp-NY Weill Cornell Med Ctr, 525 E 68th St, Payson 3, New York, NY 10065; **Phone:** 646-962-2068; **Board Cert:** Hematology 2006; Medical Oncology 2007; **Med School:** Univ VA Sch Med 1990; **Resid:** Internal Medicine, NY Hosp-Cornell Med Ctr 1993; **Fellow:** Hematology & Oncology, NY Hosp-Cornell Med Ctr 1996; **Fac Appt:** Prof Med, Cornell Univ-Weill Med Coll

Levine, Randy MD (Hem) - **Spec Exp:** Hematologic Malignancies; Bleeding/Coagulation Disorders; **Hospital:** Lenox Hill Hosp (page 106), St. Luke's - Roosevelt Hosp Ctr - Roosevelt Div (page 94); **Address:** 4 E 76th St, New York, NY 10021-2611; **Phone:** 212-717-1020; **Board Cert:** Internal Medicine 1982; Hematology 1984; Blood Banking 1985; **Med School:** SUNY Buffalo 1979; **Resid:** Internal Medicine, Montefiore Med Ctr 1982; **Fellow:** Hematology, Montefiore Med Ctr 1983; Blood Banking, Mt Sinai Hosp 1984; **Fac Appt:** Assoc Clin Prof Med, NYU Sch Med

Maslak, Peter G MD (Hem) - **Spec Exp:** Leukemia; Stem Cell Transplant; Myelodysplastic Syndromes; Clinical Trials; **Hospital:** Meml Sloan-Kettering Cancer Ctr (page 116); **Address:** 1275 York Avenue, New York, NY 10065; **Phone:** 212-639-5518; **Board Cert:** Internal Medicine 1987; Hematology 2000; Medical Oncology 1989; **Med School:** Mount Sinai Sch Med 1984; **Resid:** Internal Medicine, Univ Michigan Med Ctr 1987; **Fellow:** Hematology & Oncology, Meml Sloan Kettering Cancer Ctr 1990

Mears, John Gregory MD (Hem) - **Spec Exp:** Lymphoma; Leukemia; Multiple Myeloma; **Hospital:** NY-Presby/Columbia Univ Med Ctr, NY (page 104); **Address:** 161 Ft Washington Ave, Ste 923, New York, NY 10032; **Phone:** 212-305-3506; **Board Cert:** Internal Medicine 1976; Hematology 1978; **Med School:** Columbia P&S 1973; **Resid:** Internal Medicine, Boston Univ Med Ctr 1975; **Fellow:** Hematology & Oncology, Columbia-Presby Med Ctr 1978; **Fac Appt:** Clin Prof Med, Columbia P&S

Meyer, Richard MD (Hem) - **Spec Exp:** Lymphoma; Leukemia; Multiple Myeloma; Head & Neck Cancer; **Hospital:** Mount Sinai Med Ctr (page 102); **Address:** 1150 Park Ave, New York, NY 10128-1234; **Phone:** 212-427-7700; **Board Cert:** Internal Medicine 1975; Hematology 1978; Medical Oncology 1979; **Med School:** Mount Sinai Sch Med 1972; **Resid:** Internal Medicine, Mt Sinai Hosp 1975; Hematology, Mt Sinai Hosp 1977; **Fellow:** Medical Oncology, Mt Sinai Hosp 1977; **Fac Appt:** Assoc Clin Prof Med, Mount Sinai Sch Med

Moskovits, Tibor MD (Hem) - **Spec Exp:** Lymphoma; Breast Cancer; Lung Cancer; **Hospital:** NYU Langone Med Ctr (page 108); **Address:** NYU Clinical Cancer Center, 160 E 34th St Fl 7, New York, NY 10016; **Phone:** 212-731-5191; **Board Cert:** Internal Medicine 1988; Hematology 2003; Medical Oncology 2004; **Med School:** SUNY Downstate 1985; **Resid:** Internal Medicine, Beth Israel Med Ctr 1989; **Fellow:** Hematology & Oncology, NYU Med Ctr 1992; **Fac Appt:** Asst Clin Prof Med, NYU Sch Med

Ossias, A Lawrence MD (Hem) - **Spec Exp:** Lymphoma; Leukemia; Coagulation/Bleeding Disorders; **Hospital:** Mount Sinai Med Ctr (page 102); **Address:** 1112 Park Ave, New York, NY 10128; **Phone:** 212-427-9333; **Board Cert:** Internal Medicine 1972; Hematology 1972; Medical Oncology 1979; **Med School:** Yale Univ 1965; **Resid:** Internal Medicine, Bronx Municipal Hosp 1970; **Fellow:** Hematology, Mt Sinai Med Ctr 1972; **Fac Appt:** Asst Clin Prof Med, Mount Sinai Sch Med

Raphael, Bruce Gordon MD (Hem) - **Spec Exp:** Lymphoma; Leukemia; Multiple Myeloma; Anemia; **Hospital:** NYU Langone Med Ctr (page 108), Bellevue Hosp Ctr; **Address:** NYU Clinical Cancer Ctr, 240 E 38th St Fl 19, New York, NY 10016-6402; **Phone:** 212-731-5185; **Board Cert:** Internal Medicine 1978; Hematology 1980; Medical Oncology 1981; **Med School:** McGill Univ 1975; **Resid:** Internal Medicine, Jewish Genl Hosp 1977; **Fellow:** Medical Oncology, Meml Sloan Kettering Cancer Ctr 1978; Hematology, NYU Med Ctr 1980; **Fac Appt:** Clin Prof Med, NYU Sch Med

Savage, David G MD (Hem) - **Spec Exp:** Stem Cell Transplant; Multiple Myeloma; Lymphoma; **Hospital:** NY-Presby/Columbia Univ Med Ctr, NY (page 104); **Address:** 177 Fort Washington Ave, Fl 10, Millstein Bldg - Fl 6, rm 435, New York, NY 10032; **Phone:** 212-305-9783; **Board Cert:** Internal Medicine 1977; Hematology 1982; Medical Oncology 1985; **Med School:** Columbia P&S 1974; **Resid:** Internal Medicine, Harlem Hosp/Columbia Presby Med Ctr 1977; **Fellow:** Hematology & Oncology, Harlem Hosp/Columbia Presby Med Ctr 1982; **Fac Appt:** Prof Med, Columbia P&S

Scigliano, Eileen MD (Hem) - **Spec Exp:** Bone Marrow Transplant; **Hospital:** Mount Sinai Med Ctr (page 102); **Address:** 1 Gustave L Levy Pl, Box 1410, New York, NY 10029; **Phone:** 212-241-6021; **Board Cert:** Internal Medicine 1984; Hematology 1988; **Med School:** Israel 1981; **Resid:** Internal Medicine, Kings County Hosp 1984; **Fellow:** Medical Oncology, VA Med Ctr 1985; Hematology, Mount Sinai Hosp 1988; **Fac Appt:** Asst Clin Prof Med, Mount Sinai Sch Med

Soff, Gerald A MD (Hem) - **Spec Exp:** Bleeding/Coagulation Disorders; Thrombotic Disorders; Hematologic Disorders in Cancer Patients; Anemia; **Hospital:** Meml Sloan-Kettering Cancer Ctr (page 116); **Address:** MSKCC Div of Hematology, 1275 York Ave Fl 4 - Ste 6, New York, NY 10021; **Phone:** 212-639-2335; **Board Cert:** Internal Medicine 1984; Hematology 1988; **Med School:** Johns Hopkins Univ 1981; **Resid:** Internal Medicine, Med Coll Virginia 1984; **Fellow:** Hematology & Oncology, Beth Israel Med Ctr 1988

Tallman, Martin S MD (Hem) - **Spec Exp:** Bone Marrow Transplant; Leukemia; Hairy Cell Leukemia; **Hospital:** Meml Sloan-Kettering Cancer Ctr (page 116); **Address:** 1275 York Ave, Box 380, Ste 21-100, New York, NY 10065; **Phone:** 212-639-3842; **Board Cert:** Internal Medicine 1983; Medical Oncology 1987; Hematology 1988; **Med School:** Ros Franklin Univ/Chicago Med Sch 1980; **Resid:** Internal Medicine, Evanston Hosp 1983; **Fellow:** Medical Oncology, Fred Hutchinson Cancer Ctr 1987; **Fac Appt:** Prof Med, Cornell Univ-Weill Med Coll

Troy, Kevin M MD (Hem) - **Spec Exp:** Leukemia; Lymphoma; Multiple Myeloma; **Hospital:** Mount Sinai Med Ctr (page 102); **Address:** 1735 York Ave, Ste P2, New York, NY 10128; **Phone:** 212-860-9055; **Board Cert:** Internal Medicine 1982; Hematology 1984; **Med School:** Univ Conn 1979; **Resid:** Internal Medicine, Lenox Hill Hosp 1982; **Fellow:** Hematology, Mount Sinai Hosp 1984; **Fac Appt:** Assoc Clin Prof Med, Mount Sinai Sch Med

Vogel, James M MD (Hem) - **Spec Exp:** Breast Cancer; Colon Cancer; Leukemia & Lymphoma; Platelet Disorders; **Hospital:** Mount Sinai Med Ctr (page 102), Mount Sinai Hosp of Queens (page 102); **Address:** 1125 Park Ave, New York, NY 10128-1243; **Phone:** 212-369-4250; **Board Cert:** Internal Medicine 1969; Hematology 1972; Medical Oncology 1973; **Med School:** Columbia P&S 1962; **Resid:** Internal Medicine, Mount Sinai Hosp 1964; Internal Medicine, Mount Sinai Hosp 1967; **Fellow:** Medical Oncology, Natl Cancer Inst 1966; Hematology, Mount Sinai Hosp 1968; **Fac Appt:** Assoc Prof Med, Mount Sinai Sch Med

Wisch, Nathaniel MD (Hem) - **Spec Exp:** Lymphoma; Breast Cancer; Leukemia; Anemia-Cancer Related; **Hospital:** Lenox Hill Hosp (page 106), Mount Sinai Med Ctr (page 102); **Address:** Central Park Hematology & Oncology, 12 E 86th St, New York, NY 10028-0506; **Phone:** 212-861-6660; **Board Cert:** Internal Medicine 1965; Hematology 1972; Medical Oncology 1977; **Med School:** Northwestern Univ 1958; **Resid:** Internal Medicine, VA Hosp 1960; Internal Medicine, Montefiore Hosp 1961; **Fellow:** Hematology & Oncology, Mount Sinai Hosp 1962; **Fac Appt:** Clin Prof Med, Mount Sinai Sch Med

Wolf, David J MD (Hem) - **Spec Exp:** Hematologic Malignancies; Hematology-Benign; Solid Tumors; **Hospital:** NY-Presby/Weill Cornell Med Ctr, NY (page 104); **Address:** 115 E 61st St Fl 11, New York, NY 10065; **Phone:** 212-688-7100; **Board Cert:** Internal Medicine 1976; Hematology 1978; Medical Oncology 1979; **Med School:** SUNY Hlth Sci Ctr 1973; **Resid:** Internal Medicine, NY Hosp/Meml Hosp 1976; **Fellow:** Hematology, NY Hosp 1976; **Fac Appt:** Asst Clin Prof Med, Cornell Univ-Weill Med Coll

Hospice & Palliative Medicine

Chai, Emily MD (Hospice & Palliative Med) - **Spec Exp:** Palliative Care; **Hospital:** Mount Sinai Med Ctr (page 102); **Address:** One Gustave L Levy Pl, Box 1070, New York, NY 10029; **Phone:** 212-659-8552; **Board Cert:** Internal Medicine 2011; Geriatric Medicine 2002; Hospice & Palliative Medicine 2008; **Med School:** NYU Sch Med 1998; **Resid:** Internal Medicine, Mt Sinai Hosp 2001; **Fellow:** Geriatric Medicine, Mt Sinai Hosp 2003; **Fac Appt:** Asst Prof Med, Mount Sinai Sch Med

Portenoy, Russell MD (Hospice & Palliative Med) - **Spec Exp:** Pain Medicine; Pain-Cancer; Palliative Care; **Hospital:** Beth Israel Med Ctr - Petrie Division (page 94); **Address:** Beth Israel Med Ctr, Dept Pain Medicine/Palliative Care, First Ave at 16th St, New York, NY 10003; **Phone:** 212-844-1403; **Board Cert:** Neurology 1985; Hospice & Palliative Medicine 2008; **Med School:** Univ MD Sch Med 1980; **Resid:** Neurology, Montefiore Med Ctr 1984; **Fellow:** Pain Medicine, Meml Sloan-Kettering Cancer Ctr 1985; **Fac Appt:** Prof N, Albert Einstein Coll Med

Infectious Disease

Aberg, Judith A MD (Inf) - **Spec Exp:** AIDS/HIV; **Hospital:** Bellevue Hosp Ctr; **Address:** Bellevue C&D Bldg, 5, rm 558, 550 First Ave, New York, NY 10016; **Phone:** 212-562-4964; **Board Cert:** Infectious Disease 2006; **Med School:** Penn State Coll Med 1990; **Resid:** Internal Medicine, Cleveland Clinic Fdn 1994; **Fellow:** Infectious Disease, Washington Univ Sch Med 1996; **Fac Appt:** Prof Med, NYU Sch Med

Brause, Barry MD (Inf) - **Spec Exp:** Bone/Joint Infections; Skin/Soft Tissue Infections; Infections in Prosthetic Devices; **Hospital:** Hosp For Special Surgery (page 115), NY-Presby/Weill Cornell Med Ctr, NY (page 104); **Address:** 535 E 70th St, Ste 657W, New York, NY 10021-5718; **Phone:** 212-774-7411; **Board Cert:** Internal Medicine 1973; Infectious Disease 1976; **Med School:** Univ Pittsburgh 1970; **Resid:** Internal Medicine, NY Hosp 1973; **Fellow:** Infectious Disease, NY Hosp 1975; **Fac Appt:** Clin Prof Med, Cornell Univ-Weill Med Coll

Brown, Arthur E MD (Inf) - **Spec Exp:** Infections in Cancer Patients; Fungal Infections; Infections in Immunocompromised Patients; **Hospital:** Meml Sloan-Kettering Cancer Ctr (page 116); **Address:** 1275 York Ave, New York, NY 10065; **Phone:** 212-639-8475; **Med School:** Jefferson Med Coll 1971; **Resid:** Internal Medicine, Roosevelt Hosp 1972; Internal Medicine, USPHS Hosp-Staten Island NY & USPHS Hosp 1974; **Fellow:** Internal Medicine, Roosevelt Hosp 1976; Infectious Disease, Mem Sloan Kettering Cancer Ctr 1978; **Fac Appt:** Clin Prof Med, Cornell Univ-Weill Med Coll

Busillo, Christopher MD (Inf) - **Spec Exp:** AIDS/HIV; Travel Medicine; Lyme Disease; **Hospital:** NY Downtown Hosp; **Address:** 19 Beekman St Fl 6th, New York, NY 10038-2668; **Phone:** 212-374-2145; **Board Cert:** Internal Medicine 2000; Infectious Disease 2000; **Med School:** Italy 1986; **Resid:** Internal Medicine, Cabrini Med Ctr 1989; **Fellow:** Infectious Disease, Cabrini Med Ctr 1991

Caplivski, Daniel Simon MD (Inf) - **Spec Exp:** Travel Medicine; **Hospital:** Mount Sinai Med Ctr (page 102); **Address:** 5 E 98th St Fl 8, New York, NY 10029; **Phone:** 212-241-7468; **Board Cert:** Internal Medicine 2003; Infectious Disease 2005; **Med School:** Yale Univ 2000; **Resid:** Internal Medicine, Mt Sinai Med Ctr 2003; **Fac Appt:** Asst Prof Med, Mount Sinai Sch Med

El-Sadr, Wafaa M MD (Inf) - **Spec Exp:** AIDS/HIV; Tuberculosis; **Hospital:** Harlem Hosp Ctr; **Address:** Harlem Hospital, 506 Lenox Ave MLK Bldg - rm 3101A, New York, NY 10037; **Phone:** 212-939-2936; **Board Cert:** Internal Medicine 1979; Infectious Disease 1982; **Med School:** Egypt 1974; **Resid:** Internal Medicine, Columbia-Presby Med Ctr 1982; **Fellow:** Infectious Disease, VA Medical Ctr 1983

Flood, Mary T MD/PhD (Inf) - **Spec Exp:** Infectious Disease; HIV; Hepatitis; Herpes Simplex; **Hospital:** NY-Presby/Columbia Univ Med Ctr, NY (page 104); **Address:** 161 Fort Washington Ave, rm 346, New York, NY 10032-3702; **Phone:** 212-305-8039; **Board Cert:** Internal Medicine 2002; Infectious Disease 2004; **Med School:** Columbia P&S 1987; **Resid:** Internal Medicine, NY-Presby Hosp 1991; **Fellow:** Infectious Disease, NY-Presby Hosp 1993; **Fac Appt:** Assoc Clin Prof Med, Columbia P&S

Glesby, Marshall J MD/PhD (Inf) - **Spec Exp:** HIV/AIDS; **Hospital:** NY-Presby/Weill Cornell Med Ctr, NY (page 104); **Address:** 525 E 68th St, Baker Bldg - Fl 24, MS 97, New York, NY 10065; **Phone:** 212-746-4177; **Board Cert:** Internal Medicine 2003; Infectious Disease 2004; **Med School:** Johns Hopkins Univ 1989; **Resid:** Internal Medicine, Johns Hopkins Hosp 1992; **Fellow:** Infectious Disease, Johns Hopkins Hosp 1996; **Fac Appt:** Assoc Prof Med, Cornell Univ-Weill Med Coll

Greene, Jeffrey MD (Inf) - **Spec Exp:** AIDS/HIV; **Hospital:** NYU Langone Med Ctr (page 108); **Address:** 110 E 40th St, Ste 603, New York, NY 10016; **Phone:** 212-375-2940; **Board Cert:** Internal Medicine 1979; Infectious Disease 1982; **Med School:** NYU Sch Med 1976; **Resid:** Internal Medicine, Bellevue Hosp 1980; **Fellow:** Infectious Disease, Bellevue Hosp 1982; **Fac Appt:** Assoc Clin Prof Med, NYU Sch Med

Gumprecht, Jeffrey P MD (Inf) - **Spec Exp:** AIDS/HIV; Travel Medicine; Infections-Surgical; **Hospital:** Mount Sinai Med Ctr (page 102); **Address:** 1100 Park Ave, Ste 1C, New York, NY 10128; **Phone:** 212-427-9550; **Board Cert:** Internal Medicine 1987; Infectious Disease 2003; **Med School:** Albany Med Coll 1983; **Resid:** Internal Medicine, Mt Sinai Hosp 1987; **Fellow:** Infectious Disease, Montefiore Med Ctr 1990; **Fac Appt:** Asst Clin Prof Med, Mount Sinai Sch Med

Hammer, Glenn S MD (Inf) - **Spec Exp:** AIDS/HIV; Hospital Acquired Infections; Infections-Surgical; **Hospital:** Mount Sinai Med Ctr (page 102); **Address:** 1100 Park Ave, Ste 1C, New York, NY 10128-1202; **Phone:** 212-427-9550; **Board Cert:** Infectious Disease 1974; Internal Medicine 1973; **Med School:** NYU Sch Med 1969; **Resid:** Internal Medicine, Mount Sinai Hosp 1972; **Fellow:** Infectious Disease, Mount Sinai Hosp 1974; **Fac Appt:** Asst Clin Prof Med, Mount Sinai Sch Med

Hammer, Scott M MD (Inf) - **Spec Exp:** AIDS/HIV; **Hospital:** NY-Presby/Columbia Univ Med Ctr, NY (page 104); **Address:** 630 W 168th St, P&S Box 82, New York, NY 10032; **Phone:** 212-305-8039; **Board Cert:** Internal Medicine 1975; Infectious Disease 1980; **Med School:** Columbia P&S 1972; **Resid:** Internal Medicine, Columbia-Presby Hosp 1975; Internal Medicine, Stanford Univ Hosp 1975; **Fellow:** Infectious Disease, Mass Genl Hosp 1981; **Fac Appt:** Prof Med, Columbia P&S

Hartman, Barry J MD (Inf) - **Spec Exp:** Endocarditis; Infections-Surgical; Parasitic Infections; **Hospital:** NY-Presby/Weill Cornell Med Ctr, NY (page 104); **Address:** 407 E 70th St, Fl 4, New York, NY 10021-5302; **Phone:** 212-744-4882; **Board Cert:** Internal Medicine 1976; Infectious Disease 1980; **Med School:** Penn State Coll Med 1973; **Resid:** Internal Medicine, NY Hosp/Cornell Med Ctr 1976; **Fellow:** Infectious Disease, NY Hosp/Cornell Med Ctr 1981; **Fac Appt:** Clin Prof Med, Cornell Univ-Weill Med Coll

Helfgott, David MD (Inf) - **Spec Exp:** Infections in Immunocompromised Patients; Skin/Soft Tissue Infections; Bone/Joint Infections; Travel Medicine; **Hospital:** NY-Presby/Weill Cornell Med Ctr, NY (page 104); **Address:** 212 E 68th St, New York, NY 10065; **Phone:** 212-879-6004; **Board Cert:** Internal Medicine 1986; Infectious Disease 1988; **Med School:** Yale Univ 1983; **Resid:** Internal Medicine, NY Hosp/Cornell Med Ctr 1986; Internal Medicine, NY Hosp 1990; **Fellow:** Infectious Disease, NY Hosp/Cornell Med Ctr 1989; **Fac Appt:** Asst Clin Prof Med, Cornell Univ-Weill Med Coll

Horowitz, Harold MD (Inf) - **Spec Exp:** AIDS/HIV; Tick-borne Diseases; Travel Medicine; **Hospital:** NYU Langone Med Ctr (page 108); **Address:** NYU School Medicine, 550 First Ave, NBV 16 S 5, New York, NY 10016; **Phone:** 212-263-2115; **Board Cert:** Internal Medicine 1983; Infectious Disease 1988; **Med School:** NYU Sch Med 1979; **Resid:** Internal Medicine, Univ Wisconsin Hosp 1983; **Fellow:** Infectious Disease, New England Med Ctr 1986; **Fac Appt:** Prof Med, NYU Sch Med

Huprikar, Shirish S MD (Inf) - **Spec Exp:** Infections in Transplant Patients; Infections in Immunocompromised Patients; Infections in Transplant Patients w/HIV; **Hospital:** Mount Sinai Med Ctr (page 102); **Address:** Mt Sinai Med Ctr, 5 E 98th St Fl 12, New York, NY 10029; **Phone:** 212-241-7968; **Board Cert:** Internal Medicine 2010; Infectious Disease 2001; **Med School:** Northwestern Univ 1996; **Resid:** Internal Medicine, Mt Sinai Med Ctr 1999; **Fellow:** Infectious Disease, Mt Sinai Med Ctr 2001; **Fac Appt:** Assoc Prof Med, Mount Sinai Sch Med

Jacobs, Jonathan MD (Inf) - **Spec Exp:** AIDS/HIV; **Hospital:** NY-Presby/Weill Cornell Med Ctr, NY (page 104); **Address:** 449 E 68th St, Ground Fl, New York, NY 10065; **Phone:** 212-734-1365; **Board Cert:** Internal Medicine 1983; Infectious Disease 1986; **Med School:** Yale Univ 1980; **Resid:** Internal Medicine, NY Hosp/Cornell Med Ctr 1983; **Fellow:** Infectious Disease, NY Hosp/Cornell Med Ctr 1986; **Fac Appt:** Clin Prof Med, Cornell Univ-Weill Med Coll

Lerner, Chester W MD (Inf) - **Spec Exp:** AIDS/HIV; Travel Medicine; Sexually Transmitted Diseases; **Hospital:** NY Downtown Hosp; **Address:** 156 William St, Fl 7, New York, NY 10038-2612; **Phone:** 646-588-2500; **Board Cert:** Internal Medicine 1981; Infectious Disease 1984; **Med School:** Univ Pittsburgh 1978; **Resid:** Internal Medicine, Lenox Hill Hosp 1981; **Fellow:** Infectious Disease, Lenox Hill Hosp 1983; **Fac Appt:** Asst Clin Prof Med, Cornell Univ-Weill Med Coll

Louie, Eddie MD (Inf) - **Spec Exp:** Lyme Disease; AIDS/HIV; Hospital Acquired Infections; **Hospital:** NYU Langone Med Ctr (page 108); **Address:** 345 E 37th St, Ste 207, New York, NY 10016; **Phone:** 212-682-9202; **Board Cert:** Internal Medicine 1982; Infectious Disease 1986; **Med School:** NYU Sch Med 1979; **Resid:** Internal Medicine, Kings County Hosp 1983; **Fellow:** Infectious Disease, NYU Med Ctr 1985; **Fac Appt:** Assoc Clin Prof Med, NYU Sch Med

McMeeking, Alexander MD (Inf) - **Spec Exp:** AIDS/HIV; Hepatitis B & C; Herpes Simplex; Antibiotic Resistance; **Hospital:** NYU Langone Med Ctr (page 108); **Address:** 104 E 40th St, Ste 507, New York, NY 10016; **Phone:** 212-375-2560; **Board Cert:** Internal Medicine 1985; Infectious Disease 1988; **Med School:** UMDNJ-NJ Med Sch, Newark 1982; **Resid:** Internal Medicine, St Luke's-Roosevelt Hosp 1985; **Fellow:** Infectious Disease, Bellvue/NYU Med Ctr 1986

Mildvan, Donna MD (Inf) - **Spec Exp:** AIDS/HIV; Clinical Trials; Infectious Disease; **Hospital:** Beth Israel Med Ctr - Petrie Division (page 94); **Address:** Beth Israel Med Ctr, Div Infectious Dis, 1st Ave at 16th St, 19BH17, New York, NY 10003; **Phone:** 212-420-4005; **Board Cert:** Internal Medicine 1972; Infectious Disease 1972; **Med School:** Johns Hopkins Univ 1967; **Resid:** Internal Medicine, Mt Sinai Hosp 1970; **Fellow:** Infectious Disease, Mt Sinai Hosp 1972; **Fac Appt:** Prof Med, Albert Einstein Coll Med

Miller, Dennis K MD (Inf) - **Spec Exp:** Lyme Disease; AIDS/HIV; Travel Medicine; **Hospital:** Lenox Hill Hosp (page 106); **Address:** 4 E 76th St, New York, NY 10021-1811; **Phone:** 212-472-1237; **Board Cert:** Internal Medicine 1985; Infectious Disease 1988; **Med School:** Rush Med Coll 1982; **Resid:** Internal Medicine, Lenox Hill Hosp 1985; **Fellow:** Infectious Disease, Lenox Hill Hosp 1987

Mullen, Michael P MD (Inf) - **Spec Exp:** Osteomyelitis; AIDS/HIV; Hospital Acquired Infections; **Hospital:** Mount Sinai Med Ctr (page 102); **Address:** Mount Sinai Faculty Practice Assocs, 5 E 98th St, Fl 8, New York, NY 10029; **Phone:** 212-241-3150; **Board Cert:** Internal Medicine 1985; Infectious Disease 1986; **Med School:** Spain 1981; **Resid:** Internal Medicine, Jewish Hosp Med Ctr 1984; **Fellow:** Infectious Disease, Cabrini Med Ctr 1986; **Fac Appt:** Assoc Clin Prof Med, Mount Sinai Sch Med

Murray, Henry W MD (Inf) - **Spec Exp:** Parasitic Infections; Travel Medicine; **Hospital:** NY-Presby/Weill Cornell Med Ctr, NY (page 104); **Address:** NY Presby-Cornell Med Ctr, 525 E 68th St, Box 136, New York, NY 10065; **Phone:** 212-746-6330; **Board Cert:** Internal Medicine 1975; Infectious Disease 1978; **Med School:** Cornell Univ-Weill Med Coll 1972; **Resid:** Internal Medicine, New York Hosp 1974; Internal Medicine, Johns Hopkins Hosp 1975; **Fellow:** Infectious Disease, New York Hosp 1977; **Fac Appt:** Prof Med, Cornell Univ-Weill Med Coll

Neibart, Eric MD (Inf) - **Spec Exp:** Travel Medicine; AIDS/HIV; Fungal Infections; **Hospital:** Mount Sinai Med Ctr (page 102); **Address:** 1100 Park Ave, New York, NY 10128-1202; **Phone:** 212-427-9550; **Board Cert:** Internal Medicine 1983; Infectious Disease 1986; **Med School:** UMDNJ-NJ Med Sch, Newark 1980; **Resid:** Internal Medicine, Mt Sinai Med Ctr 1983; **Fellow:** Infectious Disease, Mt Sinai Med Ctr 1986; **Fac Appt:** Asst Prof Med, Mount Sinai Sch Med

Perlman, David MD (Inf) - **Spec Exp:** AIDS/HIV; Lyme Disease; Travel Medicine; Infectious Disease; **Hospital:** Beth Israel Med Ctr - Petrie Division (page 94), Lenox Hill Hosp (page 106); **Address:** Beth Israel Med Ctr, 120 E 16th St Fl 12, New York, NY 10003; **Phone:** 212-844-8549; **Board Cert:** Internal Medicine 1986; Infectious Disease 1988; **Med School:** Albert Einstein Coll Med 1983; **Resid:** Internal Medicine, New York Hosp/Meml-Sloan Kettering 1986; **Fellow:** Infectious Disease, Montefiore Hosp 1988; **Fac Appt:** Prof Med, Albert Einstein Coll Med

Pollock, Alan MD (Inf) - **Hospital:** Lenox Hill Hosp (page 106); **Address:** 184 E 70th St, Level B1, New York, NY 10021-5110; **Phone:** 212-988-2702; **Board Cert:** Internal Medicine 1975; Infectious Disease 1978; **Med School:** NY Med Coll 1972; **Resid:** Internal Medicine, Lenox Hill Hosp 1975; **Fellow:** Infectious Disease, Manhattan VA Hosp 1977; **Fac Appt:** Asst Clin Prof Med, NYU Sch Med

Polsky, Bruce W MD (Inf) - **Spec Exp:** AIDS/HIV; Viral Infections; Infections in Cancer Patients; AIDS Related Cancers; **Hospital:** St. Luke's - Roosevelt Hosp Ctr - Roosevelt Div (page 94), St. Luke's - Roosevelt Hosp Ctr - St Luke's Hosp (page 94); **Address:** 425 W 59th St, Ste 8A, New York, NY 10019; **Phone:** 212-523-7335; **Board Cert:** Internal Medicine 1983; Infectious Disease 1986; **Med School:** Wayne State Univ 1980; **Resid:** Internal Medicine, Montefiore Hosp 1983; **Fellow:** Infectious Disease, Meml Sloan Kettering Cancer Ctr 1986; **Fac Appt:** Prof Med, Columbia P&S

Press, Robert A MD (Inf) - **Spec Exp:** Infections-Surgical; Hospital Acquired Infections; **Hospital:** NYU Langone Med Ctr (page 108); **Address:** 530 1st Ave, Ste 4G, New York, NY 10016-6402; **Phone:** 212-263-7229; **Board Cert:** Internal Medicine 1976; **Med School:** NYU Sch Med 1973; **Resid:** Internal Medicine, Beth Israel Hosp 1975; Internal Medicine, Bellevue Hosp 1976; **Fellow:** Infectious Disease, Montefiore Hosp Med Ctr 1978; **Fac Appt:** Assoc Clin Prof Med, NYU Sch Med

Romagnoli, Mario MD (Inf) - **Spec Exp:** AIDS/HIV; Bone/Joint Infections; **Hospital:** Lenox Hill Hosp (page 106); **Address:** 903 Park Ave, New York, NY 10075; **Phone:** 212-396-3390; **Board Cert:** Internal Medicine 1979; Infectious Disease 1982; **Med School:** Columbia P&S 1976; **Resid:** Internal Medicine, Columbia-Presby Med Ctr 1979; **Fellow:** Infectious Disease, Beth Israel Med Ctr 1981; **Fac Appt:** Assoc Prof Med, Columbia P&S

Scully, Brian MD (Inf) - **Spec Exp:** Lyme Disease; **Hospital:** NY-Presby/Columbia Univ Med Ctr, NY (page 104); **Address:** 161 Fort Washington Ave, rm 346, New York, NY 10032; **Phone:** 212-305-8039; **Board Cert:** Internal Medicine 1975; Infectious Disease 1982; **Med School:** Ireland 1971; **Resid:** Internal Medicine, St Luke's-Roosevelt Hosp Ctr 1975; **Fellow:** Infectious Disease, Columbia Presby Med Ctr 1982

Sepkowitz, Kent A MD (Inf) - **Spec Exp:** Tuberculosis; Infections in Cancer Patients; Fungal Infections; **Hospital:** Meml Sloan-Kettering Cancer Ctr (page 116); **Address:** 1275 York Ave, New York, NY 10065; **Phone:** 800-525-2225; **Board Cert:** Internal Medicine 1983; Infectious Disease 2010; **Med School:** Univ Okla Coll Med 1980; **Resid:** Internal Medicine, Roosevelt Hosp 1984; **Fellow:** Infectious Disease, Meml Sloan Kettering Cancer Ctr 1991; **Fac Appt:** Prof Med, Cornell Univ-Weill Med Coll

Simberkoff, Michael S MD (Inf) - **Spec Exp:** AIDS/HIV; Pneumonia; **Hospital:** VA NY Harbor Hlthcare Sys-Manhattan Campus, NYU Langone Med Ctr (page 108); **Address:** 423 E 23rd St, 3 West Executive Office, New York, NY 10010; **Phone:** 212-951-3417; **Board Cert:** Internal Medicine 1980; Infectious Disease 1972; **Med School:** NYU Sch Med 1962; **Resid:** Internal Medicine, Bellevue Hosp 1967; **Fellow:** Infectious Disease, NYU Med Ctr 1969; **Fac Appt:** Assoc Prof Med, NYU Sch Med

Smith, Paul T MD (Inf) - **Spec Exp:** AIDS/HIV; Skin/Soft Tissue Infections; Infections in Transplant Patients; Travel Medicine; **Hospital:** NY-Presby/Weill Cornell Med Ctr, NY (page 104), Hosp For Special Surgery (page 115); **Address:** 943 Lexington Ave, New York, NY 10021; **Phone:** 212-396-4077; **Board Cert:** Internal Medicine 2005; Infectious Disease 2007; **Med School:** Hahnemann Univ 1992; **Resid:** Internal Medicine, NY Hosp-Cornell Med Ctr 1995; **Fellow:** Infectious Disease, Yale-New Haven Hosp 1997; **Fac Appt:** Asst Clin Prof Med, Cornell Univ-Weill Med Coll

Soave, Rosemary MD (Inf) - **Spec Exp:** Infections-Transplant; Parasitic Infections; Infections in Immunocompromised Patients; **Hospital:** NY-Presby/Weill Cornell Med Ctr, NY (page 104); **Address:** 450 E 69th St, New York, NY 10021; **Phone:** 212-746-9915; **Board Cert:** Internal Medicine 1979; Infectious Disease 1984; **Med School:** Cornell Univ-Weill Med Coll 1976; **Resid:** Internal Medicine, New York Hosp 1979; Internal Medicine, Meml Sloan Kettering Cancer Ctr 1980; **Fellow:** Infectious Disease, New York Hosp/Cornell Med Ctr 1982; **Fac Appt:** Assoc Prof Med, Cornell Univ-Weill Med Coll

Wallach, Frances MD (Inf) - **Spec Exp:** AIDS/HIV; Infection Control; HIV & Blood Transfusions; **Hospital:** Mount Sinai Med Ctr (page 102); **Address:** Mount Sinai Med Ctr, One Gustave L Levy Pl, New York, NY 10029; **Phone:** 212-241-7968; **Board Cert:** Internal Medicine 1989; Infectious Disease 2002; **Med School:** Albany Med Coll 1985; **Resid:** Internal Medicine, Montefiore Med Ctr 1989; **Fellow:** Nuclear Medicine, Montefiore Med Ctr 1990; Infectious Disease, NY Hosp-Cornell Med Ctr 1992; **Fac Appt:** Asst Prof Med, Mount Sinai Sch Med

Yancovitz, Stanley MD (Inf) - **Spec Exp:** Lyme Disease; AIDS/HIV; **Hospital:** Beth Israel Med Ctr - Petrie Division (page 94); **Address:** 1st Ave at 16th St, Ste 17 BH10, New York, NY 10003; **Phone:** 212-420-2600; **Board Cert:** Internal Medicine 1973; Infectious Disease 1976; **Med School:** SUNY Downstate 1967; **Resid:** Internal Medicine, Metropolitan Hosp 1969; Internal Medicine, Beth Israel Med Ctr 1972; **Fellow:** Infectious Disease, Mt Sinai Hosp 1975; **Fac Appt:** Clin Prof Med, Albert Einstein Coll Med

Internal Medicine

Aronne, Louis J MD (IM) - **Spec Exp:** Diabetes; Obesity; Weight Management; **Hospital:** NY-Presby/Weill Cornell Med Ctr, NY (page 104); **Address:** 1165 York Ave, New York, NY 10065; **Phone:** 212-583-1000; **Board Cert:** Internal Medicine 1984; **Med School:** Johns Hopkins Univ 1981; **Resid:** Internal Medicine, Bronx Muni Hosp 1984; **Fellow:** Internal Medicine, New York Hosp 1986; **Fac Appt:** Assoc Clin Prof Med, Cornell Univ-Weill Med Coll

Ascheim, Robert S MD (IM) - **Spec Exp:** Coronary Artery Disease; Congestive Heart Failure; Preventive Medicine; **Address:** 10 Rockefeller Plaza Fl 4, New York, NY 10020; **Phone:** 212-332-3774; **Board Cert:** Internal Medicine 1969; **Med School:** Tufts Univ 1962; **Resid:** Internal Medicine, Bellevue Hosp 1968; Cardiovascular Disease, Mem Sloan-Kettering Med Ctr 1967; **Fellow:** Cardiovascular Disease, New York Hosp 1970; **Fac Appt:** Assoc Prof Med, Cornell Univ-Weill Med Coll

Babitz, Lisa E MD (IM) *PCP* - **Spec Exp:** Geriatric Medicine; **Hospital:** St. Luke's - Roosevelt Hosp Ctr - Roosevelt Div (page 94); **Address:** 457 W 57th St, New York, NY 10019; **Phone:** 212-265-1471; **Board Cert:** Internal Medicine 1984; **Med School:** Yale Univ 1981; **Resid:** Internal Medicine, Yale-New Haven Hosp 1984; **Fellow:** Geriatric Medicine, NYU Med Ctr 1986; **Fac Appt:** Assoc Clin Prof Med, Columbia P&S

Barley, Christopher L MD (IM) *PCP* - **Hospital:** NY-Presby/Weill Cornell Med Ctr, NY (page 104); **Address:** 110 E 55th St Fl 9, New York, NY 10022; **Phone:** 212-758-3590; **Board Cert:** Internal Medicine 2006; **Med School:** Geo Wash Univ 1993; **Resid:** Internal Medicine, NY Hosp Cornell Med Ctr 1996; **Fac Appt:** Asst Clin Prof Med, Cornell Univ-Weill Med Coll

Baskin, David H MD (IM) *PCP* - **Spec Exp:** Preventive Medicine; Cholesterol/Lipid Disorders; **Hospital:** St. Luke's - Roosevelt Hosp Ctr - Roosevelt Div (page 94); **Address:** 185 West End Ave, Ste 1M, New York, NY 10023-5540; **Phone:** 212-595-7701; **Board Cert:** Internal Medicine 1985; **Med School:** Boston Univ 1982; **Resid:** Internal Medicine, St Lukes Roosevelt Hosp 1985; **Fac Appt:** Asst Clin Prof Med, Columbia P&S

Boxer, William MD (IM) *PCP* - **Hospital:** Lenox Hill Hosp (page 106); **Address:** Medical Associates East, 220 E 69th St, New York, NY 10021; **Phone:** 212-570-1800; **Board Cert:** Internal Medicine 2000; **Med School:** SUNY Upstate Med Univ 1997; **Resid:** Internal Medicine, Boston Univ Med Ctr 2000

Bregman, Zachary MD (IM) *PCP* - **Spec Exp:** Pulmonary Disease; AIDS/HIV; **Hospital:** Beth Israel Med Ctr - Petrie Division (page 94), NYU Langone Med Ctr (page 108); **Address:** 247 3rd Ave, Ste 304, New York, NY 10010; **Phone:** 212-505-6663; **Board Cert:** Internal Medicine 1986; **Med School:** Univ Pennsylvania 1981; **Resid:** Internal Medicine, Beth Israel Med Ctr 1984; **Fellow:** Pulmonary Disease, Beth Israel Med Ctr 1986; **Fac Appt:** Asst Prof Med, NYU Sch Med

Bush, Michael N MD (IM) *PCP* - **Spec Exp:** Preventive Medicine; **Hospital:** Lenox Hill Hosp (page 106), NYU Langone Med Ctr (page 108); **Address:** 115 E 57th St, Ste 630, New York, NY 10022; **Phone:** 212-583-2990; **Board Cert:** Internal Medicine 1981; **Med School:** SUNY Downstate 1978; **Resid:** Internal Medicine, Lenox Hill Hosp 1982; **Fac Appt:** Asst Clin Prof Med, NYU Sch Med

Case, David B MD (IM) *PCP* - **Spec Exp:** Hypertension; Preventive Cardiology; **Hospital:** NY-Presby/Columbia Univ Med Ctr, NY (page 104); **Address:** New York Physicians, 635 Madison Ave Fl 7, New York, NY 10022; **Phone:** 212-857-4660; **Board Cert:** Internal Medicine 1974; **Med School:** Columbia P&S 1968; **Resid:** Internal Medicine, Johns Hopkins Hosp 1970; **Fellow:** Cardiovascular Disease, Columbia-Presby Med Ctr 1972; **Fac Appt:** Assoc Clin Prof Med, Cornell Univ-Weill Med Coll

Charap, Mitchell MD (IM) *PCP* - **Hospital:** NYU Langone Med Ctr (page 108); **Address:** 530 1st Ave, Ste 7B, New York, NY 10016; **Phone:** 212-263-7442; **Board Cert:** Internal Medicine 2002; **Med School:** NYU Sch Med 1977; **Resid:** Internal Medicine, NYU Med Ctr 1981; **Fac Appt:** Assoc Clin Prof Med, NYU Sch Med

Charap, Peter MD (IM) *PCP* - **Spec Exp:** Preventive Medicine; **Hospital:** Mount Sinai Med Ctr (page 102); **Address:** 234 Central Park West, New York, NY 10024; **Phone:** 212-579-2200; **Board Cert:** Internal Medicine 1987; **Med School:** Mount Sinai Sch Med 1984; **Resid:** Internal Medicine, Mount Sinai Hosp 1987; **Fellow:** Public Health & Genl Preventive Med, Mount Sinai Hosp 1988; **Fac Appt:** Asst Clin Prof Med, Mount Sinai Sch Med

Cohen, Richard P MD (IM) *PCP* - **Spec Exp:** Complex Diagnosis; Preventive Medicine; **Hospital:** NY-Presby/Weill Cornell Med Ctr, NY (page 104), Hosp For Special Surgery (page 115); **Address:** 235 E 67th St, New York, NY 10021-6040; **Phone:** 212-734-6464; **Board Cert:** Internal Medicine 1978; **Med School:** Cornell Univ-Weill Med Coll 1975; **Resid:** Internal Medicine, NY Hosp 1978; **Fellow:** Infectious Disease, NY Hosp 1979; **Fac Appt:** Clin Prof Med, Cornell Univ-Weill Med Coll

Cohen, Robert L MD (IM) - ; **Address:** 314 W 14th St, FL 5, New York, NY 10014-5002; **Phone:** 212-620-0144; **Board Cert:** Internal Medicine 1978; **Med School:** Rush Med Coll 1975; **Resid:** Internal Medicine, Cook County Hosp 1979; **Fac Appt:** Asst Prof Med, Albert Einstein Coll Med

Cohn, Symra A MD (IM) *PCP* - **Spec Exp:** Women's Health; **Hospital:** NY-Presby/Weill Cornell Med Ctr, NY (page 104); **Address:** 3 E 71st St Fl 1, New York, NY 10021; **Phone:** 212-288-1302; **Board Cert:** Internal Medicine 2005; **Med School:** NY Med Coll 1991; **Resid:** Internal Medicine, NY Hosp-Cornell Med Ctr 1994; **Fac Appt:** Asst Clin Prof Med, Cornell Univ-Weill Med Coll

Constantiner, Arturo MD (IM) *PCP* - **Spec Exp:** Hypertension; Kidney Disease; Kidney Stones; Dialysis Care; **Hospital:** NY Downtown Hosp; **Address:** 19 Beekman St, Fl 6, New York, NY 10038-1522; **Phone:** 212-349-8455; **Board Cert:** Internal Medicine 1979; Nephrology 2006; **Med School:** Mexico 1975; **Resid:** Internal Medicine, Elmhurst Hosp 1979; **Fellow:** Nephrology, Mount Sinai Hosp 1981; **Fac Appt:** Asst Clin Prof Med, NYU Sch Med

Cunningham-Rundles, Ward MD (IM) *PCP* - **Spec Exp:** Allergy & Immunology; **Hospital:** NY-Presby/Weill Cornell Med Ctr, NY (page 104), Mount Sinai Med Ctr (page 102); **Address:** 240 E 68th St, New York, NY 10065-6001; **Phone:** 212-737-8973; **Board Cert:** Internal Medicine 1976; **Med School:** NYU Sch Med 1971; **Resid:** Internal Medicine, Bellevue Hosp 1973; **Fellow:** Immunology, Meml Sloan Kettering Cancer Ctr 1975; Medical Oncology, Meml Sloan Kettering Cancer Ctr 1976; **Fac Appt:** Asst Clin Prof Med, Cornell Univ-Weill Med Coll

Dhalla, Satish MD (IM) *PCP* - **Spec Exp:** Hypertension; Cholesterol/Lipid Disorders; Diabetes; Travel Medicine; **Hospital:** NYU Langone Med Ctr (page 108), NY Downtown Hosp; **Address:** 111 Broadway, Fl 2, NYU-Trinity Ctr, New York, NY 10006; **Phone:** 212-263-9700; **Board Cert:** Internal Medicine 1976; **Med School:** India 1972; **Resid:** Internal Medicine, Beekman Downtown Hosp 1976; **Fac Appt:** Assoc Clin Prof Med, NYU Sch Med

Dibner, Robin MD (IM) - **Spec Exp:** Lupus/SLE; **Hospital:** Lenox Hill Hosp (page 106), Mount Sinai Med Ctr (page 102); **Address:** 100 E 77th St, New York, NY 10021; **Phone:** 212-434-2140; **Board Cert:** Internal Medicine 1982; Rheumatology 1984; **Med School:** Wayne State Univ 1979; **Resid:** Internal Medicine, St Lukes Hosp Ctr 1982; **Fellow:** Rheumatology, SUNY Brooklyn Med Ctr 1984; **Fac Appt:** Assoc Clin Prof Med, Mount Sinai Sch Med

Dolinsky, Jason H MD (IM) *PCP* - **Hospital:** Mount Sinai Med Ctr (page 102), Beth Israel Med Ctr - Petrie Division (page 94); **Address:** 899 Lexington Ave, New York, NY 10065; **Phone:** 212-737-1102; **Board Cert:** Internal Medicine 2007; **Med School:** NYU Sch Med 1994; **Resid:** Internal Medicine, Hosp Univ Penn 1997; **Fac Appt:** Med, Albert Einstein Coll Med

Ehrlich, Martin Harvey MD (IM) *PCP* - **Spec Exp:** Complementary Medicine; Preventive Medicine; Acupuncture; **Hospital:** Beth Israel Med Ctr - Petrie Division (page 94); **Address:** Center for Health & Healing, 245 Fifth Ave Fl 2, New York, NY 10016; **Phone:** 646-935-2265; **Board Cert:** Internal Medicine 1988; **Med School:** Columbia P&S 1985; **Resid:** Internal Medicine, Harlem Hosp 1989; **Fac Appt:** Asst Prof Med, Albert Einstein Coll Med

Etingin, Orli MD (IM) *PCP* - **Spec Exp:** Preventive Medicine; Bleeding/Coagulation Disorders; Women's Health; **Hospital:** NY-Presby/Weill Cornell Med Ctr, NY (page 104); **Address:** 425 E 61st St Fl 11, New York, NY 10065; **Phone:** 212-821-0926; **Board Cert:** Internal Medicine 1984; Hematology 1988; **Med School:** Albert Einstein Coll Med 1980; **Resid:** Internal Medicine, NY Hosp 1983; **Fellow:** Hematology & Oncology, NY Hosp 1986; **Fac Appt:** Clin Prof Med, Cornell Univ-Weill Med Coll

Federman, Alex D MD (IM) *PCP* - **Spec Exp:** Preventive Medicine; Hypertension; **Hospital:** Mount Sinai Med Ctr (page 102); **Address:** Internal Medicine Assocs, 17 E 102nd St Fl 7, New York, NY 10029; **Phone:** 212-659-8551; **Board Cert:** Internal Medicine 2009; **Med School:** SUNY Downstate 1996; **Resid:** Internal Medicine, Montefiore Med Ctr 1999; **Fellow:** Research, Brigham & Women's Hosp 2001; **Fac Appt:** Assoc Prof Med, Mount Sinai Sch Med

Feltheimer, Seth MD (IM) *PCP* - **Spec Exp:** Preventive Medicine; Perioperative Medical Care; **Hospital:** NY-Presby/Columbia Univ Med Ctr, NY (page 104); **Address:** 161 Ft Washington Ave, Ste 336, New York, NY 10032; **Phone:** 212-305-8669; **Board Cert:** Internal Medicine 1984; **Med School:** Spain 1981; **Resid:** Internal Medicine, Interfaith Med Ctr 1984; **Fellow:** Internal Medicine, Columbia-Presby Med Ctr 1985; **Fac Appt:** Assoc Clin Prof Med, Columbia P&S

Feuer, Martin M MD (IM) *PCP* - **Spec Exp:** Bronchitis; Asthma; Emphysema; **Hospital:** Beth Israel Med Ctr - Petrie Division (page 94), Mount Sinai Med Ctr (page 102); **Address:** 899 Lexington Ave, New York, NY 10021-6103; **Phone:** 212-744-5433; **Board Cert:** Internal Medicine 1966; Pulmonary Disease 1972; **Med School:** NYU Sch Med 1959; **Resid:** Internal Medicine, Mount Sinai Hosp 1962; **Fellow:** Pulmonary Disease, Montefiore Med Ctr 1963; **Fac Appt:** Asst Prof Med, Albert Einstein Coll Med

Fiedler, Robert P MD (IM) *PCP* - **Spec Exp:** Thyroid Disorders; Diabetes; **Hospital:** Mount Sinai Med Ctr (page 102); **Address:** 1175 Park Ave, New York, NY 10128-1211; **Phone:** 212-289-6500; **Board Cert:** Internal Medicine 1970; Endocrinology, Diabetes & Metabolism 1972; **Med School:** Albert Einstein Coll Med 1964; **Resid:** Internal Medicine, DC Gen Hosp 1966; Internal Medicine, VA Med Ctr 1967; **Fellow:** Endocrinology, Mount Sinai Med Ctr 1969; **Fac Appt:** Assoc Clin Prof Med, Mount Sinai Sch Med

Fisher, Laura MD (IM) *PCP* - **Spec Exp:** Preventive Medicine; Lyme Disease; Women's Health; **Hospital:** NY-Presby/Weill Cornell Med Ctr, NY (page 104); **Address:** 1385 York Ave, New York, NY 10021; **Phone:** 212-717-5920; **Board Cert:** Internal Medicine 1987; **Med School:** Brown Univ 1984; **Resid:** Internal Medicine, NY Hosp-Cornell Med Ctr 1987; **Fellow:** Infectious Disease, Mass Genl Hosp 1989; **Fac Appt:** Asst Clin Prof Med, Cornell Univ-Weill Med Coll

Fried, Richard P MD (IM) *PCP* - **Spec Exp:** Lyme Disease; Fevers of Unknown Origin; Infectious Disease; **Hospital:** St. Luke's - Roosevelt Hosp Ctr - Roosevelt Div (page 94); **Address:** 15 W 72nd St, Ste 1N, New York, NY 10023; **Phone:** 212-580-4840; **Board Cert:** Internal Medicine 1972; Infectious Disease 1974; **Med School:** Columbia P&S 1968; **Resid:** Internal Medicine, St Lukes Hosp 1972; **Fellow:** Infectious Disease, Stanford Med Ctr 1974; **Fac Appt:** Assoc Clin Prof Med, Columbia P&S

Friedman, Jeffrey P MD (IM) *PCP* - **Spec Exp:** Preventive Medicine; Travel Medicine; **Hospital:** NYU Langone Med Ctr (page 108); **Address:** 317 E 34th St, Fl 10, New York, NY 10016; **Phone:** 212-726-7440; **Board Cert:** Internal Medicine 1986; **Med School:** NYU Sch Med 1983; **Resid:** Internal Medicine, Bellevue Hosp 1987; **Fac Appt:** Assoc Clin Prof Med, NYU Sch Med

Galland, Leo MD (IM) - **Spec Exp:** Nutrition; Chronic Illness; Complementary Medicine; **Address:** Foundation for Integrated Medicine, 156 Fifth Ave, Ste 519, New York, NY 10010; **Phone:** 212-989-6733; **Board Cert:** Internal Medicine 1972; **Med School:** NYU Sch Med 1968; **Resid:** Internal Medicine, Bellevue Hosp 1972; **Fellow:** Behavioral Medicine, Univ Conn Hlth Ctr 1981

Gelbard, Sandra MD (IM) *PCP* - **Hospital:** Lenox Hill Hosp (page 106); **Address:** 993 Park Ave, New York, NY 10028; **Phone:** 212-988-5303; **Board Cert:** Internal Medicine 2003; **Med School:** SUNY Stony Brook 1999; **Resid:** Internal Medicine, NYU Med Ctr 2003

Golden, Flavia A MD (IM) *PCP* - **Spec Exp:** Women's Health; **Hospital:** NY-Presby/Weill Cornell Med Ctr, NY (page 104); **Address:** 310 E 72nd St, New York, NY 10021; **Phone:** 212-396-3016; **Board Cert:** Internal Medicine 2003; **Med School:** NYU Sch Med 1990; **Resid:** Internal Medicine, New York Hosp 1993; **Fac Appt:** Asst Prof Med, Cornell Univ-Weill Med Coll

Goldin, Daniel MD (IM) *PCP* - **Hospital:** NY-Presby/Weill Cornell Med Ctr, NY (page 104); **Address:** 646 Park Ave, New York, NY 10021; **Phone:** 212-717-4884; **Board Cert:** Internal Medicine 2004; **Med School:** Cornell Univ-Weill Med Coll 2001; **Resid:** Internal Medicine, NY-Presby Hosp/Weill Cornell Med Ctr 2004

Goldstein, Paul H MD (IM) *PCP* - **Spec Exp:** Preventive Medicine; **Hospital:** NYU Langone Med Ctr (page 108); **Address:** 80 5th Ave, Ste 1601, New York, NY 10011; **Phone:** 212-645-8500; **Board Cert:** Internal Medicine 1985; **Med School:** NY Med Coll 1982; **Resid:** Internal Medicine, St Vincent's Hosp & Med Ctr 1985; **Fac Appt:** Assoc Prof Med, NY Med Coll

Greaney, Edward J MD (IM) *PCP* - **Spec Exp:** Preventive Medicine; Nutrition; **Hospital:** NYU Langone Med Ctr (page 108); **Address:** 317 E 34th St, Fl 4th, New York, NY 10016; **Phone:** 212-726-7488; **Board Cert:** Internal Medicine 2010; **Med School:** NYU Sch Med 1995; **Resid:** Internal Medicine, NYU Med Ctr-Bellevue Hosp 1999; **Fac Appt:** Asst Clin Prof Med, NYU Sch Med

Haber, Stuart MD (IM) *PCP* - **Spec Exp:** AIDS/HIV; Travel Medicine; Infectious Disease; **Address:** 12-A Sheridan Square, New York, NY 10014; **Phone:** 212-929-2370; **Board Cert:** Internal Medicine 1986; Infectious Disease 2000; **Med School:** NYU Sch Med 1983; **Resid:** Internal Medicine, Emory Univ Hosp 1986; **Fellow:** Infectious Disease, Emory Univ Hosp 1989

Hart, Catherine C MD (IM) *PCP* - **Spec Exp:** Infectious Disease; **Hospital:** NY-Presby/Weill Cornell Med Ctr, NY (page 104); **Address:** 310 E 72nd St, Fl 2, New York, NY 10021; **Phone:** 212-396-3272; **Board Cert:** Internal Medicine 1984; Infectious Disease 1986; **Med School:** Univ Pennsylvania 1980; **Resid:** Internal Medicine, New York Hosp 1983; **Fellow:** Infectious Disease, New York Hosp 1985; **Fac Appt:** Asst Clin Prof Med, Cornell Univ-Weill Med Coll

Hauptman, Allen S MD (IM) *PCP* - **Spec Exp:** Preventive Medicine; **Hospital:** NYU Langone Med Ctr (page 108); **Address:** 317 E 34th St Fl 7, New York, NY 10016-4974; **Phone:** 212-726-7494; **Board Cert:** Internal Medicine 1981; **Med School:** NYU Sch Med 1978; **Resid:** Internal Medicine, Bellevue Hosp 1982; **Fac Appt:** Asst Clin Prof Med, NYU Sch Med

Hoffman, Eileen M MD (IM) - **Spec Exp:** Women's Health; **Hospital:** NYU Langone Med Ctr (page 108); **Address:** 35 E 35 St, Ste 1J, New York, NY 10016; **Phone:** 646-424-1530; **Board Cert:** Internal Medicine 1982; **Med School:** SUNY Stony Brook 1979; **Resid:** Internal Medicine, Bellevue Hosp Ctr 1982; **Fellow:** Immunology, Rockefeller Univ 1983; **Fac Appt:** Asst Clin Prof Med, NYU Sch Med

Horbar, Gary M MD (IM) *PCP* - **Hospital:** Lenox Hill Hosp (page 106); **Address:** 6 E 85th St, New York, NY 10028; **Phone:** 212-570-9119; **Board Cert:** Internal Medicine 1979; **Med School:** NY Med Coll 1976; **Resid:** Internal Medicine, Lenox Hill Hosp 1980; **Fac Appt:** Asst Clin Prof Med, NYU Sch Med

Horovitz, Len H MD (IM) *PCP* - **Spec Exp:** Bronchoscopy; Asthma; Emphysema; Asthma; **Hospital:** Lenox Hill Hosp (page 106), Lenox Hill Hosp (Manh Eye, Ear & Throat Hosp) (page 106); **Address:** 47 E 77th St, Ste 201, New York, NY 10075; **Phone:** 212-744-3001; **Board Cert:** Internal Medicine 1980; Pulmonary Disease 1984; **Med School:** NYU Sch Med 1976; **Resid:** Internal Medicine, Lenox Hill Hosp 1980; **Fellow:** Pulmonary Disease, Lenox Hill Hosp 1982

Kaminsky, Donald L MD (IM) - **Spec Exp:** AIDS/HIV; Tropical Diseases; Travel Medicine; **Hospital:** Beth Israel Med Ctr - Petrie Division (page 94); **Address:** 10 Union Square East, Ste 5M-1, New York, NY 10003-3314; **Phone:** 212-253-6800; **Board Cert:** Internal Medicine 1982; **Med School:** Geo Wash Univ 1979; **Resid:** Internal Medicine, Beth Israel Hosp 1982; **Fellow:** Infectious Disease, Beth Israel Hosp 1984; **Fac Appt:** Asst Clin Prof Med, Albert Einstein Coll Med

Kaufman, David L MD (IM) *PCP* - **Spec Exp:** AIDS/HIV; Hepatitis C; Lyme Disease; **Hospital:** NYU Langone Med Ctr (page 108), Beth Israel Med Ctr - Petrie Division (page 94); **Address:** 37 Washington Square W, Ste 1D, MS 10011, New York, NY 10011; **Phone:** 212-982-4070; **Board Cert:** Internal Medicine 1980; **Med School:** NY Med Coll 1977; **Resid:** Internal Medicine, St Vincents Med Ctr 1980; **Fac Appt:** Asst Clin Prof Med, NYU Sch Med

Kennedy, James T MD (IM) *PCP* - **Spec Exp:** Thyroid Disorders; Diabetes; **Hospital:** NYU Langone Med Ctr (page 108); **Address:** 650 1st Ave, Fl 4th, New York, NY 10016; **Phone:** 212-689-7768; **Board Cert:** Internal Medicine 1978; **Med School:** NYU Sch Med 1972; **Resid:** Internal Medicine, Bellevue Hosp 1977; **Fac Appt:** Clin Prof Med, NYU Sch Med

Kennish, Arthur J MD (IM) *PCP* - **Spec Exp:** Mitral Valve Disease; Coronary Artery Disease; **Hospital:** Mount Sinai Med Ctr (page 102); **Address:** 108 E 96th St, New York, NY 10128-6217; **Phone:** 212-410-6610; **Board Cert:** Internal Medicine 1980; Cardiovascular Disease 1983; **Med School:** Albert Einstein Coll Med 1977; **Resid:** Internal Medicine, Mt Sinai Hosp 1980; **Fellow:** Cardiovascular Disease, Mt Sinai Hosp 1982; **Fac Appt:** Asst Clin Prof Med, Mount Sinai Sch Med

Kent, Jennifer MD (IM) *PCP* - **Hospital:** Mount Sinai Med Ctr (page 102); **Address:** Mt Sinai Medical Ctr, 5 E 98th St Fl 11, New York, NY 10029; **Phone:** 212-241-6585; **Board Cert:** Internal Medicine 2003; **Med School:** Israel 2000; **Resid:** Internal Medicine, Mt Sinai Med Ctr 2003; **Fac Appt:** Asst Prof Med, Mount Sinai Sch Med

Korenstein, Deborah R MD (IM) - **Spec Exp:** Women's Health; Eating Disorders; **Hospital:** Mount Sinai Med Ctr (page 102); **Address:** 17 E 102nd St Fl 7, New York, NY 10029; **Phone:** 212-659-8551; **Board Cert:** Internal Medicine 2006; **Med School:** Columbia P&S 1993; **Resid:** Internal Medicine, Beth Israel Hosp 1996; **Fac Appt:** Assoc Prof Med, Mount Sinai Sch Med

Lamm, Steven MD (IM) *PCP* - **Spec Exp:** Obesity; Sexual Dysfunction; Preventive Medicine; **Hospital:** NYU Langone Med Ctr (page 108), Lenox Hill Hosp (page 106); **Address:** 12 E 86th St, New York, NY 10028-0506; **Phone:** 212-988-1146; **Board Cert:** Internal Medicine 1977; **Med School:** NYU Sch Med 1974; **Resid:** Internal Medicine, NYU Med Ctr 1979; **Fellow:** Rheumatology, NYU Med Ctr 1978; **Fac Appt:** Asst Clin Prof Med, NYU Sch Med

Lee, Roberta A MD (IM) - **Spec Exp:** Complementary Medicine; **Hospital:** Beth Israel Med Ctr - Petrie Division (page 94); **Address:** Center for Health & Healing, 245 Fifth Ave Fl 2, New York, NY 10016; **Phone:** 646-935-2265; **Board Cert:** Internal Medicine 2012; **Med School:** Geo Wash Univ 1985; **Resid:** Internal Medicine, Washington Hosp Ctr 1988; **Fellow:** Complementary Medicine, Univ Arizona Med Ctr 1999

Legato, Marianne J MD (IM) *PCP* - **Spec Exp:** Cardiovascular Disease; Gender Specific Medicine; **Hospital:** Lenox Hill Hosp (page 106), St. Luke's - Roosevelt Hosp Ctr - Roosevelt Div (page 94); **Address:** 903 Park Ave, Ste 2A, New York, NY 10075; **Phone:** 212-737-5663; **Board Cert:** Internal Medicine 2003; **Med School:** NYU Sch Med 1962; **Resid:** Internal Medicine, Columbia-Presby Med Ctr 1965; **Fellow:** Cardiovascular Disease, Columbia-Presby Med Ctr 1968; **Fac Appt:** Prof Emeritus Med, NYU Sch Med

Lewin, Margaret MD (IM) *PCP* - **Spec Exp:** Preventive Medicine; Women's Health; Travel Medicine; **Hospital:** NY-Presby/Weill Cornell Med Ctr, NY (page 104), Hosp For Special Surgery (page 115); **Address:** 635 Madison Ave Fl 8, New York, NY 10022; **Phone:** 212-857-4505; **Board Cert:** Internal Medicine 1980; Hematology 1982; Medical Oncology 1983; **Med School:** Case West Res Univ 1977; **Resid:** Internal Medicine, NY Hosp/Cornell Med Ctr 1980; **Fellow:** Hematology & Oncology, NY Hosp/Cornell Med Ctr 1983; **Fac Appt:** Assoc Clin Prof Med, Cornell Univ-Weill Med Coll

Lewin, Neal A MD (IM) *PCP* - **Spec Exp:** Preventive Medicine; Headache; Migraine; Complex Diagnosis; **Hospital:** NYU Langone Med Ctr (page 108); **Address:** 120 E 36th St, Ste 1B, New York, NY 10016-3426; **Phone:** 212-889-2813; **Board Cert:** Internal Medicine 1977; Emergency Medicine 2002; Medical Toxicology 1983; **Med School:** SUNY Downstate 1974; **Resid:** Internal Medicine, NYU-Bellevue Hosp 1977; **Fac Appt:** Prof Med, NYU Sch Med

Lewin, Sharon MD (IM) *PCP* - **Spec Exp:** AIDS/HIV; Travel Medicine; Women's Health; Fevers of Unknown Origin; **Hospital:** St. Luke's - Roosevelt Hosp Ctr - Roosevelt Div (page 94); **Address:** 139 W 82nd St, New York, NY 10024-5544; **Phone:** 212-496-7200; **Board Cert:** Internal Medicine 1978; Infectious Disease 1980; **Med School:** Univ Toronto 1975; **Resid:** Internal Medicine, Wadsworth VA Hosp 1978; **Fellow:** Infectious Disease, Bellevue Hosp/NYU Med Ctr 1980; **Fac Appt:** Asst Clin Prof Med, Columbia P&S

Liguori, Michael MD (IM) *PCP* - **Spec Exp:** Geriatric Rehabilitation; AIDS/HIV; **Hospital:** NYU Langone Med Ctr (page 108); **Address:** 80 5th Ave, Ste 1601, New York, NY 10011-8002; **Phone:** 212-645-8500; **Board Cert:** Internal Medicine 1985; **Med School:** Mount Sinai Sch Med 1981; **Resid:** Internal Medicine, St Vincents Hosp 1984; **Fac Appt:** Asst Clin Prof Med, NY Med Coll

Lipton, Mark S MD (IM) *PCP* - **Spec Exp:** Preventive Cardiology; Coronary Artery Disease; Non-Invasive Cardiology; **Hospital:** NYU Langone Med Ctr (page 108); **Address:** 635 Madison Ave, Fl 3, New York, NY 10022-1009; **Phone:** 212-570-2077; **Board Cert:** Internal Medicine 1981; Cardiovascular Disease 1985; **Med School:** NYU Sch Med 1978; **Resid:** Internal Medicine, Bellevue Hosp 1981; **Fellow:** Cardiovascular Disease, NYU Med Ctr 1985; **Fac Appt:** Assoc Clin Prof Med, NYU Sch Med

Liu, George C K MD (IM) *PCP* - **Spec Exp:** Endocrinology; Chinese Community Health; Diabetes; **Hospital:** NY Downtown Hosp, NYU Langone Med Ctr (page 108); **Address:** 185 Canal St Fl 6, New York, NY 10013-4513; **Phone:** 212-343-7323; **Board Cert:** Internal Medicine 1983; **Med School:** Cornell Univ-Weill Med Coll 1978; **Resid:** Internal Medicine, NYU Med Ctr-Manhattan VA Hosp 1981; **Fellow:** Endocrinology, Stanford Univ Med Ctr 1983; **Fac Appt:** Asst Clin Prof Med, NYU Sch Med

Lodge Jr, Henry S MD (IM) *PCP* - **Spec Exp:** Preventive Medicine; **Hospital:** NY-Presby/Columbia Univ Med Ctr, NY (page 104); **Address:** New York Physicians, 635 Madison Ave Fl 8, New York, NY 10022-1009; **Phone:** 212-857-4555; **Board Cert:** Internal Medicine 1988; **Med School:** Columbia P&S 1985; **Resid:** Internal Medicine, Columbia-Presby Hosp 1988; **Fac Appt:** Assoc Clin Prof Med, Columbia P&S

Logan, Bruce D MD (IM) *PCP* - **Spec Exp:** Preventive Medicine; Hypertension; Diabetes; Cholesterol/Lipid Disorders; **Hospital:** NY Downtown Hosp, NY-Presby/Weill Cornell Med Ctr, NY (page 104); **Address:** 19 Beekman St, Fl 6, New York, NY 10038; **Phone:** 212-608-6634; **Board Cert:** Internal Medicine 1978; **Med School:** Columbia P&S 1972; **Resid:** Internal Medicine, Harlem Hosp Ctr 1978; **Fac Appt:** Assoc Clin Prof Med, Cornell Univ-Weill Med Coll

Mann, Samuel J MD (IM) - **Spec Exp:** Hypertension; **Hospital:** NY-Presby/Weill Cornell Med Ctr, NY (page 104); **Address:** Weill-Cornell Hypertension Clinic, 450 E 69th St, New York, NY 10021; **Phone:** 212-746-2200; **Board Cert:** Internal Medicine 1975; **Med School:** SUNY Downstate 1972; **Resid:** Internal Medicine, St Lukes Roosevelt Hosp 1975; **Fellow:** Hypertension, Mt Sinai Hosp 1983; **Fac Appt:** Clin Prof Med, Cornell Univ-Weill Med Coll

Minkowitz, Susan MD (IM) *PCP* - **Spec Exp:** Asthma; Emphysema; Hypertension; Chronic Obstructive Lung Disease (COPD); **Hospital:** NYU Langone Med Ctr (page 108); **Address:** 355 W 52nd St Fl 7th, New York, NY 10019; **Phone:** 646-778-5555; **Board Cert:** Internal Medicine 1988; **Med School:** NY Med Coll 1984; **Resid:** Internal Medicine, Metropolitan Hosp Ctr 1987; **Fellow:** Pulmonary Disease, Montefiore Med Ctr 1989; **Fac Appt:** Asst Prof Med, NY Med Coll

Mulvehill, Joseph MD (IM) *PCP* - **Spec Exp:** Concierge Medicine; House Calls; **Hospital:** Lenox Hill Hosp (page 106); **Address:** 10 E 78th St, Ste 1B, New York, NY 10021; **Phone:** 212-737-3136; **Board Cert:** Internal Medicine 2001; **Med School:** SUNY Stony Brook 1997; **Resid:** Internal Medicine 2000

Nelson, Deena J MD (IM) *PCP* - **Spec Exp:** Cancer Survivors-Late Effects of Therapy; Cancer Prevention; **Hospital:** NY-Presby/Weill Cornell Med Ctr, NY (page 104); **Address:** 635 Madison Ave Fl 8, New York, NY 10022-1009; **Phone:** 212-857-4670; **Board Cert:** Internal Medicine 1980; **Med School:** Albert Einstein Coll Med 1977; **Resid:** Internal Medicine, New York Hosp 1979; Internal Medicine, Barnes Hosp 1980; **Fac Appt:** Asst Clin Prof Med, Cornell Univ-Weill Med Coll

Olichney, John J MD (IM) - **Hospital:** St. Luke's - Roosevelt Hosp Ctr - Roosevelt Div (page 94); **Address:** 350 W 58th St Fl Ground, New York, NY 10019-1804; **Phone:** 212-246-9101; **Board Cert:** Internal Medicine 1974; **Med School:** Albany Med Coll 1969; **Resid:** Internal Medicine, Roosevelt Hosp 1972; **Fellow:** Hematology, St Luke's-Roosevelt Hosp Ctr 1973; **Fac Appt:** Clin Prof Med, Columbia P&S

Orsher, Stuart MD (IM) *PCP* - **Hospital:** Lenox Hill Hosp (page 106); **Address:** 9 E 79th St, New York, NY 10075; **Phone:** 212-535-7763; **Board Cert:** Internal Medicine 1983; **Med School:** Hahnemann Univ 1975; **Resid:** Internal Medicine, Lenox Hill Hosp 1978

Pecker, Mark S MD (IM) - **Spec Exp:** Hypertension; **Hospital:** NY-Presby/Weill Cornell Med Ctr, NY (page 104); **Address:** NY-Cornell Medical Ctr, Hypertension Ctr, 450 E 69th St, New York, NY 10021; **Phone:** 212-746-2210; **Board Cert:** Internal Medicine 1980; **Med School:** NYU Sch Med 1977; **Resid:** Internal Medicine, Univ Texas SW Affil Hosps 1980; **Fac Appt:** Clin Prof Med, Cornell Univ-Weill Med Coll

Postley, John E MD (IM) *PCP* - **Spec Exp:** Preventive Medicine; **Hospital:** NY-Presby/Columbia Univ Med Ctr, NY (page 104); **Address:** New York Physicians, 635 Madison Ave Fl 7, New York, NY 10022; **Phone:** 212-317-4646; **Board Cert:** Internal Medicine 1973; **Med School:** Columbia P&S 1968; **Resid:** Internal Medicine, NY-Presy/Columbia Univ Med Ctr 1973; **Fac Appt:** Asst Clin Prof Med, Columbia P&S

Primas, Ronald MD (IM) *PCP* - **Spec Exp:** Preventive Medicine; Travel Medicine; House Calls; Concierge Medicine; **Hospital:** Mount Sinai Med Ctr (page 102); **Address:** 952 5th Ave, Ste 1D, New York, NY 10021; **Phone:** 212-737-1212; **Board Cert:** Internal Medicine 2010; **Med School:** Amer Univ Caribbean 1986; **Resid:** Internal Medicine, Methodist Hosp 1990; **Fellow:** Preventive Medicine, UCSD Med Cte 1991

Rosen, Nedra J MD (IM) *PCP* - **Hospital:** Lenox Hill Hosp (page 106), NYU Langone Med Ctr (page 108); **Address:** 115 E 57th St, Ste 630, New York, NY 10022; **Phone:** 212-583-2990; **Board Cert:** Internal Medicine 1983; **Med School:** NY Med Coll 1980; **Resid:** Internal Medicine, Lenox Hill Hosp 1984

Salsitz, Edwin A MD (IM) - **Spec Exp:** Addiction/Substance Abuse; Opiate Addiction; **Hospital:** Beth Israel Med Ctr - Petrie Division (page 94); **Address:** Beth Israel Med Ctr, 1st Ave at 16th St, 10 Bernstein Pavilion, Dept Medicine, New York, NY 10003; **Phone:** 212-420-4400; **Board Cert:** Internal Medicine 1977; Pulmonary Disease 1980; **Med School:** SUNY Buffalo 1972; **Resid:** Obstetrics & Gynecology, Beth Israel Med Ctr 1974; Internal Medicine, Beth Israel Med Ctr 1977; **Fellow:** Pulmonary Disease, Beth Israel Med Ctr 1979; **Fac Appt:** Asst Clin Prof Med, Albert Einstein Coll Med

Schneider, Steven J MD (IM) *PCP* - **Spec Exp:** Travel Medicine; Occupational Medicine; Lyme Disease; **Hospital:** NYU Langone Med Ctr (page 108), Lenox Hill Hosp (page 106); **Address:** 115 E 57th St, Ste 630, New York, NY 10022; **Phone:** 212-583-2880; **Board Cert:** Internal Medicine 1979; **Med School:** Johns Hopkins Univ 1976; **Resid:** Internal Medicine, Presby Med Ctr 1979

Sherman, Iris K MD (IM) - **Spec Exp:** Diabetes; Hypertension; Preventive Cardiology; **Hospital:** Mount Sinai Med Ctr (page 102); **Address:** Westside Internal Medicine, 620 Columbus Ave, New York, NY 10024; **Phone:** 212-874-6600; **Board Cert:** Internal Medicine 2006; **Med School:** SUNY Downstate 1993; **Resid:** Internal Medicine, Mt. Sinai Hosp 1996

Siegel, Marc K MD (IM) *PCP* - **Hospital:** NYU Langone Med Ctr (page 108); **Address:** 650 First Ave Fl 7, New York, NY 10016; **Phone:** 212-532-1214; **Board Cert:** Internal Medicine 2011; **Med School:** SUNY Buffalo 1985; **Resid:** Internal Medicine, NYU-Bellvue Med Ctr 1988; **Fac Appt:** Assoc Prof Med, NYU Sch Med

Silverman, David MD (IM) *PCP* - **Spec Exp:** Infectious Disease; Preventive Medicine; **Hospital:** NYU Langone Med Ctr (page 108); **Address:** 239 Central Park West, Ste 1A-N, New York, NY 10024; **Phone:** 212-496-1929; **Board Cert:** Internal Medicine 1979; **Med School:** Columbia P&S 1976; **Resid:** Internal Medicine, NYU/Bellevue Hosp 1980; **Fellow:** Infectious Disease, NYU/Bellevue Hosp 1981; **Fac Appt:** Assoc Clin Prof Med, NYU Sch Med

Smith, Sharon E MD (IM) *PCP* - **Hospital:** Lenox Hill Hosp (page 106); **Address:** Manhattan Phys Grp, 215 E 95th St, New York, NY 10128; **Phone:** 212-491-2400; **Board Cert:** Internal Medicine 2009; **Med School:** Howard Univ 1996; **Resid:** Internal Medicine, St. Vincent's Hosp 1999

Solomon, Gregory W MD (IM) *PCP* - **Spec Exp:** Preventive Medicine; Hypertension; Cholesterol/Lipid Disorders; Concierge Medicine; **Hospital:** Mount Sinai Med Ctr (page 102); **Address:** 899 Lexington Ave, New York, NY 10065-6103; **Phone:** 212-717-9205; **Board Cert:** Internal Medicine 2005; **Med School:** NYU Sch Med 1991; **Resid:** Internal Medicine, Montefiore Med Ctr 1995; **Fac Appt:** Assoc Clin Prof Med, Mount Sinai Sch Med

Spero, Marc MD (IM) *PCP* - **Spec Exp:** Pulmonary Disease; Diving Medicine; Asthma; **Hospital:** NYU Langone Med Ctr (page 108), Lenox Hill Hosp (page 106); **Address:** 110 E 55th St Fl 17, New York, NY 10022; **Phone:** 212-355-8315; **Board Cert:** Internal Medicine 1977; Pulmonary Disease 1980; **Med School:** Albert Einstein Coll Med 1973; **Resid:** Internal Medicine, St Lukes Hosp 1977; **Fellow:** Pulmonary Disease, St Lukes Hosp 1979

Steinberg, Charles MD (IM) *PCP* - **Hospital:** NY-Presby/Weill Cornell Med Ctr, NY (page 104); **Address:** 1305 York Ave, New York, NY 10021-4870; **Phone:** 646-962-4100; **Board Cert:** Internal Medicine 1971; Infectious Disease 1974; **Med School:** Cornell Univ-Weill Med Coll 1964; **Resid:** Internal Medicine, New York Hosp 1966; Internal Medicine, New York Hosp 1969; **Fellow:** Infectious Disease, New York Hosp 1971; **Fac Appt:** Prof Med, Cornell Univ-Weill Med Coll

Strauss, Michael L MD (IM) *PCP* - **Spec Exp:** Acupuncture; **Hospital:** Beth Israel Med Ctr - Petrie Division (page 94), New York Eye & Ear Infirm (page 117); **Address:** 310 E 14th St, Fl 3 North, New York, NY 10003; **Phone:** 212-979-4204; **Board Cert:** Internal Medicine 1984; **Med School:** Belgium 1980; **Resid:** Internal Medicine, Cabrini Med Ctr 1983

Tay, Steven I MD (IM) *PCP* - **Spec Exp:** Geriatric Care; **Hospital:** Beth Israel Med Ctr - Petrie Division (page 94); **Address:** 10 Union Square E, Ste 5M-1, New York, NY 10003; **Phone:** 212-253-9322; **Board Cert:** Internal Medicine 1977; Geriatric Medicine 2004; **Med School:** SUNY Downstate 1974; **Resid:** Internal Medicine, Kings Co Hosp 1977

Underberg, James MD (IM) - **Spec Exp:** Cholesterol/Lipid Disorders; Hypertension; Preventive Cardiology; **Hospital:** NYU Langone Med Ctr (page 108); **Address:** Murray Hill Medical Group, 317 E 34th St Fl 7, New York, NY 10016-4974; **Phone:** 212-726-7430; **Board Cert:** Internal Medicine 1989; **Med School:** Univ Pennsylvania 1986; **Resid:** Internal Medicine, NYU Med Ctr/Bellevue Hosp Ctr 1993; **Fac Appt:** Asst Clin Prof Med, NYU Sch Med

Vega, Aida MD (IM) *PCP* - **Hospital:** Mount Sinai Med Ctr (page 102); **Address:** Primary Care Associates, 17 E 102nd St Fl 5 East, New York, NY 10029; **Phone:** 212-241-6585; **Board Cert:** Internal Medicine 1983; **Med School:** Boston Univ 1980; **Resid:** Internal Medicine, Univ Conn Hlth Ctr 1983; **Fac Appt:** Asst Prof Med, Univ Fla Coll Med

Wiseman, Paul E MD (IM) *PCP* - **Spec Exp:** Preventive Medicine; **Hospital:** St. Luke's - Roosevelt Hosp Ctr - Roosevelt Div (page 94); **Address:** 101 Central Park West, New York, NY 10023-4204; **Phone:** 212-496-5800; **Board Cert:** Internal Medicine 1987; **Med School:** Albert Einstein Coll Med 1981; **Resid:** Internal Medicine, Montefiore Med Ctr 1984

Witt III, Marvin MD (IM) *PCP* - **Spec Exp:** Diabetes; Hypertension; **Hospital:** Lenox Hill Hosp (page 106); **Address:** Manhattan's Physician Grp, 590 5th Ave, New York, NY 10036; **Phone:** 212-582-7117; **Board Cert:** Internal Medicine 1986; **Med School:** Germany 1983; **Resid:** Internal Medicine, Bridgeport Hosp 1986

Yaffe, Bruce MD (IM) *PCP* - **Hospital:** Lenox Hill Hosp (page 106); **Address:** 201 E 65th St, New York, NY 10065; **Phone:** 212-879-4700; **Board Cert:** Internal Medicine 1979; Gastroenterology 1981; **Med School:** Geo Wash Univ 1976; **Resid:** Internal Medicine, Mount Sinai Hosp 1979; Hepatology, Mount Sinai Hosp 1980; **Fellow:** Gastroenterology, Lenox Hill Hosp 1982

Zaremski, Benjamin MD (IM) - **Spec Exp:** Cardiovascular Disease; **Hospital:** Beth Israel Med Ctr - Petrie Division (page 94), Lenox Hill Hosp (page 106); **Address:** 510 E 80th St, New York, NY 10075; **Phone:** 212-517-0022; **Board Cert:** Internal Medicine 1986; **Med School:** Dominican Republic 1981; **Resid:** Internal Medicine, Metropolitan Hosp 1984; **Fellow:** Cardiovascular Disease, St Francis Hosp/Metropolitan Hosp 1986

Zeale, Peter J MD (IM) *PCP* - **Spec Exp:** Hypertension; Cholesterol/Lipid Disorders; **Hospital:** NYU Langone Med Ctr (page 108); **Address:** 275 7th Ave Fl 3, New York, NY 10011; **Phone:** 646-660-9998; **Board Cert:** Internal Medicine 1982; **Med School:** Georgetown Univ 1979; **Resid:** Internal Medicine, St Vincent's Hosp 1983

Interventional Cardiology

Attubato, Michael J MD (IC) - **Spec Exp:** Coronary Angioplasty/Stents; Peripheral Vascular Disease; Heart Valve Disease; **Hospital:** NYU Langone Med Ctr (page 108), Bellevue Hosp Ctr; **Address:** NYU Langone Medical Center, 530 First Ave HCC Bldg Fl 14, New York, NY 10016; **Phone:** 212-263-5656; **Board Cert:** Internal Medicine 1984; Cardiovascular Disease 1987; Interventional Cardiology 2010; **Med School:** NYU Sch Med 1981; **Resid:** Internal Medicine, NYU Med Ctr 1985; **Fellow:** Cardiovascular Disease, NYU Med Ctr 1987; **Fac Appt:** Assoc Prof Med, NYU Sch Med

Fox, John T MD (IC) - **Hospital:** Beth Israel Med Ctr - Petrie Division (page 94); **Address:** Betrh Israel Heart Inst, First Ave at 16th St, 11 Dazian, New York, NY 10003; **Phone:** 212-420-2416; **Board Cert:** Cardiovascular Disease 2007; Interventional Cardiology 2011; **Med School:** NY Med Coll 1989; **Resid:** Internal Medicine, Beth Israel Med Ctr 1993; **Fellow:** Cardiovascular Disease, Beth Israel Med Ctr 1996; Interventional Cardiology, Beth Israel Med Ctr 1997; **Fac Appt:** Asst Prof Med, Albert Einstein Coll Med

Gray, William A MD (IC) - **Spec Exp:** Peripheral Vascular Disease; Percutaneous Valve Repair; Coronary Artery Disease; Mitral Valve Surgery; **Hospital:** NY-Presby/Columbia Univ Med Ctr, NY (page 104); **Address:** Ctr for Interventional Vascular Therapy, 161 Fort Washington Ave, Fl 6th, New York, NY 10032; **Phone:** 212-305-7060; **Board Cert:** Internal Medicine 1987; Cardiovascular Disease 2002; Interventional Cardiology 2011; Vascular Medicine 2004; **Med School:** Temple Univ 1984; **Resid:** Internal Medicine, Rhode Island Hosp/Brown Univ 1988; **Fellow:** Cardiovascular Disease, Brown Univ 1992; **Fac Appt:** Assoc Prof Med, Columbia P&S

Kodali, Susheel K MD (IC) - **Spec Exp:** Cardiac Catheterization; Angioplasty & Stent Placement; Heart Valve Disease; **Hospital:** NY-Presby/Columbia Univ Med Ctr, NY (page 104); **Address:** 161 Fort Washington Ave Fl 5, New York, NY 10032; **Phone:** 212-342-3611; **Board Cert:** Internal Medicine 2001; Cardiovascular Disease 2005; Interventional Cardiology 2006; **Med School:** UCLA-David Geffen Sch Med 1998; **Resid:** Infectious Disease, UCSF Med Ctr 2001; **Fellow:** Cardiovascular Disease, NY Presby/Columbia Med Ctr 2004; Interventional Cardiology, UCSF Med Ctr 2005

Leon, Martin B MD (IC) - **Hospital:** NY-Presby/Columbia Univ Med Ctr, NY (page 104); **Address:** 161 Ft Washington Ave, Irving Pavillion Fl 6 - Ste 607, New York, NY 10032; **Phone:** 212-305-7060; **Board Cert:** Internal Medicine 1979; Cardiovascular Disease 1983; **Med School:** Yale Univ 1975; **Resid:** Internal Medicine, Yale-New Haven Hosp 1978; **Fellow:** Cardiovascular Disease, Yale-New Haven Hosp 1980

Moses, Jeffrey W MD (IC) - **Spec Exp:** Angiography-Coronary; Angioplasty & Stent Placement; Heart Valve Disease; **Hospital:** NY-Presby/Columbia Univ Med Ctr, NY (page 104); **Address:** 161 Ft Washington Ave Fl 6, New York, NY 10032; **Phone:** 212-305-7060; **Board Cert:** Internal Medicine 1977; Cardiovascular Disease 1981; Interventional Cardiology 2009; **Med School:** Univ Pennsylvania 1974; **Resid:** Internal Medicine, Penn Presby Med Ctr 1977; **Fellow:** Cardiovascular Disease, Penn Presby Med Ctr 1980

Parikh, Manish A MD (IC) - **Spec Exp:** Coronary Angioplasty/Stents; **Hospital:** Lenox Hill Hosp (page 106); **Address:** 16 E 60th St, Ste 322, New York, NY 10022; **Phone:** 212-326-8532; **Board Cert:** Cardiovascular Disease 2010; Interventional Cardiology 2010; **Med School:** UMDNJ-NJ Med Sch, Newark 1990; **Resid:** Internal Medicine, New York Hosp 1993; **Fellow:** Cardiovascular Disease, New York Hosp 1997; **Fac Appt:** Asst Prof Med, Cornell Univ-Weill Med Coll

Roubin, Gary MD/PhD (IC) - **Spec Exp:** Coronary Angioplasty/Stents; Carotid Artery Stent Placement; Peripheral Vascular Disease; **Hospital:** St. Luke's - Roosevelt Hosp Ctr - St Luke's Hosp (page 94); **Address:** 1000 10 Ave, Ste 10G, New York, NY 10019; **Phone:** 212-523-7200; **Med School:** Australia 1975; **Resid:** Internal Medicine, Royal Prince Albert Hosp 1979; Cardiovascular Disease, Hallstrom Inst of Cardiology 1981; **Fellow:** Cardiology Research, Natl Heart Fdn 1983; Interventional Cardiology, Emory Univ 1985; **Fac Appt:** Clin Prof Med, NYU Sch Med

Sharma, Samin K MD (IC) - **Spec Exp:** Angioplasty & Stent Placement; Heart Valve Disease; **Hospital:** Mount Sinai Med Ctr (page 102); **Address:** One Gustave L Levy Pl, Box 1030, New York, NY 10029; **Phone:** 212-241-4021; **Board Cert:** Internal Medicine 1986; Cardiovascular Disease 1989; **Med School:** India 1978; **Resid:** Internal Medicine, SMS Hosp 1982; Internal Medicine, NYU Downtown Hosp 1986; **Fellow:** Cardiovascular Disease, City Hosp Ctr at Elmhurst 1988; Interventional Cardiology, Mt Sinai Hosp 2000; **Fac Appt:** Prof Med, Mount Sinai Sch Med

Slater, James N MD (IC) - **Spec Exp:** Coronary Angioplasty/Stents; Heart Valve Disease; **Hospital:** NYU Langone Med Ctr (page 108), St. Luke's - Roosevelt Hosp Ctr - St Luke's Hosp (page 94); **Address:** 426 W 58th St Fl Ground, New York, NY 10019; **Phone:** 212-247-0790; **Board Cert:** Internal Medicine 1980; Cardiovascular Disease 1985; Interventional Cardiology 2010; **Med School:** Univ Rochester 1977; **Resid:** Internal Medicine, Bellevue Hosp Ctr-NYU 1981; **Fellow:** Cardiovascular Disease, Bellevue Hosp Ctr-NYU 1983; **Fac Appt:** Assoc Prof Med, NYU Sch Med

Stone, Gregg W MD (IC) - **Spec Exp:** Angioplasty & Stent Placement; Coronary Artery Disease; **Hospital:** NY-Presby/Columbia Univ Med Ctr, NY (page 104); **Address:** 161 Fort Washington Ave, Irving Pavillion Fl 6 - Ste 607, New York, NY 10032; **Phone:** 212-305-7060; **Board Cert:** Internal Medicine 1985; Cardiovascular Disease 1987; **Med School:** Johns Hopkins Univ 1982; **Resid:** Internal Medicine, NY Hosp-Cornell Medical Ctr 1985; **Fellow:** Cardiovascular Disease, Cedars-Sinai Medical Ctr 1988; Coronary Angioplasty, Mid-America Heart Inst 1989; **Fac Appt:** Prof Med, Columbia P&S

Weinberger, Judah Z MD/PhD (IC) - **Spec Exp:** Cardiac Catheterization; Peripheral Vascular Disease; Coronary Artery Disease; Heart Valve Disease; **Hospital:** NY-Presby/Columbia Univ Med Ctr, NY (page 104), NYU Langone Med Ctr (page 108); **Address:** Heart Ctr, 173 Fort Washington Ave, Ste 4-602, New York, NY 10032; **Phone:** 212-305-1581; **Board Cert:** Internal Medicine 1984; Cardiovascular Disease 1985; Interventional Cardiology 2009; **Med School:** Harvard Med Sch 1980; **Resid:** Internal Medicine, Brigham & Womens Hosp 1982; **Fellow:** Cardiovascular Disease, Brigham & Womens Hosp 1985; **Fac Appt:** Assoc Prof Med, Columbia P&S

Maternal & Fetal Medicine

Berkowitz, Richard L MD (MF) - **Spec Exp:** Fetal Therapy; Multiple Gestation; Pregnancy & Hematologic Abnormalities; **Hospital:** NY-Presby/Columbia Univ Med Ctr, NY (page 104); **Address:** 16 E 60th St, Fl 4, New York, NY 10022; **Phone:** 212-305-0197; **Board Cert:** Obstetrics & Gynecology 2005; Maternal & Fetal Medicine 2005; **Med School:** NYU Sch Med 1965; **Resid:** Obstetrics & Gynecology, NY Hosp-Cornell Med Ctr 1972; **Fac Appt:** Prof ObG, Columbia P&S

D'Alton, Mary E MD (MF) - **Spec Exp:** Pregnancy-High Risk; Multiple Gestation; Prenatal Diagnosis; **Hospital:** NY-Presby/Columbia Univ Med Ctr, NY (page 104); **Address:** 16 E 60th St, Ste 480, New York, NY 10022; **Phone:** 212-326-8951; **Board Cert:** Obstetrics & Gynecology 2010; Maternal & Fetal Medicine 2010; **Med School:** Ireland 1976; **Resid:** Obstetrics & Gynecology, Ottowa Genl Hosp 1982; **Fellow:** Maternal & Fetal Medicine, Tufts-New Eng Med Ctr 1984; **Fac Appt:** Clin Prof ObG, Columbia P&S

Eddleman, Keith A MD (MF) - **Spec Exp:** Obstetric Ultrasound; Pregnancy-High Risk; Fetal Therapy; Reproductive Genetics; **Hospital:** Mount Sinai Med Ctr (page 102); **Address:** 5 E 98th St, Box 1171, New York, NY 10029; **Phone:** 212-241-5681; **Board Cert:** Obstetrics & Gynecology 2011; Maternal & Fetal Medicine 2011; Clinical Genetics 2010; **Med School:** Wake Forest Univ 1985; **Resid:** Obstetrics & Gynecology, George Washington Univ Med Ctr 1989; **Fellow:** Maternal & Fetal Medicine, Mt Sinai Med Ctr 1991; Genetics, NY-Cornell Med Ctr 1996; **Fac Appt:** Prof ObG, Mount Sinai Sch Med

Genc, Mehmet R MD/PhD (MF) - **Spec Exp:** Amniocentesis; Hypertension in Pregnancy; Pregnancy-High Risk; Fetal Abnormalities; **Hospital:** NY-Presby/Weill Cornell Med Ctr, NY (page 104); **Address:** 525 E 68th St, Ste J-130, New York, NY 10065; **Phone:** 212-746-1604; **Board Cert:** Obstetrics & Gynecology 2011; Maternal & Fetal Medicine 2011; **Med School:** Turkey 1994; **Resid:** Obstetrics & Gynecology, NY-Presby/Weill Cornell Med Ctr 2000; **Fellow:** Maternal & Fetal Medicine, NY-Presby/Weill Cornell Med Ctr 2001; Maternal & Fetal Medicine, Brigham & Women's Hosp 2003; **Fac Appt:** Asst Prof ObG, Cornell Univ-Weill Med Coll

Grunebaum, Amos MD (MF) - **Spec Exp:** Pregnancy-High Risk; Amniocentesis; **Hospital:** NY-Presby/Weill Cornell Med Ctr, NY (page 104); **Address:** Dept Obstetrics & Gynecology, 525 E 68th St, Ste J-130, New York, NY 10065; **Phone:** 212-746-0714; **Board Cert:** Obstetrics & Gynecology 2011; Maternal & Fetal Medicine 2011; **Med School:** Germany 1974; **Resid:** Anesthesiology, Maimonides Med Ctr 1978; Obstetrics & Gynecology, Downstate Med Ctr 1982; **Fellow:** Maternal & Fetal Medicine, Downstate Med Ctr 1984; **Fac Appt:** Assoc Prof ObG, Columbia P&S

Hutson, J Milton MD (MF) - **Spec Exp:** Multiple Gestation; Pregnancy After Age 35; Amniocentesis; **Hospital:** NY-Presby/Weill Cornell Med Ctr, NY (page 104); **Address:** 523 E 72nd St Fl 9, New York, NY 10021-4099; **Phone:** 212-472-5340; **Board Cert:** Obstetrics & Gynecology 1997; Maternal & Fetal Medicine 1997; **Med School:** Univ Alabama 1975; **Resid:** Obstetrics & Gynecology, Univ Hosp 1979; **Fellow:** Maternal & Fetal Medicine, Columbia-Presby Med Ctr 1982; **Fac Appt:** Asst Clin Prof ObG, Cornell Univ-Weill Med Coll

Kalish, Robin MD (MF) - **Spec Exp:** Pregnancy-High Risk; **Hospital:** NY-Presby/Weill Cornell Med Ctr, NY (page 104); **Address:** NY Presby-Cornell Med Ctr, 525 E 68th St, Ste J130, New York, NY 10021; **Phone:** 212-746-3146; **Board Cert:** Obstetrics & Gynecology 2006; Maternal & Fetal Medicine 2006; **Med School:** Univ Tenn Coll Med 1996; **Resid:** Obstetrics & Gynecology, Winthrop Univ Hosp 2000; **Fellow:** Maternal & Fetal Medicine, NY Presby-Cornell Hosp 2003; **Fac Appt:** Asst Prof ObG, Cornell Univ-Weill Med Coll

Patrick, Sharon MD (MF) - **Spec Exp:** Pregnancy-High Risk; Premature Labor; **Hospital:** St. Luke's - Roosevelt Hosp Ctr - Roosevelt Div (page 94); **Address:** 800-A Fifth Ave, Ste 503, New York, NY 10065; **Phone:** 212-230-1785; **Board Cert:** Obstetrics & Gynecology 2011; Maternal & Fetal Medicine 2011; **Med School:** Case West Res Univ 1986; **Resid:** Obstetrics & Gynecology, Columbia Presby Hosp 1990; **Fellow:** Maternal & Fetal Medicine, Columbia Presby Hosp 1992; **Fac Appt:** Asst Clin Prof ObG, Columbia P&S

Rebarber, Andrei MD (MF) - **Spec Exp:** Pregnancy-High Risk; Ultrasound; Clotting Disorders in Pregnancy; **Hospital:** Mount Sinai Med Ctr (page 102), Valley Hosp (page 689); **Address:** 70 E 90th St, New York, NY 10128; **Phone:** 212-722-7409; **Board Cert:** Obstetrics & Gynecology 2011; Maternal & Fetal Medicine 2011; **Med School:** SUNY Hlth Sci Ctr 1991; **Resid:** Obstetrics & Gynecology, Beth Israel Med Ctr 1995; **Fellow:** Maternal & Fetal Medicine, Yale-New Haven Hosp 1997; **Fac Appt:** Assoc Prof ObG, Mount Sinai Sch Med

Roshan, Daniel MD (MF) - **Spec Exp:** Pregnancy-High Risk; Pregnancy Loss; Thrombotic Disorders; Multiple Gestation; **Hospital:** NYU Langone Med Ctr (page 108), N Shore Univ Hosp (page 106); **Address:** 213 Madison Ave, New York, NY 10016; **Phone:** 212-725-0123; **Board Cert:** Obstetrics & Gynecology 2011; Maternal & Fetal Medicine 2011; **Med School:** Israel 1992; **Resid:** Obstetrics & Gynecology, Maimonides Med Ctr 1996; **Fellow:** Maternal & Fetal Medicine, Johns Hopkins Hosp 1998; **Fac Appt:** Asst Prof ObG, NYU Sch Med

Saltzman, Daniel MD (MF) - **Spec Exp:** Pregnancy-High Risk; Prenatal Diagnosis; Ultrasound; Diabetes in Pregnancy; **Hospital:** Mount Sinai Med Ctr (page 102); **Address:** 1245 Madison Ave, New York, NY 10128; **Phone:** 212-722-7409; **Board Cert:** Obstetrics & Gynecology 2011; Maternal & Fetal Medicine 2011; **Med School:** SUNY Buffalo 1979; **Resid:** Obstetrics & Gynecology, Geo Wash Med Ctr 1983; **Fellow:** Maternal & Fetal Medicine, Brigham & Women's Hosp 1985; **Fac Appt:** Clin Prof ObG, Mount Sinai Sch Med

Stone, Joanne L MD (MF) - **Spec Exp:** Prenatal Ultrasound; Twin to Twin Transfusion Syndrome (TTTS); **Hospital:** Mount Sinai Med Ctr (page 102); **Address:** Mount Sinai Medical Ctr, 5 E 98th St, Box 1171, New York, NY 10029; **Phone:** 212-241-5681; **Board Cert:** Obstetrics & Gynecology 2011; Maternal & Fetal Medicine 2011; **Med School:** Columbia P&S 1987; **Resid:** Obstetrics & Gynecology, Mt Sinai Med Ctr 1991; **Fellow:** Maternal & Fetal Medicine, Mt Sinai Med Ctr 1993; **Fac Appt:** Assoc Prof ObG, Mount Sinai Sch Med

Wapner, Ronald J MD (MF) - **Spec Exp:** Perinatal Medicine; Genetic Disorders; Multiple Gestation; Vomiting-Cyclic; **Hospital:** NY-Presby/Columbia Univ Med Ctr, NY (page 104); **Address:** Div Maternal/Fetal Medicine, 16 E 60th St, rm 480, New York, NY 10022; **Phone:** 212-326-8951; **Board Cert:** Obstetrics & Gynecology 2000; Maternal & Fetal Medicine 2000; Clinical Genetics 2010; **Med School:** Jefferson Med Coll 1972; **Resid:** Obstetrics & Gynecology, Jefferson Univ Hosp 1976; **Fellow:** Maternal & Fetal Medicine, Jefferson Med Coll 1978; **Fac Appt:** Prof ObG, Columbia P&S

Medical Oncology

Aghajanian, Carol A MD (Onc) - **Spec Exp:** Ovarian Cancer; Gynecologic Cancer; Trophoblastic Tumors; **Hospital:** Meml Sloan-Kettering Cancer Ctr (page 116); **Address:** 300 E 66th St, New York, NY 10065; **Phone:** 646-888-4217; **Board Cert:** Internal Medicine 2002; Medical Oncology 2005; **Med School:** SUNY Downstate 1989; **Resid:** Internal Medicine, Mt Sinai Med Ctr 1993; **Fellow:** Medical Oncology, Meml Sloan Kettering Cancer Ctr 1995; **Fac Appt:** Assoc Prof Med, Cornell Univ-Weill Med Coll

Azzoli, Christopher MD (Onc) - **Spec Exp:** Lung Cancer; Lung Cancer (advanced); **Hospital:** Meml Sloan-Kettering Cancer Ctr (page 116); **Address:** 300 E 66th St, New York, NY 10065; **Phone:** 646-888-4198; **Board Cert:** Internal Medicine 2009; Medical Oncology 2001; **Med School:** Johns Hopkins Univ 1996; **Resid:** Internal Medicine, Johns Hopkins Hosp 1999; **Fellow:** Medical Oncology, Meml Sloan Kettering Cancer Ctr 2002; **Fac Appt:** Asst Prof Med, Cornell Univ-Weill Med Coll

Bajorin, Dean F MD (Onc) - **Spec Exp:** Genitourinary Cancer; Bladder Cancer; Testicular Cancer; **Hospital:** Meml Sloan-Kettering Cancer Ctr (page 116); **Address:** 1275 York Avenue, New York, NY 10065; **Phone:** 646-422-4333; **Board Cert:** Internal Medicine 1981; Medical Oncology 1985; **Med School:** NY Med Coll 1978; **Resid:** Internal Medicine, Hartford Hosp 1981; **Fellow:** Medical Oncology, Meml Sloan Kettering Ctr 1986; **Fac Appt:** Prof Med, Cornell Univ-Weill Med Coll

Barbasch, Avi MD (Onc) - **Spec Exp:** Breast Cancer; Colon & Rectal Cancer; Lung Cancer; Gastrointestinal Cancer; **Hospital:** Mount Sinai Med Ctr (page 102), Lenox Hill Hosp (page 106); **Address:** 1050 Park Ave, New York, NY 10028-1031; **Phone:** 212-860-3292; **Board Cert:** Medical Oncology 2010; **Med School:** Mexico 1975; **Resid:** Internal Medicine, Elmhurst Hosp Ctr 1980; **Fellow:** Medical Oncology, Roswell Park Cancer Inst 1982; **Fac Appt:** Assoc Clin Prof Med, Mount Sinai Sch Med

Belenkov, Elliot Michael MD (Onc) - **Spec Exp:** Solid Tumors; **Hospital:** Mount Sinai Med Ctr (page 102), Lenox Hill Hosp (page 106); **Address:** 178 E 85th St, Fl 4, New York, NY 10028; **Phone:** 212-472-5500; **Board Cert:** Internal Medicine 1987; Medical Oncology 2011; **Med School:** Russia 1976; **Resid:** Psychiatry, Metro Hospital 1983; Internal Medicine, Metro Hospital 1986; **Fellow:** Hematology, Lenox Hill Hosp 1988; **Fac Appt:** Asst Clin Prof Onc, Cornell Univ-Weill Med Coll

Berman, Ellin MD (Onc) - **Spec Exp:** Leukemia; Lymphoma; **Hospital:** Meml Sloan-Kettering Cancer Ctr (page 116); **Address:** 1275 York Ave, New York, NY 10065; **Phone:** 212-639-7762; **Board Cert:** Internal Medicine 1980; Medical Oncology 1985; Hematology 1984; **Med School:** Harvard Med Sch 1977; **Resid:** Internal Medicine, Boston Univ Med Ctr 1980; **Fellow:** Medical Oncology, Meml Sloan Kettering Cancer Ctr 1983; **Fac Appt:** Prof Med, Cornell Univ-Weill Med Coll

Blum, Ronald MD (Onc) - **Spec Exp:** Melanoma; Sarcoma; Lung Cancer; Breast Cancer; **Hospital:** Beth Israel Med Ctr - Petrie Division (page 94); **Address:** 10 Union Square East, Ste 4C, New York, NY 10003-3314; **Phone:** 212-844-8282; **Board Cert:** Internal Medicine 1975; Medical Oncology 1975; **Med School:** SUNY Buffalo 1970; **Resid:** Internal Medicine, Boston City Hosp 1974; **Fellow:** Medical Oncology, Dana-Farber Cancer Inst 1975; **Fac Appt:** Prof Med, Albert Einstein Coll Med

Bosl, George MD (Onc) - **Spec Exp:** Testicular Cancer; **Hospital:** Meml Sloan-Kettering Cancer Ctr (page 116); **Address:** 1275 York Avenue, New York, NY 10065; **Phone:** 212-639-8473; **Board Cert:** Internal Medicine 1976; Medical Oncology 1979; **Med School:** Creighton Univ 1973; **Resid:** Internal Medicine, NY Hosp 1975; Internal Medicine, Meml Sloan-Kettering Cancer Ctr 1977; **Fellow:** Medical Oncology, Univ Minn Hosps 1979; **Fac Appt:** Prof Med, Cornell Univ-Weill Med Coll

Brunckhorst, Keith R MD (Onc) - **Hospital:** Lenox Hill Hosp (page 106); **Address:** 110 E 59th St, Ste 9B, New York, NY 10022-1304; **Phone:** 212-583-2858; **Board Cert:** Internal Medicine 1979; Hematology 1982; Medical Oncology 1983; **Med School:** NY Med Coll 1976; **Resid:** Internal Medicine, Stamford Hosp 1979; **Fellow:** Hematology & Oncology, Lenox Hill Hosp 1983

Chachoua, Abraham MD (Onc) - **Spec Exp:** Lung Cancer; Thoracic Cancers; **Hospital:** NYU Langone Med Ctr (page 108); **Address:** NYU Clinical Cancer Ctr, 160 E 34th St Fl 8, New York, NY 10016; **Phone:** 212-731-5388; **Med School:** Australia 1978; **Resid:** Internal Medicine, Alfred Hosp 1982; **Fellow:** Hematology & Oncology, Alfred Hosp 1985; Hematology & Oncology, NYU Med Ctr 1988; **Fac Appt:** Assoc Prof Med, NYU Sch Med

Chapman, Paul B MD (Onc) - **Spec Exp:** Melanoma; Immunotherapy; Clinical Trials; Vaccine Therapy; **Hospital:** Meml Sloan-Kettering Cancer Ctr (page 116); **Address:** 1275 York Avenue, New York, NY 10065; **Phone:** 646-888-2378; **Board Cert:** Internal Medicine 1984; Medical Oncology 1987; **Med School:** Cornell Univ-Weill Med Coll 1981; **Resid:** Internal Medicine, Univ Chicago Hosps 1984; **Fellow:** Medical Oncology, Meml Sloan-Kettering Cancer Ctr 1987; **Fac Appt:** Prof Med, Cornell Univ-Weill Med Coll

Cohen, Seymour M MD (Onc) - **Spec Exp:** Breast Cancer; Melanoma; Lung Cancer; Lymphoma; **Hospital:** Mount Sinai Med Ctr (page 102); **Address:** 1150 5th Ave, New York, NY 10128; **Phone:** 212-249-9141; **Board Cert:** Internal Medicine 1971; Medical Oncology 1973; **Med School:** Univ Pittsburgh 1962; **Resid:** Internal Medicine, Montefiore Med Ctr 1964; Internal Medicine, Mount Sinai Med Ctr 1965; **Fellow:** Hematology, Mount Sinai Med Ctr 1966; Hematology & Oncology, LI Jewish Hosp 1969; **Fac Appt:** Assoc Clin Prof Med, Mount Sinai Sch Med

Coleman, Morton MD (Onc) - **Spec Exp:** Leukemia & Lymphoma; Hodgkin's Lymphoma; Multiple Myeloma; Waldenstrom's Macroglobulinemia; **Hospital:** NY-Presby/Weill Cornell Med Ctr, NY (page 104); **Address:** 407 E 70th St Fl 3, New York, NY 10021-5302; **Phone:** 212-517-5900; **Board Cert:** Internal Medicine 1971; Hematology 1972; Medical Oncology 1973; **Med School:** Med Coll VA 1963; **Resid:** Internal Medicine, Grady Meml Hosp-Emory 1965; Internal Medicine, NY-Presby/Cornell Univ Med Ctr 1968; **Fellow:** Hematology & Oncology, NY-Presby/Cornell Univ Med Ctr 1970; **Fac Appt:** Clin Prof Med, Cornell Univ-Weill Med Coll

Decter, Julian A MD (Onc) - **Spec Exp:** Leukemia & Lymphoma; Multiple Myeloma; Myelodysplastic Syndromes; Colon Cancer; **Hospital:** NY-Presby/Weill Cornell Med Ctr, NY (page 104); **Address:** NY Presby Hosp, Div Hem/Onc, 407 E 70th St, New York, NY 10021; **Phone:** 212-517-5900; **Board Cert:** Internal Medicine 1972; Hematology 1974; Medical Oncology 1975; **Med School:** NYU Sch Med 1966; **Resid:** Internal Medicine, Ohio State Hosps 1968; **Fellow:** Hematology, NYU Med Ctr 1970; Medical Oncology, Nat Cancer Inst 1974; **Fac Appt:** Assoc Clin Prof Onc, Cornell Univ-Weill Med Coll

Dickler, Maura N MD (Onc) - **Spec Exp:** Breast Cancer; **Hospital:** Meml Sloan-Kettering Cancer Ctr (page 116); **Address:** 1275 York Ave, New York, NY 10065; **Phone:** 646-497-9064; **Board Cert:** Medical Oncology 2008; **Med School:** Univ Chicago-Pritzker Sch Med 1991; **Resid:** Internal Medicine, Univ Chicago Hosps 1994; **Fellow:** Medical Oncology, Meml Sloan Kettering Cancer Ctr 1998; **Fac Appt:** Assoc Prof Med, Cornell Univ-Weill Med Coll

Dutcher, Janice P MD (Onc) - **Spec Exp:** Kidney Cancer; Melanoma; Breast Cancer; Lymphoma; **Hospital:** St. Luke's - Roosevelt Hosp Ctr - Roosevelt Div (page 94); **Address:** Continuum Cancer Center of NY, 1000 Tenth Ave, Ste 11C-02, New York, NY 10019; **Phone:** 212-636-3334; **Board Cert:** Internal Medicine 1979; Medical Oncology 1983; **Med School:** UC Davis 1975; **Resid:** Internal Medicine, Rush Presbyterian Med Ctr 1978; **Fellow:** Medical Oncology, National Cancer Inst 1981; **Fac Appt:** Prof Med, NY Med Coll

Feldman, Eric MD (Onc) - **Spec Exp:** Leukemia; Stem Cell Transplant; **Hospital:** NY-Presby/Weill Cornell Med Ctr, NY (page 104); **Address:** 520 E 70th St Fl 3, Weill Cornell Med Ctr Onclgy HO, New York, NY 10021; **Phone:** 646-962-2700; **Board Cert:** Internal Medicine 1984; Medical Oncology 1987; **Med School:** NY Med Coll 1981; **Resid:** Internal Medicine, Westchester Co Med Ctr 1984; **Fellow:** Medical Oncology, Westchester Co Med Ctr 1986Fred Hutchinson Cancer Rsch Ctr 1987; **Fac Appt:** Prof Med, Cornell Univ-Weill Med Coll

Fine, Robert Lance MD (Onc) - **Spec Exp:** Pancreatic Cancer; Drug Development; Neuroendocrine Tumors; Clinical Trials; **Hospital:** NY-Presby/Columbia Univ Med Ctr, NY (page 104); **Address:** 650 W 168th St Fl 20th - Ste BB20-05, New York, NY 10032; **Phone:** 212-305-1168; **Board Cert:** Internal Medicine 1983; Medical Oncology 1985; **Med School:** Univ Chicago-Pritzker Sch Med 1979; **Resid:** Internal Medicine, Stanford Univ Med Ctr 1982; **Fellow:** Medical Oncology, National Cancer Inst 1988; **Fac Appt:** Assoc Prof Med, Columbia P&S

Fornier, Monica N MD (Onc) - **Spec Exp:** Breast Cancer; **Hospital:** Meml Sloan-Kettering Cancer Ctr (page 116); **Address:** Memorial Sloan Kettering Cancer Ctr, 1275 York Ave, New York, NY 10021; **Phone:** 646-888-5240; **Med School:** Italy 1992; **Resid:** Internal Medicine, Univ Hosp; **Fellow:** Medical Oncology, Natl Cancer Inst; Medical Oncology, Meml Sloan Kettering Cancer Ctr 2002

Gabrilove, Janice MD (Onc) - **Spec Exp:** Myelodysplastic Syndromes; Leukemia; Hematologic Malignancies; Myeloproliferative Disorders; **Hospital:** Mount Sinai Med Ctr (page 102); **Address:** Mount Sinai Med Ctr, One Gustave L Levy Pl, Box 1079, Dept Hem Onc, New York, NY 10029-6574; **Phone:** 212-241-9650; **Board Cert:** Internal Medicine 1980; Medical Oncology 1983; **Med School:** Mount Sinai Sch Med 1977; **Resid:** Internal Medicine, Columbia-Presby Med Ctr 1980; **Fellow:** Hematology & Oncology, Meml Sloan-Kettering Cancer Ctr 1983; **Fac Appt:** Prof Med, Mount Sinai Sch Med

Gaynor, Mitchell MD (Onc) - **Spec Exp:** Breast Cancer; Lung Cancer; Nutrition & Cancer; Complementary Medicine; **Hospital:** NY-Presby/Weill Cornell Med Ctr, NY (page 104); **Address:** 215 E 72nd St, New York, NY 10021; **Phone:** 212-472-2828; **Board Cert:** Internal Medicine 1985; Medical Oncology 1987; Hematology 1988; **Med School:** Univ Tex SW, Dallas 1982; **Resid:** Internal Medicine, New York Hosp 1985; **Fellow:** Hematology & Oncology, New York Hosp 1988; **Fac Appt:** Asst Clin Prof Med, Cornell Univ-Weill Med Coll

Gelmann, Edward P MD (Onc) - **Spec Exp:** Prostate Cancer; Bladder Cancer; Kidney Cancer; **Hospital:** NY-Presby/Columbia Univ Med Ctr, NY (page 104); **Address:** Columbia Univ Med Ctr, Milstein Hosp Bldg 6-435, 177 Fort Washington Ave, New York, NY 10032; **Phone:** 212-305-8602; **Board Cert:** Internal Medicine 1979; Medical Oncology 1981; **Med School:** Stanford Univ 1976; **Resid:** Internal Medicine, Univ Chicago Hosps 1978; **Fellow:** Medical Oncology, National Cancer Inst 1981; **Fac Appt:** Prof Med, Columbia P&S

Goldberg, Arthur I MD (Onc) - **Spec Exp:** Breast Cancer; Prostate Cancer; Colon & Rectal Cancer; Anal Cancer; **Hospital:** Lenox Hill Hosp (page 106), Mount Sinai Med Ctr (page 102); **Address:** 121 E 79th St, New York, NY 10075; **Phone:** 212-249-0030; **Board Cert:** Internal Medicine 1974; Medical Oncology 1975; **Med School:** SUNY Hlth Sci Ctr 1969; **Resid:** Internal Medicine, New York Hosp-Cornell 1970; Internal Medicine, Bellevue Hosp 1973; **Fellow:** Cancer Immunology, Natl Cancer Inst 1972; Medical Oncology, Meml Sloan Kettering Cancer Ctr 1975

Grace, William MD (Onc) - **Spec Exp:** Breast Cancer; Liver Cancer; Pancreatic Cancer; Lung Cancer; **Hospital:** Lenox Hill Hosp (page 106); **Address:** 1384 Broadway, New York, NY 10018; **Phone:** 212-675-6826; **Board Cert:** Internal Medicine 1976; Medical Oncology 1977; **Med School:** Boston Univ 1969; **Resid:** Internal Medicine, St Vincent's Hosp & Med Ctr 1971; **Fellow:** Hematology & Oncology, Dartmouth-Hitchcock Med Ctr 1976; **Fac Appt:** Assoc Clin Prof Med, NY Med Coll

Grossbard, Michael L MD (Onc) - **Spec Exp:** Lymphoma; Gastrointestinal Cancer; Breast Cancer; **Hospital:** St. Luke's - Roosevelt Hosp Ctr - Roosevelt Div (page 94), Beth Israel Med Ctr - Petrie Division (page 94); **Address:** 1000 10th Ave, Fl 11, Ste C02, St Luke's-Roosevelt Hospital, New York, NY 10019; **Phone:** 212-523-5419; **Board Cert:** Internal Medicine 1989; Medical Oncology 2011; **Med School:** Yale Univ 1986; **Resid:** Internal Medicine, Mass Genl Hosp 1989; **Fellow:** Medical Oncology, Dana Farber Cancer Inst 1991; **Fac Appt:** Clin Prof Hem & Onc, Columbia P&S

Gulati, Subhash C MD/PhD (Onc) - **Spec Exp:** Breast Cancer; Lymphoma; Lung Cancer; **Hospital:** NY-Presby/Weill Cornell Med Ctr, NY (page 104), Wyckoff Heights Med Ctr; **Address:** 331 E 65th St, New York, NY 10065; **Phone:** 212-535-1514; **Board Cert:** Internal Medicine 1980; Medical Oncology 1983; Hematology 1986; **Med School:** Univ Miami Sch Med 1976; **Resid:** Internal Medicine, Buffalo Genl Hosp 1978; **Fellow:** Hematology & Oncology, Meml Sloan Kettering Cancer Ctr 1980; **Fac Appt:** Clin Prof Med, Cornell Univ-Weill Med Coll

Hassoun, Hani MD (Onc) - **Spec Exp:** Hematologic Malignancies; Multiple Myeloma; Lymphoma; Stem Cell Transplant; **Hospital:** Meml Sloan-Kettering Cancer Ctr (page 116); **Address:** 1275 York Ave, New York, NY 10065; **Phone:** 212-639-3228; **Board Cert:** Internal Medicine 1986; Medical Oncology 1989; **Med School:** France 1983; **Resid:** Internal Medicine, Brigham & Womens Hosp 1986; **Fellow:** Hematology & Oncology, Tufts-St Elizabeth Hosp 1991; **Fac Appt:** Assoc Prof Med, Cornell Univ-Weill Med Coll

Hershman, Dawn L MD (Onc) - **Spec Exp:** Breast Cancer; Cancer Survivors-Late Effects of Therapy; Clinical Trials; **Hospital:** NY-Presby/Columbia Univ Med Ctr, NY (page 104); **Address:** Columbia Univ Med Ctr, Hematology/Oncology, 161 Fort Washington Ave Fl 10, New York, NY 10032; **Phone:** 212-305-5098; **Board Cert:** Internal Medicine 2007; Medical Oncology 2011; **Med School:** Albert Einstein Coll Med 1994; **Resid:** Internal Medicine, Columbia Univ Med Ctr 1998; **Fellow:** Medical Oncology, Columbia Univ Med Ctr 2001; **Fac Appt:** Asst Prof Med, Columbia P&S

Hirschman, Richard J MD (Onc) - **Spec Exp:** Breast Cancer; Colon Cancer; Lung Cancer; **Hospital:** Beth Israel Med Ctr - Petrie Division (page 94); **Address:** 247 3rd Ave, Ste 401, New York, NY 10010-7455; **Phone:** 212-228-0471; **Board Cert:** Internal Medicine 1971; Hematology 1972; Medical Oncology 1973; **Med School:** Johns Hopkins Univ 1965; **Resid:** Internal Medicine, Bellevue Hosp Ctr 1967; Internal Medicine, Columbia-Presby Hosp 1970; **Fellow:** Hematology & Oncology, Columbia-Presby Hosp 1971; **Fac Appt:** Assoc Clin Prof Med, Mount Sinai Sch Med

Hirshaut, Yashar MD (Onc) - **Spec Exp:** Breast Cancer; Lung Cancer; Colon Cancer; **Hospital:** Lenox Hill Hosp (page 106), NY-Presby/Weill Cornell Med Ctr, NY (page 104); **Address:** 860 5th Ave, New York, NY 10021-5856; **Phone:** 212-861-1799; **Board Cert:** Internal Medicine 1972; Medical Oncology 1975; **Med School:** Albert Einstein Coll Med 1963; **Resid:** Internal Medicine, Montefiore Hosp Med Ctr 1965; **Fellow:** Medical Oncology, Natl Cancer Inst 1968; Medical Oncology, Meml Sloan Kettering Cancer Ctr 1970; **Fac Appt:** Assoc Clin Prof Med, Cornell Univ-Weill Med Coll

Holcombe, Randall F MD (Onc) - **Spec Exp:** Gastrointestinal Cancer; Liver Cancer; Clinical Trials; **Hospital:** Mount Sinai Med Ctr (page 102); **Address:** The Derald H. Ruttenberg Treatment Ctr, 1190 5th Ave, New York, NY 10029; **Phone:** 212-241-6756; **Board Cert:** Internal Medicine 1986; Medical Oncology 2003; Hematology 2002; **Med School:** UMDNJ-NJ Med Sch, Newark 1983; **Resid:** Internal Medicine, Brigham & Womens Hosp 1986; **Fellow:** Hematology, Harvard Med Sch; **Fac Appt:** Prof Med, Mount Sinai Sch Med

Holland, James F MD (Onc) - **Spec Exp:** Breast Cancer; Colon Cancer; Lung Cancer; Pancreatic Cancer; **Hospital:** Mount Sinai Med Ctr (page 102); **Address:** Mount Sinai Medial Center, 1 Gustave I Levy Pl, Box 1079, New York, NY 10029; **Phone:** 212-241-4495; **Board Cert:** Internal Medicine 1955; **Med School:** Columbia P&S 1947; **Resid:** Internal Medicine, Columbia-Presby Hosp 1949; Internal Medicine, Francis Delafield Hosp 1952; **Fellow:** Medical Oncology, Francis Delafield Hosp 1953; **Fac Appt:** Prof Med, Mount Sinai Sch Med

Horwitz, Steven M MD (Onc) - **Spec Exp:** Lymphoma, Cutaneous T Cell (CTCL); Hodgkin's Lymphoma; Lymphoma, Non-Hodgkin's; **Hospital:** Meml Sloan-Kettering Cancer Ctr (page 116); **Address:** Meml Sloan-Kettering Cancer Ctr, 1275 York Ave, New York, NY 10065; **Phone:** 212-639-3045; **Board Cert:** Medical Oncology 2011; **Med School:** Case West Res Univ 1993; **Resid:** Internal Medicine, Strong Memorial Hosp 1996; **Fellow:** Medical Oncology, Stanford Univ Med Ctr 1999

Hudis, Clifford A MD (Onc) - **Spec Exp:** Breast Cancer; **Hospital:** Meml Sloan-Kettering Cancer Ctr (page 116); **Address:** 1275 York Avenue, New York, NY 10065; **Phone:** 646-888-5449; **Board Cert:** Internal Medicine 1986; Medical Oncology 2001; **Med School:** Med Coll PA Hahnemann 1983; **Resid:** Internal Medicine, Hosp Med Coll Penn 1987; **Fellow:** Medical Oncology, Meml Sloan Kettering Cancer Ctr 1991; **Fac Appt:** Prof Med, Cornell Univ-Weill Med Coll

Ilson, David H MD/PhD (Onc) - **Spec Exp:** Esophageal Cancer; Colon & Rectal Cancer; Mesothelioma; Unknown Primary Cancer; **Hospital:** Meml Sloan-Kettering Cancer Ctr (page 116); **Address:** 300 E 66th St, New York, NY 10065; **Phone:** 646-888-4183; **Board Cert:** Internal Medicine 1989; Medical Oncology 2002; **Med School:** NYU Sch Med 1986; **Resid:** Internal Medicine, Bellevue-NYU Sch Med 1989; **Fellow:** Medical Oncology, Meml Sloan Kettering Hosp 1992; **Fac Appt:** Assoc Prof Med, Cornell Univ-Weill Med Coll

Jagannath, Sundar MD (Onc) - **Spec Exp:** Multiple Myeloma; **Hospital:** Mount Sinai Med Ctr (page 102); **Address:** 1 Gustave Levy Pl, PO Box 1185, New York, NY 10029; **Phone:** 212-241-7873; **Board Cert:** Internal Medicine 1980; Medical Oncology 1985; **Med School:** India 1976; **Resid:** Internal Medicine, Bronx Lebanon Hosp 1979; Internal Medicine, Harper-Grace Hosp 1980; **Fellow:** Medical Oncology, MD Anderson Cancer Ctr 1982; **Fac Appt:** Prof Med, NY Med Coll

Jakubowski, Ann MD (Onc) - **Spec Exp:** Leukemia; Bone Marrow Transplant; **Hospital:** Meml Sloan-Kettering Cancer Ctr (page 116); **Address:** 1275 York Ave, New York, NY 10065; **Phone:** 212-639-5013; **Board Cert:** Internal Medicine 1984; Medical Oncology 1987; Hematology 1986; **Med School:** Univ Conn 1981; **Resid:** Internal Medicine, Mt Sinai Hosp 1984; **Fellow:** Hematology, Montefiore Hosp 1985; Medical Oncology, Meml Sloan-Kettering Cancer Ctr 1988

Jarowski, Charles MD (Onc) - **Spec Exp:** Breast Cancer; Lung Cancer; Colon Cancer; **Hospital:** NY-Presby/Weill Cornell Med Ctr, NY (page 104), Hosp For Special Surgery (page 115); **Address:** 400 E 77th St, Ste 1A, New York, NY 10075; **Phone:** 212-794-9500; **Board Cert:** Internal Medicine 1975; Medical Oncology 1977; Hematology 1978; **Med School:** Cornell Univ-Weill Med Coll 1972; **Resid:** Internal Medicine, New York Hosp 1975; **Fellow:** Hematology & Oncology, New York Hosp 1978; **Fac Appt:** Asst Prof Med, Cornell Univ-Weill Med Coll

Jurcic, Joseph G MD (Onc) - **Spec Exp:** Leukemia; Myelodysplastic Syndromes; Clinical Trials; **Hospital:** Meml Sloan-Kettering Cancer Ctr (page 116); **Address:** 1275 York Avenue, New York, NY 10065; **Phone:** 212-639-2955; **Board Cert:** Internal Medicine 2001; Medical Oncology 2005; Hematology 2008; **Med School:** Univ Pennsylvania 1988; **Resid:** Internal Medicine, Barnes Hosp 1991; **Fellow:** Hematology & Oncology, Meml Sloan Kettering Cancer Ctr 1994; **Fac Appt:** Assoc Prof Med, Cornell Univ-Weill Med Coll

Kelsen, David Paul MD (Onc) - **Spec Exp:** Gastrointestinal Cancer; Neuroendocrine Tumors; Unknown Primary Cancer; Merkel Cell Carcinoma; **Hospital:** Meml Sloan-Kettering Cancer Ctr (page 116); **Address:** 300 E 66th St, New York, NY 10065; **Phone:** 646-888-4179; **Board Cert:** Internal Medicine 1976; Medical Oncology 1979; **Med School:** Hahnemann Univ 1972; **Resid:** Internal Medicine, Temple Univ Hosp 1976; **Fellow:** Medical Oncology, Meml Sloan Kettering Cancer Ctr 1978; **Fac Appt:** Prof Med, Cornell Univ-Weill Med Coll

Kemeny, Nancy MD (Onc) - **Spec Exp:** Colon Cancer; Rectal Cancer; Liver Cancer; **Hospital:** Meml Sloan-Kettering Cancer Ctr (page 116); **Address:** 300 E 66th St, New York, NY 10065; **Phone:** 646-888-4180; **Board Cert:** Internal Medicine 1974; Medical Oncology 1981; **Med School:** UMDNJ-NJ Med Sch, Newark 1971; **Resid:** Internal Medicine, St Luke's Hosp 1974; **Fellow:** Medical Oncology, Mem Sloan Kettering Cancer Ctr 1976; **Fac Appt:** Prof Med, Cornell Univ-Weill Med Coll

Klafter, Robert MD (Onc) - **Spec Exp:** Lymphoma; Leukemia; Breast Cancer; **Hospital:** Mount Sinai Med Ctr (page 102); **Address:** 12 E 86th St, New York, NY 10028; **Phone:** 212-861-6660; **Board Cert:** Hematology 2001; Medical Oncology 2001; **Med School:** NYU Sch Med 1994; **Resid:** Internal Medicine, NYU Med Ctr 1997; **Fellow:** Hematology & Oncology, Emory Univ Hosp 2001; **Fac Appt:** Asst Clin Prof Med, Mount Sinai Sch Med

Kozuch, Peter S MD (Onc) - **Spec Exp:** Gastrointestinal Cancer; Esophageal Cancer; Pancreatic Cancer; **Hospital:** Beth Israel Med Ctr - Petrie Division (page 94), St. Luke's - Roosevelt Hosp Ctr - St Luke's Hosp (page 94); **Address:** 10 Union Square E Fl 4 - Ste 4C, New York, NY 10003; **Phone:** 212-844-8070; **Board Cert:** Medical Oncology 2010; Hematology 2004; **Med School:** Hahnemann Univ 1994; **Resid:** Internal Medicine, Boston Med Ctr 1997; **Fellow:** Medical Oncology, UT-MD Anderson Cancer Ctr 2000; **Fac Appt:** Assoc Clin Prof Med, Albert Einstein Coll Med

Kris, Mark G MD (Onc) - **Spec Exp:** Lung Cancer; Mediastinal Tumors; Thymoma; Thoracic Cancers; **Hospital:** Meml Sloan-Kettering Cancer Ctr (page 116); **Address:** 300 E 66th St, New York, NY 10065; **Phone:** 646-888-4197; **Board Cert:** Internal Medicine 1980; Medical Oncology 1983; **Med School:** Cornell Univ-Weill Med Coll 1977; **Resid:** Internal Medicine, New York Hosp 1980; **Fellow:** Medical Oncology, Meml Sloan Kettering Cancer Ctr 1983; **Fac Appt:** Prof Med, Cornell Univ-Weill Med Coll

Krug, Lee M MD (Onc) - **Spec Exp:** Small Cell Lung Cancer; Mesothelioma; Clinical Trials; **Hospital:** Meml Sloan-Kettering Cancer Ctr (page 116); **Address:** MSKCC, Dept Thoracic Oncology, 1275 York Ave, New York, NY 10065; **Phone:** 646-888-4201; **Board Cert:** Internal Medicine 2007; Medical Oncology 2009; **Med School:** Washington Univ, St Louis 1994; **Resid:** Internal Medicine, Johns Hopkins Hosp 1997; **Fellow:** Medical Oncology, Meml Sloan Kettering Canc Ctr 1997

Kruger, Bernard M MD (Onc) - **Spec Exp:** Breast Cancer; **Hospital:** Lenox Hill Hosp (page 106); **Address:** 170 E 78th St, New York, NY 10075; **Phone:** 212-772-9222; **Board Cert:** Internal Medicine 1974; Medical Oncology 1979; **Med School:** Univ Colorado 1968; **Resid:** Internal Medicine, Boston City Hosp 1972; Internal Medicine, Georgetown Hosp 1974; **Fellow:** Medical Oncology, Mt Sinai Hosp 1976

Maki, Robert G MD/PhD (Onc) - **Spec Exp:** Sarcoma-Soft Tissue; Bone Tumors; Gastrointestinal Stromal Tumors; Desmoid Tumors; **Hospital:** Mount Sinai Med Ctr (page 102); **Address:** 1 Gustave L. Levy Pl, 1468 Madison Ave, Box 1208, New York, NY 10029-6574; **Phone:** 212-241-6756; **Board Cert:** Internal Medicine 2005; Medical Oncology 2007; **Med School:** Cornell Univ-Weill Med Coll 1992; **Resid:** Internal Medicine, Brigham & Womens Hosp 1995; **Fellow:** Medical Oncology, Dana-Farber Cancer Inst 1998; **Fac Appt:** Prof Onc, Mount Sinai Sch Med

Malamud, Stephen C MD (Onc) - **Spec Exp:** Lung Cancer; Gastrointestinal Cancer; **Hospital:** Beth Israel Med Ctr - Petrie Division (page 94), NYU Hosp For Joint Diseases (page 119); **Address:** 10 Union Square E, Ste 4B, New York, NY 10003; **Phone:** 212-844-8280; **Board Cert:** Internal Medicine 1981; Medical Oncology 1983; **Med School:** Albert Einstein Coll Med 1978; **Resid:** Internal Medicine, Beth Israel Med Ctr 1981; **Fellow:** Medical Oncology, Mt Sinai Hosp 1983; **Fac Appt:** Assoc Clin Prof Med, Albert Einstein Coll Med

Moore, Anne MD (Onc) - **Spec Exp:** Breast Cancer; **Hospital:** NY-Presby/Weill Cornell Med Ctr, NY (page 104); **Address:** Weill Cornell Breast Ctr, 425 E 61st St Fl 8, New York, NY 10065; **Phone:** 212-821-0550; **Board Cert:** Internal Medicine 1973; Hematology 1976; Medical Oncology 2008; **Med School:** Columbia P&S 1969; **Resid:** Internal Medicine, Cornell Univ Med Ctr 1973; **Fellow:** Medical Oncology, Rockefeller Univ 1973; **Fac Appt:** Prof Med, Cornell Univ-Weill Med Coll

Moskowitz, Craig H MD (Onc) - **Spec Exp:** Lymphoma; Bone Marrow Transplant; **Hospital:** Meml Sloan-Kettering Cancer Ctr (page 116); **Address:** 1275 York Ave, New York, NY 10065; **Phone:** 212-639-2696; **Board Cert:** Hematology 2002; Medical Oncology 2005; **Med School:** Wayne State Univ 1988; **Resid:** Internal Medicine, Bronx Mcpl Hosp 1992; Internal Medicine, Bronx Mcpl Hosp 1991; **Fellow:** Hematology & Oncology, Meml Sloan-Kettering Cancer Ctr

Motzer, Robert J MD (Onc) - **Spec Exp:** Kidney Cancer; Testicular Cancer; Prostate Cancer; **Hospital:** Meml Sloan-Kettering Cancer Ctr (page 116); **Address:** 1275 York Avenue, New York, NY 10065; **Phone:** 646-422-4312; **Board Cert:** Internal Medicine 1984; Medical Oncology 1987; **Med School:** Univ Mich Med Sch 1981; **Resid:** Internal Medicine, Meml Sloan Kettering Cancer Ctr 1984; **Fellow:** Medical Oncology, Meml Sloan Kettering Cancer Ctr 1987; **Fac Appt:** Assoc Prof Med, Cornell Univ-Weill Med Coll

Muggia, Franco M MD (Onc) - **Spec Exp:** Gynecologic Cancer; **Hospital:** NYU Langone Med Ctr (page 108); **Address:** NYU Clinical Cancer Ctr, 160 E 34th St Fl 4, New York, NY 10016; **Phone:** 212-731-5433; **Board Cert:** Internal Medicine 1968; Medical Oncology 1973; Hematology 1974; **Med School:** Cornell Univ-Weill Med Coll 1961; **Resid:** Internal Medicine, Hartford Hosp 1964; Internal Medicine, Francis A Delafield Hosp 1966; **Fac Appt:** Prof Med, NYU Sch Med

Nanus, David M MD (Onc) - **Spec Exp:** Prostate Cancer; Bladder Cancer; Testicular Cancer; Genitourinary Cancer; **Hospital:** NY-Presby/Weill Cornell Med Ctr, NY (page 104); **Address:** NY Hosp-Cornell Med Ctr,Payson Pavillion, 525 E 68th St Fl 3 - Ste 341, New York, NY 10021; **Phone:** 646-962-2072; **Board Cert:** Internal Medicine 1985; Medical Oncology 1987; **Med School:** Univ Hlth Scis, Chicago Med Sch 1982; **Resid:** Internal Medicine, Bronx Muni Hosp 1985; **Fellow:** Medical Oncology, Meml Sloan Kettering Canc Ctr 1989; **Fac Appt:** Prof Med, Cornell Univ-Weill Med Coll

Norton, Larry MD (Onc) - **Spec Exp:** Breast Cancer; **Hospital:** Meml Sloan-Kettering Cancer Ctr (page 116); **Address:** 300 E 66th St, BAIC Bldg Fl 9 - Ste 933, New York, NY 10065; **Phone:** 646-888-5438; **Board Cert:** Internal Medicine 1975; Medical Oncology 1977; **Med School:** Columbia P&S 1972; **Resid:** Internal Medicine, Bronx Muni Hosp 1974; **Fellow:** Medical Oncology, Natl Cancer Inst 1977; **Fac Appt:** Prof Med, Cornell Univ-Weill Med Coll

O'Connor, Owen A MD/PhD (Onc) - **Spec Exp:** Hodgkin's Lymphoma; Lymphoma, Non-Hodgkin's; Drug Development; Clinical Trials; **Hospital:** NY-Presby/Columbia Univ Med Ctr, NY (page 104); **Address:** 16 E 60th St, Ste 330, New York, NY 10065; **Phone:** 212-326-5720; **Board Cert:** Internal Medicine 2004; Medical Oncology 2005; **Med School:** UMDNJ-RW Johnson Med Sch 1994; **Resid:** Internal Medicine, NY-Presby/Weill Cornell Univ Med Ctr 1996; **Fellow:** Medical Oncology, Memorial Sloan-Kettering Cancer Ctr 2000; **Fac Appt:** Prof Med, NYU Sch Med

O'Reilly, Eileen M MD (Onc) - **Spec Exp:** Pancreatic Cancer; Liver Cancer; Biliary Cancer; Neuroendocrine Tumors; **Hospital:** Meml Sloan-Kettering Cancer Ctr (page 116); **Address:** 300 E 66th St, rm 1021, Memorial Sloan-Kettering Cancer Center, New York, NY 10065; **Phone:** 646-888-4182; **Med School:** Ireland 1990; **Resid:** Internal Medicine, St Vincent's Hosp 1994; **Fellow:** Hematology & Oncology, St Vincent's Hosp 1995; Medical Oncology, Memorial-Sloan Kettering Cancer Ctr 1997; **Fac Appt:** Assoc Prof Onc, Cornell Univ-Weill Med Coll

Offit, Kenneth MD (Onc) - **Spec Exp:** Cancer Genetics; Breast Cancer; Lymphoma; **Hospital:** Meml Sloan-Kettering Cancer Ctr (page 116); **Address:** Memorial Sloan-Kettering Cancer Center, 1275 York Ave, New York, NY 10065; **Phone:** 646-888-4050; **Board Cert:** Internal Medicine 1985; Medical Oncology 1987; **Med School:** Harvard Med Sch 1982; **Resid:** Internal Medicine, Lenox Hill Hosp 1985; **Fellow:** Hematology & Oncology, Meml Sloan Kettering Cancer Ctr 1988; **Fac Appt:** Prof Med, Cornell Univ-Weill Med Coll

Oh, William K MD (Onc) - **Spec Exp:** Genitourinary Cancer; Prostate Cancer; Testicular Cancer; Adrenal Cancer; **Hospital:** Mount Sinai Med Ctr (page 102); **Address:** Ruttenberg Treatment Center, 1190 FIfth Ave, New York, NY 10029; **Phone:** 212-659-5429; **Board Cert:** Medical Oncology 2009; **Med School:** NYU Sch Med 1992; **Resid:** Internal Medicine, Brigham & Womens Hosp 1995; **Fellow:** Medical Oncology, Dana-Farber Cancer Inst 1997; **Fac Appt:** Prof Med, Mount Sinai Sch Med

Oratz, Ruth MD (Onc) - **Spec Exp:** Breast Cancer; **Hospital:** NYU Langone Med Ctr (page 108); **Address:** 345 E 37th St, Ste 202, New York, NY 10016; **Phone:** 212-400-4904; **Board Cert:** Internal Medicine 1985; Medical Oncology 1989; **Med School:** Albert Einstein Coll Med 1982; **Resid:** Internal Medicine, NYU Med Ctr 1982; **Fellow:** Medical Oncology, NYU Med Ctr 1985; **Fac Appt:** Assoc Clin Prof Med, NYU Sch Med

Oster, Martin W MD (Onc) - **Spec Exp:** Breast Cancer; Gastrointestinal Cancer; Head & Neck Cancer; **Hospital:** NY-Presby/Columbia Univ Med Ctr, NY (page 104); **Address:** NY Presby Hosp-Columbia University Med Ctr, 161 Fort Washington Ave, New York, NY 10032-3713; **Phone:** 212-305-8231; **Board Cert:** Internal Medicine 1974; Medical Oncology 1975; **Med School:** Columbia P&S 1971; **Resid:** Internal Medicine, Mass Genl Hosp 1973; **Fellow:** Medical Oncology, Natl Cancer Inst/NIH 1976; **Fac Appt:** Assoc Clin Prof Onc, Columbia P&S

Pasmantier, Mark W MD (Onc) - **Spec Exp:** Lung Cancer; Ovarian Cancer; Breast Cancer; Lymphoma; **Hospital:** NY-Presby/Weill Cornell Med Ctr, NY (page 104); **Address:** 407 E 70th St Fl 3, New York, NY 10021-5302; **Phone:** 212-517-5900; **Board Cert:** Internal Medicine 1972; Hematology 1974; Medical Oncology 1975; **Med School:** NYU Sch Med 1966; **Resid:** Internal Medicine, Harlem Hosp 1970; **Fellow:** Hematology, Montefiore Med Ctr 1971; Medical Oncology, NY Hosp 1972; **Fac Appt:** Clin Prof Med, Cornell Univ-Weill Med Coll

Pavlick, Anna C MD (Onc) - **Spec Exp:** Melanoma; Skin Cancer; Merkel Cell Carcinoma; **Hospital:** NYU Langone Med Ctr (page 108); **Address:** 160 E 34th St, Fl 9, NYU Cancer Institute, New York, NY 10016; **Phone:** 212-731-5431; **Board Cert:** Medical Oncology 2008; **Med School:** UMDNJ Sch Osteo Med 1990; **Resid:** Internal Medicine, Hackensack Med Ctr 1993; **Fellow:** Hematology & Oncology, Meml Sloan Kettering Cancer Ctr 1996; **Fac Appt:** Assoc Prof Med, NYU Sch Med

Pfister, David G MD (Onc) - **Spec Exp:** Head & Neck Cancer; Laryngeal Cancer; Thyroid Cancer; Skin Cancer; **Hospital:** Meml Sloan-Kettering Cancer Ctr (page 116); **Address:** 300 E 66th St, New York, NY 10065; **Phone:** 646-888-4232; **Board Cert:** Internal Medicine 1985; Medical Oncology 1989; **Med School:** Univ Pennsylvania 1982; **Resid:** Internal Medicine, Hosp Univ Penn 1985; **Fellow:** Epidemiology, Yale-New Haven Hosp 1987; Hematology & Oncology, Meml Sloan Kettering Cancer Ctr 1989; **Fac Appt:** Prof Med, Cornell Univ-Weill Med Coll

Portlock, Carol S MD (Onc) - **Spec Exp:** Lymphoma; Hodgkin's Lymphoma; **Hospital:** Meml Sloan-Kettering Cancer Ctr (page 116); **Address:** 1275 York Ave, New York, NY 10065; **Phone:** 212-639-8109; **Board Cert:** Internal Medicine 1976; Medical Oncology 1978; **Med School:** Stanford Univ 1971; **Resid:** Internal Medicine, Stanford U Med Ctr 1974; **Fellow:** Medical Oncology, Stanford U Med Ctr 1976; **Fac Appt:** Clin Prof Med, Cornell Univ-Weill Med Coll

Posner, Marshall R MD (Onc) - **Spec Exp:** Head & Neck Cancer; Skin Cancer-Head & Neck; **Hospital:** Mount Sinai Med Ctr (page 102); **Address:** Mount Sinai Med Ctr, 1 Gustave L Levy Pl, Box 1128, New York, NY 10029; **Phone:** 212-241-6756; **Board Cert:** Internal Medicine 1978; Medical Oncology 1981; **Med School:** Tufts Univ 1975; **Resid:** Internal Medicine, Boston City Hosp 1978; **Fellow:** Oncology, Dana-Farber Cancer Inst 1981; **Fac Appt:** Assoc Prof Med, Mount Sinai Sch Med

Raptis, George MD (Onc) - **Spec Exp:** Breast Cancer; **Hospital:** Mount Sinai Med Ctr (page 102); **Address:** Ruttenberg Treatment Ctr, 1190 5th Ave, Box 1129, New York, NY 10029; **Phone:** 212-241-6756; **Board Cert:** Medical Oncology 2003; **Med School:** Mount Sinai Sch Med 1987; **Resid:** Internal Medicine, Mt Sinai Med Ctr 1990; **Fellow:** Hematology & Oncology, Meml Sloan-Kettering Canc Ctr 1993; **Fac Appt:** Assoc Prof Med, Mount Sinai Sch Med

Ratner, Lynn H MD (Onc) - **Spec Exp:** Breast Cancer; Carcinoid Tumors; Neuroendocrine Tumors; Gliomas; **Hospital:** Mount Sinai Med Ctr (page 102), Lenox Hill Hosp (page 106); **Address:** 112 E 83rd St, New York, NY 10028-0506; **Phone:** 212-396-0400; **Board Cert:** Internal Medicine 1977; Medical Oncology 1973; **Med School:** Albert Einstein Coll Med 1964; **Resid:** Internal Medicine, Bellevue Hosp 1966; Internal Medicine, Bellevue Hosp 1970; **Fellow:** Medical Oncology, Meml Sloan Kettering Cancer Ctr 1970

Raza, Azra MD (Onc) - **Spec Exp:** Myelodysplastic Syndromes; Leukemia; Clinical Trials; **Hospital:** NY-Presby/Columbia Univ Med Ctr, NY (page 104); **Address:** 161 Ft Washington Ave Fl 9, New York, NY 10011; **Phone:** 212-305-0566; **Board Cert:** Internal Medicine 1980; Medical Oncology 1985; **Med School:** Pakistan 1976; **Resid:** Internal Medicine, Franklin Sq Hosp 1979; Internal Medicine, Georgetown Univ/VA Med Ctr 1980; **Fellow:** Medical Oncology, Roswell Park Cancer Inst 1982

Rizvi, Naiyer A MD (Onc) - **Spec Exp:** Thoracic Cancers; Thymoma; Lung Cancer; Clinical Trials; **Hospital:** Meml Sloan-Kettering Cancer Ctr (page 116); **Address:** 300 E 66 St, New York, NY 10065; **Phone:** 646-888-4204; **Board Cert:** Internal Medicine 2002; Medical Oncology 2003; **Med School:** Canada 1987; **Resid:** Internal Medicine, University of Manitoba Med Ctr 1992; **Fellow:** Medical Oncology, Beth Israel Med Ctr 1994

Roboz, Gail J MD (Onc) - **Spec Exp:** Leukemia; Myelodysplastic Syndromes; Myeloproliferative Disorders; **Hospital:** NY-Presby/Weill Cornell Med Ctr, NY (page 104); **Address:** 525 E 68TH St, New York, NY 10021; **Phone:** 646-962-2700; **Board Cert:** Medical Oncology 2010; Hematology 2010; **Med School:** Mount Sinai Sch Med 1994; **Resid:** Internal Medicine, NY Presby Hosp/Cornell 1997; **Fellow:** Hematology & Oncology, NY Presby Hosp/Cornell 2000; **Fac Appt:** Assoc Prof Med, Cornell Univ-Weill Med Coll

Robson, Mark Emerson MD (Onc) - **Spec Exp:** Breast Cancer; Cancer Genetics; **Hospital:** Meml Sloan-Kettering Cancer Ctr (page 116); **Address:** 300 E 66th St, New York, NY 10065; **Phone:** 646-888-5434; **Board Cert:** Internal Medicine 1989; Medical Oncology 2001; Hematology 2002; **Med School:** Univ VA Sch Med 1986; **Resid:** Internal Medicine, Walter Reed AMC 1989; **Fellow:** Hematology & Oncology, Walter Reed AMC 1991

Ruggiero, Joseph T MD (Onc) - **Spec Exp:** Gastrointestinal Cancer; **Hospital:** NY-Presby/Weill Cornell Med Ctr, NY (page 104); **Address:** 1305 York Ave Fl 12, New York, NY 10021-4635; **Phone:** 646-962-6200; **Board Cert:** Internal Medicine 1980; Hematology 1982; Medical Oncology 1983; **Med School:** NYU Sch Med 1977; **Resid:** Internal Medicine, New York Hosp 1980; **Fellow:** Hematology & Oncology, New York Hosp/Cornell 1983; **Fac Appt:** Assoc Clin Prof Med, Cornell Univ-Weill Med Coll

Sabbatini, Paul J MD (Onc) - **Spec Exp:** Gynecologic Cancer; Uterine Cancer; Ovarian Cancer; **Hospital:** Meml Sloan-Kettering Cancer Ctr (page 116); **Address:** Meml Sloan Kettering Cancer Ctr, 300 E 66 St, New York, NY 10065; **Phone:** 646-888-4218; **Board Cert:** Internal Medicine 1992; Medical Oncology 1997; **Med School:** Univ Miss 1989; **Resid:** Internal Medicine, Vanderbilt Univ Med Ctr; **Fellow:** Medical Oncology, Meml Sloan-Kettering Cancer Ctr; **Fac Appt:** Asst Prof Med, Cornell Univ-Weill Med Coll

Saltz, Leonard B MD (Onc) - **Spec Exp:** Colon & Rectal Cancer; Gastrointestinal Cancer & Rare Tumors; Neuroendocrine Tumors; **Hospital:** Meml Sloan-Kettering Cancer Ctr (page 116); **Address:** Memorial Sloan Kettering Cancer Center, 300 E 66th St, rm 1049, New York, NY 10065; **Phone:** 646-888-4181; **Board Cert:** Internal Medicine 1986; Hematology 1988; Medical Oncology 1989; **Med School:** Yale Univ 1983; **Resid:** Internal Medicine, New Yor Hosp 1986; **Fellow:** Hematology & Oncology, New York Hosp-Cornell/Rockefeller Univ 1989; **Fac Appt:** Prof Med, Cornell Univ-Weill Med Coll

Sara, Gabriel MD (Onc) - **Spec Exp:** Breast Cancer; Lung Cancer; Lymphoma; Gastrointestinal Cancer; **Hospital:** St. Luke's - Roosevelt Hosp Ctr - Roosevelt Div (page 94); **Address:** 1000 10th Ave Fl 11, New York, NY 10019; **Phone:** 212-523-7580; **Board Cert:** Internal Medicine 1984; Hematology 1986; Medical Oncology 1987; **Med School:** Lebanon 1980; **Resid:** Internal Medicine, SUNY Downstate Med Ctr 1984; **Fellow:** Hematology & Oncology, St Luke's-Roosevelt Med Ctr 1986; Hematology & Oncology, Columbia-Presby Med Ctr 1987; **Fac Appt:** Asst Clin Prof Med, Columbia P&S

Scheinberg, David MD/PhD (Onc) - **Spec Exp:** Leukemia; Immunotherapy; Vaccine Therapy; **Hospital:** Meml Sloan-Kettering Cancer Ctr (page 116); **Address:** 1275 York Avenue, New York, NY 10065; **Phone:** 646-888-2190; **Board Cert:** Internal Medicine 1986; Medical Oncology 2005; **Med School:** Johns Hopkins Univ 1983; **Resid:** Internal Medicine, NY Hosp-Cornell Med Ctr 1985; **Fellow:** Medical Oncology, Meml Sloan Kettering Cancer Ctr 1987; **Fac Appt:** Prof Med, Cornell Univ-Weill Med Coll

Scher, Howard MD (Onc) - **Spec Exp:** Genitourinary Cancer; Prostate Cancer; Bladder Cancer; **Hospital:** Meml Sloan-Kettering Cancer Ctr (page 116); **Address:** 1275 York Avenue, New York, NY 10065; **Phone:** 646-422-4330; **Board Cert:** Internal Medicine 1979; Medical Oncology 1985; **Med School:** NYU Sch Med 1976; **Resid:** Internal Medicine, Bellevue Hosp 1980; **Fellow:** Medical Oncology, Meml Sloan Kettering Cancer Ctr 1983; **Fac Appt:** Prof Med, Cornell Univ-Weill Med Coll

Sherman, William H MD (Onc) - **Spec Exp:** Pancreatic Cancer; Multiple Myeloma; Melanoma; **Hospital:** NY-Presby/Columbia Univ Med Ctr, NY (page 104); **Address:** 161 Fort Washington Ave, Ste 809, New York, NY 10032-3729; **Phone:** 212-305-3856; **Board Cert:** Internal Medicine 1975; Medical Oncology 1979; **Med School:** Jefferson Med Coll 1969; **Resid:** Internal Medicine, Univ Illinois Hosp 1971; **Fellow:** Medical Oncology, Columbia-Presby Hosp 1977; **Fac Appt:** Assoc Clin Prof Med, Columbia P&S

Silverman, Lewis R MD (Onc) - **Spec Exp:** Myelodysplastic Syndromes; Leukemia & Lymphoma; Multiple Myeloma; **Hospital:** Mount Sinai Med Ctr (page 102); **Address:** Ruttenberg Treatment Ctr, 1190 5th Ave, Box 1129, New York, NY 10029; **Phone:** 212-241-6756; **Board Cert:** Internal Medicine 1981; Hematology 1986; Medical Oncology 1987; **Med School:** Belgium 1978; **Resid:** Internal Medicine, Metro Hospital 1980; Internal Medicine, Montefiore Med Ctr 1981; **Fellow:** Hematology, Montefiore Med Ctr 1982; Neoplastic Diseases, Mt Sinai Med Ctr 1984; **Fac Appt:** Assoc Prof Med, Mount Sinai Sch Med

Sklarin, Nancy T MD (Onc) - **Spec Exp:** Breast Cancer; **Hospital:** Meml Sloan-Kettering Cancer Ctr (page 116); **Address:** 300 E 66th St, New York, NY 10065; **Phone:** 646-888-5488; **Board Cert:** Internal Medicine 1984; Medical Oncology 1987; Hematology 1988; **Med School:** Albert Einstein Coll Med 1981; **Resid:** Internal Medicine, LI Jewish Med Ctr 1984; **Fellow:** Hematology & Oncology, Mount Sinai Med Ctr 1987; **Fac Appt:** Assoc Prof Med, Cornell Univ-Weill Med Coll

Slovin, Susan F MD/PhD (Onc) - **Spec Exp:** Prostate Cancer; Genitourinary Cancer; Immunotherapy; **Hospital:** Meml Sloan-Kettering Cancer Ctr (page 116), NY-Presby/Weill Cornell Med Ctr, NY (page 104); **Address:** 1275 York Ave, New York, NY 10065; **Phone:** 646-422-4470; **Board Cert:** Internal Medicine 2005; Medical Oncology 1999; **Med School:** Jefferson Med Coll 1990; **Resid:** Internal Medicine, Mt Sinai Hosp 1993; **Fellow:** Medical Oncology, Meml Sloan Kettering Cancer Ctr 1996; **Fac Appt:** Assoc Prof Med, Cornell Univ-Weill Med Coll

Smith, Julia A MD/PhD (Onc) - **Spec Exp:** Breast Cancer; Cancer Risk Assessment; **Hospital:** NYU Langone Med Ctr (page 108), Bellevue Hosp Ctr; **Address:** 160 E 34th St, Fl 3rd, MS 10016, NYU Clinical Cancer Center, New York, NY 10016; **Phone:** 212-731-5452; **Board Cert:** Internal Medicine 1985; Medical Oncology 1989; **Med School:** NYU Sch Med 1980; **Resid:** Internal Medicine, Brigham & Womens Hosp 1983; **Fellow:** Hematology & Oncology, Meml Sloan Kettering Cancer Ctr 1986; **Fac Appt:** Asst Clin Prof Med, NYU Sch Med

Speyer, James L MD (Onc) - **Spec Exp:** Ovarian Cancer; Breast Cancer; Cardiac Effects in Cancer Therapy; **Hospital:** NYU Langone Med Ctr (page 108); **Address:** 160 E 34th St, Fl 8, New York, NY 10016-4750; **Phone:** 212-731-5432; **Board Cert:** Internal Medicine 1977; Hematology 1978; Medical Oncology 1979; **Med School:** Johns Hopkins Univ 1974; **Resid:** Internal Medicine, Columbia-Presby Med Ctr 1976; Hematology, Columbia-Presby Med Ctr 1977; **Fellow:** Medical Oncology, Natl Cancer Inst 1979; **Fac Appt:** Prof Med, NYU Sch Med

Spriggs, David R MD (Onc) - **Spec Exp:** Ovarian Cancer; Drug Development; Uterine Cancer; Gynecologic Cancer; **Hospital:** Meml Sloan-Kettering Cancer Ctr (page 116); **Address:** 300 E 66th St, New York, NY 10065; **Phone:** 646-888-4223; **Board Cert:** Internal Medicine 1981; Medical Oncology 2006; **Med School:** Univ Wisc 1977; **Resid:** Internal Medicine, Columbia-Presby Hosp 1981; **Fellow:** Medical Oncology, Dana-Farber Cancer Inst 1985; **Fac Appt:** Prof Med, Cornell Univ-Weill Med Coll

Stoopler, Mark Benjamin MD (Onc) - **Spec Exp:** Lung Cancer; Esophageal Cancer; Unknown Primary Cancer; **Hospital:** NY-Presby/Columbia Univ Med Ctr, NY (page 104); **Address:** 161 Fort Washington Ave, Ste 936, New York, NY 10032-3713; **Phone:** 212-305-8230; **Board Cert:** Internal Medicine 1978; Medical Oncology 1981; **Med School:** Cornell Univ-Weill Med Coll 1975; **Resid:** Internal Medicine, North Shore Univ Hosp 1978; Internal Medicine, NY Meml Hosp 1978; **Fellow:** Medical Oncology, Meml-Sloan Kettering Cancer Ctr 1980; **Fac Appt:** Assoc Clin Prof Onc, Columbia P&S

Straus, David J MD (Onc) - **Spec Exp:** Lymphoma; Multiple Myeloma; **Hospital:** Meml Sloan-Kettering Cancer Ctr (page 116); **Address:** 1275 York Ave, Box 406, New York, NY 10065; **Phone:** 212-639-8365; **Board Cert:** Internal Medicine 1972; Hematology 1976; Medical Oncology 1977; **Med School:** Marquette Sch Med 1969; **Resid:** Internal Medicine, Montefiore Med Ctr 1972; Medical Oncology, Meml Sloan Kettering Cancer Ctr 1977; **Fellow:** Hematology, Beth Israel Hosp 1973; **Fac Appt:** Prof Onc, Cornell Univ-Weill Med Coll

Tagawa, Scott T MD (Onc) - **Spec Exp:** Prostate Cancer; Bladder Cancer; Kidney Cancer; Urologic Cancer; **Hospital:** NY-Presby/Weill Cornell Med Ctr, NY (page 104); **Address:** NY Presby-Weill Cornell Med Ctr, 525 E 68th St, Box 403, New York, NY 10065; **Phone:** 646-962-2072; **Board Cert:** Medical Oncology 2005; Hematology 2006; **Med School:** USC-Keck School of Medicine 1998; **Resid:** Internal Medicine, USC Med Ctr 2002; **Fellow:** Hematology & Oncology, USC Med Ctr 2005; **Fac Appt:** Asst Prof Hem & Onc, Cornell Univ-Weill Med Coll

Tap, William D MD (Onc) - **Spec Exp:** Sarcoma; Sarcoma-Soft Tissue; Ewing's Sarcoma; **Hospital:** Meml Sloan-Kettering Cancer Ctr (page 116); **Address:** 300 E 66th St Fl 10, New York, NY 10065; **Phone:** 646-888-4163; **Board Cert:** Internal Medicine 2003; Hematology 2006; Medical Oncology 2006; **Med School:** Thomas Jefferson Univ 2000; **Resid:** Internal Medicine, Vanderbilt Univ Med Ctr 2003; **Fellow:** Hematology & Oncology, UCLA Med Ctr 2006

Vahdat, Linda T MD (Onc) - **Spec Exp:** Breast Cancer; Breast Cancer-Novel Therapies; Clinical Trials; **Hospital:** NY-Presby/Weill Cornell Med Ctr, NY (page 104); **Address:** 425 E 61st St Fl 8, New York, NY 10065; **Phone:** 212-821-0644; **Board Cert:** Medical Oncology 2005; **Med School:** Mount Sinai Sch Med 1987; **Resid:** Internal Medicine, Mt Sinai Hosp 1990; **Fellow:** Hematology & Oncology, Meml Sloan Kettering Cancer Ctr 1994; **Fac Appt:** Prof Med, Cornell Univ-Weill Med Coll

Wolchok, Jedd D MD/PhD (Onc) - **Spec Exp:** Melanoma; Immunotherapy; Clinical Trials; Vaccine Therapy; **Hospital:** Meml Sloan-Kettering Cancer Ctr (page 116); **Address:** Meml Sloan Kettering Cancer Ctr, 1275 York Ave, New York, NY 10065; **Phone:** 646-888-2395; **Board Cert:** Medical Oncology 2011; **Med School:** NYU Sch Med 1994; **Resid:** Internal Medicine, NYU Med Ctr 1996; **Fellow:** Medical Oncology, Meml Sloan-Kettering Canc Ctr 1997

Zelenetz, Andrew D MD/PhD (Onc) - **Spec Exp:** Lymphoma; **Hospital:** Meml Sloan-Kettering Cancer Ctr (page 116); **Address:** 205 E 64th St, New York, NY 10065; **Phone:** 212-639-2656; **Board Cert:** Medical Oncology 2009; **Med School:** Harvard Med Sch 1984; **Resid:** Internal Medicine, Stanford Univ Med Ctr 1986; **Fellow:** Medical Oncology, Stanford Univ Med Ctr 1991; **Fac Appt:** Asst Prof Med, Cornell Univ-Weill Med Coll

Neonatal-Perinatal Medicine

Bateman, David MD (NP) - **Hospital:** NY-Presby/Columbia Univ Med Ctr, NY (page 104); **Address:** 3959 Broadway, CHC 1-115, New York, NY 10032; **Phone:** 212-305-5827; **Board Cert:** Pediatrics 1979; Neonatal-Perinatal Medicine 1981; **Med School:** Tufts Univ 1973; **Resid:** Pediatrics, Lincoln Hosp 1975; Pediatrics, Boston Fltg Hosp 1977; **Fellow:** Neonatal-Perinatal Medicine, Columbia-Presby Med Ctr 1982; **Fac Appt:** Assoc Prof Ped, Columbia P&S

Holzman, Ian R MD (NP) - **Spec Exp:** Neonatal Nutrition; Necrotizing Enterocolitis; Ethics; Prematurity/Low Birth Weight Infants; **Hospital:** Mount Sinai Med Ctr (page 102), Elmhurst Hosp Ctr; **Address:** Newborn Assocs, 1 Gustave L Levy Pl, Box 1508, New York, NY 10029-6500; **Phone:** 212-241-5446; **Board Cert:** Pediatrics 1974; Neonatal-Perinatal Medicine 1977; **Med School:** Univ Pittsburgh 1971; **Resid:** Pediatrics, Chldns Hosp 1975; **Fellow:** Neonatal-Perinatal Medicine, Univ Colorado Hosp 1977; **Fac Appt:** Prof Ped, Mount Sinai Sch Med

Marron-Corwin, Mary MD (NP) - **Spec Exp:** Neonatal Respiratory Care; Critical Care; Neonatal Liver Disease; **Hospital:** Harlem Hosp Ctr; **Address:** 506 Lenox Ave, MLK Pavilion, Ste 4417, New York, NY 10037; **Phone:** 212-939-8457; **Board Cert:** Neonatal-Perinatal Medicine 2008; **Med School:** Philippines 1985; **Resid:** Pediatrics, St Vincents Hosp Med Ctr 1988; **Fellow:** Neonatal-Perinatal Medicine, Babies Hosp/Colum-Presby Med Ctr 1990; **Fac Appt:** Assoc Prof Ped, Columbia P&S

Perlman, Jeffrey M MD (NP) - **Spec Exp:** Neonatal Critical Care; Prematurity/Low Birth Weight Infants; Neonatal Neurology; Lung Disease in Newborns; **Hospital:** NY-Presby/Weill Cornell Med Ctr, NY (page 104); **Address:** 525 E 68th St, Ste N 506, New York, NY 10065; **Phone:** 212-746-3530; **Board Cert:** Pediatrics 1983; Neonatal-Perinatal Medicine 1983; **Med School:** South Africa 1974; **Resid:** Pediatrics, Johannesburg Chldns Hosp 1979; Pediatrics, St Louis Chldns Hosp 1981; **Fellow:** Neonatology, St Louis Chldns Hosp 1983; **Fac Appt:** Prof Ped, Cornell Univ-Weill Med Coll

Polin, Richard A MD (NP) - **Spec Exp:** Neonatal Infections; **Hospital:** Morgan Stanley Children's Hosp of NY-Presby, NY (page 104); **Address:** 3959 Broadway CHN 1201, New York, NY 10032; **Phone:** 212-305-5827; **Board Cert:** Pediatrics 1975; Neonatal-Perinatal Medicine 1977; **Med School:** Temple Univ 1970; **Resid:** Pediatrics, Chldns Meml Hosp 1972; Pediatrics, Babies Hosp 1973; **Fellow:** Neonatal-Perinatal Medicine, Babies Hosp-Columbia 1974; **Fac Appt:** Prof Ped, Columbia P&S

Rosen, Tove S MD (NP) - **Spec Exp:** Neonatology; Substance Abuse Effects in Newborn; Ethics; **Hospital:** Morgan Stanley Children's Hosp of NY-Presby, NY (page 104); **Address:** Morgan Stanley Chldns Hosp of NY-Presby, 3959 Broadway, CHN 1201, New York, NY 10032-1559; **Phone:** 212-305-8500; **Board Cert:** Pediatrics 1971; Neonatal-Perinatal Medicine 1975; **Med School:** SUNY Hlth Sci Ctr 1965; **Resid:** Pediatrics, St Luke's Hosp 1970; **Fellow:** Neonatal-Perinatal Medicine, Columbia-Presby Med Ctr 1974; **Fac Appt:** Clin Prof Ped, Columbia P&S

Shahrivar, Farrokh MD (NP) - **Spec Exp:** Neonatology; Prematurity/Low Birth Weight Infants; **Hospital:** St. Luke's - Roosevelt Hosp Ctr - Roosevelt Div (page 94), Beth Israel Med Ctr - Petrie Division (page 94); **Address:** 1000 10th Ave NICU Fl 12, New York, NY 10019-1192; **Phone:** 212-523-3760; **Board Cert:** Pediatrics 1974; Neonatal-Perinatal Medicine 1975; **Med School:** Iran 1966; **Resid:** Pediatrics, St Luke's-Roosevelt Hosp Ctr 1971; Pediatrics, St Luke's-Roosevelt Hosp Ctr 1972; **Fellow:** Neonatal-Perinatal Medicine, St Christopher's Hosp 1973; Neonatal-Perinatal Medicine, Montefiore Med Ctr 1973; **Fac Appt:** Assoc Clin Prof Ped, Columbia P&S

Nephrology

Ames, Richard MD (Nep) - **Spec Exp:** Hypertension; Kidney Disease; Dialysis Care; **Hospital:** St. Luke's - Roosevelt Hosp Ctr - Roosevelt Div (page 94); **Address:** 200 W 57th St Fl 15, New York, NY 10019; **Phone:** 917-224-4270; **Board Cert:** Internal Medicine 1974; Nephrology 1972; Medical Oncology 1973; Hematology 1974; **Med School:** Columbia P&S 1958; **Resid:** Internal Medicine, Boston Med Ctr 1961; **Fellow:** Nephrology, Columbia-Presby Hosp 1963; **Fac Appt:** Clin Prof Med, Columbia P&S

Appel, Gerald B MD/PhD (Nep) - **Spec Exp:** Glomerulonephritis; Lupus Nephritis; Nephrotic Syndrome; **Hospital:** NY-Presby/Columbia Univ Med Ctr, NY (page 104); **Address:** 161 Fort Washington Ave Fl 2 - Ste 202, New York, NY 10032-3720; **Phone:** 212-305-0320 x3; **Board Cert:** Internal Medicine 1975; Nephrology 1978; **Med School:** Albert Einstein Coll Med 1972; **Resid:** Internal Medicine, Columbia Presby Hosp 1975; **Fellow:** Nephrology, Columbia Presby Hosp 1976; Nephrology, Yale-New Haven Hosp 1978; **Fac Appt:** Clin Prof Med, Columbia P&S

August, Phyllis MD (Nep) - **Spec Exp:** Hypertension; Hypertension in Pregnancy; Hypertension/Kidney Disease; **Hospital:** NY-Presby/Weill Cornell Med Ctr, NY (page 104); **Address:** 450 E 69th St, Hypertension Center, New York, NY 10021-4870; **Phone:** 212-746-2210; **Board Cert:** Internal Medicine 1980; Nephrology 1982; **Med School:** Yale Univ 1977; **Resid:** Internal Medicine, NY Hosp-Cornell Med Ctr 1980; **Fellow:** Nephrology, NY Hosp-Cornell Med Ctr 1983; **Fac Appt:** Prof Med, Cornell Univ-Weill Med Coll

Black, Henry R MD (Nep) - **Spec Exp:** Hypertension; **Hospital:** NYU Langone Med Ctr (page 108); **Address:** NYU Medical Ctr, 530 First Ave, SKI-9U, New York, NY 10016; **Phone:** 212-263-7751; **Board Cert:** Internal Medicine 1972; Nephrology 1974; **Med School:** NYU Sch Med 1967; **Resid:** Internal Medicine, Johns Hopkins Hosp 1971; Internal Medicine, Yale-New Haven Hosp 1972; **Fellow:** Nephrology, Yale-New Haven Hosp 1974; **Fac Appt:** Clin Prof Med, NYU Sch Med

Blumenfeld, Jon D MD (Nep) - **Spec Exp:** Polycystic Kidney Disease; Hypertension; Adrenal Disorders; **Hospital:** NY-Presby/Weill Cornell Med Ctr, NY (page 104), Rockefeller Univ; **Address:** The Rogosin Institute, 505 E 70th St Fl 2, New York, NY 10021; **Phone:** 212-746-1495; **Board Cert:** Internal Medicine 1984; Nephrology 1986; **Med School:** Yale Univ 1981; **Resid:** Internal Medicine, New York Hosp 1984; **Fellow:** Nephrology, Brigham & Womens Hosp 1988; **Fac Appt:** Prof Med, Cornell Univ-Weill Med Coll

Cohen, David J MD (Nep) - **Spec Exp:** Transplant Medicine-Kidney; Glomerulonephritis; **Hospital:** NY-Presby/Columbia Univ Med Ctr, NY (page 104); **Address:** Columbia Univ Med Ctr, 622 W 168th St, rm PH 4-124, New York, NY 10032-3720; **Phone:** 212-305-0320 x4; **Board Cert:** Internal Medicine 1980; Nephrology 1984; **Med School:** Albert Einstein Coll Med 1977; **Resid:** Internal Medicine, Mount Sinai Hosp 1980; **Fellow:** Nephrology, Columbia-Presby Hosp 1981; Transplant Immunobiology, Brigham & Womens Hosp 1983; **Fac Appt:** Clin Prof Med, Columbia P&S

DeFabritus, Albert Michael MD (Nep) - **Spec Exp:** Kidney Disease-Chronic; Hypertension; Anemia in Chronic Kidney Disease; Kidney Stones; **Hospital:** Beth Israel Med Ctr - Petrie Division (page 94); **Address:** 352 7th Ave, Ste 1003, New York, NY 10001; **Phone:** 212-807-8817; **Board Cert:** Internal Medicine 1976; Nephrology 1978; **Med School:** NY Med Coll 1973; **Resid:** Internal Medicine, St Vincent's Hosp & Med Ctr 1976; **Fellow:** Nephrology, New York Hosp 1978; **Fac Appt:** Asst Clin Prof Med, NY Med Coll

Devita, Maria V MD (Nep) - **Spec Exp:** Glomerulonephritis; Dialysis Care; Hypertension; Kidney Disease-Chronic; **Hospital:** Lenox Hill Hosp (page 106); **Address:** 130 E 77th St Fl 5, New York, NY 10075; **Phone:** 212-439-9251; **Board Cert:** Internal Medicine 1988; Nephrology 2002; **Med School:** Georgetown Univ 1984; **Resid:** Internal Medicine, Lenox Hill Hosp 1987; **Fellow:** Nephrology, Lenox Hill Hosp 1989; **Fac Appt:** Assoc Clin Prof Med, NYU Sch Med

Gardenswartz, Mark MD (Nep) - **Spec Exp:** Hypertension; Hypertension in Pregnancy; Polycystic Kidney Disease; **Hospital:** Lenox Hill Hosp (page 106), Mount Sinai Med Ctr (page 102); **Address:** 110 E 59th St, Ste 10B, New York, NY 10022; **Phone:** 212-583-2930; **Board Cert:** Internal Medicine 1978; Nephrology 1980; Critical Care Medicine 2002; **Med School:** Univ Colorado 1975; **Resid:** Internal Medicine, Columbia Presby Med Ctr 1978; **Fellow:** Nephrology, Univ Colorado Hosp 1978; **Fac Appt:** Asst Clin Prof Med, NY Med Coll

Garvey, Michael MD (Nep) - **Spec Exp:** Dialysis Care; **Hospital:** Beth Israel Med Ctr - Petrie Division (page 94); **Address:** 510-526 6th Ave, Ste 5C, New York, NY 10011; **Phone:** 212-807-7920; **Board Cert:** Internal Medicine 1979; Nephrology 1982; **Med School:** NY Med Coll 1975; **Resid:** Internal Medicine, St Vincent's Hosp & Med Ctr 1979; **Fellow:** Nephrology, NYU Med Ctr 1981

Liu, David T MD (Nep) - **Spec Exp:** Glomerulonephritis; Nephrotic Syndrome; Kidney Failure; Hypertension; **Hospital:** NYU Langone Med Ctr (page 108); **Address:** 530 1st Ave, Ste 4B, New York, NY 10016-6402; **Phone:** 212-263-0705; **Board Cert:** Internal Medicine 1980; Nephrology 1984; **Med School:** SUNY Buffalo 1977; **Resid:** Internal Medicine, Univ Miami Hosps 1980; **Fellow:** Nephrology, NYU Med Ctr 1984; **Fac Appt:** Asst Clin Prof Med, NYU Sch Med

Matalon, Robert MD (Nep) - **Spec Exp:** Dialysis Care; Kidney Failure; **Hospital:** NYU Langone Med Ctr (page 108), NY Downtown Hosp; **Address:** 530 1st Ave, Ste 4A, New York, NY 10016-6402; **Phone:** 212-263-7239; **Board Cert:** Internal Medicine 1970; Nephrology 1974; **Med School:** NYU Sch Med 1964; **Resid:** Internal Medicine, Bellevue Hosp 1967; **Fellow:** Nephrology, NYU Med Ctr 1969; **Fac Appt:** Assoc Prof Med, NYU Sch Med

Michelis, Michael F MD (Nep) - **Spec Exp:** Kidney Disease; Hypertension; Dialysis Care; **Hospital:** Lenox Hill Hosp (page 106); **Address:** 130 E 77th St, FL 5, New York, NY 10075-1851; **Phone:** 212-988-3506; **Board Cert:** Internal Medicine 1969; **Med School:** Geo Wash Univ 1963; **Resid:** Internal Medicine, Lenox Hill Hosp 1965; Internal Medicine, Hosp Med Coll Penn 1967; **Fellow:** Renal Disease, Univ Pittsburgh 1970; **Fac Appt:** Clin Prof Med, NYU Sch Med

Saal, Stuart MD (Nep) - **Spec Exp:** Transplant Medicine-Kidney; **Hospital:** NY-Presby/Weill Cornell Med Ctr, NY (page 104); **Address:** 505 E 70th St, Ste 230, New York, NY 10021-4872; **Phone:** 212-746-1553; **Board Cert:** Internal Medicine 1974; Nephrology 1978; **Med School:** NY Med Coll 1971; **Resid:** Internal Medicine, St Luke's-Roosevelt Hosp Ctr 1974; **Fellow:** Nephrology, NY Hosp 1976; **Fac Appt:** Assoc Clin Prof Med, Cornell Univ-Weill Med Coll

Sherman, Raymond MD (Nep) - **Spec Exp:** Glomerulonephritis; Hypertension; Kidney Failure-Chronic; **Hospital:** NY-Presby/Weill Cornell Med Ctr, NY (page 104); **Address:** 407 E 70th St Fl 4, New York, NY 10021-5302; **Phone:** 212-879-8245; **Board Cert:** Internal Medicine 1969; Nephrology 1974; **Med School:** SUNY Hlth Sci Ctr 1961; **Resid:** Internal Medicine, St Luke's-Roosevelt Hosp Ctr 1965; Nephrology, Strong Meml Hosp 1965; **Fellow:** Nephrology, NY Hosp/Cornell Med Ctr 1969; **Fac Appt:** Clin Prof Med, Cornell Univ-Weill Med Coll

Stern, Leonard MD (Nep) - **Spec Exp:** Kidney Failure-Chronic; Transplant Medicine-Kidney; Bone Disorders-Metabolic; Dialysis Care; **Hospital:** NY-Presby/Columbia Univ Med Ctr, NY (page 104); **Address:** 622 W 168th St, rm PH4-124, New York, NY 10032-3702; **Phone:** 212-305-3273; **Board Cert:** Internal Medicine 1978; Nephrology 1980; **Med School:** NY Med Coll 1975; **Resid:** Internal Medicine, Jacobi Med Ctr 1978; **Fellow:** Nephrology, Montefiore Med Ctr 1979; Nephrology, Yale-New Haven Hosp 1981; **Fac Appt:** Assoc Clin Prof Med, Columbia P&S

Wang, John C MD/PhD (Nep) - **Spec Exp:** Hypertension; **Hospital:** NY-Presby/Weill Cornell Med Ctr, NY (page 104); **Address:** 505 E 70th St, rm 213, New York, NY 10021; **Phone:** 212-746-3097; **Board Cert:** Internal Medicine 1985; Nephrology 1986; **Med School:** Cornell Univ-Weill Med Coll 1979; **Resid:** Internal Medicine, Laguardia Hosp 1982; **Fellow:** Nephrology, New York Hosp 1984; **Fac Appt:** Assoc Clin Prof Med, Cornell Univ-Weill Med Coll

Weisstuch, Joseph M MD (Nep) - **Hospital:** NYU Langone Med Ctr (page 108), NYU Hosp For Joint Diseases (page 119); **Address:** 530 1st Ave, Ste 4B, New York, NY 10016-6402; **Phone:** 212-263-0705; **Board Cert:** Internal Medicine 1988; Nephrology 2002; **Med School:** NYU Sch Med 1985; **Resid:** Internal Medicine, NYU Med Ctr 1989; **Fellow:** Nephrology, Bellevue Hosp 1991; **Fac Appt:** Asst Clin Prof Med, NYU Sch Med

Williams, Gail S MD (Nep) - **Spec Exp:** Kidney Failure-Chronic; Transplant Medicine-Kidney; **Hospital:** NY-Presby/Columbia Univ Med Ctr, NY (page 104); **Address:** 161 Fort Washington Ave, Ste 351, New York, NY 10032; **Phone:** 212-305-5376; **Board Cert:** Internal Medicine 1972; Nephrology 1974; **Med School:** Columbia P&S 1968; **Resid:** Internal Medicine, Columbia Presby Hosp 1973; **Fellow:** Nephrology, Columbia Presby Hosp 1974; **Fac Appt:** Assoc Clin Prof Med, Columbia P&S

Winchester, James F MD (Nep) - **Spec Exp:** Dialysis Care; Polycystic Kidney Disease; **Hospital:** Beth Israel Med Ctr - Petrie Division (page 94); **Address:** 10 Union Square E, Ste 2F, New York, NY 10003; **Phone:** 212-420-4070; **Board Cert:** Internal Medicine 2007; **Med School:** Scotland, UK 1969; **Resid:** Internal Medicine, Royal Infirmiry 1972; **Fellow:** Nephrology, Royal Infirmiry 1974

Winston, Jonathan MD (Nep) - **Spec Exp:** Kidney Disease-Chronic; Kidney Failure; HIV Related Kidney Disease; Glomerulonephritis; **Hospital:** Mount Sinai Med Ctr (page 102); **Address:** 5 E 98th St Fl 11, New York, NY 10029-6501; **Phone:** 212-241-4060; **Board Cert:** Internal Medicine 1980; Nephrology 1984; **Med School:** Geo Wash Univ 1977; **Resid:** Internal Medicine, LI Jewish Med Ctr 1980; **Fellow:** Nephrology, Mt Sinai Hosp 1982; **Fac Appt:** Assoc Prof Med, Mount Sinai Sch Med

Neurological Surgery

Anderson, Richard CE MD (NS) - **Spec Exp:** Pediatric Neurosurgery; Spinal Disorders; Brain Tumors; Peripheral Nerve Surgery; **Hospital:** Morgan Stanley Children's Hosp of NY-Presby, NY (page 104), St. Joseph's Regl Med Ctr - Paterson; **Address:** Columbia Univ/Morgan Stanley Chldn's, The Neurological Institute, 710 W 168th St, rm 213, New York, NY 10032; **Phone:** 212-305-0219; **Board Cert:** Neurological Surgery 2007; Pediatric Neurological Surgery 2008; **Med School:** Johns Hopkins Univ 1997; **Resid:** Neurological Surgery, Columbia Neuro Inst 2004; **Fellow:** Pediatric Neurological Surgery, Univ Utah; **Fac Appt:** Prof NS, Columbia P&S

Bederson, Joshua B MD (NS) - **Spec Exp:** Brain & Spinal Cord Tumors; Aneurysm-Cerebral; Meningioma; Pituitary Tumors; **Hospital:** Mount Sinai Med Ctr (page 102); **Address:** Mount Sinai Med Ctr, 1 Gustave Levy Pl, Box 1136, New York, NY 10029; **Phone:** 212-241-2377; **Board Cert:** Neurological Surgery 1993; **Med School:** UCSF 1984; **Resid:** Neurological Surgery, UCSF Med Ctr 1990; **Fellow:** Neurovascular Surgery, Barrow Neur Inst 1990; Neurovascular Surgery, Univ Hosp Zurich 1990; **Fac Appt:** Prof NS, Mount Sinai Sch Med

Bilsky, Mark H MD (NS) - **Spec Exp:** Brain & Spinal Tumors; Skull Base Tumors; Spinal Reconstructive Surgery; Spinal Cord Tumors; **Hospital:** Meml Sloan-Kettering Cancer Ctr (page 116), NY-Presby/Weill Cornell Med Ctr, NY (page 104); **Address:** 1275 York Ave MSKCC Bldg Fl c705, New York, NY 10065; **Phone:** 212-639-8526; **Board Cert:** Neurological Surgery 2010; **Med School:** Emory Univ 1988; **Resid:** Neurological Surgery, NY Hosp-Cornell Med Ctr 1994; **Fellow:** Neuro-Oncology, Louisville Univ Med Ctr 1995; **Fac Appt:** Prof NS, Cornell Univ-Weill Med Coll

Boockvar, John MD (NS) - **Spec Exp:** Brain Tumors; Gliomas; Pituitary Tumors; Minimally Invasive Surgery; **Hospital:** NY-Presby/Weill Cornell Med Ctr, NY (page 104); **Address:** 525 E 68 St, Box 99, New York, NY 10065; **Phone:** 212-746-1996; **Board Cert:** Neurological Surgery 2007; **Med School:** SUNY Downstate 1997; **Resid:** Neurological Surgery, Hosp Univ Penn 2003; **Fellow:** Neuro-Oncology, Univ Penn Cancer Ctr 2004; **Fac Appt:** Asst Prof NS, Cornell Univ-Weill Med Coll

Bruce, Jeffrey MD (NS) - **Spec Exp:** Brain Tumors; Pituitary Tumors; Skull Base Surgery; Meningioma; **Hospital:** NY-Presby/Columbia Univ Med Ctr, NY (page 104); **Address:** NY Presby Hosp, Dept Neurosurgery, 710 W 168th St N1 Bldg Fl 4 - rm 434, New York, NY 10032; **Phone:** 212-305-7346; **Board Cert:** Neurological Surgery 1993; **Med School:** UMDNJ-RW Johnson Med Sch 1983; **Resid:** Neurological Surgery, Columbia-Presby Med Ctr 1990; **Fellow:** Neurological Surgery, Nat Inst Hlth 1985; **Fac Appt:** Prof NS, Columbia P&S

Chen, Chun Siang MD (NS) - **Spec Exp:** Skull Base Tumors; Skull Base Surgery; Microsurgery; Brain & Spinal Tumors; **Hospital:** Mount Sinai Med Ctr (page 102); **Address:** Mount Sinai Med Ctr, Annenberg Bldg, One Gustave L Levy Pl Fl 8 - rm 10, New York, NY 10029; **Phone:** 212-241-8480; **Med School:** Brazil 1978; **Resid:** Neurological Surgery, Santa Casa de Misericordia of Sao Paulo Med Sch 1983; Neurological Surgery, Mt Sinai Med Ctr 2005; **Fellow:** Skull Base Surgery, St Lukes Roosevelt Hosp 2006; **Fac Appt:** Asst Prof NS, Mount Sinai Sch Med

Di Giacinto, George V MD (NS) - **Spec Exp:** Spinal Surgery; Pain Management; **Hospital:** St. Luke's - Roosevelt Hosp Ctr - Roosevelt Div (page 94); **Address:** 425 W 59th St, Ste 4E, New York, NY 10019; **Phone:** 212-523-8500; **Board Cert:** Neurological Surgery 1981; **Med School:** Harvard Med Sch 1970; **Resid:** Neurological Surgery, Columbia-Presby Hosp 1978

Feldstein, Neil A MD (NS) - **Spec Exp:** Pediatric Neurosurgery; Chiari's Deformity; Brain Tumors-Pediatric; Spinal Cord Surgery-Pediatric; **Hospital:** Morgan Stanley Children's Hosp of NY-Presby, NY (page 104), NY-Presby/Columbia Univ Med Ctr, NY (page 104); **Address:** Neurological Inst, 710 W 168th St, Fl 2, rm 213, New York, NY 10032; **Phone:** 212-305-1396; **Board Cert:** Neurological Surgery 1995; Pediatric Neurological Surgery 2007; **Med School:** NYU Sch Med 1984; **Resid:** Neurological Surgery, Baylor Coll Med 1989; **Fellow:** Pediatric Neurological Surgery, NYU Med Ctr 1991; **Fac Appt:** Assoc Prof NS, Columbia P&S

Frempong-Boadu, Anthony K MD (NS) - **Spec Exp:** Minimally Invasive Spinal Surgery; Spinal Reconstructive Surgery; Spinal Cord Tumors; Spinal Reconstructive Surgery; **Hospital:** NYU Langone Med Ctr (page 108); **Address:** 530 1st Ave, Skirball Bldg - Fl 8 - Ste S, New York, NY 10016; **Phone:** 212-263-6514; **Board Cert:** Neurological Surgery 2004; **Med School:** Temple Univ 1992; **Resid:** Neurological Surgery, NYU Med Ctr 1998; **Fellow:** Spinal Surgery, NYU Med Ctr 1999; Minimally Invasive Surgery, Univ Florida/Shands Hosp 2000; **Fac Appt:** Assoc Prof NS, NYU Sch Med

Gamache Jr, Francis W MD (NS) - **Spec Exp:** Brain & Spinal Cord Tumors; Spinal Surgery-Neck; **Hospital:** NY-Presby/Weill Cornell Med Ctr, NY (page 104), Hosp For Special Surgery (page 115); **Address:** 523 E 72nd St Fl 8, New York, NY 10021-4099; **Phone:** 212-988-5200; **Board Cert:** Neurological Surgery 1982; **Med School:** Cornell Univ-Weill Med Coll 1971; **Resid:** Surgery, NY Hosp-Cornell Med Ctr 1975; Neurological Surgery, NY Hosp-Cornell Med Ctr 1979; **Fellow:** Trauma, MD Inst Emerg Med Serv 1979; Neurovascular Surgery, Univ West Ontario 1980; **Fac Appt:** Clin Prof NS, Cornell Univ-Weill Med Coll

Ghatan, Saadi MD (NS) - **Spec Exp:** Pediatric Neurosurgery; Epilepsy; Neuro-Endoscopy; **Hospital:** St. Luke's - Roosevelt Hosp Ctr - Roosevelt Div (page 94), Beth Israel Med Ctr - Petrie Division (page 94); **Address:** 1000 Tenth Ave, Ste 5G, New York, NY 10019; **Phone:** 212-636-3204; **Board Cert:** Neurological Surgery 2007; Pediatric Neurological Surgery 2007; **Med School:** Univ Wash 1993; **Resid:** Surgery, Univ Washington Med Ctr 1994; Neurological Surgery, Univ Washington Med Ctr 2001; **Fellow:** Pediatric Neurological Surgery, Chldn's Hosp 2002; Pediatric Neurological Surgery, Great Ormond Street Hosp 2003

Golfinos, John G MD (NS) - **Spec Exp:** Brain Tumors; Acoustic Neuroma; Stereotactic Radiosurgery; Skull Base Surgery; **Hospital:** NYU Langone Med Ctr (page 108), Bellevue Hosp Ctr; **Address:** 530 First Ave, Ste 8R, New York, NY 10016; **Phone:** 212-263-2950; **Board Cert:** Neurological Surgery 1998; **Med School:** Columbia P&S 1988; **Resid:** Neurological Surgery, Barrow Neuro Inst 1995; **Fac Appt:** Assoc Prof NS, NYU Sch Med

Goodman, Robert R MD/PhD (NS) - **Spec Exp:** Parkinson's Disease/Movement Disorders; Epilepsy; Trigeminal Neuralgia; Hydrocephalus-Adult; **Hospital:** St. Luke's - Roosevelt Hosp Ctr - Roosevelt Div (page 94); **Address:** 1000 Tenth Ave, Ste 5G-80, New York, NY 10019; **Phone:** 212-636-3666; **Board Cert:** Neurological Surgery 1993; **Med School:** Johns Hopkins Univ 1982; **Resid:** Neurological Surgery, Columbia-Presby Med Ctr 1989; **Fac Appt:** Assoc Prof NS, Columbia P&S

Gutin, Philip H MD (NS) - **Spec Exp:** Brain Tumors; Meningioma; Acoustic Neuroma; **Hospital:** Meml Sloan-Kettering Cancer Ctr (page 116), NY-Presby/Weill Cornell Med Ctr, NY (page 104); **Address:** 1275 York Ave, New York, NY 10065; **Phone:** 212-639-8556; **Board Cert:** Neurological Surgery 1981; **Med School:** Univ Pennsylvania 1971; **Resid:** Neurological Surgery, UCSF Med Ctr 1979; **Fellow:** Neurological Surgery, Natl Cancer Inst 1976; **Fac Appt:** Prof NS, Cornell Univ-Weill Med Coll

Hartl, Roger MD (NS) - **Spec Exp:** Spinal Surgery-Complex; Minimally Invasive Spinal Surgery; Spinal Disc Replacement; **Hospital:** NY-Presby/Weill Cornell Med Ctr, NY (page 104); **Address:** Cornell Neurosurgery, 525 E 68th St, Starr 651, New York, NY 10065; **Phone:** 212-746-2152; **Board Cert:** Neurological Surgery 2008; **Med School:** Germany 1993; **Resid:** Neurological Surgery, NY Presby-Cornell Med Ctr 2003; **Fellow:** Spinal Surgery, Barrow Neurological Inst

Jafar, Jafar J MD (NS) - **Spec Exp:** Aneurysm-Cerebral; Brain Tumors; Skull Base Tumors; Acoustic Neuroma; **Hospital:** NYU Langone Med Ctr (page 108), Lenox Hill Hosp (page 106); **Address:** 530 1st Ave, Ste 8R, New York, NY 10016-6402; **Phone:** 212-263-6312; **Board Cert:** Neurological Surgery 1984; **Med School:** Iran 1976; **Resid:** Neurological Surgery, Univ Chicago Hosps 1982; Neurological Surgery, Natl Hosp for Nervous Disease; **Fac Appt:** Prof NS, NYU Sch Med

Kaiser, Michael G MD (NS) - **Spec Exp:** Spinal Surgery-Complex; Minimally Invasive Spinal Surgery; Spinal Disc Replacement; **Hospital:** NY-Presby/Columbia Univ Med Ctr, NY (page 104); **Address:** Neurological Institute, Dept Neurological Surgery, 710 W 168th St, New York, NY 10032; **Phone:** 212-305-0378; **Board Cert:** Neurological Surgery 2004; **Med School:** Yale Univ 1994; **Resid:** Neurological Surgery, Columbia Neuro Inst 2000; **Fellow:** Spinal Surgery, Emory Univ 2001; **Fac Appt:** Asst Prof NS, Columbia P&S

Kaplitt, Michael G MD/PhD (NS) - **Spec Exp:** Parkinson's Disease/Movement Disorders; Deep Brain Stimulation; Trigeminal Neuralgia; Hydrocephalus; **Hospital:** NY-Presby/Weill Cornell Med Ctr, NY (page 104); **Address:** 525 E 68th St, Box 99, New York, NY 10065; **Phone:** 212-746-4966; **Board Cert:** Neurological Surgery 2005; **Med School:** Cornell Univ-Weill Med Coll 1995; **Resid:** Neurological Surgery, New York Hosp 2000; **Fellow:** Stereo Neurological Surgery, Toronto Western Hosp 2001; **Fac Appt:** Assoc Prof NS, Cornell Univ-Weill Med Coll

Lavyne, Michael H MD (NS) - **Spec Exp:** Spinal Surgery; Spinal Tumors; Spinal Disorders; **Hospital:** NY-Presby/Weill Cornell Med Ctr, NY (page 104), Hosp For Special Surgery (page 115); **Address:** 110 E 55th St Fl 9, MS 10022, New York, NY 10022; **Phone:** 212-486-9100; **Board Cert:** Neurological Surgery 1982; **Med School:** Cornell Univ-Weill Med Coll 1972; **Resid:** Neurological Surgery, Mass Genl Hosp 1979; **Fellow:** Neurology, Beth Israel Hosp 1974; **Fac Appt:** Clin Prof NS, Cornell Univ-Weill Med Coll

McCormick, Paul C MD (NS) - **Spec Exp:** Spinal Surgery; Spinal Tumors; **Hospital:** NY-Presby/Columbia Univ Med Ctr, NY (page 104); **Address:** 710 W 168th St, Ste 506, New York, NY 10032-2603; **Phone:** 212-305-7976; **Board Cert:** Neurological Surgery 1993; **Med School:** Columbia P&S 1982; **Resid:** Neurological Surgery, Columbia Presby Med Ctr 1989; **Fellow:** Neurological Surgery, Natl Inst Hlth 1984; Spinal Surgery, Med Coll Wisconsin 1990; **Fac Appt:** Prof NS, Columbia P&S

McKhann II, Guy MD (NS) - **Spec Exp:** Brain Tumors; Epilepsy; **Hospital:** NY-Presby/Columbia Univ Med Ctr, NY (page 104); **Address:** 710 W 168th St, Ste 411, New York, NY 10032; **Phone:** 212-305-0052; **Board Cert:** Neurological Surgery 2004; **Med School:** Yale Univ 1990; **Resid:** Neurological Surgery, Univ Wash Med Ctr 1998; Neurological Surgery, Atkinson Morley's Hosp 1995; **Fellow:** Epilepsy, Univ Wash 1999

Patel, Aman B MD (NS) - **Spec Exp:** Interventional Neuroradiology; Endovascular Neurosurgery; Aneurysm-Cerebral; Arteriovenous Malformations; **Hospital:** Mount Sinai Med Ctr (page 102); **Address:** One Gustave L Levy Place, Box 1136, New York, NY 10029; **Phone:** 212-241-3457; **Board Cert:** Neurological Surgery 2004; **Med School:** UCLA 1993; **Resid:** Neurological Surgery, UCLA Med Ctr 1999; **Fellow:** Interventional Neuroradiology, UCLA Med Ctr 2001; **Fac Appt:** Assoc Prof NS, Mount Sinai Sch Med

Perin, Noel I MD (NS) - **Spec Exp:** Spinal Surgery-Minimally Invasive; Spinal Tumors; **Hospital:** NYU Langone Med Ctr (page 108); **Address:** NYU Langone Med Ctr, Neurosurgery, 530 First Ave, Ste 8S, New York, NY 10016; **Phone:** 212-263-5732; **Board Cert:** Neurological Surgery 1995; **Med School:** Sri Lanka 1973; **Resid:** Neurological Surgery, NYU Med Ctr 1990; **Fellow:** Spinal Surgery, NYU Med Ctr 1991; **Fac Appt:** Asst Prof NS, NYU Sch Med

Post, Kalmon MD (NS) - **Spec Exp:** Pituitary Tumors; Acoustic Neuroma; Meningioma; **Hospital:** Mount Sinai Med Ctr (page 102); **Address:** 5 E 98th St, Fl 7, New York, NY 10029-6501; **Phone:** 212-241-0933; **Board Cert:** Neurological Surgery 1978; **Med School:** NYU Sch Med 1967; **Resid:** Surgery, Bellevue Hosp 1969; Neurological Surgery, Bellevue Hosp-NYU 1975; **Fac Appt:** Prof NS, Mount Sinai Sch Med

Quest, Donald O MD (NS) - **Spec Exp:** Spinal Surgery; Neurovascular Surgery; Carotid Artery Surgery; **Hospital:** NY-Presby/Columbia Univ Med Ctr, NY (page 104), Valley Hosp (page 689); **Address:** 710 W 168th St, Ste 440, New York, NY 10032; **Phone:** 212-305-5582; **Board Cert:** Neurological Surgery 1978; **Med School:** Columbia P&S 1970; **Resid:** Surgery, Mass Genl Hosp 1972; Neurological Surgery, Columbia-Presby Hosp 1976; **Fac Appt:** Clin Prof NS, Columbia P&S

Riina, Howard A MD (NS) - **Spec Exp:** Neuroradiology; Aneurysm-Cerebral; Cerebrovascular Malformations; Stroke; **Hospital:** NYU Langone Med Ctr (page 108); **Address:** NYU Langone Med Ctr, 530 First Ave, SK1, Ste 8R, New York, NY 10016; **Phone:** 212-263-5382; **Board Cert:** Neurological Surgery 2004; **Med School:** Temple Univ 1993; **Resid:** Neurological Surgery, Hosp Univ Penn 2000; **Fellow:** Interventional Neuroradiology, Beth Israel Med Ctr 1997; Skull Base Surgery, Barrow Neuro Inst 2001; **Fac Appt:** Prof NS, NYU Sch Med

Schwartz, Theodore H MD (NS) - **Spec Exp:** Brain Tumors; Pituitary Tumors; Epilepsy; Minimally Invasive Surgery; **Hospital:** NY-Presby/Weill Cornell Med Ctr, NY (page 104); **Address:** Department of Neurosurgery, Box 99, 525 E 68th St, Starr Pavilion, rm 651, New York, NY 10065; **Phone:** 212-746-5620; **Board Cert:** Neurological Surgery 2002; **Med School:** Harvard Med Sch 1993; **Resid:** Neurological Surgery, Columbia-Presby Med Ctr 1999; **Fellow:** Neurological Surgery, Yale-New Haven Med Ctr 2000; **Fac Appt:** Prof NS, Cornell Univ-Weill Med Coll

Sen, Chandranath MD (NS) - **Spec Exp:** Brain Tumors; Skull Base Tumors; Trigeminal Neuralgia; Hemifacial Spasm; **Hospital:** NYU Langone Med Ctr (page 108); **Address:** NYU Langone Med Ctr, Dept Neurosurgery, 550 First Ave, Ste HCC-3F, New York, NY 10016; **Phone:** 212-263-5333; **Board Cert:** Neurological Surgery 1989; **Med School:** India 1976; **Resid:** Surgery, Univ Wisconsin Hosps 1980; Neurological Surgery, Univ Wisconsin Hosps 1985; **Fellow:** Microsurgery, Univ Pittsburgh Med Ctr 1986

Sisti, Michael B MD (NS) - **Spec Exp:** Acoustic Neuroma; Brain Tumors; Stereotactic Radiosurgery; Meningioma; **Hospital:** NY-Presby/Columbia Univ Med Ctr, NY (page 104); **Address:** 710 W 168th St, New York, NY 10032-2603; **Phone:** 212-305-1728; **Board Cert:** Neurological Surgery 1991; **Med School:** Columbia P&S 1981; **Resid:** Neurological Surgery, Neuro Inst-Columbia-Presby Med Ctr 1988; **Fellow:** Neurological Surgery, Natl Inst Hlth 1983; **Fac Appt:** Assoc Prof NS, Columbia P&S

Snow, Robert MD (NS) - **Spec Exp:** Spinal Surgery; Spinal Cord Tumors; Minimally Invasive Surgery; **Hospital:** NY-Presby/Weill Cornell Med Ctr, NY (page 104); **Address:** 55 E 72nd St, New York, NY 10021-4099; **Phone:** 212-717-0256; **Board Cert:** Neurological Surgery 1989; **Med School:** Stanford Univ 1981; **Resid:** Neurological Surgery, New York Hosp 1986; **Fac Appt:** Prof NS, Cornell Univ-Weill Med Coll

Solomon, Robert A MD (NS) - **Spec Exp:** Aneurysm-Cerebral; Arteriovenous Malformations; **Hospital:** NY-Presby/Columbia Univ Med Ctr, NY (page 104); **Address:** 710 W 168th St, Ste 439, New York, NY 10032; **Phone:** 212-305-4118; **Board Cert:** Neurological Surgery 1988; **Med School:** Johns Hopkins Univ 1980; **Resid:** Neurological Surgery, Neuro Inst-Columbia 1986; **Fac Appt:** Prof NS, Columbia P&S

Souweidane, Mark M MD (NS) - **Spec Exp:** Pediatric Neurosurgery; Minimally Invasive Surgery; Endoscopic Surgery; Brain Tumors-Pediatric; **Hospital:** NY-Presby/Weill Cornell Med Ctr, NY (page 104), Meml Sloan-Kettering Cancer Ctr (page 116); **Address:** 525 E 68th St, Box 99, New York, NY 10065-4870; **Phone:** 212-746-2363; **Board Cert:** Neurological Surgery 2010; Pediatric Neurological Surgery 2000; **Med School:** Wayne State Univ 1988; **Resid:** Neurological Surgery, NYU Med Ctr 1994; **Fellow:** Pediatric Neurological Surgery, Hosp Sick Chldn 1995; **Fac Appt:** Prof NS, Cornell Univ-Weill Med Coll

Stieg, Philip E MD/PhD (NS) - **Spec Exp:** Cerebrovascular Surgery; Acoustic Neuroma; Skull Base Surgery; Brain Tumors; **Hospital:** NY-Presby/Weill Cornell Med Ctr, NY (page 104); **Address:** 525 E 68th St, STARR 651, New York, NY 10021-9800; **Phone:** 212-746-4684; **Board Cert:** Neurological Surgery 1992; **Med School:** Med Coll Wisc 1983; **Resid:** Neurological Surgery, Parkland Meml Hosp/Dallas Chldns Hosp 1989; **Fellow:** Neurological Biology, Karolinska Inst 1988; **Fac Appt:** Prof NS, Cornell Univ-Weill Med Coll

Sundaresan, Narayan MD (NS) - **Spec Exp:** Spinal Surgery; Brain Tumors; Neuro-Oncology; Spinal Disorders-Degenerative; **Hospital:** Mount Sinai Med Ctr (page 102), Lincoln Med & Mental Hlth Ctr; **Address:** Central Park Neurosurgery, 1148 5th Ave, New York, NY 10128; **Phone:** 212-876-7575; **Board Cert:** Neurological Surgery 1980; **Med School:** India 1969; **Resid:** Neurological Surgery, Northwestern Meml Hosp 1975; **Fellow:** Neuro-Oncology, Meml Sloan Kettering Cancer Ctr 1977; **Fac Appt:** Prof NS, Mount Sinai Sch Med

Tabar, Viviane MD (NS) - **Spec Exp:** Brain Tumors; **Hospital:** Meml Sloan-Kettering Cancer Ctr (page 116); **Address:** 1275 York Ave, rm C711, New York, NY 10065; **Phone:** 212-639-3006; **Board Cert:** Neurological Surgery 2006; **Med School:** Amer Univ Beirut 1989; **Resid:** Neurological Surgery, Univ Mass Med Ctr 1998; **Fellow:** NIH/Natl Inst Neuro Dis & StrokeMeml Sloan Kettering Cancer Ctr

Weiner, Howard L MD (NS) - **Spec Exp:** Pediatric Neurosurgery; Epilepsy; Tuberous Sclerosis; **Hospital:** NYU Langone Med Ctr (page 108); **Address:** NYU Med Ctr, Div Pediatric Neurosurgery, 317 E 34th St, Ste 1002, New York, NY 10016; **Phone:** 212-263-6419; **Board Cert:** Neurological Surgery 2012; **Med School:** Cornell Univ 1989; **Resid:** Neurological Surgery, NYU Med Ctr 1996; **Fellow:** Pediatric Neurological Surgery, NYU Med Ctr 1997; **Fac Appt:** Prof NS, NYU Sch Med

Wisoff, Jeffrey H MD (NS) - **Spec Exp:** Pediatric Neurosurgery; Brain Tumors-Pediatric; Hydrocephalus; Chiari's Deformity; **Hospital:** NYU Langone Med Ctr (page 108), Maimonides Med Ctr (page 98); **Address:** 317 E 34th St, Ste 1002, New York, NY 10016-4974; **Phone:** 212-263-6419; **Board Cert:** Neurological Surgery 1990; Pediatric Neurological Surgery 2008; **Med School:** Geo Wash Univ 1978; **Resid:** Neurological Surgery, NYU/Bellevue Hosp 1984; **Fellow:** Pediatric Neurological Surgery, NYU Med Ctr 1985; **Fac Appt:** Assoc Prof NS, NYU Sch Med

Neurology

Apatoff, Brian R MD/PhD (N) - **Spec Exp:** Multiple Sclerosis; Neuro-Immunology; **Hospital:** NY-Presby/Weill Cornell Med Ctr, NY (page 104); **Address:** Multiple Sclerosis Institute, 401 E 55th St, New York, NY 10022; **Phone:** 212-593-6262; **Board Cert:** Neurology 1991; **Med School:** Univ Chicago-Pritzker Sch Med 1984; **Resid:** Neurology, Columbia Presby Med Ctr 1990; **Fellow:** Multiple Sclerosis, Neuro Inst-Columbia Univ 1992; **Fac Appt:** Assoc Prof N, Cornell Univ-Weill Med Coll

Belok, Lennart C MD (N) - **Spec Exp:** Carpal Tunnel Syndrome; **Hospital:** Beth Israel Med Ctr - Petrie Division (page 94); **Address:** 410 E 20th St, New York, NY 10009-8113; **Phone:** 212-254-9716; **Board Cert:** Internal Medicine 1977; Neurology 1983; **Med School:** NY Med Coll 1973; **Resid:** Internal Medicine, Beth Israel Med Ctr 1976; Neurology, NYU Med Ctr 1979

Brannagan III, Thomas H MD (N) - **Spec Exp:** Peripheral Neuropathy; Diabetic Neuropathy; **Hospital:** NY-Presby/Columbia Univ Med Ctr, NY (page 104); **Address:** Ciolumbia Univ Dept Neurology, 710 W 168th St, New York, NY 10032; **Phone:** 212-305-0405; **Board Cert:** Neurology 2005; Clinical Neurophysiology 2009; **Med School:** Univ VA Sch Med 1990; **Resid:** Neurology, Columbia-Presby Med Ctr 1994; **Fellow:** Neuromuscular Disease, Columbia-Presby Med Ctr; Neurological Immunology, Columbia-Presby Med Ctr; **Fac Appt:** Assoc Clin Prof N, Columbia P&S

Bressman, Susan MD (N) - **Spec Exp:** Parkinson's Disease; Movement Disorders; Dystonia; **Hospital:** Beth Israel Med Ctr - Petrie Division (page 94); **Address:** 10 Union Square East, Ste 5J, New York, NY 10003-3314; **Phone:** 212-844-8379; **Board Cert:** Neurology 1983; **Med School:** Columbia P&S 1977; **Resid:** Neurology, Columbia-Presby Med Ctr 1981; **Fellow:** Movement Disorders, Columbia-Presby Med Ctr 1983; **Fac Appt:** Prof N, Albert Einstein Coll Med

Britton, Carolyn B MD (N) - **Spec Exp:** Neurologic Complications-HIV/Infections; Lyme Disease; Multiple Sclerosis; **Hospital:** NY-Presby/Columbia Univ Med Ctr, NY (page 104); **Address:** 710 W 168th St, Ste 232, New York, NY 10032-2603; **Phone:** 212-305-5220; **Board Cert:** Internal Medicine 1979; Neurology 1982; **Med School:** NYU Sch Med 1975; **Resid:** Internal Medicine, Harlem Hosp 1977; Neurology, Columbia-Presby Hosp 1980; **Fellow:** Neurology, Columbia-Presby Hosp 1983; **Fac Appt:** Assoc Prof N, Columbia P&S

Bronster, David J MD (N) - **Spec Exp:** Headache; Dizziness; Seizure Disorders; **Hospital:** Mount Sinai Med Ctr (page 102); **Address:** 3 E 83rd St, New York, NY 10028-0459; **Phone:** 212-772-0008; **Board Cert:** Neurology 1984; **Med School:** Mount Sinai Sch Med 1979; **Resid:** Neurology, Mount Sinai Hosp 1983; **Fac Appt:** Assoc Clin Prof N, Mount Sinai Sch Med

Cafferty, Maureen S MD (N) - **Hospital:** St. Luke's - Roosevelt Hosp Ctr - Roosevelt Div (page 94); **Address:** St Lukes-Roosevelt Hosp-Neuro Clinic, 440 W 114th St, New York, NY 10025-1737; **Phone:** 212-523-4480; **Board Cert:** Internal Medicine 1982; Neurology 1987; **Med School:** Columbia P&S 1979; **Resid:** Internal Medicine, St Luke's-Roosevelt Hosp Ctr 1982; Neurology, Columbia-Presby Hosp 1985; **Fac Appt:** Asst Prof N, Columbia P&S

Charney, Jonathan Z MD (N) - **Spec Exp:** Headache; Stroke; **Hospital:** Mount Sinai Med Ctr (page 102); **Address:** 1111 Park Ave, Ste 1H, New York, NY 10128-1234; **Phone:** 212-831-2886; **Board Cert:** Neurology 1977; **Med School:** NY Med Coll 1969; **Resid:** Neurology, Methodist Hosp-Baylor 1971; Neurology, Columbia-Presby Med Ctr 1973; **Fac Appt:** Asst Prof N, Mount Sinai Sch Med

Coll, Raymond MD (N) - **Spec Exp:** Multiple Sclerosis; Headache; Stroke; **Hospital:** NY-Presby/Weill Cornell Med Ctr, NY (page 104); **Address:** 1365 York Ave, New York, NY 10021-4035; **Phone:** 212-249-0840; **Board Cert:** Neurology 1974; **Med School:** South Africa 1961; **Resid:** Neurology, NY Hosp 1971; **Fac Appt:** Assoc Clin Prof N, Cornell Univ-Weill Med Coll

Daras, Michael MD (N) - **Spec Exp:** Neuromuscular Disorders; **Hospital:** NY-Presby/Columbia Univ Med Ctr, NY (page 104); **Address:** 710 W 168 St, rm 246, New York, NY 10032; **Phone:** 212-305-6876; **Board Cert:** Neurology 1980; **Med School:** Greece 1969; **Resid:** Psychiatry, Elmhurst City Hosp 1976; Neurology, Metropolitan Hosp 1979; **Fellow:** Clinical Neurophysiology, Albert Einstein 1980; **Fac Appt:** Prof N, Columbia P&S

DeAngelis, Lisa M MD (N) - **Spec Exp:** Neuro-Oncology; Brain Tumors; **Hospital:** Meml Sloan-Kettering Cancer Ctr (page 116); **Address:** 1275 York Avenue, New York, NY 10065; **Phone:** 212-639-7123; **Board Cert:** Neurology 1986; **Med School:** Columbia P&S 1980; **Resid:** Neurology, Neuro Inst-Presby Hosp 1984; **Fellow:** Neuro-Oncology, Neuro Inst-Presby Hosp 1985; Neuro-Oncology, Meml Sloan-Kettering Cancer Ctr 1986; **Fac Appt:** Prof N, Cornell Univ-Weill Med Coll

Devinsky, Orrin MD (N) - **Spec Exp:** Epilepsy; Tuberous Sclerosis; Behavioral Neurology; **Hospital:** NYU Langone Med Ctr (page 108), Saint Barnabas Med Ctr; **Address:** 223 E 34th St Fl Ground, New York, NY 10016-4972; **Phone:** 646-558-0803; **Board Cert:** Neurology 1987; Clinical Neurophysiology 1990; **Med School:** Harvard Med Sch 1982; **Resid:** Neurology, NY Hosp-Cornell Med Ctr 1986; **Fellow:** Epilepsy, Natl Inst Health 1988; **Fac Appt:** Prof N, NYU Sch Med

Engel, Murray MD (N) - **Hospital:** NY-Presby/Weill Cornell Med Ctr, NY (page 104), Stamford Hosp (page 893); **Address:** 525 E 68th St, Box 91, New York, NY 10021; **Phone:** 212-746-3278; **Board Cert:** Pediatrics 1979; Neurology 1980; Clinical Neurophysiology 2005; **Med School:** Univ Chicago-Pritzker Sch Med 1972; **Resid:** Neurology, Yale-New Haven Hosp 1976; Neurology, Columbia Presby Med Ctr 1977; **Fac Appt:** Clin Prof Ped, Cornell Univ-Weill Med Coll

Fahn, Stanley MD (N) - **Spec Exp:** Movement Disorders; Parkinson's Disease; **Hospital:** NY-Presby/Columbia Univ Med Ctr, NY (page 104); **Address:** Neurological Institute, 710 W 168th St Fl 3 - rm 350, New York, NY 10032; **Phone:** 212-305-5277; **Board Cert:** Neurology 1968; **Med School:** UCSF 1958; **Resid:** Neurology, Neuro Inst-Columbia 1962; **Fellow:** Neurological Chemistry, Natl Inst Hlth 1968; **Fac Appt:** Prof N, Columbia P&S

Feinberg, Todd E MD (N) - **Spec Exp:** Alzheimer's Disease; Dementia; **Hospital:** Beth Israel Med Ctr - Petrie Division (page 94); **Address:** Beth Israel Med Ctr, Bernstein Pavilion, 10 Nathan D Perlman Pl Fl 10, New York, NY 10003; **Phone:** 212-420-4111; **Board Cert:** Psychiatry 1984; Neurology 1987; **Med School:** Mount Sinai Sch Med 1978; **Resid:** Psychiatry, Mt Sinai Med Ctr 1982; Neurology, Mt Sinai Med Ctr 1984; **Fellow:** Behavioral Neurology, Univ Florida 1986; **Fac Appt:** Clin Prof N, Albert Einstein Coll Med

Fink, Matthew E MD (N) - **Spec Exp:** Cerebrovascular Disease; Stroke; **Hospital:** NY-Presby/Weill Cornell Med Ctr, NY (page 104); **Address:** NY Cornell Med Ctr Dept Neurology, 525 E 68th St, F Bldg - Fl 6 - Ste 610, New York, NY 10065; **Phone:** 212-746-4564; **Board Cert:** Internal Medicine 1980; Neurology 1983; Vascular Neurology 2005; Neurocritical Care 2010; **Med School:** Univ Pittsburgh 1976; **Resid:** Internal Medicine, Boston Med Ctr 1980; Neurology, Columbia-Presby Hosp 1982; **Fac Appt:** Prof N, Cornell Univ

Foo, Sun-Hoo MD (N) - **Spec Exp:** Stroke; Headache; Parkinson's Disease; Dementia; **Hospital:** NYU Langone Med Ctr (page 108), NY Downtown Hosp; **Address:** 650 1st Ave, Fl 4 Floor, New York, NY 10016-3240; **Phone:** 212-213-0270; **Board Cert:** Internal Medicine 1976; Neurology 1980; **Med School:** Taiwan 1972; **Resid:** Internal Medicine, St Vincent's Hosp 1976; Neurology, NYU Med Ctr 1979; **Fac Appt:** Prof N, NYU Sch Med

Forster, George MD (N) - **Spec Exp:** Multiple Sclerosis; Parkinson's Disease; Brain Tumors; Pain-Back; **Hospital:** Mount Sinai Med Ctr (page 102); **Address:** 5 E 98 St Fl 7, New York, NY 10029; **Phone:** 212-241-7076; **Board Cert:** Neurology 1980; **Med School:** Italy 1971; **Resid:** Internal Medicine, Maimonides Med Ctr 1974; Neurology, Mt Sinai Hosp 1977; **Fac Appt:** Asst Prof N, Mount Sinai Sch Med

French, Jacqueline MD (N) - **Spec Exp:** Epilepsy/Seizure Disorders; **Hospital:** NYU Langone Med Ctr (page 108); **Address:** 223 E 34th St, New York, NY 10016; **Phone:** 646-558-0802; **Board Cert:** Neurology 1987; **Med School:** Brown Univ 1982; **Resid:** Neurology, Mount Sinai Hosp 1986; **Fellow:** Epilepsy, Mount Sinai Hosp 1988; Epilepsy, Yale-New Haven Hosp 1989; **Fac Appt:** Prof N, NYU Sch Med

Gendelman, Seymour MD (N) - **Spec Exp:** Parkinson's Disease; Dementia; Headache; **Hospital:** Mount Sinai Med Ctr (page 102); **Address:** 5 E 98th St, Fl 7, Box 1139, New York, NY 10029-6501; **Phone:** 212-241-8172; **Board Cert:** Neurology 1971; **Med School:** Geo Wash Univ 1964; **Resid:** Neurology, Mt Sinai Hosp 1968; **Fac Appt:** Clin Prof N, Mount Sinai Sch Med

Green, Mark W MD (N) - **Spec Exp:** Headache; Pain-Facial; **Hospital:** Mount Sinai Med Ctr (page 102); **Address:** Mount Sinai Sch Med, 5 E 98th St Fl 7, New York, NY 10029; **Phone:** 212-241-7076; **Board Cert:** Neurology 1979; Headache Medicine 1976; **Med School:** Albert Einstein Coll Med 1974; **Resid:** Neurology, Albert Einstein Affil Hosp 1978; **Fac Appt:** Prof N, Mount Sinai Sch Med

Gruber, Michael L MD (N) - **Spec Exp:** Neuro-Oncology; Headache; Pain-Back; **Hospital:** NYU Langone Med Ctr (page 108), Overlook Med Ctr (page 92); **Address:** NYU Clinical Cancer Ctr, 160 E 34th St Fl 7, New York, NY 10016; **Phone:** 212-731-5577; **Board Cert:** Neurology 1975; **Med School:** Temple Univ 1966; **Resid:** Pediatrics, Columbia-Presby Med Ctr 1968; Neurology, Columbia-Presby Med Ctr 1973; **Fellow:** Neuro-Oncology, Mass Genl Hosp 1990; **Fac Appt:** Prof N, NYU Sch Med

Herbert, Joseph MD (N) - **Spec Exp:** Multiple Sclerosis; Neuromuscular Disorders; Neuro-Rehabilitation; **Hospital:** NYU Hosp For Joint Diseases (page 119); **Address:** 301 E 17th St, Ste 544, New York, NY 10003; **Phone:** 212-598-6305; **Board Cert:** Neurology 1987; **Med School:** Israel 1974; **Resid:** Neurology, Longwood/Harvard U Sch Med 1983; Neuropathology, Children's Hosp 1984; **Fellow:** Clinical Genetics, Columbia Presby Med Ctr 1986; **Fac Appt:** Assoc Prof N, NYU Sch Med

Herbstein, Diego MD (N) - **Spec Exp:** Parkinson's Disease; Cerebrovascular Disease; **Hospital:** Lenox Hill Hosp (page 106), NY Hosp Queens (page 206); **Address:** 162 E 78th St, New York, NY 10075; **Phone:** 212-794-2281; **Board Cert:** Neurology 1976; **Med School:** Argentina 1968; **Resid:** Internal Medicine, Fernandez 1970; Neurology, Albert Einstein 1973; **Fellow:** Neurology, Jacobi Med Ctr 1974; **Fac Appt:** Asst Clin Prof N, Cornell Univ-Weill Med Coll

Heublum, Michael MD (N) - **Spec Exp:** Neuromuscular Disorders; Electrodiagnosis; **Hospital:** Mount Sinai Med Ctr (page 102), Beth Israel Med Ctr - Petrie Division (page 94); **Address:** 247 3rd Ave, Ste 203, New York, NY 10010; **Phone:** 212-505-9800; **Board Cert:** Internal Medicine 1989; Neurology 1993; **Med School:** SUNY Downstate 1986; **Resid:** Internal Medicine, Staten Island Univ Hosp 1989; Neurology, Mt Sinai Med Ctr 1992; **Fellow:** Neuromuscular Disease, Univ Michigan Med Ctr 1993

Hiesiger, Emile M MD (N) - **Spec Exp:** Pain-Spine; Pain-Cancer, Spine; Pain-Back; **Hospital:** NYU Langone Med Ctr (page 108), VA NY Harbor Hlthcare Sys-Manhattan Campus; **Address:** 345 37th St, Ste 320, New York, NY 10016; **Phone:** 212-263-6123; **Board Cert:** Neurology 1983; **Med School:** NY Med Coll 1978; **Resid:** Neurology, NYU Med Ctr 1982; **Fellow:** Neurology, Meml Sloan-Kettering Cancer Ctr 1984; **Fac Appt:** Assoc Clin Prof N, NYU Sch Med

Horvath, Susanna E MD (N) - **Spec Exp:** Stroke; **Hospital:** NY-Presby/Columbia Univ Med Ctr, NY (page 104), NY-Presby Hosp/The Allen Hosp (page 104); **Address:** 710 W 168th St Neurologic Bldg Fl 2, Neurological Inst-Stroke Div, MS 10032, New York, NY 10032; **Phone:** 212-305-1710; **Board Cert:** Neurology 2003; Vascular Neurology 2005; **Med School:** Hungary 1990; **Resid:** Internal Medicine, Kaleida/Millard Fillmore Hosp 1994; Neurology, SUNY-Buffalo Med Ctr 1998; **Fac Appt:** Asst Clin Prof N, Columbia P&S

Kolodny, Edwin H MD (N) - **Spec Exp:** Pediatric Neurology; Inherited Disorders of Nervous System; Gaucher Disease; Fabry's Disease; **Hospital:** NYU Langone Med Ctr (page 108), Bellevue Hosp Ctr; **Address:** 403 E 34 St Fl 2, New York, NY 10016-6402; **Phone:** 212-263-8344; **Board Cert:** Neurology 1971; Clinical Genetics 1984; Clinical Biochemical Genetics 1987; **Med School:** NYU Sch Med 1962; **Resid:** Internal Medicine, Bellevue Hosp 1964; Neurology, Mass Genl Hosp 1967; **Fellow:** Neurological Pathology, Mass Genl Hosp 1966; Neurology, Nat Inst Neurol Dis & Stroke 1970; **Fac Appt:** Prof N, NYU Sch Med

Koppel, Barbara MD (N) - **Spec Exp:** Epilepsy; Headache; Stroke; AIDS/HIV; **Hospital:** Metropolitan Hosp Ctr - NY; **Address:** Metropolitan Hosp, 1901 First Ave, rm 7C5, New York, NY 10029; **Phone:** 212-423-6144; **Board Cert:** Neurology 1983; **Med School:** Columbia P&S 1978; **Resid:** Internal Medicine, Montefiore Med Ctr 1979; Neurology, Columbia-Presby Hosp 1982; **Fac Appt:** Prof N, NY Med Coll

Kuzniecky, Ruben MD (N) - **Spec Exp:** Epilepsy/Seizure Disorders; MRI; Developmental Disorders; Brain Malformations; **Hospital:** NYU Langone Med Ctr (page 108); **Address:** 223 E 34th St Fl Ground, New York, NY 10016; **Phone:** 646-558-0806; **Board Cert:** Neurology 1990; **Med School:** Argentina 1980; **Resid:** Neurology, McGill Univ 1986; **Fellow:** Epilepsy, McGill Univ 1988; **Fac Appt:** Prof N, NYU Sch Med

Labar, Douglas R MD/PhD (N) - **Spec Exp:** Epilepsy/Seizure Disorders; **Hospital:** NY-Presby/Weill Cornell Med Ctr, NY (page 104); **Address:** Weill Cornell Epilepsy Center, 525 E 68th St, rm K-619, New York, NY 10065; **Phone:** 212-746-2359; **Board Cert:** Neurology 1987; **Med School:** Med Coll PA 1982; **Resid:** Neurology, Columbia Presby Med Ctr 1986; **Fellow:** Epilepsy, Columbia Presby Med Ctr 1988; **Fac Appt:** Prof N, Cornell Univ-Weill Med Coll

Lange, Dale J MD (N) - **Spec Exp:** Neuromuscular Disorders; Amyotrophic Lateral Sclerosis (ALS); Electromyography; **Hospital:** Hosp For Special Surgery (page 115), NY-Presby/Weill Cornell Med Ctr, NY (page 104); **Address:** Hosp For Special Surgery, 535 E 70th St, New York, NY 10021; **Phone:** 646-797-8917; **Board Cert:** Neurology 1985; Neuromuscular Medicine 2008; **Med School:** NY Med Coll 1978; **Resid:** Neurology, New England Med Ctr 1982; **Fellow:** Neuromuscular Medicine, Columbia-Presby Med Ctr 1983; **Fac Appt:** Prof N, Cornell Univ-Weill Med Coll

Latov, Norman MD/PhD (N) - **Spec Exp:** Peripheral Neuropathy; Neuro-Immunology; **Hospital:** NY-Presby/Weill Cornell Med Ctr, NY (page 104); **Address:** 1305 York Ave Fl 2 - Ste 217, New York, NY 10021; **Phone:** 646-962-3320; **Board Cert:** Neurology 1989; **Med School:** Univ Pennsylvania 1975; **Resid:** Internal Medicine, Boston City Hosp 1976; Neurology, Columbia-Presby Med Ctr 1979; **Fellow:** Immunology, Columbia-Presby Med Ctr 1981; **Fac Appt:** Prof N, Cornell Univ-Weill Med Coll

Levine, David N MD (N) - **Spec Exp:** Dementia; Stroke; Spinal Cord Disorders; Syringomyelia & Spinal Cord Diseases; **Hospital:** NYU Langone Med Ctr (page 108); **Address:** 400 E 34th St, Ste RIRM-311, New York, NY 10016-4901; **Phone:** 212-263-7744; **Board Cert:** Neurology 1976; **Med School:** Harvard Med Sch 1968; **Resid:** Neurology, Mass Genl Hosp 1974; **Fellow:** Neurology, Mass Genl Hosp 1976; **Fac Appt:** Prof N, NYU Sch Med

Lin, Michael Tai-Ju MD (N) - **Spec Exp:** Memory Disorders; Neurodegenerative Disorders; **Hospital:** NY-Presby/Weill Cornell Med Ctr, NY (page 104); **Address:** 428 E 72nd St Ground Bldg, New York, NY 10021; **Phone:** 212-746-2441; **Board Cert:** Neurology 2007; **Med School:** UCSF 1992; **Resid:** Neurology, Mass General Hosp 1996; **Fellow:** Memory Disorders, Mass General Hosp 1997; **Fac Appt:** Asst Prof N, Cornell Univ-Weill Med Coll

Louis, Elan D MD (N) - **Spec Exp:** Tremor and Dystonia; Huntington's Disease; Parkinson's Disease/Movement Disorders; **Hospital:** NY-Presby/Columbia Univ Med Ctr, NY (page 104); **Address:** Neurological Inst of New York, 710 W 168th St, Ste 350, New York, NY 10032; **Phone:** 212-305-3665; **Board Cert:** Neurology 2004; **Med School:** Yale Univ 1989; **Resid:** Neurology, NY-Presby/Columbia Univ Med Ctr 1993; **Fellow:** Movement Disorders, Neurol Inst of New York 1995; Epidemiology, Neurol Inst of New York 1995; **Fac Appt:** Prof N, Columbia P&S

Lublin, Fred D MD (N) - **Spec Exp:** Multiple Sclerosis; **Hospital:** Mount Sinai Med Ctr (page 102); **Address:** Dickinson Ctr for Multiple Sclerosis, 5 E 98th St, Box 1138, New York, NY 10029-6574; **Phone:** 212-241-6854; **Board Cert:** Neurology 1977; **Med School:** Jefferson Med Coll 1972; **Resid:** Neurology, NY Hosp/Cornell Med Ctr 1976; **Fac Appt:** Prof N, Mount Sinai Sch Med

Luciano, Daniel J MD (N) - **Spec Exp:** Epilepsy/Seizure Disorders; **Hospital:** NYU Langone Med Ctr (page 108); **Address:** NYU Comprehensive Epilepsy Center, 223 E 34th St, New York, NY 10016; **Phone:** 646-558-0805; **Board Cert:** Neurology 1992; Clinical Neurophysiology 2004; **Med School:** UMDNJ-NJ Med Sch, Newark 1984; **Resid:** Neurology, Mt Sinai Med Ctr 1988; **Fellow:** Epilepsy, Mt Sinai Med Ctr 1990; **Fac Appt:** Asst Prof N, NYU Sch Med

Marder, Karen S MD (N) - **Spec Exp:** Huntington's Disease; Alzheimer's Disease; Dementia; **Hospital:** NY-Presby/Columbia Univ Med Ctr, NY (page 104); **Address:** Neurological Institute, 710 W 168th St, Ste 104, New York, NY 10032-2603; **Phone:** 212-305-6939; **Board Cert:** Neurology 1989; **Med School:** Cornell Univ-Weill Med Coll 1983; **Resid:** Neurology, Columbia Presby Med Ctr 1987; **Fellow:** Behavioral Neurology, Columbia Presby Med Ctr 1989; **Fac Appt:** Assoc Prof N, Columbia P&S

Mauskop, Alexander MD (N) - **Spec Exp:** Headache; Migraine; Botox Therapy; **Hospital:** Beth Israel Med Ctr - Petrie Division (page 94); **Address:** New York Headache Ctr, 30 E 76th St, New York, NY 10021; **Phone:** 212-794-3550; **Board Cert:** Neurology 1987; Headache Medicine 2006; **Med School:** Ukraine 1979; **Resid:** Internal Medicine, Brookdale Hosp 1981; Neurology, Univ Hosp 1984; **Fellow:** Pain Management, Meml Sloan Kettering Cancer Ctr 1986; **Fac Appt:** Assoc Clin Prof N, SUNY Downstate

Mayer, Stephan A MD (N) - **Spec Exp:** Neurologic Critical Care; Stroke; Coma; **Hospital:** NY-Presby/Columbia Univ Med Ctr, NY (page 104); **Address:** 177 Fort Washington Ave, Ste A-300, New York, NY 10032-2603; **Phone:** 212-305-7236; **Board Cert:** Neurology 1993; **Med School:** Cornell Univ-Weill Med Coll 1988; **Resid:** Neurology, Columbia-Presby Med Ctr 1992; **Fellow:** Critical Care Neurology, Columbia-Presby Med Ctr 1993; **Fac Appt:** Assoc Prof N, Columbia P&S

Mayeux, Richard MD (N) - **Spec Exp:** Alzheimer's Disease; Dementia; **Hospital:** NY-Presby/Columbia Univ Med Ctr, NY (page 104); **Address:** 630 W 168th St, PH 19, New York, NY 10032; **Phone:** 212-305-6939; **Board Cert:** Neurology 1978; **Med School:** Univ Okla Coll Med 1972; **Resid:** Internal Medicine, Boston City Hosp 1974; Neurology, Columbia Presby Med Ctr 1977; **Fellow:** Neurology, Boston Univ 1978; **Fac Appt:** Prof N, Columbia P&S

Miller, Aaron E MD (N) - **Spec Exp:** Multiple Sclerosis; Autoimmune Disease; Optic Nerve Disorders; **Hospital:** Mount Sinai Med Ctr (page 102), Maimonides Med Ctr (page 98); **Address:** 5 E 98th St, Fl 1st, Box 1138, New York, NY 10029; **Phone:** 212-241-6854; **Board Cert:** Internal Medicine 1972; Neurology 1977; **Med School:** NYU Sch Med 1968; **Resid:** Internal Medicine, Jacobi Med Ctr 1970; Neurology, Montefiore Med Ctr 1975; **Fellow:** Neurovirology, Johns Hopkins Hosp 1977; **Fac Appt:** Prof N, Mount Sinai Sch Med

Mitsumoto, Hiroshi MD (N) - **Spec Exp:** Amyotrophic Lateral Sclerosis (ALS); Neuromuscular Disorders; Clinical Trials; **Hospital:** NY-Presby/Columbia Univ Med Ctr, NY (page 104); **Address:** Neurological Institute, 710 W 168th St Fl 9, New York, NY 10032; **Phone:** 212-305-1319; **Board Cert:** Neurology 1978; **Med School:** Japan 1968; **Resid:** Internal Medicine, Toho Univ Hosps 1972; Neurology, Univ Hosps 1976; **Fellow:** Neurological Pathology, Cleveland Clinic 1978; Neuromuscular Medicine, New England Med Ctr 1981; **Fac Appt:** Prof N, Columbia P&S

Mohr, JP MD (N) - **Spec Exp:** Stroke; Arteriovenous Malformations; Aphasia; MoyaMoya Disease; **Hospital:** NY-Presby/Columbia Univ Med Ctr, NY (page 104); **Address:** 710 W 168th St, Fl 6, rm 616, New York, NY 10032-2603; **Phone:** 212-305-8033; **Board Cert:** Neurology 1971; Vascular Neurology 2005; **Med School:** Univ VA Sch Med 1963; **Resid:** Neurology, Columbia Presby Med Ctr 1966; Neurology, Mass Genl Hosp 1968; **Fellow:** Neurology, Mass Genl Hosp 1969; **Fac Appt:** Prof N, Columbia P&S

Motiwala, Rajeev S MD (N) - **Hospital:** Mount Sinai Med Ctr (page 102); **Address:** Mount Sinai Neurology, 5 E 98 St Fl 7, New York, NY 10029; **Phone:** 212-241-7076; **Board Cert:** Neurology 1990; **Med School:** India 1979; **Resid:** Neurology, UMDMNJ Med Ctr 1988

Nealon, Nancy MD (N) - **Spec Exp:** Multiple Sclerosis; **Hospital:** NY-Presby/Weill Cornell Med Ctr, NY (page 104); **Address:** 1305 York Ave, rm Y217, New York, NY 10021; **Phone:** 646-962-9800; **Board Cert:** Internal Medicine 1978; Neurology 1984; **Med School:** Penn State Coll Med 1975; **Resid:** Neurology, NY Hosp 1981; **Fellow:** Neuromuscular Disease, Columbia-Presby Med Ctr 1982; Neuromuscular Medicine, Meml Sloan Kettering Cancer Ctr 1983; **Fac Appt:** Asst Prof N, Cornell Univ-Weill Med Coll

Neophytides, Andreas MD (N) - **Spec Exp:** Spinal Disorders; Stroke; **Hospital:** NYU Langone Med Ctr (page 108); **Address:** 650 1st Ave, New York, NY 10016; **Phone:** 212-213-9581; **Board Cert:** Neurology 1978; **Med School:** Greece 1970; **Resid:** Surgery, LIJ Med Ctr 1973; Neurology, NYU Med Ctr 1976; **Fellow:** Neurological Pharmacology, Natl Inst Hlth 1978; **Fac Appt:** Clin Prof N, NYU Sch Med

Newman, Lawrence C MD (N) - **Spec Exp:** Headache; Pain-Facial; **Hospital:** St. Luke's - Roosevelt Hosp Ctr - Roosevelt Div (page 94); **Address:** St Luke's-Roosevelt Hosp-Headache Inst, 425 W 59th St Fl 4 - Ste A, New York, NY 10019; **Phone:** 212-523-5869; **Board Cert:** Neurology 2005; Headache Medicine 2006; **Med School:** Mexico 1983; **Resid:** Internal Medicine, Elmhurst Hosp 1986; Neurology, Montefiore Med Ctr 1989; **Fellow:** Headache, Montefiore Med Ctr 1990; **Fac Appt:** Prof N, Albert Einstein Coll Med

Olanow, C Warren MD (N) - **Spec Exp:** Parkinson's Disease; Movement Disorders; **Hospital:** Mount Sinai Med Ctr (page 102); **Address:** 5 E 98 St, New York, NY 10029; **Phone:** 212-241-8435; **Med School:** Univ Toronto 1965; **Resid:** Neurology, Toronto Genl Hosp 1968; Neurology, Columbia Presby Hosp 1970; **Fellow:** Neurological Anatomy, Columbia Presby Hosp 1971; **Fac Appt:** Prof N, Mount Sinai Sch Med

Olarte, Marcelo R MD (N) - **Spec Exp:** Myasthenia Gravis; Electrodiagnosis; Headache; Neuromuscular Disorders; **Hospital:** NY-Presby/Columbia Univ Med Ctr, NY (page 104); **Address:** 903 Park Ave, New York, NY 10075; **Phone:** 212-988-3100; **Board Cert:** Neurology 1976; **Med School:** Argentina 1970; **Resid:** Neurology, St Vincent's Hosp 1974; **Fellow:** Neuromuscular Medicine, Columbia-Presby Hosp 1975; **Fac Appt:** Clin Prof N, Columbia P&S

Pacia, Steven MD (N) - **Spec Exp:** Epilepsy/Seizure Disorders; **Hospital:** NYU Langone Med Ctr (page 108), Lenox Hill Hosp (page 106); **Address:** NYU Comprehensive Epilepsy Center, 223 E 34th St, New York, NY 10016; **Phone:** 646-558-0867; **Board Cert:** Neurology 1992; Clinical Neurophysiology 2007; **Med School:** Yale Univ 1989; **Resid:** Neurology, Yale-New Haven Hosp 1992; **Fellow:** Epilepsy, Yale-New Haven Hosp 1992; **Fac Appt:** Assoc Prof N, NYU Sch Med

Pedley, Timothy A MD (N) - **Spec Exp:** Epilepsy/Seizure Disorders; **Hospital:** NY-Presby/Columbia Univ Med Ctr, NY (page 104); **Address:** The Neurological Inst of New York, 710 W 168th St, New York, NY 10032; **Phone:** 212-305-6489; **Board Cert:** Neurology 1975; **Med School:** Yale Univ 1969; **Resid:** Neurology, Stanford Univ Hosp 1973; **Fellow:** Clinical Neurophysiology, Stanford Univ Hosp 1974; Epilepsy, Stanford Univ Hosp 1975; **Fac Appt:** Prof N, Columbia P&S

Petito, Frank A MD (N) - **Spec Exp:** Multiple Sclerosis; Headache; Lyme Disease; **Hospital:** NY-Presby/Weill Cornell Med Ctr, NY (page 104); **Address:** 525 E 68th St, Ste 607, New York, NY 10065; **Phone:** 212-746-2309; **Board Cert:** Neurology 1974; **Med School:** Columbia P&S 1967; **Resid:** Neurology, New York Hosp 1971; **Fac Appt:** Prof N, Cornell Univ-Weill Med Coll

Posner, Jerome B MD (N) - **Spec Exp:** Neuro-Oncology; Brain Tumors; Paraneoplastic Syndromes; **Hospital:** Meml Sloan-Kettering Cancer Ctr (page 116); **Address:** 1275 York Ave, rm C731, New York, NY 10065; **Phone:** 212-639-7047; **Board Cert:** Neurology 1962; **Med School:** Univ Wash 1955; **Resid:** Neurology, Univ WA Affil Hosp 1959; **Fellow:** Biochemistry, Univ WA Affil Hosp 1963; **Fac Appt:** Prof N, Cornell Univ-Weill Med Coll

Rapoport, Samuel MD/PhD (N) - **Spec Exp:** Peripheral Neuropathy; Pain-Back & Neck; Electromyography; **Hospital:** NY-Presby/Weill Cornell Med Ctr, NY (page 104), Lenox Hill Hosp (page 106); **Address:** 354 E 76th St, New York, NY 10021-2505; **Phone:** 212-570-0642; **Board Cert:** Neurology 1986; **Med School:** Cornell Univ-Weill Med Coll 1976; **Resid:** Neurology, New York Hosp-Cornell 1982; **Fac Appt:** Assoc Prof N, Cornell Univ-Weill Med Coll

Relkin, Norman R MD/PhD (N) - **Spec Exp:** Alzheimer's Disease; Dementia; Memory Disorders; **Hospital:** NY-Presby/Weill Cornell Med Ctr, NY (page 104); **Address:** Weill Cornell Memory Disorders Program, 428 E 72nd St, Ste 500, New York, NY 10021; **Phone:** 212-746-2441; **Board Cert:** Neurology 1992; **Med School:** Albert Einstein Coll Med 1987; **Resid:** Neurology, New York Hosp 1991; **Fellow:** Behavioral Neurology, New York Hosp-Cornell 1992; **Fac Appt:** Asst Prof N, Cornell Univ-Weill Med Coll

Roberts, J Kirk MD (N) - **Spec Exp:** Dizziness; Stroke; **Hospital:** NY-Presby/Columbia Univ Med Ctr, NY (page 104); **Address:** Columbia University Medical Center, New York-Presbyterian Hospital, 710 W 168th St, Ste 246, New York, NY 10032; **Phone:** 212-305-6876; **Board Cert:** Neurology 2006; Vascular Neurology 2008; **Med School:** Cornell Univ-Weill Med Coll 1989; **Resid:** Internal Medicine, Columbia-Presby Med Ctr 1992; Neurology, Columbia-Presby Med Ctr 1995; **Fellow:** Stroke, Columbia-Presby Med Ctr 1997; **Fac Appt:** Assoc Clin Prof N, Columbia P&S

Sadiq, Saud MD (N) - **Spec Exp:** Multiple Sclerosis; **Hospital:** St. Luke's - Roosevelt Hosp Ctr - Roosevelt Div (page 94); **Address:** International MS Management Practice, 521 W 57th St Fl 4, New York, NY 10019; **Phone:** 212-265-8070; **Board Cert:** Neurology 2009; **Med School:** Africa 1979; **Resid:** Neurology, Univ TX Med Branch 1988; **Fellow:** Neurological Immunology, Ny Presby-Columbia Med Ctr 1991; **Fac Appt:** , Albert Einstein Coll Med

Safdieh, Joseph E MD (N) - **Spec Exp:** Headache; Migraine; Stroke; Dizziness; **Hospital:** NY-Presby/Weill Cornell Med Ctr, NY (page 104); **Address:** 520 E 70th St, Starr Pavilion, rm 607, New York, NY 10021; **Phone:** 212-746-3113; **Board Cert:** Neurology 2007; **Med School:** NYU Sch Med 2002; **Resid:** Neurology, NY Hosp-Cornell Med Ctr 2006; **Fac Appt:** Assoc Prof N, Cornell Univ-Weill Med Coll

Saunders-Pullman, Rachel MD (N) - **Spec Exp:** Movement Disorders; Parkinson's Disease; **Hospital:** Beth Israel Med Ctr - Petrie Division (page 94); **Address:** 10 Union Square E, Ste 5H, New York, NY 10003; **Phone:** 212-844-8719; **Board Cert:** Neurology 2010; **Med School:** Columbia P&S 1992; **Resid:** Neurology, Ny Presby-Columbia Med Ctr 1996

Sheinart, Kara F MD (N) - **Spec Exp:** Cerebrovascular Disease; Stroke; **Hospital:** Mount Sinai Med Ctr (page 102); **Address:** 5 E 98th St Fl 7th, New York, NY 10029; **Phone:** 212-241-7076; **Board Cert:** Neurology 2005; **Med School:** SUNY Downstate 1989; **Resid:** Internal Medicine, Mt Sinai Med Ctr 1990; Neurology, Mt Sinai Med Ctr 1993; **Fellow:** Cerebrovascular Disease, Mt Sinai Med Ctr 1995; **Fac Appt:** Asst Clin Prof N, Mount Sinai Sch Med

Shulman, Melanie MD (N) - **Spec Exp:** Memory Disorders; Epilepsy; **Hospital:** NYU Langone Med Ctr (page 108); **Address:** Barlow Center, 145 E 32 St Fl 2, New York, NY 10016; **Phone:** 212-263-3210; **Board Cert:** Neurology 2007; **Med School:** Univ Pennsylvania 1991; **Resid:** Neurology, Brigham & Women's Hosp 1995; **Fac Appt:** Asst Clin Prof N, NYU Sch Med

Simpson, David M MD (N) - **Spec Exp:** Infections-CNS; AIDS-Neurologic Complications; Peripheral Neuropathy; Neuromuscular Disorders; **Hospital:** Mount Sinai Med Ctr (page 102); **Address:** Mt Sinai Med Ctr, Dept Neurology, 1 Gustave L Levy Pl, Box 1052, Annenberg, 2nd Flr, New York, NY 10029; **Phone:** 212-241-8748; **Board Cert:** Neurology 1984; Clinical Neurophysiology 2005; Neuromuscular Medicine 2008; **Med School:** SUNY Buffalo 1979; **Resid:** Neurology, NY Hosp-Cornell Med Ctr 1983; **Fellow:** Clinical Neurophysiology, Mass Genl Hosp 1984; **Fac Appt:** Prof N, Mount Sinai Sch Med

Sivak, Mark A MD (N) - **Spec Exp:** Myasthenia Gravis; Amyotrophic Lateral Sclerosis (ALS); Neuromuscular Disorders; **Hospital:** Mount Sinai Med Ctr (page 102); **Address:** 5 E 98th St Fl 7, Box 1139, New York, NY 10029-6501; **Phone:** 212-241-8747; **Board Cert:** Neurology 1978; Neuromuscular Medicine 2008; **Med School:** Univ Louisville Sch Med 1971; **Resid:** Neurology, Mt Sinai Med Ctr 1975; **Fellow:** Electromyography, Mt Sinai Med Ctr 1976; Clinical Neurophysiology, Uppsala Univ 1986; **Fac Appt:** Asst Prof N, Mount Sinai Sch Med

Smallberg, Gerald MD (N) - **Spec Exp:** Spinal Disorders; **Hospital:** Lenox Hill Hosp (page 106), Hosp For Special Surgery (page 115); **Address:** 1010 5th Ave, New York, NY 10028-0130; **Phone:** 212-535-5348; **Board Cert:** Neurology 1977; **Med School:** Yale Univ 1969; **Resid:** Internal Medicine, Univ Mich Med Ctr 1971; Neurology, Hosp Univ Penn 1975; **Fellow:** Neurology, Columbia-Presby Med Ctr 1976

Snyder, David H MD (N) - **Spec Exp:** Multiple Sclerosis; **Hospital:** NY Hosp Queens (page 206), Lenox Hill Hosp (page 106); **Address:** 162 E 78th St, New York, NY 10075; **Phone:** 212-794-2281; **Board Cert:** Neurology 1975; **Med School:** Univ MD Sch Med 1969; **Resid:** Neurology, Univ Maryland Hosp 1973; **Fellow:** Neuropathology, Albert Einstein Med Ctr 1975; **Fac Appt:** Asst Clin Prof N, Cornell Univ-Weill Med Coll

Stuebgen, Joerg-Patrick MD (N) - **Spec Exp:** Amyotrophic Lateral Sclerosis (ALS); Peripheral Neuropathy; Neuromuscular Disorders; **Hospital:** NY-Presby/Weill Cornell Med Ctr, NY (page 104), Hosp For Special Surgery (page 115); **Address:** Dept Neur Starr 607, 520 E 70th St, New York, NY 10021; **Phone:** 212-746-2334; **Board Cert:** Neurology 2006; Clinical Neurophysiology 2009; **Med School:** South Africa 1983; **Resid:** Neurology, Univ Pretoria Med Ctr 1989; Neurology, New York Hosp 1995; **Fellow:** Clinical Neurophysiology, Menl Sloan Kettering Cancer Ctr 1995; **Fac Appt:** Prof N, Cornell Univ-Weill Med Coll

Tuchman, Alan MD (N) - **Spec Exp:** Epilepsy; Multiple Sclerosis; **Hospital:** Montefiore Med Ctr-Wakefield Campus, NY (page 100); **Address:** 975 Park Ave, New York, NY 10028; **Phone:** 212-772-9305; **Board Cert:** Neurology 1979; **Med School:** Univ Cincinnati 1972; **Resid:** Neurology, Mt Sinai Med Ctr 1976; **Fellow:** Multiple Sclerosis, Albert Einstein Med Ctr 1979; **Fac Appt:** Clin Prof N, NY Med Coll

Tuhrim, Stanley MD (N) - **Spec Exp:** Stroke; Cerebrovascular Disease; Fibromuscular Dysplasia; **Hospital:** Mount Sinai Med Ctr (page 102); **Address:** 5 E 98th St, Box 1139, New York, NY 10029-6501; **Phone:** 212-241-7076; **Board Cert:** Neurology 1984; Vascular Neurology 2005; **Med School:** Mount Sinai Sch Med 1979; **Resid:** Neurology, Mt Sinai Med Ctr 1983; **Fellow:** Cerebrovascular Disease, Univ MD Sch Med 1984; **Fac Appt:** Prof N, Mount Sinai Sch Med

Waters, Cheryl H MD (N) - **Spec Exp:** Parkinson's Disease; Movement Disorders; **Hospital:** NY-Presby/Columbia Univ Med Ctr, NY (page 104); **Address:** 710 W 168th St Fl 3, New York, NY 10032; **Phone:** 212-305-3665; **Board Cert:** Neurology 1986; **Med School:** Univ Toronto 1980; **Resid:** Internal Medicine, Univ Toronto Med Ctr 1982; Neurology, Univ Toronto Med Ctr 1985; **Fellow:** Clinical Pharmacology, Univ Toronto Med Ctr 1987; **Fac Appt:** Prof N, Columbia P&S

Weinberg, Harold J MD (N) - **Spec Exp:** Headache; Spinal Disorders; Neuromuscular Disorders; Memory Disorders; **Hospital:** NYU Langone Med Ctr (page 108); **Address:** 650 1st Ave, Fl 4, New York, NY 10016-3240; **Phone:** 212-213-9339; **Board Cert:** Neurology 1983; Electrodiagnostic Medicine 1989; **Med School:** Albert Einstein Coll Med 1978; **Resid:** Neurology, Columbia-Presby Med Ctr 1982; **Fellow:** Neuromuscular Medicine, Columbia-Presby Med Ctr 1982; **Fac Appt:** Clin Prof N, NYU Sch Med

Weinberger, Jesse MD (N) - **Spec Exp:** Stroke; **Hospital:** Mount Sinai Med Ctr (page 102); **Address:** 5 E 98th St Fl 7, New York, NY 10029-6501; **Phone:** 212-241-4529; **Board Cert:** Neurology 1976; Vascular Neurology 2005; **Med School:** Johns Hopkins Univ 1971; **Resid:** Neurology, Mt Sinai Med Ctr 1975; **Fellow:** Cerebrovascular Disease, Univ Penn 1978; **Fac Appt:** Prof N, Mount Sinai Sch Med

Neuroradiology

Berenstein, Alejandro MD (NRad) - **Spec Exp:** Interventional Neuroradiology; Aneurysm-Cerebral; Endovascular Surgery; Vascular Malformations; **Hospital:** St. Luke's - Roosevelt Hosp Ctr - Roosevelt Div (page 94); **Address:** Center for Endovascular Surgery, 1000 10th Ave, 10th Fl, Ste 10G - INN, New York, NY 10019; **Phone:** 212-636-3400; **Board Cert:** Diagnostic Radiology 1976; **Med School:** Mexico 1970; **Resid:** Diagnostic Radiology, Mt Sinai Med Ctr 1976; **Fellow:** Neuroradiology, NYU Med Ctr 1978; **Fac Appt:** Prof Rad, Albert Einstein Coll Med

Drayer, Burton P MD (NRad) - **Spec Exp:** Parkinson's Disease/Aging Brain; Alzheimer's Disease; Vascular Neurology; MRI & CT of Brain & Spine; **Hospital:** Mount Sinai Med Ctr (page 102); **Address:** 1 Gustave Levy Pl, Box 1234, New York, NY 10029; **Phone:** 212-241-6403; **Board Cert:** Neurology 1976; Diagnostic Radiology 1978; Neuroradiology 2006; **Med School:** Ros Franklin Univ/Chicago Med Sch 1971; **Resid:** Neurology, Univ Vt Med Ctr 1975; Diagnostic Radiology, Univ Pitt Hlth Ctr 1978; **Fellow:** Neuroradiology, Univ Pitt Hlth Ctr 1978; **Fac Appt:** Prof Rad, Mount Sinai Sch Med

Jahre, Caren MD (NRad) - **Spec Exp:** Cardiac CT Angiography; **Address:** Lenox Hill Radiology & Med Assocs, 61 E 77th St, New York, NY 10075; **Phone:** 212-772-3111; **Board Cert:** Diagnostic Radiology 1988; Neuroradiology 2005; **Med School:** Cornell Univ-Weill Med Coll 1982; **Resid:** Pathology, New York Hosp 1984; Diagnostic Radiology, New York Hosp 1988; **Fellow:** Neuroradiology, New York Hosp 1990; **Fac Appt:** Asst Prof Rad, NYU Sch Med

Kelly, Anna B MD (NRad) - **Hospital:** NY-Presby/Columbia Univ Med Ctr, NY (page 104); **Address:** Columbia Presby Eastside Radiology, 16 E 60th St, New York, NY 10022; **Phone:** 212-326-8518; **Board Cert:** Diagnostic Radiology 1986; Neuroradiology 2005; **Med School:** Univ Cincinnati 1982; **Resid:** Diagnostic Radiology, NY Hosp-Cornell Med Ctr 1986; **Fellow:** Neurological Radiology, NY Hosp-Cornell Med Ctr 1989

Khandji, Alexander G MD (NRad) - **Spec Exp:** Pituitary Disorders; Spine Imaging & Intervention; MRI; Headache; **Hospital:** NY-Presby/Columbia Univ Med Ctr, NY (page 104); **Address:** 177 Ft Washington Ave, Ste 4-156, New York, NY 10032-3173; **Phone:** 212-305-7669; **Board Cert:** Diagnostic Radiology 1985; Neuroradiology 2006; **Med School:** SUNY Downstate 1980; **Resid:** Surgery, MS Hershey Med Ctr 1982; Diagnostic Radiology, Columbia-Presby Med Ctr 1985; **Fellow:** Neuroradiology, Columbia-Presby Med Ctr 1987; **Fac Appt:** Prof Rad, Columbia P&S

Knopp, Edmond A MD (NRad) - **Spec Exp:** Neuroradiology; MRI; Endocrine Radiology; CT Scan; **Hospital:** NYU Langone Med Ctr (page 108); **Address:** 560 First Ave, Rusk Bldg - Fl 2nd - Ste 232A, New York, NY 10016; **Phone:** 212-263-8723; **Board Cert:** Diagnostic Radiology 1992; Neuroradiology 2005; **Med School:** SUNY Downstate 1986; **Resid:** Surgery, Maimonides Med Ctr 1988; Diagnostic Radiology, St Lukes/Roosevelt Hosp 1992; **Fellow:** Neuroradiology, NYU Med Ctr 1994; **Fac Appt:** Assoc Prof Rad, NYU Sch Med

Lis, Eric MD (NRad) - **Spec Exp:** Spinal Cord Tumors; Brain Tumors; **Hospital:** Meml Sloan-Kettering Cancer Ctr (page 116); **Address:** 1275 York Ave, Ste MRI1158, New York, NY 10065; **Phone:** 212-639-8330; **Board Cert:** Diagnostic Radiology 1995; Neuroradiology 2008; **Med School:** UMDNJ-NJ Med Sch, Newark 1990; **Resid:** Internal Medicine, Mountainside Hosp 1991; Diagnostic Radiology, UMDNJ-RW Johnson Med Sch 1995; **Fellow:** Neuroradiology, NY-Presby-Weill Cornell Med Ctr 1997

Meyers, Philip M MD (NRad) - **Spec Exp:** Interventional Neuroradiology; Endovascular Surgery; Aneurysm-Cerebral; Arteriovenous Malformations; **Hospital:** NY-Presby/Columbia Univ Med Ctr, NY (page 104), Valley Hosp (page 689); **Address:** 710 W 168 St, Ste 428, New York, NY 10032; **Phone:** 212-305-6384; **Board Cert:** Diagnostic Radiology 1997; Neuroradiology 2002; **Med School:** Case West Res Univ 1989; **Resid:** Neurological Surgery, Univ Cincinnati Med Ctr 1990; Diagnostic Radiology, Univ Cincinnati Med Ctr 1997; **Fellow:** Neurological Radiology, Univ Cincinnati Med Ctr 1998; Neurovascular Surgery, UCSF Med Ctr 2001; **Fac Appt:** Assoc Prof Rad, Columbia P&S

Nuclear Medicine

Carrasquillo, Jorge A MD (NuM) - **Spec Exp:** Radioimmunotherapy of Cancer; PET Imaging; Nuclear Endocrinology; **Hospital:** Meml Sloan-Kettering Cancer Ctr (page 116); **Address:** 1275 York Ave, Nuclear Medicine Svc, Box 77, New York, NY 10065; **Phone:** 212-639-2459; **Board Cert:** Internal Medicine 1977; Nuclear Medicine 1982; **Med School:** Univ Puerto Rico 1974; **Resid:** Internal Medicine, Univ Dist Hosp 1977; Nuclear Medicine, Univ Wash Hosp 1982; **Fac Appt:** Prof NuM, SUNY Upstate Med Univ

Fawwaz, Rashid MD/PhD (NuM) - **Spec Exp:** PET Imaging; Brain Imaging; Radioimmunotherapy of Cancer; **Hospital:** NY-Presby/Columbia Univ Med Ctr, NY (page 104); **Address:** Columbia Presby Med Ctr, Dept Rad, 177 Ft Washington Ave, MHB 3-202A, New York, NY 10032-3713; **Phone:** 212-305-7138; **Board Cert:** Nuclear Medicine 1975; **Med School:** Amer Univ Beirut 1961; **Resid:** Diagnostic Radiology, American Univ Hosp 1963; **Fellow:** Nuclear Medicine, Donner Lab-UC Berkeley 1966; **Fac Appt:** Clin Prof, Columbia P&S

Goldfarb, C Richard MD (NuM) - **Spec Exp:** Thyroid Cancer; Thyroid Disorders; **Hospital:** Beth Israel Med Ctr - Petrie Division (page 94); **Address:** Beth Israel Med Ctr, Dept Radiology, 1st Ave at 16th St, New York, NY 10003; **Phone:** 212-252-6070; **Board Cert:** Nuclear Medicine 1974; Diagnostic Radiology 1975; **Med School:** NY Med Coll 1970; **Resid:** Diagnostic Radiology, St Lukes Hosp 1974; **Fellow:** Nuclear Medicine, St Lukes Hosp 1975; **Fac Appt:** Assoc Prof NuM, Albert Einstein Coll Med

Goldsmith, Stanley J MD (NuM) - **Spec Exp:** Thyroid Cancer; PET Imaging; **Hospital:** NY-Presby/Weill Cornell Med Ctr, NY (page 104); **Address:** 525 E 68th St Starr Bldg - rm 2-21, New York, NY 10021-9800; **Phone:** 212-746-4588; **Board Cert:** Internal Medicine 1969; Nuclear Medicine 1972; Endocrinology 1972; **Med School:** SUNY Downstate 1962; **Resid:** Internal Medicine, Kings Co Hosp 1967; **Fellow:** Endocrinology, Diabetes & Metabolism, Mt Sinai Hosp 1968; Nuclear Medicine, Bronx VA Hosp 1969; **Fac Appt:** Prof Rad, Cornell Univ-Weill Med Coll

Pandit-Taskar, Neeta MD (NuM) - **Spec Exp:** Radioimmunotherapy of Cancer; Thyroid Cancer; PET Imaging; **Hospital:** Meml Sloan-Kettering Cancer Ctr (page 116); **Address:** 1275 York Ave, Molecular Imaging and Therapy Service, Dept of Radiology, Memorial Sloan Kettering Cancer Center, New York, NY 10065; **Phone:** 212-639-3046; **Board Cert:** Nuclear Medicine 2008; **Med School:** India 1990; **Resid:** Nuclear Medicine, Mt Sinai Med Ctr 1995; **Fellow:** Nuclear Medicine, Meml Sloan Kettering Cancer Ctr 2001

Sanger, Joseph J MD (NuM) - **Spec Exp:** Nuclear Cardiology; Nuclear Oncology; **Hospital:** NYU Langone Med Ctr (page 108), Bellevue Hosp Ctr; **Address:** Old Bellevue C & D Bldg, 1st Floor, rm 7, 462 First Ave, New York, NY 10016-6402; **Phone:** 212-731-5001; **Board Cert:** Nuclear Medicine 1981; **Med School:** NYU Sch Med 1977; **Resid:** Diagnostic Radiology, NYU Med Ctr 1979; **Fellow:** Nuclear Medicine, NYU Med Ctr 1981; **Fac Appt:** Assoc Prof Rad, NYU Sch Med

Santos, Elmer B MD/PhD (NuM) - **Spec Exp:** Thyroid Cancer; PET Imaging; **Hospital:** Meml Sloan-Kettering Cancer Ctr (page 116); **Address:** 1275 York Ave, New York, NY 10065; **Phone:** 212-639-7373; **Board Cert:** Nuclear Medicine 2007; **Med School:** Philippines 1991; **Resid:** Internal Medicine, Hosp St Raphael 1995; Nuclear Medicine, Meml Sloan Kettering Cancer Ctr 1997; **Fellow:** Cancer Immunology, Cambridge Univ Sch Med 2001; Radiotracer Imaging, Meml Sloan Kettering Cancer Inst 2002; **Fac Appt:** Asst Prof Rad, Cornell Univ-Weill Med Coll

Scharf, Stephen MD (NuM) - **Spec Exp:** Thyroid & Parathyroid Imaging; Kidney Imaging; Bone Imaging; CT Scan; **Hospital:** Lenox Hill Hosp (page 106); **Address:** Lenox Hill Hospital, Dept Nuclear Medicine, 100 E 77th St Fl 3, New York, NY 10075; **Phone:** 212-434-2630; **Board Cert:** Internal Medicine 1977; Nuclear Medicine 1979; **Med School:** Albert Einstein Coll Med 1974; **Resid:** Internal Medicine, Bronx Municipal Hosp 1976; Nuclear Medicine, Montefiore Med Ctr 1978; **Fellow:** Nephrology, Montefiore Med Ctr 1979; **Fac Appt:** Asst Clin Prof NuM, Albert Einstein Coll Med

Obstetrics & Gynecology

Ascher-Walsh, Charles J MD (ObG) - **Spec Exp:** Uro-Gynecology; Gynecologic Surgery; Pelvic Surgery; Robotic Surgery; **Hospital:** Mount Sinai Med Ctr (page 102); **Address:** 5 E 98th St Fl 2, New York, NY 10029; **Phone:** 212-241-7952; **Board Cert:** Obstetrics & Gynecology 2009; **Med School:** SUNY Hlth Sci Ctr 1995; **Resid:** Obstetrics & Gynecology, NY Presby Hosp-Columbia 1999; **Fellow:** Uro-Gynecology, NY Presby Hosp-Columbia 2000; **Fac Appt:** Asst Clin Prof ObG, Mount Sinai Sch Med

Bacall, Charles J MD (ObG) - **Hospital:** Mount Sinai Med Ctr (page 102); **Address:** 1150 5th Ave, Ste 1B, New York, NY 10128-2920; **Phone:** 212-996-9100; **Board Cert:** Obstetrics & Gynecology 1981; **Med School:** NY Med Coll 1975; **Resid:** Obstetrics & Gynecology, Mt Sinai Hosp 1979; **Fac Appt:** Asst Clin Prof ObG, Mount Sinai Sch Med

Berman, Alvin MD (ObG) - **Spec Exp:** Menopause Problems; Osteoporosis; Sexual Dysfunction; Women's Health over age 40; **Hospital:** Mount Sinai Med Ctr (page 102); **Address:** 111B E 88th St, New York, NY 10128; **Phone:** 212-722-5757; **Board Cert:** Obstetrics & Gynecology 1978; **Med School:** South Africa 1969; **Resid:** Obstetrics & Gynecology, Mount Sinai Hosp 1976; **Fellow:** Neonatal-Perinatal Medicine, Mount Sinai Hosp 1977; **Fac Appt:** Asst Clin Prof ObG, Mount Sinai Sch Med

Blanco, Jody MD (ObG) - **Spec Exp:** Uro-Gynecology; Uterine Fibroids; Colposcopy; **Hospital:** NY-Presby/Columbia Univ Med Ctr, NY (page 104); **Address:** 161 Ft Washington Ave Fl 4, New York, NY 10032-3713; **Phone:** 212-305-1107; **Board Cert:** Obstetrics & Gynecology 2011; **Med School:** SUNY Hlth Sci Ctr 1981; **Resid:** Obstetrics & Gynecology, Columbia-Presby Med Ctr 1985; **Fellow:** Uro-Gynecology, UC Irvine 1986; **Fac Appt:** Asst Clin Prof ObG, Columbia P&S

Brightman, Rebecca MD (ObG) - **Spec Exp:** Preconception Planning; Menopause Problems; Pregnancy-High Risk; **Hospital:** Mount Sinai Med Ctr (page 102); **Address:** 134 E 93rd St, New York, NY 10128; **Phone:** 212-348-7800; **Board Cert:** Obstetrics & Gynecology 2011; **Med School:** Mount Sinai Sch Med 1986; **Resid:** Obstetrics & Gynecology, Mt Sinai Med Ctr 1990

Brodman, Michael L MD (ObG) - **Spec Exp:** Incontinence; Laparoscopic Surgery; Pelvic Organ Prolapse Repair; Uro-Gynecology; **Hospital:** Mount Sinai Med Ctr (page 102); **Address:** Dept Gynecology/Urogynecology, 5 E 98th St Fl 2, New York, NY 10029; **Phone:** 212-241-7952; **Board Cert:** Obstetrics & Gynecology 2010; **Med School:** Mount Sinai Sch Med 1982; **Resid:** Obstetrics & Gynecology, Mt Sinai Hosp 1986; **Fellow:** Pelvic Surgery, Mt Sinai Hosp 1987; **Fac Appt:** Assoc Prof ObG, Mount Sinai Sch Med

Brustman, Lois MD (ObG) - **Spec Exp:** Prematurity/Low Birth Weight Infants; Diabetes in Pregnancy; Preconception Planning; Maternal & Fetal Medicine; **Hospital:** St. Luke's - Roosevelt Hosp Ctr - Roosevelt Div (page 94); **Address:** 1000 Tenth Ave, Ste 11A-61, New York, NY 10019-1147; **Phone:** 212-523-7579; **Board Cert:** Obstetrics & Gynecology 2011; Maternal & Fetal Medicine 2011; **Med School:** NY Med Coll 1979; **Resid:** Obstetrics & Gynecology, Montefiore Med Ctr 1984; **Fellow:** Maternal & Fetal Medicine, Montefiore Med Ctr 1988; **Fac Appt:** Assoc Prof ObG, NY Med Coll

Buterman, Irving MD (ObG) - **Spec Exp:** Women's Health; Pregnancy-High Risk; **Hospital:** Lenox Hill Hosp (page 106), Beth Israel Med Ctr - Petrie Division (page 94); **Address:** 950 Park Ave, New York, NY 10028-0320; **Phone:** 212-472-8200; **Board Cert:** Obstetrics & Gynecology 1983; **Med School:** Netherlands 1971; **Resid:** Obstetrics & Gynecology, Lenox Hill Hosp 1976; **Fellow:** Gynecologic Oncology, Lenox Hill Hosp 1977; **Fac Appt:** Asst Clin Prof ObG, NY Med Coll

Chin, Jean MD (ObG) *PCP* - **Spec Exp:** Menopause Problems; **Hospital:** Mount Sinai Med Ctr (page 102); **Address:** 785 Park Ave, New York, NY 10021; **Phone:** 212-249-7800; **Board Cert:** Obstetrics & Gynecology 1982; **Med School:** Columbia P&S 1976; **Resid:** Obstetrics & Gynecology, Mt Sinai Hosp 1980; **Fac Appt:** Asst Clin Prof ObG, Columbia P&S

Coady, Deborah MD (ObG) - **Spec Exp:** Sexual Dysfunction; Vulvar Disease; Pain-Pelvic; Uterine Fibroids; **Hospital:** NYU Langone Med Ctr (page 108); **Address:** 430 West Broadway, Fl 2, New York, NY 10012; **Phone:** 212-941-0011; **Board Cert:** Obstetrics & Gynecology 2006; **Med School:** Mount Sinai Sch Med 1980; **Resid:** Obstetrics & Gynecology, NYU-Bellevue Hosp 1984; **Fac Appt:** Asst Clin Prof ObG, NYU Sch Med

Cox, Kathryn A MD (ObG) - **Spec Exp:** Gynecology Only; Menopause Problems; Gynecologic Surgery; **Hospital:** NY-Presby/Weill Cornell Med Ctr, NY (page 104); **Address:** 449 E 68th St, Ste 8, New York, NY 10065; **Phone:** 212-535-2600; **Board Cert:** Obstetrics & Gynecology 1981; **Med School:** Univ Mich Med Sch 1975; **Resid:** Obstetrics & Gynecology, New York Hosp/Cornell 1979

Dabney, Lisa MD (ObG) - **Spec Exp:** Uro-Gynecology; Minimally Invasive Surgery; Incontinence; **Hospital:** St. Luke's - Roosevelt Hosp Ctr - St Luke's Hosp (page 94); **Address:** 425 W 59th St Fl 5 - Ste D, New York, NY 10019; **Phone:** 212-523-7570; **Board Cert:** Obstetrics & Gynecology 2011; **Med School:** UCLA 1995; **Resid:** Obstetrics & Gynecology, Beth Israel Deaconess Med Ctr 1999; **Fellow:** Uro-Gynecology, Bellvue Med Ctr 2000

Diamond, Sharon MD (ObG) *PCP* - **Spec Exp:** Menopause Problems; Pap Smear Abnormalities; Gynecology Only; **Hospital:** Mount Sinai Med Ctr (page 102); **Address:** 61 E 86th St, Ste 1, New York, NY 10028-1003; **Phone:** 212-876-2200; **Board Cert:** Obstetrics & Gynecology 2011; **Med School:** Mount Sinai Sch Med 1979; **Resid:** Obstetrics & Gynecology, Mt Sinai Med Ctr 1983; **Fac Appt:** Asst Clin Prof ObG, Mount Sinai Sch Med

Evanko, John C MD (ObG) - **Spec Exp:** Pelvic Reconstruction; Minimally Invasive Surgery; Robotic Surgery; Gynecologic Surgery-Complex; **Hospital:** NY-Presby/Columbia Univ Med Ctr, NY (page 104); **Address:** 161 Fort Washington Ave, Ste 447, New York, NY 10032; **Phone:** 212-305-1107 x6; **Board Cert:** Obstetrics & Gynecology 2008; **Med School:** NY Med Coll 1995; **Resid:** Obstetrics & Gynecology, Columbia-Presby Med Ctr 1999Meml Sloan Kettering Cancer Ctr 1998; **Fac Appt:** Assoc Clin Prof ObG, Columbia P&S

Evans, Mark I MD (ObG) - **Spec Exp:** Reproductive Genetics; Fetal Diagnosis & Therapy; Multiple Gestation; Ultrasound; **Hospital:** Mount Sinai Med Ctr (page 102); **Address:** Comprehensive Genetics, 131 E 65th St, New York, NY 10065; **Phone:** 212-288-1422; **Board Cert:** Obstetrics & Gynecology 2011; Clinical Genetics 1984; **Med School:** SUNY Downstate 1978; **Resid:** Obstetrics & Gynecology, Lying-In Hosp 1982; **Fellow:** Clinical Genetics, Natl Inst Hlth 1984; **Fac Appt:** Prof ObG, Mount Sinai Sch Med

Fishbane-Mayer, Jill MD (ObG) - **Spec Exp:** Gynecology Only; **Hospital:** Mount Sinai Med Ctr (page 102); **Address:** 4 E 95th St, Ste 1A, New York, NY 10128-0705; **Phone:** 212-348-1111; **Board Cert:** Obstetrics & Gynecology 1982; **Med School:** Mount Sinai Sch Med 1976; **Resid:** Obstetrics & Gynecology, Mount Sinai Med Ctr 1980

Friedman, Lynn S MD (ObG) - **Spec Exp:** Miscarriage-Recurrent; Infertility; Pregnancy After Age 35; Pap Smear Abnormalities; **Hospital:** Mount Sinai Med Ctr (page 102); **Address:** 885 Park Ave, Ste 1-D, New York, NY 10075; **Phone:** 212-737-3282; **Board Cert:** Obstetrics & Gynecology 2012; **Med School:** NYU Sch Med 1984; **Resid:** Obstetrics & Gynecology, Mt Sinai Med Ctr 1988; **Fac Appt:** Asst Clin Prof ObG, Mount Sinai Sch Med

Friedman Jr, Ricky MD (ObG) *PCP* - **Spec Exp:** Women's Health; Pap Smear Abnormalities; **Hospital:** Mount Sinai Med Ctr (page 102); **Address:** 47 E 88th St. 1st Fl, New York, NY 10128; **Phone:** 212-534-0200; **Board Cert:** Obstetrics & Gynecology 2011; **Med School:** SUNY Hlth Sci Ctr 1985; **Resid:** Obstetrics & Gynecology, Mount Sinai Hosp 1989; **Fac Appt:** Assoc Clin Prof ObG, Mount Sinai Sch Med

Goldman, Gary MD (ObG) - **Spec Exp:** Endometriosis; Laparoscopic Surgery-Complex; Hysterectomy Alternatives; **Hospital:** NY-Presby/Weill Cornell Med Ctr, NY (page 104); **Address:** 715 Park Ave, New York, NY 10021; **Phone:** 212-535-6100; **Board Cert:** Obstetrics & Gynecology 2011; **Med School:** SUNY Stony Brook 1986; **Resid:** Obstetrics & Gynecology, New York Hosp 1990; **Fac Appt:** Asst Clin Prof ObG, Cornell Univ-Weill Med Coll

Goldstein, Martin S MD (ObG) - **Spec Exp:** Uterine Fibroids; Laparoscopic Surgery; Pelvic Organ Prolapse Repair; Endometriosis; **Hospital:** Mount Sinai Med Ctr (page 102); **Address:** 40 E 84th St, New York, NY 10028-1314; **Phone:** 212-472-6500; **Board Cert:** Obstetrics & Gynecology 1980; **Med School:** SUNY Hlth Sci Ctr 1966; **Resid:** Obstetrics & Gynecology, Mount Sinai Hosp 1971; **Fac Appt:** Assoc Clin Prof ObG, Mount Sinai Sch Med

Goldstein, Steven R MD (ObG) - **Spec Exp:** Gynecologic Ultrasound; Menopause Problems; Uterine Fibroids; **Hospital:** NYU Langone Med Ctr (page 108); **Address:** 530 1st Av, Ste 10N, New York, NY 10016-6402; **Phone:** 212-263-7416; **Board Cert:** Obstetrics & Gynecology 2011; **Med School:** NYU Sch Med 1975; **Resid:** Obstetrics & Gynecology, NYU Affil Hosps 1980; **Fac Appt:** Prof ObG, NYU Sch Med

Gruss, Leslie MD (ObG) *PCP* - **Spec Exp:** HPV-Human Papillomavirus; Pap Smear Abnormalities; **Hospital:** NYU Langone Med Ctr (page 108); **Address:** Downtown Women Ob-Gyn Assocs, 568 Broadway, Ste 304, New York, NY 10012; **Phone:** 212-966-7600; **Board Cert:** Obstetrics & Gynecology 2011; **Med School:** Med Coll PA Hahnemann 1983; **Resid:** Obstetrics & Gynecology, Montefiore Hosp Med Ctr 1987

Gubernick, Martin MD (ObG) - **Spec Exp:** Pregnancy-High Risk; **Hospital:** NY-Presby/Weill Cornell Med Ctr, NY (page 104); **Address:** 131 E 65th St, New York, NY 10065; **Phone:** 212-288-1422; **Board Cert:** Obstetrics & Gynecology 2012; **Med School:** Northwestern Univ 1982; **Resid:** Obstetrics & Gynecology, New York Hosp 1986

Harris, Dena E MD (ObG) *PCP* - **Spec Exp:** Gynecology Only; Menopause Problems; Vulvar Disease; **Hospital:** NYU Langone Med Ctr (page 108); **Address:** 430 W Broadway, Ste 2A, New York, NY 10012; **Phone:** 212-941-0011; **Board Cert:** Obstetrics & Gynecology 2011; **Med School:** Hahnemann Univ 1976; **Resid:** Obstetrics & Gynecology, NYU Med Ctr 1980; **Fac Appt:** Asst Clin Prof ObG, NYU Sch Med

Hirsch, Lissa B MD (ObG) - **Spec Exp:** Menopause Problems; **Hospital:** Lenox Hill Hosp (page 106); **Address:** 755 Park Ave, New York, NY 10021-4255; **Phone:** 212-570-2222; **Board Cert:** Obstetrics & Gynecology 1985; **Med School:** UMDNJ-NJ Med Sch, Newark 1979; **Resid:** Obstetrics & Gynecology, NYU Med Ctr 1983

Hockstein, Steven MD (ObG) - **Spec Exp:** Uterine Fibroids; **Hospital:** NY-Presby/Weill Cornell Med Ctr, NY (page 104); **Address:** 425 E 61st St Fl 11, New York, NY 10021; **Phone:** 212-821-0810; **Board Cert:** Obstetrics & Gynecology 2011; **Med School:** Univ MD Sch Med 1993; **Resid:** Obstetrics & Gynecology, McGaw Med Ctr 1997; **Fac Appt:** Asst Clin Prof ObG, Cornell Univ-Weill Med Coll

Holland, Claudia MD (ObG) *PCP* - **Hospital:** St. Luke's - Roosevelt Hosp Ctr - Roosevelt Div (page 94); **Address:** 800A 5th Ave, Ste 503, New York, NY 10021; **Phone:** 212-230-1760; **Board Cert:** Obstetrics & Gynecology 2011; **Med School:** Mount Sinai Sch Med 1981; **Resid:** Obstetrics & Gynecology, NYU Med Ctr 1985

Karamitsos, Harry MD (ObG) - **Hospital:** Lenox Hill Hosp (page 106); **Address:** Manhattan's Physician Group, 215 E 95th St, New York, NY 10128; **Phone:** 212-996-8000; **Board Cert:** Obstetrics & Gynecology 2011; **Med School:** NY Med Coll 1993; **Resid:** Obstetrics & Gynecology, Montefiore Med Ctr 1997

Kent, Joan L MD (ObG) - **Spec Exp:** Gynecology Only; **Hospital:** NY-Presby/Weill Cornell Med Ctr, NY (page 104); **Address:** 235 E 67th St, Ste 204, New York, NY 10065; **Phone:** 212-772-2900; **Board Cert:** Obstetrics & Gynecology 2010; **Med School:** Cornell Univ-Weill Med Coll 1984; **Resid:** Obstetrics & Gynecology, New York Hosp 1988; **Fac Appt:** Assoc Prof ObG, Cornell Univ-Weill Med Coll

Kessler, Alan A MD (ObG) - **Spec Exp:** Multiple Gestation; Pregnancy-High Risk; **Hospital:** NY-Presby/Weill Cornell Med Ctr, NY (page 104); **Address:** 131 E 65th St, MS 10065, New York, NY 10065; **Phone:** 212-288-1422; **Board Cert:** Obstetrics & Gynecology 2011; **Med School:** Mexico 1978; **Resid:** Obstetrics & Gynecology, New York Hosp 1983; **Fac Appt:** Assoc Prof ObG, Cornell Univ-Weill Med Coll

Kim, Joyce M MD (ObG) *PCP* - **Spec Exp:** Pregnancy-High Risk; **Hospital:** Mount Sinai Med Ctr (page 102); **Address:** 885 Park Ave St, Ste 1D, New York, NY 10021; **Phone:** 212-737-3282; **Board Cert:** Obstetrics & Gynecology 2011; **Med School:** Mount Sinai Sch Med 1986; **Resid:** Obstetrics & Gynecology, Mount Sinai Hosp 1990

Krause, Cynthia MD (ObG) *PCP* - **Spec Exp:** Menopause Problems; Pap Smear Abnormalities; Ovarian Cancer Genetics; Breast Cancer Genetics; **Hospital:** Mount Sinai Med Ctr (page 102); **Address:** 1185 Park Ave, Ste 1L, New York, NY 10128; **Phone:** 212-369-0602; **Board Cert:** Obstetrics & Gynecology 2010; **Med School:** Duke Univ 1980; **Resid:** Internal Medicine, Baltimore City Hosp 1982; Obstetrics & Gynecology, Mount Sinai Med Ctr 1986; **Fac Appt:** Asst Clin Prof ObG, Mount Sinai Sch Med

Leiter, Gila MD (ObG) - **Spec Exp:** Osteoporosis; Multiple Gestation; Menopause Problems; Uterine Fibroids; **Hospital:** Mount Sinai Med Ctr (page 102), Beth Israel Med Ctr - Petrie Division (page 94); **Address:** Park Ave Womens Center, 1160 Park Ave, New York, NY 10028; **Phone:** 212-860-2600; **Board Cert:** Obstetrics & Gynecology 2011; **Med School:** Albert Einstein Coll Med 1983; **Resid:** Obstetrics & Gynecology, Mt Sinai Hosp 1987; **Fac Appt:** Asst Clin Prof ObG, Mount Sinai Sch Med

Levine, Richard U MD (ObG) - **Spec Exp:** Uterine Fibroids; Gynecologic Surgery; HPV-Human Papillomavirus; **Hospital:** NY-Presby/Columbia Univ Med Ctr, NY (page 104); **Address:** 16 E 60th St Fl 4 - rm 480, New York, NY 10022; **Phone:** 212-326-8491; **Board Cert:** Obstetrics & Gynecology 1994; **Med School:** Cornell Univ-Weill Med Coll 1966; **Resid:** Obstetrics & Gynecology, Columbia-Presby Med Ctr 1975; **Fellow:** Obstetrics & Gynecology, Karolinska Inst 1970; **Fac Appt:** Prof ObG, Columbia P&S

Lind, Lawrence R MD (ObG) - **Spec Exp:** Uro-Gynecology; Pelvic Reconstruction; **Hospital:** N Shore Univ Hosp (page 106), Long Island Jewish Med Ctr (page 106); **Address:** 865 Northern Blvd, Ste 202, Great Neck, NY 10021; **Phone:** 516-622-5114; **Board Cert:** Obstetrics & Gynecology 2011; **Med School:** Cornell Univ-Weill Med Coll 1990; **Resid:** Obstetrics & Gynecology, N Shore Univ Hosp 1994; **Fellow:** Gynecologic Urology, UCLA Med Ctr 1996

Lustig, Ilana MD (ObG) - **Spec Exp:** Gynecology Only; **Hospital:** NYU Langone Med Ctr (page 108); **Address:** 233 E 31st St, New York, NY 10016-6302; **Phone:** 212-696-9536; **Board Cert:** Obstetrics & Gynecology 1984; **Med School:** Geo Wash Univ 1977; **Resid:** Obstetrics & Gynecology, Yale-New Haven 1981; **Fellow:** Maternal & Fetal Medicine, Bellevue Hosp 1983; **Fac Appt:** Assoc Prof ObG, NYU Sch Med

Melnick, Hugh D MD (ObG) - **Spec Exp:** Infertility-IVF; Infertility-Male; Impotence; **Hospital:** Lenox Hill Hosp (page 106); **Address:** Advanced Fertility Services, 1625 Third Ave, Ground Fl, New York, NY 10128-3603; **Phone:** 212-369-8700; **Board Cert:** Obstetrics & Gynecology 1978; **Med School:** Temple Univ 1972; **Resid:** Obstetrics & Gynecology, Lenox Hill Hosp 1976; **Fellow:** Immunopathology, Univ Birmingham 1971

Michel, Ketly MD (ObG) - **Hospital:** Lenox Hill Hosp (page 106); **Address:** 261 E 78th St, New York, NY 10075; **Phone:** 212-249-4501; **Board Cert:** Obstetrics & Gynecology 2010; **Med School:** SUNY Upstate Med Univ 1984; **Resid:** Obstetrics & Gynecology, Metropolitan Hosp 1988

Ordorica, Steven Anthony MD (ObG) - **Spec Exp:** Pregnancy-High Risk; Miscarriage-Recurrent; Maternal & Fetal Medicine; **Hospital:** NYU Langone Med Ctr (page 108); **Address:** NYU Med Ctr, Dept OB/GYN, 530 1st Ave, Ste 10Q, New York, NY 10016-6402; **Phone:** 212-263-5982; **Board Cert:** Obstetrics & Gynecology 2011; Maternal & Fetal Medicine 2011; **Med School:** SUNY Stony Brook 1983; **Resid:** Obstetrics & Gynecology, NYU Med Ctr 1987; **Fellow:** Maternal & Fetal Medicine, NYU Med Ctr 1989; **Fac Appt:** Assoc Prof ObG, NYU Sch Med

Phillips, Robin N MD (ObG) *PCP* - **Spec Exp:** Gynecology Only; Menopause Problems; Women's Health over age 40; **Hospital:** Mount Sinai Med Ctr (page 102); **Address:** 1126 Park Ave, New York, NY 10128; **Phone:** 212-534-5300; **Board Cert:** Obstetrics & Gynecology 2000; **Med School:** Mount Sinai Sch Med 1977; **Resid:** Obstetrics & Gynecology, Mount Sinai Med Ctr 1982; **Fac Appt:** Asst Clin Prof ObG, Mount Sinai Sch Med

Rodke, Gae MD (ObG) *PCP* - **Spec Exp:** Vulvar Disease; Gynecologic Surgery; **Hospital:** St. Luke's - Roosevelt Hosp Ctr - Roosevelt Div (page 94); **Address:** 185 West End Ave, Ste 1D, New York, NY 10023-2005; **Phone:** 212-496-9800; **Board Cert:** Obstetrics & Gynecology 2011; **Med School:** Albert Einstein Coll Med 1981; **Resid:** Family Medicine, Univ Hosp 1982; Obstetrics & Gynecology, Univ Hosp 1986; **Fac Appt:** Asst Clin Prof ObG, Columbia P&S

Sadarangani, Balvinder Roy MD (ObG) - **Spec Exp:** Gynecology Only; Minimally Invasive Surgery; **Hospital:** Beth Israel Med Ctr - Petrie Division (page 94); **Address:** 247 3rd Ave, Ste 503, New York, NY 10010; **Phone:** 212-982-4100; **Board Cert:** Obstetrics & Gynecology 1980; **Med School:** India 1968; **Resid:** Obstetrics & Gynecology, St Vincent's Hosp & Med Ctr 1978

Sailon, Peter S MD (ObG) - **Spec Exp:** Gynecology Only; Hysteroscopic Surgery; Laparoscopic Surgery; **Hospital:** Lenox Hill Hosp (page 106); **Address:** 955 Park Ave, New York, NY 10028-0321; **Phone:** 212-879-9191; **Board Cert:** Obstetrics & Gynecology 1982; **Med School:** Italy 1976; **Resid:** Surgery, Univ Hosp Downstate 1977; Obstetrics & Gynecology, St Luke's-Roosevelt Hosp Ctr 1980; **Fellow:** Reproductive Endocrinology, St Luke's-Roosevelt Hosp Ctr 1981

Sassoon, Robert I MD (ObG) - **Spec Exp:** Laparoscopic Surgery; Pregnancy-High Risk; Gynecologic Surgery; **Hospital:** NY-Presby/Weill Cornell Med Ctr, NY (page 104); **Address:** 449 E 68th St Fl 2, New York, NY 10021; **Phone:** 212-628-1500; **Board Cert:** Obstetrics & Gynecology 2012; **Med School:** Cornell Univ-Weill Med Coll 1981; **Resid:** Obstetrics & Gynecology, New York Hosp 1985; **Fac Appt:** Clin Prof ObG, Cornell Univ-Weill Med Coll

Scher, Jonathan MD (ObG) - **Spec Exp:** Miscarriage-Recurrent; Pregnancy-High Risk; Infertility-IVF Failure; **Hospital:** Mount Sinai Med Ctr (page 102); **Address:** 1126 Park Ave, New York, NY 10128-1203; **Phone:** 212-427-7400; **Board Cert:** Obstetrics & Gynecology 1981; **Med School:** South Africa 1964; **Resid:** Obstetrics & Gynecology, Groote Schuur Hosp 1970; Obstetrics & Gynecology, Kings College Hosp 1972; **Fac Appt:** Asst Clin Prof ObG, Mount Sinai Sch Med

Schwartz, Judith W MD (ObG) - **Spec Exp:** Gynecologic Surgery; Menopause Problems; **Hospital:** Mount Sinai Med Ctr (page 102); **Address:** 45 E 82nd St Fl 1, New York, NY 10028; **Phone:** 212-879-5959; **Board Cert:** Obstetrics & Gynecology 2011; **Med School:** Mount Sinai Sch Med 1982; **Resid:** Obstetrics & Gynecology, Mount Sinai Hosp 1986; **Fac Appt:** Asst Clin Prof ObG, Mount Sinai Sch Med

Smilen, Scott W MD (ObG) - **Spec Exp:** Uro-Gynecology; Pelvic Organ Prolapse Repair; Minimally Invasive Surgery; Incontinence; **Hospital:** NYU Langone Med Ctr (page 108), Valley Hosp (page 689); **Address:** NYU Med Ctr, Urogynecology, 150 E 32nd St Fl 2, New York, NY 10016-6497; **Phone:** 212-263-0395; **Board Cert:** Obstetrics & Gynecology 2011; **Med School:** NYU Sch Med 1988; **Resid:** Obstetrics & Gynecology, NYU Med Ctr 1992; **Fellow:** Uro-Gynecology, NYU Med Ctr 1993; **Fac Appt:** Assoc Prof ObG, NYU Sch Med

Snyder, Jon R MD (ObG) - **Spec Exp:** Menopause Problems; Menstrual Disorders; Gynecology Only; **Hospital:** NYU Langone Med Ctr (page 108), Bellevue Hosp Ctr; **Address:** 530 1st Ave, Skirball, Ste 10N, New York, NY 10016-6402; **Phone:** 212-263-6356; **Board Cert:** Obstetrics & Gynecology 2005; **Med School:** NYU Sch Med 1972; **Resid:** Obstetrics & Gynecology, Bellevue Hosp 1976; **Fac Appt:** Assoc Clin Prof ObG, NYU Sch Med

Sullum, Stanford N MD (ObG) *PCP* - **Spec Exp:** Gynecology Only; **Hospital:** Mount Sinai Med Ctr (page 102); **Address:** 1136 5th Ave, New York, NY 10128-0122; **Phone:** 212-876-4630; **Board Cert:** Obstetrics & Gynecology 1979; **Med School:** Jefferson Med Coll 1973; **Resid:** Obstetrics & Gynecology, Mount Sinai Hosp 1977; **Fac Appt:** Asst Clin Prof ObG, Mount Sinai Sch Med

Waterstone, Melissa B MD (ObG) - **Hospital:** NY-Presby/Weill Cornell Med Ctr, NY (page 104); **Address:** Weill Cornell Med Assocs-East Side, 201 E 80th St Fl 2, New York, NY 10021; **Phone:** 646-962-7300; **Board Cert:** Obstetrics & Gynecology 2011; **Med School:** Cornell Univ-Weill Med Coll 1998; **Resid:** Obstetrics & Gynecology, George Washington Univ Hosp 2002

Yale, Suzanne I MD (ObG) - **Hospital:** Lenox Hill Hosp (page 106); **Address:** 16 E 82nd St, New York, NY 10028; **Phone:** 212-744-9300; **Board Cert:** Obstetrics & Gynecology 1984; **Med School:** UMDNJ-RW Johnson Med Sch 1977; **Resid:** Obstetrics & Gynecology, Lenox Hill Hosp 1981

Yarberry-Allen, Patricia MD (ObG) - **Spec Exp:** Gynecology Only; Menopause Problems; Women's Health; Vulvar & Vaginal Disorders; **Hospital:** NY-Presby/Weill Cornell Med Ctr, NY (page 104); **Address:** 509 Madison Ave, Ste 1212, New York, NY 10022; **Phone:** 212-410-4280; **Board Cert:** Obstetrics & Gynecology 1985; **Med School:** Univ Louisville Sch Med 1976; **Resid:** Obstetrics & Gynecology, New York Hosp 1982; **Fellow:** Infectious Disease, New York Hosp 1980; Gynecology, NEw York Hosp 1980

Young, Bruce Kenneth MD (ObG) - **Spec Exp:** Infertility; Minimally Invasive Surgery; Preventive Medicine; Miscarriage-Recurrent; **Hospital:** NYU Langone Med Ctr (page 108), Bellevue Hosp Ctr; **Address:** 530 1st Ave, HCC-5th Fl, Ste 5G, New York, NY 10016; **Phone:** 212-263-6359; **Board Cert:** Obstetrics & Gynecology 1970; Maternal & Fetal Medicine 1975; **Med School:** NYU Sch Med 1963; **Resid:** Obstetrics & Gynecology, NYU Med Ctr 1968; **Fellow:** Reproductive Endocrinology, NYU Med Ctr 1968; **Fac Appt:** Prof ObG, NYU Sch Med

Occupational Medicine

Landrigan, Philip MD (OM) - **Spec Exp:** Environmental Health in Children; **Hospital:** Mount Sinai Med Ctr (page 102); **Address:** Dept Preventive Med, One Gustave L Levy Pl, Box 1057, New York, NY 10029-6500; **Phone:** 212-824-7018; **Board Cert:** Pediatrics 1973; Public Health & Genl Preventive Med 1979; Occupational Medicine 1983; **Med School:** Harvard Med Sch 1967; **Resid:** Internal Medicine, Metro Genl Hosp 1968; Pediatrics, Chldns Hosp 1970; **Fellow:** Epidemiology, Ctrs for Disease Control 1973; Occupational Medicine, Univ London 1977; **Fac Appt:** Prof Ped, Mount Sinai Sch Med

Ophthalmology

Abramson, David H MD (Oph) - **Spec Exp:** Eye Tumors/Cancer; Orbital Tumors/Cancer; Retinoblastoma; Melanoma-Choroidal (eye); **Hospital:** Meml Sloan-Kettering Cancer Ctr (page 116), NY-Presby/Weill Cornell Med Ctr, NY (page 104); **Address:** 70 E 66th St, New York, NY 10065; **Phone:** 212-744-1700; **Board Cert:** Ophthalmology 1975; **Med School:** Albert Einstein Coll Med 1969; **Resid:** Ophthalmology, Harkness Eye Inst 1974; **Fellow:** Ocular Oncology, Columbia-Presby Med Ctr 1975; **Fac Appt:** Prof Oph, Cornell Univ-Weill Med Coll

Accardi, Frank E MD (Oph) - **Spec Exp:** Cataract Surgery; Refractive Surgery; **Hospital:** New York Eye & Ear Infirm (page 117), Lenox Hill Hosp (Manh Eye, Ear & Throat Hosp) (page 106); **Address:** 114 E 27th St, New York, NY 10016; **Phone:** 212-481-4000; **Board Cert:** Ophthalmology 1987; **Med School:** Italy 1979; **Resid:** Internal Medicine, Cabrini Med Ctr 1982; Ophthalmology, SUNY-Downstate Med Ctr 1985; **Fellow:** Cornea, SUNY-Downstate Med Ctr 1986; **Fac Appt:** Asst Clin Prof Oph, NY Med Coll

Angioletti, Louis V MD (Oph) - **Spec Exp:** Retinal Disorders; Diabetic Eye Disease/Retinopathy; Macular Degeneration; **Hospital:** New York Eye & Ear Infirm (page 117); **Address:** 7 Gramercy Park, New York, NY 10003-1759; **Phone:** 212-505-8510; **Board Cert:** Ophthalmology 1975; **Med School:** NY Med Coll 1966; **Resid:** Ophthalmology, NY Eye & Ear Infirm 1973; **Fellow:** Retina, NY Eye & Ear Infirm 1974; **Fac Appt:** Asst Clin Prof Oph, NY Med Coll

Asbell, Penny A MD (Oph) - **Spec Exp:** Corneal Disease & Transplant; LASIK-Refractive Surgery; Cataract Surgery; Keratoconus; **Hospital:** Mount Sinai Med Ctr (page 102); **Address:** 1190 Fifth Ave, Annenberg Bldg Fl 22 - Ste 22-11, New York, NY 10029; **Phone:** 212-241-7977; **Board Cert:** Ophthalmology 1980; **Med School:** SUNY Buffalo 1975; **Resid:** Ophthalmology, NYU Med Ctr 1979; **Fellow:** Immunology, NYU Med Ctr 1980; Cornea & Ext Eye Disease, LSU Eye Ctr 1982; **Fac Appt:** Prof Oph, Mount Sinai Sch Med

Auran, James D MD (Oph) - **Spec Exp:** Cataract Surgery; Cornea & External Eye Disease; Acanthamoeba Keratitis; Dry Eye Syndrome; **Hospital:** NY-Presby/Columbia Univ Med Ctr, NY (page 104); **Address:** 635 W 165th St Fl 5, New York, NY 10032-3701; **Phone:** 212-305-9535; **Board Cert:** Ophthalmology 1989; **Med School:** Cornell Univ-Weill Med Coll 1983; **Resid:** Ophthalmology, Manhattan EET Hosp 1987; **Fellow:** Ophthalmology, Manhattan EET Hosp 1988; **Fac Appt:** Clin Prof Oph, Columbia P&S

Barile, Gaetano R MD (Oph) - **Spec Exp:** Macular Disease/Degeneration; Retinal Disorders; Diabetic Eye Disease/Retinopathy; Retina/Vitreous Consultation; **Hospital:** Lenox Hill Hosp (Manh Eye, Ear & Throat Hosp) (page 106); **Address:** 210 E 64 St, New York, NY 10065; **Phone:** 212-702-7400; **Board Cert:** Ophthalmology 2008; **Med School:** Cornell Univ-Weill Med Coll 1991; **Resid:** Ophthalmology, Manhattan EET Hosp 1995; **Fellow:** Retina/Vitreous, Roosevelt Hosp/Harkness Eye Inst 1997; Retina, Moorfields Eye Hosp 1997; **Fac Appt:** Prof Oph, Columbia P&S

Barker, Barbara Ann MD (Oph) - **Spec Exp:** Glaucoma; Corneal Disease; **Hospital:** New York Eye & Ear Infirm (page 117), Beth Israel Med Ctr - Petrie Division (page 94); **Address:** 70 E 96th St, Ste 1B, New York, NY 10028; **Phone:** 212-289-2244; **Board Cert:** Ophthalmology 1981; **Med School:** Mount Sinai Sch Med 1976; **Resid:** Ophthalmology, Mt Sinai Med Ctr 1980; **Fellow:** Glaucoma, Beth Israel 1981; Cornea, Beth Israel 1983; **Fac Appt:** Asst Clin Prof Oph, Mount Sinai Sch Med

Braunstein, Richard E MD (Oph) - **Spec Exp:** LASIK-Refractive Surgery; Corneal Disease & Transplant; Cataract Surgery; **Hospital:** Lenox Hill Hosp (Manh Eye, Ear & Throat Hosp) (page 106); **Address:** MEETH Ophthalmology, 210 E 64th St, New York, NY 10065; **Phone:** 212-702-7300; **Board Cert:** Ophthalmology 2006; **Med School:** Columbia P&S 1989; **Resid:** Ophthalmology, Harkness Eye Inst 1993; **Fellow:** Cornea & Ext Eye Disease, Wilmer Inst/Johns Hopkins Hosp 1994

Buxton, Douglas F MD (Oph) - **Spec Exp:** Corneal Disease & Transplant; LASIK-Refractive Surgery; Cataract Surgery-Lens Implant; Glaucoma-Pediatric; **Hospital:** New York Eye & Ear Infirm (page 117), Lenox Hill Hosp (Manh Eye, Ear & Throat Hosp) (page 106); **Address:** 310 E 14th St, Ste 403, New York, NY 10003-4201; **Phone:** 212-979-4410; **Board Cert:** Ophthalmology 2008; Penetrating Keratoplasty 1998; Cataract/Implant Surgery 2002; Refractive Surgery(LASIK) 2002; **Med School:** Cornell Univ-Weill Med Coll 1982; **Resid:** Ophthalmology, New York Eye & Ear Infirm 1986; **Fellow:** Cornea & Ext Eye Disease, New York Eye & Ear Infirm 1988; **Fac Appt:** Assoc Clin Prof Oph, NY Med Coll

Campolattaro, Brian MD (Oph) - **Spec Exp:** Pediatric Ophthalmology; Strabismus; Tear Duct Problems; Eye Muscle Disorders; **Hospital:** New York Eye & Ear Infirm (page 117); **Address:** 30 E 40th St, Ste 405, New York, NY 10016-3507; **Phone:** 212-684-3980; **Board Cert:** Ophthalmology 2006; **Med School:** UMDNJ-NJ Med Sch, Newark 1990; **Resid:** Ophthalmology, New York Eye & Ear Infirm 1994; **Fellow:** Pediatrics, St Louis Chldns Hosp 1995; **Fac Appt:** Asst Prof Oph, NY Med Coll

Casper, Daniel S MD/PhD (Oph) - **Spec Exp:** Diabetic Eye Disease; **Hospital:** NY-Presby/Columbia Univ Med Ctr, NY (page 104); **Address:** N Berrie Diabetes Ctr-Columbia-Presby, 1150 St Nicholas Ave Fl 2, New York, NY 10032-3822; **Phone:** 212-851-5494; **Board Cert:** Ophthalmology 1991; **Med School:** Albany Med Coll 1985; **Resid:** Ophthalmology, Harkness Eye Inst-Columbia 1989; **Fellow:** Oculoplastic Surgery, Harkness Eye Inst-Columbia 1990; **Fac Appt:** Assoc Clin Prof Oph, Columbia P&S

Chaiken, Barry MD (Oph) - **Spec Exp:** Cataract Surgery; LASIK-Refractive Surgery; **Hospital:** New York Eye & Ear Infirm (page 117), Lenox Hill Hosp (Manh Eye, Ear & Throat Hosp) (page 106); **Address:** 625 Park Ave, New York, NY 10065; **Phone:** 212-249-1976; **Board Cert:** Ophthalmology 1981; **Med School:** Columbia P&S 1976; **Resid:** Ophthalmology, Mt Sinai Hosp 1980

Chang, Stanley MD (Oph) - **Spec Exp:** Retina/Vitreous Surgery; Diabetic Eye Disease/Retinopathy; Macular Disease/Degeneration; Retinal Disorders; **Hospital:** NY-Presby/Columbia Univ Med Ctr, NY (page 104); **Address:** 635 W 165th St, Box 20, New York, NY 10032; **Phone:** 212-305-9535; **Board Cert:** Ophthalmology 1979; **Med School:** Columbia P&S 1974; **Resid:** Ophthalmology, Mass Eye & Ear Infirm 1978; **Fellow:** Vitreoretinal Surgery, Bascom Palmer Eye Inst 1979; **Fac Appt:** Prof Oph, Columbia P&S

Charles, Norman MD (Oph) - **Spec Exp:** Glaucoma; Eyelid Tumors/Cancer; Contact Lenses; Cornea & External Eye Disease; **Hospital:** NYU Langone Med Ctr (page 108); **Address:** 620 Park Ave, New York, NY 10065-6561; **Phone:** 212-772-6920; **Board Cert:** Ophthalmology 1971; **Med School:** NYU Sch Med 1963; **Resid:** Ophthalmology, NYU Med Ctr 1970; **Fac Appt:** Clin Prof Oph, NYU Sch Med

Chern, Relly MD (Oph) - **Spec Exp:** Cataract Surgery; Ophthalmic Plastic Surgery; **Hospital:** New York Eye & Ear Infirm (page 117); **Address:** 923 5th Ave, New York, NY 10021; **Phone:** 212-628-0160; **Board Cert:** Ophthalmology 1983; **Med School:** Albert Einstein Coll Med 1976; **Resid:** Ophthalmology, Montefiore Hosp Med Ctr 1980; **Fac Appt:** Asst Clin Prof Oph, Albert Einstein Coll Med

Cohen, Ben Z MD (Oph) - **Spec Exp:** Retina/Vitreous Surgery; Macular Degeneration; Diabetic Eye Disease/Retinopathy; **Hospital:** New York Eye & Ear Infirm (page 117); **Address:** 140 E 80th St, FL 1, New York, NY 10075; **Phone:** 212-772-0600; **Board Cert:** Ophthalmology 1981; **Med School:** NY Med Coll 1976; **Resid:** Ophthalmology, Univ Chicago Hosps 1980; **Fellow:** Retina, Manhattan Eye & Ear Infirmary 1981; Retina, Mass Eye & Ear Infirmary 1983

Cohen, Leeber MD (Oph) - **Spec Exp:** Cataract Surgery; AIDS Related Eye Diseases; Botox Therapy; **Hospital:** New York Eye & Ear Infirm (page 117); **Address:** 11 5th Ave, Ste B Bldg, New York, NY 10003-4342; **Phone:** 212-777-1644; **Board Cert:** Ophthalmology 1989; **Med School:** SUNY Hlth Sci Ctr 1983; **Resid:** Ophthalmology, Kings Co Hosp/SUNY Downstate 1987; **Fac Appt:** Asst Clin Prof Med, SUNY Downstate

Coleman, D Jackson MD (Oph) - **Spec Exp:** Retina/Vitreous Surgery; Ultrasound-Eye; Melanoma-Choroidal (eye); **Hospital:** NY-Presby/Weill Cornell Med Ctr, NY (page 104); **Address:** 635 W 165 St Fl 1, New York, NY 10032; **Phone:** 212-305-9535; **Board Cert:** Ophthalmology 1969; **Med School:** SUNY Buffalo 1960; **Resid:** Ophthalmology, Columbia-Presby Med Ctr 1967; **Fellow:** Retina, Columbia-Presby Med Ctr 1968; **Fac Appt:** Prof Oph, Cornell Univ-Weill Med Coll

Cykiert, Robert MD (Oph) - **Spec Exp:** LASIK-Refractive Surgery; Cataract Surgery; Corneal Disease & Transplant; Keratoconus; **Hospital:** NYU Langone Med Ctr (page 108), New York Eye & Ear Infirm (page 117); **Address:** 345 E 37th St, Ste 210, New York, NY 10016-3217; **Phone:** 212-922-1430; **Board Cert:** Ophthalmology 1981; **Med School:** NY Med Coll 1976; **Resid:** Ophthalmology, Montefiore Med Ctr 1980; **Fellow:** Cornea, Wills Eye Hosp 1981; **Fac Appt:** Assoc Clin Prof Oph, NYU Sch Med

D'Amico, Donald J MD (Oph) - **Spec Exp:** Diabetic Eye Disease/Retinopathy; Retinal Detachment; Retinal Disorders; **Hospital:** NY-Presby/Weill Cornell Med Ctr, NY (page 104); **Address:** Weill Cornell Medical College, Dept of Ophthalmology, 1305 York Ave, Fl 11th, New York, NY 10021; **Phone:** 646-962-2020; **Board Cert:** Ophthalmology 1982; **Med School:** Univ IL Coll Med 1977; **Resid:** Ophthalmology, Mass Eye & Ear Infirm 1981; **Fellow:** Vitreoretinal Surgery, Bascom Palmer Eye Inst 1982; **Fac Appt:** Prof Oph, Cornell Univ-Weill Med Coll

Dayan, Alan MD (Oph) - **Spec Exp:** Retinal Dosorders; Retina/Vitreous Surgery; Macular Degeneration; Retinal Detachment; **Hospital:** New York Eye & Ear Infirm (page 117); **Address:** 310 E 14th St South Bldg - Ste 419, New York, NY 10003; **Phone:** 212-677-2000; **Board Cert:** Ophthalmology 2009; **Med School:** Mount Sinai Sch Med 1992; **Resid:** Ophthalmology, NY Eye & Ear Infirm 1996; **Fellow:** Vitreoretinal Disease, Vitreoretinal Fdn 1998

Delerme, Milton MD (Oph) - **Hospital:** Harlem Hosp Ctr; **Address:** 75 E 116th St, New York, NY 10029; **Phone:** 212-828-7700; **Board Cert:** Ophthalmology 1987; **Med School:** UMDNJ-NJ Med Sch, Newark 1978; **Resid:** Surgery, UMDNJ-Univ Hosp 1980; Ophthalmology, Harlem Hosp 1984; **Fellow:** Anterior Segment - External Disease, St Francis Hosp 1985

Della Rocca, Robert C MD (Oph) - **Spec Exp:** Orbital Tumors/Cancer; Eyelid Tumors/Cancer; Thyroid Eye Disease; Oculoplastic Surgery; **Hospital:** New York Eye & Ear Infirm (page 117), Sound Shore Med Ctr - Westchester; **Address:** 310 E 14th St, South Bldg, rm 319, New York, NY 10003; **Phone:** 212-979-4575; **Board Cert:** Ophthalmology 1975; **Med School:** Creighton Univ 1967; **Resid:** Ophthalmology, NY Eye & Ear Infirm 1973; **Fellow:** Oculoplastic Surgery, Albany Med Ctr

Dinnerstein, Stephen R MD (Oph) - **Spec Exp:** Cataract Surgery; Glaucoma; **Hospital:** New York Eye & Ear Infirm (page 117), Mount Sinai Med Ctr (page 102); **Address:** 36 E 36th St, Ste 1J, New York, NY 10016; **Phone:** 212-889-4944; **Board Cert:** Ophthalmology 1976; **Med School:** NY Med Coll 1970; **Resid:** Ophthalmology, Downstate-Kings Co Hosp Ctr 1974

Dodick, Jack M MD (Oph) - **Spec Exp:** Cataract Surgery-Lens Implant; Laser Vision Surgery; **Hospital:** NYU Langone Med Ctr (page 108), Lenox Hill Hosp (Manh Eye, Ear & Throat Hosp) (page 106); **Address:** 535 Park Ave, New York, NY 10065; **Phone:** 212-288-7638; **Board Cert:** Ophthalmology 1969; **Med School:** Univ Toronto 1963; **Resid:** Ophthalmology, Manhattan EE&T Hosp 1967; **Fellow:** Anterior Segment - External Disease, Westchester Co Med Ctr 1968; **Fac Appt:** Prof Oph, NYU Sch Med

Eggers, Howard M MD (Oph) - **Spec Exp:** Pediatric Ophthalmology; Strabismus-Adult & Pediatric; **Hospital:** NY-Presby/Columbia Univ Med Ctr, NY (page 104); **Address:** Harkness Eye Institute, 635 W 165th St, New York, NY 10032-3724; **Phone:** 212-305-5409; **Board Cert:** Ophthalmology 1978; **Med School:** Columbia P&S 1971; **Resid:** Ophthalmology, Harkness Inst-Presby Hosp 1975; **Fac Appt:** Prof Oph, Columbia P&S

Eichenbaum, Joseph MD (Oph) - **Spec Exp:** Uveitis; Glaucoma; Dry Eye Syndrome; Eye Infections; **Hospital:** Mount Sinai Med Ctr (page 102); **Address:** 1050 Park Ave, New York, NY 10028; **Phone:** 212-289-7200; **Board Cert:** Ophthalmology 1980; **Med School:** Yale Univ 1973; **Resid:** Ophthalmology, NYU Med Ctr 1977; **Fac Appt:** Assoc Clin Prof Oph, Mount Sinai Sch Med

Elahi, Ebrahim MD (Oph) - **Spec Exp:** Cosmetic & Reconstructive Surgery; Oculoplastic & Orbital Surgery; Eyelid Tumors/Cancer; Facial Plastic Surgery; **Hospital:** Mount Sinai Med Ctr (page 102), Lenox Hill Hosp (Manh Eye, Ear & Throat Hosp) (page 106); **Address:** 1034 Fifth Ave, MS 10028, New York, NY 10028; **Phone:** 212-570-0707; **Board Cert:** Ophthalmology 2001; **Med School:** Mount Sinai Sch Med 1996; **Resid:** Ophthalmology, Mt Sinai Hosp 2000; **Fellow:** Ophthalmic Plastic & Reconstructive Surgery, Manhattan EE&T Infirmary 2001; **Fac Appt:** Assoc Clin Prof Oph, Mount Sinai Sch Med

Engel, Harry MD (Oph) - **Spec Exp:** Retinal Disorders; **Hospital:** Montefiore Med Ctr-Moses Campus, NY (page 100), New York Eye & Ear Infirm (page 117); **Address:** 40 W 72nd St, New York, NY 10023; **Phone:** 212-724-2555; **Board Cert:** Ophthalmology 1981; **Med School:** NY Med Coll 1976; **Resid:** Ophthalmology, U Michigan Med Ctr 1980; **Fellow:** Eye Pathology, Wilmer Inst 1981; Retina/Vitreous, Barnes Jewish Hosp 1982; **Fac Appt:** Clin Prof Oph, Albert Einstein Coll Med

Esposito, Donna A MD (Oph) - **Spec Exp:** Glaucoma; **Hospital:** New York Eye & Ear Infirm (page 117); **Address:** 49 W 23rd St Fl 12th, New York, NY 10010; **Phone:** 212-255-4373; **Board Cert:** Ophthalmology 1991; **Med School:** NY Med Coll 1983; **Resid:** Surgery, St Vincent's Hosp 1985; Ophthalmology, St Vincent's Hosp 1989; **Fellow:** Glaucoma, NY Hosp 1990

Finger, Paul T MD (Oph) - **Spec Exp:** Eye Tumors/Cancer; Melanoma-Choroidal (eye); Retinoblastoma; Orbital Tumors/Cancer; **Hospital:** New York Eye & Ear Infirm (page 117), Lenox Hill Hosp (Manh Eye, Ear & Throat Hosp) (page 106); **Address:** 115 E 61st St Fl 5 - Ste B, New York, NY 10065; **Phone:** 212-832-8170; **Board Cert:** Ophthalmology 1990; **Med School:** Tulane Univ 1982; **Resid:** Ophthalmology, Manhattan EET Hosp 1986; **Fellow:** Ocular Oncology, N Shore Univ Hosp 1987; **Fac Appt:** Clin Prof Oph, NYU Sch Med

Fisher, Yale MD (Oph) - **Spec Exp:** Retina/Vitreous Consultation; Diabetic Eye Disease; Ocular Ultrasound; **Hospital:** Lenox Hill Hosp (Manh Eye, Ear & Throat Hosp) (page 106), NY-Presby/Weill Cornell Med Ctr, NY (page 104); **Address:** 460 Park Ave Fl 5, New York, NY 10022; **Phone:** 212-861-9797; **Board Cert:** Ophthalmology 1973; **Med School:** Cornell Univ-Weill Med Coll 1967; **Resid:** Ophthalmology, Manhattan EET Hosp 1971; **Fac Appt:** Clin Prof Oph, Cornell Univ-Weill Med Coll

Florakis, George J MD (Oph) - **Spec Exp:** Cornea Transplant; Corneal Disease; Keratoconus; Anterior Segment Trauma/Reconstruction; **Hospital:** NY-Presby/Columbia Univ Med Ctr, NY (page 104), White Plains Hosp (page 615); **Address:** Edward S Harkness Eye Inst, Columbia Univ Med Ctr/NY Presby Hosp, 635 W 165th St, Ste 303, New York, NY 10032; **Phone:** 212-927-2394; **Board Cert:** Ophthalmology 1989; **Med School:** Columbia P&S 1983; **Resid:** Ophthalmology, Harkness Eye Inst 1987; **Fellow:** Cornea & Ext Eye Disease, Univ Iowa Hosps & Clins 1988; **Fac Appt:** Clin Prof Oph, Columbia P&S

Fong, Raymond MD (Oph) - **Spec Exp:** Cataract Surgery; LASIK-Refractive Surgery; Glaucoma; **Hospital:** Lenox Hill Hosp (Manh Eye, Ear & Throat Hosp) (page 106), NY Downtown Hosp; **Address:** 109 Lafayette St Fl 4, New York, NY 10013-4154; **Phone:** 212-274-1900; **Board Cert:** Ophthalmology 1987; **Med School:** Cornell Univ 1981; **Resid:** Ophthalmology, Manhattan EET Hosp 1985

Fox, Martin L MD (Oph) - **Spec Exp:** LASIK-Refractive Surgery; Cornea Transplant; Corneal Ring Implants; **Hospital:** New York Eye & Ear Infirm (page 117); **Address:** 425 Madison Ave, Ste 1501, New York, NY 10017; **Phone:** 212-838-1053; **Board Cert:** Ophthalmology 1981; **Med School:** Hahnemann Univ 1976; **Resid:** Ophthalmology, Boston Univ Med Ctr 1980; **Fellow:** Cornea, NY Eye & Ear Infirmary 1981

Friedman, Alan H MD (Oph) - **Spec Exp:** Uveitis; Eye Tumors/Cancer; Retinal Disorders; Ophthalmic Pathology; **Hospital:** Mount Sinai Med Ctr (page 102), Lenox Hill Hosp (page 106); **Address:** 888 Park Ave, Ste 1A, New York, NY 10075; **Phone:** 212-794-2277; **Board Cert:** Ophthalmology 1971; **Med School:** NYU Sch Med 1963; **Resid:** Ophthalmology, NYU Med Ctr 1969; **Fellow:** Pathology, Hammersmith Hosp 1972; Ocular Pathology, NYU Med Ctr 1970; **Fac Appt:** Clin Prof Oph, Mount Sinai Sch Med

Friedman, Robert MD (Oph) - **Spec Exp:** Laser Refractive Surgery; Cataract Surgery; Retina/Vitreous Surgery; Macular Disease/Degeneration; **Hospital:** Lenox Hill Hosp (page 106), Mount Sinai Med Ctr (page 102); **Address:** 1001 Park Ave, New York, NY 10028-0935; **Phone:** 212-772-6202; **Board Cert:** Ophthalmology 1989; **Med School:** Albert Einstein Coll Med 1983; **Resid:** Ophthalmology, Lenox Hill Hosp 1987; **Fellow:** Vitreoretinal Surgery, Manhattan EET Hosp 1988

Fromer, Mark D MD (Oph) - **Spec Exp:** Retinal Disorders; Laser Vision Surgery; Cataract Surgery; Diabetic Eye Disease/Retinopathy; **Hospital:** New York Eye & Ear Infirm (page 117), Lenox Hill Hosp (Manh Eye, Ear & Throat Hosp) (page 106); **Address:** 550 Park Ave, New York, NY 10065; **Phone:** 212-832-9228; **Board Cert:** Ophthalmology 1989; **Med School:** UMDNJ-Rutgers Med Sch 1984; **Resid:** Ophthalmology, St Vincents Hosp 1988; **Fellow:** Vitreoretinal Surgery, Manhattan EE&T Hosp 1989; **Fac Appt:** Clin Prof Oph, NY Med Coll

Fuchs, Wayne MD (Oph) - **Spec Exp:** Diabetic Eye Disease/Retinopathy; Macular Disease/Degeneration; Retinal Disorders; Pseudoxanthoma Elasticum; **Hospital:** Mount Sinai Med Ctr (page 102), Lenox Hill Hosp (Manh Eye, Ear & Throat Hosp) (page 106); **Address:** 121 E 60th St, Ste 5B, New York, NY 10022-1186; **Phone:** 212-319-8205; **Board Cert:** Ophthalmology 1985; **Med School:** Mount Sinai Sch Med 1979; **Resid:** Ophthalmology, Mt Sinai Hosp 1983; **Fellow:** Vitreoretinal Surgery & Disease, NY Hosp-Cornell Med Ctr 1984; **Fac Appt:** Clin Prof Oph, Mount Sinai Sch Med

Gallin, Pamela F MD (Oph) - **Spec Exp:** Pediatric Ophthalmology; Amblyopia; Strabismus; Lacrimal Gland Disorders; **Hospital:** NY-Presby/Columbia Univ Med Ctr, NY (page 104), Lenox Hill Hosp (Manh Eye, Ear & Throat Hosp) (page 106); **Address:** NY Presby/Columbia Univ, 635 W 165th St, Ste 224, New York, NY 10032-3701; **Phone:** 212-305-5407; **Board Cert:** Ophthalmology 1983; **Med School:** Washington Univ, St Louis 1978; **Resid:** Ophthalmology, Mount Sinai Med Ctr 1982; **Fellow:** Pediatric Ophthalmology, Chldns Natl Med Ctr 1983; Strabismus, Columbia-Presby Med Ctr 1983; **Fac Appt:** Clin Prof Oph, Columbia P&S

Gentile, Ronald C MD (Oph) - **Spec Exp:** Retina/Vitreous Surgery; Diabetic Eye Disease/Retinopathy; Macular Degeneration; Retinal Disorders; **Hospital:** New York Eye & Ear Infirm (page 117); **Address:** 310 E 14th St, South Bldg, Ste 319, New York, NY 10003-4201; **Phone:** 212-979-4120; **Board Cert:** Ophthalmology 2008; **Med School:** SUNY Downstate 1991; **Resid:** Ophthalmology, NY Eye & Ear Infirm 1995; **Fellow:** Vitreoretinal Surgery & Disease, Kresge Eye Inst 1998; **Fac Appt:** Prof Oph, NY Med Coll

Gibralter, Richard P MD (Oph) - **Spec Exp:** Cataract Surgery; Laser Vision Surgery; Cornea Transplant; Corneal Disease & Surgery; **Hospital:** Lenox Hill Hosp (Manh Eye, Ear & Throat Hosp) (page 106), New York Eye & Ear Infirm (page 117); **Address:** 154 E 71st St, New York, NY 10021-5123; **Phone:** 212-628-2202; **Board Cert:** Ophthalmology 1981; **Med School:** Mount Sinai Sch Med 1976; **Resid:** Ophthalmology, Manhattan EE&T Hosp 1980; **Fellow:** Cornea, Manhattan EE&T Hosp 1981; **Fac Appt:** Assoc Clin Prof Oph, NYU Sch Med

Goldstein, Michael T MD (Oph) - **Spec Exp:** Corneal Disease; Keratoconus; LASIK-Refractive Surgery; **Hospital:** New York Eye & Ear Infirm (page 117), Beth Israel Med Ctr - Petrie Division (page 94); **Address:** 115 E 61st St, Ste 3A, New York, NY 10065; **Phone:** 212-371-6209; **Board Cert:** Ophthalmology 1980; **Med School:** SUNY Downstate 1974; **Resid:** Ophthalmology, Brookdale Hosp Med Ctr 1979; **Fellow:** Cornea, Manhattan Eye, Ear & Throat Hosp 1980

Grayson, Douglas K MD (Oph) - **Spec Exp:** Cataract Surgery; Glaucoma; **Hospital:** New York Eye & Ear Infirm (page 117); **Address:** 36 E 36th St, New York, NY 10016-3463; **Phone:** 212-353-0030; **Board Cert:** Ophthalmology 2006; **Med School:** Brown Univ 1989; **Resid:** Ophthalmology, NY Eye & Ear Infirm 1993; **Fellow:** Glaucoma, NY Eye & Ear Infirm 1994; **Fac Appt:** Asst Prof Oph, NY Med Coll

Guillory, Samuel L MD (Oph) - **Spec Exp:** LASIK-Refractive Surgery; PRK-Refractive Surgery; Pediatric Ophthalmology; **Hospital:** Mount Sinai Med Ctr (page 102); **Address:** 1103 Park Ave, New York, NY 10128-1236; **Phone:** 212-860-5400; **Board Cert:** Ophthalmology 1980; **Med School:** Mount Sinai Sch Med 1975; **Resid:** Ophthalmology, Mount Sinai Med Ctr 1979; **Fellow:** Ophthalmology, Cornell Med Ctr 1981; **Fac Appt:** Assoc Clin Prof Oph, Mount Sinai Sch Med

Haight, David MD (Oph) - **Spec Exp:** Laser Vision Surgery; Cornea Transplant; Cataract Surgery; **Hospital:** Lenox Hill Hosp (page 106), NY-Presby/Weill Cornell Med Ctr, NY (page 104); **Address:** 155 E 72nd St, New York, NY 10021-4371; **Phone:** 212-772-9474; **Board Cert:** Ophthalmology 1985; **Med School:** Johns Hopkins Univ 1980; **Resid:** Ophthalmology, Manhattan EE&T Hosp 1984; **Fellow:** Cornea, Manhattan EE&T Hosp 1985; **Fac Appt:** Clin Prof Oph, NYU Sch Med

Hall, Lisabeth S MD (Oph) - **Spec Exp:** Pediatric Ophthalmology; Strabismus-Adult & Pediatric; Eye Muscle Disorders; Cataract-Pediatric; **Hospital:** New York Eye & Ear Infirm (page 117); **Address:** 40 W 72nd St, New York, NY 10023; **Phone:** 212-979-4614; **Board Cert:** Ophthalmology 2009; **Med School:** SUNY Stony Brook 1992; **Resid:** Ophthalmology, Manhattan Eye & Ear Infirm 1996; **Fellow:** Pediatric Ophthalmology, Jules Stein Eye Inst 1997; **Fac Appt:** Assoc Prof Oph, NY Med Coll

Harmon, Gregory K MD (Oph) - **Spec Exp:** Cataract Surgery; Glaucoma; **Hospital:** NY-Presby/Weill Cornell Med Ctr, NY (page 104); **Address:** 205 E 64 St, Ste 101, New York, NY 10065; **Phone:** 212-888-4100; **Board Cert:** Ophthalmology 1991; **Med School:** Mount Sinai Sch Med 1982; **Resid:** Ophthalmology, NY Hosp 1986; **Fellow:** Glaucoma, NY Hosp 1987

Heinemann, Murk Hein MD (Oph) - **Hospital:** Meml Sloan-Kettering Cancer Ctr (page 116), NY-Presby/Weill Cornell Med Ctr, NY (page 104); **Address:** 1275 York Ave, rm A330, New York, NY 10065; **Phone:** 212-639-7237; **Board Cert:** Ophthalmology 1982; **Med School:** Cornell Univ-Weill Med Coll 1976; **Resid:** Ophthalmology, Yale-New Haven Hosp 1980; **Fellow:** Ophthalmology, New York Hosp 1982; **Fac Appt:** Assoc Prof Oph, Cornell Univ-Weill Med Coll

Jabs, Douglas MD (Oph) - **Spec Exp:** Uveitis; **Hospital:** Mount Sinai Med Ctr (page 102); **Address:** 1700 E 102 St 8W Bldg, New York, NY 10029; **Phone:** 212-241-6752; **Board Cert:** Ophthalmology 1982; Internal Medicine 1983; **Med School:** Johns Hopkins Univ 1977; **Resid:** Ophthalmology, Wilmer Eye Inst 1981; Internal Medicine, Johns Hopkins Hosp 1983; **Fellow:** Rheumatology, Johns Hopkins Hosp 1984; **Fac Appt:** Prof Oph, Mount Sinai Sch Med

Kazim, Michael MD (Oph) - **Spec Exp:** Thyroid Eye Disease; Oculoplastic Surgery; Orbital Tumors/Cancer; Eyelid Tumors/Cancer; **Hospital:** NY-Presby/Columbia Univ Med Ctr, NY (page 104), New York Eye & Ear Infirm (page 117); **Address:** 635 W 165th St, Ste 207, New York, NY 10032-3701; **Phone:** 212-305-5477; **Board Cert:** Ophthalmology 1989; **Med School:** Columbia P&S 1984; **Resid:** Ophthalmology, Columbia-Presby Hosp 1988; **Fellow:** Oculoplastic Surgery, Univ Penn-Childrens Hosp 1989; Orbital Surgery, Allegheny Genl Hosp 1990; **Fac Appt:** Clin Prof Oph, Columbia P&S

Kelly, Stephen E MD (Oph) - **Spec Exp:** LASIK-Refractive Surgery; Cataract Surgery; Corneal Disease; **Hospital:** New York Eye & Ear Infirm (page 117), Lenox Hill Hosp (Manh Eye, Ear & Throat Hosp) (page 106); **Address:** 154 E 71st St, New York, NY 10021-5125; **Phone:** 212-628-2202; **Board Cert:** Ophthalmology 1976; **Med School:** Washington Univ, St Louis 1970; **Resid:** Ophthalmology, NY Eye & Ear Infirmary 1975; **Fellow:** Cornea, Manhattan EET Hosp 1976

Klapper, Daniel MD (Oph) - **Spec Exp:** Laser-Refractive Surgery; Glaucoma; Cataract Surgery; **Hospital:** Lenox Hill Hosp (Manh Eye, Ear & Throat Hosp) (page 106); **Address:** 7 W 81st St, Ste 1A, New York, NY 10024; **Phone:** 212-874-2726; **Board Cert:** Ophthalmology 1991; **Med School:** Albert Einstein Coll Med 1984; **Resid:** Ophthalmology, Brookdale Univ Hosp 1988

Klein, Noah MD (Oph) - **Spec Exp:** Glaucoma; Cataract Surgery; LASIK-Refractive Surgery; **Hospital:** New York Eye & Ear Infirm (page 117), Beth Israel Med Ctr - Petrie Division (page 94); **Address:** 51 E 25th St Fl 3, New York, NY 10010; **Phone:** 212-696-9013; **Board Cert:** Ophthalmology 1985; **Med School:** Albert Einstein Coll Med 1980; **Resid:** Ophthalmology, LI Jewish Med Ctr 1985

Koplin, Richard Steven MD (Oph) - **Spec Exp:** Cataract Surgery; Laser Refractive Surgery; Eye Trauma; Eye Infections; **Hospital:** New York Eye & Ear Infirm (page 117); **Address:** 310 E 14th St South Bldg, Fl 2, MS 10003, New York, NY 10003-4201; **Phone:** 212-505-6550; **Board Cert:** Ophthalmology 1975; **Med School:** NY Med Coll 1969; **Resid:** Ophthalmology, NY Eye & Ear Infirm 1973; **Fac Appt:** Clin Prof Oph, NY Med Coll

Kupersmith, Mark J MD (Oph) - **Spec Exp:** Neuro-Ophthalmology; **Hospital:** St. Luke's - Roosevelt Hosp Ctr - Roosevelt Div (page 94); **Address:** Roosevelt Hosp, 1000 10th Ave, 10 INN Bldg, New York, NY 10019; **Phone:** 212-636-3200 x1; **Board Cert:** Ophthalmology 1981; Neurology 1981; **Med School:** Northwestern Univ 1974; **Resid:** Neurology, NYU Med Ctr 1978; Ophthalmology, NYU Med Ctr 1980; **Fac Appt:** Prof Oph, Albert Einstein Coll Med

Lauer, Simeon A MD (Oph) - **Spec Exp:** Oculoplastic Surgery; Ophthalmic Plastic Surgery; Lacrimal Gland Disorders; Orbital Surgery; **Hospital:** Hackensack Univ Med Ctr (page 96), New York Eye & Ear Infirm (page 117); **Address:** 130 E 67th St, New York, NY 10065; **Phone:** 212-879-6824; **Board Cert:** Ophthalmology 1991; **Med School:** SUNY Downstate 1984; **Resid:** Ophthalmology, Montefiore Med Ctr 1989; **Fellow:** Oculoplastic & Reconstructive Surgery, LSU Eye Ctr 1990; **Fac Appt:** Assoc Clin Prof Oph, Albert Einstein Coll Med

Lee, Carol M MD (Oph) - **Spec Exp:** Retina/Vitreous Surgery; Diabetic Eye Disease/Retinopathy; Macular Disease/Degeneration; **Hospital:** NYU Langone Med Ctr (page 108); **Address:** 161 Madison Ave, Ste 5NE, New York, NY 10016-5405; **Phone:** 212-684-2424; **Board Cert:** Ophthalmology 1991; **Med School:** SUNY Downstate 1984; **Resid:** Research, Univ Illinois E&E Inst 1986; Ophthalmology, NYU Med Ctr 1989; **Fellow:** Vitreoretinal Surgery & Disease, Washington Univ Barnes Hosp 1991; **Fac Appt:** Clin Prof Oph, NYU Sch Med

Leib, Martin L MD (Oph) - **Spec Exp:** Cataract Surgery; Laser Refractive Surgery; Oculoplastic & Orbital Surgery; Laser Surgery; **Hospital:** NY-Presby/Columbia Univ Med Ctr, NY (page 104), St. Luke's - Roosevelt Hosp Ctr - Roosevelt Div (page 94); **Address:** 635 W 165th St, Ste 230, New York, NY 10032; **Phone:** 212-305-2303; **Board Cert:** Ophthalmology 1982; **Med School:** NY Med Coll 1974; **Resid:** Surgery, Mount Sinai Med Ctr 1976; Ophthalmology, McGill Univ Affil Hosp 1979; **Fellow:** Ophthalmic Plastic Surgery, Columbia-Presby Med Ctr 1980; Orbital Surgery, Columbia-Presby Med Ctr 1980; **Fac Appt:** Clin Prof Oph, Columbia P&S

Liebmann, Jeffrey M MD (Oph) - **Spec Exp:** Glaucoma; Cataract Surgery; **Hospital:** New York Eye & Ear Infirm (page 117), Lenox Hill Hosp (Manh Eye, Ear & Throat Hosp) (page 106); **Address:** Glaucoma Associates of New York, 121 E 60th St Fl 8, New York, NY 10022; **Phone:** 212-477-7540; **Board Cert:** Ophthalmology 1989; **Med School:** Boston Univ 1983; **Resid:** Ophthalmology, SUNY Downstate Med Ctr 1987; **Fellow:** Glaucoma, New York EE Infirmary 1988; **Fac Appt:** Clin Prof Oph, NYU Sch Med

Lisman, Richard D MD (Oph) - **Spec Exp:** Oculoplastic Surgery; Eyelid/Tear Duct Reconstruction; Eyelid Cosmetic & Reconstructive Surgery; Orbital & Eyelid Tumors/Cancer; **Hospital:** NYU Langone Med Ctr (page 108), Lenox Hill Hosp (Manh Eye, Ear & Throat Hosp) (page 106); **Address:** 635 Park Ave, New York, NY 10065-6546; **Phone:** 212-585-1405; **Board Cert:** Ophthalmology 1981; **Med School:** NYU Sch Med 1976; **Resid:** Ophthalmology, Manhattan EE Hosp 1980; **Fellow:** Ophthalmic Plastic Surgery, NY Eye & Ear Infirmary 1981; Plastic Surgery, Manhattan EE&T Hosp 1982; **Fac Appt:** Clin Prof Oph, NYU Sch Med

MacKay, Cynthia J MD (Oph) - **Spec Exp:** Diabetic Eye Disease/Retinopathy; Macular Degeneration; Laser Surgery; Retinitis Pigmentosa; **Hospital:** NY-Presby/Columbia Univ Med Ctr, NY (page 104), Lenox Hill Hosp (Manh Eye, Ear & Throat Hosp) (page 106); **Address:** 315 Central Park West, Ste 1B, New York, NY 10025; **Phone:** 212-772-6050; **Board Cert:** Ophthalmology 1982; **Med School:** SUNY Hlth Sci Ctr 1977; **Resid:** Ophthalmology, Columbia-Presby Med Ctr 1981; **Fellow:** Retina, NYU Med Ctr 1982; **Fac Appt:** Clin Prof Oph, Columbia P&S

Magramm, Irene MD (Oph) - **Spec Exp:** Pediatric Ophthalmology; Strabismus; Cataract Surgery; Diplopia; **Hospital:** Lenox Hill Hosp (Manh Eye, Ear & Throat Hosp) (page 106); **Address:** 220 E 63rd St, Ste LM, New York, NY 10055; **Phone:** 212-644-5100; **Board Cert:** Ophthalmology 1987; **Med School:** Cornell Univ-Weill Med Coll 1981; **Resid:** Ophthalmology, North Shore Univ Hosp 1985; **Fellow:** Pediatric Ophthalmology, Manhattan EE&T Hosp 1986; **Fac Appt:** Asst Clin Prof Oph, Cornell Univ-Weill Med Coll

Maher, Elizabeth MD (Oph) - **Spec Exp:** Orbital Surgery; Oculoplastic Surgery; **Hospital:** New York Eye & Ear Infirm (page 117); **Address:** 36 E 36th St, New York, NY 10016; **Phone:** 212-353-0030; **Board Cert:** Ophthalmology 1989; **Med School:** Harvard Med Sch 1984; **Resid:** Ophthalmology, Manhattan EE&T Hosp 1988; **Fellow:** Ophthalmic Plastic & Reconstructive Surgery, Manhattan EE&T Hosp 1990

Mandel, Eric R MD (Oph) - **Spec Exp:** LASIK-Refractive Surgery; PRK-Refractive Surgery; Corneal Disease; **Hospital:** Lenox Hill Hosp (page 106); **Address:** 211 E 70th St, New York, NY 10021; **Phone:** 212-734-0111; **Board Cert:** Ophthalmology 1988; **Med School:** SUNY Stony Brook 1982; **Resid:** Ophthalmology, Lenox Hill Hosp 1986; **Fellow:** Cornea & Ext Eye Disease, Mass EE Infirm 1987

Mandelbaum, Sidney MD (Oph) - **Spec Exp:** Cataract Surgery; Cornea Transplant; **Hospital:** New York Eye & Ear Infirm (page 117), Long Island Jewish Med Ctr (page 106); **Address:** 178 E 71st St, New York, NY 10021; **Phone:** 212-650-0400; **Board Cert:** Ophthalmology 1982; **Med School:** Yale Univ 1976; **Resid:** Ophthalmology, Los Angeles Chldn's Hosp 1981; **Fellow:** Cornea, Bascom Palmer Eye Inst 1982; **Fac Appt:** Assoc Clin Prof Oph, Albert Einstein Coll Med

McDermott, John A MD (Oph) - **Spec Exp:** Glaucoma; Laser Vision Surgery; **Hospital:** New York Eye & Ear Infirm (page 117); **Address:** 310 E 14th St, New York, NY 10003; **Phone:** 212-979-4446; **Board Cert:** Ophthalmology 1982; **Med School:** NY Med Coll 1976; **Resid:** Ophthalmology, NY Eye & Ear Infirm 1981; Ophthalmology; **Fellow:** Glaucoma, Mass Eye & Ear Infirm 1983; **Fac Appt:** Asst Clin Prof Oph, NY Med Coll

McVeigh, Anne Marie MD (Oph) - ; **Address:** 352 7th Ave, Ste 805, New York, NY 10011; **Phone:** 212-929-3747; **Board Cert:** Ophthalmology 1989; **Med School:** NY Med Coll 1982; **Resid:** Ophthalmology, St Vincent's Hosp & Med Ctr 1986

Melton, R Christine MD (Oph) - **Hospital:** NY-Presby/Weill Cornell Med Ctr, NY (page 104); **Address:** 247 3rd Ave, Ste 202, New York, NY 10010-7454; **Phone:** 212-475-3791; **Board Cert:** Ophthalmology 1982; **Med School:** Canada 1977; **Resid:** Ophthalmology, St Vincent's Hosp & Med Ctr 1981; **Fac Appt:** Asst Clin Prof Oph, Cornell Univ-Weill Med Coll

Merhige, Kenneth E MD (Oph) - **Hospital:** St. Luke's - Roosevelt Hosp Ctr - Roosevelt Div (page 94); **Address:** St Luke's-Roosevelt Hosp Ctr, 1111 Amsterdam Ave, New York, NY 10025; **Phone:** 212-523-2562; **Board Cert:** Ophthalmology 1985; **Med School:** Cornell Univ-Weill Med Coll 1980; **Resid:** Ophthalmology, St Luke's Hosp 1984; **Fellow:** Vitreoretinal Surgery, NY Hosp-Cornell 1985

Merriam, John C MD (Oph) - **Spec Exp:** Cataract Surgery; Reconstructive Surgery; **Hospital:** NY-Presby/Columbia Univ Med Ctr, NY (page 104); **Address:** Edward S Harkness Eye Inst, 635 W 165th St, rm 305, New York, NY 10032-3724; **Phone:** 212-305-5402; **Board Cert:** Ophthalmology 1983; **Med School:** Harvard Med Sch 1977; **Resid:** Plastic Surgery, Brigham-Boston Chldns Hosp 1979; Ophthalmology, Mass Eye & Ear Infirm 1982; **Fellow:** Ophthalmology, UCSF Med Ctr 1983; Ophthalmology, Moorefields Eye Hosp; **Fac Appt:** Clin Prof Oph, Columbia P&S

Mindel, Joel S MD/PhD (Oph) - **Spec Exp:** Neuro-Ophthalmology; **Hospital:** Mount Sinai Med Ctr (page 102), James J. Peters VA Med Ctr-Bronx; **Address:** 17 E 102nd St Fl 8, New York, NY 10029; **Phone:** 212-241-0939; **Board Cert:** Ophthalmology 1970; **Med School:** Univ MD Sch Med 1964; **Resid:** Ophthalmology, Univ Michigan Med Ctr 1969; **Fellow:** Neuro-Ophthalmology, Columbia-Presby Med Ctr 1966; Ocular Pharmacology, Mount Sinai Med Ctr 1973; **Fac Appt:** Prof Oph, Mount Sinai Sch Med

Mitchell, John P MD (Oph) - **Spec Exp:** Neuro-Ophthalmology; Cataract Surgery; Glaucoma; **Hospital:** NY-Presby/Columbia Univ Med Ctr, NY (page 104); **Address:** 147 W 142 St, New York, NY 10030; **Phone:** 212-281-8400; **Board Cert:** Ophthalmology 1978; **Med School:** Cornell Univ-Weill Med Coll 1973; **Resid:** Ophthalmology, Harlem Hosp 1977; **Fellow:** Neuro-Ophthalmology, Columbia-Presby Med Ctr 1978; **Fac Appt:** Asst Prof Oph, Columbia P&S

Moazed, Kambiz T MD (Oph) - **Spec Exp:** Cataract Surgery; Eyelid/Tear Duct Reconstruction; **Hospital:** St. Luke's - Roosevelt Hosp Ctr - Roosevelt Div (page 94); **Address:** Manhattan's Physician Group, 4337 Broadway, New York, NY 10033; **Phone:** 212-712-1000; **Board Cert:** Ophthalmology 1983; **Med School:** Iran 1973; **Resid:** Ophthalmology, Mass EE Infirm 1982; **Fellow:** Eye Pathology, Stanford Univ Med Ctr 1977; Oculoplastic Surgery, Edward Harkness Eye Inst 1983; **Fac Appt:** Asst Clin Prof Oph, Columbia P&S

Moskowitz, Bruce K MD (Oph) - **Spec Exp:** Oculoplastic Surgery; Reconstructive Surgery; **Hospital:** New York Eye & Ear Infirm (page 117); **Address:** 310 E 14th St, Ste 401, New York, NY 10003; **Phone:** 212-979-4586; **Board Cert:** Ophthalmology 2012; **Med School:** SUNY Downstate 1987; **Resid:** Ophthalmology, SUNY Downstate 1991; **Fellow:** Ophthalmology, Kingsbrook Jewish Med Ctr 1992; **Fac Appt:** Asst Clin Prof Oph, NY Med Coll

Muchnick, Richard S MD (Oph) - **Spec Exp:** Pediatric Ophthalmology; Strabismus; **Hospital:** NY-Presby/Weill Cornell Med Ctr, NY (page 104), Lenox Hill Hosp (page 106); **Address:** 69 E 71st St, New York, NY 10021-4213; **Phone:** 212-744-1726; **Board Cert:** Ophthalmology 1975; **Med School:** Cornell Univ-Weill Med Coll 1967; **Resid:** Ophthalmology, NY Hosp 1973; **Fellow:** Ophthalmic Plastic Surgery, UCSF Med Ctr 1974; Pediatric Ophthalmology, Manhattan EE&T Hosp 1975; **Fac Appt:** Clin Prof Oph, Cornell Univ-Weill Med Coll

Muldoon, Thomas O MD (Oph) - **Spec Exp:** Retina/Vitreous Surgery; Macular Disease/Degeneration; Diabetic Eye Disease/Retinopathy; **Hospital:** New York Eye & Ear Infirm (page 117); **Address:** 310 E 14th St, Ste 402, New York, NY 10003-4201; **Phone:** 212-979-4595; **Board Cert:** Ophthalmology 1971; **Med School:** Univ Rochester 1962; **Resid:** Surgery, St Lukes Hosp 1966; Ophthalmology, NY EE Infirm 1969; **Fellow:** Retinal Surgery, NY EE Infirm 1970; **Fac Appt:** Assoc Clin Prof Oph, NY Med Coll

Newton, Michael MD (Oph) - **Spec Exp:** Cornea & Cataract Surgery; Refractive Surgery; Eye Infections; **Hospital:** New York Eye & Ear Infirm (page 117), Mount Sinai Med Ctr (page 102); **Address:** 799 Park Ave, New York, NY 10021-3275; **Phone:** 212-861-0146; **Board Cert:** Ophthalmology 1978; **Med School:** Tufts Univ 1971; **Resid:** Ophthalmology, Mount Sinai Hosp 1977; **Fellow:** Cornea & Ext Eye Disease, AB Nesburn MD 1978; **Fac Appt:** Assoc Clin Prof Oph, Mount Sinai Sch Med

Nightingale, Jeffrey MD (Oph) - **Spec Exp:** LASIK-Refractive Surgery; Cataract Surgery; **Hospital:** New York Eye & Ear Infirm (page 117); **Address:** 211 Central Park West, New York, NY 10024-6020; **Phone:** 212-877-7188; **Board Cert:** Ophthalmology 1977; **Med School:** SUNY Hlth Sci Ctr 1972; **Resid:** Ophthalmology, Bronx Lebanon Hosp 1976; **Fellow:** Oculoplastic Surgery, NY Eye & Ear Infirmary 1977

Obstbaum, Stephen A MD (Oph) - **Spec Exp:** Cataract Surgery; Glaucoma; **Hospital:** Lenox Hill Hosp (page 106), Lenox Hill Hosp (Manh Eye, Ear & Throat Hosp) (page 106); **Address:** 121 E 60th St Fl 2, New York, NY 10022; **Phone:** 212-477-7540; **Board Cert:** Ophthalmology 1974; **Med School:** NY Med Coll 1967; **Resid:** Ophthalmology, Flower Fifth Ave Hosp 1972; **Fellow:** Glaucoma, Washington Univ 1973; **Fac Appt:** Prof Oph, NYU Sch Med

Odel, Jeffrey G MD (Oph) - **Spec Exp:** Neuro-Ophthalmology; Retinal Disorders; Optic Nerve Disorders; **Hospital:** NY-Presby/Columbia Univ Med Ctr, NY (page 104); **Address:** Harkness Eye Institute, 635 W 165th St, rm 316, New York, NY 10032-3701; **Phone:** 212-305-5415; **Board Cert:** Ophthalmology 1981; **Med School:** Univ Rochester 1975; **Resid:** Ophthalmology, Mt Sinai Hosp 1981; **Fellow:** Ophthalmology, Bascom-Palmer Eye Inst 1977; Ophthalmology, Columbia Presby Med Ctr 1982; **Fac Appt:** Assoc Clin Prof Oph, Columbia P&S

Paccione, Jeffrey C MD (Oph) - **Spec Exp:** Retinal Disorders; Macular Degeneration; **Hospital:** Lenox Hill Hosp (Manh Eye, Ear & Throat Hosp) (page 106), New York Eye & Ear Infirm (page 117); **Address:** Retina Associates of New York, 140 E 80th St, New York, NY 10075; **Phone:** 212-772-0600; **Board Cert:** Ophthalmology 2010; **Med School:** Columbia P&S 1989; **Resid:** Ophthalmology, Manhattan EE&T Hosp 1992; **Fellow:** Vitreoretinal Disease, Mt Sinai Med Ctr 1998; **Fac Appt:** Assoc Clin Prof Oph, Mount Sinai Sch Med

Prince, Andrew MD (Oph) - **Spec Exp:** Glaucoma; Cataract Surgery; **Hospital:** New York Eye & Ear Infirm (page 117), Lenox Hill Hosp (Manh Eye, Ear & Throat Hosp) (page 106); **Address:** 178 E 71st St, New York, NY 10021-5119; **Phone:** 212-717-2200; **Board Cert:** Ophthalmology 1987; **Med School:** SUNY Downstate 1981; **Resid:** Ophthalmology, SUNY Downstate Med Ctr 1985; **Fellow:** Glaucoma, NY Eye & Ear Infirmary 1986; **Fac Appt:** Assoc Prof Oph, NYU Sch Med

Raab, Edward L MD (Oph) - **Spec Exp:** Pediatric Ophthalmology; Strabismus-Adult & Pediatric; Glaucoma-Pediatric; **Hospital:** Mount Sinai Med Ctr (page 102); **Address:** 17 E 102nd St W Fl 8th, New York, NY 10029-6501; **Phone:** 212-369-0988; **Board Cert:** Ophthalmology 1966; **Med School:** NYU Sch Med 1958; **Resid:** Ophthalmology, Mount Sinai 1964; **Fellow:** Pediatric Ophthalmology, Chldns Natl Med Ctr 1967; **Fac Appt:** Prof Oph, Mount Sinai Sch Med

Relland, Maureen MD (Oph) - **Spec Exp:** Oculoplastic Surgery; Eyelid Cosmetic Surgery; Cataract Surgery; **Hospital:** New York Eye & Ear Infirm (page 117); **Address:** 352 7th Ave, Ste 805, New York, NY 10001; **Phone:** 212-645-7771; **Board Cert:** Ophthalmology 1971; **Med School:** NY Med Coll 1964; **Resid:** Ophthalmology, St Vincent's Hosp & Med Ctr 1968; **Fac Appt:** Asst Clin Prof Oph, NY Med Coll

Ritch, Robert MD (Oph) - **Spec Exp:** Glaucoma; Complementary Medicine; **Hospital:** New York Eye & Ear Infirm (page 117); **Address:** 310 E 14th St, South Bldg - Fl 3, New York, NY 10003-4201; **Phone:** 212-477-7540; **Board Cert:** Ophthalmology 1977; **Med School:** Albert Einstein Coll Med 1972; **Resid:** Ophthalmology, Mt Sinai Hosp 1976; **Fellow:** Glaucoma, Mt Sinai Hosp 1978; **Fac Appt:** Prof Oph, NY Med Coll

Ritterband, David MD (Oph) - **Spec Exp:** Eye Infections; Corneal Disease; Refractive Surgery; **Hospital:** New York Eye & Ear Infirm (page 117); **Address:** 310 E 14th St, South Bldg Fl 2, New York, NY 10003-4201; **Phone:** 212-979-4428; **Board Cert:** Ophthalmology 2006; **Med School:** NY Med Coll 1990; **Resid:** Ophthalmology, NY Med Coll 1994; **Fellow:** Cornea & Ext Eye Disease, Eye & Ear Inst 1995

Rodgers, I Rand MD (Oph) - **Spec Exp:** Oculoplastic Surgery; Eyelid Cosmetic & Reconstructive Surgery; Eyelid/Tear Duct Disorders; **Hospital:** Mount Sinai Med Ctr (page 102), N Shore Univ Hosp (page 106); **Address:** 229 E 79 St, New York, NY 10075; **Phone:** 212-249-7600; **Board Cert:** Ophthalmology 1989; **Med School:** Mount Sinai Sch Med 1983; **Resid:** Surgery, Mt Sinai Med Ctr 1984; Ophthalmology, Mt Sinai Med Ctr 1987; **Fellow:** Ocular Oncology, Manhattan EET Hosp 1988; Ophthalmic Plastic Surgery, Mass E&E Infirm 1990; **Fac Appt:** Asst Clin Prof Oph, Mount Sinai Sch Med

Rodriguez-Sains, Rene S MD (Oph) - **Spec Exp:** Eyelid Cosmetic & Reconstructive Surgery; Eyelid Tumors/Cancer; Melanoma; Eye Tumors/Cancer; **Hospital:** New York Eye & Ear Infirm (page 117), NYU Langone Med Ctr (page 108); **Address:** 799 Park Ave, New York, NY 10021-3275; **Phone:** 212-535-0315; **Board Cert:** Ophthalmology 1982; **Med School:** NYU Sch Med 1977; **Resid:** Ophthalmology, Manhattan EET Hosp 1981; **Fellow:** Plastic Surgery, Manhattan EET Hosp 1982; Ophthalmic Oncololgy, Manhattan EET Hosp 1982; **Fac Appt:** Asst Clin Prof Oph, NYU Sch Med

Rosenthal, Jeanne L MD (Oph) - **Spec Exp:** Retina/Vitreous Surgery; Macular Degeneration; Diabetic Eye Disease/Retinopathy; **Hospital:** New York Eye & Ear Infirm (page 117); **Address:** 20 E 9th St, New York, NY 10003-5944; **Phone:** 212-674-2970; **Board Cert:** Ophthalmology 1985; **Med School:** SUNY Downstate 1979; **Resid:** Ophthalmology, NY Eye & Ear Infirm 1983; **Fellow:** Retina, NY Eye & Ear Infirm 1985; **Fac Appt:** Clin Prof Oph, NY Med Coll

Rudick Jr, A Joseph MD (Oph) - **Spec Exp:** LASIK-Refractive Surgery; Cataract Surgery; Glaucoma; Dry Eye Syndrome; **Hospital:** New York Eye & Ear Infirm (page 117), NY Downtown Hosp; **Address:** 150 Broadway, Fl 14, Ste 1401, MS 10038, New York, NY 10038; **Phone:** 212-233-2344; **Board Cert:** Ophthalmology 1989; **Med School:** Univ Pennsylvania 1983; **Resid:** Ophthalmology, Manhattan EE&T Hosp 1988

Samson, C Michael MD (Oph) - **Spec Exp:** Uveitis; Immunotherapy; Eye Infections; **Hospital:** New York Eye & Ear Infirm (page 117); **Address:** 310 E 14th St, Ste 319 S, New York, NY 10003; **Phone:** 212-979-4515; **Board Cert:** Ophthalmology 2011; **Med School:** SUNY Downstate 1994; **Resid:** Ophthalmology, NY Eye & Ear Infirm 1998; **Fellow:** Ophthalmology, Mass Eye & Ear Infirm 1999

Schiff, William M MD (Oph) - **Spec Exp:** Macular Disease/Degeneration; Diabetic Eye Disease/Retinopathy; Retinal Detachment; Macular Disease/Degeneration; **Hospital:** Lenox Hill Hosp (Manh Eye, Ear & Throat Hosp) (page 106), St. Luke's - Roosevelt Hosp Ctr - Roosevelt Div (page 94); **Address:** 210 E 64th New York, NY 10065 St, Fl 7, New York, NY 10068; **Phone:** 212-702-7400; **Board Cert:** Ophthalmology 2006; **Med School:** NYU Sch Med 1988; **Resid:** Ophthalmology, New York Eye & Ear Infirm 1994; **Fellow:** Retina/Vitreous, NY Hosp-Harkness Eye Inst 1996; **Fac Appt:** Prof Oph, Columbia P&S

Schubert, Hermann D MD (Oph) - **Spec Exp:** Diabetic Eye Disease/Retinopathy; Macular Degeneration; Retinal Disorders; Retinal Detachment; **Hospital:** NY-Presby/Columbia Univ Med Ctr, NY (page 104); **Address:** 635 W 165th St, Rm 206, New York, NY 10032-3701; **Phone:** 212-305-6534; **Board Cert:** Ophthalmology 1987; Anatomic Pathology 1981; **Med School:** Germany 1974; **Resid:** Pathology, Columbia-Presby Hosp 1979; Ophthalmology, Columbia-Presby Hosp 1985; **Fellow:** Retina, Wills Eye Hosp 1987; **Fac Appt:** Prof Oph, Columbia P&S

Schwarcz, Robert M MD (Oph) - **Spec Exp:** Oculoplastic Surgery; Cosmetic Surgery-Face; Reconstructive Surgery-Face; **Hospital:** Montefiore Med Ctr-Wakefield Campus, NY (page 100), New York Eye & Ear Infirm (page 117); **Address:** 135 E 71st St, New York, NY 10021; **Phone:** 212-396-4400; **Board Cert:** Ophthalmology 2006; **Med School:** Howard Univ 1999; **Resid:** Internal Medicine, St Luke's Roosevelt Hosp 2000; Ophthalmology, SUNY Hlth Sci Ctr 2003; **Fellow:** Facial Plastic & Reconstr Surgery, Jules Stein Eye Inst 2004; Oculoplastic Surgery, Jules Stein Eye Inst 2005; **Fac Appt:** Assoc Prof Oph, Albert Einstein Coll Med

Seedor, John A MD (Oph) - **Spec Exp:** Cornea & External Eye Disease; Laser Vision Surgery; **Hospital:** New York Eye & Ear Infirm (page 117); **Address:** 310 E 14th St, Ste 219, New York, NY 10003-4201; **Phone:** 212-979-4428; **Board Cert:** Ophthalmology 1987; **Med School:** Hahnemann Univ 1981; **Resid:** Ophthalmology, NY Eye & Ear Infirm 1985; **Fellow:** Cornea, Emory Univ Hosp 1987; **Fac Appt:** Assoc Clin Prof Oph, NY Med Coll

Serle, Janet B MD (Oph) - **Spec Exp:** Glaucoma; **Hospital:** Mount Sinai Med Ctr (page 102), Syosset Hosp (page 106); **Address:** 17 E 102 St, 8th Fl, Box 1183, New York, NY 10029; **Phone:** 212-241-0939; **Board Cert:** Ophthalmology 1987; **Med School:** Harvard Med Sch 1980; **Resid:** Ophthalmology, Mount Sinai Hosp 1985; **Fellow:** Glaucoma, Mount Sinai Hosp 1982; Glaucoma, Mount Sinai Hosp 1986; **Fac Appt:** Prof Oph, Mount Sinai Sch Med

Shabto, Uri MD (Oph) - **Spec Exp:** Retinopathy of Prematurity; Macular Disease/Degeneration; Diabetic Eye Disease/Retinopathy; Retinal Detachment; **Hospital:** New York Eye & Ear Infirm (page 117); **Address:** 310 E 14th St, South Bldg, Ste 419, New York, NY 10003-4201; **Phone:** 212-677-2000; **Board Cert:** Ophthalmology 1991; **Med School:** Harvard Med Sch 1986; **Resid:** Ophthalmology, NY Eye & Ear Infirm 1990; **Fellow:** Vitreoretinal Surgery, Montefiore Hosp 1991; **Fac Appt:** Asst Clin Prof Oph, NY Med Coll

Sherman, Spencer E MD (Oph) - **Spec Exp:** Cataract Surgery; Glaucoma; Contact Lenses; Refractive Surgery; **Hospital:** Lenox Hill Hosp (Manh Eye, Ear & Throat Hosp) (page 106), Mount Sinai Med Ctr (page 102); **Address:** 166 E 63rd St, New York, NY 10065; **Phone:** 212-753-8300; **Board Cert:** Ophthalmology 1970; **Med School:** Columbia P&S 1962; **Resid:** Ophthalmology, Mt Sinai Hosp 1968; **Fac Appt:** Asst Clin Prof Oph, Mount Sinai Sch Med

Shulman, Julius MD (Oph) - **Spec Exp:** Cataract Surgery; LASIK-Refractive Surgery; Contact Lenses; Glaucoma; **Hospital:** Mount Sinai Med Ctr (page 102); **Address:** 229 E 79th St, New York, NY 10075; **Phone:** 212-861-6200; **Board Cert:** Ophthalmology 2006; **Med School:** SUNY Hlth Sci Ctr 1969; **Resid:** Ophthalmology, Mt Sinai Med Ctr 1975; **Fac Appt:** Asst Clin Prof Oph, Mount Sinai Sch Med

Sidoti, Paul MD (Oph) - **Spec Exp:** Glaucoma; **Hospital:** New York Eye & Ear Infirm (page 117), Beth Israel Med Ctr - Petrie Division (page 94); **Address:** New York Eye & Ear Infirmary, 310 E 14th St, Ste 319, New York, NY 10003-4201; **Phone:** 212-979-4590; **Board Cert:** Ophthalmology 2005; **Med School:** Albert Einstein Coll Med 1988; **Resid:** Ophthalmology, NY Eye & Ear Infirm 1992; **Fellow:** Glaucoma, Doheny Eye Inst-USC 1994; **Fac Appt:** Prof Oph, NY Med Coll

Slakter, Jason MD (Oph) - **Spec Exp:** Retinal Disorders; Macular Degeneration; **Hospital:** Lenox Hill Hosp (Manh Eye, Ear & Throat Hosp) (page 106); **Address:** 460 Park Ave Fl 5, New York, NY 10022; **Phone:** 212-861-9797; **Board Cert:** Ophthalmology 1989; **Med School:** Albert Einstein Coll Med 1983; **Resid:** Ophthalmology, Manhattan Eye & Ear Infirm 1987; **Fellow:** Retina/Vitreous, Manhattan Eye & Ear Infirm 1988; **Fac Appt:** Clin Prof Oph, NYU Sch Med

Solomon, Joel M MD (Oph) - **Spec Exp:** Cornea & Cataract Surgery; Refractive Surgery; **Hospital:** NYU Langone Med Ctr (page 108), Bellevue Hosp Ctr; **Address:** 614 2nd Ave, Ste C, New York, NY 10016; **Phone:** 212-689-5080; **Board Cert:** Ophthalmology 1987; **Med School:** Cornell Univ-Weill Med Coll 1981; **Resid:** Internal Medicine, Albany Med Ctr 1983; Ophthalmology, NYU Med Ctr 1986; **Fellow:** Cornea & Ext Eye Disease, Med Coll Wisc 1987; **Fac Appt:** Clin Prof Oph, NYU Sch Med

Spaide, Richard MD (Oph) - **Spec Exp:** Retinal Disorders; Macular Degeneration; Diabetic Eye Disease/Retinopathy; **Hospital:** Lenox Hill Hosp (Manh Eye, Ear & Throat Hosp) (page 106); **Address:** 460 Park Ave Fl 5, New York, NY 10022; **Phone:** 212-861-9797; **Board Cert:** Ophthalmology 1987; **Med School:** Jefferson Med Coll 1981; **Resid:** Ophthalmology, St Vincent's Hosp & Med Ctr 1985; **Fellow:** Vitreoretinal Surgery & Disease, Manhattan EET Hosp 1990; **Fac Appt:** Assoc Clin Prof Oph, NY Med Coll

Starr, Michael B MD (Oph) - **Spec Exp:** LASIK-Refractive Surgery; Cornea & Cataract Surgery; Eye Infections; **Hospital:** Lenox Hill Hosp (page 106), Lenox Hill Hosp (Manh Eye, Ear & Throat Hosp) (page 106); **Address:** 67 E 78th St, New York, NY 10075; **Phone:** 212-717-0222; **Board Cert:** Ophthalmology 1978; **Med School:** Mount Sinai Sch Med 1972; **Resid:** Neurology, Mount Sinai 1974; Ophthalmology, Lenox Hill Hosp 1977; **Fellow:** Cornea, UCSF Med Ctr/ Francis Proctor Fdn 1979; **Fac Appt:** Assoc Clin Prof Oph, Mount Sinai Sch Med

Steele, Mark MD (Oph) - **Spec Exp:** Pediatric Ophthalmology; Strabismus; Eye Muscle Disorders; **Hospital:** NYU Langone Med Ctr (page 108), New York Eye & Ear Infirm (page 117); **Address:** 40 W 72nd St, New York, NY 10023; **Phone:** 212-981-9800; **Board Cert:** Ophthalmology 1991; **Med School:** NYU Sch Med 1986; **Resid:** Ophthalmology, NYU Med Ctr 1990; **Fellow:** Pediatric Ophthalmology, Wills Eye Hosp 1991; **Fac Appt:** Assoc Clin Prof Oph, NYU Sch Med

Tello, Celso MD (Oph) - **Spec Exp:** Glaucoma; **Hospital:** New York Eye & Ear Infirm (page 117); **Address:** 310 E 14th St, Ste 304, New York, NY 10003; **Phone:** 212-477-7540; **Board Cert:** Ophthalmology 2011; **Med School:** Ecuador 1988; **Resid:** Ophthalmology, NY Eye & Ear Infirm 1993; **Fellow:** Glaucoma, NY Eye & Ear Infirm 1994; **Fac Appt:** Asst Prof Oph, NYU Sch Med

Walsh, Joseph B MD (Oph) - **Spec Exp:** Diabetic Eye Disease/Retinopathy; Macular Degeneration; Retinal Disorders; **Hospital:** New York Eye & Ear Infirm (page 117); **Address:** 310 E 14th St S Bldg Fl 3 - Ste 319, New York, NY 10003-4201; **Phone:** 212-979-4282; **Board Cert:** Ophthalmology 2005; **Med School:** Georgetown Univ 1966; **Resid:** Internal Medicine, Univ Hosp 1968; Ophthalmology, NY Eye & Ear Infirm 1973; **Fellow:** Retina, Montefiore Med Ctr 1974; **Fac Appt:** Prof Oph, NY Med Coll

Wang, Frederick Mark MD (Oph) - **Spec Exp:** Pediatric Ophthalmology; Strabismus; Eye Muscle Disorders; **Hospital:** Lenox Hill Hosp (Manh Eye, Ear & Throat Hosp) (page 106), Montefiore Med Ctr-Moses Campus, NY (page 100); **Address:** 30 E 40th St, Ste 405, New York, NY 10016-1201; **Phone:** 212-684-3980; **Board Cert:** Pediatrics 1978; Ophthalmology 1980; **Med School:** Albert Einstein Coll Med 1972; **Resid:** Pediatrics, Jacobi Med Ctr 1974; Ophthalmology, Albert Einstein 1979; **Fellow:** Pediatric Ophthalmology, Children's Hosp Natl Med Ctr 1980; **Fac Appt:** Clin Prof Oph, Albert Einstein Coll Med

Warren, Floyd A MD (Oph) - **Spec Exp:** Neuro-Ophthalmology; Optic Nerve Disorders; Orbital Diseases; **Hospital:** NYU Langone Med Ctr (page 108), Lenox Hill Hosp (Manh Eye, Ear & Throat Hosp) (page 106); **Address:** Schwartz Health Care Ctr, 530 First Ave, Ste 3B, New York, NY 10016; **Phone:** 212-263-7030; **Board Cert:** Ophthalmology 1985; **Med School:** NYU Sch Med 1979; **Resid:** Ophthalmology, St Vincents Hosp 1983; **Fellow:** Neuro-Ophthalmology, Bellevue Hosp 1984; Orbital Disease, Univ Pittsburgh 1985; **Fac Appt:** Clin Prof Oph, NYU Sch Med

Weiss, Michael J MD/PhD (Oph) - **Spec Exp:** Uveitis; Retinal Disorders; Cataract Surgery; **Hospital:** NY-Presby/Columbia Univ Med Ctr, NY (page 104); **Address:** 635 W 165th St, Ste 101, New York, NY 10032-3701; **Phone:** 212-305-9925; **Board Cert:** Ophthalmology 1987; **Med School:** Columbia P&S 1981; **Resid:** Ophthalmology, Columbia-Presby Med Ctr 1985; **Fac Appt:** Clin Prof Oph, Columbia P&S

Weseley, Peter E MD (Oph) - **Spec Exp:** Retina/Vitreous Surgery; **Hospital:** New York Eye & Ear Infirm (page 117); **Address:** 310 E 14th St, Ste 419, New York, NY 10003; **Phone:** 212-979-4286; **Board Cert:** Ophthalmology 2003; **Med School:** Tulane Univ 1987; **Resid:** Ophthalmology, NY E&E Infirm 1991; **Fellow:** Vitreoretinal Surgery, Devers Eye Inst 1993

Whitmore, Wayne G MD (Oph) - **Spec Exp:** Cataract Surgery; Glaucoma; Corneal Disease; **Hospital:** NY-Presby/Weill Cornell Med Ctr, NY (page 104), Lenox Hill Hosp (Manh Eye, Ear & Throat Hosp) (page 106); **Address:** 116 E 68th St, New York, NY 10065; **Phone:** 212-249-3030; **Board Cert:** Ophthalmology 1982; **Med School:** Dartmouth Med Sch 1977; **Resid:** Ophthalmology, NY Hosp 1981; **Fellow:** Ophthalmic Oncololgy, NY Hosp 1982; **Fac Appt:** Asst Clin Prof Oph, Cornell Univ-Weill Med Coll

Wisnicki, H Jay MD (Oph) - **Spec Exp:** Strabismus; Eye Muscle Disorders; Pediatric Ophthalmology; **Hospital:** Beth Israel Med Ctr - Petrie Division (page 94), New York Eye & Ear Infirm (page 117); **Address:** Union Square Eye Care, 235 Park Ave S Fl 2, New York, NY 10003; **Phone:** 212-844-2020; **Board Cert:** Ophthalmology 1987; **Med School:** SUNY Hlth Sci Ctr 1981; **Resid:** Ophthalmology, Mount Sinai Med Ctr 1985; **Fellow:** Strabismus, Johns Hopkins Hosp 1986; **Fac Appt:** Prof Oph, Albert Einstein Coll Med

Wong, Raymond F MD (Oph) - **Spec Exp:** Diabetic Eye Disease/Retinopathy; Retinal Detachment; Macular Disease/Degeneration; **Hospital:** New York Eye & Ear Infirm (page 117); **Address:** 210 Canal St, rm 409, New York, NY 10013-4159; **Phone:** 212-227-5451; **Board Cert:** Ophthalmology 1990; **Med School:** SUNY Hlth Sci Ctr 1984; **Resid:** Ophthalmology, Yale-New Haven Hosp 1988; **Fellow:** Retina, USC-Doheny Eye Inst 1990; **Fac Appt:** Asst Clin Prof Oph, NY Med Coll

Yagoda, Arnold D MD (Oph) - **Spec Exp:** Macular Degeneration; Laser Vision Surgery; Diabetic Eye Disease/Retinopathy; **Hospital:** Lenox Hill Hosp (page 106), New York Eye & Ear Infirm (page 117); **Address:** 67 E 78th St, New York, NY 10075; **Phone:** 212-744-2513; **Board Cert:** Ophthalmology 1980; **Med School:** Cornell Univ-Weill Med Coll 1975; **Resid:** Ophthalmology, Lenox Hill Hosp 1979; **Fellow:** Vitreoretinal Disease, Montefiore Hosp Med Ctr 1980; **Fac Appt:** Asst Clin Prof Oph, Albert Einstein Coll Med

Yannuzzi, Lawrence MD (Oph) - **Spec Exp:** Retina/Vitreous Surgery; Macular Disease/Degeneration; Diabetic Eye Disease/Retinopathy; **Hospital:** NY-Presby/Columbia Univ Med Ctr, NY (page 104), Lenox Hill Hosp (Manh Eye, Ear & Throat Hosp) (page 106); **Address:** Vitreous-Retina-Macula Consultants of NY, 460 Park Ave Fl 5, New York, NY 10022; **Phone:** 212-861-9797; **Board Cert:** Ophthalmology 1970; **Med School:** Boston Univ 1964; **Resid:** Ophthalmology, Manhattan EE&T Hosp 1968; **Fellow:** Ophthalmology, Manhattan EE&T Hosp 1971; **Fac Appt:** Clin Prof Oph, Columbia P&S

Young, Joshua A MD (Oph) - **Spec Exp:** Cataract Surgery; PRK-Refractive Surgery; Contact Lenses; **Hospital:** NYU Langone Med Ctr (page 108), Lenox Hill Hosp (Manh Eye, Ear & Throat Hosp) (page 106); **Address:** 161 Madison Ave, Ste 5 SE, New York, NY 10016; **Phone:** 212-448-0101; **Board Cert:** Ophthalmology 2008; **Med School:** NYU Sch Med 1990; **Resid:** Ophthalmology, NYU Med Ctr 1994; **Fellow:** Ophthalmology, Mass Eye & Ear Infirm/Harvard 1996; **Fac Appt:** Clin Prof Oph, NYU Sch Med

Zweifach, Philip H MD (Oph) - **Spec Exp:** Cataract Surgery; Neuro-Ophthalmology; Glaucoma; **Hospital:** NY-Presby/Weill Cornell Med Ctr, NY (page 104); **Address:** 131 E 69th St, New York, NY 10021-5158; **Phone:** 212-535-1508; **Board Cert:** Ophthalmology 1968; **Med School:** Cornell Univ-Weill Med Coll 1961; **Resid:** Neurology, Boston City Hosp 1963; Ophthalmology, New York Hosp 1966; **Fellow:** Neuro-Ophthalmology, Mass Eye & Ear Infirmary 1967; **Fac Appt:** Clin Prof Oph, Cornell Univ-Weill Med Coll

Orthopaedic Surgery

Adler, Edward MD (OrS) - **Spec Exp:** Hip Replacement; Knee Replacement; Foot & Ankle Surgery; **Hospital:** NYU Hosp For Joint Diseases (page 119), NYU Langone Med Ctr (page 108); **Address:** 145 E 32nd St Fl 4, New York, NY 10016; **Phone:** 212-427-3986; **Board Cert:** Orthopaedic Surgery 2012; **Med School:** UMDNJ-NJ Med Sch, Newark 1984; **Resid:** Orthopaedic Surgery, UMDNJ-NJ Sch Med 1989; **Fellow:** Joint Replacement Surgery, Hosp for Joint Dis 1990; **Fac Appt:** Asst Clin Prof OrS, NYU Sch Med

Ahmad, Christopher S MD (OrS) - **Spec Exp:** Sports Medicine; Knee Injuries/ACL; **Hospital:** NY-Presby/Columbia Univ Med Ctr, NY (page 104); **Address:** 161 Fort Washington Ave, Fl 2, New York, NY 10032; **Phone:** 212-305-4565; **Board Cert:** Orthopaedic Surgery 2003; Orthopaedic Sports Medicine 2007; **Med School:** NYU Sch Med 1994; **Resid:** Orthopaedic Surgery, NY Orthopaedic Hosp/Columbia 2000; **Fellow:** Sports Medicine, Kerlan-Jobe Orthopaedic Clinic 2001; **Fac Appt:** Assoc Prof OrS, Columbia P&S

Alexiades, Michael M MD (OrS) - **Spec Exp:** Hip Replacement; Knee Replacement; Arthroscopic Surgery; Minimally Invasive Surgery; **Hospital:** Lenox Hill Hosp (page 106), Hosp For Special Surgery (page 115); **Address:** 523 E 72nd St Fl 7, New York, NY 10021; **Phone:** 212-774-7557; **Board Cert:** Orthopaedic Surgery 2002; **Med School:** Cornell Univ-Weill Med Coll 1983; **Resid:** Orthopaedic Surgery, Lenox Hill Hosp 1988; Surgery, Children's Hosp 1986; **Fellow:** Arthritis Surgery, Hosp for Special Surgery 1989; **Fac Appt:** Asst Prof OrS, Cornell Univ-Weill Med Coll

Bauman, Phillip A MD (OrS) - **Spec Exp:** Foot & Ankle Surgery; Knee Surgery; Dance/Sports Medicine; Arthroscopic Surgery; **Hospital:** St. Luke's - Roosevelt Hosp Ctr - Roosevelt Div (page 94), NY-Presby/Columbia Univ Med Ctr, NY (page 104); **Address:** Orthopaedic Associates of NY, 343 W 58th St, Ste 1, New York, NY 10019; **Phone:** 212-506-0228; **Board Cert:** Orthopaedic Surgery 2011; **Med School:** Columbia P&S 1981; **Resid:** Surgery, St Lukes-Roosevelt Hosp Ctr 1983; Orthopaedic Surgery, Columbia-Presby Med Ctr 1987; **Fac Appt:** Asst Prof OrS, Columbia P&S

Bendo, John A MD (OrS) - **Spec Exp:** Spinal Surgery-Minimally Invasive; Scoliosis; Spinal Disc Replacement; **Hospital:** NYU Hosp For Joint Diseases (page 119), NYU Langone Med Ctr (page 108); **Address:** Hosp for Joint Diseases-Spine Ctr, 301 E 17th St, Ste 400, New York, NY 10003; **Phone:** 212-598-6625; **Board Cert:** Orthopaedic Surgery 2008; **Med School:** Mount Sinai Sch Med 1989; **Resid:** Orthopaedic Surgery, Mt Sinai Hosp 1994; **Fellow:** Spinal Surgery, Hosp Joint Diseases 1996; **Fac Appt:** Asst Prof OrS, NYU Sch Med

Bigliani, Louis U MD (OrS) - **Spec Exp:** Shoulder Surgery; Sports Medicine; Arthroscopic Surgery; Rotator Cuff Surgery; **Hospital:** NY-Presby/Columbia Univ Med Ctr, NY (page 104); **Address:** 622 W 168th St, rm 1130, New York, NY 10032-3720; **Phone:** 212-305-0998; **Board Cert:** Orthopaedic Surgery 1994; **Med School:** Loyola Univ-Stritch Sch Med 1973; **Resid:** Surgery, Roosevelt Hosp 1974; Orthopaedic Surgery, Columbia Presby Med Ctr 1977; **Fac Appt:** Prof OrS, Columbia P&S

Bitan, Fabien D MD (OrS) - **Spec Exp:** Spinal Surgery-Pediatric & Adult; Spinal Disc Replacement; Spinal Deformity; Spinal Disorders-Degenerative; **Hospital:** Lenox Hill Hosp (page 106), Beth Israel Med Ctr - Petrie Division (page 94); **Address:** 130 E 77th St, Fl 7, New York, NY 10075; **Phone:** 212-744-8114; **Med School:** France 1981; **Resid:** Orthopaedic Surgery, Hospital Beaujon 1987; Pediatric Orthopaedic Surgery, Hosp des Enfants Malades 1990; **Fellow:** Pediatric Orthopaedic Surgery, Hosp Special Surgery 1997; Spinal Surgery, Beth Israel Med Ctr 1998

Boachie-Adjei, Oheneba MD (OrS) - **Spec Exp:** Spinal Surgery; Scoliosis; **Hospital:** Hosp For Special Surgery (page 115); **Address:** Hosp for Special Surgery, 535 E 70th St, New York, NY 10021; **Phone:** 212-606-1948; **Board Cert:** Orthopaedic Surgery 2010; **Med School:** Columbia P&S 1980; **Resid:** Surgery, St Vincents Hosp 1982; Orthopaedic Surgery, Hosp Spec Surg 1986; **Fellow:** Orthopaedic Pathology, Hosp Spec Surg 1983; Spinal Surgery, Twin Cities Scoliosis Ctr/Minn Spine Ctr 1987; **Fac Appt:** Assoc Clin Prof S, Cornell Univ-Weill Med Coll

Bosco, Joseph MD (OrS) - **Spec Exp:** Sports Medicine; Knee Surgery; Shoulder Surgery; **Hospital:** NYU Hosp For Joint Diseases (page 119), Jamaica Hosp Med Ctr; **Address:** 333 E 38th St, New York, NY 10016; **Phone:** 646-501-7223; **Board Cert:** Orthopaedic Surgery 2006; **Med School:** Univ VT Coll Med 1986; **Resid:** Orthopaedic Surgery, Univ NC Med Ctr 1991; **Fellow:** Reconstructive Surgery, Univ Ariz Coll Med 1992; **Fac Appt:** Asst Prof OrS, NYU Sch Med

Bostrom, Mathias P MD (OrS) - **Spec Exp:** Knee Replacement; Hip Replacement; Hip & Knee Reconstruction; Joint Replacement; **Hospital:** Hosp For Special Surgery (page 115), NY-Presby/Weill Cornell Med Ctr, NY (page 104); **Address:** 535 E 70th St, New York, NY 10021; **Phone:** 212-606-1674; **Board Cert:** Orthopaedic Surgery 2009; **Med School:** Johns Hopkins Univ 1989; **Resid:** Orthopaedic Surgery, Hosp for Spec Surg 1995; **Fellow:** Reconstructive Surgery, Hosp for Spec Surg 1996; **Fac Appt:** Prof OrS, Cornell Univ-Weill Med Coll

Brisson, Paul M MD (OrS) - **Spec Exp:** Spinal Surgery; **Hospital:** NY Downtown Hosp; **Address:** 51 E 25th St, Fl 6, New York, NY 10010; **Phone:** 212-813-3632; **Board Cert:** Orthopaedic Surgery 2004; **Med School:** Univ Montreal 1979; **Resid:** Orthopaedic Surgery, McGill Med Ctr 1987; **Fellow:** Spinal Surgery, Hosp Joint Diseases 1988; Spinal Surgery, Buffalo Genl Hosp 1989

Bronson, Michael J MD (OrS) - **Spec Exp:** Joint Replacement; Knee Replacement; Hip Replacement; Arthritis; **Hospital:** Mount Sinai Med Ctr (page 102); **Address:** Mt Sinai Med Ctr, Dept Orthopedic Surgery, 5 E 98th St, Box 1188, New York, NY 10029; **Phone:** 212-241-1640; **Board Cert:** Orthopaedic Surgery 1984; **Med School:** NY Med Coll 1976; **Resid:** Orthopaedic Surgery, Lenox Hill Hosp 1980; **Fellow:** Hip & Knee Surgery, Columbia-Presby Med Ctr 1981; **Fac Appt:** Assoc Prof OrS, Mount Sinai Sch Med

Buly, Robert L MD (OrS) - **Spec Exp:** Hip Replacement & Revision; Arthroscopic Surgery-Hip; Knee Replacement; Arthritis; **Hospital:** Hosp For Special Surgery (page 115), NY-Presby/Weill Cornell Med Ctr, NY (page 104); **Address:** Hospital for Special Surgery, 535 E 70th St, New York, NY 10021; **Phone:** 212-606-1971; **Board Cert:** Orthopaedic Surgery 2004; **Med School:** Cornell Univ-Weill Med Coll 1985; **Resid:** Orthopaedic Surgery, Hosp for Special Surg 1990; **Fellow:** Hip Surgery, Mueller Fdn 1991; Joint Reconstruction, Case Western Res/Univ Hosp 1992; **Fac Appt:** Assoc Prof OrS, Cornell Univ-Weill Med Coll

Cammisa Jr, Frank P MD (OrS) - **Spec Exp:** Spinal Surgery; Spinal Disc Replacement; Minimally Invasive Spinal Surgery; Scoliosis; **Hospital:** Hosp For Special Surgery (page 115); **Address:** 523 E 72nd St, Fl 3, New York, NY 10021; **Phone:** 212-606-1946; **Board Cert:** Orthopaedic Surgery 2011; **Med School:** Columbia P&S 1982; **Resid:** Surgery, Columbia-Presby Hosp 1983; Orthopaedic Surgery, Hosp for Special Surgery 1987; **Fellow:** Spinal Surgery, Jackson Meml Hosp 1988; **Fac Appt:** Assoc Prof OrS, Cornell Univ-Weill Med Coll

Casden, Andrew M MD (OrS) - **Spec Exp:** Spinal Surgery; Spinal Disc Replacement; Minimally Invasive Spinal Surgery; Scoliosis; **Hospital:** Mount Sinai Med Ctr (page 102); **Address:** Mount Sinai Med Ctr, Div Orth Surg, 17 E 102nd St Fl 5, New York, NY 10029; **Phone:** 212-241-8947; **Board Cert:** Orthopaedic Surgery 2012; **Med School:** Cornell Univ-Weill Med Coll 1983; **Resid:** Orthopaedic Surgery, Hosp Joint Diseases 1988; **Fellow:** Spinal Surgery, Rush-Presby Med Ctr 1989; **Fac Appt:** Assoc Prof OrS, Albert Einstein Coll Med

Compito, Catherine MD (OrS) - **Spec Exp:** Shoulder Surgery; Elbow Surgery; Sports Medicine; Arthroscopic Surgery; **Hospital:** Beth Israel Med Ctr - Petrie Division (page 94); **Address:** Beth Israel Orthopedics and Sports Med, 10 Union Square E, Ste 3K, New York, NY 10003; **Phone:** 212-844-8544; **Board Cert:** Orthopaedic Surgery 2009; Orthopaedic Sports Medicine 2011; **Med School:** Albert Einstein Coll Med 1986; **Resid:** Orthopaedic Surgery, Montefiore Med Ctr 1991; **Fellow:** Sports Medicine, Staten Island Univ Hosp 1992; Shoulder Surgery, NY-Presby/Columbia Univ Med Ctr 1993

Cordasco, Frank A MD (OrS) - **Spec Exp:** Sports Medicine; Arthroscopic Surgery-Knee; Arthroscopic Surgery-Shoulder; Rotator Cuff Surgery; **Hospital:** Hosp For Special Surgery (page 115); **Address:** Hospital for Special Surgery, 535 E 70th St, New York, NY 10021; **Phone:** 212-606-1636; **Board Cert:** Orthopaedic Surgery 2003; Sports Medicine 2009; **Med School:** UMDNJ-NJ Med Sch, Newark 1985; **Resid:** Orthopaedic Surgery, Columbia-Presby Hosp 1989; **Fellow:** Elbow & Shoulder Surgery, Columbia-Presby Hosp 1991; **Fac Appt:** Assoc Prof OrS, Cornell Univ-Weill Med Coll

Cornell, Charles MD (OrS) - **Spec Exp:** Trauma; Joint Replacement; Hip & Knee Replacement; **Hospital:** Hosp For Special Surgery (page 115); **Address:** 535 E 70th St, Ste 306, New York, NY 10021; **Phone:** 212-606-1414; **Board Cert:** Orthopaedic Surgery 2009; **Med School:** Cornell Univ-Weill Med Coll 1980; **Resid:** Surgery, Presby Hosp 1982; Orthopaedic Surgery, Hosp For Special Surgery 1985; **Fellow:** Orthopaedic Surgery, Univ Wash Med Ctr 1986; **Fac Appt:** Clin Prof OrS, Cornell Univ-Weill Med Coll

Craig, Edward V MD (OrS) - **Spec Exp:** Shoulder Arthroscopic Surgery; Shoulder Replacement; Sports Medicine; Elbow Surgery; **Hospital:** Hosp For Special Surgery (page 115), NY-Presby/Weill Cornell Med Ctr, NY (page 104); **Address:** 535 E 70th St, New York, NY 10021; **Phone:** 212-606-1966; **Board Cert:** Orthopaedic Surgery 1984; **Med School:** Columbia P&S 1973; **Resid:** Internal Medicine, Columbia-Presby Hosp 1976; Orthopaedic Surgery, Columbia-Presby Hosp 1980; **Fellow:** Shoulder Surgery, Columbia-Presby Hosp 1981; Hand Surgery, Columbia-Presby Hosp 1982; **Fac Appt:** Clin Prof OrS, Cornell Univ-Weill Med Coll

Cuomo, Frances MD (OrS) - **Spec Exp:** Shoulder Surgery; Elbow Surgery; Sports Medicine; **Hospital:** Beth Israel Med Ctr - Petrie Division (page 94); **Address:** Beth Israel Orthpaedics & Sports Med, 10 Union Square E, Ste 3M, New York, NY 10003; **Phone:** 212-844-6938; **Board Cert:** Orthopaedic Surgery 2012; **Med School:** NYU Sch Med 1983; **Resid:** Orthopaedic Surgery, Lenox Hill Hosp 1988; **Fellow:** Shoulder Surgery, Columbia-Presby Med Ctr 1989; **Fac Appt:** Asst Prof OrS, Albert Einstein Coll Med

Cushner, Fred D MD (OrS) - **Spec Exp:** Knee Reconstruction; Knee Injuries/Ligament Surgery; Cartilage Damage; Sports Medicine; **Hospital:** Lenox Hill Hosp (page 106), Southside Hosp (page 106); **Address:** 210 E 64th St Fl 4, New York, NY 10065; **Phone:** 212-434-4312; **Board Cert:** Orthopaedic Surgery 2007; **Med School:** Med Univ SC 1988; **Resid:** Orthopaedic Surgery, Univ SC Med Ctr 1993; **Fellow:** Knee Reconstruction, Beth Israel Med Ctr 1994

Deland, Jonathan T MD (OrS) - **Spec Exp:** Foot & Ankle Surgery; Sports Medicine; Arthritis; **Hospital:** Hosp For Special Surgery (page 115); **Address:** Hosp Spec Surg, Foot & Ankle Service, 535 E 70th St, New York, NY 10021-4099; **Phone:** 212-606-1665; **Board Cert:** Orthopaedic Surgery 2003; **Med School:** Columbia P&S 1980; **Resid:** Orthopaedic Surgery, St Luke's-Roosevelt Hosp Ctr 1982; Orthopaedic Surgery, Mass Genl Hosp 1987; **Fac Appt:** Asst Prof S, Cornell Univ-Weill Med Coll

Egol, Kenneth A MD (OrS) - **Spec Exp:** Trauma; Reconstructive Surgery; Limb Lengthening (Ilizarov Procedure); **Hospital:** NYU Hosp For Joint Diseases (page 119), Jamaica Hosp Med Ctr; **Address:** 301 E 17th St, New York, NY 10003; **Phone:** 212-598-3889; **Board Cert:** Orthopaedic Surgery 2012; **Med School:** SUNY Upstate Med Univ 1993; **Resid:** Orthopaedic Surgery, Hosp For Joint Diseases 1998; **Fellow:** Trauma, Carolinas Med Ctr 1999; **Fac Appt:** Assoc Prof OrS, NYU Sch Med

Elliott, Andrew J MD (OrS) - **Spec Exp:** Foot & Ankle Surgery; Arthroscopic Surgery; Sports Injuries; **Hospital:** Hosp For Special Surgery (page 115); **Address:** 420 E 72nd St, Fl Ground, Ste 1B, New York, NY 10021; **Phone:** 212-203-0740; **Board Cert:** Orthopaedic Surgery 2010; **Med School:** Harvard Med Sch 1991; **Resid:** Surgery, Yale/New Haven Hosp 1996; **Fellow:** Orthopaedic Surgery, Hosp For Special Surgery 1997; **Fac Appt:** Asst Clin Prof OrS, Cornell Univ-Weill Med Coll

Errico, Thomas J MD (OrS) - **Spec Exp:** Spinal Surgery; Spinal Disc Replacement; Scoliosis; **Hospital:** NYU Langone Med Ctr (page 108), NYU Hosp For Joint Diseases (page 119); **Address:** 333 E 38th St, Fl 6, MS 10016, New York, NY 10016-6402; **Phone:** 646-501-7200; **Board Cert:** Orthopaedic Surgery 2007; **Med School:** UMDNJ-NJ Med Sch, Newark 1978; **Resid:** Orthopaedic Surgery, NYU Med Ctr 1983; **Fellow:** Spinal Surgery, Toronto Genl Hosp 1984; **Fac Appt:** Assoc Prof OrS, NYU Sch Med

Fealy, Stephen MD (OrS) - **Spec Exp:** Sports Medicine; Shoulder Arthroscopic Surgery; Shoulder Replacement; Knee Replacement; **Hospital:** Hosp For Special Surgery (page 115); **Address:** Hospital for Special Surgery, 535 E 70th St, New York, NY 10021; **Phone:** 212-606-1894; **Board Cert:** Orthopaedic Surgery 2004; **Med School:** Columbia P&S 1995; **Resid:** Orthopaedic Surgery, Hosp for Special Surg 2000; **Fellow:** Sports Medicine, Hosp for Special Surg 2001; **Fac Appt:** Asst Prof OrS, Cornell Univ-Weill Med Coll

Feldman, David S MD (OrS) - **Spec Exp:** Limb Deformities; Spinal Surgery; Pediatric Orthopaedic Surgery; Scoliosis; **Hospital:** NYU Hosp For Joint Diseases (page 119), NYU Langone Med Ctr (page 108); **Address:** 67 Irving Pl Fl 8, New York, NY 10003; **Phone:** 212-533-5310; **Board Cert:** Orthopaedic Surgery 2007; **Med School:** Albert Einstein Coll Med 1988; **Resid:** Orthopaedic Surgery, Hosp for Joint Diseases 1993; **Fellow:** Pediatric Surgery, Hosp For Sick Chldn 1994; **Fac Appt:** Asst Prof OrS, NYU Sch Med

Figgie, Mark P MD (OrS) - **Spec Exp:** Joint Replacement; Minimally Invasive Surgery; Hip Surgery; Knee Surgery; **Hospital:** Hosp For Special Surgery (page 115), NY-Presby/Weill Cornell Med Ctr, NY (page 104); **Address:** 535 E 70th St, Ste 328, New York, NY 10021; **Phone:** 212-606-1932; **Board Cert:** Orthopaedic Surgery 2011; **Med School:** Case West Res Univ 1981; **Resid:** Orthopaedic Surgery, Univ Hosp-Case Western Reserve 1986; **Fellow:** Biomedical Engineering, Hosp For Special Surgery 1987; Joint Replacement Surgery, Hosp For Special Surgery 1988; **Fac Appt:** Assoc Clin Prof OrS, Cornell Univ-Weill Med Coll

Flatow, Evan L MD (OrS) - **Spec Exp:** Rotator Cuff Surgery; Shoulder Injuries; Shoulder Replacement; Shoulder Arthroscopic Surgery; **Hospital:** Mount Sinai Med Ctr (page 102); **Address:** 5 E 98th St, Fl 9, Box 1188, New York, NY 10029; **Phone:** 212-241-1663; **Board Cert:** Orthopaedic Surgery 2010; **Med School:** Columbia P&S 1981; **Resid:** Surgery, Roosevelt Hosp 1983; Orthopaedic Surgery, Columbia-Presby Med Ctr 1986; **Fellow:** Shoulder Surgery, Columbia-Presby Med Ctr 1987; **Fac Appt:** Prof OrS, Mount Sinai Sch Med

Fragomen, Austin T MD (OrS) - **Spec Exp:** Limb Deformities; Limb Lengthening; Bone Infections; Blount's Disease; **Hospital:** Hosp For Special Surgery (page 115); **Address:** 535 E 70th St, New York, NY 10021; **Phone:** 212-606-1550; **Board Cert:** Orthopaedic Surgery 2007; **Med School:** SUNY Downstate 1997; **Resid:** Surgery, Montefiore Med Ctr 1998; Orthopaedic Surgery, Westchester Med Ctr 2003; **Fac Appt:** Asst Prof OrS, Cornell Univ-Weill Med Coll

Gladstone, James N MD (OrS) - **Spec Exp:** Shoulder & Knee Surgery; Cartilage Damage; Knee-Patella Problems; Arthritis; **Hospital:** Mount Sinai Med Ctr (page 102); **Address:** Mt Sinai Med Ctr, 5 E 98th St Fl 9, Box 1188, New York, NY 10029; **Phone:** 212-241-1645; **Board Cert:** Orthopaedic Surgery 2009; Orthopaedic Sports Medicine 2007; **Med School:** Tufts Univ 1990; **Resid:** Orthopaedic Surgery, Columbia-Presby Med Ctr 1995; **Fellow:** Sports Medicine, American Sports Med Inst 1996; **Fac Appt:** Assoc Prof OrS, Mount Sinai Sch Med

Glashow, Jonathan L MD (OrS) - **Spec Exp:** Sports Medicine; Shoulder Surgery; Knee Surgery; Arthroscopic Surgery; **Hospital:** Mount Sinai Med Ctr (page 102); **Address:** 737 Park Ave, Ste 1C, New York, NY 10021; **Phone:** 212-794-5096; **Board Cert:** Orthopaedic Surgery 2004; **Med School:** Cornell Univ-Weill Med Coll 1984; **Resid:** Orthopaedic Surgery, Lenox Hill Hosp 1989; **Fellow:** Arthroscopic Surgery, S Calif Ortho Inst 1990; Shoulder Surgery, Univ Texas Med Ctr 1990; **Fac Appt:** Assoc Clin Prof OrS, Mount Sinai Sch Med

Goldstein, Jeffrey A MD (OrS) - **Spec Exp:** Spinal Surgery; Minimally Invasive Spinal Surgery; Spinal Disc Replacement; Scoliosis; **Hospital:** NYU Hosp For Joint Diseases (page 119), NYU Langone Med Ctr (page 108); **Address:** NYU Hospital for Joint Diseases, 19 Beekman St, New York, NY 10038; **Phone:** 212-513-7711; **Board Cert:** Orthopaedic Surgery 2004; **Med School:** SUNY Downstate 1990; **Resid:** Orthopaedic Surgery, Case West Univ Med Ctr 1995; **Fellow:** Spinal Surgery, Maryland Spine Ctr 1996; **Fac Appt:** Clin Prof OrS, NYU Sch Med

Goodwin, Charles MD (OrS) - **Spec Exp:** Spinal Surgery; Sports Medicine; Minimally Invasive Spinal Surgery; **Hospital:** Hosp For Special Surgery (page 115), St. Luke's - Roosevelt Hosp Ctr - Roosevelt Div (page 94); **Address:** 635 Madison Ave Fl 7, New York, NY 10022-1009; **Phone:** 212-317-4600; **Board Cert:** Orthopaedic Surgery 1985; **Med School:** Univ Cincinnati 1976; **Resid:** Surgery, St Luke's Roosevelt Hosp Ctr 1979; Orthopaedic Surgery, NY Presby Hosp/ Columbia 1982; **Fellow:** Spinal Surgery, Univ Toronto Affil Hosp 1983; **Fac Appt:** Asst Prof OrS, Cornell Univ-Weill Med Coll

Green, Steven M MD (OrS) - **Spec Exp:** Hand & Wrist Surgery; Carpal Tunnel Syndrome; Hand Surgery; **Hospital:** Mount Sinai Med Ctr (page 102), NYU Hosp For Joint Diseases (page 119); **Address:** 2 E 88th St, New York, NY 10128-0555; **Phone:** 212-348-6644; **Board Cert:** Orthopaedic Surgery 1977; **Med School:** Albert Einstein Coll Med 1970; **Resid:** Surgery, Georgia Bapt Hosp 1972; Orthopaedic Surgery, Mt Sinai Hosp 1975; **Fellow:** Hand Surgery, Thomas Jefferson Univ Hosp 1978; **Fac Appt:** Assoc Clin Prof OrS, NYU Sch Med

Greisberg, Justin K MD (OrS) - **Spec Exp:** Foot & Ankle Surgery; Ankle Replacement & Revision; Reconstructive Surgery; Trauma; **Hospital:** NY-Presby/Columbia Univ Med Ctr, NY (page 104); **Address:** NY Presbyterian-Columbia Medical Ctr, 622 W 168th St, PH-11, rm 1153, New York, NY 10032; **Phone:** 212-305-5604; **Board Cert:** Orthopaedic Surgery 2004; **Med School:** Albert Einstein Coll Med 1995; **Resid:** Orthopaedic Surgery, Rhode Island Hosp 2000; **Fellow:** Orthopaedic Trauma Surgery, Rhode Island Hosp 2001; Foot & Ankle Surgery, Harbor; **Fac Appt:** Assoc Prof OrS, Columbia P&S

Grelsamer, Ronald P MD (OrS) - **Spec Exp:** Knee-Patella Problems; Sports Medicine; Knee Reconstruction; Arthritis-Hip & Knee; **Hospital:** Mount Sinai Med Ctr (page 102); **Address:** Mount Sinai Medical Ctr, Dept Orthopaedics, 5 E 98th St, Box 1188, New York, NY 10029-6574; **Phone:** 212-241-2914; **Board Cert:** Orthopaedic Surgery 2008; **Med School:** Columbia P&S 1979; **Resid:** Orthopaedic Surgery, Columbia Presby Med Ctr 1984; **Fellow:** Hip & Knee Surgery, Columbia Presby Med Ctr 1985; **Fac Appt:** Assoc Prof OrS, Mount Sinai Sch Med

Haas, Steven B MD (OrS) - **Spec Exp:** Knee Surgery; Knee Replacement; Minimally Invasive Surgery; **Hospital:** Hosp For Special Surgery (page 115); **Address:** Hosp for Special Surgery, 535 E 70th St Fl 3, New York, NY 10021; **Phone:** 212-606-1852; **Board Cert:** Orthopaedic Surgery 2004; **Med School:** Univ Rochester 1985; **Resid:** Orthopaedic Surgery, Hosp Special Surgery 1990; **Fellow:** Knee Surgery, Hosp Special Surgery 1991; **Fac Appt:** Clin Prof OrS, Cornell Univ-Weill Med Coll

Hamilton, William G MD (OrS) - **Spec Exp:** Dance Medicine; Foot & Ankle Surgery; Sports Medicine; **Hospital:** St. Luke's - Roosevelt Hosp Ctr - Roosevelt Div (page 94), Hosp For Special Surgery (page 115); **Address:** 343 W 58th St, New York, NY 10019-1173; **Phone:** 212-765-2260; **Board Cert:** Orthopaedic Surgery 1971; **Med School:** Columbia P&S 1964; **Resid:** Surgery, St Luke's-Roosevelt Hosp Ctr 1966; Orthopaedic Surgery, Columbia-Presby Hosp 1969; **Fellow:** Pediatric Orthopaedic Surgery, Newington Chldrn's Hosp 1970; **Fac Appt:** Clin Prof OrS, Columbia P&S

Hannafin, Jo Anne MD/PhD (OrS) - **Spec Exp:** Sports Medicine-Women; Shoulder Arthroscopic Surgery; Knee Injuries/Ligament Surgery; Ligament Reconstruction; **Hospital:** Hosp For Special Surgery (page 115), NY-Presby/Weill Cornell Med Ctr, NY (page 104); **Address:** 535 E 70th St, New York, NY 10021-4872; **Phone:** 212-606-1469; **Board Cert:** Orthopaedic Surgery 2005; Orthopaedic Sports Medicine 2009; **Med School:** Albert Einstein Coll Med 1985; **Resid:** Orthopaedic Surgery, Montefiore Med Ctr 1990; **Fellow:** Sports Medicine, Hosp Special Surgery 1992; **Fac Appt:** Prof OrS, Cornell Univ-Weill Med Coll

Harwin, Steven F MD (OrS) - **Spec Exp:** Hip & Knee Replacement; Minimally Invasive Surgery; Transfusion Free Surgery; Osteonecrosis; **Hospital:** Beth Israel Med Ctr - Petrie Division (page 94); **Address:** Center for Reconstructive Joint Surgery, 910 Park Ave, New York, NY 10075; **Phone:** 212-861-9800; **Board Cert:** Orthopaedic Surgery 1976; **Med School:** SUNY Upstate Med Univ 1971; **Resid:** Orthopaedic Surgery, Albert Einstein Coll Med 1975; **Fellow:** Joint Replacement Surgery, Traveling Fellowship 1978; **Fac Appt:** Assoc Prof OrS, Albert Einstein Coll Med

Hausman, Michael R MD (OrS) - **Spec Exp:** Hand Reconstruction; Elbow Reconstruction; Reconstructive Microvascular Surgery; Arthroscopic Surgery; **Hospital:** Mount Sinai Med Ctr (page 102); **Address:** 5 E 98th St Fl 9, Box 1188, New York, NY 10029-6501; **Phone:** 212-241-1658; **Board Cert:** Orthopaedic Surgery 2010; Hand Surgery 2010; **Med School:** Yale Univ 1979; **Resid:** Surgery, Yale-New Haven Hosp 1981; Orthopaedic Surgery, Yale-New Haven Hosp 1985; **Fellow:** Hand Surgery, Roosevelt Hosp 1987; **Fac Appt:** Assoc Clin Prof OrS, Mount Sinai Sch Med

Healey, John H MD (OrS) - **Spec Exp:** Bone Tumors; Hip & Knee Replacement in Bone Tumors; Sarcoma; Sarcoma-Soft Tissue; **Hospital:** Meml Sloan-Kettering Cancer Ctr (page 116), Hosp For Special Surgery (page 115); **Address:** 1275 York Ave, New York, NY 10065; **Phone:** 212-639-7610; **Board Cert:** Orthopaedic Surgery 2007; **Med School:** Univ VT Coll Med 1978; **Resid:** Orthopaedic Surgery, Hosp Special Surg 1983; **Fellow:** Musculoskeletal Oncology, Meml Sloan Kettering Cancer Ctr 1984; Orthopaedic Surgery, Hosp Special Surgery 1984; **Fac Appt:** Prof OrS, Cornell Univ-Weill Med Coll

Hecht, Andrew MD (OrS) - **Spec Exp:** Spinal Surgery; Minimally Invasive Spinal Surgery; **Hospital:** Mount Sinai Med Ctr (page 102); **Address:** Chief Spine Surgery, Mount Sinai Med Ctr, Dept Orthopaedic Surg, 5 E 98th St, Fl 9, Box 1188, New York, NY 10029; **Phone:** 212-241-0735; **Board Cert:** Orthopaedic Surgery 2003; **Med School:** Harvard Med Sch 1994; **Resid:** Orthopaedic Surgery, Mass Genl Hosp 1999; **Fellow:** Spinal Surgery, Emory Univ Spine Ctr 2001; **Fac Appt:** Asst Prof OrS, Mount Sinai Sch Med

Helfet, David L MD (OrS) - **Spec Exp:** Fractures-Complex & Non Union; Deformity Reconstruction; Pelvic & Acetabular Fractures; Fractures-Stress; **Hospital:** Hosp For Special Surgery (page 115), NY-Presby/Weill Cornell Med Ctr, NY (page 104); **Address:** 525 E 71st St, Belaire Bldg - Fl 2, New York, NY 10021; **Phone:** 212-606-1888; **Board Cert:** Orthopaedic Surgery 1984; **Med School:** South Africa 1975; **Resid:** Surgery, Edendale Hosp 1977; Orthopaedic Surgery, Johns Hopkins Hosp 1981; **Fellow:** Orthopaedic Surgery, Inselspita Hosp 1981; Orthopaedic Surgery, UCLA Med Ctr 1982; **Fac Appt:** Prof OrS, Cornell Univ-Weill Med Coll

Hotchkiss, Robert N MD (OrS) - **Spec Exp:** Hand Surgery; Wrist Surgery; Elbow Reconstruction; Dupuytren's Contracture; **Hospital:** Hosp For Special Surgery (page 115), NY-Presby/Weill Cornell Med Ctr, NY (page 104); **Address:** 523 E 72nd St Fl 4, New York, NY 10021-4099; **Phone:** 212-606-1964; **Board Cert:** Orthopaedic Surgery 2010; Hand Surgery 2010; **Med School:** Johns Hopkins Univ 1980; **Resid:** Surgery, Johns Hopkins Hosp 1982; Orthopaedic Surgery, Johns Hopkins Hosp 1985; **Fellow:** Hand Surgery, Union Meml Hosp 1987; **Fac Appt:** Assoc Prof OrS, Cornell Univ-Weill Med Coll

Hubbard, Christopher E MD (OrS) - **Spec Exp:** Foot & Ankle Surgery; Sports Medicine; Arthroscopic Surgery; Ligament Reconstruction; **Hospital:** Beth Israel Med Ctr - Petrie Division (page 94); **Address:** Beth Israel Orthopaedics & Sports Med, 10 Union Square East, Ste 3M, New York, NY 10003-3314; **Phone:** 212-844-6940; **Board Cert:** Orthopaedic Surgery 2012; **Med School:** UMDNJ-NJ Med Sch, Newark 1994; **Resid:** Orthopaedic Surgery, Columbia-Presby Med Ctr 1999; **Fellow:** Foot & Ankle Surgery, Hosp for Special Surgery 2000; **Fac Appt:** Asst Prof OrS, Albert Einstein Coll Med

Hyman, Joshua E MD (OrS) - **Spec Exp:** Pediatric Orthopaedic Surgery; Fractures-Pediatric; Scoliosis; Clubfoot/Foot Deformities in Children; **Hospital:** Morgan Stanley Children's Hosp of NY-Presby, NY (page 104), NY-Presby/Columbia Univ Med Ctr, NY (page 104); **Address:** Children's Hosp New York, 3959 Broadway, Ste 8 North, New York, NY 10032-3784; **Phone:** 212-305-5475; **Board Cert:** Orthopaedic Surgery 2002; **Med School:** Columbia P&S 1990; **Resid:** Surgery, Beth Israel Hosp 1993; Orthopaedic Surgery, Mass Genl Hosp/Beth Israel Hosp 1998; **Fellow:** Pediatric Orthopaedic Surgery, Hosp for Sick Children 1999; **Fac Appt:** Assoc Prof OrS, Columbia P&S

Jaffe, Fredrick F MD (OrS) - **Spec Exp:** Hip Replacement; Knee Replacement; Hip & Knee Reconstruction; **Hospital:** NYU Hosp For Joint Diseases (page 119); **Address:** 333 E 38th St, New York, NY 10003-3804; **Phone:** 212-598-7605; **Board Cert:** Orthopaedic Surgery 1974; **Med School:** Tufts Univ 1968; **Resid:** Surgery, New York Hosp 1970; Orthopaedic Surgery, Hosp for Joint Diseases 1973; **Fellow:** Reconstructive Surgery, Hosp for Joint Diseases 1974; **Fac Appt:** Clin Prof OrS, NYU Sch Med

Kelly, Bryan T MD (OrS) - **Spec Exp:** Hip Surgery; Arthroscopic Surgery; Sports Medicine; **Hospital:** Hosp For Special Surgery (page 115); **Address:** 535 E 70th St, New York, NY 10021; **Phone:** 212-606-1159; **Board Cert:** Orthopaedic Surgery 2006; **Med School:** Duke Univ 1996; **Resid:** Orthopaedic Surgery, Hosp Special Surg 2001; **Fellow:** Orthopaedic Sports Medicine, Hosp Special Surg 2003; Hip Sports Injuries/Arthroscopy, Univ Pittsburgh 2004; **Fac Appt:** Assoc Prof OrS, Cornell Univ-Weill Med Coll

Kiernan, Howard MD (OrS) - **Hospital:** NY-Presby/Columbia Univ Med Ctr, NY (page 104); **Address:** 903 Park Ave, New York, NY 10075; **Phone:** 212-305-5241; **Board Cert:** Orthopaedic Surgery 1975; **Med School:** NYU Sch Med 1966; **Resid:** Surgery, Bellevue Hosp Ctr-NYU 1970; Orthopaedic Surgery, Columbia-Presby Med Ctr 1974

Lane, Joseph MD (OrS) - **Spec Exp:** Bone Disorders-Metabolic; Osteoporosis Spine-Kyphoplasty; Bone Cancer; **Hospital:** Hosp For Special Surgery (page 115), NY-Presby/Weill Cornell Med Ctr, NY (page 104); **Address:** Hosp for Special Surgery, 535 E 70th St, New York, NY 10021; **Phone:** 212-606-1172; **Board Cert:** Orthopaedic Surgery 1998; **Med School:** Harvard Med Sch 1965; **Resid:** Surgery, Hosp Univ Penn 1967; Orthopaedic Surgery, Hosp Univ Penn 1973; **Fac Appt:** Prof OrS, Cornell Univ-Weill Med Coll

Lee, Francis Y MD/PhD (OrS) - **Spec Exp:** Bone & Soft Tissue Tumors; Pediatric Orthopaedic Surgery; Bone Tumors-Metastatic; Bone Tumors-Benign; **Hospital:** Morgan Stanley Children's Hosp of NY-Presby, NY (page 104), NY-Presby/Columbia Univ Med Ctr, NY (page 104); **Address:** 3959 Broadway, Ste 800N, Columbia University Medical Center, New York, NY 10032; **Phone:** 212-305-3293; **Board Cert:** Orthopaedic Surgery 2012; **Med School:** South Korea 1986; **Resid:** Orthopaedic Surgery, NJ Med Ctr 1997; **Fellow:** Orthopaedic Oncology, Harvard Med Sch 1998; Pediatric Orthopaedic Surgery, Hosp for Sick Chldn/Univ Toronto 1999; **Fac Appt:** Assoc Prof OrS, Columbia P&S

Levine, David S MD (OrS) - **Spec Exp:** Foot & Ankle Surgery; Ankle Reconstruction; **Hospital:** Hosp For Special Surgery (page 115); **Address:** Hospital for Special Surgery, 523 E 72 St Fl 5, New York, NY 10021; **Phone:** 212-606-1940; **Board Cert:** Orthopaedic Surgery 2011; **Med School:** Cornell Univ-Weill Med Coll 1992; **Resid:** Orthopaedic Surgery, Hosp for Special Surgery 1997; **Fellow:** Foot & Ankle Surgery, Harborview Med Ctr 1998

Levy, Howard J MD (OrS) - **Spec Exp:** Knee Surgery; Shoulder Surgery; Sports Medicine; Arthroscopic Surgery; **Hospital:** Lenox Hill Hosp (page 106), Beth Israel Med Ctr - Petrie Division (page 94); **Address:** 130 E 77th St, Fl 7, New York, NY 10075; **Phone:** 212-744-8114; **Board Cert:** Orthopaedic Surgery 2004; Orthopaedic Sports Medicine 2008; **Med School:** SUNY Hlth Sci Ctr 1983; **Resid:** Orthopaedic Surgery, Jackson Meml Hosp 1989; **Fellow:** Sports Medicine, American Sports Med Inst 1989; Hand Surgery, Roosevelt Hosp 1990; **Fac Appt:** Asst Clin Prof OrS, Albert Einstein Coll Med

Lonner, Baron S MD (OrS) - **Spec Exp:** Scoliosis; Minimally Invasive Surgery; Spinal Deformity; Spinal Surgery; **Hospital:** NYU Hosp For Joint Diseases (page 119), NYU Langone Med Ctr (page 108); **Address:** 820 2nd Ave, Ste 7A, New York, NY 10017; **Phone:** 212-986-0140; **Board Cert:** Orthopaedic Surgery 2008; **Med School:** Boston Univ 1989; **Resid:** Orthopaedic Surgery, Montefiore Med Ctr 1994; **Fellow:** Orthopaedic Surgery, Hosp Special Surgery 1995; **Fac Appt:** Asst Prof OrS, NYU Sch Med

Lorich, Dean G MD (OrS) - **Spec Exp:** Trauma; Fractures-Complex; **Hospital:** Hosp For Special Surgery (page 115); **Address:** Hospital for Special Surgery, 535 E 70th St, New York, NY 10021; **Phone:** 212-746-4509; **Board Cert:** Orthopaedic Surgery 2010; **Med School:** Univ Pennsylvania 1990; **Resid:** Orthopaedic Surgery, Hosp Univ Penn 1995; **Fellow:** Orthopaedic Surgery, Hosp Special Surg 1996; **Fac Appt:** Assoc Prof OrS, Cornell Univ-Weill Med Coll

Lubliner, Jerry A MD (OrS) - **Spec Exp:** Arthroscopic Surgery; Shoulder Surgery; Knee Surgery; Rotator Cuff Surgery; **Hospital:** Beth Israel Med Ctr - Petrie Division (page 94), NYU Hosp For Joint Diseases (page 119); **Address:** New York Orthopaedics and Sports Med, 215 E 73rd St, Ste 1C, New York, NY 10021-3653; **Phone:** 212-249-8200; **Board Cert:** Orthopaedic Surgery 2009; Orthopaedic Sports Medicine 2008; **Med School:** SUNY Hlth Sci Ctr 1980; **Resid:** Orthopaedic Surgery, Hosp Joint Diseases 1985; **Fellow:** Sports Medicine, Univ West Ontario Affil Hosps 1985; **Fac Appt:** Assoc Clin Prof S, NYU Sch Med

Lyden, John MD (OrS) - **Spec Exp:** Joint Replacement; Trauma; Arthroscopic Surgery; **Hospital:** Hosp For Special Surgery (page 115), NY-Presby/Weill Cornell Med Ctr, NY (page 104); **Address:** 535 E 70th St, rm 355, New York, NY 10021-4872; **Phone:** 212-606-1126; **Board Cert:** Orthopaedic Surgery 1973; **Med School:** Columbia P&S 1965; **Resid:** Surgery, Roosevelt Hosp 1967; Orthopaedic Surgery, Hosp Special Surg 1972; **Fellow:** Hand Surgery, Hosp Special Surg 1973; **Fac Appt:** Assoc Prof OrS, NY Med Coll

Macaulay, William B MD (OrS) - **Spec Exp:** Hip Replacement; Knee Replacement; Minimally Invasive Surgery; Reconstructive Surgery; **Hospital:** NY-Presby/Columbia Univ Med Ctr, NY (page 104); **Address:** Columbia-Orthopaedics Dept, 161 Fort Washington Ave, Irving Pavilion Fl 2, New York, NY 10032; **Phone:** 212-305-6959; **Board Cert:** Orthopaedic Surgery 2012; **Med School:** Columbia P&S 1992; **Resid:** Orthopaedic Surgery, Univ Pittsburgh Med Ctr 1997; **Fellow:** Adult Reconstructive Surgery, Hosp for Special Surgery 1999; **Fac Appt:** Prof OrS, Columbia P&S

Marx, Robert G MD (OrS) - **Spec Exp:** Shoulder Surgery; Knee Injuries/Ligament Surgery; Knee Replacement; Sports Medicine; **Hospital:** Hosp For Special Surgery (page 115); **Address:** 535 E 70th St, New York, NY 10021; **Phone:** 212-606-1645; **Board Cert:** Orthopaedic Surgery 2003; **Med School:** McGill Univ 1991; **Resid:** Orthopaedic Surgery, Univ Toronto 1996; **Fellow:** Sports Medicine, Hosp Special Surgery 1998; **Fac Appt:** Prof OrS, Cornell Univ-Weill Med Coll

McCance, Sean E MD (OrS) - **Spec Exp:** Spinal Surgery; Scoliosis; **Hospital:** Mount Sinai Med Ctr (page 102), Lenox Hill Hosp (page 106); **Address:** 1155 Park Ave, Fl Ground, Ste E, New York, NY 10128; **Phone:** 212-360-6500; **Board Cert:** Orthopaedic Surgery 2010; Spine Surgery ; **Med School:** Columbia P&S 1991; **Resid:** Surgery, Strong Meml Hosp 1992; Orthopaedic Surgery, Strong Meml Hosp 1996; **Fellow:** Spinal Surgery, Twin Cities Spine Ctr 1998; **Fac Appt:** Asst Clin Prof OrS, Mount Sinai Sch Med

McCann, Peter D MD (OrS) - **Spec Exp:** Shoulder Surgery; Elbow Surgery; **Hospital:** Beth Israel Med Ctr - Petrie Division (page 94); **Address:** 10 Union Square E, Ste 3M, New York, NY 10003; **Phone:** 212-844-6735; **Board Cert:** Orthopaedic Surgery 2009; **Med School:** Columbia P&S 1980; **Resid:** Surgery, St Vincent's Hosp 1982; Orthopaedic Surgery, Columbia-Presby Med Ctr 1985; **Fellow:** Shoulder Surgery, Columbia-Presby Med Ctr 1986; **Fac Appt:** Assoc Prof OrS, Albert Einstein Coll Med

McClelland, Shearwood J MD (OrS) - **Spec Exp:** Musculoskeletal Injuries; Joint Replacement; **Hospital:** Harlem Hosp Ctr; **Address:** Harlem Hosp Ctr, Dept Ortho Surgery, 506 Lenox Ave MLK Bldg Fl 9 - rm 9122, New York, NY 10037-1889; **Phone:** 212-939-3510; **Board Cert:** Orthopaedic Surgery 2007; **Med School:** Columbia P&S 1974; **Resid:** Surgery, St. Lukes Hosp 1976; Orthopaedic Surgery, NY Ortho Hosp-Columbia 1979; **Fellow:** Joint Arthroplasty, Ohio State Univ Med Ctr 1982; **Fac Appt:** Assoc Prof OrS, Columbia P&S

Meere, Patrick MD (OrS) - **Spec Exp:** Hip Replacement & Revision; Knee Replacement & Revision; Knee Meniscal Repair; Joint Infections; **Hospital:** NYU Hosp For Joint Diseases (page 119), NYU Langone Med Ctr (page 108); **Address:** 530 1st Ave FPO Bldg - Ste 5J, New York, NY 10016; **Phone:** 212-263-2366; **Board Cert:** Orthopaedic Surgery 2008; **Med School:** McGill Univ 1988; **Resid:** Orthopaedic Surgery, McGill Univ Affil Hosp 1993; **Fellow:** Reconstructive Surgery, Hosp for Joint Diseases 1995; **Fac Appt:** Assoc Prof OrS, NYU Sch Med

Mendoza, Francis X MD (OrS) - **Spec Exp:** Shoulder & Elbow Surgery; Sports Medicine; **Hospital:** Lenox Hill Hosp (page 106); **Address:** 333 E 56th St, New York, NY 10022; **Phone:** 212-628-9600; **Board Cert:** Orthopaedic Surgery 1984; **Med School:** Columbia P&S 1976; **Resid:** Surgery, Roosevelt Hosp 1978; Orthopaedic Surgery, Columbia-Presby Hosp 1981; **Fellow:** Shoulder Surgery, Columbia-Presby Hosp 1982

Moskovich, Ronald MD (OrS) - **Spec Exp:** Scoliosis; Spinal Surgery-Pediatric & Adult; Spondylitis; Spinal Disorders; **Hospital:** NYU Hosp For Joint Diseases (page 119), NYU Langone Med Ctr (page 108); **Address:** 301 E 17th St, Ste 400, New York, NY 10003-3801; **Phone:** 212-598-6622; **Board Cert:** Orthopaedic Surgery 2012; **Med School:** South Africa 1978; **Resid:** Surgery, St George's Hosp 1984; Orthopaedic Surgery, Hosp for Joint Diseases 1988; **Fellow:** Spinal Surgery, UC Davis Med Ctr 1989; Neurological Surgery, Natl Hosp 1989; **Fac Appt:** Asst Prof OrS, NYU Sch Med

Neuwirth, Michael MD (OrS) - **Spec Exp:** Scoliosis; Spinal Surgery; **Hospital:** Beth Israel Med Ctr - Petrie Division (page 94); **Address:** Beth Israel Med Ctr - Spine Institute, 10 Union Square E, Ste 5P, New York, NY 10003-3314; **Phone:** 212-844-8692; **Board Cert:** Orthopaedic Surgery 1980; **Med School:** SUNY Hlth Sci Ctr 1974; **Resid:** Orthopaedic Surgery, Hosp for Joint Diseases 1978; **Fellow:** Spinal Surgery, Rush-Presby Med Ctr 1979; **Fac Appt:** Assoc Clin Prof OrS, NYU Sch Med

Nicholas, Stephen J MD (OrS) - **Spec Exp:** Sports Medicine; Shoulder & Knee Surgery; Arthroscopic Surgery; **Hospital:** Lenox Hill Hosp (page 106); **Address:** 130 E 77 St Fl 5, New York, NY 10075; **Phone:** 212-737-3301; **Board Cert:** Orthopaedic Surgery 2005; **Med School:** NY Med Coll 1986; **Resid:** Orthopaedic Surgery, Hosp for Special Surgery 1991; **Fellow:** Sports Medicine, Lenox Hill Hosp 1992

O'Leary, Patrick MD (OrS) - **Spec Exp:** Spinal Surgery; **Hospital:** Hosp For Special Surgery (page 115); **Address:** 1015 Madison Ave Fl 4, New York, NY 10075; **Phone:** 212-249-8100; **Board Cert:** Orthopaedic Surgery 1983; **Med School:** Ireland 1968; **Resid:** Surgery, Roosevelt Hosp 1972; Orthopaedic Surgery, Hosp Spec Surg-Cornell 1975; **Fellow:** Spinal Surgery, Univ Toronto Genl Ortho Hosp 1976; **Fac Appt:** Assoc Clin Prof OrS, Cornell Univ-Weill Med Coll

O'Malley, Martin J MD (OrS) - **Spec Exp:** Foot & Ankle Surgery; Sports Medicine; Ankle Replacement & Revision; Arthroscopic Surgery; **Hospital:** Hosp For Special Surgery (page 115), NY-Presby/Weill Cornell Med Ctr, NY (page 104); **Address:** 420 E 72nd St, Ste 1B, New York, NY 10021; **Phone:** 212-203-0740; **Board Cert:** Orthopaedic Surgery 2006; **Med School:** Case West Res Univ 1986; **Resid:** Orthopaedic Surgery, Tufts-New Eng Med Ctr 1992; **Fellow:** Foot & Ankle Surgery, Hosp for Special Surg 1993; **Fac Appt:** Assoc Prof OrS, Cornell Univ-Weill Med Coll

Padgett, Douglas E MD (OrS) - **Spec Exp:** Hip & Knee Replacement; Arthroscopic Surgery-Hip; Arthroscopic Surgery-Knee; Dance Medicine; **Hospital:** Hosp For Special Surgery (page 115); **Address:** Hosp for Special Surgery, 535 E 70 St Fl 3, New York, NY 10021; **Phone:** 212-606-1642; **Board Cert:** Orthopaedic Surgery 2003; **Med School:** NY Med Coll 1982; **Resid:** Orthopaedic Surgery, Hosp Spec Surg 1989; **Fellow:** Orthopaedic Surgery, Rush Presby Med Ctr 1990; **Fac Appt:** Assoc Prof OrS, Cornell Univ-Weill Med Coll

Parks, Michael MD (OrS) - **Spec Exp:** Hip & Knee Replacement; Joint Replacement; Reconstructive Surgery; **Hospital:** Hosp For Special Surgery (page 115), NY-Presby/Weill Cornell Med Ctr, NY (page 104); **Address:** 535 E 70th St Fl 6, New York, NY 10021; **Phone:** 646-797-8995; **Board Cert:** Orthopaedic Surgery 2010; **Med School:** Med Univ SC 1990; **Resid:** Orthopaedic Surgery, Duke Univ Med Ctr 1996; **Fellow:** Orthopaedic Surgery, Hosp for Spec Surgery 1997; **Fac Appt:** Asst Prof OrS, Cornell Univ-Weill Med Coll

Pellicci, Paul M MD (OrS) - **Spec Exp:** Hip Replacement-Young Adults; Hip Resurfacing; Knee Replacement; Joint Replacement; **Hospital:** Hosp For Special Surgery (page 115), NY-Presby/Weill Cornell Med Ctr, NY (page 104); **Address:** 535 E 70th St, New York, NY 10021-4872; **Phone:** 212-606-1010; **Board Cert:** Orthopaedic Surgery 1982; **Med School:** Cornell Univ-Weill Med Coll 1975; **Resid:** Surgery, NY Hosp 1977; Orthopaedic Surgery, Hosp Spec Surg 1980; **Fellow:** Joint Replacement Surgery, Brigham & Womens Hosp 1981; **Fac Appt:** Prof OrS, Cornell Univ-Weill Med Coll

Plancher, Kevin D MD (OrS) - **Spec Exp:** Shoulder Surgery; Elbow Surgery; Cartilage Damage & Transplant; Shoulder Replacement; **Hospital:** Beth Israel Med Ctr - Petrie Division (page 94), Lenox Hill Hosp (page 106); **Address:** 1160 Park Ave, New York, NY 10128; **Phone:** 212-876-5200; **Board Cert:** Orthopaedic Surgery 2007; Hand Surgery 2008; Orthopaedic Sports Medicine 2009; **Med School:** Georgetown Univ 1986; **Resid:** Orthopaedic Surgery, Mass Genl Hosp/Brigham & Womens Hosp 1991; **Fellow:** Hand Surgery, Indiana Hand Ctr 1993; Sports Medicine, Steadman-Hawkins Clinic 1994; **Fac Appt:** Assoc Clin Prof OrS, Albert Einstein Coll Med

Price, Andrew E MD (OrS) - **Spec Exp:** Erbs Palsy/Brachial Plexus Injuries; Cerebral Palsy; Fractures-Pediatric; Trauma-Pediatric; **Hospital:** NYU Langone Med Ctr (page 108), St. Luke's - Roosevelt Hosp Ctr - Roosevelt Div (page 94); **Address:** 129A W 20th St, New York, NY 10011; **Phone:** 212-974-7242; **Board Cert:** Orthopaedic Surgery 2011; **Med School:** NYU Sch Med 1980; **Resid:** Orthopaedic Surgery, NYU Med Ctr 1985; **Fellow:** Pediatric Orthopaedic Surgery, Newington Chldns Hosp 1986; **Fac Appt:** Assoc Prof OrS, NYU Sch Med

Rawlins, Bernard A MD (OrS) - **Spec Exp:** Scoliosis; Spinal Surgery; Chiari's Deformity; **Hospital:** Hosp For Special Surgery (page 115); **Address:** 535 E 70 St, New York, NY 10021; **Phone:** 212-606-1632; **Board Cert:** Orthopaedic Surgery 2006; **Med School:** Cornell Univ 1987; **Resid:** Orthopaedic Surgery, Columbia-Presby Hosp 1992; **Fellow:** Spinal Surgery, Minnesota Spine Ctr 1993; **Fac Appt:** Assoc Prof OrS, Cornell Univ-Weill Med Coll

Roberts, Matthew M MD (OrS) - **Spec Exp:** Foot & Ankle Surgery; Arthritis; Foot Deformities; Sports Medicine; **Hospital:** Hosp For Special Surgery (page 115); **Address:** Hospital for Special Surgery, 535 E 70th St, New York, NY 10021; **Phone:** 212-606-1181; **Board Cert:** Orthopaedic Surgery 2005; **Med School:** Univ Tex, Houston 1997; **Resid:** Orthopaedic Surgery, Hosp for Special Surg 2003; **Fellow:** Foot & Ankle Surgery, Hosp for Special Surg 2004; **Fac Appt:** Asst Prof OrS, Cornell Univ-Weill Med Coll

Rose, Donald J MD (OrS) - **Spec Exp:** Dance/Ballet Injuries; Arthroscopic Surgery; Sports Injuries; Hip Surgery; **Hospital:** NYU Hosp For Joint Diseases (page 119), NYU Langone Med Ctr (page 108); **Address:** 1095 Park Ave, New York, NY 10128-1154; **Phone:** 212-427-7750; **Board Cert:** Orthopaedic Surgery 2009; **Med School:** UMDNJ-RW Johnson Med Sch 1980; **Resid:** Surgery, Beth Israel Med Ctr 1981; Orthopaedic Surgery, Hosp for Joint Diseases 1985; **Fellow:** Sports Medicine, Temple Univ Hosp 1986; **Fac Appt:** Assoc Clin Prof OrS, NYU Sch Med

Rose, Howard A MD (OrS) - **Spec Exp:** Sports Medicine; Joint Replacement; Arthroscopic Surgery; **Hospital:** Hosp For Special Surgery (page 115), NY-Presby/Weill Cornell Med Ctr, NY (page 104); **Address:** 535 E 70th St, New York, NY 10021; **Phone:** 212-606-1278; **Board Cert:** Orthopaedic Surgery 1985; **Med School:** Geo Wash Univ 1977; **Resid:** Orthopaedic Surgery, Hosp Special Surg 1982; **Fellow:** Sports Medicine, Brigham & Womens Hosp 1983; Joint Replacement Surgery, Brigham & Womens Hosp 1983; **Fac Appt:** Asst Prof OrS, Cornell Univ-Weill Med Coll

Roye Jr, David P MD (OrS) - **Spec Exp:** Pediatric Orthopaedic Surgery; Scoliosis; Hip Disorders-Pediatric; Neuromuscular Disorders; **Hospital:** Morgan Stanley Children's Hosp of NY-Presby, NY (page 104), NY-Presby/Columbia Univ Med Ctr, NY (page 104); **Address:** Morgan Stanley Chlds Hosp NewYork-Presby, 3959 Broadway, 8 North, New York, NY 10032-1559; **Phone:** 212-305-5475; **Board Cert:** Orthopaedic Surgery 1981; **Med School:** Columbia P&S 1975; **Resid:** Orthopaedic Surgery, Columbia-Presby Med Ctr 1979; **Fellow:** Orthopaedic Surgery, Hosp for Sick Chldn 1980; **Fac Appt:** Prof OrS, Columbia P&S

Rozbruch, Jacob D MD (OrS) - **Spec Exp:** Spinal Surgery; Shoulder Surgery; Knee Surgery; **Hospital:** Beth Israel Med Ctr - Petrie Division (page 94); **Address:** 420 E 72nd St, Ste 1J, New York, NY 10021; **Phone:** 212-744-9857; **Board Cert:** Orthopaedic Surgery 1980; Pediatrics 1979; **Med School:** SUNY Buffalo 1973; **Resid:** Surgery, NY Hosp 1976; Orthopaedic Surgery, Hosp Special Surg 1979; **Fac Appt:** Asst Clin Prof OrS, Albert Einstein Coll Med

Rozbruch, S Robert MD (OrS) - **Spec Exp:** Limb Lengthening; Limb Deformities; Limb Surgery/Reconstruction; Fractures-Complex & Non Union; **Hospital:** Hosp For Special Surgery (page 115), NY-Presby/Weill Cornell Med Ctr, NY (page 104); **Address:** Hospital for Special Surgery, 535 E 70th St, River Terr Bldg - Fl 2 - Ste 204, New York, NY 10021; **Phone:** 212-606-1415; **Board Cert:** Orthopaedic Surgery 2009; **Med School:** Cornell Univ-Weill Med Coll 1990; **Resid:** Orthopaedic Surgery, Hosp Special Surgery 1995; **Fellow:** Trauma, Univ Bern Hosp 1997; Limb Lengthening, Intl Ctr Limb Length/Univ MD 1999; **Fac Appt:** Prof OrS, Cornell Univ-Weill Med Coll

Salvati, Eduardo A MD (OrS) - **Spec Exp:** Hip Replacement; Knee Replacement; **Hospital:** Hosp For Special Surgery (page 115); **Address:** Hosp for Spec Surg, 535 E 70th Street, New York, NY 10021; **Phone:** 212-606-1472; **Board Cert:** Orthopaedic Surgery 1972; **Med School:** Argentina 1963; **Resid:** Orthopaedic Surgery, Univ Florence Ortho Clinic 1965; Orthopaedic Surgery, Hosp Buenos Aires 1969; **Fellow:** Hip Surgery, Hosp For Spec Surg 1972; **Fac Appt:** Clin Prof OrS, Cornell Univ-Weill Med Coll

Sandhu, Harvinder S MD (OrS) - **Spec Exp:** Minimally Invasive Surgery; Spinal Disc Replacement; Spinal Surgery; **Hospital:** Hosp For Special Surgery (page 115); **Address:** Hosp for Special Surgery, 523 E 72nd St, New York, NY 10021; **Phone:** 212-606-1798; **Board Cert:** Orthopaedic Surgery 2007; **Med School:** Northwestern Univ 1987; **Resid:** Orthopaedic Surgery, Univ Hosp-SUNY Hlth Sci Ctr 1992; **Fellow:** Spinal Surgery, UCLA Med Ctr 1993; **Fac Appt:** Assoc Prof OrS, Cornell Univ-Weill Med Coll

Sands, Andrew K MD (OrS) - **Spec Exp:** Foot & Ankle Surgery; Ankle Replacement & Revision; Arthroscopic Surgery; Sports Medicine; **Hospital:** NY Downtown Hosp, Kingsbrook Jewish Med Ctr; **Address:** 170 William St Fl 8, New York, NY 10038; **Phone:** 212-312-5966; **Board Cert:** Orthopaedic Surgery 2003; **Med School:** NY Med Coll 1985; **Resid:** Orthopaedic Surgery, Lenox Hill Hosp 1990; **Fellow:** Foot & Ankle Surgery, Harborview Med Ctr 1994

Scher, David M MD (OrS) - **Spec Exp:** Pediatric Orthopaedic Surgery; Musculoskeletal Disorders; Trauma; Gait Disorders; **Hospital:** Hosp For Special Surgery (page 115); **Address:** Hosp for Special Surgery, 535 E 70th St, New York, NY 10021; **Phone:** 212-606-1253; **Board Cert:** Orthopaedic Surgery 2002; **Med School:** Duke Univ 1993; **Resid:** Orthopaedic Surgery, Hosp Joint Diseases 1999; **Fellow:** Pediatric Orthopaedic Surgery, Childrens Hosp 2000; **Fac Appt:** Assoc Prof OrS, Cornell Univ-Weill Med Coll

Schwab, Frank J MD (OrS) - **Spec Exp:** Spinal Surgery; Pain-Back; Spinal Deformity; Scoliosis; **Hospital:** NYU Hosp For Joint Diseases (page 119), New York Methodist Hosp (page 418); **Address:** 306 E 15th St, Ste 1F, New York, NY 10003; **Phone:** 646-794-8646; **Board Cert:** Orthopaedic Surgery 2010; **Med School:** Columbia P&S 1990; **Resid:** Surgery, NY Presby-Columbia Med Ctr 1992; Orthopaedic Surgery, NY Presby-Columbia Med Ctr 1996; **Fellow:** Orthopaedic Surgery, Hospital Lariboisiere 1991; Spinal Surgery, Maimonides Med Ctr 1997; **Fac Appt:** Clin Prof OrS, NYU Sch Med

Schwartz, Jeffrey MD (OrS) - **Hospital:** Lenox Hill Hosp (page 106); **Address:** 73 E 71st St, New York, NY 10021; **Phone:** 212-535-6600; **Board Cert:** Orthopaedic Surgery 1978; **Med School:** NY Med Coll 1972; **Resid:** Surgery, Mount Sinai Med Ctr 1973; Orthopaedic Surgery, Lenox Hill Hosp 1976

Scott, W Norman MD (OrS) - **Spec Exp:** Knee Injuries; Knee Replacement; Sports Medicine; **Hospital:** Lenox Hill Hosp (page 106); **Address:** 210 E 64th St Fl 4, New York, NY 10065; **Phone:** 646-293-7501; **Board Cert:** Orthopaedic Surgery 1978; **Med School:** Cornell Univ-Weill Med Coll 1972; **Resid:** Surgery, St Lukes-Roosevelt Hosp Ctr 1974; Orthopaedic Surgery, Hosp Special Surg 1977; **Fac Appt:** Clin Prof OrS, Cornell Univ-Weill Med Coll

Scuderi, Giles R MD (OrS) - **Spec Exp:** Knee Replacement; Knee Reconstruction; Knee Injuries/Ligament Surgery; Sports Medicine; **Hospital:** Lenox Hill Hosp (page 106), Franklin Hosp (page 106); **Address:** 210 E 64th St Fl 4, New York, NY 10065; **Phone:** 212-434-4310; **Board Cert:** Orthopaedic Surgery 2011; **Med School:** SUNY Downstate 1982; **Resid:** Orthopaedic Surgery, Lenox Hill Hosp 1987; **Fellow:** Knee Surgery, Hosp Special Surgery 1988; **Fac Appt:** Asst Clin Prof OrS, Albert Einstein Coll Med

Simon, Sheldon R MD (OrS) - **Spec Exp:** Foot & Ankle Surgery; Pediatric Orthopaedic Surgery; **Hospital:** Beth Israel Med Ctr - Petrie Division (page 94); **Address:** Beth Israel Orthopedics and Sports Med, 10 Union Square E, Ste 3K, New York, NY 10003; **Phone:** 212-844-6756; **Board Cert:** Orthopaedic Surgery 1976; **Med School:** NYU Sch Med 1966; **Resid:** Surgery, Bellevue Hosp/NYU Med Ctr 1968; Orthopaedic Surgery, Mass Genl Hosp 1973; **Fac Appt:** Clin Prof OrS, Albert Einstein Coll Med

Sink, Ernest L MD (OrS) - **Spec Exp:** Hip Surgery; Arthroscopic Surgery; Sports Medicine; **Hospital:** Hosp For Special Surgery (page 115), NY-Presby/Weill Cornell Med Ctr, NY (page 104); **Address:** 535 E 70th St, New York, NY 10021; **Phone:** 212-606-1268; **Board Cert:** Orthopaedic Surgery 2002; **Med School:** Univ Tex SW, Dallas 1994; **Resid:** Orthopaedic Surgery, Univ Tex SW Med Ctr 1999; **Fellow:** Pediatric Orthopaedic Surgery, Rady Chldn's Hosp 2000

Spivak, Jeffrey M MD (OrS) - **Spec Exp:** Spinal Surgery; Scoliosis; Sports Medicine Back Injuries; **Hospital:** NYU Hosp For Joint Diseases (page 119), NYU Langone Med Ctr (page 108); **Address:** Hosp for Joint Diseases, Spine Ctr, 301 E 17th St, Ste 400, New York, NY 10003-3804; **Phone:** 212-598-6696; **Board Cert:** Orthopaedic Surgery 2006; **Med School:** Cornell Univ-Weill Med Coll 1986; **Resid:** Orthopaedic Surgery, Hosp for Joint Diseases 1992; **Fellow:** Spinal Surgery, Thomas Jefferson Univ Hosp 1993; **Fac Appt:** Asst Prof OrS, NYU Sch Med

Strauss, Elton MD (OrS) - **Spec Exp:** Fractures; Hip & Knee Replacement; Osteomyelitis; Geriatric Orthopaedic Surgery; **Hospital:** Mount Sinai Med Ctr (page 102); **Address:** Mount Sinai Dept Orthopaedic Surgery, 5 E 98 St, Box 1188, New York, NY 10029-6501; **Phone:** 212-241-1648; **Board Cert:** Orthopaedic Surgery 1981; **Med School:** Mexico 1974; **Resid:** Orthopaedic Surgery, Bronx Lebanon Hosp 1979; **Fac Appt:** Assoc Prof OrS, Mount Sinai Sch Med

Stuchin, Steven MD (OrS) - **Spec Exp:** Hand Surgery; Arthritis; Hip & Knee Replacement; Hip Resurfacing; **Hospital:** NYU Hosp For Joint Diseases (page 119), Lenox Hill Hosp (page 106); **Address:** 333 E 38th St, New York, NY 10016; **Phone:** 212-598-6708; **Board Cert:** Orthopaedic Surgery 1984; **Med School:** Columbia P&S 1976; **Resid:** Surgery, Roosevelt Hosp 1978; Orthopaedic Surgery, Hosp for Special Surg 1981; **Fellow:** Hand Surgery, Thomas Jefferson Univ Hosp 1982; **Fac Appt:** Assoc Prof OrS, NYU Sch Med

Su, Edwin P MD (OrS) - **Spec Exp:** Hip Resurfacing; Hip Replacement; Reconstructive Surgery; **Hospital:** Hosp For Special Surgery (page 115); **Address:** Hosp for Special Surgery, 535 E 70th St, New York, NY 10021; **Phone:** 212-606-1128; **Board Cert:** Orthopaedic Surgery 2006; **Med School:** Cornell Univ-Weill Med Coll 1997; **Resid:** Orthopaedic Surgery, Hosp for Special Surgery 2002; **Fellow:** Reconstructive Surgery, Hosp for Special Surgery 2003; **Fac Appt:** Asst Prof OrS, Cornell Univ-Weill Med Coll

Tindel, Nathaniel L MD (OrS) - **Spec Exp:** Spinal Surgery; Scoliosis; Minimally Invasive Surgery; Spinal Reconstructive Surgery; **Hospital:** Lenox Hill Hosp (page 106); **Address:** NY Ctr for Spinal Disorders, 425 E 79th St, Ste 1H, New York, NY 10075; **Phone:** 212-249-3840; **Board Cert:** Orthopaedic Surgery 2009; **Med School:** Univ Pennsylvania 1989; **Resid:** Orthopaedic Surgery, Lenox Hill Hosp 1994; **Fellow:** Spinal Surgery, Univ Miami 1995; **Fac Appt:** Asst Prof OrS, Albert Einstein Coll Med

Turtel, Andrew H MD (OrS) - **Spec Exp:** Knee Surgery; Shoulder Surgery; Sports Medicine; Arthroscopic Surgery; **Hospital:** Lenox Hill Hosp (page 106), Beth Israel Med Ctr - Petrie Division (page 94); **Address:** 333 E 56th St, New York, NY 10022-3758; **Phone:** 212-319-6500; **Board Cert:** Orthopaedic Surgery 2005; **Med School:** SUNY Upstate Med Univ 1985; **Resid:** Surgery, SUNY Upstate Med Ctr 1987; Orthopaedic Surgery, LI Jewish Med Ctr 1991; **Fellow:** Sports Medicine, NYU Med Ctr 1992; **Fac Appt:** Assoc Clin Prof OrS, Albert Einstein Coll Med

Unis, George L MD (OrS) - **Spec Exp:** Sports Medicine; Arthroscopic Surgery; **Hospital:** St. Luke's - Roosevelt Hosp Ctr - Roosevelt Div (page 94), St. Luke's - Roosevelt Hosp Ctr - St Luke's Hosp (page 94); **Address:** 115 E 61st St Fl 8, New York, NY 10065; **Phone:** 212-688-3710; **Board Cert:** Orthopaedic Surgery 1973; **Med School:** UMDNJ-NJ Med Sch, Newark 1965; **Resid:** Surgery, St Lukes Roosevelt Hosp 1967; Orthopaedic Surgery, St Lukes Roosevelt Hosp 1970; **Fac Appt:** Clin Prof OrS, Columbia P&S

Vitale, Michael MD (OrS) - **Spec Exp:** Spinal Surgery-Pediatric; Scoliosis; Limb Lengthening (Ilizarov Procedure); Clubfoot/Foot Deformities in Children; **Hospital:** Morgan Stanley Children's Hosp of NY-Presby, NY (page 104), NY-Presby/Columbia Univ Med Ctr, NY (page 104); **Address:** Morgan Stanley Chldn's Hosp, 3959 Broadway, Ste 800N, New York, NY 10032; **Phone:** 212-305-5475; **Board Cert:** Orthopaedic Surgery 2003; **Med School:** Columbia P&S 1995; **Resid:** Orthopaedic Surgery, Columbia Presby Med Ctr 2000; **Fellow:** Orthopaedic Surgery, Chldn's Hosp of Los Angeles 2001

Warren, Russell MD (OrS) - **Spec Exp:** Knee Injuries/Ligament Surgery; Shoulder Surgery; Shoulder Replacement; Rotator Cuff Surgery; **Hospital:** Hosp For Special Surgery (page 115); **Address:** 535 E 70th St, New York, NY 10021-4892; **Phone:** 212-606-1178; **Board Cert:** Orthopaedic Surgery 1974; **Med School:** SUNY Upstate Med Univ 1966; **Resid:** Surgery, St Lukes Hosp 1968; Orthopaedic Surgery, Hosp For Special Surgery 1973; **Fellow:** Shoulder Surgery, Columbia-Presby Med Ctr 1977; **Fac Appt:** Prof OrS, Cornell Univ-Weill Med Coll

Weiner, Lon S MD (OrS) - **Spec Exp:** Trauma; Fractures; **Hospital:** Lenox Hill Hosp (page 106), Riverview Med Ctr; **Address:** 130 E 77th St, Black Hall, Fl 12, New York, NY 10075; **Phone:** 212-434-4880; **Board Cert:** Orthopaedic Surgery 2011; **Med School:** Mount Sinai Sch Med 1982; **Resid:** Orthopaedic Surgery, Mount Sinai Hosp 1987; **Fellow:** Pediatric Orthopaedic Surgery, Hosp Special Surg 1988

Weinfeld, Steven B MD (OrS) - **Spec Exp:** Foot & Ankle Surgery; Diabetic Leg/Foot; **Hospital:** Mount Sinai Med Ctr (page 102), Hackensack Univ Med Ctr (page 96); **Address:** 5 E 98th St Fl 9, Box 1188, New York, NY 10029; **Phone:** 212-241-1634; **Board Cert:** Orthopaedic Surgery 2009; **Med School:** Albany Med Coll 1990; **Resid:** Orthopaedic Surgery, Albany Med Ctr 1995; **Fellow:** Ankle and Foot Surgery, Union Meml Hosp 1996; **Fac Appt:** Assoc Prof OrS, Mount Sinai Sch Med

Westrich, Geoffrey H MD (OrS) - **Spec Exp:** Hip Replacement & Revision; Knee Replacement & Revision; Arthroscopic Surgery-Hip; Arthroscopic Surgery-Knee; **Hospital:** Hosp For Special Surgery (page 115), NY-Presby/Weill Cornell Med Ctr, NY (page 104); **Address:** Hospital for Special Surgery, 535 E 70th St, New York, NY 10021; **Phone:** 212-606-1510; **Board Cert:** Orthopaedic Surgery 2009; **Med School:** Tufts Univ 1990; **Resid:** Orthopaedic Surgery, Hosp for Special Surg 1995; **Fellow:** Trauma, Inselspital 1995; Adult Reconstructive Surgery, Hosp for Special Surg 1996; **Fac Appt:** Assoc Prof OrS, Cornell Univ-Weill Med Coll

Wickiewicz, Thomas L MD (OrS) - **Spec Exp:** Knee Injuries/ACL; Sports Medicine; Shoulder Surgery; Rotator Cuff Surgery; **Hospital:** Hosp For Special Surgery (page 115), NY-Presby/Weill Cornell Med Ctr, NY (page 104); **Address:** 535 E 70th St, New York, NY 10021; **Phone:** 212-606-1450; **Board Cert:** Orthopaedic Surgery 1984; **Med School:** UMDNJ-NJ Med Sch, Newark 1976; **Resid:** Orthopaedic Surgery, Hosp for Special Surg 1981; **Fellow:** Sports Medicine, UCLA Med Ctr 1982; **Fac Appt:** Clin Prof OrS, Cornell Univ-Weill Med Coll

Widmann, Roger F MD (OrS) - **Spec Exp:** Pediatric Orthopaedic Surgery; Scoliosis; Limb Lengthening; Limb Deformities; **Hospital:** Hosp For Special Surgery (page 115); **Address:** 535 E 70th St, New York, NY 10021; **Phone:** 212-606-1325; **Board Cert:** Orthopaedic Surgery 2008; **Med School:** Yale Univ 1989; **Resid:** Orthopaedic Surgery, Mass General Hosp 1994; **Fellow:** Pediatric Orthopaedic Surgery, Children's Hosp 1995; **Fac Appt:** Asst Prof OrS, Cornell Univ-Weill Med Coll

Windsor, Russell E MD (OrS) - **Spec Exp:** Knee Replacement; Hip Replacement; Knee Injuries/Ligament Surgery; **Hospital:** Hosp For Special Surgery (page 115), NY-Presby/Weill Cornell Med Ctr, NY (page 104); **Address:** Hosp for Special Surgery, 535 E 70th St, New York, NY 10021; **Phone:** 212-606-1166; **Board Cert:** Orthopaedic Surgery 2007; **Med School:** Georgetown Univ 1978; **Resid:** Orthopaedic Surgery, Hosp Univ Penn 1983; **Fellow:** Knee Surgery, Hosp For Special Surg 1984; **Fac Appt:** Prof OrS, Cornell Univ-Weill Med Coll

Wittig, James C MD (OrS) - **Spec Exp:** Bone Tumors; Sarcoma-Soft Tissue; Hip & Knee Replacement; Shoulder Tumors; **Hospital:** Mount Sinai Med Ctr (page 102), Hackensack Univ Med Ctr (page 96); **Address:** 5 E 98th St, Fl 9, New York, NY 10029; **Phone:** 212-241-1807 x4817; **Board Cert:** Orthopaedic Surgery 2003; **Med School:** NYU Sch Med 1994; **Resid:** Orthopaedic Surgery, Columbia Presby Med Ctr 1999; **Fellow:** Orthopaedic Oncology, Washington Cancer Inst 2001; Orthopaedic Oncology, NIH 2001; **Fac Appt:** Assoc Prof OrS, Mount Sinai Sch Med

Zambetti Jr, George J MD (OrS) - **Spec Exp:** Knee Reconstruction; Shoulder Surgery; Sports Medicine; Arthroscopic Surgery; **Hospital:** St. Luke's - Roosevelt Hosp Ctr - Roosevelt Div (page 94); **Address:** 343 W 58th St, New York, NY 10019-1173; **Phone:** 212-506-0236; **Board Cert:** Orthopaedic Surgery 1983; **Med School:** Albany Med Coll 1976; **Resid:** Orthopaedic Surgery, Columbia-Presby Med Ctr 1981

Zuckerman, Joseph D MD (OrS) - **Spec Exp:** Shoulder Surgery; Hip Replacement; Knee Replacement; Rotator Cuff Surgery; **Hospital:** NYU Hosp For Joint Diseases (page 119), NYU Langone Med Ctr (page 108); **Address:** NYU Hosp for Joint Diseases, Dept Ortho Surg, 301 E 17th St Fl 14 - Ste 1402, New York, NY 10003; **Phone:** 212-598-6674; **Board Cert:** Orthopaedic Surgery 2007; **Med School:** Med Coll Wisc 1978; **Resid:** Orthopaedic Surgery, Univ WA Med Ctr 1983; **Fellow:** Arthritis Surgery, Brigham & Womans Hosp 1984; Shoulder Surgery, Mayo Clinic 1984; **Fac Appt:** Prof OrS, NYU Sch Med

Otolaryngology

Amin, Milan R MD (Oto) - **Spec Exp:** Voice Disorders; Vocal Cord Disorders; Swallowing Disorders; Airway Disorders; **Hospital:** NYU Langone Med Ctr (page 108); **Address:** 345 E 37 St, Ste 306, New York, NY 10016; **Phone:** 646-754-1207; **Board Cert:** Otolaryngology 2000; **Med School:** Northwestern Univ 1994; **Resid:** Otolaryngology, Temple Univ Med Ctr 1999; **Fellow:** Wake Forest Univ Med Ctr 2000; **Fac Appt:** Asst Prof Oto, NYU Sch Med

Aviv, Jonathan MD (Oto) - **Spec Exp:** Voice Disorders; Swallowing Disorders; Cough; Endoscopy; **Hospital:** Mount Sinai Med Ctr (page 102); **Address:** 210 E 86th St, Fl 9, New York, NY 10028; **Phone:** 212-722-5570; **Board Cert:** Otolaryngology 1990; **Med School:** Columbia P&S 1985; **Resid:** Surgery, Mt Sinai Med Ctr 1987; Otolaryngology, Mt Sinai Med Ctr 1990; **Fellow:** Otolaryngology, Mt Sinai Med Ctr 1991; **Fac Appt:** Prof Oto, Mount Sinai Sch Med

Blitzer, Andrew MD/DDS (Oto) - **Spec Exp:** Voice Disorders; Swallowing Disorders; Nasal & Sinus Surgery; Botox Therapy; **Hospital:** St. Luke's - Roosevelt Hosp Ctr - Roosevelt Div (page 94); **Address:** 425 W 59th St Fl 10, New York, NY 10019-1104; **Phone:** 212-262-9500; **Board Cert:** Otolaryngology 1977; **Med School:** Mount Sinai Sch Med 1973; **Resid:** Surgery, Beth Israel Med Ctr 1974; Otolaryngology, Mt Sinai Hosp 1977; **Fac Appt:** Clin Prof Oto, Columbia P&S

Boyle, Jay O MD (Oto) - **Spec Exp:** Precancerous Lesions; Oral Cancers; Melanoma-Head & Neck; Thyroid Cancer; **Hospital:** Meml Sloan-Kettering Cancer Ctr (page 116); **Address:** Memorial Sloan Kettering Cancer Ctr, 1275 York Ave, New York, NY 10065; **Phone:** 646-639-2906; **Board Cert:** Otolaryngology 1997; **Med School:** Univ Ariz Coll Med 1990; **Resid:** Surgery, Johns Hopkins Hosp 1992; Otolaryngology, Johns Hopkins Bayview Med Ctr 1996; **Fellow:** Head and Neck Surgery, Meml Sloan Kettering Cancer Ctr 1998; **Fac Appt:** Assoc Prof Oto, Cornell Univ-Weill Med Coll

Branovan, Daniel Igor MD (Oto) - **Spec Exp:** Sinus Disorders/Surgery; Endoscopic Sinus Surgery; Thyroid Cancer; Minimally Invasive Surgery; **Hospital:** New York Eye & Ear Infirm (page 117), Beth Israel Med Ctr - Petrie Division (page 94); **Address:** 1810 Voorhies Ave, Brooklyn, NY 11235; **Phone:** 718-616-1000; **Board Cert:** Otolaryngology 1999; **Med School:** Stanford Univ 1992; **Resid:** Otolaryngology, NY E&E Infirm 1996

Carew, John F MD (Oto) - **Spec Exp:** Head & Neck Surgery; Head & Neck Cancer; **Hospital:** Lenox Hill Hosp (page 106), Mount Sinai Med Ctr (page 102); **Address:** 785 Park Ave, Ste 1A, New York, NY 10021; **Phone:** 212-744-1941; **Board Cert:** Otolaryngology 1998; **Med School:** Cornell Univ-Weill Med Coll 1991; **Resid:** Otolaryngology, Manhattan EE&T 1997; **Fellow:** Head & Neck Oncology, Meml Sloan Kettering Cancer Ctr 1998

Caruana, Salvatore M MD (Oto) - **Spec Exp:** Head & Neck Cancer; Thyroid & Parathyroid Cancer & Surgery; Nasal & Sinus Disorders; Laser Surgery; **Hospital:** NY-Presby/Columbia Univ Med Ctr, NY (page 104); **Address:** 180 Fort Washington Ave, Harkness Bldg Fl 7, New York, NY 10032; **Phone:** 212-305-5335; **Board Cert:** Otolaryngology 1996; **Med School:** Mount Sinai Sch Med 1989; **Resid:** Otolaryngology, NY EE Infirm 1995; **Fellow:** Head & Neck Surgical Oncology, Meml Sloan-Kettering Canc Ctr 1997; **Fac Appt:** Asst Prof Oto, Columbia P&S

Chandrasekhar, Sujana S MD (Oto) - **Spec Exp:** Hearing & Balance Disorders; Cochlear Implants; Acoustic Neuroma; Meniere's Disease; **Hospital:** Mount Sinai Med Ctr (page 102), New York Eye & Ear Infirm (page 117); **Address:** 210 E 64th St Fl 3, New York, NY 10021; **Phone:** 212-249-3232; **Board Cert:** Otolaryngology 1993; Neurotology 2011; **Med School:** Mount Sinai Sch Med 1986; **Resid:** Surgery, NYU Med Ctr 1988; Otolaryngology, NYU Med Ctr 1992; **Fellow:** Neurotology, House Ear Clinic 1993; **Fac Appt:** Assoc Clin Prof Oto, Mount Sinai Sch Med

Close, Lanny G MD (Oto) - **Spec Exp:** Skull Base Surgery; Head & Neck Cancer; Sinus Disorders/Surgery; Endoscopic Sinus Surgery; **Hospital:** NY-Presby/Columbia Univ Med Ctr, NY (page 104); **Address:** 16 E 60th St, Ste 470, New York, NY 10022; **Phone:** 212-326-8475; **Board Cert:** Otolaryngology 1977; **Med School:** Baylor Coll Med 1972; **Resid:** Surgery, Johns Hopkins Hosp 1974; Otolaryngology, Baylor Affil Hosps 1977; **Fellow:** Head and Neck Surgery, MD Anderson Cancer Ctr 1979; **Fac Appt:** Prof Oto, Columbia P&S

Constantinides, Minas MD (Oto) - **Spec Exp:** Rhinoplasty; Rhinoplasty Revision; Nasal Surgery; Facial Rejuvenation; **Hospital:** NYU Langone Med Ctr (page 108), Lenox Hill Hosp (page 106); **Address:** NYU Med Ctr, Div Facial Plastic Surg, 74 E 79th St, New York, NY 10075; **Phone:** 212-263-5882; **Board Cert:** Otolaryngology 1994; Facial Plastic & Reconstr Surgery 1997; **Med School:** Columbia P&S 1987; **Resid:** Surgery, Harvard Surg Svcs 1989; Otolaryngology, NYU Medical Center 1993; **Fellow:** Facial Plastic Surgery, Univ Toronto 1994; **Fac Appt:** Asst Prof Oto, NYU Sch Med

Costantino, Peter D MD (Oto) - **Spec Exp:** Skull Base Tumors; Head & Neck Cancer; Craniofacial Surgery/Reconstruction; **Hospital:** Lenox Hill Hosp (page 106); **Address:** 130 E 77th St Fl 10, New York, NY 10075; **Phone:** 212-434-4500; **Board Cert:** Otolaryngology 1990; Facial Plastic & Reconstr Surgery 2000; **Med School:** Northwestern Univ 1984; **Resid:** Surgery, Northwestern Meml Hosp 1986; Otolaryngology, Northwestern Meml Hosp 1989; **Fellow:** Head and Neck Surgery, Northwestern Meml Hosp 1990; Skull Base Surgery, Univ Pittsburgh 1991; **Fac Appt:** Prof Oto, Columbia P&S

DeLacure, Mark D MD (Oto) - **Spec Exp:** Head & Neck Cancer; Head & Neck Cancer Reconstruction; Reconstructive Microsurgery; **Hospital:** NYU Langone Med Ctr (page 108), VA NY Harbor Hlthcare Sys-Manhattan Campus; **Address:** 160 E 34th St Fl 9, New York, NY 10016; **Phone:** 212-731-5329; **Board Cert:** Otolaryngology 1992; Plastic Surgery 2012; **Med School:** Univ Fla Coll Med 1986; **Resid:** Otolaryngology, Yale Univ Sch Med 1991; Plastic/Reconstructive Surgery, UCLA Med Ctr 1993; **Fellow:** Head & Neck Oncology, Meml Sloan-Kettering Cancer Ctr 1992; **Fac Appt:** Assoc Clin Prof Oto, NYU Sch Med

Dropkin, Lloyd MD (Oto) - **Hospital:** NY-Presby/Weill Cornell Med Ctr, NY (page 104); **Address:** 449 E 68th St, Ste 11, New York, NY 10065; **Phone:** 212-535-9191; **Board Cert:** Otolaryngology 1976; **Med School:** Cornell Univ-Weill Med Coll 1970; **Resid:** Otolaryngology, New York Hosp 1976; **Fac Appt:** Assoc Prof Oto, Cornell Univ-Weill Med Coll

Edelstein, David R MD (Oto) - **Spec Exp:** Endoscopic Sinus Surgery; Nasal Reconstruction; Rhinoplasty; Sleep Disorders/Apnea; **Hospital:** Lenox Hill Hosp (Manh Eye, Ear & Throat Hosp) (page 106); **Address:** 1421 3rd Ave, Fl 4, New York, NY 10028; **Phone:** 212-452-1500; **Board Cert:** Otolaryngology 1985; **Med School:** Boston Univ 1980; **Resid:** Otolaryngology, Mount Sinai Hosp 1984; **Fac Appt:** Clin Prof Oto, Cornell Univ-Weill Med Coll

Genden, Eric M MD (Oto) - **Spec Exp:** Head & Neck Cancer & Surgery; Head & Neck Cancer Reconstruction; Airway Reconstruction; Thyroid & Parathyroid Cancer & Surgery; **Hospital:** Mount Sinai Med Ctr (page 102); **Address:** Mt Sinai Dept Otolaryngology, 1 Gustave L Levy Pl, Box 1191, New York, NY 10029; **Phone:** 212-241-9410; **Board Cert:** Otolaryngology 1999; Facial Plastic & Reconstr Surgery 2000; **Med School:** Mount Sinai Sch Med 1992; **Resid:** Otolaryngology, Barnes Jewish Hosp 1998; **Fellow:** Head and Neck Surgery, Mt Sinai Med Ctr 1999; **Fac Appt:** Assoc Prof Oto, Mount Sinai Sch Med

Godin, David A MD (Oto) - **Spec Exp:** Laryngeal & Voice Disorders; Swallowing Disorders; Sleep Disorders/Apnea; Pediatric Otolaryngology; **Hospital:** New York Eye & Ear Infirm (page 117); **Address:** 261 5th Ave, Fl 9th, Ste 901, New York, NY 10016; **Phone:** 212-679-3499; **Board Cert:** Otolaryngology 2001; **Med School:** SUNY Upstate Med Univ 1995; **Resid:** Surgery, Tulane Univ 1996; Otolaryngology, Tulane Univ 1920; **Fac Appt:** Asst Prof Oto, NYU Sch Med

Gold, Scott D MD (Oto) - **Spec Exp:** Endoscopic Sinus Surgery; Sinus Disorders/Surgery; **Hospital:** Beth Israel Med Ctr - Petrie Division (page 94), Mount Sinai Med Ctr (page 102); **Address:** 36A E 36th St, Ste 200, New York, NY 10016-3401; **Phone:** 212-889-8575; **Board Cert:** Otolaryngology 1983; **Med School:** Mount Sinai Sch Med 1979; **Resid:** Otolaryngology, Mt Sinai Med Ctr 1983; **Fac Appt:** Asst Clin Prof Oto, Mount Sinai Sch Med

Green, Robert P MD (Oto) - **Spec Exp:** Sinus Disorders; Hearing Loss/Tinnitus; Throat Disorders; **Hospital:** Mount Sinai Med Ctr (page 102); **Address:** ENT & Allergy, 210 E 86th St Fl 9, New York, NY 10028; **Phone:** 212-722-5570; **Board Cert:** Otolaryngology 1981; **Med School:** Harvard Med Sch 1977; **Resid:** Otolaryngology, Mount Sinai Hosp 1981; **Fac Appt:** Assoc Clin Prof Oto, Mount Sinai Sch Med

Guida, Robert MD (Oto) - **Spec Exp:** Rhinoplasty; Nasal Surgery; Cosmetic Surgery-Face; Skin Laser Surgery; **Hospital:** NY-Presby/Weill Cornell Med Ctr, NY (page 104), Lenox Hill Hosp (Manh Eye, Ear & Throat Hosp) (page 106); **Address:** 1175 Park Ave, Ste 1B, New York, NY 10128; **Phone:** 212-871-0900; **Board Cert:** Otolaryngology 1989; Facial Plastic & Reconstr Surgery 1994; **Med School:** Hahnemann Univ 1983; **Resid:** Surgery, Graduate Hosp 1985; Otolaryngology, NY Eye & Ear Infirm 1989; **Fellow:** Facial Plastic Surgery, Oregon Hlth Sci Ctr 1990; **Fac Appt:** Assoc Prof Oto, Cornell Univ-Weill Med Coll

Hammerschlag, Paul E MD (Oto) - **Spec Exp:** Cochlear Implants; Hearing Loss; Meniere's Disease; Balance Disorders; **Hospital:** NYU Langone Med Ctr (page 108), New York Eye & Ear Infirm (page 117); **Address:** 650 First Ave, New York, NY 10016-3240; **Phone:** 212-889-2600; **Board Cert:** Otolaryngology 1978; **Med School:** Albert Einstein Coll Med 1972; **Resid:** Surgery, Virginia Mason Hosp 1974; Otolaryngology, Mass Eye & Ear Infirm 1978; **Fellow:** Otolaryngology, Mass Eye & Ear Infirm 1978; **Fac Appt:** Assoc Clin Prof Oto, NYU Sch Med

Har-El, Gady MD (Oto) - **Spec Exp:** Head & Neck Cancer; Thyroid & Parathyroid Surgery; Sinus Tumors; Skull Base Tumors; **Hospital:** Lenox Hill Hosp (page 106), Lenox Hill Hosp (Manh Eye, Ear & Throat Hosp) (page 106); **Address:** 186 E 76th St E Fl 2, MS 10021, New York, NY 10021; **Phone:** 212-744-4368; **Board Cert:** Otolaryngology 1992; **Med School:** Israel 1982; **Resid:** Otolaryngology, SUNY Downstate Med Ctr 1991; **Fellow:** Head and Neck Surgery, Long Island Coll Hosp 1987; **Fac Appt:** Prof Oto, SUNY Hlth Sci Ctr

Hoffman, Ronald A MD (Oto) - **Spec Exp:** Cochlear Implants; Balance Disorders; Ear Disorders/Surgery; **Hospital:** New York Eye & Ear Infirm (page 117); **Address:** 380 2nd Ave Fl 9, New York, NY 10010; **Phone:** 212-614-8388; **Board Cert:** Otolaryngology 1976; **Med School:** Jefferson Med Coll 1971; **Resid:** Otolaryngology, NYU Med Ctr 1976; **Fellow:** Otology & Neurotology, Lenox Hill Hosp 1977; **Fac Appt:** Prof Oto, Albert Einstein Coll Med

Jacobs, Joseph B MD (Oto) - **Spec Exp:** Endoscopic Sinus Surgery; Sinus Disorders/Surgery; Sinus Surgery-Revision; **Hospital:** NYU Langone Med Ctr (page 108); **Address:** 345 E 37 St, Ste 306, MS 10016, Ave, New York, NY 10016-6402; **Phone:** 646-754-1203; **Board Cert:** Otolaryngology 1978; **Med School:** Albert Einstein Coll Med 1974; **Resid:** Otolaryngology, NYU Med Ctr 1978; **Fellow:** Plastic/Reconstructive Surgery, UCLA Med Ctr 1979; **Fac Appt:** Prof Oto, NYU Sch Med

Jahn, Anthony MD (Oto) - **Spec Exp:** Voice Disorders/Professional Voice Care; Hearing Loss; Otology & Neuro-Otology; **Hospital:** St. Luke's - Roosevelt Hosp Ctr - Roosevelt Div (page 94); **Address:** Head & Neck Surgical Group, 425 W 59th St, New York, NY 10019; **Phone:** 212-262-4400; **Board Cert:** Otolaryngology 1979; **Med School:** Canada 1974; **Resid:** Otolaryngology, Toronto Genl Hosp 1979; **Fac Appt:** Prof Oto, Columbia P&S

Josephson, Jordan S MD (Oto) - **Spec Exp:** Rhinoplasty Revision; Endoscopic Sinus Surgery; Nasal & Sinus Disorders; Sleep Apnea; **Hospital:** Lenox Hill Hosp (Manh Eye, Ear & Throat Hosp) (page 106); **Address:** 205 E 76th St, Ste M1, New York, NY 10021; **Phone:** 212-717-1773; **Board Cert:** Otolaryngology 1988; **Med School:** SUNY Downstate 1983; **Resid:** Otolaryngology, LI Jewish Med Ctr 1988; **Fellow:** Sinus Surgery, Johns Hopkins Hosp 1989

Kacker, Ashutosh MD (Oto) - **Spec Exp:** Sinus Surgery; **Hospital:** NY-Presby/Weill Cornell Med Ctr, NY (page 104); **Address:** 1305 York Ave Fl 5, New York, NY 10021; **Phone:** 646-962-5097; **Board Cert:** Otolaryngology 2012; **Med School:** India 1989; **Resid:** Surgery, Lenox Hill Hosp 1997; **Fellow:** Otolaryngology, Manhattan Eye, Ear & Throat 2001; **Fac Appt:** Assoc Prof Oto, Cornell Univ

Kohan, Darius MD (Oto) - **Spec Exp:** Cochlear Implants; Acoustic Neuroma; Hearing Disorders; Ear Tumors; **Hospital:** Lenox Hill Hosp (Manh Eye, Ear & Throat Hosp) (page 106), New York Eye & Ear Infirm (page 117); **Address:** 863 Park Ave, Ste 1E, New York, NY 10021; **Phone:** 212-472-1300; **Board Cert:** Otolaryngology 1990; Neurotology 2012; **Med School:** NYU Sch Med 1984; **Resid:** Surgery, Beth Israel Med Ctr 1986; Otolaryngology, NYU Med Ctr 1990; **Fellow:** Otology, NYU Med Ctr 1991; **Fac Appt:** Assoc Prof Oto, NYU Sch Med

Komisar, Arnold MD/DDS (Oto) - **Spec Exp:** Thyroid & Parathyroid Surgery; Salivary Gland Tumors; Nasal & Sinus Surgery; **Hospital:** Lenox Hill Hosp (page 106), Lenox Hill Hosp (Manh Eye, Ear & Throat Hosp) (page 106); **Address:** 1421 3rd Ave Fl 4, New York, NY 10028; **Phone:** 212-861-8888; **Board Cert:** Otolaryngology 1979; **Med School:** Hahnemann Univ 1975; **Resid:** Surgery, Beth Israel Hosp 1976; Otolaryngology, Mt Sinai Med Ctr 1979; **Fac Appt:** Clin Prof Oto, NYU Sch Med

Koufman, Jamie A MD (Oto) - **Spec Exp:** Voice Disorders; Laryngeal Disorders; **Hospital:** New York Eye & Ear Infirm (page 117); **Address:** 200 W 57th St, Ste 1203, New York, NY 10019; **Phone:** 212-463-8014; **Board Cert:** Otolaryngology 1978; **Med School:** Boston Univ 1973; **Resid:** Surgery, Hartford Hosp 1975; Otolaryngology, Boston Univ Med Ctr 1978

Kraus, Dennis H MD (Oto) - **Spec Exp:** Head & Neck Cancer; Skull Base Tumors; Thyroid & Parathyroid Surgery; Sarcoma; **Hospital:** Lenox Hill Hosp (page 106); **Address:** 130 E 77th St, Fl 10, New York, NY 10075-1851; **Phone:** 212-434-4500; **Board Cert:** Otolaryngology 1990; **Med School:** Univ Rochester 1985; **Resid:** Surgery, Cleveland Clinic 1987; Otolaryngology, Cleveland Clinic 1990; **Fellow:** Head and Neck Surgery, Meml Sloan Kettering Cancer Ctr 1991; **Fac Appt:** Prof Oto, Cornell Univ-Weill Med Coll

Krespi, Yosef P MD (Oto) - **Spec Exp:** Nasal & Sinus Cancer & Surgery; Sleep Disorders/Apnea; Head & Neck Cancer & Surgery; Snoring/Sleep Apnea; **Hospital:** Lenox Hill Hosp (Manh Eye, Ear & Throat Hosp) (page 106); **Address:** 110 E 59th St, Ste 10A, New York, NY 10019-1128; **Phone:** 212-434-4500; **Board Cert:** Otolaryngology 1981; **Med School:** Israel 1973; **Resid:** Surgery, Mt Sinai Hosp 1976; Otolaryngology, Mt Sinai Hosp 1980; **Fellow:** Surgery, Northwestern Meml Hosp 1981; **Fac Appt:** Clin Prof Oto, Columbia P&S

Krevitt, Lane MD (Oto) - **Spec Exp:** Thyroid & Parathyroid Surgery; Endoscopic Sinus Surgery; Head & Neck Cancer & Surgery; Sleep Medicine; **Hospital:** Beth Israel Med Ctr - Petrie Division (page 94); **Address:** 36A E 36th St, Ste 200, New York, NY 10016-3453; **Phone:** 212-889-8575; **Board Cert:** Otolaryngology 1999; **Med School:** Hahnemann Univ 1993; **Resid:** Surgery, Albert Einstein Univ & Affil Hosps 1994; Otolaryngology, Albert Einstein Univ & Affil Hosps 1998; **Fellow:** Head & Neck Surgical Oncology, Montefiore Med Ctr 1999

Kuhel, William I MD (Oto) - **Spec Exp:** Head & Neck Cancer & Surgery; Thyroid Cancer; Parathyroid Cancer; **Hospital:** NY-Presby/Weill Cornell Med Ctr, NY (page 104); **Address:** 1305 York Ave Fl 5, New York, NY 10021; **Phone:** 646-962-6325; **Board Cert:** Otolaryngology 1988; **Med School:** Univ Mich Med Sch 1983; **Resid:** Surgery, St Vincent's Hosp 1985; Otolaryngology, Indiana Univ 1988; **Fellow:** Head and Neck Surgery, MD Anderson Cancer Ctr 1989; **Fac Appt:** Assoc Clin Prof Oto, Cornell Univ-Weill Med Coll

Kuriloff, Daniel MD (Oto) - **Spec Exp:** Thyroid Surgery; Parathyroid Surgery; Minimally Invasive Surgery; Head & Neck Surgery; **Hospital:** Lenox Hill Hosp (page 106); **Address:** Head & Neck Inst, 110 E 59th St Fl 10 - Ste 10A, New York, NY 10022; **Phone:** 212-262-5555; **Board Cert:** Otolaryngology 1988; **Med School:** Mount Sinai Sch Med 1982; **Resid:** Surgery, Beth Israel Hosp 1984; Otolaryngology, NY Eye & Ear Infirmary 1988; **Fellow:** Head & Neck Surgical Oncology, Univ Mich Med Ctr 1990; **Fac Appt:** Assoc Prof Oto, Columbia P&S

Lalwani, Anil K MD (Oto) - **Spec Exp:** Ear Disorders/Surgery; Facial Nerve Disorders; Pediatric Otolaryngology; Skull Base Surgery; **Hospital:** NY-Presby/Columbia Univ Med Ctr, NY (page 104); **Address:** 180 Fort Washington Ave, Harkness Pavilion Fl 7, New York, NY 10032; **Phone:** 212-305-1696; **Board Cert:** Otolaryngology 1992; Neurotology 2010; **Med School:** Univ Mich Med Sch 1985; **Resid:** Surgery, Duke Univ Med Ctr 1987; Otolaryngology, UCSF Med Ctr 1991; **Fellow:** Skull Base Surgery, UCSF Med Ctr 1992; **Fac Appt:** Prof Oto, Columbia P&S

Lawson, William MD (Oto) - **Spec Exp:** Sinus Disorders/Surgery; Endoscopic Sinus Surgery; **Hospital:** Mount Sinai Med Ctr (page 102); **Address:** 5 E 98th St Fl 8, Box 1191, New York, NY 10029-6501; **Phone:** 212-241-9410; **Board Cert:** Otolaryngology 1974; **Med School:** NYU Sch Med 1965; **Resid:** Surgery, Bronx VA Hosp 1967; Otolaryngology, Mt Sinai Hosp 1973; **Fellow:** Otolaryngology, Mt Sinai Hosp 1970; **Fac Appt:** Prof Oto, Mount Sinai Sch Med

Lebovics, Robert S MD (Oto) - **Spec Exp:** Head & Neck Inflammatory Disorders; Head & Neck Autoimmune Disease; Head & Neck Infectious Disease; Relapsing Polychondritis; **Hospital:** St. Luke's - Roosevelt Hosp Ctr - Roosevelt Div (page 94); **Address:** 425 W 59th St Fl 10, New York, NY 10019; **Phone:** 212-262-2002; **Board Cert:** Otolaryngology 1988; **Med School:** SUNY Downstate 1982; **Resid:** Surgery, Montefiore-Weiler Einstein Div 1983; Otolaryngology, Montefiore-Weiler Einstein Div 1987

Lim, Jessica W MD (Oto) - **Spec Exp:** Head & Neck Cancer; Sinus Disorders; Sleep Disorders; Swallowing Disorders; **Hospital:** Lenox Hill Hosp (page 106), Lenox Hill Hosp (Manh Eye, Ear & Throat Hosp) (page 106); **Address:** 186 E 76th St, Fl 2, New York, NY 10021; **Phone:** 212-434-2323; **Board Cert:** Otolaryngology 1998; **Med School:** W VA Univ 1991; **Resid:** Surgery, NYU Med Ctr 1993; Otolaryngology, NYU Med Ctr 1997; **Fellow:** Head and Neck Surgery, Rush Univ Med Ctr 1998; **Fac Appt:** Asst Prof Oto, SUNY Downstate

Linstrom, Christopher J MD (Oto) - **Spec Exp:** Cochlear Implants; Acoustic Neuroma; Encephalocele; Cholesteatoma; **Hospital:** New York Eye & Ear Infirm (page 117); **Address:** NY Eye & Ear Infirmary, Dept Otolaryngology, 310 E 14th St, New York, NY 10003-4201; **Phone:** 212-979-4200; **Board Cert:** Otolaryngology 1987; Neurotology 2004; **Med School:** McGill Univ 1982; **Resid:** Surgery, Geo Wash Med Ctr 1984; Otolaryngology, NY Hosp 1987; **Fellow:** Otology & Neurotology, Michigan Ear Inst 1989; **Fac Appt:** Assoc Prof Oto, NY Med Coll

Markowitz, Arlene H MD (Oto) - **Hospital:** NY-Presby/Columbia Univ Med Ctr, NY (page 104), Lenox Hill Hosp (page 106); **Address:** 903 Park Ave, New York, NY 10075; **Phone:** 212-794-3999; **Board Cert:** Otolaryngology 1990; **Med School:** Columbia P&S 1984; **Resid:** Surgery, Columbia-Presby Med Ctr 1986; Otolaryngology, Columbia-Presby Med Ctr 1990; **Fac Appt:** Asst Clin Prof Oto, Columbia P&S

Miller, Philip J MD (Oto) - **Spec Exp:** Rhinoplasty; Cosmetic Surgery-Face; Facial Nerve Disorders; Facial Rejuvenation; **Hospital:** Lenox Hill Hosp (Manh Eye, Ear & Throat Hosp) (page 106), NYU Langone Med Ctr (page 108); **Address:** 60 E 56 St Fl 3, New York, NY 10022; **Phone:** 212-750-7100; **Board Cert:** Otolaryngology 1996; Facial Plastic & Reconstr Surgery 1998; **Med School:** Univ Mass Sch Med 1989; **Resid:** Otolaryngology, NYU Med Ctr 1995; **Fellow:** Facial Plastic Surgery, Oregon Health Sci Ctr 1996; **Fac Appt:** Asst Prof Oto, NYU Sch Med

Myssiorek, David MD (Oto) - **Spec Exp:** Thyroid & Parathyroid Surgery; Head & Neck Cancer; Salivary Gland Surgery; Paragangliomas; **Hospital:** NYU Langone Med Ctr (page 108), Bellevue Hosp Ctr; **Address:** 160 E 34th St, Fl 9, New York, NY 10016; **Phone:** 212-731-6085; **Board Cert:** Otolaryngology 1985; **Med School:** NYU Sch Med 1980; **Resid:** Otolaryngology, Bellevue/NYU/VA Med Ctr 1984; **Fellow:** Head & Neck Oncology, Montefiore Med Ctr 1985; **Fac Appt:** Prof Oto, NYU Sch Med

Nass, Richard L MD (Oto) - **Spec Exp:** Sinus Disorders/Surgery; Nasal Surgery; Allergy; **Hospital:** NYU Langone Med Ctr (page 108), Lenox Hill Hosp (page 106); **Address:** 1430 2nd Ave, Ste 108, New York, NY 10021; **Phone:** 212-734-4515; **Board Cert:** Otolaryngology 1979; **Med School:** NYU Sch Med 1975; **Resid:** Otolaryngology, NYU-Bellevue Hosp 1979; **Fac Appt:** Assoc Clin Prof Oto, NYU Sch Med

Parisier, Simon C MD (Oto) - **Spec Exp:** Cochlear Implants; Hearing Loss; Ear Disorders/Surgery; Cholesteatoma; **Hospital:** New York Eye & Ear Infirm (page 117); **Address:** NY Eye & Ear Infirmary - Otolaryngology, 380 2nd Ave Fl 9, New York, NY 10010; **Phone:** 212-979-4542; **Board Cert:** Otolaryngology 1967; **Med School:** Boston Univ 1961; **Resid:** Otolaryngology, Mount Sinai Hosp 1966; **Fac Appt:** Prof Oto, NY Med Coll

Persky, Mark S MD (Oto) - **Spec Exp:** Head & Neck Cancer; Skull Base Tumors; Thyroid Cancer; Vascular Lesions-Head & Neck; **Hospital:** Beth Israel Med Ctr - Petrie Division (page 94), New York Eye & Ear Infirm (page 117); **Address:** 10 Union Square East, Ste 4J, New York, NY 10003; **Phone:** 212-844-8648; **Board Cert:** Otolaryngology 1976; **Med School:** SUNY Upstate Med Univ 1972; **Resid:** Otolaryngology, Bellevue Hosp 1976; **Fellow:** Head and Neck Surgery, Beth Israel Med Ctr 1977; **Fac Appt:** Clin Prof Oto, Albert Einstein Coll Med

Pincus, Robert L MD (Oto) - **Spec Exp:** Sinus Disorders; Voice Disorders; Endoscopic Sinus Surgery; **Hospital:** Beth Israel Med Ctr - Petrie Division (page 94), Lenox Hill Hosp (page 106); **Address:** 36A E 36th St, Ste 200, New York, NY 10016-3401; **Phone:** 212-889-8575; **Board Cert:** Otolaryngology 1983; **Med School:** Univ Mich Med Sch 1978; **Resid:** Surgery, Lenox Hill Hosp 1980; Otolaryngology, Mt Sinai Med Ctr 1983; **Fac Appt:** Assoc Prof Oto, NY Med Coll

Pollack, Geoffrey MD (Oto) - **Spec Exp:** Head & Neck Surgery; **Hospital:** St. Luke's - Roosevelt Hosp Ctr - St Luke's Hosp (page 94); **Address:** 211 Central Park West, New York, NY 10024; **Phone:** 212-873-6175; **Board Cert:** Otolaryngology 1984; **Med School:** Columbia P&S 1979; **Resid:** Otolaryngology, Columbia-Presby Med Ctr 1984

Portnoy, William M MD (Oto) - **Spec Exp:** Head & Neck Cancer & Surgery; Head & Neck Cancer Reconstruction; Facial Plastic & Reconstructive Surgery; **Hospital:** Beth Israel Med Ctr - Petrie Division (page 94), New York Eye & Ear Infirm (page 117); **Address:** 160 W 18th St, New York, NY 10011; **Phone:** 212-366-0848 x201; **Board Cert:** Otolaryngology 1993; Facial Plastic & Reconstr Surgery 1993; **Med School:** Geo Wash Univ 1987; **Resid:** Otolaryngology, NY E&E Infirm 1992; Head and Neck Surgery, NY E&E Infirm 1992; **Fellow:** Head and Neck Surgery, Mercy Hosp 1993; Microvascular Surgery, Mercy Hosp 1993

Rizk, Samieh S MD (Oto) - **Spec Exp:** Facial Plastic & Reconstructive Surgery; Rhinoplasty Revision; Nasal Surgery; **Hospital:** Lenox Hill Hosp (page 106), Lenox Hill Hosp (Manh Eye, Ear & Throat Hosp) (page 106); **Address:** 1040 Park Ave, New York, NY 10028; **Phone:** 212-452-3362; **Board Cert:** Facial Plastic & Reconstr Surgery 2000; Otolaryngology 2000; **Med School:** Univ Mich Med Sch 1993; **Resid:** Otolaryngology, Manhattan EE&T Hosp 1999; **Fellow:** Facial Plastic Surgery, Facial Surgery Center 2000

Roland Sr, J Thomas MD (Oto) - **Spec Exp:** Acoustic Neuroma; Cochlear Implants; Neuro-Otology; Facial Nerve Disorders; **Hospital:** NYU Langone Med Ctr (page 108), Bellevue Hosp Ctr; **Address:** 550 First Avenue, Ste 7Q, New York, NY 10016; **Phone:** 212-263-5565; **Board Cert:** Otolaryngology 1993; Neurotology 2004; **Med School:** Temple Univ 1983; **Resid:** Otolaryngology, NYU Med Ctr 1992; **Fellow:** Neurotology, NYU Med Ctr 1993; **Fac Appt:** Assoc Prof Oto, NYU Sch Med

Romo III, Thomas MD (Oto) - **Spec Exp:** Facial Plastic & Reconstructive Surgery; Cosmetic Surgery-Face; Rhinoplasty Revision; Ear Reconstruction/Microtia; **Hospital:** Lenox Hill Hosp (page 106), Lenox Hill Hosp (Manh Eye, Ear & Throat Hosp) (page 106); **Address:** 135 E 74th St, New York, NY 10021; **Phone:** 212-288-1500; **Board Cert:** Otolaryngology 1985; Facial Plastic & Reconstr Surgery 1992; **Med School:** Baylor Coll Med 1979; **Resid:** Otolaryngology, Baylor Hosps 1982; Otolaryngology, New York Eye & Ear Infirm 1984; **Fellow:** Facial Plastic Surgery, New York Eye & Ear Infirm 1985; Facial Plastic Surgery, Tampa General Hosp 1987; **Fac Appt:** Asst Clin Prof Oto, NY Med Coll

Rosenberg, David B MD (Oto) - **Spec Exp:** Rhinoplasty Revision; Cosmetic Surgery-Face; Reconstructive Surgery; **Hospital:** Lenox Hill Hosp (Manh Eye, Ear & Throat Hosp) (page 106); **Address:** 115 E 61st St Fl 1, New York, NY 10065; **Phone:** 212-832-8595; **Board Cert:** Otolaryngology 2000; Facial Plastic & Reconstr Surgery 2002; **Med School:** Cornell Univ-Weill Med Coll 1993; **Resid:** Otolaryngology, Manhattan EE&T Hosp 1999; **Fellow:** Facial Plastic Surgery, RWJohnson Univ Hosp 2000

Rothstein, Stephen G MD (Oto) - **Spec Exp:** Voice Disorders; Swallowing Disorders; Laser Surgery; **Hospital:** NYU Langone Med Ctr (page 108); **Address:** 530 1st Ave, Ste 3C, New York, NY 10016-6402; **Phone:** 212-263-7505; **Board Cert:** Surgical Critical Care 1988; **Med School:** Ros Franklin Univ/Chicago Med Sch 1982; **Resid:** Surgery, NYU Med Ctr 1984; Otolaryngology, NYU Med Ctr 1987; **Fellow:** Head and Neck Surgery, NYU Med Ctr 1988; **Fac Appt:** Assoc Clin Prof Oto, NYU Sch Med

Sacks, Steven H MD (Oto) - **Spec Exp:** Sinus Disorders/Surgery; Thyroid & Parathyroid Surgery; Salivary Gland Tumors & Surgery; **Hospital:** Mount Sinai Med Ctr (page 102); **Address:** 210 E 86th St, Fl 9th, ENT and Allergy Associates St, New York, NY 10028; **Phone:** 212-722-5570; **Board Cert:** Otolaryngology 1981; **Med School:** Washington Univ, St Louis 1977; **Resid:** Otolaryngology, Mt Sinai Hosp 1981; **Fac Appt:** Asst Clin Prof Oto, Mount Sinai Sch Med

Schaefer, Steven D MD (Oto) - **Spec Exp:** Sinus Disorders/Surgery; Head & Neck Surgery; Endoscopic Sinus Surgery; **Hospital:** Lenox Hill Hosp (Manh Eye, Ear & Throat Hosp) (page 106), Beth Israel Med Ctr - Petrie Division (page 94); **Address:** 110 E 59th St, Fl 10, Ste 10A, New York, NY 10022; **Phone:** 212-434-4500; **Board Cert:** Otolaryngology 1978; **Med School:** UC Irvine 1972; **Resid:** Surgery, UCLA Med Ctr 1974; Otolaryngology, Stanford Med Ctr 1977; **Fac Appt:** Prof Oto, NY Med Coll

Schantz, Stimson P MD (Oto) - **Spec Exp:** Head & Neck Surgery; Head & Neck Cancer; Thyroid Cancer; **Hospital:** New York Eye & Ear Infirm (page 117), Beth Israel Med Ctr - Petrie Division (page 94); **Address:** 310 E 14th St Fl 6N, New York, NY 10003; **Phone:** 212-979-4535; **Board Cert:** Surgery 2005; **Med School:** Univ Cincinnati 1975; **Resid:** Surgery, Georgetown Univ Med CtrGeorgetown Univ Med Ctr 1982; Otolaryngology, Univ Illinois Eye & Ear Infirm 1980; **Fellow:** Surgical Oncology, MD Anderson Cancer Ctr 1984; **Fac Appt:** Prof Oto, NY Med Coll

Schley, W Shain MD (Oto) - **Spec Exp:** Nasal & Sinus Disorders; Throat Disorders; Voice Disorders; Sleep Disorders; **Hospital:** NY-Presby/Weill Cornell Med Ctr, NY (page 104); **Address:** 449 E 68th St, Fl 2, Ste DS 10, New York, NY 10065-6310; **Phone:** 212-746-2223; **Board Cert:** Otolaryngology 1973; **Med School:** Emory Univ 1966; **Resid:** Surgery, Roosevelt Hosp 1968; Otolaryngology, New York Hosp 1973; **Fac Appt:** Assoc Clin Prof Oto, Cornell Univ-Weill Med Coll

Schneider, Kenneth L MD (Oto) - **Spec Exp:** Snoring/Sleep Apnea; Nasal & Sinus Disorders; Sleep Disorders/Apnea; **Hospital:** NYU Langone Med Ctr (page 108); **Address:** 530 1st Ave, Ste 3C, New York, NY 10016-6402; **Phone:** 212-263-7505; **Board Cert:** Otolaryngology 1982; **Med School:** SUNY Hlth Sci Ctr 1978; **Resid:** Otolaryngology, NYU Med Ctr 1982; **Fellow:** Head and Neck Surgery, Montefiore Med Ctr 1983; **Fac Appt:** Assoc Clin Prof Oto, NYU Sch Med

Sclafani, Anthony P MD (Oto) - **Spec Exp:** Cosmetic Surgery-Face; Botox Therapy; Rhinoplasty; Reconstructive Surgery; **Hospital:** New York Eye & Ear Infirm (page 117), Northern Westchester Hosp (page 613); **Address:** 310 E 14th St Fl 6, New York, NY 10003; **Phone:** 212-979-4534; **Board Cert:** Otolaryngology 1996; Facial Plastic & Reconstr Surgery 1999; **Med School:** Univ Pennsylvania 1989; **Resid:** Surgery, Beth Israel Med Ctr 1991; Otolaryngology, NY Eye & Ear Infirm 1995; **Fellow:** Facial Plastic Surgery, St Louis Univ 1996; **Fac Appt:** Prof Oto, NY Med Coll

Selesnick, Samuel H MD (Oto) - **Spec Exp:** Acoustic Neuroma; Cholesteatoma; Otosclerosis; **Hospital:** NY-Presby/Weill Cornell Med Ctr, NY (page 104), Meml Sloan-Kettering Cancer Ctr (page 116); **Address:** 1305 York Ave, Fl 5, New York, NY 10021; **Phone:** 646-962-3277; **Board Cert:** Otolaryngology 1990; Neurotology 2008; **Med School:** NYU Sch Med 1985; **Resid:** Surgery, St Vincent's Med Ctr 1987; Otolaryngology, Manhattan EE&T Hosp 1990; **Fellow:** Skull Base Surgery, UCSF Med Ctr 1991; **Fac Appt:** Prof Oto, Cornell Univ-Weill Med Coll

Shemen, Larry J MD (Oto) - **Spec Exp:** Head & Neck Cancer; Thyroid Cancer; Parathyroid Cancer; Snoring/Sleep Apnea; **Hospital:** NY Hosp Queens (page 206), Lenox Hill Hosp (page 106); **Address:** 233 E 69th St, Ste 1D, New York, NY 10021; **Phone:** 212-472-8882; **Board Cert:** Otolaryngology 1983; **Med School:** Univ Toronto 1978; **Resid:** Surgery, Cedar-Sinai Med Ctr 1982; Otolaryngology, Toronto Genl Hosp 1983; **Fellow:** Head and Neck Surgery, Meml Sloan-Kettering Cancer Ctr 1984; **Fac Appt:** Assoc Clin Prof Oto, Cornell Univ-Weill Med Coll

Shugar, Joel MD (Oto) - **Spec Exp:** Hearing & Balance Disorders; Head & Neck Surgery; Nasal & Sinus Disorders; **Hospital:** Mount Sinai Med Ctr (page 102); **Address:** 55 E 87th St, Ste 1K, New York, NY 10128-1043; **Phone:** 212-289-1731; **Board Cert:** Otolaryngology 1978; **Med School:** McGill Univ 1972; **Resid:** Surgery, Jewish Genl Hosp 1974; Otolaryngology, Mount Sinai Med Ctr 1978; **Fellow:** Otolaryngology, Mount Sinai Med Ctr 1975; **Fac Appt:** Assoc Clin Prof Oto, Mount Sinai Sch Med

Singh, Bhuvanesh MD/PhD (Oto) - **Spec Exp:** Head & Neck Cancer & Surgery; Thyroid Cancer; **Hospital:** Meml Sloan-Kettering Cancer Ctr (page 116); **Address:** 1275 York Ave, MC C1073, New York, NY 10065; **Phone:** 212-639-2024; **Board Cert:** Otolaryngology 1998; **Med School:** SUNY Downstate 1991; **Resid:** Otolaryngology, SUNY Downstate Med Ctr 1997; **Fellow:** Head and Neck Surgery, Meml Sloan-Kettering Canc Ctr 1999; **Fac Appt:** Assoc Prof Oto, Cornell Univ-Weill Med Coll

Slavit, David H MD (Oto) - **Spec Exp:** Voice Disorders; Nasal & Sinus Disorders; Head & Neck Surgery; Thyroid Surgery; **Hospital:** Lenox Hill Hosp (page 106), Lenox Hill Hosp (Manh Eye, Ear & Throat Hosp) (page 106); **Address:** 787 Park Ave, New York, NY 10021-3552; **Phone:** 212-517-9177; **Board Cert:** Otolaryngology 1992; **Med School:** Mount Sinai Sch Med 1986; **Resid:** Otolaryngology, Mayo Clinic 1991; **Fac Appt:** Asst Prof Oto, SUNY Hlth Sci Ctr

Stewart, Michael G MD (Oto) - **Spec Exp:** Nasal & Sinus Disorders; Sleep Disorders/Apnea; Head & Neck Surgery; **Address:** Weill Greenberg Center, 1305 York Ave Fl 5, New York, NY 10021; **Phone:** 646-962-6673; **Board Cert:** Otolaryngology 1995; **Med School:** Johns Hopkins Univ 1988; **Resid:** Otolaryngology, Baylor Coll Med 1994; **Fac Appt:** Prof Oto, Cornell Univ-Weill Med Coll

Storper, Ian MD (Oto) - **Spec Exp:** Skull Base Surgery; Cochlear Implants; Acoustic Neuroma; **Hospital:** Lenox Hill Hosp (page 106), Lenox Hill Hosp (Manh Eye, Ear & Throat Hosp) (page 106); **Address:** 110 E 59th St, Ste 10A, New York, NY 10022; **Phone:** 212-434-4500; **Board Cert:** Otolaryngology 1995; **Med School:** Univ Pennsylvania 1988; **Resid:** Otolaryngology, UCLA Med Ctr 1994; **Fellow:** Otology & Neurotology, Ear Foundation 1995

Strome, Marshall MD (Oto) - **Spec Exp:** Voice Disorders; Swallowing Disorders; Head & Neck Cancer Reconstruction; Head & Neck Cancer & Surgery; **Hospital:** St. Luke's - Roosevelt Hosp Ctr - St Luke's Hosp (page 94), Mount Sinai Med Ctr (page 102); **Address:** 425 W 59th St, Fl 10, New York, NY 10019; **Phone:** 212-262-4444; **Board Cert:** Otolaryngology 1970; **Med School:** Univ Mich Med Sch 1964; **Resid:** Surgery, Harper Hosp 1966; Otolaryngology, Univ Michigan Hosp 1970; **Fac Appt:** Prof Oto

Sulica, Radu Lucian MD (Oto) - **Spec Exp:** Laryngeal & Vocal Cord Surgery; Voice Disorders; Vocal Cord Disorders; Botox Therapy; **Hospital:** NY-Presby/Weill Cornell Med Ctr, NY (page 104); **Address:** 1305 York Ave, Fl 5th Floor, New York, NY 10021; **Phone:** 646-962-4734; **Board Cert:** Otolaryngology 2000; **Med School:** Georgetown Univ 1993; **Resid:** Surgery, Georgetown Univ Hosp 1995; Otolaryngology, Georgetown Univ Hosp 1999; **Fellow:** Laryngology, St Lukes Roosevelt Hosp 2000; **Fac Appt:** Assoc Prof Oto, Cornell Univ-Weill Med Coll

Turk, Jon B MD (Oto) - **Spec Exp:** Facial Plastic & Reconstructive Surgery; Cosmetic Surgery-Face; **Hospital:** N Shore Univ Hosp (page 106); **Address:** 800A Fifth Ave, Ste 202, New York, NY 10065; **Phone:** 212-421-4845; **Board Cert:** Otolaryngology 1995; Facial Plastic & Reconstr Surgery 1996; **Med School:** SUNY Downstate 1988; **Resid:** Surgery, Mt Sinai Hosp 1990; Otolaryngology, Mt Sinai Hosp 1993; **Fellow:** Facial Plastic Surgery, Inselspital-Bern 1994

Urken, Mark MD (Oto) - **Spec Exp:** Head & Neck Cancer & Surgery; Head & Neck Cancer Reconstruction; Thyroid & Parathyroid Cancer & Surgery; Salivary Gland Tumors; **Hospital:** Beth Israel Med Ctr - Petrie Division (page 94); **Address:** Inst for Head, Neck & Thyroid Cancer, 10 Union Square E, Ste 5B, New York, NY 10003-3314; **Phone:** 212-844-8775; **Board Cert:** Otolaryngology 1986; **Med School:** Univ VA Sch Med 1981; **Resid:** Otolaryngology, Mt Sinai Hosp 1986; **Fellow:** Microvascular Surgery, Mercy Hosp 1987; **Fac Appt:** Prof Oto, Albert Einstein Coll Med

Volpi, David O MD (Oto) - **Spec Exp:** Sinus Disorders; Sleep Disorders; Snoring/Sleep Apnea; **Hospital:** Lenox Hill Hosp (page 106), New York Eye & Ear Infirm (page 117); **Address:** 262 Central Park West, Ste 1H, New York, NY 10024; **Phone:** 212-873-6036; **Board Cert:** Otolaryngology 1988; **Med School:** Hahnemann Univ 1982; **Resid:** Otolaryngology, NY Eye & Ear Infirm 1988

Waner, Milton MD (Oto) - **Spec Exp:** Pediatric Facial Plastic Surgery; Birthmarks/Hemangiomas; Vascular Malformations; **Hospital:** St. Luke's - Roosevelt Hosp Ctr - St Luke's Hosp (page 94), Beth Israel Med Ctr - Petrie Division (page 94); **Address:** Vascular Birthmark Institute, 126 W 60th St, New York, NY 10023; **Phone:** 212-636-3970; **Med School:** South Africa 1977; **Resid:** Surgery, Univ of Witwatersrand 1980; Otolaryngology, Univ of Witwatersrand 1984; **Fellow:** Otolaryngology, Univ Cincinnatti Med Ctr 1985

Wong, Richard J MD (Oto) - **Spec Exp:** Head & Neck Cancer; Thyroid Cancer; **Hospital:** Meml Sloan-Kettering Cancer Ctr (page 116); **Address:** 1275 York Ave, C-1069, New York, NY 10065; **Phone:** 212-639-7638; **Board Cert:** Otolaryngology 2000; **Med School:** Harvard Med Sch 1994; **Resid:** Otolaryngology, Mass General Hosp 1999; **Fellow:** Head & Neck Surgical Oncology, Meml Sloan Kettering Cancer Ctr 2000

Woo, Peak MD (Oto) - **Spec Exp:** Voice Disorders; Laryngeal Disorders; Laryngeal Cancer; **Hospital:** Mount Sinai Med Ctr (page 102); **Address:** 300 Central Park West, Ste 1-H, New York, NY 10024; **Phone:** 212-580-1004; **Board Cert:** Otolaryngology 1983; **Med School:** Boston Univ 1978; **Resid:** Otolaryngology, Boston Univ Med Ctr 1983; **Fac Appt:** Clin Prof Oto, Mount Sinai Sch Med

Zimbler, Marc S MD (Oto) - **Spec Exp:** Facial Plastic Surgery; Blepharoplasty; Rhinoplasty; **Hospital:** Beth Israel Med Ctr - Petrie Division (page 94), New York Eye & Ear Infirm (page 117); **Address:** 990 Fifth Ave, New YOrk, NY 10075; **Phone:** 212-570-9900; **Board Cert:** Otolaryngology 2001; Facial Plastic & Reconstr Surgery 2002; **Med School:** Mount Sinai Sch Med 1993; **Resid:** Surgery, NYU Med Ctr 1995; Otolaryngology, NYU Med Ctr 1999; **Fellow:** Facial Plastic Surgery, Washington Univ 2000; **Fac Appt:** Asst Prof Oto, Albert Einstein Coll Med

Pain Medicine

Bakshi, Sanjay MD (PM) - **Spec Exp:** Pain-Spine; Pain-Back & Neck; **Hospital:** Lenox Hill Hosp (page 106), Bayshore Community Hosp; **Address:** Manhattan Spine & Pain Medicine, 115 E 57th St, Ste 610, New York, NY 10022; **Phone:** 212-535-3505; **Board Cert:** Anesthesiology 1995; Pain Medicine 2007; **Med School:** India 1989; **Resid:** Anesthesiology, Brookdale Hosp Med Ctr 1994; **Fellow:** Pain Medicine, Johns Hopkins Hosp 1995

Epstein, Lawrence J MD (PM) - **Spec Exp:** Pain-Spine; Pain-Neck; Sciatica; **Hospital:** Mount Sinai Med Ctr (page 102); **Address:** Mount Sinai Medical Ctr, Pain Management, 5 E 98th St Fl 6, New York, NY 10029; **Phone:** 212-241-6372; **Board Cert:** Anesthesiology 1987; Pain Medicine 2004; **Med School:** Israel 1983; **Resid:** Anesthesiology, SUNY Brooklyn Med Ctr 1986; **Fellow:** Obstetrics & Anesthesiology, SUNY Brooklyn Med Ctr 1987; **Fac Appt:** Asst Prof Anes, Mount Sinai Sch Med

Freedman, Gordon MD (PM) - **Spec Exp:** Pain-Back & Neck; Reflex Sympathetic Dystrophy (RSD); Pain-Neuropathic; Pain-Cancer; **Hospital:** Mount Sinai Med Ctr (page 102), Mount Sinai Hosp of Queens (page 102); **Address:** 1540 York Ave, New York, NY 10028; **Phone:** 212-288-2180; **Board Cert:** Anesthesiology 1992; Pain Medicine 2004; **Med School:** Israel 1985; **Resid:** Anesthesiology, Mt Sinai Hosp 1991; **Fellow:** Pain Medicine, Mt Sinai Hosp 1991; **Fac Appt:** Assoc Prof Anes, Mount Sinai Sch Med

Gharibo, Christopher G MD (PM) - **Spec Exp:** Pain-Back & Neck; Pain-Neuropathic; Pain-Chronic; Complex Regional Pain Syndromes; **Hospital:** NYU Langone Med Ctr (page 108), NYU Hosp For Joint Diseases (page 119); **Address:** 333 E 38th St N, Fl 6, New York, NY 10016; **Phone:** 646-501-7246; **Board Cert:** Anesthesiology 1997; Pain Medicine 2009; **Med School:** UMDNJ-NJ Med Sch, Newark 1992; **Resid:** Anesthesiology, NYU Med Ctr 1997; **Fellow:** Pain Medicine, Jefferson Univ Hosp 1997; **Fac Appt:** Assoc Prof Anes, NYU Sch Med

Gusmorino, Paul MD (PM) - **Spec Exp:** Pain-Chronic; Pain Rehabilitation & Psychiatry; **Hospital:** NYU Hosp For Joint Diseases (page 119); **Address:** 246 E 20th St, New York, NY 10003; **Phone:** 212-598-6606; **Board Cert:** Psychiatry 1980; Child & Adolescent Psychiatry 1982; Pain Medicine 2006; **Med School:** Italy 1974; **Resid:** Psychiatry, Kings County Hosp 1978; **Fellow:** Child & Adolescent Psychiatry, NY Hosp 1980; **Fac Appt:** Asst Clin Prof Psyc, NYU Sch Med

Jain, Subhash MD (PM) - **Spec Exp:** Pain-Cancer; Pain-Pelvic; Reflex Sympathetic Dystrophy (RSD); Complex Regional Pain Syndromes; **Hospital:** Beth Israel Med Ctr - Petrie Division (page 94); **Address:** 360 E 72nd St, Ste C, New York, NY 10021; **Phone:** 212-439-6100; **Board Cert:** Anesthesiology 1994; Pain Medicine 1998; **Med School:** India 1968; **Resid:** Surgery, St Vincent Med Ctr 1977; Anesthesiology, New York Hosp 1979; **Fellow:** Pain Medicine, New York Hosp/Meml Sloan Kettering Cancer Ctr 1980; **Fac Appt:** Assoc Prof Anes, Cornell Univ-Weill Med Coll

Kaplan, Ronald MD (PM) - **Spec Exp:** Pain-Chronic; **Hospital:** Beth Israel Med Ctr - Petrie Division (page 94); **Address:** Pain Medicine & Palliative Care, 10 Union Square E, Ste 2R, New York, NY 10003-3314; **Phone:** 212-844-8074; **Board Cert:** Anesthesiology 2009; Pain Medicine 2004; **Med School:** Univ MD Sch Med 1974; **Resid:** Anesthesiology, Univ Maryland Hosp 1978; **Fellow:** Pediatric Anesthesiology, Chldns Hosp 1979; **Fac Appt:** Clin Prof Anes, Albert Einstein Coll Med

Kreitzer, Joel M MD (PM) - **Spec Exp:** Pain-Back; Pain-Cancer; Pain-Neuropathic; **Hospital:** Mount Sinai Med Ctr (page 102), Mount Sinai Hosp of Queens (page 102); **Address:** Upper East Side Pain Medicine, 1540 York Ave, New York, NY 10028; **Phone:** 212-288-2180; **Board Cert:** Anesthesiology 1990; Pain Medicine 2004; **Med School:** Albert Einstein Coll Med 1985; **Resid:** Anesthesiology, Mt Sinai Hosp 1989; **Fellow:** Pain Medicine, Mt Sinai Hosp 1989; **Fac Appt:** Assoc Clin Prof Anes, Mount Sinai Sch Med

Marcus, Norman J MD (PM) - **Spec Exp:** Pain-Back & Neck; Headache; Pain-Musculoskeletal; Reflex Sympathetic Dystrophy (RSD); **Hospital:** NYU Langone Med Ctr (page 108), Lenox Hill Hosp (page 106); **Address:** 30 E 40th St, Ste 1100, New York, NY 10016-1201; **Phone:** 212-532-7999; **Board Cert:** Psychiatry 1974; Pain Medicine 1993; **Med School:** SUNY Upstate Med Univ 1967; **Resid:** Psychiatry, Montefiore Med Ctr 1971; **Fellow:** Psychosomatic Medicine, Montefiore Med Ctr 1973; Pain Medicine, Lenox Hill Hosp 1995; **Fac Appt:** Assoc Clin Prof Anes, NYU Sch Med

Moqtaderi, Farideh MD (PM) - **Spec Exp:** Acupuncture; Pain-Musculoskeletal; Herpetic Neuralgia (Shingles); Fibromyalgia; **Hospital:** Mount Sinai Med Ctr (page 102); **Address:** 520 E 72nd St, Ste 1C, New York, NY 10021-4850; **Phone:** 212-426-9200; **Board Cert:** Anesthesiology 1973; **Med School:** Iran 1966; **Resid:** Anesthesiology, Mount Sinai Hosp 1969; Anesthesiology, Meml Sloan Kettering Hosp 1971; **Fellow:** Pain Medicine, Westchester Co Med Ctr 1973; **Fac Appt:** Asst Clin Prof Anes, Mount Sinai Sch Med

Ngeow, Jeffrey MD (PM) - **Spec Exp:** Pain-Musculoskeletal-Spine & Neck; Reflex Sympathetic Dystrophy (RSD); Acupuncture; Pain-Neuropathic; **Hospital:** Hosp For Special Surgery (page 115); **Address:** 635 Madison Ave Fl 5, New York, NY 10022; **Phone:** 212-224-7918; **Board Cert:** Anesthesiology 1980; Pain Medicine 2005; **Med School:** England, UK 1971; **Resid:** Anesthesiology, Peter Bent Brigham Hosp 1977; **Fellow:** Pain Medicine, Tufts New England Med Ctr 1978; **Fac Appt:** Assoc Clin Prof Anes, Cornell Univ-Weill Med Coll

Richman, Daniel MD (PM) - **Spec Exp:** Pain-Back & Neck; Complex Regional Pain Syndromes; Reflex Sympathetic Dystrophy (RSD); **Hospital:** Hosp For Special Surgery (page 115); **Address:** 535 E 70th St, New York, NY 10021-4872; **Phone:** 212-606-1768; **Board Cert:** Anesthesiology 1999; Pain Medicine 2005; **Med School:** UMDNJ-NJ Med Sch, Newark 1986; **Resid:** Anesthesiology, Hartford Hosp 1990; **Fellow:** Pain Medicine, Hosp Special Surgery 1991; **Fac Appt:** Assoc Clin Prof Anes, Cornell Univ-Weill Med Coll

Schottenstein, Douglas C MD (PM) - **Spec Exp:** Pain-Spine; Pain-Musculoskeletal; Arthritis; PRP (Regenokine); **Hospital:** NY-Presby/Columbia Univ Med Ctr, NY (page 104); **Address:** 18 E 48th St, Ste 901, New York, NY 10017; **Phone:** 212-750-1155; **Board Cert:** Neurology 2005; Pain Medicine 2006; **Med School:** Ohio State Univ 2000; **Resid:** Neurology, Emory Univ Hosps 2004; **Fellow:** Pain Medicine, NY Presby-Columbia Med Ctr 2005

Thomas, Gary P MD (PM) - **Spec Exp:** Pain-Neuropathic; Fibromyalgia; Headache; Pain-after Spinal Intervention; **Hospital:** Beth Israel Med Ctr - Petrie Division (page 94), New York Methodist Hosp (page 418); **Address:** Comprehensive Pain Mngmt, 10 Union Square E, Ste 4K, New York, NY 10003; **Phone:** 212-995-6495; **Board Cert:** Pain Medicine 2007; Anesthesiology 1996; **Med School:** Mount Sinai Sch Med 1991; **Resid:** Anesthesiology, Mount Sinai Med Ctr 1995; **Fellow:** Pain Medicine, Mount Sinai Med Ctr 1996

Waldman, Seth MD (PM) - **Spec Exp:** Pain-Spine; Pain-Neuropathic; Sciatica; **Hospital:** Hosp For Special Surgery (page 115), Burke Rehab Hosp; **Address:** Hosp For Special Surgery, 535 E 70th St, New York, NY 10021-4872; **Phone:** 212-606-1686; **Board Cert:** Anesthesiology 1994; Pain Medicine 2005; **Med School:** Albany Med Coll 1988; **Resid:** Internal Medicine, Beth Israel Med Ctr 1990; Anesthesiology, Beth Israel Hosp 1993; **Fellow:** Pain Medicine, Beth Israel Hosp/Mass Genl Hosp 1994; **Fac Appt:** Asst Clin Prof Anes, Cornell Univ-Weill Med Coll

Weinberger, Michael L MD (PM) - **Spec Exp:** Pain-Cancer; Pain-Back; Palliative Care; **Hospital:** NY-Presby/Columbia Univ Med Ctr, NY (page 104); **Address:** 630 W 168th St, PH5, rm 500, New York, NY 10032-3720; **Phone:** 212-305-7114; **Board Cert:** Internal Medicine 1986; Anesthesiology 1990; Pain Medicine 2004; Hospice & Palliative Medicine 2006; **Med School:** Columbia P&S 1983; **Resid:** Internal Medicine, St Vincent's Hosp 1986; Anesthesiology, Columbia-Presby Med Ctr 1989; **Fellow:** Pain Medicine, Meml Sloan Kettering Cancer Ctr 1990; **Fac Appt:** Assoc Prof Anes, Columbia P&S

Zou, Shengping MD (PM) - **Spec Exp:** Pain-Back; Pain-Pelvic; **Hospital:** NYU Langone Med Ctr (page 108); **Address:** 317 E 34th St Fl 9 - Ste 902, New York, NY 10016; **Phone:** 212-201-1004; **Board Cert:** Anesthesiology 1999; Pain Medicine 2012; **Med School:** China 1986; **Resid:** Anesthesiology, UMDNJ Med Ctr 1998; **Fellow:** Pain Medicine, UMDNJ Med Ctr 1999; **Fac Appt:** Asst Clin Prof Anes, NYU Sch Med

Pathology

Antonescu, Cristina R MD (Path) - **Spec Exp:** Bone Pathology; Sarcoma-Soft Tissue; Ewing's Sarcoma; **Hospital:** Meml Sloan-Kettering Cancer Ctr (page 116); **Address:** Meml Sloan Kettering Cancer Ctr, Dept Pathology, 1275 York Ave, New York, NY 10021; **Phone:** 212-639-5905; **Board Cert:** Anatomic Pathology 1998; **Med School:** Romania 1992; **Resid:** Anatomic Pathology, Lenox Hill Hosp 1996; **Fellow:** Pathology-Oncology, Meml Sloan-Kettering Canc Ctr 1997; **Fac Appt:** Assoc Prof Path, Cornell Univ-Weill Med Coll

Bleiweiss, Ira J MD (Path) - **Spec Exp:** Breast Pathology; Breast Cancer; **Hospital:** Mount Sinai Med Ctr (page 102); **Address:** Mt Sinai Med Ctr, Dept Pathology, 1 Gustave Levy Pl, Box 1194, New York, NY 10029-6504; **Phone:** 212-241-9159; **Board Cert:** Anatomic & Clinical Pathology 1988; **Med School:** West Indies 1984; **Resid:** Pathology, Mt Sinai Med Ctr 1988; **Fellow:** Surgical Pathology, Mt Sinai Med Ctr 1989; Surgical Pathology, Meml-Sloan Kettering Cancer Ctr 1990; **Fac Appt:** Prof Path, Mount Sinai Sch Med

Harpaz, Noam MD (Path) - **Spec Exp:** Gastrointestinal Pathology; **Hospital:** Mount Sinai Med Ctr (page 102); **Address:** Mount Sinai Medical Ctr, Pathology, One Gustave L Levy Pl, Box 1194, New York, NY 10029; **Phone:** 212-241-6692; **Board Cert:** Anatomic & Clinical Pathology 1986; **Med School:** Univ Miami Sch Med 1981; **Resid:** Anatomic & Clinical Pathology, Mt Sinai Med Ctr 1984; **Fac Appt:** Prof Path, Mount Sinai Sch Med

Hoda, Syed A MD (Path) - **Spec Exp:** Breast Cancer; Surgical Pathology; **Hospital:** NY-Presby/Weill Cornell Med Ctr, NY (page 104); **Address:** 525 E 68th St, 1028 Starr, New York, NY 10021-4870; **Phone:** 212-746-2700; **Board Cert:** Anatomic & Clinical Pathology 1990; Cytopathology 1991; Pathology 2001; **Med School:** Pakistan 1984; **Resid:** Anatomic & Clinical Pathology, Tulane Univ Affil Hosps 1990; **Fellow:** Cytopathology, Meml Sloan Kettering Cancer Ctr 1991; Pathology, Meml Sloan Kettering Cancer Ctr 1992; **Fac Appt:** Clin Prof Path, Cornell Univ-Weill Med Coll

Klimstra, David MD (Path) - **Spec Exp:** Gastrointestinal Pathology; Pulmonary Pathology; **Hospital:** Meml Sloan-Kettering Cancer Ctr (page 116); **Address:** Meml Sloan Kettering Canc Ctr, Dept Pathology, 1275 York Ave, New York, NY 10065; **Phone:** 212-639-2410; **Board Cert:** Anatomic Pathology 1992; **Med School:** Yale Univ 1988; **Resid:** Pathology, Yale New Haven Hosp 1991; **Fellow:** Pathology, Meml Sloan Kettering Canc Ctr 1992; **Fac Appt:** Asst Prof Path, Cornell Univ

Magro, Cynthia MD (Path) - **Spec Exp:** Cutaneous Lymphoma; **Hospital:** NY-Presby/Weill Cornell Med Ctr, NY (page 104); **Address:** 1300 York Ave, Ste F310, New York, NY 10065; **Phone:** 212-746-6434; **Board Cert:** Anatomic Pathology 1988; Dermatopathology 1990; Cytopathology 1991; **Med School:** Univ Manitoba 1984; **Resid:** Anatomic Pathology, Mass Genl Hosp 1988; **Fellow:** Cytopathology, Mass Genl Hosp 1989; Dermatology, Mass Genl Hosp 1991

Melamed, Jonathan MD (Path) - **Spec Exp:** Prostate Cancer; Tumor Banking-Prostate; **Hospital:** NYU Langone Med Ctr (page 108); **Address:** NYU Medical Ctr, Dept Pathology, TH-461, 560 First Ave, New York, NY 10016; **Phone:** 212-263-8927; **Board Cert:** Anatomic & Clinical Pathology 1992; **Med School:** South Africa 1985; **Resid:** Pathology, Lenox Hill Hosp 1991; **Fellow:** Pathology, Meml Sloan Kettering Cancer Ctr 1992; Urologic Pathology, Meml Sloan Kettering Cancer Ctr 1993; **Fac Appt:** Assoc Prof Path, NYU Sch Med

Orazi, Attilio MD (Path) - **Spec Exp:** Hematopathology; Bone Marrow Pathology; Lymph Node Pathology; Spleen Pathology; **Hospital:** NY-Presby/Weill Cornell Med Ctr, NY (page 104); **Address:** NY Presby-Cornell Medical Ctr, 525 E 68th St, Starr Pavilion, rm 707, New York, NY 10065; **Phone:** 212-746-2050; **Board Cert:** Anatomic Pathology 1997; Hematology 1998; **Med School:** Italy 1979; **Resid:** Internal Medicine, Leicester Royal Infirmary 1982; Histopathology, Northampton Genl Hosp 1983; **Fellow:** Anatomic Pathology, Natl Cancer Inst 1985; **Fac Appt:** Prof Path, Cornell Univ-Weill Med Coll

Reuter, Victor E MD (Path) - **Spec Exp:** Prostate Cancer; Genitourinary Pathology; Bladder Cancer; Testicular Cancer; **Hospital:** Meml Sloan-Kettering Cancer Ctr (page 116); **Address:** Memorial Sloan Kettering Cancer Ctr, Dept Pathology, 1275 York Ave, New York, NY 10021; **Phone:** 212-639-8225; **Board Cert:** Anatomic & Clinical Pathology 1983; **Med School:** Dominican Republic 1978; **Resid:** Anatomic Pathology, Thos Jefferson Univ Hosp 1981; Clinical Pathology, Thos Jefferson Univ Hosp 1983; **Fellow:** Surgical Pathology, Meml Sloan Kettering Cancer Ctr 1985; **Fac Appt:** Prof Path, Cornell Univ-Weill Med Coll

Rosenblum, Marc K MD (Path) - **Spec Exp:** Neuropathology; Brain Tumors; **Hospital:** Meml Sloan-Kettering Cancer Ctr (page 116); **Address:** 1275 York Ave, Meml Sloan-Kettering Cancer Ctr, New York, NY 10065; **Phone:** 212-639-3844; **Board Cert:** Anatomic Pathology 1984; Neuropathology 1988; **Med School:** Univ Miami Sch Med 1979; **Resid:** Anatomic Pathology, Mt Sinai Med Ctr 1984; **Fellow:** Pathology, Meml Sloan-Kettering Cancer Ctr 1985; Neurological Pathology, Bellevue-NYU Med Ctr 1987; **Fac Appt:** Prof Path, Cornell Univ-Weill Med Coll

Schiller, Alan L MD (Path) - **Spec Exp:** Bone & Joint Pathology; Soft Tissue Pathology; Bone Tumors; **Hospital:** Mount Sinai Med Ctr (page 102); **Address:** Mt Sinai Sch Med, Dept Pathology, 1 Gustave Levy Pl, Box 1194, New York, NY 10029-6500; **Phone:** 212-241-8014; **Board Cert:** Anatomic Pathology 1973; **Med School:** Ros Franklin Univ/Chicago Med Sch 1967; **Resid:** Pathology, Mass Genl Hosp 1972; **Fac Appt:** Prof Emeritus Path, Mount Sinai Sch Med

Soslow, Robert A MD (Path) - **Spec Exp:** Gynecologic Pathology; **Hospital:** Meml Sloan-Kettering Cancer Ctr (page 116); **Address:** 1275 York Avenue, Pathology Department, New York, NY 10065; **Phone:** 800-525-2225; **Board Cert:** Anatomic Pathology 1995; **Med School:** Univ Pennsylvania 1991; **Resid:** Anatomic Pathology, Stanford Univ Med Ctr 1994; **Fellow:** Immunopathology, Stanford Univ Med Ctr 1995; **Fac Appt:** Assoc Prof Path, Cornell Univ

Travis, William D MD (Path) - **Spec Exp:** Pulmonary Pathology; Lung Cancer; Interstitial Lung Disease; **Hospital:** Meml Sloan-Kettering Cancer Ctr (page 116); **Address:** 1275 York Ave, MSKCC Bldg, Pathology Dept, New York, NY 10065; **Phone:** 212-639-6364; **Board Cert:** Anatomic & Clinical Pathology 1985; **Med School:** Univ Fla Coll Med 1981; **Resid:** Anatomic Pathology, New England Deaconess Hosp 1983; Clinical Pathology, Mayo Clinic 1985; **Fellow:** Surgical Pathology, Mayo Clinic 1986

Wang, Beverly Y MD (Path) - **Spec Exp:** Head & Neck Pathology; **Hospital:** Beth Israel Med Ctr - Petrie Division (page 94); **Address:** Beth Israel Medical Ctr, Dept Pathology, First Avenue at 16th St, Silver Bldg Fl 11, New York, NY 10003; **Phone:** 212-844-1959; **Board Cert:** Anatomic Pathology 1998; Cytopathology 1999; **Med School:** China 1982; **Resid:** Pathology, Mount Sinai Med Ctr 1998; **Fellow:** Cytopathology, Mount Sinai Med Ctr 1999; **Fac Appt:** Prof Path, Albert Einstein Coll Med

Wenig, Bruce M MD (Path) - **Spec Exp:** Head & Neck Pathology; Surgical Pathology; Endocrine Pathology; **Hospital:** Beth Israel Med Ctr - Petrie Division (page 94), St. Luke's - Roosevelt Hosp Ctr - St Luke's Hosp (page 94); **Address:** Beth Israel Med Ctr, Dept Pathology, First Ave at 16th St, 11 Silver, Rm 34, New York, NY 10003; **Phone:** 212-420-4031; **Board Cert:** Anatomic & Clinical Pathology 2003; **Med School:** Israel 1981; **Resid:** Pathology, Mt Sinai Med Ctr 1985; Surgical Pathology, Cedars-Sinai Med Ctr 1986; **Fellow:** Head and Neck Pathology, AFIP 1987; **Fac Appt:** Prof Path, Albert Einstein Coll Med

Zagzag, David MD/PhD (Path) - **Spec Exp:** Neuropathology; Brain Tumors; Tumor Banking-Brain; **Hospital:** NYU Langone Med Ctr (page 108), Bellevue Hosp Ctr; **Address:** NYU Med Ctr, Dept Pathology, 550 First Ave, Div Neuropathology, NB-4N30, New York, NY 10016; **Phone:** 212-263-6449; **Board Cert:** Anatomic Pathology 1993; Neuropathology 1993; **Med School:** France 1984; **Resid:** Surgical Pathology, NYU Med Ctr 1990; **Fellow:** Neurological Pathology, NYU Med Ctr 1992; **Fac Appt:** Assoc Prof Path, NYU Sch Med

Pediatric Allergy & Immunology

Ehrlich, Paul M MD (PA&I) - **Spec Exp:** Asthma; Food Allergy; **Hospital:** New York Eye & Ear Infirm (page 117), NYU Langone Med Ctr (page 108); **Address:** 35 E 35th St, Ste 202, New York, NY 10016-3823; **Phone:** 212-685-4225; **Board Cert:** Pediatrics 1975; Allergy & Immunology 1977; **Med School:** NYU Sch Med 1970; **Resid:** Pediatrics, Bellevue Hosp Ctr 1973; **Fellow:** Allergy & Immunology, Walter Reed Army Med Ctr 1976; **Fac Appt:** Assoc Clin Prof Ped, NYU Sch Med

Sampson Jr, Hugh A MD (PA&I) - **Spec Exp:** Food Allergy; Eczema; Atopic Dermatitis; **Hospital:** Mount Sinai Med Ctr (page 102); **Address:** Mt Sinai Sch Med, Dept Peds, 1 Gustave Levy Pl, Box 1198, New York, NY 10029; **Phone:** 212-241-5548; **Board Cert:** Pediatrics 1980; Allergy & Immunology 1981; **Med School:** SUNY Buffalo 1975; **Resid:** Pediatrics, Chldns Meml Hosp 1979; **Fellow:** Allergy & Immunology, Duke Univ Med Ctr 1980; **Fac Appt:** Prof Ped, Mount Sinai Sch Med

Sicherer, Scott H MD (PA&I) - **Spec Exp:** Food Allergy; Drug Sensitivity; Eczema; **Hospital:** Mount Sinai Med Ctr (page 102); **Address:** 5 E 98th St Fl 10, New York, NY 10029-6500; **Phone:** 212-241-5548; **Board Cert:** Pediatrics 2008; Allergy & Immunology 2007; **Med School:** Johns Hopkins Univ 1990; **Resid:** Pediatrics, Mt Sinai Hosp 1994; **Fellow:** Allergy & Immunology, Johns Hopkins Hosp 1997; **Fac Appt:** Prof Ped, Mount Sinai Sch Med

Pediatric Cardiology

Addonizio, Linda J MD (PCd) - **Spec Exp:** Transplant Medicine-Heart; Heart Failure; Hypertrophic Cardiomyopathy; **Hospital:** Morgan Stanley Children's Hosp of NY-Presby, NY (page 104); **Address:** 3959 Broadway, Ste 229 N, New York, NY 10032; **Phone:** 212-305-6575; **Board Cert:** Pediatrics 1983; Pediatric Cardiology 1985; **Med School:** Columbia P&S 1978; **Resid:** Pediatrics, Columbia Presby/Babies Hosp 1981; **Fellow:** Pediatric Cardiology, Columbia Presby/Babies Hosp 1984; **Fac Appt:** Prof Ped, Columbia P&S

Altmann, Karen MD (PCd) - **Spec Exp:** Congenital Heart Disease; Echocardiography; **Hospital:** NY-Presby/Columbia Univ Med Ctr, NY (page 104); **Address:** 3959 Broadway, 2 North, rm 255, New York, NY 10032; **Phone:** 212-342-1560; **Board Cert:** Pediatrics 2007; Pediatric Cardiology 2011; **Med School:** Univ Pennsylvania 1988; **Resid:** Pediatrics, Morgan Stanley Chldn's Hosp 1991; **Fellow:** Pediatric Cardiology, Morgan Stanley Chldn's Hosp 1996; Pediatric Cardiology, Chldn's Hosp 1997; **Fac Appt:** Assoc Clin Prof Ped, Columbia P&S

Arnon, Rica G MD (PCd) - **Spec Exp:** Congenital Heart Disease; Exercise Physiology; **Hospital:** Mount Sinai Med Ctr (page 102), Elmhurst Hosp Ctr; **Address:** 1468 Madison Ave, Ste 3-50, New York, NY 10029-6504; **Phone:** 212-241-7672; **Board Cert:** Pediatrics 1970; Pediatric Cardiology 1973; **Med School:** SUNY Hlth Sci Ctr 1967; **Resid:** Pediatrics, Kings County Hosp 1970; **Fellow:** Pediatric Cardiology, Kings County Hosp 1973; **Fac Appt:** Assoc Prof Ped, Mount Sinai Sch Med

Borg, Morton D MD (PCd) - **Spec Exp:** Fetal Echocardiography; **Hospital:** Beth Israel Med Ctr - Petrie Division (page 94), Mount Sinai Med Ctr (page 102); **Address:** Phillips Amb Care Ctr, Dept Peds, 10 Union Square E, Ste 2J, New York, NY 10003-3314; **Phone:** 212-844-8313; **Board Cert:** Pediatrics 1986; Pediatric Cardiology 2010; **Med School:** Albert Einstein Coll Med 1981; **Resid:** Pediatrics, Brookdale Hosp 1984; **Fellow:** Pediatric Cardiology, New York Hosp 1986; **Fac Appt:** Asst Prof Ped, Albert Einstein Coll Med

Brick, David H MD (PCd) - **Spec Exp:** Fetal Echocardiography; Congenital Heart Disease; **Hospital:** NYU Langone Med Ctr (page 108); **Address:** Villiage Pediatric Cardiology, 154 W 14th St, Fl 4, New York, NY 10011; **Phone:** 212-604-7880; **Board Cert:** Pediatrics 2011; Pediatric Cardiology 2008; **Med School:** Ohio State Univ 1993; **Resid:** Pediatrics, Univ Hosp Cleveland 1996; **Fellow:** Pediatric Cardiology, NY-Presby Hosp 2000

Flynn, Patrick A MD (PCd) - **Spec Exp:** Congenital Heart Disease; Echocardiography; Kawasaki Disease; Cardiac Catheterization; **Hospital:** NY-Presby/Weill Cornell Med Ctr, NY (page 104); **Address:** 525 E 68th St, Ste F695B, New York, NY 10065; **Phone:** 212-746-3561; **Board Cert:** Pediatric Cardiology 2006; **Med School:** Univ MD Sch Med 1986; **Resid:** Pediatrics, NY Presby Hosp/Cornell Med Ctr 1990; **Fellow:** Pediatric Cardiology, NY Presby Hosp/Cornell Med Ctr 1993; **Fac Appt:** Assoc Prof Ped, Cornell Univ-Weill Med Coll

Gelb, Bruce D MD (PCd) - **Spec Exp:** Noonan Syndrome; Marfan's Syndrome; **Hospital:** Mount Sinai Med Ctr (page 102); **Address:** 1 Gustave Levy Pl, Box 1201, New York, NY 10029; **Phone:** 212-241-8592; **Board Cert:** Pediatric Cardiology 2006; **Med School:** Univ Rochester 1984; **Resid:** Pediatrics, NYPresby-Columbia Univ Med Ctr 1987; **Fellow:** Pediatric Cardiology, Baylor College Med 1991; **Fac Appt:** Prof Ped, Mount Sinai Sch Med

Love, Barry A MD (PCd) - **Spec Exp:** Cardiac Catheterization; Interventional Cardiology; Atrial Septal Defect; Arrhythmias; **Hospital:** Mount Sinai Med Ctr (page 102); **Address:** Mt Sinai Med Ctr, Div Ped Cardiology, 1468 Madison Ave, Ste 3-50, New York, NY 10029; **Phone:** 212-241-9516; **Board Cert:** Pediatrics 2004; Pediatric Cardiology 2008; **Med School:** Univ Western Ontario 1993; **Resid:** Pediatrics, Chldns Hosp Montreal 1996; **Fellow:** Pediatric Cardiology, Chldns Hosp 2000; **Fac Appt:** Asst Prof Ped, Mount Sinai Sch Med

Parness, Ira A MD (PCd) - **Spec Exp:** Echocardiography; Congenital Heart Disease; Fetal Echocardiography; **Hospital:** Mount Sinai Med Ctr (page 102), Englewood Hosp & Med Ctr; **Address:** 1 Gustave L Levy Pl, Anbg Bldg - rm 3-40, Box 1201, New York, NY 10029-6500; **Phone:** 212-241-6640; **Board Cert:** Pediatrics 1984; Pediatric Cardiology 1985; **Med School:** SUNY Downstate 1979; **Resid:** Pediatrics, Brookdale Hosp 1982; **Fellow:** Pediatric Cardiology, Chldns Hosp 1985; **Fac Appt:** Prof Ped, Mount Sinai Sch Med

Solowiejczyk, David E MD (PCd) - **Spec Exp:** Echocardiography; **Hospital:** Morgan Stanley Children's Hosp of NY-Presby, NY (page 104); **Address:** 3959 Broadway 2-North Bldg, New York, NY 10032; **Phone:** 212-305-8509; **Board Cert:** Pediatrics 2002; Pediatric Cardiology 2011; **Med School:** NYU Sch Med 1986; **Resid:** Pediatrics, Mt Sinai Med Ctr 1989; **Fellow:** Cardiovascular Disease, NY Presby Hosp-Columbia Med Ctr 1993; **Fac Appt:** Assoc Prof Ped, Columbia P&S

Sommer, Robert J MD (PCd) - **Spec Exp:** Congenital Heart Disease; Atrial Septal Defect; Cardiac Catheterization; **Hospital:** NY-Presby/Columbia Univ Med Ctr, NY (page 104), St. Joseph's Regl Med Ctr - Paterson; **Address:** 161 Fort Washington Ave Fl 6, New York, NY 10032; **Phone:** 212-342-0886; **Board Cert:** Pediatric Cardiology 2006; **Med School:** NYU Sch Med 1985; **Resid:** Pediatrics, Mt Sinai Med Ctr 1988; **Fellow:** Pediatric Cardiology, Mt Sinai Med Ctr 1991; Interventional Cardiology, Childrens Hosp 1991; **Fac Appt:** Assoc Prof Ped, Columbia P&S

Starc, Thomas J MD (PCd) - **Spec Exp:** Cholesterol/Lipid Disorders; **Hospital:** Morgan Stanley Children's Hosp of NY-Presby, NY (page 104); **Address:** NY Presby-Morgan Stanley Children's Hosp, 3959 Broadway, Ste 255 N, New York, NY 10032-1537; **Phone:** 212-305-4432; **Board Cert:** Pediatrics 1981; Pediatric Cardiology 1983; **Med School:** Mount Sinai Sch Med 1976; **Resid:** Pediatrics, USC Med Ctr 1980; **Fellow:** Pediatric Cardiology, NY Presby-Columbia Med Ctr 1984; **Fac Appt:** Clin Prof Ped, Columbia P&S

Steinberg, L Gary MD (PCd) - **Spec Exp:** Echocardiography; Congenital Heart Disease; **Hospital:** NY-Presby/Weill Cornell Med Ctr, NY (page 104); **Address:** Pediatric Cardiovascular Services, NY Presby Hosp/ Weill Cornell, 525 E 68 St, Ste F677, New York, NY 10065; **Phone:** 212-746-3561; **Board Cert:** Pediatrics 2006; Pediatric Cardiology 2006; **Med School:** Philippines 1985; **Resid:** Pediatrics, Elmhurst Hosp 1989; **Fellow:** Pediatric Cardiology, Mount Sinai Hosp 1992; **Fac Appt:** Asst Prof Ped, Cornell Univ-Weill Med Coll

Steinherz, Laurel J MD (PCd) - **Spec Exp:** Cardiac Effects of Cancer/Cancer Therapy; **Hospital:** Meml Sloan-Kettering Cancer Ctr (page 116), NY-Presby/Weill Cornell Med Ctr, NY (page 104); **Address:** 1275 York Ave, New York, NY 10021; **Phone:** 212-639-8103; **Board Cert:** Pediatrics 1976; Pediatric Cardiology 1978; **Med School:** Albert Einstein Coll Med 1970; **Resid:** Pediatrics, NY Hosp-Cornell Med Ctr 1971; Pediatrics, Chldns Hosp 1972; **Fellow:** Pediatric Cardiology, NY Hosp-Cornell Med Ctr 1975; **Fac Appt:** Prof Ped, Cornell Univ-Weill Med Coll

Pediatric Critical Care Medicine

Conway Jr, Edward E MD (PCCM) - **Spec Exp:** Neurologic Critical Care; Respiratory Failure; Head Injury; **Hospital:** Beth Israel Med Ctr - Petrie Division (page 94); **Address:** Beth Israel Med Ctr, Dept Peds, 350 E 17th St, New York, NY 10003; **Phone:** 212-420-4018; **Board Cert:** Pediatrics 2008; Pediatric Critical Care Medicine 2010; **Med School:** SUNY Hlth Sci Ctr 1984; **Resid:** Pediatrics, Montefiore Med Ctr 1988; **Fellow:** Pediatric Critical Care Medicine, Montefiore Med Ctr-Albert Einstein 1990; **Fac Appt:** Prof Ped, Albert Einstein Coll Med

Greenwald, Bruce M MD (PCCM) - **Spec Exp:** Respiratory Failure; Sepsis & Septic Shock; Asthma; Diabetes Ketoacidosis; **Hospital:** NY-Presby/Weill Cornell Med Ctr, NY (page 104), Meml Sloan-Kettering Cancer Ctr (page 116); **Address:** Div Pediatric Critical Care Med, 525 E 68th St, Ste M-508, New York, NY 10065; **Phone:** 212-746-3056; **Board Cert:** Pediatrics 1987; Pediatric Critical Care Medicine 2005; **Med School:** NYU Sch Med 1982; **Resid:** Pediatrics, NYU-Bellevue Hosp Ctr 1986; **Fellow:** Pediatric Critical Care Medicine, NY Hosp-Cornell 1988; **Fac Appt:** Prof Ped, Cornell Univ-Weill Med Coll

Sagy, Mayer MD (PCCM) - **Hospital:** NYU Langone Med Ctr (page 108); **Address:** NYU Langone Medical Ctr, Pediatric Critical Care, 550 First Ave, New York, NY 10016; **Phone:** 212-263-2377; **Board Cert:** Pediatrics 2007; Pediatric Critical Care Medicine 2007; **Med School:** Israel 1972; **Resid:** Pediatrics, Chaim Sheba Med Ctr 1982; **Fellow:** Pediatric Critical Care Medicine, Children's Hosp 1984

Pediatric Endocrinology

Fennoy, Ilene MD (PEn) - **Spec Exp:** Growth/Development Disorders; Diabetes; Klinefelter's Syndrome; Obesity; **Hospital:** Morgan Stanley Children's Hosp of NY-Presby, NY (page 104), Harlem Hosp Ctr; **Address:** 3959 Broadway, rm 106, New York, NY 10032; **Phone:** 212-305-6559; **Board Cert:** Pediatrics 1979; Pediatric Endocrinology 1980; **Med School:** UCSF 1973; **Resid:** Pediatrics, Montefiore Med Ctr 1975; **Fellow:** Nutrition, Columbia-Presby Med Ctr 1977; Endocrinology, Nat Inst Hlth 1979; **Fac Appt:** Assoc Clin Prof Ped, Columbia P&S

Franklin, Bonita H MD (PEn) - **Spec Exp:** Diabetes; Growth Disorders; Thyroid Disorders; **Hospital:** NYU Langone Med Ctr (page 108), Bellevue Hosp Ctr; **Address:** 109 Reade St, New York, NY 10013-3863; **Phone:** 212-732-2401; **Board Cert:** Pediatrics 1982; Pediatric Endocrinology 2009; **Med School:** SUNY Hlth Sci Ctr 1976; **Resid:** Pediatrics, Bronx Muni Hosp 1978; Pediatrics, Mt Sinai Hosp 1979; **Fellow:** Pediatric Endocrinology, Mt Sinai Hosp 1981; **Fac Appt:** Assoc Clin Prof Ped, NYU Sch Med

Gallagher, Mary P MD (PEn) - **Spec Exp:** Diabetes; **Hospital:** Morgan Stanley Children's Hosp of NY-Presby, NY (page 104); **Address:** 1150 St Nicholas Ave Fl 2, New York, NY 10032; **Phone:** 212-851-5494; **Board Cert:** Pediatrics 2006; Pediatric Endocrinology 2011; **Med School:** UMDNJ-NJ Med Sch, Newark 1995; **Resid:** Pediatrics, NY Presby-Columbia Med Ctr 1998; **Fellow:** Pediatric Endocrinology, NY Presby-Columbia Med Ctr 2002; **Fac Appt:** Asst Prof Ped, Columbia P&S

Kohn, Brenda MD (PEn) - **Spec Exp:** Growth Disorders; Pituitary Disorders; Thyroid Disorders; Adrenal Disorders; **Hospital:** NYU Langone Med Ctr (page 108), Lenox Hill Hosp (page 106); **Address:** 160 E 32nd St, Ste L3, New York, NY 10016-6402; **Phone:** 212-263-3185; **Board Cert:** Pediatrics 1981; Pediatric Endocrinology 1983; **Med School:** Albert Einstein Coll Med 1976; **Resid:** Pediatrics, NYU Med Ctr 1979; **Fellow:** Endocrinology, Diabetes & Metabolism, NY-Cornell Med Ctr 1983; **Fac Appt:** Assoc Prof Ped, NYU Sch Med

Maclaren, Noel K MD (PEn) - **Spec Exp:** Diabetes; Obesity; Metabolic Syndrome; **Hospital:** Lenox Hill Hosp (page 106); **Address:** Bioseek Endocrine Clinic, 200 W 57th St, Ste 610, New York, NY 10019; **Phone:** 212-371-0658; **Board Cert:** Pediatrics 1977; Pediatric Endocrinology 1978; **Med School:** New Zealand 1963; **Resid:** Pediatrics, Wellington Public Hosp 1967; **Fellow:** Pediatric Endocrinology, Johns Hopkins Hosp 1973; **Fac Appt:** Prof Ped, Cornell Univ-Weill Med Coll

New, Maria I MD (PEn) - **Spec Exp:** Adrenal Disorders; Growth/Development Disorders; **Hospital:** Mount Sinai Med Ctr (page 102); **Address:** Mount Sinai Medical Ctr, 5 E 98th St Fl 10, New York, NY 10029; **Phone:** 212-241-8210; **Board Cert:** Pediatrics 1960; **Med School:** Univ Pennsylvania 1954; **Resid:** Pediatrics, New York Hosp 1957; **Fellow:** Pediatric Endocrinology, New York Hosp 1958; Endocrinology, Diabetes & Metabolism, New York Hosp 1964; **Fac Appt:** Prof Ped, Cornell Univ-Weill Med Coll

Oberfield, Sharon E MD (PEn) - **Spec Exp:** Adrenal Disorders; Neuroendocrine Growth Disorders; Growth Disorders; **Hospital:** Morgan Stanley Children's Hosp of NY-Presby, NY (page 104); **Address:** 630 W 168th St, PH East Bldg Fl 5 East - Ste 522, New York, NY 10032; **Phone:** 212-305-6559; **Board Cert:** Pediatrics 1979; Pediatric Endocrinology 2000; **Med School:** Cornell Univ-Weill Med Coll 1974; **Resid:** Pediatrics, NY Hosp-Cornell 1976; **Fellow:** Pediatric Endocrinology, NY Hosp-Cornell 1979; **Fac Appt:** Prof Ped, Columbia P&S

Rapaport, Robert MD (PEn) - **Spec Exp:** Growth Disorders; Thyroid Disorders; Diabetes; **Hospital:** Mount Sinai Med Ctr (page 102); **Address:** 1 Gustave L Levy Pl, Annenberg Bldg - Fl 4, Box 1616, New York, NY 10029-6508; **Phone:** 212-241-8487 x4847; **Board Cert:** Pediatrics 1980; Pediatric Endocrinology 1983; **Med School:** SUNY Downstate 1974; **Resid:** Pediatrics, LIJ-Hillside Med Ctr 1977; **Fellow:** Pediatric Endocrinology, St Christopher's Hosp 1978; Pediatric Endocrinology, New York Hosp 1980; **Fac Appt:** Prof Ped, Mount Sinai Sch Med

Sklar, Charles A MD (PEn) - **Spec Exp:** Cancer Survivors-Late Effects of Therapy; Growth Disorders in Childhood Cancer; Pituitary Disorders; **Hospital:** Meml Sloan-Kettering Cancer Ctr (page 116); **Address:** 1275 York Avenue, New York, NY 10065; **Phone:** 212-639-8138; **Board Cert:** Pediatrics 1979; Pediatric Endocrinology 1980; **Med School:** USC Sch Med 1974; **Resid:** Pediatrics, Childrens Hosp 1976; **Fellow:** Pediatric Endocrinology, UCSF Med Ctr 1979; **Fac Appt:** Assoc Prof Ped, Cornell Univ-Weill Med Coll

Slonim, Alfred E MD (PEn) - **Spec Exp:** Muscular Disorders-Metabolic; Inflammatory Bowel Disease/Crohn's; Glycogen Storage Diseases; Chronic Fatigue Syndrome; **Hospital:** Morgan Stanley Children's Hosp of NY-Presby, NY (page 104); **Address:** NY Presby-Morgan Stanley Children's Hosp, 622 W 168th St, rm 517, New York, NY 10032; **Phone:** 212-305-5717; **Board Cert:** Pediatrics 1978; Pediatric Endocrinology 1986; **Med School:** Australia 1958; **Resid:** Pediatrics, Royal Chldns Hosp 1963; **Fellow:** Pediatrics, Royal Chldns Hosp 1965; Endocrinology, Hadassah Hosp 1970; **Fac Appt:** Prof Ped, Columbia P&S

Vargas-Rodriguez, Ileana MD (PEn) - **Spec Exp:** Diabetes; **Hospital:** NY-Presby/Columbia Univ Med Ctr, NY (page 104); **Address:** 1150 St Nicholas Ave Fl 2, New York, NY 10032; **Phone:** 212-851-5494; **Board Cert:** Pediatric Endocrinology 2010; **Med School:** Albert Einstein Coll Med 1986; **Resid:** Pediatrics, Babies Hosp 1989; **Fellow:** Pediatric Endocrinology, Mt Sinai Hosp 1990

Vogiatzi, Maria G MD (PEn) - **Spec Exp:** Growth Disorders; Osteoporosis; Pubertal Disorders; Adrenal Disorders; **Hospital:** NY-Presby/Weill Cornell Med Ctr, NY (page 104); **Address:** 505 E 70th St, Helmsley Tower Fl 3, New York, NY 10065; **Phone:** 212-746-3462; **Board Cert:** Pediatrics 2007; Pediatric Endocrinology 2005; **Med School:** Greece 1987; **Resid:** Pediatrics, Univ Hosp 1991; **Fellow:** Pediatric Endocrinology, New York Hosp 1993; Pediatric Endocrinology, Baylor Coll Med 1995; **Fac Appt:** Assoc Clin Prof Ped, Cornell Univ-Weill Med Coll

Pediatric Gastroenterology

Bangaru, Babu S MD (PGe) - **Spec Exp:** Ulcerative Colitis/Crohn's; Liver Disease; Nutrition; Endoscopy; **Hospital:** NYU Langone Med Ctr (page 108), Flushing Hosp Med Ctr; **Address:** NYU Medical Center, 530 First Ave, Ste 3A, New York, NY 10016; **Phone:** 212-263-7868; **Board Cert:** Pediatrics 1978; Pediatric Gastroenterology 2006; **Med School:** India 1970; **Resid:** Pediatrics, St Lukes Hosp 1976; **Fellow:** Hepatology, Albert Einstein Coll Med 1978; Gastroenterology & Nutrition, Emory Univ Sch Med 1979; **Fac Appt:** Assoc Clin Prof Ped, NYU Sch Med

Benkov, Keith J MD (PGe) - **Spec Exp:** Inflammatory Bowel Disease/Crohn's; Liver Disease; Celiac Disease; **Hospital:** Mount Sinai Med Ctr (page 102), Englewood Hosp & Med Ctr; **Address:** Mt Sinai Div Ped Gastroenterology, 5 E 98th St Fl 10, New York, NY 10029; **Phone:** 212-241-5415; **Board Cert:** Pediatrics 1984; Pediatric Gastroenterology 2005; **Med School:** Mount Sinai Sch Med 1979; **Resid:** Pediatrics, Mt Sinai Hosp 1982; **Fellow:** Pediatric Gastroenterology, Mt Sinai Hosp 1984; **Fac Appt:** Assoc Prof Ped, Mount Sinai Sch Med

Kazlow, Philip G MD (PGe) - **Spec Exp:** Inflammatory Bowel Disease; Celiac Disease; Nutrition; **Hospital:** Morgan Stanley Children's Hosp of NY-Presby, NY (page 104), Valley Hosp (page 689); **Address:** Morgan Stanley Chldns Hosp of NY-Presby, 3959 Broadway, Ste 7-718, New York, NY 10032; **Phone:** 212-305-5903; **Board Cert:** Pediatrics 1985; Pediatric Gastroenterology 2005; **Med School:** Mount Sinai Sch Med 1980; **Resid:** Pediatrics, Mt Sinai Hosp 1984; **Fellow:** Pediatric Gastroenterology, Mt Sinai Hosp 1986; **Fac Appt:** Assoc Clin Prof Ped, Columbia P&S

Levy, Joseph MD (PGe) - **Spec Exp:** Celiac Disease; Irritable Bowel Syndrome; Gastroesophageal Reflux Disease (GERD); Nutrition in Autism; **Hospital:** NYU Langone Med Ctr (page 108); **Address:** 160 E 32nd St Fl L3 Medical, New York, NY 10016; **Phone:** 212-263-5407; **Board Cert:** Pediatrics 1981; Pediatric Gastroenterology 2005; **Med School:** Israel 1973; **Resid:** Pediatrics, Beth Israel Med Ctr 1977; **Fellow:** Research, Columbia-Presby Med Ctr 1975; Pediatric Gastroenterology, Columbia-Presby Med Ctr 1979; **Fac Appt:** Prof Ped, NYU Sch Med

Sockolow, Robbyn E MD (PGe) - **Spec Exp:** Constipation; Gastroesophageal Reflux Disease (GERD); Inflammatory Bowel Disease/Crohn's; Capsule Endoscopy; **Hospital:** NY-Presby/Weill Cornell Med Ctr, NY (page 104); **Address:** Ny Presby-Cornell Med Ctr, Dept Peds, 505 E 70th St, Helmsley Tower Fl 3, New York, NY 10021; **Phone:** 646-962-3869; **Board Cert:** Pediatrics 2005; Pediatric Gastroenterology 2003; **Med School:** NY Med Coll 1986; **Resid:** Pediatrics, Montefiore Med Ctr 1989; **Fellow:** Pediatric Gastroenterology, Mt Sinai Med Ctr 1990; Pediatric Gastroenterology, Montefiore Med Ctr 1992; **Fac Appt:** Assoc Clin Prof Ped, Cornell Univ-Weill Med Coll

Spivak, William MD (PGe) - **Spec Exp:** Ulcerative Colitis; Crohn's Disease; Nutrition; Esophageal Disorders; **Hospital:** NY-Presby/Weill Cornell Med Ctr, NY (page 104), Lenox Hill Hosp (page 106); **Address:** 177 E 87th St, Ste 305, New York, NY 10128; **Phone:** 212-369-7700; **Board Cert:** Pediatrics 1981; Pediatric Gastroenterology 2005; **Med School:** Albert Einstein Coll Med 1976; **Resid:** Pediatrics, Jacobi Med Ctr/Albert Einstein Med Sch 1979; **Fellow:** Gastroenterology, Childrens Hosp 1982; Research, Brigham & Womens Hosp 1982; **Fac Appt:** Clin Prof Ped, Cornell Univ-Weill Med Coll

Pediatric Hematology-Oncology

Aledo, Alexander MD (PHO) - **Spec Exp:** Leukemia; Lymphoma; Bone Tumors; **Hospital:** NY-Presby/Weill Cornell Med Ctr, NY (page 104), NY Hosp Queens (page 206); **Address:** 525 E 68th St, rm P695, New York, NY 10021-4870; **Phone:** 212-746-3494; **Board Cert:** Pediatric Hematology-Oncology 2004; **Med School:** NYU Sch Med 1984; **Resid:** Pediatrics, NYPresby/Weill Cornell Med Ctr 1987; **Fellow:** Pediatric Hematology-Oncology, Meml Sloan Kettering Cancer Ctr 1990; **Fac Appt:** Assoc Clin Prof Ped, Cornell Univ-Weill Med Coll

Blei, Francine MD (PHO) - **Spec Exp:** Hemangiomas; Vascular Anomalies; Vascular Malformations; Lymphedema; **Hospital:** St. Luke's - Roosevelt Hosp Ctr - Roosevelt Div (page 94); **Address:** Vascular Birthmark Inst of New York, 126 W 60th St, New York, NY 10023; **Phone:** 212-523-8931; **Board Cert:** Pediatrics 1987; Pediatric Hematology-Oncology 1987; **Med School:** Israel 1982; **Resid:** Pediatrics, NYU-Bellevue 1985; **Fellow:** Pediatric Hematology-Oncology, Babies Hosp-Columbia Presby 1987; **Fac Appt:** Prof Ped, NYU Sch Med

Bussel, James MD (PHO) - **Spec Exp:** Bleeding/Coagulation Disorders; Platelet Disorders; Wiskott-Aldrich Syndrome; **Hospital:** NY-Presby/Weill Cornell Med Ctr, NY (page 104), Lenox Hill Hosp (page 106); **Address:** 525 E 68th St, rm P-695, New York, NY 10065; **Phone:** 212-746-3400; **Board Cert:** Pediatrics 1979; Pediatric Hematology-Oncology 1980; **Med School:** Columbia P&S 1975; **Resid:** Pediatrics, Chldns Hosp 1978; **Fellow:** Pediatric Hematology-Oncology, NY Presby Hosp/Cornell 1981; **Fac Appt:** Prof Ped, Cornell Univ-Weill Med Coll

Carroll, William L MD (PHO) - **Spec Exp:** Leukemia; **Hospital:** NYU Langone Med Ctr (page 108); **Address:** NYU Med Ctr, Div Ped Hem/Onc, 160 E 32nd Level L3 St, New York, NY 10016; **Phone:** 212-263-8400; **Board Cert:** Pediatrics 1984; Pediatric Hematology-Oncology 1987; **Med School:** UC Irvine 1978; **Resid:** Pediatrics, Chldns Hosp Med Ctr 1981; **Fellow:** Pediatric Hematology-Oncology, Stanford Univ 1987; **Fac Appt:** Prof Ped, NYU Sch Med

Cheung, Nai-Kong V MD/PhD (PHO) - **Spec Exp:** Neuroblastoma; **Hospital:** Meml Sloan-Kettering Cancer Ctr (page 116); **Address:** 1275 York Ave, New York, NY 10065; **Phone:** 646-888-2313; **Board Cert:** Pediatrics 1987; Pediatric Hematology-Oncology 2012; **Med School:** Harvard Med Sch 1978; **Resid:** Pediatrics, Stanford Univ Hosp 1980; **Fellow:** Pediatric Hematology-Oncology, Stanford Univ Hosp 1982; **Fac Appt:** Assoc Prof Ped, Cornell Univ-Weill Med Coll

Dunkel, Ira J MD (PHO) - **Spec Exp:** Retinoblastoma; Brain & Spinal Cord Tumors; Brain Tumors; Pediatric Cancers; **Hospital:** Meml Sloan-Kettering Cancer Ctr (page 116); **Address:** 1275 York Ave, Box 185, New York, NY 10065; **Phone:** 212-639-2153; **Board Cert:** Pediatric Hematology-Oncology 2007; **Med School:** Duke Univ 1985; **Resid:** Pediatrics, Duke Univ Med Ctr 1988; **Fellow:** Pediatric Hematology-Oncology, Memorial-Sloan Kettering 1992; **Fac Appt:** Assoc Prof Ped, Cornell Univ-Weill Med Coll

Gardner, Sharon L MD (PHO) *PCP* - **Spec Exp:** Neuro-Oncology; **Hospital:** NYU Langone Med Ctr (page 108); **Address:** Steven B Hassenfeld Childrns Ctr, 160 E 32nd St Fl 2, New York, NY 10016; **Phone:** 212-263-8400; **Board Cert:** Pediatrics 2000; Pediatric Hematology-Oncology 2000; **Med School:** Hahnemann Univ 1986; **Resid:** Pediatrics, St Christophers Hosp Chldn 1989; **Fellow:** Pediatric Hematology-Oncology, Sloan Kettering Canc Ctr 1993; **Fac Appt:** Asst Prof Ped, NYU Sch Med

Garvin Jr, James H MD/PhD (PHO) - **Spec Exp:** Brain Tumors; Pediatric Cancers; Bone Marrow Transplant; **Hospital:** Morgan Stanley Children's Hosp of NY-Presby, NY (page 104); **Address:** 161 Fort Washington Ave, Fl 7, rm 708, New York, NY 10032-3729; **Phone:** 212-305-5808; **Board Cert:** Pediatrics 1982; Pediatric Hematology-Oncology 1984; **Med School:** Jefferson Med Coll 1976; **Resid:** Pediatrics, Chldns Hosp 1978; Pediatrics, Middlesex Hosp 1979; **Fellow:** Pediatric Hematology-Oncology, Dana Farber Cancer Inst/Childrens Hosp 1982; **Fac Appt:** Clin Prof Ped, Columbia P&S

Giardina, Patricia J V MD (PHO) - **Spec Exp:** Thalassemia; **Hospital:** NY-Presby/Weill Cornell Med Ctr, NY (page 104); **Address:** 525 E 68th St, Payson Pavilion 695, New York, NY 10065; **Phone:** 212-746-3400; **Board Cert:** Pediatrics 1973; Pediatric Hematology-Oncology 1974; **Med School:** NY Med Coll 1968; **Resid:** Pediatrics, New York Hosp 1971; **Fellow:** Pediatric Hematology-Oncology, New York Hosp-Cornell 1974; **Fac Appt:** Clin Prof Ped, Cornell Univ-Weill Med Coll

Kernan, Nancy A MD (PHO) - **Spec Exp:** Leukemia; Bone Marrow Transplant; Immune Deficiency; Stem Cell Transplant; **Hospital:** Meml Sloan-Kettering Cancer Ctr (page 116); **Address:** 1275 York Ave, New York, NY 10065; **Phone:** 212-639-7250; **Board Cert:** Pediatrics 1983; Pediatric Hematology-Oncology 1984; **Med School:** Cornell Univ-Weill Med Coll 1978; **Resid:** Pediatrics, Chldns Hosp Natl Med Ctr 1981; **Fellow:** Pediatric Hematology-Oncology, Meml Sloan Kettering Cancer Ctr 1984; **Fac Appt:** Assoc Prof Ped, Cornell Univ-Weill Med Coll

Kramer, Kim MD (PHO) - **Spec Exp:** Neuroblastoma; Brain & Spinal Cord Tumors; **Hospital:** Meml Sloan-Kettering Cancer Ctr (page 116); **Address:** 1275 York, Box 429, New York, NY 10021; **Phone:** 212-639-6410; **Board Cert:** Pediatric Hematology-Oncology 2011; **Med School:** SUNY Upstate Med Univ 1989; **Resid:** Pediatrics, Strong Meml Hosp 1992; **Fellow:** Pediatric Hematology-Oncology, Meml Sloan Kettering Cancer Ctr 1994

Kushner, Brian H MD (PHO) - **Spec Exp:** Neuroblastoma; Bone Marrow Transplant; Immunotherapy; **Hospital:** Meml Sloan-Kettering Cancer Ctr (page 116); **Address:** 1275 York Avenue, New York, NY 10065; **Phone:** 212-639-6793; **Board Cert:** Pediatrics 1983; Pediatric Hematology-Oncology 1987; **Med School:** Johns Hopkins Univ 1976; **Resid:** Pediatrics, Columbia-Presby Med Ctr 1978; Pediatrics, NY Hosp 1979; **Fellow:** Pediatric Hematology-Oncology, Boston Chldns Hosp 1980; Pediatric Hematology-Oncology, Meml Sloan Kettering Cancer Ctr 1986; **Fac Appt:** Prof Ped, Cornell Univ-Weill Med Coll

Marcus, Judith R MD (PHO) - **Spec Exp:** Leukemia; Lymphoma; Bleeding/Coagulation Disorders; Solid Tumors; **Hospital:** Morgan Stanley Children's Hosp of NY-Presby, NY (page 104), White Plains Hosp (page 615); **Address:** 161 Ft Washington Ave, Ste 7I, New York, NY 10032; **Phone:** 212-305-5808; **Board Cert:** Pediatrics 1997; Pediatric Hematology-Oncology 1997; **Med School:** NYU Sch Med 1971; **Resid:** Pediatrics, Bronx Muni Hosp-Albert Einstein 1974; **Fellow:** Pediatric Hematology-Oncology, Meml Sloan Kettering Cancer Ctr 1979; **Fac Appt:** Clin Prof Ped, Columbia P&S

Meyers, Paul A MD (PHO) - **Spec Exp:** Pediatric Cancers; Bone Tumors; Sarcoma; **Hospital:** Meml Sloan-Kettering Cancer Ctr (page 116), NY-Presby/Weill Cornell Med Ctr, NY (page 104); **Address:** 1275 York Ave, New York, NY 10065; **Phone:** 212-639-5952; **Board Cert:** Pediatrics 1978; Pediatric Hematology-Oncology 1978; **Med School:** Mount Sinai Sch Med 1973; **Resid:** Pediatrics, Mt Sinai Hosp 1976; **Fellow:** Pediatric Hematology-Oncology, NY Hosp-Cornell Med Ctr 1979; **Fac Appt:** Prof Ped, Cornell Univ-Weill Med Coll

O'Reilly, Richard MD (PHO) - **Spec Exp:** Bone Marrow Transplant; **Hospital:** Meml Sloan-Kettering Cancer Ctr (page 116), NY-Presby/Weill Cornell Med Ctr, NY (page 104); **Address:** 1275 York Avenue, New York, NY 10065; **Phone:** 212-639-5957; **Board Cert:** Pediatrics 1974; **Med School:** Univ Rochester 1968; **Resid:** Pediatrics, Chldrns Hosp 1972; **Fellow:** Infectious Disease, Chldrns Hosp 1973; **Fac Appt:** Prof Ped, Cornell Univ-Weill Med Coll

Steinherz, Peter G MD (PHO) - **Spec Exp:** Leukemia & Lymphoma; Pediatric Cancers; Wilms' Tumor; **Hospital:** Meml Sloan-Kettering Cancer Ctr (page 116), NY-Presby/Weill Cornell Med Ctr, NY (page 104); **Address:** 1275 York Avenue, New York, NY 10065; **Phone:** 212-639-7951; **Board Cert:** Pediatrics 1973; Pediatric Hematology-Oncology 1978; **Med School:** Albert Einstein Coll Med 1968; **Resid:** Pediatrics, NYPresby/Weill Cornell Med Ctr 1971; **Fellow:** Pediatric Hematology-Oncology, NYPresby/Weill Cornell Med Ctr 1975; **Fac Appt:** Prof Ped, Cornell Univ-Weill Med Coll

Weiner, Michael A MD (PHO) - **Spec Exp:** Hodgkin's Lymphoma; Lymphoma; Leukemia; **Hospital:** Morgan Stanley Children's Hosp of NY-Presby, NY (page 104); **Address:** 161 Fort Washington Ave, Irving Pavilion-FL 7, New York, NY 10032-3710; **Phone:** 212-305-9770; **Board Cert:** Pediatrics 1980; Pediatric Hematology-Oncology 1980; **Med School:** SUNY Hlth Sci Ctr 1972; **Resid:** Pediatrics, Montefiore Med Ctr 1974; **Fellow:** Pediatric Hematology-Oncology, NYU Med Ctr 1976; Pediatric Hematology-Oncology, Johns Hopkins Hosp 1977; **Fac Appt:** Prof Ped, Columbia P&S

Wexler, Leonard MD (PHO) - **Spec Exp:** Rhabdomyosarcoma; Bone Cancer; Gastrointestinal Stromal Tumors; Sarcoma-Soft Tissue; **Hospital:** Meml Sloan-Kettering Cancer Ctr (page 116); **Address:** 1275 York Avenue, New York, NY 10065; **Phone:** 212-639-7990; **Board Cert:** Pediatrics 2007; Pediatric Hematology-Oncology 2007; **Med School:** Boston Univ 1985; **Resid:** Pediatrics, Montefiore Med Ctr 1988; **Fellow:** Pediatric Hematology-Oncology, National Cancer Inst 1991; **Fac Appt:** Assoc Prof Ped, Columbia P&S

Pediatric Infectious Disease

Borkowsky, William MD (PInf) - **Spec Exp:** AIDS/HIV; Congenital Infections; Immune Deficiency; **Hospital:** NYU Langone Med Ctr (page 108), Bellevue Hosp Ctr; **Address:** 550 1st Ave, Dept Pediatrics, New York, NY 10016; **Phone:** 212-263-6513; **Board Cert:** Pediatrics 1979; Pediatric Infectious Disease 2009; **Med School:** NYU Sch Med 1972; **Resid:** Pediatrics, Bellevue Hosp Ctr 1975; **Fellow:** Infectious Disease, Bellevue Hosp Ctr-NYU 1978; **Fac Appt:** Prof Ped, NYU Sch Med

Larsen, John G MD (PInf) - **Hospital:** Mount Sinai Med Ctr (page 102); **Address:** 1245 Park Ave, New York, NY 10128-1211; **Phone:** 212-427-0540; **Board Cert:** Pediatrics 1979; Pediatric Infectious Disease 2005; **Med School:** SUNY Hlth Sci Ctr 1974; **Resid:** Pediatrics, Mount Sinai Med Ctr 1977; **Fellow:** Pediatric Infectious Disease, Mount Sinai Med Ctr 1978; **Fac Appt:** Assoc Clin Prof Ped, Mount Sinai Sch Med

Neu, Natalie M MD (PInf) - **Spec Exp:** AIDS/HIV; Sexually Transmitted Diseases; **Hospital:** NY-Presby/Columbia Univ Med Ctr, NY (page 104); **Address:** 3959 Broadway, BHN 106, New York, NY 10032; **Phone:** 212-305-4558; **Board Cert:** Pediatrics 2009; Pediatric Infectious Disease 2005; **Med School:** Columbia P&S 1991; **Resid:** Pediatrics, Michigan State Med Ctr 1994; **Fellow:** Pediatric Infectious Disease, Columbia Presby Med Ctr 1997; **Fac Appt:** Assoc Clin Prof Ped, Columbia P&S

Saiman, Lisa MD (PInf) - **Spec Exp:** Cystic Fibrosis Infection; Fungal Infections; Tick-borne Diseases; Tuberculosis; **Hospital:** Morgan Stanley Children's Hosp of NY-Presby, NY (page 104); **Address:** 3959 Broadway, rm 106, New York, NY 10032; **Phone:** 212-305-4558; **Board Cert:** Pediatrics 1987; Pediatric Infectious Disease 2009; **Med School:** Albert Einstein Coll Med 1983; **Resid:** Pediatrics, Babies Hosp/NY Presby 1986; **Fellow:** Infectious Disease, Babies Hosp/NY Presby 1989; **Fac Appt:** Assoc Clin Prof Ped, Columbia P&S

Pediatric Nephrology

Benchimol, Corinne MD (PNep) - **Spec Exp:** Dialysis Care; Hemolytic Uremic Syndrome; Glomerulonephritis; **Hospital:** Mount Sinai Med Ctr (page 102); **Address:** 5 E 98 St Fl 10, New York, NY 10029; **Phone:** 212-241-6187; **Board Cert:** Pediatric Nephrology 2009; **Med School:** Southeastern Univ Coll Osteo Med 1990; **Resid:** Pediatrics, Miami Chldns Hosp 1993; **Fellow:** Pediatric Nephrology, Jacobi Med Ctr 1996; **Fac Appt:** Asst Prof Med, Mount Sinai Sch Med

Johnson, Valerie L MD/PhD (PNep) - **Spec Exp:** Nephrotic Syndrome; Glomerulonephritis; Hypertension; Transplant Medicine-Kidney; **Hospital:** NY-Presby/Weill Cornell Med Ctr, NY (page 104), Valley Hosp (page 689); **Address:** 505 E 70th St, Helmsley Tower Fl 3, New York, NY 10021; **Phone:** 646-962-4324; **Board Cert:** Pediatrics 1984; Pediatric Nephrology 1985; **Med School:** Cornell Univ-Weill Med Coll 1977; **Resid:** Pediatrics, Mt Sinai Hosp 1979; **Fellow:** Nephrology, Montefiore Med Ctr 1982; **Fac Appt:** Assoc Clin Prof Ped, Cornell Univ-Weill Med Coll

Perelstein, Eduardo MD (PNep) - **Spec Exp:** Kidney Failure; Glomerulonephritis; Hypertension; **Hospital:** NY-Presby/Weill Cornell Med Ctr, NY (page 104), NY Hosp Queens (page 206); **Address:** 505 E 70th St Fl 3, New York, NY 10021; **Phone:** 646-962-4324; **Board Cert:** Pediatrics 2011; Pediatric Nephrology 2005; **Med School:** Argentina 1974; **Resid:** Pediatrics, Chldn's Hosp 1978; **Fellow:** Pediatric Nephrology, St Christopher's Hosp for Chldn 1985; Pediatric Nephrology, NY Hosp-Cornell Med Ctr 1987; **Fac Appt:** Assoc Prof Ped, Cornell Univ-Weill Med Coll

Saland, Jeffrey M MD (PNep) - **Spec Exp:** Transplant Medicine-Kidney; Kidney Disease; Hypertension in Children; Hemolytic Uremic Syndrome; **Hospital:** Mount Sinai Med Ctr (page 102); **Address:** Mount Sinai Medical Center, 5 E 98th St, Fl 10, New York, NY 10029; **Phone:** 212-241-6187; **Board Cert:** Pediatric Nephrology 2003; **Med School:** Univ New Mexico 1995; **Resid:** Pediatrics, Chldns Hosp Med Ctr 1998; **Fellow:** Pediatric Nephrology, Univ TX-SW Med Ctr 2000; Pediatric Nephrology, Mt Sinai Med Ctr 2002; **Fac Appt:** Asst Prof Ped, Mount Sinai Sch Med

Trachtman, Howard MD (PNep) - **Spec Exp:** Electrolyte Disorders; Hypertension; Hemolytic Uremic Syndrome; Nephrotic Syndrome; **Hospital:** NYU Langone Med Ctr (page 108); **Address:** 160 E 32nd St, Level 3 Medical, New York, NY 10016; **Phone:** 212-263-5940; **Board Cert:** Pediatrics 1983; Nephrology 2003; **Med School:** Univ Pennsylvania 1978; **Resid:** Pediatrics, New England Med Ctr 1980; Pediatrics, Bronx Muni Hosp Ctr 1981; **Fellow:** Pediatric Nephrology, Albert Einstein 1983; **Fac Appt:** Prof Ped, Albert Einstein Coll Med

Pediatric Otolaryngology

April, Max M MD (PO) - **Spec Exp:** Sinus Disorders; Neck Masses; Laryngeal Disorders; Sleep Apnea; **Hospital:** NY-Presby/Weill Cornell Med Ctr, NY (page 104), Long Island Jewish Med Ctr (page 106); **Address:** 428 E 72nd St, Ste 100, New York, NY 10021; **Phone:** 646-962-2224; **Board Cert:** Otolaryngology 1990; **Med School:** Boston Univ 1985; **Resid:** Otolaryngology, Boston Univ Med Ctr 1990; **Fellow:** Pediatric Otolaryngology, Johns Hopkins Hosp 1991; **Fac Appt:** Clin Prof Oto, Cornell Univ-Weill Med Coll

Dolitsky, Jay MD (PO) - **Spec Exp:** Ear Infections; Neck Masses; Tonsil/Adenoid Disorders; Sleep Disorders; **Hospital:** New York Eye & Ear Infirm (page 117); **Address:** 261 Fifth Ave, Fl 9, Ste 901, MS 10016, New York, NY 10016; **Phone:** 212-679-3499; **Board Cert:** Otolaryngology 1990; **Med School:** SUNY Downstate 1981; **Resid:** Surgery, NYU/Bellevue Hosp 1986; Otolaryngology, Manhattan EET Hosp 1990; **Fellow:** Pediatric Otolaryngology, Children's Hosp 1992

Haddad Jr, Joseph MD (PO) - **Spec Exp:** Ear Infections; Sinus Disorders; Cleft Palate/Lip; **Hospital:** Morgan Stanley Children's Hosp of NY-Presby, NY (page 104); **Address:** Morgan Stanley Chldns Hosp of NY-Presby, 3959 Broadway, Ste 501N, New York, NY 10032-1559; **Phone:** 212-305-8933; **Board Cert:** Otolaryngology 1988; **Med School:** NYU Sch Med 1983; **Resid:** Surgery, Columbia-Presby Hosp 1985; Otolaryngology, Columbia-Presby Hosp 1988; **Fellow:** Pediatric Otolaryngology, Chldns Hosp 1990; **Fac Appt:** Clin Prof Oto, Columbia P&S

Jones, Jacqueline MD (PO) - **Spec Exp:** Sinus Disorders/Surgery; Ear Infections; **Hospital:** NY-Presby/Weill Cornell Med Ctr, NY (page 104), Lenox Hill Hosp (page 106); **Address:** 1175 Park Ave, Ste 1A, New York, NY 10128; **Phone:** 212-996-2559; **Board Cert:** Otolaryngology 1989; **Med School:** Cornell Univ-Weill Med Coll 1984; **Resid:** Otolaryngology, Hosp Univ Penn 1989; **Fellow:** Pediatric Otolaryngology, Chldns Hosp 1990; **Fac Appt:** Assoc Prof Oto, Cornell Univ-Weill Med Coll

Rothschild, Michael A MD (PO) - **Spec Exp:** Ear Disorders; Sleep Apnea; Sinusitis; **Hospital:** Mount Sinai Med Ctr (page 102); **Address:** 1175 Park Ave, Ste 1A, New York, NY 10128; **Phone:** 212-996-2995; **Board Cert:** Otolaryngology 1994; **Med School:** Yale Univ 1988; **Resid:** Surgery, Mt Sinai Med Ctr 1990; Otolaryngology, Mt Sinai Med Ctr 1993; **Fellow:** Pediatric Otolaryngology, Chldn's Hosp 1994; **Fac Appt:** Clin Prof Oto, Mount Sinai Sch Med

Ward, Robert MD (PO) - **Spec Exp:** Airway Disorders; Sinus Disorders/Surgery; Choanal Atresia; **Hospital:** NY-Presby/Weill Cornell Med Ctr, NY (page 104), Lenox Hill Hosp (Manh Eye, Ear & Throat Hosp) (page 106); **Address:** Weill Cornell Med Ctr, Otolaryngology, 428 E 72nd St, Ste 100, New York, NY 10021; **Phone:** 646-962-2224; **Board Cert:** Otolaryngology 1986; **Med School:** Cornell Univ-Weill Med Coll 1981; **Resid:** Surgery, NY Hosp 1983; Otolaryngology, NY Hosp 1986; **Fellow:** Pediatric Otolaryngology, Chldns Hosp 1986; **Fac Appt:** Assoc Clin Prof Oto, Cornell Univ-Weill Med Coll

Pediatric Pulmonology

Dimaio, Mary MD (PPul) - **Spec Exp:** Cystic Fibrosis; Asthma; Allergy; **Hospital:** NY-Presby/Weill Cornell Med Ctr, NY (page 104); **Address:** 1440 York Ave, Ste P5, New York, NY 10075; **Phone:** 212-988-5008; **Board Cert:** Pediatrics 1987; Pediatric Pulmonology 2007; Allergy & Immunology 2009; **Med School:** SUNY Hlth Sci Ctr 1981; **Resid:** Pediatrics, Kings Co Hosp/Downstate 1983; Pediatrics, N Shore Univ Hosp 1985; **Fellow:** Pediatric Pulmonology, Mt Sinai Hosp 1988

Kattan, Meyer MD (PPul) - **Spec Exp:** Asthma; Cystic Fibrosis; Chronic Lung Disease; **Hospital:** NY-Presby/Columbia Univ Med Ctr, NY (page 104), Englewood Hosp & Med Ctr; **Address:** 3959 Broadway, CHC 7-701, New York, NY 10032; **Phone:** 212-305-5122; **Board Cert:** Pediatrics 1980; Pediatric Pulmonology 2010; **Med School:** McGill Univ 1973; **Resid:** Pediatrics, Chldns Hosp 1975; Pediatrics, Hosp for Sick Chldn 1976; **Fellow:** Pulmonary Disease, Hosp for Sick Chldn 1978; **Fac Appt:** Prof Ped, Columbia P&S

Lamm, Carin MD (PPul) - **Spec Exp:** Sleep Disorders; Asthma; **Hospital:** Morgan Stanley Children's Hosp of NY-Presby, NY (page 104); **Address:** Columbia Univ Medical Ctr, 3959 Broadway Fl 7 Central, New York, NY 10032; **Phone:** 212-305-5122; **Board Cert:** Pediatrics 1980; Pediatric Pulmonology 2010; **Med School:** NYU Sch Med 1975; **Resid:** Pediatrics, Mt Sinai Med Ctr 1979; **Fellow:** Pediatric Pulmonology, Mt Sinai Med Ctr 1981; **Fac Appt:** Assoc Prof Ped, Mount Sinai Sch Med

Loughlin, Gerald M MD (PPul) - **Spec Exp:** Sleep Disorders/Apnea; Swallowing Disorders; Asthma & Chronic Lung Disease; Breathing Disorders; **Hospital:** NY-Presby/Weill Cornell Med Ctr, NY (page 104); **Address:** Cornell Med Coll, Dept Peds, 525 E 68th St, rm M-622, New York, NY 10021-4870; **Phone:** 646-962-3410; **Board Cert:** Pediatrics 1993; Pediatric Pulmonology 2012; **Med School:** Univ Rochester 1973; **Resid:** Pediatrics, Univ Ariz Med Ctr 1973; **Fellow:** Pediatric Pulmonology, Univ Ariz Med Ctr 1977; **Fac Appt:** Prof Ped, Cornell Univ-Weill Med Coll

Ting, Andrew S MD (PPul) - **Spec Exp:** Asthma; Cystic Fibrosis; Bronchoscopy; Cough; **Hospital:** Mount Sinai Med Ctr (page 102); **Address:** 5 E 98th St, Fl 8, New York, NY 10029; **Phone:** 212-241-7788; **Board Cert:** Pediatric Pulmonology 2009; **Med School:** NYU Sch Med 1987; **Resid:** Pediatrics, Mt Sinai Med Ctr 1991; **Fellow:** Pediatric Pulmonology, Mt Sinai Med Ctr 1994; **Fac Appt:** Asst Prof Ped, Mount Sinai Sch Med

Pediatric Rheumatology

Eichenfield, Andrew H MD (PRhu) - **Spec Exp:** Juvenile Arthritis; Lyme Disease; Lupus/SLE; **Hospital:** Morgan Stanley Children's Hosp of NY-Presby, NY (page 104), Nyack Hosp; **Address:** Morgan Stanley Chldns Hosp, 3959 Broadway, CHN-106, Ped Rheumatology, New York, NY 10032; **Phone:** 212-305-9304; **Board Cert:** Pediatrics 1983; Pediatric Rheumatology 2007; **Med School:** Ros Franklin Univ/Chicago Med Sch 1978; **Resid:** Pediatrics, Mt Sinai Hosp 1982; **Fellow:** Pediatric Rheumatology, Chldns Hosp 1984; **Fac Appt:** Asst Clin Prof Ped, Columbia P&S

Lazarus, Herbert MD (PRhu) - **Spec Exp:** Juvenile Arthritis; Lyme Disease; Pain-Musculoskeletal; **Hospital:** NYU Langone Med Ctr (page 108), Lenox Hill Hosp (page 106); **Address:** 390 West End Ave, Ste 1E, New York, NY 10024; **Phone:** 212-787-1444; **Board Cert:** Pediatrics 1987; Pediatric Rheumatology 2007; **Med School:** UMDNJ-NJ Med Sch, Newark 1983; **Resid:** Pediatrics, NYU Med Ctr 1986; **Fellow:** Pediatric Rheumatology, Hosp for Joint Diseases 1987; **Fac Appt:** Asst Clin Prof Ped, NYU Sch Med

Lehman, Thomas MD (PRhu) - **Spec Exp:** Arthritis; Scleroderma; Lupus/SLE; Rheumatoid Arthritis; **Hospital:** Hosp For Special Surgery (page 115), NY-Presby/Weill Cornell Med Ctr, NY (page 104); **Address:** Hospital for Special Surgery, 535 E 70 St, New York, NY 10021-4872; **Phone:** 212-606-1151; **Board Cert:** Pediatrics 1979; Pediatric Rheumatology 2007; **Med School:** Jefferson Med Coll 1974; **Resid:** Pediatrics, Chldns Hosp 1976; Pediatrics, UCSF Med Ctr 1977; **Fellow:** Pediatric Rheumatology, Chldns Hosp 1979; Rheumatology, Natl Inst Hlth 1983; **Fac Appt:** Prof Ped, Cornell Univ-Weill Med Coll

Pediatric Surgery

Bodenstein, Lawrence MD/PhD (PS) - **Hospital:** Morgan Stanley Children's Hosp of NY-Presby, NY (page 104); **Address:** 3959 Broadway, CHN-215 Fl 2 North, New York, NY 10032; **Phone:** 212-342-8586; **Board Cert:** Surgery 2003; Pediatric Surgery 2005; **Med School:** Harvard Med Sch 1986; **Resid:** Surgery, Beth Israel Hosp 1991; **Fellow:** Critical Care Medicine, Beth Israel Hosp 1992; Pediatric Surgery, Babies Hosp-Columbia Presb 1994; **Fac Appt:** Asst Prof S, Columbia P&S

Cooper, Arthur MD (PS) - **Spec Exp:** Endoscopy; Trauma; Disaster Preparedness; Child Abuse; **Hospital:** Harlem Hosp Ctr, Metropolitan Hosp Ctr - NY; **Address:** Harlem Hospital, Dept Surgery, 506 Lenox Ave, New York, NY 10037; **Phone:** 212-939-4003; **Board Cert:** Surgery 2002; Pediatric Surgery 2003; Surgical Critical Care 2004; **Med School:** Univ Pennvania 1975; **Resid:** Surgery, Hosp Univ Penn 1981; Pediatric Surgery, Childrens Hosp 1984; **Fellow:** Pediatric Nutrition, Columbia P&S-Inst Human Nutrition 1982; **Fac Appt:** Prof S, Columbia P&S

Ginsburg, Howard B MD (PS) - **Spec Exp:** Neonatal Surgery; Tumor Surgery; Pediatric Urology; Gastrointestinal Surgery; **Hospital:** NYU Langone Med Ctr (page 108), Bellevue Hosp Ctr; **Address:** 530 First Ave, Ste 10W, New York, NY 10016-6402; **Phone:** 212-263-7391; **Board Cert:** Pediatric Surgery 2001; **Med School:** Univ Cincinnati 1972; **Resid:** Surgery, NYU-Bellvue Hosp 1977; Pediatric Surgery, Columbia-Presby Med Ctr 1979; **Fellow:** Pediatric Surgery, Mass Genl Hosp 1980; **Fac Appt:** Assoc Prof PS, NYU Sch Med

La Quaglia, Michael MD (PS) - **Spec Exp:** Cancer Surgery; Neuroblastoma; Liver Cancer; Colon & Rectal Cancer; **Hospital:** Meml Sloan-Kettering Cancer Ctr (page 116), NY-Presby/Weill Cornell Med Ctr, NY (page 104); **Address:** 1275 York Ave, Ste H1315, New York, NY 10065; **Phone:** 212-639-7002; **Board Cert:** Surgery 2003; Pediatric Surgery 2007; **Med School:** UMDNJ-NJ Med Sch, Newark 1976; **Resid:** Surgery, Mass Genl Hosp 1983; **Fellow:** Cardiothoracic Surgery, Broadgreen Ctr 1984; Pediatric Surgery, Chldns Hosp 1985; **Fac Appt:** Prof S, Cornell Univ-Weill Med Coll

Middlesworth, William MD (PS) - **Hospital:** Morgan Stanley Children's Hosp of NY-Presby, NY (page 104); **Address:** Morgan Stanley Children's Hospital, Div Pediatric Surgery, 3959 Broadway, CHN 206, New York, NY 10032-1537; **Phone:** 212-342-8585; **Board Cert:** Surgery 2007; Pediatric Surgery 2007; **Med School:** UMDNJ-RW Johnson Med Sch 1989; **Resid:** Surgery, Univ Maryland Hosps 1995; **Fellow:** Pediatric Surgery, Columbia Presby Med Ctr 1997; **Fac Appt:** Asst Prof S, Columbia P&S

Quaegebeur, Jan M MD (PS) - **Spec Exp:** Arterial Switch; Heart Valve Surgery; Pediatric Cardiac Surgery; **Hospital:** Morgan Stanley Children's Hosp of NY-Presby, NY (page 104); **Address:** Morgan Stanley Chlds Hosp of NY-Presby, 3959 Broadway, Ste BN276, New York, NY 10032; **Phone:** 212-305-5975; **Med School:** Belgium 1969; **Resid:** Surgery, St Michel Clinic 1973; **Fellow:** Thoracic Surgery, Baylor Coll Med 1974; Thoracic Surgery, Univ Hosp 1978; **Fac Appt:** Prof S, Columbia P&S

Spigland, Nitsana A MD (PS) - **Spec Exp:** Congenital Anomalies; Pediatric Thoracic Surgery; Cancer Surgery; Minimally Invasive Surgery; **Hospital:** NY-Presby/Weill Cornell Med Ctr, NY (page 104); **Address:** NY Hosp-Cornell Med Ctr, 505 E 70th St, New York, NY 10021; **Phone:** 212-746-5648; **Board Cert:** Pediatric Surgery 2003; **Med School:** NY Med Coll 1982; **Resid:** Surgery, Lenox Hill Hosp 1987; **Fellow:** Pediatric Surgery, St Justine Chldn's Hosp 1989; **Fac Appt:** Assoc Prof S, Cornell Univ-Weill Med Coll

Velcek, Francisca T MD (PS) - **Spec Exp:** Anorectal Malformations; Pediatric Gynecology; Neonatal Surgery; Hernia; **Hospital:** Lenox Hill Hosp (page 106), SUNY Downstate Med Ctr (Univ Hosp of Bklyn) - LICH (page 420); **Address:** 965 5th Ave, New York, NY 10075; **Phone:** 212-744-9396; **Board Cert:** Surgery 1974; Pediatric Surgery 2007; **Med School:** Philippines 1966; **Resid:** Surgery, St Clares Hosp 1971; Pediatric Surgery, SUNY Downstate Med Ctr 1975; **Fellow:** Pediatric Surgery, SUNY Downstate Med Ctr 1973; **Fac Appt:** Prof S, SUNY Hlth Sci Ctr

Pediatrics

Allendorf, Dennis MD (Ped) *PCP* - **Spec Exp:** Congenital Anomalies; **Hospital:** Morgan Stanley Children's Hosp of NY-Presby, NY (page 104), St. Luke's - Roosevelt Hosp Ctr - Roosevelt Div (page 94); **Address:** 401 W 118th St, Ste 2, New York, NY 10027-7216; **Phone:** 212-666-4610; **Board Cert:** Pediatrics 1987; **Med School:** NY Med Coll 1970; **Resid:** Pediatrics, St Luke's-Roosevelt Hosp Ctr 1972; Pediatrics, Columbia-Presby Hosp 1973; **Fac Appt:** Asst Clin Prof Ped, Columbia P&S

Arpadi, Stephen MD (Ped) *PCP* - **Spec Exp:** AIDS/HIV; **Hospital:** St. Luke's - Roosevelt Hosp Ctr - St Luke's Hosp (page 94), NY-Presby/Columbia Univ Med Ctr, NY (page 104); **Address:** 1111 Amsterdam Ave at 114th St, New York, NY 10025; **Phone:** 212-523-3847; **Board Cert:** Pediatrics 2009; **Med School:** Geo Wash Univ 1982; **Resid:** Pediatrics, Chldns Hosp Natl Med Ctr 1985; **Fac Appt:** Assoc Prof Ped, Columbia P&S

Axelrod, Felicia B MD (Ped) - **Spec Exp:** Dysautonomia; **Hospital:** NYU Langone Med Ctr (page 108); **Address:** New York Med Ctr, 530 1St Av, Ste 9Q, New York, NY 10016-6402; **Phone:** 212-263-7225; **Board Cert:** Pediatrics 1971; **Med School:** NYU Sch Med 1966; **Resid:** Pediatrics, Bellevue/NYU Med Ctr 1969; **Fellow:** Genetics, Mt Sinai Med Ctr 1976; **Fac Appt:** Prof Ped, NYU Sch Med

Brovender, Bruce J MD (Ped) *PCP* - **Hospital:** NY-Presby/Weill Cornell Med Ctr, NY (page 104), Mount Sinai Med Ctr (page 102); **Address:** 1559 York Ave, New York, NY 10028; **Phone:** 212-585-3329; **Board Cert:** Pediatrics 2011; **Med School:** Italy 1984; **Resid:** Pediatrics, Lenox Hill Hosp 1987; **Fellow:** Pediatric Hematology-Oncology, NYU/Bellvue Hosp 1988; **Fac Appt:** Asst Clin Prof Ped, Cornell Univ-Weill Med Coll

Burstin, Harris E MD (Ped) *PCP* - **Spec Exp:** Asthma; Allergy; Critical Care; **Hospital:** NYU Langone Med Ctr (page 108); **Address:** 317 E 34th St Fl 3, New York, NY 10016-4974; **Phone:** 212-725-6300; **Board Cert:** Pediatrics 1983; **Med School:** Mexico 1977; **Resid:** Pediatrics, Bellevue Hosp Ctr 1982; **Fac Appt:** Assoc Prof Ped, NYU Sch Med

Cohen, Michel A MD (Ped) *PCP* - **Spec Exp:** Child Development; Sleep Disorders; **Hospital:** NYU Langone Med Ctr (page 108), NY-Presby/Weill Cornell Med Ctr, NY (page 104); **Address:** Tribeca Pediatrics, 46 Warren St, New York, NY 10007; **Phone:** 212-226-7666; **Board Cert:** Pediatrics 2010; **Med School:** France 1989; **Resid:** Pediatrics, New York Univ Med Ctr 1991; Pediatrics, Long Island Hosp 1993

Cross, Jennifer MD (Ped) - **Spec Exp:** Learning Disorders; Child Development; Behavioral Disorders; **Hospital:** NY-Presby/Weill Cornell Med Ctr, NY (page 104); **Address:** 525 E 68th St, New York, NY 10065; **Phone:** 646-962-4303; **Board Cert:** Pediatrics 2005; Developmental-Behavioral Pediatrics 2002; **Med School:** England, UK 1983; **Resid:** Pediatrics, Lenox Hill Hosp 1988; **Fellow:** Neonatal-Perinatal Medicine, NY Hosp 1991; Developmental-Behavioral Pediatrics, Westchester Co Med Ctr 1994; **Fac Appt:** Asst Prof Ped, Cornell Univ-Weill Med Coll

Edelstein, Gary S MD (Ped) *PCP* - **Hospital:** Morgan Stanley Children's Hosp of NY-Presby, NY (page 104), NY-Presby/Weill Cornell Med Ctr, NY (page 104); **Address:** Manhattan Pediatrics, 16 E 60th St, Ste 410, New York, NY 10022; **Phone:** 212-326-3351; **Board Cert:** Pediatrics 2008; **Med School:** NYU Sch Med 1990; **Resid:** Pediatrics, Columbia Presby Babies Hosp 1993; **Fellow:** Ambulatory Pediatrics, Columbia Presby Babies Hosp 1995

Ferrier, Genevieve E MD (Ped) *PCP* - **Spec Exp:** Developmental & Behavioral Disorders; **Hospital:** NYU Langone Med Ctr (page 108); **Address:** 46 W 11th St, New York, NY 10011-8602; **Phone:** 212-529-4330; **Board Cert:** Pediatrics 2006; **Med School:** Mount Sinai Sch Med 1988; **Resid:** Pediatrics, Chldn's Hosp 1991; **Fac Appt:** Asst Prof Ped, NY Med Coll

Freilich, Stephanie B MD (Ped) *PCP* - **Hospital:** Mount Sinai Med Ctr (page 102); **Address:** 1125 Park Ave, Ste A, New York, NY 10128-2322; **Phone:** 212-289-1400; **Board Cert:** Pediatrics 2009; **Med School:** Mount Sinai Sch Med 1991; **Resid:** Pediatrics, Mount Sinai Med Ctr 1994; **Fac Appt:** Asst Clin Prof Ped, Mount Sinai Sch Med

Goldstein, Judith MD (Ped) *PCP* - **Spec Exp:** Neonatal Care; Infectious Disease; **Hospital:** NY-Presby/Weill Cornell Med Ctr, NY (page 104), Lenox Hill Hosp (page 106); **Address:** 1559 York Ave, New York, NY 10028; **Phone:** 212-585-3329; **Board Cert:** Pediatrics 1977; **Med School:** SUNY Downstate 1972; **Resid:** Pediatrics, Lenox Hill Hosp 1975; **Fac Appt:** Asst Clin Prof Ped, Cornell Univ-Weill Med Coll

Hes, Dyan S MD (Ped) - **Spec Exp:** Obesity; Weight Management; **Hospital:** NY-Presby/Weill Cornell Med Ctr, NY (page 104), New York Methodist Hosp (page 418); **Address:** Gramercy Pediatrics, 67 Irving Pl Fl 3 South, New York, NY 10003; **Phone:** 212-473-4200; **Board Cert:** Pediatrics 2009; **Med School:** Israel 1997; **Resid:** Pediatrics, Montefiore Med Ctr 2000; **Fac Appt:** Asst Clin Prof Ped, Cornell Univ-Weill Med Coll

Inamdar, Sarla MD (Ped) *PCP* - **Spec Exp:** Rheumatology; **Hospital:** Metropolitan Hosp Ctr - NY; **Address:** 1901 1st Ave, rm 523, New York, NY 10029-7404; **Phone:** 212-423-6228; **Board Cert:** Pediatrics 1974; **Med School:** India 1969; **Resid:** Pediatrics, Metropolitan Hosp Ctr 1972; **Fac Appt:** Clin Prof Ped, NY Med Coll

Kahn, Max A MD (Ped) *PCP* - **Hospital:** NYU Langone Med Ctr (page 108), Lenox Hill Hosp (page 106); **Address:** 390 West End Ave, Ste 1E, New York, NY 10024; **Phone:** 212-787-1444; **Board Cert:** Pediatrics 1980; **Med School:** Columbia P&S 1975; **Resid:** Pediatrics, Bronx Municipal Hosp 1978; **Fac Appt:** Assoc Clin Prof Ped, NYU Sch Med

Keith, Marie B MD (Ped) *PCP* - **Hospital:** NYU Langone Med Ctr (page 108); **Address:** 552 Broadway Fl 5, New York, NY 10012; **Phone:** 212-334-3366; **Board Cert:** Pediatrics 1979; **Med School:** Mount Sinai Sch Med 1974; **Resid:** Pediatrics, NY Presby-Columbia Presby Medical Ctr 1978

Kotin, Neal M MD (Ped) *PCP* - **Spec Exp:** Asthma; Bronchitis; Sleep Disorders; Pulmonary Disease; **Hospital:** Mount Sinai Med Ctr (page 102), Lenox Hill Hosp (page 106); **Address:** Carnegie Hill Pediatrics, 1125 Park Ave, New York, NY 10128-1243; **Phone:** 212-289-1400; **Board Cert:** Pediatrics 2010; Pediatric Pulmonology 2011; **Med School:** Albany Med Coll 1982; **Resid:** Pediatrics, Johns Hopkins Hosp 1985; **Fellow:** Pediatric Pulmonology, Mt Sinai Med Ctr 1988; **Fac Appt:** Asst Clin Prof Ped, Mount Sinai Sch Med

Larson, Signe S MD (Ped) *PCP* - **Spec Exp:** Pediatric Endocrinology; **Hospital:** Mount Sinai Med Ctr (page 102); **Address:** Uptowm Padiatrics, 1245 Park Ave, New York, NY 10128; **Phone:** 212-427-0540; **Board Cert:** Pediatrics 1984; Pediatric Endocrinology 2011; **Med School:** SUNY Stony Brook 1978; **Resid:** Family Medicine, Vancouver Genl Hosp 1979; Pediatrics, St Luke's Med Ctr 1982; **Fellow:** Pediatric Endocrinology, Mt Sinai Hosp 1984

Lazarus, George M MD (Ped) *PCP* - **Hospital:** Morgan Stanley Children's Hosp of NY-Presby, NY (page 104), NY-Presby/Weill Cornell Med Ctr, NY (page 104); **Address:** 106 E 78th, New York, NY 10075-0302; **Phone:** 212-744-0840; **Board Cert:** Pediatrics 1976; **Med School:** Columbia P&S 1971; **Resid:** Pediatrics, NY Presby-Columbia Med Ctr 1974; **Fac Appt:** Assoc Clin Prof Ped, Columbia P&S

Levitzky, Susan E MD (Ped) *PCP* - **Spec Exp:** Asthma; Child Development; Adoption & Foster Care; **Hospital:** NYU Langone Med Ctr (page 108), Beth Israel Med Ctr - Petrie Division (page 94); **Address:** 161 Madison Ave, Ste 6W, New York, NY 10016-5405; **Phone:** 212-213-1960; **Board Cert:** Pediatrics 1972; **Med School:** Univ IL Coll Med 1967; **Resid:** Pediatrics, Beth Israel Hosp 1970; **Fac Appt:** Asst Clin Prof Ped, NYU Sch Med

McCarton, Cecelia MD (Ped) - **Spec Exp:** Autism; Learning Disorders; ADD/ADHD; Developmental Disorders; **Hospital:** Montefiore Med Ctr-Einstein Campus, NY (page 100); **Address:** McCarton Ctr for Developmental Pediatrics, 350 E 82nd St, New York, NY 10028; **Phone:** 212-996-9019; **Board Cert:** Pediatrics 1988; **Med School:** Albert Einstein Coll Med 1970; **Resid:** Pediatrics, Bronx Muni Hosp Ctr 1974; **Fellow:** Developmental-Behavioral Pediatrics, Montefiore Med Ctr- Weiler Einstein Div 1977; **Fac Appt:** Prof Ped, Albert Einstein Coll Med

McHugh, Margaret T MD (Ped) - **Spec Exp:** Child Abuse; Adolescent Medicine; **Hospital:** Bellevue Hosp Ctr, NYU Langone Med Ctr (page 108); **Address:** Bellevue Hosp Ctr-Pediatrics, 462 First Ave, rm GC65, New York, NY 10016; **Phone:** 212-562-5524; **Board Cert:** Pediatrics 1975; Child Abuse Pediatrics 2009; **Med School:** Georgetown Univ 1970; **Resid:** Pediatrics, Metropolitan Hosp 1973; **Fellow:** Ambulatory Pediatrics, Columbia-Presby Med Ctr 1975; **Fac Appt:** Assoc Prof Ped, NYU Sch Med

Monti, Louis G MD (Ped) *PCP* - **Spec Exp:** Infectious Disease; **Hospital:** Mount Sinai Med Ctr (page 102); **Address:** 55 E 87th St, Ste 1G, New York, NY 10128-1049; **Phone:** 212-722-0707; **Board Cert:** Pediatrics 2009; **Med School:** Mount Sinai Sch Med 1980; **Resid:** Pediatrics, Mount Sinai Hosp 1983; **Fellow:** Infectious Disease, Childrens Hosp 1984; **Fac Appt:** Asst Clin Prof Ped, Mount Sinai Sch Med

Murphy, Ramon J C MD (Ped) *PCP* - **Spec Exp:** Community Medicine; **Hospital:** Mount Sinai Med Ctr (page 102); **Address:** Uptown Pediatrics, 1245 Park Ave, New York, NY 10128; **Phone:** 212-427-0540; **Board Cert:** Pediatrics 2009; **Med School:** Northwestern Univ 1969; **Resid:** Internal Medicine, Cook Co Hosp 1970; Pediatrics, Chldns Meml Hosp 1971; **Fellow:** Pediatrics, Babies Hosp 1973; Community Medicine, Mt Sinai Med Ctr 1974; **Fac Appt:** Clin Prof Ped, Mount Sinai Sch Med

Newman-Cedar, Meryl MD (Ped) *PCP* - **Spec Exp:** Child Development; **Hospital:** NY-Presby/Weill Cornell Med Ctr, NY (page 104), Lenox Hill Hosp (page 106); **Address:** Upper East Side Pediatrics, 215 E 79th St, Ste 1C, New York, NY 10075; **Phone:** 212-737-7800; **Board Cert:** Pediatrics 1987; **Med School:** SUNY Downstate 1981; **Resid:** Pediatrics, New York Hosp 1984; **Fellow:** Developmental-Behavioral Pediatrics, New York Hosp 1987

Oeffinger, Kevin MD (Ped) - **Spec Exp:** Cancer Survivors-Late Effects of Therapy; **Hospital:** Meml Sloan-Kettering Cancer Ctr (page 116); **Address:** 300 E 66th St, New York, NY 10065; **Phone:** 646-888-4730; **Board Cert:** Family Medicine 2006; **Med School:** Univ Tex, San Antonio 1984; **Resid:** Family Medicine, Baylor Coll Med 1985; **Fellow:** Family Medicine, Fam Practice Faculty Dev Ctr 1999Natl Cancer Inst 2000

Poon, Eric Sin-Kam MD (Ped) *PCP* - **Spec Exp:** Asthma; Pediatric Cardiology; Developmental Disorders; **Hospital:** NY Downtown Hosp, NY-Presby/Weill Cornell Med Ctr, NY (page 104); **Address:** 170 William St Fl 3, New York, NY 10038-2612; **Phone:** 212-312-5350; **Board Cert:** Pediatrics 1988; **Med School:** Mexico 1982; **Resid:** Pediatrics, LI Coll Hosp 1986; **Fellow:** Pediatric Cardiology, NY Hosp-Cornell Med Ctr 1988; **Fac Appt:** Asst Clin Prof Ped, Cornell Univ-Weill Med Coll

Popper, Laura MD (Ped) *PCP* - **Hospital:** Mount Sinai Med Ctr (page 102); **Address:** 116 E 66th St, Ste 1C, New York, NY 10065; **Phone:** 212-794-2136; **Board Cert:** Pediatrics 1981; **Med School:** Columbia P&S 1974; **Resid:** Pediatrics, Babies Hosp 1976; **Fellow:** Pediatrics, Babies Hosp 1977; **Fac Appt:** Asst Clin Prof Ped, NY Coll Osteo Med

Prezioso, Paula J MD (Ped) *PCP* - **Hospital:** NYU Langone Med Ctr (page 108); **Address:** 317 E 34th St, Fl 3, New York, NY 10016-4974; **Phone:** 212-725-6300; **Board Cert:** Pediatrics 2006; **Med School:** SUNY Downstate 1987; **Resid:** Pediatrics, NYU-Bellevue Hosp 1991; **Fac Appt:** Asst Clin Prof Ped, NYU Sch Med

Prince, Alice S MD (Ped) - **Spec Exp:** Infectious Disease; **Hospital:** Morgan Stanley Children's Hosp of NY-Presby, NY (page 104); **Address:** 650 W 168th St, New York, NY 10032-3702; **Phone:** 212-305-4558; **Board Cert:** Pediatrics 1979; Pediatric Infectious Disease 2009; **Med School:** Columbia P&S 1975; **Resid:** Pediatrics, Babies Hosp 1978; **Fellow:** Infectious Disease, Columbia Univ 1981; **Fac Appt:** Prof Ped, Columbia P&S

Raucher, Harold S MD (Ped) *PCP* - **Spec Exp:** Infectious Disease; Travel Medicine; **Hospital:** Mount Sinai Med Ctr (page 102), Lenox Hill Hosp (page 106); **Address:** Carnegie Hill Pediatrics, 1125 Park Ave, New York, NY 10128-1243; **Phone:** 212-289-1400; **Board Cert:** Pediatrics 2006; Pediatric Infectious Disease 2009; **Med School:** Mount Sinai Sch Med 1978; **Resid:** Pediatrics, Mt Sinai Med Ctr 1980; **Fellow:** Pediatric Infectious Disease, Mt Sinai Med Ctr 1982; **Fac Appt:** Assoc Clin Prof Ped, Mount Sinai Sch Med

Rosello, Lori J MD (Ped) *PCP* - **Hospital:** NYU Langone Med Ctr (page 108); **Address:** 46 W 11th St, New York, NY 10011-8602; **Phone:** 212-529-4330; **Board Cert:** Pediatrics 2005; **Med School:** Albert Einstein Coll Med 1987; **Resid:** Pediatrics, Babies Hosp/Columbia 1990; **Fac Appt:** Asst Clin Prof Ped, NYU Sch Med

Rosenbaum, Michael MD (Ped) *PCP* - **Spec Exp:** Nutrition; Growth Disorders; Obesity; **Hospital:** Morgan Stanley Children's Hosp of NY-Presby, NY (page 104); **Address:** 450 W End Ave, New York, NY 10024-5307; **Phone:** 212-769-3070; **Board Cert:** Pediatrics 1988; **Med School:** Cornell Univ-Weill Med Coll 1982; **Resid:** Pediatrics, Columbia-Presby Med Ctr 1985; **Fellow:** Pediatric Endocrinology, New York Hosp 1988; **Fac Appt:** Prof Ped, Columbia P&S

Rosenfeld, Suzanne MD (Ped) *PCP* - **Spec Exp:** Developmental Disorders; Asthma; **Hospital:** NY-Presby/Weill Cornell Med Ctr, NY (page 104), Lenox Hill Hosp (page 106); **Address:** West End Pediatrics, 450 West End Ave, New York, NY 10024-5393; **Phone:** 212-769-3070; **Board Cert:** Pediatrics 1986; **Med School:** Columbia P&S 1980; **Resid:** Pediatrics, Columbia-Presby Med Ctr 1983; **Fellow:** Pediatrics, NY Hosp-Cornell Med Ctr 1984

Sacker, Ira M MD (Ped) - **Spec Exp:** Eating Disorders; Obesity; **Hospital:** NYU Langone Med Ctr (page 108); **Address:** 19 W 34th St, Penthouse Fl, New York, NY 10016; **Phone:** 212-268-4440; **Board Cert:** Pediatrics 1982; **Med School:** UCLA 1968; **Resid:** Pediatrics, Bellevue Hosp/NYU Med Ctr 1972; **Fellow:** Adolescent Medicine, Chldns Hosp 1972; **Fac Appt:** Asst Clin Prof Ped, NYU Sch Med

Sanford, Marie V MD (Ped) *PCP* - **Hospital:** NY-Presby/Weill Cornell Med Ctr, NY (page 104); **Address:** Weill Cornell Medical Associates, 12 W 72nd St, New York, NY 10023; **Phone:** 646-962-7800; **Board Cert:** Pediatrics 2009; **Med School:** Mount Sinai Sch Med 1991; **Resid:** Pediatrics, Mount Sinai Med Ctr 1995; **Fac Appt:** Asst Clin Prof Ped, Mount Sinai Sch Med

Softness, Barney MD (Ped) *PCP* - **Spec Exp:** Diabetes; **Hospital:** Morgan Stanley Children's Hosp of NY-Presby, NY (page 104), NY-Presby/Weill Cornell Med Ctr, NY (page 104); **Address:** W End Pediatrics, 450 W End Ave, New York, NY 10024-5307; **Phone:** 212-769-3070; **Board Cert:** Pediatrics 1986; Pediatric Endocrinology 1986; **Med School:** Columbia P&S 1980; **Resid:** Pediatrics, Columbia Presby Med Ctr 1983; **Fellow:** Pediatric Endocrinology, NY Cornell Med Ctr 1985; **Fac Appt:** Assoc Clin Prof Ped, Columbia P&S

Stein, Barry B MD (Ped) *PCP* - **Spec Exp:** Developmental & Behavioral Disorders; **Hospital:** Mount Sinai Med Ctr (page 102), Lenox Hill Hosp (page 106); **Address:** Carnegie Hill Pediatrics, 1125 Park Ave, New York, NY 10128-1243; **Phone:** 212-289-1400; **Board Cert:** Pediatrics 1987; **Med School:** South Africa 1980; **Resid:** Pediatrics, Mt Sinai Hosp 1986; **Fac Appt:** Asst Clin Prof Ped, Mount Sinai Sch Med

Traister, Michael R MD (Ped) *PCP* - **Spec Exp:** Adoption & Foster Care; **Hospital:** NYU Langone Med Ctr (page 108), Lenox Hill Hosp (page 106); **Address:** 390 West End Ave, Ste 1E, New York, NY 10024; **Phone:** 212-787-1444; **Board Cert:** Pediatrics 1980; **Med School:** NY Med Coll 1975; **Resid:** Pediatrics, Bronx Municipal Hosp 1978; **Fellow:** Ambulatory Pediatrics, Bellevue Hosp 1979; **Fac Appt:** Asst Clin Prof Ped, NYU Sch Med

Weinberger, Sylvain M MD (Ped) *PCP* - **Spec Exp:** Prematurity/Low Birth Weight Infants; **Hospital:** NYU Langone Med Ctr (page 108), Beth Israel Med Ctr - Petrie Division (page 94); **Address:** 51 E 25 St Fl 3, New York, NY 10010; **Phone:** 212-598-0331; **Board Cert:** Pediatrics 1982; Neonatal-Perinatal Medicine 1983; **Med School:** Belgium 1977; **Resid:** Pediatrics, LI Jewish Med Ctr 1979; **Fellow:** Neonatal-Perinatal Medicine, LI Jewish Med Ctr 1981; **Fac Appt:** Asst Clin Prof Ped, NYU Sch Med

Zimmerman, Sol S MD (Ped) *PCP* - **Spec Exp:** Growth/Development Disorders; Behavioral Disorders; Cough-Tic Syndrome; **Hospital:** NYU Langone Med Ctr (page 108); **Address:** 317 E 34th St, New York, NY 10016-4974; **Phone:** 212-725-6300; **Board Cert:** Pediatrics 1977; **Med School:** NYU Sch Med 1972; **Resid:** Pediatrics, Bellevue Hosp Ctr 1975; Pediatrics, Bellevue Hosp/NYU 1978; **Fac Appt:** Assoc Prof Ped, NYU Sch Med

Physical Medicine & Rehabilitation

Ahn, Jung Hwan MD (PMR) - **Spec Exp:** Spinal Cord Injury; Stroke Rehabilitation; Neurologic Rehabilitation; **Hospital:** NYU Langone Med Ctr (page 108); **Address:** Ambulatory Care Ctr, 240 E 38th St Fl 15, New York, NY 10016; **Phone:** 212-263-6122; **Board Cert:** Physical Medicine & Rehabilitation 1980; Spinal Cord Injury Medicine 2008; **Med School:** South Korea 1970; **Resid:** Obstetrics & Gynecology, Elmhurst City Hosp - Mt Sinai 1976; Physical Medicine & Rehabilitation, NYU Med Ctr 1979; **Fellow:** Spinal Cord Injury Medicine, NYU Med Ctr 1980; **Fac Appt:** Clin Prof PMR, NYU Sch Med

Brown, Andrew MD (PMR) - **Spec Exp:** Electromyography; **Hospital:** NY Downtown Hosp; **Address:** 19 Beekman St Fl 6, New York, NY 10038; **Phone:** 212-513-7711; **Board Cert:** Physical Medicine & Rehabilitation 1988; **Med School:** West Indies 1982; **Resid:** Pediatrics, Univ Md Hosp 1984; Physical Medicine & Rehabilitation, Mount Sinai Med Ctr 1987

Bryce, Thomas MD (PMR) - **Spec Exp:** Spinal Cord Injury; Pain-Neuropathic; **Hospital:** Mount Sinai Med Ctr (page 102); **Address:** Rehab Medicine Assocs, 5 E 98th St, Box 1240B, New York, NY 10029; **Phone:** 212-241-6321; **Board Cert:** Physical Medicine & Rehabilitation 2008; Spinal Cord Injury Medicine 2010; Pain Medicine 2002; **Med School:** Albany Med Coll 1993; **Resid:** Physical Medicine & Rehabilitation, Thomas Jefferson Univ Hosp 1997; **Fac Appt:** Assoc Prof PMR, Mount Sinai Sch Med

Dillard, James N MD (PMR) - **Spec Exp:** Pain Management; Acupuncture; Complementary Medicine; Nutrition; **Hospital:** Southampton Hosp; **Address:** 110 E 59th St, Ste 10A, New York, NY 10022; **Phone:** 212-265-4038; **Board Cert:** Physical Medicine & Rehabilitation 2005; **Med School:** Rush Med Coll 1990; **Resid:** Physical Medicine & Rehabilitation, Columbia-Presby Med Ctr 1994; **Fac Appt:** Asst Clin Prof PMR, Columbia P&S

Feinberg, Joseph H MD (PMR) - **Spec Exp:** Peripheral Neuropathy; Spinal Rehabilitation; Electrodiagnosis; Sports Medicine; **Hospital:** Hosp For Special Surgery (page 115), Kessler Inst for Rehab - W Orange; **Address:** 535 E 70th St, Hospital for Special Surgery, New York, NY 10021-4872; **Phone:** 212-606-1568; **Board Cert:** Physical Medicine & Rehabilitation 1991; Sports Medicine 2009; **Med School:** Albany Med Coll 1983; **Resid:** Surgery, Mt Sinai Hosp 1985; Physical Medicine & Rehabilitation, Rusk Inst Rehab 1990; **Fellow:** Orthopaedic Pathology, Hosp Spec Surg 1986; Orthopaedic Biomechanics, Univ Iowa Hosp & Clins 1987; **Fac Appt:** Assoc Prof PMR, Cornell Univ-Weill Med Coll

Flanagan, Steven R MD (PMR) - **Spec Exp:** Brain Injury Rehabilitation; Stroke Rehabilitation; **Hospital:** NYU Langone Med Ctr (page 108), NYU Rusk Inst (page 120); **Address:** Ambulatory Care Ctr, 240 E 38th St Fl 15, New York, NY 10016; **Phone:** 212-263-6037; **Board Cert:** Physical Medicine & Rehabilitation 2003; **Med School:** UMDNJ-NJ Med Sch, Newark 1988; **Resid:** Physical Medicine & Rehabilitation, Mt Sinai Hosp 1992; **Fac Appt:** Prof PMR, NYU Sch Med

Gold, Joan T MD (PMR) - **Spec Exp:** Cerebral Palsy; Spina Bifida; Pediatric Rehabilitation; **Hospital:** NYU Langone Med Ctr (page 108), NYU Hosp For Joint Diseases (page 119); **Address:** 400 E 34th St, Ste 518, New York, NY 10016-4901; **Phone:** 212-263-6519; **Board Cert:** Pediatrics 1979; Physical Medicine & Rehabilitation 1981; Pediatric Rehabilitation Medicine 2008; **Med School:** SUNY Downstate 1974; **Resid:** Pediatrics, Beth Israel Med Ctr 1977; Physical Medicine & Rehabilitation, Inst Rehab Med-NYU 1979; **Fac Appt:** Clin Prof PMR, NYU Sch Med

Gotlin, Robert S DO (PMR) - **Spec Exp:** Sports Medicine; Running Injuries; Pain-Coccyx; Pain-Knee & Shoulder; **Hospital:** Beth Israel Med Ctr - Petrie Division (page 94); **Address:** 245 Fifth Ave Fl 2, New York, NY 10016; **Phone:** 646-935-2255; **Board Cert:** Physical Medicine & Rehabilitation 1992; **Med School:** Southeastern Univ Coll Osteo Med 1987; **Resid:** Physical Medicine & Rehabilitation, Mount Sinai Hosp 1991; **Fac Appt:** Assoc Prof PMR, Albert Einstein Coll Med

Greenwald, Brian MD (PMR) - **Spec Exp:** Stroke Rehabilitation; Brain Injury Rehabilitation; **Hospital:** Mount Sinai Med Ctr (page 102), Elmhurst Hosp Ctr; **Address:** 5 E 98th St, Fl 6, Box 1240B, New York, NY 10029; **Phone:** 212-241-3981; **Board Cert:** Physical Medicine & Rehabilitation 2010; **Med School:** SUNY Stony Brook 1995; **Resid:** Physical Medicine & Rehabilitation, UMDNJ-NJ Med Sch 1999; **Fellow:** Physical Medicine & Rehabilitation, Med Coll Va 2000; **Fac Appt:** Asst Prof PMR, Mount Sinai Sch Med

Kim, Heakyung MD (PMR) - **Spec Exp:** Pediatric Rehabilitation; Neuromuscular Disorders; Stroke Rehabilitation; Musculoskeletal Disorders; **Hospital:** Morgan Stanley Children's Hosp of NY-Presby, NY (page 104), NY-Presby/Columbia Univ Med Ctr, NY (page 104); **Address:** 180 Fort Washington Ave, Harkness Pavilion, Ste 199, New York, NY 10032; **Phone:** 212-305-3535; **Board Cert:** Physical Medicine & Rehabilitation 2009; Pediatric Rehabilitation Medicine 2003; **Med School:** South Korea 1984; **Resid:** Physical Medicine & Rehabilitation, UMDNJ Affil Hosp 1998; **Fellow:** Physical Medicine & Rehabilitation, UMDNJ Affil Hosp 1993; **Fac Appt:** Prof PMR, Columbia P&S

Lachmann, Elisabeth A MD (PMR) - **Spec Exp:** Pain-Back; Sports Medicine; Cancer Rehabilitation; **Hospital:** NY-Presby/Weill Cornell Med Ctr, NY (page 104); **Address:** 115 E 64th St Fl 1, New York, NY 10065; **Phone:** 212-535-3005; **Board Cert:** Physical Medicine & Rehabilitation 1992; **Med School:** Med Coll PA Hahnemann 1987; **Resid:** Physical Medicine & Rehabilitation, NY-Cornell Med Ctr 1991; **Fac Appt:** Assoc Prof PMR, Cornell Univ-Weill Med Coll

Lee, Alexander J MD (PMR) - **Spec Exp:** Pain Management; **Hospital:** Beth Israel Med Ctr - Petrie Division (page 94); **Address:** 10 Union Square E, Ste 5P, Beth Israel Med Ctr, New York, NY 10003; **Phone:** 212-844-8756; **Board Cert:** Physical Medicine & Rehabilitation 2009; Pain Medicine 2003; **Med School:** Wayne State Univ 1994; **Resid:** Physical Medicine & Rehabilitation, Kessler Inst for Rehab 1998; **Fellow:** Pain Medicine, Beth Israel Med Ctr 1999

Lutz, Christopher MD (PMR) - **Spec Exp:** Pain-Low Back; Pain-Spine; Pain-Lower Back (IDET Procedure); Electromyography; **Hospital:** Hosp For Special Surgery (page 115); **Address:** Hosp for Special Surgery, 75th Street Campus, 429 E 75th St Fl 3, New York, NY 10021; **Phone:** 212-606-1494; **Board Cert:** Physical Medicine & Rehabilitation 2012; **Med School:** Georgetown Univ 1996; **Resid:** Physical Medicine & Rehabilitation, UMDNJ-Kessler Inst for Rehab 2000; **Fellow:** Sports Medicine, Hosp for Special Surgery 2001

Lutz, Gregory MD (PMR) - **Spec Exp:** Spinal Rehabilitation; Sports Medicine; Pain-Low Back; **Hospital:** Hosp For Special Surgery (page 115), Univ Med Ctr Princeton at Plainsboro; **Address:** 429 E 75 St Fl 3, New York, NY 10021; **Phone:** 212-606-1648; **Board Cert:** Physical Medicine & Rehabilitation 2003; **Med School:** Georgetown Univ 1988; **Resid:** Physical Medicine & Rehabilitation, Mayo Clinic 1992; **Fellow:** Sports Medicine, Hosp For Spec Surg 1993; **Fac Appt:** Assoc Prof PMR, Cornell Univ-Weill Med Coll

Ma, Dong M MD (PMR) - **Spec Exp:** Electromyography; Musculoskeletal Disorders; **Hospital:** NYU Rusk Inst (page 120), NYU Langone Med Ctr (page 108); **Address:** NYU Ctr for Musculoskeletal Care, 2333 E 38th St Fl 5, New York, NY 10016; **Phone:** 646-501-7277; **Board Cert:** Physical Medicine & Rehabilitation 1979; **Med School:** South Korea 1968; **Resid:** Physical Medicine & Rehabilitation, NYU Med Ctr 1975; **Fellow:** Physical Medicine & Rehabilitation, NYU Med Ctr 1977; **Fac Appt:** Clin Prof PMR, NYU Sch Med

Moldover, Jonathan MD (PMR) - **Spec Exp:** Spinal Rehabilitation; Pain-Chronic; Post Polio Syndrome/Rehabilitation; **Hospital:** Beth Israel Med Ctr - Petrie Division (page 94); **Address:** 200 W 57th St, Ste 608, New York, NY 10019-3211; **Phone:** 212-581-4488; **Board Cert:** Physical Medicine & Rehabilitation 1979; Pain Medicine 2002; **Med School:** Columbia P&S 1974; **Resid:** Internal Medicine, Strong Meml Hosp 1976; Physical Medicine & Rehabilitation, Columbia-Presby Med Ctr 1978; **Fac Appt:** Assoc Clin Prof PMR, Albert Einstein Coll Med

Neely, Michael DO (PMR) - **Spec Exp:** Pain-Knee & Shoulder; **Hospital:** St. Luke's - Roosevelt Hosp Ctr - Roosevelt Div (page 94); **Address:** 18 E 48th St, Ste 802, New York, NY 10017; **Phone:** 212-750-1110; **Board Cert:** Physical Medicine & Rehabilitation 2002; **Med School:** Ohio Univ, Coll Osteo Med 1997; **Resid:** Physical Medicine & Rehabilitation, Metro Hlth Med Ctr 2001

Ragnarsson, Kristjan T MD (PMR) - **Spec Exp:** Spinal Cord Injury; Brain Injury Rehabilitation; Pain-Back & Neck; **Hospital:** Mount Sinai Med Ctr (page 102); **Address:** 5 E 98th St, Fl 6, New York, NY 10029-6501; **Phone:** 212-659-9370; **Board Cert:** Physical Medicine & Rehabilitation 1976; **Med School:** Iceland 1969; **Resid:** Physical Medicine & Rehabilitation, NYU Med Ctr 1974; **Fellow:** Spinal Cord & Brain Injury Rehab, NYU Med Ctr 1975; **Fac Appt:** Prof PMR, Mount Sinai Sch Med

Rashbaum, Ira MD (PMR) - **Spec Exp:** Stroke Rehabilitation; **Hospital:** NYU Langone Med Ctr (page 108), NYU Rusk Inst (page 120); **Address:** 240 E 38th St Fl 15, New York, NY 10016; **Phone:** 212-263-6328; **Board Cert:** Physical Medicine & Rehabilitation 2004; **Med School:** SUNY Upstate Med Univ 1989; **Resid:** Physical Medicine & Rehabilitation, Rusk Ist Rehab Med/NYU Med Ctr 1993; **Fac Appt:** Clin Prof PMR, NYU Sch Med

Reid, Malcolm D MD (PMR) - **Hospital:** St. Luke's - Roosevelt Hosp Ctr - Roosevelt Div (page 94); **Address:** 1000 Tenth Ave, Ste 3B-20, New York, NY 10019; **Phone:** 212-523-6595; **Board Cert:** Physical Medicine & Rehabilitation 1992; **Med School:** Harvard Med Sch 1987; **Resid:** Internal Medicine, Winthrop Univ Hosp 1988; **Fellow:** Physical Medicine & Rehabilitation, Columbia-Presbyterian Med Ctr 1991; **Fac Appt:** Asst Clin Prof PMR, Columbia P&S

Rho, Dae Sik MD (PMR) - **Spec Exp:** Sports Medicine; Pain Management; **Hospital:** Lenox Hill Hosp (page 106); **Address:** 159 E 74th St, New York, NY 10021; **Phone:** 212-434-2465; **Board Cert:** Physical Medicine & Rehabilitation 1980; **Med School:** South Korea 1962; **Resid:** Physical Medicine & Rehabilitation, NYU Med Ctr 1975; **Fac Appt:** Asst Clin Prof PMR, Cornell Univ-Weill Med Coll

Sheth, Parag MD (PMR) - **Spec Exp:** Musculoskeletal Disorders; **Hospital:** Mount Sinai Med Ctr (page 102); **Address:** Mount Sinai Medical Ctr, 5 E 98th St, Box 1240B, New York, NY 10029; **Phone:** 212-241-6321; **Board Cert:** Physical Medicine & Rehabilitation 2004; Pain Medicine 2002; **Med School:** SUNY Stony Brook 1987; **Resid:** Physical Medicine & Rehabilitation, St Vincent's Med Ctr 1993; **Fac Appt:** Asst Prof PMR, Mount Sinai Sch Med

Simotas, Alexander C MD (PMR) - **Spec Exp:** Spinal Rehabilitation; **Hospital:** Hosp For Special Surgery (page 115); **Address:** 429 E 75th St Fl 4, New York, NY 10021; **Phone:** 212-606-1879; **Board Cert:** Physical Medicine & Rehabilitation 2003; **Med School:** Columbia P&S 1986; **Resid:** Physical Medicine & Rehabilitation, Rusk Inst-NYU 1991; **Fellow:** Pain Medicine, Hosp For Special Surgery 1992

Solomon, Jennifer L MD (PMR) - **Spec Exp:** Spinal Rehabilitation; **Hospital:** Hosp For Special Surgery (page 115); **Address:** 429 E 75th St Fl 4, New York, NY 10021; **Phone:** 212-606-1720; **Board Cert:** Physical Medicine & Rehabilitation 2004; **Med School:** SUNY Downstate 1999; **Resid:** Physical Medicine & Rehabilitation, UMDNJ/Kessler Rehab Inst 2003; **Fellow:** Sports Medicine, Hosp for Special Surgery 2004

Stein, Joel MD (PMR) - **Spec Exp:** Stroke Rehabilitation; **Hospital:** NY-Presby/Columbia Univ Med Ctr, NY (page 104); **Address:** 180 Fort Washington Ave, Ste 199, Harkness Pavilion, New York, NY 10032; **Phone:** 212-305-3535; **Board Cert:** Internal Medicine 1989; Physical Medicine & Rehabilitation 2003; **Med School:** Albert Einstein Coll Med 1986; **Resid:** Internal Medicine, Montefiore Med Ctr 1989; Physical Medicine & Rehabilitation, Columbia-Presby Med Ctr 1992

Strauss, Nancy E MD (PMR) - **Spec Exp:** Neuromuscular Disorders; **Hospital:** NY-Presby/Columbia Univ Med Ctr, NY (page 104), NY-Presby/Weill Cornell Med Ctr, NY (page 104); **Address:** 180 Fort Washington Ave, Ste 199, New York, NY 10032; **Phone:** 212-305-3535; **Board Cert:** Physical Medicine & Rehabilitation 2003; Electrodiagnostic Medicine 2004; **Med School:** SUNY Upstate Med Univ 1988; **Resid:** Physical Medicine & Rehabilitation, Nassau Univ Med Ctr 1992; **Fac Appt:** Clin Prof PMR, Columbia P&S

Stubblefield, Michael Dean MD (PMR) - **Spec Exp:** Cancer Rehabilitation; Pain-Cancer; Pain-Neuropathic; Pain-Musculoskeletal; **Hospital:** Meml Sloan-Kettering Cancer Ctr (page 116); **Address:** Sillerman Center for Rehabilitation, Meml Sloan-Kettering Cancer Ctr, 515 Madison Ave Fl 5, New York, NY 10022; **Phone:** 646-888-1936; **Board Cert:** Internal Medicine 2011; Physical Medicine & Rehabilitation 2012; Electrodiagnostic Medicine 2003; **Med School:** Columbia P&S 1996; **Resid:** Internal Medicine, Columbia Presby Med Ctr 2001; Physical Medicine & Rehabilitation, Columbia Presby Med Ctr 2001; **Fac Appt:** Assoc Prof PMR, Cornell Univ-Weill Med Coll

Thomas, David C MD (PMR) - **Hospital:** Mount Sinai Med Ctr (page 102); **Address:** Mount Sinai Med Ctr, 17 E 102nd St Fl 7, New York, NY 10029; **Phone:** 212-824-7210; **Board Cert:** Internal Medicine 2007; Physical Medicine & Rehabilitation 2008; **Med School:** Hahnemann Univ 1991; **Resid:** Internal Medicine, Westchester Co Med Ctr 1996; Physical Medicine & Rehabilitation, Mount Sinai Hosp 1998; **Fac Appt:** Assoc Prof Med, Mount Sinai Sch Med

Vad, Vijay B MD (PMR) - **Spec Exp:** Pain-Back; Pain-Knee & Shoulder; Sports Medicine-Golf & Tennis Injuries; Joint Pain-Minimally Invasive Therapy; **Hospital:** Hosp For Special Surgery (page 115); **Address:** 535 E 70 St, New York, NY 10021; **Phone:** 212-606-1306; **Board Cert:** Physical Medicine & Rehabilitation 2007; Sports Medicine 2007; **Med School:** Univ Okla Coll Med 1992; **Resid:** Physical Medicine & Rehabilitation, Cornell Affil Hosp 1996; **Fellow:** Sports Medicine, Hosp Special Surgery 1997; **Fac Appt:** Asst Prof PMR, Cornell Univ-Weill Med Coll

Plastic Surgery

Ahn, Christina Y MD (PlS) - **Spec Exp:** Breast Reconstruction; Cosmetic Surgery-Face & Body; Cosmetic Surgery-Breast; **Hospital:** NYU Langone Med Ctr (page 108); **Address:** 630 Third Ave Fl 6 - Ste 601, New York, NY 10017; **Phone:** 212-717-8860; **Board Cert:** Plastic Surgery 1994; **Med School:** NYU Sch Med 1983; **Resid:** Surgery, Mt Sinai Med Ctr 1988; Plastic Surgery, Univ Pittsburgh Med Ctr 1990; **Fellow:** Microvascular Surgery, UCLA Med Ctr 1991; **Fac Appt:** Assoc Prof S, NYU Sch Med

Almeyda, Elizabeth MD (PlS) - **Spec Exp:** Abdominoplasty; Cosmetic Surgery-Breast; Liposuction; **Hospital:** St. Luke's - Roosevelt Hosp Ctr - Roosevelt Div (page 94); **Address:** 75 Central Park West, New York, NY 10023-6011; **Phone:** 212-501-0600; **Board Cert:** Plastic Surgery 1988; **Med School:** Univ Rochester 1978; **Resid:** Surgery, Roosevelt Hosp 1983; **Fellow:** Plastic Surgery, New York Hosp 1985

Ascherman, Jeffrey MD (PlS) - **Spec Exp:** Breast Cosmetic & Reconstructive Surgery; Craniofacial Surgery; Cleft Palate/Lip; Cosmetic Surgery; **Hospital:** NY-Presby/Columbia Univ Med Ctr, NY (page 104), New York Eye & Ear Infirm (page 117); **Address:** 161 Ft Washington Ave, Ste 509, New York, NY 10032-3713; **Phone:** 212-305-9612; **Board Cert:** Plastic Surgery 2007; **Med School:** Columbia P&S 1988; **Resid:** Surgery, Columbia-Presby Med Ctr 1991; Plastic Surgery, Columbia-Presby Med Ctr 1994; **Fellow:** Craniofacial Surgery, Hosp Necke-Enfants Malades 1995; **Fac Appt:** Prof S, Columbia P&S

Aston, Sherrell MD (PlS) - **Spec Exp:** Cosmetic Surgery-Face & Body; Rhinoplasty; Cosmetic Surgery-Breast; Liposuction & Body Contouring; **Hospital:** Lenox Hill Hosp (page 106), NYU Langone Med Ctr (page 108); **Address:** 728 Park Ave, New York, NY 10021; **Phone:** 212-249-6000; **Board Cert:** Surgery 1974; Plastic Surgery 1978; **Med School:** Univ VA Sch Med 1968; **Resid:** Surgery, UCLA Med Ctr 1973; Plastic Surgery, NY Univ 1975; **Fellow:** Surgery, Johns Hopkins Hosp 1970; **Fac Appt:** Prof PlS, NYU Sch Med

Baker III, Daniel MD (PlS) - **Spec Exp:** Cosmetic Surgery-Face; Reconstructive Surgery-Face; Rhinoplasty; **Address:** 65 E 66th St, New York, NY 10065; **Phone:** 212-734-9695; **Board Cert:** Plastic Surgery 1978; **Med School:** Columbia P&S 1968; **Resid:** Surgery, UCSF Med Ctr 1975; Plastic Surgery, NYU Med Ctr 1977; **Fellow:** Head and Neck Surgery, NYU Med Ctr/St Vincents Hosp 1978; **Fac Appt:** Assoc Prof PlS, NYU Sch Med

Bromley, Gary S MD (PlS) - **Spec Exp:** Cosmetic Surgery; **Hospital:** NY-Presby/Weill Cornell Med Ctr, NY (page 104), Jamaica Hosp Med Ctr; **Address:** 5 E 84th St, New York, NY 10028-0407; **Phone:** 212-570-5443; **Board Cert:** Plastic Surgery 1986; **Med School:** Cornell Univ-Weill Med Coll 1978; **Resid:** Surgery, New York Hosp 1981; Plastic Surgery, New York Hosp 1983; **Fellow:** Hand Surgery, NYU Med Ctr 1984

Broumand, Stafford MD (PlS) - **Spec Exp:** Eyelid Surgery; Breast Surgery; Liposuction & Body Contouring; Craniofacial Surgery/Reconstruction; **Hospital:** Mount Sinai Med Ctr (page 102); **Address:** 740 Park Ave, New York, NY 10021-4251; **Phone:** 212-879-7900; **Board Cert:** Plastic Surgery 2006; **Med School:** Yale Univ 1985; **Resid:** Surgery, Mt Sinai Med Ctr 1990; **Fellow:** Plastic Surgery, Mass Genl Hosp 1992; Cosmetic Plastic Surgery, Cran Hosp Necker 1993; **Fac Appt:** Assoc Clin Prof PlS, Mount Sinai Sch Med

Chen, Constance MD (PlS) - **Spec Exp:** Breast Reconstruction; Microsurgery; **Hospital:** Lenox Hill Hosp (page 106), New York Eye & Ear Infirm (page 117); **Address:** 166 Fifth Ave Fl 2, New York, NY 10010; **Phone:** 212-792-6378; **Board Cert:** Plastic Surgery 2010; **Med School:** Stanford Univ 2001; **Resid:** Surgery, Univ of Washington 2004; Plastic Surgery, Univ of Washington 2005; **Fellow:** Reconstructive Microsurgery, NY Presby-Columbia Med Ctr 2008

Chiu, David T W MD (PlS) - **Spec Exp:** Hand & Microvascular Surgery; Cosmetic Surgery-Face; Peripheral Nerve Surgery; **Hospital:** NYU Langone Med Ctr (page 108), Lenox Hill Hosp (page 106); **Address:** 900 Park Ave, New York, NY 10075; **Phone:** 212-879-8880; **Board Cert:** Plastic Surgery 1982; Hand Surgery 2010; **Med School:** Columbia P&S 1973; **Resid:** Surgery, Barnes Jewish Hosp 1977; Plastic Surgery, Columbia-Presby Med Ctr 1979; **Fellow:** Hand Surgery, NYU Med Ctr 1980; **Fac Appt:** Prof PlS, NYU Sch Med

Choi, Mihye MD (PlS) - **Spec Exp:** Breast Surgery; Cosmetic Surgery; Hand Surgery; Breast Reconstruction; **Hospital:** NYU Langone Med Ctr (page 108); **Address:** KCNY Plastic Surgery, 305 E 47th St, Ste 1A, New York, NY 10017; **Phone:** 212-355-5779; **Board Cert:** Plastic Surgery 2008; Hand Surgery 2010; **Med School:** Univ Rochester 1987; **Resid:** Surgery, Beth Israel Hosp 1990; Plastic Surgery, Mt Sinai Med Ctr 1995; **Fellow:** Hand Surgery, NYU Med Ctr 1996; Research, Mass Genl Hosp 1992; **Fac Appt:** Assoc Prof S, NYU Sch Med

Colen, Helen S MD (PlS) - **Spec Exp:** Cosmetic Surgery-Face & Breast; Liposuction & Body Contouring; Vaginal Reconstruction; Poland Syndrome; **Hospital:** NYU Langone Med Ctr (page 108), Lenox Hill Hosp (Manh Eye, Ear & Throat Hosp) (page 106); **Address:** 742 Park Ave, New York, NY 10021-4251; **Phone:** 212-772-1300; **Board Cert:** Plastic Surgery 1983; **Med School:** NYU Sch Med 1972; **Resid:** Surgery, Univ Colorado Med Ctr 1979; Plastic Surgery, St Lukes Hosp 1981; **Fellow:** Microsurgery, NYU Med Ctr 1982; **Fac Appt:** Assoc Clin Prof PlS, NYU Sch Med

Cordeiro, Peter G MD (PlS) - **Spec Exp:** Reconstructive Surgery; Breast Reconstruction; Facial Plastic & Reconstructive Surgery; **Hospital:** Meml Sloan-Kettering Cancer Ctr (page 116), Lenox Hill Hosp (Manh Eye, Ear & Throat Hosp) (page 106); **Address:** 1275 York Ave, New York, NY 10065; **Phone:** 212-639-2521; **Board Cert:** Surgery 2008; Plastic Surgery 2007; **Med School:** Harvard Med Sch 1983; **Resid:** Surgery, New Engl Deaconess Hosp-Harvard 1989; Plastic Surgery, NYU Med Ctr 1991; **Fellow:** Microsurgery, Meml Sloan-Kettering Cancer Ctr. 1992; Craniofacial Surgery, Univ Miami 1992; **Fac Appt:** Prof S, Cornell Univ-Weill Med Coll

Diktaban, Theodore MD (PlS) - **Spec Exp:** Liposuction & Body Contouring; Rhinoplasty; Breast Augmentation; Facial Rejuvenation; **Hospital:** Lenox Hill Hosp (page 106), Lenox Hill Hosp (Manh Eye, Ear & Throat Hosp) (page 106); **Address:** 635 Madison Ave, Fl 4th, New York, NY 10022; **Phone:** 212-206-0023; **Board Cert:** Otolaryngology 1981; Plastic Surgery 1988; **Med School:** NY Med Coll 1976; **Resid:** Otolaryngology, Mount Sinai Hosp 1981; Plastic Surgery, Lenox Hill Hosp 1983; **Fellow:** Reconstructive Microsurgery, Univ Louisville 1984; **Fac Appt:** Clin Prof PlS, NY Med Coll

Disa, Joseph MD (PlS) - **Spec Exp:** Cancer Reconstruction; Breast Reconstruction; Head & Neck Reconstruction; Microsurgery; **Hospital:** Meml Sloan-Kettering Cancer Ctr (page 116); **Address:** 1275 York Ave, New York, NY 10065; **Phone:** 212-639-5022; **Board Cert:** Surgery 2005; Plastic Surgery 2009; **Med School:** Univ Mass Sch Med 1988; **Resid:** Surgery, Univ Md Med Ctr 1994; Plastic Surgery, Johns Hopkins Univ 1996; **Fellow:** Reconstructive Microsurgery, Meml Sloan-Kettering Cancer Ctr.; **Fac Appt:** Prof PlS, Cornell Univ-Weill Med Coll

Forley, Bryan G MD (PlS) - **Spec Exp:** Cosmetic Surgery; Reconstructive Surgery; **Hospital:** Beth Israel Med Ctr - Petrie Division (page 94), New York Eye & Ear Infirm (page 117); **Address:** 5 E 82nd St, New York, NY 10028-0342; **Phone:** 212-861-3757; **Board Cert:** Plastic Surgery 2008; **Med School:** Mount Sinai Sch Med 1984; **Resid:** Surgery, NYU Med Ctr & Mt Sinai Med Ctr 1989; Plastic Surgery, Saint Francis Meml Hosp 1992; **Fellow:** Craniofacial Surgery, Hosp for Sick Children, Great Ormond St 1993

Foster, Craig A MD (PlS) - **Spec Exp:** Cosmetic Surgery-Face & Nose; Cosmetic Surgery-Breast; Rhinoplasty Revision; **Hospital:** Lenox Hill Hosp (page 106); **Address:** 850 Park Ave, Ste 1A, New York, NY 10075; **Phone:** 212-744-5746; **Board Cert:** Otolaryngology 1980; Plastic Surgery 1984; **Med School:** Univ Minn 1974; **Resid:** Otolaryngology, Univ Minn Hosps 1980; Plastic Surgery, NYU Med Ctr 1982

Freund, Robert M MD (PlS) - **Spec Exp:** Cosmetic Surgery-Face & Neck; Cosmetic Surgery-Breast; Rhinoplasty Revision; **Hospital:** Lenox Hill Hosp (page 106), Long Island Jewish Med Ctr (page 106); **Address:** 171 East End Ave, Ste CS, New York, NY 10128; **Phone:** 212-583-1200; **Board Cert:** Plastic Surgery 2008; **Med School:** Cornell Univ-Weill Med Coll 1987; **Resid:** Surgery, NYU Med Ctr 1993; Plastic Surgery, NYU Med Ctr 1995; **Fellow:** Microvascular Surgery, NYU Med Ctr 1991

Friedman, David J MD (PlS) - **Spec Exp:** Cosmetic Surgery-Face; Liposuction & Body Contouring; Abdominoplasty; Breast Reconstruction; **Hospital:** Beth Israel Med Ctr - Petrie Division (page 94), Lenox Hill Hosp (page 106); **Address:** 630 Park Ave, New York, NY 10065; **Phone:** 212-439-1600; **Board Cert:** Plastic Surgery 2008; **Med School:** Albany Med Coll 1988; **Resid:** Surgery, Beth Israel Med Ctr 1993; Plastic Surgery, Mt Sinai Med Ctr 1994

Gayle, Lloyd MD (PlS) - **Spec Exp:** Breast Reconstruction & Augmentation; Hand Surgery; Cosmetic Surgery-Body; **Hospital:** NY-Presby/Weill Cornell Med Ctr, NY (page 104), Maimonides Med Ctr (page 98); **Address:** 50 E 69th St, New York, NY 10021; **Phone:** 212-452-5121; **Board Cert:** Plastic Surgery 1993; **Med School:** NYU Sch Med 1983; **Resid:** Surgery, NYU Med Ctr 1988; Plastic Surgery, NY Hosp-Cornell Univ 1990; **Fellow:** Hand & Microvascular Surgery, Davies Med Ctr 1991; **Fac Appt:** Assoc Prof S, Cornell Univ-Weill Med Coll

Ginsberg, Gerald D MD (PlS) - **Spec Exp:** Cosmetic Surgery; Reconstructive Plastic Surgery; **Hospital:** NY Downtown Hosp; **Address:** Dept of Surgery, 170 William St Fl 5, New York, NY 10038; **Phone:** 212-452-3421; **Board Cert:** Plastic Surgery 1984; **Med School:** Northwestern Univ 1974; **Resid:** Surgery, NYU Med Ctr 1980; Plastic Surgery, NYU Med Ctr 1982; **Fellow:** Hand Surgery, NYU Med Ctr 1983; **Fac Appt:** Assoc Clin Prof PlS, NYU Sch Med

Godfrey, Norman V MD (PlS) - **Spec Exp:** Rhinoplasty; Nasal Reconstruction; Nasal Surgery; **Hospital:** NY-Presby/Weill Cornell Med Ctr, NY (page 104), NY Hosp Queens (page 206); **Address:** 1158 5th Ave, New York, NY 10029; **Phone:** 212-628-6600; **Board Cert:** Plastic Surgery 1984; **Med School:** Harvard Med Sch 1973; **Resid:** Surgery, Bellevue Hosp 1978; Plastic Surgery, Bellevue Hosp 1980; **Fellow:** Microvascular Surgery, Bellevue Hosp 1981; **Fac Appt:** Asst Clin Prof S, Cornell Univ-Weill Med Coll

Godfrey, Philip M MD/DMD (PlS) - **Spec Exp:** Breast Cosmetic & Reconstructive Surgery; Liposuction & Body Contouring; Abdominoplasty; Congenital Breast Anomalies; **Hospital:** NY-Presby/Weill Cornell Med Ctr, NY (page 104); **Address:** 1158 5th Ave, New York, NY 10029; **Phone:** 212-628-6600; **Board Cert:** Plastic Surgery 1988; **Med School:** Med Coll PA 1981; **Resid:** Surgery, Hartford Hosp 1984; Plastic Surgery, New York Hosp 1986; **Fellow:** Plastic Surgery, Meml Sloan Kettering Cancer Ctr 1987; **Fac Appt:** Asst Clin Prof S, Cornell Univ-Weill Med Coll

Grant, Robert T MD (PlS) - **Spec Exp:** Breast Reconstruction; Cosmetic Surgery; Reconstructive Plastic Surgery; **Hospital:** NY-Presby/Columbia Univ Med Ctr, NY (page 104), NY-Presby/Weill Cornell Med Ctr, NY (page 104); **Address:** 161 Fort Washington Ave, rm 511, 50 E 69th St, New York, NY 10032; **Phone:** 212-305-3103; **Board Cert:** Surgery 2011; Plastic Surgery 2013; **Med School:** Albany Med Coll 1983; **Resid:** Surgery, NY Hosp 1988; Plastic Surgery, NY Hosp 1990; **Fellow:** Microvascular Surgery, NYU Med Ctr/Bellevue Hosp 1991; **Fac Appt:** Clin Prof PlS, Columbia P&S

Hidalgo, David A MD (PlS) - **Spec Exp:** Cosmetic Surgery-Face; Cosmetic Surgery-Breast; Rhinoplasty; Reconstructive Surgery; **Hospital:** NY-Presby/Weill Cornell Med Ctr, NY (page 104), Lenox Hill Hosp (page 106); **Address:** 655 Park Ave, New York, NY 10065; **Phone:** 212-517-9777; **Board Cert:** Plastic Surgery 1987; **Med School:** Georgetown Univ 1978; **Resid:** Surgery, NYU Med Ctr 1983; Plastic Surgery, NYU Med Ctr 1985; **Fellow:** Microsurgery, NYU Med Ctr 1986; **Fac Appt:** Clin Prof S, Cornell Univ-Weill Med Coll

Hoffman, Lloyd A MD (PlS) - **Spec Exp:** Cosmetic Surgery-Face; Liposuction & Body Contouring; Breast Reconstruction; Facial Rejuvenation; **Hospital:** NY-Presby/Weill Cornell Med Ctr, NY (page 104), Lenox Hill Hosp (page 106); **Address:** 12A E 68th St, New York, NY 10021; **Phone:** 212-861-1640; **Board Cert:** Plastic Surgery 1989; **Med School:** Northwestern Univ 1978; **Resid:** Surgery, New York Hosp 1983; Plastic Surgery, NYU Med Ctr 1986; **Fellow:** Hand Surgery, NYU Med Ctr 1987; **Fac Appt:** Assoc Prof PlS, Cornell Univ-Weill Med Coll

Hunter, John G MD (PlS) - **Spec Exp:** Female Genital Cosmetic Surgery; Cosmetic Surgery-Breast; Cosmetic Surgery-Body; **Hospital:** NY-Presby/Weill Cornell Med Ctr, NY (page 104), New York Methodist Hosp (page 418); **Address:** 47 E 63rd St, New York, NY 10065; **Phone:** 212-751-4444; **Board Cert:** Plastic Surgery 1991; **Med School:** SUNY Downstate 1983; **Resid:** Surgery, Mount Sinai Hosp 1986; **Fellow:** Plastic Surgery, Univ Hosp-SUNY Downstate 1988; **Fac Appt:** Assoc Clin Prof S, Cornell Univ-Weill Med Coll

Imber, Gerald MD (PlS) - **Spec Exp:** Cosmetic Surgery-Face; Eyelid Surgery; **Hospital:** NY-Presby/Weill Cornell Med Ctr, NY (page 104); **Address:** 121A E 83rd St, New York, NY 10028; **Phone:** 212-472-1800; **Board Cert:** Plastic Surgery 1976; **Med School:** SUNY Downstate 1966; **Resid:** Surgery, LI Jewish Med Ctr 1972; Plastic Surgery, NY Hosp 1974; **Fac Appt:** Asst Clin Prof S, Cornell Univ-Weill Med Coll

Jacobs, Elliot W MD (PlS) - **Spec Exp:** Cosmetic Surgery-Face & Breast; Gynecomastia; Body Contouring; Rhinoplasty; **Hospital:** New York Eye & Ear Infirm (page 117), Beth Israel Med Ctr - Petrie Division (page 94); **Address:** 815 Park Ave, New York, NY 10021-3276; **Phone:** 212-570-6080; **Board Cert:** Plastic Surgery 1982; **Med School:** Mount Sinai Sch Med 1970; **Resid:** Surgery, Mt Sinai Med Ctr 1974; Plastic Surgery, Mt Sinai Med Ctr 1977

Karp, Nolan MD (PlS) - **Spec Exp:** Breast Cosmetic & Reconstructive Surgery; Liposuction & Body Contouring; Skin Cancer; **Hospital:** NYU Langone Med Ctr (page 108); **Address:** KCNY Plastic Surgery, 305 E 47th St, Ste 1A, New York, NY 10017; **Phone:** 212-355-5779; **Board Cert:** Plastic Surgery 1994; **Med School:** Northwestern Univ 1983; **Resid:** Surgery, NYU Med Ctr 1988; **Fellow:** Plastic Surgery, NYU Med Ctr 1991; **Fac Appt:** Assoc Prof PlS, NYU Sch Med

Karpinski, Richard H S MD (PlS) - **Spec Exp:** Cosmetic Surgery-Face; Liposuction; Rhinoplasty; Hyperhidrosis; **Hospital:** St. Luke's - Roosevelt Hosp Ctr - Roosevelt Div (page 94); **Address:** 200 Central Park South, Ste 108, New York, NY 10019-1436; **Phone:** 212-977-9797; **Board Cert:** Plastic Surgery 1983; **Med School:** Harvard Med Sch 1971; **Resid:** Surgery, Boston City Hosp 1973; Surgery, New England Deaconess 1977; **Fellow:** Plastic Surgery, NYU Med Ctr 1981; **Fac Appt:** Asst Clin Prof PlS, Columbia P&S

Kolker, Adam R MD (PlS) - **Spec Exp:** Cosmetic Surgery-Breast; Breast Reconstruction; Abdominoplasty; Body Contouring after Weight Loss; **Hospital:** Mount Sinai Med Ctr (page 102), Lenox Hill Hosp (page 106); **Address:** 710 Park Ave, New York, NY 10021; **Phone:** 212-744-6500; **Board Cert:** Plastic Surgery 2011; Surgery 2005; **Med School:** Albany Med Coll 1990; **Resid:** Surgery, St Vincent's Hosp 1995; Plastic/Reconstructive Surgery, Beth Israel Deaconess Med Ctr 1998; **Fellow:** Microsurgery, NYU Med Ctr 1996; Craniofacial Surgery, Univ Melbourne Chldns Hosp 2000; **Fac Appt:** Assoc Clin Prof S, Mount Sinai Sch Med

Lesesne, Carroll B MD (PlS) - **Spec Exp:** Cosmetic Surgery-Face; Rhinoplasty; Abdominoplasty; Skin Cancer; **Hospital:** Lenox Hill Hosp (Manh Eye, Ear & Throat Hosp) (page 106), Northern Westchester Hosp (page 613); **Address:** 620 Park Ave, New York, NY 10021-6591; **Phone:** 212-570-6318; **Board Cert:** Plastic Surgery 1987; **Med School:** Duke Univ 1980; **Resid:** Surgery, Stanford Univ Med Ctr 1983; Plastic Surgery, New York Hosp 1985; **Fellow:** Plastic Surgery, Meml Sloan Kettering Cancer Ctr 1985; **Fac Appt:** Asst Clin Prof PlS, NYU Sch Med

Levine, Joshua L MD (PlS) - **Spec Exp:** Breast Reconstruction; Microsurgery; **Hospital:** New York Eye & Ear Infirm (page 117), Montefiore Med Ctr-Einstein Campus, NY (page 100); **Address:** 1776 Broadway at 57th St, Ste 1200, New York, NY 10019; **Phone:** 212-245-8140; **Board Cert:** Plastic Surgery 2005; **Med School:** Med Coll GA 1994; **Resid:** Plastic Surgery, Montefiore Med Ctr 2000; Plastic Surgery, Montefiore Med Ctr 2001; **Fellow:** Cosmetic Plastic Surgery, NY Eye & Ear Infirm 2003; Reconstructive Microsurgery, Louisiana State Univ 2004

Matarasso, Alan MD (PlS) - **Spec Exp:** Cosmetic Surgery-Face & Eyes; Rhinoplasty; Liposuction; Abdominoplasty; **Hospital:** Lenox Hill Hosp (Manh Eye, Ear & Throat Hosp) (page 106); **Address:** 1009 Park Ave, New York, NY 10028-0936; **Phone:** 212-249-7500; **Board Cert:** Plastic Surgery 1986; **Med School:** Univ Miami Sch Med 1979; **Resid:** Surgery, Montefiore Med Ctr 1983; Plastic Surgery, Montefiore Med Ctr 1985; **Fellow:** Plastic Surgery, Manhattan EET Hosp/NYU 1985; **Fac Appt:** Clin Prof PlS, Albert Einstein Coll Med

McCarthy, Joseph G MD (PlS) - **Spec Exp:** Craniofacial Surgery-Pediatric; Reconstructive Surgery-Face; Cosmetic Surgery-Face; **Hospital:** NYU Langone Med Ctr (page 108), Lenox Hill Hosp (Manh Eye, Ear & Throat Hosp) (page 106); **Address:** 722 Park Ave, New York, NY 10021-4954; **Phone:** 212-628-4420; **Board Cert:** Surgery 1972; Plastic Surgery 1978; **Med School:** Columbia P&S 1964; **Resid:** Surgery, Columbia-Presby Med Ctr 1971; Plastic Surgery, NYU Med Ctr 1973; **Fac Appt:** Prof PlS, NYU Sch Med

Mehrara, Babak J MD (PlS) - **Spec Exp:** Breast Reconstruction; Cancer Reconstruction; Microsurgery; Reconstructive Surgery-Face; **Hospital:** Meml Sloan-Kettering Cancer Ctr (page 116); **Address:** 1275 York Ave, New York, NY 10065; **Phone:** 212-639-8639; **Board Cert:** Plastic Surgery 2003; **Med School:** Columbia P&S 1993; **Resid:** Surgery, NYU Med Ctr 1996; Plastic Surgery, NYU Med Ctr 2001; **Fellow:** Microsurgery, UCLA Med Ctr 2002; **Fac Appt:** Assoc Prof S, Cornell Univ-Weill Med Coll

Monasebian, Douglas M MD/DMD (PlS) - **Spec Exp:** Cosmetic Surgery-Face; Facial Plastic & Reconstructive Surgery; **Hospital:** Mount Sinai Med Ctr (page 102), St. Luke's - Roosevelt Hosp Ctr - St Luke's Hosp (page 94); **Address:** 784 Park Ave, New York, NY 10021; **Phone:** 212-472-8700; **Board Cert:** Plastic Surgery 2009; **Med School:** Univ Nebr Coll Med 1992; **Resid:** Surgery, Univ Nebraska Med Ctr 1995; **Fellow:** Plastic Surgery, Montefiore Med Ctr 1997; **Fac Appt:** Asst Clin Prof PlS, Mount Sinai Sch Med

Perrotti, John A MD (PlS) - **Spec Exp:** Liposuction & Body Contouring; Cosmetic Surgery-Face & Breast; Abdominoplasty; **Hospital:** Lenox Hill Hosp (Manh Eye, Ear & Throat Hosp) (page 106), Lenox Hill Hosp (page 106); **Address:** 330 E 63rd St, New York, NY 10065; **Phone:** 212-258-2200; **Board Cert:** Plastic Surgery 2010; **Med School:** NY Med Coll 1991; **Resid:** Surgery, Westchester Medical Ctr 1996; Plastic Surgery, Cleveland Clinic 1998; **Fac Appt:** Asst Clin Prof S, NY Med Coll

Pitman, Gerald H MD (PlS) - **Spec Exp:** Cosmetic Surgery-Face; Liposuction; Abdominoplasty; **Hospital:** Lenox Hill Hosp (Manh Eye, Ear & Throat Hosp) (page 106), NYU Langone Med Ctr (page 108); **Address:** 170 E 73rd St, New York, NY 10021; **Phone:** 212-517-2600; **Board Cert:** Plastic Surgery 1978; **Med School:** Univ Pennsylvania 1968; **Resid:** Surgery, Columbia-Presby Hosp 1975; Plastic Surgery, NYU Med Ctr 1977; **Fellow:** Microsurgery, NYU Med Ctr 1981; **Fac Appt:** Clin Prof PlS, NYU Sch Med

Razaboni, Rosa MD (PlS) - **Spec Exp:** Cosmetic Surgery; Breast Reconstruction; Body Contouring after Weight Loss; **Hospital:** Lenox Hill Hosp (page 106), Mount Sinai Med Ctr (page 102); **Address:** 14-A E 68th St, New York, NY 10021-5847; **Phone:** 212-772-0200; **Board Cert:** Plastic Surgery 1993; **Med School:** Brazil 1975; **Resid:** Surgery, St Vincents Hosp 1985; Plastic Surgery, NYU Med Ctr 1988; **Fellow:** Surgery, Hospital Trousseau 1986; **Fac Appt:** Asst Prof PlS, Mount Sinai Sch Med

Romita, Mauro C MD (PlS) - **Spec Exp:** Cosmetic Surgery-Face; Liposuction & Body Contouring; Reconstructive Plastic Surgery; **Hospital:** Lenox Hill Hosp (page 106); **Address:** 853 5th Ave, New York, NY 10065; **Phone:** 212-772-3220; **Board Cert:** Plastic Surgery 1983; **Med School:** Univ Miami Sch Med 1973; **Resid:** Surgery, NYU Med Ctr 1978; Plastic Surgery, NYU Med Ctr 1980; **Fellow:** Craniofacial Surgery, NYU Med Ctr 1981; Microsurgery, NYU Med Ctr 1982; **Fac Appt:** Asst Prof S, NY Med Coll

Rose, Elliott H MD (PlS) - **Spec Exp:** Facial Plastic & Reconstructive Surgery; Cosmetic Surgery-Face & Body; Facial Paralysis Reconstruction; Burns-Reconstructive Plastic Surgery; **Hospital:** Mount Sinai Med Ctr (page 102); **Address:** The Aesthetic Surgery Center, 895 Park Ave, New York, NY 10021-0327; **Phone:** 212-639-1346; **Board Cert:** Plastic Surgery 1979; **Med School:** Univ Tex Med Br, Galveston 1970; **Resid:** Surgery, Johns Hopkins Hosp 1973; Plastic Surgery, Stanford Univ Med Ctr 1977; **Fellow:** Hand & Microvascular Surgery, UCSF Med Ctr 1978; **Fac Appt:** Assoc Clin Prof PlS, Mount Sinai Sch Med

Rosenblatt, William B MD (PlS) - **Spec Exp:** Nasal Surgery; Cosmetic Surgery-Face & Body; Cosmetic Surgery-Breast; Rhinoplasty; **Hospital:** Lenox Hill Hosp (page 106), Lenox Hill Hosp (Manh Eye, Ear & Throat Hosp) (page 106); **Address:** 308 E 79th St, Ste 1D, New York, NY 10075; **Phone:** 212-570-6100; **Board Cert:** Otolaryngology 1977; Plastic Surgery 1980; **Med School:** NY Med Coll 1973; **Resid:** Otolaryngology, Metropolitan Hosp 1977; Plastic Surgery, Lenox Hill Hosp 1979

Sabry, M Zakir MD (PlS) - **Spec Exp:** Cosmetic Surgery; Breast Reconstruction; Craniofacial Surgery; Cleft Palate/Lip; **Hospital:** Lenox Hill Hosp (page 106); **Address:** 936 5th Ave, Office 2, New York, NY 10021; **Phone:** 212-737-1308; **Board Cert:** Plastic Surgery 2004; **Med School:** NY Med Coll 1993; **Resid:** Surgery, St Vincents Hosp 1999; Plastic Surgery, Med Coll Virginia 2001; **Fellow:** Craniofacial Surgery, Barnes Jewish Hosp 2002; **Fac Appt:** Asst Clin Prof PlS, Med Coll VA

Schulman, Matthew R MD (PlS) - **Spec Exp:** Body Contouring; Cosmetic Surgery-Breast; Liposuction; Liposuction; **Hospital:** Mount Sinai Med Ctr (page 102), Westchester Med Ctr; **Address:** 950 Park Ave, New York, NY 10028; **Phone:** 212-289-1851; **Board Cert:** Plastic Surgery 2007; **Med School:** Jefferson Med Coll 2000; **Resid:** Surgery, Mt Sinai Med Ctr 2003; **Fellow:** Plastic Surgery, Mt Sinai Med Ctr 2006; **Fac Appt:** Assoc Prof PlS, Mount Sinai Sch Med

Schulman, Norman H MD (PlS) - **Spec Exp:** Cosmetic Surgery-Face & Body; Breast Cosmetic & Reconstructive Surgery; Nasal Surgery; Tuberous Breast; **Hospital:** Lenox Hill Hosp (page 106), Lenox Hill Hosp (Manh Eye, Ear & Throat Hosp) (page 106); **Address:** 308 E 79th St, New York, NY 10075; **Phone:** 212-861-5004; **Board Cert:** Surgery 1973; Plastic Surgery 1976; **Med School:** Tufts Univ 1965; **Resid:** Surgery, Jacobi Med Ctr 1972; Plastic Surgery, Lenox Hill Hosp 1974; **Fellow:** Plastic Surgery, Roswell Park Cancer Inst 1975; **Fac Appt:** Clin Prof PlS, Cornell Univ-Weill Med Coll

Scott, Susan Craig MD (PlS) - **Spec Exp:** Eyelid Surgery/Blepharoplasty; Hand Surgery; **Hospital:** NYU Hosp For Joint Diseases (page 119), Lenox Hill Hosp (page 106); **Address:** 150 E 77th St, New York, NY 10075; **Phone:** 212-288-9922; **Board Cert:** Plastic Surgery 1987; Hand Surgery 2005; **Med School:** Columbia P&S 1974; **Resid:** Surgery, St Luke's-Roosevelt Hosp Ctr 1979; Plastic Surgery, NYU Med Ctr 1981; **Fellow:** Hand Surgery, St Luke's-Roosevelt Hosp Ctr 1982; **Fac Appt:** Asst Clin Prof PlS, Columbia P&S

Sherman, John E MD (PlS) - **Spec Exp:** Cosmetic Surgery-Face; Liposuction & Body Contouring; Facial Plastic & Reconstructive Surgery; Cosmetic Surgery-Breast; **Hospital:** NY-Presby/Weill Cornell Med Ctr, NY (page 104), Lenox Hill Hosp (page 106); **Address:** 1016 Fifth Ave, New York, NY 10028-0132; **Phone:** 212-535-2300; **Board Cert:** Plastic Surgery 1984; **Med School:** NY Med Coll 1975; **Resid:** Surgery, Montefiore Med Ctr 1978; Plastic Surgery, NY Hosp/Meml Sloan Kettering Cancer Ctr 1980; **Fac Appt:** Asst Clin Prof S, Cornell Univ-Weill Med Coll

Silich, Robert C MD (PlS) - **Spec Exp:** Cosmetic Surgery-Face & Eyes; Blepharoplasty; Rhinoplasty; **Hospital:** NY-Presby/Weill Cornell Med Ctr, NY (page 104), Lenox Hill Hosp (page 106); **Address:** 121 E 83rd St, Ste A, MS 10028, New York, NY 10028; **Phone:** 212-628-6800; **Board Cert:** Plastic Surgery 2011; **Med School:** Georgetown Univ 1993; **Resid:** Surgery, Cornell Med Ctr 1997; Plastic Surgery, Cornell Med Ctr 1999; **Fac Appt:** Asst Clin Prof PlS, Cornell Univ-Weill Med Coll

Silver, Lester MD (PlS) - **Spec Exp:** Cleft Palate/Lip; Pediatric Plastic Surgery; Reconstructive Surgery; **Hospital:** Mount Sinai Med Ctr (page 102); **Address:** 5 E 98th St, Box 1259, New York, NY 10029-6574; **Phone:** 212-241-1968; **Board Cert:** Plastic Surgery 1978; **Med School:** Ros Franklin Univ/Chicago Med Sch 1960; **Resid:** Surgery, Montefiore Med Ctr 1966; Plastic Surgery, Mt Sinai Med Ctr 1969; **Fac Appt:** Prof PlS, Mount Sinai Sch Med

Skolnik, Richard A MD (PlS) - **Spec Exp:** Cosmetic Surgery-Face; Cosmetic Surgery-Breast; Liposuction & Body Contouring; **Hospital:** Mount Sinai Med Ctr (page 102); **Address:** 21 E 87th St, New York, NY 10128-0506; **Phone:** 212-722-1977; **Board Cert:** Plastic Surgery 1983; **Med School:** Cornell Univ-Weill Med Coll 1976; **Resid:** Surgery, Mt Sinai Hosp 1979; Plastic Surgery, Mt Sinai Hosp 1982; **Fac Appt:** Assoc Clin Prof PlS, Mount Sinai Sch Med

Spector, Jason A MD (PlS) - **Spec Exp:** Cosmetic Surgery; **Hospital:** NY-Presby/Weill Cornell Med Ctr, NY (page 104); **Address:** New York Presby-Weill Cornell, 520 E 70th St, Star Pavilion, 8th Fl, New York, NY 10065-4870; **Phone:** 212-746-4532; **Board Cert:** Plastic Surgery 2007; **Med School:** NYU Sch Med 1996; **Resid:** Surgery, NYU Med Ctr 2002; Plastic Surgery, NYU Med Ctr 2005; **Fellow:** Plastic Surgery, NYU Med Ctr 2006; Microsurgery, NYU Med Ctr 2006; **Fac Appt:** Asst Prof S, Cornell Univ-Weill Med Coll

Spinelli, Henry M MD (PlS) - **Spec Exp:** Cosmetic Surgery-Face; Craniofacial Surgery/Reconstruction; Oculoplastic & Orbital Surgery; Eyelid Surgery/Blepharoplasty; **Hospital:** NY-Presby/Weill Cornell Med Ctr, NY (page 104), Lenox Hill Hosp (Manh Eye, Ear & Throat Hosp) (page 106); **Address:** 875 Fifth Ave, New York, NY 10021-4952; **Phone:** 212-570-6235; **Board Cert:** Ophthalmology 1987; Plastic Surgery 1993; **Med School:** NYU Sch Med 1981; **Resid:** Ophthalmology, Manhattan EET Hosp 1985; Plastic/Reconstructive Surgery, NYU-Bellevue Hosp 1990; **Fellow:** Craniofacial Surgery, NYU Med Ctr 1991; **Fac Appt:** Clin Prof S, Cornell Univ-Weill Med Coll

Staffenberg, David A MD (PlS) - **Spec Exp:** Craniofacial Surgery/Reconstruction; Pediatric Plastic Surgery; Ear Reconstruction/Microtia; Cosmetic Surgery-Face; **Hospital:** NYU Langone Med Ctr (page 108); **Address:** NYU Med Ctr, 305 E 33rd St, New York, NY 10016; **Phone:** 212-263-8065; **Board Cert:** Plastic Surgery 2009; **Med School:** NY Med Coll 1989; **Resid:** Surgery, Maimonides Med Ctr 1995; Plastic Surgery, Emory Univ Med Ctr 1997; **Fellow:** Craniofacial Surgery, UCLA Med Ctr 1998; **Fac Appt:** Assoc Prof PlS, Albert Einstein Coll Med

Sultan, Mark R MD (PlS) - **Spec Exp:** Breast Reconstruction; Cosmetic Surgery-Breast; Cosmetic Surgery-Face; Liposuction & Body Contouring; **Hospital:** St. Luke's - Roosevelt Hosp Ctr - Roosevelt Div (page 94); **Address:** 1100 Park Ave, New York, NY 10128; **Phone:** 212-360-0700; **Board Cert:** Plastic Surgery 1992; **Med School:** Columbia P&S 1982; **Resid:** Surgery, Columbia-Presby Hosp 1987; Plastic Surgery, Columbia-Presby Hosp 1990; **Fellow:** Head and Neck Surgery, Emory Univ Hosp 1989; **Fac Appt:** Assoc Prof S, Columbia P&S

Tabbal, Nicolas MD (PlS) - **Spec Exp:** Rhinoplasty; Cosmetic Surgery-Face; Eyelid Surgery; **Hospital:** Lenox Hill Hosp (Manh Eye, Ear & Throat Hosp) (page 106), NYU Langone Med Ctr (page 108); **Address:** 521 Park Ave, rm 1, New York, NY 10021-8140; **Phone:** 212-644-5800; **Board Cert:** Plastic Surgery 1980; **Med School:** Lebanon 1972; **Resid:** Surgery, Am Univ Med Ctr 1976; Plastic Surgery, Akron City Hosp 1979; **Fellow:** Surgery, Upstate Med Ctr 1977; Reconstructive Microsurgery, NYU Med Ctr 1980

Talmor, Mia MD (PlS) - **Spec Exp:** Breast Reconstruction; Reconstructive Surgery; Cosmetic Surgery; Nipple Sparing Mastectomy; **Hospital:** NY-Presby/Weill Cornell Med Ctr, NY (page 104); **Address:** New York Presbyterian Hospital, 425 E 61st St, Fl 10, New York, NY 10065; **Phone:** 212-821-0933; **Board Cert:** Plastic Surgery 2012; Surgery 2011; **Med School:** Cornell Univ 1993; **Resid:** Surgery, NY Hosp-Cornell Med Ctr 1999; Plastic Surgery, NY Hosp-Cornell Med Ctr 2001; **Fac Appt:** Assoc Clin Prof PlS, Cornell Univ-Weill Med Coll

Taub, Peter J MD (PlS) - **Spec Exp:** Pediatric Plastic Surgery; Craniofacial Surgery; Cosmetic Surgery; Maxillofacial Surgery; **Hospital:** Mount Sinai Med Ctr (page 102), Westchester Med Ctr; **Address:** 5 E 98th St, Fl 14th, Ste B, New York, NY 10029-6574; **Phone:** 212-241-4178; **Board Cert:** Surgery 2009; Plastic Surgery 2003; **Med School:** Albert Einstein Coll Med 1993; **Resid:** Surgery, Mt Sinai Med Ctr 1999; Plastic Surgery, UCLA Med Ctr 2001; **Fellow:** Craniofacial Surgery, UCLA Med Ctr 2002; **Fac Appt:** Prof S, Mount Sinai Sch Med

Thorne, Charles H MD (PlS) - **Spec Exp:** Cosmetic Surgery-Face; Ear Reconstruction/Microtia; Craniofacial Surgery; Rhinoplasty; **Hospital:** NYU Langone Med Ctr (page 108), Lenox Hill Hosp (Manh Eye, Ear & Throat Hosp) (page 106); **Address:** 812 Park Ave, New York, NY 10021-2759; **Phone:** 212-794-0044; **Board Cert:** Plastic Surgery 2007; **Med School:** UCLA 1981; **Resid:** Surgery, Mass Genl Hosp 1986; Plastic Surgery, NYU Med Ctr 1988; **Fellow:** Craniofacial Surgery, NYU Med Ctr 1989; **Fac Appt:** Assoc Prof PlS, NYU Sch Med

Ting, Jess MD (PlS) - **Spec Exp:** Breast Reconstruction; Cosmetic Surgery; **Hospital:** Mount Sinai Med Ctr (page 102), Mount Sinai Hosp of Queens (page 102); **Address:** 5 E 98th St, Fl 14, Ste B, Box 1259, New York, NY 10029; **Phone:** 212-241-4410; **Board Cert:** Plastic Surgery 2002; Hand Surgery 2003; **Med School:** Columbia P&S 1995; **Resid:** Surgery, Columbia Presby Med Ctr 1998; Plastic Surgery, Univ Pittsburgh Med Ctr 2000; **Fellow:** Hand Surgery, Hosp Special Surgery 2001; **Fac Appt:** Asst Prof S, Mount Sinai Sch Med

Verga, Michele MD (PlS) - **Spec Exp:** Cosmetic Surgery-Face; Liposuction; Body Contouring; Reconstructive Surgery; **Hospital:** Mount Sinai Med Ctr (page 102); **Address:** 1010 5th Ave, New York, NY 10028-0130; **Phone:** 212-535-0470; **Board Cert:** Plastic Surgery 1984; **Med School:** Italy 1974; **Resid:** Surgery, Mt Sinai Hosp 1978; Surgery, Lutheran Med Ctr 1980; **Fellow:** Plastic Surgery, Mt Sinai Hosp 1983; **Fac Appt:** Asst Clin Prof S, Mount Sinai Sch Med

Vickery, Carlin MD (PlS) - **Spec Exp:** Breast Cosmetic & Reconstructive Surgery; Cosmetic Surgery-Body; Cosmetic Surgery-Face; **Hospital:** Mount Sinai Med Ctr (page 102); **Address:** 1125 5th Ave, New York, NY 10128; **Phone:** 212-288-9800; **Board Cert:** Plastic Surgery 1987; **Med School:** NYU Sch Med 1977; **Resid:** Surgery, New York Univ Med Ctr 1982; **Fellow:** Microsurgery, New York Univ Med Ctr 1985; **Fac Appt:** Assoc Clin Prof S, Mount Sinai Sch Med

Weiss, Paul R MD (PlS) - **Spec Exp:** Breast Cosmetic & Reconstructive Surgery; Cosmetic Surgery-Face; Cosmetic Surgery-Body; **Hospital:** Montefiore Med Ctr-Moses Campus, NY (page 100), Montefiore Med Ctr-Einstein Campus, NY (page 100); **Address:** 1049 5th Ave, Ste 2D, New York, NY 10028-0115; **Phone:** 212-861-8000; **Board Cert:** Surgery 1975; Plastic Surgery 2010; **Med School:** Tulane Univ 1969; **Resid:** Surgery, Montefiore Med Ctr/Bronx Muni Hosp 1974; Plastic Surgery, Montefiore Med Ctr 1976; **Fac Appt:** Clin Prof S, Albert Einstein Coll Med

Wells, Scott B MD (PlS) - **Spec Exp:** Cosmetic Surgery-Face; Abdominoplasty; Breast Augmentation; **Hospital:** Winthrop Univ Hosp (page 504); **Address:** 655 Park Ave, New York, NY 10065; **Phone:** 212-794-3900; **Board Cert:** Plastic Surgery 2005; **Med School:** NY Med Coll 1985; **Resid:** Surgery, Beth Israel Med Ctr 1990; Plastic/Reconstructive Surgery, SUNY Hlth Sci Ctr 1992

Zevon, Scott MD (PlS) - **Spec Exp:** Breast Augmentation; Breast Surgery; Body Contouring; Liposuction; **Hospital:** St. Luke's - Roosevelt Hosp Ctr - Roosevelt Div (page 94), SUNY Downstate Med Ctr (Univ Hosp of Bklyn) - LICH (page 420); **Address:** 75 Central Park W, Ste 1AB, New York, NY 10023; **Phone:** 212-496-6600; **Board Cert:** Plastic Surgery 1989; **Med School:** Boston Univ 1979; **Resid:** Surgery, St Luke's-Roosevelt Hosp Ctr 1984; Plastic Surgery, Nassau Co Med Ctr 1986; **Fellow:** Craniofacial Surgery, Mayo Clinic 1987

Zide, Barry M MD/DMD (PlS) - **Spec Exp:** Facial Surgery-Chin & Lip; Birthmarks/Hemangiomas; Reconstructive Plastic Surgery; Melanoma; **Hospital:** NYU Langone Med Ctr (page 108), Lenox Hill Hosp (page 106); **Address:** 420 E 55th St, Ste 1D, New York, NY 10022-5140; **Phone:** 212-421-2424; **Board Cert:** Plastic Surgery 1981; **Med School:** Tufts Univ 1973; **Resid:** Surgery, Stanford Med Ctr 1976; Plastic Surgery, Univ NC Hosp 1978; **Fellow:** Head & Neck Oncology, Roswell Park Cancer Inst 1979; Craniofacial Surgery, NYU Med Ctr 1980; **Fac Appt:** Prof PlS, NYU Sch Med

Preventive Medicine

Cahill, John MD (PrM) - **Spec Exp:** Tropical Diseases; Travel Medicine; Parasitic Infections; International Health; **Hospital:** St. Luke's - Roosevelt Hosp Ctr - Roosevelt Div (page 94); **Address:** 425 W 59th St, Ste 8A, New York, NY 10019; **Phone:** 212-492-5500; **Board Cert:** Emergency Medicine 2011; **Med School:** Mount Sinai Sch Med 1996; **Resid:** Emergency Medicine, Rhode Island Hosp 1997; Emergency Medicine, Rhode Island Hosp 2000; **Fellow:** Tropical Medicine, Royal Coll Surgeons 1998; **Fac Appt:** Asst Clin Prof Med, Columbia P&S

Cahill, Kevin M MD (PrM) - **Spec Exp:** Tropical Diseases; International Health; Parasitic Infections; Tropical Diseases; **Hospital:** Lenox Hill Hosp (page 106); **Address:** 850 5th Ave, New York, NY 10065; **Phone:** 212-434-2477; **Board Cert:** Public Health & Genl Preventive Med 1970; **Med School:** Cornell Univ-Weill Med Coll 1961; **Resid:** Internal Medicine, US Navy Med Res Unit 1965; Public Health & Genl Preventive Med, US Navy Med Res Unit 1965; **Fac Appt:** Clin Prof Med, NYU Sch Med

Hoffman, Robert S MD (PrM) - **Spec Exp:** Poison Control; Disaster Preparedness; **Hospital:** NYU Langone Med Ctr (page 108), Bellevue Hosp Ctr; **Address:** NY Poison Control Ctr, 455 1st Ave, rm 123, New York, NY 10016; **Phone:** 212-340-4494; **Board Cert:** Internal Medicine 1987; Emergency Medicine 2005; Medical Toxicology 2008; **Med School:** NYU Sch Med 1984; **Resid:** Internal Medicine, NYU Med Ctr 1987; **Fellow:** Medical Toxicology, NYU Med Ctr 1989; **Fac Appt:** Assoc Prof Med, NYU Sch Med

Psychiatry

Adler, Lenard A MD (Psyc) - **Spec Exp:** ADD/ADHD; Psychopharmacology; **Hospital:** NYU Langone Med Ctr (page 108); **Address:** 650 First Ave Fl 7, New York, NY 10016; **Phone:** 212-263-3580; **Board Cert:** Psychiatry 1987; **Med School:** Emory Univ 1982; **Resid:** Psychiatry, NYU Med Ctr 1986; **Fac Appt:** Prof Psyc, NYU Sch Med

Almeleh, Jack MD (Psyc) - **Spec Exp:** Cognitive Psychotherapy; Anxiety & Depression; **Hospital:** Mount Sinai Med Ctr (page 102); **Address:** 340 E 52nd St, New York, NY 10022; **Phone:** 212-355-4250; **Board Cert:** Psychiatry 1977; **Med School:** SUNY Buffalo 1969; **Resid:** Psychiatry, Temple Univ Hosp 1073; **Fac Appt:** Asst Clin Prof Psyc, Mount Sinai Sch Med

Alper, Kenneth R MD (Psyc) - **Spec Exp:** Psychopharmacology; **Hospital:** NYU Langone Med Ctr (page 108); **Address:** 150 E 58th St Fl 25, New York, NY 10155; **Phone:** 212-966-3506; **Board Cert:** Psychiatry 1989; **Med School:** Univ Tex, San Antonio 1984; **Resid:** Psychiatry, NYU Med Ctr 1988; **Fellow:** Clinical Neurophysiology, NYU Med Ctr 1990; **Fac Appt:** Assoc Prof Psyc, NYU Sch Med

Appelbaum, Paul S MD (Psyc) - **Spec Exp:** Forensic Psychiatry; Depression; Anxiety & Mood Disorders; **Hospital:** NY-Presby/Columbia Univ Med Ctr, NY (page 104); **Address:** NY State Psychiatric Inst, 1051 Riverside Drive, rm 6714, Box 122, New York, NY 10032; **Phone:** 212-543-4184; **Board Cert:** Psychiatry 1981; Forensic Psychiatry 2004; **Med School:** Harvard Med Sch 1976; **Resid:** Psychiatry, Mass Mental Health Ctr 1980; **Fac Appt:** Prof Psyc, Columbia P&S

Arkow, Stan D MD (Psyc) - **Spec Exp:** Psychotherapy; Psychopharmacology; **Hospital:** NY-Presby/Columbia Univ Med Ctr, NY (page 104); **Address:** 740 W End Ave, Ste 5-A, New York, NY 10025; **Phone:** 212-663-5185; **Board Cert:** Psychiatry 1985; **Med School:** Columbia P&S 1977; **Resid:** Psychiatry, Columbia-Presby Med Ctr/Psych Inst 1981; **Fac Appt:** Assoc Clin Prof Psyc, Columbia P&S

Aronoff, Michael S MD (Psyc) - **Spec Exp:** Stress Management; Anxiety & Depression; Sleep Disorders; Family & Couples Therapy; **Hospital:** Lenox Hill Hosp (page 106), NYU Langone Med Ctr (page 108); **Address:** 60 Riverside Drive, Ste 16E, New York, NY 10024-6171; **Phone:** 212-799-8257; **Board Cert:** Psychiatry 1977; **Med School:** Univ Pennsylvania 1966; **Resid:** Psychiatry, NY State Psych Inst/Columbia Univ 1972; **Fellow:** Psychoanalysis, Columbia-Presby Hosp 1976; **Fac Appt:** Clin Prof Psyc, NYU Sch Med

Attia, Evelyn MD (Psyc) - **Spec Exp:** Eating Disorders; Mood Disorders; **Hospital:** NY-Presby/Weill Cornell Med Ctr, NY (page 104), NY State Psychiatric Inst; **Address:** NYS Psychiatric Inst, Box 98, 1051 Riverside Drive, New York, NY 10032; **Phone:** 914-997-5732; **Board Cert:** Psychiatry 1992; **Med School:** Columbia P&S 1986; **Resid:** Psychiatry, Hosp Univ Penn 1987; Psychiatry, NY State Psych Inst 1990; **Fac Appt:** Assoc Clin Prof Psyc, Columbia P&S

Barbuto, Joseph MD (Psyc) - **Spec Exp:** Psychiatry in Cancer; Anxiety & Mood Disorders; Personality Disorders; **Hospital:** NY-Presby/Weill Cornell Med Ctr, NY (page 104), Meml Sloan-Kettering Cancer Ctr (page 116); **Address:** 945 Fifth Ave Ave, Ste 5, New York, NY 10021; **Phone:** 212-724-7366; **Board Cert:** Psychiatry 1983; **Med School:** Albert Einstein Coll Med 1978; **Resid:** Psychiatry, NY Hosp 1982; **Fellow:** Psychiatric Oncology, Meml Sloan-Kettering Cancer Ctr 1986; **Fac Appt:** Assoc Clin Prof Psyc, Cornell Univ-Weill Med Coll

Basch, Samuel MD (Psyc) - **Spec Exp:** Psychopharmacology; Psychiatry in Physical Illness; Psychiatry in Cancer; Psychoanalysis; **Hospital:** Mount Sinai Med Ctr (page 102); **Address:** 10 E 85th St, Ste 1B, New York, NY 10028; **Phone:** 212-427-0344; **Board Cert:** Psychiatry 1970; **Med School:** Hahnemann Univ 1961; **Resid:** Psychiatry, Mount Sinai Hosp 1965; **Fellow:** Psychoanalysis, Columbia Presby Hosp 1976; **Fac Appt:** Prof Psyc, Mount Sinai Sch Med

Bialer, Philip MD (Psyc) - **Spec Exp:** Psychiatry in Physical Illness; Psychiatry in Head & Neck Cancer; **Hospital:** Meml Sloan-Kettering Cancer Ctr (page 116); **Address:** 305 1st Ave, New York, NY 10022; **Phone:** 646-888-0009; **Board Cert:** Psychiatry 1989; Psychosomatic Medicine 2005; **Med School:** Ohio State Univ 1977; **Resid:** Internal Medicine, Mt Sinai Med Ctr 1978; Psychiatry, SUNY Hlth Sci Ctr 1988; **Fellow:** Psychosomatic Medicine, Beth Israel Med Ctr 1989; **Fac Appt:** Assoc Clin Prof Psyc, Cornell Univ-Weill Med Coll

Bone, Stanley MD (Psyc) - **Spec Exp:** Psychotherapy; Psychoanalysis; **Hospital:** NY-Presby/Columbia Univ Med Ctr, NY (page 104); **Address:** 1155 Park Ave, New York, NY 10128-1209; **Phone:** 212-831-0917; **Board Cert:** Psychiatry 1979; **Med School:** Mount Sinai Sch Med 1974; **Resid:** Psychiatry, Columbia Presby 1978; **Fellow:** Psychoanalysis, Columbia Univ 1983; **Fac Appt:** Clin Prof Psyc, Columbia P&S

Borbely, Antal MD (Psyc) - **Spec Exp:** Career Related Problems; Relationship Problems; Creativity Enhancement; **Address:** 675 W End Ave, Ste 1A, New York, NY 10025; **Phone:** 212-222-1678; **Board Cert:** Psychiatry 1976; **Med School:** Switzerland 1968; **Resid:** Psychiatry, NY State Psyc Inst 1972; Psychiatry, Albert Einstein Affil Hosp 1973; **Fellow:** Community Psychiatry, Albert Einstein Affil Hosp 1975

Breitbart, William MD (Psyc) - **Spec Exp:** Psychiatry in Cancer; AIDS Related Cancers; Pain-Cancer; Palliative Care; **Hospital:** Meml Sloan-Kettering Cancer Ctr (page 116); **Address:** 1275 York Ave, New York, NY 10065; **Phone:** 646-888-0100; **Board Cert:** Internal Medicine 1982; Psychiatry 1986; Psychosomatic Medicine 2005; **Med School:** Albert Einstein Coll Med 1978; **Resid:** Internal Medicine, Bronx Muni Hosp Ctr 1982; Psychiatry, Bronx Muni Hosp Ctr 1984; **Fellow:** Psychiatric Oncology, Meml Sloan Kettering Cancer Ctr 1986; **Fac Appt:** Prof Psyc, Cornell Univ-Weill Med Coll

Brodie, Jonathan D MD (Psyc) - **Spec Exp:** Psychopharmacology; Anxiety & Depression; Neuro-Psychiatry; **Hospital:** NYU Langone Med Ctr (page 108); **Address:** 155 E 38th St, Ste 3L, New York, NY 10016; **Phone:** 212-986-6693; **Board Cert:** Psychiatry 1979; **Med School:** NYU Sch Med 1975; **Resid:** Psychiatry, NYU Med Ctr/Bellevue Hosp 1978; **Fac Appt:** Prof Psyc, NYU Sch Med

Bronheim, Harold E MD (Psyc) - **Spec Exp:** Psychiatry in Body Image Awareness; Relationship Problems; Psychiatry in Physical Illness; Anxiety & Depression; **Hospital:** Mount Sinai Med Ctr (page 102); **Address:** 1155 Park Ave, New York, NY 10028; **Phone:** 212-996-5777; **Board Cert:** Psychiatry 1985; Internal Medicine 1986; Psychosomatic Medicine 2005; Geriatric Psychiatry 2011; **Med School:** SUNY Downstate 1980; **Resid:** Psychiatry, Mount Sinai Hosp 1984; **Fellow:** Internal Medicine, Beth Israel Hosp 1985; **Fac Appt:** Clin Prof Psyc, Mount Sinai Sch Med

Brown, Richard P MD (Psyc) - **Spec Exp:** Psychopharmacology; Complementary Medicine; **Hospital:** NY-Presby/Columbia Univ Med Ctr, NY (page 104); **Address:** 30 East End Ave, Ste 1B, New York, NY 10028-7053; **Phone:** 212-737-0821; **Board Cert:** Psychiatry 1983; **Med School:** Columbia P&S 1977; **Resid:** Psychiatry, New York Hosp 1982; **Fellow:** Psychopharmacology, New York Hosp 1984; **Fac Appt:** Assoc Prof Psyc, Columbia P&S

Bukberg, Judith MD (Psyc) - **Spec Exp:** Psychotherapy; Psychoanalysis; **Address:** 3 E 10th St, Ste 1A, New York, NY 10003; **Phone:** 212-614-0312; **Board Cert:** Psychiatry 1979; **Med School:** Mount Sinai Sch Med 1974; **Resid:** Psychiatry, Mount Sinai Hosp 1978; **Fellow:** Liaison Psychiatry, Meml Sloan Kettering Cancer Ctr 1980; Psychoanalysis, NY Psych Inst 1996; **Fac Appt:** Assoc Clin Prof Psyc, NY Med Coll

Cabaniss, Deborah L MD (Psyc) - **Spec Exp:** Psychoanalysis; Psychodynamic Psychotherapy; **Hospital:** NY State Psychiatric Inst; **Address:** NY State Psychiatric Inst, 1051 Riverside Dr, Unit 63 rm 1300E, New York, NY 10032; **Phone:** 212-543-5666; **Board Cert:** Psychiatry 1993; **Med School:** Columbia P&S 1988; **Resid:** Psychiatry, New York State Psy Inst 1992; **Fellow:** Psychoanalysis, NY Presby/Columbia Univ Med Ctr 1996; **Fac Appt:** Clin Prof Psyc, Columbia P&S

Caligor, Eve MD (Psyc) - **Spec Exp:** Psychoanalysis; Personality Disorders; **Hospital:** NYU Langone Med Ctr (page 108); **Address:** 19 E 88th St, Ste 1D, MS 10128, New York, NY 10128; **Phone:** 212-996-5285; **Board Cert:** Psychiatry 1987; **Med School:** Harvard Med Sch 1982; **Resid:** Psychiatry, NY Presby/Columbia Univ Med Ctr 1986; **Fellow:** Psychiatry, NY Presby/Columbia Univ Med Ctr 1987; **Fac Appt:** Clin Prof Psyc, NYU Sch Med

Cherry, Sabrina MD (Psyc) - **Spec Exp:** Psychoanalysis; Psychotherapy; **Hospital:** NY State Psychiatric Inst; **Address:** 285 Central Park W, New York, NY 10024; **Phone:** 212-721-2869; **Board Cert:** Psychiatry 1992; **Med School:** Columbia P&S 1987; **Resid:** Psychiatry, NY Presby/Columbia Univ Med Ctr 1991; **Fellow:** Psychoanalysis, Columbia Univ Ctr for Psychoanalytic Training 1998; **Fac Appt:** Assoc Clin Prof Psyc, Columbia P&S

Chung, Henry MD (Psyc) - **Spec Exp:** Depression; Anxiety Disorders; **Hospital:** Montefiore Med Ctr-Moses Campus, NY (page 100), NYU Langone Med Ctr (page 108); **Address:** 85 Fifth Ave, Ste 907, New York, NY 10003; **Phone:** 917-533-6908; **Board Cert:** Psychiatry 2004; **Med School:** SUNY Buffalo 1989; **Resid:** Psychiatry, NY Hosp 1994; **Fellow:** Research, NY Hosp 1995; **Fac Appt:** Assoc Clin Prof Psyc, NYU Sch Med

Cohen, Arnold R MD (Psyc) - **Spec Exp:** Psychotherapy; ADD/ADHD; Autism; **Hospital:** Mount Sinai Med Ctr (page 102); **Address:** 64 E 94th St, Apt 1A, New York, NY 10128; **Phone:** 212-289-6800; **Board Cert:** Psychiatry 1969; **Med School:** SUNY Hlth Sci Ctr 1963; **Resid:** Psychiatry, Mount Sinai Hosp 1966; **Fellow:** Child & Adolescent Psychiatry, Mount Sinai Hosp 1970; **Fac Appt:** Asst Clin Prof Psyc, Mount Sinai Sch Med

Devlin, Michael James MD (Psyc) - **Spec Exp:** Eating Disorders; Obesity; **Hospital:** NY-Presby/Columbia Univ Med Ctr, NY (page 104); **Address:** New York State Psyc Inst, 1051 Riverside, New York, NY 10032; **Phone:** 212-543-5748; **Board Cert:** Psychiatry 1987; **Med School:** Columbia P&S 1982; **Resid:** Psychiatry, NY State Psych Inst-Columbia P&S 1986; **Fellow:** Biological Psychiatry, NY State Psych Inst-Columbia P&S 1989; **Fac Appt:** Clin Prof Psyc, Columbia P&S

Douglas, Carolyn Jory MD (Psyc) - **Spec Exp:** Depression; Anxiety Disorders; Relationship Problems; **Hospital:** NY-Presby/Columbia Univ Med Ctr, NY (page 104), NY-Presby/Weill Cornell Med Ctr, NY (page 104); **Address:** 345 E 84th St, New York, NY 10028-4434; **Phone:** 212-396-9808; **Board Cert:** Psychiatry 1985; **Med School:** Harvard Med Sch 1980; **Resid:** Psychiatry, NY Hosp-Payne Whitney Clinic 1984; **Fac Appt:** Assoc Clin Prof Psyc, Columbia P&S

Fallon, Brian A MD (Psyc) - **Spec Exp:** Lyme Disease-Neuro Complications; Psychosomatic Disorders; Obsessive-Compulsive Disorder; Psychiatry in Physical Illness; **Hospital:** NY-Presby/Columbia Univ Med Ctr, NY (page 104); **Address:** NYS Psychiatric Institute, 1051 Riverside Drive, Room 3724, Unit/Box 69, New York, NY 10032; **Phone:** 212-543-5487; **Board Cert:** Psychiatry 1991; **Med School:** Columbia P&S 1985; **Resid:** Psychiatry, NYS Psychiatric Inst 1989; **Fellow:** Psychiatric Research, NYS Psychiatric Inst 1992; Psychodynamic Psychotherapy, Columbia Univ Psychoanalytic Inst 1990; **Fac Appt:** Prof Psyc, Columbia P&S

Ferran Jr, Ernesto MD (Psyc) - **Spec Exp:** Cultural Psychiatry; Child & Adolescent Psychiatry; Mood Disorders; Couples Therapy; **Hospital:** NYU Langone Med Ctr (page 108); **Address:** 15 Charles St, Ste 6H, New York, NY 10014-3024; **Phone:** 212-924-2673; **Board Cert:** Psychiatry 1983; Child & Adolescent Psychiatry 1986; **Med School:** Albert Einstein Coll Med 1976; **Resid:** Psychiatry, Bellevue Hosp/NYU Med Ctr 1979; **Fellow:** Child & Adolescent Psychiatry, Bellevue Hosp/NYU Med Ctr 1981; **Fac Appt:** Clin Prof Psyc, NYU Sch Med

Finkel, Jay MD (Psyc) - **Spec Exp:** Anxiety Disorders; Mood Disorders; **Hospital:** Mount Sinai Med Ctr (page 102); **Address:** 108 E 91st St, New York, NY 10128-1657; **Phone:** 212-289-2077; **Board Cert:** Psychiatry 1985; **Med School:** NY Med Coll 1980; **Resid:** Psychiatry, Mount Sinai Hosp 1984; **Fac Appt:** Asst Clin Prof Psyc, Mount Sinai Sch Med

First, Michael B MD (Psyc) - **Spec Exp:** Psychotherapy; Psychopharmacology; Forensic Psychiatry; Sexual Addiction; **Hospital:** NY-Presby/Columbia Univ Med Ctr, NY (page 104); **Address:** NY State Psychiatric Inst, Unit 60, 1051 Riverside Drive, New York, NY 10032; **Phone:** 212-543-5531; **Board Cert:** Psychiatry 1989; **Med School:** Univ Pittsburgh 1983; **Resid:** Psychiatry, NY State Psych Inst 1987; **Fellow:** Psychiatric Research, NY State Psych Inst 1988; **Fac Appt:** Clin Prof Psyc, Columbia P&S

Fox, Herbert A MD (Psyc) - **Spec Exp:** Electroconvulsive Therapy (ECT); Psychotherapy; Psychopharmacology; **Hospital:** Lenox Hill Hosp (page 106), Gracie Square Hosp; **Address:** 416 E 76th St, New York, NY 10021-4032; **Phone:** 212-674-8622; **Board Cert:** Psychiatry 1976; **Med School:** Albert Einstein Coll Med 1969; **Resid:** Psychiatry, Montefiore Med Ctr 1973; **Fac Appt:** Assoc Prof Psyc, Cornell Univ-Weill Med Coll

Friedman, Richard Alan MD (Psyc) - **Spec Exp:** Psychopharmacology; Anxiety & Mood Disorders; Depression; **Hospital:** NY-Presby/Weill Cornell Med Ctr, NY (page 104); **Address:** 525 E 68th St, Box 140, New York, NY 10021-4870; **Phone:** 212-746-5775; **Board Cert:** Psychiatry 1989; **Med School:** UMDNJ-RW Johnson Med Sch 1982; **Resid:** Psychiatry, Mount Sinai 1987; **Fac Appt:** Prof Psyc, Cornell Univ-Weill Med Coll

Fyer, Abby J MD (Psyc) - **Spec Exp:** Anxiety Disorders; Panic Disorder; **Hospital:** NY State Psychiatric Inst; **Address:** 1051 Riverside Dr, Box 82, New York, NY 10032; **Phone:** 212-543-5372; **Board Cert:** Psychiatry 1980; **Med School:** NYU Sch Med 1973; **Resid:** Psychiatry, Montefiore Med Ctr 1978; **Fac Appt:** Prof Psyc, Columbia P&S

Fyer, Minna R MD (Psyc) - **Spec Exp:** Anxiety Disorders; Mood Disorders; Menopause Problems; **Hospital:** NY-Presby/Weill Cornell Med Ctr, NY (page 104); **Address:** 242 E 72nd St, New York, NY 10021-4574; **Phone:** 212-861-2586; **Board Cert:** Psychiatry 1985; **Med School:** SUNY Hlth Sci Ctr 1980; **Resid:** Psychiatry, NY Hosp/Payne Whitney Cl 1984; **Fellow:** Psychopharmacology, NY State Psych Inst/Columbia 1986; **Fac Appt:** Asst Prof Psyc, Cornell Univ-Weill Med Coll

Goff, Donald C MD (Psyc) - **Spec Exp:** Schizophrenia; Psychopharmacology; **Hospital:** NYU Langone Med Ctr (page 108); **Address:** 1 Park Ave Fl 8 - rm 8-212, New York, NY 10016; **Phone:** 646-754-4843; **Board Cert:** Psychiatry 1986; **Med School:** UCLA 1980; **Resid:** Psychiatry, Mass Genl Hosp 1984; **Fellow:** Psychopharmacology, Tufts-New England Med Ctr 1985; **Fac Appt:** Assoc Clin Prof Psyc, NYU Sch Med

Goldenberg, David B MD (Psyc) - **Spec Exp:** HIV Psychiatry; Psychoanalysis; Gender Issues; Psychiatry in Cancer; **Hospital:** NY-Presby/Weill Cornell Med Ctr, NY (page 104); **Address:** 35 E 85th St, New York, NY 10028; **Phone:** 212-717-4834; **Board Cert:** Psychiatry 2007; Psychosomatic Medicine 2005; **Med School:** Univ MD Sch Med 1991; **Resid:** Psychiatry, Yale-New Haven Hosp 1996; **Fellow:** Psychiatry, Meml Sloan Kettering Cancer Ctr 1997

Goldman, Neil S MD (Psyc) - **Spec Exp:** Mood Disorders; Anxiety Disorders; Addiction/Substance Abuse; **Hospital:** N Shore Univ Hosp (page 106); **Address:** 235 W 48th St, Ste 26H, New York, NY 10036; **Phone:** 212-929-4395; **Board Cert:** Psychiatry 1981; **Med School:** Ros Franklin Univ/Chicago Med Sch 1970; **Resid:** Psychiatry, Brookdale Hosp 1974; **Fellow:** Addiction Psychiatry, St Vincents Hosp 1979; **Fac Appt:** Asst Prof Psyc, NY Med Coll

Goldstein, Susanna K MD (Psyc) - **Spec Exp:** Psychopharmacology; Anxiety Disorders; **Hospital:** Lenox Hill Hosp (page 106); **Address:** 65 Central Park West, Ste 1BR, New York, NY 10023; **Phone:** 212-362-6657; **Board Cert:** Psychiatry 1985; **Med School:** Israel 1975; **Resid:** Psychiatry, Rambam Med Ctr 1980; Neurology, Rambam Med Ctr 1981; **Fellow:** Biological Psychiatry, Montefiore Med Ctr 1983; **Fac Appt:** Asst Clin Prof Psyc, NYU Sch Med

Gorman, Lauren K MD (Psyc) - **Spec Exp:** Psychopharmacology; Anxiety & Mood Disorders; **Hospital:** Mount Sinai Med Ctr (page 102); **Address:** 685 West End Ave, Ste 1AF, New York, NY 10025; **Phone:** 212-580-7713; **Board Cert:** Psychiatry 1983; **Med School:** Columbia P&S 1977; **Resid:** Ophthalmology, Bellevue Hosp 1979; Psychiatry, Mt Sinai Hosp 1982; **Fellow:** Biological Psychiatry, Montefiore Hosp Med Ctr 1984; **Fac Appt:** Asst Clin Prof Psyc, Mount Sinai Sch Med

Heller, Stanley S MD (Psyc) - **Spec Exp:** Panic Disorder; Depression; **Address:** 1136 Fifth Ave, New York, NY 10128; **Phone:** 212-831-5919; **Board Cert:** Psychiatry 1975; **Med School:** Columbia P&S 1960; **Resid:** Psychiatry, NYS Psych Inst-Columbia 1966; **Fac Appt:** Assoc Clin Prof Psyc, Columbia P&S

Hoffman, Joel MD (Psyc) - **Spec Exp:** Psychopharmacology; Depression; Treatment Resistant Mental Illness; **Hospital:** Lenox Hill Hosp (page 106), NY-Presby/Weill Cornell Med Ctr, NY (page 104); **Address:** 1236 Park Ave, New York, NY 10128-1717; **Phone:** 212-722-3004; **Board Cert:** Psychiatry 1977; **Med School:** Columbia P&S 1963; **Resid:** Internal Medicine, Univ Michigan Med Ctr 1967; Psychiatry, NYS Psychiatric Inst 1972; **Fac Appt:** Asst Clin Prof Psyc, Columbia P&S

Hollander, Eric MD (Psyc) - **Spec Exp:** Obsessive-Compulsive Disorder; Anxiety Disorders; Autism; Body Dysmorphic Disorder (BDD); **Hospital:** Montefiore Med Ctr-Moses Campus, NY (page 100), Lenox Hill Hosp (page 106); **Address:** 901 Fifth Ave, New York, NY 10021; **Phone:** 212-873-4051; **Board Cert:** Psychiatry 1987; **Med School:** SUNY Hlth Sci Ctr 1982; **Resid:** Internal Medicine, Mount Sinai Hosp 1983; Psychiatry, Mount Sinai Hosp 1986; **Fellow:** Psychiatry, Columbia-Presby Med Ctr 1988; **Fac Appt:** Prof Psyc, Albert Einstein Coll Med

Kahn, David A MD (Psyc) - **Spec Exp:** Anxiety & Mood Disorders; Psychopharmacology; Psychotherapy; Schizophrenia; **Hospital:** NY-Presby/Columbia Univ Med Ctr, NY (page 104); **Address:** 180 Fort Washington Ave, rm HP240, New York, NY 10032; **Phone:** 212-472-0100; **Board Cert:** Psychiatry 1984; **Med School:** Columbia P&S 1979; **Resid:** Psychiatry, NY State Psych Inst 1983; **Fellow:** Biological Psychiatry, NY State Psych Inst 1984; **Fac Appt:** Clin Prof Psyc, Columbia P&S

Kalinich, Lila J MD (Psyc) - **Spec Exp:** Psychoanalysis; Psychotherapy; Adolescent Psychiatry; **Hospital:** NY-Presby/Columbia Univ Med Ctr, NY (page 104), NY State Psychiatric Inst; **Address:** 333 Central Park W, Ste 12, New York, NY 10025-7104; **Phone:** 212-866-0200; **Board Cert:** Psychiatry 1975; **Med School:** Northwestern Univ 1969; **Resid:** Psychiatry, Columbia-Presby Hosp 1973; **Fac Appt:** Clin Prof Psyc, Columbia P&S

Karasu, Sylvia R MD (Psyc) - **Spec Exp:** Weight Management; Eating Disorders; **Hospital:** NY-Presby/Weill Cornell Med Ctr, NY (page 104); **Address:** 2 E 88th St, New York, NY 10128; **Phone:** 212-534-7822; **Board Cert:** Psychiatry 1981; Child & Adolescent Psychiatry 1982; **Med School:** Albert Einstein Coll Med 1976; **Resid:** Psychiatry, Payne Whitney-Cornell Univ 1979; **Fellow:** Child Psychiatry, Payne Whitney-Cornell Univ 1981; **Fac Appt:** Assoc Clin Prof Psyc

Karasu, T Byram MD (Psyc) - **Spec Exp:** Depression; Personality Disorders; Psychotherapy; **Hospital:** Montefiore Med Ctr-Moses Campus, NY (page 100); **Address:** 2 E 88th St, New York, NY 10128-0555; **Phone:** 212-426-5208; **Board Cert:** Psychiatry 1972; **Med School:** Turkey 1959; **Resid:** Psychiatry, Yale-New Haven Hosp 1969; **Fac Appt:** Prof Psyc, Albert Einstein Coll Med

Kaufmann, Charles A MD (Psyc) - **Spec Exp:** Schizophrenia; Bipolar/Mood Disorders; Genetic Counseling-Psychiatric; **Hospital:** NY-Presby/Columbia Univ Med Ctr, NY (page 104), NY State Psychiatric Inst; **Address:** 161 Fort Washington Ave, Ste 348, New York, NY 10032; **Phone:** 914-238-7909; **Board Cert:** Psychiatry 1982; **Med School:** Columbia P&S 1977; **Resid:** Psychiatry, NY Hosp 1981; **Fellow:** Research, Natl Inst Hlth 1985; Research, Ctr for Neurobio & Behavior 1988; **Fac Appt:** Assoc Prof Psyc, Columbia P&S

Kavey, Neil B MD (Psyc) - **Spec Exp:** Sleep Medicine; Narcolepsy; Sleep Disorders/Apnea; **Hospital:** NY-Presby/Columbia Univ Med Ctr, NY (page 104), Rockefeller Univ; **Address:** The Sleep Disorders Center, Columbia University Medical Center, 161 Fort Washington Ave, Irving Pav Bldg, New York, NY 10032; **Phone:** 212-305-1860; **Board Cert:** Psychiatry 1976; Sleep Medicine 2003; **Med School:** Columbia P&S 1969; **Resid:** Psychiatry, Columbia Presby Med Ctr 1973; **Fac Appt:** Clin Prof Psyc, Columbia P&S

Kocsis, James MD (Psyc) - **Spec Exp:** Psychopharmacology; Mood Disorders; Anxiety Disorders; **Hospital:** NY-Presby/Weill Cornell Med Ctr, NY (page 104); **Address:** 525 E 68th St, Box 140, New York, NY 10021-4885; **Phone:** 212-746-5913; **Board Cert:** Psychiatry 1977; **Med School:** Cornell Univ-Weill Med Coll 1968; **Resid:** Psychiatry, New York Hosp 1975; **Fac Appt:** Prof Psyc, Cornell Univ-Weill Med Coll

Kowallis, George MD (Psyc) - **Spec Exp:** Depression; Anxiety Disorders; ADD/ADHD; **Address:** 162 W 56th St, Ste 407, New York, NY 10019-3831; **Phone:** 212-757-0324; **Board Cert:** Psychiatry 1977; Child & Adolescent Psychiatry 1978; **Med School:** Univ Pennsylvania 1969; **Resid:** Psychiatry, St Luke's-Roosevelt Hosp Ctr 1974; **Fac Appt:** Asst Clin Prof Psyc, NY Med Coll

Kranzler, Elliot MD (Psyc) - **Spec Exp:** Anxiety & Depression; Bereavement/Traumatic Grief; ADD/ADHD; **Hospital:** NY-Presby/Columbia Univ Med Ctr, NY (page 104); **Address:** 451 West End Ave, New York, NY 10024-5329; **Phone:** 212-580-9758; **Board Cert:** Psychiatry 1984; Child & Adolescent Psychiatry 1986; **Med School:** Albert Einstein Coll Med 1978; **Resid:** Psychiatry, Payne-Whitney Clinic 1982; **Fellow:** Child & Adolescent Psychiatry, Columbia-Presby 1984; Research, Columbia-Presby/NIMH; **Fac Appt:** Asst Prof Psyc, Columbia P&S

Kremberg, M Roy MD (Psyc) - **Spec Exp:** Mood Disorders; Anxiety Disorders; ADD/ADHD; **Hospital:** St. Luke's - Roosevelt Hosp Ctr - Roosevelt Div (page 94), NY-Presby/Columbia Univ Med Ctr, NY (page 104); **Address:** 2109 Broadway, Ste 8144, New York, NY 10023-2106; **Phone:** 212-875-8568; **Board Cert:** Psychiatry 1980; Child & Adolescent Psychiatry 1982; **Med School:** Columbia P&S 1976; **Resid:** Psychiatry, St Luke's-Roosevelt Hosp Ctr 1978; **Fellow:** Child & Adolescent Psychiatry, St Luke's-Roosevelt Hosp Ctr 1980

Krueger, Richard B MD (Psyc) - **Spec Exp:** Sexual Behavior-Compulsive; **Hospital:** NY-Presby/Columbia Univ Med Ctr, NY (page 104); **Address:** 210 E 68th St, Ste 1H, New York, NY 10021-6047; **Phone:** 212-517-6624; **Board Cert:** Psychiatry 1984; Internal Medicine 1980; Addiction Psychiatry 2007; Forensic Psychiatry 2006; **Med School:** Harvard Med Sch 1977; **Resid:** Internal Medicine, Boston VA Hosp 1980; **Fellow:** Psychiatry, Boston Univ Hosp 1983; **Fac Appt:** Assoc Prof Psyc, Columbia P&S

Levitan, Stephan MD (Psyc) - **Spec Exp:** Psychotherapy; Psychopharmacology; Couples Therapy; Psychoanalysis; **Hospital:** NY-Presby/Columbia Univ Med Ctr, NY (page 104); **Address:** 185 E 85th St, Ste 29J, New York, NY 10028-2143; **Phone:** 212-722-4311; **Board Cert:** Psychiatry 1974; **Med School:** SUNY Buffalo 1965; **Resid:** Psychiatry, Hillside Hosp 1969; **Fellow:** Psychoanalysis, Columbia Presby Med Ctr 1973; **Fac Appt:** Clin Prof Psyc, Columbia P&S

Lindenmayer, Jean-Pierre MD (Psyc) - **Spec Exp:** Psychopharmacology; Schizophrenia; Bipolar/Mood Disorders; **Address:** 18 E 77th St, Ste B, New York, NY 10021-1700; **Phone:** 212-249-2720; **Board Cert:** Psychiatry 1975; **Med School:** Switzerland 1967; **Resid:** Psychiatry, Univ Hosp-Geneva Med Sch 1969; Psychiatry, SUNY Downstate Med Ctr 1973; **Fellow:** Research, SUNY Downstate Med Ctr 1975; **Fac Appt:** Clin Prof Psyc, NYU Sch Med

Lipton, Brian P MD (Psyc) - **Spec Exp:** Psychotherapy; Psychopharmacology; Anxiety & Mood Disorders; Psychosomatic Disorders; **Hospital:** Lenox Hill Hosp (page 106); **Address:** 1111 Park Ave, Ste 1A, New York, NY 10128-1234; **Phone:** 212-427-4499; **Board Cert:** Psychiatry 1970; **Med School:** SUNY Hlth Sci Ctr 1964; **Resid:** Psychiatry, Hillside Hosp 1968; **Fac Appt:** Asst Clin Prof Psyc, NYU Sch Med

Malaspina, Dolores MD (Psyc) - **Spec Exp:** Schizophrenia; Treatment Resistant Mental Illness; **Hospital:** NYU Langone Med Ctr (page 108); **Address:** 136 E 57th St, Ste 1201, New York, NY 10022; **Phone:** 718-877-5708; **Board Cert:** Psychiatry 1989; **Med School:** UMDNJ-NJ Med Sch, Newark 1983; **Resid:** Psychiatry, NY-Presby/Columbia Univ Med Ctr 1987; **Fellow:** Psychiatry, NY State Psych Inst 1989; **Fac Appt:** Prof Psyc, NYU Sch Med

Manevitz, Alan MD (Psyc) - **Spec Exp:** Marital/Family/Sex Therapy; Depression-TMS Therapy; ADD/PTSD; Frbromyalgia Syndrome (FMS); **Hospital:** NY-Presby/Weill Cornell Med Ctr, NY (page 104), Lenox Hill Hosp (page 106); **Address:** 60 Sutton Place South, Ste 1CN, New York, NY 10022; **Phone:** 212-751-5072; **Board Cert:** Psychiatry 1987; **Med School:** Columbia P&S 1980; **Resid:** Psychiatry, NY Hosp 1984; **Fellow:** Psychopharmacology, NY Hosp 1985; **Fac Appt:** Assoc Clin Prof Psyc, Cornell Univ-Weill Med Coll

Mann, J John MD/PhD (Psyc) - **Spec Exp:** Mood Disorders; Clinical Trials; Suicide; **Hospital:** NY-Presby/Columbia Univ Med Ctr, NY (page 104); **Address:** NYS Psychiatric Institute, 1051 Riverside Drive, Box 42, New York, NY 10032; **Phone:** 212-543-5571; **Board Cert:** Psychiatry 1980; **Med School:** Australia 1978; **Resid:** Psychiatry, Royal Melbourne Hosp 1976; **Fac Appt:** Prof Psyc, Columbia P&S

Marin, Deborah B MD (Psyc) - **Spec Exp:** Memory Disorders; Depression; Depression in the Elderly; Geriatric Psychiatry; **Hospital:** Mount Sinai Med Ctr (page 102); **Address:** 1 Gustave Levy Pl, Box 1068, MS 10029, New York, NY 10029; **Phone:** 212-659-8092; **Board Cert:** Psychiatry 1990; **Med School:** Mount Sinai Sch Med 1984; **Resid:** Psychiatry, Mount Sinai Hosp 1988; **Fellow:** Psychiatry, NY Hosp-Cornell Med Ctr 1991; **Fac Appt:** Prof Psyc, Mount Sinai Sch Med

Markowitz, John C MD (Psyc) - **Spec Exp:** Depression; Post Traumatic Stress Disorder; Cognitive Psychotherapy; Psychopharmacology; **Hospital:** NY-Presby/Columbia Univ Med Ctr, NY (page 104), NY State Psychiatric Inst; **Address:** 40 E 83rd St, New York, NY 10028; **Phone:** 212-288-3070; **Board Cert:** Psychiatry 1987; **Med School:** Columbia P&S 1982; **Resid:** Psychiatry, Payne Whitney Clin/New York Hosp 1987; **Fac Appt:** Prof Psyc, Columbia P&S

McGrath, Patrick J MD (Psyc) - **Spec Exp:** Psychopharmacology-Consultation; Depression-Consultation; **Hospital:** NY-Presby/Columbia Univ Med Ctr, NY (page 104), NY State Psychiatric Inst; **Address:** 161 Fort Washington Ave, New York, NY 10032-3713; **Phone:** 212-543-5764; **Board Cert:** Psychiatry 1979; **Med School:** Columbia P&S 1974; **Resid:** Psychiatry, NY State Psych Inst 1978; **Fac Appt:** Assoc Clin Prof Psyc, Columbia P&S

McMullen Jr, Robert MD (Psyc) - **Spec Exp:** Psychopharmacology; Anxiety Disorders; Bipolar/Mood Disorders; Pain-Facial (TMJ); **Address:** 171 W 79th St, Ste 2, New York, NY 10024-6449; **Phone:** 212-362-9635; **Board Cert:** Psychiatry 1982; **Med School:** Georgetown Univ 1976; **Resid:** Psychiatry, Columbia-Presby Med Ctr 1980; **Fac Appt:** Asst Prof Psyc, Columbia P&S

Mellman, Lisa A MD (Psyc) - **Spec Exp:** Anxiety & Depression; Relationship Problems; Work Problems; **Hospital:** NY-Presby/Columbia Univ Med Ctr, NY (page 104), NY State Psychiatric Inst; **Address:** Columbia Univ Med Ctr, 161 Ft Washington Ave, New York, NY 10032; **Phone:** 917-620-6010; **Board Cert:** Psychiatry 1986; **Med School:** Case West Res Univ 1981; **Resid:** Psychiatry, Psych Inst/Columbia-Presby Med Ctr 1985; **Fellow:** Psychoanalysis, Columbia Univ 1991; **Fac Appt:** Clin Prof Psyc, Columbia P&S

Michels, Robert MD (Psyc) - **Spec Exp:** Psychoanalysis; **Hospital:** NY-Presby/Weill Cornell Med Ctr, NY (page 104); **Address:** 418 E 71st St, New York, NY 10021-4894; **Phone:** 212-746-6001; **Board Cert:** Psychiatry 1964; **Med School:** Northwestern Univ 1958; **Resid:** Psychiatry, Columbia-Presby Hosp 1962; **Fac Appt:** Prof Psyc, Cornell Univ-Weill Med Coll

Moore, Joanne MD (Psyc) - **Spec Exp:** Depression; Anxiety Disorders; **Hospital:** NY-Presby/Columbia Univ Med Ctr, NY (page 104); **Address:** 635 W 165th St, Ste 303, New York, NY 10032; **Phone:** 212-305-9499; **Board Cert:** Psychiatry 1988; Addiction Psychiatry 2006; **Med School:** Harvard Med Sch 1982; **Resid:** Psychiatry, Columbia-Presby Med Ctr 1987; **Fellow:** Geriatric Psychiatry, Columbia-Presby Med Ctr 1984; **Fac Appt:** Assoc Prof Psyc, Columbia P&S

Muhlbauer, Helen G MD (Psyc) - **Spec Exp:** Women's Health-Mental Health; Addiction/Substance Abuse; Psychosomatic Disorders; **Hospital:** NY-Presby/Columbia Univ Med Ctr, NY (page 104); **Address:** NY Presby Hosp-Dept Psychiatry, Allen Pavillion, 3 River E, 5141 Broadway, New York, NY 10034; **Phone:** 212-932-4642; **Board Cert:** Psychiatry 1991; Addiction Psychiatry 2008; Psychosomatic Medicine 2006; **Med School:** Albert Einstein Coll Med 1977; **Resid:** Psychiatry, Albert Einstein Affil Hosp 1981; **Fac Appt:** Asst Prof Psyc, Columbia P&S

Muskin, Philip R MD (Psyc) - **Spec Exp:** Psychopharmacology; Anxiety & Depression; Psychiatry in Physical Illness; **Hospital:** NY-Presby/Columbia Univ Med Ctr, NY (page 104); **Address:** 1700 York Ave, New York, NY 10128-7820; **Phone:** 212-722-8438; **Board Cert:** Psychiatry 1979; Geriatric Psychiatry 2011; Psychosomatic Medicine 2005; **Med School:** NY Med Coll 1974; **Resid:** Psychiatry, NYS Psych Inst 1978; **Fellow:** Psychosomatic Medicine, Columbia-Presby Hosp 1979; Psychopharmacology, NY State Psych Inst 1979; **Fac Appt:** Prof Psyc, Columbia P&S

Nininger, James MD (Psyc) - **Spec Exp:** Psychotherapy; Psychopharmacology; Geriatric Psychiatry; **Hospital:** NY-Presby/Weill Cornell Med Ctr, NY (page 104); **Address:** 10 E 78th St, Ste 5A, New York, NY 10075; **Phone:** 212-879-8338; **Board Cert:** Psychiatry 1978; **Med School:** Univ Cincinnati 1974; **Resid:** Psychiatry, Mount Sinai Hosp 1977; **Fac Appt:** Assoc Clin Prof Psyc, Cornell Univ-Weill Med Coll

Nunes, Edward MD (Psyc) - **Spec Exp:** Depression; Substance Abuse; **Hospital:** NY State Psychiatric Inst, NY-Presby/Columbia Univ Med Ctr, NY (page 104); **Address:** 1051 Riverside Drive, #51, New York, NY 10032-1007; **Phone:** 212-579-0339; **Board Cert:** Psychiatry 1986; Addiction Psychiatry 2002; **Med School:** Univ Conn 1981; **Resid:** Psychiatry, Columbia-Presby/NYS Psyc Inst 1985; **Fellow:** Psychopharmacology, Columbia-Presby/NYS Psyc Inst 1988; **Fac Appt:** Prof Psyc, Columbia P&S

Oberfield, Richard MD (Psyc) - **Spec Exp:** Child & Adolescent Psychiatry; Divorce/Family Issues; ADD/ADHD; **Hospital:** NYU Langone Med Ctr (page 108); **Address:** 200 E 33rd St, Ste 2J, New York, NY 10016-4874; **Phone:** 212-684-0148; **Board Cert:** Psychiatry 1979; Child & Adolescent Psychiatry 1980; **Med School:** Mount Sinai Sch Med 1974; **Resid:** Psychiatry, Bellevue Hosp 1976; **Fellow:** Child & Adolescent Psychiatry, Bellevue Hosp 1978; **Fac Appt:** Clin Prof Psyc, NYU Sch Med

Olds, David D MD (Psyc) - **Spec Exp:** Psychoanalysis; Psychotherapy; **Hospital:** NY-Presby/Columbia Univ Med Ctr, NY (page 104); **Address:** 108 E 96th St, Ste 6F, New York, NY 10128; **Phone:** 212-427-9688; **Board Cert:** Psychiatry 1975; **Med School:** Columbia P&S 1967; **Resid:** Psychiatry, NY State Psych Inst 1971; **Fellow:** Psychiatry, Columbia-Psych Ctr 1977; **Fac Appt:** Clin Prof Psyc, Columbia P&S

Papp, Laszlo A MD (Psyc) - **Spec Exp:** Anxiety & Mood Disorders; Depression; Panic Disorder; Psychopharmacology; **Hospital:** NY-Presby/Columbia Univ Med Ctr, NY (page 104); **Address:** 124 E 84th St, Ste 1B, New York, NY 10028; **Phone:** 212-360-5750; **Board Cert:** Psychiatry 1993; **Med School:** Hungary 1978; **Resid:** Internal Medicine, Natl Inst of Rheumatology 1981; Psychiatry, Beth Israel Med Ctr 1986; **Fellow:** Psychopharmacology, Columbia Univ 1989; **Fac Appt:** Assoc Prof Psyc, Columbia P&S

Pawel, Michael A MD (Psyc) - **Spec Exp:** Adolescent Psychiatry; **Hospital:** St. Luke's - Roosevelt Hosp Ctr - St Luke's Hosp (page 94); **Address:** 15 W 72nd St, Ste 1J, New York, NY 10023; **Phone:** 212-873-9170; **Board Cert:** Psychiatry 1977; **Med School:** Albert Einstein Coll Med 1971; **Resid:** Psychiatry, Montefiore Hosp Med Ctr 1974; **Fac Appt:** Asst Prof Psyc, Columbia P&S

Pfeffer, Cynthia R MD (Psyc) - **Spec Exp:** Child & Adolescent Psychiatry; Bereavement/Traumatic Grief; Anxiety & Depression; ADD/ADHD; **Hospital:** NY-Presby/Weill Cornell Med Ctr, NY (page 104), NYU Langone Med Ctr (page 108); **Address:** 1100 Park Ave, Ste 1B, MS 10128, New York, NY 10128; **Phone:** 212-717-2334; **Board Cert:** Psychiatry 1975; Child & Adolescent Psychiatry 1976; **Med School:** NYU Sch Med 1968; **Resid:** Psychiatry, Montefiore Med Ctr 1973; **Fellow:** Child & Adolescent Psychiatry, Montefiore Med Ctr 1973; **Fac Appt:** Prof Psyc, Cornell Univ-Weill Med Coll

Pines, Jeffrey M. MD (Psyc) - **Spec Exp:** Substance Abuse; **Hospital:** NY-Presby/Columbia Univ Med Ctr, NY (page 104); **Address:** NY Presbyterian Hosp, 161 Fort Washington Ave, New York, NY 10032; **Phone:** 212-579-1913; **Board Cert:** Psychiatry 1982; **Med School:** Columbia P&S 1973; **Resid:** Internal Medicine, Presby Hosp 1976; Psychiatry, NY State Psych Inst 1980; **Fellow:** Rheumatology, Hosp For Special Surg 1977; Liaison Psychiatry, Columbia-Presby Med Ctr 1981; **Fac Appt:** Assoc Clin Prof Psyc, Columbia P&S

Preven, David W MD (Psyc) - **Spec Exp:** Forensic Psychiatry; Psychopharmacology; Psychotherapy; **Hospital:** Montefiore Med Ctr-Moses Campus, NY (page 100); **Address:** 52 Riverside Drive, New York, NY 10024-6501; **Phone:** 212-799-4907; **Board Cert:** Psychiatry 1969; Forensic Psychiatry 2005; **Med School:** Harvard Med Sch 1963; **Resid:** Psychiatry, Jacobi Hosp/ Albert Einstein 1967; **Fellow:** Psychiatry, NIMH-Albert Einstein Affil Hosp 1971; **Fac Appt:** Clin Prof Psyc, Albert Einstein Coll Med

Rees, Ellen MD (Psyc) - **Spec Exp:** Psychoanalysis; Psychotherapy; **Hospital:** NY-Presby/Weill Cornell Med Ctr, NY (page 104); **Address:** 108 E 96th St Fl 7 - Ste F, New York, NY 10128-6217; **Phone:** 212-722-5988; **Board Cert:** Psychiatry 1979; **Med School:** Albert Einstein Coll Med 1974; **Resid:** Psychiatry, Mt Sinai Hosp 1977; **Fellow:** Psychiatry, New York Hosp-Cornell 1978; Psychoanalysis, Columbia Univ Ctr Psych Trng 1991; **Fac Appt:** Assoc Clin Prof Psyc, Cornell Univ-Weill Med Coll

Roose, Steven MD (Psyc) - **Spec Exp:** Depression in the Elderly; **Hospital:** NY-Presby/Columbia Univ Med Ctr, NY (page 104); **Address:** NY State Psychiatric Institute, 1051 Riverside Drive, New York, NY 10032; **Phone:** 212-831-8644; **Board Cert:** Psychiatry 1979; **Med School:** Mount Sinai Sch Med 1974; **Resid:** Psychiatry, NY Psychiatric Inst 1978; **Fellow:** Research, Columbia-Presby Med Ctr 1981; **Fac Appt:** Clin Prof Psyc, Columbia P&S

Rosen, Arnold M MD (Psyc) - **Spec Exp:** Depression; Psychopharmacology; **Address:** 200 E 78th St, New York, NY 10075; **Phone:** 212-288-6380; **Board Cert:** Psychiatry 1976; **Med School:** Univ Tex SW, Dallas 1968; **Resid:** Psychiatry, Metropolitan Hosp Ctr 1970; Psychiatry, Metropolitan Hosp Ctr 1974; **Fellow:** Psychiatry, Metropolitan Hosp Ctr 1975

Rosenthal, Jesse S MD (Psyc) - **Spec Exp:** ADD/ADHD; Anxiety Disorders; Depression; **Hospital:** Beth Israel Med Ctr - Petrie Division (page 94); **Address:** 21 E 93rd St, New York, NY 10128-0609; **Phone:** 212-876-3080; **Board Cert:** Psychiatry 1978; **Med School:** Geo Wash Univ 1973; **Resid:** Psychiatry, Mount Sinai Hosp 1976; **Fac Appt:** Asst Clin Prof Psyc, Mount Sinai Sch Med

Rosenthal, Richard N MD (Psyc) - **Spec Exp:** Anxiety & Mood Disorders; Addiction/Substance Abuse; **Hospital:** St. Luke's - Roosevelt Hosp Ctr - Roosevelt Div (page 94), Beth Israel Med Ctr - Petrie Division (page 94); **Address:** 1090 Amerstdam Ave, Fl 16, Ste G, New York, NY 10025; **Phone:** 212-523-5366; **Board Cert:** Psychiatry 1985; Addiction Psychiatry 2012; **Med School:** SUNY Hlth Sci Ctr 1980; **Resid:** Psychiatry, Mount Sinai Hosp 1984; **Fac Appt:** Prof Psyc, Columbia P&S

Rosner, Richard MD (Psyc) - **Spec Exp:** Adolescent Psychiatry; Forensic Psychiatry; Addiction/Substance Abuse; **Hospital:** NYU Langone Med Ctr (page 108), Bellevue Hosp Ctr; **Address:** 140 E 83rd St, Ste 6A, New York, NY 10028-1928; **Phone:** 212-988-6014; **Board Cert:** Psychiatry 1974; Forensic Psychiatry 2004; Addiction Psychiatry 2004; **Med School:** NYU Sch Med 1966; **Resid:** Psychiatry, Mount Sinai Hosp 1970; **Fac Appt:** Clin Prof Psyc, NYU Sch Med

Ross, Steven G MD (Psyc) - **Spec Exp:** Addiction/Substance Abuse; Alcohol Abuse; Adolescent Psychiatry; Psychiatry in Cancer; **Hospital:** NYU Langone Med Ctr (page 108), Bellevue Hosp Ctr; **Address:** 462 1st Ave, rm NBV 10E-7, New York, NY 10016; **Phone:** 212-562-4097; **Board Cert:** Psychiatry 2009; **Med School:** Mexico 1980; **Resid:** Psychiatry, Maimonides Med Ctr 1986; **Fac Appt:** Asst Prof Psyc, NYU Sch Med

Roth, Andrew J MD (Psyc) - **Spec Exp:** Psychiatry of Prostate Cancer; Geriatric Psychiatry; **Hospital:** Meml Sloan-Kettering Cancer Ctr (page 116); **Address:** 641 Lexington Ave Fl 7, New York, NY 10022; **Phone:** 646-888-0024; **Board Cert:** Psychiatry 1993; Geriatric Psychiatry 2007; Psychosomatic Medicine 2005; **Med School:** NY Med Coll 1988; **Resid:** Psychiatry, Mt Sinai Med Ctr 1992; **Fellow:** Liaison Psychiatry, Meml Sloan-Kettering Canc Ctr 1994; **Fac Appt:** Clin Prof Psyc, Cornell Univ-Weill Med Coll

Rubinstein, Mort MD (Psyc) - **Spec Exp:** Psychopharmacology; **Hospital:** VA NY Harbor Hlthcare Sys-Manhattan Campus; **Address:** 423 E 23rd St, New York, NY 10010-5013; **Phone:** 212-686-7500 x7991; **Board Cert:** Psychiatry 1988; **Med School:** NY Med Coll 1976; **Resid:** Psychiatry, NYU-Bellevue Hosp 1979; **Fellow:** Psychiatry, Mount Sinai Med Ctr 1980; **Fac Appt:** Assoc Clin Prof Psyc, NYU Sch Med

Sacks, Michael MD (Psyc) - **Spec Exp:** Personality Disorders; Relationship Problems; Anxiety & Depression; **Hospital:** NY-Presby/Weill Cornell Med Ctr, NY (page 104); **Address:** 525 E 68th St, Box 140, New York, NY 10021-4870; **Phone:** 212-746-3710; **Board Cert:** Psychiatry 1973; **Med School:** NYU Sch Med 1967; **Resid:** Psychiatry, NY State Psych Inst 1971; **Fellow:** Psychiatry, Natl Inst Mental Health 1973; **Fac Appt:** Prof Psyc, Cornell Univ-Weill Med Coll

Sadock, Virginia MD (Psyc) - **Spec Exp:** Psychotherapy; Sexual Dysfunction; Anxiety & Depression; Marital/Family/Sex Therapy; **Hospital:** NYU Langone Med Ctr (page 108); **Address:** 4 E 89th St, Ste 1E, New York, NY 10128; **Phone:** 212-427-0885; **Board Cert:** Psychiatry 1975; **Med School:** NY Med Coll 1970; **Resid:** Psychiatry, Metropolitan Hosp 1973; **Fac Appt:** Clin Prof Psyc, NYU Sch Med

Samberg, Eslee MD (Psyc) - **Spec Exp:** Psychoanalysis; **Hospital:** NY-Presby/Weill Cornell Med Ctr, NY (page 104); **Address:** 165 W End Ave, Ste 1M, New York, NY 10024; **Phone:** 212-874-7725; **Board Cert:** Psychiatry 1983; **Med School:** Cornell Univ-Weill Med Coll 1978; **Resid:** Psychiatry, NY Hosp-Cornell Med Ctr 1982; **Fac Appt:** Assoc Clin Prof Psyc, Cornell Univ-Weill Med Coll

Sawyer, David MD (Psyc) - **Spec Exp:** Psychoanalysis; Child & Adolescent Psychiatry; Stress Management; **Hospital:** NY-Presby/Weill Cornell Med Ctr, NY (page 104); **Address:** 1 W 64th St, Ste 1C, New York, NY 10023; **Phone:** 212-787-8260; **Board Cert:** Psychiatry 1982; Child & Adolescent Psychiatry 1984; **Med School:** NY Med Coll 1977; **Resid:** Psychiatry, NY Hosp-Cornell-Westchester 1980; **Fellow:** Child & Adolescent Psychiatry, NY Hosp-Cornell-Westchester 1982

Scharf, Robert D MD (Psyc) - **Spec Exp:** Psychotherapy; Psychopharmacology; Psychoanalysis; **Hospital:** St. Luke's - Roosevelt Hosp Ctr - Roosevelt Div (page 94); **Address:** 207 E 74th St, Ste 1L, New York, NY 10021-3341; **Phone:** 212-988-4145; **Board Cert:** Psychiatry 1976; **Med School:** Albert Einstein Coll Med 1960; **Resid:** Internal Medicine, Barnes Hosp/Straight Ward Med 1961; Psychiatry, Kings Co Hosp 1964; **Fellow:** Psychoanalysis, NY Psychoanalytic Inst 1973; **Fac Appt:** Asst Clin Prof Psyc, Columbia P&S

Schein, Jonah MD (Psyc) - **Spec Exp:** Depression; Anxiety Disorders; **Hospital:** NY-Presby/Weill Cornell Med Ctr, NY (page 104); **Address:** 1349 Lexington Ave, Ste 1E, New York, NY 10128-1514; **Phone:** 212-876-2324; **Board Cert:** Psychiatry 1975; **Med School:** NYU Sch Med 1969; **Resid:** Psychiatry, NY State Psych Inst 1973; **Fac Appt:** Assoc Clin Prof Psyc, Cornell Univ-Weill Med Coll

Schore, Arthur MD (Psyc) - **Spec Exp:** Depression; Sexual Dysfunction; Eating Disorders; **Hospital:** NY-Presby/Columbia Univ Med Ctr, NY (page 104); **Address:** 905 5th Ave, New York, NY 10021-4156; **Phone:** 212-535-6070; **Board Cert:** Psychiatry 1980; **Med School:** Ros Franklin Univ/Chicago Med Sch 1965; **Resid:** Columbia-Presby 1969; **Fellow:** NYS Psychiatric Inst 1975; **Fac Appt:** Psyc, Cornell Univ-Weill Med Coll

Seaman, Cheryl MD (Psyc) - **Spec Exp:** Anxiety Disorders; Depression; Psychopharmacology; Psychotherapy; **Address:** 286 Madison Ave, PH, New York, NY 10017; **Phone:** 917-687-8901; **Board Cert:** Psychiatry 1986; Geriatric Psychiatry 2001; **Med School:** Columbia P&S 1979; **Resid:** Psychiatry, NY Hosp-Westchester Div 1983

Shapiro, Peter A MD (Psyc) - **Spec Exp:** Depression; Psychiatry in Physical Illness; Liaison Psychiatry; **Hospital:** NY-Presby/Columbia Univ Med Ctr, NY (page 104); **Address:** 239 Central Park West, Ste 1-BW, New York, NY 10024-6038; **Phone:** 212-874-6030; **Board Cert:** Psychiatry 1985; Psychosomatic Medicine 2005; **Med School:** Columbia P&S 1980; **Resid:** Psychiatry, NY State Psych Inst 1984; **Fellow:** Liaison Psychiatry, Columbia-Presby Med Ctr 1986; **Fac Appt:** Prof Psyc, Columbia P&S

Shaw, Ronda R MD (Psyc) - **Spec Exp:** Psychoanalysis; Psychotherapy; **Hospital:** Mount Sinai Med Ctr (page 102); **Address:** 35 E 85th St, Profl, Ste 2, New York, NY 10028-0954; **Phone:** 212-772-0321; **Board Cert:** Psychiatry 1977; **Med School:** Wayne State Univ 1966; **Resid:** Psychiatry, Einstein Hosp 1970; **Fac Appt:** Assoc Clin Prof Psyc, Mount Sinai Sch Med

Shinbach, Kent MD (Psyc) - **Spec Exp:** Depression; Psychopharmacology; Geriatric Psychiatry; **Hospital:** Gracie Square Hosp, NY Downtown Hosp; **Address:** 14 EAST 75 E 75th St, Ste 1A, MS 10021, New York, NY 10021; **Phone:** 212-744-7100; **Board Cert:** Psychiatry 1970; **Med School:** Jefferson Med Coll 1963; **Resid:** Psychiatry, NY Med Coll 1968; **Fac Appt:** Asst Clin Prof Psyc, Cornell Univ-Weill Med Coll

Siever, Larry J MD (Psyc) - **Spec Exp:** Psychopharmacology; Depression; Personality Disorders; **Hospital:** Mount Sinai Med Ctr (page 102), James J. Peters VA Med Ctr-Bronx; **Address:** 1 Gustave L Levy Pl, Box 1230, New York, NY 10029-6500; **Phone:** 212-774-1722; **Board Cert:** Psychiatry 1980; **Med School:** Stanford Univ 1975; **Resid:** Psychiatry, McLean Hosp 1978; **Fellow:** Biological Psychiatry, Natl Inst Mntl Hlth 1982; **Fac Appt:** Prof Psyc, Mount Sinai Sch Med

Silver, Jonathan M MD (Psyc) - **Spec Exp:** Neuro-Psychiatry; Psychopharmacology; Brain Injury; **Hospital:** Lenox Hill Hosp (page 106); **Address:** 40 E 83rd St, Ste 1E, New York, NY 10028; **Phone:** 212-874-6453; **Board Cert:** Psychiatry 1984; Behavioral Neurology & Neuropsychiatry 2006; **Med School:** Albert Einstein Coll Med 1979; **Resid:** Psychiatry, NY State Psych Inst 1983; **Fellow:** Research, NY State Psych Inst 1985; **Fac Appt:** Clin Prof Psyc, NYU Sch Med

Snyder, Stephen L MD (Psyc) - **Spec Exp:** Sexual Dysfunction; Relationship Problems; Couples Therapy; **Hospital:** Mount Sinai Med Ctr (page 102); **Address:** 115 Central Park W, Ste 15, New York, NY 10023; **Phone:** 212-875-9800; **Board Cert:** Psychiatry 1989; **Med School:** UCSF 1983; **Resid:** Internal Medicine, UCSF Med Ctr-Mt Zion 1984; Psychiatry, Payne Whitney Psy Clinic 1987; **Fellow:** Behavioral Medicine, Mt Sinai Med Ctr 1989; **Fac Appt:** Assoc Clin Prof Psyc, Mount Sinai Sch Med

Spitz, Henry MD (Psyc) - **Spec Exp:** Family & Couples Therapy; Addiction/Substance Abuse; Anxiety Disorders; **Hospital:** NY-Presby/Columbia Univ Med Ctr, NY (page 104); **Address:** 101 Central Park West, Ste 1C, New York, NY 10023; **Phone:** 212-873-1415; **Board Cert:** Psychiatry 1973; **Med School:** NY Med Coll 1965; **Resid:** Psychiatry, NY Med Coll 1969; **Fellow:** Psychiatry, NY Med Coll 1971; **Fac Appt:** Clin Prof Psyc, Columbia P&S

Stein, Stefan MD (Psyc) - **Spec Exp:** Couples Therapy; Psychotherapy & Psychopharmacology; **Hospital:** NY-Presby/Weill Cornell Med Ctr, NY (page 104); **Address:** 850 Park Ave, Ste 1E, New York, NY 10075; **Phone:** 212-249-0200; **Board Cert:** Psychiatry 1970; **Med School:** NYU Sch Med 1963; **Resid:** Internal Medicine, Boston City Hosp 1964; Psychiatry, Albert Einstein Coll Med 1968; **Fellow:** Psychiatry, Mass Genl Hosp 1965; Psychoanalysis, NY Psychoan Inst 1974; **Fac Appt:** Prof Psyc, Cornell Univ-Weill Med Coll

Stone, Michael H MD (Psyc) - **Spec Exp:** Personality Disorders; Psychoanalysis; Forensic Psychiatry; Addiction/Substance Abuse; **Address:** 225 Central Park West, Ste 114, New York, NY 10024-6027; **Phone:** 212-758-2000; **Board Cert:** Psychiatry 1971; **Med School:** Cornell Univ-Weill Med Coll 1958; **Resid:** Internal Medicine, Bellevue Hosp 1961; Psychiatry, NYS Psych Inst 1966; **Fellow:** Hematology, Meml Sloan Kettering Cancer Ctr 1962; Medical Oncology, Meml Sloan Kettering Cancer Ctr 1963; **Fac Appt:** Prof Emeritus Psyc, Columbia P&S

Strain, James J MD (Psyc) - **Spec Exp:** Psychiatry in Physical Illness; Psychoanalysis; **Hospital:** Mount Sinai Med Ctr (page 102); **Address:** 1425 Madison Ave, Ste 6-24, New York, NY 10029; **Phone:** 212-659-8728; **Board Cert:** Psychiatry 1969; **Med School:** Case West Res Univ 1962; **Resid:** Psychiatry, Univ Hosps 1966; **Fellow:** Psychiatric Research, Univ Hosps 1967; Psychoanalysis, New York Psychoanal Inst 1972; **Fac Appt:** Prof Psyc, Mount Sinai Sch Med

Sussman, Norman MD (Psyc) - **Spec Exp:** Psychopharmacology; Anxiety & Mood Disorders; Bipolar/Mood Disorders; **Hospital:** NYU Langone Med Ctr (page 108); **Address:** 150 E 58th St, Fl 27, New York, NY 10155; **Phone:** 212-588-9722; **Board Cert:** Psychiatry 1980; **Med School:** NY Med Coll 1975; **Resid:** Psychiatry, Metropolitan Hosp Ctr 1977; Psychiatry, Westchester Co Med Ctr 1978; **Fac Appt:** Prof Psyc, NYU Sch Med

Swiller, Hillel MD (Psyc) - **Spec Exp:** Psychotherapy; Couples Therapy; **Hospital:** Mount Sinai Med Ctr (page 102); **Address:** 108 E 96th St, Ste 9F, New York, NY 10128; **Phone:** 212-534-5588; **Board Cert:** Psychiatry 1972; **Med School:** Cornell Univ-Weill Med Coll 1965; **Resid:** Psychiatry, Albert Einstein Coll Med 1969; **Fac Appt:** Clin Prof Psyc, Mount Sinai Sch Med

Tancredi, Laurence R MD (Psyc) - **Spec Exp:** Forensic Psychiatry; Anxiety & Depression; **Hospital:** Lenox Hill Hosp (page 106); **Address:** 129B E 71st St, New York, NY 10021-4201; **Phone:** 212-288-5197; **Board Cert:** Psychiatry 1979; **Med School:** Univ Pennsylvania 1966; **Resid:** Psychiatry, NYS Psych Inst 1975; Psychiatry, Yale-New Haven Hosp 1977; **Fac Appt:** Clin Prof Psyc, NYU Sch Med

Tardiff, Kenneth J MD (Psyc) - **Spec Exp:** Psychopharmacology; Forensic Psychiatry; Psychotherapy; **Hospital:** NY-Presby/Weill Cornell Med Ctr, NY (page 104); **Address:** Payne Whitney Clinic-NY Hosp, Dept Psyc, 525 E 68th St, Psy Box 140, New York, NY 10021-4870; **Phone:** 212-746-3871; **Board Cert:** Psychiatry 1976; **Med School:** Tulane Univ 1969; **Resid:** Psychiatry, Mass Genl Hosp 1973; **Fellow:** Public Health, Harvard Sch Public Hlth 1973; **Fac Appt:** Prof Psyc, Cornell Univ-Weill Med Coll

Taylor, Noel MD (Psyc) - **Spec Exp:** Anxiety Disorders; Mood Disorders; **Address:** 150 E 58 St, Fl 27, New York, NY 10155; **Phone:** 212-888-9038; **Board Cert:** Psychiatry 1985; **Med School:** Johns Hopkins Univ 1980; **Resid:** Psychiatry, Johns Hopkins Hosp 1984; **Fellow:** Psychiatry, Beth Israel Med Ctr 1986; **Fac Appt:** Asst Prof Psyc, Albert Einstein Coll Med

Teusink, J Paul MD (Psyc) - **Spec Exp:** Geriatric Psychiatry; Depression; Dementia; **Hospital:** Beth Israel Med Ctr - Petrie Division (page 94); **Address:** 88 University Pl, Ste 705, New York, NY 10003; **Phone:** 347-466-2521; **Board Cert:** Psychiatry 1976; Geriatric Psychiatry 2001; **Med School:** Univ Mich Med Sch 1969; **Resid:** Psychiatry, Topeka State Hosp 1971; Psychiatry, CF Menninger Meml Hosp 1973; **Fac Appt:** Assoc Prof Psyc, Albert Einstein Coll Med

Tolchin, Joan MD (Psyc) - **Spec Exp:** Child & Adolescent Psychiatry; Psychotherapy; **Hospital:** NY-Presby/Weill Cornell Med Ctr, NY (page 104); **Address:** 35 E 84th St, New York, NY 10028-0871; **Phone:** 212-744-1446; **Board Cert:** Psychiatry 1979; Child & Adolescent Psychiatry 1982; **Med School:** NYU Sch Med 1972; **Resid:** Psychiatry, Bronx Municipal Hosp 1975; **Fellow:** Child & Adolescent Psychiatry, NY Presby Hosp 1977; **Fac Appt:** Assoc Clin Prof Psyc, Cornell Univ-Weill Med Coll

Wachtel, Alan B MD (Psyc) - **Spec Exp:** ADD/ADHD; Mood Disorders; Learning Disorders; **Hospital:** NYU Langone Med Ctr (page 108); **Address:** 201 E 87th St, Ste 16J, New York, NY 10128; **Phone:** 212-348-0175; **Board Cert:** Psychiatry 1977; **Med School:** Mount Sinai Sch Med 1972; **Resid:** Psychiatry, Mt Sinai Hosp 1976; **Fellow:** Liaison Psychiatry, NY Hosp-Cornell Med Ctr 1977; **Fac Appt:** Assoc Clin Prof Psyc, NYU Sch Med

Wager, Steven G MD (Psyc) - **Spec Exp:** Psychopharmacology; Depression; Anxiety Disorders; **Address:** 145 W 86th St, Ste 1B, New York, NY 10024-3421; **Phone:** 212-769-9620; **Board Cert:** Psychiatry 1986; **Med School:** Case West Res Univ 1980; **Resid:** Psychiatry, Columbia-Presby Med Ctr 1984; **Fellow:** Psychopharmacology, Columbia-Presby Med Ctr 1986

Wallack, Joel J MD (Psyc) - **Spec Exp:** Psychopharmacology; Psychiatry in Physical Illness; Anxiety & Depression; **Hospital:** Beth Israel Med Ctr - Petrie Division (page 94), Mount Sinai Med Ctr (page 102); **Address:** Beth Israel Med Ctr, 10 Union Square E, New York, NY 10003; **Phone:** 212-420-2398; **Board Cert:** Psychiatry 1979; Psychosomatic Medicine 2005; **Med School:** UMDNJ-NJ Med Sch, Newark 1974; **Resid:** Psychiatry, St Lukes Hosp 1978; **Fellow:** Consultation Psychiatry, Montefiore Med Ctr 1979; Psychosomatic Medicine, Mt Sinai Hosp 1980; **Fac Appt:** Prof Psyc, Mount Sinai Sch Med

Walsh, B Timothy MD (Psyc) - **Spec Exp:** Eating Disorders; **Hospital:** NY State Psychiatric Inst, NY-Presby/Columbia Univ Med Ctr, NY (page 104); **Address:** NY State Psychiatric Inst-Unit 98, 1051 Riverside Dr, New York, NY 10032-2695; **Phone:** 212-543-5739; **Board Cert:** Psychiatry 1978; **Med School:** Harvard Med Sch 1972; **Resid:** Internal Medicine, Dartmouth Affil Hosps 1973; Psychiatry, Bronx Muni Hosp Ctr 1977; **Fac Appt:** Prof Psyc, Columbia P&S

Weill, Terry L MD (Psyc) - **Spec Exp:** Bipolar/Mood Disorders; Psychiatry in Physical Illness; **Hospital:** Mount Sinai Med Ctr (page 102), Beth Israel Med Ctr - Petrie Division (page 94); **Address:** 350 Central Park West, New York, NY 10023-6547; **Phone:** 212-316-5818; **Board Cert:** Psychiatry 1985; **Med School:** Hahnemann Univ 1980; **Resid:** Psychiatry, Mount Sinai Med Ctr 1984; **Fellow:** Psychoanalysis, NYS Psyc Inst 1991; **Fac Appt:** Asst Prof Psyc, Mount Sinai Sch Med

Welsh, Howard K MD (Psyc) - **Spec Exp:** Psychotherapy; Psychoanalysis; **Hospital:** NYU Langone Med Ctr (page 108); **Address:** 27 W 86th St, Ste 1 C, New York, NY 10024-3615; **Phone:** 212-362-5846; **Board Cert:** Psychiatry 1976; **Med School:** Albert Einstein Coll Med 1971; **Resid:** Psychiatry, Kings County Hosp 1974; **Fac Appt:** Clin Prof Psyc, NYU Sch Med

Wilner, Philip MD (Psyc) - **Hospital:** NY-Presby/Weill Cornell Med Ctr, NY (page 104); **Address:** 525 E 68th St, Box 140, New York, NY 10065; **Phone:** 212-746-3705; **Board Cert:** Psychiatry 1989; **Med School:** Columbia P&S 1983; **Resid:** Psychiatry, NY Hosp 1987; **Fellow:** Psychopharmacology, NY Hosp 1991; **Fac Appt:** Assoc Prof Psyc, Cornell Univ-Weill Med Coll

Winters, Richard A MD (Psyc) - **Spec Exp:** Psychopharmacology; Crisis Intervention; Psychodynamic Psychotherapy; **Address:** 201 E 87th St, Ste 12-B, New York, NY 10128; **Phone:** 212-744-1346; **Board Cert:** Psychiatry 1977; **Med School:** NY Med Coll 1972; **Resid:** Psychiatry, Metropolitan Hosp Ctr 1975; **Fac Appt:** Asst Prof Psyc, NY Med Coll

Zimberg, Sheldon MD (Psyc) - **Spec Exp:** Geriatric Psychiatry; Hypnosis; Addiction Psychiatry; **Hospital:** St. Luke's - Roosevelt Hosp Ctr - St Luke's Hosp (page 94), Beth Israel Med Ctr - Petrie Division (page 94); **Address:** 245-A E 61st St, New York, NY 10065; **Phone:** 212-988-5139; **Board Cert:** Psychiatry 1969; Addiction Psychiatry 2004; **Med School:** SUNY Hlth Sci Ctr 1961; **Resid:** Psychiatry, NYS Psych Inst/Colum-Presby Med Ctr 1965; **Fellow:** Community Psychiatry, Columbia Univ Sch Pub Hlth 1966; **Fac Appt:** Clin Prof Psyc, Columbia P&S

Pulmonary Disease

Acquista, Angelo J MD (Pul) - **Spec Exp:** Asthma; Disaster Preparedness; **Hospital:** Lenox Hill Hosp (page 106); **Address:** Madison Medical, 110 E 59th St, Ste 9C, New York, NY 10022; **Phone:** 212-583-2850; **Board Cert:** Internal Medicine 1984; Pulmonary Disease 1986; **Med School:** NYU Sch Med 1981; **Resid:** Internal Medicine, Lenox Hill Hosp 1984; **Fellow:** Pulmonary Disease, Lenox Hill Hosp 1986

Adams, Francis V MD (Pul) - **Spec Exp:** Asthma; Chronic Obstructive Lung Disease (COPD); Pulmonary Fibrosis; Sarcoidosis; **Hospital:** NYU Langone Med Ctr (page 108); **Address:** 650 First Ave, New York, NY 10016-3240; **Phone:** 212-447-0088; **Board Cert:** Internal Medicine 1974; Pulmonary Disease 1976; **Med School:** Cornell Univ-Weill Med Coll 1971; **Resid:** Internal Medicine, Georgetown Univ Hosp 1973; **Fellow:** Pulmonary Disease, Bellevue Hosp 1975; **Fac Appt:** Asst Prof Med, NYU Sch Med

Addrizzo-Harris, Doreen MD (Pul) - **Spec Exp:** Bronchoscopy; Tuberculosis; Lung Cancer; Interstitial Lung Disease; **Hospital:** NYU Langone Med Ctr (page 108), Bellevue Hosp Ctr; **Address:** 530 First Ave Fl 5 - Ste 5E, New York, NY 10016; **Phone:** 212-263-7951; **Board Cert:** Internal Medicine 2002; Pulmonary Disease 2006; Critical Care Medicine 2007; **Med School:** NYU Sch Med 1989; **Resid:** Internal Medicine, Bellevue Hosp/NYU Med Ctr 1992; **Fellow:** Pulmonary Critical Care Medicine, Bellevue Hosp/NYU Med Ctr 1996; **Fac Appt:** Assoc Prof Med, NYU Sch Med

Adler, Jack MD (Pul) - **Spec Exp:** Asthma; Chronic Obstructive Lung Disease (COPD); Tuberculosis; **Hospital:** Mount Sinai Med Ctr (page 102), Lenox Hill Hosp (page 106); **Address:** 210 E 86th St, New York, NY 10028; **Phone:** 212-535-3622; **Board Cert:** Internal Medicine 1970; Pulmonary Disease 1971; **Med School:** Univ Chicago-Pritzker Sch Med 1962; **Resid:** Internal Medicine, Philadelphia Genl Hosp 1967; Internal Medicine, Michael Reese Hosp Med Ctr 1968; **Fellow:** Pulmonary Disease, Bronx Municipal Hosp Ctr 1971; **Fac Appt:** Assoc Prof Med, Mount Sinai Sch Med

Arcasoy, Selim M MD (Pul) - **Spec Exp:** Transplant Medicine-Lung; Chronic Obstructive Lung Disease (COPD); Interstitial Lung Disease; Pulmonary Embolism; **Hospital:** NY-Presby/Columbia Univ Med Ctr, NY (page 104); **Address:** Ctr for Advanced Lung Dis/Transp, 622 W 168th St PH Bldg Fl 14E - rm 104, New York, NY 10032-3720; **Phone:** 212-305-6589; **Board Cert:** Internal Medicine 2003; Pulmonary Disease 2006; Critical Care Medicine 2007; **Med School:** Turkey 1990; **Resid:** Internal Medicine, SUNY Downstate Med Ctr 1994; **Fellow:** Pulmonary Critical Care Medicine, Univ Pittsburgh Med Ctr 1998; **Fac Appt:** Prof Med, Columbia P&S

Baskin, Martin MD (Pul) - **Spec Exp:** Asthma; Pneumonia; Emphysema; **Hospital:** St. Luke's - Roosevelt Hosp Ctr - Roosevelt Div (page 94); **Address:** 185 W End Ave, Ste 1M, New York, NY 10023-5567; **Phone:** 212-595-7701; **Board Cert:** Internal Medicine 1985; Pulmonary Disease 1988; **Med School:** Mount Sinai Sch Med 1981; **Resid:** Internal Medicine, Beth Israel Med Ctr 1984; **Fellow:** Pulmonary Disease, St Luke's Roosevelt Hosp Ctr 1988; Critical Care Medicine, St Luke's Roosevelt Hosp Ctr 1989; **Fac Appt:** Asst Clin Prof Med, Columbia P&S

Basner, Robert C MD (Pul) - **Spec Exp:** Sleep Disorders/Apnea; **Hospital:** NY-Presby/Columbia Univ Med Ctr, NY (page 104); **Address:** 622 W 168th, Ste 859, Columbia University Medical Center, New York, NY 10032; **Phone:** 212-305-7591; **Board Cert:** Internal Medicine 1986; Pulmonary Disease 1988; Sleep Medicine 2009; **Med School:** Columbia P&S 1983; **Resid:** Internal Medicine, Beth Israel Hosp 1986; **Fellow:** Pulmonary Disease, Brigham & Women's Hosp 1989; **Fac Appt:** Assoc Clin Prof Med, Columbia P&S

Bevelaqua, Frederick MD (Pul) - **Spec Exp:** Asthma; Lung Cancer; Chronic Obstructive Lung Disease (COPD); Sarcoidosis; **Hospital:** NYU Langone Med Ctr (page 108); **Address:** 35A E 35th St, Ste 204, New York, NY 10016; **Phone:** 212-213-6796; **Board Cert:** Internal Medicine 1978; Pulmonary Disease 1980; **Med School:** NYU Sch Med 1974; **Resid:** Internal Medicine, NYU Med Ctr 1978; **Fellow:** Pulmonary Disease, NYU Med Ctr 1980; **Fac Appt:** Asst Clin Prof Med, NYU Sch Med

Blair, Lester W MD (Pul) - **Spec Exp:** Asthma; Sarcoidosis; Bronchitis; Chronic Obstructive Lung Disease (COPD); **Hospital:** NY Downtown Hosp; **Address:** 170 William St Fl 7, New York, NY 10038; **Phone:** 646-588-2500; **Board Cert:** Internal Medicine 1987; Pulmonary Disease 1980; Critical Care Medicine 2009; **Med School:** Columbia P&S 1974; **Resid:** Internal Medicine, Columbia-Presby Med Ctr 1977; **Fellow:** Pulmonary Disease, Bellevue Hosp 1979; **Fac Appt:** Assoc Clin Prof Med, Cornell Univ-Weill Med Coll

Burschtin, Omar E MD (Pul) - **Spec Exp:** Sleep Disorders/Apnea; Airway Disorders; Asthma; **Hospital:** NYU Langone Med Ctr (page 108); **Address:** Sleep Medicine Assocs NYC, 11 E 26th St Fl 13, New York, NY 10010; **Phone:** 212-481-1818; **Board Cert:** Pulmonary Disease 2008; Sleep Medicine 2009; **Med School:** Uruguay 1988; **Resid:** Internal Medicine, NYU Downtown Hosp 1994; **Fellow:** Pulmonary Critical Care Medicine, NYU 1998; **Fac Appt:** Asst Prof Med, NYU Sch Med

Cooke, Joseph T MD (Pul) - **Spec Exp:** Asthma; Lung Cancer; Critical Care; Emphysema; **Hospital:** NY-Presby/Weill Cornell Med Ctr, NY (page 104); **Address:** Weill Greenberg Center, Pulmonary/Critical Care Medicine, 1305 York Ave Fl 4, New York, NY 10021; **Phone:** 646-962-2333; **Board Cert:** Internal Medicine 1989; Pulmonary Disease 2002; Critical Care Medicine 2003; **Med School:** SUNY Downstate 1985; **Resid:** Internal Medicine, New York Hosp 1988; **Fellow:** Pulmonary Intensive Care, New York Hosp 1991; **Fac Appt:** Assoc Clin Prof Med, Cornell Univ-Weill Med Coll

DiFabrizio, Larry MD (Pul) - **Hospital:** Lenox Hill Hosp (page 106); **Address:** 5 E 98th St, New York, NY 10029; **Phone:** 212-241-5656; **Board Cert:** Internal Medicine 1987; Critical Care Medicine 2002; Pulmonary Disease 2000; Sleep Medicine 2009; **Med School:** Washington Univ, St Louis 1984; **Resid:** Internal Medicine, Brigham & Womens Hosp 1987; **Fellow:** Pulmonary Critical Care Medicine, Brigham & Womens Hosp 1988; Rheumatology, Columbia-Presby Med Ctr 1990

Eden, Edward MD (Pul) - **Spec Exp:** Emphysema; Asthma; Sarcoidosis; Emphysema/Alpha-1 Antitrypsin Deficiency; **Hospital:** St. Luke's - Roosevelt Hosp Ctr - Roosevelt Div (page 94); **Address:** 425 W 59th St, Ste 8A, New York, NY 10019-1104; **Phone:** 212-492-5500; **Board Cert:** Internal Medicine 1980; Pulmonary Disease 1982; Critical Care Medicine 2007; **Med School:** England, UK 1975; **Resid:** Internal Medicine, Wayne State Univ Affil Hosp 1978; Internal Medicine, Univ Hosp 1980; **Fellow:** Pulmonary Disease, Mount Sinai Hosp 1982; Pulmonary Disease, Columbia-Presby Med Ctr 1985; **Fac Appt:** Assoc Prof Med, Columbia P&S

Fishman, Donald MD (Pul) - **Spec Exp:** Asthma; Chronic Obstructive Lung Disease (COPD); Bronchoscopy; Interstitial Lung Disease; **Hospital:** St. Luke's - Roosevelt Hosp Ctr - Roosevelt Div (page 94), Lenox Hill Hosp (page 106); **Address:** 200 W 57th St, Ste 1201, New York, NY 10019; **Phone:** 212-765-5151; **Board Cert:** Internal Medicine 1976; Pulmonary Disease 1978; **Med School:** Univ Pennsylvania 1973; **Resid:** Internal Medicine, Univ Mich Med Ctr 1976; **Fellow:** Pulmonary Disease, NYU Med Ctr 1978; **Fac Appt:** Asst Clin Prof Med, Columbia P&S

Garay, Stuart M MD (Pul) - **Spec Exp:** Asthma; Chronic Obstructive Lung Disease (COPD); Sleep Apnea; **Hospital:** NYU Langone Med Ctr (page 108); **Address:** New York Pulmonary Associates, 463 Third Ave Fl 2, New York, NY 10016-6025; **Phone:** 212-685-6001; **Board Cert:** Internal Medicine 1977; Pulmonary Disease 1980; **Med School:** Harvard Med Sch 1974; **Resid:** Internal Medicine, Mt Sinai Hosp 1977; **Fellow:** Pulmonary Disease, Bellevue Hosp 1979; **Fac Appt:** Clin Prof Med, NYU Sch Med

Kaplan, Rana MD (Pul) - **Spec Exp:** Asthma; Cystic Fibrosis; **Hospital:** Meml Sloan-Kettering Cancer Ctr (page 116), NY-Presby/Weill Cornell Med Ctr, NY (page 104); **Address:** 1275 York Ave, Ste A3, New York, NY 10065; **Phone:** 212-639-8025; **Board Cert:** Pulmonary Disease 2002; Critical Care Medicine 2004; **Med School:** Cornell Univ-Weill Med Coll 1996; **Resid:** Internal Medicine, New Eng Med Ctr 1999; **Fellow:** Pulmonary Critical Care Medicine, NY Presby Hosp 2003

Klapholz, Ari MD (Pul) - **Spec Exp:** Lung Cancer; Sleep Disorders/Apnea; Emphysema; Asthma; **Hospital:** Beth Israel Med Ctr - Petrie Division (page 94); **Address:** 275 7th Ave Fl 3, New York, NY 10001; **Phone:** 646-660-9999; **Board Cert:** Internal Medicine 1987; Pulmonary Disease 2010; Critical Care Medicine 2011; Sleep Medicine 2007; **Med School:** NY Med Coll 1984; **Resid:** Internal Medicine, Beth Israel Med Ctr 1987; **Fellow:** Pulmonary Disease, Beth Israel Med Ctr 1989; Critical Care Medicine, Mount Sinai Med Ctr 1990; **Fac Appt:** Asst Prof Med, Mount Sinai Sch Med

Kolodny, Erwin MD (Pul) - **Spec Exp:** Asthma; Emphysema; Bronchitis; **Hospital:** NYU Langone Med Ctr (page 108); **Address:** 650 1st Ave, New York, NY 10016-3240; **Phone:** 212-213-0090; **Board Cert:** Internal Medicine 1977; Pulmonary Disease 1978; **Med School:** NYU Sch Med 1973; **Resid:** Internal Medicine, Bellevue Hosp 1976; **Fellow:** Pulmonary Disease, NYU Med Ctr 1978; **Fac Appt:** Asst Clin Prof Med, NYU Sch Med

Krieger, Ana C MD (Pul) - **Spec Exp:** Sleep Disorders/Apnea; Narcolepsy; Pulmonary Hypertension; **Hospital:** NY-Presby/Weill Cornell Med Ctr, NY (page 104); **Address:** Weill Cornell Center for Sleep Medicine, 425 E 61st St Fl 5, New York, NY 10065; **Phone:** 646-962-7378; **Board Cert:** Internal Medicine 2011; Pulmonary Disease 2011; Sleep Medicine 2000; **Med School:** Brazil 1992; **Resid:** Internal Medicine, Univ Chicago Hosps 1996; **Fellow:** Critical Care Medicine, Finch/Chicago Med Sch 1998; Pulmonary Disease, NYU 2000; **Fac Appt:** Assoc Prof Med, Cornell Univ-Weill Med Coll

Lederer, David MD (Pul) - **Spec Exp:** Transplant-Lung; Pulmonary Fibrosis; Interstitial Lung Disease; **Hospital:** NY-Presby/Columbia Univ Med Ctr, NY (page 104); **Address:** 622 W 168t St, PH-14, Room 104, New York, NY 10032; **Phone:** 212-305-7771; **Board Cert:** Pulmonary Disease 2005; Internal Medicine 2002; Critical Care Medicine 2006; **Med School:** SUNY Downstate 1999; **Resid:** Internal Medicine, NY Presby/Columbia Med Ctr 2003; **Fellow:** Pulmonary Critical Care Medicine, NY Presby/Columbia Med Ctr 2006; **Fac Appt:** Asst Prof Med, Columbia P&S

Lee, Marjorie MD (Pul) - **Spec Exp:** Asthma; Emphysema; Sarcoidosis; **Hospital:** Beth Israel Med Ctr - Petrie Division (page 94); **Address:** 247 3rd Ave, Ste 403, New York, NY 10010-7455; **Phone:** 212-533-1185; **Board Cert:** Internal Medicine 1976; Pulmonary Disease 1978; **Med School:** SUNY Hlth Sci Ctr 1973; **Resid:** Internal Medicine, Kaiser Hosp 1976; Pulmonary Disease, Cabrini Hosp 1977; **Fellow:** Pulmonary Disease, Yale-New Haven Hosp 1979

Libby, Daniel M MD (Pul) - **Spec Exp:** Asthma; Lung Cancer; Interstitial Lung Disease; Chronic Obstructive Lung Disease (COPD); **Hospital:** NY-Presby/Weill Cornell Med Ctr, NY (page 104); **Address:** 635 Madison Ave, Ste 1101, New York, NY 10022; **Phone:** 212-628-6611; **Board Cert:** Internal Medicine 1977; Pulmonary Disease 1980; **Med School:** Baylor Coll Med 1974; **Resid:** Internal Medicine, NY Hosp 1977; **Fellow:** Pulmonary Disease, NY Hosp 1979; **Fac Appt:** Clin Prof Med, Cornell Univ-Weill Med Coll

Lowy, Joseph MD (Pul) - **Spec Exp:** Lung Cancer; Asthma; Chronic Obstructive Lung Disease (COPD); **Hospital:** NYU Langone Med Ctr (page 108); **Address:** 530 First Ave, HCC-Suite 4F, New York, NY 10016; **Phone:** 212-263-6202; **Board Cert:** Internal Medicine 1983; Pulmonary Disease 1986; Hospice & Palliative Medicine 2008; **Med School:** Univ Rochester 1980; **Resid:** Internal Medicine, Bellevue Hosp 1983; **Fellow:** Pulmonary Disease, UCSD Med Ctr 1986; **Fac Appt:** Assoc Clin Prof Med, NYU Sch Med

Maxfield, Roger A MD (Pul) - **Spec Exp:** Emphysema & Asthma; Occupational Lung Disease; Lung Cancer; Bronchoscopy; **Hospital:** NY-Presby/Columbia Univ Med Ctr, NY (page 104); **Address:** Columbia Presbyterian Eastside, 16 E 60th St, Ste 320, New York, NY 10022-1002; **Phone:** 212-326-8415; **Board Cert:** Internal Medicine 1980; Pulmonary Disease 1986; **Med School:** Brown Univ 1977; **Resid:** Internal Medicine, Georgetown Univ Hosp 1980; **Fellow:** Pulmonary Disease, Bellevue-NYU Med Ctr 1985; **Fac Appt:** Clin Prof Med, Columbia P&S

Miller, Rachel L MD (Pul) - **Spec Exp:** Asthma; **Hospital:** NY-Presby/Columbia Univ Med Ctr, NY (page 104); **Address:** 622 W 168th St - PH8, New York, NY 10032; **Phone:** 212-305-0631; **Board Cert:** Internal Medicine 1993; Pulmonary Disease 1996; Critical Care Medicine 1997; Allergy & Immunology 1999; **Med School:** NYU Sch Med 1990; **Resid:** Internal Medicine, NY Presby/Columbia Med Ctr 1993; **Fellow:** Pulmonary Critical Care Medicine, NY Presby/Columbia Med Ctr 1995

Nash, Thomas MD (Pul) - **Spec Exp:** Asthma; Cough; Pneumonia; **Hospital:** NY-Presby/Weill Cornell Med Ctr, NY (page 104), Hosp For Special Surgery (page 115); **Address:** 310 E 72nd St, New York, NY 10021-4726; **Phone:** 212-734-6612; **Board Cert:** Internal Medicine 1981; Infectious Disease 1984; Pulmonary Disease 1988; **Med School:** NYU Sch Med 1978; **Resid:** Internal Medicine, New York Hosp-Cornell 1981; **Fellow:** Infectious Disease, New York Hosp-Cornell 1983; Pulmonary Disease, Meml Sloan Kettering Cancer Ctr 1985; **Fac Appt:** Assoc Clin Prof Med, NYU Sch Med

Nelson, Judith E MD (Pul) - **Spec Exp:** Palliative Care; Critical Care; **Hospital:** Mount Sinai Med Ctr (page 102); **Address:** Mt Sinai Medical Ctr, One Gustave Levy Pl, Box 1232, New York, NY 10029; **Phone:** 212-241-2587; **Board Cert:** Internal Medicine 1989; Pulmonary Disease 2002; Critical Care Medicine 2003; Hospice & Palliative Medicine 2005; **Med School:** NYU Sch Med 1986; **Resid:** Internal Medicine, Mt Sinai Med Ctr 1989; **Fellow:** Pulmonary Critical Care Medicine, Mt Sinai Med Ctr 1992; **Fac Appt:** Assoc Prof Med, Mount Sinai Sch Med

Padilla, Maria L MD (Pul) - **Spec Exp:** Pulmonary Fibrosis; Transplant Medicine-Lung; Sarcoidosis; Pulmonary Hypertension; **Hospital:** Mount Sinai Med Ctr (page 102); **Address:** Mt Sinai Med Ctr, Div Pulmonology, One Gustave L Levy Pl, Box 1232, New York, NY 10029-6574; **Phone:** 212-241-5656; **Board Cert:** Internal Medicine 1978; Pulmonary Disease 1980; **Med School:** Mount Sinai Sch Med 1975; **Resid:** Internal Medicine, Mt Sinai Hosp 1978; **Fellow:** Pulmonary Disease, Mt Sinai Hosp 1980; Critical Care Medicine, Mt Sinai Hosp 1991; **Fac Appt:** Prof Med, Mount Sinai Sch Med

Posner, David H MD (Pul) - **Spec Exp:** Interstitial Lung Disease; Lung Cancer; Sarcoidosis; Pulmonary Fibrosis; **Hospital:** Lenox Hill Hosp (page 106), NY-Presby/Weill Cornell Med Ctr, NY (page 104); **Address:** 178 E 85th St, Fl 3, New York, NY 10028-2119; **Phone:** 212-737-0470; **Board Cert:** Internal Medicine 1984; Pulmonary Disease 1988; **Med School:** NY Med Coll 1981; **Resid:** Internal Medicine, Lenox Hill Hosp 1985; **Fellow:** Pulmonary Disease, LI Jewish Med Ctr 1987; **Fac Appt:** Assoc Clin Prof Med, NYU Sch Med

Prager, Kenneth MD (Pul) - **Spec Exp:** Lung Disease; Asthma; Ethics; **Hospital:** NY-Presby/Columbia Univ Med Ctr, NY (page 104); **Address:** 161 Ft Washington Ave, Ste 310, New York, NY 10032; **Phone:** 212-305-5535; **Board Cert:** Internal Medicine 1973; **Med School:** Harvard Med Sch 1968; **Resid:** Internal Medicine, Columbia-Presby Med Ctr 1972; Internal Medicine, Billings Hosp 1973; **Fac Appt:** Clin Prof Med, Columbia P&S

Rapoport, David M MD (Pul) - **Spec Exp:** Sleep Disorders/Apnea; Sleep Medicine; Hepatopulmonary Syndrome; **Hospital:** Bellevue Hosp Ctr, NYU Langone Med Ctr (page 108); **Address:** 462 1st Ave, rm 7W54, New York, NY 10016-6402; **Phone:** 212-263-6407; **Board Cert:** Internal Medicine 1977; Pulmonary Disease 1980; Sleep Medicine 2007; **Med School:** Albert Einstein Coll Med 1974; **Resid:** Internal Medicine, Roosevelt Hosp 1977; **Fellow:** Pulmonary Disease, NYU/Bellevue Med Ctr 1979; **Fac Appt:** Assoc Prof Med, NYU Sch Med

Raskin, Jonathan MD (Pul) - **Spec Exp:** Asthma; Chronic Obstructive Lung Disease (COPD); Pulmonary Rehabilitation; **Hospital:** Beth Israel Med Ctr - Petrie Division (page 94), Lenox Hill Hosp (page 106); **Address:** 1000 Park Ave, New York, NY 10028-0934; **Phone:** 212-288-4600; **Board Cert:** Internal Medicine 1982; Pulmonary Disease 1984; **Med School:** Mexico 1978; **Resid:** Internal Medicine, Beth Israel Med Ctr 1982; **Fellow:** Pulmonary Disease, Mount Sinai Hosp 1985; **Fac Appt:** Asst Clin Prof Med, Albert Einstein Coll Med

Sanders, Abraham MD (Pul) - **Hospital:** NY-Presby/Weill Cornell Med Ctr, NY (page 104), Hosp For Special Surgery (page 115); **Address:** 1305 York Ave Fl 4, New York, NY 10021; **Phone:** 646-962-2333; **Board Cert:** Internal Medicine 1979; Pulmonary Disease 1982; Critical Care Medicine 2008; **Med School:** SUNY Downstate 1976; **Resid:** Internal Medicine, Univ Hosp/Kings County Hosp 1980; **Fellow:** Pulmonary Disease, Kings County Hosp 1980; Pulmonary Disease, Royal Postgraduate Sch Med 1981; **Fac Appt:** Assoc Prof Med, Cornell Univ-Weill Med Coll

Schluger, Neil MD (Pul) - **Spec Exp:** Tuberculosis; **Hospital:** NY-Presby/Columbia Univ Med Ctr, NY (page 104); **Address:** Div Pulm, Allergy & Crit Care Med, 630 W 168th St, PH-8 East, Rm 101, New York, NY 10032; **Phone:** 212-305-1544; **Board Cert:** Internal Medicine 1988; Pulmonary Disease 2003; **Med School:** Univ Pennsylvania 1985; **Resid:** Internal Medicine, St Lukes Hosp 1989; **Fellow:** Pulmonary Critical Care Medicine, NY Hosp-Cornell 1992; **Fac Appt:** Prof Med, Columbia P&S

Steiger, David MD (Pul) - **Spec Exp:** Rheumatologic Diseases of the Lung; Thromboembolic Disorders; Pulmonary Hypertension; Critical Care; **Hospital:** NYU Hosp For Joint Diseases (page 119), NYU Langone Med Ctr (page 108); **Address:** 305 2nd Ave, Ste 16, New York, NY 10003; **Phone:** 212-598-6422; **Board Cert:** Internal Medicine 1987; Pulmonary Disease 2002; Critical Care Medicine 2005; **Med School:** England, UK 1981; **Resid:** Internal Medicine, St Thomas's Hosp 1984; Internal Medicine, St Lukes Hosp 1989; **Fellow:** Pulmonary Disease, UCSF Med Ctr 1994; **Fac Appt:** Asst Prof Med, NYU Sch Med

Stein, Sidney MD (Pul) - **Spec Exp:** Asthma; Bronchitis; Emphysema; Hiccups-Chronic; **Hospital:** Beth Israel Med Ctr - Petrie Division (page 94); **Address:** 55 E 34th St Fl 6, New York, NY 10016-4337; **Phone:** 212-879-7777; **Board Cert:** Internal Medicine 1982; Pulmonary Disease 1988; **Med School:** SUNY Hlth Sci Ctr 1979; **Resid:** Internal Medicine, Beth Israel Med Ctr 1982; **Fellow:** Pulmonary Disease, Beth Israel Med Ctr 1984; **Fac Appt:** Asst Clin Prof Med, Albert Einstein Coll Med

Stover-Pepe, Diane E MD (Pul) - **Spec Exp:** Interstitial Lung Disease; Pulmonary Infections; Pulmonary Disease/Immunocompromised; Bronchiolitis Obliterans; **Hospital:** Meml Sloan-Kettering Cancer Ctr (page 116); **Address:** 1275 York Ave, New York, NY 10065; **Phone:** 212-639-8380; **Board Cert:** Internal Medicine 1975; Pulmonary Disease 1978; **Med School:** Albert Einstein Coll Med 1970; **Resid:** Internal Medicine, Harlem Hosp Ctr 1972; Internal Medicine, NY Hosp-Cornell Med Ctr 1975; **Fellow:** Pulmonary Disease, Montefiore Med Ctr 1977; **Fac Appt:** Prof Med, Cornell Univ-Weill Med Coll

Sukumaran, Muthiah MD (Pul) - **Spec Exp:** Asthma; Chronic Obstructive Lung Disease (COPD); Lung Cancer; Tuberculosis; **Hospital:** NY Downtown Hosp, NYU Langone Med Ctr (page 108); **Address:** Trinty Medical Centre, 111 Broadway, New York, NY 10006; **Phone:** 212-263-9700; **Board Cert:** Internal Medicine 1976; Pulmonary Disease 1980; **Med School:** India 1973; **Resid:** Internal Medicine, Elmhurst City Hosp 1976; **Fellow:** Pulmonary Disease, Elmhurst City Hosp 1977; **Fac Appt:** Assoc Clin Prof Med, NY Med Coll

Thomashow, Byron MD (Pul) - **Spec Exp:** Emphysema; Asthma; Respiratory Failure; Chronic Obstructive Lung Disease (COPD); **Hospital:** NY-Presby/Columbia Univ Med Ctr, NY (page 104); **Address:** 161 Fort Washington Ave, rm 311, New York, NY 10032; **Phone:** 212-305-5261; **Board Cert:** Internal Medicine 1977; Pulmonary Disease 1980; **Med School:** Columbia P&S 1974; **Resid:** Internal Medicine, Roosevelt Hosp 1977; Pulmonary Disease, Roosevelt Hosp 1978; **Fellow:** Pulmonary Disease, Harlem Hosp Ctr 1979; **Fac Appt:** Clin Prof Med, Columbia P&S

Villamena, Patricia C MD (Pul) - **Spec Exp:** Lung Cancer; Chronic Obstructive Lung Disease (COPD); Critical Care; **Hospital:** Beth Israel Med Ctr - Petrie Division (page 94); **Address:** Beth Israel Med Ctr, 1st Ave & 16th St, Dazian Bldg, 7th Fl, Pulm Div, New York, NY 10003; **Phone:** 212-420-2377; **Board Cert:** Internal Medicine 1989; Pulmonary Disease 2006; **Med School:** NY Med Coll 1977; **Resid:** Internal Medicine, Metropolitan Hosp 1980; **Fellow:** Pulmonary Disease, Beth Israel Med Ctr 1986; **Fac Appt:** Asst Prof Med, Albert Einstein Coll Med

Yip, Chun MD (Pul) - **Spec Exp:** Asthma; Emphysema; Chronic Obstructive Lung Disease (COPD); **Hospital:** NY-Presby/Columbia Univ Med Ctr, NY (page 104); **Address:** 67 Hudson St Fl 1A, New York, NY 10013; **Phone:** 212-305-8548; **Board Cert:** Internal Medicine 1979; Pulmonary Disease 1984; **Med School:** Albert Einstein Coll Med 1976; **Resid:** Internal Medicine, Columbia-Presby Med Ctr 1979; **Fellow:** Pulmonary Disease, Bellevue Hosp Ctr 1981; **Fac Appt:** Clin Prof Med, Columbia P&S

Radiation Oncology

Chadha, Manjeet MD (RadRO) - **Spec Exp:** Breast Cancer; Gynecologic Cancer; **Hospital:** Beth Israel Med Ctr - Petrie Division (page 94), St. Luke's - Roosevelt Hosp Ctr - St Luke's Hosp (page 94); **Address:** Charles & Bernice Blitman Dept, Div of Radiation Oncology, 10 Union Square E, Ste 4G, New York, NY 10003; **Phone:** 212-844-8022; **Board Cert:** Therapeutic Radiology 1985; **Med School:** India 1980; **Resid:** Radiation Oncology, Columbia Presby Med Ctr 1983; Radiation Oncology, Meml Sloan Kettering Cancer Ctr 1985; **Fellow:** Radiation Oncology, Meml Sloan Kettering Cancer Ctr 1986; **Fac Appt:** Assoc Prof RadRO, Albert Einstein Coll Med

Chao, KS Clifford MD (RadRO) - **Spec Exp:** Intensity Modulated Radiotherapy (IMRT); **Hospital:** NY-Presby/Weill Cornell Med Ctr, NY (page 104); **Address:** 622 W 168th St, New York, NY 10032; **Phone:** 212-305-9987; **Board Cert:** Radiation Oncology 2010; **Med School:** Taiwan 1982; **Resid:** Radiation Oncology, Mallinckrodt Inst Rad-Wash Med Ctr 1993; **Fellow:** Radiation Oncology, Mallinckrodt Inst Rad-Wash Med Ctr 1994; **Fac Appt:** Prof RadRO, Cornell Univ-Weill Med Coll

Ennis, Ronald D MD (RadRO) - **Spec Exp:** Prostate Cancer; Brachytherapy; Breast Cancer; Stereotactic Radiosurgery; **Hospital:** St. Luke's - Roosevelt Hosp Ctr - Roosevelt Div (page 94), Beth Israel Med Ctr - Petrie Division (page 94); **Address:** 1000 10th Ave, Lower Level, Dept Radiation Oncology, Roosevelt Hospital, New York, NY 10019; **Phone:** 212-523-7165; **Board Cert:** Radiation Oncology 2004; **Med School:** Yale Univ 1990; **Resid:** Therapeutic Radiology, Yale-New Haven Hosp 1994; **Fac Appt:** Assoc Prof RadRO, Albert Einstein Coll Med

Formenti, Silvia C MD (RadRO) - **Spec Exp:** Breast Cancer; Chemo-Radiation Combined Therapy; **Hospital:** NYU Langone Med Ctr (page 108); **Address:** NYU Med Ctr, Dept Radiation Oncology, 160 E 34th St, New York, NY 10016; **Phone:** 212-263-2601; **Board Cert:** Radiation Oncology 1991; **Med School:** Italy 1980; **Resid:** Internal Medicine, San Carlo Borromeo Hosp 1983; Medical Oncology, Univ of Pavia Med Ctr 1985; **Fellow:** Radiation Oncology, USC Med Ctr 1990; **Fac Appt:** Prof RadRO, NYU Sch Med

Harrison, Louis B MD (RadRO) - **Spec Exp:** Brachytherapy; Head & Neck Cancer; Radiation Therapy-Intraoperative; **Hospital:** Beth Israel Med Ctr - Petrie Division (page 94), St. Luke's - Roosevelt Hosp Ctr - Roosevelt Div (page 94); **Address:** Beth Israel Med Ctr, Dept Rad Onc, 10 Union Square East, Ste 4G, New York, NY 10003-3314; **Phone:** 212-844-8087; **Board Cert:** Therapeutic Radiology 1986; **Med School:** SUNY Downstate 1982; **Resid:** Therapeutic Radiology, Yale-New Haven Hosp 1986; **Fac Appt:** Prof RadRO, Albert Einstein Coll Med

Hayes, Mary Katherine MD (RadRO) - **Spec Exp:** Breast Cancer; **Hospital:** NY-Presby/Weill Cornell Med Ctr, NY (page 104); **Address:** 525 E 68th St, Box 575, New York, NY 10065; **Phone:** 212-746-3679; **Board Cert:** Radiation Oncology 1988; **Med School:** Dominica 1984; **Resid:** Radiation Oncology, Meml Sloan Kettering Cancer Ctr 1988; **Fac Appt:** Assoc Clin Prof RadRO, Cornell Univ

Isaacson, Steven R MD (RadRO) - **Spec Exp:** Brain Tumors; Neuro-Oncology; Stereotactic Radiosurgery; Gliomas; **Hospital:** NY-Presby/Columbia Univ Med Ctr, NY (page 104); **Address:** NY Presbyterian-Columbia Med Ctr, Dept Radiation Oncology, 622 W 168th St BHN Bldg - rm B-11, New York, NY 10032-3720; **Phone:** 212-305-2611; **Board Cert:** Radiation Oncology 1988; Otolaryngology 1978; **Med School:** Jefferson Med Coll 1973; **Resid:** Otolaryngology, Hosp Univ Penn 1978; Radiation Oncology, SUNY Hlth Sci Ctr 1988; **Fac Appt:** Clin Prof RadRO, Columbia P&S

Lee, Nancy MD (RadRO) - **Spec Exp:** Intensity Modulated Radiotherapy (IMRT); Head & Neck Cancer; Skin Cancer; **Hospital:** Meml Sloan-Kettering Cancer Ctr (page 116); **Address:** MSKCC, Dept Rad Onc, 1275 York Ave, New York, NY 10065; **Phone:** 212-639-3341; **Board Cert:** Radiation Oncology 2000; **Med School:** UMDNJ-NJ Med Sch, Newark 1995; **Resid:** Radiation Oncology, NY-Presby/Columbia Med Ctr 2001

McCormick, Beryl MD (RadRO) - **Spec Exp:** Breast Cancer; Eye Tumors/Cancer; **Hospital:** Meml Sloan-Kettering Cancer Ctr (page 116); **Address:** 1275 York Avenue, New York, NY 10065; **Phone:** 212-639-6828; **Board Cert:** Therapeutic Radiology 1977; **Med School:** UMDNJ-NJ Med Sch, Newark 1973; **Resid:** Therapeutic Radiology, Meml Sloan Kettering Cancer Ctr 1977; **Fac Appt:** Prof RadRO, Cornell Univ-Weill Med Coll

Ng, John Paul Tracy MD (RadRO) - **Spec Exp:** Prostate Cancer; Head & Neck Cancer; **Address:** 408 Broadway, New York, NY 10013; **Phone:** 212-925-8882; **Board Cert:** Radiation Oncology 1993; **Med School:** Albert Einstein Coll Med 1988; **Resid:** Radiation Oncology, Meml Sloan Kettering Cancer Ctr 1992; **Fac Appt:** Asst Prof RadRO, NY Med Coll

Nori, Dattatreyudu MD (RadRO) - **Spec Exp:** Prostate Cancer; Brachytherapy; Lung Cancer; Breast Cancer; **Hospital:** NY-Presby/Weill Cornell Med Ctr, NY (page 104), NY Hosp Queens (page 206); **Address:** 525 E 68th St, Box 575, New York, NY 10065; **Phone:** 212-746-3679; **Board Cert:** Therapeutic Radiology 1979; **Med School:** India 1970; **Resid:** Radiation Oncology, Meml Sloan Kettering Cancer Ctr 1975; **Fellow:** Radiation Oncology, Meml Sloan Kettering Cancer Ctr 1978; **Fac Appt:** Prof RadRO, Cornell Univ-Weill Med Coll

Parashar, Bhupesh MD (RadRO) - **Spec Exp:** Head & Neck Cancer; Lung Cancer; Breast Cancer; Gastrointestinal Cancer; **Hospital:** NY-Presby/Weill Cornell Med Ctr, NY (page 104); **Address:** NY Presbyterian-Cornell Med Ctr, 525 E 68th St, rm N046, New York, NY 10065; **Phone:** 212-746-3612; **Board Cert:** Radiation Oncology 2006; **Med School:** India 1994; **Resid:** Radiation Oncology, Montefiore-Weiler Einstein Med Ctr 2005; **Fac Appt:** Asst Clin Prof Rad, Cornell Univ-Weill Med Coll

Rosenbaum, Alfred MD (RadRO) - **Spec Exp:** Breast Cancer; Prostate Cancer; Intensity Modulated Radiotherapy (IMRT); **Hospital:** Mount Sinai Med Ctr (page 102), Lenox Hill Hosp (page 106); **Address:** Rosetta Radiology, 1421 Third Ave, New York, NY 10028; **Phone:** 212-744-5538; **Board Cert:** Diagnostic Radiology 1973; **Med School:** Germany 1966; **Resid:** Diagnostic Radiology, Maimonides Med Ctr 1970; Radiation Oncology, Mount Sinai Hosp 1972; **Fellow:** Diagnostic Radiology, Montefiore Med Ctr 1973; **Fac Appt:** Asst Clin Prof, Mount Sinai Sch Med

Schiff, Peter B MD/PhD (RadRO) - **Spec Exp:** Prostate Cancer; Gynecologic Cancer; Lung Cancer; **Hospital:** NYU Langone Med Ctr (page 108); **Address:** NYU Clinical Cancer Ctr, 160 E 34th St Fl 1, New York, NY 10016; **Phone:** 212-731-5003; **Board Cert:** Radiation Oncology 1990; **Med School:** Albert Einstein Coll Med 1984; **Resid:** Radiation Oncology, Meml Sloan Kettering Cancer Ctr 1988; **Fac Appt:** Prof RadRO, NYU Sch Med

Sherr, David L MD (RadRO) - **Spec Exp:** Intensity Modulated Radiotherapy (IMRT); Stereotactic Radiosurgery; Image Guided Radiotherapy (IGRT); **Hospital:** Mount Sinai Med Ctr (page 102); **Address:** Rosetta Radiology, 1421 Third Ave, New York, NY 10028; **Phone:** 212-744-5538; **Board Cert:** Radiation Oncology 1987; **Med School:** Albert Einstein Coll Med 1981; **Resid:** Internal Medicine, Brookdale Hosp Med Ctr 1983; Radiation Oncology, Columbia-Presby Med Ctr 1986

Stock, Richard MD (RadRO) - **Spec Exp:** Prostate Cancer; Urologic Cancer; **Hospital:** Mount Sinai Med Ctr (page 102); **Address:** Dept Radiation Oncology, 1184 5th Ave, Box 1236, New York, NY 10029; **Phone:** 212-241-7502; **Board Cert:** Radiation Oncology 1993; **Med School:** Mount Sinai Sch Med 1988; **Resid:** Radiation Oncology, Meml Sloan Kettering Cancer Ctr 1992; **Fac Appt:** Prof RadRO, Mount Sinai Sch Med

Yahalom, Joachim MD (RadRO) - **Spec Exp:** Lymphoma; Hodgkin's Lymphoma; Multiple Myeloma; **Hospital:** Meml Sloan-Kettering Cancer Ctr (page 116); **Address:** 1275 York Ave, SM03, Dept Radiation Onc, New York, NY 10065; **Phone:** 212-639-5999; **Board Cert:** Radiation Oncology 1988; **Med School:** Israel 1976; **Resid:** Internal Medicine, Hadassah Hosp 1979; Radiation Oncology, Hadassah Hosp 1984; **Fellow:** Radiation Oncology, Meml Sloan Kettering Canc Ctr 1986; **Fac Appt:** Prof RadRO, Cornell Univ-Weill Med Coll

Zelefsky, Michael J MD (RadRO) - **Spec Exp:** Prostate Cancer; Brachytherapy; Head & Neck Cancer; **Hospital:** Meml Sloan-Kettering Cancer Ctr (page 116); **Address:** 1275 York Ave, New York, NY 10065; **Phone:** 212-639-6802; **Board Cert:** Radiation Oncology 1991; **Med School:** Albert Einstein Coll Med 1986; **Resid:** Radiation Oncology, Meml Sloan Kettering Cancer Ctr 1990; **Fac Appt:** Prof RadRO, Cornell Univ-Weill Med Coll

Reproductive Endocrinology

Chang, Peter L MD (RE) - **Spec Exp:** Infertility-IVF; Polycystic Ovarian Syndrome; **Hospital:** Beth Israel Med Ctr - Petrie Division (page 94); **Address:** 10 Union Square East, Ste 2E, New York, NY 10003; **Phone:** 212-844-8587; **Board Cert:** Obstetrics & Gynecology 2011; Reproductive Endocrinology/Infertility 2011; **Med School:** Univ Tex, San Antonio 1992; **Resid:** Obstetrics & Gynecology, Univ TX Hlth Sci Ctr 1996; **Fellow:** Reproductive Endocrinology, Columbia P&S 1998; **Fac Appt:** Asst Prof ObG, Albert Einstein Coll Med

Cholst, Ina N MD (RE) - **Spec Exp:** Laparoscopic Surgery; Infertility-IVF; Menopause Problems; **Hospital:** NY-Presby/Weill Cornell Med Ctr, NY (page 104); **Address:** Ctr for Reproductive Med & Infertility, 1305 York Ave Fl 6, New York, NY 10021; **Phone:** 646-962-3025; **Board Cert:** Obstetrics & Gynecology 1984; Reproductive Endocrinology 1985; **Med School:** NYU Sch Med 1977; **Resid:** Obstetrics & Gynecology, Yale-New Haven Hosp 1981; **Fellow:** Reproductive Endocrinology, Columbia-Presby Med Ctr 1983; **Fac Appt:** Assoc Prof ObG, Cornell Univ-Weill Med Coll

Copperman, Alan B MD (RE) - **Spec Exp:** Infertility-IVF; Fertility Preservation in Cancer; Hysteroscopic Surgery; **Hospital:** Mount Sinai Med Ctr (page 102); **Address:** 635 Madison Ave, Fl 10, New York, NY 10022; **Phone:** 212-756-5777; **Board Cert:** Obstetrics & Gynecology 2011; Reproductive Endocrinology 2011; **Med School:** NY Med Coll 1989; **Resid:** Obstetrics & Gynecology, Yale-New Haven Hosp 1993; **Fellow:** Reproductive Endocrinology, Mt Sinai Med Ctr 1995; **Fac Appt:** Clin Prof ObG, Mount Sinai Sch Med

David, Sami MD (RE) - **Spec Exp:** Infertility; Miscarriage-Recurrent; Endometriosis; Uterine Fibroids; **Hospital:** Mount Sinai Med Ctr (page 102); **Address:** 1045 Fifth Ave, Ste 1A, New York, NY 10028-1002; **Phone:** 212-831-0430; **Board Cert:** Obstetrics & Gynecology 1980; **Med School:** Columbia P&S 1971; **Resid:** Obstetrics & Gynecology, New York Hosp 1976; **Fellow:** Reproductive Endocrinology, Hosp Univ Penn 1978; **Fac Appt:** Prof ObG, Mount Sinai Sch Med

Davis, Owen K MD (RE) - **Spec Exp:** Infertility-IVF; Reproductive Surgery; **Hospital:** NY-Presby/Weill Cornell Med Ctr, NY (page 104); **Address:** 1305 York Ave, Fl 6, New York, NY 10021-4872; **Phone:** 646-962-3765; **Board Cert:** Obstetrics & Gynecology 2011; Reproductive Endocrinology/Infertility 2011; **Med School:** Wake Forest Univ 1982; **Resid:** Obstetrics & Gynecology, NY Hosp 1986; **Fellow:** Reproductive Endocrinology, Brigham & Women's Hosp 1988; **Fac Appt:** Prof ObG, Cornell Univ-Weill Med Coll

Fateh, Majid MD (RE) - **Spec Exp:** Endometriosis; Laparoscopic Surgery; Infertility; **Hospital:** Lenox Hill Hosp (page 106); **Address:** 1016 5th Ave, New York, NY 10028-0132; **Phone:** 212-734-5555; **Board Cert:** Obstetrics & Gynecology 2010; **Med School:** West Indies 1980; **Resid:** Obstetrics & Gynecology, Lenox Hill Hosp 1984; **Fellow:** Reproductive Endocrinology, Univ Penn 1986

Grifo, James A MD/PhD (RE) - **Spec Exp:** Preimplantation Genetic Diagnosis; Fertility Preservation in Cancer; Hysteroscopic Surgery; Laparoscopic Surgery; **Hospital:** NYU Langone Med Ctr (page 108); **Address:** 660 1st Ave, Fl 5, New York, NY 10016; **Phone:** 212-263-7978; **Board Cert:** Obstetrics & Gynecology 2011; Reproductive Endocrinology 2011; **Med School:** Case West Res Univ 1984; **Resid:** Obstetrics & Gynecology, NY Hosp-Cornell Med Ctr 1988; **Fellow:** Reproductive Endocrinology, Yale-New Haven Hosp 1990; **Fac Appt:** Prof ObG, NYU Sch Med

Grunfeld, Lawrence MD (RE) - **Spec Exp:** Infertility-IVF; Hysteroscopic Surgery; Laparoscopic Surgery; **Hospital:** Mount Sinai Med Ctr (page 102), Lenox Hill Hosp (page 106); **Address:** 635 Madison Ave, Fl 10, New York, NY 10022-1009; **Phone:** 212-756-5777; **Board Cert:** Obstetrics & Gynecology 2011; Reproductive Endocrinology 2011; **Med School:** Mount Sinai Sch Med 1979; **Resid:** Obstetrics & Gynecology, Montefiore Med Ctr 1984; **Fellow:** Reproductive Endocrinology, Montefiore Med Ctr 1987; **Fac Appt:** Assoc Clin Prof ObG, Mount Sinai Sch Med

Keefe, David Lawrence MD (RE) - **Spec Exp:** Infertility-IVF; Infertility-Advanced Maternal Age; **Hospital:** NYU Langone Med Ctr (page 108); **Address:** 660 First Ave Fl 5, New York, NY 10016; **Phone:** 212-263-8990; **Board Cert:** Obstetrics & Gynecology 2011; Reproductive Endocrinology 2011; **Med School:** Georgetown Univ 1980; **Resid:** Psychiatry, Harvard Psych Srv/Camb Hosp 1983; Obstetrics & Gynecology, Yale New Haven Hosp 1989; **Fellow:** Psychiatry, Univ Chicago Hosp & Clins 1985; Reproductive Endocrinology, Yale New Haven Hosp 1991; **Fac Appt:** Prof ObG, Univ S Fla Coll Med

Keltz, Martin D MD (RE) - **Spec Exp:** Infertility-IVF; Pregnancy Loss-Recurrent; **Hospital:** St. Luke's - Roosevelt Hosp Ctr - Roosevelt Div (page 94); **Address:** 425 W 59th St, Ste 5A, New York, NY 10019; **Phone:** 212-523-7751; **Board Cert:** Obstetrics & Gynecology 2010; Reproductive Endocrinology 2010; **Med School:** NYU Sch Med 1989; **Resid:** Obstetrics & Gynecology, NYU/Bellevue Hosp 1993; **Fellow:** Reproductive Endocrinology, Yale-New Haven Hosp 1996; **Fac Appt:** Assoc Clin Prof ObG, Columbia P&S

Licciardi, Frederick L MD (RE) - **Spec Exp:** Infertility-IVF; Infertility; Fertility Preservation in Cancer; **Hospital:** NYU Langone Med Ctr (page 108); **Address:** NYU Medical Ctr, 660 First Ave, 5th Fl, New York, NY 10016; **Phone:** 212-263-7754; **Board Cert:** Obstetrics & Gynecology 2007; Reproductive Endocrinology 2007; **Med School:** UMDNJ-Rutgers Med Sch 1986; **Resid:** Obstetrics & Gynecology, St Barnabas Med Ctr 1990; **Fellow:** Reproductive Endocrinology, NY Hosp-Cornell Med Ctr 1992; **Fac Appt:** Assoc Prof ObG, NYU Sch Med

Matera, Cristina MD (RE) - **Spec Exp:** Infertility; Miscarriage-Recurrent; Laparoscopic Surgery; Menopause Problems; **Hospital:** NY-Presby/Columbia Univ Med Ctr, NY (page 104); **Address:** 50 E 77th St, New York, NY 10075; **Phone:** 212-639-9122; **Board Cert:** Obstetrics & Gynecology 2011; Reproductive Endocrinology 2011; **Med School:** NYU Sch Med 1986; **Resid:** Obstetrics & Gynecology, Columbia-Presby Hosp 1990; **Fellow:** Reproductive Endocrinology, Columbia-Presby Hosp 1992; **Fac Appt:** Asst Clin Prof ObG, Columbia P&S

Mukherjee, Tanmoy MD (RE) - **Spec Exp:** Infertility-IVF; Endometriosis; Uterine Fibroids; **Hospital:** Mount Sinai Med Ctr (page 102); **Address:** 635 Madison Ave, Fl 10, New York, NY 10022; **Phone:** 212-756-5777; **Board Cert:** Obstetrics & Gynecology 2011; Reproductive Endocrinology 2011; **Med School:** Albert Einstein Coll Med 1990; **Resid:** Obstetrics & Gynecology, Montefiore Med Ctr 1994; **Fellow:** Reproductive Endocrinology, Mt Sinai Hosp 1996; **Fac Appt:** Asst Clin Prof ObG, Mount Sinai Sch Med

Noyes, Nicole MD (RE) - **Spec Exp:** Infertility-IVF; Fertility Preservation in Cancer; Reproductive Surgery; **Hospital:** NYU Langone Med Ctr (page 108); **Address:** NYU Fertility Clinic, 660 First Ave, 5th FL, New York, NY 10016; **Phone:** 212-263-7981; **Board Cert:** Obstetrics & Gynecology 2011; Reproductive Endocrinology 2011; **Med School:** Univ VT Coll Med 1986; **Resid:** Obstetrics & Gynecology, NY Hosp-Cornell Med Ctr 1990; **Fellow:** Reproductive Endocrinology, NY Hosp-Cornell Med Ctr 1992; **Fac Appt:** Assoc Prof ObG, NYU Sch Med

Quagliarello, John MD (RE) - **Spec Exp:** Infertility; Gynecologic Surgery; Uterine Fibroids; Endometriosis; **Hospital:** NYU Langone Med Ctr (page 108), Bellevue Hosp Ctr; **Address:** 530 1st Ave SKB Bldg - Ste 10Q, New York, NY 10016-6402; **Phone:** 212-263-6358; **Board Cert:** Obstetrics & Gynecology 1979; Reproductive Endocrinology 1981; **Med School:** McGill Univ 1970; **Resid:** Obstetrics & Gynecology, NYU Med Ctr 1977; **Fellow:** Reproductive Endocrinology, NYU Med Ctr 1979; **Fac Appt:** Assoc Prof ObG, NYU Sch Med

Rosenwaks, Zev MD (RE) - **Spec Exp:** Infertility-IVF; Genetic Disorders; Fertility Preservation in Cancer; **Hospital:** NY-Presby/Weill Cornell Med Ctr, NY (page 104); **Address:** Ctr For Reproductive Medicine & Infertility, 1305 York Ave Fl 6, New York, NY 10021-4872; **Phone:** 646-962-3743; **Board Cert:** Obstetrics & Gynecology 1978; Reproductive Endocrinology 1981; **Med School:** SUNY Downstate 1972; **Resid:** Obstetrics & Gynecology, LI Jewish Med Ctr 1976; **Fellow:** Reproductive Endocrinology, Johns Hopkins Hosp 1978; **Fac Appt:** Prof ObG, Cornell Univ-Weill Med Coll

Sandler, Benjamin MD (RE) - **Spec Exp:** Infertility-IVF; Reproductive Surgery; **Hospital:** Mount Sinai Med Ctr (page 102); **Address:** 635 Madison Ave Fl 10, RMA of New York, New York, NY 10022-1009; **Phone:** 212-756-5777; **Board Cert:** Obstetrics & Gynecology 2011; **Med School:** Mexico 1982; **Resid:** Obstetrics & Gynecology, Michael Reese Hosp 1987; **Fellow:** Reproductive Endocrinology, Mt Sinai Hosp 1989; **Fac Appt:** Asst Clin Prof ObG, Mount Sinai Sch Med

Sauer, Mark V MD (RE) - **Spec Exp:** Infertility-IVF; **Hospital:** NY-Presby/Columbia Univ Med Ctr, NY (page 104); **Address:** 1790 Broadway, Fl 2, New York, NY 10019; **Phone:** 646-756-8282; **Board Cert:** Obstetrics & Gynecology 2011; Reproductive Endocrinology 2011; **Med School:** Univ IL Coll Med 1980; **Resid:** Obstetrics & Gynecology, Univ Illinois Med Ctr 1984; **Fellow:** Reproductive Endocrinology, Harbor-UCLA Med Ctr 1986; **Fac Appt:** Prof ObG, Columbia P&S

Schattman, Glenn L MD (RE) - **Spec Exp:** Infertility; Robotic Assisted Laparoscopic Surgery; Minimally Invasive Surgery; Congenital Anomalies-Gynecologic; **Hospital:** NY-Presby/Weill Cornell Med Ctr, NY (page 104); **Address:** New York Hosp Cornell Med Ctr, Center for Reproductive Medicine, 1305 York Ave Fl 6, New York, NY 10021; **Phone:** 646-962-3836; **Board Cert:** Obstetrics & Gynecology 2011; Reproductive Endocrinology 2011; **Med School:** SUNY Downstate 1987; **Resid:** Obstetrics & Gynecology, Geo Wash Univ Med Ctr 1991; **Fellow:** Reproductive Endocrinology, New York Hosp/Cornell 1993; **Fac Appt:** Assoc Prof ObG, Cornell Univ-Weill Med Coll

Schmidt-Sarosi, Cecilia MD (RE) - **Spec Exp:** Infertility-IVF; Menopause Problems; Polycystic Ovarian Syndrome; Uterine Fibroids; **Hospital:** NYU Langone Med Ctr (page 108); **Address:** 51 E 67th St, New York, NY 10065; **Phone:** 212-535-5350; **Board Cert:** Obstetrics & Gynecology 2009; Reproductive Endocrinology/Infertility 2009; **Med School:** NYU Sch Med 1976; **Resid:** Obstetrics & Gynecology, NYU Med Ctr 1980; **Fellow:** Reproductive Endocrinology, NYU Med Ctr 1982; **Fac Appt:** Prof ObG, NYU Sch Med

Spandorfer, Steven MD (RE) - **Spec Exp:** Infertility-IVF; **Hospital:** NY-Presby/Weill Cornell Med Ctr, NY (page 104); **Address:** 1305 York Ave Fl 6, New York, NY 10021; **Phone:** 646-962-3638; **Board Cert:** Obstetrics & Gynecology 2011; Reproductive Endocrinology 2011; **Med School:** Emory Univ 1988; **Resid:** Obstetrics & Gynecology, Univ Penn Med Ctr 1996; **Fellow:** Reproductive Endocrinology, NY Hosp 1998; **Fac Appt:** Asst Prof ObG, Cornell Univ-Weill Med Coll

Stein, Daniel MD (RE) *PCP* - **Hospital:** Northern Westchester Hosp (page 613), St. Luke's - Roosevelt Hosp Ctr - Roosevelt Div (page 94); **Address:** 425 W 59th St Ste. 5A, New York, NY 10019; **Phone:** 212-523-7751; **Board Cert:** Reproductive Endocrinology/Infertility 2011; Obstetrics & Gynecology 2011; **Med School:** NY Med Coll 1989; **Resid:** Obstetrics & Gynecology, Thomas Jefferson Univ Hosp 1995; Reproductive Endocrinology, NJ Med Sch 1997

Sultan, Khalid M MD (RE) - **Spec Exp:** Infertility-IVF; Laparoscopic Surgery; **Hospital:** Lenox Hill Hosp (page 106); **Address:** 1016 5th Ave, New York, NY 10028-0132; **Phone:** 212-734-5555; **Board Cert:** Obstetrics & Gynecology 2010; Reproductive Endocrinology 2010; **Med School:** NY Med Coll 1988; **Resid:** Obstetrics & Gynecology, Lenox Hill Hosp 1992; **Fellow:** Reproductive Endocrinology, New York Hosp 1994; **Fac Appt:** Asst Clin Prof ObG, NYU Sch Med

Tortoriello, Drew MD (RE) - **Spec Exp:** Infertility-IVF; Polycystic Ovarian Syndrome; **Hospital:** St. Luke's - Roosevelt Hosp Ctr - Roosevelt Div (page 94); **Address:** 425 5th Ave, Fl 3, New York, NY 10016; **Phone:** 646-792-7476; **Board Cert:** Obstetrics & Gynecology 2007; Reproductive Endocrinology 2007; **Med School:** SUNY Downstate 1992; **Resid:** Obstetrics & Gynecology, NY Presby Hosp/Cornell 1996; **Fellow:** Reproductive Endocrinology, UMDNJ Affil Hosp 1998; Reproductive Endocrinology, Mass Genl Hosp

Warren, Michelle MD (RE) - **Spec Exp:** Menopause Problems; Infertility; Menstrual Disorders; Women's Health; **Hospital:** NY-Presby/Columbia Univ Med Ctr, NY (page 104); **Address:** 134 E 73rd St, New York, NY 10021; **Phone:** 212-737-4664; **Board Cert:** Internal Medicine 1972; Endocrinology 1973; **Med School:** Cornell Univ-Weill Med Coll 1965; **Resid:** Internal Medicine, Bellevue Hosp Ctr 1968; Internal Medicine, Meml Sloan Kettering Canc Ctr 1968; **Fellow:** Endocrinology, Columbia Presby Med Ctr 1971; **Fac Appt:** Prof ObG, Columbia P&S

Rheumatology

Adlersberg, Jay B MD (Rhu) - **Spec Exp:** Rheumatoid Arthritis; Osteoarthritis; Psoriatic Arthritis; Sports Medicine; **Hospital:** Lenox Hill Hosp (page 106), NYU Hosp For Joint Diseases (page 119); **Address:** 220 E 69th St, Ground Fl, New York, NY 10021-5737; **Phone:** 212-570-1800; **Board Cert:** Internal Medicine 1972; Rheumatology 1980; **Med School:** Univ Pennsylvania 1969; **Resid:** Internal Medicine, Bellevue Hosp 1972; **Fellow:** Rheumatology, Bellevue Hosp 1974; **Fac Appt:** Asst Prof Med, Mount Sinai Sch Med

Agus, Bertrand MD (Rhu) - **Spec Exp:** Lupus/SLE; Rheumatoid Arthritis; Sarcoidosis; Gout; **Hospital:** NYU Langone Med Ctr (page 108); **Address:** 251 E 33rd St, Fl 4, New York, NY 10016-4804; **Phone:** 212-779-8421; **Board Cert:** Internal Medicine 1972; Rheumatology 1972; **Med School:** NYU Sch Med 1965; **Resid:** Internal Medicine, NYU Med Ctr 1970; **Fellow:** Rheumatology, NYU Med Ctr 1972; **Fac Appt:** Assoc Clin Prof Med, NYU Sch Med

Ali, Yousaf MD (Rhu) - **Spec Exp:** Gout; Osteoporosis; Behcet's Syndrome; **Hospital:** Mount Sinai Med Ctr (page 102); **Address:** Mount Sinai Medical Center, Mount Sinai Faculty Practice Associates, 5 E 98th St, New York, NY 10029; **Phone:** 212-241-1671; **Board Cert:** Internal Medicine 2008; Rheumatology 2009; **Med School:** England, UK 1992; **Resid:** Internal Medicine, OR Hlth & Sci Univ Hosp 1997; **Fellow:** Rheumatology, Yale-New Haven Hosp 1999; **Fac Appt:** Asst Prof Med, Mount Sinai Sch Med

Bauer, Bertha A MD (Rhu) - **Spec Exp:** Fibromyalgia; Osteoporosis; **Hospital:** NYU Langone Med Ctr (page 108); **Address:** 1185 Park Ave, Ste 1L, New York, NY 10128-6217; **Phone:** 212-828-7933; **Board Cert:** Internal Medicine 1980; **Med School:** Columbia P&S 1977; **Resid:** Internal Medicine, New England Deaconess Hosp 1980; **Fellow:** Rheumatology, Yale-New Haven Hosp 1982; **Fac Appt:** Asst Clin Prof Med, NYU Sch Med

Belmont, H Michael MD (Rhu) - **Spec Exp:** Lupus/SLE; Antiphospholipid Syndrome (APS); Wegener's Granulomatosis; Rheumatoid Arthritis; **Hospital:** NYU Hosp For Joint Diseases (page 119), NYU Langone Med Ctr (page 108); **Address:** 333 E 30th St, Fl 4, MS 10016, New York, NY 10016; **Phone:** 646-501-7400 x7213; **Board Cert:** Internal Medicine 1983; Rheumatology 1986; **Med School:** Univ Pittsburgh 1980; **Resid:** Internal Medicine, Mt Sinai Hosp 1983; **Fellow:** Rheumatology, NYU/Bellevue Hosp 1985; **Fac Appt:** Assoc Prof Med, NYU Sch Med

Blume, Ralph S MD (Rhu) - **Spec Exp:** Vasculitis; Lupus/SLE; Rheumatoid Arthritis; **Hospital:** NY-Presby/Columbia Univ Med Ctr, NY (page 104); **Address:** 161 Fort Washington Ave, Ste 537, New York, NY 10032-3713; **Phone:** 212-305-5512; **Board Cert:** Internal Medicine 1972; Rheumatology 1974; **Med School:** Columbia P&S 1964; **Resid:** Internal Medicine, NY-Presby/Columbia Univ Med Ctr 1968; **Fellow:** Rheumatology, NY-Presby/Columbia Univ Med Ctr 1970; **Fac Appt:** Clin Prof Med, Columbia P&S

Buyon, Jill P MD (Rhu) - **Spec Exp:** Lupus/SLE in Pregnancy; Lupus/SLE in Menopause; **Hospital:** NYU Hosp For Joint Diseases (page 119), NYU Langone Med Ctr (page 108); **Address:** Ctr for Musculoskeletal Care, 333 E 38th St, New York, NY 10016; **Phone:** 646-501-7400; **Board Cert:** Internal Medicine 1981; Rheumatology 1984; **Med School:** Albert Einstein Coll Med 1978; **Resid:** Internal Medicine, Montefiore Med Ctr 1981; **Fellow:** Rheumatology, NYU Med Ctr 1983; **Fac Appt:** Prof Med, NYU Sch Med

Crane, Richard MD (Rhu) - **Spec Exp:** Rheumatoid Arthritis; Gout; Osteoarthritis; Arthritis; **Hospital:** Mount Sinai Med Ctr (page 102); **Address:** 1088 Park Ave, New York, NY 10128-1132; **Phone:** 212-860-4000; **Board Cert:** Internal Medicine 1984; Rheumatology 1986; **Med School:** Mount Sinai Sch Med 1981; **Resid:** Internal Medicine, Mt Sinai Hosp 1984; **Fellow:** Rheumatology, Mt Sinai Hosp 1986

Faller, Jason MD (Rhu) - **Spec Exp:** Lyme Disease; Rheumatoid Arthritis; Gout; Lupus/SLE; **Hospital:** St. Luke's - Roosevelt Hosp Ctr - Roosevelt Div (page 94), Lenox Hill Hosp (page 106); **Address:** 333 W 57th St, Ste 104, New York, NY 10019-3115; **Phone:** 212-307-6880; **Board Cert:** Internal Medicine 1980; Rheumatology 1982; **Med School:** Univ Pennsylvania 1977; **Resid:** Internal Medicine, Rush Presby St Lukes Hosp 1980; **Fellow:** Rheumatology, Univ Mich 1982; **Fac Appt:** Asst Clin Prof Med, Columbia P&S

Fields, Theodore R MD (Rhu) - **Spec Exp:** Gout; Rheumatoid Arthritis; Osteoarthritis; **Hospital:** Hosp For Special Surgery (page 115), NY-Presby/Weill Cornell Med Ctr, NY (page 104); **Address:** 535 E 70th St, Fl 8, Ste 848F, New York, NY 10021-4872; **Phone:** 212-606-1286; **Board Cert:** Internal Medicine 1979; Rheumatology 1982; **Med School:** SUNY Downstate 1976; **Resid:** Internal Medicine, Nassau Co Med Ctr 1979; **Fellow:** Rheumatology, Univ Hosp 1982; **Fac Appt:** Clin Prof Med, Cornell Univ-Weill Med Coll

Fischer, Harry MD (Rhu) - **Spec Exp:** Lupus/SLE; Rheumatoid Arthritis; Vasculitis; **Hospital:** Beth Israel Med Ctr - Petrie Division (page 94); **Address:** 10 Union Square East, Ste 3D Bldg, New York, NY 10003-3314; **Phone:** 212-844-8101; **Board Cert:** Internal Medicine 1983; Rheumatology 2010; **Med School:** Mount Sinai Sch Med 1979; **Resid:** Internal Medicine, Beth Israel Med Ctr 1983; **Fellow:** Rheumatology, Hosp Joint Diseases 1985; **Fac Appt:** Assoc Clin Prof Med, Albert Einstein Coll Med

Gibofsky, Allan MD (Rhu) - **Spec Exp:** Rheumatic Fever; Rheumatoid Arthritis; Inflammatory Arthritis; Behcet's Syndrome; **Hospital:** Hosp For Special Surgery (page 115), NY-Presby/Weill Cornell Med Ctr, NY (page 104); **Address:** 535 E 70th St, New York, NY 10021-4872; **Phone:** 212-606-1423; **Board Cert:** Internal Medicine 1977; Rheumatology 1980; **Med School:** Cornell Univ-Weill Med Coll 1973; **Resid:** Pathology, NY-Cornell Med Ctr 1974; Internal Medicine, NY-Cornell Med Ctr 1977; **Fellow:** Rheumatology/Immunology, Hosp for Special Surgery 1979; **Fac Appt:** Prof Med, Cornell Univ-Weill Med Coll

Goodman, Susan M MD (Rhu) - **Spec Exp:** Lupus Nephritis; Rheumatoid Arthritis; Psoriatic Arthritis; **Hospital:** Hosp For Special Surgery (page 115), NY-Presby/Weill Cornell Med Ctr, NY (page 104); **Address:** 535 E 70th St, New York, NY 10021; **Phone:** 212-606-1163; **Board Cert:** Internal Medicine 1980; Rheumatology 1982; **Med School:** Univ Cincinnati 1977; **Resid:** Internal Medicine, Lenox Hill Hosp 1980; **Fellow:** Rheumatology, Columbia Presby Hosp 1983; **Fac Appt:** Asst Clin Prof Med, Cornell Univ-Weill Med Coll

Gorevic, Peter D MD (Rhu) - **Spec Exp:** Autoimmune Disease; Amyloidosis/Joint Disease; Cryoglobulinemia; **Hospital:** Mount Sinai Med Ctr (page 102), Huntington Hosp (page 106); **Address:** 5 E 98th St Fl 11, New York, NY 10029; **Phone:** 212-241-1671; **Board Cert:** Internal Medicine 1973; Rheumatology 1976; Allergy & Immunology 1977; Diagnostic Lab Immunology 1986; **Med School:** NYU Sch Med 1970; **Resid:** Internal Medicine, NYU Med Ctr 1973; **Fellow:** Rheumatology, NYU Med Ctr 1975; Allergy & Immunology, NYU Med Ctr 1977; **Fac Appt:** Prof Med, Mount Sinai Sch Med

Greisman, Stewart G MD (Rhu) - **Spec Exp:** Lupus/SLE; Rheumatoid Arthritis; **Hospital:** St. Luke's - Roosevelt Hosp Ctr - Roosevelt Div (page 94), Hosp For Special Surgery (page 115); **Address:** 457 W 57th St, Ste 106, New York, NY 10019-1701; **Phone:** 212-265-1471; **Board Cert:** Internal Medicine 1984; Rheumatology 1986; **Med School:** Yale Univ 1981; **Resid:** Internal Medicine, Yale-New Haven Hosp 1984; **Fellow:** Rheumatology, Hosp Special Surg 1986; **Fac Appt:** Assoc Clin Prof Med, Columbia P&S

Honig, Stephen MD (Rhu) - **Spec Exp:** Osteoporosis; Rheumatoid Arthritis; Osteoarthritis; Lupus/SLE; **Hospital:** NYU Hosp For Joint Diseases (page 119), NYU Langone Med Ctr (page 108); **Address:** 301 E 17th St, Ste 1100, New York, NY 10003-3804; **Phone:** 212-598-6367; **Board Cert:** Internal Medicine 1975; Rheumatology 1978; **Med School:** Univ Tenn Coll Med 1972; **Resid:** Internal Medicine, St Vincent's Hosp Med Ctr 1975; **Fellow:** Rheumatology, NYU Med Ctr 1977; **Fac Appt:** Assoc Clin Prof Med, NYU Sch Med

Horowitz, Mark D MD (Rhu) - **Spec Exp:** Lupus/SLE; Rheumatoid Arthritis; Fibromyalgia; **Hospital:** Mount Sinai Med Ctr (page 102); **Address:** 21 E 90th St, Ground Fl, New York, NY 10128-0654; **Phone:** 212-860-3077; **Board Cert:** Internal Medicine 1986; **Med School:** NE Ohio Univ 1983; **Resid:** Internal Medicine, Mt Sinai Med Ctr 1986; **Fellow:** Rheumatology, Mt Sinai Med Ctr 1989

Kerr, Leslie D MD (Rhu) - **Spec Exp:** Rheumatoid Arthritis; Scleroderma; Lupus/SLE; Geriatric Rheumatology; **Hospital:** Mount Sinai Med Ctr (page 102); **Address:** Mount Sinai Med Ctr, 1 Gustave Levy Pl, Box 1244, New York, NY 10029; **Phone:** 212-241-1671; **Board Cert:** Internal Medicine 1983; Rheumatology 1986; **Med School:** Columbia P&S 1980; **Resid:** Internal Medicine, Mt Sinai Hospital 1983; **Fellow:** Rheumatology, Mt Sinai Hospital 1985; **Fac Appt:** Assoc Prof Med, Mount Sinai Sch Med

Lee, Sicy H MD (Rhu) - **Spec Exp:** Rheumatoid Arthritis; Psoriatic Arthritis; Lupus/SLE; **Hospital:** NYU Hosp For Joint Diseases (page 119), NYU Langone Med Ctr (page 108); **Address:** 333 E 38th St Fl 4, New York, NY 10016; **Phone:** 646-501-7400; **Board Cert:** Internal Medicine 1982; Rheumatology 1984; **Med School:** Univ Cincinnati 1979; **Resid:** Internal Medicine, Good Samaritan 1982; **Fellow:** Rheumatology, Hosp for Joint Diseases 1984; **Fac Appt:** Asst Clin Prof Med, NYU Sch Med

Magid, Steven K MD (Rhu) - **Spec Exp:** Rheumatoid Arthritis; Osteoarthritis; Lyme Disease; Polymyalgia Rheumatica; **Hospital:** Hosp For Special Surgery (page 115); **Address:** 535 E 70th St, Fl 7, New York, NY 10021; **Phone:** 212-606-1060; **Board Cert:** Internal Medicine 1979; Rheumatology 1984; **Med School:** Cornell Univ-Weill Med Coll 1976; **Resid:** Internal Medicine, New York Hosp 1979; **Fellow:** Rheumatology, Hosp For Special Surgery 1981; **Fac Appt:** Clin Prof Med, Cornell Univ-Weill Med Coll

Marchetta, Paula MD (Rhu) - **Spec Exp:** Rheumatoid Arthritis; Psoriatic Arthritis; Sjogren's Syndrome; Osteoarthritis; **Hospital:** NYU Langone Med Ctr (page 108); **Address:** Concorde Med Grp, 40 Park Ave, New York, NY 10016-3467; **Phone:** 212-696-5415; **Board Cert:** Internal Medicine 1986; Rheumatology 2010; **Med School:** NYU Sch Med 1983; **Resid:** Internal Medicine, Bellevue Hosp-NYU Med Ctr 1987; **Fellow:** Rheumatology, NYU Med Ctr-Bellevue Hosp 1989; **Fac Appt:** Asst Clin Prof Med, NYU Sch Med

Markenson, Joseph A MD (Rhu) - **Spec Exp:** Rheumatoid Arthritis; Lupus/SLE; Osteoarthritis; **Hospital:** Hosp For Special Surgery (page 115), NY-Presby/Weill Cornell Med Ctr, NY (page 104); **Address:** Hosp for Special Surgery, 535 E 70th St, Ste 659W, New York, NY 10021-4892; **Phone:** 212-606-1261; **Board Cert:** Internal Medicine 1976; Rheumatology 1978; **Med School:** SUNY Downstate 1970; **Resid:** Internal Medicine, New York Hosp 1975; **Fellow:** Rheumatology, Hosp For Special Surg 1976; **Fac Appt:** Clin Prof Med, Cornell Univ-Weill Med Coll

Meed, Steven D MD (Rhu) - **Spec Exp:** Lyme Disease; Chronic Fatigue Syndrome; Acupuncture; Fibromyalgia; **Hospital:** Lenox Hill Hosp (page 106), St. Luke's - Roosevelt Hosp Ctr - Roosevelt Div (page 94); **Address:** 150 E 58th St Fl 18, New York, NY 10155; **Phone:** 212-583-2960; **Board Cert:** Internal Medicine 1979; Rheumatology 1986; **Med School:** NYU Sch Med 1975; **Resid:** Internal Medicine, Brookdale Hosp 1977; **Fellow:** Rheumatology, Barnes Hosp-Wash Univ 1979; **Fac Appt:** Asst Clin Prof Med, NYU Sch Med

Mitnick, Hal J MD (Rhu) - **Spec Exp:** Rheumatoid Arthritis; Psoriatic Arthritis; Osteoporosis; Dermatomyositis; **Hospital:** NYU Langone Med Ctr (page 108); **Address:** 333 E 34th St, Ste 1C, New York, NY 10016-4977; **Phone:** 212-889-7217; **Board Cert:** Internal Medicine 1976; Rheumatology 1978; **Med School:** NYU Sch Med 1972; **Resid:** Internal Medicine, Bellevue Hosp 1976; **Fellow:** Rheumatology, NYU Med Ctr 1978; **Fac Appt:** Clin Prof Med, NYU Sch Med

Nickerson, Katherine G MD (Rhu) - **Hospital:** NY-Presby/Columbia Univ Med Ctr, NY (page 104); **Address:** 161 Ft Washington Ave, Irving Bldg, rm 346, New York, NY 10032-3713; **Phone:** 212-305-8039; **Board Cert:** Internal Medicine 1984; Rheumatology 1986; **Med School:** UCSF 1981; **Resid:** Internal Medicine, Beth Israel Hosp 1984; **Fellow:** Rheumatology, Columbia-Presby Med Ctr 1986; **Fac Appt:** Assoc Prof Med, Columbia P&S

Ornstein, Matthew MD (Rhu) - **Spec Exp:** Arthritis; **Hospital:** Mount Sinai Med Ctr (page 102); **Address:** 65 E 96th St, Ste 1B, New York, NY 10128-1307; **Phone:** 212-722-7157; **Board Cert:** Rheumatology 2004; **Med School:** SUNY Stony Brook 1988; **Resid:** Internal Medicine, Mt Sinai Med Ctr 1991; **Fellow:** Rheumatology, Mt Sinai Med Ctr 1993

Paget, Stephen MD (Rhu) - **Spec Exp:** Rheumatoid Arthritis; Lupus/SLE; Vasculitis; Connective Tissue Disorders; **Hospital:** Hosp For Special Surgery (page 115); **Address:** 535 E 70th St Fl 7, New York, NY 10021; **Phone:** 212-606-1845; **Board Cert:** Internal Medicine 1974; Rheumatology 2009; **Med School:** SUNY Downstate 1971; **Resid:** Internal Medicine, Johns Hopkins Hosp 1973; **Fellow:** Rheumatology, Hosp Special Surg 1975; **Fac Appt:** Prof Med, Cornell Univ-Weill Med Coll

Parrish, Edward MD (Rhu) - **Spec Exp:** Immune Deficiency; **Hospital:** Hosp For Special Surgery (page 115), NY-Presby/Weill Cornell Med Ctr, NY (page 104); **Address:** 535 E 70th St Fl 6, New York, NY 10021; **Phone:** 212-606-1743; **Board Cert:** Internal Medicine 1983; Rheumatology 1986; **Med School:** Wake Forest Univ 1980; **Resid:** Internal Medicine, Columbia-Presby Med Ctr 1983; **Fellow:** Rheumatology/Immunology, Columbia-Presby Med Ctr 1985

Rackoff, Paula MD (Rhu) - **Spec Exp:** Osteoporosis; Sjogren's Syndrome; Arthritis; **Hospital:** Beth Israel Med Ctr - Petrie Division (page 94); **Address:** 10 Union Square East, Ste 3D, New York, NY 10003-3314; **Phone:** 212-844-8101; **Board Cert:** Internal Medicine 1989; Rheumatology 2004; **Med School:** Yale Univ 1986; **Resid:** Internal Medicine, Yale-New Haven Hosp 1989; **Fellow:** Rheumatology, Yale-New Haven Hosp 1992; **Fac Appt:** Asst Prof Med, Albert Einstein Coll Med

Radin, Allen R MD (Rhu) - **Spec Exp:** Rheumatoid Arthritis; Lupus/SLE; Osteoarthritis; Scleroderma; **Hospital:** Lenox Hill Hosp (page 106), NY-Presby/Weill Cornell Med Ctr, NY (page 104); **Address:** 50 E 81st St, Ste 1, New York, NY 10028; **Phone:** 212-289-6855; **Board Cert:** Internal Medicine 1980; Rheumatology 1982; **Med School:** NYU Sch Med 1977; **Resid:** Internal Medicine, Univ Hosp 1980; **Fellow:** Rheumatology, NYU Med Ctr 1982

Salmon, Jane E MD (Rhu) - **Spec Exp:** Lupus/SLE; Antiphospholipid Syndrome (APS); Rheumatoid Arthritis; **Hospital:** Hosp For Special Surgery (page 115); **Address:** 535 E 70th St, New York, NY 10021-4872; **Phone:** 212-606-1728; **Board Cert:** Internal Medicine 1981; Rheumatology 1984; **Med School:** Columbia P&S 1978; **Resid:** Internal Medicine, New York Hosp 1981; **Fellow:** Rheumatology, Hosp Special Surgery 1983; **Fac Appt:** Prof Med, Cornell Univ-Weill Med Coll

Samuels, Jonathan MD (Rhu) - **Spec Exp:** Scleroderma; Dermatomyositis; Gout; Osteoarthritis; **Hospital:** NYU Langone Med Ctr (page 108); **Address:** Center for Musculoskeletal Care, 333 E 38th St, New York, NY 10016; **Phone:** 646-501-7400; **Board Cert:** Internal Medicine 2002; Rheumatology 2004; **Med School:** Cornell Univ 1999; **Resid:** Internal Medicine, University Hosp 2002; **Fellow:** Rheumatology, Weill-Cornell Med Ctr 2005; **Fac Appt:** Asst Prof Med, NYU Sch Med

Schwartzfarb, Lanny MD (Rhu) - **Spec Exp:** Rheumatoid Arthritis; Psoriatic Arthritis; Sapho Syndrome; **Hospital:** Beth Israel Med Ctr - Petrie Division (page 94), NYU Langone Med Ctr (page 108); **Address:** 315 E 69th St, Lobby J, New York, NY 10021; **Phone:** 212-734-5670; **Board Cert:** Internal Medicine 1975; Rheumatology 1978; **Med School:** NYU Sch Med 1972; **Resid:** Internal Medicine, Beth Israel Med Ctr 1975; **Fellow:** Rheumatology, Columbia-Presby Med Ctr 1977

Schwartzman, Sergio MD (Rhu) - **Spec Exp:** Lupus/SLE; Raynaud's Disease; Uveitis; Vasculitis; **Hospital:** Hosp For Special Surgery (page 115); **Address:** Hosp for Special Surgery, 535 E 70th St, New York, NY 10021-4892; **Phone:** 212-606-1557; **Board Cert:** Internal Medicine 1985; Rheumatology 1988; **Med School:** Mount Sinai Sch Med 1982; **Resid:** Internal Medicine, LI Jewish Med Ctr 1985; **Fellow:** Rheumatology, Hosp Special Surgery 1987; **Fac Appt:** Assoc Prof Med, Cornell Univ-Weill Med Coll

Smiles, Stephen MD (Rhu) - **Spec Exp:** Arthritis; Osteoporosis; Lupus/SLE; Gout; **Hospital:** NYU Langone Med Ctr (page 108); **Address:** Ctr for Arthritis & Autoimmunity, 333 E 38th St Fl 4, New York, NY 10016; **Phone:** 212-473-3280; **Board Cert:** Internal Medicine 1977; Rheumatology 1980; **Med School:** SUNY Buffalo 1973; **Resid:** Internal Medicine, Bellevue Hosp Ctr 1977; **Fellow:** Rheumatology, Bellevue Hosp Ctr 1979; **Fac Appt:** Asst Clin Prof Med, NYU Sch Med

Solitar, Bruce M MD (Rhu) - **Spec Exp:** Arthritis; Fibromyalgia; Reiter's Syndrome; Retroperitoneal Fibrosis; **Hospital:** NYU Langone Med Ctr (page 108), NYU Hosp For Joint Diseases (page 119); **Address:** 333 E 34th St, New York, NY 10016; **Phone:** 212-889-7217; **Board Cert:** Internal Medicine 2012; Rheumatology 2004; **Med School:** NYU Sch Med 1988; **Resid:** Internal Medicine, NYU/Bellevue Med Ctr 1992; **Fellow:** Rheumatology, NYU/Bellevue Med Ctr 1994; **Fac Appt:** Assoc Clin Prof Med, NYU Sch Med

Solomon, Gary MD (Rhu) - **Spec Exp:** Psoriatic Arthritis; Rheumatoid Arthritis; Autoimmune Disease; **Hospital:** NYU Hosp For Joint Diseases (page 119), NYU Langone Med Ctr (page 108); **Address:** Ctr for Musculoskeletal Care, 333 E 38th St, New York, NY 10016; **Phone:** 646-501-7400; **Board Cert:** Internal Medicine 1980; Rheumatology 1982; **Med School:** Mount Sinai Sch Med 1977; **Resid:** Internal Medicine, Mt Sinai Med Ctr 1980; **Fellow:** Rheumatology, Montefiore Med Ctr 1982; **Fac Appt:** Assoc Clin Prof Med, NYU Sch Med

Spiera, Harry MD (Rhu) - **Spec Exp:** Lupus/SLE; Scleroderma; Vasculitis; Behcet's Syndrome; **Hospital:** Mount Sinai Med Ctr (page 102), NY-Presby/Weill Cornell Med Ctr, NY (page 104); **Address:** Rheumatology Assocs, 1088 Park Ave, New York, NY 10128-1132; **Phone:** 212-860-4000 x2; **Board Cert:** Internal Medicine 1965; Rheumatology 1972; **Med School:** NYU Sch Med 1958; **Resid:** Internal Medicine, VA Med Ctr 1960; Internal Medicine, Mt Sinai Hosp 1961; **Fellow:** Rheumatology, Columbia-Presby Med Ctr 1963; **Fac Appt:** Clin Prof Med, Mount Sinai Sch Med

Spiera, Robert MD (Rhu) - **Spec Exp:** Vasculitis; Lupus/SLE; Scleroderma; **Hospital:** Hosp For Special Surgery (page 115), Mount Sinai Med Ctr (page 102); **Address:** 1088 Park Ave, New York, NY 10128-1132; **Phone:** 212-860-2100; **Board Cert:** Internal Medicine 2002; Rheumatology 2004; **Med School:** Yale Univ 1989; **Resid:** Internal Medicine, New York Hosp 1992; **Fellow:** Rheumatology, Hosp Special Surg 1995; **Fac Appt:** Assoc Clin Prof Med, Cornell Univ-Weill Med Coll

Stern, Richard MD (Rhu) - **Spec Exp:** Rheumatoid Arthritis; Osteoporosis; Osteoarthritis; Polymyalgia Rheumatica; **Hospital:** Hosp For Special Surgery (page 115), NY-Presby/Weill Cornell Med Ctr, NY (page 104); **Address:** 475 E 72nd St, New York, NY 10021-4458; **Phone:** 212-879-2282; **Board Cert:** Internal Medicine 1973; Rheumatology 1976; **Med School:** Tufts Univ 1970; **Resid:** Internal Medicine, NY Hosp 1973; **Fellow:** Immunology, Rockefeller Univ Hosp 1975; Rheumatology, Hosp Special Surgery 1975; **Fac Appt:** Assoc Clin Prof Med, Cornell Univ-Weill Med Coll

Whitman III, Hendricks H MD (Rhu) - **Spec Exp:** Rheumatoid Arthritis; Scleroderma; **Hospital:** Hosp For Special Surgery (page 115); **Address:** Hospital for Special Surgery, 535 E 70th St Fl 6, New York, NY 10021; **Phone:** 212-774-2802; **Board Cert:** Internal Medicine 1978; Rheumatology 1980; **Med School:** Univ NC Sch Med 1975; **Resid:** Internal Medicine, NY Hosp-Cornell 1978; **Fellow:** Rheumatology, NY Hosp-Cornell 1980; **Fac Appt:** Asst Clin Prof Med, Cornell Univ-Weill Med Coll

Yee, Arthur M F MD/PhD (Rhu) - **Spec Exp:** Sarcoidosis; Gout; Rheumatoid Arthritis; Psoriatic Arthritis; **Hospital:** Hosp For Special Surgery (page 115), NY-Presby/Weill Cornell Med Ctr, NY (page 104); **Address:** Hosp for Special Surgery, 535 E 70th St, New York, NY 10021; **Phone:** 212-606-1171; **Board Cert:** Internal Medicine 2004; Rheumatology 2006; **Med School:** NYU Sch Med 1991; **Resid:** Internal Medicine, NY Hosp-Cornell Med Ctr 1993; **Fellow:** Rheumatology, NY Hosp-Cornell Med Ctr 1995; **Fac Appt:** Asst Prof Med, Cornell Univ-Weill Med Coll

Sports Medicine

Altchek, David MD (SM) - **Spec Exp:** Shoulder Surgery; Elbow Surgery; Knee Surgery; Arthroscopic Surgery; **Hospital:** Hosp For Special Surgery (page 115), NY-Presby/Weill Cornell Med Ctr, NY (page 104); **Address:** Hospital for Special Surgery, 535 E 70th St, New York, NY 10021; **Phone:** 212-606-1909; **Board Cert:** Orthopaedic Surgery 2011; **Med School:** Cornell Univ-Weill Med Coll 1982; **Resid:** Orthopaedic Surgery, Hosp for Special Surg 1987; **Fellow:** Sports Medicine, Hosp for Special Surg 1988; **Fac Appt:** Assoc Prof OrS, Cornell Univ-Weill Med Coll

Callahan, Lisa MD (SM) - **Spec Exp:** Primary Care Sports Medicine; Sports Medicine-Women; Fractures-Stress; **Hospital:** Hosp For Special Surgery (page 115), NY-Presby/Weill Cornell Med Ctr, NY (page 104); **Address:** Hospital for Special Surgery, 535 E 70th St, New York, NY 10021; **Phone:** 212-606-1532; **Board Cert:** Family Medicine 2004; Sports Medicine 2003; **Med School:** E Carolina Univ 1987; **Resid:** Family Medicine, San Jose Med Ctr 1990; **Fellow:** Sports Medicine, Stanford Univ 1991; **Fac Appt:** Assoc Prof FMed, Cornell Univ-Weill Med Coll

Halpern, Brian MD (SM) - **Spec Exp:** Primary Care Sports Medicine; Knee Injuries; Shoulder Injuries; **Hospital:** Hosp For Special Surgery (page 115); **Address:** 535 E 70th St, New York, NY 10021; **Phone:** 212-606-1329; **Board Cert:** Family Medicine 2008; Sports Medicine 2004; **Med School:** Cornell Univ-Weill Med Coll 1981; **Resid:** Family Medicine, Univ Md Med Ctr 1984; **Fellow:** Sports Medicine, Hughston Ortho Clinic 1985; **Fac Appt:** Asst Clin Prof Med, Cornell Univ-Weill Med Coll

Hamner, Daniel MD (SM) - **Spec Exp:** Running Injuries; Acupuncture; Primary Care Sports Medicine; **Address:** 80 E 11th St, Ste 619, New York, NY 10003; **Phone:** 212-260-5999; **Board Cert:** Physical Medicine & Rehabilitation 1986; **Med School:** NY Med Coll 1976; **Resid:** Physical Medicine & Rehabilitation, New York Hosp-Cornell Med Ctr 1979; **Fellow:** Cardiac Rehabilitation, Emory Med Ctr 1980

Hershman, Elliott MD (SM) - **Spec Exp:** Knee Injuries; Knee Surgery; Arthroscopic Surgery; Ligament Reconstruction; **Hospital:** Lenox Hill Hosp (page 106); **Address:** 130 E 77th St Fl 7, New York, NY 10075; **Phone:** 212-744-8114; **Board Cert:** Orthopaedic Surgery 2008; **Med School:** Univ Rochester 1979; **Resid:** Orthopaedic Surgery, Lenox Hill Hosp 1984; **Fellow:** Sports Medicine, Cleveland Clin 1985; **Fac Appt:** Asst Clin Prof OrS, Mount Sinai Sch Med

Krinick, Ronald M MD (SM) - **Spec Exp:** Knee Injuries; Shoulder Injuries; **Hospital:** NY Downtown Hosp; **Address:** 19 Beekman St Fl 5, New York, NY 10038; **Phone:** 212-513-7711; **Board Cert:** Orthopaedic Surgery 2008; **Med School:** NYU Sch Med 1979; **Resid:** Orthopaedic Surgery, NYU/Bellvue Med Ctr 1984; **Fellow:** Sports Medicine, NYU Med Ctr 1985; **Fac Appt:** Assoc Clin Prof OrS, NYU Sch Med

Levine, William N MD (SM) - **Spec Exp:** Arthroscopic Surgery; Shoulder & Elbow Surgery; Knee Injuries; **Hospital:** NY-Presby/Columbia Univ Med Ctr, NY (page 104); **Address:** 622 W 168th St, Fl PH-11, rm 1117, New York, NY 10032; **Phone:** 212-305-0762; **Board Cert:** Orthopaedic Surgery 2010; Orthopaedic Sports Medicine 2008; **Med School:** Case West Res Univ 1990; **Resid:** Surgery, Beth Israel Hosp 1991; Orthopaedic Surgery, New Eng Med Ctr Hosps 1995; **Fellow:** Shoulder Surgery, Columbia-Presby Med Ctr 1996; Sports Medicine, Univ MD Med Ctr 1998; **Fac Appt:** Clin Prof OrS, Columbia P&S

Maharam, Lewis G MD (SM) - **Spec Exp:** Primary Care Sports Medicine; Running Injuries; Pain-Back; **Hospital:** Mount Sinai Med Ctr (page 102); **Address:** 24 W 57th St, Ste 509, New York, NY 10019-3918; **Phone:** 212-765-5763; **Board Cert:** Sports Medicine 1991; **Med School:** Emory Univ 1985; **Resid:** Internal Medicine, Danbury Hosp 1987; Internal Medicine, NY Infirm/Beekman Downtown 1989; **Fellow:** Sports Medicine, Pascack Valley Hosp 1990; **Fac Appt:** Asst Clin Prof OrS, NYU Sch Med

Metzl, Jordan D MD (SM) - **Spec Exp:** Adolescent Sports Medicine; Running Injuries; Dance/Ballet Injuries; **Hospital:** Hosp For Special Surgery (page 115); **Address:** 519 E 72nd St, Ste 206, New York, NY 10021; **Phone:** 212-606-1678; **Board Cert:** Sports Medicine 2011; **Med School:** Univ MO-Columbia Sch Med 1993; **Resid:** Pediatrics, Tufts-New Engl Med Ctr 1996; **Fellow:** Sports Medicine, Vanderbilt Univ Med Ctr 1997; Sports Medicine, Harvard Med Sch 1998; **Fac Appt:** Assoc Prof Ped, Cornell Univ-Weill Med Coll

Nisonson, Barton MD (SM) - **Spec Exp:** Shoulder & Knee Surgery; Arthroscopic Surgery; Knee Replacement; **Hospital:** Lenox Hill Hosp (page 106); **Address:** 130 E 77th St Fl 8, New York, NY 10021-1851; **Phone:** 212-570-9120; **Board Cert:** Orthopaedic Surgery 1974; **Med School:** Columbia P&S 1966; **Resid:** Surgery, Columbia-Presby Med Ctr 1968; Orthopaedic Surgery, Columbia-Presby Med Ctr 1973

Noy, Ron MD (SM) - **Hospital:** Beth Israel Med Ctr - Petrie Division (page 94); **Address:** 424 Madison Ave Fl 9, New York, NY 10017; **Phone:** 646-862-0180; **Board Cert:** Orthopaedic Surgery 2003; Orthopaedic Sports Medicine 2008; **Med School:** UMDNJ-NJ Med Sch, Newark 1991; **Resid:** Surgery, Lenox Hill Med Ctr 1992; Orthopaedic Surgery, Kingsbrook Jewish Med Ctr 2000; **Fellow:** Orthopaedic Sports Medicine, Indiana Univ Med Ctr 2001

Rodeo, Scott A MD (SM) - **Spec Exp:** Knee Injuries; Cartilage Damage; **Hospital:** Hosp For Special Surgery (page 115); **Address:** Hosp for Special Surgery, 535 E 70th St, New York, NY 10021; **Phone:** 212-606-1513; **Board Cert:** Orthopaedic Surgery 2009; Orthopaedic Sports Medicine 2007; **Med School:** Cornell Univ-Weill Med Coll 1989; **Resid:** Orthopaedic Surgery, Hosp Special Surgery 1994; **Fellow:** Sports Medicine, Hosp Special Surgery 1996; **Fac Appt:** Assoc Clin Prof OrS, Cornell Univ-Weill Med Coll

Roth, Neil S MD (SM) - **Hospital:** Lenox Hill Hosp (page 106), White Plains Hosp (page 615); **Address:** Lenox Hill Hospital, 130 E 77th St, Black Hall Fl 8, New York, NY 10021; **Phone:** 212-861-2300; **Board Cert:** Orthopaedic Surgery 2001; Orthopaedic Sports Medicine 2008; **Med School:** Duke Univ 1991; **Resid:** Orthopaedic Surgery, Columbia Presby Med Ctr 1997; **Fellow:** Sports Medicine, Kerlan-Jobe Orth Clin 1999

Williams, Riley J MD (SM) - **Spec Exp:** Cartilage Damage & Transplant; Shoulder Arthroscopic Surgery; Knee Injuries/ACL; Knee Surgery; **Hospital:** Hosp For Special Surgery (page 115), NY-Presby/Weill Cornell Med Ctr, NY (page 104); **Address:** Hosp Special Surgery, 535 E 70th St Fl Blair 1, New York, NY 10021; **Phone:** 212-606-1855; **Board Cert:** Orthopaedic Sports Medicine 2009; **Med School:** Stanford Univ 1992; **Resid:** Orthopaedic Surgery, Hosp Special Surgery 1997; **Fellow:** Sports Medicine & Shoulder Surgery, Hosp Special Surgery 1998; **Fac Appt:** Assoc Prof OrS, Cornell Univ-Weill Med Coll

Surgery

Amory, Spencer E MD (S) - **Spec Exp:** Laparoscopic Surgery; Gastrointestinal Surgery; Hernia; **Hospital:** NY-Presby Hosp/The Allen Hosp (page 104); **Address:** 5141 Broadway, Ste 3-178, New York, NY 10034; **Phone:** 212-305-5221; **Board Cert:** Surgery 2010; **Med School:** Johns Hopkins Univ 1983; **Resid:** Surgery, Columbia Presby Med Ctr 1989; **Fellow:** Emergency Medicine, Peninsula Hosp 1990; **Fac Appt:** Assoc Clin Prof S, Columbia P&S

Attiyeh, Fadi F MD (S) - **Spec Exp:** Colon & Rectal Cancer; Hepatobiliary Surgery; Pancreatic Surgery; **Hospital:** St. Luke's - Roosevelt Hosp Ctr - Roosevelt Div (page 94); **Address:** 425 W 59th St, Ste 8B-1, New York, NY 10019; **Phone:** 212-307-1144; **Board Cert:** Surgery 1975; Colon & Rectal Surgery 1982; **Med School:** Amer Univ Beirut 1969; **Resid:** Surgery, Amer Univ Hosp 1973; **Fellow:** Surgical Oncology, Meml Sloan Kettering Canc Ctr 1976; **Fac Appt:** Assoc Clin Prof S, Columbia P&S

Axelrod, Deborah MD (S) - **Spec Exp:** Breast Cancer; Breast Disease; **Hospital:** NYU Langone Med Ctr (page 108); **Address:** NYU Clinical Cancer Ctr, 160 E 34th St Fl 3, New York, NY 10016; **Phone:** 212-731-5366; **Board Cert:** Surgery 2008; **Med School:** Israel 1982; **Resid:** Surgery, Beth Israel Med Ctr 1988; **Fellow:** Surgical Oncology, Meml Sloan Kettering Cancer Ctr 1986; **Fac Appt:** Assoc Prof S, NYU Sch Med

Barie, Philip MD (S) - **Spec Exp:** Trauma; Critical Care; Hernia; Gastrointestinal Surgery; **Hospital:** NY-Presby/Weill Cornell Med Ctr, NY (page 104), Hosp For Special Surgery (page 115); **Address:** Weill Med College-Cornell Univ, 525 E 68th St, Box 206, New York, NY 10065; **Phone:** 212-746-5401; **Board Cert:** Surgery 2004; Surgical Critical Care 2005; **Med School:** Boston Univ 1977; **Resid:** Surgery, NY Hosp-Cornell Med Ctr 1984; **Fellow:** Trauma, Albany Med Coll 1981; **Fac Appt:** Prof S, Cornell Univ-Weill Med Coll

Berman, Russell MD (S) - **Spec Exp:** Melanoma; **Hospital:** NYU Langone Med Ctr (page 108); **Address:** NYU Clinical Cancer Ctr, 160 E 34th St Fl 9, New York, NY 10016; **Phone:** 212-731-5415; **Board Cert:** Surgery 2007; **Med School:** NYU Sch Med 1990; **Resid:** Surgery, NYU Med Ctr/Bellevue Hosp 1997; **Fellow:** Surgical Oncology, Meml Sloan Kettering Cancer Ctr 1994; Surgical Oncology, UT MD Anderson Cancer Ctr 2000; **Fac Appt:** Asst Prof S, NYU Sch Med

Bernik, Stephanie F MD (S) - **Spec Exp:** Breast Cancer & Surgery; Breast Disease; Phyllodes Tumors; Angiosarcoma; **Hospital:** Lenox Hill Hosp (page 106); **Address:** Lenox Hill Hosp, 100 E 77th St Wollman Bldg Fl 3, New York, NY 10075; **Phone:** 212-434-6900; **Board Cert:** Surgery 2011; **Med School:** Yale Univ 1993; **Resid:** Surgery, St Vincents Hosp 1999; **Fellow:** Breast Surgery, Meml Sloan Kettering Cancer Ctr 2000

Bessey, Palmer Q MD (S) - **Spec Exp:** Burn Care; Wound Healing/Care; Nutrition; **Hospital:** NY-Presby/Weill Cornell Med Ctr, NY (page 104); **Address:** 525 E 68th St, Box 137, New York, NY 10065; **Phone:** 212-746-0242; **Board Cert:** Surgery 2011; Surgical Critical Care 2005; **Med School:** Univ VT Coll Med 1975; **Resid:** Surgery, Univ Alabama Hosp 1981; **Fellow:** Metabolism, Brigham & Women's Hosp 1983; **Fac Appt:** Prof S, Cornell Univ-Weill Med Coll

Bessler, Marc MD (S) - **Spec Exp:** Obesity/Bariatric Surgery; Laparoscopic Surgery; Gastrointestinal Metabolic Surgery; Natural Orifice Surgery (NOTES); **Hospital:** NY-Presby/Columbia Univ Med Ctr, NY (page 104); **Address:** NY Presby Med Ctr, Dept of Surgery, 161 Fort Washington Ave Fl 5 - rm 524, New York, NY 10032; **Phone:** 212-305-9506; **Board Cert:** Surgery 2007; **Med School:** NYU Sch Med 1989; **Resid:** Surgery, Columbia Presby Med Ctr 1995; **Fac Appt:** Clin Prof S, Columbia P&S

Bloom, Norman D MD (S) - **Spec Exp:** Breast Cancer; Sarcoma; Cancer Surgery; **Hospital:** Beth Israel Med Ctr - Petrie Division (page 94), NYU Langone Med Ctr (page 108); **Address:** The Gramercy, 61 Irving Pl @ 18th St, Ste LLB, New York, NY 10003; **Phone:** 212-505-6167; **Board Cert:** Surgery 2010; **Med School:** SUNY Downstate 1974; **Resid:** Surgery, Maimonides Med Ctr 1978; **Fellow:** Surgical Oncology, Meml Sloan Kettering Canc Ctr 1979; **Fac Appt:** Clin Prof S, NYU Sch Med

Boolbol, Susan K MD (S) - **Spec Exp:** Breast Surgery; **Hospital:** Beth Israel Med Ctr - Petrie Division (page 94); **Address:** 10 Union Square East, Ste 4E, New York, NY 10003; **Phone:** 212-844-6231; **Board Cert:** Surgery 2003; **Med School:** Geo Wash Univ 1994; **Resid:** Surgery, New York Hosp 2000; **Fellow:** Breast Surgery, Meml Sloan Kettering Cancer Ctr 2001

Brady, Mary Sue MD (S) - **Spec Exp:** Melanoma; Merkel Cell Carcinoma; Sarcoma-Soft Tissue; **Hospital:** Meml Sloan-Kettering Cancer Ctr (page 116); **Address:** 1275 York Ave, rm H1211, New York, NY 10065; **Phone:** 212-639-8347; **Board Cert:** Surgery 2009; **Med School:** Univ Miami Sch Med 1983; **Resid:** Surgery, NY Hosp-Cornell Med Ctr 1988; **Fellow:** Surgical Oncology, Meml Sloan-Kettering Cancer Ctr 1990; Immunology, Meml Sloan-Kettering Cancer Ctr 1992; **Fac Appt:** Assoc Prof S, Cornell Univ-Weill Med Coll

Cassell, Lauren S MD (S) - **Spec Exp:** Breast Surgery; Breast Cancer; Nipple Sparing Mastectomy; **Hospital:** Lenox Hill Hosp (page 106); **Address:** 114A E 78th St, New York, NY 10075; **Phone:** 212-535-4040; **Board Cert:** Surgery 2003; **Med School:** NY Med Coll 1977; **Resid:** Surgery, Lenox Hill Hosp 1982

Chabot, John A MD (S) - **Spec Exp:** Liver & Biliary Surgery; Pancreatic Cancer; Pancreatic Surgery; Thyroid & Parathyroid Surgery; **Hospital:** NY-Presby/Columbia Univ Med Ctr, NY (page 104); **Address:** NY Presby-Columbia Medical Ctr, 161 Ft Washington Ave Fl 8 - Ste 819, New York, NY 10032; **Phone:** 212-305-9468; **Board Cert:** Surgery 2010; **Med School:** Dartmouth Med Sch 1983; **Resid:** Surgery, Columbia-Presby Med Ctr 1990; **Fac Appt:** Prof S, Columbia P&S

Cherqui, Daniel MD (S) - **Spec Exp:** Liver Cancer; Transplant-Liver; Hepatobiliary Surgery; Minimally Invasive Surgery; **Hospital:** NY-Presby/Weill Cornell Med Ctr, NY (page 104); **Address:** 525 E 68th St, Box 287, New York, NY 10065; **Phone:** 212-746-2127; **Med School:** France 1980; **Resid:** Surgery, Hospitaux de Paris 1986; **Fellow:** Hepatobiliary Surgery, Paul Brousse Hosp 1987; Transplant Surgery, Univ Chicago Med Ctr; **Fac Appt:** Prof S, Cornell Univ-Weill Med Coll

Cioroiu, Michael G MD (S) - **Spec Exp:** Breast Disease; Wound Healing/Care; Endoscopy; **Hospital:** Mount Sinai Hosp of Queens (page 102), Beth Israel Med Ctr - Petrie Division (page 94); **Address:** 247 3rd Ave, Ste L 3, New York, NY 10010-7453; **Phone:** 212-995-8099; **Board Cert:** Surgery 2004; **Med School:** Romania 1971; **Resid:** Surgery, Cabrini Med Ctr 1985; **Fac Appt:** Assoc Clin Prof S, Mount Sinai Sch Med

Coit, Daniel G MD (S) - **Spec Exp:** Melanoma; Pancreatic Cancer; Stomach Cancer; **Hospital:** Meml Sloan-Kettering Cancer Ctr (page 116); **Address:** 1275 York Avenue, New York, NY 10065; **Phone:** 646-497-9072; **Board Cert:** Surgery 2004; **Med School:** Univ Cincinnati 1976; **Resid:** Internal Medicine, New Eng Deaconess Hosp 1978; Surgery, New Eng Deaconess Hosp 1983; **Fellow:** Surgical Oncology, Meml Sloan Kettering Canc Ctr 1985; **Fac Appt:** Prof S, Cornell Univ-Weill Med Coll

Edye, Michael MD (S) - **Spec Exp:** Laparoscopic Abdominal Surgery; Colon Cancer; Diverticulitis; Obesity/Bariatric Surgery; **Hospital:** Mount Sinai Med Ctr (page 102); **Address:** 17 E 102nd St Fl 5, Ctr for Advanced Medicine Bldg, New York, NY 10029; **Phone:** 212-241-0872; **Med School:** Australia 1977; **Resid:** Surgery, St Vincents Hosp 1980; Surgery, Royal N Shore Hosp 1984; **Fellow:** Laparoscopic Surgery, Univ Bordeaux 1992; **Fac Appt:** Assoc Clin Prof S, Mount Sinai Sch Med

El-Tamer, Mahmoud B MD (S) - **Spec Exp:** Breast Cancer; **Hospital:** Meml Sloan-Kettering Cancer Ctr (page 116); **Address:** Meml Sloan Kettering Cancer Ctr, 300 E 66th St, New York, NY 10032; **Phone:** 646-888-4753; **Board Cert:** Surgery 2001; **Med School:** Amer Univ Beirut 1981; **Resid:** Surgery, American Univ Hosp 1985; Surgery, SUNY Downstate Med Ctr 1992; **Fellow:** Surgical Oncology, Meml Sloan Kettering Cancer Ctr 1989; **Fac Appt:** Assoc Prof S, Columbia P&S

Emond, Jean C MD (S) - **Spec Exp:** Transplant-Liver; Liver Cancer; Liver & Biliary Cancer; Hepatobiliary Surgery; **Hospital:** NY-Presby/Columbia Univ Med Ctr, NY (page 104), Holy Name Med Ctr (page 688); **Address:** 622 W 168th St, PH - Fl 14, New York, NY 10032; **Phone:** 212-305-9691; **Board Cert:** Surgery 2006; **Med School:** Univ Chicago-Pritzker Sch Med 1979; **Resid:** Surgery, Cook Cty Hosp 1984; **Fellow:** Surgery, Hopital P Brousse/Univ de Paris Sud 1985; Transplant Surgery, Univ Chicago Hosps 1987; **Fac Appt:** Prof S, Columbia P&S

Estabrook, Alison MD (S) - **Spec Exp:** Breast Cancer; Breast Disease; Breast Cancer-High Risk Women; **Hospital:** St. Luke's - Roosevelt Hosp Ctr - Roosevelt Div (page 94); **Address:** Comprehensive Breast Center, 425 W 59th St Fl 7 - Ste 7A, New York, NY 10019-1104; **Phone:** 212-523-7500; **Board Cert:** Surgery 2004; **Med School:** NYU Sch Med 1978; **Resid:** Surgery, Columbia Presby Med Ctr 1984; **Fellow:** Surgical Oncology, Columbia Presby Med Ctr 1982; **Fac Appt:** Prof S, Columbia P&S

Fahey III, Thomas J MD (S) - **Spec Exp:** Endocrine Surgery; Pheochromocytoma; Pancreatic Cancer; Minimally Invasive Surgery; **Hospital:** NY-Presby/Weill Cornell Med Ctr, NY (page 104); **Address:** NY Presby Cornell Med Ctr, Dept Surgery, 525 E 68 St, rm Starr 8, Box 249, New York, NY 10065; **Phone:** 212-746-5130; **Board Cert:** Surgery 2002; **Med School:** Cornell Univ-Weill Med Coll 1986; **Resid:** Surgery, New York Hosp 1992; **Fellow:** Endocrine Surgery, Royal North Shore Hosp 1993; **Fac Appt:** Prof S, Cornell Univ-Weill Med Coll

Feldman, Sheldon M MD (S) - **Spec Exp:** Breast Surgery; Breast Cancer; Complementary Medicine; **Hospital:** NY-Presby/Columbia Univ Med Ctr, NY (page 104); **Address:** NY Presbyterian-Columbia Med Ctr, Div Surgical Oncology, 161 Fort Washington Ave, Fl 10, Ste 1005, New York, NY 10032; **Phone:** 212-305-9676; **Board Cert:** Surgery 2011; **Med School:** NYU Sch Med 1975; **Resid:** Surgery, NYU-Bellevue Med Ctr 1980; **Fellow:** Peripheral Vascular Surgery, Beth Israel Med Ctr 1981; **Fac Appt:** Assoc Clin Prof S, Columbia P&S

Fielding, George MD (S) - **Spec Exp:** Obesity/Bariatric Surgery; Hernia; Laparoscopic Surgery; **Hospital:** NYU Langone Med Ctr (page 108); **Address:** 530 First Ave, Ste 10-S, New York, NY 10016; **Phone:** 212-263-3166; **Med School:** Australia 1980; **Resid:** Surgery, Royal Brisbane & Women's Hosp 1986; Surgery, Glasgow Royal Infirmary 1988; **Fac Appt:** Assoc Prof S, NYU Sch Med

Fong, Yuman MD (S) - **Spec Exp:** Pancreatic Cancer; Liver & Biliary Cancer; Stomach Cancer; **Hospital:** Meml Sloan-Kettering Cancer Ctr (page 116), NY-Presby/Weill Cornell Med Ctr, NY (page 104); **Address:** 1275 York Ave, rm C887, New York, NY 10065; **Phone:** 212-639-2016; **Board Cert:** Surgery 2002; **Med School:** Cornell Univ-Weill Med Coll 1984; **Resid:** Surgery, NY Hosp-Cornell Med Ctr 1992; **Fellow:** Surgical Oncology, Meml Sloan-Kettering Cancer Ctr 1994; **Fac Appt:** Prof S, Cornell Univ-Weill Med Coll

Geller, Peter MD (S) - **Spec Exp:** Gastrointestinal Surgery; Hernia; Breast Cancer; Sentinel Node Surgery; **Hospital:** NY-Presby/Columbia Univ Med Ctr, NY (page 104); **Address:** Columbia Eastside, 16 E 60 St, rm 330, New York, NY 10022; **Phone:** 212-305-6657; **Board Cert:** Surgery 2004; **Med School:** Columbia P&S 1980; **Resid:** Surgery, Columbia-Presby Med Ctr 1985; **Fellow:** Vascular Surgery, Columbia-Presby Med Ctr 1986; **Fac Appt:** Assoc Prof S, Columbia P&S

Gouge, Thomas H MD (S) - **Spec Exp:** Esophageal Cancer; Pancreatic Cancer; Gastroesophageal Reflux Disease (GERD); **Hospital:** Bellevue Hosp Ctr; **Address:** 336 Central Park W, New York, NY 10025; **Phone:** 212-951-3366; **Board Cert:** Surgery 2007; **Med School:** Yale Univ 1970; **Resid:** Surgery, NYU Med Ctr 1975; **Fac Appt:** Prof S, NYU Sch Med

Heerdt, Alexandra S MD (S) - **Spec Exp:** Breast Cancer; **Hospital:** Meml Sloan-Kettering Cancer Ctr (page 116); **Address:** 300 E 66th St, New York, NY 10065; **Phone:** 646-888-5253; **Board Cert:** Surgery 2002; **Med School:** Jefferson Med Coll 1987; **Resid:** Surgery, NY Hosp-Cornell Med Ctr 1992; **Fellow:** Surgical Oncology, Meml Sloan Kettering Cancer Ctr 1993

Heller, Keith S MD (S) - **Spec Exp:** Thyroid & Parathyroid Surgery; Minimally Invasive Surgery; Head & Neck Tumors; Endocrine Surgery; **Hospital:** NYU Langone Med Ctr (page 108); **Address:** 530 First Ave, Ste 6H, New York, NY 10016; **Phone:** 212-263-7710; **Board Cert:** Surgery 2006; **Med School:** NYU Sch Med 1971; **Resid:** Surgery, NYU-Bellevue Hosp 1976; **Fellow:** Surgical Oncology, Meml Sloan Kettering Cancer Ctr 1978; **Fac Appt:** Prof S, NYU Sch Med

Herron, Daniel M MD (S) - **Spec Exp:** Obesity/Bariatric Surgery; Laparoscopic Surgery; Endoscopic Surgery; **Hospital:** Mount Sinai Med Ctr (page 102); **Address:** 17 E 102nd St, CAM Bldg - Fl 5, New York, NY 10029; **Phone:** 212-824-7891; **Board Cert:** Surgery 2008; **Med School:** Univ Pennsylvania 1992; **Resid:** Surgery, New England Med Ctr 1998; **Fellow:** Laparoscopic Surgery, Oregon Univ Hlth Sci Ctr 1999; **Fac Appt:** Prof S, Mount Sinai Sch Med

Hiotis, Spiros P MD/PhD (S) - **Spec Exp:** Liver Cancer; Gallbladder & Biliary Cancer; Pancreatic Cancer; Stomach Cancer; **Hospital:** Mount Sinai Med Ctr (page 102); **Address:** Surgical Oncology Assocs, 5 E 98th St Fl 12, Box 1259, New York, NY 100 129; **Phone:** 212-241-2891; **Board Cert:** Surgery 2010; **Med School:** Univ MD Sch Med 1992; **Resid:** Surgery, USF Med Ctr 1998; **Fellow:** Surgical Oncology, Meml Sloan Kettering Cancer Ctr 2000; **Fac Appt:** Asst Prof S, Mount Sinai Sch Med

Inabnet, William B MD (S) - **Spec Exp:** Thyroid Surgery; Adrenal Surgery; Pancreatic Surgery; Minimally Invasive Surgery; **Hospital:** Mount Sinai Med Ctr (page 102); **Address:** 5 E 98th St Fl 14, Box 1259, New York, NY 10029; **Phone:** 212-241-6918; **Board Cert:** Surgery 2007; **Med School:** Univ NC Sch Med 1991; **Resid:** Surgery, Rush Presby-St Lukes Med Ctr 1996; **Fellow:** Endocrine Surgery, Cochin Hosp 1997; **Fac Appt:** Asst Prof S, Columbia P&S

Jacob, Brian MD (S) - **Spec Exp:** Hernia; Obesity/Bariatric Surgery; **Hospital:** Mount Sinai Med Ctr (page 102); **Address:** 1010 Fifth Ave, New York, NY 10028; **Phone:** 212-879-6677; **Board Cert:** Surgery 2005; **Med School:** Wayne State Univ 1998; **Resid:** Surgery, Mt Sinai Sch Med 2004; **Fellow:** Minimally Invasive Surgery, NY Presby/Columbia Med Ctr 2005; **Fac Appt:** Assoc Clin Prof S, Mount Sinai Sch Med

Jarnagin, William MD (S) - **Spec Exp:** Hepatobiliary Surgery; Liver Cancer; Pancreatic Cancer; Gallbladder & Biliary Cancer; **Hospital:** Meml Sloan-Kettering Cancer Ctr (page 116); **Address:** 1275 York Ave, New York, NY 10065; **Phone:** 212-639-7601; **Board Cert:** Surgery 2006; **Med School:** Rush Med Coll 1988; **Resid:** Surgery, Univ Calif San Francisco 1996; **Fellow:** Hepatopancreatobiliary Surgery, Meml Sloan-Kettering Cancer Ctr 1997; **Fac Appt:** Prof S, Cornell Univ

Kapur, Sandip MD (S) - **Spec Exp:** Transplant-Kidney; Pancreatic Islet Cell Transplant; Transplant-Pancreas; **Hospital:** NY-Presby/Weill Cornell Med Ctr, NY (page 104), NY-Presby/Columbia Univ Med Ctr, NY (page 104); **Address:** 525 E 68th St, Baker Bldg Fl 19 - Ste F1919, Box 98, New York, NY 10065; **Phone:** 212-746-5330; **Board Cert:** Surgery 2007; **Med School:** Cornell Univ-Weill Med Coll 1990; **Resid:** Surgery, Cornell Univ Med Ctr 1996; **Fellow:** Research, The Rogosin Inst 1994; Transplant Surgery, Thomas E Starzl Transplant Inst 1998; **Fac Appt:** Assoc Prof S, Cornell Univ-Weill Med Coll

Karpeh Jr, Martin S MD (S) - **Spec Exp:** Gastrointestinal Cancer; Esophageal Cancer; Pancreatic Cancer; Liver Cancer; **Hospital:** Beth Israel Med Ctr - Petrie Division (page 94); **Address:** Beth Israel Medical Center, Philips Ambulatory Care Center, 10 Union Square E, Ste 4D, New York, NY 10003; **Phone:** 212-420-4041; **Board Cert:** Surgery 2006; **Med School:** Penn State Coll Med 1983; **Resid:** Surgery, Hosp Univ Penn 1989; **Fellow:** Surgical Oncology, Meml Sloan Kettering Cancer Ctr 1991; **Fac Appt:** Prof S, Mount Sinai Sch Med

Kato, Tomoaki MD (S) - **Spec Exp:** Transplant-Liver; Transplant Surgery-Pediatric; Transplant-Multi Organ; Transplant-Auto Transplantation; **Hospital:** NY-Presby/Columbia Univ Med Ctr, NY (page 104); **Address:** Columbia Univ Med Ctr, 622 W 168th St PH 14 Bldg - rm 105, New York, NY 10032; **Phone:** 212-305-5101; **Med School:** Japan 1991; **Resid:** Surgery, Itami City Hospital 1995; **Fellow:** Transplant Surgery, Jackson Meml Hosp 1997; **Fac Appt:** Prof S, Columbia P&S

Kimmelstiel, Fred M MD (S) - **Spec Exp:** Laparoscopic Surgery; Breast Surgery; Cancer Surgery; Hernia; **Hospital:** St. Luke's - Roosevelt Hosp Ctr - Roosevelt Div (page 94); **Address:** 225 W 71st St, New York, NY 10023; **Phone:** 212-362-6060; **Board Cert:** Surgery 2006; **Med School:** NY Med Coll 1980; **Resid:** Surgery, St Lukes Roosevelt Hosp Ctr 1985; **Fellow:** Transplant Surgery, Univ Hosp 1986; **Fac Appt:** Asst Clin Prof S, Columbia P&S

Labow, Daniel M MD (S) - **Spec Exp:** Pancreatic Cancer; Gastrointestinal Cancer; Liver Cancer; **Hospital:** Mount Sinai Med Ctr (page 102); **Address:** 1 Gustave L Levy Pl, Box 1259, New York, NY 10029; **Phone:** 212-241-2891; **Board Cert:** Surgery 2003; **Med School:** Brown Univ 1995; **Resid:** Surgery, Univ Chicago Hosps 1997; Research, NY Presby/Cornell Med Ctr 1999; **Fellow:** Surgical Oncology, Sloan Kettering Cancer Ctr 2004; **Fac Appt:** Asst Prof S, Mount Sinai Sch Med

Lee, James A MD (S) - **Spec Exp:** Adrenal Surgery; Endocrine Surgery; Thyroid & Parathyroid Surgery; Pancreatic Surgery; **Hospital:** NY-Presby/Columbia Univ Med Ctr, NY (page 104); **Address:** Columbia Univ Med Ctr, Irving Pavilion, 161 Fort Washington Ave, rm 808, New York, NY 10032; **Phone:** 212-305-0444; **Board Cert:** Surgery 2005; **Med School:** Columbia P&S 1999; **Resid:** Surgery, NY Presby Hosp 2005; Research, NY Presby Hosp 2003; **Fellow:** Endocrine Surgery, UCSF Med Ctr 2006; **Fac Appt:** Asst Prof S, Columbia P&S

Lieberman, Michael D MD (S) - **Spec Exp:** Gastrointestinal Cancer; Colon & Rectal Cancer & Surgery; Hepatobiliary Surgery; Pancreatic Cancer; **Hospital:** NY-Presby/Weill Cornell Med Ctr, NY (page 104); **Address:** 1315 York Ave, Box 216, New York, NY 10021; **Phone:** 212-746-5434; **Board Cert:** Surgery 2003; **Med School:** UMDNJ-NJ Med Sch, Newark 1985; **Resid:** Surgery, Hosp Univ Penn 1992; **Fellow:** Surgical Oncology, Hosp Univ Penn 1990; Surgical Oncology, Meml Sloan-Kettering Cancer Ctr 1994; **Fac Appt:** Assoc Prof S, Cornell Univ-Weill Med Coll

Michelassi, Fabrizio MD (S) - **Spec Exp:** Gastrointestinal Cancer; Crohn's Disease; Ulcerative Colitis; Colon Cancer; **Hospital:** NY-Presby/Weill Cornell Med Ctr, NY (page 104); **Address:** 525 E 68th St Fl 7 - rm F-739, Box 129, New York, NY 10065; **Phone:** 212-746-6006; **Board Cert:** Surgery 2002; **Med School:** Italy 1975; **Resid:** Surgery, NYU Med Ctr 1981; **Fellow:** Research, Mass Genl Hosp 1983; **Fac Appt:** Prof S, Cornell Univ-Weill Med Coll

Mills, Christopher B MD (S) - **Spec Exp:** Breast Surgery; Cancer Surgery; **Hospital:** Beth Israel Med Ctr - Petrie Division (page 94); **Address:** 325 W 15th St, New York, NY 10011; **Phone:** 212-604-6006; **Board Cert:** Surgery 2009; **Med School:** UMDNJ-NJ Med Sch, Newark 1973; **Resid:** Surgery, St Vincent's Hosp & Med Ctr 1978; **Fellow:** Nutrition & Metabolism, Ravenswood Hosp Med Ctr 1979; **Fac Appt:** Asst Prof S, NY Med Coll

Morrow, Monica MD (S) - **Spec Exp:** Breast Cancer; **Hospital:** Meml Sloan-Kettering Cancer Ctr (page 116); **Address:** 300 E 66th St Fl 4, New York, NY 10065; **Phone:** 646-888-5354; **Board Cert:** Surgery 2011; **Med School:** Jefferson Med Coll 1976; **Resid:** Surgery, Med Ctr Hosp Vermont 1981; **Fellow:** Surgical Oncology, Meml Sloan Kettering Cancer Ctr 1983; **Fac Appt:** Prof S, Cornell Univ-Weill Med Coll

Newman, Elliot MD (S) - **Spec Exp:** Gastrointestinal Cancer; Robotic Surgery; Liver & Biliary Cancer; Colon & Rectal Cancer; **Hospital:** NYU Langone Med Ctr (page 108); **Address:** NYU Clinical Cancer Ctr, 160 E 34th St, New York, NY 10016; **Phone:** 212-731-5466; **Board Cert:** Surgery 2004; **Med School:** NYU Sch Med 1986; **Resid:** Surgery, NYU Med Ctr 1989; Surgery, NYU Med Ctr 1993; **Fellow:** Research, Meml Sloan Kettering Cancer Ctr 1991; Surgical Oncology, Meml Sloan Kettering Cancer Ctr 1995; **Fac Appt:** Assoc Prof S, NYU Sch Med

Nowak, Eugene J MD (S) - **Spec Exp:** Breast Cancer; Hernia; Sentinel Node Surgery; Gastrointestinal Surgery; **Hospital:** NY-Presby/Weill Cornell Med Ctr, NY (page 104); **Address:** 325 E 79th St, Ground Fl, New York, NY 10075-0954; **Phone:** 212-517-6693; **Board Cert:** Surgery 2002; **Med School:** UMDNJ-NJ Med Sch, Newark 1975; **Resid:** Surgery, New York Hosp 1980; **Fac Appt:** Asst Clin Prof S, Cornell Univ-Weill Med Coll

Osborne, Michael P MD (S) - **Spec Exp:** Breast Cancer & Surgery; Breast Disease; Breast Reconstruction; **Hospital:** Beth Israel Med Ctr - Petrie Division (page 94); **Address:** 325 W 15 St, Beth Israel Comprehensive Cancer Center, New York, NY 10011; **Phone:** 212-367-0133; **Med School:** England, UK 1970; **Resid:** Surgery, Charing Cross Hosp 1977; Surgery, Royal Marsden Hosp 1980; **Fellow:** Surgical Oncology, Meml Sloan-Kettering Canc Ctr 1981; **Fac Appt:** Prof S, Cornell Univ-Weill Med Coll

Pachter, H Leon MD (S) - **Spec Exp:** Adrenal Surgery; Gastrointestinal Surgery; Pancreatic Cancer; Hernia; **Hospital:** NYU Langone Med Ctr (page 108), Bellevue Hosp Ctr; **Address:** 530 1st Ave, Ste 6C, New York, NY 10016; **Phone:** 212-263-7302; **Board Cert:** Surgery 2009; **Med School:** NYU Sch Med 1971; **Resid:** Surgery, NYU Med Ctr 1976; **Fac Appt:** Prof S, NYU Sch Med

Paty, Philip B MD (S) - **Spec Exp:** Colon & Rectal Cancer; Gastrointestinal Cancer; Pelvic Tumors; **Hospital:** Meml Sloan-Kettering Cancer Ctr (page 116); **Address:** 1275 York Avenue, New York, NY 10065; **Phone:** 646-497-9065; **Board Cert:** Surgery 2001; **Med School:** Stanford Univ 1983; **Resid:** Surgery, UCSF Med Ctr 1990; **Fellow:** Surgical Oncology, Meml Sloan Kettering Cancer Ctr 1992; **Fac Appt:** Prof S, Cornell Univ-Weill Med Coll

Pomp, Alfons MD (S) - **Spec Exp:** Obesity/Bariatric Surgery; Laparoscopic Abdominal Surgery; Hernia; **Hospital:** NY-Presby/Weill Cornell Med Ctr, NY (page 104); **Address:** Weill Cornell College of Medicine, 525 E 68th St, Box 294, New York, NY 10065; **Phone:** 212-746-5294; **Board Cert:** Surgery 2010; **Med School:** Univ Sherbrooke 1980; **Resid:** Surgery, Univ Montreal Med Ctr 1985; **Fellow:** Nutrition, Rhode Island Hosp 1988; **Fac Appt:** Prof S, Cornell Univ-Weill Med Coll

Port, Elisa R MD (S) - **Spec Exp:** Breast Cancer & Surgery; Sentinel Node Surgery; Nipple Sparing Mastectomy; **Hospital:** Mount Sinai Med Ctr (page 102); **Address:** 1176 5th Ave, New York, NY 10029; **Phone:** 212-241-3806; **Board Cert:** Surgery 2000; **Med School:** Mount Sinai Sch Med 1992; **Resid:** Surgery, Cedars Sinai Med Ctr 1995; Surgery, LIJ Med Ctr 1997; **Fac Appt:** Assoc Prof S, Mount Sinai Sch Med

Ratner, Lloyd E MD (S) - **Spec Exp:** Transplant-Kidney; Transplant-Pancreas; Pancreatic Surgery; **Hospital:** NY-Presby/Columbia Univ Med Ctr, NY (page 104); **Address:** Columbia University, PH 14, 622 W 168th St, rm 408, New York, NY 10032; **Phone:** 212-305-6469; **Board Cert:** Surgery 2009; **Med School:** Hahnemann Univ 1983; **Resid:** Surgery, LIJ Med Ctr 1988; **Fellow:** Transplant Surgery, Barnes Jewish Hosp 1990; **Fac Appt:** Assoc Prof S, Columbia P&S

Reiner, Mark A MD (S) - **Spec Exp:** Laparoscopic Surgery; Hernia; Esophageal Surgery; Pancreatic Surgery; **Hospital:** Mount Sinai Med Ctr (page 102); **Address:** 1010 5th Ave, Ste 82 & 83, New York, NY 10028-0130; **Phone:** 212-879-6677; **Board Cert:** Surgery 2011; **Med School:** SUNY Downstate 1974; **Resid:** Surgery, Mt Sinai Hosp 1979; **Fac Appt:** Clin Prof S, Mount Sinai Sch Med

Ren-Fielding, Christine J MD (S) - **Spec Exp:** Obesity/Bariatric Surgery; Laparoscopic Surgery; **Hospital:** NYU Langone Med Ctr (page 108); **Address:** NYU Med Ctr, 530 First Ave, Ste 10-S, New York, NY 10016; **Phone:** 212-263-3166; **Board Cert:** Surgery 2010; **Med School:** Tufts Univ 1993; **Resid:** Surgery, NYU Med Ctr 1999; **Fellow:** Bariatric Surgery, NYU Med Ctr 2000; **Fac Appt:** Asst Prof S, NYU Sch Med

Rosenberg, Vladimiro MD (S) - **Spec Exp:** Breast Cancer; Melanoma; Thyroid & Parathyroid Surgery; Sarcoma-Soft Tissue; **Hospital:** Mount Sinai Med Ctr (page 102), Lenox Hill Hosp (page 106); **Address:** 1440 York Ave, Ste P-10, New York, NY 10075; **Phone:** 212-772-0010; **Med School:** Argentina 1965; **Resid:** Surgery, Mt Sinai Hosp 1977; **Fellow:** Surgical Oncology, MD Anderson Cancer Ctr 1978; **Fac Appt:** Asst Clin Prof S, Mount Sinai Sch Med

Roses, Daniel F MD (S) - **Spec Exp:** Breast Cancer; Melanoma; Thyroid Cancer; Parathyroid Cancer; **Hospital:** NYU Langone Med Ctr (page 108); **Address:** 530 First Ave, Ste 6B, New York, NY 10016-6402; **Phone:** 212-263-7329; **Board Cert:** Surgery 1975; **Med School:** NYU Sch Med 1969; **Resid:** Surgery, NYU-Bellevue Hosp 1974; **Fellow:** Surgical Oncology, NYU-Bellevue Hosp 1978; **Fac Appt:** Prof Surg & Onc, NYU Sch Med

Rubino, Francesco MD (S) - **Spec Exp:** Gastrointestinal Metabolic Surgery; Diabetes Surgery-Rubino's Procedure; Obesity/Bariatric Surgery; **Hospital:** NY-Presby/Weill Cornell Med Ctr, NY (page 104); **Address:** NY Presbyterian Hosp/Weill Cornell, 525 E 68th St, rm P714, New York, NY 10021; **Phone:** 212-746-5925; **Med School:** Italy 1994; **Resid:** Surgery, Catholic Univ/Policlinico Gemelli; **Fellow:** Laparoscopic Surgery, European Inst of Telesurgery; Research, Catholic Univ; **Fac Appt:** Asst Prof S, Cornell Univ-Weill Med Coll

Salky, Barry A MD (S) - **Spec Exp:** Laparoscopic Abdominal Surgery; Gastroesophageal Reflux Disease (GERD); Colon Cancer; Ulcerative Colitis; **Hospital:** Mount Sinai Med Ctr (page 102); **Address:** Mt Sinai Medical Center, Div of Laparoscopic Surgery, 5 E 98th St Fl 14 - Ste C, Box 1259, New York, NY 10029; **Phone:** 212-241-6156; **Board Cert:** Surgery 2010; **Med School:** Univ Tenn Coll Med 1970; **Resid:** Surgery, Mount Sinai Hosp 1973; Surgery, Mount Sinai Hosp 1978; **Fac Appt:** Prof S, Mount Sinai Sch Med

Schnabel, Freya MD (S) - **Spec Exp:** Breast Cancer; Breast Cancer-High Risk Women; **Hospital:** NYU Langone Med Ctr (page 108); **Address:** 160 E 34th St Fl 3, New York, NY 10016; **Phone:** 212-731-5367; **Board Cert:** Surgery 2008; **Med School:** NYU Sch Med 1982; **Resid:** Surgery, NYU Med Ctr 1987; **Fellow:** Research, SUNY Hlth Sci Ctr 1988; **Fac Appt:** Prof S, NYU Sch Med

Schwartz, Myron E MD (S) - **Spec Exp:** Gastrointestinal Cancer; Liver Cancer; Hepatobiliary Surgery; **Hospital:** Mount Sinai Med Ctr (page 102); **Address:** Mount Sinai Med Ctr, 5 E 98th St Fl 12, Box 1104, New York, NY 10029; **Phone:** 212-659-8084; **Board Cert:** Surgery 2009; **Med School:** Jefferson Med Coll 1976; **Resid:** Surgery, Mt Sinai Hosp 1986; Vascular Surgery, Mt Sinai Hosp 1987; **Fac Appt:** Prof S, Mount Sinai Sch Med

Shah, Jatin P MD/PhD (S) - **Spec Exp:** Head & Neck Cancer & Surgery; Thyroid Cancer; Skull Base Tumors; Salivary Gland Tumors & Surgery; **Hospital:** Meml Sloan-Kettering Cancer Ctr (page 116); **Address:** 1275 York Ave, New York, NY 10065; **Phone:** 646-497-9161; **Board Cert:** Surgery 1975; **Med School:** India 1964; **Resid:** Surgery, SSG Hosp 1967; Surgery, NY Eye & Ear Infirm 1974; **Fellow:** Head & Neck Surgical Oncology, Meml Sloan-Kettering Hosp 1972; **Fac Appt:** Prof S, Cornell Univ-Weill Med Coll

Shah, Paresh C MD (S) - **Spec Exp:** Laparoscopic Surgery; Obesity/Bariatric Surgery; Minimally Invasive Surgery; **Hospital:** Lenox Hill Hosp (page 106); **Address:** 186 E 76 St Fl 1, New York, NY 10021; **Phone:** 212-434-3285; **Board Cert:** Surgery 2010; **Med School:** SUNY Downstate 1991; **Resid:** Surgery, SUNY- Downstate Med Ctr 1993; Surgery, Mass General Hosp 1995; **Fellow:** Laparoscopic Surgery, Lahey Clinic 1999

Shapiro, Richard L MD (S) - **Spec Exp:** Breast Cancer; Melanoma; Thyroid & Parathyroid Surgery; Cancer Surgery; **Hospital:** NYU Langone Med Ctr (page 108); **Address:** NYU Medical Clinical Cancer Center, 160 E 34th St Fl 4, New York, NY 10016; **Phone:** 212-731-5347; **Board Cert:** Surgery 2004; **Med School:** NYU Sch Med 1988; **Resid:** Surgery, NYU Langone Med Ctr 1993; **Fellow:** Surgical Oncology, NYU Langone Med Ctr 1995; **Fac Appt:** Assoc Prof S, NYU Sch Med

Simmons, Rache M MD (S) - **Spec Exp:** Breast Cancer & Surgery; Minimally Invasive Surgery; **Hospital:** NY-Presby/Weill Cornell Med Ctr, NY (page 104); **Address:** Weill Cornell Breast Ctr, 425 E 61st St Fl 10, New York, NY 10065; **Phone:** 212-821-0853; **Board Cert:** Surgery 2005; **Med School:** Duke Univ 1988; **Resid:** Surgery, Univ NC Hosp 1993; **Fellow:** Surgical Oncology, NY Hosp-Cornell Hosp 1994; **Fac Appt:** Assoc Prof S, Cornell Univ-Weill Med Coll

Singer, Samuel MD (S) - **Spec Exp:** Sarcoma-Soft Tissue; **Hospital:** Meml Sloan-Kettering Cancer Ctr (page 116); **Address:** 1275 York Ave, Ste H1210, New York, NY 10065; **Phone:** 646-497-9072; **Board Cert:** Surgery 2010; **Med School:** Harvard Med Sch 1982; **Resid:** Surgery, Brigham & Women's Hosp 1988; **Fellow:** Surgical Oncology, Dana Farber Cancer Inst 1990; **Fac Appt:** Assoc Prof S, Cornell Univ-Weill Med Coll

Slater, Gary MD (S) - **Spec Exp:** Gastrointestinal Surgery; Laparoscopic Surgery; Hernia; **Hospital:** Mount Sinai Med Ctr (page 102); **Address:** 5 E 98th St Fl 14, Ste C, New York, NY 10029-6501; **Phone:** 212-241-9281; **Board Cert:** Surgery 1975; **Med School:** NYU Sch Med 1968; **Resid:** Surgery, Mount Sinai Hosp 1974; **Fac Appt:** Prof S, Mount Sinai Sch Med

Swistel, Alexander J MD (S) - **Spec Exp:** Breast Cancer & Surgery; Cancer Reconstruction; Nipple Sparing Mastectomy; **Hospital:** NY-Presby/Weill Cornell Med Ctr, NY (page 104), St. Luke's - Roosevelt Hosp Ctr - Roosevelt Div (page 94); **Address:** 425 E 61st St, Fl 10, New York, NY 10065; **Phone:** 212-821-0602; **Board Cert:** Surgery 2005; **Med School:** Brown Univ 1975; **Resid:** Surgery, St Luke's Roosevelt Hosp Ctr 1981; **Fellow:** Surgical Oncology, Meml Sloan Kettering Canc Ctr 1983; **Fac Appt:** Assoc Clin Prof S, Cornell Univ-Weill Med Coll

Tartter, Paul MD (S) - **Spec Exp:** Breast Cancer; Breast Cancer in Elderly; Sentinel Node Surgery; **Hospital:** St. Luke's - Roosevelt Hosp Ctr - Roosevelt Div (page 94); **Address:** 425 W 59th St, Ste 7A, New York, NY 10019-1104; **Phone:** 212-523-7500; **Board Cert:** Surgery 2011; **Med School:** Brown Univ 1977; **Resid:** Surgery, Mt Sinai Hosp 1982; **Fac Appt:** Assoc Prof S, Columbia P&S

Teperman, Lewis W MD (S) - **Spec Exp:** Transplant-Liver; Transplant-Kidney; Liver Cancer; Hepatobiliary Surgery; **Hospital:** NYU Langone Med Ctr (page 108); **Address:** NYU Transplant Associates, 403 E 34th St Fl 3, New York, NY 10016; **Phone:** 212-263-8134; **Board Cert:** Surgery 2007; **Med School:** Mount Sinai Sch Med 1981; **Resid:** Surgery, Columbia Presby Med Ctr 1984; Surgery, LI Jewish Med Ctr 1986; **Fellow:** Transplant Surgery, Univ Pittsburgh 1988; **Fac Appt:** Assoc Prof S, NYU Sch Med

Tousimis, Eleni MD (S) - **Spec Exp:** Breast Cancer & Surgery; Breast Disease; Minimally Invasive Surgery; **Hospital:** NY-Presby/Weill Cornell Med Ctr, NY (page 104); **Address:** 425 E 61st St, Fl 10, New York, NY 10065; **Phone:** 212-821-0850; **Board Cert:** Surgery 2002; **Med School:** Albany Med Coll 1996; **Resid:** Surgery, Guthrie Clin-Robert Packer Hosp 2001; **Fellow:** Surgery, Meml Sloan Kettering Canc Ctr 2002; **Fac Appt:** Asst Prof S, Cornell Univ-Weill Med Coll

Van Zee, Kimberly J MD (S) - **Spec Exp:** Breast Cancer; **Hospital:** Meml Sloan-Kettering Cancer Ctr (page 116); **Address:** Meml Sloan Kettering Cancer Ctr, Evelyn H Lauder Breast Center, 300 E 66th St, New York, NY 10065; **Phone:** 800-525-2225; **Board Cert:** Surgery 2003; **Med School:** Harvard Med Sch 1987; **Resid:** Surgery, NY Hosp-Cornell Univ Med Ctr 1990; Surgery, NY Hosp-Cornell Univ Med Ctr 1994; **Fellow:** Research, NY Hosp-Cornell Univ Med Ctr 1993; **Fac Appt:** Prof S, Cornell Univ-Weill Med Coll

Vine, Anthony J MD (S) - **Spec Exp:** Laparoscopic Abdominal Surgery; Gastroesophageal Reflux Disease (GERD); Colon & Rectal Surgery; **Hospital:** Mount Sinai Med Ctr (page 102); **Address:** 1010 5th Ave, New York, NY 10028-0130; **Phone:** 212-879-6677; **Board Cert:** Surgery 2009; **Med School:** Vanderbilt Univ 1989; **Resid:** Surgery, Mt Sinai Med Ctr 1996; **Fellow:** Colon & Rectal Surgery, Mass Genl Hosp 1994; **Fac Appt:** Asst Clin Prof S, Mount Sinai Sch Med

Wallack, Marc MD (S) - **Spec Exp:** Melanoma; Breast Surgery; **Hospital:** Metropolitan Hosp Ctr - NY; **Address:** 1901 1st Ave, rm 12A-1, New York, NY 10029; **Phone:** 212-423-6614; **Board Cert:** Surgery 2011; **Med School:** Univ Pittsburgh 1970; **Resid:** Surgery, Hosp Univ Penn 1977; **Fellow:** Medical Oncology, Wistar Inst Anatomy & Biology 1977; **Fac Appt:** Prof S, NY Med Coll

Wedderburn, Raymond MD (S) - **Hospital:** St. Luke's - Roosevelt Hosp Ctr - Roosevelt Div (page 94); **Address:** 1111 Amsterdam Ave Muhlenberg Bldg, Fl 2 - Ste M2 Section D, New York, NY 10025; **Phone:** 212-523-5295; **Board Cert:** Surgery 2002; Surgical Critical Care 2003; **Med School:** Cornell Univ-Weill Med Coll 1986; **Resid:** Surgery, St Luke's-Roosevelt Hosp Ctr 1991; **Fellow:** Surgical Critical Care, Jackson Meml Hosp 1993; **Fac Appt:** Asst Clin Prof S, Columbia P&S

Yurt, Roger W MD (S) - **Spec Exp:** Burn Care; Wound Healing/Care; Hyperbaric Medicine; Critical Care; **Hospital:** NY-Presby/Weill Cornell Med Ctr, NY (page 104); **Address:** 525 E 68th St, rm L706, New York, NY 10021-4885; **Phone:** 212-746-5410; **Board Cert:** Surgery 2008; **Med School:** Univ Miami Sch Med 1972; **Resid:** Surgery, Parkland Meml Hosp 1974; Surgery, New York Hosp-Cornell Med Ctr 1980; **Fellow:** Internal Medicine, Brigham & Womens Hosp 1978; **Fac Appt:** Prof S, Cornell Univ-Weill Med Coll

Zarnegar, Rasa MD (S) - **Spec Exp:** Minimally Invasive Surgery; Endocrine Surgery; Gallbladder & Biliary Disease; Stomach Cancer; **Hospital:** NY-Presby/Weill Cornell Med Ctr, NY (page 104); **Address:** 525 E 68th St, Starr 8, New York, NY 10065; **Phone:** 212-746-5130; **Board Cert:** Surgery 2006; **Med School:** Univ Chicago-Pritzker Sch Med; **Resid:** Surgery, Univ Chicago Hosps 2003; Surgery, Univ Hosps Case Med Ctr 2005; **Fellow:** Endocrine Surgery, UCSF Med Ctr 2006; Minimally Invasive Surgery, UCSF Med Ctr 2006; **Fac Appt:** Asst Prof S, Cornell Univ-Weill Med Coll

Thoracic & Cardiac Surgery

Adams, David H MD (T&CS) - **Spec Exp:** Mitral Valve Surgery; Heart Valve Surgery; Minimally Invasive Cardiac Surgery; Aortic Surgery; **Hospital:** Mount Sinai Med Ctr (page 102); **Address:** The Mount Sinai Medical Center, Department of Cardiothoracic Surgery, 1190 Fifth Ave, MS 1028, New York, NY 10029; **Phone:** 212-659-6820; **Board Cert:** Thoracic Surgery 2003; **Med School:** Duke Univ 1983; **Resid:** Surgery, Brigham & Women's Hosp 1990; Thoracic & Cardiac Surgery, Brigham & Women's Hosp/Chldn's Hosp 1992; **Fellow:** Research, Harvard Med Sch 1988; Surgery, Harvard Med Sch 1992; **Fac Appt:** Prof T&CS, Mount Sinai Sch Med

Altorki, Nasser K MD (T&CS) - **Spec Exp:** Esophageal Cancer; Lung Cancer; Thoracic Cancers; Vaccine Therapy; **Hospital:** NY-Presby/Weill Cornell Med Ctr, NY (page 104); **Address:** 525 E 68th St, M-404, New York, NY 10065; **Phone:** 212-746-5156; **Board Cert:** Surgery 2006; Thoracic Surgery 2007; **Med School:** Egypt 1978; **Resid:** Surgery, Univ Chicago Hosps 1985; **Fellow:** Cardiothoracic Surgery, Univ Chicago Hosps 1987; **Fac Appt:** Prof S, Cornell Univ-Weill Med Coll

Argenziano, Michael MD (T&CS) - **Spec Exp:** Robotic Cardiac Surgery; Coronary Artery Surgery; Maze Procedure for Atrial Fibrillation; **Hospital:** NY-Presby/Columbia Univ Med Ctr, NY (page 104); **Address:** NY Presby Med Ctr, Milstein Bldg, 177 Fort Washington Ave, rm 7-435, New York, NY 10032; **Phone:** 212-305-5888; **Board Cert:** Thoracic Surgery 2002; **Med School:** Columbia P&S 1992; **Resid:** Surgery, Columbia Presby Med Ctr 1998; **Fellow:** Cardiothoracic Surgery, Columbia Presby Med Ctr 1999; **Fac Appt:** Asst Prof S, Columbia P&S

Bacha, Emile A MD (T&CS) - **Spec Exp:** Pediatric Cardiac Surgery; Congenital Heart Surgery; Neonatal & Infant Cardiac Surgery; Minimally Invasive Cardiac Surgery; **Hospital:** NY-Presby/Columbia Univ Med Ctr, NY (page 104), Morgan Stanley Children's Hosp of NY-Presby, NY (page 104); **Address:** Morgan Stanley Chldns Hosp North, Columbia Univ Medical Ctr, 3959 Broadway, rm 274, New York, NY 10032; **Phone:** 212-305-2688; **Board Cert:** Thoracic & Cardiac Surgery 2009; Congenital Cardiac Surgery 2009; **Med School:** Germany 1989; **Resid:** Thoracic Surgery, Mass Genl Hosp 1993; Surgery, Emory Univ Med Ctr 1995; **Fellow:** Pediatric Cardiac Surgery, Hosp Marie Lanne Longe 1996; Pediatric Cardiac Surgery, Mass Genl Hosp 1998; **Fac Appt:** Prof S, Columbia P&S

Bains, Manjit MD (T&CS) - **Spec Exp:** Cardiothoracic Surgery; Esophageal Cancer; Lung Cancer; **Hospital:** Meml Sloan-Kettering Cancer Ctr (page 116); **Address:** 1275 York Ave, rm C861, New York, NY 10065; **Phone:** 212-639-7450; **Board Cert:** Surgery 1971; Thoracic Surgery 1972; **Med School:** India 1963; **Resid:** Surgery, Rochester Genl Hosp 1970; **Fellow:** Thoracic Surgery, Sloan Kettering Cancer Ctr 1972; **Fac Appt:** Clin Prof S, Cornell Univ-Weill Med Coll

Camunas, Jorge Luis MD (T&CS) - **Spec Exp:** Lung Cancer; Pacemakers; Defibrillators; Thymoma; **Hospital:** Mount Sinai Med Ctr (page 102), James J. Peters VA Med Ctr-Bronx; **Address:** 16 E 98th St, Fl 1, Ste F, New York, NY 10029; **Phone:** 212-423-5817; **Board Cert:** Thoracic & Cardiac Surgery 2002; **Med School:** Georgetown Univ 1970; **Resid:** Surgery, Harlem Hosp 1976; Cardiothoracic Surgery, Mount Sinai Hosp 1980; **Fellow:** Cardiothoracic Surgery, St Lukes-Roosevelt Med Ctr 1978; **Fac Appt:** Assoc Prof TS, Mount Sinai Sch Med

Chen, Jonathan M MD (T&CS) - **Spec Exp:** Pediatric Cardiothoracic Surgery; Arrhythmias; Congenital Heart Disease; **Hospital:** Morgan Stanley Children's Hosp of NY-Presby, NY (page 104), NY-Presby/Columbia Univ Med Ctr, NY (page 104); **Address:** NY Presbyterian-Weill Cornell Med Ctr, 525 E 68th St, Ste M404, New York, NY 10065; **Phone:** 212-746-5014; **Board Cert:** Surgery 2001; Thoracic Surgery 2003; **Med School:** Columbia P&S 1994; **Resid:** Surgery, NY Columbia Presby Hosp 2000; **Fellow:** Cardiothoracic Surgery, NY Columbia Presby Hosp 2001; **Fac Appt:** Asst Prof S, Columbia P&S

Ciaburri, Daniel G MD (T&CS) - **Spec Exp:** Coronary Artery Surgery; Heart Valve Surgery; **Hospital:** New York Methodist Hosp (page 418); **Address:** 525 E 26 St Fl 4, Brooklyn, NY 10065; **Phone:** 212-746-5172; **Board Cert:** Thoracic Surgery 2009; Surgery 2009; **Med School:** Univ Conn 1983; **Resid:** Surgery, NY Presby-Cornell Med Ctr 1988; **Fellow:** Cardiothoracic Surgery, NY Presby-Cornell Med Ctr 1990; **Fac Appt:** Asst Prof TS, Cornell Univ-Weill Med Coll

Connery, Cliff MD (T&CS) - **Spec Exp:** Thoracic Cancers; Mediastinal Tumors; Minimally Invasive Surgery; Lung Cancer; **Hospital:** St. Luke's - Roosevelt Hosp Ctr - Roosevelt Div (page 94), Beth Israel Med Ctr - Petrie Division (page 94); **Address:** 1000 Tenth Ave, Ste 2B-07, New York, NY 10019; **Phone:** 212-523-7475; **Board Cert:** Surgery 2010; Thoracic & Cardiac Surgery 2003; Surgical Critical Care 2003; **Med School:** Eastern VA Med Sch 1984; **Resid:** Surgery, Univ Hosp 1989; Thoracic Surgery, Strong Meml Hosp 1992; **Fac Appt:** Asst Prof S, Columbia P&S

Crawford, Bernard MD (T&CS) - **Spec Exp:** Lung Cancer; Minimally Invasive Surgery; Esophageal Cancer; **Hospital:** NYU Langone Med Ctr (page 108); **Address:** 160 E 34th St, Fl 8, New York, NY 10016; **Phone:** 212-731-5580; **Board Cert:** Thoracic & Cardiac Surgery 2009; **Med School:** Geo Wash Univ 1980; **Resid:** Surgery, NYU Med Ctr 1985; **Fellow:** Cardiothoracic Surgery, NYU Med Ctr 1987; **Fac Appt:** Asst Prof TS, NYU Sch Med

Culliford III, Alfred T MD (T&CS) - **Spec Exp:** Mitral Valve Minimally Invasive Surgery; Coronary Artery Surgery; **Hospital:** NYU Langone Med Ctr (page 108); **Address:** NYU Medical Ctr, 530 1st Ave, Ste 9V, New York, NY 10016; **Phone:** 212-263-7288; **Board Cert:** Surgery 1974; Thoracic & Cardiac Surgery 2007; **Med School:** NY Med Coll 1969; **Resid:** Surgery, NYU Med Ctr 1974; **Fellow:** Thoracic Surgery, NYU Med Ctr 1976; **Fac Appt:** Prof TS, NYU Sch Med

DeAnda Jr, Abelardo MD (T&CS) - **Spec Exp:** Aneurysm-Aortic; Heart Valve Surgery; Cardiothoracic Surgery; Marfan's Syndrome; **Hospital:** NYU Langone Med Ctr (page 108), Bellevue Hosp Ctr; **Address:** NYU Medical Ctr, Cardiothoracic Surgery, 530 First Ave, Ste 9V, New York, NY 10016; **Phone:** 212-263-6516; **Board Cert:** Thoracic Surgery 2002; **Med School:** Stanford Univ 1990; **Resid:** Surgery, Stanford Med Ctr 1997; **Fellow:** Thoracic Surgery, Stanford Med Ctr 2000; **Fac Appt:** Assoc Prof TS, NYU Sch Med

Downey, Robert J MD (T&CS) - **Spec Exp:** Lung Cancer; Thoracic Cancers; **Hospital:** Meml Sloan-Kettering Cancer Ctr (page 116); **Address:** 1275 York Avenue, New York, NY 10065; **Phone:** 212-639-8124; **Board Cert:** Surgery 2002; Surgical Critical Care 2006; Thoracic & Cardiac Surgery 2005; **Med School:** Columbia P&S 1985; **Resid:** Surgery, Columbia-Presby Med Ctr 1991; **Fellow:** Thoracic Surgery, Mayo Clinic 1992; Thoracic Surgery, Columbia-Presby Med Ctr 1994

Filsoufi, Farzan MD (T&CS) - **Spec Exp:** Mitral Valve Surgery; Minimally Invasive Heart Valve Surgery; Heart Valve Surgery; Robotic Cardiac Surgery; **Hospital:** Mount Sinai Med Ctr (page 102), Elmhurst Hosp Ctr; **Address:** Mt Sinai Med Ctr, Dept Cardiothoracic Surg, 1190 5th Ave, Box 1028, New York, NY 10029; **Phone:** 212-659-6813; **Med School:** France 1991; **Resid:** Surgery, Univ Paris Hosps 1994; Thoracic Surgery, Hospital Broussais/U of Paris 1995; **Fellow:** Cardiothoracic Surgery, Hospital Broussais/U of Paris 1996; Heart Valve Surgery, Brigham & Women's Hosp 2000; **Fac Appt:** Prof TS, Mount Sinai Sch Med

Flores, Raja M MD (T&CS) - **Spec Exp:** Mesothelioma; Lung Cancer; Video Assisted Thoracic Surgery (VATS); Esophageal Cancer; **Hospital:** Mount Sinai Med Ctr (page 102); **Address:** Mt. Sinai Medical Ctr, 1440 Madison Ave, New York, NY 10029; **Phone:** 212-241-9466; **Board Cert:** Surgery 2009; Thoracic & Cardiac Surgery 2010; **Med School:** Albert Einstein Coll Med 1992; **Resid:** Surgery, Columbia Presby Med Ctr 1997; **Fellow:** Thoracic Surgery, Brigham & Womens Hosp/Dana Faber Cancer Inst 2000; **Fac Appt:** Assoc Prof TS, Cornell Univ-Weill Med Coll

Fontana, Gregory MD (T&CS) - **Spec Exp:** Minimally Invasive Surgery; Cardiac Surgery-Pediatric; Mitral Valve Surgery; Coronary Artery Surgery; **Hospital:** Lenox Hill Hosp (page 106); **Address:** Lenox Hill Hosp, Cardiothoracic Dept, 130 E 77th St Fl 4, New York, NY 10075; **Phone:** 212-434-3792; **Board Cert:** Thoracic Surgery 2004; **Med School:** UCLA 1984; **Resid:** Surgery, Duke Univ Med Ctr 1990; Thoracic Surgery, Duke Univ Med Ctr 1993; **Fellow:** Pediatric Cardiac Surgery, UCLA Med Ctr; Pediatric Cardiac Surgery, Chldns Hosp; **Fac Appt:** Clin Prof S, UCLA

Galloway, Aubrey MD (T&CS) - **Spec Exp:** Minimally Invasive Heart Valve Surgery; Mitral Valve Surgery; Coronary Artery Surgery; Robotic Surgery; **Hospital:** NYU Langone Med Ctr (page 108); **Address:** 530 1st Ave, Ste 9V, New York, NY 10016-6402; **Phone:** 212-263-7185; **Board Cert:** Thoracic Surgery 2006; **Med School:** Tulane Univ 1978; **Resid:** Surgery, Univ Colo Hlth Sci Ctr 1983; Cardiovascular Surgery, NYU Med Ctr 1985; **Fellow:** Research, Boston Chldns Hosp 1981; Cardiothoracic Surgery, NYU Med Ctr 1985; **Fac Appt:** Prof TS, NYU Sch Med

Ginsburg, Mark E MD (T&CS) - **Spec Exp:** Lung Cancer; Transplant-Lung; Emphysema-Lung Volume Reduction; **Hospital:** NY-Presby/Columbia Univ Med Ctr, NY (page 104), Good Samaritan Hosp - Suffern; **Address:** 161 Ft Washington Ave Fl 3 - Ste 301, New York, NY 10032; **Phone:** 212-305-3408; **Board Cert:** Surgery 2005; Thoracic Surgery 2006; **Med School:** Tufts Univ 1980; **Resid:** Surgery, Strong Meml Hosp 1985; **Fellow:** Thoracic Surgery, Strong Meml Hosp 1987; **Fac Appt:** Asst Clin Prof S, Columbia P&S

Girardi, Leonard N MD (T&CS) - **Spec Exp:** Aneurysm-Aortic; Cardiac Surgery; Marfan's Syndrome; Cardiothoracic Surgery; **Hospital:** NY-Presby/Weill Cornell Med Ctr, NY (page 104); **Address:** Cardiothoracic Surgery Dept, 525 E 68th St, Ste M404, New York, NY 10065; **Phone:** 212-746-5194; **Board Cert:** Surgery 2005; Thoracic Surgery 2007; **Med School:** Cornell Univ-Weill Med Coll 1989; **Resid:** Surgery, NY Presby/Cornell Univ Med Ctr 1994; **Fellow:** Cardiothoracic Surgery, NY Presby Hosp/Cornell Univ Med Ctr 1996; Cardiothoracic Surgery, Baylor Coll Med 1997; **Fac Appt:** Assoc Prof TS, Cornell Univ-Weill Med Coll

Gorenstein, Lyall MD (T&CS) - **Spec Exp:** Thoracic Cancers; Esophageal Surgery; Minimally Invasive Thoracic Surgery; Hyperhidrosis-Palmar; **Hospital:** NY-Presby/Columbia Univ Med Ctr, NY (page 104); **Address:** 161 Fort Washington Ave, New York, NY 10032; **Phone:** 212-305-3408; **Board Cert:** Surgery 2009; Thoracic Surgery 2001; **Med School:** Univ Toronto 1983; **Resid:** Radiation Therapy, Univ Toronto 1988; Thoracic Surgery, Univ Toronto 1992; **Fellow:** Thoracic Surgery, MD Anderson Cancer Ctr 1990; **Fac Appt:** Asst Clin Prof S, Columbia P&S

Grossi, Eugene A MD (T&CS) - **Spec Exp:** Minimally Invasive Cardiac Surgery; Mitral Valve Surgery; Cardiac Tumors, Myxomas; **Hospital:** NYU Langone Med Ctr (page 108); **Address:** NYU Langone Med Ctr, 530 1st Ave, Ste 9V, New York, NY 10016-6402; **Phone:** 212-263-7452; **Board Cert:** Thoracic Surgery 2011; **Med School:** Columbia P&S 1981; **Resid:** Surgery, NYU Med Ctr 1987; Thoracic Surgery, NYU Med Ctr 1991; **Fac Appt:** Prof S, NYU Sch Med

Hoffman, Darryl M MD (T&CS) - **Spec Exp:** Cardiac Surgery; Maze Procedure for Atrial Fibrillation; Pacemakers/Defibrillators; **Hospital:** Beth Israel Med Ctr - Petrie Division (page 94), St. Luke's - Roosevelt Hosp Ctr - Roosevelt Div (page 94); **Address:** Division of Cardiac Surgery, 317 E 17th St, Fierman Hall, 11th Fl, New York, NY 10003; **Phone:** 212-420-2584; **Med School:** South Africa 1983; **Resid:** Surgery 1989Edinburgh Royal Infirm; **Fellow:** Cardiac Surgery, Allegheny Genl Hosp 1993; Cardiac Surgery, Mayo Clinic 1994; **Fac Appt:** Asst Prof S, Albert Einstein Coll Med

Isom, O Wayne MD (T&CS) - **Spec Exp:** Cardiac Surgery; Coronary Artery Surgery; Heart Valve Surgery; **Hospital:** NY-Presby/Weill Cornell Med Ctr, NY (page 104), NY Hosp Queens (page 206); **Address:** 525 E 68th St, rm M-404, New York, NY 10065; **Phone:** 212-746-5151; **Board Cert:** Surgery 1971; Thoracic Surgery 1972; **Med School:** Univ Tex, Houston 1965; **Resid:** Surgery, Parkland Meml Hosp 1970; **Fellow:** Thoracic Surgery, NYU Med Ctr 1972; **Fac Appt:** Prof TS, Cornell Univ-Weill Med Coll

Krellenstein, Daniel J MD/PhD (T&CS) - **Spec Exp:** Lung Cancer; Minimally Invasive Thoracic Surgery; Asbestos-related Lung Disease; **Hospital:** Mount Sinai Med Ctr (page 102), Lenox Hill Hosp (page 106); **Address:** 16 E 98th St, Ste 1F, New York, NY 10029-6545; **Phone:** 212-423-9311; **Board Cert:** Surgery 1974; Thoracic & Cardiac Surgery 2006; **Med School:** SUNY Buffalo 1964; **Resid:** Surgery, SUNY Downstate Med Ctr 1971; **Fellow:** Thoracic & Cardiac Surgery, Kings County Hosp Ctr 1972; **Fac Appt:** Assoc Clin Prof TS, Mount Sinai Sch Med

Krieger, Karl H MD (T&CS) - **Spec Exp:** Heart Valve Surgery; Coronary Artery Surgery; Cardiac Surgery-Adult; **Hospital:** NY-Presby/Weill Cornell Med Ctr, NY (page 104), NY Hosp Queens (page 206); **Address:** Cardiothoracic Surgery Dept, 525 E 68th St, Ste M404, New York, NY 10065; **Phone:** 212-746-5152; **Board Cert:** Thoracic Surgery 2004; **Med School:** Johns Hopkins Univ 1975; **Resid:** Surgery, Johns Hopkins 1976Bellevue Hosp 1979; **Fellow:** Thoracic Surgery, NYU Med Ctr 1981; **Fac Appt:** Prof S, Cornell Univ-Weill Med Coll

Lazzaro, Richard S MD (T&CS) - **Spec Exp:** Robotic Surgery; Minimally Invasive Surgery; Thoracic Surgery; **Hospital:** Lenox Hill Hosp (page 106), N Shore Univ Hosp (page 106); **Address:** Lenox Hill Hospital, Dept Cardiothoracic Surgery, 130 E 77th St, Black Hall-4th Fl, New York, NY 10075; **Phone:** 212-434-3000; **Board Cert:** Surgery 2006; Thoracic & Cardiac Surgery 2007; **Med School:** Albany Med Coll 1988; **Resid:** Surgery, North Shore Univ Hosp 1994; **Fellow:** Cardiothoracic Surgery, SUNY Downstate Med Ctr 1997; Thoracic Surgery, Univ Pittsburgh 1998

Loulmet, Didier F MD (T&CS) - **Spec Exp:** Heart Valve Surgery; Robotic Cardiac Surgery; Minimally Invasive Cardiac Surgery; Aneurysm-Aortic; **Hospital:** NYU Langone Med Ctr (page 108); **Address:** NYU Medical Ctr, Cardiothoracic Surgery, 530 1st Ave, Ste 9V, New York, NY 10016; **Phone:** 212-263-2329; **Med School:** France 1984; **Resid:** Cardiothoracic Surgery, Paris Univ Hosp 1990; Cardiothoracic Surgery, Brigham & Women's Hosp 1991; **Fellow:** Pediatric Cardiac Surgery, Children's Hosp 1992; **Fac Appt:** Assoc Prof TS, NYU Sch Med

Mosca, Ralph S MD (T&CS) - **Spec Exp:** Cardiothoracic Surgery; Congenital Heart Disease-Adult & Child; Pediatric Cardiac Surgery; **Hospital:** NYU Langone Med Ctr (page 108); **Address:** 530 1st Ave, Ste 9V, New York, NY 10016; **Phone:** 212-263-5989; **Board Cert:** Thoracic Surgery 2011; **Med School:** SUNY Upstate Med Univ 1985; **Resid:** Surgery, SUNY Hlth Sci Ctr 1990; **Fellow:** Cardiothoracic Surgery, Columbia-Presby Med Ctr 1992; Pediatric Cardiac Surgery, Univ Mich Med Ctr 1993; **Fac Appt:** Prof TS, NYU Sch Med

Naka, Yoshifumi MD/PhD (T&CS) - **Spec Exp:** Transplant-Heart & Lung; Ventricular Assist Device (LVAD); Heart Failure & Ventricular Containment; Mitral Valve Surgery; **Hospital:** NY-Presby/Columbia Univ Med Ctr, NY (page 104); **Address:** 177 Fort Washington Ave, MHB Bldg Fl 7 - rm 435, New York, NY 10032; **Phone:** 212-305-0828; **Med School:** Japan 1984; **Resid:** Surgery, Osaka Police Hosp 1991; **Fellow:** Cardiovascular Surgery, Osaka Police Hosp 1993; Cardiothoracic Surgery, Columbia Univ Med Ctr 1998; **Fac Appt:** Asst Prof S, Columbia P&S

Nguyen, Khanh H MD (T&CS) - **Spec Exp:** Pediatric Cardiac Surgery; **Hospital:** Mount Sinai Med Ctr (page 102); **Address:** Mount Sinai Med Ctr, 1190 5th Ave, Box 1028, New York, NY 10029; **Phone:** 212-659-9472; **Board Cert:** Thoracic Surgery 2006; **Med School:** UC Irvine 1985; **Resid:** Surgery, Flushing Hosp 1992; Thoracic Surgery, Mt Sinai Med Ctr 1995

Oz, Mehmet C MD (T&CS) - **Spec Exp:** Transplant-Heart; Heart Valve Surgery; Minimally Invasive Cardiac Surgery; **Hospital:** NY-Presby/Columbia Univ Med Ctr, NY (page 104); **Address:** NY Presby Hosp, Dept Cardiothoracic Surg, 177 Ft Washington Ave, MHB- Rm 7, GN435, New York, NY 10032; **Phone:** 212-305-4434; **Board Cert:** Thoracic Surgery 2003; **Med School:** Univ Pennsylvania 1986; **Resid:** Surgery, Columbia Presby Med Ctr 1991; **Fellow:** Cardiothoracic Surgery, Columbia Presby Med Ctr 1993; **Fac Appt:** Prof S, Columbia P&S

Pass, Harvey I MD (T&CS) - **Spec Exp:** Lung Cancer; Mesothelioma; Clinical Trials; Robotic Surgery; **Hospital:** NYU Langone Med Ctr (page 108); **Address:** NYU Cancer Ctr, 160 E 34th St, Fl 8, New York, NY 10016; **Phone:** 212-731-5414; **Board Cert:** Thoracic & Cardiac Surgery 2001; **Med School:** Duke Univ 1973; **Resid:** Surgery, Duke Univ Med Ctr 1975; Surgery, Univ Miss Med Ctr 1980; **Fellow:** Cardiothoracic Surgery, MUSC Med Ctr 1982; Thoracic Oncology, Natl Cancer Inst 1985; **Fac Appt:** Prof T&CS, NYU Sch Med

Plestis, Konstadinos MD (T&CS) - **Spec Exp:** Aortic Surgery; Heart Valve Surgery; Aneurysm-Aortic; Aneurysm-Abdominal Aortic; **Hospital:** Lenox Hill Hosp (page 106); **Address:** Lenox Hill, Aortic Wellness Ctr, 130 E 77th St Fl 4th, New York, NY 10075; **Phone:** 212-434-6030; **Board Cert:** Surgery 2003; Vascular Surgery 2005; Thoracic Surgery 2008; **Med School:** Greece 1987; **Resid:** Surgery, Brooklyn Hosp Ctr 1993; Vascular Surgery, Baylor Univ Med Ctr 1995; **Fellow:** Cardiothoracic Surgery, Montefiore Med Ctr 1999; **Fac Appt:** Asst Prof S, Mount Sinai Sch Med

Port, Jeffrey L MD (T&CS) - **Spec Exp:** Cardiothoracic Surgery; Lung Cancer; Esophageal Cancer; **Hospital:** NY-Presby/Weill Cornell Med Ctr, NY (page 104); **Address:** 525 E 68th St, Ste M404, New York, NY 10065; **Phone:** 212-746-5197; **Board Cert:** Surgery 2009; Thoracic & Cardiac Surgery 2009; **Med School:** NYU Sch Med 1991; **Resid:** Surgery, NYU Med Ctr 1998; **Fellow:** Thoracic Surgery, NY Presby Hosp 2000; **Fac Appt:** Assoc Prof TS, Cornell Univ-Weill Med Coll

Rusch, Valerie MD (T&CS) - **Spec Exp:** Mesothelioma; Lung Cancer; Esophageal Cancer; **Hospital:** Meml Sloan-Kettering Cancer Ctr (page 116); **Address:** 1275 York Ave, New York, NY 10021-6094; **Phone:** 212-639-5873; **Board Cert:** Surgery 2011; Thoracic Surgery 2003; **Med School:** Columbia P&S 1975; **Resid:** Surgery, Univ Wash Med Ctr 1980; Cardiothoracic Surgery, Univ Wash Med Ctr 1982; **Fac Appt:** Prof TS, Cornell Univ-Weill Med Coll

Smith, Craig R MD (T&CS) - **Spec Exp:** Mitral Valve Surgery; Transplant-Heart; Minimally Invasive Cardiac Surgery; Robotic Cardiac Surgery; **Hospital:** NY-Presby/Columbia Univ Med Ctr, NY (page 104); **Address:** Columbia Presbyterian Med Ctr, 177 Fort Washington Ave Fl 7 - Ste 435, New York, NY 10032; **Phone:** 212-305-8312; **Board Cert:** Thoracic Surgery 2004; **Med School:** Case West Res Univ 1977; **Resid:** Surgery, Strong Meml Hosp 1982; **Fellow:** Cardiothoracic Surgery, Columbia Presby Med Ctr 1984; **Fac Appt:** Prof S, Columbia P&S

Sonett, Joshua R MD (T&CS) - **Spec Exp:** Minimally Invasive Thoracic Surgery; Transplant-Lung; Thoracic Cancers; Emphysema-Lung Volume Reduction; **Hospital:** NY-Presby/Columbia Univ Med Ctr, NY (page 104); **Address:** 161 Fort Washington Ave, Ste 301, New York, NY 10032; **Phone:** 212-305-8086; **Board Cert:** Surgery 2004; Thoracic Surgery 2007; **Med School:** E Carolina Univ 1988; **Resid:** Surgery, Univ Mass Med Ctr 1993; **Fellow:** Cardiothoracic Surgery, Univ Pittsburgh Med Ctr 1994; Thoracic Surgery, Meml Sloan Kettering Cancer Ctr; **Fac Appt:** Prof S, Columbia P&S

Spotnitz, Henry MD (T&CS) - **Spec Exp:** Pacemakers/Defibrillators; Heart Valve Surgery; **Hospital:** NY-Presby/Columbia Univ Med Ctr, NY (page 104); **Address:** 622 W 168th St, Ste 1422, New York, NY 10032; **Phone:** 212-305-6191; **Board Cert:** Surgery 1974; Thoracic Surgery 2005; **Med School:** Columbia P&S 1966; **Resid:** Surgery, Columbia-Presby Med Ctr 1973; Thoracic Surgery, Columbia-Presby Med Ctr 1975; **Fellow:** Research, Natl Inst Hlth 1969; **Fac Appt:** Prof S, Columbia P&S

Stelzer, Paul MD (T&CS) - **Spec Exp:** Heart Valve Surgery; Aneurysm-Thoracic Aortic; Ross Procedure/Aortic Valve Disease; **Hospital:** Mount Sinai Med Ctr (page 102); **Address:** 1190 5th Ave, Box 1028, New York, NY 10029; **Phone:** 212-659-6871; **Board Cert:** Thoracic Surgery 2000; **Med School:** Columbia P&S 1972; **Resid:** Surgery, St Luke's Roosevelt Hosp 1977; Thoracic Surgery, NY Hosp 1981; **Fac Appt:** Assoc Clin Prof TS, Albert Einstein Coll Med

Stewart, Allan MD (T&CS) - **Spec Exp:** Heart Valve Surgery-Aortic; Aneurysm-Aortic; Aortic Surgery; **Hospital:** NY-Presby/Columbia Univ Med Ctr, NY (page 104); **Address:** 177 Fort Washington Ave, Milstein Hosp Bldg Fl 7 - rm 435, New York, NY 10030; **Phone:** 212-305-4980; **Board Cert:** Surgery 2003; Thoracic Surgery 2006; **Med School:** UMDNJ-NJ Med Sch, Newark 1995; **Resid:** Surgery, Univ PA Hlth Sys 2002; **Fellow:** Thoracic Surgery, NY Presby Hosp 2004; **Fac Appt:** Asst Prof TS, Columbia P&S

Swistel, Daniel MD (T&CS) - **Spec Exp:** Coronary Artery Surgery; Minimally Invasive Surgery; Heart Valve Surgery; Hypertrophic Cardiomyopathy; **Hospital:** St. Luke's - Roosevelt Hosp Ctr - St Luke's Hosp (page 94); **Address:** 1111 Amsterdam Ave, MU 2 Section A, New York, NY 10025; **Phone:** 212-523-4088; **Board Cert:** Thoracic Surgery 2006; **Med School:** UMDNJ-RW Johnson Med Sch 1979; **Resid:** Surgery, St Lukes-Roosevelt Hosp 1984; Cardiothoracic Surgery, Montefiore Med Ctr 1986; **Fac Appt:** Assoc Clin Prof TS, Columbia P&S

Tranbaugh, Robert MD (T&CS) - **Spec Exp:** Coronary Artery Surgery; Heart Valve Surgery; Aneurysm-Thoracic Aortic; **Hospital:** Beth Israel Med Ctr - Petrie Division (page 94), St. Luke's - Roosevelt Hosp Ctr - Roosevelt Div (page 94); **Address:** 317 E 17th St, Fl 11, Division of Cardiac Surgery, Beth Israel Medical Center, New York, NY 10003; **Phone:** 212-420-2584; **Board Cert:** Thoracic Surgery 2004; **Med School:** Univ Pennsylvania 1976; **Resid:** Surgery, UCSF Med Ctr 1983; Cardiothoracic Surgery, UCSF Med Ctr 1985; **Fac Appt:** Assoc Prof T&CS, Albert Einstein Coll Med

Williams, Mathew R MD (T&CS) - **Spec Exp:** Interventional Cardiology; Heart Valve Surgery; **Hospital:** NY-Presby/Columbia Univ Med Ctr, NY (page 104); **Address:** Milstein Hospital Bldg Fl 7 - rm 435, 177 Fort Washington Ave, New York, NY 10032; **Phone:** 212-305-9320; **Board Cert:** Thoracic Surgery 2007; **Med School:** Columbia P&S 1996; **Resid:** Surgery, UCLA Med Ctr 1998; Surgery, NY Presby Hosp/Columbia 2003; **Fellow:** Cardiothoracic Surgery, NY Presby Hosp/Columbia 2005; Interventional Cardiology, NY Presby Hosp/Columbia 2006; **Fac Appt:** Asst Prof S, Columbia P&S

Urology

Armenakas, Noel MD (U) - **Spec Exp:** Genitourinary Reconstruction; Erectile Dysfunction; **Hospital:** Lenox Hill Hosp (page 106), NY-Presby/Weill Cornell Med Ctr, NY (page 104); **Address:** 880 5th Ave, New York, NY 10021-4951; **Phone:** 212-535-1950; **Board Cert:** Urology 2012; **Med School:** Greece 1985; **Resid:** Urology, Monmouth Med Ctr 1987; Urology, Lenox Hill Hosp 1991; **Fellow:** Trauma, UCSF Med Ctr 1992; Reconstructive Surgery, UCSF Med Ctr 1992; **Fac Appt:** Assoc Clin Prof U, Cornell Univ-Weill Med Coll

Bar-Chama, Natan MD (U) - **Spec Exp:** Infertility-Male; Erectile Dysfunction; Vasectomy Reversal; Varicocele Microsurgery; **Hospital:** Mount Sinai Med Ctr (page 102); **Address:** Center for Male Reproductive Health, 635 Madison Ave Fl 10, New York, NY 10022; **Phone:** 212-756-5777; **Board Cert:** Urology 2006; **Med School:** Albert Einstein Coll Med 1987; **Resid:** Urology, Montefiore Med Ctr 1993; **Fellow:** Male Infertility, Baylor Coll Med 1994; **Fac Appt:** Assoc Prof U, Mount Sinai Sch Med

Benson, Mitchell C MD (U) - **Spec Exp:** Prostate Cancer/Robotic Surgery; Bladder Cancer; Kidney Cancer; Continent Urinary Diversions; **Hospital:** NY-Presby/Columbia Univ Med Ctr, NY (page 104); **Address:** 161 Fort Washington Ave, Ste 1102, New York, NY 10032-3713; **Phone:** 212-305-5201; **Board Cert:** Urology 1984; **Med School:** Columbia P&S 1977; **Resid:** Surgery, Mount Sinai Med Ctr 1979; Urology, Columbia-Presby Hosp 1982; **Fellow:** Oncology, Johns Hopkins Hosp 1984; **Fac Appt:** Prof U, Columbia P&S

Berman, Steven MD (U) - **Spec Exp:** Prostate Cancer; Kidney Stones; **Hospital:** Beth Israel Med Ctr - Petrie Division (page 94); **Address:** 201 E 19th St, New York, NY 10003; **Phone:** 212-673-7300; **Board Cert:** Urology 2006; **Med School:** SUNY Downstate 1981; **Resid:** Surgery, Montefiore Med Ctr 1983; Urology, Montefiore Med Ctr 1986

Birkhoff, John MD (U) - **Spec Exp:** Urologic Cancer; Kidney Stones; **Hospital:** NY-Presby/Columbia Univ Med Ctr, NY (page 104); **Address:** 161 Fort Washington Ave, rm 1142, New York, NY 10032; **Phone:** 212-305-5421; **Board Cert:** Urology 1976; **Med School:** Columbia P&S 1969; **Resid:** Urology, Columbia-Presby 1975; **Fac Appt:** Asst Clin Prof Med, Columbia P&S

Birns, Douglas R MD (U) - **Spec Exp:** Prostate Cancer; Kidney Cancer; Bladder Cancer; **Hospital:** Mount Sinai Med Ctr (page 102), Beth Israel Med Ctr - Petrie Division (page 94); **Address:** 157 E 72nd St, New York, NY 10021-4331; **Phone:** 212-744-8700; **Board Cert:** Urology 2006; **Med School:** SUNY Downstate 1981; **Resid:** Surgery, Mount Sinai Hosp 1982; Urology, Mount Sinai Hosp 1986; **Fac Appt:** Asst Clin Prof U, Mount Sinai Sch Med

Blaivas, Jerry G MD (U) - **Spec Exp:** Uro-Gynecology; Urology-Female; Neurogenic Bladder; Incontinence after Prostate Cancer; **Hospital:** NY-Presby/Weill Cornell Med Ctr, NY (page 104), Lenox Hill Hosp (page 106); **Address:** 445 E 77th St, New York, NY 10075; **Phone:** 212-772-3900; **Board Cert:** Urology 1978; **Med School:** Tufts Univ 1968; **Resid:** Surgery, Boston Med Ctr 1971; Urology, New England Med Ctr 1976; **Fac Appt:** Clin Prof U, Cornell Univ-Weill Med Coll

Bochner, Bernard MD (U) - **Spec Exp:** Bladder Cancer; Urinary Reconstruction; **Hospital:** Meml Sloan-Kettering Cancer Ctr (page 116); **Address:** MSKCC, Dept Urology, 353 E 68 St, New York, NY 10065; **Phone:** 646-422-4387; **Board Cert:** Urology 2011; **Med School:** UCLA 1990; **Resid:** Surgery, LAC/USC Med Ctr 1992; Urology, LAC/USC Med Ctr 1996; **Fellow:** Urologic Oncology, USC/Norris Comp Cancer Ctr 1999

Boczko, Stanley MD (U) - **Spec Exp:** Prostate Cancer; Impotence; Prostate Disease; **Hospital:** Montefiore Med Ctr-Moses Campus, NY (page 100), Lenox Hill Hosp (page 106); **Address:** 23 E 79th St, New York, NY 10021; **Phone:** 212-628-1800; **Board Cert:** Urology 1981; **Med School:** Albert Einstein Coll Med 1973; **Resid:** Surgery, Montefiore Med Ctr 1975; Urology, Montefiore Med Ctr 1979; **Fellow:** Transplant Surgery, Montefiore Med Ctr 1975; **Fac Appt:** Assoc Prof U, Albert Einstein Coll Med

Brodherson, Michael MD (U) - **Spec Exp:** Urologic Cancer; Kidney Stones; **Hospital:** Lenox Hill Hosp (page 106); **Address:** 4 E 76th St, New York, NY 10021-2611; **Phone:** 212-794-2749; **Board Cert:** Urology 1981; **Med School:** SUNY Downstate 1973; **Resid:** Internal Medicine, Lenox Hill Hosp 1976; Urology, Lenox Hill Hosp 1979

DelPizzo, Joseph J MD (U) - **Spec Exp:** Laparoscopic Kidney Surgery; Robotic Surgery; Minimally Invasive Surgery; Kidney Stones; **Hospital:** NY-Presby/Weill Cornell Med Ctr, NY (page 104); **Address:** NY Presby-Cornell Med Ctr, Dept Urology, 525 E 68th St Fl 9, New York, NY 10021; **Phone:** 212-746-5250; **Board Cert:** Urology 2003; **Med School:** Albert Einstein Coll Med 1994; **Resid:** Surgery, Mercy Med Ctr 1996; Urology, Univ Maryland Med System 2000; **Fac Appt:** Assoc Prof U, Cornell Univ-Weill Med Coll

Dillon, Robert W MD (U) - **Spec Exp:** Kidney Stones; Urologic Cancer; Urology-Female; **Hospital:** Mount Sinai Med Ctr (page 102); **Address:** 58-A E 79th St, New York, NY 10075; **Phone:** 212-794-9000; **Board Cert:** Urology 1980; **Med School:** NY Med Coll 1973; **Resid:** Surgery, Mt Sinai Hosp 1975; Urology, Mt Sinai Hosp 1978; **Fac Appt:** Asst Clin Prof U, Mount Sinai Sch Med

Droller, Michael J MD (U) - **Spec Exp:** Urologic Cancer; Bladder Cancer; Prostate Cancer; Kidney Cancer; **Hospital:** Mount Sinai Med Ctr (page 102); **Address:** 5 E 98th St, Fl 6, Box 1272, New York, NY 10029-6501; **Phone:** 212-241-3868; **Board Cert:** Urology 2001; **Med School:** Harvard Med Sch 1968; **Resid:** Surgery, Peter Bent Brigham Hosp 1970; Urology, Stanford Univ Med Ctr 1976; **Fellow:** Immunology, Univ Stockholm 1977; **Fac Appt:** Prof U, Mount Sinai Sch Med

Eastham, James MD (U) - **Spec Exp:** Prostate Cancer; Prostate Cancer/Robotic Surgery; **Hospital:** Meml Sloan-Kettering Cancer Ctr (page 116); **Address:** 1275 York Ave, New York, NY 10065; **Phone:** 646-422-4390; **Board Cert:** Urology 2005; **Med School:** USC Sch Med 1987; **Resid:** Urology, USC Med Ctr 1993

Fine, Eugene M MD (U) - **Spec Exp:** Prostate Cancer; Kidney Stones; Erectile Dysfunction; Prostate Disease; **Hospital:** Mount Sinai Med Ctr (page 102), Lenox Hill Hosp (page 106); **Address:** 12 E 86th St, New York, NY 10028; **Phone:** 212-517-9555; **Board Cert:** Urology 2005; **Med School:** Mexico 1978; **Resid:** Surgery, Downstate Med Ctr Univ Hosp 1981; Urology, Mount Sinai Hosp 1985; **Fac Appt:** Asst Clin Prof U, Mount Sinai Sch Med

Fisch, Harry MD (U) - **Spec Exp:** Infertility-Male; Microsurgery; Vasectomy Reversal; **Hospital:** NY-Presby/Weill Cornell Med Ctr, NY (page 104), Lenox Hill Hosp (page 106); **Address:** 944 Park Ave, Ste 1C, New York, NY 10028; **Phone:** 212-879-0800; **Board Cert:** Urology 2010; **Med School:** Mount Sinai Sch Med 1983; **Resid:** Surgery, Montefiore Med Ctr 1985; Urology, Montefiore Med Ctr 1989; **Fac Appt:** Prof U, Columbia P&S

Fracchia, John MD (U) - **Spec Exp:** Urologic Cancer; **Hospital:** Lenox Hill Hosp (page 106), NY-Presby/Weill Cornell Med Ctr, NY (page 104); **Address:** 245 E 54th St, Ste 2N, New York, NY 10022; **Phone:** 212-570-6800 x185; **Board Cert:** Urology 1981; **Med School:** UMDNJ-NJ Med Sch, Newark 1973; **Resid:** Urology, New York Hosp 1978; **Fac Appt:** Assoc Clin Prof S, Cornell Univ-Weill Med Coll

Glassberg, Kenneth MD (U) - **Spec Exp:** Pediatric Urology; Genital Reconstruction; Varicocele in Adolescents; **Hospital:** Morgan Stanley Children's Hosp of NY-Presby, NY (page 104), NY-Presby/Columbia Univ Med Ctr, NY (page 104); **Address:** Morgan Stanley Chlds Hosp of NY-Presby, 3959 Broadway, rm 1117, New York, NY 10032; **Phone:** 212-305-9918; **Board Cert:** Urology 1977; Pediatric Urology 2009; **Med School:** SUNY Downstate 1968; **Resid:** Surgery, Montefiore Hosp Med Ctr 1972; Urology, Univ Hosp 1975; **Fellow:** Pediatric Urology, Adler Hey Chldns Hosp 1976; Pediatric Urology, Hosp For Sick Chldn 1976; **Fac Appt:** Prof U, Columbia P&S

Goldstein, Marc MD (U) - **Spec Exp:** Infertility-Male; Varicocele Microsurgery; Vasectomy & Vasectomy Reversal; Erectile Dysfunction; **Hospital:** NY-Presby/Weill Cornell Med Ctr, NY (page 104); **Address:** Cornell Inst for Reproductive Med, 525 E 68th St, Box 269, New York, NY 10065-4870; **Phone:** 212-746-5470; **Board Cert:** Urology 1982; **Med School:** SUNY Downstate 1972; **Resid:** Surgery, Columbia-Presby Med Ctr 1974; Urology, SUNY Downstate Med Ctr 1980; **Fellow:** Microsurgery, Rockefeller Univ 1982; Reproductive Medicine, Rockefeller Univ 1982; **Fac Appt:** Prof U, Cornell Univ-Weill Med Coll

Grasso III, Michael MD (U) - **Spec Exp:** Urologic Cancer; Laparoscopic Surgery; Kidney Stones; Testicular Cancer; **Hospital:** Lenox Hill Hosp (page 106), Westchester Med Ctr; **Address:** 100 E 77 th St, East Bldg - Fl 4th, New York, NY 10075; **Phone:** 212-434-6300; **Board Cert:** Urology 2004; **Med School:** Jefferson Med Coll 1986; **Resid:** Surgery, Jefferson Univ Hosp 1988; Urology, Jefferson Univ Hosp 1992; **Fac Appt:** Prof U, NY Med Coll

Gribetz, Michael MD (U) - **Spec Exp:** Prostate Disease; Urology-Female; Sexual Dysfunction; Kidney Stones; **Hospital:** Mount Sinai Med Ctr (page 102); **Address:** 1155 Park Ave, New York, NY 10128-1209; **Phone:** 212-831-1300; **Board Cert:** Urology 1980; **Med School:** Albert Einstein Coll Med 1973; **Resid:** Surgery, Montefiore Med Ctr 1975; Urology, Mt Sinai Hosp 1978; **Fac Appt:** Asst Clin Prof U, Mount Sinai Sch Med

Gupta, Mantu MD (U) - **Spec Exp:** Kidney Stones; **Hospital:** NY-Presby/Columbia Univ Med Ctr, NY (page 104); **Address:** Dept Urology, 161 Fort Washington Ave Fl 11, New York, NY 10019; **Phone:** 212-305-0114; **Board Cert:** Urology 2007; **Med School:** Northwestern Univ 1989; **Resid:** Urology, UCSF Med Ctr 1995; **Fellow:** Endourology, LI Jewish Hosp 1996; **Fac Appt:** Assoc Prof U, Columbia P&S

Hall, Simon J MD (U) - **Spec Exp:** Urologic Cancer; Minimally Invasive Urologic Surgery; Continent Urinary Diversions; Prostate Cancer; **Hospital:** Mount Sinai Med Ctr (page 102); **Address:** 5 E 98th St, Box 1272, New York, NY 10029; **Phone:** 212-241-4812; **Board Cert:** Urology 2009; **Med School:** Columbia P&S 1988; **Resid:** Surgery, Mt Sinai Med Ctr 1990; Urology, Boston Univ 1994; **Fellow:** Urology, Baylor Coll Med 1996; **Fac Appt:** Assoc Prof U, Mount Sinai Sch Med

Hensle, Terry MD (U) - **Spec Exp:** Pediatric Urology; Hypospadias; Urinary Reconstruction; Wilms' Tumor; **Hospital:** Hackensack Univ Med Ctr (page 96); **Address:** 699 Teaneck Rd, Ste 103, Teaneck, NJ 07616; **Phone:** 201-645-3362; **Board Cert:** Urology 1978; **Med School:** Cornell Univ-Weill Med Coll 1968; **Resid:** Surgery, Boston City Hosp 1973; Urology, Mass Genl Hosp 1976; **Fellow:** Pediatric Urology, Mass Genl Hosp 1977; Pediatric Urology, Great Ormond St Hosp 1978; **Fac Appt:** Prof U, Columbia P&S

Herr, Harry W MD (U) - **Spec Exp:** Bladder Cancer; Prostate Cancer; Testicular Cancer; **Hospital:** Meml Sloan-Kettering Cancer Ctr (page 116), NY-Presby/Weill Cornell Med Ctr, NY (page 104); **Address:** 1275 York Avenue, New York, NY 10021; **Phone:** 800-525-2225; **Board Cert:** Urology 1976; **Med School:** UCSF 1969; **Resid:** Urology, UC Irvine Med Ctr 1974; **Fellow:** Urology, Meml Sloan Kettering Cancer Ctr 1976; **Fac Appt:** Assoc Prof S, Cornell Univ-Weill Med Coll

Kaminetsky, Jed MD (U) - **Spec Exp:** Sexual Dysfunction; Prostate Cancer; Kidney Stones; Prostate Disease; **Hospital:** NYU Langone Med Ctr (page 108); **Address:** 215 Lexington Ave Fl 20, New York, NY 10016; **Phone:** 212-686-9015; **Board Cert:** Urology 2010; **Med School:** NYU Sch Med 1984; **Resid:** Urology, NYU Med Ctr 1990; **Fac Appt:** Asst Clin Prof U, NYU Sch Med

Kaplan, Steven A MD (U) - **Spec Exp:** Urodynamics; Voiding Dysfunction; Incontinence after Prostate Cancer; Incontinence; **Hospital:** NY-Presby/Weill Cornell Med Ctr, NY (page 104); **Address:** 425 E 61 St, Fl 12, New York, NY 10065; **Phone:** 646-962-4811; **Board Cert:** Urology 2011; **Med School:** Mount Sinai Sch Med 1982; **Resid:** Surgery, Mount Sinai Hosp 1984; Urology, Columbia Presby Med Ctr 1988; **Fellow:** Urology, Columbia Presby Med Ctr 1990; **Fac Appt:** Prof U, Cornell Univ-Weill Med Coll

Kirschenbaum, Alexander M MD (U) - **Spec Exp:** Prostate Cancer; Bladder Cancer; Kidney Cancer; **Hospital:** Mount Sinai Med Ctr (page 102); **Address:** 229 E 79th St, Ste 1A, New York, NY 10075; **Phone:** 646-422-0926; **Board Cert:** Urology 2006; **Med School:** Mount Sinai Sch Med 1980; **Resid:** Surgery, Mt Sinai Hosp 1982; Urology, Mt Sinai Hosp 1985; **Fellow:** Urologic Oncology, Mt Sinai Hosp 1987; **Fac Appt:** Assoc Prof U, Mount Sinai Sch Med

Klein, George MD (U) - **Spec Exp:** Kidney Stones; Sexual Dysfunction; Prostate Cancer; **Hospital:** Mount Sinai Med Ctr (page 102), Lenox Hill Hosp (page 106); **Address:** 157 E 72nd St, Ground Fl, New York, NY 10021; **Phone:** 212-744-8700; **Board Cert:** Urology 1983; **Med School:** Cornell Univ-Weill Med Coll 1976; **Resid:** Surgery, North Shore Univ Hosp 1978; Urology, Mount Sinai Hosp 1981; **Fac Appt:** Asst Prof U, Mount Sinai Sch Med

Lepor, Herbert MD (U) - **Spec Exp:** Prostate Cancer; **Hospital:** NYU Langone Med Ctr (page 108); **Address:** 150 E 32nd St, Fl 2, NYU Urology Assocaites, New York, NY 10016; **Phone:** 646-825-6327; **Board Cert:** Urology 2006; **Med School:** Johns Hopkins Univ 1975; **Resid:** Urology, Johns Hopkins Hosp 1986; **Fac Appt:** Prof U, NYU Sch Med

Lizza, Eli F MD (U) - **Spec Exp:** Impotence; Infertility-Male; **Hospital:** Lenox Hill Hosp (page 106), NY-Presby/Weill Cornell Med Ctr, NY (page 104); **Address:** New York Urological Assocs, 245 E 54th St, Ste 2N, New York, NY 10022; **Phone:** 212-570-6800 x180; **Board Cert:** Urology 2006; **Med School:** UMDNJ-NJ Med Sch, Newark 1979; **Resid:** Surgery, Lenox Hill Hosp 1981; Urology, W VA Med Ctr 1984; **Fellow:** Infertility, Columbia Presby Med Ctr 1985

Loo, Marcus Hsieu-Hong MD (U) - **Spec Exp:** Prostate Disease; Kidney Stones; Voiding Dysfunction; Prostate Cancer; **Hospital:** NY-Presby/Weill Cornell Med Ctr, NY (page 104); **Address:** 254 Canal St, Ste 3001, New York, NY 10013-3501; **Phone:** 212-925-8388; **Board Cert:** Urology 2008; **Med School:** Cornell Univ-Weill Med Coll 1981; **Resid:** Surgery, NY Hosp-Cornell Med Ctr 1983; Urology, NY Hosp-Cornell Med Ctr 1988; **Fellow:** Urology, NY Hosp-Cornell Med Ctr 1984; **Fac Appt:** Clin Prof U, Cornell Univ-Weill Med Coll

Lowe, Franklin Charles MD (U) - **Spec Exp:** Prostate Disease; Complementary Medicine; Prostate Cancer; Kidney Stones; **Hospital:** St. Luke's - Roosevelt Hosp Ctr - Roosevelt Div (page 94), NY-Presby/Columbia Univ Med Ctr, NY (page 104); **Address:** 425 W 59th St, Ste 3A, New York, NY 10019-1104; **Phone:** 212-523-7790; **Board Cert:** Urology 2006; **Med School:** Columbia P&S 1979; **Resid:** Surgery, Johns Hopkins Hosp 1981; Urology, Johns Hopkins Hosp 1984; **Fac Appt:** Clin Prof U, Columbia P&S

Marks, Jon O MD (U) - **Spec Exp:** Kidney Stones; Interstitial Cystitis; **Hospital:** Beth Israel Med Ctr - Petrie Division (page 94); **Address:** 201 E 19th St, New York, NY 10003; **Phone:** 212-673-7300; **Board Cert:** Urology 1983; **Med School:** NY Med Coll 1976; **Resid:** Surgery, Lenox Hill Hosp 1978; Urology, Lenox Hill Hosp 1981

McGovern, Thomas P MD (U) - **Spec Exp:** Bladder Cancer; Prostate Cancer; **Hospital:** NY-Presby/Weill Cornell Med Ctr, NY (page 104), Lenox Hill Hosp (page 106); **Address:** 449 E 68 St Fl 2 - Ste 8, New York, NY 10065-6310; **Phone:** 212-772-7411; **Board Cert:** Urology 1983; **Med School:** Cornell Univ-Weill Med Coll 1974; **Resid:** Surgery, Mass Genl Hosp 1976; Urology, New York Hosp 1980; **Fac Appt:** Asst Clin Prof U, Cornell Univ-Weill Med Coll

McKiernan, James M MD (U) - **Spec Exp:** Kidney Cancer; Bladder Cancer; Prostate Cancer; Testicular Cancer; **Hospital:** NY-Presby/Columbia Univ Med Ctr, NY (page 104); **Address:** Dept Urology, 161 Ft Washington Ave Fl 11, New York, NY 10032; **Phone:** 212-305-0114; **Board Cert:** Urology 2003; **Med School:** Columbia P&S 1993; **Resid:** Surgery, Columbia Presby Med Ctr 1995; Urology, Columbia Presby Med Ctr 1999; **Fellow:** Urologic Oncology, Meml Sloan-Kettering Cancer Ctr 2001; **Fac Appt:** Asst Prof U, Columbia P&S

Mulhall, John P MD (U) - **Spec Exp:** Erectile Dysfunction; Peyronie's Disease; Penile Prostheses; Infertility-Male; **Hospital:** Meml Sloan-Kettering Cancer Ctr (page 116); **Address:** Kimmel Center, MSKCC, 353 E 68th St, Fl 5, New York, NY 10021; **Phone:** 646-422-4359; **Board Cert:** Urology 2008; **Med School:** Ireland 1985; **Resid:** Urology, Univ Conn Health Ctr 1995; **Fellow:** Urology, Boston Univ Med Ctr 1996; **Fac Appt:** Prof U, Cornell Univ-Weill Med Coll

Nagler, Harris M MD (U) - **Spec Exp:** Vasectomy Reversal; Infertility-Male; Varicocele Microsurgery; Erectile Dysfunction; **Hospital:** Beth Israel Med Ctr - Petrie Division (page 94); **Address:** Beth Israel Med Ctr, Dept Urology, 10 Union Square E, Ste 3A, New York, NY 10003-3314; **Phone:** 212-844-8700; **Board Cert:** Urology 1982; **Med School:** Temple Univ 1975; **Resid:** Urology, Columbia Presby Med Ctr 1980; **Fellow:** Reproductive Medicine, Columbia Presby Med Ctr 1981; **Fac Appt:** Prof U, Albert Einstein Coll Med

Nitti, Victor MD (U) - **Spec Exp:** Urology-Female; Incontinence-Male & Female; Urodynamics; Voiding Dysfunction; **Hospital:** NYU Langone Med Ctr (page 108); **Address:** NYU Urology Assocs, 150 E 32nd St, 2nd Fl, New York, NY 10016; **Phone:** 646-825-6324; **Board Cert:** Urology 2002; **Med School:** UMDNJ-NJ Med Sch, Newark 1985; **Resid:** Surgery, Univ Hosp 1987; Urology, Univ Hosp 1991; **Fellow:** Female Urology, UCLA Med Ctr 1992; **Fac Appt:** Prof U, NYU Sch Med

Palese, Michael A MD (U) - **Spec Exp:** Kidney Cancer; Laparoscopic Surgery; Robotic Surgery; Kidney Stones; **Hospital:** Mount Sinai Med Ctr (page 102); **Address:** 5 E 98th St Fl 6, New York, NY 10029; **Phone:** 212-241-3868; **Board Cert:** Urology 2006; **Med School:** Mount Sinai Sch Med 1997; **Resid:** Surgery, Univ MD Med Ctr 1999; Urology, Univ MD Med Ctr 2003; **Fellow:** Urologic Oncology, NY Presby-Cornell Med Ctr 2004; Robotic Surgery, NY Presby-Cornell Med Ctr 2004; **Fac Appt:** Assoc Prof U, Mount Sinai Sch Med

Peng, Benjamin C. H. MD (U) - **Spec Exp:** Prostate Disease; Kidney Stones; Urologic Cancer; **Hospital:** NY Downtown Hosp, NYU Langone Med Ctr (page 108); **Address:** 168 Canal St, Ste 510, New York, NY 10013-4503; **Phone:** 212-226-2200; **Board Cert:** Urology 2011; **Med School:** Columbia P&S 1984; **Resid:** Surgery, Mount Sinai Hosp 1986; Urology, Columbia-Presby Hosp 1990; **Fac Appt:** Asst Clin Prof U, NYU Sch Med

Poppas, Dix P MD (U) - **Spec Exp:** Genital Reconstruction-Pediatric; Robotic Surgery-Pediatric; Minimally Invasive Surgery-Pediatric; Pediatric Urology; **Hospital:** NY-Presby/Weill Cornell Med Ctr, NY (page 104); **Address:** Inst for Pediatric Urology, NY Presby Hosp-Weill Cornell, 525 E 68th St, rm F931, Box 94, New York, NY 10065; **Phone:** 212-746-5337; **Board Cert:** Urology 2008; Pediatric Urology 2008; **Med School:** Eastern VA Med Sch 1988; **Resid:** Urology, NY Hosp-Cornell Med Ctr 1994; **Fellow:** Pediatric Urology, Chldns Hosp Harvard Med Sch 1996; **Fac Appt:** Prof U, Cornell Univ-Weill Med Coll

Provet, John A MD (U) - **Spec Exp:** Urologic Cancer; Kidney Stones; Prostate Disease; **Hospital:** NYU Langone Med Ctr (page 108); **Address:** 215 Lexington Ave Fl 20, New York, NY 10016; **Phone:** 212-686-9015; **Board Cert:** Urology 2009; **Med School:** NYU Sch Med 1983; **Resid:** Surgery, NYU/VA Med Ctr/Bellevue Hosp 1985; Urology, NYU/VA Med Ctr/Bellevue Hosp 1989; **Fac Appt:** Assoc Clin Prof U, NYU Sch Med

Reckler, Jon M MD (U) - **Hospital:** NY-Presby/Weill Cornell Med Ctr, NY (page 104), Lenox Hill Hosp (page 106); **Address:** New York Urological Associates, 880 5th Ave, New York, NY 10021; **Phone:** 212-535-1950; **Board Cert:** Urology 1976; **Med School:** Harvard Med Sch 1966; **Resid:** Surgery, Univ Hosp 1968; Urology, Peter Bent Brigham Hosp 1974; **Fac Appt:** Assoc Clin Prof U, Cornell Univ-Weill Med Coll

Romas, Nicholas A MD (U) - **Spec Exp:** Prostate Disease; Prostate Cancer; Erectile Dysfunction; **Hospital:** St. Luke's - Roosevelt Hosp Ctr - Roosevelt Div (page 94), NY-Presby/Columbia Univ Med Ctr, NY (page 104); **Address:** 425 W 59th St, Ste 3A, New York, NY 10019-1104; **Phone:** 212-523-7788; **Board Cert:** Urology 1974; **Med School:** Columbia P&S 1962; **Resid:** Surgery, New York Hosp-Cornell 1964; Urology, Columbia-Presby Med Ctr 1968; **Fac Appt:** Clin Prof U, Columbia P&S

Russo, Paul MD (U) - **Spec Exp:** Kidney Cancer; Prostate Cancer; Penile Cancer; **Hospital:** Meml Sloan-Kettering Cancer Ctr (page 116); **Address:** 1275 York Ave, New York, NY 10065; **Phone:** 800-525-2225; **Board Cert:** Urology 2004; **Med School:** Columbia P&S 1979; **Resid:** Urology, Barnes Hosp-Wash Univ 1984; **Fellow:** Urologic Oncology, Mem Sloan Kettering Cancer Ctr 1988; **Fac Appt:** Assoc Prof U, Cornell Univ-Weill Med Coll

Samadi, David B MD (U) - **Spec Exp:** Prostate Cancer/Robotic Surgery; Kidney Cancer; Bladder Cancer; Urologic Cancer; **Hospital:** Mount Sinai Med Ctr (page 102); **Address:** 625 Madison Ave, Fl 2, New York, NY 10022; **Phone:** 212-241-8779; **Board Cert:** Urology 2004; **Med School:** SUNY Stony Brook 1994; **Resid:** Surgery, Montefiore Med Ctr 1996; Urology, Montefiore Med Ctr 2000; **Fellow:** Urologic Oncology, Meml Sloan Kettering Cancer Ctr 2001; Laparoscopic Surgery, Henri Mondor Hosp 2003; **Fac Appt:** Asst Prof U, Mount Sinai Sch Med

Scardino, Peter T MD (U) - **Spec Exp:** Prostate Cancer; Bladder Cancer; Urologic Cancer; Urinary Reconstruction; **Hospital:** Meml Sloan-Kettering Cancer Ctr (page 116); **Address:** 1275 York Avenue, New York, NY 10065; **Phone:** 646-422-4329; **Board Cert:** Urology 1981; **Med School:** Duke Univ 1971; **Resid:** Surgery, Mass Genl Hosp 1973; Urology, UCLA Med Ctr 1979; **Fellow:** Urology, Natl Cancer Inst 1976; **Fac Appt:** Prof U, Cornell Univ-Weill Med Coll

Scherr, Douglas S MD (U) - **Spec Exp:** Prostate Cancer/Robotic Surgery; Bladder Cancer; Robotic Surgery; Testicular Cancer; **Hospital:** NY-Presby/Weill Cornell Med Ctr, NY (page 104); **Address:** Brady Urologic Health Ctr, 525 E 68th St Starr 900, New York, NY 10021; **Phone:** 212-746-5788; **Board Cert:** Urology 2003; **Med School:** Geo Wash Univ 1994; **Resid:** Urology, NY Hosp-Cornell Med Ctr 1999; **Fellow:** Urologic Oncology, Meml Sloan-Kettering Canc Ctr 2002; **Fac Appt:** Assoc Prof U, Cornell Univ-Weill Med Coll

Schiff, Howard I MD (U) - **Spec Exp:** Prostate Benign Disease; Infertility-Male; Prostate Cancer; Lupus Cystitis; **Hospital:** Mount Sinai Med Ctr (page 102), NY-Presby/Weill Cornell Med Ctr, NY (page 104); **Address:** 1120 Park Ave, Ste 1E, New York, NY 10128-1242; **Phone:** 212-996-6660; **Board Cert:** Urology 1982; **Med School:** W VA Univ 1975; **Resid:** Surgery, Montefiore Hosp Med Ctr 1977; Urology, Mount Sinai Hosp 1980; **Fac Appt:** Asst Clin Prof U, Mount Sinai Sch Med

Schlegel, Peter N MD (U) - **Spec Exp:** Prostate Cancer; Infertility-Male; **Hospital:** NY-Presby/Weill Cornell Med Ctr, NY (page 104), Hosp For Special Surgery (page 115); **Address:** Brady Urologic Health Ctr, 525 E 68th St Starr Bldg Fl 9 - Ste 900, New York, NY 10021-4870; **Phone:** 212-746-5491; **Board Cert:** Urology 2011; **Med School:** Univ Mass Sch Med 1983; **Resid:** Surgery, Johns Hopkins Hosp 1985; Urology, Johns Hopkins Hosp 1989; **Fellow:** Medical Oncology, Johns Hopkins Hosp 1987; Male Reproduction, NY Hosp-Cornell Med Ctr 1991; **Fac Appt:** Prof U, Cornell Univ-Weill Med Coll

Schlussel, Richard MD (U) - **Spec Exp:** Pediatric Urology; Hypospadias; Robotic Surgery; Reconstructive Surgery; **Hospital:** NY-Presby/Weill Cornell Med Ctr, NY (page 104), Englewood Hosp & Med Ctr; **Address:** 65 E 96th St, Ste 1B, New York, NY 10128; **Phone:** 203-359-4211; **Board Cert:** Urology 2010; Pediatric Urology 2010; **Med School:** Albert Einstein Coll Med 1986; **Resid:** Urology, Mt Sinai Med Ctr 1992; **Fellow:** Urology, Harvard Univ/Chldns Hosp 1994; **Fac Appt:** Asst Prof U, Columbia P&S

Shapiro, Ellen MD (U) - **Spec Exp:** Pediatric Urology; **Hospital:** NYU Langone Med Ctr (page 108), Hackensack Univ Med Ctr (page 96); **Address:** 150 E 32nd St Fl 2, New York, NY 10016; **Phone:** 646-825-6326; **Board Cert:** Urology 2008; Pediatric Urology 2008; **Med School:** Univ Nebr Coll Med 1978; **Resid:** Surgery, Johns Hopkins Hosp 1980; Urology, Johns Hopkins Hosp 1986; **Fellow:** Pediatric Urology, Chldns Hosp Michigan 1987; **Fac Appt:** Prof U, NYU Sch Med

Sheinfeld, Joel MD (U) - **Spec Exp:** Testicular Cancer; Fertility Preservation in Cancer; **Hospital:** Meml Sloan-Kettering Cancer Ctr (page 116); **Address:** 353 E 68th St, New York, NY 10065; **Phone:** 646-422-4311; **Board Cert:** Urology 2009; **Med School:** Univ Fla Coll Med 1981; **Resid:** Urology, Strong Meml Hosp 1986; **Fellow:** Urologic Oncology, Meml Sloan Kettering Cancer Ctr 1989; **Fac Appt:** Assoc Prof U, Cornell Univ-Weill Med Coll

Silva, Jose V MD (U) - **Spec Exp:** Urologic Cancer; **Hospital:** St. Luke's - Roosevelt Hosp Ctr - Roosevelt Div (page 94), Montefiore Med Ctr-Moses Campus, NY (page 100); **Address:** 425 W 59th St, Ste 3A, New York, NY 10019; **Phone:** 212-582-3421; **Board Cert:** Urology 1983; **Med School:** India 1970; **Resid:** Surgery, Beth Israel Med Ctr 1978; Urology, St Luke's-Roosevelt Hosp Ctr 1981; **Fellow:** Surgery, Meml Sloan Kettering Cancer Ctr 1982

Sogani, Pramod MD (U) - **Spec Exp:** Prostate Cancer; Testicular Cancer; Bladder Cancer; Kidney Cancer; **Hospital:** Meml Sloan-Kettering Cancer Ctr (page 116); **Address:** 1275 York Ave, New York, NY 10065; **Phone:** 646-422-4395; **Board Cert:** Urology 1976; **Med School:** India 1960; **Resid:** Urology, NYU Med Ctr 1969; Urology, Geo Wash Univ Med Ctr 1971; **Fellow:** Surgical Oncology, Meml Sloan Kettering Cancer Ctr 1973; **Fac Appt:** Prof U, Cornell Univ-Weill Med Coll

Stifelman, Michael D MD (U) - **Spec Exp:** Robotic Surgery; Urologic Cancer; Urinary Reconstruction; Retroperitoneal Fibrosis; **Hospital:** NYU Langone Med Ctr (page 108), Bellevue Hosp Ctr; **Address:** 150 E 32nd St Fl 2, New York, NY 10016-6024; **Phone:** 646-825-6325; **Board Cert:** Urology 2011; **Med School:** Albert Einstein Coll Med 1993; **Resid:** Surgery, Columbia-Presby Med Ctr 1995; Urology, Columbia-Presby Med Ctr 1999; **Fellow:** Laparoscopic Surgery, NY Hosp 2000; **Fac Appt:** Asst Prof U, NYU Sch Med

Taneja, Samir S MD (U) - **Spec Exp:** Prostate Cancer; Kidney Cancer; Bladder Cancer; **Hospital:** NYU Langone Med Ctr (page 108); **Address:** NYU Urology Associates, 150 E 32nd St, Fl 2, New York, NY 10016-6024; **Phone:** 646-825-6321; **Board Cert:** Urology 2009; **Med School:** Northwestern Univ 1990; **Resid:** Urology, UCLA Med Ctr 1996; **Fellow:** Urologic Oncology, NYU Med Ctr 1998; **Fac Appt:** Prof U, NYU Sch Med

Te, Alexis E MD (U) - **Spec Exp:** Prostate Benign Disease; Prostate Surgery; Incontinence; **Hospital:** NY-Presby/Weill Cornell Med Ctr, NY (page 104); **Address:** Weill Medical College, Brady Prostate Center, 425 E 61th St, New York, NY 10065; **Phone:** 212-746-4811; **Board Cert:** Urology 2006; **Med School:** Cornell Univ-Weill Med Coll 1988; **Resid:** Urology, NY Presbyterian-Columbia Presby Med Ctr 1994; **Fellow:** Urodynamics, NY Presbyterian-Columbia Presby Med Ctr 1995; **Fac Appt:** Assoc Prof U, Cornell Univ-Weill Med Coll

Tewari, Ashutosh K MD (U) - **Spec Exp:** Prostate Cancer/Robotic Surgery; **Hospital:** NY-Presby/Weill Cornell Med Ctr, NY (page 104); **Address:** Brady Urologic Health Center, 525 E 68th St, Starr 900, New York, NY 10021; **Phone:** 212-746-5638; **Board Cert:** Urology 2006; **Med School:** India 1984; **Resid:** Surgery, GSVM Medical College 1990; Urology, Henry Ford Hosp 2003; **Fellow:** Transplant Surgery, Liverpool Univ Med Ctr 1993; Urologic Oncology, Shands Healthcare 1995; **Fac Appt:** Assoc Prof U, Cornell Univ-Weill Med Coll

Vapnek, Jonathan M MD (U) - **Spec Exp:** Incontinence; Urology-Female; Neurogenic Bladder; Urodynamics; **Hospital:** Mount Sinai Med Ctr (page 102); **Address:** 229 E 79th St, Ste 1A, New York, NY 10075; **Phone:** 212-717-9500; **Board Cert:** Urology 2005; **Med School:** UCSD 1986; **Resid:** Surgery, UCSD Med Ctr 1988; Urology, UCSF Med Ctr 1992; **Fellow:** Neurourology, UC Davis Med Ctr 1993; **Fac Appt:** Assoc Clin Prof U, Mount Sinai Sch Med

Williams, John J MD (U) - **Spec Exp:** Genitourinary Cancer; Prostate Disease; Kidney Stones; **Hospital:** NY-Presby/Weill Cornell Med Ctr, NY (page 104), Lenox Hill Hosp (page 106); **Address:** 820 Park Ave, New York, NY 10021-2758; **Phone:** 212-861-1100; **Board Cert:** Urology 1976; **Med School:** Georgetown Univ 1966; **Resid:** Surgery, Strong Meml Hosp 1968; Urology, NY Hosp 1974

Young, George P H MD (U) - **Spec Exp:** Incontinence-Female; Urologic Cancer; Urology-Female; **Hospital:** Lenox Hill Hosp (page 106), Mount Sinai Med Ctr (page 102); **Address:** 1060 5th Ave Fl 1EF, New York, NY 10128; **Phone:** 212-876-9811; **Board Cert:** Urology 2006; **Med School:** Brazil 1983; **Resid:** Surgery, Staten Island Univ Hosp 1989; Urology, New York Hosp 1993; **Fellow:** Microsurgery, Population Council, Rockefeller Univ 1985; Female Urology, UCLA Med Ctr 1994; **Fac Appt:** Assoc Prof U, Cornell Univ-Weill Med Coll

Vascular & Interventional Radiology

Brown, Karen T MD (VIR) - **Spec Exp:** Liver Cancer; Radiofrequency Tumor Ablation; **Hospital:** Meml Sloan-Kettering Cancer Ctr (page 116); **Address:** 1275 York Ave, New York, NY 10065; **Phone:** 212-639-5882; **Board Cert:** Diagnostic Radiology 1984; Vascular & Interventional Radiology 2004; **Med School:** Boston Univ 1979; **Resid:** Diagnostic Radiology, Mass Genl Hosp 1984; **Fellow:** Vascular & Interventional Radiology, Mass Genl Hosp 1985; **Fac Appt:** Prof Rad, Cornell Univ-Weill Med Coll

Covey, Anne M MD (VIR) - **Spec Exp:** Liver Tumors; Chemoembolization & Tumor Ablation; Biliary Surgery; **Hospital:** Meml Sloan-Kettering Cancer Ctr (page 116); **Address:** MSKCC, Interventional Radiology, 1275 York Ave, New York, NY 10065; **Phone:** 212-639-6746; **Board Cert:** Diagnostic Radiology 1999; Vascular & Interventional Radiology 2001; **Med School:** Columbia P&S 1994; **Resid:** Diagnostic Radiology, Yale-New Haven Hosp 1998; **Fellow:** Vascular & Interventional Radiology, Yale-New Haven Hosp 2001

Getrajdman, George I MD (VIR) - **Hospital:** Meml Sloan-Kettering Cancer Ctr (page 116); **Address:** Memorial Sloan Kettering Cancer Ctr, 1275 York Ave, New York, NY 10021; **Phone:** 212-639-2598; **Board Cert:** Diagnostic Radiology 1988; **Med School:** Johns Hopkins Univ 1980; **Resid:** Surgery, NY Presby/Columbia Med Ctr 1985; Diagnostic Radiology, NY Presby/Columbia Med Ctr 1988; **Fellow:** Vascular & Interventional Radiology, NY Presby/Columbia Med Ctr

Javit, Daniel J MD (VIR) - **Hospital:** Lenox Hill Hosp (page 106); **Address:** Lenox Hill Hospital, Dept Radiology, 100 E 77th St, New York, NY 10021; **Phone:** 212-434-2908; **Board Cert:** Diagnostic Radiology 1993; Vascular & Interventional Radiology 1995; **Med School:** Cornell Univ-Weill Med Coll 1988; **Resid:** Diagnostic Radiology, Mt Sinai Hosp 1993; **Fellow:** Interventional Radiology, NY-Cornell Med Ctr 1994

Khilnani, Neil M MD (VIR) - **Spec Exp:** Vein Disorders; Varicose Veins; Uterine Fibroid Embolization; **Hospital:** NY-Presby/Weill Cornell Med Ctr, NY (page 104); **Address:** Cornell Vascular Assocs, 416 E 55th St, Main Floor, New York, NY 10022; **Phone:** 212-752-7999; **Board Cert:** Diagnostic Radiology 1991; Vascular & Interventional Radiology 2008; **Med School:** Mount Sinai Sch Med 1986; **Resid:** Radiology, Columbia Presby Med Ctr 1991; **Fellow:** Vascular & Interventional Radiology, Columbia Presby Med Ctr 1992; **Fac Appt:** Assoc Prof Rad, Cornell Univ-Weill Med Coll

Lookstein, Robert A MD (VIR) - **Spec Exp:** Peripheral Vascular Disease; Renovascular Disease; Vein Disorders; **Hospital:** Mount Sinai Med Ctr (page 102); **Address:** Mt Sinai Med Ctr, 1176 Fifth Ave, New York, NY 10029; **Phone:** 212-241-7409; **Board Cert:** Diagnostic Radiology 2001; Vascular & Interventional Radiology 2003; **Med School:** SUNY Downstate 1995; **Resid:** Diagnostic Radiology, Mt Sinai Med Ctr 2001; **Fellow:** Vascular & Interventional Radiology, Mt Sinai Med Ctr 2002; **Fac Appt:** Assoc Prof Rad, Mount Sinai Sch Med

Rosen, Robert J MD (VIR) - **Spec Exp:** Vascular Malformations; Aneurysm-Aortic; Chemoembolization & Tumor Ablation; **Hospital:** Lenox Hill Hosp (page 106); **Address:** Lenox Hill Heart & Vascular Inst, 130 E 77th St Fl 9, New York, NY 10075; **Phone:** 212-434-2606; **Board Cert:** Diagnostic Radiology 1980; **Med School:** Hahnemann Univ 1976; **Resid:** Diagnostic Radiology, Hahnemann Med Coll 1979; **Fellow:** Vascular & Interventional Radiology, Hosp Univ Penn 1980; **Fac Appt:** Assoc Prof Rad, NYU Sch Med

Saboeiro, Gregory R MD (VIR) - **Spec Exp:** Musculoskeletal Imaging; Ultrasound; Spinal Imaging & Intervention; **Hospital:** Hosp For Special Surgery (page 115); **Address:** Hosp for Special Surgery, 535 E 70th St Fl 3, New York, NY 10021; **Phone:** 212-606-1566; **Board Cert:** Diagnostic Radiology 1993; **Med School:** St Louis Univ 1989; **Resid:** Radiology, St Louis Univ Hosp 1993; **Fellow:** Interventional Radiology, Mallinckrodt Inst 1994; Musculoskeletal Imaging, Hosp Special Surgery 2005; **Fac Appt:** Asst Prof Rad, Cornell Univ-Weill Med Coll

Shams, Joseph N MD (VIR) - **Spec Exp:** Peripheral Vascular Disease; Uterine Fibroids; Liver Tumors; Vascular Disease; **Hospital:** Beth Israel Med Ctr - Petrie Division (page 94), St. Luke's - Roosevelt Hosp Ctr - Roosevelt Div (page 94); **Address:** 144 4th Ave, New York, NY 10003; **Phone:** 212-420-2509; **Board Cert:** Diagnostic Radiology 1993; Vascular & Interventional Radiology 2006; **Med School:** SUNY Downstate 1988; **Resid:** Diagnostic Radiology, Beth Israel Med Ctr 1993; **Fellow:** Vascular & Interventional Radiology, Yale-New Haven Hosp 1994; **Fac Appt:** Asst Prof Rad, Albert Einstein Coll Med

Solomon, Stephen B MD (VIR) - **Spec Exp:** Radiofrequency Tumor Ablation; Kidney Cancer; Liver Cancer; Lung Cancer; **Hospital:** Meml Sloan-Kettering Cancer Ctr (page 116); **Address:** Meml Sloan-Kettering Cancer Ctr, Ctr for Image Guided Intervention, 1275 York Ave, New York, NY 10021; **Phone:** 212-639-5012; **Board Cert:** Diagnostic Radiology 1998; **Med School:** Yale Univ 1993; **Resid:** Diagnostic Radiology, Johns Hopkins Hosp 1998

Weintraub, Joshua L MD (VIR) - **Spec Exp:** Gastrointestinal Cancer; Chemoembolization & Tumor Ablation; Uterine Fibroid Embolization; Vascular Malformations; **Hospital:** NY-Presby/Columbia Univ Med Ctr, NY (page 104); **Address:** NY Presbyterian-Columbia Med Ctr, Dept Radiology, 622 W 168th St, New York, NY 10032; **Phone:** 212-305-7094; **Board Cert:** Diagnostic Radiology 1996; Vascular & Interventional Radiology 1998; **Med School:** Wayne State Univ 1991; **Resid:** Diagnostic Radiology, Beth Israel Hosp 1996; **Fellow:** Vascular & Interventional Radiology, Hosp Univ Penn 1997; **Fac Appt:** Assoc Prof Rad, Columbia P&S

Vascular Surgery

Adelman, Mark MD (VascS) - **Spec Exp:** Carotid Artery Surgery; Aneurysm-Abdominal Aortic; Vein Disorders; Endovascular Surgery; **Hospital:** NYU Langone Med Ctr (page 108), Bellevue Hosp Ctr; **Address:** 530 1st Ave, Ste 6F, MS 10016, New York, NY 10016-6402; **Phone:** 212-263-7311; **Board Cert:** Surgery 1999; Vascular Surgery 2001; **Med School:** NYU Sch Med 1985; **Resid:** Surgery, NYU Med Ctr 1990; **Fellow:** Vascular Surgery, NYU Med Ctr 1991; **Fac Appt:** Prof VascS, NYU Sch Med

Benvenisty, Alan I MD (VascS) - **Spec Exp:** Renovascular Disease; Aneurysm-Aortic; Endovascular Surgery; Minimally Invasive Vascular Surgery; **Hospital:** St. Luke's - Roosevelt Hosp Ctr - St Luke's Hosp (page 94), St. Luke's - Roosevelt Hosp Ctr - Roosevelt Div (page 94); **Address:** 1090 Amsterdam Ave Fl 12, New York, NY 10025; **Phone:** 212-523-4706; **Board Cert:** Surgery 2004; Vascular Surgery 2009; **Med School:** Columbia P&S 1978; **Resid:** Surgery, Columbia-Presby Med Ctr 1983; **Fellow:** Vascular Surgery, Columbia-Presby Med Ctr 1984; Transplant Surgery, Columbia-Presby Med Ctr 1984; **Fac Appt:** Clin Prof S, Columbia P&S

Bernik, Thomas R MD (VascS) - **Spec Exp:** Carotid Artery Surgery; Aortic Surgery; Peripheral Vascular Disease; Chemoembolization & Tumor Ablation; **Hospital:** Beth Israel Med Ctr - Petrie Division (page 94), Lenox Hill Hosp (page 106); **Address:** Beth Israel Med Ctr, Div Vasc Surg, 1st Ave at 16th St, 12 Fierman Hall, New York, NY 10003; **Phone:** 212-844-5555; **Board Cert:** Surgery 2001; Vascular Surgery 2005; **Med School:** Geo Wash Univ 1994; **Resid:** Surgery, St Vincent's Hosp 2000; **Fellow:** Vascular Surgery, N Shore Univ Hosp 2002; Endovascular Surgery, Strong Meml Hosp 2002; **Fac Appt:** Asst Prof VascS, NY Med Coll

Carroccio, Alfio MD (VascS) - **Spec Exp:** Aneurysm-Aortic; Minimally Invasive Surgey; **Hospital:** Lenox Hill Hosp (page 106); **Address:** 130 E 77 St Fl 13, New York, NY 10075; **Phone:** 212-434-3420; **Board Cert:** Surgery 2010; Vascular Surgery 2005; **Med School:** Mount Sinai Sch Med 1996; **Resid:** Surgery, Mount Sinai Hosp 2001; **Fellow:** Vascular Surgery, Mount Sinai Hosp 2003

Cayne, Neal S MD (VascS) - **Spec Exp:** Endovascular Surgery; Aneurysm-Abdominal & Thoracic Aortic; Carotid Artery Surgery; **Hospital:** NYU Langone Med Ctr (page 108); **Address:** 530 First Ave, Fl 6, Ste F, New York, NY 10016; **Phone:** 212-263-5626; **Board Cert:** Surgery 2010; Vascular Surgery 2003; **Med School:** NY Med Coll 1995; **Resid:** Surgery, Montefiore Med Ctr 2000; **Fellow:** Vascular Surgery, Montefiore Med Ctr 2002; **Fac Appt:** Asst Prof VascS, NYU Sch Med

Chideckel, Norman MD (VascS) - **Spec Exp:** Vein Disorders; Wound Healing/Care; Laser Surgery; **Hospital:** Beth Israel Med Ctr - Petrie Division (page 94); **Address:** 380 2nd Ave, Ste 1004, New York, NY 10010; **Phone:** 212-473-1877; **Board Cert:** Surgery 2007; **Med School:** SUNY Downstate 1979; **Resid:** Surgery, Beth Israel Med Ctr 1984; **Fellow:** Vascular Surgery, Lutheran Med Ctr 1985; **Fac Appt:** Asst Clin Prof S, Albert Einstein Coll Med

Ellozy, Sharif Hamed MD (VascS) - **Spec Exp:** Endovascular Surgery; Aneurysm-Aortic; **Hospital:** Mount Sinai Med Ctr (page 102); **Address:** 5 E 98th St Fl 14 - Ste Floor, Box 1273, New York, NY 10029; **Phone:** 212-241-5315; **Board Cert:** Surgery 2004; Vascular Surgery 2005; **Med School:** NYU Sch Med 1996; **Resid:** Surgery, Mt Sinai Med Ctr 2002; **Fellow:** Vascular Surgery, Mt Sinai Med Ctr 2003; **Fac Appt:** Assoc Prof S, Mount Sinai Sch Med

Fantini, Gary A MD (VascS) - **Spec Exp:** Spinal Access Surgery; **Hospital:** Hosp For Special Surgery (page 115), NY-Presby/Weill Cornell Med Ctr, NY (page 104); **Address:** 635 Madison Ave, Fl 7, New York, NY 10022; **Phone:** 212-317-4550; **Board Cert:** Surgery 2012; Vascular Surgery 2010; **Med School:** Albert Einstein Coll Med 1983; **Resid:** Surgery, NY Hosp-Cornell Med Ctr 1989; **Fellow:** Vascular Surgery, UCSF Med Ctr 1990; **Fac Appt:** Assoc Prof S, Cornell Univ-Weill Med Coll

Faries, Peter L MD (VascS) - **Spec Exp:** Aneurysm-Abdominal Aortic; Peripheral Vascular Disease; Renovascular Disease; Carotid Artery Surgery; **Hospital:** Mount Sinai Med Ctr (page 102); **Address:** 5 E 98th St, Ste 415, New York, NY 10029; **Phone:** 212-241-5386; **Board Cert:** Surgery 2008; Vascular Surgery 2009; **Med School:** Univ Pennsylvania 1992; **Resid:** Surgery, Montefiore Med Ctr 1998; **Fellow:** Vascular Surgery, Beth Israel Deaconess Med Ctr 2000; **Fac Appt:** Assoc Prof S, Cornell Univ-Weill Med Coll

Green, Richard M MD (VascS) - **Spec Exp:** Aneurysm-Abdominal Aortic; Carotid Artery Surgery; Percutaneous Vascular Interventions; **Hospital:** Lenox Hill Hosp (page 106); **Address:** 130 E 77th St, Fl 13, New York, NY 10075; **Phone:** 212-434-3420; **Board Cert:** Vascular Surgery 2003; **Med School:** Univ Rochester 1970; **Resid:** Surgery, Strong Meml Hosp 1976

New York (Manhattan)
Vascular Surgery

Grossi, Robert J MD (VascS) - **Spec Exp:** Carotid Artery Surgery; Aneurysm-Abdominal Aortic; Wound Healing/Care; **Hospital:** Beth Israel Med Ctr - Petrie Division (page 94), NY Downtown Hosp; **Address:** Beth Israel Med Ctr, Div Vasc Surg, 1st Ave at 16th St, 12 Fierman Hall, New York, NY 10003; **Phone:** 212-844-5559; **Board Cert:** Surgery 2006; Vascular Surgery 2008; **Med School:** UMDNJ-NJ Med Sch, Newark 1981; **Resid:** Surgery, St Vincent's Hosp 1986; **Fellow:** Vascular Surgery, Temple Univ Hosp 1987

Harrington, Elizabeth MD (VascS) - **Spec Exp:** Carotid Artery Surgery; Aneurysm-Aortic; Arterial Bypass Surgery-Leg; **Hospital:** Mount Sinai Med Ctr (page 102); **Address:** 2 E 93rd St, New York, NY 10128; **Phone:** 212-876-7400; **Board Cert:** Surgery 2009; Vascular Surgery 2006; **Med School:** NY Med Coll 1975; **Resid:** Surgery, Mt Sinai Hosp 1980; **Fellow:** Vascular Surgery, Mt Sinai Hosp 1981; **Fac Appt:** Assoc Prof VascS, Mount Sinai Sch Med

Harrington, Martin MD (VascS) - **Spec Exp:** Carotid Artery Surgery; Aneurysm-Aortic; Arterial Bypass Surgery-Leg; **Hospital:** Mount Sinai Med Ctr (page 102); **Address:** 2 E 93rd St, New York, NY 10128; **Phone:** 212-876-7400; **Board Cert:** Internal Medicine 1978; Hematology 1980; Surgery 2003; Vascular Surgery 2007; **Med School:** Harvard Med Sch 1975; **Resid:** Internal Medicine, St Luke's Roosevelt Hosp Ctr 1979; Surgery, Mt Sinai Hosp 1984; **Fellow:** Surgical Oncology, Meml Sloan Kettering Cancer Ctr 1986; Vascular Surgery, Mt Sinai Hosp 1989

Jacobowitz, Glenn R MD (VascS) - **Spec Exp:** Vein Disorders; Minimally Invasive Vascular Surgery; Aneurysm-Abdominal Aortic; Carotid Artery Surgery; **Hospital:** NYU Langone Med Ctr (page 108), Bellevue Hosp Ctr; **Address:** Schwartz Health Care Ctr, 530 First Ave, Ste 6F, New York, NY 10016; **Phone:** 212-263-7311; **Board Cert:** Surgery 2006; Vascular Surgery 2005; **Med School:** NYU Sch Med 1989; **Resid:** Surgery, NYU Med Ctr 1995; **Fellow:** Vascular Surgery, NYU Med Ctr 1996; **Fac Appt:** Assoc Prof VascS, NYU Sch Med

Karwowski, John MD (VascS) - **Spec Exp:** Carotid Artery Surgery; Minimally Invasive Vascular Surgery; Carotid Artery Stent Placement; **Hospital:** NY-Presby/Weill Cornell Med Ctr, NY (page 104); **Address:** 525 E 68th St, Starr 8, New York, NY 10065; **Phone:** 212-746-5567; **Board Cert:** Surgery 2004; Vascular Surgery 2008; **Med School:** Tufts Univ 1995; **Resid:** Surgery, Stanford Univ Hosp & Clinics 2003; **Fellow:** Vascular Neurology, Stanford Univ Hosp & Clinics 2005; **Fac Appt:** Asst Prof VascS, Cornell Univ-Weill Med Coll

Maldonado, Thomas MD (VascS) - **Spec Exp:** Aortic Stent Grafts; Endovascular Surgery; **Hospital:** NYU Langone Med Ctr (page 108), Bellevue Hosp Ctr; **Address:** NYU Medical Ctr, Univ Vascular Assocs, 530 First Ave, Ste 6F, New York, NY 10016; **Phone:** 212-263-5626; **Board Cert:** Surgery 2003; Vascular Surgery 2005; **Med School:** NYU Sch Med 1995; **Resid:** Surgery, NYU Med Ctr 1998; Surgery, NYU Med Ctr 2002; **Fellow:** Research, NYU Med Ctr 2000; Vascular Surgery, NYU Med Ctr 2003; **Fac Appt:** Assoc Prof S, NYU Sch Med

Marin, Michael L MD (VascS) - **Spec Exp:** Aneurysm-Aortic; Peripheral Vascular Disease; Limb Sparing Surgery; Endovascular Surgery; **Hospital:** Mount Sinai Med Ctr (page 102); **Address:** Mount Sinai Medical Ctr, 5 E 98th St, Box 1273, New York, NY 10029; **Phone:** 212-241-5315; **Board Cert:** Surgery 2011; **Med School:** Mount Sinai Sch Med 1984; **Resid:** Surgery, Columbia-Presby Med Ctr 1990; **Fellow:** Transplant Surgery, Columbia-Presby Med Ctr 1988; Vascular Surgery, Montefiore Med Ctr 1992; **Fac Appt:** Prof S, Mount Sinai Sch Med

McKinsey, James F MD (VascS) - **Spec Exp:** Aneurysm-Abdominal Aortic; Endovascular Surgery; Carotid Artery Surgery; **Hospital:** NY-Presby/Columbia Univ Med Ctr, NY (page 104); **Address:** NY Presby Hosp/Columbia U Med Ctr, Irving Pavilion Fl 5, 161 Fort Washington Ave, New York, NY 10032; **Phone:** 212-342-3255; **Board Cert:** Surgery 2001; Vascular Surgery 2003; **Med School:** Univ Fla Coll Med 1987; **Resid:** Surgery, Georgia Baptist Med Ctr 1992; **Fellow:** Vascular Surgery, Univ Chicago Hosps 1993; **Fac Appt:** Assoc Clin Prof S, Columbia P&S

Mendes, Donna M MD (VascS) - **Spec Exp:** Varicose Veins; Aneurysm-Aortic; Limb Sparing Surgery; **Hospital:** St. Luke's - Roosevelt Hosp Ctr - Roosevelt Div (page 94), Lenox Hill Hosp (page 106); **Address:** 10 W 66th St, New York, NY 10023; **Phone:** 212-636-4990; **Board Cert:** Surgery 2004; Vascular Surgery 2011; **Med School:** Columbia P&S 1977; **Resid:** Surgery, St Luke's-Roosevelt Hosp Ctr 1982; **Fellow:** Vascular Surgery, Englewood Hosp 1984; **Fac Appt:** Asst Clin Prof S, Columbia P&S

Morrissey, Nicholas J MD (VascS) - **Spec Exp:** Minimally Invasive Vascular Surgery; Aneurysm-Abdominal & Thoracic Aortic; Carotid Artery Surgery; **Hospital:** NY-Presby/Columbia Univ Med Ctr, NY (page 104); **Address:** 161 Fort Washington Ave, Herbert Irving Pavilion, rm 538, New York, NY 10032; **Phone:** 212-342-2929; **Board Cert:** Surgery 2009; Vascular Surgery 2003; **Med School:** Univ Rochester 1992; **Resid:** Surgery, Strong Meml Hosp 1999; **Fellow:** Vascular Surgery, Mount Sinai Hosp 2001; **Fac Appt:** Assoc Prof S, Columbia P&S

Nalbandian, Matthew M MD (VascS) - **Spec Exp:** Spinal Access Surgery; Endovascular Surgery; Varicose Veins; Vein Disorders; **Hospital:** NYU Langone Med Ctr (page 108), Holy Name Med Ctr (page 688); **Address:** 247 Third Ave, Ste L1, New York, NY 10010; **Phone:** 212-254-6882; **Board Cert:** Surgery 2009; Vascular Surgery 2008; **Med School:** UMDNJ-NJ Med Sch, Newark 1993; **Resid:** Surgery, Boston Med Ctr 1998; **Fellow:** Vascular Surgery, NYU Med Ctr 2000; **Fac Appt:** Asst Prof VascS, NYU Sch Med

Riles, Thomas MD (VascS) - **Spec Exp:** Aneurysm-Aortic-Medical Management; Carotid Artery Medical Management; **Hospital:** NYU Langone Med Ctr (page 108); **Address:** NYU Med Ctr, Univ Vascular Assoc, 530 1st Ave, Ste 6F, New York, NY 10016; **Phone:** 212-263-6360; **Board Cert:** Vascular Surgery 2003; **Med School:** Baylor Coll Med 1969; **Resid:** Surgery, NYU Med Ctr 1976; **Fellow:** Vascular Surgery, NYU Med Ctr 1977; **Fac Appt:** Prof S, NYU Sch Med

Rockman, Caron B MD (VascS) - **Spec Exp:** Carotid Artery Surgery; Aneurysm-Abdominal Aortic; Peripheral Vascular Disease; Vein Disorders; **Hospital:** NYU Langone Med Ctr (page 108); **Address:** 530 1st Ave Fl 6 - Ste F, MS 10016, New York, NY 10016; **Phone:** 212-263-7311; **Board Cert:** Surgery 2006; Vascular Surgery 2007; **Med School:** NYU Sch Med 1990; **Resid:** Surgery, NYU Med Ctr 1995; **Fellow:** Vascular Surgery, NYU Med Ctr 1997; **Fac Appt:** Assoc Prof S, NYU Sch Med

Schneider, Darren B MD (VascS) - **Spec Exp:** Endovascular Surgery; Minimally Invasive Vascular Surgery; Aneurysm-Aortic; Peripheral Vascular Disease; **Hospital:** NY-Presby/Weill Cornell Med Ctr, NY (page 104); **Address:** Weill Cornell Dept Vascular Surgery, 525 E 68th St, New York, NY 10021; **Phone:** 212-746-5192; **Board Cert:** Surgery 2001; Vascular Surgery 2003; **Med School:** UCSD 1992; **Resid:** Surgery, UCSF Med Ctr 2000; **Fellow:** Interventional Radiology, UCSF Med Ctr 2001; Vascular Surgery, UCSF Med Ctr 2002; **Fac Appt:** Assoc Prof S, Cornell Univ-Weill Med Coll

Stein, Jeffrey S MD (VascS) - **Spec Exp:** Aneurysm-Aortic; Arterial Disease; Varicose Veins; **Hospital:** Mount Sinai Med Ctr (page 102), Lenox Hill Hosp (page 106); **Address:** 12 E 97th St, Ste 1C, New York, NY 10029; **Phone:** 212-396-0500; **Board Cert:** Surgery 2009; Vascular Surgery 2002; Surgical Critical Care 2001; **Med School:** Washington Univ, St Louis 1982; **Resid:** Surgery, Mt Sinai Hosp 1988; **Fellow:** Surgical Critical Care, Mt Sinai Hosp 1989; Vascular Surgery, Mt Sinai Hosp 1990; **Fac Appt:** Asst Clin Prof S, Mount Sinai Sch Med

Teodorescu, Victoria MD (VascS) - **Spec Exp:** Endovascular Surgery; Aneurysm; Diabetic Leg/Foot; Peripheral Vascular Disease; **Hospital:** Mount Sinai Med Ctr (page 102); **Address:** 5 E 98th St, Fl 3, New York, NY 10029; **Phone:** 212-241-5315; **Board Cert:** Surgery 2011; Vascular Surgery 2003; **Med School:** NYU Sch Med 1985; **Resid:** Surgery, Mt Sinai Hosp 1991; **Fellow:** Vascular Surgery, Mt Sinai Hosp 1992; **Fac Appt:** Assoc Prof S, Mount Sinai Sch Med

Todd, George MD (VascS) - **Spec Exp:** Minimally Invasive Vascular Surgery; Aneurysm-Abdominal Aortic; Carotid Artery Surgery; **Hospital:** St. Luke's - Roosevelt Hosp Ctr - Roosevelt Div (page 94); **Address:** St Luke's-Roosevelt Hosp Ctr, Dept Surg, 1000 10th Ave, rm 5G77, New York, NY 10019; **Phone:** 212-523-7481; **Board Cert:** Surgery 2010; Vascular Surgery 2006; **Med School:** Penn State Coll Med 1974; **Resid:** Surgery, Columbia-Presby Med Ctr 1979; **Fellow:** Vascular Surgery, Columbia-Presby Med Ctr 1980; **Fac Appt:** Prof S, Columbia P&S

Bronx

Bronx

Adolescent Medicine

Alderman, Elizabeth MD (AM) - **Spec Exp:** Adolescent Gynecology; Eating Disorders; Parenting Issues; **Hospital:** Montefiore Med Ctr-Moses Campus, NY (page 100); **Address:** Chldn's Hosp Montefiore, Dept Adolescent Med, 3415 Bainbridge Rd, Bronx, NY 10467; **Phone:** 718-920-6614; **Board Cert:** Pediatrics 2005; Adolescent Medicine 2009; **Med School:** SUNY Stony Brook 1987; **Resid:** Pediatrics, Montefiore Med Ctr 1990; **Fellow:** Adolescent Medicine, Montefiore Med Ctr 1992; **Fac Appt:** Clin Prof Ped, Albert Einstein Coll Med

Coupey, Susan MD (AM) - **Spec Exp:** Adolescent Gynecology; Menstrual Disorders; Reproductive Endocrinology; Uterine/Vaginal Agenisis; **Hospital:** Montefiore Med Ctr-Moses Campus, NY (page 100); **Address:** Chldn's Hosp Montefiore, Dept Adolescent Medicine, 3415 Bainbridge Rd, Bronx, NY 10467; **Phone:** 718-920-6781; **Board Cert:** Pediatrics 1979; Adolescent Medicine 2009; **Med School:** Canada 1975; **Resid:** Pediatrics, Chldns Hosp 1978; **Fellow:** Adolescent Medicine, Montefiore Hosp Med Ctr 1979; **Fac Appt:** Prof Ped, Albert Einstein Coll Med

Rieder, Jessica MD (AM) - **Spec Exp:** Obesity; Vaccines; Eating Disorders; **Hospital:** Montefiore Med Ctr-Moses Campus, NY (page 100); **Address:** Chldn's Hosp Montefiore, 3415 Bainbridge Ave, Bronx, NY 10467; **Phone:** 718-920-2897; **Board Cert:** Pediatrics 2006; Adolescent Medicine 2009; **Med School:** Univ Alberta 1994; **Resid:** Pediatrics, Montefiore Med Ctr 1998; **Fellow:** Adolescent Medicine, Albert Einstein Coll Med 2001; **Fac Appt:** Assoc Clin Prof Ped, Albert Einstein Coll Med

Allergy & Immunology

Bernstein, Larry J MD (A&I) - **Spec Exp:** Asthma; Immune Deficiency; Sinus Disorders; Food Allergy; **Hospital:** Montefiore Med Ctr-Moses Campus, NY (page 100); **Address:** 118 Morris Park Ave Fl 3, Bronx, NY 10461; **Phone:** 718-863-8465; **Board Cert:** Pediatrics 1981; Allergy & Immunology 1985; **Med School:** Albert Einstein Coll Med 1977; **Resid:** Pediatrics, Jacobi Med Ctr 1981; **Fellow:** Allergy & Immunology, Albert Einstein Coll Med 1983; **Fac Appt:** Assoc Clin Prof Ped, Albert Einstein Coll Med

Kaufman, Alan MD (A&I) - **Spec Exp:** Asthma; Sinus Disorders; Urticaria; Immunodeficiency Disorders; **Hospital:** Montefiore Med Ctr-Moses Campus, NY (page 100), Lawrence Hosp Ctr; **Address:** 3626 E Tremont Ave, Ste 202, Bronx, NY 10465-2030; **Phone:** 718-597-9000; **Board Cert:** Internal Medicine 1988; Allergy & Immunology 2009; **Med School:** West Indies 1984; **Resid:** Internal Medicine, Metropolitan Hosp Ctr 1987; **Fellow:** Allergy & Immunology, Montefiore Med Ctr 1989

Lehach, Joan G MD (A&I) - **Spec Exp:** Asthma; **Hospital:** St. Barnabas Hosp - Bronx, Montefiore Med Ctr-Einstein Campus, NY (page 100); **Address:** 1488 Metropolitan Ave, Ste 12, Bronx, NY 10462; **Phone:** 718-918-1991; **Board Cert:** Internal Medicine 2010; **Med School:** Chile 1985; **Resid:** Internal Medicine, St Barnabas Med Ctr 1988; **Fellow:** Allergy & Immunology, Albert Einstein Med Ctr 1990

Rosenstreich, David L MD (A&I) - **Spec Exp:** Urticaria; Sinusitis; Atopic Dermatitis; **Hospital:** Montefiore Med Ctr-Moses Campus, NY (page 100), Jacobi Med Ctr; **Address:** 1515 Blondell Ave, Fl 2, Ste 220, Bronx, NY 10461; **Phone:** 866-633-8255; **Board Cert:** Internal Medicine 1972; Allergy & Immunology 1975; Clinical & Laboratory Immunology 1990; **Med School:** NYU Sch Med 1967; **Resid:** Internal Medicine, Albert Einstein Med Ctr 1969; **Fellow:** Allergy & Immunology, Natl Inst Hlth 1972; **Fac Appt:** Prof Med, Albert Einstein Coll Med

Rubinstein, Arye MD/PhD (A&I) - **Spec Exp:** Immune Deficiency; Asthma; Allergy; **Hospital:** Montefiore Med Ctr-Moses Campus, NY (page 100), Montefiore Med Ctr-Einstein Campus, NY (page 100); **Address:** 1180 Morris Park Ave Fl 3, Bronx, NY 10461; **Phone:** 718-863-8465; **Board Cert:** Pediatrics 1976; Allergy & Immunology 1977; **Med School:** Switzerland 1962; **Resid:** Pediatrics, Tel Aviv Univ Hosp 1967; **Fellow:** Allergy & Immunology, Univ Bern 1969; Allergy & Immunology, Harvard Med Sch 1973; **Fac Appt:** Prof Ped, Albert Einstein Coll Med

Cardiac Electrophysiology

Ferrick, Kevin J MD (CE) - **Spec Exp:** Arrhythmias; Sudden Death Prevention; **Hospital:** Montefiore Med Ctr-Moses Campus, NY (page 100), Stamford Hosp (page 893); **Address:** Montefiore Medical Center, Arrhythmia Service, 111 E 210th St, Bronx, NY 10467; **Phone:** 718-920-4148; **Board Cert:** Internal Medicine 1981; Cardiovascular Disease 1983; Cardiac Electrophysiology 2002; **Med School:** Med Coll Wisc 1977; **Resid:** Internal Medicine, Montefiore Hospital 1980; **Fellow:** Cardiovascular Disease, Columbia-Presby Med Ctr 1981; Cardiac Electrophysiology, Columbia-Presby Med Ctr 1983; **Fac Appt:** Prof Med, Albert Einstein Coll Med

Gross, Jay MD (CE) - **Spec Exp:** Pacemakers; **Hospital:** Montefiore Med Ctr-Einstein Campus, NY (page 100); **Address:** 111 E 210th St, Arrhythmia Service, Bronx, NY 10467-2490; **Phone:** 718-920-4291; **Board Cert:** Internal Medicine 1986; Cardiovascular Disease 1989; Cardiac Electrophysiology 2002; **Med School:** Albert Einstein Coll Med 1983; **Resid:** Internal Medicine, Montefiore Med Ctr 1986; **Fellow:** Cardiovascular Disease, Montrfiore Med Ctr 1988; **Fac Appt:** Prof Med, Albert Einstein Coll Med

Krumerman, Andrew K MD (CE) - **Spec Exp:** Atrial Fibrillation; Arrhythmias; **Hospital:** Montefiore Med Ctr-Moses Campus, NY (page 100); **Address:** Arrhythmia Service, 111 E 210th St Fl 2, Bronx, NY 10467; **Phone:** 718-920-4776; **Board Cert:** Cardiovascular Disease 2003; Cardiac Electrophysiology 2004; **Med School:** Israel 1996; **Resid:** Internal Medicine, Montefiore Med Ctr 1999; **Fellow:** Cardiovascular Disease, N Shore Univ Hosp 2001; Cardiac Electrophysiology, Montefiore Med Ctr 2002

Cardiovascular Disease

Garcia, Mario J MD (Cv) - **Spec Exp:** Echocardiography-Transesophageal; **Hospital:** Montefiore Med Ctr-Moses Campus, NY (page 100); **Address:** Montefiore Einstein Heart/Cardiovascular Care, 111 E 210th St, Bronx, NY 10467; **Phone:** 718-920-4172; **Board Cert:** Internal Medicine 2003; Cardiovascular Disease 2003; **Med School:** Dominican Republic 1986; **Resid:** Internal Medicine, St Vincent's Med Ctr 1990; **Fellow:** Nuclear Cardiology, Mass Genl Hosp 1994; Cardiovascular Disease, Cleveland Clinic 1996; **Fac Appt:** Prof Med, Albert Einstein Coll Med

Greenberg, Mark A MD (Cv) - **Spec Exp:** Interventional Cardiology; Cardiac Catheterization; Heart Valve Disease; **Hospital:** Montefiore Med Ctr-Moses Campus, NY (page 100); **Address:** 111 E 210th St, Division of Cardiology, Bronx, NY 10467; **Phone:** 718-920-4212; **Board Cert:** Internal Medicine 1976; Cardiovascular Disease 1979; **Med School:** Univ IL Coll Med 1973; **Resid:** Internal Medicine, Montefiore Med Ctr 1976; **Fellow:** Cardiovascular Disease, Montefiore Med Ctr 1978; **Fac Appt:** Clin Prof Med, Albert Einstein Coll Med

Kaufman, David B MD (Cv) - **Spec Exp:** Nuclear Cardiology; **Hospital:** Montefiore Med Ctr-Einstein Campus, NY (page 100); **Address:** Riverdale Heart Ctr, 2600 Netherland Ave, Ste 121, Riverdale, NY 10463; **Phone:** 718-548-1590; **Board Cert:** Internal Medicine 1980; Cardiovascular Disease 1983; **Med School:** Cornell Univ-Weill Med Coll 1977; **Resid:** Internal Medicine, Montefiore Med Ctr 1980; **Fellow:** Cardiovascular Disease, Montefiore Med Ctr 1983

Keller, Peter Karl MD (Cv) - **Spec Exp:** Congestive Heart Failure; Coronary Artery Disease; Arrhythmias; **Hospital:** Montefiore Med Ctr-Einstein Campus, NY (page 100), NY Westchester Sq Med Ctr; **Address:** 1578 Williamsbridge Rd, Bronx, NY 10461-6265; **Phone:** 718-892-7817; **Board Cert:** Internal Medicine 1988; Cardiovascular Disease 2011; **Med School:** Mount Sinai Sch Med 1985; **Resid:** Internal Medicine, Bronx Municipal Hosp 1988; **Fellow:** Cardiovascular Disease, Bronx Municipal Hosp 1991; **Fac Appt:** Assoc Clin Prof Med, Albert Einstein Coll Med

Lucariello, Richard MD (Cv) - **Spec Exp:** Congestive Heart Failure; Angina; Hypertension; **Hospital:** Montefiore Med Ctr-Wakefield Campus, NY (page 100); **Address:** 600 E 233 St, Bronx, NY 10466; **Phone:** 718-920-9256; **Board Cert:** Internal Medicine 1987; Cardiovascular Disease 2011; **Med School:** NY Med Coll 1984; **Resid:** Internal Medicine, Westchester Med Ctr 1987; **Fellow:** Cardiovascular Disease, St Vincent's Hosp & Med Ctr 1989; Cardiovascular Disease, Westchester Med Ctr 1990; **Fac Appt:** Assoc Clin Prof Med, NY Med Coll

Menegus, Mark A MD (Cv) - **Spec Exp:** Acute Coronary Syndromes; Cardiac Catheterization; Interventional Cardiology; Heart Valve Disease; **Hospital:** Montefiore Med Ctr-Moses Campus, NY (page 100), St. Barnabas Hosp - Bronx; **Address:** Montefiore Medical Center-Div Cardiology, 111 E 210th St, Bronx, NY 10467-2401; **Phone:** 718-920-5528; **Board Cert:** Internal Medicine 1984; Cardiovascular Disease 1987; **Med School:** UMDNJ-RW Johnson Med Sch 1981; **Resid:** Internal Medicine, Montefiore Med Ctr 1984; **Fellow:** Cardiovascular Disease, Montefiore Med Ctr 1987; **Fac Appt:** Clin Prof Med, Albert Einstein Coll Med

Monrad, E Scott MD (Cv) - **Spec Exp:** Coronary Artery Disease; Heart Valve Disease; Cardiac Catheterization; **Hospital:** Montefiore Med Ctr-Einstein Campus, NY (page 100), Jacobi Med Ctr; **Address:** 1825 Eastchester Rd, Bronx, NY 10461; **Phone:** 646-670-5120; **Board Cert:** Internal Medicine 1982; Cardiovascular Disease 1985; **Med School:** McGill Univ 1979; **Resid:** Internal Medicine, New England Med Ctr 1982; **Fellow:** Cardiovascular Disease, Beth Israel Med Ctr 1985; **Fac Appt:** Clin Prof Med, Albert Einstein Coll Med

Neuberg, Gerald W MD (Cv) - **Spec Exp:** Congestive Heart Failure; **Hospital:** NY-Presby/Columbia Univ Med Ctr, NY (page 104), NY-Presby Hosp/The Allen Hosp (page 104); **Address:** 3050 Corlear Ave, Ste 204, Bronx, NY 10463; **Phone:** 718-601-8720; **Board Cert:** Internal Medicine 1986; Cardiovascular Disease 1989; **Med School:** Columbia P&S 1983; **Resid:** Internal Medicine, NY Presby Hosp 1986; **Fellow:** Cardiovascular Disease, Westchester Med Ctr 1988; Cardiovascular Disease, Mt Sinai Med Ctr 1989; **Fac Appt:** Assoc Clin Prof Med, Columbia P&S

Phillips, Malcolm C MD (Cv) - **Spec Exp:** Preventive Cardiology; Echocardiography; Cardiac Stress Testing; **Hospital:** St. Barnabas Hosp - Bronx; **Address:** 4422 3rd Ave, Bronx, NY 10457-2545; **Phone:** 718-960-6205; **Board Cert:** Internal Medicine 1979; Cardiovascular Disease 1981; **Med School:** Columbia P&S 1976; **Resid:** Internal Medicine, New York Hosp 1978; **Fellow:** Cardiovascular Disease, New York Hosp 1980; **Fac Appt:** Asst Clin Prof Med, Cornell Univ-Weill Med Coll

Sahar, David I MD (Cv) - **Spec Exp:** Arrhythmias; Atrial Fibrillation; Heart Valve Disease; Coronary Artery Disease; **Hospital:** NY-Presby/Columbia Univ Med Ctr, NY (page 104); **Address:** 2600 Netherland Ave, Ste 106, Bronx, NY 10463-4813; **Phone:** 212-305-4567; **Board Cert:** Internal Medicine 1983; Cardiovascular Disease 1987; **Med School:** Columbia P&S 1980; **Resid:** Internal Medicine, Ohio State Univ 1983; **Fellow:** Cardiovascular Disease, St Lukes Hosp 1985; Cardiac Electrophysiology, Columbia Presby Hosp 1987; **Fac Appt:** Assoc Prof Med, Columbia P&S

Schick, David MD (Cv) - **Hospital:** Montefiore Med Ctr-Moses Campus, NY (page 100); **Address:** 3201 Grand Concourse, Ste 1J, Bronx, NY 10468-1226; **Phone:** 718-933-2244; **Board Cert:** Internal Medicine 1972; Cardiovascular Disease 1975; **Med School:** Albert Einstein Coll Med 1966; **Resid:** Internal Medicine, Montefiore Hosp 1971; Cardiovascular Disease, Montefiore Hosp 1973; **Fac Appt:** Asst Clin Prof Med, Albert Einstein Coll Med

Silverman, Rubin MD (Cv) - **Spec Exp:** Echocardiography; **Hospital:** St. Barnabas Hosp - Bronx, Montefiore Med Ctr-Einstein Campus, NY (page 100); **Address:** 1180 Morris Park Ave Fl 2, Bronx, NY 10461-1925; **Phone:** 718-409-3335; **Board Cert:** Internal Medicine 1981; Cardiovascular Disease 1983; **Med School:** Albert Einstein Coll Med 1978; **Resid:** Internal Medicine, Jacobi Med Ctr 1981; **Fellow:** Cardiovascular Disease, Montefiore Med Ctr 1983; **Fac Appt:** Asst Prof Med, Albert Einstein Coll Med

Child & Adolescent Psychiatry

Gerbino-Rosen, Ginny M MD (ChAP) - **Spec Exp:** Child & Adolescent Psychiatry; Aggression Disorders; **Hospital:** Bronx Children's Psych Ctr; **Address:** Bronx Chldns Psych Ctr, 1000 Waters Pl, House 8, Bronx, NY 10461-2701; **Phone:** 718-239-3600; **Board Cert:** Psychiatry 1981; Child & Adolescent Psychiatry 1987; Forensic Psychiatry 2009; **Med School:** Creighton Univ 1976; **Resid:** Psychiatry, Bellevue-NYU Med Ctr 1979; **Fellow:** Child & Adolescent Psychiatry, Bellevue-NYU Med Ctr 1981; **Fac Appt:** Asst Prof Psyc, Albert Einstein Coll Med

Lomonaco, Salvatore MD (ChAP) - **Hospital:** Montefiore Med Ctr-Moses Campus, NY (page 100); **Address:** Albert Einstein College Med, 1300 Morris Park Ave, Belfer Bldg - rm 405, Bronx, NY 10461; **Phone:** 718-430-2020; **Board Cert:** Psychiatry 1976; **Med School:** SUNY Downstate 1966; **Resid:** Psychiatry, Montefiore Med Ctr 1971; Child Psychiatry, Montefiore Med Ctr 1972; **Fac Appt:** Assoc Prof Psyc, Albert Einstein Coll Med

Child Neurology

Moshe, Solomon L MD (ChiN) - **Spec Exp:** Epilepsy/Seizure Disorders; **Hospital:** Montefiore Med Ctr-Moses Campus, NY (page 100); **Address:** 3415 Bainbridge Ave Fl 4, Bronx, NY 10467; **Phone:** 718-920-4378; **Board Cert:** Pediatrics 1978; Child Neurology 1979; Clinical Neurophysiology 2006; **Med School:** Greece 1972; **Resid:** Pediatrics, Univ MD Hosp 1975; Pediatric Neurology, Albert Einstein 1978; **Fellow:** Neurology, Albert Einstein 1979; **Fac Appt:** Prof N, Albert Einstein Coll Med

Shinnar, Shlomo MD/PhD (ChiN) - **Spec Exp:** Epilepsy/Seizure Disorders; Headache; **Hospital:** Montefiore Med Ctr-Moses Campus, NY (page 100); **Address:** Montefiore Med Ctr, Dept Neurophsiology, Pediatric Neurology, 111 E 210th St Fl 4, Bronx, NY 10467; **Phone:** 718-920-4378; **Board Cert:** Neurology 1984; Pediatrics 1984; Clinical Neurophysiology 2005; **Med School:** Albert Einstein Coll Med 1978; **Resid:** Pediatrics, Johns Hopkins Hosp 1980; Neurology, Johns Hopkins Hosp 1983; **Fac Appt:** Prof N, Albert Einstein Coll Med

Clinical Genetics

Marion, Robert W MD (CG) - **Spec Exp:** Spina Bifida; Williams Syndrome; Marfan's Syndrome; Down Syndrome; **Hospital:** Montefiore Med Ctr-Moses Campus, NY (page 100), Blythedale Children's Hosp; **Address:** 3415 Bainbridge Ave, Bronx, NY 10467; **Phone:** 718-741-2323; **Board Cert:** Pediatrics 1985; Clinical Genetics 1987; **Med School:** Albert Einstein Coll Med 1979; **Resid:** Pediatrics, Montefiore Med Ctr 1982; **Fellow:** Clinical Genetics, Montefiore Med Ctr 1984; **Fac Appt:** Prof Ped, Albert Einstein Coll Med

Ostrer, Harry MD (CG) - **Spec Exp:** Genetic Disorders; Hereditary Cancer; **Hospital:** Montefiore Med Ctr-Wakefield Campus, NY (page 100); **Address:** Albert Einstein College of Medicine, 1300 Morris Park Ave, Ullman Bldg, rm 819, Bronx, NY 10461; **Phone:** 718-430-8605; **Board Cert:** Clinical Genetics 1984; Pediatrics 1985; Clinical Cytogenetics 1990; Clinical Molecular Genetics 2010; **Med School:** Columbia P&S 1976; **Resid:** Pediatrics, Johns Hopkins Hosp 1978; Clinical Genetics, Johns Hopkins Hosp 1984; **Fellow:** Molecular Genetics, Natl Inst Health 1981; **Fac Appt:** Prof Path, Albert Einstein Coll Med

Critical Care Medicine

Siegel, Robert MD (CCM) - **Spec Exp:** Pneumonia; Infectious Disease; **Hospital:** James J. Peters VA Med Ctr-Bronx, Mount Sinai Med Ctr (page 102); **Address:** 130 W Kingsbridge Rd, Ste 8C, Bronx, NY 10468-3992; **Phone:** 718-584-9000 x6723; **Board Cert:** Internal Medicine 1982; Pulmonary Disease 1986; Critical Care Medicine 2009; **Med School:** Columbia P&S 1979; **Resid:** Internal Medicine, St Luke's Hosp 1982; Internal Medicine, Booth Meml Hosp 1983; **Fellow:** Pulmonary Disease, Bronx Municipal Hosp 1985; **Fac Appt:** Assoc Prof Med, Mount Sinai Sch Med

Dermatology

Cohen, Steven R MD (D) - **Spec Exp:** Occupational Dermatology; Contact Dermatitis; Psoriasis; **Hospital:** Montefiore Med Ctr-Moses Campus, NY (page 100); **Address:** 3514 Bainbridge Ave, Bronx, NY 10467; **Phone:** 866-633-8255; **Board Cert:** Dermatology 2009; **Med School:** Univ Pennsylvania 1971; **Resid:** Dermatology, Yale-New Haven Hosp 1977; **Fac Appt:** Prof D, Albert Einstein Coll Med

Liteplo, Ronald R MD (D) - **Spec Exp:** Melanoma; Skin Diseases-Immunologic; **Hospital:** Montefiore Med Ctr-Moses Campus, NY (page 100); **Address:** 3176 Bainbridge Ave, Bronx, NY 10467; **Phone:** 718-515-0200; **Board Cert:** Internal Medicine 1975; Dermatology 1978; **Med School:** NYU Sch Med 1972; **Resid:** Internal Medicine, Univ Hosp 1975; Dermatology, Univ Hosp 1978; **Fellow:** Immunology, Univ Hosp 1976; **Fac Appt:** Asst Clin Prof Med, Albert Einstein Coll Med

Rosen, Douglas MD (D) - **Spec Exp:** Skin Cancer; Hair Removal-Laser; Acne; **Hospital:** NY Westchester Sq Med Ctr; **Address:** 3620 E Tremont Ave, FL 2, Bronx, NY 10465; **Phone:** 718-792-4700; **Board Cert:** Dermatology 1984; **Med School:** Albert Einstein Coll Med 1980; **Resid:** Dermatology, Montefiore Hosp Med Ctr 1984; **Fac Appt:** Assoc Prof D, Albert Einstein Coll Med

Rudikoff, Donald MD (D) - **Spec Exp:** AIDS Related Skin Disorders; Skin Infections; Smallpox; **Hospital:** Bronx Lebanon Hosp Ctr; **Address:** 2739 3rd Ave, Bronx, NY 10451; **Phone:** 718-838-1016; **Board Cert:** Internal Medicine 1980; Dermatology 2009; **Med School:** NY Med Coll 1973; **Resid:** Internal Medicine, Beth Israel Med Ctr 1980; Dermatology, Mount Sinai Med Ctr 1982; **Fac Appt:** Assoc Prof D, Mount Sinai Sch Med

Diagnostic Radiology

Amis Jr, E Stephen MD (DR) - **Spec Exp:** Urologic Imaging; **Hospital:** Montefiore Med Ctr-Moses Campus, NY (page 100); **Address:** Montefiore Med Ctr, Dept Radiology, 111 E 210th St, Bronx, NY 10467; **Phone:** 718-920-5113; **Board Cert:** Urology 1975; Diagnostic Radiology 1979; **Med School:** Northwestern Univ 1967; **Resid:** Urology, US Naval Hosp 1972; Diagnostic Radiology, US Naval Hosp 1978; **Fellow:** Urologic Radiology, Mass General Hosp 1981; **Fac Appt:** Prof, Albert Einstein Coll Med

Friedman, Stanley N MD (DR) - **Hospital:** NY Westchester Sq Med Ctr; **Address:** NY Westchester Sq Med Ctr, Dept Rad, 2475 St Raymond Ave, Bronx, NY 10461-3124; **Phone:** 718-430-7321; **Board Cert:** Diagnostic Radiology 1974; **Med School:** NY Med Coll 1968; **Resid:** Diagnostic Radiology, Mt Sinai Hosp 1970; Radiation Oncology, Albert Einstein 1972; **Fellow:** Diagnostic Radiology, Mt Sinai Hosp 1973; **Fac Appt:** Asst Clin Prof, Cornell Univ-Weill Med Coll

Haramati, Linda B MD (DR) - **Spec Exp:** AIDS/HIV; Lung Cancer; **Hospital:** Montefiore Med Ctr-Moses Campus, NY (page 100), Jacobi Med Ctr; **Address:** Montefiore Med Ctr, Dept Radiology, 111 E 210th St, Bronx, NY 10467-2401; **Phone:** 718-920-7458; **Board Cert:** Diagnostic Radiology 1990; **Med School:** Albert Einstein Coll Med 1985; **Resid:** Diagnostic Radiology, Montefiore Med Ctr 1990; **Fellow:** Thoracic Radiology, Columbia-Presby Med Ctr 1991; **Fac Appt:** Prof, Albert Einstein Coll Med

Haramati, Nogah MD (DR) - **Spec Exp:** Orthopaedic Imaging; Rheumatology; Musculoskeletal Imaging; **Hospital:** Montefiore Med Ctr-Moses Campus, NY (page 100), Jacobi Med Ctr; **Address:** 1825 Eastchester Rd, rm 3-006, Bronx, NY 10461; **Phone:** 718-904-2965; **Board Cert:** Diagnostic Radiology 1990; **Med School:** SUNY Hlth Sci Ctr 1985; **Resid:** Diagnostic Radiology, Montefiore Hosp Med Ctr 1990; **Fellow:** Musculoskeletal Imaging, Columbia-Presby Med Ctr 1991; **Fac Appt:** Clin Prof Rad, Albert Einstein Coll Med

Koenigsberg, Mordecai MD (DR) - **Spec Exp:** Ultrasound; **Hospital:** Montefiore Med Ctr-Einstein Campus, NY (page 100); **Address:** Montefiore Med Ctr-Weiler Einstein, 1825 Eastchester Rd, rm 3035, Bronx, NY 10461; **Phone:** 718-904-2322; **Board Cert:** Pediatrics 1970; Nuclear Medicine 1973; Diagnostic Radiology 1974; **Med School:** Albert Einstein Coll Med 1963; **Resid:** Pediatrics, Jacobi Med Ctr 1966; Diagnostic Radiology, Jacobi Med Ctr 1974; **Fac Appt:** Prof Rad, Albert Einstein Coll Med

Laks, Mitchell MD (DR) - **Spec Exp:** MRI; Ultrasound; CT Body Scan; **Hospital:** Montefiore Med Ctr-Moses Campus, NY (page 100); **Address:** Montefiore Med Ctr, Dept Rad, 111 E 210th St, Bronx, NY 10467; **Phone:** 718-920-4396; **Board Cert:** Diagnostic Radiology 1990; **Med School:** Harvard Med Sch 1985; **Resid:** Diagnostic Radiology, Einstein Affil Hosp 1990; **Fellow:** Magnetic Resonance Imaging, Brigham & Womens Hosp 1991; **Fac Appt:** Asst Prof Rad, Albert Einstein Coll Med

Morehouse, Helen MD (DR) - **Spec Exp:** Genitourinary Imaging; MRI; Ultrasound; **Hospital:** Bronx Lebanon Hosp Ctr; **Address:** Bronx-Lebanon Hosp, Dept Radiology, 1650 Grand Concourse, Bronx, NY 10457-7606; **Phone:** 718-590-1800; **Board Cert:** Diagnostic Radiology 1976; **Med School:** Univ KY Coll Med 1971; **Resid:** Diagnostic Radiology, Rochester Genl Hosp 1975; **Fellow:** Diagnostic Radiology, Downstate Med Ctr 1976; **Fac Appt:** Prof Rad, Albert Einstein Coll Med

Rozenblit, Alla MD (DR) - **Spec Exp:** Liver Disease; CT Scan; MRI; **Hospital:** Montefiore Med Ctr-Moses Campus, NY (page 100); **Address:** 111 E 210th St, Bronx, NY 10467-2401; **Phone:** 718-920-4396; **Board Cert:** Diagnostic Radiology 1984; **Med School:** Russia 1971; **Resid:** Diagnostic Radiology, Queens Hosp Ctr 1984; **Fellow:** Ultrasound/CT, LI Jewish Med Ctr 1985; **Fac Appt:** Clin Prof Rad, Albert Einstein Coll Med

Spindola-Franco, Hugo MD (DR) - **Spec Exp:** Cardiac Imaging; Congenital Heart Disease; Thoracic Radiology; **Hospital:** Montefiore Med Ctr-Moses Campus, NY (page 100); **Address:** 111 E 210th St, Bronx, NY 10467-2401; **Phone:** 718-920-4872; **Board Cert:** Diagnostic Radiology 1970; **Med School:** Mexico 1966; **Resid:** Diagnostic Radiology, Montefiore Hosp Med Ctr 1970; **Fellow:** Cardiovascular Radiology, Peter Bent Brigham Hosp/Harvard Med Sch 1971; **Fac Appt:** Prof, Albert Einstein Coll Med

Stern, Harvey MD (DR) - **Spec Exp:** Nuclear Medicine; **Hospital:** Bronx Lebanon Hosp Ctr; **Address:** Bronx-Lebanon Hosp, Dept Radiology, 1650 Grand Concourse, Bronx, NY 10457-7606; **Phone:** 718-901-8142; **Board Cert:** Diagnostic Radiology 1975; Nuclear Radiology 1978; **Med School:** Albert Einstein Coll Med 1971; **Resid:** Diagnostic Radiology, Bronx Muni Hosp 1975; **Fac Appt:** Asst Prof Rad, Albert Einstein Coll Med

Wolf, Ellen L MD (DR) - **Spec Exp:** Gastrointestinal Imaging; Abdominal Imaging; **Hospital:** Montefiore Med Ctr-Moses Campus, NY (page 100); **Address:** 111 E 210th St, Bronx, NY 10467; **Phone:** 718-920-4851; **Board Cert:** Diagnostic Radiology 1976; **Med School:** Mount Sinai Sch Med 1972; **Resid:** Diagnostic Radiology, Columbia-Presby 1974; Diagnostic Radiology, Johns Hopkins 1976; **Fellow:** Pediatric Radiology, Columbia-Presby 1977; **Fac Appt:** Clin Prof Rad, Albert Einstein Coll Med

Endocrinology, Diabetes & Metabolism

Cohen, Charmian MD (EDM) - **Spec Exp:** Diabetes; Thyroid Disorders; Obesity; **Hospital:** Montefiore Med Ctr-Einstein Campus, NY (page 100); **Address:** 1200 Waters Pl, Ste M105, Bronx, NY 10461; **Phone:** 718-892-7033; **Board Cert:** Internal Medicine 1987; Endocrinology, Diabetes & Metabolism 1989; **Med School:** South Africa 1977; **Resid:** Internal Medicine, G Schuer Hosp 1984; **Fellow:** Endocrinology, Diabetes & Metabolism, Albert Einstein 1986; **Fac Appt:** Asst Prof Med, Albert Einstein Coll Med

Grajower, Martin M MD (EDM) - **Spec Exp:** Diabetes; Osteoporosis; Thyroid Disorders; Metabolic Disorders; **Hospital:** Montefiore Med Ctr-Moses Campus, NY (page 100); **Address:** 3736 Henry Hudson Pkwy E, Riverdale, NY 10463; **Phone:** 718-549-6268; **Board Cert:** Internal Medicine 1987; Endocrinology, Diabetes & Metabolism 1981; **Med School:** Albert Einstein Coll Med 1973; **Resid:** Internal Medicine, Montefiore Hosp Med Ctr 1975; Internal Medicine, Boston Med Ctr 1976; **Fellow:** Endocrinology, Diabetes & Metabolism, Montefiore Hosp Med Ctr 1978; **Fac Appt:** Asst Prof Med, Albert Einstein Coll Med

Guzman, Rodolfo MD (EDM) - **Spec Exp:** Endocrinology; Diabetes; Thyroid Disorders; **Hospital:** Bronx Lebanon Hosp Ctr; **Address:** 860 Grand Concourse, Ste 1K, Bronx, NY 10451; **Phone:** 718-585-5060; **Board Cert:** Internal Medicine 2000; Endocrinology, Diabetes & Metabolism 2000; **Med School:** Dominican Republic 1979; **Resid:** Internal Medicine, Bronx-Lebanon Hosp 1990; **Fellow:** Endocrinology, Diabetes & Metabolism, Lincoln Med Ctr 1992

Shamoon, Harry MD (EDM) - **Hospital:** Montefiore Med Ctr-Einstein Campus, NY (page 100); **Address:** 1575 Blondell Ave, Ste 200, Bronx, NY 10461-2601; **Phone:** 718-405-8260; **Board Cert:** Internal Medicine 1977; Endocrinology, Diabetes & Metabolism 1979; **Med School:** Yale Univ 1974; **Resid:** Internal Medicine, Jacobi Med Ctr 1977; **Fellow:** Endocrinology, Diabetes & Metabolism, Yale-New Haven Hosp 1979; **Fac Appt:** Prof Med, Albert Einstein Coll Med

Surks, Martin I MD (EDM) - **Spec Exp:** Thyroid Disorders; **Hospital:** Montefiore Med Ctr-Moses Campus, NY (page 100), N Central Bronx Hosp; **Address:** 3400 Bainbridge Ave Fl 2, Bronx, NY 10467; **Phone:** 866-633-8255; **Board Cert:** Internal Medicine 1967; Endocrinology, Diabetes & Metabolism 1977; **Med School:** NYU Sch Med 1960; **Resid:** Internal Medicine, Montefiore Hosp Med Ctr 1962; Internal Medicine, VA Hosp 1964; **Fellow:** Research, Natl Inst Arthritis-Metabolic Disease 1964; **Fac Appt:** Prof Med, Albert Einstein Coll Med

Zonszein, Joel MD (EDM) - **Spec Exp:** Thyroid Disorders; Diabetes; **Hospital:** Montefiore Med Ctr-Moses Campus, NY (page 100); **Address:** 1575 Blondell Ave, Ste 200, Bronx, NY 10461; **Phone:** 866-633-8255; **Board Cert:** Nuclear Medicine 1976; Internal Medicine 1977; Endocrinology 1977; **Med School:** Mexico 1969; **Resid:** Internal Medicine, Maimonides Med Ctr 1972; Internal Medicine, Jacobi Med Ctr 1973; **Fellow:** Endocrinology, Northwestern Univ Med Sch 1974; Endocrinology, Georgetown Univ Hosp 1975; **Fac Appt:** Assoc Prof Med, Albert Einstein Coll Med

Family Medicine

Biagiotti, Wendy MD (FMed) *PCP* - **Hospital:** Montefiore Med Ctr-Moses Campus, NY (page 100); **Address:** 3101 E Tremont Ave, Bronx, NY 10461; **Phone:** 718-863-7925; **Board Cert:** Family Medicine 2009; **Med School:** Mexico 1988; **Resid:** Family Medicine, St Joseph's Hosp&Med Ctr 1994

Coloka-Kump, Rodika DO (FMed) *PCP* - **Spec Exp:** Preventive Medicine; **Hospital:** Saint Joseph's Med Ctr - Yonkers, St. John's Riverside Hosp-Andrus Pavil; **Address:** 530 W 236th St, rm #1D, Bronx, NY 10463; **Phone:** 718-548-4560; **Board Cert:** Family Medicine 2004; **Med School:** NY Coll Osteo Med 1988; **Resid:** Family Medicine, St Joseph's Med Ctr 1989

Cordero, Evelyn MD (FMed) *PCP* - **Hospital:** Montefiore Med Ctr-Wakefield Campus, NY (page 100), NY Westchester Sq Med Ctr; **Address:** 941 Castle Hill Ave, Bronx, NY 10473; **Phone:** 718-792-3117; **Board Cert:** Family Medicine 2003; **Med School:** SUNY Hlth Sci Ctr 1979; **Resid:** Family Medicine, St Joseph's Med Ctr 1982

Delaney, Brian MD (FMed) *PCP* - **Spec Exp:** Geriatric Care; **Hospital:** Montefiore Med Ctr-Moses Campus, NY (page 100), St. Barnabas Hosp - Bronx; **Address:** 2371 Arthur Ave, Bronx, NY 10458; **Phone:** 718-364-6199; **Board Cert:** Family Medicine 2007; Geriatric Medicine 2012; **Med School:** Albert Einstein Coll Med 1983; **Resid:** Family Medicine, Montefiore Med Ctr 1986; **Fac Appt:** Asst Prof FMed, Albert Einstein Coll Med

Franzetti, Carl J DO (FMed) *PCP* - **Spec Exp:** Diabetes; **Hospital:** Saint Joseph's Med Ctr - Yonkers, NY-Presby/Columbia Univ Med Ctr, NY (page 104); **Address:** 3050 Corlear Ave, Ste 201, Bronx, NY 10463-3897; **Phone:** 718-543-2700; **Board Cert:** Family Medicine 2005; **Med School:** NY Coll Osteo Med 1984; **Resid:** Family Medicine, Warren Hosp 1987

Maselli, Frank J MD (FMed) *PCP* - **Spec Exp:** Diving Medicine; Hyperbaric Medicine; **Hospital:** Saint Joseph's Med Ctr - Yonkers, NY-Presby/Columbia Univ Med Ctr, NY (page 104); **Address:** 3050 Corlear Ave, Ste 201, Bronx, NY 10463; **Phone:** 718-543-2700; **Board Cert:** Family Medicine 2004; **Med School:** Israel 1983; **Resid:** Family Medicine, Univ Hosp 1986; **Fac Appt:** Asst Prof FMed, SUNY Downstate

Morrow, Robert MD (FMed) *PCP* - **Spec Exp:** Preventive Medicine; Geriatric Medicine; Autism; **Hospital:** Montefiore Med Ctr-Moses Campus, NY (page 100), Saint Joseph's Med Ctr - Yonkers; **Address:** 5997 Riverdale Ave, Bronx, NY 10471-1602; **Phone:** 718-884-9803; **Board Cert:** Family Medicine 2009; **Med School:** Mount Sinai Sch Med 1974; **Resid:** Family Medicine, Montefiore Med Ctr 1977; **Fac Appt:** Assoc Clin Prof FMed, Albert Einstein Coll Med

Soloway, Bruce H MD (FMed) *PCP* - **Spec Exp:** AIDS/HIV; **Hospital:** Montefiore Med Ctr-Moses Campus, NY (page 100); **Address:** Montefiore Medical Center, 360 E 193 St, Bronx, NY 10458; **Phone:** 718-933-2400; **Board Cert:** Family Medicine 2007; **Med School:** Albert Einstein Coll Med 1985; **Resid:** Family Medicine, Montefiore Med Ctr 1988; **Fac Appt:** Assoc Prof FMed, Albert Einstein Coll Med

Gastroenterology

Abelow, Arthur MD (Ge) - **Spec Exp:** Endoscopy; Nutrition; **Hospital:** Montefiore Med Ctr-Einstein Campus, NY (page 100), NY Westchester Sq Med Ctr; **Address:** New York Associates in Gastroenterology, 1250 Waters Pl Fl 12, Bronx, NY 10461; **Phone:** 718-863-7397; **Board Cert:** Internal Medicine 1983; Gastroenterology 1985; **Med School:** Albert Einstein Coll Med 1980; **Resid:** Internal Medicine, Bronx Muni Hosp Ctr 1983; **Fellow:** Gastroenterology, Montefiore Med Ctr 1985; **Fac Appt:** Asst Clin Prof Med, Albert Einstein Coll Med

Antony, Michael MD (Ge) - **Spec Exp:** Colonoscopy; Endoscopy; Liver Disease; **Hospital:** Montefiore Med Ctr-Einstein Campus, NY (page 100), NY Westchester Sq Med Ctr; **Address:** 1842 Williamsbridge Rd, Bronx, NY 10461; **Phone:** 718-828-0100; **Board Cert:** Internal Medicine 1985; Gastroenterology 1989; **Med School:** SUNY Hlth Sci Ctr 1982; **Resid:** Internal Medicine, Bronx Muni Hosp 1985; **Fellow:** Gastroenterology, Montefiore Med Ctr 1988; **Fac Appt:** Assoc Clin Prof Med, Albert Einstein Coll Med

Brandt, Lawrence MD (Ge) - **Spec Exp:** Inflammatory Bowel Disease; Clostridium Difficile Disease; **Hospital:** Montefiore Med Ctr-Moses Campus, NY (page 100); **Address:** 3400 Bainbridge Ave Fl 2, Bronx, NY 10467-2401; **Phone:** 866-633-8255; **Board Cert:** Internal Medicine 1972; Gastroenterology 2006; **Med School:** SUNY Downstate 1968; **Resid:** Internal Medicine, Mt Sinai Hosp 1972; **Fellow:** Gastroenterology, Mt Sinai Hosp 1972; **Fac Appt:** Prof Emeritus Med, Albert Einstein Coll Med

Frager, Joseph MD (Ge) - **Spec Exp:** Colon Cancer; Endoscopy; Laser Surgery; **Hospital:** Montefiore Med Ctr-Moses Campus, NY (page 100), NY Hosp Queens (page 206); **Address:** 277 Van Cortlandt Ave E, Bronx, NY 10467-3011; **Phone:** 718-798-8867; **Board Cert:** Internal Medicine 1983; Gastroenterology 1985; **Med School:** Univ Pennsylvania 1980; **Resid:** Internal Medicine, Montefiore Med Ctr 1983; **Fellow:** Gastroenterology, Montefiore Med Ctr 1985; **Fac Appt:** Asst Clin Prof Med, Albert Einstein Coll Med

Gaglio Sr, Paul J MD (Ge) - **Spec Exp:** Transplant Medicine-Liver; Liver Disease; **Hospital:** Montefiore Med Ctr-Moses Campus, NY (page 100); **Address:** 111 E 210th St, Rosenthal Bldg - Fl 2, Bronx, NY 10467; **Phone:** 718-920-6240; **Board Cert:** Internal Medicine 2001; Gastroenterology 2003; Transplant Hepatology 2006; **Med School:** UMDNJ-NJ Med Sch, Newark 1988; **Resid:** Infectious Disease, Mt Sinai Med Ctr 1991; **Fellow:** Gastroenterology, UMDNJ Affil Hosp 1993; **Fac Appt:** Prof Med, Albert Einstein Coll Med

Greenwald, David A MD (Ge) - **Spec Exp:** Endoscopy; Gastroesophageal Reflux Disease (GERD); Peptic Ulcer Disease; **Hospital:** Montefiore Med Ctr-Moses Campus, NY (page 100), Montefiore Med Ctr-Einstein Campus, NY (page 100); **Address:** Montefiore Med Ctr, Div Gastroenterology, 111 E 210th St, Bronx, NY 10467; **Phone:** 866-633-8255; **Board Cert:** Internal Medicine 1989; Gastroenterology 2003; **Med School:** Albert Einstein Coll Med 1986; **Resid:** Internal Medicine, Columbia Presby Med Ctr 1989; **Fellow:** Gastroenterology, Columbia Presby Med Ctr 1993; **Fac Appt:** Assoc Prof Med, Albert Einstein Coll Med

Gupta, Sanjeev MD (Ge) - **Spec Exp:** Hepatitis; Liver Disease; Gastrointestinal Disorders; Liver Failure; **Hospital:** Montefiore Med Ctr-Einstein Campus, NY (page 100); **Address:** 1515 Blondell Ave, Ste 220, Bronx, NY 10461-2601; **Phone:** 866-633-8255; **Board Cert:** Internal Medicine 1989; **Med School:** India 1976; **Resid:** Internal Medicine, PGIMER 1980; Internal Medicine, Hammersmith Hosp 1982; **Fellow:** Gastroenterology, Hammersmith Hosp 1985; Hepatology, LAC-USC Med Ctr 1987; **Fac Appt:** Prof Med, Albert Einstein Coll Med

Gutwein, Isadore P MD (Ge) - **Spec Exp:** Pancreatic/Biliary Endoscopy (ERCP); Colonoscopy; Hepatitis; Inflammatory Bowel Disease/Crohn's; **Hospital:** Montefiore Med Ctr-Moses Campus, NY (page 100); **Address:** 3765 Riverdale Ave, Bronx, NY 10463-1845; **Phone:** 718-543-3636; **Board Cert:** Internal Medicine 1976; Gastroenterology 1979; **Med School:** Albert Einstein Coll Med 1973; **Resid:** Internal Medicine, Montefiore Hosp Med Ctr 1976; **Fellow:** Gastroenterology, St Luke's Hosp 1978; **Fac Appt:** Asst Prof Med, Albert Einstein Coll Med

Hertan, Hilary I MD (Ge) - **Spec Exp:** Endoscopic Ultrasound; **Hospital:** Montefiore Med Ctr-Wakefield Campus, NY (page 100); **Address:** Dept Gastroenterology, 600 E 233rd St Fl 4, Bronx, NY 10466; **Phone:** 718-920-9887; **Board Cert:** Internal Medicine 1986; Gastroenterology 1989; **Med School:** NY Med Coll 1982; **Resid:** Internal Medicine, North Shore Univ Hosp 1985; **Fellow:** Gastroenterology, Our Lady of Mercy Med Ctr 1990; **Fac Appt:** Asst Prof Med, NY Med Coll

Ho, Sammy MD (Ge) - **Spec Exp:** Pancreatic/Biliary Endoscopy (ERCP); Endoscopic Ultrasound; Endoscopy; **Hospital:** Montefiore Med Ctr-Moses Campus, NY (page 100); **Address:** 111 E 210th St, Bronx, NY 10467; **Phone:** 866-633-8255; **Board Cert:** Gastroenterology 2005; **Med School:** SUNY Stony Brook 1998; **Resid:** Internal Medicine, Kaiser Fdn Hosp 2001; **Fellow:** Gastroenterology, Winthrop Univ Hosp 2004; **Fac Appt:** Asst Prof Med, Albert Einstein Coll Med

Korsten, Mark A MD (Ge) - **Spec Exp:** Constipation; Gastrointestinal Motility Disorders; Spinal Cord Injury & Colonic Motility; Liver Disease; **Hospital:** James J. Peters VA Med Ctr-Bronx; **Address:** 130 W Kingsbridge Rd, Ste 3H, Bronx, NY 10468; **Phone:** 718-584-9000 x6753; **Board Cert:** Internal Medicine 1973; Gastroenterology 1975; **Med School:** Yale Univ 1970; **Resid:** Internal Medicine, Mt Sinai Hosp 1973; **Fellow:** Gastroenterology, Mt Sinai Hosp 1975; **Fac Appt:** Prof Med, Mount Sinai Sch Med

Mehta, Rekha MD (Ge) - **Spec Exp:** Palliative Care; **Hospital:** Calvary Hosp (page 114); **Address:** 1740 Eastchester Rd, Bronx, NY 10461; **Phone:** 718-518-2208; **Board Cert:** Internal Medicine 1984; Gastroenterology 1987; **Med School:** India 1972; **Resid:** Internal Medicine, New Rochelle Med Ctr 1977; **Fellow:** Gastroenterology, Univ of South Carolina 1981; Nutrition, Univ of Pitt Sch of Med 1989; **Fac Appt:** Asst Clin Prof Med, NY Med Coll

Remy, Prospere MD (Ge) - **Spec Exp:** Liver Disease; **Hospital:** Bronx Lebanon Hosp Ctr; **Address:** 860 Grand Concourse, Ste 1K, Bronx, NY 10451-2815; **Phone:** 718-585-5060; **Board Cert:** Internal Medicine 2004; Gastroenterology 2004; **Med School:** Mexico 1984; **Resid:** Internal Medicine, Bronx-Lebanon Hosp 1990; **Fellow:** Gastroenterology, Bronx-Lebanon Hosp 1992; **Fac Appt:** Asst Prof Med, Albert Einstein Coll Med

Sable, Robert A MD (Ge) - **Spec Exp:** Hepatitis B & C; Gastroesophageal Reflux Disease (GERD); Inflammatory Bowel Disease; Irritable Bowel Syndrome; **Hospital:** Montefiore Med Ctr-Moses Campus, NY (page 100), St. Barnabas Hosp - Bronx; **Address:** 3765 Riverdale Ave, Ste 7, Bronx, NY 10463-1845; **Phone:** 718-543-3636; **Board Cert:** Internal Medicine 1987; Gastroenterology 2000; **Med School:** Albert Einstein Coll Med 1973; **Resid:** Internal Medicine, Montefiore Hosp Med Ctr 1976; **Fellow:** Gastroenterology, NY Med Coll 1978; **Fac Appt:** Asst Prof Med, Albert Einstein Coll Med

Schweitzer, Philip E MD (Ge) - **Spec Exp:** Liver Disease; Gastrointestinal Disorders; Esophageal Disorders; **Hospital:** Montefiore Med Ctr-Moses Campus, NY (page 100), Montefiore Med Ctr-Wakefield Campus, NY (page 100); **Address:** 3184 Grand Concourse, Ste 2D, Bronx, NY 10458-1007; **Phone:** 718-584-0404; **Board Cert:** Internal Medicine 1972; Gastroenterology 1977; **Med School:** Cornell Univ-Weill Med Coll 1967; **Resid:** Internal Medicine, St Lukes-Roosevelt Hosp 1972; **Fellow:** Gastroenterology, Mount Sinai Hosp 1974

Sherman, Howard I MD (Ge) - **Spec Exp:** Colonoscopy; Biliary Disease; **Hospital:** Montefiore Med Ctr-Einstein Campus, NY (page 100), NY Westchester Sq Med Ctr; **Address:** 1250 Waters Pl Fl 12, Ste 1201, Bronx, NY 10461-3000; **Phone:** 718-863-7397; **Board Cert:** Internal Medicine 1976; Gastroenterology 1979; **Med School:** Albert Einstein Coll Med 1973; **Resid:** Internal Medicine, Emory Univ Hosp 1976; **Fellow:** Gastroenterology, Emory Univ Hosp 1978; **Fac Appt:** Assoc Clin Prof Med, Albert Einstein Coll Med

Stein, David F MD (Ge) - **Spec Exp:** Liver Disease; Hepatitis B & C; HIV & Hepatitis co-infection; Endoscopy; **Hospital:** Montefiore Med Ctr-Moses Campus, NY (page 100), St. Barnabas Hosp - Bronx; **Address:** Riverdale Gastro & Liver Diseases, 3765 Riverdale Ave, Ste 7, Bronx, NY 10463; **Phone:** 718-543-3636; **Board Cert:** Gastroenterology 2008; **Med School:** SUNY Downstate 1990; **Resid:** Internal Medicine, NYU/Bellvue Med Ctr/VA Med Ctr 1994; **Fellow:** Gastroenterology, NYU Med Ctr/Bellevue Med Ctr/VA Med Ctr 1996; **Fac Appt:** Asst Clin Prof Med, Albert Einstein Coll Med

Geriatric Medicine

Dharmarajan, Thiruvinvamvalai MD (Ger) - **Spec Exp:** Kidney Disease; **Hospital:** Montefiore Med Ctr-Wakefield Campus, NY (page 100); **Address:** 3250 Westchester Ave, Ste 101, Bronx, NY 10461; **Phone:** 718-518-9304; **Board Cert:** Internal Medicine 1977; Geriatric Medicine 2010; Nephrology 1980; **Med School:** India 1967; **Resid:** Internal Medicine, Misericordia Hosp 1977; **Fellow:** Nephrology, Misericordia Hosp 1979; **Fac Appt:** Prof Med, NY Med Coll

Ehrlich, Amy R MD (Ger) - **Spec Exp:** Preventive Medicine; **Hospital:** Montefiore Med Ctr-Wakefield Campus, NY (page 100); **Address:** Montefiore Div Geriatric Medicine, 111 E 210th St, Bronx, NY 10467; **Phone:** 866-633-8255; **Board Cert:** Internal Medicine 1988; Geriatric Medicine 2004; **Med School:** Harvard Med Sch 1985; **Resid:** Internal Medicine, Beth Israel Hosp 1988; **Fac Appt:** Assoc Clin Prof Med, Albert Einstein Coll Med

Goldberg, Roy J MD (Ger) *PCP* - **Spec Exp:** Long Term Care; Medications in the Elderly; Palliative Care; **Hospital:** Montefiore Med Ctr-Einstein Campus, NY (page 100), Sound Shore Med Ctr - Westchester; **Address:** Director-Kings Harbor Multicare Ctr, 2000 E Gunhill Rd, Bronx, NY 10469; **Phone:** 718-405-3535; **Board Cert:** Internal Medicine 1985; Geriatric Medicine 2002; **Med School:** Albert Einstein Coll Med 1982; **Resid:** Internal Medicine, Montefiore Med Ctr 1985; **Fac Appt:** Assoc Clin Prof Med, Albert Einstein Coll Med

Jacobs, Laurie G MD (Ger) *PCP* - **Spec Exp:** Vein Disorders; **Hospital:** Montefiore Med Ctr-Moses Campus, NY (page 100); **Address:** Montefiore Med Ctr, Dept Geriatrics, 3400 Bainbridge Ave, Bronx, NY 10467; **Phone:** 866-633-8255; **Board Cert:** Internal Medicine 1988; Geriatric Medicine 2012; **Med School:** Columbia P&S 1985; **Resid:** Internal Medicine, Montefiore Med Ctr 1988; **Fellow:** Geriatric Medicine, Montefiore Med Ctr 1990; **Fac Appt:** Prof Med, Albert Einstein Coll Med

Malik, Rubina MD (Ger) *PCP* - **Spec Exp:** Osteoporosis; **Hospital:** Montefiore Med Ctr-Moses Campus, NY (page 100); **Address:** MMC Greene Med Arts, Pavilion, 3400 Bainbridge Ave, Bronx, NY 10467; **Phone:** 866-633-8255; **Board Cert:** Internal Medicine 2006; Geriatric Medicine 2009; **Med School:** SUNY Stony Brook 1992; **Resid:** Internal Medicine, Univ Hosp 1993; Gastroenterology, Univ Hosp 1996; **Fac Appt:** , Albert Einstein Coll Med

Russell, Robin MD (Ger) - **Spec Exp:** Kidney Failure; Kidney Disease; Geriatric Dialysis; **Hospital:** Montefiore Med Ctr-Wakefield Campus, NY (page 100); **Address:** 4234 Bronx Blvd, Bronx, NY 10466; **Phone:** 347-341-4340; **Board Cert:** Internal Medicine 1974; Nephrology 1980; Geriatric Medicine 2002; **Med School:** Univ New Mexico 1971; **Resid:** Internal Medicine, Harlem Hosp 1974; **Fellow:** Nephrology, Harlem Hosp 1976; **Fac Appt:** Asst Prof Med, NY Med Coll

Geriatric Psychiatry

Kennedy, Gary MD (GerPsy) - **Spec Exp:** Alzheimer's Disease; Dementia; Depression; **Hospital:** Montefiore Med Ctr-Moses Campus, NY (page 100); **Address:** Dept of Psychiatry & Behavioral Sciences, Montefiore Medical Center, 111 E 210th St, Bronx, NY 10467-2490; **Phone:** 718-920-6270; **Board Cert:** Psychiatry 1980; Geriatric Psychiatry 2010; Psychosomatic Medicine 2005; **Med School:** Univ Tex, San Antonio 1975; **Resid:** Psychiatry, VA Hosp-Univ Texas 1979; **Fellow:** Geriatric Psychiatry, Montefiore Med Ctr 1981; Psychosomatic Medicine, Montefiore Med Ctr 1983; **Fac Appt:** Prof Psyc, Albert Einstein Coll Med

Gynecologic Oncology

Einstein, Mark H MD (GO) - **Spec Exp:** Cervical Cancer; HPV-Human Papilloma Virus; **Hospital:** Montefiore Med Ctr-Moses Campus, NY (page 100); **Address:** 1695 Eastchester Rd, rm 601, Bronx, NY 10461; **Phone:** 718-405-8082; **Board Cert:** Obstetrics & Gynecology 2005; Gynecologic Oncology 2005; **Med School:** Univ Miami Sch Med 1995; **Resid:** Obstetrics & Gynecology, St Barnabas Med Ctr 1999; **Fellow:** Gynecologic Oncology, Albert Einstein Affil Hosp 2002; **Fac Appt:** Asst Prof ObG, Albert Einstein Coll Med

Goldberg, Gary L MD (GO) - **Spec Exp:** Ovarian Cancer; Uterine Cancer; **Hospital:** Montefiore Med Ctr-Moses Campus, NY (page 100); **Address:** 1695 Eastchester Rd, Ste L2, Bronx, NY 10461; **Phone:** 718-405-8082; **Board Cert:** Obstetrics & Gynecology 1997; Gynecologic Oncology 1997; **Med School:** South Africa 1975; **Resid:** Obstetrics & Gynecology, Groote Schuur Hosp 1981; **Fellow:** Gynecologic Oncology, Groote Schuur Hosp 1983; **Fac Appt:** Assoc Prof ObG, Albert Einstein Coll Med

Smith, Harriet O MD (GO) - **Spec Exp:** Uterine Cancer; Pelvic Reconstruction; Ovarian Cancer; **Hospital:** Montefiore Med Ctr-Moses Campus, NY (page 100), Jacobi Med Ctr; **Address:** 1695 Eastchester Rd, Ste 601, Bronx, NY 10461; **Phone:** 718-405-8082; **Board Cert:** Obstetrics & Gynecology 2011; Gynecologic Oncology 2011; **Med School:** Med Coll GA 1981; **Resid:** Obstetrics & Gynecology, Med Coll Georgia 1985; Gynecologic Oncology, MD Anderson Cancer Ctr 1988; **Fellow:** Reconstructive Pelvic Surgery, Emory Univ Hosp 1989; Gynecologic Oncology, Montefiore Med Ctr 1990

Smotkin, David MD (GO) - **Spec Exp:** Gynecologic Cancer; Gynecologic Cancer-Rare; **Hospital:** Montefiore Med Ctr-Moses Campus, NY (page 100); **Address:** Montefiore Women's Ctr, 3332 Rochambeau Ave, Bronx, NY 10467; **Phone:** 718-920-4794; **Board Cert:** Obstetrics & Gynecology 2011; Gynecologic Oncology 2011; **Med School:** Yale Univ 1980; **Resid:** Obstetrics & Gynecology, Univ Colorado Hosp 1984; **Fellow:** Gynecologic Oncology, UCLA Med Ctr 1987; **Fac Appt:** Asst Prof ObG, Albert Einstein Coll Med

Hand Surgery

Kulick, Roy G MD (HS) - **Spec Exp:** Carpal Tunnel Syndrome; Arthritis; Tendon Surgery; Hand & Upper Extremity Surgery; **Hospital:** Montefiore Med Ctr-Einstein Campus, NY (page 100); **Address:** Dept Orthopaedic Surgery, 1250 Waters Pl Fl 11, Bronx, NY 10461; **Phone:** 718-920-2060; **Board Cert:** Orthopaedic Surgery 1980; Hand Surgery 2011; **Med School:** Cornell Univ-Weill Med Coll 1973; **Resid:** Surgery, St Lukes-Roosevelt Hosp 1975; Orthopaedic Surgery, NY Presby Hosp/Columbia Univ Med Ctr 1978; **Fellow:** Hand Surgery, Hosp for Special Surgery 1979; **Fac Appt:** Assoc Prof OrS, Albert Einstein Coll Med

Hematology

Billett, Henny H MD (Hem) - **Spec Exp:** Bleeding/Coagulation Disorders; Thrombotic Disorders; Platelet Disorders; Sickle Cell Disease; **Hospital:** Montefiore Med Ctr-Einstein Campus, NY (page 100), Montefiore Med Ctr-Moses Campus, NY (page 100); **Address:** 1515 Blondell Ave, Ste 220, Bronx, NY 10461-2601; **Phone:** 718-405-8323; **Board Cert:** Internal Medicine 1979; Hematology 1982; **Med School:** Mount Sinai Sch Med 1974; **Resid:** Internal Medicine, Montefiore Hosp Med Ctr 1979; **Fellow:** Tropical Medicine, London Sch Hygiene/Trop Med 1977; Hematology, Montefiore Hosp Med Ctr 1981; **Fac Appt:** Prof Med, Albert Einstein Coll Med

Landau, Leon MD (Hem) - **Hospital:** Montefiore Med Ctr-Moses Campus, NY (page 100), Comm Hosp - Dobbs Ferry; **Address:** 75 E Gun Hill Rd, Bronx, NY 10467-2103; **Phone:** 718-655-3932; **Board Cert:** Internal Medicine 1977; Hematology 1978; Medical Oncology 1981; **Med School:** Albert Einstein Coll Med 1971; **Resid:** Internal Medicine, Montefiore Med Ctr 1973; Internal Medicine, Metropolitan Hosp Ctr 1974; **Fellow:** Hematology, Montefiore Med Ctr 1978; Medical Oncology, Montefiore Med Ctr 1978; **Fac Appt:** Asst Prof Med, Albert Einstein Coll Med

Infectious Disease

Berger, Judith MD (Inf) - **Spec Exp:** AIDS/HIV; Travel Medicine; **Hospital:** St. Barnabas Hosp - Bronx; **Address:** St Barnabas Hosp, Dept Med, 4422 Third Ave, Bronx, NY 10457; **Phone:** 718-960-6205; **Board Cert:** Internal Medicine 1984; Infectious Disease 1986; **Med School:** Mount Sinai Sch Med 1980; **Resid:** Internal Medicine, Brookdale Hosp 1984; **Fellow:** Infectious Disease, Downstate Med Ctr 1986; **Fac Appt:** Asst Clin Prof Med, Cornell Univ-Weill Med Coll

Corpuz, Marilou MD (Inf) - **Spec Exp:** Hospital Acquired Infections; **Hospital:** Montefiore Med Ctr-Wakefield Campus, NY (page 100); **Address:** Montefiore North Division, 4234 Bronx Blvd, Bronx, NY 10466-2604; **Phone:** 347-341-4340; **Board Cert:** Internal Medicine 1988; Infectious Disease 2002; **Med School:** Philippines 1985; **Resid:** Internal Medicine, Griffin Hosp 1988; **Fellow:** Infectious Disease, LI Jewish Med Ctr 1991; **Fac Appt:** Assoc Prof Med, NY Med Coll

Robbins, Noah MD (Inf) - **Spec Exp:** AIDS/HIV; Sexually Transmitted Diseases; **Hospital:** Montefiore Med Ctr-Moses Campus, NY (page 100); **Address:** 3400 Bainbridge Ave Fl 8, Bronx, NY 10467-2490; **Phone:** 718-920-8888; **Board Cert:** Internal Medicine 1974; Infectious Disease 1980; **Med School:** McGill Univ 1969; **Resid:** Internal Medicine, Albany Med Ctr 1975; **Fellow:** Infectious Disease, Montefiore Hosp Med Ctr 1976; **Fac Appt:** Clin Prof Med, Albert Einstein Coll Med

Saltzman, Simone MD (Inf) - **Hospital:** Montefiore Med Ctr-Einstein Campus, NY (page 100); **Address:** 1575 Blondell Ave, Ste 200, Bronx, NY 10461-1915; **Phone:** 866-633-8255; **Board Cert:** Internal Medicine 1977; Infectious Disease 1980; **Med School:** SUNY Downstate 1973; **Resid:** Internal Medicine, Montefiore Hosp Med Ctr 1976; **Fellow:** Infectious Disease, Montefiore Hosp Med Ctr 1979; **Fac Appt:** Asst Prof Med, Albert Einstein Coll Med

Tanowitz, Herbert B MD (Inf) - **Spec Exp:** Parasitic Infections; Tropical Diseases; **Hospital:** Montefiore Med Ctr-Einstein Campus, NY (page 100), Jacobi Med Ctr; **Address:** 1300 Morris Park Ave Bldg F - rm 504, Bronx, NY 10461-1926; **Phone:** 718-430-3342; **Board Cert:** Internal Medicine 1974; Infectious Disease 1976; **Med School:** Albert Einstein Coll Med 1967; **Resid:** Internal Medicine, Lincoln Hosp 1971; **Fellow:** Infectious Disease, Albert Einstein 1973; **Fac Appt:** Prof Med, Albert Einstein Coll Med

Telzak, Edward E MD (Inf) - **Spec Exp:** AIDS/HIV; Tuberculosis; Infections-Opportunistic; **Hospital:** Bronx Lebanon Hosp Ctr; **Address:** 1650 Selwyn Ave, Milstein Bldg, Ste 10C, Bronx, NY 10457-7606; **Phone:** 718-960-1212; **Board Cert:** Internal Medicine 1983; Infectious Disease 1988; **Med School:** Albert Einstein Coll Med 1980; **Resid:** Internal Medicine, New England Med Ctr 1983; **Fellow:** Infectious Disease, Brigham & Women's Hosp 1985; Tropical Medicine, New England Med Ctr 1986; **Fac Appt:** Prof Med, Albert Einstein Coll Med

Weiss, Louis MD (Inf) - **Spec Exp:** Parasitic Infections; AIDS/HIV; **Hospital:** Montefiore Med Ctr-Einstein Campus, NY (page 100); **Address:** 1575 Blondell Ave, Ste 200, Bronx, NY 10461; **Phone:** 718-405-8311; **Board Cert:** Internal Medicine 1985; Infectious Disease 1988; **Med School:** Johns Hopkins Univ 1982; **Resid:** Internal Medicine, Univ Chicago 1985; **Fellow:** Infectious Disease, Montefiore Med Ctr 1989; **Fac Appt:** Prof Med, Albert Einstein Coll Med

Internal Medicine

Berman, Daniel S MD (IM) *PCP* - **Spec Exp:** Infectious Disease; **Hospital:** NY Westchester Sq Med Ctr; **Address:** 2475 St Raymonds Ave, Bronx, NY 10461; **Phone:** 914-524-8138; **Board Cert:** Internal Medicine 1985; Infectious Disease 1988; **Med School:** NYU Sch Med 1982; **Resid:** Internal Medicine, NYU Med Ctr 1985; **Fellow:** Infectious Disease, NYU Med Ctr 1989

Buatti, Elizabeth MD (IM) *PCP* - **Hospital:** Montefiore Med Ctr-Moses Campus, NY (page 100); **Address:** 3444 Kossuth, Bronx, NY 10467; **Phone:** 718-920-5903; **Board Cert:** Internal Medicine 1981; **Med School:** Georgetown Univ 1978; **Resid:** Internal Medicine, St Vincent's Hosp 1981; **Fac Appt:** Asst Prof Med, Albert Einstein Coll Med

Ernst, Jerome MD (IM) *PCP* - **Spec Exp:** AIDS/HIV; **Hospital:** Bronx Lebanon Hosp Ctr; **Address:** BronxCare-Avalon Med Ctr, 1770 Grand Concourse Fl 2, Bronx, NY 10457; **Phone:** 718-518-5581; **Board Cert:** Internal Medicine 1978; Pulmonary Disease 1982; **Med School:** Israel 1969; **Resid:** Internal Medicine, Montefiore Med Ctr 1972; **Fellow:** Pulmonary Disease, Montefiore Med Ctr 1977; **Fac Appt:** Assoc Prof Med, Albert Einstein Coll Med

Fojas, Antonio MD (IM) *PCP* - **Hospital:** Montefiore Med Ctr-Wakefield Campus, NY (page 100); **Address:** 4234 Bronx Blvd, Bronx, NY 10466; **Phone:** 347-341-4300; **Board Cert:** Internal Medicine 2003; **Med School:** Philippines 1984; **Resid:** Internal Medicine, Our Lady of Mercy Med Ctr 1987; **Fellow:** Internal Medicine, Our Lady of Mercy Med Ctr 1988; **Fac Appt:** Asst Prof Med, NY Med Coll

Mojtabai, Shaparak MD (IM) *PCP* - **Spec Exp:** Women's Health-Geriatric; Diabetes; Hypertension; **Hospital:** St. Barnabas Hosp - Bronx; **Address:** 2016 Bronxdale Ave, Ste 302, Bronx Park Medical Pavilion, Bronx, NY 10462-3389; **Phone:** 718-822-1515; **Board Cert:** Internal Medicine 1989; Geriatric Medicine 2004; **Med School:** Iran 1982; **Resid:** Internal Medicine, St Barnabas Hosp-Cornell 1988; **Fellow:** Internal Medicine, St Barnabas Hosp-Cornell 1989

Sander Jr, Norbert W MD (IM) *PCP* - **Spec Exp:** Preventive Medicine; Sports Medicine; **Hospital:** Sound Shore Med Ctr - Westchester; **Address:** 340 City Island Ave, Bronx, NY 10464; **Phone:** 718-885-0333; **Board Cert:** Internal Medicine 1981; **Med School:** Albert Einstein Coll Med 1971; **Resid:** Internal Medicine, Metropolitan Hosp Ctr 1974

Selwyn, Peter MD (IM) - **Spec Exp:** AIDS/HIV; Palliative Care; Addiction/Substance Abuse; **Hospital:** Montefiore Med Ctr-Moses Campus, NY (page 100); **Address:** Montfiore Family Hlth Ctr, 360 E 193rd St Fl 2, Bronx, NY 10458; **Phone:** 718-933-2400; **Board Cert:** Family Medicine 2005; Hospice & Palliative Medicine 2006; **Med School:** Harvard Med Sch 1981; **Resid:** Family Medicine, Montefiore Med Ctr 1984; **Fac Appt:** Prof Med, Albert Einstein Coll Med

Swiderski, Deborah M MD (IM) *PCP* - **Hospital:** Montefiore Med Ctr-Moses Campus, NY (page 100); **Address:** MMG-Comprehensive Heath Care Ctr, 305 E 161 St, Bronx, NY 10451; **Phone:** 718-579-2500; **Board Cert:** Internal Medicine 1986; **Med School:** Columbia P&S 1980; **Resid:** Internal Medicine, Montefiore Hosp 1983; **Fac Appt:** Asst Prof Med, Albert Einstein Coll Med

Teffera, Fassil MD (IM) *PCP* - **Spec Exp:** Diabetes; Hypertension; Preventive Medicine; **Hospital:** Montefiore Med Ctr-Wakefield Campus, NY (page 100), Montefiore Med Ctr-Moses Campus, NY (page 100); **Address:** 2426 Eastchester Rd, Ste 101, Bronx, NY 10469; **Phone:** 718-708-4726; **Board Cert:** Internal Medicine 2003; **Med School:** Ethiopia 1976; **Resid:** Internal Medicine, Our Lady of Mercy Med Ctr 1993; **Fac Appt:** Asst Clin Prof Med, NY Med Coll

Walker, Yvette MD (IM) *PCP* - **Spec Exp:** Diabetes; Hypertension; **Address:** Morris Heights Hlth Ctr, 85 W Burnside Ave, Bronx, NY 10453; **Phone:** 718-716-4400; **Board Cert:** Internal Medicine 1986; **Med School:** SUNY Downstate 1983; **Resid:** Internal Medicine, Kings Co Hosp 1986; **Fac Appt:** Asst Prof Med, Albert Einstein Coll Med

Maternal & Fetal Medicine

Chazotte, Cynthia MD (MF) - **Spec Exp:** Pregnancy-High Risk; Asthma in Pregnancy; **Hospital:** Montefiore Med Ctr-Einstein Campus, NY (page 100); **Address:** 1695 Eastchester Rd, Ste L2, Bronx, NY 10461; **Phone:** 718-405-8200; **Board Cert:** Obstetrics & Gynecology 2011; Maternal & Fetal Medicine 2011; **Med School:** NY Med Coll 1981; **Resid:** Obstetrics & Gynecology, Montefiore Med Ctr 1985; **Fellow:** Maternal & Fetal Medicine, Montefiore Med Ctr 1987; **Fac Appt:** Prof ObG, Albert Einstein Coll Med

Henderson, Cassandra E MD (MF) - **Spec Exp:** Pregnancy-High Risk; Diabetes in Pregnancy; **Hospital:** Montefiore Med Ctr-Wakefield Campus, NY (page 100); **Address:** 2604 Third Ave, Bronx, NY 10454; **Phone:** 718-920-9600; **Board Cert:** Obstetrics & Gynecology 2011; Maternal & Fetal Medicine 2011; **Med School:** Loyola Univ-Stritch Sch Med 1980; **Resid:** Obstetrics & Gynecology, Univ Chicago Hosp 1984; **Fellow:** Maternal & Fetal Medicine, Montefiore Med Ctr-Einstein Div 1986; **Fac Appt:** Assoc Prof ObG, Albert Einstein Coll Med

Medical Oncology

Bruckner, Howard W MD (Onc) - **Spec Exp:** Pancreatic Cancer; **Hospital:** NY Downtown Hosp; **Address:** 2330 Eastchester Rd, Bronx, NY 10469; **Phone:** 718-732-4050; **Board Cert:** Internal Medicine 1972; Medical Oncology 1973; **Med School:** Albert Einstein Coll Med 1966; **Resid:** Internal Medicine, Montefiore/Weiler-Einstein Div 1970; **Fellow:** Medical Oncology, Yale-New Haven Hosp 1971

Camacho, Fernando J MD (Onc) - **Spec Exp:** Breast Cancer; Lymphoma; Bladder Cancer; **Hospital:** Montefiore Med Ctr-Moses Campus, NY (page 100), Saint Joseph's Med Ctr - Yonkers; **Address:** 60 E 208th St, Bronx, NY 10467-2702; **Phone:** 718-405-1700; **Board Cert:** Internal Medicine 1976; Hematology 1978; Medical Oncology 1981; **Med School:** SUNY Buffalo 1973; **Resid:** Internal Medicine, Montefiore Med Ctr 1976; Hematology, Montefiore Med Ctr 1977; **Fellow:** Medical Oncology, Sloan-Kettering Cancer Ctr 1979; **Fac Appt:** Asst Clin Prof Med, Albert Einstein Coll Med

Fuks, Joachim MD (Onc) - **Spec Exp:** Lung Cancer; Breast Cancer; Colon Cancer; **Hospital:** NY Westchester Sq Med Ctr, Montefiore Med Ctr-Einstein Campus, NY (page 100); **Address:** 1578 Williamsbridge Rd Fl 2, Bronx, NY 10461-6265; **Phone:** 718-931-2290; **Board Cert:** Internal Medicine 1981; Medical Oncology 1983; **Med School:** Spain 1975; **Resid:** Internal Medicine, Mt Sinai Hosp 1978; **Fellow:** Medical Oncology, Natl Cancer Ctr 1981

Perez-Soler, Roman MD (Onc) - **Spec Exp:** Lung Cancer; Mesothelioma; Drug Development; **Hospital:** Montefiore Med Ctr-Einstein Campus, NY (page 100), Montefiore Med Ctr-Moses Campus, NY (page 100); **Address:** Montefiore Med Ctr, Dept Oncology, 111 E 210th St, Hoffheimer Main-Rm 100, Bronx, NY 10467; **Phone:** 718-920-4001; **Board Cert:** Internal Medicine 1987; Medical Oncology 1989; **Med School:** Spain 1977; **Resid:** Internal Medicine, Univ Autonoma Med Ctr 1982; **Fellow:** Medical Oncology, MD Anderson Hosp 1985; **Fac Appt:** Prof Med, Albert Einstein Coll Med

Ramirez, Mark Anthony MD (Onc) - **Spec Exp:** Lymphoma, Non-Hodgkin's; Breast Cancer; Lung Cancer; **Hospital:** Montefiore Med Ctr-Moses Campus, NY (page 100), Saint Joseph's Med Ctr - Yonkers; **Address:** 60 E 208th St, Bronx, NY 10467; **Phone:** 718-405-1700; **Board Cert:** Internal Medicine 1985; Medical Oncology 1989; Hematology 2005; **Med School:** Cornell Univ-Weill Med Coll 1982; **Resid:** Internal Medicine, Montefiore Med Ctr 1985; **Fellow:** Hematology & Oncology, Montefiore Med Ctr 1988; **Fac Appt:** Asst Clin Prof Med, Albert Einstein Coll Med

Sparano, Joseph A MD (Onc) - **Spec Exp:** Breast Cancer; Lymphoma; **Hospital:** Montefiore Med Ctr-Einstein Campus, NY (page 100); **Address:** 1825 Eastchester Rd Fl 2 - Ste 2S-48, Bronx, NY 10461; **Phone:** 718-904-2555; **Board Cert:** Internal Medicine 1986; Medical Oncology 1989; **Med School:** NY Med Coll 1982; **Resid:** Internal Medicine, St Vincents Hosp 1986; **Fellow:** Medical Oncology, Montefiore Med Ctr 1988; **Fac Appt:** Prof Med, Albert Einstein Coll Med

Vogl, Steven E MD (Onc) - **Spec Exp:** Breast Cancer; Lung Cancer; **Hospital:** Montefiore Med Ctr-Einstein Campus, NY (page 100), White Plains Hosp (page 615); **Address:** 2220 Tiemann Ave, Bronx, NY 10469; **Phone:** 718-519-7774; **Board Cert:** Internal Medicine 1975; Medical Oncology 1975; **Med School:** Cornell Univ-Weill Med Coll 1970; **Resid:** Internal Medicine, Jacobi Med Ctr 1972; **Fellow:** Medical Oncology, Mt Sinai Med Ctr 1975

Neonatal-Perinatal Medicine

Campbell, Deborah MD (NP) - **Spec Exp:** Prematurity/Low Birth Weight Infants; Neurodevelopmental Disabilities; **Hospital:** Montefiore Med Ctr-Einstein Campus, NY (page 100); **Address:** 1825 Eastchester Rd, Bronx, NY 10461-2301; **Phone:** 718-904-4105; **Board Cert:** Pediatrics 1983; Neonatal-Perinatal Medicine 1985; **Med School:** SUNY Buffalo 1978; **Resid:** Pediatrics, Montefiore Med Ctr 1981; **Fellow:** Neonatal-Perinatal Medicine, Montefiore Med Ctr 1983; **Fac Appt:** Clin Prof Ped, Albert Einstein Coll Med

Nephrology

Charytan, Chaim MD (Nep) - **Spec Exp:** Hypertension; Diabetic Kidney Disease; Kidney Stones; Nephrotic Syndrome; **Hospital:** NY Hosp Queens (page 206); **Address:** 1874 Pelham Pkwy South, Bronx, NY 10461-3733; **Phone:** 718-931-5800; **Board Cert:** Internal Medicine 1969; Nephrology 1974; **Med School:** Albert Einstein Coll Med 1964; **Resid:** Internal Medicine, Bronx Municipal Hosp 1967; **Fellow:** Nephrology, Boston Univ Hosp 1968; **Fac Appt:** Clin Prof Med, Cornell Univ-Weill Med Coll

Coco, Maria MD (Nep) - **Spec Exp:** Hypertension; Kidney Disease; **Hospital:** Montefiore Med Ctr-Moses Campus, NY (page 100); **Address:** 111 E 210th St, Bronx, NY 10467-2401; **Phone:** 718-920-4136; **Board Cert:** Internal Medicine 1985; Nephrology 1988; **Med School:** Italy 1982; **Resid:** Internal Medicine, Bronx Lebanon Hosp 1985; **Fellow:** Nephrology, Montefiore Hosp Med Ctr 1988; **Fac Appt:** Prof Med, Albert Einstein Coll Med

Croll, James MD (Nep) - **Spec Exp:** Dialysis Care; Hypertension; Kidney Failure-Chronic; **Hospital:** St. Barnabas Hosp - Bronx; **Address:** 4422 3rd Ave, Bronx, NY 10457; **Phone:** 718-960-6295; **Board Cert:** Internal Medicine 1978; Nephrology 1982; **Med School:** Belgium 1975; **Resid:** Internal Medicine, Genesee Hosp 1978; **Fellow:** Nephrology, VA Med Ctr 1981

Gorkin, Janet U MD (Nep) - **Spec Exp:** Hypertension; Diabetic Kidney Disease; Kidney Failure; **Hospital:** Montefiore Med Ctr-Moses Campus, NY (page 100); **Address:** 3327 Bainbridge Ave, Bronx, NY 10467; **Phone:** 718-881-5100; **Board Cert:** Internal Medicine 1976; Nephrology 1980; **Med School:** Mount Sinai Sch Med 1973; **Resid:** Internal Medicine, Mt Sinai Hosp 1976; **Fellow:** Nephrology, Mt Sinai Hosp 1978; **Fac Appt:** Prof Med, Albert Einstein Coll Med

Laitman, Robert MD (Nep) - **Spec Exp:** Diabetic Kidney Disease; Cholesterol/Lipid Disorders; **Hospital:** Montefiore Med Ctr-Einstein Campus, NY (page 100); **Address:** 2510 Westchester Ave, Ste 106, Bronx, NY 10461-2606; **Phone:** 718-518-1276; **Board Cert:** Internal Medicine 1986; Nephrology 1988; Geriatric Medicine 2010; **Med School:** Washington Univ, St Louis 1983; **Resid:** Internal Medicine, Jacobi Med Ctr 1986; **Fellow:** Nephrology, Montefiore Hosp Med Ctr 1988

Lynn, Robert I MD (Nep) - **Spec Exp:** Hypertension; Dialysis Care; **Hospital:** Montefiore Med Ctr-Einstein Campus, NY (page 100); **Address:** 1200 Waters Pl, Ste M104, Bronx, NY 10461; **Phone:** 718-794-1200; **Board Cert:** Internal Medicine 1977; Nephrology 1980; **Med School:** Columbia P&S 1974; **Resid:** Internal Medicine, Columbia-Presby Med Ctr 1977; **Fellow:** Nephrology, Yale-New Haven Hosp 1979; **Fac Appt:** Assoc Prof Med, Albert Einstein Coll Med

Uday, Kalpana MD (Nep) - **Spec Exp:** Hypertension; **Hospital:** Bronx Lebanon Hosp Ctr; **Address:** 1650 Grand Concourse, Fl 2, Bronx, NY 10457-7606; **Phone:** 718-992-7669; **Board Cert:** Internal Medicine 1989; Nephrology 2003; **Med School:** India 1980; **Resid:** Internal Medicine, Jamaica Med Ctr 1989; **Fellow:** Nephrology, Montefiore Med Ctr 1991; **Fac Appt:** Asst Prof Med, Albert Einstein Coll Med

Yoo, Jinil MD (Nep) - **Spec Exp:** Kidney Disease; Hypertension; Diabetes; **Hospital:** Montefiore Med Ctr-Wakefield Campus, NY (page 100); **Address:** 600 E 233rd St, Bronx, NY 10466; **Phone:** 347-341-4340; **Board Cert:** Internal Medicine 1974; Nephrology 1976; **Med School:** South Korea 1967; **Resid:** Internal Medicine, Joslin Diabetes Center 1973; Internal Medicine, Metropolitan Hosp Ctr 1974; **Fellow:** Nephrology, NY Med Coll/Metro Hosp 1976; **Fac Appt:** Prof Med, NY Med Coll

Neurological Surgery

Flamm, Eugene S MD (NS) - **Spec Exp:** Aneurysm-Cerebral; Brain Tumors; Cerebrovascular Neurosurgery; **Hospital:** Montefiore Med Ctr-Moses Campus, NY (page 100); **Address:** 3316 Rochambeau Ave, Bronx, NY 10467-2841; **Phone:** 718-920-2339; **Board Cert:** Neurological Surgery 1973; **Med School:** SUNY Buffalo 1962; **Resid:** Surgery, New York Hosp 1964; Neurological Surgery, NYU Med Ctr 1970; **Fellow:** Neurological Surgery, Univ Zurich 1971; **Fac Appt:** Prof NS, Albert Einstein Coll Med

LaSala, Patrick MD (NS) - **Spec Exp:** Brain Tumors; Epilepsy; Stereotactic Radiosurgery; **Hospital:** Montefiore Med Ctr-Moses Campus, NY (page 100); **Address:** Dept Neurosurgery, 3316 Rochambeau Ave, Bronx, NY 10467-2803; **Phone:** 718-920-7466; **Board Cert:** Neurological Surgery 1991; **Med School:** Columbia P&S 1980; **Resid:** Neurological Surgery, Columbia-Presby Med Ctr 1987; **Fac Appt:** Assoc Prof NS, Albert Einstein Coll Med

Neurology

Cohen, Joel S MD (N) - **Spec Exp:** Epilepsy; Headache; Stroke; Parkinson's Disease; **Hospital:** Montefiore Med Ctr-Moses Campus, NY (page 100), Montefiore Med Ctr-Einstein Campus, NY (page 100); **Address:** 1610 Williamsbridge Rd Fl 2, Bronx, NY 10461-2601; **Phone:** 718-597-8000; **Board Cert:** Neurology 1992; **Med School:** Albert Einstein Coll Med 1983; **Resid:** Neurology, Montefiore Med Ctr 1987; **Fellow:** Neurology, Montefiore Med Ctr 1988; **Fac Appt:** Assoc Prof N, Albert Einstein Coll Med

Freddo, Lorenza MD (N) - **Spec Exp:** Pain Management; Multiple Sclerosis; Peripheral Neuropathy; **Hospital:** St. Barnabas Hosp - Bronx; **Address:** Belmont Medical Associates, 2371 Arthur Ave, Bronx, NY 10458; **Phone:** 718-364-6199; **Board Cert:** Neurology 1992; **Med School:** Italy 1980; **Resid:** Neurology, Italy 1984; Neurology, Columbia Presby Hosp 1990; **Fellow:** Columbia Presby Hosp 1986

Grenell, Steven L MD (N) - **Spec Exp:** Pain Management; Headache; **Hospital:** Montefiore Med Ctr-Moses Campus, NY (page 100), Lawrence Hosp Ctr; **Address:** 3975 Sedgewick Ave, Ste 1-F, Bronx, NY 10463; **Phone:** 718-796-6055; **Board Cert:** Neurology 1989; **Med School:** UMDNJ-Rutgers Med Sch 1977; **Resid:** Internal Medicine, Montefiore Hosp 1979; Neurology, Montefiore Hosp 1982; **Fellow:** Internal Medicine, Montefiore Hosp 1982; **Fac Appt:** Asst Prof N, Albert Einstein Coll Med

Herskovitz, Steven MD (N) - **Spec Exp:** Electromyography; Neuromuscular Disorders; Peripheral Neuropathy; **Hospital:** Montefiore Med Ctr-Moses Campus, NY (page 100); **Address:** 111 E 210th St, Bronx, NY 10467-2401; **Phone:** 718-920-4930; **Board Cert:** Internal Medicine 1983; Neurology 1987; Neuromuscular Medicine 2008; **Med School:** Cornell Univ-Weill Med Coll 1980; **Resid:** Internal Medicine, Montefiore Med Ctr 1983; Neurology, Montefiore Med Ctr 1986; **Fellow:** Electromyography, Montefiore Med Ctr 1987; **Fac Appt:** Prof N, Albert Einstein Coll Med

Kaufman, David Myland MD (N) - **Spec Exp:** Movement Disorders; **Hospital:** Montefiore Med Ctr-Moses Campus, NY (page 100); **Address:** 3400 Bainbridge Ave, Main Fl, Bronx, NY 10467; **Phone:** 718-920-4730; **Board Cert:** Internal Medicine 1972; Neurology 1976; **Med School:** Univ Chicago-Pritzker Sch Med 1968; **Resid:** Internal Medicine, Montefiore Med Ctr 1971; Neurology, Montefiore Med Ctr 1974; **Fac Appt:** Prof N, Albert Einstein Coll Med

Lipton, Richard MD (N) - **Spec Exp:** Headache; Clinical Trials; **Hospital:** Montefiore Med Ctr-Einstein Campus, NY (page 100); **Address:** Montefiore Headache Ctr, 1575 Blondell Ave, Ste 225, Bronx, NY 10461-2662; **Phone:** 718-405-8360; **Board Cert:** Neurology 1985; **Med School:** Univ Chicago-Pritzker Sch Med 1980; **Resid:** Neurology, Montefiore Med Ctr 1984; **Fellow:** Neurological Physiology, Montefiore Med Ctr 1985; NeuroEpidemiology, Columbia Univ 1990; **Fac Appt:** Prof N, Albert Einstein Coll Med

Sparr, Steven MD (N) - **Hospital:** Montefiore Med Ctr-Moses Campus, NY (page 100); **Address:** Montefiore Med Ctr, 111 E 210th St, Bronx, NY 10467; **Phone:** 718-920-6402; **Board Cert:** Internal Medicine 1984; Neurology 1987; Vascular Neurology 2008; **Med School:** SUNY Buffalo 1980; **Resid:** Internal Medicine, Boston City Hosp 1983; Neurology, Albert Einstein 1986; **Fellow:** Neurological Rehabilitation, Burke Rehabilitation Hosp 1987; **Fac Appt:** Assoc Prof N, Albert Einstein Coll Med

Swerdlow, Michael L MD (N) - **Spec Exp:** Myasthenia Gravis; Spinal Disorders; Multiple Sclerosis; **Hospital:** Montefiore Med Ctr-Moses Campus, NY (page 100); **Address:** 3400 Bainbridge Ave, Bronx, NY 10467-2401; **Phone:** 718-920-4178; **Board Cert:** Neurology 1975; **Med School:** Univ Pennsylvania 1967; **Resid:** Internal Medicine, Mount Sinai Hosp 1969; Neurology, Montefiore Med Ctr 1972; **Fellow:** Neurology, Natl Inst Hlth 1974; **Fac Appt:** Prof N, Albert Einstein Coll Med

Neuroradiology

Bello, Jacqueline A MD (NRad) - **Spec Exp:** Aneurysm-Cerebral; Pain-Back; **Hospital:** Montefiore Med Ctr-Moses Campus, NY (page 100); **Address:** Montefiore Med Ctr, 111 E 210th St, Red Zone, Bronx, NY 10467; **Phone:** 718-920-4030; **Board Cert:** Diagnostic Radiology 1984; Neuroradiology 2010; **Med School:** Columbia P&S 1980; **Resid:** Diagnostic Radiology, Columbia-PresbyMed Ctr 1984; **Fellow:** Neuroradiology, Neuro Inst/Columbia-Presby Med Ctr 1986; **Fac Appt:** Prof Rad, Albert Einstein Coll Med

Nuclear Medicine

Freeman, Leonard M MD (NuM) - **Spec Exp:** Nuclear Oncology; Gastrointestinal Disorders; PET Imaging; CT Scan; **Hospital:** Montefiore Med Ctr-Moses Campus, NY (page 100); **Address:** 111 E 210th St Foreman Bldg Fl 4, Bronx, NY 10467-2401; **Phone:** 718-920-6060; **Board Cert:** Diagnostic Radiology 1966; Nuclear Medicine 1972; Nuclear Radiology 1974; **Med School:** Ros Franklin Univ/Chicago Med Sch 1961; **Resid:** Diagnostic Radiology, Bronx Municipal Hosp 1965; **Fac Appt:** Prof NuM, Albert Einstein Coll Med

Milstein, David M MD (NuM) - **Hospital:** Montefiore Med Ctr-Einstein Campus, NY (page 100), Montefiore Med Ctr-Moses Campus, NY (page 100); **Address:** Montefiore Medical Park, 1695A Eastchester Rd, Bronx, NY 10461; **Phone:** 718-405-8455; **Board Cert:** Nuclear Medicine 1972; Diagnostic Radiology 1972; **Med School:** Albert Einstein Coll Med 1967; **Resid:** Diagnostic Radiology, Bronx Muni Hosp Ctr 1972; **Fellow:** Diagnostic Radiology, Bronx Muni Hosp Ctr 1972; **Fac Appt:** Prof NuM, Albert Einstein Coll Med

Obstetrics & Gynecology

Levy, Judith MD (ObG) *PCP* - **Hospital:** Montefiore Med Ctr-Einstein Campus, NY (page 100); **Address:** 1695 Eastchester Rd, Ste L2, Bronx, NY 10461; **Phone:** 718-405-8200; **Board Cert:** Obstetrics & Gynecology 2011; **Med School:** Albert Einstein Coll Med 1981; **Resid:** Obstetrics & Gynecology, Bronx Muni Hosp 1985; **Fac Appt:** Asst Prof ObG, Albert Einstein Coll Med

Reilly, Kevin D MD (ObG) *PCP* - **Spec Exp:** Menopause Problems; **Hospital:** Montefiore Med Ctr-Wakefield Campus, NY (page 100); **Address:** 600 E 233rd St, Bronx, NY 10466-2604; **Phone:** 718-920-9648; **Board Cert:** Obstetrics & Gynecology 1976; **Med School:** Univ Mich Med Sch 1969; **Resid:** Obstetrics & Gynecology, St Vincent's Hosp & Med Ctr 1974; **Fac Appt:** Assoc Prof ObG, NY Med Coll

Young, Constance MD (ObG) - **Spec Exp:** Gynecology Only; Pelvic Surgery; Menopause Problems; **Hospital:** Jacobi Med Ctr; **Address:** Jacobi Med Ctr, 1400 Pelham Pkwy S Bldg 1 - rm 3W6, Bronx, NY 10461; **Phone:** 718-918-5700; **Board Cert:** Obstetrics & Gynecology 2012; **Med School:** Cornell Univ-Weill Med Coll 1983; **Resid:** Obstetrics & Gynecology, North Shore Univ Hosp 1987

Ophthalmology

Chess, Jeremy MD (Oph) - **Spec Exp:** Retina/Vitreous Surgery; **Hospital:** Montefiore Med Ctr-Moses Campus, NY (page 100); **Address:** 2221 Boston Rd, Bronx, NY 10467; **Phone:** 718-798-3030; **Board Cert:** Ophthalmology 1977; **Med School:** Boston Univ 1970; **Resid:** Ophthalmology, Boston Univ Med Ctr 1974; **Fellow:** Vitreoretinal Surgery, Boston Univ Med Ctr 1983; **Fac Appt:** Assoc Clin Prof Oph, Albert Einstein Coll Med

Hayworth, Robin S MD (Oph) - **Spec Exp:** Cataract Surgery; Glaucoma; **Hospital:** Lenox Hill Hosp (Manh Eye, Ear & Throat Hosp) (page 106), Montefiore Med Ctr-Einstein Campus, NY (page 100); **Address:** 787 Lydig Ave, Bronx, NY 10462-2144; **Phone:** 718-863-7774; **Board Cert:** Ophthalmology 1985; **Med School:** Cornell Univ-Weill Med Coll 1978; **Resid:** Surgery, NY Hosp 1980; Ophthalmology, Manhattan EET Hosp 1983

Mayers, Martin MD (Oph) - **Spec Exp:** Cataract Surgery; Cornea Transplant; Eye Infections; **Hospital:** Bronx Lebanon Hosp Ctr, Montefiore Med Ctr-Wakefield Campus, NY (page 100); **Address:** Bronx-Lebanon Hosp Ctr, 1650 Grand Concourse, Milstein Bldg - rm 1C, Bronx, NY 10456; **Phone:** 718-518-8008; **Board Cert:** Ophthalmology 1985; **Med School:** Albert Einstein Coll Med 1979; **Resid:** Ophthalmology, SUNY Downstate Med Ctr 1983; **Fellow:** Cornea, Proctor Fdn-UCSF 1984; **Fac Appt:** Assoc Prof Oph, Albert Einstein Coll Med

Medow, Norman MD (Oph) - **Spec Exp:** Cataract-Pediatric; Glaucoma-Pediatric; Corneal Disease-Pediatric; **Hospital:** Montefiore Med Ctr-Moses Campus, NY (page 100); **Address:** Montefiore Hosp Ctr, Dept Ophthalmology, 3400 Bainbridge Ave, Bronx, NY 10467; **Phone:** 718-920-2020; **Board Cert:** Ophthalmology 1975; **Med School:** SUNY Hlth Sci Ctr 1966; **Resid:** Ophthalmology, Manhattan EE&T Hosp 1972; **Fellow:** Cataract/Lens Implant Surgery, Charles Kelman, MD 1973; **Fac Appt:** Assoc Clin Prof Oph, Cornell Univ-Weill Med Coll

Rosenbaum, Pearl S MD (Oph) - **Spec Exp:** Cataract Surgery; Glaucoma; Diabetic Eye Disease; Ophthalmic Pathology; **Hospital:** Montefiore Med Ctr-Moses Campus, NY (page 100), Bronx Lebanon Hosp Ctr; **Address:** 1250 Waters Pl, Ste 502, Bronx, NY 10461; **Phone:** 718-518-0060; **Board Cert:** Ophthalmology 1988; **Med School:** Albert Einstein Coll Med 1982; **Resid:** Ophthalmology, Albert Einstein 1986; **Fellow:** Ophthalmic Pathology, Baylor Coll of Med 1988; Ophthalmic Oncololgy, Baylor Coll of Med 1988; **Fac Appt:** Prof Oph, Albert Einstein Coll Med

Slamovits, Thomas L MD (Oph) - **Spec Exp:** Neuro-Ophthalmology; Optic Nerve Disorders; Vision Loss-Unexplained Loss; Diabetic Eye Disease/Retinopathy; **Hospital:** Montefiore Med Ctr-Moses Campus, NY (page 100), Hackensack Univ Med Ctr (page 96); **Address:** 1250 Pelham Pkwy S, Bronx, NY 10461; **Phone:** 718-794-1500; **Board Cert:** Ophthalmology 1980; **Med School:** Ohio State Univ 1975; **Resid:** Ophthalmology, Univ Pitts Eye & Ear 1979; **Fellow:** Neuro-Ophthalmology, Washington Univ-Barnes Hosp 1980; **Fac Appt:** Clin Prof Oph, Albert Einstein Coll Med

Tiwari, Ram MD (Oph) - **Spec Exp:** Diabetic Eye Disease/Retinopathy; Glaucoma; Cataract Surgery; **Hospital:** Montefiore Med Ctr-Wakefield Campus, NY (page 100), NY-Presby/Columbia Univ Med Ctr, NY (page 104); **Address:** 1739 Williamsbridge Rd, Bronx, NY 10461-6203; **Phone:** 718-824-1560; **Board Cert:** Ophthalmology 1977; **Med School:** India 1966; **Resid:** Ophthalmology, Maulana Azad Med Coll 1971; **Fellow:** Retina, Columbia-Presby Med Ctr 1978; **Fac Appt:** Asst Clin Prof Oph, Columbia P&S

Wolf, Kenneth J MD (Oph) - **Spec Exp:** Diabetic Eye Disease/Retinopathy; Cataract Surgery; **Address:** 1180 Morris Park Ave Fl 2, Bronx, NY 10461-1925; **Phone:** 718-892-6110; **Board Cert:** Ophthalmology 1980; **Med School:** Albert Einstein Coll Med 1974; **Resid:** Ophthalmology, Montefiore Hosp Med Ctr 1978; **Fac Appt:** Asst Clin Prof Oph, Albert Einstein Coll Med

Orthopaedic Surgery

Cobelli, Neil MD (OrS) - **Spec Exp:** Knee Replacement; Hip Replacement; **Hospital:** Montefiore Med Ctr-Einstein Campus, NY (page 100); **Address:** 1250 Waters Pl Fl 11, Bronx, NY 10461; **Phone:** 718-920-2060; **Board Cert:** Orthopaedic Surgery 1985; **Med School:** Dartmouth Med Sch 1976; **Resid:** Orthopaedic Surgery, Montefiore Med Ctr 1983; **Fac Appt:** Assoc Prof OrS, Albert Einstein Coll Med

Geller, David S MD (OrS) - **Spec Exp:** Bone Cancer; Sarcoma; Sarcoma-Soft Tissue; **Hospital:** Montefiore Med Ctr-Moses Campus, NY (page 100); **Address:** MMC Medical Arts Pavilion, 3400 Bainbridge Ave Fl 6, Bronx, NY 10467; **Phone:** 718-920-5722; **Board Cert:** Orthopaedic Surgery 2008; **Med School:** Israel 2000; **Resid:** Orthopaedic Surgery, Montefiore Med Ctr 2005; **Fellow:** Orthopaedic Oncology, Mass General Hosp 2006; **Fac Appt:** Asst Prof OrS, Albert Einstein Coll Med

Kleinman, Paul G MD (OrS) - **Spec Exp:** Pediatric Orthopaedic Surgery; Hand Surgery; Trauma; Sports Medicine; **Hospital:** St. Barnabas Hosp - Bronx; **Address:** 2016 Bronxdale Ave, Ste 202, Bronx, NY 10462-3365; **Phone:** 718-863-8695; **Board Cert:** Orthopaedic Surgery 2009; **Med School:** Stanford Univ 1979; **Resid:** Surgery, St Lukes Hosp 1981; Orthopaedic Surgery, Columbia-Presby Hosp 1985; **Fellow:** Hand Surgery, Allegheny Genl Hosp 1986; Pediatric Orthopaedic Surgery, Hosp Joint Diseases 1990

Kulsakdinun, Chaiyaporn MD (OrS) - **Spec Exp:** Foot & Ankle Surgery; Fractures; Sports Injuries; **Hospital:** Montefiore Med Ctr-Einstein Campus, NY (page 100); **Address:** 1250 Waters Pl Fl 11, Bronx, NY 10461; **Phone:** 718-920-2060; **Board Cert:** Orthopaedic Surgery 2003; **Med School:** Yale Univ 1993; **Resid:** Orthopaedic Surgery, Yale-New Haven Hosp 1998; **Fellow:** Foot & Ankle Surgery, Hosp Special Surgery 1999; **Fac Appt:** Asst Prof OrS, Albert Einstein Coll Med

Levy, I Martin MD (OrS) - **Spec Exp:** Sports Medicine; Arthroscopic Surgery; **Hospital:** Montefiore Med Ctr-Einstein Campus, NY (page 100); **Address:** 1250 Waters Pl Fl 11, Bronx, NY 10461; **Phone:** 347-577-4411; **Board Cert:** Orthopaedic Surgery 1982; **Med School:** NY Med Coll 1976; **Resid:** Orthopaedic Surgery, Bronx Municipal Hosps 1980; **Fellow:** Sports Medicine, Hosp for Special Surg 1981

Olsewski, John M MD (OrS) - **Spec Exp:** Spinal Reconstructive Surgery; Scoliosis; Spinal Surgery-Neck; Cervical Myelopathy; **Hospital:** Montefiore Med Ctr-Einstein Campus, NY (page 100), Sound Shore Med Ctr - Westchester; **Address:** 2157 Tomlinson Ave, Bronx, NY 10461; **Phone:** 718-794-2501; **Board Cert:** Orthopaedic Surgery 2007; **Med School:** SUNY Buffalo 1986; **Resid:** Orthopaedic Surgery, SUNY Buffalo 1992; **Fellow:** Spinal Surgery, Twin Cities Scoliosis/Spine Ctr 1994; **Fac Appt:** Assoc Clin Prof OrS, Albert Einstein Coll Med

Wilson, Arnold B MD (OrS) - **Spec Exp:** Hip Replacement; Knee Replacement; Knee Injuries/Ligament Surgery; Sports Medicine; **Hospital:** Montefiore Med Ctr-Moses Campus, NY (page 100), NYU Hosp For Joint Diseases (page 119); **Address:** Wilson Orthopaedics, 75 E Gun Hill Rd, Bronx, NY 10467-2103; **Phone:** 718-798-1000; **Board Cert:** Orthopaedic Surgery 2007; **Med School:** UMDNJ-Univ Med Dent NJ 1987; **Resid:** Orthopaedic Surgery, Catholic Med Ctr of Brooklyn & Queens 1993; **Fellow:** Sports Medicine/Knee Surgery, Beth Israel Med Ctr 1994

Otolaryngology

Feghali, Joseph G MD (Oto) - **Spec Exp:** Ear Disorders/Surgery; Acoustic Neuroma; Hearing Disorders; Neuro-Otology; **Hospital:** Montefiore Med Ctr-Moses Campus, NY (page 100); **Address:** 182 E 210th St, Bronx, NY 10467; **Phone:** 718-881-3277; **Board Cert:** Otolaryngology 1990; **Med School:** Lebanon 1978; **Resid:** Otolaryngology, American Univ Beirut 1982; Otolaryngology, Montefiore Med Ctr 1990; **Fellow:** Otology & Neurotology, House Ear Inst 1983; Neurological Surgery, Meml Sloan Kettering Cancer Ctr 1984; **Fac Appt:** Clin Prof Oto, Albert Einstein Coll Med

Fried, Marvin P MD (Oto) - **Spec Exp:** Endoscopic Sinus Surgery; Head & Neck Tumors; Laryngeal & Voice Disorders; Sinus Disorders/Surgery; **Hospital:** Montefiore Med Ctr-Moses Campus, NY (page 100), Montefiore Med Ctr-Einstein Campus, NY (page 100); **Address:** 3400 Bainbridge Ave, Fl 3, Bronx, NY 10467; **Phone:** 718-920-4646; **Board Cert:** Otolaryngology 1975; **Med School:** Tufts Univ 1969; **Resid:** Surgery, Jewish Hosp 1971; Otolaryngology, Barnes Hosp 1975; **Fellow:** Stroke, Washington Univ 1976; **Fac Appt:** Prof Oto, Albert Einstein Coll Med

Goldstein, Steven I MD (Oto) - **Spec Exp:** Sinus Surgery; Nasal Surgery; Facial Plastic Surgery; Rhinoplasty; **Hospital:** NY Westchester Sq Med Ctr, Montefiore Med Ctr-Wakefield Campus, NY (page 100); **Address:** 1200 Waters Pl, Bronx, NY 10461; **Phone:** 718-863-4366; **Board Cert:** Otolaryngology 1987; **Med School:** SUNY Buffalo 1982; **Resid:** Surgery, NYU Med Ctr 1984; Otolaryngology, NYU Med Ctr 1987; **Fellow:** Facial Plastic Surgery, Mt Sinai Hosp 1988; **Fac Appt:** Clin Prof Oto, Albert Einstein Coll Med

Smith, Richard V MD (Oto) - **Spec Exp:** Head & Neck Cancer; Thyroid & Parathyroid Surgery; Salivary Gland Tumors; Robotic Surgery; **Hospital:** Montefiore Med Ctr-Moses Campus, NY (page 100), Montefiore Med Ctr-Einstein Campus, NY (page 100); **Address:** Medical Arts Pavilion, 3400 Bainbridge Ave, Fl 3, Bronx, NY 10467; **Phone:** 718-920-4646; **Board Cert:** Otolaryngology 1996; **Med School:** Univ VT Coll Med 1990; **Resid:** Otolaryngology, Georgetown Univ Hosp 1995; **Fac Appt:** Clin Prof Oto, Albert Einstein Coll Med

Yankelowitz, Stanley M MD (Oto) - **Spec Exp:** Nasal & Sinus Surgery; Pediatric Otolaryngology; **Hospital:** Montefiore Med Ctr-Moses Campus, NY (page 100), NY Westchester Sq Med Ctr; **Address:** 1200 Waters Pl, Ste 110, Bronx, NY 10461; **Phone:** 718-863-4366; **Med School:** South Africa 1974; **Resid:** Otolaryngology, Univ Stellenbosch 1985; Otolaryngology, Univ Cape Town 1987; **Fellow:** Pediatric Otolaryngology, Montefiore Med Ctr-Weiler Div 1988

Pediatric Allergy & Immunology

Wiznia, Andrew A MD (PA&I) - **Spec Exp:** AIDS/HIV; **Hospital:** Jacobi Med Ctr, N Central Bronx Hosp; **Address:** Jacobi Medical Ctr, Bldg 1, 1400 Pelham Pkwy S, rm 1W5-8, Bronx, NY 10461; **Phone:** 718-918-5222; **Board Cert:** Pediatrics 1986; **Med School:** Columbia P&S 1980; **Resid:** Pediatrics, Bronx Muni Hosp Ctr 1983; Pediatrics, Bronx-Lebanon Hosp Ctr 1984; **Fellow:** Allergy & Immunology, Montefiore-Weiler Einstein Div 1986; **Fac Appt:** Prof Ped, Albert Einstein Coll Med

Pediatric Cardiology

Hsu, Daphne MD (PCd) - **Spec Exp:** Interventional Cardiology; Heart Failure; Transplant Medicine-Heart; **Hospital:** Montefiore Med Ctr-Moses Campus, NY (page 100); **Address:** Chldn's Hosp at Montefiore, 3415 Bainbridge Ave, Bronx, NY 10467; **Phone:** 718-741-2315; **Board Cert:** Pediatrics 1988; Pediatric Cardiology 2010; **Med School:** Yale Univ 1982; **Resid:** Pediatrics, Columbia Babies & Chldn's Hosp 1985; **Fellow:** Pediatric Cardiology, Columbia Babies & Chldn's Hosp 1988; **Fac Appt:** Prof Ped, Albert Einstein Coll Med

Pass, Robert H MD (PCd) - **Spec Exp:** Arrhythmias; Cardiac Electrophysiology; Cardiac Catheterization; **Hospital:** Montefiore Med Ctr-Moses Campus, NY (page 100); **Address:** Chldn's Hosp at Montefiore, 3415 Bainbridge Ave, Bronx, NY 10467; **Phone:** 718-741-2183; **Board Cert:** Pediatric Cardiology 2006; **Med School:** Boston Univ 1991; **Resid:** Pediatrics, NY Presby/Cornell Med Ctr 1994; **Fellow:** Cardiovascular Disease, Chldn's Hosp 1998

Schiller, Myles S MD (PCd) - **Spec Exp:** Congenital Heart Disease & Acquired; Exercise Physiology; **Hospital:** Montefiore Med Ctr-Moses Campus, NY (page 100), St. Barnabas Hosp - Bronx; **Address:** Children's Hosp Montefiore, 3415 Bainbridge Ave, Bronx, NY 10467; **Phone:** 718-741-2254; **Board Cert:** Pediatrics 1978; Pediatric Cardiology 1979; **Med School:** Ros Franklin Univ/Chicago Med Sch 1973; **Resid:** Pediatrics, New York Hosp-Cornell 1975; **Fellow:** Pediatric Cardiology, New York Hosp-Cornell 1977; **Fac Appt:** Assoc Clin Prof Ped, Albert Einstein Coll Med

Shenoy, Rajesh U MD (PCd) - **Spec Exp:** Echocardiography; Fetal Echocardiography; Congenital Heart Disease; **Hospital:** Montefiore Med Ctr-Moses Campus, NY (page 100), St. Barnabas Hosp - Bronx; **Address:** Chldn's Hosp at Montefiore, 3415 Bainbridge Ave, Bronx, NY 10467; **Phone:** 718-741-2370; **Board Cert:** Pediatrics 2006; Pediatric Cardiology 2008; **Med School:** India 1995; **Resid:** Pediatrics, Univ Illinois Affil Hosp 1996; **Fellow:** Pediatric Cardiology, N Shore Hosp 2000; **Fac Appt:** Asst Prof Ped, Albert Einstein Coll Med

Walsh, Christine A MD (PCd) - **Spec Exp:** Arrhythmias; Congenital Heart Disease; Sudden Infant Death Syndrome (SIDS); **Hospital:** Montefiore Med Ctr-Moses Campus, NY (page 100); **Address:** 3415 Bainbridge Ave Fl 5, Bronx, NY 10467-2401; **Phone:** 718-741-2343; **Board Cert:** Pediatrics 1978; Pediatric Cardiology 1983; Pediatric Critical Care Medicine 2003; **Med School:** Yale Univ 1973; **Resid:** Pediatrics, Columbia-Presby Med Ctr 1976; **Fellow:** Pediatric Cardiology, Columbia-Presby Med Ctr 1978; Cardiac Electrophysiology, Columbia P&S 1980; **Fac Appt:** Prof Ped, Albert Einstein Coll Med

Pediatric Critical Care Medicine

Singer, Lewis Philip MD (PCCM) - **Spec Exp:** Respiratory Failure; Airway Disorders; **Hospital:** Montefiore Med Ctr-Moses Campus, NY (page 100); **Address:** 3415 Bainbridge Ave, Bronx, NY 10467-2401; **Phone:** 718-741-2440; **Board Cert:** Pediatrics 1981; Neonatal-Perinatal Medicine 1983; Pediatric Critical Care Medicine 2005; **Med School:** UMDNJ-NJ Med Sch, Newark 1977; **Resid:** Pediatrics, Montefiore Hosp Med Ctr 1981; **Fellow:** Neonatology, Montefiore Hosp Med Ctr 1983; **Fac Appt:** Prof Ped, Albert Einstein Coll Med

Ushay, H Michael MD/PhD (PCCM) - **Spec Exp:** Respiratory Failure; Sepsis & Septic Shock; Cardiac Critical Care; **Hospital:** Montefiore Med Ctr-Moses Campus, NY (page 100); **Address:** CHAM, Div Critical Care Med, 3415 Bainbridge Ave, Bronx, NY 10467; **Phone:** 718-741-2440; **Board Cert:** Pediatrics 2005; Pediatric Critical Care Medicine 2009; **Med School:** UMDNJ-NJ Med Sch, Newark 1986; **Resid:** Pediatrics, Montefiore/Bronx Muni Hosp 1990; **Fellow:** Pediatric Pulmonology, Montefiore Med Ctr 1991; Pediatric Critical Care Medicine, NY Hosp-Cornell Univ Med Ctr 1993; **Fac Appt:** Clin Prof Ped, Albert Einstein Coll Med

Weingarten, Jacqueline MD (PCCM) - **Spec Exp:** Heart Disease; Lung Disease; Nutrition; **Hospital:** Montefiore Med Ctr-Moses Campus, NY (page 100); **Address:** 111 E 210th St, Children's Hospital at Montefiore, Rosenthal Bldg - Fl 4, Bronx, NY 10467; **Phone:** 718-741-2440; **Board Cert:** Pediatrics 2010; Pediatric Critical Care Medicine 2010; **Med School:** Cornell Univ-Weill Med Coll 1986; **Resid:** Pediatrics, Columbia-Presby Med Ctr 1989; Pediatrics, Columbia-Presby Med Ctr 1990; **Fellow:** Pediatric Critical Care Medicine, Cornell/NY Hosp 1996; **Fac Appt:** Assoc Prof Ped, Albert Einstein Coll Med

Pediatric Endocrinology

Agarwal, Chhavi MD (PEn) - **Spec Exp:** Diabetes; Rett Syndrome; Calcium Disorders; **Hospital:** Montefiore Med Ctr-Moses Campus, NY (page 100); **Address:** Children's Hospital at Montefiore, 3415 Bainbridge Ave, Bronx, NY 10467; **Phone:** 718-920-4664; **Board Cert:** Pediatrics 2011; Pediatric Endocrinology 2007; **Med School:** India 1990; **Resid:** Pediatrics, Flushing Hosp Med Ctr 2004; **Fellow:** Pediatric Endocrinology, NY-Presby/Columbia Med Ctr 2007; **Fac Appt:** Asst Prof Ped, Albert Einstein Coll Med

Pediatric Gastroenterology

Thompson, John F MD (PGe) - **Spec Exp:** Inflammatory Bowel Disease/Crohn's; Short Bowel Syndrome; Transplant Medicine-Bowel; **Hospital:** Montefiore Med Ctr-Moses Campus, NY (page 100); **Address:** Children's Hosp at Montefiore, 3415 Bainbridge Ave, Bronx, NY 10467; **Phone:** 718-741-2450; **Board Cert:** Pediatrics 1983; Pediatric Gastroenterology 2005; **Med School:** Loyola Univ-Stritch Sch Med 1977; **Resid:** Pediatrics, Wylers Chldns Hosp-Univ Chicago 1980; **Fellow:** Pediatric Gastroenterology, Babies Hosp-Columbia Univ 1985; **Fac Appt:** Prof Ped, Univ Miami Sch Med

Pediatric Hematology-Oncology

Dasgupta, Indira K MD (PHO) - **Spec Exp:** Sickle Cell Disease; Anemia; **Hospital:** Montefiore Med Ctr-Wakefield Campus, NY (page 100); **Address:** 600 E 233rd St, Fl 4, Bronx, NY 10466-2697; **Phone:** 718-920-9014; **Board Cert:** Pediatrics 1981; Pediatric Hematology-Oncology 1984; **Med School:** India 1967; **Resid:** Pediatrics, New York Methodist Hosp 1974; **Fellow:** Pediatric Hematology-Oncology, Meml Sloan Kettering Cancer Ctr 1979; Pediatric Hematology-Oncology, Mount Sinai Hosp 1980; **Fac Appt:** Assoc Clin Prof Ped, NY Med Coll

Gorlick, Richard MD (PHO) - **Spec Exp:** Bone Tumors; Sarcoma; Solid Tumors; **Hospital:** Montefiore Med Ctr-Moses Campus, NY (page 100); **Address:** 111 E 210th St, Rosenthal 3, Bronx, NY 10467-2940; **Phone:** 718-741-2342; **Board Cert:** Pediatrics 2008; Pediatric Hematology-Oncology 2011; **Med School:** SUNY Downstate 1990; **Resid:** Pediatrics, Columbia-Presby Med Ctr 1993; **Fellow:** Pediatric Hematology-Oncology, Meml Sloan Kettering Cancer Ctr 1995

Levy, Adam S MD (PHO) - **Spec Exp:** Brain Tumors; Neuro-Oncology; **Hospital:** Montefiore Med Ctr-Moses Campus, NY (page 100); **Address:** Chldns Hosp at Montefiore, 3415 Bainbridge Ave, Bronx, NY 10467; **Phone:** 718-741-2342; **Board Cert:** Pediatrics 2005; Pediatric Hematology-Oncology 2010; **Med School:** NYU Sch Med 1994; **Resid:** Pediatrics, Mt Sinai Hosp 1998; **Fellow:** Pediatric Hematology-Oncology, Meml Sloan Kettering Cancer Ctr 2001; **Fac Appt:** Assoc Prof Ped, Albert Einstein Coll Med

Moulton, Thomas MD (PHO) - **Spec Exp:** Sickle Cell Disease; **Hospital:** Bronx Lebanon Hosp Ctr; **Address:** Bronx-Lebanon Hosp Ctr, 1650 Selwyn Ave, Ste 6D, Bronx, NY 10457; **Phone:** 718-579-7337; **Board Cert:** Pediatric Hematology-Oncology 2012; **Med School:** Loyola Univ-Stritch Sch Med 1984; **Resid:** Pediatrics, Rainbow Babies-Chldns Hosp 1987; **Fellow:** Pediatric Hematology-Oncology, Babies Hosp 1990; **Fac Appt:** Asst Prof Ped, Albert Einstein Coll Med

Pediatric Infectious Disease

Herold, Betsy C MD (PInf) - **Hospital:** Montefiore Med Ctr-Einstein Campus, NY (page 100); **Address:** 1300 Morris Park Ave, Forchheimer Bldg, Ste 702, Bronx, NY 10461; **Phone:** 718-741-2470; **Board Cert:** Pediatrics 1986; Pediatric Infectious Disease 2005; **Med School:** Univ Pennsylvania 1982; **Resid:** Pediatrics, Northwestern Meml Hosp 1985; **Fellow:** Infectious Disease, Northwestern Meml Hosp 1989; **Fac Appt:** Prof Ped, Albert Einstein Coll Med

Litman, Nathan MD (PInf) - **Spec Exp:** Infections in Immunocompromised Patients; Hospital Acquired Infections; **Hospital:** Montefiore Med Ctr-Moses Campus, NY (page 100); **Address:** Montefiore Med Ctr, Div Ped Infectious Disease, 111 E 210th St Fl 4, Bronx, NY 10467-2401; **Phone:** 718-741-2470; **Board Cert:** Pediatrics 1978; Pediatric Infectious Disease 2009; **Med School:** Albert Einstein Coll Med 1971; **Resid:** Pediatrics, Montefiore Med Ctr 1974; **Fellow:** Infectious Disease, Montefiore Med Ctr 1978; **Fac Appt:** Prof Ped, Albert Einstein Coll Med

Pediatric Nephrology

Kaskel, Frederick J MD/PhD (PNep) - **Spec Exp:** Transplant Medicine-Kidney; Nephrotic Syndrome; Kidney Disease-Chronic; Dialysis Care; **Hospital:** Montefiore Med Ctr-Moses Campus, NY (page 100), Bronx Lebanon Hosp Ctr; **Address:** Children's Hospital at Montefiore, 111 E 210th St, Bronx, NY 10467-2401; **Phone:** 718-655-1120; **Board Cert:** Pediatrics 1980; Pediatric Nephrology 1982; **Med School:** Univ Cincinnati 1975; **Resid:** Pediatrics, Montefiore Med Ctr 1977; **Fellow:** Pediatric Nephrology, Montefiore Med Ctr 1981; **Fac Appt:** Prof Ped, Albert Einstein Coll Med

Pediatric Otolaryngology

Bent, John P MD (PO) - **Spec Exp:** Airway Reconstruction; Sinus Disorders/Surgery; Hearing Loss; **Hospital:** Montefiore Med Ctr-Moses Campus, NY (page 100); **Address:** Children's Hospital at Montefiore, Dept Otolaryngology, Head & Neck Surgery, 3400 Bainbridge Ave Fl 3, Bronx, NY 10467-2490; **Phone:** 718-920-4646; **Board Cert:** Otolaryngology 1995; **Med School:** Wake Forest Univ 1989; **Resid:** Otolaryngology, Med Coll Georgia 1994; **Fellow:** Pediatric Otolaryngology, Univ Iowa Hosp & Clins 1995; **Fac Appt:** Assoc Prof Oto, Albert Einstein Coll Med

Pediatric Pulmonology

Arens, Raanan MD (PPul) - **Spec Exp:** Sleep Disorders/Apnea; **Hospital:** Montefiore Med Ctr-Einstein Campus, NY (page 100); **Address:** Chldns Hosp at Montefiore, Respiratory & Sleep Medicine, 3415 Bainbridge Ave, Bronx, NY 10467; **Phone:** 718-515-2330 x225; **Board Cert:** Pediatrics 2010; Pediatric Pulmonology 2011; Sleep Medicine 2009; **Med School:** Israel 1986; **Resid:** Pediatrics, Shera Med Ctr 1990; Pediatrics, Chldns Hosp 1995; **Fellow:** Pediatric Pulmonology, Chldns Hosp 1994; **Fac Appt:** Assoc Prof Ped, Albert Einstein Coll Med

Pediatric Rheumatology

Ilowite, Norman T MD (PRhu) - **Spec Exp:** Juvenile Arthritis; Lyme Disease; Lupus/SLE; Dermatomyositis; **Hospital:** Montefiore Med Ctr-Moses Campus, NY (page 100), Jacobi Med Ctr; **Address:** Chldns Hosp-Montefiore, Rheumatology, 3415 Bainbridge Ave Fl Rosenthal3, Bronx, NY 10467; **Phone:** 718-741-2456; **Board Cert:** Pediatrics 1985; Clinical & Laboratory Immunology 1990; Pediatric Rheumatology 2007; **Med School:** SUNY Downstate 1979; **Resid:** Pediatrics, Chldns Hosp Natl Med Ctr 1982; **Fellow:** Pediatric Rheumatology, Univ WA Med Ctr 1984; **Fac Appt:** Prof Ped, Albert Einstein Coll Med

Pediatric Surgery

Weinberg, Gerard MD (PS) - **Spec Exp:** Abdominal Wall Reconstruction; Trauma; Neonatal Surgery; **Hospital:** Montefiore Med Ctr-Moses Campus, NY (page 100); **Address:** 3355 Bainbridge Ave, Bronx, NY 10467; **Phone:** 718-920-7200; **Board Cert:** Surgery 2009; Pediatric Surgery 2009; **Med School:** Albert Einstein Coll Med 1973; **Resid:** Surgery, Albert Einstein Affil Hosps 1976; Pediatric Surgery, Childrens Hosp 1977; **Fellow:** Pediatric Surgery, Univ of Miami Hosps 1979; **Fac Appt:** Prof S, Albert Einstein Coll Med

Pediatrics

Andrade, Joseph MD (Ped) *PCP* - **Spec Exp:** Asthma; **Hospital:** Montefiore Med Ctr-Wakefield Campus, NY (page 100); **Address:** 1163 Manor Ave, Bronx, NY 10472; **Phone:** 718-589-3501; **Board Cert:** Pediatrics 2007; Internal Medicine 2011; **Med School:** Ecuador 1981; **Resid:** Pediatrics, Our Lady of Mercy Med Ctr 1986; Internal Medicine, Our Lady of Mercy Med Ctr 1988

Arnstein, Ellis MD (Ped) *PCP* - **Spec Exp:** Developmental Disorders; **Hospital:** Bronx Lebanon Hosp Ctr; **Address:** Bronx Lebanon Hosp Ctr, 1650 Selwyn Ave, Ste 6D, Bronx, NY 10457; **Phone:** 718-579-7337; **Board Cert:** Pediatrics 1975; Neurodevelopmental Disabilities 2012; **Med School:** SUNY Downstate 1969; **Resid:** Pediatrics, Univ Wash Med Ctr 1973; **Fellow:** Child & Adolescent Psychiatry, Tufts-New England Med Ctr 1974; **Fac Appt:** Asst Prof Ped, NY Med Coll

Balk, Sophie J MD (Ped) *PCP* - **Spec Exp:** Environmental Medicine; **Hospital:** Montefiore Med Ctr-Moses Campus, NY (page 100), Montefiore Med Ctr-Einstein Campus, NY (page 100); **Address:** 1621 Eastchester Road, Bronx, NY 10461-2604; **Phone:** 718-405-8090; **Board Cert:** Pediatrics 1979; **Med School:** Albert Einstein Coll Med 1974; **Resid:** Pediatrics, Montefiore Hosp Med Ctr 1977; **Fac Appt:** Assoc Prof Ped, Albert Einstein Coll Med

Belamarich, Peter F MD (Ped) - **Spec Exp:** Cholesterol/Lipid Disorders; **Hospital:** Montefiore Med Ctr-Einstein Campus, NY (page 100); **Address:** Children's Hospital at Montefiore, 3415 Bainbridge Ave, Fl 4, Bronx, NY 10467; **Phone:** 718-741-2432; **Board Cert:** Pediatrics 1987; **Med School:** Boston Univ 1983; **Resid:** Pediatrics, Brookdale Hosp 1986; **Fellow:** Pediatric Gastroenterology, Columbia Presby Hosp 1989

Bloomfield, Diane MD (Ped) *PCP* - **Hospital:** Montefiore Med Ctr-Moses Campus, NY (page 100); **Address:** 3444 Kossuth Ave, DTC Bldg, FL 1B, Bronx, NY 10467-2461; **Phone:** 718-920-5873; **Board Cert:** Pediatrics 1987; **Med School:** Cornell Univ-Weill Med Coll 1982; **Resid:** Pediatrics, NY Hosp 1985; **Fellow:** Ambulatory Pediatrics, NY Hosp 1986; **Fac Appt:** Asst Prof Ped, Cornell Univ-Weill Med Coll

Cahill, Linda T MD (Ped) - **Spec Exp:** Child Abuse; **Hospital:** Montefiore Med Ctr-Moses Campus, NY (page 100); **Address:** Butler Child Advocacy Ctr, Chldns Hosp-Montefiore, 3314 Steuben Ave, Bronx, NY 10467; **Phone:** 718-920-5833; **Board Cert:** Pediatrics 1975; Child Abuse Pediatrics 2009; **Med School:** Med Coll PA 1969; **Resid:** Pediatrics, Beth Israel Med Ctr 1972; **Fellow:** Pediatric Infectious Disease, Mt Sinai Hosp 1974; **Fac Appt:** Assoc Prof Ped, Albert Einstein Coll Med

Esteban-Cruciani, Nora MD (Ped) - **Spec Exp:** Chronic Illness; Nutrition; Metabolic Disorders; **Hospital:** Montefiore Med Ctr-Moses Campus, NY (page 100); **Address:** 3415 Bainbridge Ave, Department of Pediatrics, Rosenthal-4, Bronx, NY 10467; **Phone:** 718-741-2257; **Board Cert:** Pediatrics 2008; **Med School:** Argentina 1980; **Resid:** Pediatrics, Italian Hosp 1983; Pediatrics, Albert Einstein Coll Med 1993; **Fellow:** Research, Nat Inst Hlth 1991; Research, Albert Einstein Coll Med 2005; **Fac Appt:** Assoc Prof Ped, Albert Einstein Coll Med

Haber, Patricia MD (Ped) *PCP* - **Hospital:** Montefiore Med Ctr-Moses Campus, NY (page 100); **Address:** 1500 Astor Ave Fl 2, Bronx, NY 10469-5900; **Phone:** 718-881-0100; **Board Cert:** Pediatrics 2009; Pediatric Rheumatology 2011; **Med School:** Johns Hopkins Univ 1976; **Resid:** Pediatrics, Johns Hopkins Hosp 1979; **Fellow:** Immunology, Univ Alabama Hosp 1982; Pediatric Rheumatology, Univ Alabama Hosp 1984; **Fac Appt:** Asst Prof Ped, Albert Einstein Coll Med

Hirschman, Alan MD (Ped) *PCP* - **Spec Exp:** Asthma; **Hospital:** Montefiore Med Ctr-Moses Campus, NY (page 100); **Address:** 3765 Riverdale Ave, Ste 4, Bronx, NY 10463-1845; **Phone:** 718-548-7300; **Board Cert:** Pediatrics 1981; **Med School:** UMDNJ-NJ Med Sch, Newark 1976; **Resid:** Pediatrics, Montefiore Med Ctr 1980; **Fac Appt:** Asst Clin Prof, Albert Einstein Coll Med

Igel, Gerard MD (Ped) *PCP* - **Spec Exp:** Chronic Illness; Behavioral Disorders; Developmental Disorders; Foster Care; **Hospital:** Montefiore Med Ctr-Moses Campus, NY (page 100), Jacobi Med Ctr; **Address:** 1613 Tenbroeck Ave, Bronx, NY 10461-2007; **Phone:** 718-828-9060; **Board Cert:** Pediatrics 1986; **Med School:** Israel 1981; **Resid:** Pediatrics, Jacobi Med Ctr 1984; **Fac Appt:** Asst Clin Prof Ped, Albert Einstein Coll Med

Kaminer, Ruth MD (Ped) - **Spec Exp:** Developmental & Behavioral Disorders; **Hospital:** Montefiore Med Ctr-Moses Campus, NY (page 100); **Address:** Rose F Kennedy Ctr, 1410 Pelham Pkwy S, rm 108, Bronx, NY 10461-1101; **Phone:** 718-430-2100; **Board Cert:** Pediatrics 1971; Developmental-Behavioral Pediatrics 2002; **Med School:** NYU Sch Med 1962; **Resid:** Pediatrics, Chldn's Hops 1964Bronx Munipal Hosp 1968; **Fellow:** Developmental-Behavioral Pediatrics, Albert Einstein Affil Hosp 1974; **Fac Appt:** Clin Prof Ped, Albert Einstein Coll Med

Katzenstein, Martin S MD (Ped) - **Spec Exp:** Neonatal Nutrition; Ethics; Neonatal Respiratory Care; **Hospital:** Montefiore Med Ctr-Wakefield Campus, NY (page 100), Westchester Med Ctr; **Address:** 4350 Van Cortlandt Park E, Bronx, NY 10470; **Phone:** 374-982-2181; **Board Cert:** Pediatrics 2004; **Med School:** NY Med Coll 1978; **Resid:** Pediatrics, New York Hosp 1981; **Fellow:** Neonatal-Perinatal Medicine, New York Hosp-Cornell 1982; Neonatal-Perinatal Medicine, Westchester Co Med Ctr 1984; **Fac Appt:** Assoc Clin Prof Ped, NY Med Coll

Mayers, Marguerite MD (Ped) *PCP* - **Spec Exp:** Tuberculosis; AIDS/HIV; Travel Medicine; **Hospital:** Montefiore Med Ctr-Moses Campus, NY (page 100); **Address:** Montefiore Medical Group, 3444 Kossuth Ave, Bronx, NY 10467-2401; **Phone:** 718-920-5871; **Board Cert:** Pediatrics 1977; Pediatric Infectious Disease 2009; **Med School:** Albert Einstein Coll Med 1971; **Resid:** Pediatrics, Montefiore Hosp Med Ctr 1974; **Fellow:** Infectious Disease, Montefiore Hosp Med Ctr 1976; **Fac Appt:** Clin Prof Ped, Albert Einstein Coll Med

Oppedisano, Carlyn Ann MD (Ped) *PCP* - **Spec Exp:** Parenting Issues; **Hospital:** Morgan Stanley Children's Hosp of NY-Presby, NY (page 104); **Address:** 2600 Netherland Ave, Ste 120, Riverdale, NY 10463-4813; **Phone:** 718-796-3580; **Board Cert:** Pediatrics 2009; **Med School:** Columbia P&S 1981; **Resid:** Pediatrics, Babies Hosp 1985; **Fac Appt:** Assoc Clin Prof Ped, Columbia P&S

Schechter, Miriam MD (Ped) *PCP* - **Spec Exp:** Asthma; Vaccines; **Hospital:** Montefiore Med Ctr-Moses Campus, NY (page 100); **Address:** 1621 Eastchester Rd, Ste 115, Bronx, NY 10461-2604; **Phone:** 718-405-8040; **Board Cert:** Pediatrics 2007; **Med School:** NYU Sch Med 1989; **Resid:** Pediatrics, Mount Sinai 1992; Pediatrics, Mount Sinai 1993; **Fac Appt:** Asst Prof Ped, Albert Einstein Coll Med

Stein, Ruth E K MD (Ped) *PCP* - **Spec Exp:** Chronic Illness; Developmental & Behavioral Disorders; **Hospital:** Montefiore Med Ctr-Moses Campus, NY (page 100); **Address:** 1300 Morris Park Ave, VE Bldg Fl 6 - Ste B27, Bronx, NY 10461; **Phone:** 718-862-1721; **Board Cert:** Pediatrics 1971; Developmental-Behavioral Pediatrics 2004; **Med School:** Albert Einstein Coll Med 1966; **Resid:** Pediatrics, Bronx Muni Hosp 1968; Pediatrics, Chldns Hosp Natl Med Ctr 1969; **Fellow:** Community Medicine, Chldns Hosp Natl Med Ctr 1969; **Fac Appt:** Prof Ped, Albert Einstein Coll Med

Strassberg, Barbara E MD (Ped) *PCP* - **Spec Exp:** Developmental Disorders; **Hospital:** Morgan Stanley Children's Hosp of NY-Presby, NY (page 104); **Address:** 2600 Netherland Ave, Ste 120, Bronx, NY 10463-4813; **Phone:** 718-796-3580; **Board Cert:** Pediatrics 2009; **Med School:** SUNY Upstate Med Univ 1981; **Resid:** Pediatrics, Columbia-Presby Hosp 1984; **Fac Appt:** Assoc Clin Prof Ped, Columbia P&S

Weiner, Richard L MD (Ped) *PCP* - **Spec Exp:** Adolescent Medicine; **Hospital:** Montefiore Med Ctr-Moses Campus, NY (page 100), Montefiore Med Ctr-Einstein Campus, NY (page 100); **Address:** 2300 Westchester Ave, Bronx, NY 10462; **Phone:** 718-409-8000; **Board Cert:** Pediatrics 1991; **Med School:** Albert Einstein Coll Med 1975; **Resid:** Pediatrics, Jacobi Med Ctr 1978; **Fac Appt:** Assoc Prof Ped, Albert Einstein Coll Med

Zoltan, Irving MD (Ped) *PCP* - **Spec Exp:** Diagnostic Problems; Infectious Disease; Asthma; **Hospital:** Montefiore Med Ctr-Moses Campus, NY (page 100), Montefiore Med Ctr-Einstein Campus, NY (page 100); **Address:** 1613 Tenbroeck Ave, Bronx, NY 10461; **Phone:** 718-828-9060; **Board Cert:** Pediatrics 1979; **Med School:** Albert Einstein Coll Med 1974; **Resid:** Pediatrics, Jacobi Med Ctr 1978; **Fac Appt:** Asst Clin Prof Ped, Albert Einstein Coll Med

Physical Medicine & Rehabilitation

DeAraujo, Maria MD (PMR) - **Spec Exp:** Arthritis; Pain-Low Back; Electromyography; Pain-Musculoskeletal; **Hospital:** Montefiore Med Ctr-Wakefield Campus, NY (page 100); **Address:** Dept of Phy Med & Rehab, 600 E 233rd St, Bronx, NY 10466-2604; **Phone:** 718-920-9171; **Board Cert:** Physical Medicine & Rehabilitation 1989; **Med School:** Brazil 1972; **Resid:** Physical Medicine & Rehabilitation, St Vincent's Hosp & Med Ctr 1981; **Fellow:** Physical Medicine & Rehabilitation, Westchester Med Ctr 1989; **Fac Appt:** Clin Prof PMR, NY Med Coll

Levin, Sheryl MD (PMR) - **Spec Exp:** Neuro-Rehabilitation; Pain-Musculoskeletal; Arthritis; **Hospital:** Montefiore Med Ctr-Moses Campus, NY (page 100); **Address:** 3435 Dekalb Ave, Bronx, NY 10467-2301; **Phone:** 718-547-8899; **Board Cert:** Physical Medicine & Rehabilitation 1989; **Med School:** Cornell Univ-Weill Med Coll 1984; **Resid:** Physical Medicine & Rehabilitation, New York Hosp 1988; **Fac Appt:** Assoc Clin Prof PMR, Albert Einstein Coll Med

Thomas, Mark Alvin MD (PMR) - **Hospital:** Montefiore Med Ctr-Moses Campus, NY (page 100); **Address:** 150 E 210th St, Fl 2, Bronx, NY 10467; **Phone:** 718-920-2753; **Board Cert:** Physical Medicine & Rehabilitation 1988; **Med School:** Mexico 1982; **Resid:** Physical Medicine & Rehabilitation, Nassau Co Med Ctr 1986; **Fac Appt:** Assoc Prof PMR, Albert Einstein Coll Med

Plastic Surgery

Goldstein, Robert D MD (PlS) - **Spec Exp:** Breast Surgery; Nasal Surgery; Abdominoplasty; **Hospital:** Montefiore Med Ctr-Einstein Campus, NY (page 100), Montefiore Med Ctr-Moses Campus, NY (page 100); **Address:** 2425 Eastchester Rd, Bronx, NY 10469; **Phone:** 718-405-7500; **Board Cert:** Plastic Surgery 1985; **Med School:** Penn State Coll Med 1977; **Resid:** Surgery, Montefiore Med Ctr 1981; Plastic Surgery, Montefiore Med Ctr 1984; **Fellow:** Hand Surgery, Montefiore Med Ctr-Einstein Div 1982; **Fac Appt:** Assoc Clin Prof PlS, Albert Einstein Coll Med

Greenstein, Bruce MD (PlS) - **Spec Exp:** Burn Care; Burns-Reconstructive Plastic Surgery; **Hospital:** Jacobi Med Ctr, N Central Bronx Hosp; **Address:** Jacobi Med Ctr, Dept Plastic Surgery, 1400 Pelham Pkwy S, rm 209, Bronx, NY 10461; **Phone:** 718-918-5970; **Board Cert:** Plastic Surgery 1984; **Med School:** SUNY Upstate Med Univ 1975; **Resid:** Surgery, Montefiore Hosp Med Ctr 1980; Plastic Surgery, Montefiore Hosp Med Ctr 1982; **Fellow:** Hand Surgery, Montefiore Hosp Med Ctr 1983; **Fac Appt:** Assoc Clin Prof PlS, Albert Einstein Coll Med

Liebling, Ralph W MD (PlS) - **Spec Exp:** Reconstructive Surgery; Microsurgery; Hand Surgery; Burn Care; **Hospital:** Jacobi Med Ctr, N Central Bronx Hosp; **Address:** Jacobi Med Ctr, Dept Plastic Recons Surg, 1400 Pelham Parkway South, Bronx, NY 10461; **Phone:** 718-918-7000; **Board Cert:** Plastic Surgery 1988; **Med School:** Albert Einstein Coll Med 1977; **Resid:** Surgery, Montefiore Med Ctr 1981; Plastic Surgery, Montefiore Med Ctr 1983; **Fellow:** Reconstructive Microsurgery, NYU/Bellevue Hosp Ctr 1984; **Fac Appt:** Assoc Prof S, Albert Einstein Coll Med

Psychiatry

Asnis, Gregory M MD (Psyc) - **Spec Exp:** Psychopharmacology; Mood Disorders; Anxiety Disorders; Depression; **Hospital:** Montefiore Med Ctr-Moses Campus, NY (page 100), Phelps Meml Hosp Ctr (page 614); **Address:** 111 E 210th St, Bronx, NY 10467-2401; **Phone:** 718-920-4287; **Board Cert:** Psychiatry 1978; **Med School:** Hahnemann Univ 1972; **Resid:** Psychiatry, Mt Sinai Hosp 1976; **Fellow:** Psychiatry, Columbia-Presby Med Ctr 1981; **Fac Appt:** Prof Psyc, Albert Einstein Coll Med

Gelfand, Janice MD (Psyc) - **Spec Exp:** Depression; Anxiety Disorders; Psychosomatic Disorders; Personality Disorders; **Hospital:** NY-Presby/Columbia Univ Med Ctr, NY (page 104); **Address:** 3765 Riverdale Ave, Bronx, NY 10463-1845; **Phone:** 718-361-3482; **Board Cert:** Psychiatry 1990; **Med School:** NYU Sch Med 1985; **Resid:** Psychiatry, NYU Med Ctr 1989; **Fellow:** Psychiatry, Beth Israel Med Ctr 1991; **Fac Appt:** Asst Prof Psyc, Columbia P&S

Heiman, Peter L MD (Psyc) - **Spec Exp:** Psychiatry in Physical Illness; **Hospital:** Montefiore Med Ctr-Moses Campus, NY (page 100); **Address:** 4465 Douglas Ave, Bronx, NY 10471; **Phone:** 212-472-8885; **Board Cert:** Psychiatry 1975; **Med School:** Albert Einstein Coll Med 1968; **Resid:** Psychiatry, Montefiore Hosp Med Ctr 1972; **Fac Appt:** Asst Clin Prof Psyc, Albert Einstein Coll Med

Lebinger, Martin B MD (Psyc) - **Spec Exp:** Depression; Anxiety Disorders; Panic Disorder; **Hospital:** Bronx Psych Ctr; **Address:** 1540 Pelham Pkwy S, Ste 1A, Bronx, NY 10461-1130; **Phone:** 718-518-0222; **Board Cert:** Psychiatry 1980; **Med School:** Albert Einstein Coll Med 1976; **Resid:** Psychiatry, Montefiore Med Ctr 1979; **Fellow:** Psychiatry, LI Jewish-Hillside Med Ctr 1981; **Fac Appt:** Asst Clin Prof Psyc, Albert Einstein Coll Med

Osei-Tutu, John MD (Psyc) - **Spec Exp:** Anxiety & Depression; Addiction/Substance Abuse; **Hospital:** Bronx Lebanon Hosp Ctr; **Address:** 1276 Fulton Ave, Bronx, NY 10456; **Phone:** 718-901-6133; **Board Cert:** Psychiatry 1990; Addiction Psychiatry 2003; **Med School:** Ghana 1976; **Resid:** Psychiatry, Bronx-Lebanon Hosp 1983; **Fac Appt:** Asst Prof Psyc, Albert Einstein Coll Med

Schwartz, Bruce J MD (Psyc) - **Spec Exp:** Depression; Bipolar/Mood Disorders; Schizophrenia; Anxiety & Depression; **Hospital:** Montefiore Med Ctr-Moses Campus, NY (page 100); **Address:** Montefiore Medical Ctr, Dept Psychiatry, 111 E 210th St, Bronx, NY 10467-2490; **Phone:** 718-920-4040; **Board Cert:** Psychiatry 1980; **Med School:** SUNY Downstate 1975; **Resid:** Psychiatry, Bronx Muni Hosp 1979; **Fac Appt:** Clin Prof Psyc, Albert Einstein Coll Med

Wyszynski, Bernard MD (Psyc) - **Hospital:** Montefiore Med Ctr-Moses Campus, NY (page 100); **Address:** Montefore Medical Ctr, KLAU 2, 111 E 210th St, Bronx, NY 10467; **Phone:** 718-920-4737; **Board Cert:** Psychiatry 1987; Neurology 1985; **Med School:** Univ Pennsylvania 1980; **Resid:** Neurology, Mount Sinai Med Ctr 1984; Psychiatry, Mount Sinai Med Ctr 1987; **Fac Appt:** Assoc Prof Psyc, Albert Einstein Coll Med

Pulmonary Disease

Aldrich, Thomas K MD (Pul) - **Spec Exp:** Asthma; Chronic Obstructive Lung Disease (COPD); Sickle Cell Disease-Lung; Sarcoidosis; **Hospital:** Montefiore Med Ctr-Moses Campus, NY (page 100); **Address:** 3400 Bainbridge Ave, Fl 2nd, Bronx, NY 10467-2401; **Phone:** 718-920-6087; **Board Cert:** Internal Medicine 1978; Pulmonary Disease 1980; **Med School:** Univ Minn 1975; **Resid:** Internal Medicine, UC Irvine Med Ctr 1978; **Fellow:** Pulmonary Disease, Univ Virginia Med Ctr 1980; Physiology, Univ Penn 1982; **Fac Appt:** Prof Med, Albert Einstein Coll Med

Appel, David MD (Pul) - **Spec Exp:** Sleep Disorders/Apnea; Asthma; Smoking Cessation; **Hospital:** Montefiore Med Ctr-Moses Campus, NY (page 100); **Address:** 111 E 210th St, Pulmonary Div, Bronx, NY 10467; **Phone:** 718-920-6055; **Board Cert:** Internal Medicine 1976; Sleep Medicine 2002; **Med School:** Albert Einstein Coll Med 1973; **Resid:** Internal Medicine, Bronx Municipal Hosp 1976; **Fellow:** Pulmonary Disease, Bronx Municipal Hosp 1978; **Fac Appt:** Assoc Prof Med, Albert Einstein Coll Med

Casper, Theodore MD (Pul) - **Spec Exp:** Critical Care Medicine; **Hospital:** NY Westchester Sq Med Ctr, Montefiore Med Ctr-Einstein Campus, NY (page 100); **Address:** 1250 Waters Pl, Ste 506, Bronx, NY 10461; **Phone:** 718-892-1200; **Board Cert:** Internal Medicine 1983; Pulmonary Disease 1986; **Med School:** Columbia P&S 1980; **Resid:** Internal Medicine, St Luke's Hosp 1983; **Fellow:** Pulmonary Disease, St Luke's Hosp 1985

Karetzky, Monroe MD (Pul) - **Spec Exp:** Asthma; Sleep Disorders; **Hospital:** Hackensack Univ Med Ctr (page 96), Englewood Hosp & Med Ctr; **Address:** Bronx Pulmonary Center, 441 E Tremont Ave, Bronx, NY 10457; **Phone:** 718-583-9240; **Board Cert:** Internal Medicine 1971; Pulmonary Disease 1974; Critical Care Medicine 1989; Geriatric Medicine 2002; **Med School:** Cornell Univ-Weill Med Coll 1963; **Resid:** Internal Medicine, Mary I Bassett Hosp 1966; **Fellow:** Cardiopulmonary Disease, Mary I Bassett Hosp 1967; **Fac Appt:** Assoc Clin Prof Med, UMDNJ-NJ Med Sch, Newark

Klapper, Philip MD (Pul) - **Spec Exp:** Asthma; Emphysema; Chronic Obstructive Lung Disease (COPD); **Hospital:** Montefiore Med Ctr-Moses Campus, NY (page 100), Lawrence Hosp Ctr; **Address:** 3322 Bainbridge Ave, Bronx, NY 10467; **Phone:** 718-884-2000; **Board Cert:** Internal Medicine 1986; Pulmonary Disease 2010; Critical Care Medicine 2003; **Med School:** Albert Einstein Coll Med 1983; **Resid:** Internal Medicine, Montefiore Hosp Med Ctr 1986; **Fellow:** Pulmonary Disease, SUNY Downstate Med Ctr 1990; Critical Care Medicine, Montefiore Hosp Med Ctr 1991; **Fac Appt:** Asst Clin Prof Med, Albert Einstein Coll Med

Loganathan, Raghunandan S MD (Pul) - **Spec Exp:** Critical Care; Pneumonia; Asthma; Chronic Obstructive Lung Disease (COPD); **Hospital:** Lincoln Med & Mental Hlth Ctr; **Address:** Lincoln Medical & Mental Health Ctr, 234 E 149th St, Ste 820, Bronx, NY 10451; **Phone:** 914-330-1302; **Board Cert:** Pulmonary Disease 2002; Critical Care Medicine 2003; **Med School:** India 1994; **Resid:** Internal Medicine, Bronx-Lebanon Hosp 2000; **Fellow:** Pulmonary Disease, Meml Sloan Kettering Cancer Ctr 2002; Critical Care Medicine, Montefiore Med Ctr 2003

Marino, William MD (Pul) - **Spec Exp:** Respiratory Failure; Asthma; Bronchoscopy; **Hospital:** Montefiore Med Ctr-Wakefield Campus, NY (page 100); **Address:** 4234 Bronx Blvd Fl 2, Bronx, NY 10466; **Phone:** 347-341-4300; **Board Cert:** Internal Medicine 1980; Pulmonary Disease 1984; Critical Care Medicine 2007; **Med School:** Albert Einstein Coll Med 1977; **Resid:** Internal Medicine, Montefiore Hosp Med Ctr 1980; **Fellow:** Pulmonary Disease, Columbia-Presby Med ctr 1982; **Fac Appt:** Assoc Clin Prof Med, NY Med Coll

Prezant, David MD (Pul) - **Spec Exp:** Asthma; **Hospital:** Montefiore Med Ctr-Moses Campus, NY (page 100); **Address:** 111 E 210th St, Bronx, NY 10467-2401; **Phone:** 718-920-6095; **Board Cert:** Internal Medicine 1984; Pulmonary Disease 1986; **Med School:** Albert Einstein Coll Med 1981; **Resid:** Internal Medicine, Harlem Hosp 1984; **Fellow:** Pulmonary Disease, Montefiore Hosp Med Ctr 1986; **Fac Appt:** Assoc Prof Med, Albert Einstein Coll Med

Sender, Joel MD (Pul) - **Spec Exp:** Asthma; Sarcoidosis; **Hospital:** St. Barnabas Hosp - Bronx; **Address:** 2016 Bronxdale Ave, Ste 301, Bronx, NY 10462-3300; **Phone:** 718-409-2222; **Board Cert:** Internal Medicine 1978; Pulmonary Disease 1980; Geriatric Medicine 2005; **Med School:** Albany Med Coll 1975; **Resid:** Internal Medicine, Mount Sinai Hosp 1978; **Fellow:** Pulmonary Disease, Mount Sinai Hosp 1980

Radiation Oncology

Bodner, William R MD (RadRO) - **Spec Exp:** Brachytherapy; Stereotactic Radiosurger; **Hospital:** Montefiore Med Ctr-Einstein Campus, NY (page 100); **Address:** 1625 Poplar St, MS 10461, Bronx, NY 10461; **Phone:** 718-405-8550; **Board Cert:** Radiation Oncology 2005; **Med School:** Wake Forest Univ 1987; **Resid:** Radiation Oncology, NY Med Coll Affil Hosp 1995; **Fac Appt:** Assoc Prof RadRO, Albert Einstein Coll Med

Kalnicki, Shalom MD (RadRO) - **Spec Exp:** Lung Cancer; Head & Neck Cancer; Gynecologic Cancer; Prostate Cancer; **Hospital:** Montefiore Med Ctr-Moses Campus, NY (page 100), Montefiore Med Ctr-Einstein Campus, NY (page 100); **Address:** Montefiore Medical Group, 1625 Poplar St Fl 2, Bronx, NY 10461; **Phone:** 718-920-5280; **Board Cert:** Therapeutic Radiology 1979; **Med School:** Israel 1974; **Resid:** Radiation Therapy, Montefiore Med Ctr 1978; **Fac Appt:** Clin Prof Rad, Albert Einstein Coll Med

Rheumatology

Efthimiou, Petros MD (Rhu) - **Hospital:** Lincoln Med & Mental Hlth Ctr, Rockefeller Univ; **Address:** 234 E 149 St Fl 9 - Ste 28, Bronx, NY 10451; **Phone:** 718-579-6131; **Board Cert:** Internal Medicine 2011; Rheumatology 2003; **Med School:** Greece 1996; **Resid:** Internal Medicine, Brown Univ-Rhode Island Hosp 2001; **Fellow:** Rheumatology, NY-Presby/Weill Cornell Med Ctr 2004; **Fac Appt:** Assoc Prof Med, Cornell Univ-Weill Med Coll

Fomberstein, Barry MD (Rhu) - **Spec Exp:** Rheumatoid Arthritis; Gout; **Hospital:** Montefiore Med Ctr-Wakefield Campus, NY (page 100); **Address:** Montefiore Med Ctr-North Div, 600 E 233rd St, Bronx, NY 10466-2697; **Phone:** 718-920-9168; **Board Cert:** Internal Medicine 1979; Rheumatology 1982; **Med School:** Albert Einstein Coll Med 1976; **Resid:** Internal Medicine, LIJ Med Ctr 1979; **Fellow:** Rheumatology, LIJ Med Ctr 1981; **Fac Appt:** Assoc Clin Prof Med, NY Med Coll

Keiser, Harold D MD (Rhu) - **Spec Exp:** Rheumatoid Arthritis; Lupus/SLE; **Hospital:** Montefiore Med Ctr-Einstein Campus, NY (page 100), Jacobi Med Ctr; **Address:** 1575 Blondell Ave, Ste 200, Bronx, NY 10461-2662; **Phone:** 866-633-8255; **Board Cert:** Internal Medicine 1972; Rheumatology 1972; **Med School:** NYU Sch Med 1964; **Resid:** Internal Medicine, Clevelnd Metro Genl Hosp 1968; **Fellow:** Rheumatology, Albert Einstein Coll Med 1972; **Fac Appt:** Prof Med, Albert Einstein Coll Med

Weinstein, Joshua W MD (Rhu) - **Spec Exp:** Lupus/SLE; Rheumatoid Arthritis; Gout; **Hospital:** Montefiore Med Ctr-Einstein Campus, NY (page 100), NY Hosp Queens (page 206); **Address:** 7235 112 St, Forest Hills, NY 11375; **Phone:** 718-575-0649; **Board Cert:** Internal Medicine 1975; Rheumatology 1978; **Med School:** SUNY Downstate 1972; **Resid:** Internal Medicine, Maimonides Med Ctr 1975; **Fellow:** Rheumatology, Montefiore Med Ctr 1977; **Fac Appt:** Asst Prof Med, Albert Einstein Coll Med

Surgery

Agarwal, Nanakram MD (S) - **Spec Exp:** Breast Surgery; Colon & Rectal Surgery; **Hospital:** Montefiore Med Ctr-Wakefield Campus, NY (page 100); **Address:** 600 E 233rd St Fl 4, Bronx, NY 10466; **Phone:** 718-920-9143; **Board Cert:** Surgery 2001; Critical Care Medicine 2005; **Med School:** India 1973; **Resid:** Surgery, Our Lady of Mercy Med Ctr 1981; **Fellow:** Critical Care Medicine, Westchester Co Med Ctr 1982; **Fac Appt:** Prof S, NY Med Coll

Bellemare, Sarah MD (S) - **Spec Exp:** Hepatobiliary Surgery; Transplant-Liver; Robotic Surgery; Laparoscopic Surgery; **Hospital:** Montefiore Med Ctr-Einstein Campus, NY (page 100), Montefiore Med Ctr-Moses Campus, NY (page 100); **Address:** Montefiore Med Ctr - Weiler Div, 111 E 210th St, Rosenthal 2, Bronx, NY 10467; **Phone:** 718-904-2047; **Board Cert:** Surgery 2001; **Med School:** Canada 1996; **Resid:** Surgery, Montreal Univ Med Ctr 2001; **Fellow:** Hepatobiliary Surgery, NY Presby-Columbia Med Ctr 2003; Transplant Surgery, NY Presby-Columbia Med Ctr 2004; **Fac Appt:** Asst Clin Prof S, Albert Einstein Coll Med

Cosgrove, John M MD (S) - **Spec Exp:** Laparoscopic Surgery; Endoscopy; Biliary Surgery; Gastrointestinal Surgery; **Hospital:** Bronx Lebanon Hosp Ctr, N Shore Univ Hosp (page 106); **Address:** 1650 Selwyn Ave, Ste 4A, Bronx, NY 10457; **Phone:** 718-960-1227; **Board Cert:** Surgery 2008; **Med School:** NY Med Coll 1983; **Resid:** Surgery, Beth Israel Med Ctr 1988; **Fac Appt:** Assoc Prof S, Albert Einstein Coll Med

Greenstein, Stuart MD (S) - **Spec Exp:** Laparoscopic Surgery; Dialysis Access Surgery; Transplant-Kidney; **Hospital:** Montefiore Med Ctr-Moses Campus, NY (page 100); **Address:** 111 E 210th St, Bronx, NY 10467; **Phone:** 877-287-3536; **Board Cert:** Surgery 2003; **Med School:** Harvard Med Sch 1979; **Resid:** Surgery, UMDNJ Med Ctr 1984; **Fellow:** Vascular Surgery, Hosp Univ Penn 1985; Transplant Surgery, SUNY Downstate 1986; **Fac Appt:** Prof S, Albert Einstein Coll Med

Kennedy, Timothy J MD (S) - **Spec Exp:** Laparoscopic Surgery; Pancreatic Cancer; Stomach Cancer; **Hospital:** Montefiore Med Ctr-Einstein Campus, NY (page 100), Montefiore Med Ctr-Moses Campus, NY (page 100); **Address:** 1575 Blondell Ave Fl 2 - Ste 125, Bronx, NY 10461; **Phone:** 718-405-8240; **Board Cert:** Surgery 2007; **Med School:** Georgetown Univ 1999; **Resid:** Surgery, Northwestern Meml Hosp 2006; **Fellow:** Surgical Oncology, Meml Sloan Kettering Cancer Ctr 2008

Kinkhabwala, Milan M MD (S) - **Spec Exp:** Transplant-Liver; Hepatobiliary Surgery; Liver & Biliary Surgery; Liver & Biliary Cancer; **Hospital:** Montefiore Med Ctr-Moses Campus, NY (page 100), Montefiore Med Ctr-Einstein Campus, NY (page 100); **Address:** 111 E 210th St, Bronx, NY 10467; **Phone:** 718-920-6659; **Board Cert:** Surgery 2004; **Med School:** Cornell Univ-Weill Med Coll 1989; **Resid:** Surgery, NY Presby/Weil Cornell 1994; **Fellow:** Hepatobiliary Surgery, UCLA Med Ctr; **Fac Appt:** Prof S, Albert Einstein Coll Med

Libutti, Steven K MD (S) - **Spec Exp:** Liver Cancer; Neuroendocrine Tumors; Gastrointestinal Cancer; **Hospital:** Montefiore Med Ctr-Einstein Campus, NY (page 100), Montefiore Med Ctr-Moses Campus, NY (page 100); **Address:** Montefiore-Einstein Ctr for Cancer Care, 1521 Jarret Pl, Bronx, NY 10461; **Phone:** 718-862-8840; **Board Cert:** Surgery 2004; **Med School:** Columbia P&S 1990; **Resid:** Surgery, Columbia Presby Med Ctr 1995; **Fellow:** Surgical Oncology, Natl Cancer Inst 1996; **Fac Appt:** Prof S, Albert Einstein Coll Med

Sas, Norman S MD (S) - **Spec Exp:** Breast Cancer; Laparoscopic Surgery; Hernia; **Hospital:** Montefiore Med Ctr-Moses Campus, NY (page 100), Lawrence Hosp Ctr; **Address:** 3220 Fairfield Ave, Riverdale, NY 10463-3240; **Phone:** 718-549-0700; **Board Cert:** Surgery 2009; **Med School:** NY Med Coll 1974; **Resid:** Surgery, Montefiore Med Ctr 1978; **Fac Appt:** Asst Clin Prof S, Albert Einstein Coll Med

Shamamian, Peter MD (S) - **Spec Exp:** Pancreatic Cancer; Gastrointestinal Cancer; **Hospital:** Montefiore Med Ctr-Moses Campus, NY (page 100), Montefiore Med Ctr-Einstein Campus, NY (page 100); **Address:** 3400 Bainbridge St Fl 4, Bronx, NY 10467; **Phone:** 718-920-4089; **Board Cert:** Surgery 2005; **Med School:** UMDNJ-RW Johnson Med Sch 1989; **Resid:** Surgery, NYU Med Ctr 1995; **Fellow:** Surgical Oncology, Natl Inst Hlth 1993; **Fac Appt:** Prof S, Albert Einstein Coll Med

Thoracic & Cardiac Surgery

D'Alessandro, David A MD (T&CS) - **Spec Exp:** Cardiac Surgery; Transplant-Heart; Mechanical Assist Devices; **Hospital:** Montefiore Med Ctr-Moses Campus, NY (page 100), Montefiore Med Ctr-Einstein Campus, NY (page 100); **Address:** 3400 Bainbridge Ave, MAP Bldg - Fl 5th, Bronx, NY 10467; **Phone:** 718-920-6515; **Board Cert:** Surgery 2004; Thoracic Surgery 2006; **Med School:** Columbia P&S 1997; **Resid:** Surgery, NY Presby-Columbia Med Ctr 2002; Thoracic Surgery, NY Presby-Columbia Med Ctr 2004; **Fac Appt:** Asst Prof TS, Albert Einstein Coll Med

DeRose Jr, Joseph J MD (T&CS) - **Spec Exp:** Robotic Cardiac Surgery; Minimally Invasive Cardiac Surgery; Aortic Surgery; Mitral Valve Surgery; **Hospital:** Montefiore Med Ctr-Einstein Campus, NY (page 100), Montefiore Med Ctr-Moses Campus, NY (page 100); **Address:** Montefiore-Weiler Medical Ctr, Dept Cardiothoracic Surgery, 1575 Blondell Ave, Ste 125, Bronx, NY 10461; **Phone:** 718-405-8371; **Board Cert:** Thoracic Surgery 2002; **Med School:** Columbia P&S 1993; **Resid:** Surgery, Columbia Presby Med Ctr 1999; **Fellow:** Cardiothoracic Surgery, Columbia Presby Med Ctr 2001; **Fac Appt:** Assoc Prof TS, Albert Einstein Coll Med

Goldstein, Daniel J MD (T&CS) - **Spec Exp:** Transplant-Heart; **Hospital:** Montefiore Med Ctr-Moses Campus, NY (page 100); **Address:** 3400 Bainbridge Avenue MAP-5, Bronx, NY 10467; **Phone:** 718-920-2144; **Board Cert:** Thoracic Surgery 2010; **Med School:** Mount Sinai Sch Med 1991; **Resid:** Surgery, Columbia Presby Med Ctr 1997; **Fellow:** Cardiothoracic Surgery, Columbia Presby Med Ctr 1999

Keller, Steven M MD (T&CS) - **Spec Exp:** Lung Cancer; Esophageal Cancer; Mediastinal Tumors; Hyperhidrosis-Palmar; **Hospital:** Montefiore Med Ctr-Moses Campus, NY (page 100), Montefiore Med Ctr-Einstein Campus, NY (page 100); **Address:** Montefiore-Einstein Medical Ctr, 1575 Blondell Ave, Ste 125, Bronx, NY 10461; **Phone:** 718-405-8378; **Board Cert:** Thoracic Surgery 2007; **Med School:** Albany Med Coll 1977; **Resid:** Surgery, Mount Sinai Hosp 1985; Thoracic Surgery, Mem Sloan Kettering Cancer Ctr 1987; **Fellow:** Surgical Oncology, NIH/National Cancer Inst 1983; **Fac Appt:** Prof TS, Albert Einstein Coll Med

Michler, Robert E MD (T&CS) - **Spec Exp:** Heart Valve Surgery; Coronary Artery Surgery; Minimally Invasive Surgery; Atrial Fibrillation; **Hospital:** Montefiore Med Ctr-Moses Campus, NY (page 100), Montefiore Med Ctr-Einstein Campus, NY (page 100); **Address:** Montefiore, Dept Cardio/Thoracic Surgery, Green Medical Arts Pavilion, 3400 Bainbridge Ave, Ste 5, New York, NY 10467; **Phone:** 718-920-2100; **Board Cert:** Thoracic Surgery 2010; **Med School:** Dartmouth Med Sch 1981; **Resid:** Surgery, Columbia Presby Med Ctr 1987; **Fellow:** Cardiothoracic Surgery, Columbia Presby Med Ctr 1989; Congenital Heart Surgery, Boston Children's Hosp 1990; **Fac Appt:** Prof S, Albert Einstein Coll Med

Weinstein, Samuel MD (T&CS) - **Spec Exp:** Pediatric Cardiac Surgery; Congenital Heart Disease-Adult; Transplant-Heart; **Hospital:** Montefiore Med Ctr-Moses Campus, NY (page 100), Montefiore Med Ctr-Einstein Campus, NY (page 100); **Address:** Montefiore Med Ctr, Moses Div, Dept Cardiothoracic Surgery, 3400 Bainbridge Ave Fl 5 - Ste 5A, Bronx, NY 10467; **Phone:** 718-920-7745; **Board Cert:** Surgery 2004; Thoracic Surgery 2007; Congenital Cardiac Surgery 2009; **Med School:** SUNY Stony Brook 1989; **Resid:** Surgery, Columbia Presby Med Ctr 1996; Cardiothoracic Surgery, Columbia Presby Med Ctr 1998; **Fellow:** Pediatric Cardiothoracic Surgery, Chldns Hosp 1999; **Fac Appt:** Assoc Prof TS, Albert Einstein Coll Med

Urology

Ghavamian, Reza MD (U) - **Spec Exp:** Urologic Cancer; Prostate Cancer/Robotic Surgery; Minimally Invasive Surgery; **Hospital:** Montefiore Med Ctr-Moses Campus, NY (page 100); **Address:** MMC Medical Arts Pavilion, 3400 Bainbridge Ave, Bronx, NY 10467; **Phone:** 718-920-8475; **Board Cert:** Urology 2008; **Med School:** Boston Univ 1991; **Resid:** Urology, Univ Mass Med Ctr 1997; **Fellow:** Urologic Oncology, Mayo Clinic 1998; **Fac Appt:** Clin Prof U, Albert Einstein Coll Med

Stein, Mark MD (U) - **Spec Exp:** Incontinence; Impotence; **Hospital:** Beth Israel Med Ctr - Petrie Division (page 94), NY Westchester Sq Med Ctr; **Address:** 3594 E Tremont Ave, Ste 320, Bronx, NY 10465; **Phone:** 718-518-1108; **Board Cert:** Urology 2011; **Med School:** Yale Univ 1984; **Resid:** Surgery, Montefiore Med Ctr 1985; Urology, Montefiore Med Ctr 1990; **Fac Appt:** Asst Prof U, NY Med Coll

Vascular & Interventional Radiology

Cynamon, Jacob MD (VIR) - **Spec Exp:** Peripheral Vascular Disease; Uterine Fibroids; Liver Cancer; Dialysis Access; **Hospital:** Montefiore Med Ctr-Moses Campus, NY (page 100); **Address:** Montefiore Med Ctr, Dept Interventional Radiology, 111 E 210th St, Bronx, NY 10467; **Phone:** 718-920-5729; **Board Cert:** Diagnostic Radiology 1987; Vascular & Interventional Radiology 2004; **Med School:** Albert Einstein Coll Med 1983; **Resid:** Surgery, Montefiore Hosp Med Ctr 1984; Diagnostic Radiology, Montefiore Hosp Med Ctr 1987; **Fellow:** Vascular & Interventional Radiology, New York Hosp-Cornell 1988; **Fac Appt:** Clin Prof Rad, Albert Einstein Coll Med

Vascular Surgery

Lipsitz, Evan C MD (VascS) - **Spec Exp:** Aneurysm-Abdominal & Thoracic Aortic; Endovascular Surgery; Limb Sparing Surgery; Carotid Artery Surgery; **Hospital:** Montefiore Med Ctr-Moses Campus, NY (page 100), Montefiore Med Ctr-Einstein Campus, NY (page 100); **Address:** 111 E 210 St, MAP Bldg - Fl 4, Bronx, NY 10467; **Phone:** 718-920-2016; **Board Cert:** Vascular Surgery 2008; **Med School:** Columbia P&S 1990; **Resid:** Surgery, Columbia Presby Hosp 1996; **Fellow:** Vascular Surgery, Montefiore Med Ctr 1999; **Fac Appt:** Assoc Prof VascS, Albert Einstein Coll Med

Kings (Brooklyn)

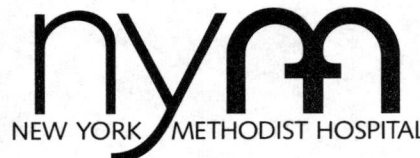

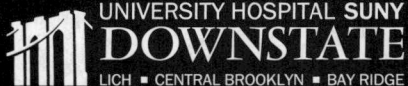

UNIVERSITY HOSPITAL SUNY
DOWNSTATE
LICH ■ CENTRAL BROOKLYN ■ BAY RIDGE

SUNY Downstate Central Brooklyn
University Hospital of Brooklyn

SUNY Downstate Medical Center is Brooklyn's only academic medical center and one of the nation's leading urban medical centers. University Hospital of Brooklyn, Downstate's flagship hospital, is the hub of an educational network of 30 affiliated hospitals.

We provide a full array of services, with over 150 clinical specialties and subspecialties, including:

Advanced Endoscopy • Allergy & Immunology • Cardiovascular Medicine

Dialysis Treatment Center • Emergency Medicine

Endocrinology/Metabolism/Diabetes • Epilepsy Center • Family Practice

Digestive Disease Center • Geriatric Medicine • Hematology & Oncology

Infectious Diseases • Interventional Pain Management

Neurology • Obstetrics/Gynecology • Ophthalmology • Orthopaedics

Otolaryngology • Pediatrics/Pediatric Subspecialties

Pulmonary/Critical Care Medicine • Rehabilitation Medicine

Renal Diseases • Rheumatology • Sleep Disorders Center

Sports Medicine • Stroke Center

Surgery • Transplantation • Urology

Providing advanced care to the borough of Brooklyn at three major locations:

SUNY Downstate Central Brooklyn	**SUNY Downstate Long Island College Hospital**	**SUNY Downstate Bay Ridge**
450 Clarkson Avenue	339 Hicks Street	699 92nd Street
Brooklyn, NY 11203	Brooklyn, NY 11201	Brooklyn, NY 11228
Phone (718) 270-1000	Phone (718) 780-1000	Phone (718) 567-1234

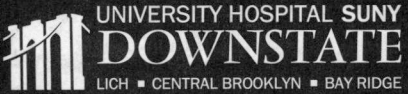

Adolescent Medicine

Hayes, Leslie Allyson MD (AM) - **Spec Exp:** Nutrition; Adolescent Gynecology; **Hospital:** New York Methodist Hosp (page 418); **Address:** New York Methodist Hosp, Dept Peds, 506 6th St, Brooklyn, NY 11215; **Phone:** 718-780-5268; **Board Cert:** Adolescent Medicine 2012; **Med School:** Mount Sinai Sch Med 1986; **Resid:** Pediatrics, Chldns Hosp Natl Med Ctr 1989; **Fellow:** Adolescent Medicine, Univ Hosp-UMDNJ 1991

Allergy & Immunology

Greeley, Norman H MD (A&I) - **Spec Exp:** Asthma; **Hospital:** SUNY Downstate Med Ctr (Univ Hosp of Bklyn) - LICH (page 420); **Address:** 140 Clinton St Fl 1, Brooklyn, NY 11201-4701; **Phone:** 718-624-4465; **Board Cert:** Internal Medicine 1985; Allergy & Immunology 1987; Clinical & Laboratory Immunology 1988; **Med School:** Mexico 1980; **Resid:** Internal Medicine, Long Island Coll Hosp 1985; **Fellow:** Allergy & Immunology, Downstate Med Ctr 1987

Klein, Norman MD (A&I) - **Spec Exp:** Asthma; Food Allergy; Hay Fever; Immune Deficiency; **Hospital:** Brookdale Univ Hosp Med Ctr, Brooklyn Hosp Ctr-Downtown; **Address:** 1648 E 14th St, Brooklyn, NY 11229-1175; **Phone:** 718-627-0183; **Board Cert:** Pediatrics 1981; Allergy & Immunology 1983; **Med School:** SUNY Hlth Sci Ctr 1976; **Resid:** Pediatrics, Brookdale Univ Hosp 1979; **Fellow:** Allergy & Immunology, Montefiore Med Ctr 1980; **Fac Appt:** Asst Prof Ped, SUNY Hlth Sci Ctr

Rao, Yalamanchi K MD (A&I) - **Spec Exp:** Pediatric Allergy & Immunology; **Hospital:** New York Methodist Hosp (page 418); **Address:** 565 Bay Ridge Pkwy, Brooklyn, NY 11209; **Phone:** 718-748-7551; **Board Cert:** Pediatrics 1978; Allergy & Immunology 1989; **Med School:** India 1968; **Resid:** Pediatrics, Long Island Coll Hosp 1977; Allergy & Immunology, Long Island Coll Hosp 1979

Richheimer, Michael Steven MD (A&I) - **Spec Exp:** Asthma; Skin Allergies; Sinus Disorders; Immunodeficiency Disorders; **Hospital:** Stony Brook Univ Med Ctr, New York Methodist Hosp (page 418); **Address:** 1855 Union Blvd, 724 E Park Ave, 1029 Manhattan Ave, Brooklyn, NY 11209; **Phone:** 631-665-6363; **Board Cert:** Allergy & Immunology 2006; **Med School:** Grenada 1985; **Resid:** Internal Medicine, St Joseph's Hosp-Seton Hall Univ 1988; **Fellow:** Allergy & Immunology, SUNY Stony Brook Med Ctr 1990; **Fac Appt:** Assoc Clin Prof A&I, SUNY Stony Brook

Schneider, Arlene T MD (A&I) - **Spec Exp:** Asthma; Sinusitis; Food Allergy; **Hospital:** SUNY Downstate Med Ctr (Univ Hosp of Bklyn) - LICH (page 420); **Address:** Allergy & Asthma Care Ctr, 159 Clinton St, Brooklyn, NY 11201-4601; **Phone:** 718-624-6495; **Board Cert:** Pediatrics 1974; Allergy & Immunology 1975; **Med School:** SUNY Downstate 1968; **Resid:** Pediatrics, LI Coll Hosp 1972; **Fellow:** Allergy & Immunology, LI Coll Hosp 1974; **Fac Appt:** Asst Clin Prof Ped, SUNY Hlth Sci Ctr

Silverman, Bernard A MD (A&I) - **Spec Exp:** Asthma & Allergy; Food Allergy; Urticaria; Atopic Dermatitis; **Hospital:** Mount Sinai Med Ctr (page 102), SUNY Downstate Med Ctr (Univ Hosp of Bklyn) - LICH (page 420); **Address:** 2044 Ocean Ave, Ste A7, Brooklyn, NY 11230; **Phone:** 718-998-5556; **Board Cert:** Pediatrics 1984; Allergy & Immunology 1985; **Med School:** Wayne State Univ 1979; **Resid:** Pediatrics, Brookdale Hosp Med Ctr 1982; **Fellow:** Allergy & Immunology, Montefiore-Weiler Einstein Div 1984; **Fac Appt:** Asst Clin Prof Ped, Mount Sinai Sch Med

Cardiac Electrophysiology

Kassotis, John MD (CE) - **Spec Exp:** Arrhythmias; Atrial Fibrillation; Ventricular Tachycardia Ablation; Congenital Heart Disease; **Hospital:** SUNY Downstate Med Ctr (Univ Hosp of Bklyn) (page 419); **Address:** 450 Clarkson Ave, Box 1199, Brooklyn, NY 11203; **Phone:** 718-270-4147; **Board Cert:** Internal Medicine 2007; Cardiovascular Disease 2008; Cardiac Electrophysiology 2009; **Med School:** Columbia P&S 1990; **Resid:** Internal Medicine, Columbia-Presby Med Ctr 1993; **Fellow:** Cardiovascular Disease, Columbia-Presby Med Ctr 1996; Cardiac Electrophysiology, Columbia-Presby Med Ctr 1997; **Fac Appt:** Assoc Prof Med, SUNY Downstate

Turitto, Gioia MD (CE) - **Spec Exp:** Pacemakers; Defibrillators; Arrhythmias; **Hospital:** New York Methodist Hosp (page 418); **Address:** NY Methodist Hosp, Div Cardiology, 506 Sixth St, Fl 2, Brooklyn, NY 11215; **Phone:** 718-780-3626; **Board Cert:** Internal Medicine 2002; Cardiovascular Disease 2003; Cardiac Electrophysiology 2004; **Med School:** Italy 1981; **Resid:** Internal Medicine, SUNY Downstate Med Ctr 1992; **Fellow:** Cardiovascular Disease, SUNY Downstate Med Ctr 1987; **Fac Appt:** Assoc Prof Med, SUNY Downstate

Wilbur, Sabrina L MD (CE) - **Spec Exp:** Arrhythmias; Pacemakers/Defibrillators; **Hospital:** SUNY Downstate Med Ctr (Univ Hosp of Bklyn) - LICH (page 420), New York Methodist Hosp (page 418); **Address:** 185 Montague St Fl 3, Brooklyn, NY 11201; **Phone:** 718-855-7223; **Board Cert:** Cardiovascular Disease 2005; Cardiac Electrophysiology 2009; **Med School:** Dominican Republic 1987; **Resid:** Internal Medicine, Episcopal Hosp 1991; **Fellow:** Cardiovascular Disease, Episcopal Hosp 1994; Cardiac Electrophysiology, Hosp Univ Penn 1995

Cardiovascular Disease

Borer, Jeffrey S MD (Cv) - **Spec Exp:** Heart Valve Disease; Heart Failure; Nuclear Cardiology; **Hospital:** SUNY Downstate Med Ctr (Univ Hosp of Bklyn) (page 419), NY-Presby/Weill Cornell Med Ctr, NY (page 104); **Address:** SUNY Downstate Med Ctr, Div Cardiology, 445 Lenox Rd, Brooklyn, NY 11226; **Phone:** 212-289-7777; **Board Cert:** Internal Medicine 1973; Cardiovascular Disease 1975; **Med School:** Cornell Univ-Weill Med Coll 1969; **Resid:** Internal Medicine, Mass Genl Hosp 1971; **Fellow:** Cardiovascular Disease, Natl Heart, Lung & Blood Inst 1974; Cardiovascular Disease, Guy's Hosp 1975; **Fac Appt:** Prof Med, SUNY Downstate

Charnoff, Judah A MD (Cv) - **Spec Exp:** Coronary Artery Disease; Congestive Heart Failure; Cholesterol/Lipid Disorders; **Hospital:** Maimonides Med Ctr (page 98), Beth Israel Med Ctr- Kings Hwy Div (page 94); **Address:** 1262 Ocean Pkwy, Brooklyn, NY 11230-5102; **Phone:** 718-859-5843; **Board Cert:** Internal Medicine 1987; Cardiovascular Disease 2005; **Med School:** NYU Sch Med 1984; **Resid:** Internal Medicine, Brookdale Hosp 1987; **Fellow:** Cardiovascular Disease, Maimonides Med Ctr 1989; **Fac Appt:** Asst Prof Med, SUNY Downstate

Dilmanian, Hajir E MD (Cv) - **Spec Exp:** Echocardiography; Diagnostic Problems; **Hospital:** New York Methodist Hosp (page 418); **Address:** NY Methodist Hosp, Div Cardiology, 506 6th Ave Fl 2, Brooklyn, NY 11215; **Phone:** 718-780-7830; **Board Cert:** Internal Medicine 2004; Cardiovascular Disease 2007; **Med School:** SUNY Downstate 2001; **Resid:** Internal Medicine, NYU Med Ctr 2004; **Fellow:** Cardiovascular Disease, Westchester Med Ctr 2007

Feit, Alan MD (Cv) - **Spec Exp:** Interventional Cardiology; **Hospital:** SUNY Downstate Med Ctr (Univ Hosp of Bklyn) (page 419); **Address:** SUNY, Dept Cardiology, 450 Clarkson Ave, Box 1199, Brooklyn, NY 11203-2012; **Phone:** 718-270-2631; **Board Cert:** Internal Medicine 1978; Cardiovascular Disease 1981; Interventional Cardiology 2009; **Med School:** Columbia P&S 1975; **Resid:** Internal Medicine, Roosevelt Hosp 1978; **Fellow:** Cardiovascular Disease, Roosevelt Hosp Ctr 1980; **Fac Appt:** Prof Med, SUNY Downstate

Gelbfish, Joseph S MD (Cv) - **Spec Exp:** Preventive Cardiology; Heart Valve Disease; **Hospital:** New York Methodist Hosp (page 418), NY-Presby/Columbia Univ Med Ctr, NY (page 104); **Address:** 2500 Avenue I, Brooklyn, NY 11210; **Phone:** 718-951-0100; **Board Cert:** Internal Medicine 1986; Cardiovascular Disease 1989; **Med School:** NYU Sch Med 1980; **Resid:** Surgery, Maimonides Medical Ctr 1984; Internal Medicine, Maimonides Medical Ctr 1985; **Fellow:** Cardiovascular Disease, Maimonides Medical Ctr 1988; Cardiovascular Disease, Beth Israel 1989

Gelles, Jeremiah MD (Cv) - **Spec Exp:** Heart Failure; Hypertension; Arrhythmias; Preventive Cardiology; **Hospital:** New York Methodist Hosp (page 418), Maimonides Med Ctr (page 98); **Address:** 263 7th Ave, Ste 5H, Brooklyn, NY 11215-3690; **Phone:** 718-832-1818; **Board Cert:** Internal Medicine 1972; Cardiovascular Disease 1975; **Med School:** NYU Sch Med 1966; **Resid:** Internal Medicine, Mount Sinai Hosp 1970; Internal Medicine, Montefiore Med Ctr 1969; **Fellow:** Cardiovascular Disease, Mount Sinai Hosp 1971; Cardiac Electrophysiology, Columbia Presby Med Ctr 1973; **Fac Appt:** Asst Clin Prof Med, Cornell Univ-Weill Med Coll

Greengart, Alvin MD (Cv) - **Spec Exp:** Echocardiography; Non-Invasive Cardiology; **Hospital:** Maimonides Med Ctr (page 98); **Address:** Maimonides Med Ctr, Dept Cardiology, 4802 Tenth Ave, Brooklyn, NY 11219; **Phone:** 718-283-6257; **Board Cert:** Internal Medicine 1977; Cardiovascular Disease 1979; **Med School:** Mount Sinai Sch Med 1974; **Resid:** Internal Medicine, Brookdale Med Ctr 1977; **Fellow:** Cardiovascular Disease, Brookdale Med Ctr 1979

Gupta, Prem MD (Cv) - **Spec Exp:** Heart Valve Disease; Congestive Heart Failure; Atrial Fibrillation; **Hospital:** Maimonides Med Ctr (page 98); **Address:** 4709 Fort Hamilton Pkwy, Brooklyn, NY 11219-2927; **Phone:** 718-633-4244; **Board Cert:** Internal Medicine 1971; Cardiovascular Disease 1973; **Med School:** India 1964; **Resid:** Internal Medicine, VA Med Ctr 1968; Internal Medicine, VA Med Ctr 1969; **Fellow:** Cardiovascular Disease, VA Med Ctr 1971; **Fac Appt:** Clin Prof Med, SUNY Downstate

Hanley, Gerard MD (Cv) - **Hospital:** Beth Israel Med Ctr- Kings Hwy Div (page 94), New York Methodist Hosp (page 418); **Address:** 3131 Kings Hwy, Ste B1, Brooklyn, NY 11234; **Phone:** 718-421-1212; **Board Cert:** Internal Medicine 1989; **Med School:** SUNY Stony Brook 1984; **Resid:** Internal Medicine, Univ Hosp 1987; **Fellow:** Cardiovascular Disease, Univ Hosp 1990; Cardiovascular Disease, Westchester Co Med Ctr 1991

Heitner, John F MD (Cv) - **Spec Exp:** Nuclear Cardiology; Cardiac MRI; **Hospital:** New York Methodist Hosp (page 418); **Address:** Div Cardiology, 506 Sixth St, Brooklyn, NY 11215; **Phone:** 718-780-5037; **Board Cert:** Cardiovascular Disease 2004; **Med School:** Albert Einstein Coll Med 1997; **Resid:** Internal Medicine, Duke Univ Hosps 2000; **Fellow:** Cardiovascular Disease, Emory Univ Hosp 2002; Cardiovascular Disease, Duke Univ Hosps 2004

Hollander, Gerald MD (Cv) - **Spec Exp:** Coronary Artery Disease; Heart Failure; **Hospital:** Maimonides Med Ctr (page 98); **Address:** 4802 10th Ave, Professional Bldg, Div Cardiology, Brooklyn, NY 11219-2844; **Phone:** 718-283-7643; **Board Cert:** Internal Medicine 1976; Cardiovascular Disease 1979; **Med School:** SUNY Downstate 1973; **Resid:** Internal Medicine, Brookdale Hosp 1976; **Fellow:** Cardiovascular Disease, Brookdale Hosp 1978; **Fac Appt:** Clin Prof Med, SUNY Hlth Sci Ctr

Kang, Pritpal S MD (Cv) - **Hospital:** Lutheran Med Ctr - Brooklyn; **Address:** 705 86th St, Ste M3, Brooklyn, NY 11228-3625; **Phone:** 718-836-0600; **Board Cert:** Internal Medicine 1979; Cardiovascular Disease 1981; **Med School:** India 1972; **Resid:** Internal Medicine, Methodist Hosp-SUNY Downstate 1978; **Fellow:** Cardiovascular Disease, VA Med Ctr 1980

Kantrowitz, Niki E MD (Cv) - **Spec Exp:** Interventional Cardiology; Congestive Heart Failure; **Hospital:** SUNY Downstate Med Ctr (Univ Hosp of Bklyn) - LICH (page 420), Beth Israel Med Ctr - Petrie Division (page 94); **Address:** 339 Hicks St, Brooklyn, NY 11201; **Phone:** 718-780-4626; **Board Cert:** Internal Medicine 1981; Cardiovascular Disease 1987; Interventional Cardiology 2009; **Med School:** Wayne State Univ 1977; **Resid:** Internal Medicine, Columbia-Presby Med Ctr 1980; **Fellow:** Cardiovascular Disease, Stanford Univ Med Ctr 1983; **Fac Appt:** Assoc Clin Prof Med, NY Med Coll

Kerstein, Joshua MD (Cv) - **Spec Exp:** Atrial Fibrillation; Coronary Artery Disease; Brugada Syndrome; Long QT Syndrome; **Hospital:** Maimonides Med Ctr (page 98); **Address:** Maimonides Med Ctr, Div Cardiology, 4802 10th Ave Fl 4, Brooklyn, NY 11219; **Phone:** 718-283-8614; **Board Cert:** Cardiovascular Disease 2005; Nuclear Cardiology 2002; **Med School:** SUNY Downstate 1989; **Resid:** Internal Medicine, Maimonides Med Ctr 1992; **Fellow:** Cardiovascular Disease, Maimonides Med Ctr 1995; **Fac Appt:** Asst Prof Med, SUNY Downstate

Kleeman, Harris J MD (Cv) - **Spec Exp:** Hypertension; Coronary Artery Disease; **Hospital:** Maimonides Med Ctr (page 98); **Address:** 1660 E 14th St, Brooklyn, NY 11229; **Phone:** 718-375-6969; **Board Cert:** Internal Medicine 1982; Cardiovascular Disease 1985; **Med School:** SUNY Hlth Sci Ctr 1979; **Resid:** Internal Medicine, Staten Island Hosp 1983; **Fellow:** Cardiovascular Disease, Maimonides Med Ctr 1985

Konka, Sudarsanam MD (Cv) - **Hospital:** SUNY Downstate Med Ctr (Univ Hosp of Bklyn) - LICH (page 420), New York Methodist Hosp (page 418); **Address:** 100 Clinton St, Ste 20, Brooklyn, NY 11201; **Phone:** 718-935-9837; **Board Cert:** Internal Medicine 1974; Cardiovascular Disease 1977; **Med School:** India 1970; **Resid:** Internal Medicine, Long Island Coll Hosp 1974; **Fellow:** Cardiovascular Disease, Nassau County Med Ctr 1975; Cardiovascular Disease, Long Island Coll Hosp 1976

Moskovits, Norbert MD (Cv) - **Spec Exp:** Heart Failure; Coronary Artery Disease; Cardiac Catheterization; Cholesterol/Lipid Disorders; **Hospital:** Maimonides Med Ctr (page 98); **Address:** Maimonides Med Ctr, Div Cardiology, 4802 10 Ave Fl 4, Brooklyn, NY 11219; **Phone:** 718-283-7948; **Board Cert:** Internal Medicine 2002; Cardiovascular Disease 2005; **Med School:** Germany 1986; **Resid:** Internal Medicine, Maimonides Med Ctr 1992; **Fellow:** Cardiovascular Disease, Beth Israel Med Ctr 1995; **Fac Appt:** Asst Prof Med, Mount Sinai Sch Med

Paiusco, A Dino MD (Cv) - **Spec Exp:** Preventive Cardiology; **Hospital:** Beth Israel Med Ctr- Kings Hwy Div (page 94), New York Methodist Hosp (page 418); **Address:** Univ Heart Associates, 3131 Kings Hwy, Ste A7, Brooklyn, NY 11234; **Phone:** 718-998-2323; **Board Cert:** Internal Medicine 1989; **Med School:** Mexico 1984; **Resid:** Internal Medicine, Univ Hosp 1989; **Fellow:** Cardiovascular Disease, SUNY Hlth Sci Ctr 1992

Prabhu, H Sudhakar MD (Cv) - **Spec Exp:** Echocardiography; Nuclear Cardiology; **Hospital:** SUNY Downstate Med Ctr (Univ Hosp of Bklyn) - LICH (page 420), Lutheran Med Ctr - Brooklyn; **Address:** 6999 92nd St, Brooklyn, NY 11228; **Phone:** 718-833-2620; **Board Cert:** Internal Medicine 1978; Cardiovascular Disease 1981; Nuclear Cardiology 2006; Echocardiography 2008; **Med School:** India 1971; **Resid:** Internal Medicine, LI Coll Hosp 1976; **Fellow:** Cardiovascular Disease, LI Coll Hosp 1978; **Fac Appt:** Clin Prof Med, SUNY Downstate

Traube, Charles MD (Cv) - **Hospital:** Beth Israel Med Ctr- Kings Hwy Div (page 94); **Address:** 2270 Kimball St, Ste 210, Brooklyn, NY 11234; **Phone:** 718-692-2700; **Board Cert:** Internal Medicine 1978; Cardiovascular Disease 1981; **Med School:** Albert Einstein Coll Med 1975; **Resid:** Internal Medicine, Brookdale Hosp 1978; **Fellow:** Cardiovascular Disease, Brookdale Hosp 1980; **Fac Appt:** Asst Clin Prof Med, Albert Einstein Coll Med

Wein, Paul K MD (Cv) - **Spec Exp:** Preventive Cardiology; Hypertension; Cholesterol/Lipid Disorders; Coronary Artery Disease; **Hospital:** Beth Israel Med Ctr- Kings Hwy Div (page 94), Long Island Jewish Med Ctr (page 106); **Address:** 3131 Kings Hwy, Ste D6, Brooklyn, NY 11234-2642; **Phone:** 718-338-2283; **Board Cert:** Internal Medicine 1979; Cardiovascular Disease 1983; **Med School:** SUNY Hlth Sci Ctr 1976; **Resid:** Internal Medicine, Norwalk Hosp 1979; **Fellow:** Cardiovascular Disease, LI Jewish Medical Ctr 1981

Zaloom, Robert MD (Cv) - **Spec Exp:** Cardiac Catheterization; Angiography-Coronary; Nutrition; **Hospital:** Lutheran Med Ctr - Brooklyn, Lenox Hill Hosp (page 106); **Address:** 217 Ovington Ave, Brooklyn, NY 11209-1204; **Phone:** 718-238-0098; **Board Cert:** Internal Medicine 1986; Cardiovascular Disease 1989; **Med School:** France 1983; **Resid:** Internal Medicine, Lutheran Med Ctr 1986; **Fellow:** Cardiovascular Disease, Univ Hosp 1988

Child & Adolescent Psychiatry

Engel, Lenore MD (ChAP) - **Hospital:** Kings County Hosp Ctr, SUNY Downstate Med Ctr (Univ Hosp of Bklyn) (page 419); **Address:** 115 Henry St, Ste 1G, Brooklyn, NY 11201-2562; **Phone:** 718-855-8911; **Board Cert:** Psychiatry 1983; Child & Adolescent Psychiatry 1985; Forensic Psychiatry 2008; **Med School:** SUNY Downstate 1978; **Resid:** Psychiatry, Kings Co Hosp 1982; **Fellow:** Child & Adolescent Psychiatry, SUNY Downstate 1984; **Fac Appt:** Asst Clin Prof Psyc, SUNY Downstate

Holzer, Barry D MD (ChAP) - **Spec Exp:** ADD/ADHD; Behavioral Disorders; Bipolar/Mood Disorders; **Address:** 2350 Ocean Ave, Ste 2J, Brooklyn, NY 11229; **Phone:** 718-743-7600; **Board Cert:** Psychiatry 1990; **Med School:** Albert Einstein Coll Med 1984; **Resid:** Internal Medicine, Maimonides Med Ctr 1985; **Fellow:** Psychiatry, Hillside Hosp-LIJ 1988; Child & Adolescent Psychiatry, Schneider Chldns Hosp-LIJ 1990

Child Neurology

Cracco, Joan B MD (ChiN) - **Spec Exp:** Spina Bifida; Epilepsy; Neurophysiology; **Hospital:** SUNY Downstate Med Ctr (Univ Hosp of Bklyn) (page 419), Kings County Hosp Ctr; **Address:** SUNY Downstate Med Ctr, 450 Clarkson Ave, Box 118, Brooklyn, NY 11203-2056; **Phone:** 718-270-2042; **Board Cert:** Pediatrics 1968; Neurology 1972; Clinical Neurophysiology 2011; **Med School:** UMDNJ-NJ Med Sch, Newark 1963; **Resid:** Pediatrics, Mayo Clinic 1966; Neurology, Thomas Jefferson Univ Hosp 1969; **Fac Appt:** Prof N, SUNY Hlth Sci Ctr

Pavlakis, Steven G MD (ChiN) - **Spec Exp:** Cerebrovascular Disease-Pediatric; Stroke; ADD/ADHD; Neurogenetics; **Hospital:** Maimonides Med Ctr (page 98), Mount Sinai Med Ctr (page 102); **Address:** Pediatric Faculty Practice- Neurology, 977 48th St, Brooklyn, NY 11219; **Phone:** 718-283-8260; **Board Cert:** Pediatrics 1985; Child Neurology 1987; Neurodevelopmental Disabilities 2011; **Med School:** Brown Univ 1979; **Resid:** Pediatrics, Columbia-Presby Med Ctr 1981; **Fellow:** Pediatric Neurology, Columbia-Presby Med Ctr 1984; **Fac Appt:** Prof N, Mount Sinai Sch Med

Schubert, Romaine MD (ChiN) - **Spec Exp:** Epilepsy/Seizure Disorders; Developmental Disorders; Tourette's Syndrome; **Hospital:** New York Methodist Hosp (page 418); **Address:** 263 7th Ave, Ste 4A, Brooklyn, NY 11215; **Phone:** 718-246-8590; **Board Cert:** Child Neurology 1991; Pediatrics 2003; Clinical Neurophysiology 2010; Neurodevelopmental Disabilities 2002; **Med School:** Germany 1984; **Resid:** Pediatrics, SUNY Downstate/Kings Co Med Ctr 1987; **Fellow:** Child Neurology, SUNY Downstate/Kings Co Med Ctr 1990; **Fac Appt:** Asst Clin Prof Ped, Cornell Univ-Weill Med Coll

Clinical Genetics

Gilbert, Fred MD (CG) - **Spec Exp:** Cancer Genetics; Prenatal Diagnosis; **Hospital:** NY-Presby/Weill Cornell Med Ctr, NY (page 104); **Address:** 240 Willoughby St, Brooklyn, NY 11201; **Phone:** 718-250-6911; **Board Cert:** Clinical Genetics 1982; Clinical Cytogenetics 1982; **Med School:** Albert Einstein Coll Med 1966; **Resid:** Internal Medicine, Barnes Hosp 1968; Internal Medicine, Natl Inst Hlth 1971; **Fellow:** Clinical Genetics, Yale-New Haven Hosp 1974; **Fac Appt:** Assoc Prof Ped, Cornell Univ-Weill Med Coll

Colon & Rectal Surgery

Asarian, Armand P MD (CRS) - **Spec Exp:** Colon Cancer; Breast Cancer; **Hospital:** Brooklyn Hosp Ctr-Downtown; **Address:** Brooklyn Hosp Ctr, 121 DeKalb Ave, Dept Surg, Brooklyn, NY 11201; **Phone:** 718-250-6088; **Board Cert:** Surgery 2005; Colon & Rectal Surgery 2009; **Med School:** SUNY Downstate 1991; **Resid:** Surgery, Brooklyn Hosp Ctr 1996; **Fellow:** Colon & Rectal Surgery, Baylor Univ Med Ctr 1997; **Fac Appt:** Asst Clin Prof S, Cornell Univ-Weill Med Coll

Fleischer, Marian MD (CRS) - **Spec Exp:** Colonoscopy; Colon & Rectal Cancer; Pelvic & Perineal Surgery; Pelvic Organ Prolapse Repair; **Hospital:** Maimonides Med Ctr (page 98), St. John's Riverside Hosp-Andrus Pavil; **Address:** 9707 4 Ave, Brooklyn, NY 11209-8129; **Phone:** 718-836-3603; **Board Cert:** Colon & Rectal Surgery 1984; **Med School:** Italy 1972; **Resid:** Surgery, Maimonides Med Ctr 1981; Colon & Rectal Surgery, Baltimore Med Ctr 1982

Lacqua, Frank MD (CRS) - **Spec Exp:** Colonoscopy; Colon Cancer; Anal Disorders & Reconstruction; **Hospital:** Lutheran Med Ctr - Brooklyn; **Address:** 1220 Avenue P, Brooklyn, NY 11229; **Phone:** 718-376-1004; **Board Cert:** Colon & Rectal Surgery 2011; Surgery 2009; **Med School:** SUNY Buffalo 1985; **Resid:** Surgery, St Lukes-Roosevelt Hosp 1990; **Fellow:** Colon & Rectal Surgery, Univ Tex Hlth Sci Ctr 1991

Dermatology

Baldwin, Hilary MD (D) - **Spec Exp:** Acne & Rosacea; Cosmetic Dermatology; **Hospital:** SUNY Downstate Med Ctr (Univ Hosp of Bklyn) (page 419), Kings County Hosp Ctr; **Address:** 142 Joralemon St, Brooklyn, NY 11201; **Phone:** 718-797-3340; **Board Cert:** Dermatology 1988; **Med School:** Boston Univ 1984; **Resid:** Dermatology, NYU Med Ctr 1988; **Fac Appt:** Assoc Prof D, SUNY Downstate

Berry, Richard MD (D) - **Spec Exp:** Skin Cancer; Hair Removal-Laser; Botox Therapy; **Hospital:** SUNY Downstate Med Ctr (Univ Hosp of Bklyn) (page 419); **Address:** 2820 Ocean Pkwy, Brooklyn, NY 11235-7958; **Phone:** 718-996-3000; **Board Cert:** Dermatology 1978; **Med School:** SUNY Hlth Sci Ctr 1974; **Resid:** Internal Medicine, Roosevelt Hosp 1975; Dermatology, SUNY Downstate Med Ctr 1978; **Fac Appt:** Asst Clin Prof D, SUNY Hlth Sci Ctr

Biro, David MD/PhD (D) - **Spec Exp:** Mohs' Surgery; Skin Laser Surgery; Cosmetic Dermatology; **Hospital:** SUNY Downstate Med Ctr (Univ Hosp of Bklyn) (page 419); **Address:** 9921 4th Ave Fl 1, Brooklyn, NY 11209-8347; **Phone:** 718-833-7616; **Board Cert:** Dermatology 2004; **Med School:** Columbia P&S 1991; **Resid:** Dermatology, SUNY Hlth Sci Ctr 1995; **Fac Appt:** Asst Clin Prof D, SUNY Hlth Sci Ctr

Brancaccio, Ronald R MD (D) - **Spec Exp:** Contact Dermatitis; Skin Laser Surgery; Cosmetic Dermatology; **Hospital:** Lutheran Med Ctr - Brooklyn, NYU Langone Med Ctr (page 108); **Address:** Skin Inst NY, 7901 4 Ave, Brooklyn, NY 11209-3957; **Phone:** 718-491-5800; **Board Cert:** Dermatology 1977; **Med School:** Geo Wash Univ 1972; **Resid:** Dermatology, Univ Oregon Hlth Sci Ctr 1976; **Fellow:** Tropical Medicine, Univ Sao Paulo 1976; **Fac Appt:** Clin Prof D, NYU Sch Med

Danziger, Stephen MD (D) - **Spec Exp:** Skin Cancer & Moles; Acne & Rosacea; Psoriasis/Eczema; Warts; **Hospital:** New York Methodist Hosp (page 418), SUNY Downstate Med Ctr (Univ Hosp of Bklyn) - LICH (page 420); **Address:** 20 Plaza St E, Ste A17, Brooklyn, NY 11238; **Phone:** 718-638-3640; **Board Cert:** Dermatology 1975; **Med School:** SUNY Downstate 1968; **Resid:** Internal Medicine, St. Luke's - Roosevelt Hosp Ctr 1969; Dermatology, SUNY Downstate Med Ctr/Kings County Med Ctr 1974; **Fac Appt:** Asst Clin Prof D, SUNY Downstate

Deitz, Marcia MD (D) - **Spec Exp:** Acne; Psoriasis; Warts; Eczema; **Hospital:** Coney Island Hosp; **Address:** 1486 Ocean Pkwy, Brooklyn, NY 11230-6453; **Phone:** 718-627-3024; **Board Cert:** Dermatology 1984; **Med School:** SUNY Downstate 1980; **Resid:** Internal Medicine, Brookdale Hosp 1981; Dermatology, NY Med Coll Affil Hosps 1984; **Fac Appt:** Asst Clin Prof Med, NY Coll Osteo Med

Feldman, Philip MD (D) - **Spec Exp:** Acne; Eczema; Skin Tumors; **Hospital:** SUNY Downstate Med Ctr (Univ Hosp of Bklyn) - LICH (page 420); **Address:** 142 Joralemon St, Ste 4B, Brooklyn, NY 11201-4709; **Phone:** 718-237-0404; **Board Cert:** Dermatology 1970; **Med School:** Switzerland 1963; **Resid:** Dermatology, NY Presby Hosp/Columbia 1967; **Fac Appt:** Asst Clin Prof D, SUNY Downstate

Glick, Sharon A MD (D) - **Spec Exp:** Pediatric Dermatology; **Hospital:** SUNY Downstate Med Ctr (Univ Hosp of Bklyn) (page 419), Kings County Hosp Ctr; **Address:** SUNY Downstate Med Ctr, Dept Dermatology, 450 Clarkson Ave, Box 46, Brooklyn, NY 11203; **Phone:** 718-270-1230; **Board Cert:** Dermatology 2001; Pediatric Dermatology 2004; **Med School:** Albert Einstein Coll Med 1988; **Resid:** Pediatrics, Yale-New Haven Hosp 1991; Dermatology, Yale-New Haven Hosp 1994; **Fac Appt:** Assoc Prof D, SUNY Downstate

Simon, Steven I MD (D) - **Spec Exp:** Skin Cancer; Botox Therapy; Laser Hair Removal; **Hospital:** SUNY Downstate Med Ctr (Univ Hosp of Bklyn) (page 419), Franklin Hosp (page 106); **Address:** 2270 Kimball St, Brooklyn, NY 11234-5139; **Phone:** 718-253-4550; **Board Cert:** Dermatology 1981; **Med School:** Mexico 1975; **Resid:** Internal Medicine, Brookdale Hosp 1978; Dermatology, Downstate Med Ctr 1981; **Fac Appt:** Assoc Clin Prof D, SUNY Hlth Sci Ctr

Diagnostic Radiology

Amodio, John B MD (DR) - **Spec Exp:** Pediatric Radiology; **Hospital:** Kings County Hosp Ctr, SUNY Downstate Med Ctr (Univ Hosp of Bklyn) (page 419); **Address:** SUNY Downstate Med Ctr, Dept Radiology, 450 Clarkson Ave, Box 1198, Brooklyn, NY 11203; **Phone:** 718-270-1603; **Board Cert:** Diagnostic Radiology 1984; Pediatric Radiology 2005; **Med School:** NY Med Coll 1980; **Resid:** Diagnostic Radiology, Montefiore Med Ctr 1984; **Fellow:** Pediatric Radiology, Columbia-Presby Med Ctr 1985

Garner, Steven Charles MD (DR) - **Spec Exp:** Trauma Radiology; **Hospital:** New York Methodist Hosp (page 418); **Address:** 506 6th St, Brooklyn, NY 11215; **Phone:** 718-780-5870; **Board Cert:** Diagnostic Radiology 1984; **Med School:** Ros Franklin Univ/Chicago Med Sch 1976; **Resid:** Diagnostic Radiology, Mt Sinai Hosp 1983

Lerman, Jay E MD (DR) - **Spec Exp:** Urologic Imaging; Musculoskeletal Imaging; **Address:** Lerman Diagnostic Imaging, 6511 Fort Hamilton Pkwy, Brooklyn, NY 11219; **Phone:** 718-491-4545; **Board Cert:** Diagnostic Radiology 1991; **Med School:** Albert Einstein Coll Med 1986; **Resid:** Diagnostic Radiology, Montefiore Med Ctr 1991; **Fellow:** Cross Sectional Imaging, Thom Jefferson Hosp 1992

Reede, Deborah MD (DR) - **Spec Exp:** Head & Neck Imaging; Chest Radiology; **Hospital:** SUNY Downstate Med Ctr (Univ Hosp of Bklyn) - LICH (page 420); **Address:** 339 Hicks St, Brooklyn, NY 11201; **Phone:** 718-780-1793; **Board Cert:** Diagnostic Radiology 1980; **Med School:** SUNY Upstate Med Univ 1976; **Resid:** Diagnostic Radiology, SUNY Upstate Med Ctr 1979; Diagnostic Radiology, NYU Med Ctr 1980; **Fellow:** Head & Neck Radiology, NYU Med Ctr 1981

Endocrinology, Diabetes & Metabolism

Brickman, Alan MD (EDM) - **Spec Exp:** Diabetes; Thyroid Disorders; Cholesterol/Lipid Disorders; Calcium Disorders; **Hospital:** Maimonides Med Ctr (page 98); **Address:** 1318 52 St, Brooklyn, NY 11219-3802; **Phone:** 718-436-9898; **Board Cert:** Internal Medicine 1979; Endocrinology, Diabetes & Metabolism 1981; **Med School:** Albert Einstein Coll Med 1976; **Resid:** Internal Medicine, Maimonides Med Ctr 1979; **Fellow:** Endocrinology, Diabetes & Metabolism, Yale-New Haven Hosp 1981

Giegerich, Edmund W MD (EDM) - **Spec Exp:** Thyroid Disorders; Diabetes; **Hospital:** New York Methodist Hosp (page 418); **Address:** 263 7th Ave, Ste 5A, Brooklyn, NY 11215; **Phone:** 718-246-8600; **Board Cert:** Internal Medicine 1980; Endocrinology, Diabetes & Metabolism 1983; **Med School:** SUNY Downstate 1977; **Resid:** Internal Medicine, Rhode Island Hosp 1980; **Fellow:** Endocrinology, Diabetes & Metabolism, Mount Sinai Hosp 1982; **Fac Appt:** Assoc Clin Prof Med, SUNY Hlth Sci Ctr

Goldman, Joel M MD (EDM) - **Spec Exp:** Thyroid Disorders; Diabetes; Calcium Disorders; **Hospital:** Brookdale Univ Hosp Med Ctr, Beth Israel Med Ctr- Kings Hwy Div (page 94); **Address:** 1 Brookdale Plaza, rm 101A-SBSI, Brooklyn, NY 11212-3132; **Phone:** 718-240-5378; **Board Cert:** Internal Medicine 1976; Endocrinology, Diabetes & Metabolism 1979; **Med School:** Univ Ariz Coll Med 1973; **Resid:** Internal Medicine, UMDNJ-Newark Affil Hosps 1975; Internal Medicine, Albert Einstein Coll Med 1976; **Fellow:** Endocrinology, Diabetes & Metabolism, NIAMDD-Natl Inst Hlth 1979; **Fac Appt:** Assoc Prof Med, SUNY Downstate

Resta, Christine MD (EDM) - **Spec Exp:** Diabetes; Thyroid Disorders; Osteoporosis; **Hospital:** Maimonides Med Ctr (page 98); **Address:** 984 50th St, Brooklyn, NY 11219; **Phone:** 718-283-8846; **Board Cert:** Internal Medicine 2002; Endocrinology, Diabetes & Metabolism 2005; **Med School:** Albert Einstein Coll Med 1989; **Resid:** Internal Medicine, Montefiore Med Ctr 1992; **Fellow:** Endocrinology, Diabetes & Metabolism, Montefiore Med Ctr 1995; **Fac Appt:** Asst Clin Prof Med, Albert Einstein Coll Med

Silverberg, Arnold MD (EDM) - **Spec Exp:** Thyroid Disorders; Osteoporosis; Diabetes; **Hospital:** Maimonides Med Ctr (page 98); **Address:** 908 48th St, Fl 1, Brooklyn, NY 11219-2918; **Phone:** 718-283-6200; **Board Cert:** Internal Medicine 1968; Endocrinology 1977; **Med School:** Albert Einstein Coll Med 1961; **Resid:** Internal Medicine, Montefiore Hosp Med Ctr 1965; Internal Medicine, Mount Sinai Hosp 1964; **Fellow:** Endocrinology, Diabetes & Metabolism, Mount Sinai Hosp 1968; **Fac Appt:** Assoc Clin Prof Med, Mount Sinai Sch Med

Warman, Jacob MD (EDM) - **Spec Exp:** Pituitary Disorders; Calcium Disorders; Thyroid Disorders; **Hospital:** Brooklyn Hosp Ctr-Downtown; **Address:** 121 DeKalb Ave, Brooklyn, NY 11201; **Phone:** 718-250-8995; **Board Cert:** Internal Medicine 1976; Endocrinology, Diabetes & Metabolism 1979; **Med School:** SUNY Downstate 1973; **Resid:** Internal Medicine, Maimonides Med Ctr 1976; **Fellow:** Endocrinology, Diabetes & Metabolism, Jewish Hosp 1978; **Fac Appt:** Asst Prof Med, SUNY Downstate

Family Medicine

Athanail, Steven MD (FMed) *PCP* - **Spec Exp:** Sports Medicine; **Hospital:** Lutheran Med Ctr - Brooklyn; **Address:** 268 Bay Ridge Pkwy, Ste 1B, Brooklyn, NY 11209; **Phone:** 718-748-7272; **Board Cert:** Family Medicine 2008; **Med School:** Howard Univ 1979; **Resid:** Family Medicine, Montefiore Hosp Med Ctr 1983

Krotowski, Mark MD (FMed) *PCP* - **Spec Exp:** Caribbean Health Care; Hypertension; Diabetes; **Hospital:** Brookdale Univ Hosp Med Ctr, SUNY Downstate Med Ctr (Univ Hosp of Bklyn) (page 419); **Address:** 8923 Avenue A, Brooklyn, NY 11236-1206; **Phone:** 718-385-8181; **Board Cert:** Family Medicine 2008; **Med School:** Israel 1976; **Resid:** Pediatrics, Brookdale Univ Hosp 1977; Family Medicine, Brookdale Univ Hosp 1979; **Fac Appt:** Assoc Clin Prof FMed, SUNY Downstate

Lopez, Clark MD (FMed) *PCP* - **Spec Exp:** Geriatric Care; **Hospital:** New York Methodist Hosp (page 418), Lutheran Med Ctr - Brooklyn; **Address:** 60 Plaza St E, Brooklyn, NY 11238; **Phone:** 718-783-3919; **Board Cert:** Family Medicine 2003; **Med School:** SUNY Downstate 1972; **Resid:** Family Medicine, Kings County Hosp 1976; **Fellow:** Family Medicine, Kings County Hosp 1977; **Fac Appt:** Asst Prof FMed, SUNY Downstate

Moskowitz, George MD (FMed) *PCP* - **Spec Exp:** Geriatric Medicine; Obesity; Preventive Medicine; **Hospital:** Maimonides Med Ctr (page 98), Beth Israel Med Ctr- Kings Hwy Div (page 94); **Address:** 1318 42 St, Brooklyn, NY 11219-1405; **Phone:** 718-436-2496; **Board Cert:** Family Medicine 2005; **Med School:** Belgium 1973; **Resid:** Family Medicine, St Vincents Hosp 1976; Family Medicine, Med Coll S Carolina 1978

Sadovsky, Richard MD (FMed) *PCP* - **Spec Exp:** Preventive Medicine; Diabetes; Hepatitis; Thyroid Disorders; **Hospital:** SUNY Downstate Med Ctr (Univ Hosp of Bklyn) (page 419); **Address:** 450 Clarkson Ave, Box 67, Brooklyn, NY 11203-2012; **Phone:** 718-270-2697; **Board Cert:** Family Medicine 2008; **Med School:** SUNY Hlth Sci Ctr 1974; **Resid:** Family Medicine, SUNY Hosp 1977; **Fac Appt:** Assoc Prof FMed, SUNY Hlth Sci Ctr

Schiowitz, Emanuel DO (FMed) *PCP* - **Hospital:** Maimonides Med Ctr (page 98); **Address:** 1701 59 St, Brooklyn, NY 11204-2254; **Phone:** 718-259-0222; **Board Cert:** Family Medicine 1968; **Med School:** Philadelphia Coll Osteo Med 1963; **Resid:** Family Medicine, Interboro Med Ctr 1964; **Fac Appt:** Asst Clin Prof FMed, NY Coll Osteo Med

Sheridan, Bernadette L MD (FMed) *PCP* - **Spec Exp:** Geriatric Cardiology; Women's Health; Adolescent Medicine; **Hospital:** New York Methodist Hosp (page 418); **Address:** 1222 E 96 St Fl 2, Brooklyn, NY 11236; **Phone:** 718-257-3355; **Board Cert:** Family Medicine 2004; **Med School:** SUNY Buffalo 1979; **Resid:** Family Medicine, Brookdale Hosp 1982

Vincent, Miriam MD/PhD (FMed) *PCP* - **Spec Exp:** Diabetes; Arthritis; Preventive Medicine; Osteoporosis; **Hospital:** SUNY Downstate Med Ctr (Univ Hosp of Bklyn) (page 419), Kings County Hosp Ctr; **Address:** 470 Clarkson Ave, Box 67, Brooklyn, NY 11203-2012; **Phone:** 718-270-2697; **Board Cert:** Family Medicine 2008; **Med School:** SUNY Hlth Sci Ctr 1985; **Resid:** Family Medicine, Univ Hosp 1988; **Fac Appt:** Prof FMed, SUNY Hlth Sci Ctr

Gastroenterology

Erber, William MD (Ge) - **Spec Exp:** Endoscopy; Inflammatory Bowel Disease/Crohn's; Gastrointestinal Cancer; Capsule Endoscopy; **Hospital:** Maimonides Med Ctr (page 98), Beth Israel Med Ctr - Petrie Division (page 94); **Address:** 591 Ocean Pkwy, Brooklyn, NY 11218-5913; **Phone:** 718-972-8500; **Board Cert:** Internal Medicine 1975; Gastroenterology 1979; **Med School:** Ros Franklin Univ/Chicago Med Sch 1967; **Resid:** Internal Medicine, Maimonides Med Ctr 1969; Internal Medicine, Maimonides Med Ctr 1973; **Fellow:** Research, Hadassah Hosp 1972; Gastroenterology, Albert Einstein Coll Med 1975; **Fac Appt:** Asst Clin Prof Med, SUNY Downstate

Gamss, Jeffrey S MD (Ge) - **Spec Exp:** Colonoscopy; **Hospital:** Beth Israel Med Ctr- Kings Hwy Div (page 94); **Address:** 1630 E 14th St, Brooklyn, NY 11229; **Phone:** 718-692-1198; **Board Cert:** Internal Medicine 1986; Gastroenterology 1989; **Med School:** SUNY Downstate 1983; **Resid:** Internal Medicine, Brookdale Hosp 1986; **Fellow:** Gastroenterology, SUNY Downstate 1988

Gettenberg, Gary S MD (Ge) - **Spec Exp:** Gastrointestinal Cancer; Colon Cancer Screening; Gastroesophageal Reflux Disease (GERD); Celiac Disease; **Hospital:** Maimonides Med Ctr (page 98), New York Methodist Hosp (page 418); **Address:** 1630 E 14th St, Brooklyn, NY 11229-1104; **Phone:** 718-339-0391; **Board Cert:** Internal Medicine 1987; Gastroenterology 1989; **Med School:** NY Med Coll 1983; **Resid:** Internal Medicine, Maimonides Med Ctr 1986; **Fellow:** Gastroenterology, Maimonides Med Ctr 1988

Gress, Frank G MD (Ge) - **Spec Exp:** Endoscopy; Pancreatic/Biliary Endoscopy (ERCP); Pancreatic Disease; Barrett's Esophagus; **Hospital:** SUNY Downstate Med Ctr (Univ Hosp of Bklyn) (page 419), VA NY Harbor Hlthcr Sys-Brooklyn Campus; **Address:** SUNY Downstate Medical Center, Digestive Disease Center, 760 Parkside Ave, Brooklyn, NY 11226; **Phone:** 718-270-1113; **Board Cert:** Gastroenterology 2012; **Med School:** Mount Sinai Sch Med 1988; **Resid:** Internal Medicine, Montefiore Med Ctr 1991; **Fellow:** Gastroenterology, SUNY Brooklyn & Meth Hosp 1993; Advanced Endoscopy, Indiana Univ Med Ctr 1994; **Fac Appt:** Prof Med, SUNY Downstate

Grosman, Irwin M MD (Ge) - **Spec Exp:** Colon Cancer Screening; Irritable Bowel Syndrome; Liver Disease; **Hospital:** SUNY Downstate Med Ctr (Univ Hosp of Bklyn) - LICH (page 420); **Address:** 339 Hicks St, Othmer Bldg - Fl 6, Brooklyn, NY 11201-5514; **Phone:** 718-780-1468; **Board Cert:** Internal Medicine 1987; Gastroenterology 1989; **Med School:** SUNY Stony Brook 1984; **Resid:** Internal Medicine, Montefiore Hosp Med Ctr 1987; **Fellow:** Gastroenterology, Montefiore Hosp Med Ctr 1989; **Fac Appt:** Assoc Clin Prof Med, SUNY Hlth Sci Ctr

Gupta, Jagdish MD (Ge) - **Spec Exp:** Colon Cancer; Hepatitis; Peptic Ulcer Disease; **Hospital:** SUNY Downstate Med Ctr (Univ Hosp of Bklyn) - LICH (page 420); **Address:** 207 Berkeley Pl, Brooklyn, NY 11217; **Phone:** 718-638-3150; **Board Cert:** Internal Medicine 1975; Gastroenterology 1977; **Med School:** India 1970; **Resid:** Internal Medicine, LI Coll Hosp 1975; **Fellow:** Gastroenterology, LI Coll Hosp 1977; **Fac Appt:** Asst Clin Prof Med, SUNY Downstate

Iswara, Kadirawelpillai MD (Ge) - **Spec Exp:** Pancreatic/Biliary Endoscopy (ERCP); Colonoscopy; Endoscopy; Hepatitis; **Hospital:** Maimonides Med Ctr (page 98), Coney Island Hosp; **Address:** 2511 Ocean Ave, Ste 104, Brooklyn, NY 11225; **Phone:** 718-615-0400; **Board Cert:** Internal Medicine 1980; Gastroenterology 1975; **Med School:** Sri Lanka 1968; **Resid:** Internal Medicine, Coney Island Hosp 1972; Internal Medicine, Bronx VA Hosp 1973; **Fellow:** Gastroenterology, Maimonides Med Ctr 1976; **Fac Appt:** Asst Clin Prof Med, Mount Sinai Sch Med

Leb, Alvin D MD (Ge) - **Spec Exp:** Endoscopy; **Hospital:** Beth Israel Med Ctr- Kings Hwy Div (page 94); **Address:** 2985 Quentin Rd, Brooklyn, NY 11229; **Phone:** 718-336-2218; **Board Cert:** Internal Medicine 1985; Gastroenterology 1989; **Med School:** SUNY Downstate 1982; **Resid:** Internal Medicine, Brookdale Univ Hosp 1985; **Fellow:** Gastroenterology, Brookdale Univ Hosp 1988

Maizel, Barry MD (Ge) - **Spec Exp:** Endoscopy; Inflammatory Bowel Disease; Liver Disease; **Hospital:** New York Methodist Hosp (page 418), NY Hosp Queens (page 206); **Address:** 90 8th Ave, Brooklyn, NY 11215-1553; **Phone:** 718-622-8255; **Board Cert:** Internal Medicine 1979; Gastroenterology 1981; **Med School:** Italy 1975; **Resid:** Internal Medicine, Jewish Hosp 1978; **Fellow:** Gastroenterology, NY Med Coll-Metropolitan Hosp 1980

Mayer, Ira E MD (Ge) - **Spec Exp:** Inflammatory Bowel Disease/Crohn's; Gastroesophageal Reflux Disease (GERD); Gastrointestinal Motility Disorders; **Hospital:** Maimonides Med Ctr (page 98); **Address:** 575 Kings Hwy, Brooklyn, NY 11223; **Phone:** 718-891-0100; **Board Cert:** Internal Medicine 1978; Gastroenterology 1981; **Med School:** NY Med Coll 1975; **Resid:** Internal Medicine, Metropolitan Hosp Ctr 1978; **Fellow:** Gastroenterology, Emory Univ Hosp 1980; **Fac Appt:** Asst Clin Prof Med, Mount Sinai Sch Med

Notar-Francesco, Vincent J MD (Ge) - **Hospital:** New York Methodist Hosp (page 418); **Address:** 263 7th Ave, Ste 5A, Brooklyn, NY 11215; **Phone:** 718-246-8600; **Board Cert:** Internal Medicine 1989; Gastroenterology 2001; **Med School:** Mount Sinai Sch Med 1986; **Resid:** Internal Medicine, Stony Brook Univ Hosp 1989; **Fellow:** Gastroenterology, SUNY Downstate Med Ctr 1991

Piccione, Paul MD (Ge) - **Hospital:** Lutheran Med Ctr - Brooklyn; **Address:** 560 Bay Ridge Pkwy, Brooklyn, NY 11209-2702; **Phone:** 718-748-5219; **Board Cert:** Internal Medicine 1985; Gastroenterology 1987; **Med School:** Italy 1981; **Resid:** Internal Medicine, Lutheran Med Ctr 1985; **Fellow:** Gastroenterology, St Luke's-Roosevelt Hosp 1986

Shike, Moshe MD (Ge) - **Spec Exp:** Gastrointestinal Cancer; Nutrition & Cancer Prevention; Endoscopy; **Hospital:** Meml Sloan-Kettering Cancer Ctr (page 116); **Address:** 1275 York Ave, New York, NY 10065; **Phone:** 212-639-7230; **Board Cert:** Internal Medicine 1977; Gastroenterology 1981; **Med School:** Israel 1975; **Resid:** Internal Medicine, Mt Auburn Hosp 1977; **Fellow:** Gastroenterology, Toronto Genl Hosp 1981; **Fac Appt:** Prof Med, Cornell Univ-Weill Med Coll

Sohn, Won MD (Ge) - **Spec Exp:** Endoscopy; Pancreatic/Biliary Endoscopy (ERCP); **Hospital:** New York Methodist Hosp (page 418); **Address:** 213-33 39th Ave, Ste 428, Bayside, NY 11361; **Phone:** 718-428-5333; **Board Cert:** Internal Medicine 2010; Gastroenterology 2010; **Med School:** SUNY Downstate 1994; **Resid:** Internal Medicine, Yale New Haven Hosp 1997; **Fellow:** Gastroenterology, NY Presby Hosp 2000

Sorra, Toomas MD (Ge) - **Spec Exp:** Colon & Rectal Cancer; Hepatitis; Gastroesophageal Reflux Disease (GERD); **Hospital:** SUNY Downstate Med Ctr (Univ Hosp of Bklyn) - LICH (page 420); **Address:** 166 Clinton St, Brooklyn, NY 11201-4618; **Phone:** 718-834-0100; **Board Cert:** Internal Medicine 1981; Gastroenterology 1983; **Med School:** Mexico 1975; **Resid:** Internal Medicine, LI Coll Hosp 1980; **Fellow:** Gastroenterology, LI Coll Hosp 1982; **Fac Appt:** Asst Prof Med, SUNY Downstate

Zimbalist, Eliot MD (Ge) - **Spec Exp:** Colon Cancer Screening; Hepatitis C; Irritable Bowel Syndrome; Inflammatory Bowel Disease; **Hospital:** Maimonides Med Ctr (page 98), Lutheran Med Ctr - Brooklyn; **Address:** 452 77 St, Brooklyn, NY 11209-3206; **Phone:** 718-921-5548; **Board Cert:** Internal Medicine 1983; Gastroenterology 1985; **Med School:** Mount Sinai Sch Med 1980; **Resid:** Internal Medicine, Maimonides Med Ctr 1983; **Fellow:** Gastroenterology, Meml Sloan Kettering Cancer Ctr 1985; **Fac Appt:** Assoc Prof Med, Mount Sinai Sch Med

Geriatric Medicine

Baccash, Emil MD (Ger) *PCP* - **Hospital:** New York Methodist Hosp (page 418); **Address:** 20 8th Ave, Brooklyn, NY 11217; **Phone:** 718-622-7000; **Board Cert:** Internal Medicine 1981; Geriatric Medicine 2005; **Med School:** Italy 1978; **Resid:** Internal Medicine, NY Methodist Hosp 1981

Paris, Barbara E MD (Ger) - **Spec Exp:** Preventive Medicine; Frail Elderly; **Hospital:** Maimonides Med Ctr (page 98), Mount Sinai Med Ctr (page 102); **Address:** Maimonides Medical Center, Division of Geriatrics, 4802 10th Ave, Brooklyn, NY 11219; **Phone:** 718-283-7071; **Board Cert:** Internal Medicine 1982; Geriatric Medicine 2008; Hospice & Palliative Medicine 2007; **Med School:** SUNY Downstate 1977; **Resid:** Internal Medicine, St Vincents Hosp 1980; **Fellow:** Geriatric Medicine, Mt Sinai Hosp 1986; **Fac Appt:** Clin Prof Med, Mount Sinai Sch Med

Geriatric Psychiatry

Amin, Ravindra MD (GerPsy) - **Spec Exp:** Alzheimer's Disease; Anxiety Disorders; Depression; Memory Disorders; **Hospital:** SUNY Downstate Med Ctr (Univ Hosp of Bklyn) - LICH (page 420); **Address:** 161 Atlantic Ave, Brooklyn, NY 11201; **Phone:** 718-313-2994; **Board Cert:** Psychiatry 1993; Geriatric Psychiatry 2004; Addiction Psychiatry 2006; **Med School:** India 1985; **Resid:** Psychiatry, Elmhurst Hosp 1992; **Fellow:** Geriatric Psychiatry, Mt Sinai Med Ctr 1994

Cohen, Carl MD (GerPsy) - **Spec Exp:** Alzheimer's Disease; Schizophrenia; Depression in the Elderly; **Hospital:** SUNY Downstate Med Ctr (Univ Hosp of Bklyn) (page 419); **Address:** SUNY Health Science Center Assocs, 370 Lenox Rd, Brooklyn, NY 11226-2206; **Phone:** 718-287-4806; **Board Cert:** Psychiatry 1977; Geriatric Psychiatry 2009; **Med School:** SUNY Buffalo 1971; **Resid:** Psychiatry, NYU Med Ctr 1974; **Fellow:** Community Psychiatry, NYU Med Ctr 1975; **Fac Appt:** Prof Psyc, SUNY Hlth Sci Ctr

Greenberg, Robert M MD (GerPsy) - **Spec Exp:** Electroconvulsive Therapy (ECT); Neuro-Psychiatry; **Hospital:** Lutheran Med Ctr - Brooklyn, Hoboken Univ Med Ctr - Hoboken; **Address:** Lutheran Medical Ctr, 150 55th St, Brooklyn, NY 11220; **Phone:** 718-630-6079; **Board Cert:** Psychiatry 1986; Geriatric Psychiatry 2001; **Med School:** Mount Sinai Sch Med 1978; **Resid:** Psychiatry, New York Hosp-Westchester Div 1983

Rosen, Evelyn MD (GerPsy) - **Hospital:** New York Methodist Hosp (page 418); **Address:** 583 5th St, Brooklyn, NY 11215-3503; **Phone:** 212-813-9410; **Board Cert:** Psychiatry 1992; **Med School:** Mexico 1986; **Resid:** Psychiatry, Univ Hosp 1991; **Fellow:** Geriatric Psychiatry, Univ Hosp 1992

Gynecologic Oncology

Chambers, Joseph MD/PhD (GO) - **Spec Exp:** Uterine Cancer; Pelvic Surgery; **Hospital:** SUNY Downstate Med Ctr (Univ Hosp of Bklyn) - LICH (page 420); **Address:** 97 Amity St, rm H320, Brooklyn, NY 11201-5509; **Phone:** 718-780-2984; **Board Cert:** Obstetrics & Gynecology 2011; Gynecologic Oncology 2011; **Med School:** Georgetown Univ 1977; **Resid:** Obstetrics & Gynecology, Univ Virginia Hosp 1981; **Fellow:** Gynecologic Oncology, Yale-New Haven Hosp 1984; **Fac Appt:** Clin Prof ObG, SUNY Downstate

Economos, Katherine MD (GO) - **Spec Exp:** Ovarian Cancer; Cervical Cancer; Uterine Cancer; Vulvar & Vaginal Cancer; **Hospital:** New York Methodist Hosp (page 418); **Address:** 263 7th Ave, Ste 3A, Brooklyn, NY 11215; **Phone:** 718-780-3090; **Board Cert:** Gynecologic Oncology 2011; Obstetrics & Gynecology 2011; **Med School:** SUNY Downstate 1986; **Resid:** Obstetrics & Gynecology, Maimonides Med Ctr 1990; **Fellow:** Gynecologic Oncology, Univ Texas SW Med Ctr 1993; **Fac Appt:** Assoc Clin Prof ObG, Cornell Univ-Weill Med Coll

Khulpateea, Neekianund MD (GO) - **Spec Exp:** Hysterectomy Alternatives; Gynecologic Cancer; **Hospital:** Maimonides Med Ctr (page 98); **Address:** Maimonides Med Ctr, Div Gyn, 953 49th St Fl 2, Brooklyn, NY 11219-2923; **Phone:** 718-283-7370; **Board Cert:** Obstetrics & Gynecology 1981; **Med School:** Israel 1972; **Resid:** Obstetrics & Gynecology, Meth Hosp 1976; **Fellow:** Gynecologic Oncology, Univ Hosp Downstate 1978; **Fac Appt:** Asst Clin Prof ObG, SUNY Downstate

Serur, Eli MD (GO) - **Spec Exp:** Nutrition & Cancer; Laparoscopic Surgery; Gynecologic Cancer; Minimally Invasive Surgery; **Hospital:** Brooklyn Hosp Ctr-Downtown, Richmond Univ Med Ctr; **Address:** 240 Willoughby St, Ste 3A, Brooklyn, NY 11201; **Phone:** 718-250-8106; **Board Cert:** Obstetrics & Gynecology 2011; Gynecologic Oncology 2011; **Med School:** NYU Sch Med 1985; **Resid:** Obstetrics & Gynecology, Kings County Hosp 1989; **Fellow:** Gynecologic Oncology, Kings County Hosp 1991; **Fac Appt:** Asst Clin Prof ObG, Cornell Univ-Weill Med Coll

Hand Surgery

Caligiuri, Daniel A MD (HS) - **Spec Exp:** Hand & Wrist Surgery; Nerve & Tendon Reconstruction; **Hospital:** SUNY Downstate Med Ctr (Univ Hosp of Bklyn) - LICH (page 420); **Address:** Long Island Coll Hosp, 97 Amity St, Brooklyn, NY 11201; **Phone:** 718-780-4700; **Board Cert:** Orthopaedic Surgery 2005; Hand Surgery 2005; **Med School:** SUNY Downstate 1986; **Resid:** Orthopaedic Surgery, SUNY Downstate 1991; **Fellow:** Hand Surgery, Thomas Jefferson Univ Hosp 1992; **Fac Appt:** Asst Clin Prof OrS, SUNY Downstate

Choueka, Jack MD (HS) - **Spec Exp:** Hand & Upper Extremity Surgery; Rotato Cuff Surgery; Wrist Surgery; Shoulder Surgery; **Hospital:** Maimonides Med Ctr (page 98); **Address:** Maimonedes Orthopedics, 1301 57th St, Brooklyn, NY 11219; **Phone:** 718-283-7362; **Board Cert:** Orthopaedic Surgery 2011; Hand Surgery 2011; **Med School:** SUNY Hlth Sci Ctr 1991; **Resid:** Orthopaedic Surgery, Hosp Joint Diseases 1996; Hand Surgery, Univ Chicago Hosps 1998

Solomon, Ronald MD (HS) - **Hospital:** SUNY Downstate Med Ctr (Univ Hosp of Bklyn) - LICH (page 420), Brooklyn Hosp Ctr-Downtown; **Address:** 142 Joralemon St, Ste 12A, Brooklyn, NY 11201-4742; **Phone:** 718-625-4975; **Board Cert:** Hand Surgery 2004; **Med School:** Univ Rochester 1977; **Resid:** Surgery, NY Med Coll/Metropolitan Hosp 1982; **Fellow:** Hand Surgery, NY Med Coll/ Metropolitan Hosp 1983

Hematology

Dosik, Harvey MD (Hem) - **Spec Exp:** Leukemia & Lymphoma; Anemia; Multiple Myeloma; **Hospital:** New York Methodist Hosp (page 418); **Address:** 506 6th St, Ste 1J, Brooklyn, NY 11215-3609; **Phone:** 718-780-5240; **Board Cert:** Internal Medicine 1970; Hematology 1976; **Med School:** NYU Sch Med 1963; **Resid:** Internal Medicine, Kings County Hosp 1967; **Fellow:** Hematology, Maimonides Med Ctr 1969; **Fac Appt:** Prof Med, Cornell Univ-Weill Med Coll

Hyde, Phyllis MD (Hem) - **Hospital:** SUNY Downstate Med Ctr (Univ Hosp of Bklyn) - LICH (page 420); **Address:** 46 Livingston St, Brooklyn, NY 11201; **Phone:** 718-855-1124; **Board Cert:** Internal Medicine 1983; Hematology 1986; Medical Oncology 1987; **Med School:** SUNY Downstate 1980; **Resid:** Internal Medicine, Columbia-Presby 1983; **Fellow:** Hematology & Oncology, NYU Med Ctr 1986

Infectious Disease

Asnis, Deborah S MD (Inf) - **Spec Exp:** West Nile Virus; AIDS/HIV; Meningitis; **Hospital:** Flushing Hosp Med Ctr; **Address:** 90 Brighton 11th St, Brooklyn, NY 11235; **Phone:** 718-332-7770; **Board Cert:** Internal Medicine 1985; Infectious Disease 1988; **Med School:** Northwestern Univ 1981; **Resid:** Ophthalmology, LI Jewish Hosp 1983; Internal Medicine, LI Jewish Hosp 1985; **Fellow:** Infectious Disease, LI Jewish Hosp 1987; **Fac Appt:** Asst Clin Prof Med, Cornell Univ-Weill Med Coll

Augenbraun, Michael MD (Inf) - **Spec Exp:** AIDS/HIV; Sexually Transmitted Diseases; **Hospital:** SUNY Downstate Med Ctr (Univ Hosp of Bklyn) (page 419); **Address:** 450 Clarkson Ave, Box 56, Brooklyn, NY 11203; **Phone:** 718-270-1432; **Board Cert:** Internal Medicine 1988; Infectious Disease 2010; **Med School:** Univ Rochester 1985; **Resid:** Internal Medicine, North Shore Univ Hosp 1988; Internal Medicine, Meml Sloan Kettering Cancer Ctr 1988; **Fellow:** Infectious Disease, SUNY Downstate Med Ctr 1990; **Fac Appt:** Prof Med, SUNY Downstate

Berkowitz, Leonard B MD (Inf) - **Spec Exp:** AIDS/HIV; **Hospital:** Brooklyn Hosp Ctr-Downtown; **Address:** 121 DeKalb Ave, Ste 5H, Brooklyn, NY 11201-5425; **Phone:** 718-250-6922; **Board Cert:** Internal Medicine 1980; Infectious Disease 1984; **Med School:** SUNY Downstate 1977; **Resid:** Internal Medicine, Kings Co Med Ctr 1981; **Fellow:** Infectious Disease, Kings Co Med Ctr 1983; **Fac Appt:** Asst Clin Prof Med, SUNY Hlth Sci Ctr

Chapnick, Edward MD (Inf) - **Spec Exp:** AIDS/HIV; Travel Medicine; Antibiotic Resistance; **Hospital:** Maimonides Med Ctr (page 98); **Address:** Maimonides Med Ctr, Infectious Disease, 4802 10th Ave, Brooklyn, NY 11219-2844; **Phone:** 718-283-7492; **Board Cert:** Internal Medicine 1988; Infectious Disease 2002; **Med School:** SUNY Downstate 1985; **Resid:** Internal Medicine, Maimonides Med Ctr 1989; **Fellow:** Infectious Disease, Maimonides Med Ctr 1991; **Fac Appt:** Assoc Prof Med, Mount Sinai Sch Med

Cofsky, Richard MD (Inf) - **Hospital:** Brookdale Univ Hosp Med Ctr; **Address:** Brookdale Univ Hosp, 1 Brookdale Plaza, rm 596, Brooklyn, NY 11212-3139; **Phone:** 718-240-5096; **Board Cert:** Internal Medicine 1981; Infectious Disease 1984; **Med School:** Univ MD Sch Med 1978; **Resid:** Internal Medicine, Maimonides Med Ctr 1981; **Fellow:** Infectious Disease, Downstate Med Ctr 1984

Landesman, Sheldon MD (Inf) - **Hospital:** SUNY Downstate Med Ctr (Univ Hosp of Bklyn) (page 419); **Address:** SUNY Downstate, 450 Clarkson Ave, Box 97, Brooklyn, NY 11203; **Phone:** 718-270-3034; **Board Cert:** Internal Medicine 1976; **Med School:** SUNY Downstate 1972; **Resid:** Interventional Cardiology, Tufts-New England Med Ctr 1976; **Fellow:** Research, Baltimore Cancer Rsrch Inst/NCI 1975; Infectious Disease, Tufts-New England Med Ctr 1977

Lutwick, Larry I MD (Inf) - **Spec Exp:** Hepatitis; Infectious Mononucleosis; Epstein-Barr Virus; **Hospital:** VA NY Harbor Hlthcr Sys-Brooklyn Campus, Maimonides Med Ctr (page 98); **Address:** Brooklyn VA Medical Ctr, 800 Poly Pl, rm 12-125, Brooklyn, NY 11209; **Phone:** 718-836-6600 x3728; **Board Cert:** Internal Medicine 1975; Infectious Disease 1976; **Med School:** SUNY Downstate 1972; **Resid:** Internal Medicine, Barnes Hosp-Washington Univ 1974; **Fellow:** Infectious Disease, Barnes Hosp-Washington Univ 1976; **Fac Appt:** Prof Med, SUNY Downstate

Pujol-Morato, Fernando MD (Inf) - **Spec Exp:** AIDS/HIV; **Hospital:** New York Methodist Hosp (page 418); **Address:** 20 8th Ave, Brooklyn, NY 11217; **Phone:** 718-636-7400; **Board Cert:** Internal Medicine 1986; Infectious Disease 1988; **Med School:** Dominican Republic 1979; **Resid:** Internal Medicine, LI College Hosp 1985; **Fellow:** Infectious Disease, LI College Hosp 1987; **Fac Appt:** Asst Prof Med, Cornell Univ-Weill Med Coll

Sepkowitz, Douglas MD (Inf) - **Spec Exp:** AIDS/HIV; Tuberculosis; **Hospital:** SUNY Downstate Med Ctr (Univ Hosp of Bklyn) - LICH (page 420); **Address:** 339 Hicks St, Brooklyn, NY 11201; **Phone:** 718-780-1435; **Board Cert:** Internal Medicine 1982; Infectious Disease 1986; **Med School:** Univ Okla Coll Med 1979; **Resid:** Internal Medicine, Maimonides Medical Ctr 1982; **Fellow:** Infectious Disease, Long Island Coll Hosp 1986

Stein, Alan J MD (Inf) - **Spec Exp:** AIDS/HIV; Travel Medicine; **Hospital:** New York Methodist Hosp (page 418), Brooklyn Hosp Ctr-Downtown; **Address:** 348 13th St, Ste 5F, Brooklyn, NY 11215; **Phone:** 718-369-4850; **Board Cert:** Internal Medicine 1976; Infectious Disease 1978; **Med School:** NY Med Coll 1972; **Resid:** Internal Medicine, Lenox Hill Hosp 1974; Internal Medicine, Metro Hosp Ctr 1976; **Fellow:** Infectious Disease, NYU Med Ctr 1978; **Fac Appt:** Assoc Clin Prof Med, NYU Sch Med

Internal Medicine

Behm, Dutsi MD (IM) *PCP* - **Hospital:** New York Methodist Hosp (page 418), Maimonides Med Ctr (page 98); **Address:** 421 Ocean Pkwy, Ste 2A, Brooklyn, NY 11218-2408; **Phone:** 718-438-8585; **Med School:** Ukraine 1973; **Resid:** Internal Medicine, NY Methodist Hosp 1983

Berman, Sandra MD (IM) *PCP* - **Hospital:** SUNY Downstate Med Ctr (Univ Hosp of Bklyn) - LICH (page 420); **Address:** 100 Clinton St, Brooklyn, NY 11201; **Phone:** 718-797-5339; **Board Cert:** Internal Medicine 2006; **Med School:** Mexico 1979; **Resid:** Internal Medicine, LI Jewish Med Ctr 1996

Bharathan, Thayyullathil MD (IM) *PCP* - **Spec Exp:** Alzheimer's Disease; Dementia; Palliative Care; Pain Management; **Hospital:** New York Methodist Hosp (page 418); **Address:** 263 7th Ave, Ste 4H, Brooklyn, NY 11215-3691; **Phone:** 718-246-8561; **Board Cert:** Internal Medicine 1976; **Med School:** India 1962; **Resid:** Internal Medicine, New York Methodist Hosp 1972; **Fac Appt:** Asst Clin Prof Med, Cornell Univ-Weill Med Coll

Butt, Ahmar A MD (IM) *PCP* - **Spec Exp:** Stroke; Hypertension; Congestive Heart Failure; **Hospital:** Brooklyn Hosp Ctr-Downtown; **Address:** 121 DeKalb Ave, Brooklyn, NY 11201-5465; **Phone:** 718-250-6120; **Board Cert:** Internal Medicine 2005; **Med School:** Pakistan 1983; **Resid:** Internal Medicine, Brooklyn Hosp 1994; **Fac Appt:** Asst Clin Prof Med, Cornell Univ-Weill Med Coll

Cohen, Barry A MD (IM) *PCP* - **Hospital:** Beth Israel Med Ctr- Kings Hwy Div (page 94); **Address:** 151A West End Ave, Brooklyn, NY 11235-4808; **Phone:** 718-934-1222; **Board Cert:** Internal Medicine 1986; **Med School:** Dominican Republic 1982; **Resid:** Internal Medicine, Elmhurst Hosp/Mt Sinai 1986

Ditchek, Alan MD (IM) *PCP* - **Spec Exp:** Chronic Fatigue Syndrome; Diabetes; Lyme Disease; Hypertension; **Hospital:** Beth Israel Med Ctr- Kings Hwy Div (page 94); **Address:** 2516 Ocean Ave, Brooklyn, NY 11229-3916; **Phone:** 718-769-0444; **Board Cert:** Internal Medicine 1986; Infectious Disease 2007; **Med School:** Mexico 1981; **Resid:** Internal Medicine, Luthern Med Ctr 1985; **Fellow:** Infectious Disease, Nassau Co Med Ctr 1986; Infectious Disease, SUNY Downstate 1995; **Fac Appt:** Asst Clin Prof Med, SUNY Hlth Sci Ctr

Ellis, Earl A MD (IM) *PCP* - **Spec Exp:** Geriatric Rehabilitation; **Hospital:** Brooklyn Hosp Ctr-Downtown, SUNY Downstate Med Ctr (Univ Hosp of Bklyn) (page 419); **Address:** 66 Rutland Rd, Brooklyn, NY 11225-5313; **Phone:** 718-282-4412; **Board Cert:** Internal Medicine 1984; Geriatric Medicine 2000; **Med School:** Howard Univ 1980; **Resid:** Internal Medicine, Elmhurst Hosp 1983

Gambarin, Boris L MD/PhD (IM) *PCP* - **Spec Exp:** Cardiovascular Disease; Diabetes; **Hospital:** New York Methodist Hosp (page 418); **Address:** 5923 16th Ave, Brooklyn, NY 11204; **Phone:** 718-259-6122; **Board Cert:** Internal Medicine 2005; **Med School:** Russia 1969; **Resid:** Internal Medicine, Interfaith Med Ctr 1995; **Fac Appt:** Asst Prof Med, Cornell Univ-Weill Med Coll

Grunzweig, Milton J MD (IM) *PCP* - **Hospital:** Brookdale Univ Hosp Med Ctr, Beth Israel Med Ctr - Petrie Division (page 94); **Address:** 2000 Ocean Ave, Brooklyn, NY 11230; **Phone:** 718-769-7900; **Board Cert:** Internal Medicine 1989; **Med School:** SUNY Hlth Sci Ctr 1986; **Resid:** Internal Medicine, Brookdale Hosp 1989

Hsuih, Terence CH MD (IM) *PCP* - **Hospital:** Lutheran Med Ctr - Brooklyn; **Address:** 775 57th St, Brooklyn, NY 11220; **Phone:** 718-439-6163; **Board Cert:** Internal Medicine 2008; **Med School:** Mount Sinai Sch Med 1995; **Resid:** Internal Medicine, New York Hosp 1998

Hyman, Jeffrey S MD (IM) *PCP* - **Hospital:** Staten Island Univ Hosp - North (page 106); **Address:** 8012 3rd Ave, Brooklyn, NY 11209; **Phone:** 718-745-5600; **Board Cert:** Internal Medicine 2007; **Med School:** Mexico 1980; **Resid:** Internal Medicine, Maimonides Med Ctr 1984

Joy, Mark MD (IM) *PCP* - **Spec Exp:** Diabetes; Thyroid Disorders; **Hospital:** VA NY Harbor Hlthcr Sys-Brooklyn Campus; **Address:** 800 Poly Pl, Dept of Medicine, Brooklyn, NY 11209; **Phone:** 718-630-3766; **Board Cert:** Internal Medicine 1983; **Med School:** W VA Univ 1979; **Resid:** Internal Medicine, Mercy Hosp 1982; **Fac Appt:** Asst Clin Prof Med, NY Med Coll

Kaiser, Stephen MD (IM) *PCP* - **Spec Exp:** Diabetes; Hypertension; **Hospital:** Maimonides Med Ctr (page 98); **Address:** 1335 Ocean Pkwy, Brooklyn, NY 11218-5152; **Phone:** 718-382-8900; **Board Cert:** Internal Medicine 1972; **Med School:** SUNY Buffalo 1964; **Resid:** Internal Medicine, Kings County Hosp 1967; **Fellow:** Hematology, Maimonides Med Ctr 1969

Katzenelenbogen, Moshe MD (IM) *PCP* - **Hospital:** Beth Israel Med Ctr- Kings Hwy Div (page 94); **Address:** 3901 Nostrand Ave, Brooklyn, NY 11235; **Phone:** 718-646-1422; **Board Cert:** Internal Medicine 1984; **Med School:** Romania 1980; **Resid:** Internal Medicine, Coney Island Hosp 1984

Kazdin, Hal J MD (IM) *PCP* - **Spec Exp:** Osteoarthritis; Rheumatoid Arthritis; Pain Management; **Hospital:** New York Comm Hosp, Beth Israel Med Ctr- Kings Hwy Div (page 94); **Address:** 90 Brighton 11th St, Brooklyn, NY 11235-5304; **Phone:** 718-332-7770; **Board Cert:** Internal Medicine 1982; **Med School:** Philippines 1977; **Resid:** Internal Medicine, Elmhurst Hosp 1981; **Fellow:** Rheumatology, LI Jewish Hosp 1983

Levey, Robert MD (IM) *PCP* - **Spec Exp:** Chronic Obstructive Lung Disease (COPD); Alzheimer's Disease; **Hospital:** SUNY Downstate Med Ctr (Univ Hosp of Bklyn) - LICH (page 420); **Address:** 349 Henry St Fl 5th, Brooklyn, NY 11201; **Phone:** 718-780-2838; **Board Cert:** Internal Medicine 1977; **Med School:** Univ Mich Med Sch 1970; **Resid:** Internal Medicine, Long Island Coll Hosp 1977

Lu, Bing MD/PhD (IM) *PCP* - **Spec Exp:** Chinese Community Health; Acupuncture; Sinusitis; Irritable Bowel Syndrome; **Hospital:** Maimonides Med Ctr (page 98), SUNY Downstate Med Ctr (Univ Hosp of Bklyn) (page 419); **Address:** Universial Medical Service, 4506 8th Ave, Brooklyn, NY 11220; **Phone:** 718-972-1233; **Board Cert:** Internal Medicine 2007; **Med School:** China 1982; **Resid:** Internal Medicine, Miriam Hosp 1997; **Fac Appt:** Asst Prof Med, SUNY Hlth Sci Ctr

Malik, Asim R MD (IM) *PCP* - **Spec Exp:** Peptic Acid Disorders; **Hospital:** New York Methodist Hosp (page 418); **Address:** 1224 8th Ave, Brooklyn, NY 11215; **Phone:** 718-788-5588; **Board Cert:** Internal Medicine 2004; Gastroenterology 2007; **Med School:** Pakistan 1976; **Resid:** Surgery, New York Methodist Hosp 1978; Internal Medicine, New York Methodist Hosp 1981; **Fellow:** Gastroenterology, Wayne Cnty Genl Hosp 1983

Marush, Arthur MD (IM) *PCP* - **Hospital:** Beth Israel Med Ctr- Kings Hwy Div (page 94); **Address:** 2270 Kimball St, Ste 210, Brooklyn, NY 11234-5139; **Phone:** 718-692-2700; **Board Cert:** Internal Medicine 1981; **Med School:** Albert Einstein Coll Med 1978; **Resid:** Internal Medicine, Brookdale

Sherman, Frederic MD (IM) *PCP* - **Spec Exp:** Cardiovascular Disease; Alzheimer's Disease; **Hospital:** SUNY Downstate Med Ctr (Univ Hosp of Bklyn) - LICH (page 420), Lutheran Med Ctr - Brooklyn; **Address:** 8672 Bay Pkwy, Brooklyn, NY 11214-4102; **Phone:** 718-372-2234; **Board Cert:** Internal Medicine 1976; **Med School:** NY Med Coll 1972; **Resid:** Internal Medicine, Mount Sinai HospLong Island Coll Hosp 1976; **Fellow:** Cardiovascular Disease, Long Island Coll Hosp 1977

Simon, Todd L MD (IM) *PCP* - **Spec Exp:** Preventive Medicine; Asthma; **Hospital:** New York Methodist Hosp (page 418); **Address:** 263 7th Ave, Ste 4H, Brooklyn, NY 11215; **Phone:** 718-246-8561; **Board Cert:** Internal Medicine 2006; **Med School:** NYU Sch Med 1991; **Resid:** Internal Medicine, Mt Sinai Hosp 1994; **Fac Appt:** Assoc Prof Med, Cornell Univ-Weill Med Coll

Tal, Avraham MD (IM) *PCP* - **Spec Exp:** Hypertension; Cholesterol/Lipid Disorders; Diabetes; **Hospital:** Coney Island Hosp; **Address:** 2601 Ocean Pkwy, Ste 4N39, Brooklyn, NY 11235-7745; **Phone:** 718-616-3881; **Board Cert:** Internal Medicine 1983; **Med School:** Italy 1975; **Resid:** Internal Medicine, Kingsbrook Jewish Med Ctr 1979; Internal Medicine, Long Island Coll Hosp 1977

Vieira, Jeffrey MD (IM) *PCP* - **Spec Exp:** Infectious Disease; AIDS/HIV; Chronic Fatigue Syndrome; **Hospital:** SUNY Downstate Med Ctr (Univ Hosp of Bklyn) - LICH (page 420); **Address:** 349 Henry St Fl 5, Brooklyn, NY 11201; **Phone:** 718-857-3237; **Board Cert:** Internal Medicine 1980; **Med School:** NY Med Coll 1977; **Resid:** Internal Medicine, St Elizabeth's Med Ctr 1980; **Fellow:** Infectious Disease, Univ Hosp 1982; **Fac Appt:** Assoc Prof Med, SUNY Downstate

Walfish, Jacob S MD (IM) *PCP* - **Spec Exp:** Gastrointestinal Disorders; Irritable Bowel Syndrome; Diagnostic Problems; **Hospital:** NYU Langone Med Ctr (page 108); **Address:** NYU-Williamsburg, 101 Broadway, Ste 301, Brooklyn, NY 11249; **Phone:** 718-384-5179; **Board Cert:** Internal Medicine 1977; Gastroenterology 1979; **Med School:** Harvard Med Sch 1974; **Resid:** Internal Medicine, Mount Sinai Hosp 1977; **Fellow:** Gastroenterology, Mount Sinai Hosp 1979; **Fac Appt:** Asst Clin Prof Med, NYU Sch Med

Ziemba, David MD (IM) *PCP* - **Hospital:** SUNY Downstate Med Ctr (Univ Hosp of Bklyn) - LICH (page 420); **Address:** 1458 47th St, Brooklyn, NY 11219-2634; **Phone:** 718-438-0600; **Board Cert:** Internal Medicine 1983; **Med School:** SUNY Downstate 1979; **Resid:** Internal Medicine, Coney Island Hosp 1983

Interventional Cardiology

Brener, Sorin MD (IC) - **Spec Exp:** Angioplasty & Stent Placement; **Hospital:** New York Methodist Hosp (page 418); **Address:** New York Methodist Hosp, 506 6th St, Brooklyn, NY 11215; **Phone:** 718-780-7830; **Board Cert:** Internal Medicine 2002; Cardiovascular Disease 2005; Interventional Cardiology 2009; **Med School:** Israel 1984; **Resid:** Internal Medicine, Cleveland Clinic 1992; **Fellow:** Cardiovascular Disease, Cleveland Clinic 1996

Sacchi, Terrence J MD (IC) - **Spec Exp:** Arrhythmias; Cardiac Catheterization; Coronary Angioplasty/Stents; Percutaneous Coronary Intervention; **Hospital:** New York Methodist Hosp (page 418); **Address:** NY Methodist Hospital, 506 6th St, Brooklyn, NY 11215; **Phone:** 718-780-7830; **Board Cert:** Internal Medicine 1979; Cardiovascular Disease 1981; Interventional Cardiology 2009; **Med School:** Albany Med Coll 1976; **Resid:** Internal Medicine, St Vincents Hosp 1979; **Fellow:** Cardiovascular Disease, Georgetown Univ Hosp 1981; Interventional Cardiology, Mercy Hosp 1987; **Fac Appt:** Assoc Clin Prof Med, SUNY Downstate

Shani, Jacob MD (IC) - **Spec Exp:** Cardiac Catheterization; Angioplasty & Stent Placement; Percutaneous Valve Repair; **Hospital:** Maimonides Med Ctr (page 98); **Address:** Maimonides Med Ctr, Cardiac Cath Lab, 4802 10th Ave, Brooklyn, NY 11219-2844; **Phone:** 718-283-7480; **Board Cert:** Internal Medicine 1981; Cardiovascular Disease 1983; Interventional Cardiology 2009; **Med School:** Israel 1977; **Resid:** Internal Medicine, Maimonides Med Ctr 1981; **Fellow:** Cardiovascular Disease, Beth Israel Hosp 1983; **Fac Appt:** Prof Med, NYU Sch Med

Maternal & Fetal Medicine

Bush, Jacqueline MD (MF) - **Spec Exp:** Pregnancy-High Risk; Diabetes in Pregnancy; **Hospital:** New York Methodist Hosp (page 418); **Address:** 263 7th Ave, Ste 3A, Brooklyn, NY 11215; **Phone:** 718-246-8500; **Board Cert:** Obstetrics & Gynecology 2007; **Med School:** SUNY Stony Brook 1989; **Resid:** Obstetrics & Gynecology, Univ Hosp-SUNY Hlth Scis Ctr; Obstetrics & Gynecology, Kings Co Hosp Ctr

Chandra, Prasanta C MD (MF) - **Spec Exp:** Pregnancy-High Risk; Premature Labor; Pregnancy-Teenage; **Hospital:** Wyckoff Heights Med Ctr; **Address:** 220A Saint Nicholas Ave, Brooklyn, NY 11237; **Phone:** 718-418-8745; **Board Cert:** Obstetrics & Gynecology 1979; Maternal & Fetal Medicine 1980; **Med School:** India 1969; **Resid:** Surgery, Bronx Muni Hosp-Albert Einstein Med Ctr 1972; Obstetrics & Gynecology, Bronx Muni Hosp-Albert Einstein Med Ctr 1976; **Fellow:** Maternal & Fetal Medicine, Bronx Muni Hosp-Albert Einstein Med Ctr 1978

Medical Oncology

Astrow, Alan B MD (Onc) - **Spec Exp:** Ovarian Cancer; Breast Cancer; Lymphoma; **Hospital:** Maimonides Med Ctr (page 98); **Address:** MMC Hematology/Oncology, 6300 8th Ave, Brooklyn, NY 11220; **Phone:** 718-765-2653; **Board Cert:** Internal Medicine 1983; Hematology 1986; Medical Oncology 1987; **Med School:** Yale Univ 1980; **Resid:** Internal Medicine, Boston City Hosp 1983; **Fellow:** Hematology & Oncology, NYU Med Ctr 1986; **Fac Appt:** Assoc Clin Prof Med, NY Med Coll

Bashevkin, Michael MD (Onc) - **Spec Exp:** Solid Tumors; Bleeding/Coagulation Disorders; Hematologic Malignancies; **Hospital:** Maimonides Med Ctr (page 98); **Address:** 1660 E 14st St, Ste 501, Brooklyn, NY 11229; **Phone:** 718-382-8500 x501; **Board Cert:** Internal Medicine 1976; Hematology 1978; Medical Oncology 1979; **Med School:** SUNY Downstate 1973; **Resid:** Internal Medicine, VA Med Ctr 1976; **Fellow:** Hematology & Oncology, Maimonides Med Ctr 1979

Chandra, Pradeep MD (Onc) - **Spec Exp:** Gastrointestinal Cancer; Colon Cancer; Breast Cancer; **Hospital:** Interfaith Med Ctr; **Address:** 1545 Atlantic Ave, Brooklyn, NY 11213; **Phone:** 718-613-6588; **Board Cert:** Internal Medicine 1980; Hematology 1974; Medical Oncology 1983; **Med School:** India 1966; **Resid:** Internal Medicine, Wyckoff Heights Hosp 1969; Internal Medicine, Bronx Lebanon Hosp 1971; **Fellow:** Hematology, LIJ Med Ctr 1973; **Fac Appt:** Prof Med, Cornell Univ-Weill Med Coll

Dosik, David MD (Onc) - **Spec Exp:** Breast Cancer; Lung Cancer; Colon Cancer; **Hospital:** New York Methodist Hosp (page 418), New York Comm Hosp; **Address:** NY Methodist Hosp - Dept Medicine, 501 6th St, Ste 1J, Brooklyn, NY 11215; **Phone:** 718-780-5240; **Board Cert:** Hematology 2006; Medical Oncology 2007; **Med School:** SUNY Downstate 1990; **Resid:** Internal Medicine, Staten Island Univ Hosp 1993; **Fellow:** Hematology & Oncology, NYU Med Ctr 1996

Geraghty, Michael MD (Onc) - **Hospital:** SUNY Downstate Med Ctr (Univ Hosp of Bklyn) - LICH (page 420); **Address:** 349 Henry St, Brooklyn, NY 11201; **Phone:** 718-780-4803; **Board Cert:** Internal Medicine 1972; Hematology 1974; Medical Oncology 2009; **Med School:** Georgetown Univ 1966; **Resid:** Internal Medicine, Bellevue Hosp 1971; **Fellow:** Hematology, Bellevue Hosp 1973; **Fac Appt:** Asst Clin Prof Med, SUNY Hlth Sci Ctr

Lebowicz, Joseph MD (Onc) - **Spec Exp:** Lung Cancer; Breast Cancer; Gastrointestinal Cancer; **Hospital:** Maimonides Med Ctr (page 98); **Address:** 1660 E 14th St, Ste 501, Brooklyn, NY 11229; **Phone:** 718-382-8500; **Board Cert:** Internal Medicine 1978; Hematology 1980; Medical Oncology 1981; **Med School:** Albert Einstein Coll Med 1975; **Resid:** Internal Medicine, Maimonides Med Ctr 1978; **Fellow:** Hematology & Oncology, Maimonides Med Ctr 1981

Lichter, Stephen M MD (Onc) - **Spec Exp:** Breast Cancer; Lung Cancer; Gastrointestinal Cancer; Prostate Cancer; **Hospital:** Beth Israel Med Ctr- Kings Hwy Div (page 94), New York Methodist Hosp (page 418); **Address:** 2935 Ave S, Brooklyn, NY 11229; **Phone:** 718-616-0801; **Board Cert:** Internal Medicine 1978; Medical Oncology 1981; **Med School:** Ros Franklin Univ/Chicago Med Sch 1975; **Resid:** Internal Medicine, Brookdale Hosp 1978; **Fellow:** Hematology & Oncology, Brookdale Hosp 1980; **Fac Appt:** Asst Clin Prof Med, SUNY Hlth Sci Ctr

Solomon, William B MD (Onc) - **Spec Exp:** Lung Cancer; Urologic Cancer; Clinical Trials; **Hospital:** Maimonides Med Ctr (page 98); **Address:** Maimonides Med Ctr, Hem/Onc Dept, 6300 8th Ave Fl 2, Brooklyn, NY 11220; **Phone:** 718-765-2613; **Board Cert:** Internal Medicine 1978; Hematology 1982; Medical Oncology 1985; **Med School:** Columbia P&S 1975; **Resid:** Internal Medicine, Montefiore Hosp Med Ctr 1978; **Fellow:** Hematology, Beth Israel Hosp 1981; Molecular Biology, Mass Inst Tech; **Fac Appt:** Prof Med, SUNY Downstate

Neonatal-Perinatal Medicine

Gudavalli, Madhu R MD (NP) - **Spec Exp:** Prematurity/Low Birth Weight Infants; **Hospital:** New York Methodist Hosp (page 418); **Address:** New York Methodist Hosp, Dept Pediatrics, 506 6th St, Brooklyn, NY 11215; **Phone:** 718-780-3727; **Board Cert:** Pediatrics 1980; Neonatal-Perinatal Medicine 2009; **Med School:** India 1972; **Resid:** Pediatrics, NY Infirm 1976; Pediatrics, Booth Meml Hosp 1977; **Fellow:** Neonatal-Perinatal Medicine, Bellevue Hosp 1979

Koenig, Eli MD (NP) - **Hospital:** SUNY Downstate Med Ctr (Univ Hosp of Bklyn) - LICH (page 420); **Address:** 339 Hicks St, Brooklyn, NY 11201-5509; **Phone:** 718-670-1536; **Board Cert:** Pediatrics 1986; Neonatal-Perinatal Medicine 2007; **Med School:** Italy 1979; **Resid:** Pediatrics, Beth Israel Med Ctr 1982; **Fellow:** Neonatal-Perinatal Medicine, Babies Hosp 1984; **Fac Appt:** Asst Prof Ped, SUNY Downstate

Siracuse, Jeffrey F MD (NP) - **Spec Exp:** Necrotizing Enterocolitis; Respiratory Distress Syndrome; Neonatology; **Hospital:** SUNY Downstate Med Ctr (Univ Hosp of Bklyn) - LICH (page 420); **Address:** 339 Hicks St Fl 4, Brooklyn, NY 11201; **Phone:** 718-780-1832; **Board Cert:** Pediatrics 1985; Neonatal-Perinatal Medicine 1985; **Med School:** Italy 1977; **Resid:** Pediatrics, St Vincents Hosp 1980; **Fellow:** Neonatal-Perinatal Medicine, Columbia-Presby Med Ctr 1982; **Fac Appt:** Asst Prof Ped, NY Med Coll

Sokal, Myron MD (NP) - **Spec Exp:** Neonatal Care; **Hospital:** Brookdale Univ Hosp Med Ctr; **Address:** 1 Brookdale Plaza, 244-Strausberg Bldg, Brooklyn, NY 11212; **Phone:** 718-240-5629; **Board Cert:** Pediatrics 1972; Neonatal-Perinatal Medicine 1975; **Med School:** Albert Einstein Coll Med 1967; **Resid:** Pediatrics, Yale-New Haven Hosp 1969; **Fellow:** Neonatal-Perinatal Medicine, Columbia-Presby Med Ctr 1971; **Fac Appt:** Prof Ped, SUNY Hlth Sci Ctr

Nephrology

Chou, Shyan-Yih MD (Nep) - **Spec Exp:** Kidney Disease; Hypertension; Dialysis Care; **Hospital:** Brookdale Univ Hosp Med Ctr; **Address:** 1 Brookdale Plaza, rm 169-CHC, Brooklyn, NY 11212-3139; **Phone:** 718-240-5615; **Board Cert:** Internal Medicine 1972; Nephrology 1974; **Med School:** Taiwan 1966; **Resid:** Internal Medicine, Brookdale Hosp 1970; Internal Medicine, Brookdale Hosp 1970; **Fellow:** Nephrology, Brookdale Hosp 1973; **Fac Appt:** Prof Med, SUNY Downstate

Delano, Barbara MD (Nep) - **Spec Exp:** Dialysis Care; Kidney Failure-Chronic; Kidney Disease-Acute; **Hospital:** SUNY Downstate Med Ctr (Univ Hosp of Bklyn) (page 419), Kings County Hosp Ctr; **Address:** 450 Clarkson Ave, Box 52, Brooklyn, NY 11203-2056; **Phone:** 718-270-1584; **Board Cert:** Internal Medicine 2010; **Med School:** SUNY Hlth Sci Ctr 1965; **Resid:** Internal Medicine, SUNY Downstate Med Ctr 1967; **Fellow:** Nephrology, SUNY Downstate Med Ctr 1969; **Fac Appt:** Prof Med, SUNY Downstate

Lipner, Henry I MD (Nep) - **Spec Exp:** Kidney Disease; Hypertension; Dialysis Care; **Hospital:** Maimonides Med Ctr (page 98); **Address:** 1435 86th St, Brooklyn, NY 11228; **Phone:** 718-648-0101; **Board Cert:** Internal Medicine 1974; Nephrology 1976; **Med School:** NYU Sch Med 1968; **Resid:** Internal Medicine, Jewish Hosp 1971; **Fellow:** Nephrology, Montefiore Hosp Med Ctr 1972

Markell, Mariana S MD (Nep) - **Spec Exp:** Transplant Medicine-Kidney; Complementary Medicine; **Hospital:** SUNY Downstate Med Ctr (Univ Hosp of Bklyn) (page 419), Kings County Hosp Ctr; **Address:** 450 Clarkson Ave, Box 52, Brooklyn, NY 11203; **Phone:** 718-270-1584; **Board Cert:** Internal Medicine 1984; Nephrology 1986; **Med School:** NY Med Coll 1981; **Resid:** Internal Medicine, Columbia-Presby 1984; **Fellow:** Nephrology, Columbia-Presby 1985UCLA Med Ctr 1986; **Fac Appt:** Assoc Prof Med, SUNY Downstate

Mittman, Neal MD (Nep) - **Spec Exp:** Lupus Nephritis; Dialysis Care; Hypertension; **Hospital:** SUNY Downstate Med Ctr (Univ Hosp of Bklyn) - LICH (page 420); **Address:** 115 Remsen St, Brooklyn, NY 11201-4212; **Phone:** 718-852-4949; **Board Cert:** Internal Medicine 1980; Nephrology 1982; **Med School:** NY Med Coll 1977; **Resid:** Internal Medicine, Metropolitan Hosp Ctr 1980; **Fellow:** Nephrology, Albert Einstein Coll Med 1982; **Fac Appt:** Assoc Prof Med, SUNY Hlth Sci Ctr

Neelakantappa, Kotresha H MD (Nep) - **Spec Exp:** Kidney Disease; Hypertension; **Hospital:** New York Methodist Hosp (page 418); **Address:** 9920 4th Ave, Ste 309, Brooklyn, NY 11209; **Phone:** 718-745-3079; **Board Cert:** Internal Medicine 1977; Nephrology 1978; **Med School:** India 1969; **Resid:** Internal Medicine, NY Methodist Hosp 1974; **Fellow:** Nephrology, NYU Med Ctr 1976; **Fac Appt:** Asst Prof Med, NYU Sch Med

Pannone, John MD (Nep) - **Spec Exp:** Dialysis Care; Kidney Disease-Chronic; Hypertension; **Hospital:** Lutheran Med Ctr - Brooklyn; **Address:** 61 Oliver St, Ste PR-1, Brooklyn, NY 11209; **Phone:** 718-238-4980; **Board Cert:** Internal Medicine 1978; Nephrology 1980; **Med School:** Italy 1974; **Resid:** Internal Medicine, Lutheran Med Ctr 1977; **Fellow:** Nephrology, Brookdale Hosp Med Ctr 1979; Nephrology, New York Hosp-Cornell Med Ctr 1980

Parnes, Eliezer MD (Nep) - **Spec Exp:** Hypertension; Dialysis Care; Diabetic Kidney Disease; **Hospital:** Beth Israel Med Ctr- Kings Hwy Div (page 94); **Address:** 3131 Kings Hwy, rm D-5, Brooklyn, NY 11234-2643; **Phone:** 718-338-2283; **Board Cert:** Internal Medicine 1989; Nephrology 2003; **Med School:** SUNY Downstate 1986; **Resid:** Internal Medicine, Brookdale Hosp Med Ctr 1989; **Fellow:** Nephrology, Brookdale Hosp Med Ctr 1992

Salifu, Moro MD (Nep) - **Spec Exp:** Kidney Disease; **Hospital:** SUNY Downstate Med Ctr (Univ Hosp of Bklyn) (page 419); **Address:** SUNY Downstate, 450 Clarkson Ave, Box 52, Brooklyn, NY 11203; **Phone:** 718-270-3174; **Board Cert:** Internal Medicine 2009; Nephrology 2010; **Med School:** Turkey 1994; **Resid:** Internal Medicine, SUNY Hlth Sci Ctr 1998; **Fellow:** Nephrology, SUNY Hlth Sci Ctr 2001

Shapiro, Warren B MD (Nep) - **Spec Exp:** Kidney Failure-Chronic; Kidney Failure; Hypertension; Dialysis Care; **Hospital:** Brookdale Univ Hosp Med Ctr; **Address:** 1 Brookdale Plaza, rm 169-CHC, Brooklyn, NY 11212-3139; **Phone:** 718-240-5615; **Board Cert:** Internal Medicine 1972; Nephrology 1974; **Med School:** Ros Franklin Univ/Chicago Med Sch 1966; **Resid:** Internal Medicine, UCSF Med Ctr 1967; Internal Medicine, NY Med Coll 1970; **Fellow:** Nephrology, NY Med Coll 1971; **Fac Appt:** Assoc Clin Prof Med, SUNY Downstate

Shein, Leon MD (Nep) - **Spec Exp:** Hypertension; Diabetic Kidney Disease; Electrolyte Disorders; Nutrition; **Hospital:** New York Methodist Hosp (page 418), Interfaith Med Ctr; **Address:** NY Methodist Hosp, 446 McDonald Ave, Brooklyn, NY 11218; **Phone:** 718-972-4200; **Board Cert:** Internal Medicine 1989; Nephrology 2003; **Med School:** Philippines 1983; **Resid:** Internal Medicine, Woodhull Med Ctr 1986; **Fellow:** Nephrology, Brookdale Hosp 1988

Spitalewitz, Samuel MD (Nep) - **Spec Exp:** Diabetic Kidney Disease; Hypertension; **Hospital:** Brookdale Univ Hosp Med Ctr; **Address:** 1 Brookdale Plaza, Ste 169-CHC, Brooklyn, NY 11212-3139; **Phone:** 718-240-5615; **Board Cert:** Internal Medicine 1978; Nephrology 1980; **Med School:** NYU Sch Med 1975; **Resid:** Internal Medicine, Brookdale Hosp 1978; **Fellow:** Nephrology, Brookdale Hosp 1981; **Fac Appt:** Assoc Clin Prof Med, SUNY Downstate

Stam, Lawrence MD (Nep) - **Spec Exp:** Dialysis Care; Plasmapheresis; **Hospital:** New York Methodist Hosp (page 418); **Address:** 506 6th St, Brooklyn, NY 11215-3609; **Phone:** 718-830-7109; **Board Cert:** Internal Medicine 1981; Nephrology 1984; **Med School:** SUNY Stony Brook 1978; **Resid:** Internal Medicine, St Elizabeth Hosp 1981; **Fellow:** Nephrology, Jewish Hosp 1982; **Fac Appt:** Asst Clin Prof Med, Cornell Univ-Weill Med Coll

Neurological Surgery

Cardoso, Erico R MD (NS) - **Spec Exp:** Pituitary Tumors; Spinal Cord Disorders; Hydrocephalus; **Hospital:** Kingsbrook Jewish Med Ctr; **Address:** Kingsbrook Jewish Med Ctr, 585 Schenectady Ave, Brooklyn, NY 11203; **Phone:** 718-604-5500; **Board Cert:** Neurological Surgery 1994; **Med School:** Brazil 1973; **Resid:** Surgery, Ottawa Civic Hosp 1976; Neurological Surgery, Ottawa Civic Hosp 1980; **Fellow:** Neurological Surgery, Clin Rsch Fellowship Univ Hosp 1981; Neurological Surgery, Inst Neurol Scis 1982; **Fac Appt:** Assoc Prof NS, SUNY Downstate

Hirschfeld, Alan D MD (NS) - **Spec Exp:** Brain Tumors; **Hospital:** Lutheran Med Ctr - Brooklyn; **Address:** 8413 13th Ave, Brooklyn, NY 11228; **Phone:** 718-234-0979; **Board Cert:** Neurological Surgery 1986; **Med School:** NYU Sch Med 1977; **Resid:** Surgery, NYU-Bellevue Hosp 1978; Neurological Surgery, NYU-Bellevue Hosp 1982; **Fac Appt:** Assoc Prof S, NY Med Coll

Schwartz, Amit Y MD (NS) - **Hospital:** Maimonides Med Ctr (page 98), Mount Sinai Med Ctr (page 102); **Address:** Maimonides Med Ctr, 948 48th St, rm 228, Brooklyn, NY 11219; **Phone:** 718-283-7219; **Board Cert:** Neurological Surgery 2005; **Med School:** Mount Sinai Sch Med 1995; **Resid:** Neurological Surgery, Mt Sinai Med Ctr 2001; **Fellow:** Skull Base Surgery, Jackson Meml Hosp 2002; **Fac Appt:** Asst Clin Prof NS, Mount Sinai Sch Med

Zonenshayn, Martin MD (NS) - **Spec Exp:** Parkinson's Disease; Stereotactic Radiosurgery; Carpal Tunnel Syndrome; Trigeminal Neuralgia; **Hospital:** New York Methodist Hosp (page 418); **Address:** 263 Seventh Ave, Ste 4D, Brooklyn, NY 11215; **Phone:** 718-246-8660; **Board Cert:** Neurological Surgery 2008; **Med School:** NYU Sch Med 1996; **Resid:** Neurological Surgery, NY Presby Cornell Med Ctr/MSKCC 2002; **Fellow:** Stereo Neurological Surgery, NYU Hosp Joint Diseases 2003; **Fac Appt:** Assoc Clin Prof NS, Cornell Univ-Weill Med Coll

Neurology

Azhar, Salman MD (N) - **Spec Exp:** Stroke; Neuro-Rehabilitation; Dementia; Spasticity Management; **Hospital:** Lutheran Med Ctr - Brooklyn; **Address:** 8714 5th Ave, Brooklyn, NY 11209; **Phone:** 718-630-8600; **Board Cert:** Neurology 2008; Vascular Neurology 2008; **Med School:** Med Coll VA 1993; **Resid:** Neurology, Med Coll Va Hosp 1995; Neurology, Mt Sinai Med Ctr 1997; **Fellow:** Stroke, NINDS/NIH 1999; **Fac Appt:** Asst Prof N, SUNY Downstate

Bodis-Wollner, Ivan MD (N) - **Spec Exp:** Parkinson's Disease; Neuro-Ophthalmology; Behavioral Neurology; **Hospital:** SUNY Downstate Med Ctr (Univ Hosp of Bklyn) (page 419), Kings County Hosp Ctr; **Address:** 470 Clarkson Ave, Ste A, Box 35, Brooklyn, NY 11203; **Phone:** 718-270-2734; **Board Cert:** Neurology 1977; **Med School:** Austria 1965; **Resid:** Neurology, Mount Sinai Hosp 1974; **Fellow:** Clinical Neurophysiology, Mass Genl Hosp 1974; **Fac Appt:** Prof N, SUNY Downstate

Buckner, Cary D MD (N) - **Spec Exp:** Neuromuscular Disorders; Clinical Neurophysiology; **Hospital:** New York Methodist Hosp (page 418); **Address:** NYMH Division of Neurology, 263 7th Ave, Ste 4A, Brooklyn, NY 11215; **Phone:** 718-246-8614; **Board Cert:** Neurology 2009; Clinical Neurophysiology 2001; **Med School:** Georgetown Univ 1994; **Resid:** Neurology, Columbia Presby Med Ctr 1998; **Fellow:** Neuromuscular Disease, Columbia Presby Med Ctr 1999

Crystal, Howard MD (N) - **Spec Exp:** Alzheimer's Disease; Dementia; **Hospital:** SUNY Downstate Med Ctr (Univ Hosp of Bklyn) (page 419), Kings County Hosp Ctr; **Address:** 470 Clarkson Ave, Box 1274, Brooklyn, NY 11203-2056; **Phone:** 718-270-6388; **Board Cert:** Neurology 1981; **Med School:** Univ Pennsylvania 1976; **Resid:** Neurology, Montefiore Med Ctr 1980; **Fellow:** Neurological Pathology, Montefiore Med Ctr 1982; **Fac Appt:** Prof N, SUNY Downstate

Drexler, Ellen MD (N) - **Spec Exp:** Headache; **Hospital:** Maimonides Med Ctr (page 98); **Address:** 883 65th St, Brooklyn, NY 11210-4737; **Phone:** 718-283-7470; **Board Cert:** Neurology 1983; Headache Medicine 2006; **Med School:** SUNY Downstate 1978; **Resid:** Neurology, Montefiore Med Ctr 1982; **Fac Appt:** Assoc Prof N, Mount Sinai Sch Med

Kay, Arthur D MD (N) - **Spec Exp:** Alzheimer's Disease; Parkinson's Disease; Dementia; Stroke; **Hospital:** Brookdale Univ Hosp Med Ctr, Flushing Hosp Med Ctr; **Address:** 1 Brookdale Plaza, Ste 475, Brooklyn, NY 11212-3139; **Phone:** 718-240-5622; **Board Cert:** Neurology 1983; **Med School:** SUNY Downstate 1978; **Resid:** Internal Medicine, Brookdale Hosp 1979; Neurology, Mount Sinai Hosp 1982; **Fellow:** Natl Inst Hlth 1984; **Fac Appt:** Assoc Prof N, SUNY Downstate

Keilson, Marshall MD (N) - **Spec Exp:** Alzheimer's Disease; Epilepsy; **Hospital:** Maimonides Med Ctr (page 98); **Address:** 2044 Ocean Ave, Ste A6, Brooklyn, NY 11230; **Phone:** 718-759-6065; **Board Cert:** Neurology 1982; **Med School:** Albert Einstein Coll Med 1977; **Resid:** Internal Medicine, Montefiore Hosp Med Ctr 1978; Neurology, Albert Einstein 1981; **Fellow:** Clinical Neurophysiology, Univ Hosp 1983

Levine, Steven R MD (N) - **Spec Exp:** Stroke; Cerebrovascular Disease; **Hospital:** SUNY Downstate Med Ctr (Univ Hosp of Bklyn) (page 419); **Address:** SUNY Downstate Medical Center, 470 Clarkson Ave, Box 1213, Brooklyn, NY 11203; **Phone:** 718-221-5188; **Board Cert:** Neurology 1986; Vascular Neurology 2005; **Med School:** Med Coll Wisc 1981; **Resid:** Neurology, Univ Mich Hosps 1985; **Fellow:** Cerebrovascular Disease, Henry Ford Hosp 1987; **Fac Appt:** Prof N, Mount Sinai Sch Med

Maccabee, Paul J MD (N) - **Spec Exp:** Neuromuscular Disorders; Electromyography; Peripheral Neuropathy; **Hospital:** SUNY Downstate Med Ctr (Univ Hosp of Bklyn) (page 419); **Address:** SUNY Downstate Med Ctr, 470 Clarkson Ave, Box 35, Brooklyn, NY 11203; **Phone:** 718-270-2502; **Board Cert:** Neurology 1977; Clinical Neurophysiology 2003; **Med School:** Boston Univ 1970; **Resid:** Neurology, Boston Univ Med Ctr 1976; **Fellow:** Clinical Neurophysiology, Mass Genl Hosp 1978; Clinical Neurophysiology, Mt Sinai Hosp 1979; **Fac Appt:** Prof N, SUNY Hlth Sci Ctr

Maniscalco, Anthony MD (N) - **Spec Exp:** Movement Disorders; Cerebrovascular Disease; Neuromuscular Disorders; **Hospital:** Maimonides Med Ctr (page 98), Lutheran Med Ctr - Brooklyn; **Address:** Brooklyn Neurology, 117 70th St, Brooklyn, NY 11209-1113; **Phone:** 718-836-8800; **Board Cert:** Internal Medicine 1982; Neurology 1988; **Med School:** Italy 1978; **Resid:** Internal Medicine, Maimonides Medical Ctr 1981; Neurology, St Vincent's Hosp & Med Ctr 1984; **Fac Appt:** Assoc Clin Prof N, SUNY Downstate

Nouri, Shahin MD (N) - **Spec Exp:** Epilepsy/Seizure Disorders; **Hospital:** New York Methodist Hosp (page 418); **Address:** NY Methodist Hosp, Dept Neurology, 263 7th Ave, Ste 4A, Brooklyn, NY 11215; **Phone:** 718-246-8614; **Board Cert:** Neurology 2004; Clinical Neurophysiology 2005; **Med School:** Germany 1994; **Resid:** Internal Medicine, Staten Island Univ Hosp 1998; Neurology, Georgetown Univ Med Ctr 2001; **Fellow:** Clinical Neurophysiology, NYU Med Ctr 2002

Roohi, Fereydoon MD (N) - **Spec Exp:** Electromyography; Neuromuscular Disorders; **Hospital:** SUNY Downstate Med Ctr (Univ Hosp of Bklyn) - LICH (page 420); **Address:** Long Island Coll Hosp, Dept Neurology, 339 Hicks St, Brooklyn, NY 11201-5509; **Phone:** 718-780-1124; **Board Cert:** Neurology 1980; **Med School:** Iran 1967; **Resid:** Neurology, Kings Co Hosp 1975; **Fellow:** Neuromuscular Medicine, NY Presby Hosp 1976; **Fac Appt:** Assoc Prof N, SUNY Downstate

Rosenbaum, Daniel MD (N) - **Spec Exp:** Stroke; **Hospital:** SUNY Downstate Med Ctr (Univ Hosp of Bklyn) (page 419), Kings County Hosp Ctr; **Address:** SUNY Downstate, Dept Neurology, 450 Clarkson Ave, Box 1213, Brooklyn, NY 11203; **Phone:** 718-270-2051; **Board Cert:** Neurology 1988; Vascular Neurology 2005; **Med School:** Albert Einstein Coll Med 1982; **Resid:** Internal Medicine, Brookdale Hosp 1983; Neurology, Albert Einstein 1986; **Fellow:** Stroke, Univ Tex Med Sch 1988; **Fac Appt:** Prof N, SUNY Downstate

Rudolph, Steven H MD (N) - **Spec Exp:** Stroke; Neuro-Ophthalmology; **Hospital:** Maimonides Med Ctr (page 98), Mount Sinai Med Ctr (page 102); **Address:** 948 48th St, Brooklyn, NY 11219; **Phone:** 718-283-7670; **Board Cert:** Neurology 1981; Vascular Neurology 2005; **Med School:** SUNY Hlth Sci Ctr 1976; **Resid:** Neurology, Mt Sinai Hosp 1980; **Fellow:** Neuro-Ophthalmology, Mt Sinai Hosp 1982; **Fac Appt:** Asst Clin Prof N, Mount Sinai Sch Med

Salgado, Miran W MD (N) - **Spec Exp:** Movement Disorders; Parkinson's Disease; Botox Therapy; Headache; **Hospital:** New York Methodist Hosp (page 418); **Address:** Center for Neurology, 263 7th Ave, Ste 4A, Brooklyn, NY 11215; **Phone:** 718-246-8614; **Board Cert:** Neurology 2004; Vascular Neurology 2006; **Med School:** Sri Lanka 1990; **Resid:** Neurology, SUNY Downstate Med Ctr 1994; **Fellow:** Movement Disorders, Columbia Presby Med Ctr 1995

Sobol, Norman J MD (N) - **Spec Exp:** Headache; Stroke; Parkinson's Disease; **Hospital:** Beth Israel Med Ctr- Kings Hwy Div (page 94), Maimonides Med Ctr (page 98); **Address:** 3131 Kings Hwy, Ste C7, Brooklyn, NY 11234-2642; **Phone:** 718-677-0009; **Board Cert:** Neurology 1980; Internal Medicine 1977; **Med School:** Univ Chicago-Pritzker Sch Med 1974; **Resid:** Internal Medicine, Kings County Hosp 1976; Neurology, Kings County Hosp 1978; **Fellow:** Clinical Neurophysiology, Kings County Hosp 1980; **Fac Appt:** Asst Prof N, SUNY Downstate

Vas, George A MD (N) - **Spec Exp:** Stroke; Multiple Sclerosis; **Hospital:** SUNY Downstate Med Ctr (Univ Hosp of Bklyn) (page 419), Kings County Hosp Ctr; **Address:** 450 Clarkson Ave N, Ste A, Brooklyn, NY 11203-2056; **Phone:** 718-270-2502; **Board Cert:** Internal Medicine 1973; Neurology 1977; Clinical Neurophysiology 2002; **Med School:** Univ Pittsburgh 1970; **Resid:** Internal Medicine, New York Hosp 1972; Neurology, New York Hosp 1975; **Fac Appt:** Prof N, SUNY Downstate

Yellin, Joseph C DO (N) - **Spec Exp:** Headache; Memory Disorders; Dementia; **Hospital:** New York Comm Hosp, Lenox Hill Hosp (page 106); **Address:** 2502 Kings Hwy, Brooklyn, NY 11229; **Phone:** 718-377-2223; **Med School:** Univ Osteo Med & Hlth Sci, Des Moines 1978; **Resid:** Neurology, Kings Co Hosp 1982

Nuclear Medicine

Strashun, Arnold M MD (NuM) - **Spec Exp:** Neurologic Imaging; Nuclear Cardiology; Thyroid Disorders; PET Imaging-Brain; **Hospital:** SUNY Downstate Med Ctr (Univ Hosp of Bklyn) (page 419), Kings County Hosp Ctr; **Address:** 450 Clarkson Ave, Box 1210, Dept Radiology, Brooklyn, NY 11203; **Phone:** 718-270-1603; **Board Cert:** Internal Medicine 1977; Nuclear Medicine 1979; **Med School:** Baylor Coll Med 1974; **Resid:** Internal Medicine, Texas Med Ctr 1977; **Fellow:** Nuclear Medicine, VA Med Ctr 1978; Nuclear Medicine, Mount Sinai Hosp 1979; **Fac Appt:** Prof NuM, SUNY Downstate

Obstetrics & Gynecology

Barzegar, Hooshang MD (ObG) *PCP* - **Spec Exp:** Gynecology Only; **Hospital:** Brookdale Univ Hosp Med Ctr; **Address:** 1636 E 14th St, Ste 124, Brooklyn, NY 11229-1100; **Phone:** 718-998-3500; **Board Cert:** Obstetrics & Gynecology 1999; **Med School:** Iran 1960; **Resid:** Obstetrics & Gynecology, Brooklyn Cumberland Hosp 1968; Obstetrics & Gynecology, Montefiore Med Ctr 1970; **Fac Appt:** Asst Clin Prof ObG, SUNY Downstate

Comrie, Millicent MD (ObG) *PCP* - **Spec Exp:** Menopause Problems; Uterine Fibroids; **Hospital:** SUNY Downstate Med Ctr (Univ Hosp of Bklyn) - LICH (page 420); **Address:** 148 Pierrepont St, Brooklyn, NY 11201; **Phone:** 718-852-9180; **Board Cert:** Obstetrics & Gynecology 1983; **Med School:** SUNY Hlth Sci Ctr 1976; **Resid:** Obstetrics & Gynecology, Long Island Coll Hosp 1980; **Fellow:** Public Health, Columbia Univ 1981; **Fac Appt:** Asst Clin Prof ObG, SUNY Hlth Sci Ctr

Dor, Nathan MD (ObG) - **Spec Exp:** Pregnancy-High Risk; **Hospital:** Maimonides Med Ctr (page 98); **Address:** 943 48th St, Brooklyn, NY 11219-2919; **Phone:** 718-853-1535; **Board Cert:** Obstetrics & Gynecology 2011; Maternal & Fetal Medicine 2011; **Med School:** Israel 1973; **Resid:** Obstetrics & Gynecology, Montefiore Med Ctr 1977; **Fellow:** Perinatal Medicine, Westchester Co Med Ctr 1979; **Fac Appt:** Asst Prof ObG, SUNY Downstate

Haratz-Rubinstein, Natan MD (ObG) - **Spec Exp:** Obstetric Ultrasound; Pregnancy-High Risk; **Hospital:** NY Methodist Hosp (page 418); **Address:** NY Methodist Hosp, Dept Ob/Gyn, 506 6th St Fl 4, Brooklyn, NY 11215; **Phone:** 718-780-5799; **Board Cert:** Obstetrics & Gynecology 2010; **Med School:** Venezuela 1989; **Resid:** Obstetrics & Gynecology, Conception Palacio Maternity Hosp 1994; Obstetrics & Gynecology, NY Presby-Columbia Med Ctr 1997; **Fac Appt:** Asst Prof ObG, SUNY Downstate

Lederman, Sanford MD (ObG) - **Spec Exp:** Pregnancy-High Risk; Ultrasound; Prenatal Diagnosis; **Hospital:** New York Methodist Hosp (page 418); **Address:** 506 6th St, Brooklyn, NY 11215; **Phone:** 718-780-3272; **Board Cert:** Obstetrics & Gynecology 1982; **Med School:** Mexico 1974; **Resid:** Obstetrics & Gynecology, Long Island Coll Hosp 1979; **Fellow:** Maternal & Fetal Medicine, UC-Irvine Mem Hosp 1981; **Fac Appt:** Assoc Clin Prof ObG, SUNY Downstate

Maher, John T MD (ObG) - **Hospital:** New York Methodist Hosp (page 418); **Address:** Brooklyn Women's Healthcare, 110 4th Ave, Brooklyn, NY 11217; **Phone:** 718-852-5810; **Board Cert:** Obstetrics & Gynecology 2009; **Med School:** UMDNJ-NJ Med Sch, Newark 1989; **Resid:** Obstetrics & Gynecology, NY Hosp-Cornell Med Ctr 1993

Minkoff, Howard L MD (ObG) - **Spec Exp:** AIDS/HIV in Pregnancy-Consultation; Pregnancy-High Risk, Consultation; **Hospital:** Maimonides Med Ctr (page 98), SUNY Downstate Med Ctr (Univ Hosp of Bklyn) (page 419); **Address:** Maimonides Med Ctr, Dept Ob-Gyn, 4802 Tenth Ave, Brooklyn, NY 11219; **Phone:** 718-283-7973; **Board Cert:** Obstetrics & Gynecology 1995; Maternal & Fetal Medicine 1995; **Med School:** Penn State Coll Med 1975; **Resid:** Obstetrics & Gynecology, Kings Co Hosp Ctr 1979; Obstetrics & Gynecology, SUNY Hlth Sci Ctr 1981; **Fellow:** Maternal & Fetal Medicine, Kings Co Hosp Ctr 1981; **Fac Appt:** Prof ObG, SUNY Hlth Sci Ctr

Reizis, Igal MD (ObG) - **Spec Exp:** Gynecology Only; **Hospital:** Maimonides Med Ctr (page 98); **Address:** 5925 15th Ave, Brooklyn, NY 11219-5009; **Phone:** 718-972-2700; **Board Cert:** Obstetrics & Gynecology 1984; **Med School:** Israel 1977; **Resid:** Obstetrics & Gynecology, Maimonides Med Ctr

Ophthalmology

Ackerman, Jacob L MD (Oph) - **Spec Exp:** Glaucoma; Cataract Surgery-Lens Implant; Eyelid Cosmetic Surgery; **Hospital:** Brookdale Univ Hosp Med Ctr, New York Methodist Hosp (page 418); **Address:** 1987 Utica Ave, Fl 1, Brooklyn, NY 11234-3213; **Phone:** 718-968-8700; **Board Cert:** Ophthalmology 1976; **Med School:** Albert Einstein Coll Med 1971; **Resid:** Ophthalmology, LI Jewish Hillside Med Ctr 1975; **Fac Appt:** Asst Prof Oph, SUNY Hlth Sci Ctr

Berman, David H MD (Oph) - **Spec Exp:** Retinal Detachment; Diabetic Eye Disease/Retinopathy; Macular Degeneration; **Hospital:** SUNY Downstate Med Ctr (Univ Hosp of Bklyn) - LICH (page 420), Brooklyn Hosp Ctr-Downtown; **Address:** 185 Montague St, Ste PH, Brooklyn, NY 11201; **Phone:** 718-222-3050; **Board Cert:** Ophthalmology 1989; **Med School:** SUNY Downstate 1982; **Resid:** Internal Medicine, Kings Co Hosp 1984; Ophthalmology, Kings Co Hosp 1987; **Fellow:** Ophthalmology, Kings Co Hosp 1988; Retina/Vitreous, Hermann Eye Ctr 1989; **Fac Appt:** Assoc Clin Prof Oph, SUNY Downstate

Brecher, Rubin MD (Oph) - **Spec Exp:** Diabetic Eye Disease/Retinopathy; Macular Degeneration; **Hospital:** Maimonides Med Ctr (page 98); **Address:** 736 Ocean Pkwy, Brooklyn, NY 11230-1116; **Phone:** 718-851-1186; **Board Cert:** Ophthalmology 1991; **Med School:** Albert Einstein Coll Med 1984; **Resid:** Ophthalmology, Montefiore Med Ctr 1988; **Fellow:** Medical Retina, Moorefields Eye Hosp 1989

Deutsch, James A MD (Oph) - **Spec Exp:** Strabismus; Cataract Surgery; **Hospital:** SUNY Downstate Med Ctr (Univ Hosp of Bklyn) - LICH (page 420); **Address:** 110 Remsen St, Ste 1B, Brooklyn, NY 11201-4261; **Phone:** 718-855-8700; **Board Cert:** Ophthalmology 1989; **Med School:** NYU Sch Med 1984; **Resid:** Ophthalmology, Mt Sinai Hosp 1988; **Fellow:** Pediatric Ophthalmology, Wills Eye Hosp 1989; **Fac Appt:** Asst Clin Prof Oph, Mount Sinai Sch Med

Douros, Stella MD (Oph) - **Spec Exp:** Diabetic Eye Disease/Retinopathy; Macular Degeneration; Retina/Vitreous Surgery; **Hospital:** New York Eye & Ear Infirm (page 117), Lenox Hill Hosp (Manh Eye, Ear & Throat Hosp) (page 106); **Address:** 7501 6th Ave, Brooklyn, NY 11209; **Phone:** 718-238-2336; **Board Cert:** Ophthalmology 2009; **Med School:** Albert Einstein Coll Med 1991; **Resid:** Ophthalmology, Lenox Hill Hosp 1995; **Fellow:** Vitreoretinal Surgery, Joslin Diabetes Ctr 1996; **Fac Appt:** Clin Prof Oph, Mount Sinai Sch Med

Dweck, Monica MD (Oph) - **Spec Exp:** Eyelid Surgery; Tear Duct Problems; Orbital Diseases; Tear Duct Problems; **Hospital:** SUNY Downstate Med Ctr (Univ Hosp of Bklyn) (page 419), SUNY Downstate Med Ctr (Univ Hosp of Bklyn) - LICH (page 420); **Address:** 339 Hicks St, Othmer Bldg - Fl 4, MS 11201, Brooklyn, NY 11201; **Phone:** 718-780-1530; **Board Cert:** Ophthalmology 2008; **Med School:** SUNY Downstate 1986; **Resid:** Ophthalmology, NY Eye & Ear Infirm 1990; **Fellow:** Oculoplastic Surgery, The Cleveland Clinic 1991; **Fac Appt:** Asst Prof Oph, SUNY Hlth Sci Ctr

Feinstein, Neil C MD (Oph) - **Spec Exp:** Cataract Surgery; Glaucoma; Diabetic Eye Disease/Retinopathy; Macular Degeneration; **Hospital:** Maimonides Med Ctr (page 98), Lenox Hill Hosp (Manh Eye, Ear & Throat Hosp) (page 106); **Address:** 919 48th St, Brooklyn, NY 11219-2919; **Phone:** 718-435-1800; **Board Cert:** Ophthalmology 1979; **Med School:** Albert Einstein Coll Med 1974; **Resid:** Ophthalmology, SUNY Downstate Med Ctr 1978

Freedman, Jeffrey MD/PhD (Oph) - **Spec Exp:** Glaucoma; Uveitis; Cornea Transplant; **Hospital:** SUNY Downstate Med Ctr (Univ Hosp of Bklyn) - LICH (page 420), Interfaith Med Ctr; **Address:** 161 Atlantic Ave, Ste 203, Brooklyn, NY 11201-6720; **Phone:** 718-596-9086; **Board Cert:** Ophthalmology 1975; **Med School:** South Africa 1964; **Resid:** Internal Medicine, Baragwanat Genl Hosp 1966; Ophthalmology, Transvaal General Hosp 1967; **Fellow:** Ophthalmology, SUNY Downstate Med Ctr 1970; **Fac Appt:** Prof Oph, SUNY Downstate

Hyman, George F MD (Oph) - **Spec Exp:** Laser Vision Surgery; Corneal Disease; Cornea & Cataract Surgery; **Hospital:** Brookdale Univ Hosp Med Ctr; **Address:** 2460 Flatbush Ave, Ste 4, Brooklyn, NY 11234-5000; **Phone:** 718-252-1200; **Board Cert:** Ophthalmology 1976; **Med School:** Univ MD Sch Med 1968; **Resid:** Ophthalmology, Univ Hosp/Downstate Med Ctr 1974; **Fellow:** Anterior Segment - External Disease, Univ Witwatersrand 1975; **Fac Appt:** Asst Prof Oph, SUNY Hlth Sci Ctr

Jaffe, Herbert MD (Oph) - **Spec Exp:** Cataract Surgery; Glaucoma; **Hospital:** Beth Israel Med Ctr- Kings Hwy Div (page 94); **Address:** 2128 Ocean Ave, Brooklyn, NY 11229-1406; **Phone:** 718-339-7469; **Board Cert:** Ophthalmology 1983; **Med School:** Belgium 1968; **Resid:** Ophthalmology, SUNY Downstate Med Ctr 1972

Lazzaro, Douglas MD (Oph) - **Spec Exp:** Corneal Disease; Cataract Surgery; **Hospital:** SUNY Downstate Med Ctr (Univ Hosp of Bklyn) (page 419); **Address:** 7901 4th Ave, Brooklyn, NY 11209; **Phone:** 718-748-1334; **Board Cert:** Ophthalmology 2007; **Med School:** SUNY Downstate 1990; **Resid:** Ophthalmology, SUNY Downstate Med Ctr 1994; **Fellow:** Cornea & Refractive Surgery, Manhattan Eye & Ear Infirmary 1995; **Fac Appt:** Prof Oph, SUNY Downstate

Lebowitz, Mark A MD (Oph) - **Spec Exp:** LASIK-Refractive Surgery; Cataract Surgery; Corneal Disease & Surgery; **Hospital:** Lenox Hill Hosp (Manh Eye, Ear & Throat Hosp) (page 106); **Address:** 1301 Avenue J, Brooklyn, NY 11230-3605; **Phone:** 718-284-1921; **Board Cert:** Ophthalmology 2006; **Med School:** NYU Sch Med 1982; **Resid:** Ophthalmology, SUNY Downstate Med Ctr 1986; **Fellow:** Cornea & Ext Eye Disease, Manhattan EET Hosp 1987

Lieberman, David M MD (Oph) - **Spec Exp:** Contact Lenses; Corneal Disease; **Hospital:** New York Methodist Hosp (page 418); **Address:** 9 Prospect Park West, Ste 1-B, Brooklyn, NY 11215; **Phone:** 718-622-8900; **Board Cert:** Ophthalmology 1973; **Med School:** SUNY Downstate 1965; **Resid:** Ophthalmology, Univ Hosp 1970

Lombardo, James MD (Oph) - **Spec Exp:** Diabetic Eye Disease/Retinopathy; Glaucoma; **Hospital:** New York Eye & Ear Infirm (page 117); **Address:** 7801 4th Ave, Brooklyn, NY 11209-3701; **Phone:** 718-836-6661; **Board Cert:** Ophthalmology 1982; **Med School:** NYU Sch Med 1976; **Resid:** Internal Medicine, St Vincent's Hosp & Med Ctr 1977; Ophthalmology, NY Eye & Ear Infirmary 1980

Mogil, Laurey G MD (Oph) - **Spec Exp:** Glaucoma; **Hospital:** Mount Sinai Med Ctr (page 102); **Address:** KLM Ophthalmology, 1301 Avenue J, Brooklyn, NY 11230-3605; **Phone:** 718-645-0600; **Board Cert:** Ophthalmology 2006; **Med School:** Albert Einstein Coll Med 1980; **Resid:** Ophthalmology, Mt Sinai Med Ctr 1984; **Fellow:** Glaucoma, Mt Sinai Med Ctr 1985; **Fac Appt:** Asst Clin Prof Oph, Mount Sinai Sch Med

Pearlstein, Eric MD (Oph) - **Spec Exp:** Cataract Surgery; Corneal Disease; **Hospital:** SUNY Downstate Med Ctr (Univ Hosp of Bklyn) - LICH (page 420); **Address:** 430 Bay Ridge Pkwy, Brooklyn, NY 11209; **Phone:** 718-680-0600; **Board Cert:** Ophthalmology 1988; **Med School:** SUNY Hlth Sci Ctr 1983; **Resid:** Ophthalmology, LI Jewish Med Ctr 1987; **Fellow:** Cornea & Ext Eye Disease, Univ Minn-Duluth Sch Med 1988

Reich, Raymond MD (Oph) - **Spec Exp:** Cataract Surgery; Ophthalmic Plastic Surgery; Laser Refractive Surgery; **Hospital:** SUNY Downstate Med Ctr (Univ Hosp of Bklyn) - LICH (page 420), Maimonides Med Ctr (page 98); **Address:** 118 West End Ave, Brooklyn, NY 11235; **Phone:** 718-332-6200; **Board Cert:** Ophthalmology 1978; **Med School:** Albert Einstein Coll Med 1973; **Resid:** Ophthalmology, Univ Hosp 1977; **Fellow:** Ophthalmic Plastic Surgery, Harvard-Mass EE Infirm 1978; **Fac Appt:** Asst Prof Oph, SUNY Hlth Sci Ctr

Saffra, Norman MD (Oph) - **Spec Exp:** Microsurgery; Retinal Disorders; Cataract Surgery; **Hospital:** Maimonides Med Ctr (page 98); **Address:** 902 49th St, Brooklyn, NY 11219-2922; **Phone:** 718-283-8000; **Board Cert:** Ophthalmology 2005; **Med School:** Albert Einstein Coll Med 1988; **Resid:** Ophthalmology, Montefiore Med Ctr 1992; **Fellow:** Retina, SUNY Hlth Sci Ctr 1993; Neuro-Ophthalmology, Kingsbrook Jewish Med Ctr; **Fac Appt:** Clin Prof Oph, Mount Sinai Sch Med

Sciortino, Patrick MD (Oph) - **Spec Exp:** LASIK-Refractive Surgery; Cataract Surgery; **Hospital:** New York Comm Hosp, SUNY Downstate Med Ctr (Univ Hosp of Bklyn) - LICH (page 420); **Address:** 914 Bay Ridge Pkwy, Brooklyn, NY 11228-2302; **Phone:** 718-748-5700; **Board Cert:** Ophthalmology 2009; **Med School:** NY Med Coll 1978; **Resid:** Ophthalmology, St Vincents Hosp 1980; Ophthalmology, Catholic Med Ctr; **Fellow:** Ophthalmology, Univ Hosp 1984

Seidman, Mitchell DO (Oph) - **Spec Exp:** Cataract Surgery; **Hospital:** New York Methodist Hosp (page 418); **Address:** 2989 Ocean Pkwy, Brooklyn, NY 11235; **Phone:** 718-332-2020; **Board Cert:** Ophthalmology 1979; **Med School:** Philadelphia Coll Osteo Med 1974; **Resid:** Ophthalmology, Temple Univ Hosp 1978; **Fellow:** Anterior Segment - External Disease 1979

Sherman, Steven I DO (Oph) - **Spec Exp:** Glaucoma; Anterior Segment Surgery; **Hospital:** New York Methodist Hosp (page 418), Interfaith Med Ctr; **Address:** 2303 Avenue Z Fl 1, Brooklyn, NY 11235-2805; **Phone:** 718-934-6600; **Board Cert:** Ophthalmology 1990; **Med School:** Univ Osteo Med & Hlth Sci, Des Moines 1977; **Resid:** Internal Medicine, Coney Island Hosp 1979; Ophthalmology, UHPHS Hosp 1982; **Fellow:** Glaucoma, SUNY Downstate Med Ctr 1983; **Fac Appt:** Asst Clin Prof Oph, Touro Coll Osteopathic Med-NY

Silberman, Deborah MD (Oph) - **Spec Exp:** Laser Vision Surgery; Cataract Surgery; **Address:** 1335 Linden Blvd, Brooklyn, NY 11212-4751; **Phone:** 718-240-5557; **Board Cert:** Ophthalmology 1990; **Med School:** SUNY Buffalo 1984; **Resid:** Internal Medicine, St Luke's-Roosevelt Hosp Ctr 1985; Ophthalmology, Brookdale Hosp Med Ctr 1988

Smith, Edward MD (Oph) - **Spec Exp:** Cataract Surgery; Neuro-Ophthalmology; **Hospital:** SUNY Downstate Med Ctr (Univ Hosp of Bklyn) (page 419), Kingsbrook Jewish Med Ctr; **Address:** Downstate Ophthalmology Assocs, 11 Plaza St West, Brooklyn, NY 11217; **Phone:** 718-638-2020; **Board Cert:** Ophthalmology 1989; **Med School:** SUNY Downstate 1984; **Resid:** Ophthalmology, Univ Hosp 1988; **Fellow:** Neuro-Ophthalmology, Univ Hosp 1989; **Fac Appt:** Assoc Prof Oph, SUNY Downstate

Stein, Arnold MD (Oph) - **Spec Exp:** Retinal Disorders; Glaucoma; Cataract Surgery; Laser Surgery; **Hospital:** Beth Israel Med Ctr- Kings Hwy Div (page 94), Long Island Jewish Med Ctr (page 106); **Address:** 1226 Ocean Pkwy, Lobby Lvl, Ste 1, Brooklyn, NY 11230; **Phone:** 718-692-0400; **Board Cert:** Ophthalmology 1987; **Med School:** SUNY Downstate 1982; **Resid:** Ophthalmology, LI Jewish Med Ctr 1986; **Fac Appt:** Asst Clin Prof Oph, Albert Einstein Coll Med

Unterricht, Sam L MD (Oph) - **Spec Exp:** Macular Disease/Degeneration; Retinal Disorders; Optic Nerve Disorders; Neuro-Ophthalmology; **Hospital:** New York Methodist Hosp (page 418), Kingsbrook Jewish Med Ctr; **Address:** 20 Plaza St E, Brooklyn, NY 11238-4955; **Phone:** 718-622-5800; **Board Cert:** Ophthalmology 1982; **Med School:** SUNY Downstate 1976; **Resid:** Ophthalmology, Univ Hosp 1980; **Fellow:** Neuro-Ophthalmology, Kingsbrook Jewish MC 1981; Retina/Vitreous, Univ Hosp 1982; **Fac Appt:** Asst Clin Prof Oph, SUNY Hlth Sci Ctr

Zellner, James H MD (Oph) - **Spec Exp:** Laser Refractive Surgery; Cataract Surgery; **Hospital:** New York Eye & Ear Infirm (page 117); **Address:** 7817 5th Ave, Brooklyn, NY 11209-2702; **Phone:** 718-748-2020; **Board Cert:** Ophthalmology 1982; **Med School:** Albert Einstein Coll Med 1977; **Resid:** Ophthalmology, Kings County Hosp Ctr 1981

Orthopaedic Surgery

Mani, John Vijay MD (OrS) - **Spec Exp:** Hip Replacement; Knee Replacement; **Hospital:** SUNY Downstate Med Ctr (Univ Hosp of Bklyn) - LICH (page 420); **Address:** 161 Atlantic Ave, Brooklyn, NY 11201-6720; **Phone:** 718-855-0088; **Board Cert:** Orthopaedic Surgery 1977; **Med School:** India 1970; **Resid:** Orthopaedic Surgery, Brookdale Hosp 1976; **Fellow:** Orthopaedic Surgery, Hosp for Special Surgery 1978; **Fac Appt:** Assoc Clin Prof OrS, SUNY Hlth Sci Ctr

Menezes, Placido MD (OrS) - **Spec Exp:** Hip Replacement; Knee Replacement; Fractures; **Hospital:** New York Methodist Hosp (page 418), Brooklyn Hosp Ctr-Downtown; **Address:** 543 2nd St, Brooklyn, NY 11215-2607; **Phone:** 718-788-7600; **Board Cert:** Orthopaedic Surgery 1980; **Med School:** India 1970; **Resid:** Surgery, NY Methodist Hosp 1975; Orthopaedic Surgery, Brooklyn Jewish Hosp & Med Ctr 1978; **Fac Appt:** Asst Clin Prof OrS, SUNY Downstate

Merola, Andrew A MD (OrS) - **Spec Exp:** Spinal Surgery; Scoliosis; **Hospital:** New York Methodist Hosp (page 418), Mount Sinai Med Ctr (page 102); **Address:** 567 1st St, Brooklyn, NY 11215; **Phone:** 718-783-5542; **Board Cert:** Orthopaedic Surgery 2009; **Med School:** Howard Univ 1990; **Resid:** Orthopaedic Surgery, Kings Co Hosp/SUNY Downstate 1995; **Fellow:** Spinal Surgery, Univ Colorado Med Ctr 1996; **Fac Appt:** Assoc Prof OrS, SUNY Downstate

Morgan, Daniel J MD (OrS) - **Spec Exp:** Sports Medicine; Joint Replacement; Arthroscopic Surgery; Shoulder Surgery; **Hospital:** Beth Israel Med Ctr- Kings Hwy Div (page 94); **Address:** Kings Hwy Orthopedic Assocs, Brooklyn, NY 11234; **Phone:** 718-258-2588; **Board Cert:** Orthopaedic Surgery 2011; **Med School:** Univ MD Sch Med 1985; **Resid:** Surgery, Washington Hosp Ctr 1986; Orthopaedic Surgery, Kingsbrook Jewish Med Ctr 1997

Soifer, Todd MD (OrS) - **Spec Exp:** Arthritis; Knee Injuries; Arthroscopic Surgery; Rotator Cuff Surgery; **Hospital:** Beth Israel Med Ctr- Kings Hwy Div (page 94); **Address:** Kings Hwy Orthopedic Assocs, 3131 Kings Hwy, Ste C11, Brooklyn, NY 11234-2643; **Phone:** 718-258-2588 x0; **Board Cert:** Orthopaedic Surgery 2007; **Med School:** Mount Sinai Sch Med 1989; **Resid:** Orthopaedic Surgery, Beth Israel Med Ctr/Kingsbrook Jewish Med Ctr 1994

Spero, Charles R MD (OrS) - **Spec Exp:** Pediatric Orthopaedic Surgery; **Hospital:** SUNY Downstate Med Ctr (Univ Hosp of Bklyn) (page 419), Kings County Hosp Ctr; **Address:** SUNY Downstate Medical Center, 450 Clarkson Ave, Box 30, Brooklyn, NY 11203; **Phone:** 718-270-2055; **Board Cert:** Orthopaedic Surgery 1981; **Med School:** Geo Wash Univ 1973; **Resid:** Orthopaedic Surgery, Lenox Hill Hosp 1978; **Fellow:** Pediatric Orthopaedic Surgery, Hosp for Special Surgery 1979; **Fac Appt:** Assoc Prof OrS, SUNY Downstate

Splain, Shepard H DO (OrS) - **Spec Exp:** Arthroscopic Surgery; Shoulder & Knee Reconstruction; Sports Medicine; Joint Replacement; **Hospital:** Brookdale Univ Hosp Med Ctr; **Address:** 1 Brookdale Plaza, Ste 152, Brooklyn, NY 11212; **Phone:** 718-240-5888; **Board Cert:** Orthopaedic Surgery 1980; **Med School:** Mich State Univ Coll Osteo Med 1973; **Resid:** Orthopaedic Surgery, Brookdale Hosp 1978; **Fellow:** Sports Medicine, Oklahoma Hlth Scis Ctr 1979; **Fac Appt:** Assoc Clin Prof OrS, SUNY Downstate

Tepler, Melvin MD (OrS) - **Spec Exp:** Fractures; **Hospital:** Maimonides Med Ctr (page 98); **Address:** 1252 E 9th St, Brooklyn, NY 11230-5180; **Phone:** 718-677-6000; **Board Cert:** Orthopaedic Surgery 2009; **Med School:** NY Med Coll 1980; **Resid:** Surgery, Maimonides Med Ctr 1981; Orthopaedic Surgery, Maimonides Med Ctr 1985

Urban, William P MD (OrS) - **Spec Exp:** Sports Medicine; **Hospital:** SUNY Downstate Med Ctr (Univ Hosp of Bklyn) (page 419); **Address:** SUNY Downstate Medical Ctr, Dept Orthopaedics & Rehab Medicine, 450 Clarkson Ave, Box 30, Brooklyn, NY 11203; **Phone:** 718-270-4673; **Board Cert:** Orthopaedic Surgery 2009; **Med School:** SUNY Downstate 1990; **Resid:** Orthopaedic Surgery, SUNY Downstate Medical Ctr 1994; **Fellow:** Sports Medicine, Univ Kentucky Med Ctr 1995; **Fac Appt:** Assoc Prof OrS, SUNY Downstate

Walsh, Raymond B MD (OrS) - **Hospital:** Lutheran Med Ctr - Brooklyn; **Address:** 6900 4th Ave, Brooklyn, NY 11209-1453; **Phone:** 718-238-6400; **Board Cert:** Orthopaedic Surgery 1981; **Med School:** England, UK 1974; **Resid:** Surgery, Maimonides Med Ctr 1976; Orthopaedic Surgery, Maimonides Med Ctr 1979

Wert, Sanford MD (OrS) - **Hospital:** New York Comm Hosp; **Address:** 3075 Brighton 13th St, Brooklyn, NY 11235-5607; **Phone:** 718-332-4747; **Board Cert:** Orthopaedic Surgery 1985; **Med School:** Mexico 1974; **Resid:** Orthopaedic Surgery, Maimonides Med Ctr 1975; Orthopaedic Surgery, LIJ Hosp 1979

Otolaryngology

Chaudhry, M Rashid MD (Oto) - **Spec Exp:** Cosmetic Surgery-Face; Sinus Surgery; **Hospital:** Brookdale Univ Hosp Med Ctr; **Address:** 1 Brookdale Plaza, Ste 157-CHC, Brooklyn, NY 11212; **Phone:** 718-240-6366; **Board Cert:** Otolaryngology 1978; **Med School:** Pakistan 1969; **Resid:** Otolaryngology, Downstate Med Ctr-Kings Co 1978; **Fac Appt:** Asst Prof Oto, SUNY Downstate

Hanson, Matthew B MD (Oto) - **Spec Exp:** Otology; **Hospital:** SUNY Downstate Med Ctr (Univ Hosp of Bklyn) (page 419), SUNY Downstate Med Ctr (Univ Hosp of Bklyn) - LICH (page 420); **Address:** 470 Clarkson Ave, Box 126, Brooklyn, NY 11203; **Phone:** 718-270-4701; **Board Cert:** Otolaryngology 1997; Neurotology 2008; **Med School:** Univ Iowa Coll Med 1989; **Resid:** Otolaryngology, Columbia-Presby Med Ctr 1995; **Fellow:** Neurotology, Baptist Hosp 1997; **Fac Appt:** Asst Prof Oto, SUNY Downstate

Lagmay, Victor MD (Oto) - **Spec Exp:** Thyroid & Parathyroid Surgery; Head & Neck Cancer & Surgery; Endoscopic Sinus Surgery; **Hospital:** Maimonides Med Ctr (page 98); **Address:** 919 49th St, Brooklyn, NY 11219; **Phone:** 718-283-6260; **Board Cert:** Otolaryngology 1999; **Med School:** NYU Sch Med 1992; **Resid:** Otolaryngology, NYU Med Ctr 1998; **Fellow:** Head and Neck Surgery, Beth Israel Med Ctr 1999; **Fac Appt:** Asst Clin Prof S, SUNY Downstate

Sperling, Neil M MD (Oto) - **Spec Exp:** Otosclerosis; Hearing Loss; Meniere's Disease; **Hospital:** SUNY Downstate Med Ctr (Univ Hosp of Bklyn) - LICH (page 420), New York Eye & Ear Infirm (page 117); **Address:** New York Otolaryngology Group, 134 Atlantic Ave, Brooklyn, NY 11201; **Phone:** 718-780-1498; **Board Cert:** Otolaryngology 1990; **Med School:** NY Med Coll 1985; **Resid:** Surgery, Beth Israel Med Ctr 1986; Otolaryngology, NY Eye & Ear Infirm 1990; **Fellow:** Otology, Minnesota Ear Clinic 1991; **Fac Appt:** Assoc Prof Oto, SUNY Downstate

Vastola, A Paul MD (Oto) - **Spec Exp:** Throat Disorders; **Hospital:** Maimonides Med Ctr (page 98); **Address:** 919 49th St, Brooklyn, NY 11219-2916; **Phone:** 718-283-6260; **Board Cert:** Otolaryngology 1995; **Med School:** Boston Univ 1988; **Resid:** Otolaryngology, Manhattan Eye, Ear & Throat Hospital 1993; **Fellow:** Pediatric Otolaryngology, Texas Chldn's Hosp 1994; **Fac Appt:** Asst Clin Prof Oto, SUNY Hlth Sci Ctr

Pain Medicine

Lefkowitz, Mathew MD (PM) - **Spec Exp:** Pain-Low Back; Pain-after Spinal Intervention; Sciatica; Pain-Back & Neck; **Hospital:** New York Methodist Hosp (page 418); **Address:** 185 Montague St Fl 6, Brooklyn, NY 11201; **Phone:** 718-625-4244; **Board Cert:** Anesthesiology 1993; Pain Medicine 2005; **Med School:** Belgium 1983; **Resid:** Anesthesiology, Mount Sinai Hosp 1986; **Fellow:** Pain Medicine, Mount Sinai Hosp 1987

Pathology

Mirra, Suzanne S MD (Path) - **Spec Exp:** Neuropathology; Alzheimer's Disease; **Hospital:** SUNY Downstate Med Ctr (Univ Hosp of Bklyn) (page 419), Kings County Hosp Ctr; **Address:** SUNY Health Science Ctr, Dept Pathology, 450 Clarkson Ave, Box 25, Brooklyn, NY 11203; **Phone:** 718-270-4599; **Board Cert:** Anatomic Pathology 1973; Neuropathology 1973; **Med School:** SUNY Downstate 1967; **Resid:** Anatomic Pathology, Kings Co Hosp 1970; Neuropathology, Montefiore Med Ctr 1971; **Fellow:** Neuropathology, Yale Univ 1973; **Fac Appt:** Prof Path, SUNY Downstate

Vigorita, Vincent J MD (Path) - **Spec Exp:** Bone Pathology; Surgical Pathology; **Hospital:** Maimonides Med Ctr (page 98), SUNY Downstate Med Ctr (Univ Hosp of Bklyn) (page 419); **Address:** 4802 Tenth Ave, Brooklyn, NY 11219; **Phone:** 917-648-5945; **Board Cert:** Anatomic Pathology 1980; **Med School:** NY Med Coll 1976; **Resid:** Pathology, Johns Hopkins Hosp 1978; **Fellow:** Pathology, Meml Sloan Kettering Cancer Ctr 1979; **Fac Appt:** Prof Path, SUNY Downstate

Pediatric Cardiology

Kaplovitz, Harry S MD (PCd) - **Spec Exp:** Syncope; Echocardiography; Heart Failure; **Hospital:** Maimonides Med Ctr (page 98); **Address:** Maimonides Med Ctr, 4802 Tenth Ave, rm K106, Brooklyn, NY 11219; **Phone:** 718-283-7501; **Board Cert:** Pediatrics 1988; Pediatric Cardiology 2007; **Med School:** Albert Einstein Coll Med 1981; **Resid:** Pediatrics, North Shore Univ Hosp 1984; **Fellow:** Pediatric Cardiology, NYU Med Ctr 1986

Presti, Salvatore MD (PCd) - **Spec Exp:** Fetal Echocardiography; Congenital Heart Disease; Kawasaki Disease; **Hospital:** Lenox Hill Hosp (page 106), NYU Langone Med Ctr (page 108); **Address:** 25 Schermerhorn St, Brooklyn, NY 11201-4824; **Phone:** 718-923-1123; **Board Cert:** Pediatrics 1984; Pediatric Cardiology 2010; **Med School:** Italy 1978; **Resid:** Pediatrics, Lenox Hill Hosp 1982; **Fellow:** Pediatric Cardiology, NYU Med Ctr 1984; **Fac Appt:** Assoc Clin Prof Ped, NYU Sch Med

Ramaswamy, Prema MD (PCd) - **Spec Exp:** Fetal Echocardiography; Congenital Heart Disease; **Hospital:** Maimonides Med Ctr (page 98); **Address:** 4802 10th Ave, rm K106, Brooklyn, NY 11219-2844; **Phone:** 718-283-7501; **Board Cert:** Pediatrics 2009; Pediatric Cardiology 2011; **Med School:** India 1986; **Resid:** Pediatrics, M Y Hosp 1990; Pediatrics, Montefiore Med Ctr 1993; **Fellow:** Pediatric Cardiology, NY Hosp-Cornell 1996; **Fac Appt:** Asst Prof Ped, Mount Sinai Sch Med

Pediatric Endocrinology

Agdere, Levon MD (PEn) - **Spec Exp:** Diabetes; Short Stature in Children; Thyroid Disorders; **Hospital:** New York Methodist Hosp (page 418); **Address:** 263 7th Ave, Ste 3B, Brooklyn, NY 11215; **Phone:** 718-246-8540; **Board Cert:** Pediatric Endocrinology 2006; **Med School:** Turkey 1981; **Resid:** Pediatrics, Lutheran Med Ctr 1986; **Fellow:** Pediatric Endocrinology, NY Hosp-Cornell Med Ctr 1989

Avruskin, Theodore W MD (PEn) - **Spec Exp:** Growth Disorders; Diabetes; Thyroid Disorders; **Hospital:** Brookdale Univ Hosp Med Ctr, SUNY Downstate Med Ctr (Univ Hosp of Bklyn) (page 419); **Address:** 1 Brookdale Plaza, Aaron Bldg, rm 222, Brooklyn, NY 11212; **Phone:** 718-240-5960; **Board Cert:** Pediatrics 1965; **Med School:** Univ Toronto 1960; **Resid:** Pediatrics, Montreal Chldns Hosp 1962; Pediatrics, Chldns Hosp Med Ctr 1964; **Fellow:** Pediatric Endocrinology, Chldns Hosp Med Ctr 1968; **Fac Appt:** Prof Ped, SUNY Downstate

Pediatric Gastroenterology

Jelin, Abraham MD (PGe) - **Spec Exp:** Nutrition; Breast Feeding Problems; Gastroesophageal Reflux Disease (GERD); Constipation; **Hospital:** Brooklyn Hosp Ctr-Downtown, New York Methodist Hosp (page 418); **Address:** Bklyn Hosp Ctr, Dept Peds, 121 DeKalb Ave, Brooklyn, NY 11201-5425; **Phone:** 718-250-6277; **Board Cert:** Pediatrics 1977; Pediatric Gastroenterology 2012; **Med School:** NYU Sch Med 1972; **Resid:** Pediatrics, Grady Meml Hosp 1973; Pediatrics, Montefiore Med Ctr 1974; **Fellow:** Pediatric Gastroenterology, Emory Univ Hosp 1977; **Fac Appt:** Asst Clin Prof Ped, NYU Sch Med

McFarlane-Ferreira, Yvonne B MD (PGe) - **Spec Exp:** Pain-Abdominal Recurrent; Failure to Thrive; Constipation; Inflammatory Bowel Disease; **Hospital:** New York Methodist Hosp (page 418), Brooklyn Hosp Ctr-Downtown; **Address:** Park Slope Pediatrics, 263 7th Ave, Ste 3B, Brooklyn, NY 11215; **Phone:** 718-246-8515; **Board Cert:** Pediatrics 2005; Pediatric Gastroenterology 2010; **Med School:** West Indies 1983; **Resid:** Anesthesiology, Princess Margaret Hosp 1986; Pediatrics, Brooklyn Hosp 1989; **Fellow:** Pediatric Gastroenterology, Mt Sinai Hosp 1992; **Fac Appt:** Asst Clin Prof Ped, Cornell Univ-Weill Med Coll

Narwal, Shivinder MD (PGe) - **Spec Exp:** Nutrition; **Hospital:** Maimonides Med Ctr (page 98); **Address:** 948 48th St Fl 3, Brooklyn, NY 11219; **Phone:** 718-283-8260; **Board Cert:** Pediatric Gastroenterology 2007; **Med School:** India 1983; **Resid:** Pediatrics, Kings Co Hosp Ctr 1993; **Fellow:** Pediatric Gastroenterology, Babies Hosp 1996; **Fac Appt:** Asst Prof Ped, SUNY Hlth Sci Ctr

Rabinowitz, Simon S MD/PhD (PGe) - **Spec Exp:** Inflammatory Bowel Disease; Hepatitis; Gastroesophageal Reflux Disease (GERD); Gastrointestinal Disorders; **Hospital:** SUNY Downstate Med Ctr (Univ Hosp of Bklyn) (page 419); **Address:** SUNY Downstate Med Ctr, 445 Lenox Rd, Box 49, Brooklyn, NY 11203; **Phone:** 718-270-4714; **Board Cert:** Pediatrics 2009; Pediatric Gastroenterology 2007; **Med School:** Univ Miami Sch Med 1983; **Resid:** Pediatrics, Mount Sinai Hosp 1985; **Fellow:** Pediatric Gastroenterology, Mount Sinai Hosp 1987; **Fac Appt:** Clin Prof Ped, NY Med Coll

Schwarz, Steven M MD (PGe) - **Spec Exp:** Gastroesophageal Reflux Disease (GERD); Nutrition; Endoscopy; Inflammatory Bowel Disease; **Hospital:** SUNY Downstate Med Ctr (Univ Hosp of Bklyn) (page 419), Beth Israel Med Ctr - Petrie Division (page 94); **Address:** Children's Hosp at SUNY Downstate, 445 Lenox Rd, Box 49, Brooklyn, NY 11203; **Phone:** 718-270-4714; **Board Cert:** Pediatrics 1979; Pediatric Gastroenterology 2005; **Med School:** Columbia P&S 1974; **Resid:** Pediatrics, Columbia-Presby Med Ctr 1977; **Fellow:** Pediatric Gastroenterology, Stanford Univ Med Ctr 1978; Pediatric Gastroenterology, Columbia-Presby Med Ctr 1980; **Fac Appt:** Prof Ped, SUNY Downstate

Wetzler, Graciela MD (PGe) - **Spec Exp:** Peptic Ulcer Disease; Gastroesophageal Reflux Disease (GERD); Irritable Bowel Syndrome; Inflammatory Bowel Disease/Crohn's; **Hospital:** Maimonides Med Ctr (page 98); **Address:** Maimonides Med Ctr, Dept Peds GE, 4802 10th Ave, Brooklyn, NY 11219; **Phone:** 718-283-8260; **Board Cert:** Pediatric Gastroenterology 2003; **Med School:** Argentina 1984; **Resid:** Pediatrics, Montefiore Med Ctr 1992; **Fellow:** Pediatric Gastroenterology, NY Hosp-Cornell Med Ctr 1995; **Fac Appt:** Assoc Clin Prof Ped, SUNY Downstate

Pediatric Hematology-Oncology

Guarini, Ludovico MD (PHO) - **Spec Exp:** Leukemia; Solid Tumors; Sickle Cell Disease; **Hospital:** Maimonides Med Ctr (page 98); **Address:** MMC Dept of Pediatrics, 6300 Eighth Ave Fl 2, Brooklyn, NY 11220; **Phone:** 718-765-2671; **Board Cert:** Pediatrics 1984; Pediatric Hematology-Oncology 2007; **Med School:** Italy 1974; **Resid:** Pediatrics, Beth Israel Hosp 1981; **Fellow:** Pediatric Hematology-Oncology, Columbia-Presby Med Ctr 1984; **Fac Appt:** Assoc Prof Ped, SUNY Hlth Sci Ctr

Kulpa, Jolanta MD (PHO) - **Spec Exp:** Sickle Cell Disease; Leukemia; Thalassemia; Bleeding/Coagulation Disorders; **Hospital:** New York Methodist Hosp (page 418); **Address:** 502 8th Ave, Brooklyn, NY 11215; **Phone:** 718-780-3066; **Board Cert:** Pediatrics 1983; Pediatric Hematology-Oncology 1984; **Med School:** Med Coll PA 1972; **Resid:** Pediatrics, Lenox Hill Hosp 1975; **Fellow:** Blood Banking Transfusion Medicine, NY Blood Center 1977; Pediatric Hematology-Oncology, NY Hosp/Cornell/Sloan Kettering 1979; **Fac Appt:** Asst Clin Prof Ped, SUNY Hlth Sci Ctr

Miller, Scott T MD (PHO) - **Spec Exp:** Sickle Cell Disease; **Hospital:** SUNY Downstate Med Ctr (Univ Hosp of Bklyn) (page 419), Kings County Hosp Ctr; **Address:** Univ Hosp Brooklyn, 450 Clarkson Ave, Box 49, Brooklyn, NY 11203-2056; **Phone:** 718-270-4714; **Board Cert:** Pediatrics 1981; Pediatric Hematology-Oncology 1982; **Med School:** Albert Einstein Coll Med 1976; **Resid:** Pediatrics, Montefiore Med Ctr 1979; **Fellow:** Pediatric Hematology-Oncology, Ny Hosp-Cornell Med Ctr 1981; **Fac Appt:** Prof Ped, SUNY Downstate

Sadanandan, Swayam MD (PHO) - **Spec Exp:** Sickle Cell Disease; Bleeding/Coagulation Disorders; Anemia; Pediatric Cancers; **Hospital:** Brooklyn Hosp Ctr-Downtown; **Address:** 121 DeKalb Ave, Brooklyn, NY 11201; **Phone:** 718-250-6074; **Board Cert:** Pediatrics 1980; Pediatric Hematology-Oncology 1984; **Med School:** India 1972; **Resid:** Pediatrics, St Vincent's Hosp & Med Ctr 1979; **Fellow:** Pediatric Hematology-Oncology, NYU Med Ctr 1981; **Fac Appt:** Asst Clin Prof Ped, NYU Sch Med

Sundaram, Revathy MD (PHO) - **Spec Exp:** Thalassemia; Sickle Cell Disease; Leukemia; **Hospital:** SUNY Downstate Med Ctr (Univ Hosp of Bklyn) - LICH (page 420), New York Methodist Hosp (page 418); **Address:** 502 8th Ave, Brooklyn, NY 11215; **Phone:** 718-780-3066; **Board Cert:** Pediatrics 1980; Pediatric Hematology-Oncology 1984; **Med School:** India 1973; **Resid:** Pediatrics, Rutgers Univ Hosp 1978; Pediatrics, Long Island Hosp 1980; **Fellow:** Pediatric Hematology-Oncology, Long Island Hosp 1983; **Fac Appt:** Asst Prof Ped, SUNY Hlth Sci Ctr

Viswanathan, Kusum MD (PHO) - **Spec Exp:** Sickle Cell Disease; Pediatric Cancers; Anemia; **Hospital:** Brookdale Univ Hosp Med Ctr; **Address:** 1 Brookdale Plaza, rm 346-CHC, Brooklyn, NY 11212-3139; **Phone:** 718-240-5904; **Board Cert:** Pediatrics 1986; Pediatric Hematology-Oncology 1987; **Med School:** India 1980; **Resid:** Pediatrics, Long Island Coll Hosp 1984; **Fellow:** Pediatric Hematology-Oncology, Long Island Coll Hosp 1986; **Fac Appt:** Assoc Clin Prof Ped, SUNY Hlth Sci Ctr

Pediatric Infectious Disease

Gesner, Matthew J MD (PInf) - **Spec Exp:** AIDS/HIV; Kawasaki Disease; **Hospital:** Kings County Hosp Ctr, SUNY Downstate Med Ctr (Univ Hosp of Bklyn) (page 419); **Address:** Kings County Hosp, 451 Clarkson Ave, Box 294, Brooklyn, NY 11203; **Phone:** 718-245-2562; **Board Cert:** Pediatrics 2006; Pediatric Infectious Disease 2009; **Med School:** SUNY Downstate 1988; **Resid:** Pediatrics, Chldns Hosp 1991; **Fellow:** Pediatric Infectious Disease, Bellevue Hosp Ctr 1994; **Fac Appt:** Asst Prof Ped, SUNY Downstate

Pediatric Nephrology

Kaplan, Matthew MD (PNep) - **Spec Exp:** Hypertension; Glomerulonephritis; **Hospital:** SUNY Downstate Med Ctr (Univ Hosp of Bklyn) - LICH (page 420), Coney Island Hosp; **Address:** Brooklyn Hosp, 121 Dekalb Ave Fl 9, Brooklyn, NY 11201; **Phone:** 718-250-6911; **Board Cert:** Pediatrics 1974; Pediatric Nephrology 1976; **Med School:** SUNY Downstate 1968; **Resid:** Pediatrics, NY Hosp-Cornell Med Ctr 1972; **Fellow:** Pediatric Nephrology, NY Hosp-Cornell Med Ctr 1976; **Fac Appt:** Assoc Clin Prof Ped, SUNY Downstate

Schoeneman, Morris J MD (PNep) - **Spec Exp:** Hypertension; Kidney Failure-Chronic; Urinary Tract Infections; Dialysis Care; **Hospital:** SUNY Downstate Med Ctr (Univ Hosp of Bklyn) (page 419), Richmond Univ Med Ctr; **Address:** SUNY Downstate Med Ctr, 470 Clarkson Ave, Box 49, Brooklyn, NY 11203; **Phone:** 718-270-4714; **Board Cert:** Pediatrics 1974; Pediatric Nephrology 1974; **Med School:** Georgetown Univ 1969; **Resid:** Pediatrics, Univ NC Hosp 1970; Pediatrics, Univ MD Hosp 1972; **Fellow:** Pediatric Nephrology, Montefiore Med Ctr 1975; **Fac Appt:** Prof Ped, SUNY Hlth Sci Ctr

Pediatric Otolaryngology

Goldsmith, Ari J MD (PO) - **Spec Exp:** Voice Disorders; Airway Disorders; Hearing Loss; Sleep Apnea; **Hospital:** SUNY Downstate Med Ctr (Univ Hosp of Bklyn) - LICH (page 420); **Address:** 921 49th St, Brooklyn, NY 11209; **Phone:** 718-283-6260; **Board Cert:** Otolaryngology 1994; **Med School:** Albert Einstein Coll Med 1988; **Resid:** Otolaryngology, LI Jewish Hosp 1993; **Fellow:** Pediatric Otolaryngology, Chldns Hosp 1994; **Fac Appt:** Assoc Prof Oto, SUNY Hlth Sci Ctr

Rosenfeld, Richard M MD (PO) - **Spec Exp:** Sinus Disorders/Surgery; Head & Neck Surgery; Ear Disorders/Surgery; **Hospital:** SUNY Downstate Med Ctr (Univ Hosp of Bklyn) (page 419), SUNY Downstate Med Ctr (Univ Hosp of Bklyn) - LICH (page 420); **Address:** Univ Otolaryngologists, 134 Atlantic Ave, Brooklyn, NY 11201; **Phone:** 718-780-1498; **Board Cert:** Otolaryngology 1989; **Med School:** SUNY Buffalo 1984; **Resid:** Surgery, Mount Sinai Med Ctr 1986; Otolaryngology, Mount Sinai Med Ctr 1989; **Fellow:** Pediatric Otolaryngology, Chldn's Hosp 1991; **Fac Appt:** Prof Oto, SUNY Downstate

Pediatric Pulmonology

Giusti, Robert J MD (PPul) - **Spec Exp:** Cystic Fibrosis; Asthma; Cough-Chronic; **Hospital:** NYU Langone Med Ctr (page 108); **Address:** NYU Pediatric Pulmonology, 160 E 32nd St, L-3 Medical, New York, NY 10016; **Phone:** 212-263-5940; **Board Cert:** Pediatrics 1987; Pediatric Pulmonology 2011; **Med School:** SUNY Downstate 1981; **Resid:** Pediatrics, Bellevue Hosp 1985; **Fac Appt:** Asst Prof Ped, NYU Sch Med

Lee, Haesoon MD (PPul) - **Spec Exp:** Asthma; Lung Injuries - RSV Related; Sleep Apnea; Tuberculosis; **Hospital:** SUNY Downstate Med Ctr (Univ Hosp of Bklyn) (page 419), Kings County Hosp Ctr; **Address:** SUNY-Downstate Med Ctr, Dept Pediatrics, 450 Clarkson Ave, Box 49, Brooklyn, NY 11203-2056; **Phone:** 718-221-5316; **Board Cert:** Pediatrics 1979; Pediatric Pulmonology 2011; **Med School:** South Korea 1972; **Resid:** Pediatrics, St Francis Hosp 1975; **Fellow:** Pediatric Pulmonology, Albert Einstein Affil Hosp 1977; **Fac Appt:** Assoc Prof Ped, SUNY Downstate

Marcus, Michael MD (PPul) - **Spec Exp:** Asthma; Sleep Apnea; Chronic Lung Disease; Gastroesophageal Reflux Disease (GERD); **Hospital:** Maimonides Med Ctr (page 98); **Address:** 4802 10th Ave, brooklyn, NY 11219; **Phone:** 718-980-5864; **Board Cert:** Pediatrics 1984; Allergy & Immunology 1987; Pediatric Pulmonology 2009; **Med School:** SUNY Stony Brook 1980; **Resid:** Pediatrics, Nassau County Med Ctr 1983; **Fellow:** Pediatric Pulmonology, Chldn's Hosp 1985; Allergy & Immunology, Chldn's Hosp 1985; **Fac Appt:** Asst Clin Prof Ped, SUNY Downstate

Narula, Pramod MD (PPul) - **Spec Exp:** Asthma; Chronic Lung Disease; **Hospital:** New York Methodist Hosp (page 418); **Address:** 502 8th Ave, Brooklyn, NY 11215-3609; **Phone:** 718-780-3066; **Board Cert:** Pediatrics 2005; Pediatric Pulmonology 2009; **Med School:** India 1977; **Resid:** Pediatrics, Winthrop Univ Hosp 1989; **Fellow:** Pediatric Pulmonology, Columbia-Presby Med Ctr 1994; **Fac Appt:** Assoc Clin Prof Ped, Cornell Univ-Weill Med Coll

Pediatric Surgery

Kessler, Edmund MD (PS) - **Spec Exp:** Neck Masses; Tumor Surgery; Gallbladder Surgery-Pediatric; Neonatal Surgery; **Hospital:** Steven & Alexandra Cohen Chldn's Med Ctr of NY (page 106), New York Methodist Hosp (page 418); **Address:** 263 7th Ave, Ste 4E, Brooklyn, NY 11215; **Phone:** 516-498-9000; **Med School:** South Africa 1968; **Resid:** Surgery, Univ Witwatersrand 1970; **Fellow:** Pediatric Surgery, Univ Witwatersrand 1977; **Fac Appt:** Asst Clin Prof S, Columbia P&S

Pediatrics

Ajl, Stephen MD (Ped) *PCP* - **Hospital:** Brooklyn Hosp Ctr-Downtown; **Address:** 121 DeKalb Ave, Brooklyn, NY 11201; **Phone:** 718-250-8764; **Board Cert:** Pediatrics 1980; Child Abuse Pediatrics 2009; **Med School:** Temple Univ 1975; **Resid:** Pediatrics, NY-Presby Hosp/Cornell 1978; **Fellow:** Ambulatory Pediatrics, Mount Sinai Med Ctr 1979; **Fac Appt:** Assoc Clin Prof Ped, SUNY Downstate

Fernandes, David R MD (Ped) *PCP* - **Hospital:** New York Methodist Hosp (page 418); **Address:** 126 95th St, Brooklyn, NY 11209-7203; **Phone:** 718-238-7842; **Board Cert:** Pediatrics 1980; **Med School:** SUNY Downstate 1972; **Resid:** Pediatrics, Kings County Hosp 1974; Pediatrics, N Shore Univ Hosp 1976; **Fellow:** Ambulatory Pediatrics, NYU-Bellevue Hosp 1977; **Fac Appt:** Asst Clin Prof Ped, SUNY Downstate

Gately, Adrian C MD (Ped) *PCP* - **Hospital:** New York Methodist Hosp (page 418); **Address:** 300 Park Pl, Brooklyn, NY 11238; **Phone:** 718-622-0469; **Board Cert:** Pediatrics 1983; **Med School:** Albert Einstein Coll Med 1975; **Resid:** Pediatrics, Jacobi Med Ctr 1978

Glaser, Amy MD (Ped) *PCP* - **Hospital:** SUNY Downstate Med Ctr (Univ Hosp of Bklyn) - LICH (page 420), NYU Langone Med Ctr (page 108); **Address:** 60 8th Ave, Brooklyn, NY 11217-3902; **Phone:** 718-636-0019; **Board Cert:** Pediatrics 1985; **Med School:** Mount Sinai Sch Med 1979; **Resid:** Pediatrics, Montefiore Hosp Med Ctr 1982; **Fellow:** Adolescent Medicine, Mt Sinai Hosp 1983

Jackson, Rosemary M MD (Ped) *PCP* - **Spec Exp:** Diabetes; Obesity; **Hospital:** SUNY Downstate Med Ctr (Univ Hosp of Bklyn) (page 419), SUNY Downstate Med Ctr (Univ Hosp of Bklyn) - LICH (page 420); **Address:** 86 E 49th St, Ste G, Brooklyn, NY 11203; **Phone:** 718-363-6646; **Board Cert:** Pediatrics 2008; **Med School:** SUNY Upstate Med Univ 1985; **Resid:** Pediatrics, Downstate Med Ctr 1988; **Fac Appt:** Asst Clin Prof Ped, SUNY Downstate

Oghia, Hady MD (Ped) *PCP* - **Spec Exp:** Neonatal Care; **Hospital:** Richmond Univ Med Ctr; **Address:** 7506 16th Ave, Brooklyn, NY 11214-1064; **Phone:** 718-331-3166; **Med School:** Mexico 1979; **Resid:** Pediatrics, St Vincent's Hosp & Med Ctr 1983

Preis, Oded MD (Ped) *PCP* - **Spec Exp:** Prematurity/Low Birth Weight Infants; **Hospital:** Maimonides Med Ctr (page 98), New York Methodist Hosp (page 418); **Address:** 1729 E 12th St, Brooklyn, NY 11229; **Phone:** 718-339-4919; **Board Cert:** Pediatrics 1978; Neonatal-Perinatal Medicine 1981; **Med School:** Israel 1971; **Resid:** Pediatrics, Maimonides Med Ctr 1975; **Fellow:** Neonatal-Perinatal Medicine, SUNY - Downstate Med Ctr 1977; **Fac Appt:** Assoc Clin Prof Ped, SUNY Downstate

Sergiou, Harry G MD (Ped) *PCP* - **Hospital:** SUNY Downstate Med Ctr (Univ Hosp of Bklyn) - LICH (page 420); **Address:** 554 Henry St, Brooklyn, NY 11231; **Phone:** 718-625-5591; **Board Cert:** Pediatrics 2011; **Med School:** Greece 1979; **Resid:** Pediatrics, Long Island Coll Hosp 1985

Wu, Jason J MD/PhD (Ped) *PCP* - **Spec Exp:** Chinese Community Health; **Hospital:** Maimonides Med Ctr (page 98); **Address:** 781 47th St, Brooklyn, NY 11220; **Phone:** 718-435-5980; **Board Cert:** Pediatrics 2010; **Med School:** China 1982; **Resid:** Pediatrics, Maimonides Med Ctr 2001; **Fac Appt:** Asst Clin Prof Ped, Mount Sinai Sch Med

Physical Medicine & Rehabilitation

Atakent, Pinar E MD (PMR) - **Spec Exp:** Pain Management; Stroke Rehabilitation; Electrodiagnosis; Acupuncture; **Hospital:** SUNY Downstate Med Ctr (Univ Hosp of Bklyn) (page 419); **Address:** LI Coll Hosp, 339 Hicks St, Brooklyn, NY 11201-5509; **Phone:** 718-780-4685; **Board Cert:** Physical Medicine & Rehabilitation 1982; **Med School:** Turkey 1971; **Resid:** Physical Medicine & Rehabilitation, Jacobi Med Ctr 1981

Gifford, Irina MD (PMR) - **Spec Exp:** Musculoskeletal Disorders; Neurologic Rehabilitation; Pediatric Rehabilitation; **Hospital:** Kingsbrook Jewish Med Ctr; **Address:** 585 Schenectady Ave, Brooklyn, NY 11203-1822; **Phone:** 718-604-5341; **Board Cert:** Physical Medicine & Rehabilitation 1990; **Med School:** Romania 1960; **Resid:** Physical Medicine & Rehabilitation, Mount Sinai Hosp 1989; **Fellow:** Pediatric Rehabilitation Medicine, Albert Einstein Med Sch 1990

Ross, Marc MD (PMR) - **Spec Exp:** Sports Medicine; Pain-Back; Gait Disorders; **Hospital:** Kingsbrook Jewish Med Ctr, Mount Sinai Med Ctr (page 102); **Address:** Kingsbrook Jewish Med Ctr, Dept Physical Med & Rehab, 585 Schenectady Ave, Brooklyn, NY 11203; **Phone:** 718-604-5341; **Board Cert:** Physical Medicine & Rehabilitation 2004; **Med School:** NY Med Coll 1989; **Resid:** Physical Medicine & Rehabilitation, Mt Sinai Med Ctr 1993; **Fac Appt:** Asst Prof PMR, Mount Sinai Sch Med

Stein, Perry MD (PMR) - **Spec Exp:** Pain Management; **Hospital:** Mercy Med Ctr - Rockville Centre, Maimonides Med Ctr (page 98); **Address:** 383 Ocean Pkwy, Brooklyn, NY 11218; **Phone:** 718-941-6000; **Board Cert:** Physical Medicine & Rehabilitation 1991; **Med School:** Mexico 1985; **Resid:** Physical Medicine & Rehabilitation, Univ Hosp 1990

Vallarino, Ramon MD (PMR) - **Spec Exp:** Pain Management; Functional Ability Loss; Electromyography; Musculoskeletal Disorders; **Hospital:** New York Methodist Hosp (page 418); **Address:** 164 20 St, Brooklyn, NY 11232; **Phone:** 516-418-0675; **Board Cert:** Physical Medicine & Rehabilitation 1977; **Med School:** Peru 1966; **Resid:** Physical Medicine & Rehabilitation, Mount Sinai Hosp 1968; **Fellow:** Rheumatology, Mount Sinai Hosp 1968; **Fac Appt:** Asst Clin Prof PMR, SUNY Hlth Sci Ctr

Psychiatry

Berkowitz, Howard L MD (Psyc) - **Spec Exp:** Anxiety Disorders; Depression; Geriatric Psychiatry; **Hospital:** Maimonides Med Ctr (page 98); **Address:** 910 48th St, Brooklyn, NY 11219-2927; **Phone:** 718-633-2025; **Board Cert:** Psychiatry 1977; Geriatric Psychiatry 2004; **Med School:** Albert Einstein Coll Med 1972; **Resid:** Internal Medicine, Beth Israel Hosp 1973; Psychiatry, Kings County Hosp 1976; **Fellow:** Consultation Psychiatry, Kings County Hosp 1977; **Fac Appt:** Assoc Clin Prof Psyc, SUNY Downstate

Coplan, Jeremy MD (Psyc) - **Spec Exp:** Anxiety Disorders; Psychosomatic Disorders; Bipolar/Mood Disorders; **Hospital:** SUNY Downstate Med Ctr (Univ Hosp of Bklyn) (page 419); **Address:** 450 Clarkson Ave, Box 1203, Brooklyn, NY 11203; **Phone:** 718-270-2023; **Board Cert:** Psychiatry 1990; **Med School:** South Africa 1983; **Resid:** Psychiatry, SUNY-Downstate Med Ctr 1989; **Fellow:** Biological Psychiatry, Columbia-Presby Med Ctr 1990; **Fac Appt:** Prof Psyc, SUNY Downstate

Eitan, Noam MD (Psyc) - **Spec Exp:** Anxiety Disorders; Depression; Gay & Lesbian Issues; **Hospital:** Woodhull Med & Mental Hlth Ctr; **Address:** 760 Broadway, Brooklyn, NY 11206; **Phone:** 718-963-5793; **Board Cert:** Psychiatry 2008; **Med School:** Israel 1986; **Resid:** Psychiatry, Shalvata Hosp 1991; **Fellow:** Psychoanalysis, Sackler Sch Med 1995

Goldberg, Jeffrey DO (Psyc) - **Spec Exp:** Geriatric Psychiatry; Anxiety & Depression; Mood Disorders; **Hospital:** Coney Island Hosp; **Address:** 5025 Ft Hamilton Pkwy, Brooklyn, NY 11219; **Phone:** 718-633-8183; **Board Cert:** Psychiatry 1986; Geriatric Psychiatry 2006; **Med School:** NY Coll Osteo Med 1981; **Resid:** Psychiatry, Maimonides Med Ctr 1985; **Fac Appt:** Asst Clin Prof Psyc, SUNY Downstate

Heisman, Alexander MD (Psyc) - **Spec Exp:** Addiction/Substance Abuse; Liaison Psychiatry; Pain-Chronic; **Hospital:** Beth Israel Med Ctr- Kings Hwy Div (page 94), New York Methodist Hosp (page 418); **Address:** 3045 Ocean Pkwy, Ste 1A, Brooklyn, NY 11235; **Phone:** 718-449-1705; **Board Cert:** Psychiatry 2007; Psychosomatic Medicine 2008; **Med School:** Russia 1976; **Resid:** Psychiatry, Montefiore Med Ctr 1996

Idupuganti, Sudharam MD (Psyc) - **Spec Exp:** Depression; Electroconvulsive Therapy (ECT); Panic Disorder; **Hospital:** Maimonides Med Ctr (page 98); **Address:** 585 Bayridge Pkwy, Brooklyn, NY 11209-3309; **Phone:** 718-921-1001; **Board Cert:** Psychiatry 1981; **Med School:** India 1974; **Resid:** Psychiatry, Maimonides Med Ctr 1979; **Fac Appt:** Asst Prof Psyc, SUNY Downstate

Licht, Arnold Lawrence MD (Psyc) - **Spec Exp:** Geriatric Psychiatry; Mood Disorders; Addiction/Substance Abuse; **Hospital:** SUNY Downstate Med Ctr (Univ Hosp of Bklyn) - LICH (page 420), New York Methodist Hosp (page 418); **Address:** 161 Atlantic Ave, Fl 1, Ste 1, Brooklyn, NY 11201; **Phone:** 718-935-0986; **Board Cert:** Psychiatry 1975; Geriatric Psychiatry 2001; **Med School:** SUNY Hlth Sci Ctr 1969; **Resid:** Psychiatry, Albert Einstein 1973; **Fac Appt:** Asst Prof Psyc, SUNY Downstate

Viswanathan, Ramaswamy MD (Psyc) - **Spec Exp:** Depression; Anxiety Disorders; **Hospital:** SUNY Downstate Med Ctr (Univ Hosp of Bklyn) (page 419), Kings County Hosp Ctr; **Address:** 450 Clarkson Ave, Ste A3-474, Brooklyn, NY 11203-2098; **Phone:** 718-270-2352; **Board Cert:** Psychiatry 1978; Internal Medicine 1989; Geriatric Psychiatry 2002; Addiction Psychiatry 2003; **Med School:** India 1972; **Resid:** Internal Medicine, Queens Hosp Ctr 1974; Psychiatry, SUNY Hlth Sci Ctr 1977; **Fellow:** Psychiatry, SUNY Hlth Sci Ctr 1978; **Fac Appt:** Assoc Clin Prof Psyc, SUNY Hlth Sci Ctr

Pulmonary Disease

Abott, Michael L MD (Pul) - **Spec Exp:** Asthma; Emphysema; **Hospital:** New York Methodist Hosp (page 418), Lutheran Med Ctr - Brooklyn; **Address:** 7124 18th Ave, Brooklyn, NY 11204-5203; **Phone:** 718-234-3333; **Board Cert:** Internal Medicine 1983; Pulmonary Disease 1986; **Med School:** Mexico 1978; **Resid:** Internal Medicine, Coney Island Hosp 1982; **Fellow:** Pulmonary Disease, Montefiore Med Ctr 1984

Amin, Hossam H MD (Pul) - **Spec Exp:** Asthma & Allergy; Critical Care; **Hospital:** Metropolitan Hosp Ctr - NY, New York Methodist Hosp (page 418); **Address:** 6903 4th Ave, Brooklyn, NY 11209; **Phone:** 718-238-6161; **Board Cert:** Internal Medicine 2006; Pulmonary Disease 2008; Critical Care Medicine 2009; **Med School:** Egypt 1988; **Resid:** Internal Medicine, Interfaith Med Ctr 1996; **Fellow:** Pulmonary Disease, Interfaith Med Ctr 1998; Critical Care Medicine, Mt Sinai Med Ctr 1999; **Fac Appt:** Assoc Prof Med, NY Med Coll

Bernstein, Chaim MD (Pul) - **Spec Exp:** Asthma; Chronic Obstructive Lung Disease (COPD); Emphysema; **Hospital:** Beth Israel Med Ctr- Kings Hwy Div (page 94); **Address:** 3131 Kings Hwy, Ste D10, Brooklyn, NY 11234-2643; **Phone:** 718-252-3590; **Board Cert:** Internal Medicine 1977; Pulmonary Disease 1982; Critical Care Medicine 2007; **Med School:** NYU Sch Med 1974; **Resid:** Internal Medicine, Brookdale Med Ctr 1977; Pulmonary Disease, Manhattan VA Hosp 1979; **Fellow:** Pulmonary Disease, Bellevue Hosp-NYU 1979

Bondi, Elliott MD (Pul) - **Spec Exp:** Asthma; Tuberculosis; Pneumonia; **Hospital:** Brookdale Univ Hosp Med Ctr; **Address:** Brookdale Hospital, Pulmonary Medicine, 1 Brookdale Plaza, rm A107, Brooklyn, NY 11212; **Phone:** 718-240-5236; **Board Cert:** Internal Medicine 1987; Pulmonary Disease 1982; **Med School:** Univ MD Sch Med 1971; **Resid:** Internal Medicine, Maimonides Medical Ctr 1973; Internal Medicine, Bronx Muni Hosp 1974; **Fellow:** Pulmonary Disease, Bronx Muni Hosp 1976; **Fac Appt:** Assoc Clin Prof Med, SUNY Downstate

Demetis, Spiro MD (Pul) - **Spec Exp:** Sarcoidosis; Lung Cancer; Asthma & Emphysema; Pulmonary Hypertension; **Hospital:** SUNY Downstate Med Ctr (Univ Hosp of Bklyn) (page 419), Lutheran Med Ctr - Brooklyn; **Address:** 450 Clarkson Ave, Box 19, Brooklyn, NY 11203; **Phone:** 718-270-1821; **Board Cert:** Internal Medicine 1989; Pulmonary Disease 2005; Critical Care Medicine 2005; **Med School:** Mexico 1983; **Resid:** Internal Medicine, Univ Hosp 1988; **Fellow:** Pulmonary Disease, Univ Hosp 1990; Critical Care Medicine, Univ Hosp 1991; **Fac Appt:** Assoc Prof Med, SUNY Hlth Sci Ctr

George, Liziamma MD (Pul) - **Spec Exp:** Sleep Disorders; Smoking Cessation; **Hospital:** New York Methodist Hosp (page 418); **Address:** 263 7th St, Ste 5A, Brooklyn, NY 11215; **Phone:** 718-246-8600; **Board Cert:** Internal Medicine 1987; Critical Care Medicine 1999; Pulmonary Disease 2010; Sleep Medicine 2009; **Med School:** India 1980; **Resid:** Internal Medicine, St Joseph's Med Ctr 1987; **Fellow:** Pulmonary Disease, St Joseph's Med Ctr 1989; **Fac Appt:** Assoc Clin Prof Med, Cornell Univ-Weill Med Coll

Gulrajani, Ramesh MD (Pul) - **Spec Exp:** Asthma; Sarcoidosis; Lung Cancer; **Hospital:** Brooklyn Hosp Ctr-Downtown; **Address:** 121 DeKalb Ave, Dept Internal Med, Ste 7E, Brooklyn, NY 11201-5425; **Phone:** 718-250-6950; **Board Cert:** Internal Medicine 1979; Pulmonary Disease 1984; **Med School:** India 1974; **Resid:** Internal Medicine, Brooklyn Cumberland Med Ctr 1979; **Fellow:** Pulmonary Disease, Brooklyn Cumberland Med Ctr 1981; **Fac Appt:** Assoc Clin Prof Med, Cornell Univ-Weill Med Coll

Hammer, Arthur MD (Pul) - **Spec Exp:** Asthma; Sleep Disorders; Pulmonary Fibrosis; **Hospital:** Beth Israel Med Ctr- Kings Hwy Div (page 94); **Address:** 3131 Kings Hwy, Ste D10, Brooklyn, NY 11234-2643; **Phone:** 718-252-3590; **Board Cert:** Internal Medicine 2006; Pulmonary Disease 2009; **Med School:** Mexico 1970; **Resid:** Internal Medicine, Brookdale Hosp 1974; **Fellow:** Pulmonary Disease, NYU 1976

Kupfer, Yizhak MD (Pul) - **Spec Exp:** Sleep & Snoring Disorders; Cough; Mechanical Ventilation; **Hospital:** Maimonides Med Ctr (page 98); **Address:** Div Pulmonary & Critical Care Medicine, 953 49th St, Ste 511, Brooklyn, NY 11219-2923; **Phone:** 718-283-8380; **Board Cert:** Internal Medicine 1989; Pulmonary Disease 2000; Critical Care Medicine 2000; Sleep Medicine 2007; **Med School:** SUNY Downstate 1986; **Resid:** Internal Medicine, Maimonides Med Ctr 1989; **Fellow:** Pulmonary Disease, Maimonides Med Ctr 1991; Critical Care Medicine, Maimonides Med Ctr 1992; **Fac Appt:** Assoc Clin Prof Med, SUNY Downstate

Lombardo, Gerard T MD (Pul) - **Spec Exp:** Sleep Apnea; Sleep & Snoring Disorders; **Hospital:** New York Methodist Hosp (page 418); **Address:** 9101 4th Ave, Brooklyn, NY 11209; **Phone:** 718-745-1156; **Board Cert:** Internal Medicine 1984; Pulmonary Disease 1986; Sleep Medicine 2009; **Med School:** Grenada 1981; **Resid:** Internal Medicine, NY Methodist Hosp 1984; **Fellow:** Pulmonary Disease, NY Methodist Hosp 1986; **Fac Appt:** Asst Clin Prof Med, Cornell Univ-Weill Med Coll

Miarrostami, Rameen M MD (Pul) - **Spec Exp:** Asthma; Chronic Obstructive Lung Disease (COPD); Emphysema; Cough; **Hospital:** New York Methodist Hosp (page 418), Lutheran Med Ctr - Brooklyn; **Address:** 7124 18th Ave, Brooklyn, NY 11204-5203; **Phone:** 718-234-3333; **Board Cert:** Internal Medicine 2011; Pulmonary Disease 2004; **Med School:** Dominican Republic 1985; **Resid:** Internal Medicine, Lincoln Med Ctr 1991; **Fellow:** Pulmonary Disease, LI Coll Hosp 1993

Raoof, Suhail MD (Pul) - **Spec Exp:** Critical Care Medicine; Chronic Obstructive Lung Disease (COPD); Mechanical Ventilation; Lung Disease; **Hospital:** New York Methodist Hosp (page 418); **Address:** Div, Pulmonary & Critical Care, 506 6th St, Brooklyn, NY 11215; **Phone:** 718-780-5835; **Board Cert:** Internal Medicine 2002; Pulmonary Disease 2003; Critical Care Medicine 2004; **Med School:** India 1982; **Resid:** Internal Medicine, LIJ Med Ctr 1989; Internal Medicine, Nassau County Med Ctr 1991; **Fellow:** Pulmonary Critical Care Medicine, Stony Brook Affil Hosps 1992; **Fac Appt:** Prof Med, Cornell Univ-Weill Med Coll

Saleh, Anthony MD (Pul) - **Spec Exp:** Asthma; Interstitial Lung Disease; Lung Cancer; **Hospital:** New York Methodist Hosp (page 418); **Address:** 7206 7th Ave, Brooklyn, NY 11209; **Phone:** 718-745-1200; **Board Cert:** Internal Medicine 1988; Pulmonary Disease 2010; **Med School:** Grenada 1985; **Resid:** Internal Medicine, NY Methodist Hosp 1988; **Fellow:** Pulmonary Disease, NY Methodist Hosp 1990; **Fac Appt:** Asst Clin Prof Med, Cornell Univ-Weill Med Coll

Smith, Peter R MD (Pul) - **Spec Exp:** Chronic Obstructive Lung Disease (COPD); Smoking Cessation; Sarcoidosis; Wegener's Granulomatosis; **Hospital:** SUNY Downstate Med Ctr (Univ Hosp of Bklyn) - LICH (page 420); **Address:** Long Island Coll Hosp, Div Pulmonology, 339 Hicks St, Brooklyn, NY 11201; **Phone:** 718-780-1416; **Board Cert:** Internal Medicine 1973; Pulmonary Disease 1974; Critical Care Medicine 2009; **Med School:** Columbia P&S 1968; **Resid:** Internal Medicine, Downstate Med Ctr 1970; Internal Medicine, Jacobi Med Ctr 1971; **Fellow:** Pulmonary Disease, Downstate Med Ctr 1974; **Fac Appt:** Clin Prof Med, SUNY Hlth Sci Ctr

Tessler, Sidney MD (Pul) - **Spec Exp:** Cough; Asthma; Mechanical Ventilation; **Hospital:** Maimonides Med Ctr (page 98); **Address:** 953 49th St, Fl 5, rm 511, Div Pul & Critical Care Med, Brooklyn, NY 11219-2923; **Phone:** 718-283-8380; **Board Cert:** Internal Medicine 1977; Pulmonary Disease 1980; Critical Care Medicine 2007; **Med School:** SUNY Hlth Sci Ctr 1970; **Resid:** Internal Medicine, Coney Island Hosp 1972; Internal Medicine, Maimonides Med Ctr 1976; **Fellow:** Pulmonary Disease, Maimonides Med Ctr 1977; **Fac Appt:** Clin Prof Med, SUNY Hlth Sci Ctr

Radiation Oncology

Ashamalla, Hani MD (RadRO) - **Spec Exp:** Brachytherapy; Prostate Cancer; Gastrointestinal Cancer; Breast Cancer; **Hospital:** New York Methodist Hosp (page 418), Wyckoff Heights Med Ctr; **Address:** NY Methodist Hosp, Dept Rad Oncology, 506 6th St, Brooklyn, NY 11215; **Phone:** 718-780-3677; **Board Cert:** Radiation Oncology 2004; **Med School:** Egypt 1983; **Resid:** Radiation Oncology, NY Methodist Hosp 1994; **Fellow:** Radiation Oncology, NY Methodist Hosp 1995; Radiation Oncology, Chldns Hosp 1995; **Fac Appt:** Assoc Clin Prof RadRO, Cornell Univ-Weill Med Coll

Cooper, Jay MD (RadRO) - **Spec Exp:** Head & Neck Cancer; Skin Cancer; Chemo-Radiation Combined Therapy; Intensity Modulated Radiotherapy (IMRT); **Hospital:** Maimonides Med Ctr (page 98); **Address:** 6300 8th Ave, Brooklyn, NY 11220; **Phone:** 718-765-2700; **Board Cert:** Therapeutic Radiology 1977; **Med School:** NYU Sch Med 1973; **Resid:** Radiation Oncology, NYU Med Ctr 1977; **Fac Appt:** Prof RadRO, Albert Einstein Coll Med

Donahue, Bernadine R MD (RadRO) - **Spec Exp:** Brain Tumors; Gastrointestinal Cancer; Pediatric Cancers; Solid Tumors; **Hospital:** Maimonides Med Ctr (page 98); **Address:** Maimonides Med Ctr, Dept Radiation Oncology, 6300 8th Ave, Lower Level, Brooklyn, NY 11220; **Phone:** 718-765-2700; **Board Cert:** Internal Medicine 1987; Radiation Oncology 1991; **Med School:** Boston Univ 1984; **Resid:** Internal Medicine, Boston Univ Med Ctr 1987; **Fellow:** Radiation Oncology, NYU Med Ctr 1990

Gliedman, Paul R MD (RadRO) - **Spec Exp:** Breast Cancer; Prostate Cancer; Brain Tumors; Stereotactic Radiosurgery; **Hospital:** St. Luke's - Roosevelt Hosp Ctr - Roosevelt Div (page 94), Beth Israel Med Ctr- Kings Hwy Div (page 94); **Address:** Brooklyn Radiation Oncology, 2101 Avenue X, Brooklyn, NY 11235; **Phone:** 718-512-2160; **Board Cert:** Radiation Oncology 1987; **Med School:** Columbia P&S 1983; **Resid:** Radiation Oncology, NYU Med Ctr 1987

Rotman, Marvin Z MD (RadRO) - **Spec Exp:** Bladder Cancer; Gynecologic Cancer; Eye Tumors/Cancer; Prostate Cancer; **Hospital:** SUNY Downstate Med Ctr (Univ Hosp of Bklyn) (page 419), SUNY Downstate Med Ctr (Univ Hosp of Bklyn) - LICH (page 420); **Address:** 450 Clarkson Ave, Box 1211, Brooklyn, NY 11203-2056; **Phone:** 718-270-2181; **Board Cert:** Diagnostic Radiology 1966; Radiation Oncology 1999; **Med School:** Jefferson Med Coll 1958; **Resid:** Internal Medicine, Albert Einstein Med Ctr 1960; Radiation Oncology, Montefiore Hosp Med Ctr 1965; **Fac Appt:** Prof RadRO, SUNY Downstate

Reproductive Endocrinology

Grazi, Richard MD (RE) - **Spec Exp:** Infertility-IVF; Preimplantation Genetic Diagnosis; Fertility Preservation in Cancer; **Hospital:** Maimonides Med Ctr (page 98), Richmond Univ Med Ctr; **Address:** 1355 84th St, Brooklyn, NY 11228-3030; **Phone:** 718-283-8600; **Board Cert:** Obstetrics & Gynecology 2006; Reproductive Endocrinology/Infertility 2006; **Med School:** SUNY Buffalo 1981; **Resid:** Obstetrics & Gynecology, NYU Med Ctr 1985; **Fellow:** Reproductive Endocrinology, UMDNJ Med Ctr 1987; **Fac Appt:** Assoc Clin Prof ObG, Mount Sinai Sch Med

Kofinas, George D MD (RE) - **Spec Exp:** Infertility-IVF; Fertility Preservation; Robotic Assisted Laparoscopic Surgery; Hysteroscopic Surgery; **Hospital:** New York Methodist Hosp (page 418); **Address:** 506 6th St WP Bldg Fl 4, Brooklyn, NY 11215-3609; **Phone:** 718-780-5065; **Board Cert:** Obstetrics & Gynecology 2011; Reproductive Endocrinology 2011; **Med School:** Greece 1975; **Resid:** Obstetrics & Gynecology, NY Methodist Hosp 1982; Obstetrics & Gynecology, Brooklyn Hosp 1984; **Fellow:** Reproductive Endocrinology, Univ Hosp 1986; **Fac Appt:** Asst Prof ObG, SUNY Hlth Sci Ctr

Seifer, David B MD (RE) - **Spec Exp:** Infertility-IVF; Infertility-Advanced Maternal Age; Fertility Preservation in Cancer; **Hospital:** Maimonides Med Ctr (page 98), Richmond Univ Med Ctr; **Address:** 1355 84th St, Brooklyn, NY 11228; **Phone:** 718-283-8600; **Board Cert:** Obstetrics & Gynecology 2011; Reproductive Endocrinology/Infertility 2011; **Med School:** Univ IL Coll Med 1981; **Resid:** Obstetrics & Gynecology, Stanford Univ Hosp 1985; **Fellow:** Reproductive Endocrinology, Yale-New Haven Hosp 1991; **Fac Appt:** Prof ObG, Mount Sinai Sch Med

Rheumatology

Bernstein, Lawrence J MD (Rhu) - **Spec Exp:** Rheumatoid Arthritis; Polymyositis; Scleroderma; **Hospital:** Brookdale Univ Hosp Med Ctr; **Address:** Dept Rehab Medicine, 1 Brookdale Plaza, rm 344 CHC, Brooklyn, NY 11212; **Phone:** 718-240-6126; **Board Cert:** Internal Medicine 1965; Physical Medicine & Rehabilitation 1968; Rheumatology 1972; **Med School:** NYU Sch Med 1958; **Resid:** Internal Medicine, Bellevue Hosp 1961; **Fellow:** Rheumatology, NYU Med Ctr 1962

Bienenstock, Harry MD (Rhu) - **Spec Exp:** Rheumatoid Arthritis; Musculoskeletal Disorders; **Hospital:** Beth Israel Med Ctr- Kings Hwy Div (page 94), Hosp For Special Surgery (page 115); **Address:** 4015 Avenue U, Brooklyn, NY 11234-5117; **Phone:** 718-252-8181; **Board Cert:** Internal Medicine 1965; Rheumatology 1972; **Med School:** Ros Franklin Univ/Chicago Med Sch 1957; **Resid:** Internal Medicine, VA Med Ctr 1960; **Fellow:** Rheumatology, Hosp For Special Surgery 1962; **Fac Appt:** Assoc Clin Prof Med, Cornell Univ-Weill Med Coll

Garner, Bruce MD (Rhu) - **Spec Exp:** Rheumatoid Arthritis; Osteoporosis; Osteoarthritis; Lupus/SLE; **Hospital:** Lutheran Med Ctr - Brooklyn; **Address:** 7901 4th Ave, Ste A5, Brooklyn, NY 11209-3915; **Phone:** 718-921-5239; **Board Cert:** Internal Medicine 1987; Rheumatology 1988; **Med School:** Mexico 1981; **Resid:** Internal Medicine, Lutheran Med Ctr 1985; **Fellow:** Rheumatology, Washington Hosp Ctr 1987; **Fac Appt:** Asst Clin Prof Med, SUNY Downstate

Green, Stuart MD (Rhu) - **Spec Exp:** Rheumatoid Arthritis; Osteoporosis; Lupus/SLE; **Hospital:** Brooklyn Hosp Ctr-Downtown; **Address:** 121 DeKalb Ave Fl 7, Brooklyn, NY 11201-5425; **Phone:** 718-250-6921; **Board Cert:** Internal Medicine 1982; Rheumatology 1986; **Med School:** Georgetown Univ 1979; **Resid:** Internal Medicine, St Luke's/Roosevelt Hosp Ctr 1982; **Fellow:** Rheumatology, SUNY Downstate Med Ctr 1985; **Fac Appt:** Asst Clin Prof Med, NYU Sch Med

Lesser, Robert S MD (Rhu) - **Spec Exp:** Polymyalgia Rheumatica; Rheumatoid Arthritis; Lupus/SLE; **Hospital:** Beth Israel Med Ctr- Kings Hwy Div (page 94); **Address:** 4015 Avenue U, Brooklyn, NY 11234-5117; **Phone:** 718-252-5151; **Board Cert:** Internal Medicine 1985; Rheumatology 1988; **Med School:** Ros Franklin Univ/Chicago Med Sch 1982; **Resid:** Internal Medicine, Hahnemann Univ Hosp 1985; **Fellow:** Rheumatology, Hahnemann Univ Hosp 1987; **Fac Appt:** Assoc Clin Prof Med, SUNY Hlth Sci Ctr

Patel, Jitendra K MD (Rhu) - **Spec Exp:** Arthritis; Fibromyalgia; Pain-Back; **Hospital:** Kingsbrook Jewish Med Ctr, Beth Israel Med Ctr- Kings Hwy Div (page 94); **Address:** 3420 Ave N, Brooklyn, NY 11234-2607; **Phone:** 718-258-7019; **Board Cert:** Internal Medicine 1979; Rheumatology 1982; **Med School:** India 1975; **Resid:** Internal Medicine, Mem U Newfoundland 1979; **Fellow:** Rheumatology, Georgetown Univ Hosp 1982

Schiff, Carl F MD (Rhu) - **Spec Exp:** Rheumatoid Arthritis; Osteoporosis; **Hospital:** Maimonides Med Ctr (page 98); **Address:** Maimonides Med Ctr, 4802 10th Ave, Ste E352, Brooklyn, NY 11219; **Phone:** 718-283-8519; **Board Cert:** Internal Medicine 1983; Rheumatology 1986; **Med School:** Yale Univ 1980; **Resid:** Internal Medicine, Mt Sinai Hosp 1983; **Fellow:** Rheumatology, Columbia-Presby Med Ctr 1986; **Fac Appt:** Asst Clin Prof Med, SUNY Hlth Sci Ctr

Surgery

Adler, Harry MD (S) - **Spec Exp:** Biliary Surgery; Laparoscopic Surgery; Hernia; Colon Surgery; **Hospital:** Maimonides Med Ctr (page 98); **Address:** 948 48th St Fl 3, Brooklyn, NY 11219; **Phone:** 718-283-7952; **Board Cert:** Surgery 2005; Surgical Critical Care 2008; **Med School:** NYU Sch Med 1980; **Resid:** Surgery, Bellevue Hosp/NYU Med Ctr 1985; **Fellow:** Surgical Critical Care, Maimonides Med Ctr 1986; **Fac Appt:** Asst Clin Prof S, SUNY Downstate

Alfonso II, Antonio E MD (S) - **Spec Exp:** Thyroid Cancer; Head & Neck Surgery; Breast Cancer; **Hospital:** SUNY Downstate Med Ctr (Univ Hosp of Bklyn) - LICH (page 420), SUNY Downstate Med Ctr (Univ Hosp of Bklyn) (page 419); **Address:** Long Island Coll Hosp, 339 Hicks St, Brooklyn, NY 11201; **Phone:** 718-875-3244; **Board Cert:** Surgery 1973; **Med School:** Philippines 1968; **Resid:** Surgery, Temple Univ Hosp 1972; **Fellow:** Surgical Oncology, Meml Sloan Kettering Cancer Ctr 1974; **Fac Appt:** Prof Emeritus S, SUNY Downstate

Bernstein, Michael O MD (S) - **Spec Exp:** Breast Cancer; Hernia; Gastrointestinal Surgery; **Hospital:** SUNY Downstate Med Ctr (Univ Hosp of Bklyn) - LICH (page 420); **Address:** 350 Henry St, Brooklyn, NY 11201; **Phone:** 718-780-1563; **Board Cert:** Surgery 2007; **Med School:** Penn State Coll Med 1983; **Resid:** Surgery, SUNY-Kings Co Hosp 1988; **Fac Appt:** Asst Prof S, SUNY Downstate

Borgen, Patrick I MD (S) - **Spec Exp:** Breast Cancer; Breast Cancer & Surgery; **Hospital:** Maimonides Med Ctr (page 98); **Address:** Maimonides Breast Ctr, 6300 8th Ave, Brooklyn, NY 11220; **Phone:** 718-765-2570; **Board Cert:** Surgery 2002; **Med School:** Louisiana State U, New Orleans 1984; **Resid:** Surgery, Ochsner Fdn Hosp 1989; **Fellow:** Surgical Oncology, Meml Sloan Kettering Canc Ctr 1990; **Fac Appt:** Prof S, Cornell Univ-Weill Med Coll

Borriello, Raffaele MD (S) - **Spec Exp:** Breast Surgery; Hernia; Gastrointestinal Surgery; **Hospital:** SUNY Downstate Med Ctr (Univ Hosp of Bklyn) - LICH (page 420), New York Methodist Hosp (page 418); **Address:** 100 Clinton St, Ste 2, Brooklyn, NY 11201; **Phone:** 718-625-0767; **Board Cert:** Surgery 2005; **Med School:** SUNY Downstate 1981; **Resid:** Surgery, Kings Co Hosp 1986; **Fac Appt:** Assoc Prof S, SUNY Downstate

Chiariello, Mario MD (S) - **Spec Exp:** Cancer Surgery; **Hospital:** New York Methodist Hosp (page 418); **Address:** 1479 73rd St, Brooklyn, NY 11228-2111; **Phone:** 718-331-4938; **Board Cert:** Surgery 2010; **Med School:** Italy 1978; **Resid:** Surgery, Brooklyn Cumberland Hosp 1984

Dresner, Lisa S MD (S) - **Spec Exp:** Breast Surgery; Critical Care; **Hospital:** SUNY Downstate Med Ctr (Univ Hosp of Bklyn) (page 419); **Address:** SUNY HSC, Dept Surg, 450 Clarkson Ave, Box 40, Brooklyn, NY 11203-2056; **Phone:** 718-270-1973; **Board Cert:** Surgery 2011; Surgical Critical Care 2003; **Med School:** SUNY Downstate 1985; **Resid:** Surgery, SUNY Downstate Med Ctr 1992; **Fellow:** Surgical Critical Care, Jackson Meml Hosp 1993; **Fac Appt:** Assoc Prof S, SUNY Downstate

Fahoum, Bashar MD (S) - **Spec Exp:** Laparoscopic Surgery; Critical Care; Trauma; **Hospital:** New York Methodist Hosp (page 418); **Address:** 506 6th St, Brooklyn, NY 11215-3609; **Phone:** 718-780-3288; **Board Cert:** Surgery 2003; Surgical Critical Care 2004; **Med School:** Syria 1987; **Resid:** Surgery, New York Methodist Hosp 1993; **Fellow:** Surgical Critical Care, New York Med Coll 2003; **Fac Appt:** Asst Prof S, Cornell Univ-Weill Med Coll

Fogler, Richard MD (S) - **Spec Exp:** Breast Surgery; Colon & Rectal Surgery; Gastrointestinal Surgery; **Hospital:** Brookdale Univ Hosp Med Ctr; **Address:** 1 Brookdale Plaza, rm 122, Brooklyn, NY 11212-3139; **Phone:** 718-240-5437; **Board Cert:** Surgery 1975; **Med School:** NY Med Coll 1968; **Resid:** Surgery, Brookdale Hosp 1973; **Fac Appt:** Clin Prof S, SUNY Hlth Sci Ctr

Genato, Romulo MD (S) - **Spec Exp:** Breast Surgery; Laparoscopic Surgery; Hernia; **Hospital:** Brooklyn Hosp Ctr-Downtown; **Address:** Brooklyn Hosp Ctr, Dept Surg, 121 DeKalb Ave, Brooklyn, NY 11201-5425; **Phone:** 718-250-8970; **Board Cert:** Surgery 2010; **Med School:** Philippines 1972; **Resid:** Surgery, Brooklyn Hosp 1979; **Fac Appt:** Asst Clin Prof S, Cornell Univ-Weill Med Coll

Gorecki, Piotr J MD (S) - **Spec Exp:** Laparoscopic Surgery; Obesity/Bariatric Surgery; Gastrointestinal Surgery; **Hospital:** New York Methodist Hosp (page 418); **Address:** 263 7th Ave Fl 5A, Brooklyn, NY 11215; **Phone:** 718-246-8600; **Board Cert:** Surgery 2009; **Med School:** Poland 1991; **Resid:** Surgery, NY Methodist Hosp 1998; **Fellow:** Laparoscopic Surgery, Mayo Clinic 1999; **Fac Appt:** Asst Prof S, Cornell Univ-Weill Med Coll

Hong, Joon Ho MD (S) - **Spec Exp:** Vascular Surgery; **Hospital:** SUNY Downstate Med Ctr (Univ Hosp of Bklyn) (page 419); **Address:** SUNY Downstate Med Ctr, 450 Clarkson Ave, Box 40, Brooklyn, NY 11203; **Phone:** 718-270-1898; **Board Cert:** Surgery 2009; **Med School:** South Korea 1967; **Resid:** Surgery, Downstate Med Ctr 1979; **Fac Appt:** Prof S, SUNY Downstate

Kaleya, Ronald MD (S) - **Spec Exp:** Pancreatic Cancer; Breast Cancer; Colon & Rectal Cancer; **Hospital:** Maimonides Med Ctr (page 98); **Address:** 948 48th St, Brooklyn, NY 11219; **Phone:** 718-283-7602; **Board Cert:** Surgery 2008; **Med School:** Cornell Univ-Weill Med Coll 1980; **Resid:** Surgery, Albert Einstein Med Ctr 1985; **Fellow:** Surgical Oncology, Meml Sloan Kettering Cancer Ctr 1987

Lewis, Theophilus MD (S) - **Spec Exp:** Breast Cancer & Surgery; **Hospital:** SUNY Downstate Med Ctr (Univ Hosp of Bklyn) (page 419); **Address:** 451 Clarkson Ave, rm 4101, Box 40, Brooklyn, NY 11203-0040; **Phone:** 718-270-2155; **Board Cert:** Surgery 2003; **Med School:** SUNY Downstate 1978; **Resid:** Surgery, Kings Co Hosp 1983

Lois, William A MD (S) - **Spec Exp:** Dialysis Access Surgery; Vascular Surgery; Wound Healing/Care; **Hospital:** Kingsbrook Jewish Med Ctr; **Address:** 5723 Avenue N, Brooklyn, NY 11234; **Phone:** 718-251-1111; **Board Cert:** Surgery 1999; **Med School:** Spain 1982; **Resid:** Surgery, Interfaith Med Ctr 1987

Manasseh, Donna-Marie MD (S) - **Spec Exp:** Breast Surgery; **Hospital:** Maimonides Med Ctr (page 98); **Address:** 745 64th St, Brooklyn, NY 11220; **Phone:** 718-765-2570; **Board Cert:** Surgery 2005; **Med School:** Harvard Med Sch 1996; **Resid:** Surgery, NY Presby Hosp 2002; **Fellow:** Surgical Breast Oncology, Meml Sloan Kettering Cancer Ctr 2005; **Fac Appt:** Asst Clin Prof S, Columbia P&S

Rajpal, Sanjeev MD (S) - **Spec Exp:** Cancer Surgery; Laparoscopic Surgery; Breast Surgery; **Hospital:** Beth Israel Med Ctr- Kings Hwy Div (page 94), Brookdale Univ Hosp Med Ctr; **Address:** 9413 Flatlands Ave, Ste 203E, Brooklyn, NY 11236-5233; **Phone:** 718-251-1212; **Board Cert:** Surgery 2002; **Med School:** India 1975; **Resid:** Surgery, Brookdale Hosp Med Ctr 1980; **Fellow:** Surgical Oncology, Roswell Park Meml Inst 1982; Laparoscopic Surgery, Yale Univ 2001; **Fac Appt:** Asst Prof S, SUNY Downstate

Schwartzman, Alexander MD (S) - **Spec Exp:** Breast Cancer; Colon Surgery; Laparoscopic Surgery; Hernia; **Hospital:** SUNY Downstate Med Ctr (Univ Hosp of Bklyn) (page 419); **Address:** 470 Clarkson Ave, Box 40, Brooklyn, NY 11203; **Phone:** 718-270-1791; **Board Cert:** Surgery 2010; **Med School:** Dominican Republic 1983; **Resid:** Surgery, Brooklyn Hosp 1988

Steiner, Henry MD (S) - **Spec Exp:** Breast Surgery; **Hospital:** Maimonides Med Ctr (page 98); **Address:** 8105 Bay Pkwy, Brooklyn, NY 11214; **Phone:** 718-331-7314; **Board Cert:** Surgery 2001; **Med School:** SUNY Downstate 1976; **Resid:** Surgery, Maimonides Med Ctr 1980; **Fellow:** Vascular Surgery, Maimonides Med Ctr 1981

Wright, Albert M MD (S) - **Spec Exp:** Breast Disease; Colon & Rectal Surgery; Thyroid Surgery; **Hospital:** Interfaith Med Ctr, New York Methodist Hosp (page 418); **Address:** 1 Plaza St, Ste 1B, Brooklyn, NY 11217; **Phone:** 718-638-1971; **Board Cert:** Surgery 2010; **Med School:** England, UK 1970; **Resid:** Surgery, Mt Sinai Hosp 1977; **Fac Appt:** Asst Clin Prof S, Cornell Univ-Weill Med Coll

Thoracic & Cardiac Surgery

Abrol, Sunil MD (T&CS) - **Spec Exp:** Cardiac Surgery; Aneurysm-Thoracic Aortic; Heart Valve Surgery; Aortic Surgery; **Hospital:** Maimonides Med Ctr (page 98), Jamaica Hosp Med Ctr; **Address:** Maimonides Med Ctr, Cardiothoracic Surg, 4802 10th Ave Fl 4 - rm D, Brooklyn, NY 11219; **Phone:** 718-283-7686; **Board Cert:** Surgery 2009; Thoracic Surgery 2002; **Med School:** India 1986; **Resid:** Surgery, Maimonides Med Ctr 1998; **Fellow:** Thoracic Surgery, SUNY Hlth Sci Ctr 2001; **Fac Appt:** Asst Prof S, Mount Sinai Sch Med

Burack, Joshua H MD (T&CS) - **Spec Exp:** Cardiothoracic Surgery; **Hospital:** SUNY Downstate Med Ctr (Univ Hosp of Bklyn) (page 419), Kings County Hosp Ctr; **Address:** SUNY Downstate, Dept Cardiothor Surg, 450 Clarkson Ave, Box 40, Brooklyn, NY 11203; **Phone:** 718-270-1981; **Board Cert:** Thoracic Surgery 2009; **Med School:** Albert Einstein Coll Med 1982; **Resid:** Surgery, Montefiore Med Ctr 1987; **Fellow:** Cardiothoracic Surgery, Univ Hosp 1989; **Fac Appt:** Assoc Prof S, SUNY Downstate

Harris, Loren MD (T&CS) - **Spec Exp:** Thoracic Cancers; Esophageal Cancer; **Hospital:** Maimonides Med Ctr (page 98); **Address:** 4802 Tenth Ave, Brooklyn, NY 11219; **Phone:** 718-283-7686; **Board Cert:** Thoracic Surgery 2006; **Med School:** NYU Sch Med 1987; **Resid:** Surgery, NYU Med Ctr 1994; **Fellow:** Cardiovascular Surgery, NYU Med Ctr 1996; **Fac Appt:** Asst Prof S, Albert Einstein Coll Med

Tortolani, Anthony J MD (T&CS) - **Spec Exp:** Transfusion Free Surgery; Heart Valve Surgery; Coronary Artery Surgery; **Hospital:** New York Methodist Hosp (page 418), NY-Presby/Weill Cornell Med Ctr, NY (page 104); **Address:** New York Methodist Hosp, Dept Surgery, 506 6th St Fl 6, Brooklyn, NY 11215; **Phone:** 718-780-5990; **Board Cert:** Surgery 1975; Thoracic Surgery 2009; **Med School:** Geo Wash Univ 1969; **Resid:** Surgery, N Shore Univ Hosp 1974; **Fellow:** Cardiothoracic Surgery, NYU Med Ctr 1978; **Fac Appt:** Assoc Prof S, Cornell Univ-Weill Med Coll

Urology

Friedman, Steven C MD (U) - **Spec Exp:** Pediatric Urology; Urinary Tract Infections; Robotic Urologic Surgery; Urinary Reconstruction; **Hospital:** Maimonides Med Ctr (page 98), Steven & Alexandra Cohen Chldn's Med Ctr of NY (page 106); **Address:** 909 49th St, Brooklyn, NY 11219; **Phone:** 718-283-7743; **Board Cert:** Urology 2010; Pediatric Urology 2010; **Med School:** SUNY Downstate 1983; **Resid:** Surgery, Beth Israel 1985; Urology, Maimonides Med Ctr 1988; **Fellow:** Pediatric Urology, Chldns Hosp 1991

Grunberger, Ivan MD (U) - **Spec Exp:** Prostate Cancer; Impotence; Minimally Invasive Surgery; Kidney Stones; **Hospital:** New York Methodist Hosp (page 418), SUNY Downstate Med Ctr (Univ Hosp of Bklyn) - LICH (page 420); **Address:** One Prospect Park West, Ste C, Brooklyn, NY 11215; **Phone:** 718-230-7788; **Board Cert:** Urology 2007; **Med School:** NYU Sch Med 1980; **Resid:** Surgery, N Shore Univ Hosp 1982; Urology, NYU Med Ctr 1986; **Fac Appt:** Clin Prof U, Cornell Univ-Weill Med Coll

Horowitz, Mark MD (U) - **Spec Exp:** Pediatric Urology; **Hospital:** SUNY Downstate Med Ctr (Univ Hosp of Bklyn) (page 419), NY Hosp Queens (page 206); **Address:** 256 Mason Ave C Bldg Fl 3, Staten Island, NY 10305; **Phone:** 718-226-1271; **Board Cert:** Urology 2006; **Med School:** NY Med Coll 1986; **Resid:** Urology, SUNY Downstate Med Ctr 1992; **Fellow:** Pediatric Urology, Chldns Hosp & Med Ctr 1994; **Fac Appt:** Assoc Prof U, SUNY Downstate

Irwin, Mark MD (U) - **Spec Exp:** Prostate Disease; Erectile Dysfunction; Kidney Stones; **Hospital:** SUNY Downstate Med Ctr (Univ Hosp of Bklyn) - LICH (page 420); **Address:** LI Coll Hosp, Dept Urology, 339 Hicks St Fl 7, Brooklyn, NY 11201; **Phone:** 718-780-1520; **Board Cert:** Urology 2009; **Med School:** Med Coll Wisc 1982; **Resid:** Surgery, Kings County Hosp 1985; Urology, Kings County Hosp 1988; **Fac Appt:** Assoc Clin Prof U, SUNY Downstate

Lindsay, Gaius K MD (U) - **Hospital:** Maimonides Med Ctr (page 98); **Address:** 3121 Ocean Ave, Brooklyn, NY 11235; **Phone:** 718-283-7741; **Board Cert:** Urology 1976; **Med School:** India 1967; **Resid:** Surgery, NY Methodist Hosp 1970; Urology, Maimonides Med Ctr 1973; **Fac Appt:** Asst Clin Prof U, SUNY Downstate

Meisenberg, Gene MD (U) - **Spec Exp:** Prostate Disease; Kidney Stones; Impotence; **Hospital:** NY-Presby/Weill Cornell Med Ctr, NY (page 104), SUNY Downstate Med Ctr (Univ Hosp of Bklyn) - LICH (page 420); **Address:** 1523 Voorhies Ave, Fl 5th, MS 11235, Brooklyn, NY 11235; **Phone:** 718-743-2200; **Board Cert:** Urology 2011; **Med School:** Russia 1981; **Resid:** Surgery, Beth Israel Hosp 1993; Urology, RW Johnson Univ Hosp 1997

Rosenthal, Sheldon MD (U) - **Spec Exp:** Kidney Stones; Prostate Disease; **Hospital:** Wyckoff Heights Med Ctr; **Address:** 359 Stockholm St Fl 1, Brooklyn, NY 11237; **Phone:** 718-821-3200; **Board Cert:** Urology 1977; **Med School:** Ros Franklin Univ/Chicago Med Sch 1967; **Resid:** Surgery, Albert Einstein 1970; Urology, NY Med Coll 1973

Saada, Simon MD (U) - **Spec Exp:** Kidney Stones; Prostate Cancer; Kidney Cancer; **Hospital:** Maimonides Med Ctr (page 98), Richmond Univ Med Ctr; **Address:** 705 86th St, Ste M2, Brooklyn, NY 11228-3219; **Phone:** 718-238-1075; **Board Cert:** Urology 1981; **Med School:** Egypt 1970; **Resid:** Surgery, LI Coll Med Ctr 1974; Urology, Charleston Area Med Ctr 1977

Shabsigh, Ridwan MD (U) - **Spec Exp:** Erectile Dysfunction; Hypogonadism; Clinical Trials; **Hospital:** Maimonides Med Ctr (page 98); **Address:** 3121 Ocean Ave, Brooklyn, NY 11235; **Phone:** 718-283-7746; **Board Cert:** Urology 2011; **Med School:** Syria 1976; **Resid:** Urology, Seepark Hosp 1983; Urology, Baylor Affil Hsop 1990; **Fellow:** Urology, Baylor Affil Hosp 1987; **Fac Appt:** Clin Prof U, Columbia P&S

Silver, David A MD (U) - **Spec Exp:** Laparoscopic Surgery; Urologic Cancer; Robotic Surgery; Continent Urinary Diversions; **Hospital:** Maimonides Med Ctr (page 98), Lutheran Med Ctr - Brooklyn; **Address:** 6323 7th Ave, Brooklyn, NY 11220; **Phone:** 718-283-7153; **Board Cert:** Urology 2007; **Med School:** Albert Einstein Coll Med 1989; **Resid:** Surgery, Maimonides Med Ctr 1995; **Fellow:** Urology, Meml Sloan-Kettering Canc Ctr 1997

Wainstein, Sasha MD (U) - **Spec Exp:** Impotence; Voiding Dysfunction; Endourology; **Hospital:** Maimonides Med Ctr (page 98), Forest Hills Hosp (page 106); **Address:** 4720 Fort Hamilton Pkwy, Brooklyn, NY 11219-2500; **Phone:** 718-436-3900; **Board Cert:** Urology 1977; **Med School:** Colombia 1969; **Resid:** Urology, Maimonides Medical Ctr 1975

Vascular & Interventional Radiology

Sclafani, Salvatore JA MD (VIR) - **Spec Exp:** Uterine Fibroid Embolization; Varicocele Embolization; Trauma; Vascular Malformations; **Hospital:** SUNY Downstate Med Ctr (Univ Hosp of Bklyn) (page 419); **Address:** American Access Care Physicians, 577 Prospect Ave, Brooklyn, NY 11215; **Phone:** 718-369-1444; **Board Cert:** Diagnostic Radiology 1976; Vascular & Interventional Radiology 2009; **Med School:** SUNY Upstate Med Univ 1972; **Resid:** Diagnostic Radiology, Univ Hosp-SUNY 1976; **Fac Appt:** Prof Rad, SUNY Downstate

Vascular Surgery

Ascher, Enrico MD (VascS) - **Spec Exp:** Endovascular Surgery; Carotid Artery Surgery; Limb Sparing Surgery; Aneurysm; **Hospital:** Lutheran Med Ctr - Brooklyn; **Address:** 960 50 St, Brooklyn, NY 11219; **Phone:** 718-438-3800; **Board Cert:** Vascular Surgery 2004; **Med School:** Brazil 1974; **Resid:** Surgery, NY Med Coll 1981; **Fellow:** Vascular Surgery, Montefiore Med Ctr 1982; **Fac Appt:** Prof S, SUNY Downstate

D'Ayala, Marcus D MD (VascS) - **Spec Exp:** Endovascular Surgery; Aneurysm-Abdominal Aortic; Carotid Artery Surgery; Peripheral Vascular Disease; **Hospital:** New York Methodist Hosp (page 418); **Address:** NY Methodist Hospital, Dept Surgery, 506 Sixth St, Brooklyn, NY 11215; **Phone:** 718-780-3288; **Board Cert:** Surgery 2008; Vascular Surgery 2009; **Med School:** Univ Wisc 1992; **Resid:** Surgery, Montefiore Med Ctr 1997; **Fellow:** Vascular Surgery, Mt Sinai Med Ctr 1998; **Fac Appt:** Assoc Clin Prof S, Cornell Univ-Weill Med Coll

Weiser, Robert MD (VascS) - **Spec Exp:** Lower Limb Arterial Disease; Carotid Artery Surgery; Lower Limb Ulcers; **Hospital:** SUNY Downstate Med Ctr (Univ Hosp of Bklyn) - LICH (page 420), New York Methodist Hosp (page 418); **Address:** 186 Joralemon St Fl 7, Brooklyn, NY 11201-4326; **Phone:** 718-797-1101; **Board Cert:** Surgery 2005; **Med School:** Albert Einstein Coll Med 1977; **Resid:** Surgery, Montefiore Med Ctr 1982; **Fellow:** Vascular Surgery, Montefiore Med Ctr 1983

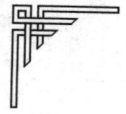

The Best in American Medicine
www.CastleConnolly.com

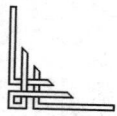

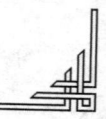

Queens

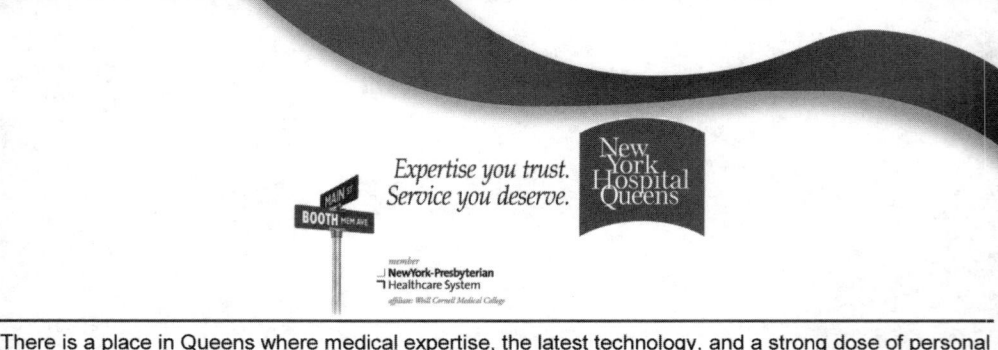

There is a place in Queens where medical expertise, the latest technology, and a strong dose of personal service help people feel better and return to daily living faster. A place where you can find remarkable medicine and remarkable results – results that show our care is among the very best you can find.

A place where we use sophisticated diagnostic and surgical procedures every day. Here, we treat everything from heart conditions and childhood obesity…to diabetes and dental disease…to tough cancers, high-risk pregnancies and serious emergencies. Even your aching knees can find relief here.

And, when you are *our* patient, we treat you like a member of our own family.
This is New York Hospital Queens. Right here, in Queens.

Designations, Affiliations & Accomplishments
- 535-bed tertiary care facility and community teaching hospital, accredited by the Joint Commission
- Member of the New York-Presbyterian Healthcare System, affiliated with the Joan & Sanford I. Weill Medical College of Cornell University
- West Building opened in 2010, adding 80 certified beds, a state-of-the-art ambulatory surgery center and interventional procedure area with a hybrid operating room
- One of the largest employers in Queens County with 3,500+ employees and 1,600+ voluntary attending physicians
- Recognized by Thomson Reuters as one of the Thomson Top 100 performance improvement leader among major teaching hospitals in the U.S. in 2007 and 2008
- Designated New York State Level 1 Regional Trauma Center and Emergency Heart Care Station
- Designated New York State Stroke Center
- Designated Level 3 Neonatal Intensive Care Unit
- Cancer Center accredited by the American College of Surgeon's Commission on Cancer
- Theresa and Eugene M. Lang Center for Research and Education with 200+ ongoing clinical trials

Expertise You Can Trust
13 Clinical Departments:
- Surgery
- Cardiothoracic Surgery
- Orthopaedics & Rehabilitation
- Anesthesiology
- Medicine
- Emergency Medicine
- Obstetrics & Gynecology
- Pediatrics
- Community Health
- Dental & Oral Medicine
- Pathology & Clinical Laboratories
- Radiation Oncology
- Radiology
- Plus numerous sub-specialties…
- And, 18 community health centers throughout Queens

2011 Operating Statistics
- 36,086 patient discharges
- 4,139 deliveries
- 121,466 emergency room encounters
- 14,330 surgical procedures
- 15,294 ambulatory surgery/endoscopy procedures
- 3,789 cardiac catheterizations & PCI
- 141,264 ambulatory care visits
- 1,919,572 laboratory procedures

New in 2012
- Opened Urgent Care Center and expanded the Emergency Room
- Opened Transitional Care Unit
- Opened NYHQ Center for Wound Healing @ Silvercrest Center for Nursing and Rehabilitation

Allergy & Immunology

Fine, Stanley MD (A&I) - **Spec Exp:** Asthma; Drug Sensitivity; Latex Allergy; **Hospital:** NY Hosp Queens (page 206), Flushing Hosp Med Ctr; **Address:** 37-31 149th St, Flushing, NY 11354-4841; **Phone:** 718-358-5565; **Board Cert:** Internal Medicine 1964; Allergy & Immunology 1972; **Med School:** Columbia P&S 1957; **Resid:** Internal Medicine, Jacobi Med Ctr 1959; Internal Medicine, Montefiore Hosp Med Ctr 1962; **Fellow:** Allergy & Immunology, St Luke's-Roosevelt Hosp Ctr 1963; **Fac Appt:** Asst Clin Prof Med, Cornell Univ-Weill Med Coll

Menchell, David L MD (A&I) - **Spec Exp:** Asthma; Nasal & Sinus Disorders; **Hospital:** NY Hosp Queens (page 206); **Address:** 73-03 198th St, Fresh Meadows, NY 11366-1818; **Phone:** 718-465-4100; **Board Cert:** Internal Medicine 1980; Allergy & Immunology 1983; **Med School:** NYU Sch Med 1977; **Resid:** Internal Medicine, NY Hosp Med Ctr 1980; **Fellow:** Allergy & Immunology, NY Hosp Med Ctr 1983

Cardiovascular Disease

Akinboboye, Olakunle MD (Cv) - **Spec Exp:** Diabetes & Heart Disease; Nuclear Stress Testing; Hypertension; Coronary Artery Disease; **Address:** Laurelton Heart Specialists, 236 Merrick Blvd, Rosedale, NY 11413; **Phone:** 718-949-9400; **Board Cert:** Internal Medicine 2005; Cardiovascular Disease 2005; Nuclear Cardiology 1996; **Med School:** Nigeria 1984; **Resid:** Internal Medicine, Nassau County Med Ctr 1991; **Fellow:** Cardiovascular Disease, Columbia Presby Med Ctr 1995; Nuclear Cardiology, Columbia Presby Med Ctr 1994; **Fac Appt:** Assoc Prof Med, SUNY Stony Brook

Hsueh, John Tzu-Lang MD (Cv) - **Spec Exp:** Coronary Artery Disease; Heart Valve Disease; **Hospital:** NY Hosp Queens (page 206), Flushing Hosp Med Ctr; **Address:** 136-17 39th Ave Fl 4 - Ste CFE, Flushing, NY 11354; **Phone:** 718-559-3600; **Board Cert:** Internal Medicine 1987; Cardiovascular Disease 1979; **Med School:** Taiwan 1970; **Resid:** Internal Medicine, Flushing Hosp Med Ctr 1976; **Fellow:** Cardiovascular Disease, Wayne State Univ 1978

Kirtane, Sanjay S MD (Cv) - **Spec Exp:** Coronary Artery Disease; Nuclear Cardiology; Heart Failure; Nuclear Cardiology; **Hospital:** St. John's Epis Hosp - S Shore, South Nassau Comm Hosp; **Address:** 114-12 Beach Channel Drive, Ste 7, Rockaway Park, NY 11694; **Phone:** 718-318-1029; **Board Cert:** Internal Medicine 1980; Cardiovascular Disease 1983; Nuclear Cardiology 2009; **Med School:** India 1974; **Resid:** Internal Medicine, St John's Episcopal Hosp 1980; **Fellow:** Cardiovascular Disease, LI Jewish Med Ctr/St John's Episcopal Hosp 1982

Qadir, Shuja MD (Cv) - **Spec Exp:** Heart Failure; Arrhythmias; Coronary Artery Disease; **Hospital:** NY Hosp Queens (page 206), N Shore Univ Hosp (page 106); **Address:** 85-04 67th Rd, Rego Park, NY 11374; **Phone:** 718-275-6061; **Board Cert:** Internal Medicine 1984; Cardiovascular Disease 1987; **Med School:** Pakistan 1977; **Resid:** Internal Medicine, Catholic Med Ctr 1985; **Fellow:** Cardiovascular Disease, Catholic Med Ctr 1987; **Fac Appt:** Asst Prof Med, NY Med Coll

Robbins, Michael J MD (Cv) - **Spec Exp:** Echocardiography; Non-Invasive Cardiology; **Hospital:** Mount Sinai Med Ctr (page 102); **Address:** 94-36 58th Ave, Ste G4, Rego Park, NY 11373-5149; **Phone:** 718-760-0011; **Board Cert:** Internal Medicine 1984; Cardiovascular Disease 1987; **Med School:** Cornell Univ 1981; **Resid:** Internal Medicine, Bronx Muni Hosp/Albert Einstein Coll Med 1985; **Fellow:** Cardiovascular Disease, Mt Sinai Hosp 1987; **Fac Appt:** Assoc Prof Med, Mount Sinai Sch Med

Rydzinski, Mayer MD (Cv) - **Spec Exp:** Echocardiography; **Hospital:** NY Hosp Queens (page 206), Forest Hills Hosp (page 106); **Address:** 80-02 Kew Gardens Road, Ste 323, Kew Gardens, NY 11415; **Phone:** 718-268-7633; **Board Cert:** Internal Medicine 1979; Cardiovascular Disease 1981; Echocardiography 2008; **Med School:** Albert Einstein Coll Med 1976; **Resid:** Internal Medicine, Metropolitan Hosp Ctr 1977; Internal Medicine, Montefiore Hosp Med Ctr 1979; **Fellow:** Cardiovascular Disease, LI Jewish Hosp 1981

Siskind, Steven J MD (Cv) - **Spec Exp:** Angina; Heart Failure; Arrhythmias; **Hospital:** NY Hosp Queens (page 206), Lenox Hill Hosp (page 106); **Address:** 142-42 Booth Memorial Ave, Flushing, NY 11355; **Phone:** 718-353-4004; **Board Cert:** Internal Medicine 1979; Cardiovascular Disease 1981; **Med School:** Albert Einstein Coll Med 1976; **Resid:** Internal Medicine, Jacobi Med Ctr 1979; **Fellow:** Cardiovascular Disease, Albert Einstein 1981; **Fac Appt:** Asst Prof, Cornell Univ-Weill Med Coll

Child & Adolescent Psychiatry

Fornari, Victor MD (ChAP) - **Spec Exp:** Eating Disorders; Trauma Psychiatry; Post Traumatic Stress Disorder; **Hospital:** Zucker Hillside Hosp (page 106); **Address:** Zucker Hillside Hospital, Ambulatory Care Pavilion Lower Level, 75-59 263rd St, Glen Oaks, NY 11004; **Phone:** 718-470-3510; **Board Cert:** Psychiatry 1984; Child & Adolescent Psychiatry 1985; **Med School:** SUNY Downstate 1979; **Resid:** Psychiatry, Hosp Univ Penn 1982; **Fellow:** Child & Adolescent Psychiatry, LIJ Med Ctr 1984; **Fac Appt:** Prof Psyc, NYU Sch Med

Kafantaris, Vivian P MD (ChAP) - **Spec Exp:** Bipolar/Mood Disorders; ADD/ADHD; Aggression Disorders; Clinical Trials; **Hospital:** Zucker Hillside Hosp (page 106); **Address:** The Zucker Hillside Hospital, Psychiatry Rsch, 75-59 263rd St, Glen Oaks, NY 11004; **Phone:** 718-470-8556; **Board Cert:** Psychiatry 1989; Child & Adolescent Psychiatry 1990; Addiction Psychiatry 2007; **Med School:** Albert Einstein Coll Med 1983; **Resid:** Psychiatry, Albert Einstein Coll Med 1987; **Fellow:** Child & Adolescent Psychiatry, NYU/Bellevue Hosp Ctr 1989; Psychopharmacology, Dr Magda Campbell 1989; **Fac Appt:** Assoc Prof Psyc, Albert Einstein Coll Med

Colon & Rectal Surgery

Tiszenkel, Howard I MD (CRS) - **Spec Exp:** Colon Cancer; **Hospital:** NY Hosp Queens (page 206); **Address:** 56-45 Main St, rm WLL300, Flushing, NY 11355-5000; **Phone:** 718-445-0220; **Board Cert:** Surgery 2006; Colon & Rectal Surgery 1988; **Med School:** NY Med Coll 1981; **Resid:** Surgery, St Luke's Hosp 1986; Colon & Rectal Surgery, Carle Clinic 1987

Critical Care Medicine

Nierman, David M MD (CCM) - **Spec Exp:** Critical Illness-Prolonged; Respiratory Failure; Sepsis; **Hospital:** Mount Sinai Hosp of Queens (page 102), Mount Sinai Med Ctr (page 102); **Address:** 25-10 30th Ave, Astoria, NY 11102; **Phone:** 718-267-4293; **Board Cert:** Internal Medicine 1984; Pulmonary Disease 1988; Critical Care Medicine 2002; **Med School:** Israel 1981; **Resid:** Internal Medicine, LIJ-Hillside Med Ctr 1984; Emergency Medicine, LIJ-Hillside Med Ctr 1984; **Fellow:** Pulmonary Disease, St Lukes-Roosevelt Hosp 1988; **Fac Appt:** Assoc Prof CCM, Mount Sinai Sch Med

Dermatology

Beyda, Bernadette A MD (D) - **Hospital:** NY Hosp Queens (page 206); **Address:** 141-23 59th Ave, Flushing, NY 11355-5304; **Phone:** 718-445-0566; **Board Cert:** Dermatology 1982; **Med School:** France 1976; **Resid:** Pathology, Booth Meml Med Ctr 1979; Dermatology, NY Hosp 1982

Gladstein, Michael J MD (D) - ; **Address:** 3062 36th Street, Astoria, NY 11103-4798; **Phone:** 718-728-8979; **Board Cert:** Dermatology 1987; **Med School:** NYU Sch Med 1979; **Resid:** Dermatology, NYU Med Ctr 1985

Pereira, Frederick A MD (D) - **Spec Exp:** Skin Cancer; Geriatric Dermatology; **Hospital:** NY Hosp Queens (page 206), Mount Sinai Med Ctr (page 102); **Address:** 51-14 Kissena Blvd, Flushing, NY 11355-4163; **Phone:** 718-359-4425; **Board Cert:** Dermatology 2009; **Med School:** UMDNJ-NJ Med Sch, Newark 1968; **Resid:** Dermatology, Mt Sinai Hosp 1974; Dermatology, Metro Hosp 1975

Diagnostic Radiology

Mollin, Joel MD (DR) - **Spec Exp:** Ultrasound; CT Scan; **Hospital:** Elmhurst Hosp Ctr; **Address:** 79-01 Broadway, E1-18, Radiology, Elmhurst, NY 11373; **Phone:** 718-334-2052; **Board Cert:** Diagnostic Radiology 1985; Psychiatry 1976; **Med School:** SUNY Downstate 1969; **Resid:** Diagnostic Radiology, USPHS Hosp-Staten Island 1981; Diagnostic Radiology, Mt Sinai Hosp 1983; **Fac Appt:** Asst Clin Prof, Mount Sinai Sch Med

Tartell, Jay D MD (DR) - **Hospital:** Mount Sinai Hosp of Queens (page 102); **Address:** Advanced Radiological Imaging, 89-40 56th Ave, Elmhurst, NY 11373-4943; **Phone:** 718-335-5532; **Board Cert:** Diagnostic Radiology 1987; **Med School:** NY Med Coll 1982; **Resid:** Diagnostic Radiology, Bronx Muni Hosp 1986; **Fellow:** Ultrasound/CT/MRI, North Shore Univ Hosp 1987

Youner, Craig J MD (DR) - **Hospital:** Mount Sinai Hosp of Queens (page 102); **Address:** Advanced Radiological Imaging, 29-16 Astoria Blvd, Astoria, NY 11102-1742; **Phone:** 718-204-5800; **Board Cert:** Diagnostic Radiology 1978; **Med School:** Albany Med Coll 1973; **Resid:** Internal Medicine, N Shore Univ Hosp 1975; Diagnostic Radiology, N Shore Univ Hosp 1978; **Fac Appt:** Asst Clin Prof Rad, Mount Sinai Sch Med

Endocrinology, Diabetes & Metabolism

Lorber, Daniel L MD (EDM) - **Spec Exp:** Diabetes; **Hospital:** NY Hosp Queens (page 206); **Address:** 59-45 161st St, Fresh Meadows, NY 11365-1414; **Phone:** 718-762-3111; **Board Cert:** Internal Medicine 1987; Endocrinology, Diabetes & Metabolism 1977; **Med School:** Albert Einstein Coll Med 1972; **Resid:** Internal Medicine, Jacobi Med Ctr 1975; **Fellow:** Endocrinology, Diabetes & Metabolism, Vanderbilt Univ Hosp 1977; **Fac Appt:** Assoc Clin Prof Med, Cornell Univ-Weill Med Coll

Rosman, Lawrence D MD (EDM) - **Spec Exp:** Thyroid Disorders; Osteoporosis; Diabetes; Pituitary Disorders; **Hospital:** NY Hosp Queens (page 206), NYU Langone Med Ctr (page 108); **Address:** 112-03 Queens Blvd, Ste 207, Forest Hills, NY 11375-5550; **Phone:** 718-263-3718; **Board Cert:** Internal Medicine 1978; Endocrinology 1983; **Med School:** NYU Sch Med 1975; **Resid:** Internal Medicine, NYU Med Ctr 1978; **Fellow:** Endocrinology, Diabetes & Metabolism, NYU Med Ctr 1980; **Fac Appt:** Asst Clin Prof Med, NYU Sch Med

Tibaldi, Joseph M MD (EDM) - **Spec Exp:** Diabetes; Thyroid Disorders; Geriatric Endocrinology; **Hospital:** NY Hosp Queens (page 206); **Address:** 59-45 161st St, Flushing, NY 11365-1414; **Phone:** 718-762-3111; **Board Cert:** Internal Medicine 1982; Endocrinology, Diabetes & Metabolism 1985; **Med School:** Mount Sinai Sch Med 1979; **Resid:** Internal Medicine, Mount Sinai Med Ctr 1982; **Fellow:** Endocrinology, Montefiore Med Ctr 1984; **Fac Appt:** Asst Clin Prof Med, Albert Einstein Coll Med

Family Medicine

Fisher, George C MD (FMed) *PCP* - **Spec Exp:** Preventive Medicine; Hypertension; Cholesterol/Lipid Disorders; Diabetes; **Hospital:** Mount Sinai Hosp of Queens (page 102), Mount Sinai Med Ctr (page 102); **Address:** 22-33 33rd St, Astoria, NY 11105; **Phone:** 718-726-1000; **Board Cert:** Family Medicine 2008; **Med School:** England, UK 1979; **Resid:** Family Medicine, St Joseph Med Ctr 1993

Istrico, Richard A DO (FMed) *PCP* - **Spec Exp:** Sports Injuries; Nutrition; Preventive Medicine; **Hospital:** Long Island Jewish Med Ctr (page 106); **Address:** 158-01 Crossbay Blvd, Jamaica, NY 11414-3137; **Phone:** 718-738-9115; **Board Cert:** Family Medicine 1981; **Med School:** Philadelphia Coll Osteo Med 1978; **Resid:** Family Medicine, Interboro Hosp 1979; Sports Medicine, Baptist Med Ctr 1980

Molnar, Thomas G MD (FMed) *PCP* - **Spec Exp:** Hypertension; Diabetes; **Hospital:** NY Hosp Queens (page 206), Flushing Hosp Med Ctr; **Address:** 83-39 Daniels St, Jamaica, NY 11435-1208; **Phone:** 718-291-5151; **Board Cert:** Family Medicine 2007; **Med School:** Hungary 1982; **Resid:** Surgery, Flushing Hosp 1985; Family Medicine, Univ Hosp 1988

Muraca, Glenn DO (FMed) *PCP* - **Spec Exp:** Sports Medicine; Nutrition; **Hospital:** Flushing Hosp Med Ctr; **Address:** 104-01 Corona Ave, Corona, NY 11368; **Phone:** 718-271-2020; **Board Cert:** Family Medicine 1994; **Med School:** NY Coll Osteo Med 1990; **Resid:** Family Medicine, Peninsula Hosp 1994

Reddy, Mallikarjuna D MD (FMed) *PCP* - **Spec Exp:** Geriatric Care; **Hospital:** NY Hosp Queens (page 206); **Address:** 72-18 164th St, Flushing, NY 11365-4222; **Phone:** 718-969-6640; **Board Cert:** Family Medicine 2009; **Med School:** India 1982; **Resid:** Family Medicine, Catholic Med Ctr 1990

Roth, Alan R DO (FMed) *PCP* - **Spec Exp:** Palliative Care; Diabetes; Hypertension; **Hospital:** Jamaica Hosp Med Ctr, Flushing Hosp Med Ctr; **Address:** 11940 Metropolitan Ave, Kew Gardens, NY 11415; **Phone:** 718-849-0624; **Board Cert:** Family Medicine 2009; Hospice & Palliative Medicine 2008; **Med School:** NY Coll Osteo Med 1986; **Resid:** Family Medicine, Jamaica Hosp Med Ctr 1989; **Fac Appt:** Asst Clin Prof FMed, Albert Einstein Coll Med

Gastroenterology

Esposito, Stephen P MD (Ge) - **Hospital:** NY Hosp Queens (page 206), NY-Presby/Columbia Univ Med Ctr, NY (page 104); **Address:** 26-19 Francis Lewis Blvd, Bayside, NY 11358; **Phone:** 718-224-7186; **Board Cert:** Internal Medicine 1989; Gastroenterology 2002; **Med School:** SUNY Upstate Med Univ 1986; **Resid:** Internal Medicine, LI Jewish Hosp 1989; **Fellow:** Gastroenterology, Booth Meml Hosp 1991

Harooni, Robert B MD (Ge) - **Spec Exp:** Colonoscopy; Peptic Ulcer Disease; Capsule Endoscopy; **Hospital:** NY Hosp Queens (page 206); **Address:** 55-16 Main St, Lower Level, Flushing, NY 11355; **Phone:** 718-461-6161; **Board Cert:** Internal Medicine 1981; Gastroenterology 1985; **Med School:** Iran 1973; **Resid:** Internal Medicine, Booth Meml Hosp 1982; **Fellow:** Gastroenterology, Booth Meml Hosp 1984; **Fac Appt:** Med, Cornell Univ-Weill Med Coll

Nussbaum, Michel E MD (Ge) - **Spec Exp:** Endoscopy & Colonoscopy; Colon Cancer Screening; Inflammatory Bowel Disease; Peptic Ulcer Disease; **Hospital:** NY Hosp Queens (page 206), Flushing Hosp Med Ctr; **Address:** 142-43 Booth Memorial Ave, Flushing, NY 11355-5343; **Phone:** 718-886-1919; **Board Cert:** Internal Medicine 1981; Gastroenterology 1983; **Med School:** Belgium 1977; **Resid:** Internal Medicine, NY Hosp Queens 1980; **Fellow:** Gastroenterology, NY Hosp Queens 1982; **Fac Appt:** Assoc Clin Prof Med, Cornell Univ-Weill Med Coll

Ramgopal, Mekala MD (Ge) - **Spec Exp:** Peptic Acid Disorders; Inflammatory Bowel Disease; Colon & Rectal Cancer Detection; Hepatitis; **Hospital:** St. John's Epis Hosp - S Shore; **Address:** 21-24 Camp Rd, Far Rockaway, NY 11691; **Phone:** 718-327-0207; **Board Cert:** Internal Medicine 1978; Gastroenterology 1979; **Med School:** India 1974; **Resid:** Internal Medicine, Jersey City Med Ctr 1976; Internal Medicine, VA Med Ctr 1977; **Fellow:** Gastroenterology, Univ of Med/Dentistry 1979

Rand, James A MD (Ge) - **Spec Exp:** Colonoscopy; Endoscopy; **Hospital:** NY Hosp Queens (page 206); **Address:** 200-12 44th Ave, Bayside, NY 11361; **Phone:** 718-224-7454; **Board Cert:** Internal Medicine 1978; Gastroenterology 1981; **Med School:** Albert Einstein Coll Med 1975; **Resid:** Internal Medicine, Strong Meml Hosp 1977; Internal Medicine, Columbia-Presby 1978; **Fellow:** Gastroenterology, Montefiore Hosp Med Ctr 1980

Vogelman, Arthur MD (Ge) - **Spec Exp:** Colon Cancer; Peptic Ulcer Disease; Gastroesophageal Reflux Disease (GERD); **Hospital:** Forest Hills Hosp (page 106), NY Hosp Queens (page 206); **Address:** 7146 110th St, Forest Hills, NY 11375-4842; **Phone:** 718-261-2500; **Board Cert:** Internal Medicine 1979; Gastroenterology 1981; **Med School:** Univ Pittsburgh 1975; **Resid:** Internal Medicine, Mt Sinai Hosp 1978; **Fellow:** Gastroenterology, Mt Sinai Hosp 1980

Weg, Arnold MD (Ge) - **Spec Exp:** Endoscopy; Inflammatory Bowel Disease/Crohn's; **Hospital:** NY-Presby/Weill Cornell Med Ctr, NY (page 104); **Address:** 71-36 110th St, Ste 1G, Forest Hills, NY 11375-4836; **Phone:** 718-520-2210; **Board Cert:** Internal Medicine 1985; Gastroenterology 1987; **Med School:** NYU Sch Med 1982; **Resid:** Internal Medicine, Columbia-Presby 1985; **Fellow:** Gastroenterology, NY Hosp 1986

Geriatric Medicine

Brody, Samuel MD (Ger) - **Spec Exp:** Frail Elderly; **Hospital:** Forest Hills Hosp (page 106); **Address:** 69-15 Yellowstone Blvd, Forest Hills, NY 11375; **Phone:** 718-268-4500; **Board Cert:** Internal Medicine 1980; Gastroenterology 1983; Geriatric Medicine 2008; **Med School:** Vanderbilt Univ 1977; **Resid:** Internal Medicine, Vanderbilt Med Ctr 1980; **Fellow:** Gastroenterology, Temple Univ Hosp 1982

Geriatric Psychiatry

Greenwald, Blaine MD (GerPsy) - **Spec Exp:** Depression; Dementia; **Hospital:** Zucker Hillside Hosp (page 106), N Shore Univ Hosp (page 106); **Address:** Zucker Hillside Hospital - ACP 2102, North Shore-Long Island Jewish Health System, 75-59 263rd St, Glen Oaks, NY 11004; **Phone:** 718-470-8159; **Board Cert:** Psychiatry 1983; Geriatric Psychiatry 2000; **Med School:** NY Med Coll 1978; **Resid:** Psychiatry, Mt Sinai Hosp 1982; **Fellow:** Geriatric Psychiatry, Mt Sinai Hosp/Bronx VA Hosp 1983; **Fac Appt:** Assoc Prof Psyc, Hofstra N Shore-LIJ Sch Med

Gynecologic Oncology

Welshinger, Marie MD (GO) - **Spec Exp:** Gynecologic Cancer; **Hospital:** NY Hosp Queens (page 206); **Address:** 56-45 Main St, West Wing, lower level, rm 100, Flushing, NY 11355; **Phone:** 718-670-1170; **Board Cert:** Obstetrics & Gynecology 2010; Gynecologic Oncology 2010; **Med School:** Univ Minn 1988; **Resid:** Obstetrics & Gynecology, SUNY Stony Brook Hosp 1992; **Fellow:** Gynecologic Oncology, Meml Sloan Kett Cancer Ctr 1996

Infectious Disease

Masci, Joseph MD (Inf) - **Spec Exp:** AIDS/HIV; Tropical Diseases; Disaster Preparedness; **Hospital:** Elmhurst Hosp Ctr; **Address:** Elmhurst Hosp, Dept Med, 79-01 Broadway, rm C 6-10, Elmhurst, NY 11373; **Phone:** 718-334-3446; **Board Cert:** Internal Medicine 1979; Infectious Disease 1982; **Med School:** NYU Sch Med 1976; **Resid:** Internal Medicine, Boston City Hosp 1979; **Fellow:** Infectious Disease, Mt Sinai Hosp 1982; **Fac Appt:** Prof Med, Mount Sinai Sch Med

Segal-Maurer, Sorana MD (Inf) - **Spec Exp:** AIDS/HIV; **Hospital:** NY Hosp Queens (page 206); **Address:** 56-45 Main St, Infectious Disease Section, Flushing, NY 11355-5000; **Phone:** 718-670-1525; **Board Cert:** Internal Medicine 2000; Infectious Disease 2000; **Med School:** Mount Sinai Sch Med 1988; **Resid:** Internal Medicine, Bronx Muni Hosp Ctr 1991; **Fellow:** Infectious Disease, Montefiore Med Ctr 1993

Internal Medicine

Amin, Mahendra MD (IM) *PCP* - **Hospital:** NY Hosp Queens (page 206), Long Island Jewish Med Ctr (page 106); **Address:** 89-02 Springfield Blvd, Queens Village, NY 11427-2514; **Phone:** 718-776-4444; **Board Cert:** Internal Medicine 1984; **Med School:** India 1978; **Resid:** Internal Medicine, Metro Hosp Ctr 1982; **Fellow:** Internal Medicine, Metro Hosp Ctr 1985

Beyda, Allan E MD (IM) *PCP* - **Spec Exp:** Preventive Medicine; Cholesterol/Lipid Disorders; **Hospital:** NY Hosp Queens (page 206), N Shore Univ Hosp (page 106); **Address:** 141-23 59th Ave, Flushing, NY 11355-5304; **Phone:** 718-359-7406; **Board Cert:** Internal Medicine 1979; **Med School:** France 1976; **Resid:** Internal Medicine, New York Hosp Med Ctr 1979

Blum, Daniel N MD (IM) *PCP* - **Spec Exp:** Geriatric Care; Hypertension; Diabetes; **Hospital:** NY Hosp Queens (page 206); **Address:** 13806 Jewel Ave, Flushing, NY 11367-1933; **Phone:** 718-520-0248; **Board Cert:** Internal Medicine 1984; **Med School:** Albert Einstein Coll Med 1980; **Resid:** Internal Medicine, NY Hosp of Queens 1984

Brewer, Marlon E MD (IM) *PCP* - **Spec Exp:** Diabetes; Hypertension; **Hospital:** Elmhurst Hosp Ctr; **Address:** 79-01 Broadway, rm A116, Elmhurst, NY 11373; **Phone:** 718-334-2424; **Board Cert:** Internal Medicine 2004; **Med School:** Spain 1986; **Resid:** Internal Medicine, Elmhurst Hosp 1992; **Fac Appt:** Asst Clin Prof Med, Mount Sinai Sch Med

Fukilman, Oscar J MD (IM) *PCP* - **Spec Exp:** Preventive Medicine; **Hospital:** Mount Sinai Hosp of Queens (page 102); **Address:** 25-31 30th Road, Ste 1A, Astoria, NY 11102; **Phone:** 718-267-1102; **Board Cert:** Internal Medicine 1979; **Med School:** Argentina 1968; **Resid:** Internal Medicine, Elmhurst Hosp/Mt Sinai Hosp Svc 1972

Joseph, John L MD (IM) _PCP_ - **Spec Exp:** Rheumatology; Osteoporosis; Arthritis; **Hospital:** Forest Hills Hosp (page 106), NY Hosp Queens (page 206); **Address:** 66-20 108th St, Forest Hills, NY 11375; **Phone:** 718-896-8920; **Board Cert:** Internal Medicine 1983; **Med School:** Mexico 1977; **Resid:** Internal Medicine, Coney Island Hosp 1982; **Fellow:** Rheumatology, Long Island Coll Hosp 1984

Messana, Ida MD (IM) _PCP_ - **Hospital:** Long Island Jewish Med Ctr (page 106), N Shore Univ Hosp (page 106); **Address:** 109-33 71st Rd, Ste 2E, Forest Hills, NY 11375; **Phone:** 718-263-4345; **Board Cert:** Internal Medicine 1988; **Med School:** SUNY Stony Brook 1984; **Resid:** Internal Medicine, Montefiore Med Ctr 1987; **Fellow:** Geriatric Medicine, Montefiore Med Ctr 1989

Pasquale, Jack MD (IM) - **Spec Exp:** Nutrition; Nutrition & Cancer Prevention/Control; Nutrition in Cancer Therapy; **Hospital:** NY Hosp Queens (page 206), Jamaica Hosp Med Ctr; **Address:** Clinical Nutrition Service, 73-03 198th St, Fresh Meadows, NY 11366-1818; **Phone:** 718-465-0041; **Board Cert:** Internal Medicine 1987; **Med School:** Grenada 1981; **Resid:** Internal Medicine, Millard Fillmore Hosp 1984; **Fellow:** Nutrition, Hosp Univ Penn 1985

Reilly, Thomas MD (IM) _PCP_ - **Hospital:** NY Hosp Queens (page 206); **Address:** 86-27 Forest Pkwy, Woodhaven, NY 11421-1143; **Phone:** 718-805-2404; **Board Cert:** Internal Medicine 1984; **Med School:** SUNY Hlth Sci Ctr 1979; **Resid:** Internal Medicine, Staten Island Hosp 1982; **Fellow:** Hematology, St Vincent's Hosp & Med Ctr 1985

Somogyi, Anthony MD (IM) _PCP_ - **Hospital:** NY Hosp Queens (page 206); **Address:** 42-23 Francis Lewis Blvd, Ste 201, Bayside, NY 11361; **Phone:** 718-224-5687; **Board Cert:** Internal Medicine 1979; **Med School:** Belgium 1976; **Resid:** Internal Medicine, NY Hosp Queens 1980

Interventional Cardiology

Papadakos, Stylianos P MD (IC) - **Spec Exp:** Cardiac Catheterization; Percutaneous Myocardial Revasc (PMR); **Hospital:** Lenox Hill Hosp (page 106), NY Hosp Queens (page 206); **Address:** CV Assocs NY & Bayside, 44-01 Francis Lewis Blvd, Level 3, Bayside, NY 11361; **Phone:** 718-423-3355; **Board Cert:** Cardiovascular Disease 2004; Interventional Cardiology 1999; **Med School:** Greece 1985; **Resid:** Internal Medicine, Booth Meml Med Ctr 1989; Internal Medicine, Mt Sinai Hosp 1990; **Fellow:** Cardiovascular Disease, Univ Conn Hosp 1994; **Fac Appt:** Asst Clin Prof Med, Cornell Univ-Weill Med Coll

Maternal & Fetal Medicine

Inglis, Steven R MD (MF) - **Spec Exp:** Pregnancy-High Risk; Obstetric Ultrasound; Prenatal Diagnosis; **Hospital:** Jamaica Hosp Med Ctr; **Address:** Jamaica Hospital, Dept OB/GYN, 89-06 135th St, Ste 6A, Jamaica, NY 11418; **Phone:** 718-206-7642; **Board Cert:** Obstetrics & Gynecology 2012; Maternal & Fetal Medicine 2012; **Med School:** NY Med Coll 1986; **Resid:** Obstetrics & Gynecology, Albany Med Ctr 1990; **Fellow:** Maternal & Fetal Medicine, New York Hosp 1992; **Fac Appt:** Assoc Prof ObG, Cornell Univ-Weill Med Coll

Skupski, Daniel MD (MF) - **Spec Exp:** Fetal Therapy; Multiple Gestation; **Hospital:** NY Hosp Queens (page 206), NY-Presby/Weill Cornell Med Ctr, NY (page 104); **Address:** 56-45 Main St, Flushing, NY 11355-5060; **Phone:** 718-670-1534; **Board Cert:** Obstetrics & Gynecology 2010; Maternal & Fetal Medicine 2010; **Med School:** Univ Mich Med Sch 1985; **Resid:** Obstetrics & Gynecology, Hurley Med Ctr 1989; **Fellow:** Maternal & Fetal Medicine, NY Hosp Cornell Med Ctr 1994; **Fac Appt:** Assoc Prof ObG, Cornell Univ-Weill Med Coll

Medical Oncology

Abramowitz, Avram L MD (Onc) - **Spec Exp:** Bone Marrow Transplant; **Hospital:** Mount Sinai Hosp of Queens (page 102), Long Island Jewish Med Ctr (page 106); **Address:** 176-60 Union Tpke, Ste 360, Fresh Meadows, NY 11366; **Phone:** 718-460-2300; **Board Cert:** Internal Medicine 1987; Hematology 2004; Medical Oncology 2004; **Med School:** NY Med Coll 1984; **Resid:** Internal Medicine, Roosevelt Hosp 1987; **Fellow:** Hematology & Oncology, Roosevelt Hosp 1989; Bone Marrow Transplant, Mount Sinai Med Ctr 1993

Benisovich, Vladimir I MD (Onc) - **Spec Exp:** Breast Cancer; Lung Cancer; Colon Cancer; **Hospital:** Elmhurst Hosp Ctr, Mount Sinai Med Ctr (page 102); **Address:** 79-01 Broadway, Ste H2-04, Elmhurst, NY 11373-1329; **Phone:** 718-334-3723; **Board Cert:** Internal Medicine 1982; Hematology 1984; Medical Oncology 1985; **Med School:** Russia 1966; **Resid:** Internal Medicine, Bronx Lebanon Med Ctr 1980; **Fellow:** Hematology, NYU Med Ctr 1982; Medical Oncology, Mt Sinai Med Ctr 1983

Cortes, Engracio P MD (Onc) - **Spec Exp:** Breast Cancer; Gastrointestinal Cancer; Lung Cancer; Lymphoma; **Hospital:** NY Hosp Queens (page 206), Long Island Jewish Med Ctr (page 106); **Address:** 200-20 44th Ave, Bayside, NY 11361; **Phone:** 718-279-9101; **Board Cert:** Internal Medicine 1976; Medical Oncology 1977; **Med School:** Philippines 1964; **Resid:** Internal Medicine, Lemuel Shattuck Hosp 1968; **Fellow:** Medical Oncology, Roswell Park Cancer Inst 1971; **Fac Appt:** Assoc Clin Prof Med, Cornell Univ-Weill Med Coll

Daly, Jane E MD (Onc) - **Hospital:** NY Hosp Queens (page 206); **Address:** 87-23 Myrtle Ave, Glendale, NY 11385-7431; **Phone:** 718-441-5581; **Board Cert:** Internal Medicine 1978; Hematology 1980; Medical Oncology 1981; **Med School:** NY Med Coll 1975; **Resid:** Internal Medicine, Kings County Hosp 1978; **Fellow:** Hematology, LI Jewish Med Ctr 1980; Medical Oncology, Albert Einstein 1981

Greenberg, Howard J MD (Onc) - **Spec Exp:** Breast Cancer; Colon Cancer; Lymphoma; Coagulation/Bleeding Disorders; **Hospital:** Mount Sinai Hosp of Queens (page 102), Mount Sinai Med Ctr (page 102); **Address:** 2715 30th Ave, Astoria, NY 11102; **Phone:** 718-278-3569; **Board Cert:** Internal Medicine 1976; Hematology 1978; Medical Oncology 1979; **Med School:** SUNY Downstate 1973; **Resid:** Internal Medicine, Mt Sinai Hosp 1976; **Fellow:** Hematology, Mt Sinai Hosp 1978; Medical Oncology, Meml Sloan Kettering Cancer Ctr 1979; **Fac Appt:** Asst Clin Prof Med, Mount Sinai Sch Med

Shum, Kee Y MD (Onc) - **Spec Exp:** Breast Cancer; Lung Cancer; Colon Cancer; **Hospital:** NY Hosp Queens (page 206), Flushing Hosp Med Ctr; **Address:** 136-25 Maple Ave, Ste 205, Flushing, NY 11355-3891; **Phone:** 718-463-2245; **Board Cert:** Internal Medicine 1984; Medical Oncology 1987; **Med School:** Cornell Univ-Weill Med Coll 1981; **Resid:** Internal Medicine, Kings County Hosp 1985; **Fellow:** Medical Oncology, Meml Sloan Kettering Cancer Ctr 1987

Neonatal-Perinatal Medicine

Hand, Ivan L MD (NP) - **Spec Exp:** Respiratory Distress Syndrome; Prematurity/Low Birth Weight Infants; Nutrition; Breast Feeding Problems; **Hospital:** Kings County Hosp Ctr, Queens Hosp Ctr - Jamaica; **Address:** Director, Division of Neonatology, 451 Clarkson Ave, Brooklyn, NY 11203; **Phone:** 718-245-4753; **Board Cert:** Pediatrics 1986; Neonatal-Perinatal Medicine 2004; **Med School:** Albert Einstein Coll Med 1982; **Resid:** Pediatrics, Montefiore Med Ctr 1985; Pediatrics, Bronx Lebanon Hosp 1986; **Fellow:** Neonatal-Perinatal Medicine, NY Hosp-Cornell Med Ctr 1988; **Fac Appt:** Assoc Prof Ped, SUNY Downstate

Nephrology

Galler, Marilyn MD (Nep) - **Spec Exp:** Hypertension; Kidney Disease; **Hospital:** NY Hosp Queens (page 206); **Address:** 56-45 Main St, rm M201, Flushing, NY 11355; **Phone:** 718-670-1151; **Board Cert:** Internal Medicine 1979; Nephrology 1984; **Med School:** NYU Sch Med 1975; **Resid:** Internal Medicine, Bronx Municipal Hosp 1979; **Fellow:** Nephrology, Montefiore Med Ctr 1981; **Fac Appt:** Asst Clin Prof Med, Cornell Univ-Weill Med Coll

Mattoo, Nirmal K MD (Nep) - **Spec Exp:** Kidney Failure; Hypertension; Dialysis Care; **Hospital:** Wyckoff Heights Med Ctr, Forest Hills Hosp (page 106); **Address:** 385 Seneca Ave, Ridgewood, NY 11385; **Phone:** 347-312-3041; **Board Cert:** Internal Medicine 1974; Nephrology 1978; **Med School:** India 1967; **Resid:** Internal Medicine, Queens Hosp Ctr 1971; Internal Medicine, Catholic Med Ctr 1972; **Fellow:** Nephrology, Elmhurst Hosp Ctr 1975

Scott III, David MD (Nep) - **Spec Exp:** Hypertension; Kidney Disease; Diabetes; **Hospital:** NY Hosp Queens (page 206), NY-Presby/Weill Cornell Med Ctr, NY (page 104); **Address:** 1 Cross Island Plaza, Rosedale, NY 11422; **Phone:** 718-276-4750; **Board Cert:** Internal Medicine 2003; Nephrology 2005; **Med School:** Tufts Univ 1985; **Resid:** Internal Medicine, Harlem Hosp 1988; **Fellow:** Nephrology, Harlem Hosp 1990

Spinowitz, Bruce S MD (Nep) - **Spec Exp:** Diabetic Kidney Disease; Hypertension; Kidney Stones; **Hospital:** NY Hosp Queens (page 206), Montefiore Med Ctr-Einstein Campus, NY (page 100); **Address:** 56-45 Main St, rm M201, Flushing, NY 11355-5045; **Phone:** 718-670-1151; **Board Cert:** Internal Medicine 1976; Nephrology 1978; **Med School:** NYU Sch Med 1973; **Resid:** Internal Medicine, Bellevue Hosp 1976; **Fellow:** Nephrology, Bellevue Hosp 1978; **Fac Appt:** Assoc Clin Prof Med, Cornell Univ-Weill Med Coll

Neurology

Appelbaum, Jeffrey C DO (N) - **Spec Exp:** Multiple Sclerosis; Peripheral Neuropathy; **Hospital:** NY Hosp Queens (page 206), Long Island Jewish Med Ctr (page 106); **Address:** 59-07 175 Pl, Flushing, NY 11365; **Phone:** 718-939-0800; **Board Cert:** Neurology 1982; **Med School:** Philadelphia Coll Osteo Med 1977; **Resid:** Neurology, Downstate Med Ctr 1981; **Fac Appt:** Assoc Prof N, NY Coll Osteo Med

Casson, Ira MD (N) - **Spec Exp:** Sports Neurology; Headache; Head Injury; Concussion; **Hospital:** Long Island Jewish Med Ctr (page 106); **Address:** 112-03 Queens Blvd, Ste 201, Forest Hills, NY 11375-5550; **Phone:** 718-544-6633; **Board Cert:** Neurology 1980; **Med School:** NYU Sch Med 1975; **Resid:** Neurology, NYU Med Ctr 1979; **Fac Appt:** Asst Prof N, Albert Einstein Coll Med

Oribe, Emilio M MD (N) - **Spec Exp:** Movement Disorders; Stroke; **Hospital:** NY Hosp Queens (page 206), NY-Presby/Weill Cornell Med Ctr, NY (page 104); **Address:** 27-47 Crescent St, Astoria, NY 11102; **Phone:** 718-606-9193; **Board Cert:** Therapeutic Radiology 1986; Neurology 1991; **Med School:** Uruguay 1981; **Resid:** Internal Medicine, NYU Downtown Hosp 1986; Neurology, Mt Sinai Med Ctr 1989; **Fellow:** Movement Disorders, Mt Sinai Med Ctr 1991

Obstetrics & Gynecology

Benedicto, Milagros A MD (ObG) - **Hospital:** Wyckoff Heights Med Ctr; **Address:** 68-52 Fresh Pond Rd, Ridgewood, NY 11385; **Phone:** 718-381-7016; **Board Cert:** Obstetrics & Gynecology 2011; **Med School:** Philippines 1964; **Resid:** Obstetrics & Gynecology, Wyckoff Heights Hosp 1969; **Fellow:** Obstetrics & Gynecology, Wyckoff Heights Hosp 1971

Olanescu, Andrea D MD (ObG) - **Spec Exp:** Laparoscopic Surgery; Uterine Fibroids; Pelvic Organ Prolapse Repair; **Hospital:** Mount Sinai Hosp of Queens (page 102), Flushing Hosp Med Ctr; **Address:** 23-22 30th Rd, Ste 1F, Astoria, NY 11102; **Phone:** 718-278-0888; **Board Cert:** Obstetrics & Gynecology 2012; **Med School:** Romania 1992; **Resid:** Obstetrics & Gynecology, Jersey City Med Ctr 2002

Ophthalmology

Aharon, Raphael MD (Oph) - **Hospital:** Montefiore Med Ctr-Moses Campus, NY (page 100), NY Hosp Queens (page 206); **Address:** 108-37 71st Ave, Forest Hills, NY 11375-4566; **Phone:** 718-268-6120; **Board Cert:** Ophthalmology 1987; **Med School:** Albert Einstein Coll Med 1980; **Resid:** Internal Medicine, Brookdale Hosp 1981; Ophthalmology, Albert Einstein Coll Med 1984; **Fac Appt:** Asst Clin Prof Oph, Albert Einstein Coll Med

Fishman, Allen J MD (Oph) - **Spec Exp:** Cataract Surgery-Lens Implant; LASIK-Refractive Surgery; **Hospital:** Flushing Hosp Med Ctr; **Address:** 92-29 Queens Blvd, Ste 2I, Rego Park, NY 11374; **Phone:** 718-261-7007; **Board Cert:** Ophthalmology 1981; **Med School:** Ros Franklin Univ/Chicago Med Sch 1976; **Resid:** Surgery, Beth Israel Med Ctr 1977; Ophthalmology, Brookdale Hosp 1980

Grasso, Cono M MD (Oph) - **Spec Exp:** Cataract Surgery; Glaucoma; Oculoplastic Surgery; **Hospital:** Jamaica Hosp Med Ctr, Flushing Hosp Med Ctr; **Address:** 83-05 Grand Ave, Elmhurst, NY 11373-4104; **Phone:** 718-429-0300; **Board Cert:** Ophthalmology 1979; **Med School:** NY Med Coll 1974; **Resid:** Ophthalmology, Wills Eye 1978; **Fac Appt:** Assoc Prof Oph, NY Med Coll

Mackool, Richard J MD (Oph) - **Spec Exp:** Cataract Surgery; LASIK-Refractive Surgery; Lens Implants-Multifocal; Corneal Disease & Surgery; **Hospital:** New York Eye & Ear Infirm (page 117); **Address:** Mackool Eye Institute, 31-24 41st St, Astoria, NY 11103; **Phone:** 718-728-3400; **Board Cert:** Ophthalmology 2011; **Med School:** Boston Univ 1968; **Resid:** Ophthalmology, New York EE Infirm 1973; **Fac Appt:** Clin Prof Oph, NYU Sch Med

Winterkorn, Jacqueline MD/PhD (Oph) - **Spec Exp:** Neuro-Ophthalmology; Brain Tumors; Eye Muscle Disorders; **Hospital:** NY-Presby/Weill Cornell Med Ctr, NY (page 104); **Address:** 161-10 Union Tpke, Flushing, NY 11366; **Phone:** 718-380-5346; **Board Cert:** Ophthalmology 1989; **Med School:** Cornell Univ-Weill Med Coll 1983; **Resid:** Ophthalmology, Mount Sinai Med Ctr 1987; **Fellow:** Neuro-Ophthalmology, Columbia Presby Med Ctr 1988; **Fac Appt:** Clin Prof Oph, Cornell Univ-Weill Med Coll

Orthopaedic Surgery

Besser, Walter A MD (OrS) - **Spec Exp:** Joint Replacement; Fractures; **Hospital:** Mount Sinai Hosp of Queens (page 102), NY Hosp Queens (page 206); **Address:** 30-71 29th St, Astoria, NY 11102; **Phone:** 718-204-7752; **Board Cert:** Orthopaedic Surgery 1977; **Med School:** Spain 1968; **Resid:** Orthopaedic Surgery, LI Jewish Hosp 1971; Orthopaedic Surgery, Brooklyn Jewish Hosp 1974; **Fellow:** Orthopaedic Surgery, Hosp Special Surg 1977; **Fac Appt:** Asst Clin Prof OrS, NYU Sch Med

Schwartz, Evan MD (OrS) - **Spec Exp:** Sports Medicine; Shoulder Surgery; Knee Surgery; Joint Replacement; **Hospital:** Lenox Hill Hosp (page 106); **Address:** 72-41 Grand Ave, Maspeth, NY 11378; **Phone:** 718-558-1975; **Board Cert:** Orthopaedic Surgery 2010; **Med School:** SUNY Buffalo 1981; **Resid:** Orthopaedic Surgery, Montefiore Med Ctr 1986; **Fellow:** Sports Medicine, Hosp Special Surg 1987; **Fac Appt:** Asst Prof OrS, NY Med Coll

Touliopoulos, Steven J MD (OrS) - **Spec Exp:** Sports Medicine; **Hospital:** Mount Sinai Hosp of Queens (page 102), NY Downtown Hosp; **Address:** 23-18 31st St, Ste 210, Astoria, NY 11105; **Phone:** 718-777-1885; **Board Cert:** Orthopaedic Surgery 2010; Orthopaedic Sports Medicine 2007; **Med School:** SUNY Downstate 1991; **Resid:** Orthopaedic Surgery, SUNY Hlth Sci Ctr 1996; **Fellow:** Orthopaedic Sports Medicine, Lenox Hill Hosp/Nicholas Inst 1997; **Fac Appt:** Asst Prof OrS, Mount Sinai Sch Med

Otolaryngology

Huo, Jerry MD (Oto) - **Spec Exp:** Endoscopic Sinus Surgery; Thyroid Surgery; Parotid Gland Surgery; Vocal Cord Disorders; **Hospital:** NY Hosp Queens (page 206); **Address:** 136-20 38th Ave, Ste 7J, Flushing, NY 11354; **Phone:** 718-670-0006; **Board Cert:** Otolaryngology 1998; **Med School:** Mount Sinai Sch Med 1991; **Resid:** Surgery, Lenox Hill Hosp 1993; Otolaryngology, Manhattan EE&T Hosp 1997; **Fac Appt:** Asst Clin Prof Oto, Cornell Univ-Weill Med Coll

La Marca, Charles MD (Oto) - **Hospital:** NS-LIJ Hlth Sys (page 106); **Address:** 75-06 Eliot Ave, Middle Village, NY 11379-1207; **Phone:** 718-335-2224; **Board Cert:** Otolaryngology 1984; **Med School:** Mexico 1977; **Resid:** Otolaryngology, Downstate Med Ctr 1982

Snyder, Gary M MD (Oto) - **Spec Exp:** Cosmetic Surgery-Face; Endoscopic Sinus Surgery; Voice Disorders; Sinus Surgery; **Hospital:** Flushing Hosp Med Ctr, N Shore Univ Hosp (page 106); **Address:** 26-01 Corporal Kennedy St, FL 1 Bldg, Bayside, NY 11360-2452; **Phone:** 718-423-4091; **Board Cert:** Otolaryngology 1983; **Med School:** NY Med Coll 1979; **Resid:** Surgery, North Shore Univ Hosp 1980; Otolaryngology, Manhattan EET Hosp 1983

Pediatric Cardiology

Rutkovsky, Lisa E MD (PCd) - **Spec Exp:** Congenital Heart Disease; Arrhythmias; **Hospital:** NY Hosp Queens (page 206); **Address:** 142-23 Booth Memorial Ave, Flushing, NY 11355; **Phone:** 718-460-9776; **Board Cert:** Pediatrics 2007; Pediatric Cardiology 2007; **Med School:** NYU Sch Med 1986; **Resid:** Pediatrics, N Shore Univ Hosp 1989; **Fellow:** Pediatric Cardiology, NYU-Bellevue Hosp 1989; **Fac Appt:** Asst Clin Prof Ped, NYU Sch Med

Pediatrics

Abularrage, Joseph J MD (Ped) *PCP* - **Hospital:** NY Hosp Queens (page 206); **Address:** 56-45 Main St, Dept of Pediatrics, Flushing, NY 11355-5045; **Phone:** 718-670-1033; **Board Cert:** Pediatrics 1981; **Med School:** NYU Sch Med 1975; **Resid:** Pediatrics, NYU-Bellevue Hosp 1979; **Fellow:** Public Health & Genl Preventive Med, Columbia-Presby Med Ctr 1981

Goldstein, Steven J MD (Ped) *PCP* - **Spec Exp:** Nutrition; Asthma; **Hospital:** Long Island Jewish Med Ctr (page 106), NY Hosp Queens (page 206); **Address:** 141-49 70th Rd, Flushing, NY 11367; **Phone:** 718-268-5282; **Board Cert:** Pediatrics 1983; **Med School:** SUNY Hlth Sci Ctr 1978; **Resid:** Pediatrics, LI Jewish Med Ctr 1981

Psychiatry

Brenner, Ronald MD (Psyc) - **Spec Exp:** Depression; Dementia; Panic Disorder; **Hospital:** St. John's Epis Hosp - S Shore, Mercy Med Ctr - Rockville Centre; **Address:** 327 Beach 19th St, Far Rockaway, NY 11691; **Phone:** 718-869-7248; **Board Cert:** Psychiatry 1979; Geriatric Psychiatry 2006; **Med School:** Spain 1974; **Resid:** Psychiatry, St Luke's Hosp 1978; **Fellow:** Pharmacology, New York Univ Med Ctr 1979; **Fac Appt:** Clin Prof Psyc, SUNY Hlth Sci Ctr

Kalash, Glenn DO (Psyc) - **Spec Exp:** Psychiatry in Physical Illness; Psychosomatic Disorders; Forensic Psychiatry; Liaison Psychiatry; **Hospital:** Jamaica Hosp Med Ctr, St. Francis Hosp - The Heart Ctr (page 121); **Address:** Jamaica Hosp, Dept Psychiatry, 8900 Van Wyck Expressway, Jamaica, NY 11418; **Phone:** 718-206-7167; **Board Cert:** Psychiatry 2008; Forensic Psychiatry 2009; Psychosomatic Medicine 2005; **Med School:** NY Coll Osteo Med 1992; **Resid:** Psychiatry, LIJ Med Ctr 1996; **Fellow:** Liaison Psychiatry, Meml Sloan Kettering Cancer Ctr 1997

Mendelowitz, Alan MD (Psyc) - **Spec Exp:** Schizophrenia; Psychopharmacology; **Hospital:** Zucker Hillside Hosp (page 106); **Address:** 75-59 263rd St, rm 208, Glen Oaks, NY 11004; **Phone:** 718-470-8397; **Board Cert:** Psychiatry 1992; **Med School:** UMDNJ-Rutgers Med Sch 1987; **Resid:** Psychiatry, Hillside Hosp-LIJ Med Ctr 1991; **Fac Appt:** Asst Prof Psyc, Albert Einstein Coll Med

Selzer, Jeffrey A MD (Psyc) - **Spec Exp:** Mood Disorders; Depression; Addiction/Substance Abuse; **Hospital:** Zucker Hillside Hosp (page 106), N Shore Univ Hosp (page 106); **Address:** 75-59 263rd St, Glen Oaks, NY 11004-1150; **Phone:** 718-470-8023; **Board Cert:** Psychiatry 1985; Addiction Psychiatry 2003; **Med School:** Univ Mich Med Sch 1979; **Resid:** Psychiatry, UCLA Med Ctr 1983; **Fac Appt:** Assoc Prof Psyc, Albert Einstein Coll Med

Siris, Samuel G MD (Psyc) - **Spec Exp:** Schizophrenia; Depression in Schizophrenia; Panic Disorder in Schizophrenia; **Hospital:** Zucker Hillside Hosp (page 106); **Address:** 7559 263rd St, Glen Oaks, NY 11004-1150; **Phone:** 718-470-8138; **Board Cert:** Psychiatry 1976; **Med School:** Columbia P&S 1970; **Resid:** Psychiatry, NY State Psychiatric Inst 1974; **Fellow:** Biological Psychiatry, Nat Inst Mental Hlth 1976; Psychoanalysis, Columbia Univ 1982; **Fac Appt:** Prof Psyc, Albert Einstein Coll Med

Sullivan, Ann Marie MD (Psyc) - **Spec Exp:** Psychotherapy; Psychopharmacology; **Hospital:** Elmhurst Hosp Ctr, Mount Sinai Med Ctr (page 102); **Address:** Elmhurst Hosp Ctr, 79-01 Broadway, rm D8, Elmhurst, NY 11373; **Phone:** 718-334-1141; **Board Cert:** Psychiatry 1978; **Med School:** NYU Sch Med 1974; **Resid:** Psychiatry, Bellevue Hosp 1978; **Fac Appt:** Assoc Prof Psyc, Mount Sinai Sch Med

Vivek, Seeth MD (Psyc) - **Spec Exp:** Depression; Panic Disorder; Obsessive-Compulsive Disorder; Liaison Psychiatry; **Hospital:** Jamaica Hosp Med Ctr, Flushing Hosp Med Ctr; **Address:** 75-58 113th St, Ste 1A, Forest Hills, NY 11375-7429; **Phone:** 718-268-9595; **Board Cert:** Psychiatry 1980; Psychosomatic Medicine 2005; **Med School:** India 1972; **Resid:** Psychiatry, Natl Inst Mental Hlth 1976; Psychiatry, Mount Sinai Hosp 1979; **Fellow:** Liaison Psychiatry, Montefiore Hosp 1981; **Fac Appt:** Prof Psyc, NY Coll Osteo Med

Pulmonary Disease

Chadha, Jang B S MD (Pul) - **Spec Exp:** Sleep Disorders; Asthma; Emphysema; Critical Care Medicine; **Hospital:** Flushing Hosp Med Ctr, Forest Hills Hosp (page 106); **Address:** 11203 Queens Blvd, Ste 201, Forest Hills, NY 11375; **Phone:** 718-544-6660; **Board Cert:** Internal Medicine 1982; Pulmonary Disease 1984; Critical Care Medicine 2008; Sleep Medicine 2007; **Med School:** India 1976; **Resid:** Internal Medicine, Lincoln Hosp 1982; **Fellow:** Pulmonary Disease, NY Med Coll 1984

Donath, Joseph MD (Pul) - **Spec Exp:** Asthma; Lung Cancer; Critical Care; **Hospital:** NY Hosp Queens (page 206), Flushing Hosp Med Ctr; **Address:** 112-41 Queens Blvd, Ste 101A, Forest Hills, NY 11375-5564; **Phone:** 718-380-1553; **Board Cert:** Internal Medicine 1980; Pulmonary Disease 1982; Critical Care Medicine 2009; **Med School:** Hungary 1972; **Resid:** Internal Medicine, VA Med Ctr 1980; **Fellow:** Pulmonary Disease, Mt Sinai Hosp 1982; **Fac Appt:** Asst Clin Prof Med, NY Med Coll

Fleischman, Jean K MD (Pul) - **Hospital:** Queens Hosp Ctr - Jamaica; **Address:** Queens Hosp Ctr, Dept Medicine, 82-68 164th St, N Bldg Fl 7, Jamaica, NY 11432-1140; **Phone:** 718-883-4050; **Board Cert:** Internal Medicine 1985; Pulmonary Disease 1988; **Med School:** NYU Sch Med 1982; **Resid:** Internal Medicine, Manhattan VA/NYU Med Ctr 1985; **Fellow:** Pulmonary Disease, NYU Med Ctr 1987; **Fac Appt:** Assoc Clin Prof Med, Mount Sinai Sch Med

Kassapidis, Sotirios MD (Pul) - **Hospital:** Mount Sinai Hosp of Queens (page 102), N Shore Univ Hosp (page 106); **Address:** 22-31 33rd Street, Astoria, NY 11105; **Phone:** 718-278-6595; **Board Cert:** Critical Care Medicine 2010; **Med School:** Grenada 1987; **Resid:** Internal Medicine, SUNY Hlth Sci Ctr 1993; **Fellow:** Pulmonary Disease, SUNY Hlth Sci Ctr 1995; Critical Care Medicine, SUNY Hlth Sci Ctr 1996; **Fac Appt:** Asst Clin Prof Med, NYU Sch Med

Nath, Sunil MD (Pul) - **Spec Exp:** Asthma; Emphysema; Lung Cancer; **Hospital:** NY Hosp Queens (page 206); **Address:** 55-14 Main St, Flushing, NY 11355-5044; **Phone:** 718-359-3131; **Board Cert:** Internal Medicine 1980; Pulmonary Disease 1982; **Med School:** India 1976; **Resid:** Internal Medicine, NY Hosp Med Ctr 1980; **Fellow:** Pulmonary Disease, NY Hosp Med Ctr 1982

Silverman, Joel R MD (Pul) - **Spec Exp:** Emphysema; Asthma; Pulmonary Rehabilitation; Sarcoidosis; **Hospital:** Flushing Hosp Med Ctr, N Shore Univ Hosp (page 106); **Address:** 111-20 Queens Blvd, Forest Hills, NY 11375-6341; **Phone:** 718-544-4224; **Board Cert:** Internal Medicine 1977; Pulmonary Disease 1980; Critical Care Medicine 2005; **Med School:** Univ Okla Coll Med 1974; **Resid:** Internal Medicine, N Shore Univ Hosp 1977; **Fellow:** Pulmonary Disease, Bellevue Hosp 1979

Thurm, Craig A MD (Pul) - **Spec Exp:** Asthma; Chronic Obstructive Lung Disease (COPD); Interstitial Lung Disease; Pulmonary Fibrosis; **Hospital:** Jamaica Hosp Med Ctr; **Address:** Jamaica Hospital, Div Pulmonology, 134-20 Jamaica Ave Fl 1, Jamaica, NY 11418; **Phone:** 718-206-8776; **Board Cert:** Internal Medicine 2000; Pulmonary Disease 2000; Critical Care Medicine 2000; **Med School:** Albert Einstein Coll Med 1987; **Resid:** Internal Medicine, Francis Scott Key Med Ctr 1990; **Fellow:** Pulmonary Critical Care Medicine, Univ Maryland 1993

Radiation Oncology

Dalton, Jack F MD (RadRO) - **Spec Exp:** Brain Tumors; Head & Neck Cancer; Breast Cancer; **Hospital:** Mount Sinai Med Ctr (page 102), Lenox Hill Hosp (page 106); **Address:** 106-14 70th Ave, Forest Hills, NY 11375-4253; **Phone:** 718-520-6620; **Board Cert:** Internal Medicine 1974; Hematology 1976; Medical Oncology 1981; Therapeutic Radiology 1983; **Med School:** Univ Pittsburgh 1970; **Resid:** Hematology, Mt Sinai Hosp 1975; Diagnostic Radiology, Mt Sinai Hosp 1981; **Fac Appt:** Asst Clin Prof Med, Mount Sinai Sch Med

Katz, Alan J MD (RadRO) - **Spec Exp:** Brachytherapy; Prostate Cancer; Intensity Modulated Radiotherapy (IMRT); **Address:** 40-20 Main St, Queens, NY 11354; **Phone:** 888-880-6646; **Board Cert:** Therapeutic Radiology 1981; **Med School:** NYU Sch Med 1977; **Resid:** Therapeutic Radiology, NYU Med Ctr 1981

Lipsztein, Roberto MD (RadRO) - **Hospital:** Lenox Hill Hosp (page 106), Mount Sinai Med Ctr (page 102); **Address:** 106-14 70th Ave, Forest Hills, NY 11375-4253; **Phone:** 718-520-6620; **Board Cert:** Therapeutic Radiology 1982; **Med School:** Brazil 1974; **Resid:** Internal Medicine, Mount Sinai Hosp 1979; **Fellow:** Radiation Oncology, Mount Sinai Hosp 1981

Varsos, George MD (RadRO) - **Spec Exp:** Gynecologic Cancer; Urologic Cancer; **Hospital:** Mount Sinai Hosp of Queens (page 102), Mount Sinai Med Ctr (page 102); **Address:** 23-22 30th Ave, Astoria, NY 11102; **Phone:** 718-267-2763; **Board Cert:** Radiation Oncology 1992; **Med School:** Mount Sinai Sch Med 1985; **Resid:** Surgery, Univ Hosp-SUNY 1987; Radiation Oncology, SUNY Hlth Sci Ctr 1991; **Fellow:** Radiation Oncology, Meml Sloan-Kettering Cancer Ctr 1992; **Fac Appt:** Asst Clin Prof RadRO, Mount Sinai Sch Med

Rheumatology

Sharon, Ezra MD (Rhu) - **Spec Exp:** Rheumatoid Arthritis; Lupus/SLE; Fibromyalgia; Gout; **Hospital:** Mount Sinai Hosp of Queens (page 102), Mount Sinai Hosp of Queens (page 102); **Address:** 70-31 108 St, Forest Hills, NY 11375; **Phone:** 718-793-6832; **Board Cert:** Internal Medicine 1973; Rheumatology 1974; **Med School:** Israel 1967; **Resid:** Internal Medicine, Mt Sinai Med Ctr 1971; Rheumatology, SUNY Downstate Med Ctr 1973

Sonpal, Girish K M MD (Rhu) - **Spec Exp:** Osteoporosis; Rheumatoid Arthritis; Lupus/SLE; Autoimmune Disease; **Hospital:** NY Hosp Queens (page 206), Flushing Hosp Med Ctr; **Address:** 149-65 24th Ave, Flushing, NY 11357-3646; **Phone:** 718-445-0500; **Board Cert:** Internal Medicine 1974; Rheumatology 1976; **Med School:** India 1969; **Resid:** Internal Medicine, Catholic Med Ctr 1974; **Fellow:** Rheumatology, Worcester City Hosp 1975; Rheumatology, Queens Hosp Ctr 1976; **Fac Appt:** Asst Prof Med, Cornell Univ-Weill Med Coll

Sports Medicine

Rosen, Jeffrey E MD (SM) - **Spec Exp:** Pediatric Sports Medicine; **Hospital:** NY Hosp Queens (page 206), NYU Hosp For Joint Diseases (page 119); **Address:** NYHQ Ctr Orthopaedic & Rehab Medicine, 163-03 Horace Harding Expressway Fl 2, Fresh Meadows, NY 11365; **Phone:** 866-670-6824; **Board Cert:** Orthopaedic Surgery 2012; **Med School:** Columbia P&S 1993; **Resid:** Orthopaedic Surgery, Hosp for Joint Diseases 1998; **Fellow:** Sports Medicine & Arthroscopic Surgery, Kerlan-Jobe Orthopaedic Clinic 1999; **Fac Appt:** Asst Prof OrS, NYU Sch Med

Surgery

Biviano, Bernard J MD (S) - **Spec Exp:** Critical Care; **Hospital:** Mount Sinai Hosp of Queens (page 102); **Address:** 25-10 30th Ave, Astoria, NY 11102; **Phone:** 718-267-4363; **Board Cert:** Surgery 2006; Surgical Critical Care 2007; **Med School:** UMDNJ-RW Johnson Med Sch 1990; **Resid:** Surgery, Cabrini Med Ctr 1995; **Fellow:** Surgical Critical Care, Metropolitan Hosp 1996; **Fac Appt:** S, Mount Sinai Sch Med

Kemeny, M Margaret MD (S) - **Spec Exp:** Liver Cancer; Pancreatic Cancer; Colon & Rectal Cancer; Cancer Surgery; **Hospital:** Queens Hosp Ctr - Jamaica, N Shore Univ Hosp (page 106); **Address:** Queens Cancer Ctr at Queens Hosp, 82-68 164th St, Jamaica, NY 11432-1140; **Phone:** 718-883-4031; **Board Cert:** Surgery 2003; **Med School:** Columbia P&S 1972; **Resid:** Surgery, Columbia-Presby Hosp 1974; Surgery, Univ Colorado Med Ctr 1976; **Fellow:** Surgery, Meml Sloan Kettering Cancer Ctr 1977; Surgical Oncology, National Cancer Inst 1981; **Fac Appt:** Prof S, Mount Sinai Sch Med

Mendoza, Ernesto MD (S) - **Spec Exp:** Parathyroid Surgery; Throat Disorders; Head & Neck Surgery; **Hospital:** New York Methodist Hosp (page 418); **Address:** 40-45 78th St, Elmhurst, NY 11373-1152; **Phone:** 718-397-9058; **Board Cert:** Surgery 2009; **Med School:** Peru 1974; **Resid:** Surgery, Jewish Hosp 1983; **Fellow:** Head and Neck Surgery, Tulane Univ 1985; Surgical Oncology, Roswell Park Meml Inst 1986

Pace, Benjamin W MD (S) - **Spec Exp:** Breast Surgery; Breast Cancer; **Hospital:** Queens Hosp Ctr - Jamaica; **Address:** Queens Hosp, Department of Surgery, 82-68 164th St, rm A-365, Jamaica, NY 11432-1140; **Phone:** 718-883-4640; **Board Cert:** Surgery 2004; **Med School:** Mexico 1977; **Resid:** Surgery, LI Jewish Med Ctr 1983; **Fac Appt:** Assoc Prof S, Mount Sinai Sch Med

Siegel, Beth M MD (S) - **Spec Exp:** Breast Cancer; Breast Disease; **Hospital:** NYU Langone Med Ctr (page 108); **Address:** NYU Columbus Medical, 97-85 Queens Blvd, Rego Park, NY 11374; **Phone:** 718-261-9100; **Board Cert:** Surgery 2011; **Med School:** Dominica 1982; **Resid:** Surgery, NY Med Ctr of Queens 1988; **Fac Appt:** Asst Prof S, NYU Sch Med

Sung, Kap-Jae MD (S) - **Spec Exp:** Breast Cancer; Laparoscopic Surgery; **Hospital:** Forest Hills Hosp (page 106), NY Hosp Queens (page 206); **Address:** 66-83 70 St, Middle Village, NY 11379-1130; **Phone:** 718-651-2929; **Board Cert:** Surgery 2005; **Med School:** South Korea 1973; **Resid:** Surgery, Wyckoff Heights Hosp 1986; **Fac Appt:** Asst Prof S, NY Med Coll

Zeitlin, Alan P MD (S) - **Spec Exp:** Vascular Surgery; Breast Cancer; Laparoscopic Abdominal Surgery; Gastrointestinal Surgery; **Hospital:** Flushing Hosp Med Ctr, Mount Sinai Hosp of Queens (page 102); **Address:** 69-60 108th St, Forest Hills, NY 11375-4323; **Phone:** 718-544-0442; **Board Cert:** Surgery 2002; **Med School:** Univ Miami Sch Med 1974; **Resid:** Surgery, Montefiore Med Ctr 1979; **Fac Appt:** Asst Clin Prof S, Mount Sinai Sch Med

Thoracic & Cardiac Surgery

Graver, L Michael MD (T&CS) - **Spec Exp:** Minimally Invasive Heart Valve Surgery; Coronary Artery Surgery; Aortic Surgery; Heart Valve Surgery; **Hospital:** Long Island Jewish Med Ctr (page 106); **Address:** 270-05 76th Ave, Ste O-4000, Long Island Jewish Med Ctr, New Hyde Park, NY 11040-1433; **Phone:** 718-470-7460; **Board Cert:** Surgery 2003; Thoracic Surgery 2004; **Med School:** Albany Med Coll 1977; **Resid:** Surgery, St Luke's-Roosevelt Hosp Ctr 1982; Cardiovascular Surgery, Deaconness Hosp 1983; **Fellow:** Cardiovascular Pathology, NY Hosp-Cornell Med Ctr 1985; **Fac Appt:** Prof TS, Hofstra N Shore-LIJ Sch Med

Lang, Samuel J MD (T&CS) - **Spec Exp:** Minimally Invasive Cardiac Surgery; Heart Valve Surgery; Cardiothoracic Surgery; **Hospital:** NY Hosp Queens (page 206); **Address:** 56-45 Main St, rm 387, Flushing, NY 11355; **Phone:** 718-670-1137; **Board Cert:** Thoracic Surgery 2006; **Med School:** Univ Alabama 1978; **Resid:** Surgery, UCLA Med Ctr 1982; Thoracic Surgery, NYU Med Ctr 1983; **Fellow:** Cardiothoracic Surgery, UCLA Med Ctr 1985; Pediatric Cardiac Surgery, Hosp for Sick Chldn 1986

Lee, Paul C MD (T&CS) - **Spec Exp:** Lung Cancer; Esophageal Cancer; Gastroesophageal Reflux Disease (GERD); Minimally Invasive Thoracic Surgery; **Hospital:** NY Hosp Queens (page 206), NY-Presby/Weill Cornell Med Ctr, NY (page 104); **Address:** 56-45 Main St, Ste WA-100, Flushing, NY 11355; **Phone:** 718-670-2707; **Board Cert:** Surgery 2002; Thoracic Surgery 2004; **Med School:** Johns Hopkins Univ 1995; **Resid:** Cardiothoracic Surgery, NY Presby Hosp-Cornell 2003; Thoracic Surgery, Meml Sloan Kettering Cancer Ctr 2003; **Fellow:** Minimally Invasive Surgery, Meml SUniv Pittsburgh 2003; **Fac Appt:** Asst Prof S, Cornell Univ-Weill Med Coll

Urology

Farrell, Robert M MD (U) - **Spec Exp:** Endourology; Urologic Cancer; **Hospital:** NY Hosp Queens (page 206), Flushing Hosp Med Ctr; **Address:** 58-42 Main St, Flushing, NY 11355; **Phone:** 718-353-3710; **Board Cert:** Urology 1976; **Med School:** Cornell Univ-Weill Med Coll 1966; **Resid:** Surgery, NY Hosp 1968; Urology, NY Hosp 1975

Sandhaus, Jeffrey MD (U) - **Spec Exp:** Prostate Cancer; Minimally Invasive Surgery; Vasectomy-Scalpelless; **Hospital:** Mount Sinai Hosp of Queens (page 102), NY-Presby/Weill Cornell Med Ctr, NY (page 104); **Address:** 36-01 31st Ave Fl 1, Astoria, NY 11106-1051; **Phone:** 718-932-3535; **Board Cert:** Urology 1976; **Med School:** NY Med Coll 1966; **Resid:** Urology, Univ Hosp 1973; **Fellow:** Nephrology, Univ Hosp 1970; **Fac Appt:** Asst Clin Prof U, Mount Sinai Sch Med

Tarasuk, Albert P MD (U) - **Spec Exp:** Prostate Disease; Bladder Surgery; Kidney Stones; **Hospital:** NY Hosp Queens (page 206), Flushing Hosp Med Ctr; **Address:** 58-42 Main St, Flushing, NY 11355-5336; **Phone:** 718-353-3710; **Board Cert:** Urology 1972; **Med School:** Geo Wash Univ 1964; **Resid:** Urology, Beth Israel Med Ctr 1969

Tillem, Steven MD (U) - **Hospital:** Mount Sinai Hosp of Queens (page 102), NY Hosp Queens (page 206); **Address:** 31-19 Newton Ave, Ste 801, Astoria, NY 11102; **Phone:** 718-777-2111; **Board Cert:** Urology 2009; **Med School:** UMDNJ-NJ Med Sch, Newark 1992; **Resid:** Surgery, LI Jewish Med Ctr 1994; Urology, LI Jewish Med Ctr 1998

Vascular & Interventional Radiology

Rogers, David M MD (VIR) - **Hospital:** NY Hosp Queens (page 206), Wyckoff Heights Med Ctr; **Address:** 56-45 Main St, Flushing, NY 11355; **Phone:** 718-670-1050; **Board Cert:** Diagnostic Radiology 1987; **Med School:** Columbia P&S 1981; **Resid:** Diagnostic Radiology, Mt Sinai Med Ctr 1987; **Fellow:** Vascular & Interventional Radiology, NYU Med Ctr 1988

Vascular Surgery

Landis, Gregg MD (VascS) - **Spec Exp:** Endovascular Sugery; Carotid Artery Surgery; Aortic Surgery; **Hospital:** NY Hosp Queens (page 206), NY-Presby/Weill Cornell Med Ctr, NY (page 104); **Address:** 56-45 Main St, Flushing, NY 11355; **Phone:** 718-445-0220; **Board Cert:** Surgery 2009; Vascular Surgery 2011; **Med School:** UMDNJ-NJ Med Sch, Newark 1995; **Resid:** Surgery, Montefiore Med Ctr 2000; **Fellow:** Vascular Surgery, SUNY Downstate Med Ctr 2002; **Fac Appt:** Assoc Clin Prof VascS, Cornell Univ-Weill Med Coll

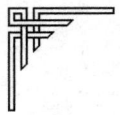

The Best in American Medicine
www.CastleConnolly.com

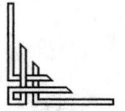
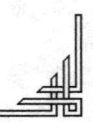

Richmond (Staten Island)

Richmond (Staten Island)

Adolescent Medicine

Lee, April C MD (AM) - **Hospital:** Staten Island Univ Hosp - North (page 106), NS-LIJ Hlth Sys (page 106); **Address:** 242 Mason Ave, Staten Island, NY 10305; **Phone:** 718-226-6294; **Board Cert:** Pediatrics 1986; Adolescent Medicine 2009; **Med School:** NYU Sch Med 1980; **Resid:** Pediatrics, NYU Med Ctr 1983; **Fellow:** Adolescent Medicine, Brookdale Hosp 1986; **Fac Appt:** Asst Clin Prof Ped, SUNY Hlth Sci Ctr

Allergy & Immunology

Rao, Yalamanchili A K MD (A&I) - **Hospital:** Staten Island Univ Hosp - North (page 106), Richmond Univ Med Ctr; **Address:** 896 Targee St, Staten Island, NY 10304; **Phone:** 718-816-8200; **Board Cert:** Internal Medicine 1977; Allergy & Immunology 1977; **Med School:** India 1968; **Resid:** Allergy & Immunology, Long Island Coll Hosp 1975; Internal Medicine, Long Island Coll Hosp 1977; **Fac Appt:** Asst Clin Prof Med, SUNY Downstate

Cardiovascular Disease

Besser, Louis M MD (Cv) - **Spec Exp:** Coronary Artery Disease; Arrhythmias; **Hospital:** Richmond Univ Med Ctr, Staten Island Univ Hosp - North (page 106); **Address:** 11 Ralph Pl, Ste 310, Staten Island, NY 10304-4419; **Phone:** 718-442-1777; **Board Cert:** Internal Medicine 1988; Cardiovascular Disease 1989; **Med School:** Mexico 1981; **Resid:** Internal Medicine, St Vincents Med Ctr 1986; **Fellow:** Cardiovascular Disease, St Vincents Med Ctr 1988; **Fac Appt:** Asst Clin Prof Med, NY Med Coll

Bogin, Marc MD (Cv) - **Spec Exp:** Echocardiography; Cardiac Catheterization; **Hospital:** Staten Island Univ Hosp - North (page 106), Richmond Univ Med Ctr; **Address:** Heart, Lung & Surgery Ctr, 501 Seaview Ave, Ste 200, Staten Island, NY 10305; **Phone:** 718-663-6400; **Board Cert:** Internal Medicine 1989; Cardiovascular Disease 2003; **Med School:** Mexico 1985; **Resid:** Internal Medicine, Booth Meml Hosp 1990; **Fellow:** Cardiovascular Disease, St Vincent's Hosp & Med Ctr 1993; **Fac Appt:** Asst Clin Prof Med, NY Med Coll

Grodman, Richard S MD (Cv) - **Spec Exp:** Echocardiography; Cardiac Catheterization; **Hospital:** Richmond Univ Med Ctr; **Address:** Richmond University Medical Center, 355 Bard Ave, Staten Island, NY 10310-1664; **Phone:** 718-818-4642; **Board Cert:** Internal Medicine 1976; Cardiovascular Disease 1979; **Med School:** SUNY Downstate 1973; **Resid:** Internal Medicine, SUNY Downstate 1976; Critical Care Medicine, SUNY Downstate 1977; **Fellow:** Cardiovascular Disease, Rhode Island Hosp-Brown 1979; **Fac Appt:** Assoc Clin Prof Med, NY Med Coll

Lafferty, James C MD (Cv) - **Spec Exp:** Electrophysiologic Testing; **Hospital:** Staten Island Univ Hosp - North (page 106); **Address:** Staten Island Heart, 501 Seaview Ave, Ste 300, Staten Island, NY 10305; **Phone:** 718-663-7000 x6; **Board Cert:** Internal Medicine 1985; Cardiovascular Disease 1987; Cardiac Electrophysiology 2006; **Med School:** SUNY Hlth Sci Ctr 1982; **Resid:** Internal Medicine, Staten Island Hosp 1985; **Fellow:** Cardiovascular Disease, Univ Hosp 1987; **Fac Appt:** Assoc Prof Med, SUNY Downstate

Schwartz, Charles A MD (Cv) - **Spec Exp:** Echocardiography; Cardiac Catheterization; Transesophageal Echocardiogram (TEE); **Hospital:** Staten Island Univ Hosp - North (page 106); **Address:** 501 Seaview Ave, Ste 300, Staten Island, NY 10305; **Phone:** 718-663-7000; **Board Cert:** Internal Medicine 1983; Cardiovascular Disease 1985; Echocardiography 2011; **Med School:** SUNY Downstate 1980; **Resid:** Internal Medicine, Staten Island Hosp 1983; **Fellow:** Cardiovascular Disease, St Vincent's Hosp & Med Ctr 1985; **Fac Appt:** Asst Clin Prof Med, SUNY Downstate

Vazzana, Thomas MD (Cv) - **Spec Exp:** Invasive Cardiology; Non-Invasive Cardiology; Interventional Cardiology; **Hospital:** Staten Island Univ Hosp - North (page 106), Richmond Univ Med Ctr; **Address:** Heart, Lung & Surgery Ctr, 501 Seaview Ave, Ste 200, Staten Island, NY 10305; **Phone:** 718-663-6400; **Board Cert:** Internal Medicine 1989; Cardiovascular Disease 2011; Interventional Cardiology 2002; **Med School:** Grenada 1985; **Resid:** Internal Medicine, St Joseph's Hosp & Med Ctr 1989; **Fellow:** Cardiovascular Disease, St Vincent's Hosp & Med Ctr 1991; **Fac Appt:** Asst Prof Med, NY Med Coll

Winter, Steven MD (Cv) - **Spec Exp:** Cholesterol/Lipid Disorders; Preventive Cardiology; Non-Invasive Cardiology; **Hospital:** Staten Island Univ Hosp - North (page 106), Richmond Univ Med Ctr; **Address:** 2627 Hylan Blvd, Bldg B, Staten Island, NY 10306-4339; **Phone:** 718-351-5600; **Board Cert:** Internal Medicine 1979; Cardiovascular Disease 1981; **Med School:** UMDNJ-NJ Med Sch, Newark 1976; **Resid:** Internal Medicine, N Shore Univ Hosp 1979; Internal Medicine, Meml Sloan Kettering Cancer Ctr 1979; **Fellow:** Cardiovascular Disease, Rhode Island Hosp 1981; **Fac Appt:** Asst Clin Prof Med, SUNY Hlth Sci Ctr

Child Neurology

De Carlo, Regina MD (ChiN) - **Spec Exp:** Autism & Developmental Disorders; Headache; Learning Disorders; ADD/ADHD; **Hospital:** Richmond Univ Med Ctr, NYU Langone Med Ctr (page 108); **Address:** 2550 Victory Blvd, Staten Island, NY 10314-6635; **Phone:** 718-983-0923; **Board Cert:** Pediatrics 1984; Child Neurology 1984; **Med School:** UMDNJ-NJ Med Sch, Newark 1977; **Resid:** Pediatrics, NYU Med Ctr 1980; Neurology, NYU Med Ctr 1983; **Fellow:** Child Neurology, NYU Med Ctr 1984; **Fac Appt:** Asst Clin Prof N, NYU Sch Med

Dermatology

Bernstein, Charles MD (D) - **Hospital:** Staten Island Univ Hosp - North (page 106); **Address:** 244 Buel Ave Fl 2, Staten Island, NY 10305; **Phone:** 718-980-5767; **Board Cert:** Internal Medicine 1983; Dermatology 1987; **Med School:** SUNY Downstate 1980; **Resid:** Internal Medicine, Staten Island Hosp 1984; Dermatology, Downstate Med Ctr 1987; **Fac Appt:** Assoc Clin Prof D, SUNY Hlth Sci Ctr

Lederman, Josiane MD (D) - **Spec Exp:** Cosmetic Dermatology; Skin Cancer; Laser Surgery; **Address:** 116 Lamberts Ln, Staten Island, NY 10314-7210; **Phone:** 718-370-0422; **Board Cert:** Dermatology 1986; **Med School:** France 1981; **Resid:** Dermatology, Saint Louis Hosp 1983; **Fellow:** Dermatology, Mass Genl Hosp-Harvard 1986

McCormack, Patricia C MD (D) - **Spec Exp:** Psoriasis; Skin Cancer; Skin Laser Surgery; **Hospital:** Richmond Univ Med Ctr; **Address:** 1550 Richmond Ave, Ste 207, Staten Island, NY 10314; **Phone:** 718-698-1616; **Board Cert:** Dermatology 1985; **Med School:** UMDNJ-Rutgers Med Sch 1981; **Resid:** Dermatology, Westchester Med Ctr/NY Med Coll 1985

Urbanek, Richard W MD (D) - **Spec Exp:** Liposuction; Laser Surgery; Botox Therapy; **Address:** 1324 Victory Blvd, Staten Island, NY 10301; **Phone:** 718-448-4488; **Board Cert:** Dermatology 1977; **Med School:** Cornell Univ-Weill Med Coll 1972; **Resid:** Dermatology, Temple Univ Hosp 1976; **Fac Appt:** Asst Prof D, NYU Sch Med

Endocrinology, Diabetes & Metabolism

Cohen, Neil D MD (EDM) - **Spec Exp:** Diabetes; Thyroid Disorders; Osteoporosis; **Hospital:** Staten Island Univ Hosp - North (page 106), Staten Island Univ Hosp - South (page 106); **Address:** 1460 Victory Blvd, Staten Island, NY 10301-3914; **Phone:** 718-442-0300; **Board Cert:** Internal Medicine 2003; Endocrinology, Diabetes & Metabolism 2005; **Med School:** Med Coll PA Hahnemann 1990; **Resid:** Internal Medicine, N Shore Univ Hosp 1993; **Fellow:** Endocrinology, Diabetes & Metabolism, Montefiore Med Ctr 1995; **Fac Appt:** Assoc Clin Prof Med, SUNY Downstate

Das, Seshadri MD (EDM) - **Spec Exp:** Diabetes; Thyroid Disorders; **Hospital:** Richmond Univ Med Ctr, Staten Island Univ Hosp - South (page 106); **Address:** 45 Little Clove Rd, Staten Island, NY 10301; **Phone:** 718-273-5522; **Board Cert:** Internal Medicine 1983; Endocrinology, Diabetes & Metabolism 2008; **Med School:** India 1968; **Resid:** Internal Medicine, North Middlesex Hosp 1975; Internal Medicine, Whittington Hosp/Royal Free Hosp 1977; **Fellow:** Endocrinology, Diabetes & Metabolism, SUNY Downstate 1980

Hoffman, Richard S MD (EDM) - **Spec Exp:** Diabetes; Thyroid Disorders; Parathyroid Disorders; Adrenal Disorders; **Hospital:** Staten Island Univ Hosp - North (page 106); **Address:** 1460 Victory Blvd, Staten Island, NY 10301; **Phone:** 718-442-0300; **Board Cert:** Internal Medicine 1971; Endocrinology, Diabetes & Metabolism 1975; **Med School:** SUNY Hlth Sci Ctr 1965; **Resid:** Internal Medicine, Long Island Coll Hosp 1967; Internal Medicine, Boston City Hosp 1968; **Fellow:** Endocrinology, Boston City Hosp 1970; **Fac Appt:** Assoc Clin Prof Med, SUNY Downstate

Rothman, Jeffrey G MD (EDM) - **Spec Exp:** Diabetes; Osteoporosis; Thyroid Disorders; **Hospital:** Staten Island Univ Hosp - North (page 106), Staten Island Univ Hosp - South (page 106); **Address:** 1460 Victory Blvd, Staten Island, NY 10301-3914; **Phone:** 718-442-0300; **Board Cert:** Internal Medicine 1973; Endocrinology, Diabetes & Metabolism 1977; **Med School:** SUNY Buffalo 1970; **Resid:** Internal Medicine, Hosp Univ Penn 1973; **Fellow:** Endocrinology, Diabetes & Metabolism, Hosp Univ Penn 1977; **Fac Appt:** Asst Clin Prof Med, SUNY Downstate

Family Medicine

Nepola, Neil MD (FMed) *PCP* - **Hospital:** Staten Island Univ Hosp - South (page 106); **Address:** 217 Rose Ave, Staten Island, NY 10306-2918; **Phone:** 718-667-6767; **Board Cert:** Family Medicine 2004; **Med School:** Philippines 1979; **Resid:** Family Medicine, UMDNJ-St Peter's Hosp 1983

Gastroenterology

Bruckstein, Alex MD (Ge) - **Spec Exp:** Colonoscopy; Gastroscopy; Gastroesophageal Reflux Disease (GERD); **Hospital:** Staten Island Univ Hosp - North (page 106), Staten Island Univ Hosp - South (page 106); **Address:** 2627 Hylan Blvd, Staten Island, NY 10306-4339; **Phone:** 718-667-3200; **Board Cert:** Internal Medicine 1979; Gastroenterology 1983; **Med School:** Albert Einstein Coll Med 1975; **Resid:** Internal Medicine, Roosevelt Hosp 1977; Internal Medicine, St Luke's Hosp 1978; **Fellow:** Gastroenterology, VA Med Ctr-NYU 1980; **Fac Appt:** Asst Clin Prof Med, SUNY Downstate

Fazio, Richard MD (Ge) - **Spec Exp:** Colonoscopy; Gastroesophageal Reflux Disease (GERD); **Hospital:** Richmond Univ Med Ctr; **Address:** 78 Todt Hill Rd, Ste 203, Staten Island, NY 10314-4528; **Phone:** 718-448-1122; **Board Cert:** Internal Medicine 1982; Gastroenterology 1983; **Med School:** Italy 1978; **Resid:** Internal Medicine, Maimonides Med Ctr 1981; **Fellow:** Gastroenterology, St Vincent's Med Ctr 1983; **Fac Appt:** Prof Med, SUNY Downstate

Wickremesinghe, Prasanna C MD (Ge) - **Spec Exp:** Inflammatory Bowel Disease/Crohn's; Hepatitis; Endoscopy; **Hospital:** Richmond Univ Med Ctr; **Address:** 481 Bard Ave, Staten Island, NY 10310; **Phone:** 718-448-0865; **Board Cert:** Internal Medicine 1980; Gastroenterology 1975; **Med School:** Sri Lanka 1968; **Resid:** Internal Medicine, Coney Island Hosp 1972; **Fellow:** Gastroenterology, Maimonides Medical Ctr 1975; **Fac Appt:** Asst Prof Med, NY Med Coll

Geriatric Medicine

Seminara, Donna MD (Ger) - **Hospital:** Staten Island Univ Hosp - North (page 106); **Address:** Island Internists, 420 Lyndale Ave, Staten Island, NY 10312-6131; **Phone:** 718-967-5630; **Board Cert:** Internal Medicine 2010; Geriatric Medicine 2000; **Med School:** Mexico 1986; **Resid:** Internal Medicine, Staten Island Univ Hosp 1990

Gynecologic Oncology

Maiman, Mitchell MD (GO) - **Spec Exp:** Cervical Cancer; Ovarian Cancer; Uterine Cancer; **Hospital:** Staten Island Univ Hosp - North (page 106); **Address:** 256 Mason Ave Fl C, Staten Island, NY 10305-3408; **Phone:** 718-226-6400; **Board Cert:** Obstetrics & Gynecology 2011; Gynecologic Oncology 2011; **Med School:** SUNY Hlth Sci Ctr 1981; **Resid:** Obstetrics & Gynecology, Montefiore Med Ctr 1985; **Fellow:** Gynecologic Oncology, SUNY Downstate Med Ctr 1987; **Fac Appt:** Prof ObG, SUNY Downstate

Infectious Disease

Glaser, Jordan MD (Inf) - **Spec Exp:** AIDS/HIV; **Hospital:** Staten Island Univ Hosp - North (page 106), Staten Island Univ Hosp - South (page 106); **Address:** 1408 Richmond Rd, Staten Island, NY 10304; **Phone:** 718-816-3362; **Board Cert:** Internal Medicine 1982; Infectious Disease 1984; **Med School:** SUNY Hlth Sci Ctr 1979; **Resid:** Internal Medicine, Staten Island Hosp 1980; Infectious Disease, Staten Island Hosp 1982; **Fellow:** Infectious Disease, Univ Hosp 1984; **Fac Appt:** Assoc Clin Prof Med, SUNY Hlth Sci Ctr

Internal Medicine

Fulop, Robert MD (IM) *PCP* - **Spec Exp:** Diagnostic Problems; Geriatric Medicine; **Hospital:** Richmond Univ Med Ctr, Staten Island Univ Hosp - North (page 106); **Address:** 476 Klondike Ave, Staten Island, NY 10314-6216; **Phone:** 718-761-1156; **Board Cert:** Internal Medicine 1982; Geriatric Medicine 2005; **Med School:** SUNY Upstate Med Univ 1978; **Resid:** Internal Medicine, Brookdale Hosp 1981; **Fac Appt:** Asst Clin Prof Med, NY Med Coll

Gazzara, Paul MD (IM) *PCP* - **Spec Exp:** Complementary Medicine; Acupuncture; Addiction/Substance Abuse; **Hospital:** Staten Island Univ Hosp - North (page 106); **Address:** 3589 Hylan Blvd, Staten Island, NY 10308-3513; **Phone:** 718-966-3700; **Board Cert:** Internal Medicine 1986; **Med School:** SUNY Downstate 1983; **Resid:** Internal Medicine, Staten Island Hosp 1986; **Fac Appt:** Asst Clin Prof Med, SUNY Hlth Sci Ctr

Hendricks, Judith MD (IM) *PCP* - **Spec Exp:** Hypertension; Cholesterol/Lipid Disorders; **Hospital:** Staten Island Univ Hosp - North (page 106); **Address:** 1870 Richmond Rd, Staten Island, NY 10306; **Phone:** 718-667-5400; **Board Cert:** Internal Medicine 1978; **Med School:** Univ Okla Coll Med 1975; **Resid:** Internal Medicine, Staten Island Hosp 1978; **Fac Appt:** Asst Clin Prof Med, SUNY Hlth Sci Ctr

Malach, Barbara MD (IM) *PCP* - **Spec Exp:** Geriatric Medicine; **Hospital:** Staten Island Univ Hosp - North (page 106); **Address:** 2627B Hylan Blvd, Staten Island, NY 10306-4339; **Phone:** 718-987-6000; **Board Cert:** Internal Medicine 1983; Geriatric Medicine 2008; **Med School:** SUNY Downstate 1979; **Resid:** Internal Medicine, Staten Island Hosp 1982

Strange, Theodore MD (IM) *PCP* - **Spec Exp:** Geriatric Medicine; **Hospital:** Staten Island Univ Hosp - South (page 106), Staten Island Univ Hosp - North (page 106); **Address:** 68 Seguine Ave, Staten Island, NY 10309-3723; **Phone:** 718-356-6500; **Board Cert:** Internal Medicine 2001; Geriatric Medicine 2002; **Med School:** SUNY Hlth Sci Ctr 1985; **Resid:** Internal Medicine, Staten Island Univ Hosp 1988; **Fac Appt:** Assoc Clin Prof Med, SUNY Downstate

Interventional Cardiology

Malpeso, James V MD (IC) - **Spec Exp:** Cardiac Catheterization; Angioplasty & Stent Placement; Cardiac CT Angiography; **Hospital:** Staten Island Univ Hosp - North (page 106); **Address:** 501 Seaview Ave HLS Bldg Fl 3 - Ste 302, Staten Island, NY 10305; **Phone:** 718-226-9600; **Board Cert:** Internal Medicine 1979; Cardiovascular Disease 1981; Cardiovascular Computed Tomography 2008; **Med School:** Albert Einstein Coll Med 1975; **Resid:** Internal Medicine, Kings County Hosp 1978; **Fellow:** Cardiovascular Disease, St Vincent's Hosp & Med Ctr 1980; **Fac Appt:** Asst Prof Med, SUNY Downstate

Medical Oncology

Forlenza, Thomas J MD (Onc) - **Spec Exp:** Palliative Care; Bleeding/Coagulation Disorders; Breast Cancer; Lung Cancer; **Hospital:** Richmond Univ Med Ctr; **Address:** 102 Hart Blvd, Staten Island, NY 10301-2615; **Phone:** 718-816-4949; **Board Cert:** Internal Medicine 1981; Hematology 1984; Blood Banking 1984; Medical Oncology 1985; **Med School:** Boston Univ 1977; **Resid:** Internal Medicine, Univ Kentucky Med Ctr 1980; **Fellow:** Hematology, NYU Med Ctr 1982; Medical Oncology, Kings County Hosp 1983; **Fac Appt:** Asst Prof Med, NYU Sch Med

Friscia, Philip MD (Onc) - **Spec Exp:** Lung Cancer; Colon Cancer; Hematology; **Hospital:** Staten Island Univ Hosp - North (page 106), Staten Island Univ Hosp - South (page 106); **Address:** 256 Mason Ave, C Bldg, Nalitt Inst, Staten Island, NY 10305; **Phone:** 718-226-6400; **Board Cert:** Internal Medicine 1978; Medical Oncology 1981; **Med School:** Italy 1972; **Resid:** Internal Medicine, Long Island Coll Hosp 1976; **Fellow:** Hematology & Oncology, Long Island Coll Hosp 1979; **Fac Appt:** Asst Clin Prof Med, SUNY Downstate

Odaimi, Marcel MD (Onc) - **Spec Exp:** Brain Tumors; **Hospital:** Staten Island Univ Hosp - South (page 106), Staten Island Univ Hosp - North (page 106); **Address:** 256 Mason Ave C Bldg, Nalitt Inst, Staten Island, NY 10305-3408; **Phone:** 718-226-6400; **Board Cert:** Internal Medicine 1987; Medical Oncology 1989; **Med School:** Amer Univ Beirut 1981; **Resid:** Internal Medicine, Amer Univ Beirut 1983; Internal Medicine, Staten Island Hosp 1987; **Fellow:** Medical Oncology, MD Anderson Hosp 1985

Terjanian, Terenig O MD (Onc) - **Hospital:** Staten Island Univ Hosp - North (page 106); **Address:** 256 Mason Ave C Bldg Fl 1, Nalitt Inst, Staten Island, NY 10305-3408; **Phone:** 718-226-6400; **Board Cert:** Internal Medicine 1984; Medical Oncology 1987; Hematology 1988; **Med School:** France 1978; **Resid:** Anatomic Pathology, Amer Univ Beirut 1981; Internal Medicine, Staten Island Univ Hosp 1984; **Fellow:** Medical Oncology, UT MD Anderson Cancer Ctr 1986; Hematology, NYU Med Ctr 1988

Neonatal-Perinatal Medicine

Roth, Philip MD/PhD (NP) - **Spec Exp:** Neonatal Infections/Immunity; Breast Feeding Problems; **Hospital:** Staten Island Univ Hosp - North (page 106); **Address:** 475 Seaview Ave Fl 4 East, Staten Island, NY 10305-3436; **Phone:** 718-226-9796; **Board Cert:** Pediatrics 1987; Neonatal-Perinatal Medicine 2011; **Med School:** Columbia P&S 1982; **Resid:** Pediatrics, Chldns Hosp 1986; **Fellow:** Neonatal-Perinatal Medicine, Hosp Univ Penn 1988; **Fac Appt:** Assoc Prof Ped, SUNY Downstate

Nephrology

Grossman, Susan D MD (Nep) - **Hospital:** Richmond Univ Med Ctr; **Address:** 1366 Victory Blvd, Staten Island, NY 10310; **Phone:** 718-273-3400; **Board Cert:** Internal Medicine 1980; Nephrology 1982; **Med School:** UMDNJ-NJ Med Sch, Newark 1977; **Resid:** Internal Medicine, Univ Hosp 1980; **Fellow:** Nephrology, New England Med Ctr 1982

Kleiner, Morton MD (Nep) - **Spec Exp:** Hypertension; Kidney Disease; **Hospital:** Staten Island Univ Hosp - North (page 106); **Address:** 347 Edison St, Staten Island, NY 10306-3034; **Phone:** 718-987-5942; **Board Cert:** Internal Medicine 1977; Nephrology 1982; **Med School:** NY Med Coll 1974; **Resid:** Internal Medicine, N Shore Univ Hosp 1977; **Fellow:** Nephrology, NY Hosp-Cornell Med Ctr 1979; **Fac Appt:** Asst Clin Prof Med, SUNY Downstate

Pepe, John M MD (Nep) - **Spec Exp:** Transplant Medicine-Kidney; **Hospital:** Richmond Univ Med Ctr, Staten Island Univ Hosp - South (page 106); **Address:** 1550 Richmond Ave, Ste 205, Staten Island, NY 10314-1519; **Phone:** 718-982-7800; **Board Cert:** Internal Medicine 1978; Nephrology 1980; **Med School:** Med Coll PA Hahnemann 1975; **Resid:** Internal Medicine, Univ Hosp 1978; **Fellow:** Nephrology, Bronx Muni Hosp/ Einstein 1980; **Fac Appt:** Asst Prof Med, NY Med Coll

Neurology

Jutkowitz, Robert S MD (N) - **Spec Exp:** Headache; Seizure Disorders; **Hospital:** Richmond Univ Med Ctr; **Address:** 78 Todt Hill Rd, Ste 205, Staten Island, NY 10314-4528; **Phone:** 718-442-7133; **Board Cert:** Neurology 1976; **Med School:** Univ Louisville Sch Med 1968; **Resid:** Internal Medicine, St Viincents Hosp 1970; Neurology, Mt Sinai Hosp 1974

Najjar, Souhel MD (N) - **Spec Exp:** Epilepsy; Seizure Disorders; **Hospital:** Staten Island Univ Hosp - North (page 106), NYU Langone Med Ctr (page 108); **Address:** 501 Seaview Ave, Ste 104, Staten Island, NY 10305; **Phone:** 718-683-3766; **Board Cert:** Neurology 1993; **Med School:** Syria 1983; **Resid:** Pathology, Albany Med Ctr 1988; Neurology, Albany Med Ctr 1992; **Fellow:** Neurological Pathology, NYU Med Ctr 1994; **Fac Appt:** Assoc Clin Prof N, NYU Sch Med

Obstetrics & Gynecology

Ponterio, Jane M MD (ObG) *PCP* - **Spec Exp:** Menopause Problems; Hysterectomy Alternatives; Adolescent Gynecology; **Hospital:** Richmond Univ Med Ctr, Staten Island Univ Hosp - North (page 106); **Address:** 1583 Richmond Ave, Staten Island, NY 10314; **Phone:** 718-983-0204; **Board Cert:** Obstetrics & Gynecology 2011; **Med School:** NY Med Coll 1981; **Resid:** Obstetrics & Gynecology, St Luke's-Roosevelt Hosp Ctr 1985; **Fac Appt:** Asst Prof ObG, NY Med Coll

Reilly, James G DO (ObG) - **Spec Exp:** Colposcopy; Laparoscopic Surgery; Hysterectomy Alternatives; **Hospital:** Richmond Univ Med Ctr, Staten Island Univ Hosp - North (page 106); **Address:** 668 Castleton Ave, Staten Island, NY 10301-2044; **Phone:** 718-448-4300; **Board Cert:** Obstetrics & Gynecology 2011; **Med School:** NY Coll Osteo Med 1991; **Resid:** Obstetrics & Gynecology, St Vincent Cath Med Ctr 1995; **Fac Appt:** Asst Clin Prof ObG, NY Coll Osteo Med

Ophthalmology

Derespinis, Patrick MD (Oph) - **Spec Exp:** Eye Muscle Disorders; Pediatric Ophthalmology; Eye Disorders-Congenital; **Hospital:** Staten Island Univ Hosp - South (page 106), Univ Hosp-UMDNJ—Newark; **Address:** Pediatric Eye Care, 2504 Richmond Rd, Staten Island, NY 10306; **Phone:** 718-667-1010; **Board Cert:** Ophthalmology 1989; **Med School:** Mexico 1981; **Resid:** Internal Medicine, Booth Meml Med Ctr 1983; Ophthalmology, UMDNJ 1987; **Fellow:** Pediatric Ophthalmology, Manhattan EE&T Hosp 1988; **Fac Appt:** Assoc Clin Prof Oph, UMDNJ-NJ Med Sch, Newark

Kramer, Philip W MD (Oph) - **Spec Exp:** Diabetic Eye Disease/Retinopathy; Cataract Surgery; Glaucoma; **Hospital:** Staten Island Univ Hosp - South (page 106), New York Eye & Ear Infirm (page 117); **Address:** 1460 Victory Blvd, Staten Island, NY 10301-3914; **Phone:** 718-447-0022; **Board Cert:** Ophthalmology 1985; **Med School:** Temple Univ 1980; **Resid:** Ophthalmology, NY Eye & Ear Infirmary 1984

Zerykier, Abraham L MD (Oph) - **Spec Exp:** Cataract Surgery; Diabetic Eye Disease/Retinopathy; Glaucoma; **Hospital:** Staten Island Univ Hosp - South (page 106), Beth Israel Med Ctr- Kings Hwy Div (page 94); **Address:** 16 Ross Ave, Staten Island, NY 10306-2216; **Phone:** 718-667-4444; **Board Cert:** Ophthalmology 1980; **Med School:** Hahnemann Univ 1975; **Resid:** Internal Medicine, Brookdale Hosp 1976; Ophthalmology, Jewish Hosp 1979; **Fac Appt:** Asst Clin Prof Oph, SUNY Downstate

Orthopaedic Surgery

Drucker, David A MD (OrS) - **Spec Exp:** Hip & Knee Replacement; **Hospital:** Staten Island Univ Hosp - North (page 106), Beth Israel Med Ctr- Kings Hwy Div (page 94); **Address:** New York Hip & Knee, 11 Ralph Pl, Ste 103A, Staten Island, NY 10304; **Phone:** 718-727-6945; **Board Cert:** Orthopaedic Surgery 2004; **Med School:** Univ Chicago-Pritzker Sch Med 1983; **Resid:** Orthopaedic Surgery, UNDMJ Univ Hosp 1989; **Fellow:** Hip & Knee Surgery, Indiana Univ 1990; **Fac Appt:** Asst Clin Prof OrS, UMDNJ-NJ Med Sch, Newark

Flynn, Maryirene MD (OrS) - **Spec Exp:** Arthroscopic Surgery; Sports Medicine; **Hospital:** Richmond Univ Med Ctr, Staten Island Univ Hosp - North (page 106); **Address:** Staten Island Orthopedics, 2052 Richmond Rd, Staten Island, NY 10306; **Phone:** 718-351-6500; **Board Cert:** Orthopaedic Surgery 2005; **Med School:** Albert Einstein Coll Med 1986; **Resid:** Orthopaedic Surgery, Montefiore Hosp Med Ctr 1991; **Fellow:** Sports Medicine, Staten Island Hosp 1992

Jayaram, Nadubeethi MD (OrS) - **Spec Exp:** Hand Surgery; **Hospital:** Richmond Univ Med Ctr; **Address:** 11 Ralph Pl, Ste 102, Staten Island, NY 10304; **Phone:** 718-447-6545; **Board Cert:** Orthopaedic Surgery 2003; **Med School:** India 1973; **Resid:** Surgery, Univ Hosp 1981; Orthopaedic Surgery, Univ Hosp 1985; **Fellow:** Vascular Surgery, Lutheran Med Ctr 1982; Hand Surgery, Univ Alabama Hosp 1988

Reilly, John P MD (OrS) - **Spec Exp:** Sports Medicine; Trauma; **Hospital:** Staten Island Univ Hosp - North (page 106); **Address:** 3311 Hylan Blvd, Staten Island, NY 10308; **Phone:** 718-667-7500; **Board Cert:** Orthopaedic Surgery 2010; **Med School:** SUNY Downstate 1981; **Resid:** Orthopaedic Surgery, Lenox Hill Hosp 1986; Orthopaedic Surgery, Chldns Hosp; **Fellow:** Orthopaedic Surgery, Univ MD Hosp 1987

Sherman, Mark F MD (OrS) - **Spec Exp:** Sports Medicine; Knee Injuries; **Hospital:** Richmond Univ Med Ctr, Staten Island Univ Hosp - North (page 106); **Address:** Staten Island Orthopedics, 2052 Richmond Rd, Staten Island, NY 10304; **Phone:** 718-351-6500; **Board Cert:** Orthopaedic Surgery 1981; **Med School:** NYU Sch Med 1975; **Resid:** Surgery, Bellevue Hosp 1976; Orthopaedic Surgery, Bellevue Hosp 1979; **Fellow:** Sports Medicine, Hosp for Special Surgery 1980

Otolaryngology

Castellano, Bartolomeo MD (Oto) - **Hospital:** Mount Sinai Med Ctr (page 102); **Address:** 78 Todt Hill Rd, Ste 204, Staten Island, NY 10314-4528; **Phone:** 718-273-2626; **Board Cert:** Otolaryngology 1985; **Med School:** Mexico 1979; **Resid:** Otolaryngology, NYU Med Ctr 1984; **Fellow:** Facial Plastic Surgery, Mt Sinai Med Ctr 1985; **Fac Appt:** Asst Prof Oto, NYU Sch Med

Sinnreich, Abraham MD (Oto) - **Spec Exp:** Sinus Disorders; Sleep Disorders/Apnea; **Hospital:** SUNY Downstate Med Ctr (Univ Hosp of Bklyn) - LICH (page 420), Mount Sinai Med Ctr (page 102); **Address:** 1887 Richmond Ave, Ste 5, Staten Island, NY 10314; **Phone:** 718-370-0072; **Board Cert:** Otolaryngology 1984; **Med School:** Albert Einstein Coll Med 1979; **Resid:** Otolaryngology, Mount Sinai Hosp 1983; **Fac Appt:** Asst Clin Prof Oto, SUNY Downstate

Pain Medicine

Diwan, Sudhir MD (PM) - **Spec Exp:** Pain-after Spinal Intervention; Pain-Musculoskeletal; Pain-Neuropathic; Pain-Cancer; **Hospital:** Staten Island Univ Hosp - North (page 106); **Address:** Spine & Pain Inst of New York, 1534 Victory Blvd, Staten Island, NY 10314; **Phone:** 718-667-3577; **Board Cert:** Anesthesiology 2012; Pain Medicine 2002; **Med School:** India 1983; **Resid:** Surgery, St Luke's-Roosevelt Hosp Ctr 1994; Anesthesiology, St Luke's-Roosevelt Hosp Ctr 1997; **Fellow:** Pain Medicine, NY Presby Hosp 1998

Stilwell, Anne Marie MD (PM) - **Spec Exp:** Pain-Spine; Pain-after Spinal Intervention; **Hospital:** Richmond Univ Med Ctr; **Address:** 45 McLean Ave, Staten Island, NY 10305; **Phone:** 718-448-6373; **Board Cert:** Anesthesiology 2009; Pain Medicine 2007; **Med School:** Univ Rochester 1990; **Resid:** Anesthesiology, NY Hosp-Cornell Med Ctr 1994; **Fellow:** Pain Management, NY Hosp-Cornell Med Ctr 1996

Pediatric Endocrinology

Torrado-Jule, Carmen MD (PEn) - **Spec Exp:** Diabetes; Thyroid Disorders; Growth Disorders; Obesity; **Hospital:** Staten Island Univ Hosp - North (page 106), N Shore Univ Hosp (page 106); **Address:** 584 Forest Ave, Staten Island, NY 10310-2512; **Phone:** 718-226-5619; **Board Cert:** Pediatrics 2008; Pediatric Endocrinology 2005; **Med School:** Dominican Republic 1983; **Resid:** Pediatrics, Kings County Hosp 1987; **Fellow:** Pediatric Endocrinology, Kings County Hosp 1990; **Fac Appt:** Asst Prof Ped, SUNY Hlth Sci Ctr

Pediatrics

Bastawros, Mary N MD (Ped) *PCP* - **Hospital:** Richmond Univ Med Ctr, Staten Island Univ Hosp - North (page 106); **Address:** 314 Seaview Ave, Staten Island, NY 10305; **Phone:** 718-668-3417; **Board Cert:** Pediatrics 1985; **Med School:** Egypt 1966; **Resid:** Pediatrics, Methodist Hosp 1974

Duchnowska, Alicja B MD (Ped) *PCP* - **Hospital:** Staten Island Univ Hosp - North (page 106); **Address:** 934 Ionia Ave, Staten Island, NY 10309-2308; **Phone:** 718-984-5255; **Board Cert:** Pediatrics 1985; **Med School:** Poland 1965; **Resid:** Pediatrics, Natl Inst of Mother & Child 1970; Pediatrics, Staten Island Hosp 1982; **Fellow:** Pediatrics, Staten Island Hosp 1984

Short, Joan MD (Ped) *PCP* - **Hospital:** Richmond Univ Med Ctr, Staten Island Univ Hosp - North (page 106); **Address:** 32 2nd St, Staten Island, NY 10306; **Phone:** 718-979-7472; **Board Cert:** Pediatrics 1982; **Med School:** Univ Tenn Coll Med 1966; **Resid:** Pediatrics, City of Memphis Hosp; **Fellow:** Pediatric Oncology, St Jude Chldns Hosp

Visconti, Ernest MD (Ped) *PCP* - **Spec Exp:** Infectious Disease; **Hospital:** Lutheran Med Ctr - Brooklyn, Richmond Univ Med Ctr; **Address:** 314 Seaview Ave, Staten Island, NY 10305-2246; **Phone:** 718-668-3417; **Board Cert:** Pediatrics 1992; Pediatric Infectious Disease 2009; **Med School:** SUNY Upstate Med Univ 1971; **Resid:** Pediatrics, New York Hosp 1974; **Fellow:** Infectious Disease, Rhode Island Hosp 1978

Physical Medicine & Rehabilitation

Weinberg, Jeffrey B MD (PMR) - **Spec Exp:** Geriatric Rehabilitation; Musculoskeletal Injuries; **Hospital:** Staten Island Univ Hosp - North (page 106); **Address:** Staten Island Univ Hosp, Dept Rehab Med, 475 Seaview Ave, Staten Island, NY 10305; **Phone:** 718-226-6362; **Board Cert:** Physical Medicine & Rehabilitation 1985; **Med School:** NY Med Coll 1980; **Resid:** Physical Medicine & Rehabilitation, NYU Med Ctr 1983; **Fellow:** Geriatric Medicine, NYU Med Ctr 1986; **Fac Appt:** Asst Clin Prof PMR, SUNY Downstate

Weiner, Kevin H MD (PMR) - ; **Address:** 262 Nelson Ave, Staten Island, NY 10308; **Phone:** 718-442-4422; **Board Cert:** Physical Medicine & Rehabilitation 2009; **Med School:** Ros Franklin Univ/Chicago Med Sch 1994; **Resid:** Physical Medicine & Rehabilitation, NYU Med Ctr 1998

Plastic Surgery

Cherofsky, Alan MD (PlS) - **Spec Exp:** Breast Surgery; Pediatric Plastic Surgery; Cosmetic Surgery-Body; **Hospital:** Staten Island Univ Hosp - South (page 106), Richmond Univ Med Ctr; **Address:** 4546 Hylan Blvd, Staten Island, NY 10312-6400; **Phone:** 718-967-3300; **Board Cert:** Plastic Surgery 1993; **Med School:** SUNY Hlth Sci Ctr 1982; **Resid:** Surgery, Staten Island Univ Hosp 1987; Plastic Surgery, Univ Missouri Hosp 1989

Cutolo Jr, Louis C MD (PlS) - **Spec Exp:** Breast Augmentation; Liposuction; Eyelid Surgery; Cosmetic Surgery-Face & Neck; **Hospital:** Staten Island Univ Hosp - North (page 106), SUNY Downstate Med Ctr (Univ Hosp of Bklyn) - LICH (page 420); **Address:** 1557 Victory Blvd, Staten Island, NY 10314; **Phone:** 718-720-9400; **Board Cert:** Plastic Surgery 2003; **Med School:** SUNY Downstate 1985; **Resid:** Surgery, Staten Island Hosp 1990; **Fellow:** Plastic Surgery, Univ Florida/Shands Hosp 1992

Psychiatry

Di Buono, Mark MD (Psyc) - **Spec Exp:** Geriatric Psychiatry; Depression; Autism; **Address:** Richmond Behavioral Assocs, 4349 Hylan Blvd, Staten Island, NY 10312; **Phone:** 718-227-1897; **Board Cert:** Psychiatry 1990; Geriatric Psychiatry 2008; **Med School:** Mexico 1981; **Resid:** Psychiatry, Stony Brook Univ Hosp 1986; **Fac Appt:** Asst Clin Prof Psyc, SUNY Downstate

Pulmonary Disease

Castellano, Michael A MD (Pul) - **Spec Exp:** Asthma; Emphysema; **Hospital:** Staten Island Univ Hosp - North (page 106); **Address:** 501 Seaview Ave, Ste 102, Staten Island, NY 10305; **Phone:** 718-980-5700; **Board Cert:** Internal Medicine 1974; Pulmonary Disease 1978; Critical Care Medicine 2007; Geriatric Medicine 2004; **Med School:** Italy 1968; **Resid:** Internal Medicine, Staten Island Hosp 1972; **Fellow:** Pulmonary Disease, NYU-Bellvue Hosp 1974; **Fac Appt:** Asst Prof Med, SUNY Downstate

Maniatis, Theodore MD (Pul) - **Spec Exp:** Asthma; Lung Cancer; Chronic Obstructive Lung Disease (COPD); Interstitial Lung Disease; **Hospital:** Staten Island Univ Hosp - North (page 106), Staten Island Univ Hosp - South (page 106); **Address:** 501 Seaview Ave, Ste 102, Staten Island, NY 10305; **Phone:** 718-980-5700; **Board Cert:** Internal Medicine 1983; Pulmonary Disease 1986; Critical Care Medicine 2007; **Med School:** SUNY Hlth Sci Ctr 1980; **Resid:** Internal Medicine, Staten Island Univ Hosp 1983; **Fellow:** Pulmonary Disease, UMDNJ Med Ctr 1985; **Fac Appt:** Asst Clin Prof Med, SUNY Downstate

Martins, Publius MD (Pul) - **Spec Exp:** Asthma; Emphysema; **Hospital:** Richmond Univ Med Ctr; **Address:** 283 Bard Ave, Staten Island, NY 10310-1664; **Phone:** 718-816-8068; **Board Cert:** Internal Medicine 1984; **Med School:** Portugal 1975; **Resid:** Internal Medicine, St Vincent's Hosp 1981; **Fellow:** Pulmonary Disease, Meml Hosp 1983; **Fac Appt:** Assoc Clin Prof Med, NY Med Coll

Sasso, Louis MD (Pul) - **Spec Exp:** Asthma; Chronic Obstructive Lung Disease (COPD); Interstitial Lung Disease; **Hospital:** Staten Island Univ Hosp - North (page 106); **Address:** 501 Seaview Ave, Staten Island, NY 10305-3400; **Phone:** 718-980-5700; **Board Cert:** Internal Medicine 1976; Pulmonary Disease 1978; Critical Care Medicine 2005; Geriatric Medicine 2009; **Med School:** UMDNJ-NJ Med Sch, Newark 1972; **Resid:** Internal Medicine, St Vincent's Hosp & Med Ctr 1974; Internal Medicine, CMDNJ-Martland Hosp 1975; **Fellow:** Pulmonary Disease, Bellevue Hosp/NYU Med Ctr 1977; **Fac Appt:** Asst Clin Prof Med, SUNY Downstate

Radiation Oncology

Adams, Marc MD (RadRO) - **Spec Exp:** Prostate Cancer; Breast Cancer; Lung Cancer; Brain Tumors; **Hospital:** Richmond Univ Med Ctr; **Address:** 360 Bard Ave, Staten Island, NY 10310; **Phone:** 718-876-2023; **Board Cert:** Radiation Oncology 1990; **Med School:** Univ Alabama 1985; **Resid:** Radiation Oncology, St Barnabas Hosp 1989; **Fac Appt:** Asst Prof RadRO, NY Med Coll

Rheumatology

Goldstein, Mark A MD (Rhu) - **Spec Exp:** Rheumatoid Arthritis; Osteoporosis; Lupus/SLE; **Hospital:** Staten Island Univ Hosp - South (page 106), Richmond Univ Med Ctr; **Address:** 1534 Victory Blvd, Staten Island, NY 10314; **Phone:** 718-447-0055; **Board Cert:** Internal Medicine 1982; Rheumatology 1988; **Med School:** NY Med Coll 1979; **Resid:** Internal Medicine, Montefiore Med Ctr 1980; Internal Medicine, Montefiore Med Ctr 1982; **Fellow:** Critical Care Medicine, Montefiore Med Ctr 1983; Rheumatology, Montefiore Med Ctr 1987

Jarrett, Mark MD (Rhu) - **Spec Exp:** Lupus/SLE; Osteoporosis; Rheumatoid Arthritis; **Hospital:** Staten Island Univ Hosp - North (page 106); **Address:** 145 Community Drive, Great Neck, NY 11021; **Phone:** 516-465-3214; **Board Cert:** Internal Medicine 1978; Rheumatology 1980; Geriatric Medicine 2008; **Med School:** NYU Sch Med 1975; **Resid:** Internal Medicine, Montefiore Med Ctr 1978; **Fellow:** Rheumatology, Montefiore Med Ctr 1980; **Fac Appt:** Asst Clin Prof Med, SUNY Downstate

Surgery

D'Anna, John MD (S) - **Spec Exp:** Vascular Surgery; **Hospital:** Staten Island Univ Hosp - North (page 106), Staten Island Univ Hosp - South (page 106); **Address:** 375 Seguine Ave, Staten Island, NY 10305; **Phone:** 718-226-2950; **Board Cert:** Surgery 2011; **Med School:** Georgetown Univ 1977; **Resid:** Surgery, St Vincent's Hosp Med Ctr 1982; **Fellow:** Vascular Surgery, St Vincent's Hosp Med Ctr 1983; **Fac Appt:** Assoc Clin Prof S, SUNY Downstate

Hornyak, Stephen W MD (S) - **Spec Exp:** Breast Surgery; Laparoscopic Surgery; Gastrointestinal Surgery; **Hospital:** Staten Island Univ Hosp - North (page 106), Richmond Univ Med Ctr; **Address:** 1130 Victory Blvd, Staten Island, NY 10301; **Phone:** 718-442-3400; **Board Cert:** Surgery 2010; **Med School:** SUNY Hlth Sci Ctr 1974; **Resid:** Surgery, Kings County Hosp 1979; **Fellow:** Research, Meml Sloan Kettering Cancer Ctr 1980; **Fac Appt:** Asst Clin Prof S, SUNY Downstate

Pahuja, Murlidhar MD (S) - **Spec Exp:** Breast Cancer; Laparoscopic Surgery; Wound Healing/Care; **Hospital:** Staten Island Univ Hosp - North (page 106), Staten Island Univ Hosp - South (page 106); **Address:** 4287 Richmond Ave, Staten Island, NY 10312; **Phone:** 718-967-6230; **Board Cert:** Surgery 2004; **Med School:** Pakistan 1971; **Resid:** Surgery, Stamford Hosp 1978; Surgery, Staten Island Hosp 1982; **Fellow:** Burn Surgery, NY Hosp 1980

Thoracic & Cardiac Surgery

McGinn Jr, Joseph MD (T&CS) - **Spec Exp:** Cardiothoracic Surgery; **Hospital:** Staten Island Univ Hosp - North (page 106), Richmond Univ Med Ctr; **Address:** 501 Seaview Ave, Ste 202, Staten Island, NY 10305; **Phone:** 718-226-1612; **Board Cert:** Surgery 2009; Thoracic Surgery 2009; Surgical Critical Care 2003; **Med School:** SUNY Downstate 1981; **Resid:** Surgery, Downstate Med Ctr 1985; Thoracic Surgery, LIJ Med Ctr 1987; **Fellow:** Cardiothoracic Surgery, LIJ Med Ctr 1988; **Fac Appt:** Asst Clin Prof S, SUNY Downstate

Rosell, Frank M MD (T&CS) - **Hospital:** Staten Island Univ Hosp - North (page 106); **Address:** 501 Seaview Ave, Ste 202, Staten Island, NY 10305; **Phone:** 718-226-1612; **Board Cert:** Surgery 2006; Thoracic Surgery 2010; **Med School:** NYU Sch Med 1992; **Resid:** Surgery, NY Med Coll 1997; **Fellow:** Thoracic Surgery, Long Island Jewish Med Ctr 2000

Urology

Lessing, Jeffrey MD (U) - **Spec Exp:** Prostate Disease; Impotence; Kidney Stones; Infertility-Male; **Hospital:** Staten Island Univ Hosp - North (page 106), Staten Island Univ Hosp - South (page 106); **Address:** 78 Todt Hill Rd, Ste 112, Staten Island, NY 10314; **Phone:** 718-448-3880; **Board Cert:** Urology 1982; **Med School:** NYU Sch Med 1975; **Resid:** Surgery, New York Univ Med Ctr 1977; Urology, Mount Sinai Hosp 1980

Raboy, Adley MD (U) - **Spec Exp:** Prostate Disease; Kidney Stones; Minimally Invasive Surgery; **Hospital:** Staten Island Univ Hosp - North (page 106), Staten Island Univ Hosp - South (page 106); **Address:** Staten Island Urological Assocs, 1460 Victory Blvd, Staten Island, NY 10301-3914; **Phone:** 718-273-8100; **Board Cert:** Urology 2012; **Med School:** SUNY Downstate 1984; **Resid:** Surgery, Staten Island Hosp 1986; **Fellow:** Urology, Univ Hosp 1990; **Fac Appt:** Asst Clin Prof U, SUNY Downstate

Savino, Michael MD (U) - **Spec Exp:** Robotic Surgery; Prostate Cancer; Kidney Stones; Laparoscopic Surgery; **Hospital:** Staten Island Univ Hosp - South (page 106), Maimonides Med Ctr (page 98); **Address:** 375 Seguine Ave Fl 1, Staten Island, NY 10309; **Phone:** 718-226-2950; **Board Cert:** Urology 2007; **Med School:** Mexico 1979; **Resid:** Surgery, Maimonides Med Ctr 1982; Urology, Maimonides Med Ctr 1985

Vascular Surgery

Deitch, Jonathan MD (VascS) - **Spec Exp:** Aneurysm-Aortic; Carotid Artery Surgery; Endovascular Surgery; **Hospital:** Staten Island Univ Hosp - North (page 106); **Address:** 256 Mason Ave B Bldg Fl 2, Staten Island, NY 10305; **Phone:** 718-226-6800; **Board Cert:** Vascular Surgery 2009; **Med School:** NY Med Coll 1991; **Resid:** Surgery, Montefiore Med Ctr 1996; **Fellow:** Vascular Surgery, Wake Forest Univ 1998; Endovascular Surgery, UMDNJ 1998

Rodino, William MD (VascS) - **Hospital:** New York Methodist Hosp (page 418); **Address:** 2025 Richmond Ave, Staten Island, NY 10314; **Phone:** 718-259-3436; **Board Cert:** Surgery 2006; Vascular Surgery 2007; **Med School:** SUNY Downstate 1990; **Resid:** Surgery, SUNY Hlth Sci Ctr 1995; **Fellow:** Vascular Surgery, SUNY Hlth Sci Ctr 1997

Nassau

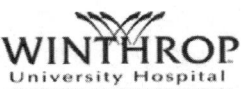

WINTHROP
University Hospital

Your Health Means Everything.™

259 First Street, Mineola, NY 11501
www.winthrop.org
For Physician Referral:
1-866-WINTHROP

Sponsorship: Voluntary, Not-for-Profit
Beds: 591
Accreditation: The Joint Commission

GENERAL OVERVIEW

Founded in 1896 by a group of local physicians and concerned citizens, Winthrop-University Hospital is Long Island's first voluntary and second largest hospital. The university-affiliated medical center and New York State-designated Regional Trauma Center offers sophisticated diagnostic and therapeutic care in virtually every specialty and subspecialty of medicine and surgery.

Winthrop has earned many prestigious accreditations, including designations as a New York State (NYS) Stroke Center and NYS Regional Perinatal Center, and is known across the State for its excellent outcomes in interventional cardiology and cardiac surgery. In addition to its leading cardiology and specialty care services such as Orthopaedics, Winthrop boasts several specialized Centers that are dedicated to Cancer Care, Digestive Disorders, Family Care including Women's and Children's Health Services, Lung Care and Neurosciences.

Patient care, academics and research are the three components of Winthrop's mission. Because research is so essential, Winthrop has initiated the creation of a new four-floor, 95,000-square-foot Diabetes and Obesity Research Institute which will house basic science research, clinical/translational research, outcomes research, medical education classrooms and support services.

STAFF

The Hospital employs 6,000 dedicated and caring individuals, including nearly 1,500 nurses. Winthrop's medical staff – which includes more than 1,300 full-time and voluntary attending physicians – cared for more than 37,000 inpatients, handled more than 68,000 emergency visits, and conducted more than 800,000 outpatient appointments in 2011.

ACADEMIC AND CLINICAL AFFILIATIONS

Winthrop is an affiliated member of the New York-Presbyterian Healthcare System and is the Regional Clinical Campus of Stony Brook University School of Medicine.

SPECIAL PROGRAMS AND SERVICES

Advances in Neuroscience:
At Winthrop's Department of Neuroscience, an interdisciplinary team of healthcare professionals are pioneering the use of advanced approaches for diagnosis and treatment, including computerized imaging systems, state-of-the-art surgical interventions such as deep brain stimulation and the latest generation of medication therapies. In addition to a 14-bed Neurosciences Special Care Unit, the Department boasts comprehensive resources for the diagnosis and treatment of a wide range of conditions, including aneurysms, blood clots and tumors and special programs for conditions including Multiple Sclerosis, Movement Disorders, and Epilepsy.

Innovative Prostate Cancer Treatment:
At Winthrop, prostate cancer patients are offered a full array of treatment options. Minimally invasive surgery using the daVinci Surgical Robot System is available, as well as intensity-modulated radiation therapy (IMRT), cryotherapy, and more. In addition, Winthrop pioneered the use of CyberKnife for prostate cancer – a technology that takes radiotherapy to new levels of accuracy. Winthrop is the second largest site in the world for treating prostate cancer with CyberKnife and is a designated CyberKnife training site.

Excellence in Women's Healthcare:
Winthrop is a nationally recognized, regional leader in women's health services. The experts at the Winthrop Breast Health Center – the only center in Nassau County to earn accreditation by the National Accreditation Program for Breast Centers (NAPBC) – provide comprehensive risk assessment, diagnosis, treatment and follow-up care to patients. Winthrop is also the only site in the tri-state area to earn accreditation by the American Institute of Ultrasound in Medicine (AIUM) for fetal echocardiograms. Winthrop was the only hospital in New York State to simultaneously receive the HealthGrades Maternity Care Excellence Award, the HealthGrades Gynecologic Surgery Excellence Award, and the HealthGrades Women's Health Excellence Award in 2011.

No Place Like Home:
Winthrop's award-winning certified home health care agency offers nursing, as well as physical, speech and occupational therapies in conjunction with medical social work and home health aide services to Nassau County residents. In 2011, our home health agency was named for the fifth consecutive year to the HomeCare Elite™ – a compilation of the top-performing home health agencies in the United States, attesting to the impressive care provided by our home care professionals.

SELECT NATIONAL PERFORMANCE RECOGNITIONS

Healthgrades® Distinguished Hospital for Clinical Excellence™, 2009-2012

Healthgrades® America's 100 Best Hospitals for Cardiac Care™, 2010-2012

2012-13 Best Regional Hospitals in the New York Metro Area - *U.S. News & World Report* with 11 high-performing specialties

2012-13 Best Children's Hospitals - *U.S. News & World Report* for excellence in pediatric diabetes & endocrinology and pediatric urology

"100 Hospitals with Great Women's Health Programs" - *Becker's Hospital Review*

"Most Wired" Hospital by *Hospitals & Health Networks* Magazine

NAEC Level 4 Epilepsy Center

HCM Center of Excellence by The National Hypertrophic Cardiomyopathy Association

NAPBC National Breast Center

New York State Designated Regional Trauma Center

New York State Regional Perinatal Center

New York State Stroke Center

The Joint Commission: *Accreditation – Hospital, Certified Home Health Agency*

WINTHROP'S mission is founded upon the basic core value of "**YOUR HEALTH MEANS EVERYTHING**" and all of its employees are committed to ensuring the integrity, comfort and well-being of every individual.

Adolescent Medicine

Arden, Martha MD (AM) - **Spec Exp:** Adolescent Gynecology; Nutrition; Eating Disorders; **Hospital:** Steven & Alexandra Cohen Chldn's Med Ctr of NY (page 106), N Shore Univ Hosp (page 106); **Address:** 2001 Marcus Ave, Ste N204, New Hyde Park, NY 11040; **Phone:** 347-882-1321; **Board Cert:** Pediatrics 2010; Adolescent Medicine 2009; **Med School:** Yale Univ 1984; **Resid:** Pediatrics, Babies Hosp 1987; **Fellow:** Adolescent Medicine, Schneider Chldn's Hosp 1990; **Fac Appt:** Assoc Clin Prof Ped, Albert Einstein Coll Med

Fisher, Martin M MD (AM) - **Spec Exp:** Eating Disorders; Chronic Fatigue Syndrome; **Hospital:** Steven & Alexandra Cohen Chldn's Med Ctr of NY (page 106), N Shore Univ Hosp (page 106); **Address:** 410 Lakeville Rd, Ste 108, New Hyde Park, NY 11040; **Phone:** 516-465-3270; **Board Cert:** Pediatrics 1979; Adolescent Medicine 2009; **Med School:** Albert Einstein Coll Med 1975; **Resid:** Pediatrics, LIJ Med Ctr 1978; **Fellow:** Adolescent Medicine, LIJ Med Ctr 1980; **Fac Appt:** Prof Ped, NYU Sch Med

Jacobson, Marc S MD (AM) - **Spec Exp:** Cholesterol/Lipid Disorders; Obesity; Preventive Cardiology; **Hospital:** NS-LIJ Hlth Sys (page 106); **Address:** 3 ProHealth Plaza, Ste 200, Lake Success, NY 11042; **Phone:** 516-304-3950; **Board Cert:** Pediatrics 1983; Adolescent Medicine 2009; **Med School:** Univ Kansas 1973; **Resid:** Pediatrics, Univ Kansas Med Ctr 1976; **Fellow:** Adolescent Medicine, Univ Maryland Hosp 1979; **Fac Appt:** Prof Ped, Albert Einstein Coll Med

Levin Carmine, Linda MD (AM) - **Spec Exp:** Eating Disorders; **Hospital:** Steven & Alexandra Cohen Chldn's Med Ctr of NY (page 106); **Address:** Division of Adolescent Medicine, 410 Lakeville Rd, Ste 108, New Hyde Park, NY 11042; **Phone:** 516-465-3270; **Board Cert:** Pediatrics 1987; Adolescent Medicine 2009; **Med School:** NYU Sch Med 1982; **Resid:** Pediatrics, Montefiore Med Ctr 1985; **Fellow:** Adolescent Medicine, Montefiore Med Ctr 1986; **Fac Appt:** Assoc Prof Ped, Hofstra N Shore-LIJ Sch Med

Swedler, Jane MD (AM) - **Spec Exp:** Adolescent Gynecology; **Hospital:** Winthrop Univ Hosp (page 504); **Address:** 222 Station Plaza N, Ste 611, Mineola, NY 11501; **Phone:** 516-663-2532; **Board Cert:** Family Medicine 2009; Adolescent Medicine 2011; **Med School:** McGill Univ 1987; **Resid:** Family Medicine, Queen Elizabeth Hosp. 1989; Family Medicine, SUNY Stonybrook 1990; **Fellow:** Adolescent Medicine, Montefiore Med Ctr 1992; **Fac Appt:** Asst Prof Med, Mount Sinai Sch Med

Allergy & Immunology

Boxer, Mitchell MD (A&I) - **Spec Exp:** Asthma; Drug Sensitivity; Allergic Aspergillosis; Churg-Strauss Vasculitis; **Hospital:** Long Island Jewish Med Ctr (page 106); **Address:** 2001 Marcus Ave, Ste N220, Lake Success, NY 11042; **Phone:** 516-482-0910; **Board Cert:** Internal Medicine 1984; Allergy & Immunology 1987; **Med School:** NY Med Coll 1981; **Resid:** Internal Medicine, LI Jewish Med Ctr 1984; **Fellow:** Allergy & Immunology, Northwestern Meml Med Ctr 1987; **Fac Appt:** Asst Clin Prof Med, Albert Einstein Coll Med

Corriel, Robert N MD (A&I) - **Spec Exp:** Asthma & Allergy; Sinus Disorders; Rhinitis; Food Allergy; **Hospital:** N Shore Univ Hosp (page 106), Long Island Jewish Med Ctr (page 106); **Address:** 1129 Northern Blvd, Ste 300, Manhasset, NY 11030-3527; **Phone:** 516-365-6077; **Board Cert:** Pediatrics 1983; Allergy & Immunology 1985; **Med School:** Wake Forest Univ 1976; **Resid:** Pediatrics, N Shore Univ Hosp 1979; **Fellow:** Allergy & Immunology, Univ Tex Hlth Sci Ctr 1981; **Fac Appt:** Asst Clin Prof Ped, Hofstra N Shore-LIJ Sch Med

Edwards, Bruce L MD (A&I) - **Spec Exp:** Asthma; Sinus Disorders; Food Allergy; **Hospital:** Long Island Jewish Med Ctr (page 106), Plainview Hosp (page 106); **Address:** 700 Old Country Rd, Ste 105, Plainview, NY 11803-4932; **Phone:** 516-933-1125; **Board Cert:** Allergy & Immunology 2009; **Med School:** Case West Res Univ 1984; **Resid:** Pediatrics, Babies Hosp/Columbia Presby 1987; **Fellow:** Allergy & Immunology, Schneider Chldns Hosp-LIJ 1989

Fonacier, Luz MD (A&I) - **Spec Exp:** Skin Allergies; Drug Sensitivity; Asthma & Allergy; **Hospital:** Winthrop Univ Hosp (page 504); **Address:** 120 Mineola Blvd, Ste 410, Mineola, NY 11501; **Phone:** 516-663-2097; **Board Cert:** Internal Medicine 1989; Allergy & Immunology 2011; **Med School:** Philippines 1978; **Resid:** Dermatology, Univ Philippines 1983; Internal Medicine, Lutheran Med Ctr 1989; **Fellow:** Dermatology, NYU Med Ctr 1986; Allergy & Immunology, NY Hosp-Cornell Med Ctr 1991; **Fac Appt:** Clin Prof A&I, SUNY Stony Brook

Frieri, Marianne MD/PhD (A&I) - **Spec Exp:** Asthma; Food Allergy; Immune Deficiency; Rhinitis; **Hospital:** N Shore Univ Hosp (page 106), Nassau Univ Med Ctr; **Address:** 566 Broadway, Massapequa, NY 11758; **Phone:** 516-541-6262; **Board Cert:** Internal Medicine 1984; Allergy & Immunology 1985; Clinical & Laboratory Immunology 1990; **Med School:** Loyola Univ-Stritch Sch Med 1978; **Resid:** Internal Medicine, St Josephs Hosp 1980; **Fellow:** Allergy & Immunology, NIH/NIAID 1983; **Fac Appt:** Prof Med, SUNY Stony Brook

Goldstein, Stanley MD (A&I) - **Spec Exp:** Asthma; Pulmonary Disease; **Hospital:** Long Island Jewish Med Ctr (page 106), Mercy Med Ctr - Rockville Centre; **Address:** 242 Merrick Rd, Ste 401, Rockville Centre, NY 11570; **Phone:** 516-536-7336; **Board Cert:** Pediatrics 1979; Allergy & Immunology 1981; Pediatric Pulmonology 2011; **Med School:** NY Med Coll 1975; **Resid:** Pediatrics, LI Jewish Med Ctr 1978; **Fellow:** Allergy & Immunology, Chldns Hosp 1982

Lang, Paul MD (A&I) - **Spec Exp:** Asthma; Food Allergy; Insect Allergies; **Hospital:** N Shore Univ Hosp (page 106), Winthrop Univ Hosp (page 504); **Address:** One Hollow Ln, Ste 110, New Hyde Park, NY 11042; **Phone:** 516-365-6666; **Board Cert:** Pediatrics 1978; Allergy & Immunology 1979; **Med School:** Cornell Univ-Weill Med Coll 1973; **Resid:** Pediatrics, USC Med Ctr 1975; Allergy & Immunology, Roosevelt Hosp 1977; **Fac Appt:** Assoc Clin Prof Ped, NYU Sch Med

Markovics, Sharon B MD (A&I) - **Spec Exp:** Allergy; Asthma; Rhinitis; Sinus Disorders; **Hospital:** N Shore Univ Hosp (page 106), Long Island Jewish Med Ctr (page 106); **Address:** 1129 Northern Blvd, Ste 300, Manhasset, NY 11030-3527; **Phone:** 516-365-6077; **Board Cert:** Pediatrics 1979; Allergy & Immunology 1981; **Med School:** Albert Einstein Coll Med 1975; **Resid:** Pediatrics, Bellevue Hosp 1977; **Fellow:** Allergy & Immunology, Montreal Chldns Hosp 1979; **Fac Appt:** Asst Clin Prof Ped, NYU Sch Med

Novick, Brian MD (A&I) - **Spec Exp:** Asthma-Adult & Pediatric; Sinus Disorders; Food Allergy; Hives; **Hospital:** Montefiore Med Ctr-Moses Campus, NY (page 100), Lenox Hill Hosp (page 106); **Address:** 30 Newbridge Rd, Ste 101, East Meadow, NY 11554; **Phone:** 516-731-5740; **Board Cert:** Pediatrics 1984; Allergy & Immunology 2012; **Med School:** Mexico 1978; **Resid:** Pediatrics, Albert Einstein Coll Med 1982; **Fellow:** Allergy & Immunology, Albert Einstein Coll Med 1984; **Fac Appt:** Asst Clin Prof A&I, Albert Einstein Coll Med

Sicklick, Marc MD (A&I) - **Spec Exp:** Asthma; Allergy; Immune Deficiency; **Hospital:** N Shore Univ Hosp (page 106), Long Island Jewish Med Ctr (page 106); **Address:** 123 Grove Ave, Ste 110, Cedarhurst, NY 11516-2302; **Phone:** 516-569-5550; **Board Cert:** Pediatrics 1979; Allergy & Immunology 1987; **Med School:** Albert Einstein Coll Med 1974; **Resid:** Pediatrics, Bronx Muni Hosp Ctr 1977; **Fellow:** Allergy & Immunology, Montefiore Med Ctr 1979; **Fac Appt:** Assoc Clin Prof Ped, Albert Einstein Coll Med

Weinstock, Gary A MD (A&I) - **Spec Exp:** Asthma; Allergy; Hives; **Hospital:** N Shore Univ Hosp (page 106), Glen Cove Hosp (page 106); **Address:** 310 E Shore Rd, Ste 207, Great Neck, NY 11023-2432; **Phone:** 516-487-1073; **Board Cert:** Internal Medicine 1982; Pulmonary Disease 1984; Allergy & Immunology 1985; **Med School:** Albany Med Coll 1979; **Resid:** Internal Medicine, North Shore Univ/Meml Sloan Kettering Cancer Ctr 1982; **Fellow:** Pulmonary Disease, SUNY-Stony Brook 1983; Allergy & Immunology, SUNY-Stony Brook 1986; **Fac Appt:** Asst Clin Prof Med, NYU Sch Med

Wertheim, David MD (A&I) - **Spec Exp:** Pediatric Allergy & Immunology; **Hospital:** NS-LIJ Hlth Sys (page 106), St. Francis Hosp - The Heart Ctr (page 121); **Address:** 2800 Marcus Ave, Ste 202, Lake Success, NY 11042; **Phone:** 516-608-2898; **Board Cert:** Allergy & Immunology 2006; **Med School:** Med Coll PA 1988; **Resid:** Pediatrics, Schneider Chldns Hosp 1992; **Fellow:** Allergy & Immunology, Long Island Jewish Med Ctr 1994; **Fac Appt:** Asst Clin Prof Ped, Albert Einstein Coll Med

Cardiac Electrophysiology

Jadonath, Ram L MD (CE) - **Spec Exp:** Arrhythmias; Atrial Fibrillation; Pacemakers; Defibrillators; **Hospital:** N Shore Univ Hosp (page 106); **Address:** 300 Community Drive, Manhasset, NY 11030; **Phone:** 516-562-2300; **Board Cert:** Internal Medicine 1989; Cardiovascular Disease 2006; Cardiac Electrophysiology 2006; **Med School:** Columbia P&S 1986; **Resid:** Internal Medicine, St Lukes Hosp 1989; **Fellow:** Cardiovascular Disease, St Lukes/Roosevelt Hosps 1992; Cardiac Electrophysiology, /Philadelphia Heart Inst 1993; **Fac Appt:** Assoc Prof Med, Albert Einstein Coll Med

Levine, Joseph H MD (CE) - **Spec Exp:** Arrhythmias; Sudden Death Prevention; Atrial Fibrillation; Pacemakers; **Hospital:** St. Francis Hosp - The Heart Ctr (page 121); **Address:** 100 Port Washington Blvd, Roslyn, NY 11576; **Phone:** 516-622-1011; **Board Cert:** Internal Medicine 1983; Cardiovascular Disease 1987; Cardiac Electrophysiology 2003; **Med School:** Univ Rochester 1980; **Resid:** Internal Medicine, Yale-New Haven Hosp 1983; **Fellow:** Cardiovascular Disease, Johns Hopkins Hosp 1986; Cardiac Electrophysiology, Hosp Univ Penn 1986

Cardiovascular Disease

Anto, Maliakal Joseph MD (Cv) - **Spec Exp:** Hypertension; Coronary Artery Disease; Non-Invasive Cardiology; Congestive Heart Failure; **Hospital:** Syosset Hosp (page 106), Plainview Hosp (page 106); **Address:** 8 Greenfield Rd, Syosset, NY 11791; **Phone:** 516-496-7900; **Board Cert:** Internal Medicine 1980; Cardiovascular Disease 1989; **Med School:** India 1974; **Resid:** Internal Medicine, Our Lady of Mercy Med Ctr 1979; **Fellow:** Cardiovascular Disease, Nassau County Med Ctr 1981

Bhansali, Rohan Dilip MD (Cv) *PCP* - **Spec Exp:** Echocardiography; Nuclear Cardiology; Nuclear Stress Testing; **Hospital:** Long Island Jewish Med Ctr (page 106); **Address:** 27-05 76th Ave Fl 4, Oncology Building, New Hyde Park, NY 11040; **Phone:** 718-470-7330; **Board Cert:** Internal Medicine 2011; Cardiovascular Disease 2001; **Med School:** SUNY Upstate Med Univ 1998; **Resid:** Internal Medicine, Long Island Jewish Med Ctr 2001; **Fellow:** Cardiovascular Disease, Long Island Jewish Med Ctr 2004

Breen, William John MD (Cv) - **Spec Exp:** Echocardiography; **Hospital:** Plainview Hosp (page 106); **Address:** 43 Crossways Park Drive, Woodbury, NY 11797; **Phone:** 516-938-3000; **Board Cert:** Internal Medicine 1980; Cardiovascular Disease 1983; **Med School:** NY Med Coll 1977; **Resid:** Internal Medicine, North Shore Univ Hosp 1980; **Fellow:** Cardiovascular Disease, North Shore Univ Hosp 1982; **Fac Appt:** Assoc Prof Med, NYU Sch Med

Chadda, Kul MD (Cv) - **Hospital:** South Nassau Comm Hosp, Wyckoff Heights Med Ctr; **Address:** South Nassau Comm Hosp, Electrophysiology Svcs, 1 Healthy Way, Oceanside, NY 11572; **Phone:** 516-632-3418; **Board Cert:** Internal Medicine 1974; Cardiovascular Disease 1977; **Med School:** India 1966; **Resid:** Internal Medicine, Elmhurst City Hosp 1972; Cardiovascular Disease, Prebyterian Hosp 1973; **Fac Appt:** Clin Prof Med, SUNY Stony Brook

Chen, Timothy T MD (Cv) - **Spec Exp:** Congestive Heart Failure; Cardiovascular Disease/Young Adult; Pacemakers; **Hospital:** South Nassau Comm Hosp, N Shore Univ Hosp (page 106); **Address:** South Shore Heart Assocs, 242 Merrick Rd, Ste 402, Rockville Center, NY 11570; **Phone:** 516-763-2800; **Board Cert:** Cardiovascular Disease 2004; Echocardiography 2004; Nuclear Cardiology 2004; **Med School:** Columbia P&S 1998; **Resid:** Internal Medicine, Montefiore Med Ctr. 2001; **Fellow:** Cardiovascular Disease, Montefiore Med Ctr. 2004

Chesner, Michael D MD (Cv) - **Spec Exp:** Preventive Cardiology; Cholesterol/Lipid Disorders; Cardiac Stress Testing; **Hospital:** Long Beach Med Ctr; **Address:** 325 W Park Ave, Long Beach, NY 11561-3223; **Phone:** 516-432-2004; **Board Cert:** Internal Medicine 2004; Cardiovascular Disease 2007; **Med School:** Albert Einstein Coll Med 1987; **Resid:** Internal Medicine, Bronx Municipal Hosp 1990; **Fellow:** Cardiovascular Disease, LI Jewish Hosp 1993; **Fac Appt:** Assoc Prof Med, NY Coll Osteo Med

Cramer, Marvin MD (Cv) - **Spec Exp:** Coronary Artery Disease; Echocardiography; Stress Echocardiography; **Hospital:** N Shore Univ Hosp (page 106), St. Francis Hosp - The Heart Ctr (page 121); **Address:** 225 Community Drive, Ste 130, Great Neck, NY 11021; **Phone:** 516-504-0474; **Board Cert:** Internal Medicine 1974; Cardiovascular Disease 1977; Nuclear Cardiology 2005; Echocardiography 2007; **Med School:** Jefferson Med Coll 1969; **Resid:** Internal Medicine, St Lukes Med Ctr 1973; **Fellow:** Cardiovascular Disease, Columbia-Presby Med Ctr 1976; **Fac Appt:** Assoc Clin Prof Med, NYU Sch Med

D'Agostino, Ronald DO (Cv) - **Spec Exp:** Hypertension; Cholesterol/Lipid Disorders; Mitral Valve Disease; **Hospital:** Long Island Jewish Med Ctr (page 106), N Shore Univ Hosp (page 106); **Address:** 1129 Northern Blvd, Ste 408, Manhasset, NY 11030-3022; **Phone:** 516-627-2121; **Board Cert:** Internal Medicine 2000; Cardiovascular Disease 2011; **Med School:** NY Coll Osteo Med 1985; **Resid:** Internal Medicine, Long Island Jewish Hosp 1989; Internal Medicine, Long Island Jewish Hosp 1993; **Fellow:** Cardiovascular Disease, Long Island Jewish Hosp 1992; **Fac Appt:** Asst Prof Med, NY Coll Osteo Med

Dresdale, Robert J MD (Cv) - **Spec Exp:** Heart Disease in Women; Pulmonary Hypertension; **Hospital:** N Shore Univ Hosp (page 106), St. Francis Hosp - The Heart Ctr (page 121); **Address:** 225 Community Drive, Ste 130, Great Neck, NY 11021-5506; **Phone:** 516-504-0474; **Board Cert:** Internal Medicine 1975; Cardiovascular Disease 1977; **Med School:** Columbia P&S 1972; **Resid:** Internal Medicine, Columbia-Presby Med Ctr 1974; **Fellow:** Cardiovascular Disease, Columbia-Presby Med Ctr 1976; **Fac Appt:** Assoc Clin Prof Med, NYU Sch Med

Ezratty, Ari M MD (Cv) - **Spec Exp:** Interventional Cardiology; **Hospital:** St. Francis Hosp - The Heart Ctr (page 121); **Address:** 100 Port Washington Blvd, Roslyn, NY 11576; **Phone:** 516-570-6907; **Board Cert:** Internal Medicine 1988; Cardiovascular Disease 2002; **Med School:** Mount Sinai Sch Med 1985; **Resid:** Internal Medicine, Mt Sinai Hosp 1989; **Fellow:** Cardiovascular Disease, Brigham & Womens Hosp 1992; Interventional Cardiology, Mt Sinai Hosp 1994; **Fac Appt:** Med, Mount Sinai Sch Med

Fein, Frederick S MD (Cv) - **Spec Exp:** Heart Disease; **Hospital:** Winthrop Univ Hosp (page 504); **Address:** 120 Mineola Blvd, Ste 500, Mineola, NY 11501; **Phone:** 516-663-4480; **Board Cert:** Internal Medicine 1975; Cardiovascular Disease 1977; **Med School:** NYU Sch Med 1972; **Resid:** Internal Medicine, Montefiore Hosp Med Ctr 1975; **Fellow:** Cardiovascular Disease, Montefiore Hosp Med Ctr 1977; **Fac Appt:** Assoc Prof Med, Albert Einstein Coll Med

Gindea, Aaron J MD (Cv) - **Spec Exp:** Heart Valve Disease; Congestive Heart Failure; Congenital Heart Disease; **Hospital:** N Shore Univ Hosp (page 106), St. Francis Hosp - The Heart Ctr (page 121); **Address:** 800 Community Drive, Manhasset, NY 11030-3803; **Phone:** 516-627-6622; **Board Cert:** Internal Medicine 1985; Cardiovascular Disease 1989; **Med School:** NYU Sch Med 1982; **Resid:** Internal Medicine, Bellevue Hosp 1985; **Fellow:** Cardiovascular Disease, Bellevue Hosp 1987; **Fac Appt:** Assoc Clin Prof Med, NYU Sch Med

Gleckel, Louis W MD (Cv) *PCP* - **Spec Exp:** Preventive Cardiology; Cardiac Stress Testing; Cholesterol/Lipid Disorders; Hypertension; **Hospital:** Long Island Jewish Med Ctr (page 106); **Address:** 2 Ohio Drive, Fl 2, Lake Success, NY 11042-1052; **Phone:** 516-622-6060; **Board Cert:** Internal Medicine 1986; **Med School:** SUNY Hlth Sci Ctr 1983; **Resid:** Internal Medicine, LI Jewish Hosp 1986; **Fellow:** Cardiovascular Disease, LI Jewish Hosp 1989; **Fac Appt:** Asst Clin Prof Med, SUNY Downstate

Goldberg, Steven Mark MD (Cv) - **Spec Exp:** Cholesterol/Lipid Disorders; Preventive Cardiology; **Hospital:** N Shore Univ Hosp (page 106); **Address:** 1010 Northern Blvd, Ste 110, Great Neck, NY 11021-5306; **Phone:** 516-390-2430; **Board Cert:** Internal Medicine 1982; Cardiovascular Disease 1985; **Med School:** Univ Pennsylvania 1979; **Resid:** Internal Medicine, N Shore Univ Hosp 1982; **Fellow:** Cardiovascular Disease, N Shore Univ Hosp 1984; **Fac Appt:** Assoc Prof Med, NYU Sch Med

Gomez, Henry Esteban MD (Cv) - **Spec Exp:** Echocardiography; Non-Invasive Cardiology; **Hospital:** N Shore Univ Hosp (page 106); **Address:** Long Island Cardiovascular, 1129 Northen Blvd, Ste 408, Manhasset, NY 11030; **Phone:** 516-627-2121; **Board Cert:** Internal Medicine 2004; Cardiovascular Disease 2008; **Med School:** Mount Sinai Sch Med 1990; **Resid:** Internal Medicine, Montefiore Med Ctr 1993; **Fellow:** Cardiovascular Disease, Long Island Jewish Med Ctr 1996

Goodman, Mark A MD (Cv) - **Spec Exp:** Cholesterol/Lipid Disorders; Pacemakers/Defibrillators; Coronary Artery Disease; Congestive Heart Failure; **Hospital:** Winthrop Univ Hosp (page 504), N Shore Univ Hosp (page 106); **Address:** 975 Stewart Ave, Garden City, NY 11530-4816; **Phone:** 516-222-8610; **Board Cert:** Internal Medicine 1972; Cardiovascular Disease 1973; **Med School:** SUNY Upstate Med Univ 1967; **Resid:** Internal Medicine, Montefiore Med Ctr 1969; Internal Medicine, Mt Sinai Hosp 1970; **Fellow:** Cardiovascular Disease, Montefiore Med Ctr 1972; **Fac Appt:** Assoc Clin Prof Med, SUNY Stony Brook

Green, Stephen J MD (Cv) - **Spec Exp:** Heart Attack; Angioplasty; Cholesterol/Lipid Disorders; Interventional Cardiology; **Hospital:** N Shore Univ Hosp (page 106), Long Island Jewish Med Ctr (page 106); **Address:** 300 Community Drive, Department of Cardiology, Manhasset, NY 11030; **Phone:** 516-562-4100; **Board Cert:** Internal Medicine 1983; Cardiovascular Disease 1985; Interventional Cardiology 2009; **Med School:** Tufts Univ 1980; **Resid:** Internal Medicine, N Shore Univ Hosp 1983; **Fellow:** Cardiovascular Disease, N Shore Univ Hosp 1985; **Fac Appt:** Assoc Prof Med, Hofstra N Shore-LIJ Sch Med

Greenberg, Steven M MD (Cv) - **Spec Exp:** Pacemakers/Defibrillators; Arrhythmias; Congestive Heart Failure; **Hospital:** St. Francis Hosp - The Heart Ctr (page 121); **Address:** Arrhythmia Center, 100 Port Washington Blvd, Roslyn, NY 11576-1353; **Phone:** 516-562-6672; **Board Cert:** Internal Medicine 1986; Cardiovascular Disease 1989; **Med School:** Albany Med Coll 1983; **Resid:** Internal Medicine, Bronx Muni Hosp Ctr 1987; **Fellow:** Cardiovascular Disease, Mt Sinai Med Ctr 1990

Hershman, Ronnie MD (Cv) - **Spec Exp:** Invasive Cardiology; **Hospital:** St. Francis Hosp - The Heart Ctr (page 121); **Address:** 1 Hollow Ln, Ste 103, Lake Success, NY 11042; **Phone:** 516-869-5400; **Board Cert:** Internal Medicine 1985; Cardiovascular Disease 1987; **Med School:** Mount Sinai Sch Med 1982; **Resid:** Internal Medicine, Mt Sinai Med Ctr 1985; **Fellow:** Cardiovascular Disease, Mt Sinai Med Ctr 1989

Jauhar, Rajiv MD (Cv) - **Spec Exp:** Angioplasty & Stent Placement; Cardiac Catheterization; Cardiac Imaging; **Hospital:** Long Island Jewish Med Ctr (page 106); **Address:** 270-05 76 Ave Fl 4, New Hyde Park, NY 11040; **Phone:** 718-470-7330; **Board Cert:** Internal Medicine 1994; Cardiovascular Disease 2009; Interventional Cardiology 2010; **Med School:** Univ Chicago-Pritzker Sch Med 1991; **Resid:** Internal Medicine, UCSD Med Ctr 1994; **Fellow:** Cardiovascular Disease, NY-Presby/Weill Cornell Med Ctr 1999

Jelveh, Mansoor MD (Cv) - **Hospital:** N Shore Univ Hosp (page 106), St. Joseph's Hosp-Nassau; **Address:** 875 Old Country Rd, Ste 102, Plainview, NY 11803; **Phone:** 516-935-8877; **Board Cert:** Internal Medicine 1975; Cardiovascular Disease 1977; **Med School:** Iran 1968; **Resid:** Internal Medicine, Nassau County Med Ctr 1975; **Fellow:** Cardiovascular Disease, Beth Israel 1977

Kaplan, Barry M MD (Cv) - **Spec Exp:** Interventional Cardiology; **Hospital:** Long Island Jewish Med Ctr (page 106); **Address:** LI Jewish Med Ctr/Div Cardiology, 270-05 76 Ave, New Hyde Park, NY 11040; **Phone:** 718-470-7330; **Board Cert:** Cardiovascular Disease 2005; Interventional Cardiology 1999; **Med School:** Israel 1987; **Resid:** Internal Medicine, NYU/VA Med Ctr 1991; **Fellow:** Cardiovascular Disease, Montefiore Med Ctr 1994; Interventional Cardiology, William Beaumont Hosp; **Fac Appt:** Asst Prof Med, NYU Sch Med

Kobren, Steven M MD (Cv) - **Spec Exp:** Heart Failure; Mitral Valve Prolapse; Nuclear Stress Testing; **Hospital:** NYU Langone Med Ctr (page 108), Long Island Jewish Med Ctr (page 106); **Address:** NYU Great Neck Medical, 488 Great Neck Rd, Great Neck, NY 11021-4308; **Phone:** 516-482-6747; **Board Cert:** Internal Medicine 1986; Cardiovascular Disease 1989; Critical Care Medicine 2001; Echocardiography 2007; **Med School:** SUNY Downstate 1983; **Resid:** Internal Medicine, LIJ Medical Ctr 1987; **Fellow:** Cardiovascular Disease, LIJ Medical Ctr 1990; **Fac Appt:** Asst Prof Med, Albert Einstein Coll Med

Koss, Jerome MD (Cv) - **Spec Exp:** Interventional Cardiology; Heart Valve Disease; Nuclear Cardiology; Atrial Fibrillation; **Hospital:** Long Island Jewish Med Ctr (page 106), St. Francis Hosp - The Heart Ctr (page 121); **Address:** 3003 New Hyde Park Rd, Ste 406, New Hyde Park, NY 11042; **Phone:** 516-358-5401; **Board Cert:** Internal Medicine 1977; Cardiovascular Disease 1981; Interventional Cardiology 2010; **Med School:** Albert Einstein Coll Med 1974; **Resid:** Internal Medicine, Jacobi Med Ctr 1978; **Fellow:** Cardiovascular Disease, Montefiore Med Ctr 1980; **Fac Appt:** Asst Prof Med, Albert Einstein Coll Med

Lachmann, Justine S MD (Cv) - **Spec Exp:** Heart Failure; Pulmonary Hypertension; **Hospital:** Winthrop Univ Hosp (page 504); **Address:** 120 Mineola Blvd, Ste 500, Mineola, NY 11501; **Phone:** 516-663-4481; **Board Cert:** Cardiovascular Disease 2001; **Med School:** UMDNJ-RW Johnson Med Sch 1995; **Resid:** Internal Medicine, NYU Med Ctr 1998; **Fellow:** Cardiovascular Disease, Montefiore Med Ctr 1998

Mintz, Guy L MD (Cv) - **Spec Exp:** Preventive Cardiology; Cholesterol/Lipid Disorders; Coronary Artery Disease; Hypertension; **Hospital:** N Shore Univ Hosp (page 106), St. Francis Hosp - The Heart Ctr (page 121); **Address:** 287 Northern Blvd, Ste 211, Great Neck, NY 11021; **Phone:** 516-482-3401; **Board Cert:** Internal Medicine 1987; Cardiovascular Disease 2003; **Med School:** Boston Univ 1984; **Resid:** Internal Medicine, N Shore Univ Hosp 1987; **Fellow:** Cardiovascular Disease, N Shore Univ Hosp 1989; **Fac Appt:** Assoc Prof Med, NYU Sch Med

Nash, Ira S MD (Cv) - **Spec Exp:** Preventive Cardiology; Coronary Artery Disease; **Hospital:** NS-LIJ Hlth Sys (page 106); **Address:** Physician & Ambulatory Network Services, North Shore-LIJ, 600 Community Drive, Ste 302, Manhasset, NY 11030; **Phone:** 212-835-6340 x203; **Board Cert:** Internal Medicine 1987; Cardiovascular Disease 1989; **Med School:** Harvard Med Sch 1984; **Resid:** Internal Medicine, Beth Israel Hosp 1987; **Fellow:** Cardiovascular Disease, Beth Israel Hosp 1990; **Fac Appt:** Assoc Prof Med, Mount Sinai Sch Med

Nicosia, Thomas A MD (Cv) - **Spec Exp:** Coronary Artery Disease; Congestive Heart Failure; **Hospital:** St. Francis Hosp - The Heart Ctr (page 121), N Shore Univ Hosp (page 106); **Address:** 1615 Northern Blvd, Ste 301, Manhasset, NY 11030; **Phone:** 516-627-9355; **Board Cert:** Internal Medicine 1979; Cardiovascular Disease 1981; **Med School:** Univ Cincinnati 1974; **Resid:** Internal Medicine, University Hosp 1978; **Fellow:** Cardiovascular Disease, Bellevue Hosp 1980

Pappas, Thomas W MD (Cv) - **Spec Exp:** Interventional Cardiology; Coronary Angioplasty/Stents; Angiography-Coronary; Cardiac Imaging; **Hospital:** St. Francis Hosp - The Heart Ctr (page 121); **Address:** 1155 Northern Blvd, Ste 330, Manhasset, NY 11030; **Phone:** 516-726-7575; **Board Cert:** Internal Medicine 1986; Cardiovascular Disease 1989; Interventional Cardiology 2010; **Med School:** Cornell Univ-Weill Med Coll 1983; **Resid:** Internal Medicine, New York Hosp 1986; **Fellow:** Cardiovascular Disease, New York Hosp-Cornell 1988; Interventional Cardiology, NYU Med Ctr 1990

Ragno, Philip D MD (Cv) - **Spec Exp:** Cholesterol/Lipid Disorders; Congestive Heart Failure; **Hospital:** Winthrop Univ Hosp (page 504), N Shore Univ Hosp (page 106); **Address:** 1401 Franklin Ave, Garden City, NY 11501; **Phone:** 516-877-2626; **Board Cert:** Internal Medicine 1987; Cardiovascular Disease 1989; **Med School:** SUNY Stony Brook 1984; **Resid:** Internal Medicine, Winthrop Univ Hosp 1987; **Fellow:** Cardiovascular Disease, Winthrop Univ Hosp 1989

Rutkovsky, Edward V MD (Cv) - **Spec Exp:** Nuclear Stress Testing; Echocardiography; **Hospital:** N Shore Univ Hosp (page 106), St. Francis Hosp - The Heart Ctr (page 121); **Address:** 2035 Lakeville Rd, Ste 101, New Hyde Park, NY 11040-1661; **Phone:** 516-328-9797; **Board Cert:** Internal Medicine 1987; Cardiovascular Disease 1989; **Med School:** NYU Sch Med 1984; **Resid:** Internal Medicine, NYU Med Ctr 1987; **Fellow:** Cardiovascular Disease, N Shore Univ Hosp 1989; **Fac Appt:** Asst Clin Prof Med, NYU Sch Med

Schreiber, Carl MD (Cv) - **Spec Exp:** Coronary Artery Disease; Nuclear Cardiology; Non-Invasive Cardiology; **Hospital:** Glen Cove Hosp (page 106), N Shore Univ Hosp (page 106); **Address:** 70 Glen St, Glen Cove, NY 11542-2853; **Phone:** 516-484-7893; **Board Cert:** Internal Medicine 1982; Cardiovascular Disease 1985; **Med School:** Med Coll GA 1979; **Resid:** Internal Medicine, Columbia-Presby Med Ctr 1982; **Fellow:** Cardiovascular Disease, Westchester Med Ctr 1984

Shayani, Steven S MD (Cv) - **Spec Exp:** Coronary Artery Disease; Congestive Heart Failure; Nuclear Cardiology; **Hospital:** Mount Sinai Med Ctr (page 102), St. Francis Hosp - The Heart Ctr (page 121); **Address:** 200 Old Country Rd, Ste 278, Mineola, NY 11501; **Phone:** 516-877-0977; **Board Cert:** Internal Medicine 2002; Cardiovascular Disease 2005; **Med School:** SUNY Upstate Med Univ 1988; **Resid:** Internal Medicine, Winthrop Univ Hosp 1991; **Fellow:** Cardiovascular Disease, Winthrop Univ Hosp 1994; **Fac Appt:** Asst Clin Prof Med, Mount Sinai Sch Med

Shlofmitz, Richard A MD (Cv) - **Spec Exp:** Interventional Cardiology; Cardiac Catheterization; **Hospital:** St. Francis Hosp - The Heart Ctr (page 121); **Address:** 100 Port Washington Blvd, Ste 105, Vizza Pavilion, Roslyn, NY 11576; **Phone:** 516-390-9640; **Board Cert:** Internal Medicine 1984; Cardiovascular Disease 1987; **Med School:** NYU Sch Med 1980; **Resid:** Internal Medicine, North Shore Univ Hosp 1984; **Fellow:** Cardiovascular Disease, Columbia Presby Med Ctr 1987

Sokol, Sergio MD (Cv) - **Spec Exp:** Echocardiography; **Hospital:** St. John's Epis Hosp - S Shore; **Address:** Five Towns Heart Imaging, 650 Central Ave, Ste K, Cedarhurst, NY 11516; **Phone:** 516-804-8590; **Board Cert:** Internal Medicine 2001; Cardiovascular Disease 2004; **Med School:** Israel 1994; **Resid:** Internal Medicine, Montefiore Med Ctr 1998; **Fellow:** Cardiovascular Disease, N Shore Univ Hosp 2001

Spadaro, Louise A MD (Cv) - **Spec Exp:** Preventive Cardiology; Heart Disease in Women; **Hospital:** St. Francis Hosp - The Heart Ctr (page 121); **Address:** 100 Port Washington Blvd, Vizza Bldg Fl 1 - Ste 101, Roslyn, NY 11576; **Phone:** 516-562-6653; **Board Cert:** Internal Medicine 1987; Cardiovascular Disease 1989; **Med School:** NYU Sch Med 1984; **Resid:** Internal Medicine, Bellevue Hosp 1987; **Fellow:** Cardiovascular Disease, Bellevue Hosp/NYU Med Ctr 1989

Tenet, William MD (Cv) - **Spec Exp:** Congestive Heart Failure; Coronary Artery Disease; **Hospital:** N Shore Univ Hosp (page 106), Lenox Hill Hosp (page 106); **Address:** 1155 Northern Blvd, Ste 330, Manhasset, NY 11030; **Phone:** 516-627-4330; **Board Cert:** Internal Medicine 1983; Cardiovascular Disease 1987; **Med School:** Italy 1980; **Resid:** Internal Medicine, Booth Meml Med Ctr 1984; **Fellow:** Cardiovascular Disease, Univ Conn Hlth Ctr 1986; **Fac Appt:** Asst Clin Prof Med, Cornell Univ-Weill Med Coll

Weg, Ira L MD (Cv) - **Spec Exp:** Congestive Heart Failure; Coronary Artery Disease; **Hospital:** South Nassau Comm Hosp; **Address:** 158 Hempstead Ave, Lynbrook, NY 11563; **Phone:** 516-593-3541; **Board Cert:** Internal Medicine 1979; Cardiovascular Disease 1981; **Med School:** SUNY Hlth Sci Ctr 1976; **Resid:** Internal Medicine, Kings County Hosp 1979; **Fellow:** Cardiovascular Disease, Montefiore Med Ctr 1981; **Fac Appt:** Asst Clin Prof Med, Albert Einstein Coll Med

Zeldis, Steven M MD (Cv) - **Spec Exp:** Echocardiography; Cardiac Stress Testing; Cardiac Imaging; **Hospital:** Winthrop Univ Hosp (page 504); **Address:** 200 Old Country Rd, Ste 278, Mineola, NY 11501-4298; **Phone:** 516-877-0977; **Board Cert:** Internal Medicine 1975; Cardiovascular Disease 1977; **Med School:** Yale Univ 1972; **Resid:** Internal Medicine, Yale Med Ctr 1975; **Fellow:** Cardiovascular Disease, Hosp Univ Penn 1977; **Fac Appt:** Assoc Prof Med, SUNY Stony Brook

Child & Adolescent Psychiatry

Foley, Carmel A MD (ChAP) - **Spec Exp:** Mood Disorders; **Hospital:** Steven & Alexandra Cohen Chldn's Med Ctr of NY (page 106); **Address:** 420 Lakeville Rd, 1st Floor, New Hyde Park, NY 11040; **Phone:** 718-470-3550; **Board Cert:** Psychiatry 1979; Child & Adolescent Psychiatry 1981; Psychosomatic Medicine 2009; **Med School:** Ireland 1972; **Resid:** Psychiatry, St Patrick's Hosp 1976; Psychiatry, Lafayette Clinic 1977; **Fellow:** Child & Adolescent Psychiatry, Lafayette Clinic 1979; **Fac Appt:** Assoc Prof Psyc, Albert Einstein Coll Med

Williams, Daniel T MD (ChAP) - **Spec Exp:** Neuro-Psychiatry; Psychopharmacology; Psychosomatic Disorders; **Hospital:** NY-Presby/Columbia Univ Med Ctr, NY (page 104), NS-LIJ Hlth Sys (page 106); **Address:** 3003 New Hyde Park Rd, Ste 204, New Hyde Park, NY 11042; **Phone:** 516-488-3636; **Board Cert:** Psychiatry 1975; Child & Adolescent Psychiatry 1976; **Med School:** Cornell Univ-Weill Med Coll 1969; **Resid:** Psychiatry, Mount Sinai Hosp 1972; **Fellow:** Child & Adolescent Psychiatry, Columbia-Presby Hosp 1974

Child Neurology

Atluru, Vijaya MD (ChiN) - **Spec Exp:** Epilepsy; Seizure Disorders; Migraine; **Hospital:** Winthrop Univ Hosp (page 504); **Address:** Winthrop Child Neurology Assocs, 120 Mineola Blvd, Ste 430, Mineola, NY 11501; **Phone:** 516-663-9494; **Board Cert:** Pediatrics 1979; Child Neurology 1983; **Med School:** India 1973; **Resid:** Pediatrics, Nassau Co Med Ctr 1977; **Fellow:** Child Neurology, Stony Brook Univ Med Ctr 1980; **Fac Appt:** Assoc Prof N, SUNY Stony Brook

Bergtraum, Marcia MD (ChiN) - **Hospital:** Long Island Jewish Med Ctr (page 106); **Address:** 3003 New Hyde Park Rd, Ste 204, New Hyde Park, NY 11042-1214; **Phone:** 516-488-2323; **Board Cert:** Pediatrics 1981; Child Neurology 1988; **Med School:** Georgetown Univ 1974; **Resid:** Pediatric Hematology-Oncology, LI Jewish Hosp 1978; Pediatric Neurology, LI Jewish Hosp 1982; **Fellow:** Child Neurology, Neur Inst/Columbia-Presby 1983

LaJoie, Josiane M MD (ChiN) *PCP* - **Spec Exp:** Epilepsy/Seizure Disorders; Neurophysiology; **Hospital:** NS-LIJ Hlth Sys (page 106), Steven & Alexandra Cohen Chldn's Med Ctr of NY (page 106); **Address:** Steven & Alexandra Cohen Chldns Med Ctr, Div of Pediatric Neurology, 410 Lakeview Rd, Ste 105, New Hyde Park, NY 11042; **Phone:** 516-465-5255; **Board Cert:** Pediatrics 2005; Child Neurology 2012; Clinical Neurophysiology 2005; **Med School:** Univ Pennsylvania 1996; **Resid:** Pediatric Neurology, Albert Einstein Med Ctr 2000; **Fellow:** Clinical Neurophysiology, Albert Einstein Med Ctr 2001; **Fac Appt:** Asst Prof N, NYU Sch Med

Maytal, Joseph MD (ChiN) - **Spec Exp:** Epilepsy/Seizure Disorders; Migraine; **Hospital:** Steven & Alexandra Cohen Chldn's Med Ctr of NY (page 106); **Address:** Div Pediatric Neurology, 410 Lakeville Rd, Ste 105, Lake Success, NY 11042; **Phone:** 516-465-5255; **Board Cert:** Pediatrics 1986; Child Neurology 1988; **Med School:** Israel 1979; **Resid:** Pediatrics, Brookdale Hosp 1983; Child Neurology, Montefiore Med Ctr 1986; **Fellow:** Neurological Physiology, Albert Einstein Med Coll 1987; **Fac Appt:** Clin Prof N, Albert Einstein Coll Med

Smith, Robin E MD (ChiN) - **Spec Exp:** Cerebral Palsy; Neuromuscular Disorders; Headache; Epilepsy/Seizure Disorders; **Hospital:** Steven & Alexandra Cohen Chldn's Med Ctr of NY (page 106); **Address:** NRAD Medical Assocs, 105 Froehlich Farm Blvd, Woodbury, NY 11797; **Phone:** 516-222-2022 x7776; **Board Cert:** Pediatrics 2006; Child Neurology 2008; **Med School:** South Africa 1985; **Resid:** Pediatrics, Johannesburg Hosp 1993; Pediatrics, Schneider Childrens Hosp 1998; **Fellow:** Child Neurology, Schneider Childrens Hosp 1997; **Fac Appt:** Asst Prof N, Hofstra N Shore-LIJ Sch Med

Clinical Genetics

Bialer, Martin G MD/PhD (CG) - **Spec Exp:** Marfan's Syndrome; Neurofibromatosis; Metabolic Genetic Disorders; Cancer Genetics; **Hospital:** Steven & Alexandra Cohen Chldn's Med Ctr of NY (page 106), NS-LIJ Hlth Sys (page 106); **Address:** 1554 Northern Blvd, Ste 204, Manhasset, NY 11030; **Phone:** 516-365-3996; **Board Cert:** Pediatrics 1987; Clinical Biochemical Genetics 1990; Clinical Genetics 1990; **Med School:** Med Univ SC 1983; **Resid:** Pediatrics, N Shore Univ Hosp 1986; **Fellow:** Clinical Genetics, Univ VA Hlth Sci Ctr 1989; **Fac Appt:** Clin Prof Ped, NYU Sch Med

Fox, Joyce MD (CG) - **Hospital:** Long Island Jewish Med Ctr (page 106), Steven & Alexandra Cohen Chldn's Med Ctr of NY (page 106); **Address:** 1554 Northern Blvd, Ste 204, Manhasset, NY 11030; **Phone:** 516-365-3996; **Board Cert:** Pediatrics 1986; Clinical Genetics 1987; **Med School:** Columbia P&S 1980; **Resid:** Pediatrics, Case Western Univ Hosp 1983; **Fellow:** Clinical Genetics, Yale-New Haven Hosp 1986; **Fac Appt:** , Albert Einstein Coll Med

Colon & Rectal Surgery

Greenwald, Marc MD (CRS) - **Spec Exp:** Laparoscopic Surgery; Colonoscopy; Anorectal Disorders; Colon & Rectal Cancer; **Hospital:** N Shore Univ Hosp (page 106), St. Francis Hosp - The Heart Ctr (page 121); **Address:** 310 E Shore Rd, Ste 203, Great Neck, NY 11023-2432; **Phone:** 516-482-8657; **Board Cert:** Surgery 2009; Colon & Rectal Surgery 2011; **Med School:** Albert Einstein Coll Med 1985; **Resid:** Surgery, Montefiore Hosp Med Ctr 1990; **Fellow:** Colon & Rectal Surgery, St Francis Hosp 1991

Moseson, Michael J MD (CRS) - **Spec Exp:** Anorectal Disorders; Colonoscopy/Polypectomy; **Hospital:** St. Francis Hosp - The Heart Ctr (page 121), N Shore Univ Hosp (page 106); **Address:** 3 Vermont Drive, Lake Success, NY 11042; **Phone:** 516-608-6848; **Board Cert:** Colon & Rectal Surgery 1982; Surgery 2002; **Med School:** Spain 1975; **Resid:** Surgery, North Shore Univ Hosp 1980; Colon & Rectal Surgery, UMDNJ-RWJohnson Med Ctr 1981; **Fac Appt:** Asst Clin Prof S, Cornell Univ-Weill Med Coll

Procaccino Jr, John A MD (CRS) - **Spec Exp:** Inflammatory Bowel Disease/Crohn's; Colon & Rectal Cancer; Anorectal Disorders; Colon & Rectal Cancer-Familial Polyposis; **Hospital:** N Shore Univ Hosp (page 106), Long Island Jewish Med Ctr (page 106); **Address:** Chief, Division of Colon & Rectal Surg, 900 Northern Blvd, Ste 100, Great Neck, NY 11021; **Phone:** 516-730-2100; **Board Cert:** Surgery 2009; Colon & Rectal Surgery 2011; **Med School:** NYU Sch Med 1984; **Resid:** Surgery, N Shore Univ Hosp 1989; **Fellow:** Colon & Rectal Surgery, Cleveland Clinic 1990; **Fac Appt:** Asst Clin Prof S, Cornell Univ-Weill Med Coll

Sullivan III, James D MD (CRS) - **Spec Exp:** Cancer Surgery; Colon & Rectal Cancer & Surgery; **Hospital:** N Shore Univ Hosp (page 106), St. Francis Hosp - The Heart Ctr (page 121); **Address:** North Shore Oncology Associates, 600 Northern Blvd, Ste 111, Great Neck, NY 11021; **Phone:** 516-941-1213; **Board Cert:** Surgery 2004; Colon & Rectal Surgery 2005; **Med School:** NY Med Coll 1987; **Resid:** Surgery, N Shore Univ Hosp 1992; **Fellow:** Colon & Rectal Surgery, Cleveland Clinic 1993

Dermatology

Aprile, Georgette MD (D) - **Spec Exp:** Acne; Atopic Dermatitis; **Hospital:** Glen Cove Hosp (page 106); **Address:** 8 Med Plaza, Lower Level, Ste 103, Glen Cove, NY 11542; **Phone:** 516-759-9200; **Board Cert:** Dermatology 1978; **Med School:** NY Med Coll 1974; **Resid:** Dermatology, New York Hosp 1978

Bruckstein, Robert MD (D) - **Spec Exp:** Acne; Skin Cancer; Cosmetic Dermatology; Skin Laser Surgery; **Hospital:** St. John's Epis Hosp - S Shore; **Address:** 290 Central Ave, Ste 206, Lawrence, NY 11559-8507; **Phone:** 516-239-2332; **Board Cert:** Dermatology 1977; **Med School:** NYU Sch Med 1972; **Resid:** Dermatology, Bellevue Hosp Ctr 1975; **Fac Appt:** Asst Clin Prof D, NYU Sch Med

De Pietro, William MD (D) - **Spec Exp:** Skin Laser Surgery; Dermatologic Surgery; **Hospital:** Glen Cove Hosp (page 106); **Address:** 10 Medical Plaza, Ste 102, Glen Cove, NY 11542; **Phone:** 516-671-1780; **Board Cert:** Dermatology 1980; **Med School:** Georgetown Univ 1976; **Resid:** Dermatology, St Luke's Hosp 1980

Demento, Frank MD (D) - **Spec Exp:** Dermatologic Surgery; Skin Cancer; **Hospital:** Winthrop Univ Hosp (page 504), NY-Presby/Columbia Univ Med Ctr, NY (page 104); **Address:** 520 Franklin Ave, Ste 229, Garden City, NY 11530; **Phone:** 516-746-1227; **Board Cert:** Dermatology 1969; **Med School:** UMDNJ-NJ Med Sch, Newark 1964; **Resid:** Dermatology, USPHS Hosp 1966; **Fellow:** Dermatology, Columbia-Presby Hosp 1968

Dolitsky, Charisse MD (D) - **Spec Exp:** Acne; Skin Cancer; Botox Therapy; Facial Rejuvenation; **Hospital:** Long Beach Med Ctr; **Address:** 604 E Park Ave, Long Beach, NY 11561; **Phone:** 516-432-0011; **Board Cert:** Dermatology 1989; **Med School:** SUNY Downstate 1985; **Resid:** Dermatology, Univ Hosp 1989

Falcon, Ronald MD (D) - **Spec Exp:** Skin Cancer; Acne; Psoriasis; **Hospital:** Long Beach Med Ctr; **Address:** 604 E Park Ave, Long Beach, NY 11561; **Phone:** 516-432-0011; **Board Cert:** Dermatology 1989; **Med School:** SUNY Downstate 1985; **Resid:** Dermatology, SUNY Downstate 1989

Franck, Jeanne M MD (D) - **Spec Exp:** Mohs' Surgery; **Hospital:** Winthrop Univ Hosp (page 504), NY-Presby/Columbia Univ Med Ctr, NY (page 104); **Address:** 520 Franklin Ave, Ste 207, Garden City, NY 11530; **Phone:** 516-741-1055; **Board Cert:** Dermatology 2004; **Med School:** Columbia P&S 1991; **Resid:** Dermatology, Columbia Presby Med Ctr 1995; **Fellow:** Mohs Surgery, Univ Minn Med Ctr

Hefter, Harold MD (D) - **Spec Exp:** Cosmetic Dermatology; Dermatologic Surgery; Acne; **Hospital:** Franklin Hosp (page 106), Jacobi Med Ctr; **Address:** 135 Rockaway Tpke, Ste 100, Lawrence, NY 11559-1033; **Phone:** 516-371-1600; **Board Cert:** Dermatology 1985; **Med School:** Albert Einstein Coll Med 1981; **Resid:** Dermatology, Albert Einstein 1985; **Fac Appt:** Asst Prof D, Albert Einstein Coll Med

Hisler, Barbara M MD (D) - **Spec Exp:** Skin Cancer; Acne; Psoriasis; **Hospital:** Long Island Jewish Med Ctr (page 106); **Address:** 1300 Union Tpke, Ste 303, New Hyde Park, NY 11040-1759; **Phone:** 516-326-0333; **Board Cert:** Internal Medicine 1986; Dermatology 1989; **Med School:** NY Med Coll 1983; **Resid:** Internal Medicine, LI Jewish Med Ctr 1985; Dermatology, Detroit Med Ctr 1988; **Fac Appt:** Asst Prof Med, Albert Einstein Coll Med

Levine, Laurie J MD (D) - **Spec Exp:** Skin Laser Surgery; Botox Therapy; Cosmetic Dermatology; **Hospital:** Winthrop Univ Hosp (page 504); **Address:** 200 Old Country Rd, Ste 140, Mineola, NY 11501-4237; **Phone:** 516-742-6136; **Board Cert:** Dermatology 1988; **Med School:** SUNY Stony Brook 1984; **Resid:** Dermatology, T Jefferson Univ Hosp 1988; **Fellow:** Dermatologic Surgery, T Jefferson Univ Hosp 1989; **Fac Appt:** Asst Clin Prof D, SUNY Stony Brook

Paltzik, Robert L MD (D) - **Spec Exp:** Pediatric Dermatology; Dermatologic Surgery; **Hospital:** N Shore Univ Hosp (page 106), Winthrop Univ Hosp (page 504); **Address:** 2 Hillside Ave, Ste G, Williston Park, NY 11596-2335; **Phone:** 516-747-2230; **Board Cert:** Dermatology 1977; Pediatrics 1976; **Med School:** NYU Sch Med 1971; **Resid:** Pediatrics, Yale-New Haven Hosp 1973; Dermatology, SUNY Downstate Med Ctr 1977; **Fac Appt:** Asst Prof D, NYU Sch Med

Sarnoff, Deborah S MD (D) - **Spec Exp:** Mohs' Surgery; Skin Cancer; Dermatologic Surgery; Skin Laser Surgery; **Hospital:** NYU Langone Med Ctr (page 108); **Address:** 31 N Blvd, Greenvale, NY 11548; **Phone:** 516-484-9000; **Board Cert:** Dermatology 2009; **Med School:** Geo Wash Univ 1980; **Resid:** Dermatology, NYU Med Ctr 1984; **Fellow:** Dermatologic Surgery, NYU Med Ctr 1986; **Fac Appt:** Clin Prof D, NYU Sch Med

Silverman, Mark K MD (D) - **Spec Exp:** Melanoma; Skin Cancer; Skin Laser Surgery; **Hospital:** South Nassau Comm Hosp; **Address:** 258 Merrick Rd, Oceanside, NY 11572; **Phone:** 516-766-0345; **Board Cert:** Internal Medicine 1989; Dermatology 2001; **Med School:** Tufts Univ 1986; **Resid:** Internal Medicine, Montefiore Med Ctr 1989; Dermatology, Montefiore Med Ctr 1994; **Fellow:** Research, NYU 1991

Sklar, Jeffrey Alan MD (D) - **Spec Exp:** Facial Rejuvenation; Cosmetic Dermatology; Laser Surgery; **Hospital:** NY-Presby/Columbia Univ Med Ctr, NY (page 104), Syosset Hosp (page 106); **Address:** 800 Woodbury Rd, Ste A, Woodbury, NY 11797-2503; **Phone:** 516-496-9400; **Board Cert:** Dermatology 1986; **Med School:** Columbia P&S 1982; **Resid:** Dermatology, Columbia Presby Hosp 1986; **Fac Appt:** Asst Clin Prof D, Columbia P&S

Spinowitz, Alan MD (D) - **Spec Exp:** Skin Cancer; Mohs' Surgery; **Hospital:** Franklin Hosp (page 106); **Address:** 877 Stewart Ave, Ste 27, Garden City, NY 11530-4803; **Phone:** 516-745-0606; **Board Cert:** Dermatology 1985; **Med School:** SUNY Hlth Sci Ctr 1981; **Resid:** Dermatology, Univ Illinois Med Ctr 1985; **Fellow:** Dermatologic Surgery, Univ Illinois Med Ctr 1987

Walczyk, John MD (D) - **Spec Exp:** Cosmetic Dermatology; **Hospital:** NY-Presby/Columbia Univ Med Ctr, NY (page 104), Plainview Hosp (page 106); **Address:** 1165 Northern Blvd, Ste 405, Manhasset, NY 11030; **Phone:** 516-365-8030; **Board Cert:** Dermatology 2003; **Med School:** Columbia P&S 1990; **Resid:** Internal Medicine, N Shore Univ Hosp 1991; Dermatology, Columbia Presby Hosp 1994

Diagnostic Radiology

Goodman, Kenneth J MD (DR) - **Spec Exp:** Urologic Imaging; Ultrasound; CT Scan; **Hospital:** St. Francis Hosp - The Heart Ctr (page 121); **Address:** St Francis Hosp-The Heart Ctr, Dept Radiology, 100 Port Washington Blvd, Roslyn, NY 11576-1353; **Phone:** 516-562-6500; **Board Cert:** Diagnostic Radiology 1977; **Med School:** Univ Tex, San Antonio 1972; **Resid:** Diagnostic Radiology, Cornell Med Ctr 1977; **Fellow:** Diagnostic Radiology, Cornell Med Ctr 1978

Hammel, Jay D MD (DR) - **Spec Exp:** MRI; **Hospital:** N Shore Univ Hosp (page 106), Syosset Hosp (page 106); **Address:** 4277 Hempstead Tpke, Ste 200, Bethpage, NY 11714; **Phone:** 516-796-4340; **Board Cert:** Diagnostic Radiology 1989; **Med School:** SUNY Upstate Med Univ 1984; **Resid:** Diagnostic Radiology, St Vincent's Med Ctr 1989

Hoffman, Janet C MD (DR) - **Hospital:** Long Island Jewish Med Ctr (page 106); **Address:** 270-05 76th Ave, rm C-204, New Hyde Park, NY 11040; **Phone:** 718-470-3456; **Board Cert:** Diagnostic Radiology 1978; **Med School:** SUNY Downstate 1974; **Resid:** Diagnostic Radiology, Colum Presby Hosp 1978; **Fellow:** Ultrasound, NY Hosp-Cornell Med Ctr 1979

Khan, Arfa MD (DR) - **Spec Exp:** Thoracic Radiology; **Hospital:** Long Island Jewish Med Ctr (page 106), NS-LIJ Hlth Sys (page 106); **Address:** 270-05 76th Ave, rm C204, New Hyde Park, NY 11040; **Phone:** 718-470-7164; **Board Cert:** Diagnostic Radiology 1971; **Med School:** India 1964; **Resid:** Diagnostic Radiology, Queens Hosp 1970; **Fellow:** Diagnostic Radiology, LI Jewish Med Ctr 1971; **Fac Appt:** Assoc Prof Rad, Albert Einstein Coll Med

Luchs, Jonathan S MD (DR) - ; **Address:** 224 Seventh St, Garden City, NY 11530; **Phone:** 516-747-0161; **Board Cert:** Diagnostic Radiology 2003; **Med School:** Israel 1996; **Resid:** Surgery, Maimonides Med Ctr 1999; **Fellow:** Diagnostic Radiology, Winthrop Univ Hosp 2003; Musculoskeletal Imaging, Hosp for Special Surgery

Port, Abraham MD (DR) - **Spec Exp:** Breast Cancer; Mammography; **Hospital:** South Nassau Comm Hosp; **Address:** Complete Women's Imaging, 990 Stewart Ave, Ste 100, Garden City, NY 11530; **Phone:** 516-222-4294; **Board Cert:** Diagnostic Radiology 1985; **Med School:** Albert Einstein Coll Med 1981; **Resid:** Diagnostic Radiology, Montefiore Med Ctr 1985; **Fellow:** Body Imaging, NY Hosp-Cornell Med Ctr 1986

Rossi, Dennis R MD (DR) - **Spec Exp:** MRI; **Hospital:** Long Beach Med Ctr; **Address:** Elmont MRI, 545 Elmont Rd, Elmont, NY 11003; **Phone:** 516-328-7200; **Board Cert:** Diagnostic Radiology 1973; **Med School:** SUNY Downstate 1968; **Resid:** Diagnostic Radiology, Montefiore Hosp Med Ctr 1972; **Fac Appt:** Assoc Clin Prof, SUNY Stony Brook

Sherman, Scott J MD (DR) - **Spec Exp:** CT Scan; PET Imaging; **Hospital:** St. Francis Hosp - The Heart Ctr (page 121), St. Joseph's Hosp-Nassau; **Address:** 100 Port Washington Blvd, Roslyn, NY 11576; **Phone:** 516-562-6500; **Board Cert:** Diagnostic Radiology 1983; Nuclear Medicine 1984; **Med School:** Northwestern Univ 1979; **Resid:** Diagnostic Radiology, NY Hosp 1983; Nuclear Medicine, NY Hosp 1984; **Fellow:** Ultrasound, NY Hosp 1985

Weck, Steven MD (DR) - **Spec Exp:** Interventional Radiology; **Hospital:** Glen Cove Hosp (page 106); **Address:** 101 St. Andrews Ln, Fl 1st, Glen Cove, NY 11542; **Phone:** 516-674-7540; **Board Cert:** Diagnostic Radiology 1977; **Med School:** NYU Sch Med 1973; **Resid:** Diagnostic Radiology, NYU Med Ctr 1977

Yoon, Sydney S MD (DR) - **Spec Exp:** MRI; CT Scan; Neuroradiology; Neuroradiology; **Hospital:** South Nassau Comm Hosp; **Address:** 1 Healthy Way, Dept of Radiology, Oceanside, NY 11572; **Phone:** 516-632-4660; **Board Cert:** Internal Medicine 1989; Diagnostic Radiology 1993; Vascular & Interventional Radiology 2011; Neuroradiology 2006; **Med School:** Univ Chicago-Pritzker Sch Med 1986; **Resid:** Internal Medicine, Johns Hopkins Hosp 1989; Diagnostic Radiology, UCLA Med Ctr 1993; **Fellow:** Neuroradiology, Columbia Presby Med Ctr 1995; Vascular & Interventional Radiology, UCLA Med Ctr 1997

Endocrinology, Diabetes & Metabolism

Aloia, John MD (EDM) - **Spec Exp:** Osteoporosis; **Hospital:** Winthrop Univ Hosp (page 504); **Address:** 1300 Franklin Ave, Ste ML6, Garden City, NY 11530; **Phone:** 516-663-3511; **Board Cert:** Internal Medicine 1969; Endocrinology 1972; **Med School:** Creighton Univ 1962; **Resid:** Internal Medicine, Meadowbrook Hosp 1966; Internal Medicine, Harrisburg Hosp 1967; **Fellow:** Endocrinology, Diabetes & Metabolism, Jefferson Univ Med Ctr 1969; **Fac Appt:** Prof Med, SUNY Stony Brook

Bhatt, Anjani A MD (EDM) - **Spec Exp:** Thyroid Disorders; Diabetes; **Address:** 871 E Park Ave, Long Beach, NY 11561; **Phone:** 516-889-8853; **Board Cert:** Internal Medicine 1983; Endocrinology, Diabetes & Metabolism 1985; **Med School:** India 1976; **Resid:** Internal Medicine, Brooklyn Hosp 1981; **Fellow:** Endocrinology, Brooklyn Hosp 1984

Bitton, Rachelle N MD (EDM) - **Spec Exp:** Osteoporosis; Thyroid Disorders; Diabetes; Pituitary Disorders; **Hospital:** Long Island Jewish Med Ctr (page 106), N Shore Univ Hosp (page 106); **Address:** ProHealth Care Assocs, 2 ProHealth Plaza, Ste 201, Lake Success, NY 11042; **Phone:** 516-390-5760; **Board Cert:** Internal Medicine 1981; Endocrinology, Diabetes & Metabolism 1985; **Med School:** SUNY Downstate 1978; **Resid:** Internal Medicine, Brookdale Hosp 1981; **Fellow:** Endocrinology, Diabetes & Metabolism, Univ Hosp 1984

Friedman, Seth G MD (EDM) - **Spec Exp:** Thyroid Disorders; Pituitary Disorders; Diabetes; Osteoporosis; **Hospital:** N Shore Univ Hosp (page 106), Long Island Jewish Med Ctr (page 106); **Address:** 560 Northern Blvd, Ste 207, Great Neck, NY 11021; **Phone:** 516-466-6165; **Board Cert:** Internal Medicine 2002; Endocrinology, Diabetes & Metabolism 2003; **Med School:** Mount Sinai Sch Med 1988; **Resid:** Internal Medicine, LI Jewish Med Ctr 1991; **Fellow:** Endocrinology, Diabetes & Metabolism, Albert Einstein 1993

Gordon, Jeffrey H MD (EDM) - **Spec Exp:** Diabetes; Thyroid Disorders; Pituitary Disorders; **Hospital:** St. Francis Hosp - The Heart Ctr (page 121), N Shore Univ Hosp (page 106); **Address:** 3 School St, Ste 306, Glen Cove, NY 11542-2548; **Phone:** 516-759-2420; **Board Cert:** Internal Medicine 1972; Endocrinology, Diabetes & Metabolism 1973; **Med School:** Cornell Univ-Weill Med Coll 1965; **Resid:** Internal Medicine, Bellevue Hosp 1967; **Fellow:** Endocrinology, Duke Univ Med Ctr 1970; Endocrinology, VA Hosp 1972; **Fac Appt:** Asst Clin Prof Med, NYU Sch Med

Greenfield, Martin MD (EDM) - **Spec Exp:** Diabetes; Thyroid Disorders; Osteoporosis; Adrenal Disorders; **Hospital:** Long Island Jewish Med Ctr (page 106), N Shore Univ Hosp (page 106); **Address:** ProHealth Care Assocs, 2 ProHealth Plaza, Ste 201, Lake Success, NY 11042; **Phone:** 516-608-6823; **Board Cert:** Internal Medicine 1987; Endocrinology, Diabetes & Metabolism 1979; **Med School:** SUNY Downstate 1968; **Resid:** Internal Medicine, LI Jewish Med Ctr 1971; **Fellow:** Endocrinology, Diabetes & Metabolism, Brigham & Womens Hosp 1975; **Fac Appt:** Asst Clin Prof Med, Albert Einstein Coll Med

Hupart, Kenneth H MD (EDM) - **Spec Exp:** Thyroid Disorders; Osteoporosis; Diabetes; Cholesterol/Lipid Disorders; **Hospital:** Nassau Univ Med Ctr; **Address:** Nassau Univ Med Ctr, Div Endocrinology, 2201 Heampstead Tpke, East Meadow, NY 11554; **Phone:** 516-572-4848; **Board Cert:** Internal Medicine 1985; Endocrinology 1989; **Med School:** SUNY Stony Brook 1982; **Resid:** Internal Medicine, Montefiore Hosp Med Ctr 1986; **Fellow:** Endocrinology, Diabetes & Metabolism, Montefiore Hosp Med Ctr 1988; **Fac Appt:** Assoc Clin Prof Med, Albert Einstein Coll Med

Kaplan, Jonathan MD (EDM) - **Spec Exp:** Diabetes; **Hospital:** N Shore Univ Hosp (page 106); **Address:** 1000 Northern Blvd, Ste 240, Great Neck, NY 11021; **Phone:** 516-829-0802; **Board Cert:** Internal Medicine 2006; Endocrinology, Diabetes & Metabolism 2008; **Med School:** Israel 1990; **Resid:** Internal Medicine, Rambam Med Ctr 1994; Internal Medicine, N Shore Univ Hosp 1996; **Fellow:** Endocrinology, Diabetes & Metabolism, Albert Einstein 1998

Lomasky, Steven MD (EDM) - **Spec Exp:** Diabetes; Cholesterol/Lipid Disorders; Thyroid Disorders; **Hospital:** South Nassau Comm Hosp; **Address:** 242 Merrick Rd, rm 403, Rockville Ctr, NY 11570; **Phone:** 516-536-3700; **Board Cert:** Endocrinology, Diabetes & Metabolism 1989; Internal Medicine 1985; **Med School:** Israel 1982; **Resid:** Internal Medicine, Montefiore Med Ctr 1986; **Fellow:** Endocrinology, Diabetes & Metabolism, Montefiore Med Ctr 1987; **Fac Appt:** Asst Clin Prof Med, Albert Einstein Coll Med

Margulies, Paul MD (EDM) - **Spec Exp:** Thyroid Disorders; Adrenal Disorders; Pituitary Disorders; Addison's Disease; **Hospital:** N Shore Univ Hosp (page 106); **Address:** 444 Community, Ste 312, Manhasset, NY 11030-3820; **Phone:** 516-627-1366; **Board Cert:** Internal Medicine 1975; Endocrinology, Diabetes & Metabolism 1977; **Med School:** Univ Chicago-Pritzker Sch Med 1970; **Resid:** Internal Medicine, New York Hosp 1975; **Fellow:** Endocrinology, Diabetes & Metabolism, New York Hosp 1976; **Fac Appt:** Assoc Prof Med, NYU Sch Med

Rosenthal, David S MD (EDM) - **Spec Exp:** Thyroid Disorders; Pituitary Disorders; Adrenal Disorders; Osteoporosis; **Hospital:** Nassau Univ Med Ctr; **Address:** Nassau Univ Med Ctr, Div Endocrinology, 2201 Hempstead Tpke, Box 49, East Meadow, NY 11554; **Phone:** 516-572-4848; **Board Cert:** Internal Medicine 1969; Endocrinology, Diabetes & Metabolism 1972; **Med School:** NYU Sch Med 1963; **Resid:** Internal Medicine, Wilford Hall USAF Med Ctr 1967; **Fellow:** Endocrinology, Diabetes & Metabolism, Boston Univ Med Ctr 1972; Nuclear Medicine, Boston Univ Med Ctr 1972; **Fac Appt:** Asst Prof Med, SUNY Stony Brook

Shapiro, Lawrence E MD (EDM) - **Spec Exp:** Thyroid Disorders; Diabetes; **Hospital:** Winthrop Univ Hosp (page 504); **Address:** 1300 Franklin Ave, Ste ML6, Garden City, NY 11530; **Phone:** 516-663-3511; **Board Cert:** Internal Medicine 1975; Endocrinology 1977; **Med School:** SUNY Downstate 1971; **Resid:** Internal Medicine, Bellevue Hosp 1974; **Fellow:** Endocrinology, Diabetes & Metabolism, NYU Med Ctr 1975; **Fac Appt:** Prof Med, SUNY Stony Brook

Vaswani, Ashok N MD (EDM) - **Spec Exp:** Osteoporosis; Obesity; **Hospital:** Winthrop Univ Hosp (page 504); **Address:** 901 Stewart Ave, Ste 204, Garden City, NY 11530; **Phone:** 516-739-0414; **Board Cert:** Internal Medicine 1977; Endocrinology, Diabetes & Metabolism 1983; **Med School:** India 1970; **Resid:** Internal Medicine, Nassau County Med Ctr 1974; **Fac Appt:** Asst Prof Med, SUNY Stony Brook

Weinerman, Stuart MD (EDM) - **Spec Exp:** Osteoporosis; Calcium Disorders; Paget's Disease of Bone; **Hospital:** N Shore Univ Hosp (page 106), Long Island Jewish Med Ctr (page 106); **Address:** 2800 Marcus Ave, Ste 200, Lake Success, NY 11021-5310; **Phone:** 516-708-2540; **Board Cert:** Internal Medicine 1987; Endocrinology, Diabetes & Metabolism 1989; **Med School:** Albert Einstein Coll Med 1984; **Resid:** Internal Medicine, N Shore Univ Hosp 1987; **Fellow:** Endocrinology, Diabetes & Metabolism, NY Hosp/Meml Sloan Kettering Cancer Ctr 1989; **Fac Appt:** Asst Prof Med, NYU Sch Med

Family Medicine

Arcati, Anthony T MD (FMed) *PCP* - **Hospital:** Winthrop Univ Hosp (page 504); **Address:** 530 Hicksville Rd, Bethpage, NY 11714; **Phone:** 516-937-5000; **Board Cert:** Family Medicine 2003; **Med School:** Mexico 1975; **Resid:** Family Medicine, Nassau Co Med Ctr 1979

Arcati, Robert J MD (FMed) *PCP* - **Hospital:** Winthrop Univ Hosp (page 504); **Address:** 530 Hicksville Rd, Bethpage, NY 11714; **Phone:** 516-937-5000; **Board Cert:** Family Medicine 2008; **Med School:** Mount Sinai Sch Med 1986; **Resid:** Family Medicine, Somerset Med Ctr 1989

Capobianco, Luigi MD (FMed) *PCP* - **Spec Exp:** Geriatric Care; **Hospital:** Glen Cove Hosp (page 106); **Address:** One School St, Ste 203, Glen Cove, NY 11542; **Phone:** 516-671-9800; **Board Cert:** Family Medicine 2007; Geriatric Medicine 2008; **Med School:** Italy 1984; **Resid:** Family Medicine, N Shore Univ Hosp 1988

Edelstein, Martin P MD (FMed) *PCP* - **Spec Exp:** Preventive Medicine; **Hospital:** N Shore Univ Hosp (page 106); **Address:** 11 Beverly Rd, Great Neck, NY 11021-1320; **Phone:** 516-487-1614; **Board Cert:** Family Medicine 2008; **Med School:** McGill Univ 1971; **Resid:** Family Medicine, Jewish Genl Hosp 1973; **Fac Appt:** Asst Clin Prof FMed, NYU Sch Med

Moynihan, Brian T DO (FMed) *PCP* - **Spec Exp:** Hypertension; Diabetes; Skin Diseases; **Hospital:** St. Joseph's Hosp-Nassau, N Shore Univ Hosp (page 106); **Address:** 2840 Jerusalem Ave, Wantagh, NY 11793-2017; **Phone:** 516-781-1141; **Med School:** NY Coll Osteo Med 1983; **Resid:** Family Medicine, Massapequa Genl Hosp 1984; Family Medicine, Kennedy Meml Hosp 1985; **Fac Appt:** Asst Prof FMed, NY Coll Osteo Med

Rechter, Lesley MD (FMed) *PCP* - **Spec Exp:** Women's Health; **Hospital:** Stony Brook Univ Med Ctr; **Address:** 54 Birchwood Park Drive, Jericho, NY 11753-2202; **Phone:** 516-933-6850; **Board Cert:** Family Medicine 2003; **Med School:** NY Med Coll 1976; **Resid:** Family Medicine, Nassau County Med Ctr 1979; **Fac Appt:** Assoc Clin Prof FMed, SUNY Stony Brook

Soskel, Neil DO (FMed) *PCP* - **Spec Exp:** Sports Medicine; **Hospital:** South Nassau Comm Hosp; **Address:** 185 Merrick Rd, Ste 1B, Lynbrook, NY 11563; **Phone:** 516-887-0077; **Board Cert:** Family Medicine 2008; **Med School:** NY Coll Osteo Med 1986; **Resid:** Family Medicine, S Nassau Comm Hosp 1989; **Fac Appt:** Assoc Prof FMed, NY Coll Osteo Med

Gastroenterology

Bartolomeo, Robert S MD (Ge) - **Spec Exp:** Colonoscopy; Inflammatory Bowel Disease; Gastroesophageal Reflux Disease (GERD); Colon Cancer Screening; **Hospital:** Winthrop Univ Hosp (page 504); **Address:** 1103 Stewart Ave, Ste 300, Garden City, NY 11530; **Phone:** 516-248-3737; **Board Cert:** Internal Medicine 1974; Gastroenterology 1977; **Med School:** NY Med Coll 1971; **Resid:** Internal Medicine, Metropolitan Hosp Ctr 1973; Internal Medicine, Beth Israel Hosp 1974; **Fellow:** Gastroenterology, Bridgeport Hosp 1976

Bernstein, David E MD (Ge) - **Spec Exp:** Liver Disease; Hepatitis; Colonoscopy; **Hospital:** N Shore Univ Hosp (page 106); **Address:** North Shore Univ Hosp, Div Gastroenterology, 300 Community Drive, Manhasset, NY 11030-3816; **Phone:** 516-562-4281; **Board Cert:** Internal Medicine 2011; Gastroenterology 2003; **Med School:** SUNY Stony Brook 1988; **Resid:** Internal Medicine, Montefiore Med Ctr 1991; **Fellow:** Gastroenterology, Jackson Meml Hosp 1993; **Fac Appt:** Assoc Prof Med, NYU Sch Med

Blumstein, Meyer MD (Ge) - **Spec Exp:** Endoscopy; Gastroesophageal Reflux Disease (GERD); Inflammatory Bowel Disease; **Hospital:** Long Island Jewish Med Ctr (page 106), South Nassau Comm Hosp; **Address:** 158 Hempstead Ave, Lynbrook, NY 11563-1605; **Phone:** 516-593-3541; **Board Cert:** Internal Medicine 1989; **Med School:** SUNY Hlth Sci Ctr 1986; **Resid:** Internal Medicine, LI Jewish Med Ctr 1989; **Fellow:** Gastroenterology, LI Jewish Med Ctr 1991; **Fac Appt:** Asst Prof Med, Albert Einstein Coll Med

Caccese, William MD (Ge) - **Spec Exp:** Endoscopy; Colon Cancer; **Hospital:** Plainview Hosp (page 106); **Address:** 700 Old Country Rd, Ste 206, Plainview, NY 11803-4932; **Phone:** 516-681-1200; **Board Cert:** Internal Medicine 1981; Gastroenterology 1983; **Med School:** SUNY Hlth Sci Ctr 1978; **Resid:** Internal Medicine, N Shore Univ Hosp 1981; **Fellow:** Gastroenterology, N Shore Univ Hosp 1983

Cerulli, Maurice A MD (Ge) - **Spec Exp:** Inflammatory Bowel Disease; Gastroesophageal Reflux Disease (GERD); Colon Cancer Screening; Hepatitis B & C; **Hospital:** Long Island Jewish Med Ctr (page 106), N Shore Univ Hosp (page 106); **Address:** 270-05 76th Ave, rm B202, 410 Lakeville Rd, Ste 107, New Hyde Park, NY 11040; **Phone:** 718-470-7281; **Board Cert:** Internal Medicine 1975; Gastroenterology 1977; **Med School:** SUNY Hlth Sci Ctr 1972; **Resid:** Internal Medicine, Kings County Hosp 1975; **Fellow:** Gastroenterology, Johns Hopkins Hosp 1977; **Fac Appt:** Assoc Clin Prof Med, Hofstra N Shore-LIJ Sch Med

DeVito, Bethany S MD (Ge) - **Spec Exp:** Women's Health; Capsule Endoscopy; **Hospital:** N Shore Univ Hosp (page 106), Long Island Jewish Med Ctr (page 106); **Address:** N Shore Univ Hospital, 4 Levitt Pavilion, 300 Community Drive, Manhasset, NY 11030; **Phone:** 516-562-4281; **Board Cert:** Gastroenterology 2007; **Med School:** SUNY Upstate Med Univ 1992; **Resid:** Internal Medicine, St Vincents Hosp 1995; **Fellow:** Gastroenterology, NY Hosp 1997

Eskreis, David MD (Ge) - **Spec Exp:** Ulcerative Colitis/Crohn's; **Hospital:** NS-LIJ Hlth Sys (page 106); **Address:** 2001 Marcus Ave, Ste W85, Lake Success, NY 11042; **Phone:** 516-326-2700; **Board Cert:** Internal Medicine 1986; Gastroenterology 1987; **Med School:** Geo Wash Univ 1982; **Resid:** Internal Medicine, Bronx Muni Hosp Ctr 1985; **Fellow:** Gastroenterology, Bronx Muni Hosp Ctr 1987

Farber, Charles MD (Ge) - **Spec Exp:** Colon Cancer; Gastroesophageal Reflux Disease (GERD); **Hospital:** Plainview Hosp (page 106); **Address:** 146A Manetto Hill Rd, Ste 205, Plainview, NY 11803; **Phone:** 516-822-4404; **Board Cert:** Internal Medicine 1981; Gastroenterology 1983; **Med School:** SUNY Hlth Sci Ctr 1978; **Resid:** Internal Medicine, N Shore Univ Hosp 1981; **Fellow:** Gastroenterology, Albert Einstein 1983

Goldblum, Lester DO (Ge) - **Spec Exp:** Endoscopy; Colon Cancer; Capsule Endoscopy; **Hospital:** St. Joseph's Hosp-Nassau, Plainview Hosp (page 106); **Address:** Massapequa Gastroenterology, 850 Hicksville Rd, Ste 100, Seaford, NY 11783; **Phone:** 516-796-9000; **Board Cert:** Internal Medicine 1983; **Med School:** Univ Osteo Med & Hlth Sci, Des Moines 1979; **Resid:** Internal Medicine, Nassau County Med Ctr 1983; **Fellow:** Gastroenterology, Nassau County Med Ctr 1985; **Fac Appt:** Asst Clin Prof Med, NY Coll Osteo Med

Gastroenterology

Goldman, Ira S MD (Ge) - **Spec Exp:** Endoscopy & Colonoscopy; Colon Cancer Screening; **Hospital:** N Shore Univ Hosp (page 106), St. Francis Hosp - The Heart Ctr (page 121); **Address:** 310 E Shore Rd, Ste 206, Great Neck, NY 11023-2432; **Phone:** 516-487-7677; **Board Cert:** Internal Medicine 1980; Gastroenterology 1983; **Med School:** Columbia P&S 1977; **Resid:** Internal Medicine, Columbia-Presby Med Ctr 1980; **Fellow:** Gastroenterology, UCSF Med Ctr 1983; **Fac Appt:** Assoc Prof Med, Hofstra N Shore-LIJ Sch Med

Gould, Perry M MD (Ge) - **Spec Exp:** Ulcerative Colitis; Colon & Rectal Cancer; Gastroesophageal Reflux Disease (GERD); Capsule Endoscopy; **Hospital:** Winthrop Univ Hosp (page 504); **Address:** 1103 Stewart Ave, Ste 300, Garden City, NY 11530; **Phone:** 516-248-3737; **Board Cert:** Internal Medicine 1980; Gastroenterology 1983; **Med School:** NY Med Coll 1977; **Resid:** Internal Medicine, LI Jewish Hosp 1980; **Fellow:** Gastroenterology, NY Med Coll 1983; **Fac Appt:** Asst Clin Prof Med, SUNY Stony Brook

Greenberg, Ronald MD (Ge) - **Spec Exp:** Inflammatory Bowel Disease; Peptic Acid Disorders; **Hospital:** Long Island Jewish Med Ctr (page 106); **Address:** 270-05 76th Ave, rm B 202, New Hyde Park, NY 11040; **Phone:** 718-470-7281; **Board Cert:** Internal Medicine 1982; Gastroenterology 1985; **Med School:** Hahnemann Univ 1979; **Resid:** Internal Medicine, Albany Med Ctr 1982; **Fellow:** Gastroenterology, St Luke's Hosp 1985; **Fac Appt:** Assoc Clin Prof Med, Albert Einstein Coll Med

Grendell, James H MD (Ge) - **Spec Exp:** Pancreatic Disease; Nutrition; Liver Disease; **Hospital:** Winthrop Univ Hosp (page 504); **Address:** 222 Station Plaza N, Ste 428, Mineola, NY 11501-3819; **Phone:** 516-663-2066; **Board Cert:** Internal Medicine 1978; Gastroenterology 1981; **Med School:** Ohio State Univ 1975; **Resid:** Internal Medicine, Beth Israel Hosp 1978; **Fellow:** Gastroenterology, UCSF Med Ctr 1981; **Fac Appt:** Prof Med, SUNY Stony Brook

Katz, Seymour MD (Ge) - **Spec Exp:** Inflammatory Bowel Disease; Colonoscopy; Endoscopy; **Hospital:** N Shore Univ Hosp (page 106), Long Island Jewish Med Ctr (page 106); **Address:** 1000 Northern Blvd, Ste 140, Great Neck, NY 11021; **Phone:** 516-466-2340; **Board Cert:** Internal Medicine 1971; Gastroenterology 1972; **Med School:** NYU Sch Med 1964; **Resid:** Internal Medicine, Albert Einstein Sch Med 1966; Internal Medicine, Jacobi Med Ctr 1969; **Fellow:** Gastroenterology, NY Hosp 1971; **Fac Appt:** Asst Clin Prof Med, Cornell Univ-Weill Med Coll

McKinley, Matthew MD (Ge) - **Spec Exp:** Gastroesophageal Reflux Disease (GERD); Barrett's Esophagus; Biliary Disease; **Hospital:** N Shore Univ Hosp (page 106); **Address:** 2800 Marcus Ave, Ste 201, Lake Success, NY 11042; **Phone:** 516-622-6076; **Board Cert:** Internal Medicine 1978; Gastroenterology 1981; **Med School:** Creighton Univ 1975; **Resid:** Internal Medicine, N Shore Univ Hosp 1978; Internal Medicine, Meml Sloan Kettering Cancer Ctr 1978; **Fellow:** Gastroenterology, Yale-New Haven Hosp 1980; **Fac Appt:** Assoc Prof Med, NYU Sch Med

Miller, Seth MD (Ge) - **Hospital:** Long Beach Med Ctr; **Address:** 206 West Park Ave, Long Beach, NY 11561; **Phone:** 516-432-8021; **Board Cert:** Internal Medicine 1983; Gastroenterology 1987; **Med School:** Mount Sinai Sch Med 1980; **Resid:** Internal Medicine, Beth Israel Med Ctr 1983; **Fellow:** Gastroenterology, Beth Israel Med Ctr 1985

Milman, Perry J MD (Ge) - **Spec Exp:** Gastroesophageal Reflux Disease (GERD); Colon Cancer; Inflammatory Bowel Disease; Endoscopy; **Hospital:** Long Island Jewish Med Ctr (page 106), N Shore Univ Hosp (page 106); **Address:** 2001 Marcus Ave, Ste N18, Lake Success, NY 11042-1011; **Phone:** 516-775-7770; **Board Cert:** Internal Medicine 1976; Gastroenterology 1979; **Med School:** SUNY Downstate 1973; **Resid:** Internal Medicine, LI Jewish Med Ctr 1976; **Fellow:** Gastroenterology, VA Hosp/NYU 1978; **Fac Appt:** Asst Clin Prof Med, Albert Einstein Coll Med

Schwartz, Gary MD (Ge) - **Spec Exp:** Colon Cancer Screening; Gastroesophageal Reflux Disease (GERD); **Hospital:** Winthrop Univ Hosp (page 504); **Address:** 1103 Stewart Ave, Ste 300, Garden City, NY 11530; **Phone:** 516-248-3737; **Board Cert:** Internal Medicine 1985; Gastroenterology 1987; **Med School:** Mexico 1979; **Resid:** Internal Medicine, Winthrop Univ Hosp 1983; **Fellow:** Gastroenterology, Univ Hosp 1986

Talansky, Arthur L MD (Ge) - **Spec Exp:** Crohn's Disease; Ulcerative Colitis; Colonoscopy; **Hospital:** N Shore Univ Hosp (page 106), St. Francis Hosp - The Heart Ctr (page 121); **Address:** 233 E Shore Rd, Ste 101, Great Neck, NY 11023-2433; **Phone:** 516-487-2444; **Board Cert:** Internal Medicine 1980; Gastroenterology 1983; **Med School:** Mount Sinai Sch Med 1977; **Resid:** Internal Medicine, Meml Sloan Kettering Cancer Ctr 1980; **Fellow:** Gastroenterology, Mount Sinai Hosp 1982; **Fac Appt:** Asst Clin Prof Med, NYU Sch Med

Weissman, Gary S MD (Ge) - **Spec Exp:** Gastrointestinal Cancer; Inflammatory Bowel Disease; Esophageal Disorders; **Hospital:** N Shore Univ Hosp (page 106), Long Island Jewish Med Ctr (page 106); **Address:** 2800 Marcus Ave, Ste 201, Lake Success, NY 11042; **Phone:** 516-622-6076; **Board Cert:** Internal Medicine 1980; Gastroenterology 1983; **Med School:** NY Med Coll 1976; **Resid:** Internal Medicine, North Shore Univ Hosp 1980; **Fellow:** Gastroenterology, Meml Sloan Kettering Cancer Ctr 1982; **Fac Appt:** Assoc Clin Prof Med, NYU Sch Med

Geriatric Medicine

Berger, Jeffrey MD (Ger) *PCP* - **Spec Exp:** Ethics; Palliative Care; Geriatric Care; **Hospital:** Winthrop Univ Hosp (page 504); **Address:** 222 Station Plaza North, Ste 518, Mineola, NY 11501-3893; **Phone:** 516-663-2588; **Board Cert:** Internal Medicine 2001; Hospice & Palliative Medicine 2008; **Med School:** SUNY Stony Brook 1988; **Resid:** Internal Medicine, Winthrop Univ Hosp 1991; **Fac Appt:** Assoc Prof Med, SUNY Stony Brook

Gomolin, Irving MD (Ger) - **Spec Exp:** Medications in the Elderly; Dementia; **Hospital:** Winthrop Univ Hosp (page 504); **Address:** 222 Station Plaza N, Fl 5, Ste 518, Mineola, NY 11501; **Phone:** 516-663-2588; **Board Cert:** Internal Medicine 1979; Geriatric Medicine 2008; **Med School:** McGill Univ 1976; **Resid:** Internal Medicine, Jewish Genl Hosp 1978; Internal Medicine, Beth Israel Hosp 1981; **Fellow:** Clinical Pharmacology, Harvard Med Sch 1980; **Fac Appt:** Clin Prof Med, SUNY Stony Brook

Guzik, Howard MD (Ger) *PCP* - **Hospital:** N Shore Univ Hosp (page 106); **Address:** 2800 Marcus Ave Ste 200, New Hyde Park, NY 11042; **Phone:** 516-708-2510; **Board Cert:** Internal Medicine 1981; Geriatric Medicine 2008; Hospice & Palliative Medicine 2010; **Med School:** Albert Einstein Coll Med 1984; **Resid:** Internal Medicine, Montefiore Med Ctr 1985; **Fellow:** Geriatric Medicine, Montefiore Med Ctr 1986

Lanman, Geraldine MD (Ger) *PCP* - **Spec Exp:** Geriatric Medicine; **Hospital:** Long Island Jewish Med Ctr (page 106); **Address:** 1 Delaware Drive, Ste 48, New Hyde Park, NY 11042; **Phone:** 516-326-5320; **Board Cert:** Internal Medicine 1983; **Med School:** Univ Calgary 1980; **Resid:** Internal Medicine, LIJ Med Ctr 1986; **Fellow:** Geriatric Medicine, LIJ Med Ctr 1988; **Fac Appt:** Asst Clin Prof Med, Albert Einstein Coll Med

Macina, Lucy MD (Ger) *PCP* - **Spec Exp:** Frail Elderly; Dementia; **Hospital:** Winthrop Univ Hosp (page 504); **Address:** 222 Station Plaza N, Ste 518, Mineola, NY 11501-3893; **Phone:** 516-663-2588; **Board Cert:** Internal Medicine 1982; Geriatric Medicine 2002; **Med School:** Loyola Univ-Stritch Sch Med 1978; **Resid:** Internal Medicine, VA Hosp 1980; Internal Medicine, Loyola Univ Med Ctr 1982; **Fellow:** Geriatric Medicine, Roger Williams Hosp 1985; **Fac Appt:** Asst Clin Prof Med, SUNY Stony Brook

Wolf-Klein, Gisele MD (Ger) *PCP* - **Spec Exp:** Dementia; Falls in the Elderly; Alzheimer's Disease; **Hospital:** Long Island Jewish Med Ctr (page 106); **Address:** 2800 Marcus Ave, Lake Success, NY 11042; **Phone:** 516-708-2520; **Board Cert:** Internal Medicine 1984; Geriatric Medicine 2012; **Med School:** Switzerland 1975; **Resid:** Internal Medicine, Long Island Hosp 1978; **Fellow:** Geriatric Medicine, LI Jewish Med Ctr 1979; **Fac Appt:** Prof Med, Hofstra N Shore-LIJ Sch Med

Gynecologic Oncology

Chalas, Eva MD (GO) - **Spec Exp:** Gynecologic Cancer; Minimally Invasive Surgery; **Hospital:** Winthrop Univ Hosp (page 504); **Address:** 200 Old Country Rd, Ste 365, Mineola, NY 11501; **Phone:** 516-294-5440; **Board Cert:** Obstetrics & Gynecology 2011; Gynecologic Oncology 2011; **Med School:** SUNY Stony Brook 1981; **Resid:** Obstetrics & Gynecology, Univ Hosp 1985; **Fellow:** Gynecologic Oncology, Meml Sloan Kettering Cancer Ctr 1987; **Fac Appt:** Prof ObG, SUNY Stony Brook

Lovecchio, John L MD (GO) - **Spec Exp:** Ovarian Cancer; Uterine Cancer; Cervical Cancer; Vulvar Disease/Cancer; **Hospital:** N Shore Univ Hosp (page 106), Long Island Jewish Med Ctr (page 106); **Address:** North Shore Hospital, 10 Monti, 300 Community Drive, Manhasset, NY 11030-3816; **Phone:** 516-562-4438; **Board Cert:** Obstetrics & Gynecology 2005; Gynecologic Oncology 2005; **Med School:** SUNY Buffalo 1975; **Resid:** Obstetrics & Gynecology, Univ Hosp Case West Res 1979; **Fellow:** Gynecologic Oncology, Jackson Meml Hosp 1982; **Fac Appt:** Prof ObG, NYU Sch Med

Menzin, Andrew William MD (GO) - **Spec Exp:** Uterine Cancer; Ovarian Cancer; Cervical Cancer; **Hospital:** N Shore Univ Hosp (page 106), Long Island Jewish Med Ctr (page 106); **Address:** 300 Community Drive, 10 Monti, Manhasset, NY 11030-3816; **Phone:** 516-562-4438; **Board Cert:** Obstetrics & Gynecology 2011; Gynecologic Oncology 2011; **Med School:** NYU Sch Med 1989; **Resid:** Obstetrics & Gynecology, Hosp Univ Penn 1993; **Fellow:** Gynecologic Oncology, Hosp Univ Penn 1995; **Fac Appt:** Prof ObG, Hofstra N Shore-LIJ Sch Med

Hand Surgery

Gluck, Robert I MD (HS) - **Spec Exp:** Microvascular Surgery; Dupuytren's Contracture; Carpal Tunnel Syndrome; Minimally Invasive Surgery; **Hospital:** NS-LIJ Hlth Sys (page 106), Long Island Jewish Med Ctr (page 106); **Address:** Hand Center Long Island NY, 410 Lakeville Rd, Ste 310, New Hyde Park, NY 11042; **Phone:** 516-280-5844; **Board Cert:** Hand Surgery 2002; **Med School:** Albert Einstein Coll Med 1982; **Resid:** Surgery, Long Island Jewish Hosp 1987; **Fellow:** Hand & Microvascular Surgery, Stony Brook Univ Med Ctr 1989; **Fac Appt:** Asst Clin Prof S, Albert Einstein Coll Med

Kamler, Kenneth M MD (HS) - **Spec Exp:** Carpal Tunnel Syndrome; Arthritis; Fractures; **Hospital:** NS-LIJ Hlth Sys (page 106); **Address:** 410 Lakeville Rd, Ste 303, New Hyde Park, NY 11042; **Phone:** 516-326-2266; **Med School:** France 1975; **Resid:** Orthopaedic Surgery, LI Jewish Med Ctr 1979; **Fellow:** Hand Surgery, Columbia-Presby Med Ctr 1981

Lane, Lewis B MD (HS) - **Spec Exp:** Carpal Tunnel Syndrome; Arthritis; Sports Injuries; Hand Reconstruction; **Hospital:** N Shore Univ Hosp (page 106), St. Francis Hosp - The Heart Ctr (page 121); **Address:** University Orthopaedics, 611 Northern Blvd, Ste 200, Great Neck, NY 11021; **Phone:** 516-723-2663; **Board Cert:** Orthopaedic Surgery 1981; Hand Surgery 2010; **Med School:** Columbia P&S 1974; **Resid:** Surgery, NY Hosp 1975; Orthopaedic Surgery, Hosp for Special Surg 1979; **Fellow:** Research, Hosp for Special Surg 1976; Hand Surgery, St Luke's-Roosevelt Hosp Ctr 1980; **Fac Appt:** Assoc Clin Prof OrS, Albany Med Coll

Teplitz, Glenn A MD (HS) - **Spec Exp:** Carpal Tunnel Syndrome; Fractures; Sports Injuries; Wrist/Hand Injuries; **Hospital:** Winthrop Univ Hosp (page 504); **Address:** Winthrop Orthopaedic Assocs, 1300 Franklin Ave, Ste UL-3A, Garden City, NY 11530; **Phone:** 516-747-8900; **Board Cert:** Orthopaedic Surgery 2007; **Med School:** Tulane Univ 1987; **Resid:** Orthopaedic Surgery, UMDNJ Med Ctr 1993; **Fellow:** Hand Surgery, Hosp for Special Surgery 1994; **Fac Appt:** Asst Clin Prof OrS, SUNY Stony Brook

Tuckman, David MD (HS) - **Hospital:** NS-LIJ Hlth Sys (page 106), St. Francis Hosp - The Heart Ctr (page 121); **Address:** 600 Northern Blvd Ste 300, Great Neck, NY 11021; **Phone:** 516-627-8717; **Board Cert:** Orthopaedic Surgery 2007; Hand Surgery 2009; **Med School:** Albert Einstein Coll Med 1998; **Resid:** Orthopaedic Surgery, Long Island Jewish Med Ctr 2003; **Fellow:** Sports Medicine & Shoulder Surgery, Hosp for Joint Diseases 2004; Hand Surgery, Hosp for Joint Diseases 2005

Hematology

Allen, Steven Lee MD (Hem) - **Spec Exp:** Bleeding/Coagulation Disorders; Leukemia & Lymphoma; Multiple Myeloma; Gaucher Disease; **Hospital:** N Shore Univ Hosp (page 106), Long Island Jewish Med Ctr (page 106); **Address:** Monter Cancer Ctr, 450 Lakeville Rd, Lake Success, NY 11042; **Phone:** 516-734-8959; **Board Cert:** Internal Medicine 1980; Hematology 1982; Medical Oncology 1983; **Med School:** Johns Hopkins Univ 1977; **Resid:** Internal Medicine, NY Hosp-Cornell 1980; **Fellow:** Hematology & Oncology, NY Hosp-Cornell 1983; **Fac Appt:** Prof Med, Hofstra N Shore-LIJ Sch Med

Kolitz, Jonathan E MD (Hem) - **Spec Exp:** Leukemia & Lymphoma; Hodgkin's Lymphoma; Multiple Myeloma; Myelodysplastic Syndromes; **Hospital:** N Shore Univ Hosp (page 106); **Address:** 450 Lakeville Rd, Lake Success, NY 11042; **Phone:** 516-734-8970; **Board Cert:** Internal Medicine 1982; Medical Oncology 1985; Hematology 1988; **Med School:** Yale Univ 1979; **Resid:** Internal Medicine, N Shore Univ Hosp 1982; **Fellow:** Hematology & Oncology, Meml Sloan Kettering Cancer Ctr 1985; **Fac Appt:** Prof Hem & Onc, Hofstra N Shore-LIJ Sch Med

Rai, Kanti R MD (Hem) - **Spec Exp:** Leukemia; Lymphoma; Multiple Myeloma; **Hospital:** Long Island Jewish Med Ctr (page 106); **Address:** 410 Lakeville Rd, Ste 212, Long Island Jewish Med Ctr, Div of Hem-Onc, New Hyde Park, NY 10042; **Phone:** 718-470-4050; **Board Cert:** Pediatrics 1959; **Med School:** India 1955; **Resid:** Pediatrics, Lincoln Hosp 1958; Pediatrics, North Shore Univ Hosp 1959; **Fellow:** Hematology, LI Jewish Med Ctr 1960; **Fac Appt:** Prof Med, Albert Einstein Coll Med

Staszewski, Harry MD (Hem) - **Spec Exp:** Hematologic Malignancies; **Hospital:** Winthrop Univ Hosp (page 504); **Address:** 200 Old Country Rd, Ste 450, Mineola, NY 11501; **Phone:** 516-663-9500; **Board Cert:** Internal Medicine 1981; Medical Oncology 1983; Hematology 1984; **Med School:** Yale Univ 1978; **Resid:** Internal Medicine, N Shore Univ Hosp 1981; **Fellow:** Medical Oncology, Meml Sloan Kettering Cancer Ctr 1983; Hematology, LI Jewish Hosp 1984; **Fac Appt:** Asst Prof Med, SUNY Stony Brook

Infectious Disease

Cervia, Joseph S MD (Inf) - **Spec Exp:** AIDS/HIV; Travel Medicine; Pediatric Infections; Immune Deficiency; **Hospital:** N Shore Univ Hosp (page 106), Steven & Alexandra Cohen Chldn's Med Ctr of NY (page 106); **Address:** North Shore-LIJ Health System, 300 Community Drive, Manhasset, NY 11030; **Phone:** 516-562-4280; **Board Cert:** Internal Medicine 1989; Pediatrics 2003; Infectious Disease 2010; Pediatric Infectious Disease 2009; **Med School:** NY Med Coll 1984; **Resid:** Internal Medicine & Pediatrics, Brookdale Hosp 1988; **Fellow:** Infectious Disease, New York Hosp/Cornell 1990; **Fac Appt:** Clin Prof Med, Albert Einstein Coll Med

Cunha, Burke A MD (Inf) - **Spec Exp:** Infections in Immunocompromised Patients; Fevers of Unknown Origin; Pneumonia; Chronic Fatigue Syndrome; **Hospital:** Winthrop Univ Hosp (page 504); **Address:** 222 Station Plz N, Ste 432, Mineola, NY 11501; **Phone:** 516-663-2507; **Board Cert:** Internal Medicine 1977; Infectious Disease 1978; **Med School:** Penn State Coll Med 1972; **Resid:** Internal Medicine, Hartford Hosp 1975; **Fellow:** Infectious Disease, Hartford Hosp 1977; **Fac Appt:** Prof Med, SUNY Stony Brook

Farber, Bruce MD (Inf) - **Hospital:** NS-LIJ Hlth Sys (page 106); **Address:** N Shore Univ Hosp, Div Infectious Dis, 400 Community Drive, Manhasset, NY 11030; **Phone:** 516-562-4280; **Board Cert:** Internal Medicine 1979; Infectious Disease 1984; **Med School:** Northwestern Univ 1976; **Resid:** Internal Medicine, Univ Va Hosp 1979; **Fellow:** Infectious Disease, Mass Genl Hosp 1982

Hirsch, Bruce E MD (Inf) - **Spec Exp:** Infectious Disease in Elderly; **Hospital:** NS-LIJ Hlth Sys (page 106), Long Island Jewish Med Ctr (page 106); **Address:** N Shore Univ Hosp, Infectious Disease, 400 Community Drive, Manhasset, NY 11030; **Phone:** 516-562-4280; **Board Cert:** Internal Medicine 1986; Geriatric Medicine 2007; Infectious Disease 2004; **Med School:** Cornell Univ-Weill Med Coll 1982; **Resid:** Internal Medicine, N Shore Univ Hosp 1986; Geriatric Medicine, NY-Presby/Weill Cornell Med Ctr 1988; **Fellow:** Infectious Disease, Jacobi Med Ctr 1989; Infectious Disease, N Shore Univ Hosp 1994

Johnson, Diane H MD (Inf) - **Spec Exp:** AIDS/HIV; Sexually Transmitted Diseases; Travel Medicine; **Hospital:** Winthrop Univ Hosp (page 504); **Address:** 222 Station Plaza N, Ste 432, Mineola, NY 11501; **Phone:** 516-663-2507; **Board Cert:** Internal Medicine 2004; Infectious Disease 2004; **Med School:** Univ VT Coll Med 1989; **Resid:** Internal Medicine, Winthrop Univ Hosp 1992; **Fellow:** Infectious Disease, Winthrop Univ Hosp 1994; **Fac Appt:** Asst Prof Med, SUNY Stony Brook

Klein, Natalie MD (Inf) - **Hospital:** Winthrop Univ Hosp (page 504); **Address:** 222 Station Plaza N, Ste 432, Mineola, NY 11501-3957; **Phone:** 516-663-2507; **Board Cert:** Internal Medicine 1982; Infectious Disease 1984; **Med School:** Jefferson Med Coll 1979; **Resid:** Internal Medicine, Mount Sinai Hosp 1982; **Fellow:** Infectious Disease, Mount Sinai Hosp 1984; **Fac Appt:** Assoc Prof Med, SUNY Stony Brook

McGowan, Joseph MD (Inf) - **Spec Exp:** AIDS/HIV; HIV in Pregnancy; HIV & Hepatitis co-infection; AIDS/HIV in Elderly; **Hospital:** NS-LIJ Hlth Sys (page 106); **Address:** 400 Community Drive, Manhasset, NY 11030; **Phone:** 516-562-4280; **Board Cert:** Internal Medicine 2002; Infectious Disease 2002; **Med School:** Mount Sinai Sch Med 1987; **Resid:** Internal Medicine, Montefiore Med Ctr 1990; **Fellow:** Infectious Disease, Montefiore Med Ctr 1993

Scheer, Max MD (Inf) - **Spec Exp:** Skin/Soft Tissue Infections; Infections-Respiratory; Sexually Transmitted Diseases; **Hospital:** N Shore Univ Hosp (page 106); **Address:** 15 Irving Pl, Woodmere, NY 11598-1229; **Phone:** 516-374-6750; **Board Cert:** Internal Medicine 1979; Infectious Disease 1982; **Med School:** SUNY Downstate 1975; **Resid:** Family Medicine, Kings Co Hosp-SUNY 1978; Internal Medicine, Morristown Meml Hosp 1979; **Fellow:** Infectious Disease, Mt Sinai Hosp 1981; **Fac Appt:** Asst Clin Prof Med, NYU Sch Med

Internal Medicine

Ammazzalorso, Michael MD (IM) _PCP_ - **Spec Exp:** Hypertension; Diabetes; **Hospital:** Winthrop Univ Hosp (page 504); **Address:** 222 Station Plz N, Ste 310, Mineola, NY 11501-3893; **Phone:** 516-663-2051; **Board Cert:** Internal Medicine 2010; Geriatric Medicine 1999; **Med School:** SUNY Downstate 1987; **Resid:** Internal Medicine, Staten Island Hosp 1991; **Fac Appt:** Asst Prof Med, SUNY Stony Brook

Berbari, Nicholas E MD (IM) *PCP* - **Hospital:** Winthrop Univ Hosp (page 504); **Address:** 222 Station Plaza N, Ste 310, Mineola, NY 11501; **Phone:** 516-663-2051; **Board Cert:** Internal Medicine 2006; **Med School:** SUNY Stony Brook 1993; **Resid:** Internal Medicine, Winthrop Univ Hosp 1997; **Fac Appt:** Asst Prof Med, SUNY Stony Brook

Corapi, Mark MD (IM) *PCP* - **Hospital:** Winthrop Univ Hosp (page 504); **Address:** 222 Station Plaza N, Ste 310, Mineola, NY 11501; **Phone:** 516-663-2051; **Board Cert:** Internal Medicine 1985; **Med School:** SUNY Downstate 1982; **Resid:** Internal Medicine, Long Island Jewish Med Ctr 1985; **Fellow:** Internal Medicine, Long Island Jewish Med Ctr 1986; **Fac Appt:** Assoc Prof Med, SUNY Stony Brook

Cusumano, Stephen P MD (IM) *PCP* - **Spec Exp:** Hypertension; Asthma; **Hospital:** St. Joseph's Hosp-Nassau, Winthrop Univ Hosp (page 504); **Address:** 850 Hicksville Rd, Ste 104, Seaford, NY 11783; **Phone:** 516-735-5454; **Board Cert:** Internal Medicine 1988; **Med School:** Univ Hlth Scis, Chicago Med Sch 1985; **Resid:** Internal Medicine, Winthrop Univ Hosp 1988

Federbush, Richard MD (IM) *PCP* - **Spec Exp:** Hypertension; Cholesterol/Lipid Disorders; Diabetes; **Hospital:** Plainview Hosp (page 106), Syosset Hosp (page 106); **Address:** 175 Jericho Tpke, Ste 216, Syosset, NY 11791; **Phone:** 516-364-9800; **Board Cert:** Internal Medicine 2012; **Med School:** Mexico 1985; **Resid:** Internal Medicine, Univ Hosp-SUNY 1989; **Fac Appt:** Asst Clin Prof Med, Hofstra N Shore-LIJ Sch Med

Gelberg, Burt MD (IM) *PCP* - **Spec Exp:** Preventive Medicine; Colonoscopy; Gastroscopy; **Hospital:** Franklin Hosp (page 106); **Address:** 401 Franklin Ave, Franklin Square, Franklin Square, NY 11010-1227; **Phone:** 516-326-2255; **Board Cert:** Internal Medicine 1975; **Med School:** SUNY Hlth Sci Ctr 1972; **Resid:** Internal Medicine, Lenox Hill Hosp 1975; **Fellow:** Gastroenterology, Lenox Hill Hosp 1977

Goodman, Michael MD (IM) - **Hospital:** South Nassau Comm Hosp; **Address:** 2495 Newbridge Rd, Bellmore, NY 11710; **Phone:** 516-826-1200; **Board Cert:** Internal Medicine 1980; **Med School:** Italy 1975; **Resid:** Internal Medicine, Nassau County Med Ctr 1978

Gorski, Lydia E MD (IM) *PCP* - **Spec Exp:** Women's Health; Geriatric Medicine; Preventive Medicine; **Hospital:** Winthrop Univ Hosp (page 504), N Shore Univ Hosp (page 106); **Address:** 820 Jericho Tpke, New Hyde Park, NY 11040-4514; **Phone:** 516-352-0430; **Board Cert:** Internal Medicine 1988; **Med School:** Poland 1982; **Resid:** Internal Medicine, St Vincent's Catholic Med Ctrs 1987

Gottridge, Joanne MD (IM) *PCP* - **Hospital:** N Shore Univ Hosp (page 106), Long Island Jewish Med Ctr (page 106); **Address:** 865 Northern Blvd, Ste 102, Great Neck, NY 11021; **Phone:** 516-622-5001; **Board Cert:** Internal Medicine 1983; **Med School:** Case West Res Univ 1980; **Resid:** Internal Medicine, N Shore Univ Hosp 1983; **Fac Appt:** Assoc Prof Med, NYU Sch Med

Hotchkiss, Edward MD (IM) *PCP* - **Hospital:** South Nassau Comm Hosp; **Address:** 158 Hempstead Ave, Lynbrook, NY 11563; **Phone:** 516-593-3541; **Board Cert:** Internal Medicine 1972; **Med School:** SUNY Hlth Sci Ctr 1965; **Resid:** Internal Medicine, LI Jewish Med Ctr 1972; **Fellow:** Psychiatry, Univ Hosp 1971; **Fac Appt:** Assoc Prof Med, Albert Einstein Coll Med

Leong, Pauline MD (IM) *PCP* - **Hospital:** N Shore Univ Hosp (page 106); **Address:** 865 Northern Blvd, Ste 102, Great Neck, NY 11021-5310; **Phone:** 516-622-5000; **Board Cert:** Internal Medicine 1988; **Med School:** NYU Sch Med 1983; **Resid:** Internal Medicine, New York Hosp 1988

Pollak, Harvey MD (IM) *PCP* - **Spec Exp:** Hypertension; Heart Disease; Cholesterol/Lipid Disorders; **Hospital:** N Shore Univ Hosp (page 106); **Address:** 2 Prohealth Plaza Fl 1st - Ste 101, Lake Success, NY 11042; **Phone:** 516-622-6020; **Board Cert:** Internal Medicine 1974; **Med School:** Ros Franklin Univ/Chicago Med Sch 1971; **Resid:** Internal Medicine, Meml Sloan Kettering Cancer Ctr 1973; Internal Medicine, N Shore Univ Hosp 1975; **Fac Appt:** Clin Prof Med, NYU Sch Med

Rakowitz, Frederic MD (IM) *PCP* - **Spec Exp:** Preventive Medicine; **Hospital:** N Shore Univ Hosp (page 106); **Address:** 295 Northern Blvd, Ste 208, Great Neck, NY 11021-4701; **Phone:** 516-482-4940; **Board Cert:** Internal Medicine 1981; **Med School:** Albany Med Coll 1978; **Resid:** Internal Medicine, North Shore Univ Hosp 1981

Rubenstein, Jack MD (IM) *PCP* - **Spec Exp:** Complex Diagnosis; Kidney Failure-Chronic; Geriatric Care; Dialysis Care; **Hospital:** Franklin Hosp (page 106), N Shore Univ Hosp (page 106); **Address:** 70 Glen Cove Rd, Ste 301, Roslyn Heights, NY 11577-1731; **Phone:** 516-621-1502; **Board Cert:** Internal Medicine 2008; Nephrology 2009; Geriatric Medicine 2008; **Med School:** NY Med Coll 1976; **Resid:** Internal Medicine, North Shore Univ Hosp 1979; Nephrology, North Shore Univ Hosp 1980; **Fellow:** Nephrology, NYU Med Ctr 1982; **Fac Appt:** Assoc Clin Prof Med, NYU Sch Med

Rucker, Steve MD (IM) *PCP* - **Spec Exp:** Hypertension; Kidney Disease; Kidney Stones; **Hospital:** St. Francis Hosp - The Heart Ctr (page 121), Long Island Jewish Med Ctr (page 106); **Address:** 1999 Marcus Ave, Ste 216, Lake Success, NY 11042; **Phone:** 516-775-4545; **Board Cert:** Internal Medicine 1986; Nephrology 1988; **Med School:** Univ Pittsburgh 1983; **Resid:** Internal Medicine, LI Jewish Med Ctr 1986; **Fellow:** Nephrology, Mount Sinai Med Ctr 1988

Taubman, Lowell MD (IM) *PCP* - **Spec Exp:** Dementia; Alzheimer's Disease; **Hospital:** Long Beach Med Ctr; **Address:** 206 Riverside Blvd, Long Beach, NY 11561; **Phone:** 516-432-5670; **Board Cert:** Internal Medicine 1988; **Med School:** Mexico 1980; **Resid:** Internal Medicine, Montefiore Hosp 1983; Internal Medicine, St Clares Hosp 1984; **Fellow:** Geriatric Medicine, Jewish Inst Geriatric Care 1986

Timpone, Leonard MD (IM) *PCP* - **Spec Exp:** Geriatric Medicine; Headache; **Hospital:** Franklin Hosp (page 106), Mercy Med Ctr - Rockville Centre; **Address:** 1051 Adams Ave, Franklin Square, NY 11010-2251; **Phone:** 516-354-4858; **Board Cert:** Internal Medicine 2004; **Med School:** France 1984; **Resid:** Internal Medicine, NY Downtown Hosp 1988

Weinstein, Jay MD (IM) *PCP* - **Hospital:** Lenox Hill Hosp (page 106); **Address:** 865 Northern Blvd, Ste 102, Great Neck, NY 11021; **Phone:** 516-622-5000 x8; **Board Cert:** Internal Medicine 2000; **Med School:** Hahnemann Univ 1987; **Resid:** Internal Medicine, St Vincents Hosp Med Ctr 1990

Weinstein, Mark J MD (IM) *PCP* - **Spec Exp:** Hypertension; Diabetes; Cholesterol/Lipid Disorders; **Hospital:** Plainview Hosp (page 106), St. Joseph's Hosp-Nassau; **Address:** 4045 Hempstead Tpke Fl 3, Bethpage, NY 11714-5706; **Phone:** 516-731-7770; **Board Cert:** Internal Medicine 1978; Infectious Disease 1980; **Med School:** Harvard Med Sch 1975; **Resid:** Internal Medicine, Univ Hosp 1978; **Fellow:** Infectious Disease, Univ Hosp 1980

Wolff, Edward MD (IM) *PCP* - **Spec Exp:** Asthma; Heart Disease; **Hospital:** St. Francis Hosp - The Heart Ctr (page 121), N Shore Univ Hosp (page 106); **Address:** 107 Northern Blvd, Ste 404, Great Neck, NY 11021; **Phone:** 516-498-1818; **Board Cert:** Internal Medicine 1987; **Med School:** Georgetown Univ 1966; **Resid:** Internal Medicine, Metro Hosp Ctr 1970; **Fellow:** Pulmonary Disease, Metro Hosp Ctr 1971; **Fac Appt:** Med, Cornell Univ-Weill Med Coll

Interventional Cardiology

Abittan, Meyer H MD (IC) - **Spec Exp:** Angiography-Coronary; Preventive Cardiology; **Hospital:** St. Francis Hosp - The Heart Ctr (page 121); **Address:** St Francis Hosp, The Heart Ctr, 100 Port Washington Blvd, Ste G-03, Roslyn, NY 11576; **Phone:** 516-627-1155; **Board Cert:** Internal Medicine 1989; **Med School:** Mount Sinai Sch Med 1986; **Resid:** Internal Medicine, Brookdale Univ Hosp Med Ctr 1989; **Fellow:** Cardiovascular Disease, Mt Sinai Med Ctr 1990

Berke, Andrew D MD (IC) - **Hospital:** St. Francis Hosp - The Heart Ctr (page 121), South Nassau Comm Hosp; **Address:** 100 Port Washington Blvd, Roslyn, NY 11576; **Phone:** 516-365-2211; **Board Cert:** Internal Medicine 1982; Cardiovascular Disease 1985; Interventional Cardiology 2009; **Med School:** Brown Univ 1979; **Resid:** Internal Medicine, Columbia-Presby Med Ctr 1982; **Fellow:** Cardiovascular Disease, Columbia-Presby Med Ctr 1985; **Fac Appt:** Asst Clin Prof Med, Columbia P&S

Lituchy, Andrew MD (IC) - **Spec Exp:** Coronary Artery Disease; Angioplasty & Stent Placement; Peripheral Vascular Disease; Interventional Cardiology; **Hospital:** St. Francis Hosp - The Heart Ctr (page 121), South Nassau Comm Hosp; **Address:** 100 Port Washington Blvd, Ste G-05, Roslyn, NY 11576-1353; **Phone:** 516-365-4888; **Board Cert:** Cardiovascular Disease 2005; **Med School:** Hahnemann Univ 1988; **Resid:** Internal Medicine, Bronx Muni/Albert Einstein Med Ctr 1991; **Fellow:** Cardiovascular Disease, NY-Cornell Med Ctr 1994; Interventional Cardiology, NY-Cornell Med Ctr 1995

Petrossian, George A MD (IC) - **Spec Exp:** Carotid Artery Stent Placement; Peripheral Vascular Disease; Coronary Angioplasty/Stents; Renovascular Disease; **Hospital:** St. Francis Hosp - The Heart Ctr (page 121), South Nassau Comm Hosp; **Address:** 1405 Old Northern Blvd, 1st Floor, Roslyn, NY 11576-1353; **Phone:** 516-484-6777; **Board Cert:** Internal Medicine 1986; Cardiovascular Disease 1989; Interventional Cardiology 2010; **Med School:** Mount Sinai Sch Med 1983; **Resid:** Internal Medicine, Columbia-Presby Med Ctr 1987; **Fellow:** Cardiovascular Disease, Columbia -Presby Med Ctr 1989; Interventional Cardiology, Mass Genl Hosp 1990

Zisfein, Jerome B MD (IC) - **Spec Exp:** Coronary Angioplasty/Stents; Pacemakers; Cardiac Cathetherization; **Hospital:** N Shore Univ Hosp (page 106), Winthrop Univ Hosp (page 504); **Address:** South Shore Heart Assocs, 242 Merrick Rd, Ste 402, Rockville Centre, NY 11570-5254; **Phone:** 516-763-2800; **Board Cert:** Internal Medicine 1984; Cardiovascular Disease 1987; Interventional Cardiology 2010; **Med School:** NY Med Coll 1981; **Resid:** Internal Medicine, Rhode Island Hosp 1984; **Fellow:** Cardiovascular Disease, Mass Gen Hosp 1989

Maternal & Fetal Medicine

Fleischer, Adiel MD (MF) - **Spec Exp:** Pregnancy-High Risk; **Hospital:** Long Island Jewish Med Ctr (page 106), N Shore Univ Hosp (page 106); **Address:** LIJ Med Ctr, Dept ObGyn, 270-05 76th Ave, rm 471, New Hyde Park, NY 11040-1433; **Phone:** 718-470-5466; **Board Cert:** Obstetrics & Gynecology 1999; Maternal & Fetal Medicine 1999; **Med School:** Romania 1972; **Resid:** Obstetrics & Gynecology, Maimonides Med Ctr 1975; **Fellow:** Maternal & Fetal Medicine, Montefiore Med Ctr 1976; **Fac Appt:** Assoc Prof ObG, Hofstra N Shore-LIJ Sch Med

Klein, Victor R MD (MF) - **Spec Exp:** Multiple Gestation; Pregnancy-High Risk; Genetic Disorders; **Hospital:** N Shore Univ Hosp (page 106), Long Island Jewish Med Ctr (page 106); **Address:** 825 Northern Blvd, Ste 301, Great Neck, NY 11021-5302; **Phone:** 516-472-5700; **Board Cert:** Obstetrics & Gynecology 2011; Maternal & Fetal Medicine 2011; Clinical Genetics 2004; **Med School:** SUNY Downstate 1980; **Resid:** Internal Medicine, Kings Co Hosp Ctr 1981; Obstetrics & Gynecology, Johns Hopkins Hosp 1985; **Fellow:** Clinical Genetics, Univ Texas SW Med Ctr 1987; Maternal & Fetal Medicine, Univ Texas SW Med Ctr 1987; **Fac Appt:** Assoc Clin Prof ObG, NYU Sch Med

Meirowitz, Natalie MD (MF) - **Spec Exp:** Prenatal Diagnosis; Pregnancy Loss; Pregnancy-High Risk; **Hospital:** NS-LIJ Hlth Sys (page 106); **Address:** LIJ Med Ctr, Dept Ob/Gyn, 270-05 76th Ave, rm 471, New Hyde Park, NY 11040; **Phone:** 516-470-7636; **Board Cert:** Obstetrics & Gynecology 2011; Maternal & Fetal Medicine 2011; **Med School:** Harvard Med Sch 1993; **Resid:** Obstetrics & Gynecology, North Shore Univ Med Ctr 1997; **Fellow:** Maternal & Fetal Medicine, UMDNJ Med Ctr 2000; **Fac Appt:** Asst Prof ObG, Albert Einstein Coll Med

Rochelson, Burton L MD (MF) - **Spec Exp:** Pregnancy-High Risk; Ultrasound; Prenatal Diagnosis; **Hospital:** N Shore Univ Hosp (page 106); **Address:** 300 Community Drive, Levitt Bldg - Fl 3, Manhasset, NY 11030-3876; **Phone:** 516-562-2892; **Board Cert:** Obstetrics & Gynecology 2011; Maternal & Fetal Medicine 2011; **Med School:** Univ Mich Med Sch 1978; **Resid:** Obstetrics & Gynecology, LI Jewish Med Ctr 1982; **Fellow:** Maternal & Fetal Medicine, Univ Hosp 1986; **Fac Appt:** Prof ObG, Hofstra N Shore-LIJ Sch Med

Vintzileos, Anthony M MD (MF) - **Spec Exp:** Ultrasound; Fetal Therapy; **Hospital:** Winthrop Univ Hosp (page 504); **Address:** Women's Contemporary Care Assocs, 120 Mineola Blvd Ste 100, Mineola, NY 11501; **Phone:** 516-663-8657; **Board Cert:** Obstetrics & Gynecology 1999; Maternal & Fetal Medicine 1999; **Med School:** Greece 1975; **Resid:** Obstetrics & Gynecology, St Josephs Hosp Med Ctr 1981; **Fellow:** Maternal & Fetal Medicine, Univ Conn Hlth Ctr 1983; **Fac Appt:** Prof ObG, UMDNJ-RW Johnson Med Sch

Medical Oncology

Arena, Francis P MD (Onc) - **Spec Exp:** Breast Cancer; **Hospital:** NS-LIJ Hlth Sys (page 106), NYU Langone Med Ctr (page 108); **Address:** 1999 Marcus Ave, Ste 120, Lake Success, NY 11042; **Phone:** 516-466-6611; **Board Cert:** Internal Medicine 1978; Medical Oncology 2006; **Med School:** Cornell Univ-Weill Med Coll 1975; **Resid:** Internal Medicine, NY Hosp-Cornell Med Ctr 1979; **Fellow:** Hematology & Oncology, Meml Sloan Kettering Cancer Ctr 1980; **Fac Appt:** Assoc Clin Prof Med, Cornell Univ-Weill Med Coll

Bradley, Thomas P MD (Onc) - **Spec Exp:** Bladder Cancer; Prostate Cancer; Kidney Cancer; **Hospital:** N Shore Univ Hosp (page 106); **Address:** Monter Cancer Center, 450 Lakeville Rd, Lake Success, NY 11042; **Phone:** 516-734-8900; **Board Cert:** Internal Medicine 1987; Medical Oncology 2011; Hematology 2002; **Med School:** Mexico 1982; **Resid:** Internal Medicine, Univ Hosp-SUNY Downstate 1988; **Fellow:** Hematology & Oncology, Univ Hosp-SUNY Downstate 1991; **Fac Appt:** Assoc Prof Med, Albert Einstein Coll Med

Budman, Daniel MD (Onc) - **Spec Exp:** Breast Cancer; Lymphoma; Drug Discovery & Development; Psychopharmacology; **Hospital:** N Shore Univ Hosp (page 106); **Address:** 450 Lakeville Road Rd, Monter Cancer Center, Lake Success, NY 11042; **Phone:** 516-734-8900; **Board Cert:** Internal Medicine 1975; Hematology 1978; Medical Oncology 1979; **Med School:** Albert Einstein Coll Med 1972; **Resid:** Internal Medicine, Hosp Univ Penn 1974; Hematology, Natl Inst Hlth 1976; **Fellow:** Medical Oncology, Sloan Kettering Cancer Ctr 1977; Hematology, NYU Med Ctr 1978; **Fac Appt:** Prof Med, NYU Sch Med

Citron, Marc L MD (Onc) - **Spec Exp:** Breast Cancer; Lung Cancer; **Hospital:** Long Island Jewish Med Ctr (page 106); **Address:** ProHealth Care Assocs, Div Oncology, 2800 Marcus Ave, Ste 205, Lake Success, NY 11042-1008; **Phone:** 516-622-6150; **Board Cert:** Internal Medicine 1977; Medical Oncology 1979; **Med School:** Wayne State Univ 1974; **Resid:** Internal Medicine, Georgetown Univ Hosp 1977; **Fellow:** Medical Oncology, Georgetown Univ Hosp 1979; **Fac Appt:** Clin Prof Med, Albert Einstein Coll Med

Hindenburg, Alexander A MD (Onc) - **Spec Exp:** Pancreatic Cancer; Breast Cancer; Gynecologic Cancer; Myelodysplastic Syndromes; **Hospital:** Winthrop Univ Hosp (page 504); **Address:** Winthrop Oncology/Hematology Assocs, 200 Old Country Rd, Ste 450, Mineola, NY 11501; **Phone:** 516-663-9500; **Board Cert:** Internal Medicine 1981; Medical Oncology 1983; Hematology 1988; **Med School:** UMDNJ-RW Johnson Med Sch 1978; **Resid:** Internal Medicine, Mt Sinai Hosp 1981; **Fellow:** Hematology & Oncology, Columbia-Presby Med Ctr 1984; **Fac Appt:** Asst Prof Med, SUNY Stony Brook

Kappel, Bruce I MD (Onc) - **Spec Exp:** Breast Cancer; Colon Cancer; **Hospital:** Plainview Hosp (page 106), St. Joseph's Hosp-Nassau; **Address:** 40 Crossways Park Drive, Ste 103, Woodbury, NY 11797; **Phone:** 516-921-5533; **Board Cert:** Internal Medicine 1985; Medical Oncology 1987; Hematology 1988; **Med School:** Emory Univ 1982; **Resid:** Internal Medicine, Emory Univ Hosp 1985; **Fellow:** Medical Oncology, Columbia-Presby Med Ctr 1988

Kessler, Leonard MD (Onc) - **Hospital:** South Nassau Comm Hosp, Mercy Med Ctr - Rockville Centre; **Address:** 242 Merrick Rd, Ste 301, Rockville Centre, NY 11570; **Phone:** 516-536-1455; **Board Cert:** Internal Medicine 1979; Medical Oncology 1981; Hematology 1982; **Med School:** Albert Einstein Coll Med 1975; **Resid:** Internal Medicine, Montefiore Hosp Med Ctr 1977; **Fellow:** Hematology, Montefiore Hosp Med Ctr 1981; Medical Oncology, Meml Sloan Kettering Cancer Ctr 1980

Marino, John S MD (Onc) - **Spec Exp:** Breast Cancer; Colon Cancer; Lung Cancer; **Hospital:** N Shore Univ Hosp (page 106), St. Francis Hosp - The Heart Ctr (page 121); **Address:** 2001 Marcus Ave, Ste S265, Lake Success, NY 11042; **Phone:** 516-883-0122; **Board Cert:** Internal Medicine 1982; Medical Oncology 1985; **Med School:** NY Med Coll 1979; **Resid:** Internal Medicine, N Shore Univ Hosp 1982; **Fellow:** Medical Oncology, Jacobi Med Ctr 1983; Medical Oncology, N Shore Univ Hosp 1984; **Fac Appt:** Asst Clin Prof Med, NYU Sch Med

Mehrotra, Bhoomi MD (Onc) - **Spec Exp:** Lung Cancer; Head & Neck Cancer; Gastrointestinal Cancer; **Hospital:** Long Island Jewish Med Ctr (page 106); **Address:** Dept Hematology/Oncology, 270-05 76th Ave, New Hyde Park, NY 11040; **Phone:** 718-470-8934; **Board Cert:** Internal Medicine 2000; Medical Oncology 2003; Hematology 2004; **Med School:** India 1986; **Resid:** Internal Medicine, LI Jewish Medical Ctr 1990; **Fellow:** Hematology & Oncology, UCSD Med Ctr 1993; **Fac Appt:** Assoc Clin Prof Med, Albert Einstein Coll Med

Schwartz, Paula R MD (Onc) - **Spec Exp:** Breast Cancer; Colon Cancer; **Hospital:** N Shore Univ Hosp (page 106), Long Island Jewish Med Ctr (page 106); **Address:** 3003 New Hyde Park Rd, Ste 401, New Hyde Park, NY 11042; **Phone:** 516-354-5700; **Board Cert:** Internal Medicine 1986; Hematology 1988; **Med School:** SUNY Downstate 1980; **Resid:** Internal Medicine, LI Jewish Med Ctr 1981; Internal Medicine, LI Jewish Med Ctr 1983; **Fellow:** Hematology, Mt Sinai Hosp 1985; Hematology, N Shore Univ Hosp 1989

Tomao, Frank A MD (Onc) - **Spec Exp:** Lung Cancer; Breast Cancer; **Hospital:** NS-LIJ Hlth Sys (page 106), St. Francis Hosp - The Heart Ctr (page 121); **Address:** 2001 Marcus Ave, Ste S265, Lake Success, NY 11042; **Phone:** 516-883-0122; **Board Cert:** Internal Medicine 1974; Medical Oncology 1975; **Med School:** Cornell Univ-Weill Med Coll 1965; **Resid:** Medical Oncology, Meml Sloan Kettering Cancer Ctr 1967; Medical Oncology, Bellevue Hosp 1968; **Fellow:** Medical Oncology, Meml Sloan Kettering Cancer Ctr 1969

Vinciguerra, Vincent P MD (Onc) - **Spec Exp:** Breast Cancer; Gastrointestinal Cancer; Lung Cancer; Cancer Prevention; **Hospital:** N Shore Univ Hosp (page 106); **Address:** Monter Cancer Ctr, 450 Lakeville Rd, Lake Success, NY 11042; **Phone:** 516-734-8954; **Board Cert:** Internal Medicine 1971; Hematology 1974; Medical Oncology 1975; **Med School:** Georgetown Univ 1966; **Resid:** Internal Medicine, NY Hosp-Cornell 1969; Internal Medicine, N Shore Univ Hosp 1971; **Fellow:** Hematology & Oncology, NY Hosp-Cornell 1970; Hematology & Oncology, N Shore Univ Hosp 1974; **Fac Appt:** Prof Med, NYU Sch Med

Weiselberg, Lora MD (Onc) - **Spec Exp:** Breast Cancer; Cancer Prevention; **Hospital:** N Shore Univ Hosp (page 106), Long Island Jewish Med Ctr (page 106); **Address:** Monter Cancer Center, 450 Lakeville Rd, Lake Success, NY 11042; **Phone:** 516-734-8963; **Board Cert:** Internal Medicine 1978; Medical Oncology 1981; Hematology 1982; **Med School:** NY Med Coll 1975; **Resid:** Internal Medicine, Stamford Hosp 1978; **Fellow:** Medical Oncology, N Shore Univ Hosp 1980; Hematology, N Shore Univ Hosp 1980; **Fac Appt:** Assoc Prof Med, Hofstra N Shore-LIJ Sch Med

Weiss, Rita MD/PhD (Onc) - **Hospital:** St. Francis Hosp - The Heart Ctr (page 121), N Shore Univ Hosp (page 106); **Address:** 107 Northern Blvd, Ste 306, Great Neck, NY 11021-4309; **Phone:** 516-482-0080; **Board Cert:** Internal Medicine 1984; Medical Oncology 1989; **Med School:** Mexico 1977; **Resid:** Internal Medicine, Winthrop Univ Hosp 1980; **Fellow:** Medical Oncology, Mount Sinai 1982; **Fac Appt:** Asst Clin Prof Onc, NYU Sch Med

Neonatal-Perinatal Medicine

Boxer, Harriet MD (NP) - **Spec Exp:** Prematurity/Low Birth Weight Infants; Chronic Obstructive Lung Disease (COPD); **Hospital:** Nassau Univ Med Ctr; **Address:** Nassau Univ Med Ctr, Div Neonatology, 2201 Hempstead Tpke, Box 30, East Meadow, NY 11554; **Phone:** 516-572-3319; **Board Cert:** Pediatrics 1977; Neonatal-Perinatal Medicine 1977; **Med School:** SUNY Downstate 1972; **Resid:** Pediatrics, Babies Hosp 1974; Pediatrics, Children's Hosp 1975; **Fellow:** Neonatal-Perinatal Medicine, LI Jewish-Hillside Med Ctr 1977; **Fac Appt:** Asst Prof Ped, SUNY Stony Brook

Schanler, Richard J MD (NP) - **Spec Exp:** Nutrition; Breast Feeding Problems; **Hospital:** N Shore Univ Hosp (page 106), Steven & Alexandra Cohen Chldn's Med Ctr of NY (page 106); **Address:** 300 Community Drive, Dept Neonatal-Perinatal Medicine, Manhasset, NY 11030; **Phone:** 516-562-4665; **Board Cert:** Pediatrics 1979; Neonatal-Perinatal Medicine 2009; **Med School:** UMDNJ-NJ Med Sch, Newark 1974; **Resid:** Pediatrics, Univ Colorado Hlth Sci Ctr 1977; **Fellow:** Neonatology, Brown Univ 1980; **Fac Appt:** Prof Ped, Albert Einstein Coll Med

Steele, Andrew M MD (NP) - **Spec Exp:** Lung Disease in Newborns; Sudden Infant Death Syndrome (SIDS); Breathing Disorders; **Hospital:** Steven & Alexandra Cohen Chldn's Med Ctr of NY (page 106), N Shore Univ Hosp (page 106); **Address:** Steven & Alexandra Cohen Chldn's Hosp, 269-01 76th Ave, New Hyde Park, NY 11040-1433; **Phone:** 718-470-3013; **Board Cert:** Pediatrics 1981; Neonatal-Perinatal Medicine 2009; **Med School:** SUNY Hlth Sci Ctr 1976; **Resid:** Pediatrics, LI Jewish Med Ctr 1978; **Fellow:** Neonatal-Perinatal Medicine, LI Jewish Med Ctr 1980; **Fac Appt:** Assoc Prof Ped, Hofstra N Shore-LIJ Sch Med

Nephrology

Bellucci, Alessandro G MD (Nep) - **Spec Exp:** Hypertension; Kidney Stones; Kidney Disease; Kidney Failure; **Hospital:** N Shore Univ Hosp (page 106); **Address:** North Shore Univ Hosp, Dept Nephrology, 300 Community Drive, Manhasset, NY 11030; **Phone:** 516-562-4312; **Board Cert:** Internal Medicine 1979; Nephrology 1982; **Med School:** Italy 1975; **Resid:** Internal Medicine, Cabrini Med Ctr 1979; **Fellow:** Nephrology, N Shore Univ Hosp 1982; **Fac Appt:** Assoc Prof Med, NYU Sch Med

Bourla, Steven L MD (Nep) - **Spec Exp:** Kidney Disease; **Hospital:** Plainview Hosp (page 106), St. Joseph's Hosp-Nassau; **Address:** Island Medical Group, 789 Old Country Rd, Plainview, NY 11803; **Phone:** 516-433-3600; **Board Cert:** Internal Medicine 1979; Nephrology 1982; **Med School:** NY Med Coll 1975; **Resid:** Internal Medicine, LI Jewish Med Ctr 1978; **Fellow:** Nephrology, NYU Med Ctr 1981

Mailloux, Lionel U MD (Nep) - **Spec Exp:** Hypertension; Dialysis Care; **Hospital:** N Shore Univ Hosp (page 106), Glen Cove Hosp (page 106); **Address:** 50 Seaview Blvd, Port Washington, NY 11050; **Phone:** 516-484-6093; **Board Cert:** Internal Medicine 1977; Nephrology 1972; **Med School:** Hahnemann Univ 1962; **Resid:** Internal Medicine, Hartford Hosp 1965; **Fellow:** Nephrology, Hahnemann Hosp 1966; **Fac Appt:** Assoc Prof Med, NYU Sch Med

Mattana, Joseph MD (Nep) - **Spec Exp:** Diabetic Kidney Disease; Hypertension; Glomerulonephritis; **Hospital:** Long Island Jewish Med Ctr (page 106), N Shore Univ Hosp (page 106); **Address:** 100 Community Drive Fl 2, Great Neck, NY 11021; **Phone:** 516-465-3010; **Board Cert:** Nephrology 2004; **Med School:** SUNY Hlth Sci Ctr 1987; **Resid:** Internal Medicine, LI Jewish Hosp 1990; **Fellow:** Nephrology, LI Jewish Hosp 1993; **Fac Appt:** Prof Med, Albert Einstein Coll Med

Singhal, Pravin C MD (Nep) - **Spec Exp:** Hypertension; Diabetic Kidney Disease; **Hospital:** Long Island Jewish Med Ctr (page 106), N Shore Univ Hosp (page 106); **Address:** 100 Community Drive Fl 2, Great Neck, NY 11021; **Phone:** 516-465-3010; **Board Cert:** Internal Medicine 1983; Nephrology 1986; **Med School:** India 1970; **Resid:** Internal Medicine, Postgrad Inst Med Ed. 1972; Internal Medicine, Brigham Womens Hosp 1983; **Fellow:** Nephrology, Montefiore Med Ctr 1985; **Fac Appt:** Prof Med, Albert Einstein Coll Med

Wagner, John D MD (Nep) - **Spec Exp:** Hypertension; Dialysis Care; Kidney Failure-Chronic; **Hospital:** Long Island Jewish Med Ctr (page 106), N Shore Univ Hosp (page 106); **Address:** 100 Community Drive Fl 2, Great Neck, NY 11021; **Phone:** 516-465-3010; **Board Cert:** Internal Medicine 1981; Nephrology 1984; **Med School:** Yale Univ 1978; **Resid:** Internal Medicine, Bellevue-NYU 1982; **Fellow:** Nephrology, Bellevue-NYU-VAMC 1984; **Fac Appt:** Assoc Clin Prof Med, Albert Einstein Coll Med

Neurological Surgery

Brisman, Jonathan L MD (NS) - **Spec Exp:** Interventional Neuroradiology; Vascular Neurosurgery; Arteriovenous Malformations; Endovascular Surgery; **Hospital:** Winthrop Univ Hosp (page 504), South Nassau Comm Hosp; **Address:** Neurological Surgery, 100 Merrick Rd, Ste 200, Rockville Ctr, NY 11570; **Phone:** 516-255-9031; **Board Cert:** Neurological Surgery 2008; **Med School:** Columbia P&S 1995; **Resid:** Surgery, Mass Genl Hosp 1996; Neurological Surgery, Mass Genl Hosp 2002; **Fellow:** Interventional Neuroradiology, Roosevelt Hosp 2003

Brown, Jeffrey A MD (NS) - **Spec Exp:** Trigeminal Neuralgia; Pain-Chronic; **Hospital:** Winthrop Univ Hosp (page 504), N Shore Univ Hosp (page 106); **Address:** 600 Northern Blvd, Ste 118, Great Neck, NY 11021-5200; **Phone:** 516-478-0008; **Board Cert:** Neurological Surgery 1986; **Med School:** Univ Chicago-Pritzker Sch Med 1976; **Resid:** Surgery, Univ Chicago Hosps 1977; Neurological Surgery, Univ Chicago Hosps 1982; **Fac Appt:** Prof NS, Wayne State Univ

Eisenberg, Mark MD (NS) - **Spec Exp:** Skull Base Surgery; Spinal Surgery-Minimally Invasive; Pituitary Tumors; Brain Tumors; **Hospital:** Long Island Jewish Med Ctr (page 106); **Address:** 900 Northern Blvd, Ste 260, Great Neck, NY 11021; **Phone:** 516-773-7737; **Board Cert:** Neurological Surgery 2010; **Med School:** Univ Miami Sch Med 1988; **Resid:** Neurological Surgery, Mount Sinai Med Ctr 1994; **Fellow:** Skull Base Surgery, Univ Arkansas Med Ctr 1995; **Fac Appt:** Asst Clin Prof NS, NYU Sch Med

Epstein, Nancy E MD (NS) - **Spec Exp:** Spinal Surgery; Spinal Surgery-Neck; Transfusion Free Surgery; **Hospital:** Winthrop Univ Hosp (page 504); **Address:** 410 Lakeville Rd, Ste 204, New Hyde Park, NY 11042-1199; **Phone:** 516-354-3401; **Board Cert:** Neurological Surgery 1984; **Med School:** Columbia P&S 1976; **Resid:** Neurological Surgery, Bellevue Hosp Ctr-NYU 1981; **Fac Appt:** Clin Prof NS, Albert Einstein Coll Med

Holtzman, Robert N MD (NS) - **Spec Exp:** Brain & Spinal Cord Tumors; Spinal Surgery; Aneurysm-Cerebral; Chiari's Deformity; **Hospital:** Lenox Hill Hosp (page 106); **Address:** 1991 Marcus Ave, Ste 108, Lake Success, NY 11042; **Phone:** 212-529-3580; **Board Cert:** Neurology 1978; Neurological Surgery 1980; **Med School:** Columbia P&S 1969; **Resid:** Surgery, Harbor Genl Hosp 1973; Neurological Surgery, New York Neurological Inst 1977; **Fac Appt:** Assoc Clin Prof NS, Columbia P&S

Langer, David J MD (NS) - **Spec Exp:** Neurovascular Surgery; Arteriovenous Malformations; Aneurysm-Cerebral; Carotid Artery Surgery; **Hospital:** N Shore Univ Hosp (page 106); **Address:** 300 Community Drive, Tower 9, Manhasset, NY 11030; **Phone:** 516-562-3023; **Board Cert:** Neurological Surgery 2003; **Med School:** Univ Pennsylvania 1991; **Resid:** Neurological Surgery, Hosp Univ Penn 1998; **Fellow:** Neurovascular Surgery, Beth Israel Med Ctr 1999; **Fac Appt:** Asst Prof NS, Albert Einstein Coll Med

Levine, Mitchell E MD (NS) - **Spec Exp:** Brain Tumors; **Hospital:** N Shore Univ Hosp (page 106); **Address:** 900 Northern Blvd, Ste 260, Great Neck, NY 11021; **Phone:** 516-773-7737; **Board Cert:** Neurological Surgery 1987; **Med School:** Mount Sinai Sch Med 1977; **Resid:** Surgery, Mt Sinai Hosp 1978; Neurological Surgery, Mt Sinai Hosp 1983

Mittler, Mark A MD (NS) - **Spec Exp:** Pediatric Neurosurgery; Brain & Spinal Cord Tumors; Vascular Malformations; Hydrocephalus; **Hospital:** Steven & Alexandra Cohen Chldn's Med Ctr of NY (page 106), N Shore Univ Hosp (page 106); **Address:** LI Neurosurgical Assocs, 410 Lakeville Rd, Ste 204, New Hyde Park, NY 11042; **Phone:** 516-354-3401; **Board Cert:** Neurological Surgery 2001; Pediatric Neurological Surgery 2001; **Med School:** Univ Rochester 1991; **Resid:** Neurological Surgery, RI Hosp/Brown Univ 1998; **Fellow:** Pediatric Neurological Surgery, Children's Hosp 1999; **Fac Appt:** Asst Prof NS, Hofstra N Shore-LIJ Sch Med

Onesti, Stephen T MD (NS) - **Spec Exp:** Spinal Surgery; Minimally Invasive Spinal Surgery; Spinal Disorders-Degenerative; Pain-Chronic; **Hospital:** South Nassau Comm Hosp; **Address:** 1991 Marcus Ave, Ste 108, Lake Success, NY 11042; **Phone:** 516-255-9031; **Board Cert:** Neurological Surgery 1995; **Med School:** Harvard Med Sch 1986; **Resid:** Neurological Surgery, Columbia-Presby Med Ctr 1993; **Fellow:** Neurological Science, Columbia-Presby Med Ctr 1988; **Fac Appt:** Prof NS, SUNY Downstate

Rekate, Harold MD (NS) - **Spec Exp:** Chiari's Deformity; Hydrocephalus; Pediatric Neurosurgery; Brain Tumors; **Hospital:** N Shore Univ Hosp (page 106); **Address:** 865 Northern Blvd, Ste 302, Great Neck, NY 11021; **Phone:** 516-570-4408; **Board Cert:** Neurological Surgery 1980; Pediatric Neurological Surgery 1996; **Med School:** Med Coll VA 1970; **Resid:** Neurological Surgery, Univ Hosps-Case West Res 1978; **Fac Appt:** Prof NS, Hofstra N Shore-LIJ Sch Med

Schulder, Michael MD (NS) - **Spec Exp:** Brain Tumors; Movement Disorders; Skull Base Surgery; **Hospital:** N Shore Univ Hosp (page 106), Long Island Jewish Med Ctr (page 106); **Address:** North Shore University Hospital, 300 Community Drive, Tower 9, Manhasset, NY 11030; **Phone:** 516-562-3062; **Board Cert:** Neurological Surgery 1991; **Med School:** Columbia P&S 1982; **Resid:** Neurological Surgery, Montefiore Hosp Med Ctr/Albert Einstein 1988; **Fac Appt:** , UMDNJ-NJ Med Sch, Newark

Neurology

Blanck, Richard H MD (N) - **Spec Exp:** Multiple Sclerosis; Pain-Back; **Hospital:** N Shore Univ Hosp (page 106), St. Francis Hosp - The Heart Ctr (page 121); **Address:** 1991 Marcus Ave, Ste 110, Lake Success, NY 11042; **Phone:** 516-466-4700; **Board Cert:** Internal Medicine 1976; Neurology 1980; **Med School:** UMDNJ-NJ Med Sch, Newark 1973; **Resid:** Internal Medicine, N Shore Univ Hosp 1975; Neurology, N Shore Univ Hosp 1977; **Fac Appt:** Assoc Clin Prof N, NYU Sch Med

Ettinger, Alan MD (N) - **Spec Exp:** Epilepsy; Seizure Disorders; **Hospital:** Winthrop Univ Hosp (page 504), Huntington Hosp (page 106); **Address:** Neurological Surgery, PC, 1991 Marcus Ave, Ste 108, Lake Success, NY 11042; **Phone:** 516-442-2250; **Board Cert:** Neurology 1989; **Med School:** Boston Univ 1983; **Resid:** Internal Medicine, Hartford Hosp 1985; Neurology, Montefiore Med Ctr 1988; **Fellow:** Epilepsy, Montefiore Med Ctr 1989; **Fac Appt:** Prof N, Albert Einstein Coll Med

Gordon, Marc L MD (N) - **Spec Exp:** Dementia; Headache; Multiple Sclerosis; Alzheimer's Disease; **Hospital:** Long Island Jewish Med Ctr (page 106); **Address:** 611 Northern Blvd, Ste 150, Great Neck, NY 11021-5207; **Phone:** 516-325-7000; **Board Cert:** Neurology 1990; **Med School:** Columbia P&S 1985; **Resid:** Neurology, Jacobi Med Ctr 1989; **Fellow:** Neuropsychopharmacology, Albert Einstein Coll Med 1990; **Fac Appt:** Assoc Clin Prof N, Albert Einstein Coll Med

Haimovic, Itzhak C MD (N) - **Spec Exp:** Spinal Disorders; Epilepsy; Headache; **Hospital:** N Shore Univ Hosp (page 106), Long Island Jewish Med Ctr (page 106); **Address:** 170 Great Neck Rd, Great Neck, NY 11021; **Phone:** 516-487-4464; **Board Cert:** Neurology 1981; Clinical Neurophysiology 2010; **Med School:** NY Med Coll 1975; **Resid:** Neurology, N Shore Univ Hosp 1977; Neurology, NY Hosp-Cornell Univ 1980; **Fellow:** Neurological Physiology, Columbia-Presby 1981; **Fac Appt:** Assoc Clin Prof N, NYU Sch Med

Hainline, Brian MD (N) - **Spec Exp:** Pain-Chronic; Spinal Disorders; Reflex Sympathetic Dystrophy (RSD); **Hospital:** N Shore Univ Hosp (page 106); **Address:** 3 Delaware Drive, Lake Success, NY 11042; **Phone:** 516-622-6088; **Board Cert:** Neurology 1987; Pain Medicine 2011; **Med School:** Univ Chicago-Pritzker Sch Med 1982; **Resid:** Neurology, NY Hosp 1986; **Fac Appt:** Assoc Clin Prof N, NYU Sch Med

Harden, Cynthia L MD (N) - **Spec Exp:** Epilepsy/Seizure Disorders; **Hospital:** NS-LIJ Hlth Sys (page 106); **Address:** LIJ Cushing Neuroscience Inst, 611 Northern Blvd, Ste 150, Great Neck, NY 11021; **Phone:** 516-325-7000; **Board Cert:** Neurology 1989; **Med School:** Univ Wisc 1983; **Resid:** Internal Medicine, St Luke's Roosevelt Hosp 1985; Neurology, Mt Sinai Hosp 1988; **Fellow:** Clinical Neurophysiology, Albert Einstein Med Coll 1989

Kanner, Ronald MD (N) - **Spec Exp:** Headache; Pain-Chronic; Migraine; **Hospital:** Long Island Jewish Med Ctr (page 106); **Address:** 270-05 76th Ave, rm M2006, Dept Neurology, New Hyde Park, NY 11040; **Phone:** 718-470-7311; **Board Cert:** Neurology 1980; **Med School:** Spain 1975; **Resid:** Internal Medicine, Philadelphia Genl Hosp 1976; Neurology, Montefiore Med Ctr 1979; **Fellow:** Neurology, Meml Sloan-Kettering Cancer Ctr 1981; **Fac Appt:** Prof N, Albert Einstein Coll Med

Kelemen, John MD (N) - **Spec Exp:** Electromyography; Neuromuscular Disorders; Botox for Muscle Overactivity; Dystonia; **Hospital:** Plainview Hosp (page 106); **Address:** Island Neurological Assocs, 824 Old Country Rd, Plainview, NY 11803-4935; **Phone:** 516-822-2230; **Board Cert:** Neurology 1979; **Med School:** Georgetown Univ 1974; **Resid:** Internal Medicine, Nassau County Med Ctr 1978; **Fellow:** Neuromuscular Medicine, New England Med Ctr 1980

Kessler, Jeffrey T MD (N) - **Spec Exp:** Parkinson's Disease; Dementia; Pain-Facial; **Hospital:** N Shore Univ Hosp (page 106), St. Francis Hosp - The Heart Ctr (page 121); **Address:** 1991 Marcus Ave, Ste 110, Lake Success, NY 11042; **Phone:** 516-466-4700; **Board Cert:** Internal Medicine 1974; Neurology 1976; **Med School:** Cornell Univ-Weill Med Coll 1969; **Resid:** Internal Medicine, NY Hosp-Cornell Med Ctr 1971; **Fellow:** Neurology, NY Hosp-Cornell Med Ctr 1974; **Fac Appt:** Assoc Clin Prof N, NYU Sch Med

Kula, Roger W MD (N) - **Spec Exp:** Neuromuscular Disorders; Myasthenia Gravis; Syringomyelia & Spinal Cord Diseases; Chiari's Deformity; **Hospital:** N Shore Univ Hosp (page 106), Steven & Alexandra Cohen Chldn's Med Ctr of NY (page 106); **Address:** 611 Northern Blvd, Ste 150, Great Neck, NY 11021; **Phone:** 516-570-4425; **Board Cert:** Internal Medicine 1975; Neurology 1977; Neuromuscular Medicine 2008; **Med School:** Johns Hopkins Univ 1970; **Resid:** Internal Medicine, New York Hosp 1972; Neurology, UCSF Med Ctr 1974; **Fellow:** Neuromuscular Medicine, Natl Inst Hlth 1977; **Fac Appt:** Assoc Prof N, Hofstra N Shore-LIJ Sch Med

Levy, Lewis MD (N) - **Spec Exp:** Tourette's Syndrome; Parkinson's Disease; **Hospital:** South Nassau Comm Hosp; **Address:** Long Island Neurology Consultants, 777 Sunrise Hwy, Ste 200, Lynbrook, NY 11563; **Phone:** 516-887-3516; **Board Cert:** Neurology 1979; **Med School:** SUNY Downstate 1973; **Resid:** Neurology, Albert Einstein 1977; **Fac Appt:** Asst Clin Prof N, Albert Einstein Coll Med

Libman, Richard MD (N) - **Spec Exp:** Stroke; **Hospital:** Long Island Jewish Med Ctr (page 106); **Address:** 270-05 76th Ave, Ste M2006, New Hyde Park, NY 11040-1433; **Phone:** 718-470-7311; **Board Cert:** Neurology 1991; Vascular Neurology 2005; **Med School:** McGill Univ 1986; **Resid:** Neurology, Montefiore Med Ctr 1990; **Fellow:** Stroke, Columbia-Presby Med Ctr 1993; **Fac Appt:** Assoc Prof N, Albert Einstein Coll Med

Newman, Stephen M MD (N) - **Spec Exp:** Multiple Sclerosis; Migraine; **Hospital:** Plainview Hosp (page 106); **Address:** Island Neurological Assocs, 824 Old Country Rd, Plainview, NY 11803; **Phone:** 516-822-2230; **Board Cert:** Neurology 1978; **Med School:** SUNY Buffalo 1972; **Resid:** Neurology, Nassau County Med Ctr 1976

Ragone, Philip S MD (N) - **Spec Exp:** Electromyography; **Hospital:** St. Francis Hosp - The Heart Ctr (page 121), N Shore Univ Hosp (page 106); **Address:** 1010 Northern Blvd, Ste 136, Great Neck, NY 11021; **Phone:** 516-482-4100; **Board Cert:** Internal Medicine 1985; Neurology 1989; Electrodiagnostic Medicine 1990; **Med School:** NY Med Coll 1982; **Resid:** Internal Medicine, Lenox Hill Hosp 1985; Neurology, Albert Einstein 1988; **Fellow:** Electromyography, Albert Einstein 1989

Schaul, Neil S MD (N) - **Spec Exp:** Epilepsy/Seizure Disorders; Electrodiagnosis; **Hospital:** NY Hosp Queens (page 206); **Address:** 1575 Hillside Ave, Ste 100, New Hyde Park, NY 11040; **Phone:** 516-616-6286; **Board Cert:** Neurology 1976; **Med School:** SUNY Hlth Sci Ctr 1966; **Resid:** Internal Medicine, DC General Hosp 1968; Neurology, Montreal Neur Inst 1974; **Fellow:** Neurological Physiology, Montreal Neur Inst 1977; **Fac Appt:** Assoc Prof Med, Cornell Univ-Weill Med Coll

Turner, Ira MD (N) - **Spec Exp:** Headache; **Hospital:** Plainview Hosp (page 106); **Address:** Island Neurological Assocs, 824 Old Country Rd, Plainview, NY 11803; **Phone:** 516-822-2230; **Board Cert:** Neurology 1978; Headache Medicine 2007; **Med School:** SUNY Downstate 1972; **Resid:** Neurology, Nassau Co Med Ctr 1976

Neuroradiology

Ortiz, Orlando MD (NRad) - **Spec Exp:** Interventional Neuroradiology; Spine Imaging & Intervention; **Hospital:** Winthrop Univ Hosp (page 504); **Address:** 259 First St, Mineola, NY 11501; **Phone:** 516-663-2123; **Board Cert:** Diagnostic Radiology 1990; Neuroradiology 2006; **Med School:** Harvard Med Sch 1985; **Resid:** Diagnostic Radiology, LIJ Med Ctr 1990; **Fellow:** Neurological Radiology, NY Presby-Columbia Med Ctr 1992

Pile-Spellman, John MD (NRad) - **Spec Exp:** Interventional Neuroradiology; Cerebrovascular Disease; Aneurysm; Arteriovenous Malformations; **Hospital:** Winthrop Univ Hosp (page 504); **Address:** Neurological Surgery, 1991 Marcus Ave, Ste 108, Lake Success, NY 11042; **Phone:** 516-442-2250; **Board Cert:** Diagnostic Radiology 1984; **Med School:** Tufts Univ 1978; **Resid:** Neurological Surgery, New England Med Ctr 1981; Neurological Radiology, Mass Genl Hosp 1984; **Fellow:** Interventional Neuroradiology, NYU Med Ctr 1986; **Fac Appt:** Prof Rad, Columbia P&S

Setton, Avi MD (NRad) - **Spec Exp:** Cerebrovascular Disease; Stroke; **Hospital:** N Shore Univ Hosp (page 106); **Address:** N Shore Univ Hospital, 300 Community Drive, 9 Tower, Manhasset, NY 11030; **Phone:** 516-562-3021; **Med School:** Israel 1978; **Resid:** Diagnostic Radiology, Bellevue Med Ctr 1991; **Fellow:** Neurological Radiology, NYU Med Ctr 1992

Nuclear Medicine

Palestro, Christopher MD (NuM) - **Spec Exp:** Pain after Joint Replacement; Diabetic Leg/Foot Infections; AIDS Related Infections; **Hospital:** Long Island Jewish Med Ctr (page 106), N Shore Univ Hosp (page 106); **Address:** Nuclear Medicine, 270-05 76th Ave Fl 4, New Hyde Park, NY 11040-1402; **Phone:** 718-470-7080; **Board Cert:** Nuclear Medicine 1982; **Med School:** Mexico 1975; **Resid:** Diagnostic Radiology, Roosevelt Hosp 1980; **Fellow:** Nuclear Medicine, Meml Sloan Kettering Cancer Ctr 1982; **Fac Appt:** Prof NuM, Albert Einstein Coll Med

Yung, Elizabeth MD (NuM) - **Spec Exp:** PET Imaging; **Hospital:** Winthrop Univ Hosp (page 504); **Address:** 259 First St, Mineola, NY 11501; **Phone:** 516-663-2778; **Board Cert:** Diagnostic Radiology 1984; Nuclear Radiology 1991; **Med School:** Tufts Univ 1980; **Resid:** Diagnostic Radiology, St Vincent's Hosp & Med Ctr 1984; **Fellow:** Nuclear Medicine, Yale-New Haven Hosp 1991

Obstetrics & Gynecology

Benedict, Leonard A MD (ObG) - **Spec Exp:** Pregnancy-High Risk; Gynecologic Surgery; **Hospital:** N Shore Univ Hosp (page 106); **Address:** 433 Uniondale Ave, Uniondale, NY 11553; **Phone:** 516-483-8798; **Board Cert:** Obstetrics & Gynecology 1981; **Med School:** Scotland, UK 1972; **Resid:** Obstetrics & Gynecology, Brooklyn Jewish Hosp 1978; **Fac Appt:** Asst Clin Prof ObG, NYU Sch Med

Haselkorn, Joan MD (ObG) *PCP* - **Spec Exp:** Laparoscopic Surgery; Hysteroscopic Surgery; Uterine Fibroids; Gynecology Only; **Hospital:** South Nassau Comm Hosp; **Address:** 556 Merrick Rd, Ste 200, Rockville Centre, NY 11570; **Phone:** 516-255-2044; **Board Cert:** Obstetrics & Gynecology 2012; **Med School:** Israel 1982; **Resid:** Obstetrics & Gynecology, NYU Med Ctr 1986

Jacob, Jessica MD (ObG) *PCP* - **Hospital:** N Shore Univ Hosp (page 106); **Address:** 3003 New Hyde Park Rd, Ste 407, New Hyde Park, NY 11042-1214; **Phone:** 516-488-8145; **Board Cert:** Obstetrics & Gynecology 2011; **Med School:** NYU Sch Med 1983; **Resid:** Obstetrics & Gynecology, N Shore Univ Hosp 1987; **Fac Appt:** Asst Clin Prof ObG, NYU Sch Med

Krim, Eileen MD (ObG) - **Spec Exp:** Menopause Problems; Adolescent Gynecology; Osteoporosis; Laparoscopic Surgery; **Hospital:** N Shore Univ Hosp (page 106); **Address:** 3111 New Hyde Park Rd, North Hills, NY 11040-3500; **Phone:** 516-365-6100; **Board Cert:** Obstetrics & Gynecology 1982; **Med School:** NY Med Coll 1975; **Resid:** Obstetrics & Gynecology, Beth Israel 1979; **Fellow:** Maternal & Fetal Medicine, N Shore Univ Hosp 1981; **Fac Appt:** Assoc Clin Prof ObG, NYU Sch Med

Leong, Mary MD (ObG) - **Spec Exp:** Pelvic Reconstruction; Menopause Problems; Uterine Fibroids; **Hospital:** Long Island Jewish Med Ctr (page 106); **Address:** Womens Comprehensive Hlth Ctr, 1554 Northern Blvd Fl 5th, Manhasset, NY 11030; **Phone:** 516-390-9242; **Board Cert:** Obstetrics & Gynecology 2011; **Med School:** NYU Sch Med 1978; **Resid:** Obstetrics & Gynecology, Bellevue Hosp Ctr 1982; **Fac Appt:** Asst Prof ObG, Albert Einstein Coll Med

Mack, Laurence F MD (ObG) *PCP* - **Spec Exp:** Infertility; Pregnancy-High Risk; Autoimmune Disease in Pregnancy; Pap Smear Abnormalities; **Hospital:** Plainview Hosp (page 106), Mercy Med Ctr - Rockville Centre; **Address:** 1130 N Broadway, PO Box 1550, North Massapequa, NY 11758-0910; **Phone:** 516-799-3462; **Board Cert:** Obstetrics & Gynecology 2011; **Med School:** Univ Hlth Scis, Chicago Med Sch 1985; **Resid:** Obstetrics & Gynecology, Brookdale Hosp 1989

Nimaroff, Michael MD (ObG) *PCP* - **Spec Exp:** Laparoscopic Surgery; Hysterectomy Alternatives; Hysteroscopic Surgery; **Hospital:** N Shore Univ Hosp (page 106), Long Island Jewish Med Ctr (page 106); **Address:** 825 Northern Blvd Fl 3 - Ste 301, Great Neck, NY 11021; **Phone:** 516-472-5700; **Board Cert:** Obstetrics & Gynecology 2011; **Med School:** UMDNJ-NJ Med Sch, Newark 1987; **Resid:** Obstetrics & Gynecology, N Shore Univ Hosp 1991; **Fac Appt:** Asst Clin Prof ObG, NYU Sch Med

Toles, Allen W MD (ObG) - **Spec Exp:** Pregnancy-High Risk; **Hospital:** Long Island Jewish Med Ctr (page 106); **Address:** 1554 Northern Blvd Fl 5, Manhasset, NY 11030; **Phone:** 516-390-9242; **Board Cert:** Obstetrics & Gynecology 2011; **Med School:** Meharry Med Coll 1986; **Resid:** Obstetrics & Gynecology, Howard Univ Hosp 1990; **Fac Appt:** Asst Prof ObG, Albert Einstein Coll Med

Vasudeva, Kusum MD (ObG) - **Spec Exp:** Pregnancy-High Risk; Menopause Problems; **Hospital:** N Shore Univ Hosp (page 106); **Address:** 2 Ohio Drive, Pro Health Plaza, Lake Success, NY 11042; **Phone:** 516-608-6800; **Board Cert:** Obstetrics & Gynecology 1975; **Med School:** India 1968; **Resid:** Obstetrics & Gynecology, N Shore Univ Hosp 1974; **Fellow:** Maternal & Fetal Medicine, N Shore Univ Hosp 1976

Veloso Jr, Manuel A MD (ObG) - **Spec Exp:** Gynecology Only; Gynecologic Ultrasound; Hysteroscopic Surgery; HPV-Human Papillomavirus; **Hospital:** Long Beach Med Ctr; **Address:** 303 E Park Ave, Long Beach, NY 11561; **Phone:** 516-431-2828; **Board Cert:** Obstetrics & Gynecology 1979; **Med School:** Philippines 1966; **Resid:** Obstetrics & Gynecology, Kings Co Hosp 1972

Occupational Medicine

Mendelsohn, Sara L MD (OM) - **Spec Exp:** Travel Medicine; Occupational Disease & Injury; Preventive Medicine; **Address:** 800 Woodbury Rd, Ste K, Woodbury, NY 11797; **Phone:** 516-682-9142; **Board Cert:** Occupational Medicine 1993; **Med School:** Boston Univ 1988; **Resid:** Occupational Medicine, Univ of Illinois Med Ctr 1991; **Fac Appt:** Asst Clin Prof Med, SUNY Stony Brook

Ophthalmology

Berke, Stanley J MD (Oph) - **Spec Exp:** Glaucoma; Cataract Surgery-Lens Implant; Laser Surgery; **Hospital:** Mercy Med Ctr - Rockville Centre; **Address:** 901 Stewart Ave, Ste 255, Garden City, NY 11530; **Phone:** 516-794-2020; **Board Cert:** Ophthalmology 1987; **Med School:** SUNY Buffalo 1981; **Resid:** Ophthalmology, Nassau Med Ctr 1985; **Fellow:** Anterior Segment - External Disease, Mass Eye & Ear Infirmary 1986; **Fac Appt:** Assoc Clin Prof Oph, Albert Einstein Coll Med

Boniuk, Vivien MD (Oph) - **Spec Exp:** Diagnostic Problems; **Hospital:** Queens Hosp Ctr - Jamaica; **Address:** 600 Northern Blvd, Ste 214, Great Neck, NY 11021; **Phone:** 516-470-2020; **Board Cert:** Ophthalmology 1969; **Med School:** Dalhousie Univ 1964; **Resid:** Ophthalmology, Barnes Hosp-Washington Univ 1967; **Fellow:** Ophthalmological Pathology, Baylor Coll Affil Hosp 1968; **Fac Appt:** Assoc Prof Oph, Albert Einstein Coll Med

D'Aversa, Gerard MD (Oph) - **Spec Exp:** Cataract Surgery; Laser-Refractive Surgery; Cornea Transplant; **Hospital:** Long Island Jewish Med Ctr (page 106); **Address:** 65 Roosevelt Ave, rm 204, Valley Stream, NY 11580-1106; **Phone:** 516-374-4199; **Board Cert:** Ophthalmology 2006; **Med School:** Albert Einstein Coll Med 1989; **Resid:** Ophthalmology, LI Jewish Med Ctr 1993; **Fellow:** Univ Florida 1994; **Fac Appt:** Asst Prof Oph, Albert Einstein Coll Med

Fastenberg, David M MD (Oph) - **Spec Exp:** Retina/Vitreous Surgery; Macular Degeneration; Diabetic Eye Disease/Retinopathy; **Hospital:** Syosset Hosp (page 106), Long Island Jewish Med Ctr (page 106); **Address:** 600 Northern Blvd, rm 216, Great Neck, NY 11021; **Phone:** 516-466-0390; **Board Cert:** Ophthalmology 1981; **Med School:** NY Med Coll 1976; **Resid:** Ophthalmology, Northwestern Univ Med Ctr 1980; **Fellow:** Retina, USC-Doheny Eye Inst 1982; **Fac Appt:** Assoc Clin Prof Oph, Albert Einstein Coll Med

Ferrone, Philip J MD (Oph) - **Spec Exp:** Retinal Disorders; **Hospital:** Syosset Hosp (page 106), Long Island Jewish Med Ctr (page 106); **Address:** 600 Northern Blvd, Ste 216, Great Neck, NY 11021; **Phone:** 516-466-0390; **Board Cert:** Ophthalmology 2006; **Med School:** Harvard Med Sch 1989; **Resid:** Ophthalmology, Duke Univ Med Ctr 1993; **Fellow:** Vitreoretinal Surgery, Associated Retinal Consultants 1995

Garber, Perry F MD (Oph) - **Spec Exp:** Ophthalmic Plastic Surgery; Blepharoplasty; Lacrimal Gland Disorders; Tear Duct Problems; **Hospital:** St. Francis Hosp - The Heart Ctr (page 121), Long Island Jewish Med Ctr (page 106); **Address:** 800 Community Drive, Ste 304, Manhasset, NY 11030; **Phone:** 516-627-6630; **Board Cert:** Ophthalmology 1976; **Med School:** SUNY Downstate 1968; **Resid:** Surgery, Mount Sinai Hosp 1970; Ophthalmology, Bellevue Hosp 1975; **Fellow:** Ophthalmic Plastic Surgery, NY Eye & Ear Infirmary 1976; **Fac Appt:** Assoc Clin Prof Oph, Albert Einstein Coll Med

Girardi, Anthony MD (Oph) - **Spec Exp:** Cataract Surgery; Glaucoma; **Hospital:** Glen Cove Hosp (page 106); **Address:** 8 Medical Plaza, Ste 201, Glen Cove, NY 11542; **Phone:** 516-676-4596; **Board Cert:** Ophthalmology 1985; **Med School:** SUNY Stony Brook 1980; **Resid:** Ophthalmology, Kings Co Hosp 1984; **Fac Appt:** Asst Clin Prof Oph, SUNY Downstate

Goldberg, Leslie P MD (Oph) - **Spec Exp:** Cataract Surgery; LASIK-Refractive Surgery; Eyelid Cosmetic Surgery; **Hospital:** St. Francis Hosp - The Heart Ctr (page 121), N Shore Univ Hosp (page 106); **Address:** Long Island Eye Surgeons, 2110 Northern Blvd, Ste 208, Manhasset, NY 11030-3500; **Phone:** 516-627-5113; **Board Cert:** Ophthalmology 1977; **Med School:** Ros Franklin Univ/Chicago Med Sch 1970; **Resid:** Ophthalmology, NYU Med Ctr 1976; **Fac Appt:** Asst Clin Prof Oph, NYU Sch Med

Hatsis, Alexander MD (Oph) - **Spec Exp:** LASIK-Refractive Surgery; Cataract Surgery; Corneal Disease & Surgery; Keratoconus; **Hospital:** South Nassau Comm Hosp, Nassau Univ Med Ctr; **Address:** 2 Lincoln Ave, Ste 401, Rockville Centre, NY 11570; **Phone:** 516-763-4106; **Board Cert:** Ophthalmology 2003; **Med School:** Italy 1978; **Resid:** Surgery, Nassau County Med Ctr 1980; Ophthalmology, Nassau County Med Ctr 1981; **Fellow:** Ophthalmology, Nassau County Med Ctr 1983

Kasper, William S MD (Oph) - **Spec Exp:** Cataract Surgery; Glaucoma; Cornea & External Eye Disease; **Hospital:** Winthrop Univ Hosp (page 504), Nassau Univ Med Ctr; **Address:** 520 Franklin Ave, Ste L9, Garden City, NY 11040; **Phone:** 516-742-3937; **Board Cert:** Ophthalmology 1974; **Med School:** Belgium 1967; **Resid:** Ophthalmology, Nassau Co Med Ctr 1971

Malik, Sajid MD (Oph) - **Spec Exp:** Cataract Surgery; Lens Implants-Multifocal; **Hospital:** Winthrop Univ Hosp (page 504); **Address:** Woodbury Optical, 185 Woodbury Rd, Hicksville, NY 11801; **Phone:** 516-681-3937; **Board Cert:** Ophthalmology 2010; **Med School:** SUNY Stony Brook 1989; **Resid:** Ophthalmology, Harlem Hosp 1994

Marks, Alan B MD (Oph) - **Spec Exp:** Cataract Surgery; Laser-Refractive Surgery; Eyelid Cosmetic Surgery; **Hospital:** St. Francis Hosp - The Heart Ctr (page 121), Syosset Hosp (page 106); **Address:** Long Island Eye Surgeons, 2110 Northern Blvd, Ste 208, Manhasset, NY 11030; **Phone:** 516-627-5113; **Board Cert:** Ophthalmology 1983; **Med School:** NY Med Coll 1978; **Resid:** Ophthalmology, N Shore Univ Hosp 1982

Nauheim, Richard MD (Oph) - **Spec Exp:** Corneal Disease; Cataract Surgery; **Hospital:** South Nassau Comm Hosp; **Address:** 2025 Merrick Ave, Merrick, NY 11566; **Phone:** 516-868-7110; **Board Cert:** Ophthalmology 1989; **Med School:** SUNY Buffalo 1984; **Resid:** Ophthalmology, Nassau Univ Med Ctr 1988; **Fellow:** Cornea & Ext Eye Disease, Eye & Ear Inst - UPMC 1989; **Fac Appt:** Asst Prof Oph, SUNY Stony Brook

Nelson, David B MD (Oph) - **Spec Exp:** Cataract Surgery; Glaucoma; **Hospital:** Mercy Med Ctr - Rockville Centre; **Address:** 2000 N Village Ave, Ste 402, Rockville Center, NY 11570-1001; **Phone:** 516-766-2519; **Board Cert:** Ophthalmology 1977; **Med School:** SUNY Hlth Sci Ctr 1972; **Resid:** Ophthalmology, NY Eye & Ear Infirmary 1976; **Fac Appt:** Asst Prof Oph, SUNY Stony Brook

Packer, Samuel MD (Oph) - **Spec Exp:** Ethics; **Hospital:** N Shore Univ Hosp (page 106), Long Island Jewish Med Ctr (page 106); **Address:** 600 Northern Blvd, Ste 214, Great Neck, NY 11021; **Phone:** 516-465-8400; **Board Cert:** Ophthalmology 1973; **Med School:** SUNY Hlth Sci Ctr 1966; **Resid:** Ophthalmology, Yale-New Haven Hosp 1971; **Fac Appt:** Prof Oph, NYU Sch Med

Perry, Henry MD (Oph) - **Spec Exp:** Laser-Refractive Surgery; Cornea Transplant; Cataract Surgery; Eyelid/Tear Duct Disorders; **Hospital:** Mercy Med Ctr - Rockville Centre; **Address:** 2000 N Village Ave, Ste 402, Rockville Centre, NY 11570-1001; **Phone:** 516-766-2519; **Board Cert:** Ophthalmology 1977; **Med School:** Univ Cincinnati 1971; **Resid:** Ophthalmology, Nassau County Med Ctr 1975; Ophthalmology, Hosp Univ Penn 1974; **Fellow:** Cornea, Mass Eye & Ear Infirmary 1977; Ophthalmic Pathology, Armed Forces Inst of Pathology 1976; **Fac Appt:** Assoc Clin Prof Oph, Cornell Univ-Weill Med Coll

Prywes, Arnold S MD (Oph) - **Spec Exp:** Glaucoma; Cataract Surgery; **Hospital:** N Shore Univ Hosp (page 106); **Address:** 4212 Hempstead Tpke, Bethpage, NY 11714-5709; **Phone:** 516-731-4800; **Board Cert:** Ophthalmology 1978; **Med School:** Mount Sinai Sch Med 1972; **Resid:** Ophthalmology, Mount Sinai Hosp 1977; **Fellow:** Ophthalmology, Mount Sinai Hosp 1974; **Fac Appt:** Asst Clin Prof Oph, Albert Einstein Coll Med

Rosenthal, Kenneth J MD (Oph) - **Spec Exp:** Corneal Disease; Cataract Surgery; **Hospital:** St. Francis Hosp - The Heart Ctr (page 121), Syosset Hosp (page 106); **Address:** 310 E Shore Rd, rm 102, Great Neck, NY 11023; **Phone:** 516-466-8989; **Board Cert:** Ophthalmology 1986; **Med School:** Albany Med Coll 1978; **Resid:** Ophthalmology, N Shore Univ Hosp 1983

Rubin, Laurence MD (Oph) - **Spec Exp:** Cataract Surgery; Intraocular Lenses; Glaucoma; **Hospital:** St. Joseph's Hosp-Nassau, Syosset Hosp (page 106); **Address:** Mid-Island Eye Phys & Surgeons, 4277 Hempstead Tpke, Ste 109, Bethpage, NY 11714-5706; **Phone:** 516-796-4030; **Board Cert:** Ophthalmology 1987; **Med School:** NY Med Coll 1980; **Resid:** Ophthalmology, New York Eye & Ear Infirm 1984

Rubin, Steven E MD (Oph) - **Spec Exp:** Strabismus; Pediatric Ophthalmology; Amblyopia; **Hospital:** N Shore Univ Hosp (page 106), Long Island Jewish Med Ctr (page 106); **Address:** 600 Northern Blvd, Ste 220, Great Neck, NY 11021-5200; **Phone:** 516-465-8444; **Board Cert:** Ophthalmology 1983; **Med School:** SUNY Downstate 1978; **Resid:** Ophthalmology, Univ Penn-Scheie Eye Inst 1982; **Fellow:** Pediatric Ophthalmology, Wills Eye Hosp 1983; **Fac Appt:** Prof Oph, NYU Sch Med

Schlessinger, David A MD (Oph) - **Spec Exp:** Eyelid Cosmetic & Reconstructive Surgery; Oculoplastic Surgery; Neuro-Ophthalmology; **Hospital:** Syosset Hosp (page 106), Winthrop Univ Hosp (page 504); **Address:** 75 Froehlich Farm Blvd, Woodbury, NY 11797; **Phone:** 516-496-2122; **Board Cert:** Ophthalmology 2005; **Med School:** Univ Pittsburgh 1988; **Resid:** Ophthalmology, Interfaith Med Ctr 1992; **Fellow:** Ophthalmic Plastic & Reconstructive Surgery, Univ Minnesota Hosp 1993; Neuro-Ophthalmology, Univ Minnesota Hosp 1993

Sturm, Richard T MD (Oph) - **Spec Exp:** Glaucoma; Cataract Surgery; **Address:** 360 Merrick Rd Fl 3, Lynbrook, NY 11563; **Phone:** 516-593-7709; **Board Cert:** Ophthalmology 1989; **Med School:** NY Med Coll 1983; **Resid:** Ophthalmology, St Luke's-Roosevelt Hosp Ctr 1987; **Fellow:** Glaucoma, Mass Eye & Ear Infirm 1988

Svitra, Paul MD (Oph) - **Spec Exp:** Diabetic Eye Disease/Retinopathy; Macular Degeneration; Retinal Detachment; Retinal Disorders; **Hospital:** N Shore Univ Hosp (page 106), Winthrop Univ Hosp (page 504); **Address:** 3003 New Hyde Park Rd, Ste 203, New Hyde Park, NY 11042; **Phone:** 516-327-0505; **Board Cert:** Ophthalmology 1990; **Med School:** Cornell Univ-Weill Med Coll 1984; **Resid:** Ophthalmology, Mass Eye & Ear Infirmary 1989; **Fellow:** Retina/Vitreous, Duke Eye Ctr 1990; Ophthalmic Pathology, Mass Eye & Ear Infirmary 1986; **Fac Appt:** Asst Prof Oph, Cornell Univ-Weill Med Coll

Udell, Ira J MD (Oph) - **Spec Exp:** Cornea Transplant; Corneal Disease; Tear Duct Problems; **Hospital:** Long Island Jewish Med Ctr (page 106), N Shore Univ Hosp (page 106); **Address:** LI Jewish Med Ctr, Dept Ophthalmology, 600 Northern Blvd, Ste 214, Great Neck, NY 11021-5200; **Phone:** 516-470-2020; **Board Cert:** Ophthalmology 1980; **Med School:** Tulane Univ 1974; **Resid:** Ophthalmology, LI Jewish Med Ctr 1979; **Fellow:** Cornea, Mass Eye & Ear Infirm 1981; **Fac Appt:** Prof Oph, Albert Einstein Coll Med

Weinstein, Joseph MD (Oph) - **Spec Exp:** Cataract Surgery; Refractive Surgery; Contact Lenses; **Hospital:** N Shore Univ Hosp (page 106), Syosset Hosp (page 106); **Address:** 4212 Hempstead Tpke, Eye Care Assoc, Bethpage, NY 11714-5712; **Phone:** 516-731-4800; **Board Cert:** Ophthalmology 1982; **Med School:** Albert Einstein Coll Med 1977; **Resid:** Ophthalmology, Long Island Jewish Med Ctr 1981

Orthopaedic Surgery

Asnis, Stanley MD (OrS) - **Spec Exp:** Hip Replacement; Knee Replacement; **Hospital:** N Shore Univ Hosp (page 106), St. Francis Hosp - The Heart Ctr (page 121); **Address:** 611 Northern Blvd, Ste 200, Great Neck, NY 11021; **Phone:** 516-723-2663; **Board Cert:** Orthopaedic Surgery 1976; **Med School:** Washington Univ, St Louis 1968; **Resid:** Surgery, NY Hosp 1971; Orthopaedic Surgery, Hosp for Special Surg 1975; **Fellow:** Research, Hosp for Special Surg 1972; **Fac Appt:** Assoc Clin Prof OrS, Albert Einstein Coll Med

Capozzi, James MD (OrS) - **Spec Exp:** Joint Replacement; Fractures in the Elderly; Arthroscopic Surgery; **Hospital:** Winthrop Univ Hosp (page 504); **Address:** 1300 Franklin Ave, Ste UL3A, Garden City, NY 11530; **Phone:** 516-747-8900; **Board Cert:** Orthopaedic Surgery 2010; **Med School:** Mount Sinai Sch Med 1981; **Resid:** Orthopaedic Surgery, Mount Sinai Hosp 1986; **Fellow:** Joint Replacement Surgery, New England Baptist Hosp 1987; **Fac Appt:** Assoc Clin Prof OrS, Mount Sinai Sch Med

D'Agostino, Richard J MD (OrS) - **Spec Exp:** Sports Medicine; Knee Surgery; Shoulder Surgery; **Hospital:** St. Francis Hosp - The Heart Ctr (page 121), N Shore Univ Hosp (page 106); **Address:** 600 Northern Blvd, Ste 300, Great Neck, NY 11021; **Phone:** 516-627-8717; **Board Cert:** Orthopaedic Surgery 2011; **Med School:** Mount Sinai Sch Med 1982; **Resid:** Orthopaedic Surgery, Mt Sinai Med Ctr 1987; **Fellow:** Sports Medicine, New Eng Baptist Hosp 1988; **Fac Appt:** Asst Prof OrS, Cornell Univ-Weill Med Coll

Dines, David M MD (OrS) - **Spec Exp:** Shoulder Surgery; Sports Medicine; Shoulder Replacement; **Hospital:** Long Island Jewish Med Ctr (page 106), Hosp For Special Surgery (page 115); **Address:** 935 Northern Blvd, Ste 303, Great Neck, NY 11021-5309; **Phone:** 516-482-1037; **Board Cert:** Orthopaedic Surgery 1980; **Med School:** UMDNJ-NJ Med Sch, Newark 1974; **Resid:** Surgery, NY Hosp-Cornell Med Ctr 1976; Orthopaedic Surgery, Hosp Special Surg 1979; **Fac Appt:** Clin Prof OrS, Albert Einstein Coll Med

Kenan, Samuel MD (OrS) - **Spec Exp:** Bone Tumors; **Hospital:** Lenox Hill Hosp (page 106); **Address:** 300 Old Country Rd, Ste 221, Mineola, NY 11501; **Phone:** 516-280-3733; **Med School:** Israel 1976; **Resid:** Orthopaedic Surgery, Hadassah Univ Hosp 1984; **Fellow:** Orthopaedic Pathology, Hosp for Joint Diseases 1987; **Fac Appt:** Prof OrS, NYU Sch Med

Levitz, Craig L MD (OrS) - **Spec Exp:** Sports Medicine; Shoulder Surgery; Knee Injuries/ACL; Cartilage Damage & Transplant; **Hospital:** South Nassau Comm Hosp; **Address:** 36 Lincoln Ave Fl 3, Rockville Centre, NY 11570; **Phone:** 516-536-2800; **Board Cert:** Orthopaedic Surgery 2011; Orthopaedic Sports Medicine 2007; **Med School:** Univ Pennsylvania 1992; **Resid:** Orthopaedic Surgery, Hosp Univ Penn 1997; **Fellow:** Sports Medicine, Amer Sports Med Inst 1998

Mauri, Thomas MD (OrS) - **Spec Exp:** Spinal Surgery; **Hospital:** NS-LIJ Hlth Sys (page 106); **Address:** 611 Northern Blvd, Ste 200, Great Neck, NY 11021; **Phone:** 516-723-2663; **Board Cert:** Orthopaedic Surgery 2009; **Med School:** Albany Med Coll 1980; **Resid:** Neurological Surgery, North Shore Univ Hosp 1982; Orthopaedic Surgery, Hosp for Special Surgery 1985; **Fellow:** Spinal Surgery, Rancho Los Amigos Natl Rehab Ctr 1986

Montero, Carlos F MD (OrS) - **Spec Exp:** Hand Surgery; **Hospital:** St. Joseph's Hosp-Nassau, Plainview Hosp (page 106); **Address:** ProHealth Orthopedics, 2920 Hempstead Tpke, Levittown, NY 11756; **Phone:** 516-735-4048; **Board Cert:** Orthopaedic Surgery 1974; **Med School:** Argentina 1968; **Resid:** Surgery, Bronx VA Hosp 1970; Orthopaedic Surgery, Nassau County Med Ctr 1973; **Fellow:** Hand Surgery, Nassau County Med Ctr 1974; **Fac Appt:** Asst Clin Prof OrS, SUNY Stony Brook

Rich, Daniel Stephen MD (OrS) - **Spec Exp:** Knee Replacement; Hip Replacement; **Hospital:** Hosp For Special Surgery (page 115), St. Francis Hosp - The Heart Ctr (page 121); **Address:** 585 Plandome Rd, Ste 103, Manhasset, NY 11030-1971; **Phone:** 516-627-1525; **Board Cert:** Orthopaedic Surgery 1984; **Med School:** Harvard Med Sch 1977; **Resid:** Surgery, St Luke's-Roosevelt Hosp Ctr 1979; Orthopaedic Surgery, Hosp for Special Surgery 1982; **Fac Appt:** Asst Clin Prof OrS, Cornell Univ-Weill Med Coll

Sgaglione, Nicholas MD (OrS) - **Spec Exp:** Sports Medicine; **Hospital:** N Shore Univ Hosp (page 106); **Address:** 611 Northern Blvd, Ste 200, Great Neck, NY 11021; **Phone:** 516-723-2663; **Board Cert:** Orthopaedic Surgery 2012; **Med School:** Mount Sinai Sch Med 1983; **Resid:** Orthopaedic Surgery, Hosp Special Surg 1988; **Fellow:** Sports Medicine, Southern Cal Ortho Inst 1989; **Fac Appt:** Assoc Clin Prof OrS, Albert Einstein Coll Med

Shebairo, Raymond MD (OrS) - **Spec Exp:** Arthroscopic Surgery; Shoulder & Knee Surgery; Joint Replacement; **Hospital:** Long Island Jewish Med Ctr (page 106); **Address:** 1575 Hillside Ave, Ste 303, New Hyde Park, NY 11040; **Phone:** 516-437-5500; **Board Cert:** Orthopaedic Surgery 1982; **Med School:** Med Coll Wisc 1973; **Resid:** Orthopaedic Surgery, LIJ Med Ctr 1977

Simonson, Barry G MD (OrS) - **Spec Exp:** Sports Medicine; Arthroscopic Surgery; Hip & Knee Reconstruction; Hip & Knee Replacement; **Hospital:** Glen Cove Hosp (page 106); **Address:** 825 Northern Blvd, Ste 201, Great Neck, NY 11021-5323; **Phone:** 516-773-7500; **Board Cert:** Orthopaedic Surgery 2004; **Med School:** Mount Sinai Sch Med 1984; **Resid:** Orthopaedic Surgery, LI Jewish Med Ctr 1990; **Fellow:** Sports Medicine, New York Univ Med Ctr 1991

Ticker, Jonathan MD (OrS) - **Spec Exp:** Shoulder Surgery; Rotator Cuff Surgery; Shoulder Arthroscopic Surgery; Sports Medicine; **Hospital:** South Nassau Comm Hosp, Long Island Jewish Med Ctr (page 106); **Address:** Orlin & Cohen Orthopaedic Assocs, 1728 Sunrise Hwy, Merrick, NY 11566; **Phone:** 516-992-4700; **Board Cert:** Orthopaedic Surgery 2008; **Med School:** UMDNJ-NJ Med Sch, Newark 1988; **Resid:** Orthopaedic Surgery, NY Presby-Columbia Med Ctr 1994; **Fellow:** Shoulder Surgery, NY Presby-Columbia Med Ctr 1991; Sports Medicine & Shoulder Surgery, Univ Pittsburgh 1995; **Fac Appt:** Asst Prof OrS, Columbia P&S

Otolaryngology

Durante, Anthony J MD (Oto) - **Hospital:** Winthrop Univ Hosp (page 504); **Address:** 134 Mineola Blvd, Ste 201, Mineola, NY 11501; **Phone:** 516-294-9363; **Board Cert:** Otolaryngology 1975; **Med School:** Italy 1967; **Resid:** Surgery, Nassau Hosp 1970; Otolaryngology, Albert Einstein Coll Med 1975; **Fac Appt:** Asst Clin Prof S, SUNY Stony Brook

Frank, Douglas K MD (Oto) - **Spec Exp:** Head & Neck Cancer & Surgery; Thyroid & Parathyroid Surgery; Salivary Gland Tumors & Surgery; Skull Base Surgery; **Hospital:** Long Island Jewish Med Ctr (page 106), N Shore Univ Hosp (page 106); **Address:** 430 Lakeville Rd, New Hyde Park, NY 11042; **Phone:** 718-470-7552; **Board Cert:** Otolaryngology 1997; **Med School:** Univ Pennsylvania 1990; **Resid:** Surgery, St Vincent Hosp 1992; Otolaryngology, NY Ear & Ear Infirm 1996; **Fellow:** Head and Neck Surgery, UT MD Anderson Cancer Ctr 1999; **Fac Appt:** Assoc Prof Oto, Albert Einstein Coll Med

Gordon, Michael A MD (Oto) - **Spec Exp:** Balance Disorders; Hearing Disorders; Otosclerosis; Ear Surgery; **Hospital:** Long Island Jewish Med Ctr (page 106); **Address:** 990 Stewart Ave, Ste 610, Garden City, NY 11530; **Phone:** 516-222-1881; **Board Cert:** Otolaryngology 1993; **Med School:** Albert Einstein Coll Med 1986; **Resid:** Otolaryngology, Montrfiore Hosp Med Ctr 1992; **Fellow:** Otology & Neurotology, Ear Research Foundation 1993; **Fac Appt:** Asst Prof Oto, Albert Einstein Coll Med

Grosso, John MD (Oto) - **Spec Exp:** Pediatric Otolaryngology; Otology; **Hospital:** Plainview Hosp (page 106), Syosset Hosp (page 106); **Address:** Long Island ENT Assocs, 875 Old Country Rd, Ste 200, Plainview, NY 11803-4934; **Phone:** 516-931-5552; **Board Cert:** Otolaryngology 1993; **Med School:** SUNY Upstate Med Univ 1986; **Resid:** Otolaryngology, Univ Hosp 1992

Jacono, Andrew A MD (Oto) *PCP* - **Spec Exp:** Cosmetic Surgery-Face; Rhinoplasty; **Hospital:** NS-LIJ Hlth Sys (page 106), New York Eye & Ear Infirm (page 117); **Address:** 440 Northern Blvd, Great Neck, NY 11021; **Phone:** 516-773-4646; **Board Cert:** Otolaryngology 2002; Facial Plastic & Reconstr Surgery 2004; **Med School:** Albert Einstein Coll Med 1996; **Resid:** Otolaryngology, New York Eye & Ear Infirmary 2001; **Fellow:** Facial Plastic Surgery, Univ of Rochester 2002; **Fac Appt:** Asst Clin Prof Oto, NY Med Coll

Mattucci, Kenneth MD (Oto) - **Spec Exp:** Otology; Neuro-Otology; Nasal & Sinus Disorders; **Hospital:** St. Francis Hosp - The Heart Ctr (page 121), N Shore Univ Hosp (page 106); **Address:** 29 Barstow Rd, Ste 203, Great Neck, NY 11021; **Phone:** 516-482-7960; **Board Cert:** Otolaryngology 1970; **Med School:** Wake Forest Univ 1964; **Resid:** Surgery, New York Hosp 1966; Otolaryngology, NY Eye & Ear Infirm 1969; **Fellow:** Otolaryngology, New York Hosp 1970; **Fac Appt:** Clin Prof Oto, NY Med Coll

Moisa, Idel MD (Oto) - **Spec Exp:** Thyroid Surgery; Sinusitis; Snoring/Sleep Apnea; Endoscopic Sinus Surgery; **Hospital:** Glen Cove Hosp (page 106); **Address:** 3 School St, Rm 304 Bldg, 3 School St, Rm 304 Bldg, Glen Cove, NY 11542-2548; **Phone:** 516-671-0085; **Board Cert:** Otolaryngology 1988; **Med School:** Albert Einstein Coll Med 1983; **Resid:** Otolaryngology, Montefiore Med Ctr 1988; **Fellow:** Head and Neck Surgery, Montefiore Med Ctr 1990; **Fac Appt:** Asst Clin Prof Oto, NYU Sch Med

Perlman, Philip W MD (Oto) - **Spec Exp:** Pediatric & Adult Otolaryngology; Endoscopic Sinus Surgery; Head & Neck Surgery; Snoring/Sleep Apnea; **Hospital:** St. Francis Hosp - The Heart Ctr (page 121), N Shore Univ Hosp (page 106); **Address:** Progressive Ear, Nose & Throat Assocs, 333 E Shore Rd, Ste 102, Manhasset, NY 11030-2911; **Phone:** 516-466-5100; **Board Cert:** Otolaryngology 1988; Facial Plastic & Reconstr Surgery 1994; **Med School:** SUNY Downstate 1983; **Resid:** Surgery, Staten Island Hosp 1985; Otolaryngology, Albany Meml Hosp 1988; **Fellow:** Facial Plastic & Reconstr Surgery, AAFPRS 1989

Rosner, Louis M MD (Oto) - **Spec Exp:** Rhinoplasty; Endoscopic Sinus Surgery; Head & Neck Cancer; **Hospital:** South Nassau Comm Hosp, Mercy Med Ctr - Rockville Centre; **Address:** 176 N Village Ave, Ste 1A, Rockville Centre, NY 11570-3800; **Phone:** 516-678-0303; **Board Cert:** Otolaryngology 1982; **Med School:** Ros Franklin Univ/Chicago Med Sch 1978; **Resid:** Otolaryngology, NY Eye & Ear Infirm 1982

Setzen, Michael MD (Oto) - **Spec Exp:** Nasal & Sinus Surgery; Rhinoplasty; Sleep Disorders/Apnea; Snoring/Sleep Apnea; **Hospital:** N Shore Univ Hosp (page 106), St. Francis Hosp - The Heart Ctr (page 121); **Address:** 600 Northern Blvd, Ste 312, Great Neck, NY 11021-5200; **Phone:** 516-829-0045; **Board Cert:** Otolaryngology 1982; **Med School:** South Africa 1974; **Resid:** Surgery, Cleveland Clinic Fdn 1978; Otolaryngology, Barnes Jewish Hosp 1982; **Fac Appt:** Assoc Clin Prof Oto, NYU Sch Med

Shikowitz, Mark J MD (Oto) - **Spec Exp:** Sleep Apnea; Facial Plastic & Reconstructive Surgery; Rhinoplasty; Otoplasty; **Hospital:** Long Island Jewish Med Ctr (page 106), Steven & Alexandra Cohen Chldn's Med Ctr of NY (page 106); **Address:** Hearing & Speech Bldg, 430 Lakeville Rd, New Hyde Park, NY 11042; **Phone:** 718-470-7552; **Board Cert:** Otolaryngology 1987; **Med School:** Dominica 1981; **Resid:** Otolaryngology, LI Jewish Med Ctr 1986; **Fac Appt:** Assoc Prof Oto, Albert Einstein Coll Med

Soletic, Raymond MD (Oto) - **Spec Exp:** Endoscopic Sinus Surgery; Cosmetic Surgery-Face; **Hospital:** St. Francis Hosp - The Heart Ctr (page 121); **Address:** 1615 Northern Blvd, Ste 201, Manhasset, NY 11030; **Phone:** 516-365-7952; **Board Cert:** Otolaryngology 1990; **Med School:** Mexico 1982; **Resid:** Surgery, Baystate/Tufts 1985; Otolaryngology, Manhattan EE&T Hosp 1989

Tawfik, Bernard MD (Oto) - **Spec Exp:** Thyroid Disorders; Sinus Disorders; Snoring/Sleep Apnea; Sleep Disorders/Apnea; **Hospital:** Glen Cove Hosp (page 106), Winthrop Univ Hosp (page 504); **Address:** 3 School St, Ste 304, Glen Cove, NY 11542; **Phone:** 516-671-0085; **Board Cert:** Otolaryngology 1977; **Med School:** Johns Hopkins Univ 1971; **Resid:** Otolaryngology, Manhattan Eye & Ear 1977

Vambutas, Andrea MD (Oto) - **Spec Exp:** Hearing & Balance Disorders; Pediatric Otolaryngology; Cochlear Implants; **Hospital:** Long Island Jewish Med Ctr (page 106); **Address:** Hearing and Speech Ctr, 430 Lakeville Rd, New Hyde Park, NY 11042; **Phone:** 718-470-7552; **Board Cert:** Otolaryngology 1998; **Med School:** Albert Einstein Coll Med 1992; **Resid:** Otolaryngology, LIJ Med Ctr 1998; **Fellow:** Otology, Fairview Univ Med Ctr 1999; **Fac Appt:** Asst Prof Oto, Albert Einstein Coll Med

Youngerman, Jay MD (Oto) - **Spec Exp:** Head & Neck Surgery; Sleep & Snoring Disorders; Ear Disorders/Surgery; Pediatric Otolaryngology; **Hospital:** Plainview Hosp (page 106), Syosset Hosp (page 106); **Address:** Long Island ENT Assocs, 875 Old Country Rd, Ste 200, Plainview, NY 11803-4934; **Phone:** 516-931-5552; **Board Cert:** Otolaryngology 1984; **Med School:** Med Coll VA 1979; **Resid:** Otolaryngology, LI Jewish Med Ctr 1983

Zahtz, Gerald MD (Oto) - **Spec Exp:** Sinus Disorders/Surgery; Pediatric Otolaryngology; **Hospital:** Long Island Jewish Med Ctr (page 106); **Address:** 430 Lakeville Rd, New Hyde Park, NY 11042; **Phone:** 718-470-7552; **Board Cert:** Otolaryngology 1981; **Med School:** St Louis Univ 1977; **Resid:** Surgery, LIJ-Hillside Med Ctr 1978; Otolaryngology, LIJ-Hillside Med Ctr 1981; **Fac Appt:** Assoc Prof Oto, Albert Einstein Coll Med

Zelman, Warren H MD (Oto) - **Spec Exp:** Head & Neck Surgery; Sinus Disorders/Surgery; Pediatric & Adult Otolaryngology; **Hospital:** Winthrop Univ Hosp (page 504); **Address:** 990 Stewart Ave, Ste 610, Garden City, NY 11530; **Phone:** 516-739-3999; **Board Cert:** Otolaryngology 1987; **Med School:** Ros Franklin Univ/Chicago Med Sch 1982; **Resid:** Surgery, Univ Hosp-SUNY 1984; Otolaryngology, Manhattan EE&T Hosp 1987

Pain Medicine

Agin, Carole MD (PM) - **Spec Exp:** Acupuncture; Complex Regional Pain Syndromes; Pain-Neuropathic; Pain-Back; **Hospital:** NS-LIJ Hlth Sys (page 106); **Address:** 3 Delaware Drive, Lake Success, NY 11042; **Phone:** 516-622-6105; **Board Cert:** Anesthesiology 1991; Pain Medicine 2004; **Med School:** Ros Franklin Univ/Chicago Med Sch 1986; **Resid:** Anesthesiology, Beth Israel Med Ctr 1990; **Fellow:** Pain Medicine, Meml Sloan Kettering Cancer Ctr 1991

Pinsky, Steven MD (PM) - **Hospital:** Mercy Med Ctr - Rockville Centre; **Address:** 176 N Village Ave, Ste 2D, Rockville Centre, NY 11570; **Phone:** 516-764-4875; **Board Cert:** Anesthesiology 1994; Pain Medicine 2007; **Med School:** Albert Einstein Coll Med 1989; **Resid:** Anesthesiology, SUNY Downstate 1993; **Fellow:** Pain Medicine, St Lukes Roosevelt Med Ctr 1994

Pathology

Crawford, James M MD/PhD (Path) - **Spec Exp:** Liver Pathology; Gastrointestinal Pathology; Gastrointestinal Cancer; **Hospital:** N Shore Univ Hosp (page 106), Long Island Jewish Med Ctr (page 106); **Address:** N Shore-LIJ Laboratories, 10 Nevada Drive, Lake Success, NY 11042-1114; **Phone:** 516-719-1060; **Board Cert:** Anatomic Pathology 1987; **Med School:** Duke Univ 1982; **Resid:** Pathology, Brigham & Women's Hosp 1984; **Fellow:** Gastrointestinal Pathology, Brigham & Women's Hosp 1987; Pathology, Royal Free hosp 1989

Kahn, Leonard B MD (Path) - **Spec Exp:** Bone Pathology; Head & Neck Pathology; Soft Tissue Tumors; Jaw Tumors; **Hospital:** Long Island Jewish Med Ctr (page 106), N Shore Univ Hosp (page 106); **Address:** 6 Ohio Drive, Ste 202, rm 621, Lake Success, NY 10042; **Phone:** 516-304-7264; **Board Cert:** Anatomic Pathology 1980; **Med School:** South Africa 1960; **Resid:** Pathology, Univ Cape Town 1966; **Fellow:** Pathology, Washington Univ 1969; **Fac Appt:** Prof Path, Albert Einstein Coll Med

Pediatric Allergy & Immunology

Bonagura, Vincent R MD (PA&I) - **Spec Exp:** AIDS/HIV; **Hospital:** Steven & Alexandra Cohen Chldn's Med Ctr of NY (page 106), Long Island Jewish Med Ctr (page 106); **Address:** 865 Northern Blvd, Ste 101, Great Neck, NY 11021; **Phone:** 516-622-5070; **Board Cert:** Pediatrics 1979; Allergy & Immunology 1981; Clinical & Laboratory Immunology 1986; **Med School:** Columbia P&S 1975; **Resid:** Pediatrics, Columbia Presby Hosp 1978; **Fellow:** Allergy & Immunology, Columbia Presby Hosp 1983; **Fac Appt:** Prof Ped, Albert Einstein Coll Med

Fagin, James MD (PA&I) - **Spec Exp:** Asthma; Allergy; Immunodeficiency Disorders; Rhinitis; **Hospital:** Steven & Alexandra Cohen Chldn's Med Ctr of NY (page 106), N Shore Univ Hosp (page 106); **Address:** 865 Northern Blvd, Ste 101, MS 11021, Div of Allergy/Immunology, Great Neck, NY 11021-5303; **Phone:** 516-622-5070; **Board Cert:** Pediatrics 1980; Allergy & Immunology 1983; **Med School:** Belgium 1976; **Resid:** Pediatrics, N Shore Univ Hosp 1979; **Fellow:** Allergy & Immunology, Chldns Hosp of Pittsburgh 1981; **Fac Appt:** Asst Prof Ped, NYU Sch Med

Pediatric Cardiology

Better, Donna J MD (PCd) - **Spec Exp:** Echocardiography; Fetal Echocardiography; Congenital Heart Disease; **Hospital:** Winthrop Univ Hosp (page 504), Morgan Stanley Children's Hosp of NY-Presby, NY (page 104); **Address:** 120 Mineola Blvd, Ste 210, Mineola, NY 11501; **Phone:** 516-663-4600; **Board Cert:** Pediatric Cardiology 2011; **Med School:** Albert Einstein Coll Med 1989; **Resid:** Pediatrics, Mt Sinai Hosp 1992; **Fellow:** Pediatric Cardiology, Columbia-Presby Med Ctr 1995; **Fac Appt:** Asst Clin Prof Ped, Columbia P&S

Blaufox, Andrew D MD (PCd) - **Hospital:** Steven & Alexandra Cohen Chldn's Med Ctr of NY (page 106); **Address:** Steven & Alexandra Cohen Children's Med Ctr, 269-01 76th Ave, New Hyde Park, NY 11040; **Phone:** 718-470-7350; **Board Cert:** Pediatrics 2004; Pediatric Cardiology 2000; **Med School:** Albert Einstein Coll Med 1993; **Resid:** Pediatrics, Mt Sinai Med Ctr 1996; **Fellow:** Pediatric Cardiology, Mt Sinai Med Ctr 1999; **Fac Appt:** Asst Prof Ped, Cornell Univ-Weill Med Coll

Cooper, Rubin MD (PCd) - **Spec Exp:** Congenital Heart Disease; Rheumatic Heart Disease; Kawasaki Disease; **Hospital:** Steven & Alexandra Cohen Chldn's Med Ctr of NY (page 106); **Address:** Steven & Alexandra Cohen Chldns Med Ctr, 269-01 76th Ave, Ste 139, New Hyde Park, NY 11040; **Phone:** 718-470-3661; **Board Cert:** Pediatrics 1976; Pediatric Cardiology 1979; **Med School:** NY Med Coll 1971; **Resid:** Pediatrics, Strong Meml Hosp 1973; **Fellow:** Pediatric Cardiology, Strong Meml Hosp 1975; **Fac Appt:** Prof Ped, Cornell Univ-Weill Med Coll

Levchuck, Sean G MD (PCd) - **Spec Exp:** Interventional Cardiology; Congenital Heart Disease; Atrial Septal Defect; **Hospital:** St. Francis Hosp - The Heart Ctr (page 121), Steven & Alexandra Cohen Chldn's Med Ctr of NY (page 106); **Address:** 100 Port Washington Blvd, Ste 108, Roslyn, NY 11576-1353; **Phone:** 516-365-3340; **Board Cert:** Pediatrics 2008; Pediatric Cardiology 2011; **Med School:** West Indies 1989; **Resid:** Pediatrics, Winthrop Univ Hosp 1992; **Fellow:** Pediatric Cardiology, St Christophers Hosp 1995

Romano, Angela MD (PCd) - **Spec Exp:** Echocardiography; Marfan's Syndrome; Kawasaki Disease; **Hospital:** Steven & Alexandra Cohen Chldn's Med Ctr of NY (page 106); **Address:** Dept Pediatric Cardiology, 269-01 76th Ave Fl 1 - rm 139, New Hyde Park, NY 11040; **Phone:** 718-470-7350; **Board Cert:** Pediatrics 1984; Pediatric Cardiology 2010; **Med School:** Columbia P&S 1980; **Resid:** Pediatrics, Babies Hosp/Columbia Univ Med Ctr 1984; **Fellow:** Pediatric Cardiology, Children's Hosp 1987; **Fac Appt:** Asst Prof Ped, Albert Einstein Coll Med

Schiff, Russell J MD (PCd) - **Spec Exp:** Echocardiography; Fetal Echocardiography; Cardiomyopathy; Congenital Heart Disease; **Hospital:** Huntington Hosp (page 106), Steven & Alexandra Cohen Chldn's Med Ctr of NY (page 106); **Address:** 43 Crossways Park Drive W, Woodbury, NY 11797; **Phone:** 516-992-5205; **Board Cert:** Pediatrics 1986; Pediatric Cardiology 2010; **Med School:** SUNY Stony Brook 1981; **Resid:** Pediatrics, Schneider Chldns Hosp 1984; **Fellow:** Pediatric Cardiology, Schneider Chldns Hosp 1986; **Fac Appt:** Asst Prof Ped, NYU Sch Med

Shapir, Yehuda MD (PCd) - **Spec Exp:** Congenital Heart Disease & Acquired; Echocardiography; Fetal Echocardiography; **Hospital:** Steven & Alexandra Cohen Chldn's Med Ctr of NY (page 106); **Address:** Steven & Alexandra Cohen Chldn's Med Ctr, 269-01 76th Ave, Ste 139, New Hyde Park, NY 11040-1433; **Phone:** 718-470-7350; **Board Cert:** Pediatric Cardiology 2006; **Med School:** Israel 1977; **Resid:** Pediatrics, Rambam Med Ctr 1981; **Fellow:** Pediatric Cardiology, UCLA Med Ctr 1985; **Fac Appt:** Assoc Prof Ped, Albert Einstein Coll Med

Vallone, Ambrose M MD (PCd) - **Spec Exp:** Cardiac Catheterization; Syncope; Fetal Echocardiography; **Hospital:** St. Francis Hosp - The Heart Ctr (page 121), NS-LIJ Hlth Sys (page 106); **Address:** 100 Port Washington Blvd, Ste 108, Roslyn, NY 11576-1353; **Phone:** 516-365-3340; **Board Cert:** Pediatrics 1983; Pediatric Cardiology 2010; **Med School:** Johns Hopkins Univ 1977; **Resid:** Pediatrics, Johns Hopkins Hosp 1980; **Fellow:** Pediatric Cardiology, Yale-New Haven Hosp 1983; Pediatric Critical Care Medicine, Yale-New Haven Hosp 1983

Pediatric Endocrinology

Accacha, Siham D MD (PEn) - **Spec Exp:** Diabetes; Growth Disorders; Metabolic Syndrome; **Hospital:** Winthrop Univ Hosp (page 504); **Address:** 120 Mineola Blvd, Ste 210, Mineola, NY 11501; **Phone:** 516-663-4600; **Board Cert:** Pediatric Endocrinology 2005; **Med School:** France 1993; **Resid:** Pediatrics, Westchester Med Ctr 2001; **Fellow:** Pediatric Endocrinology, Winthrop Univ Hosp 2005

Carey, Dennis MD (PEn) - **Spec Exp:** Diabetes; Calcium Disorders; Growth Disorders; Thyroid Disorders; **Hospital:** Steven & Alexandra Cohen Chldn's Med Ctr of NY (page 106); **Address:** 1991 Marcus Ave, Ste M100, Lake Success, NY 11042-2057; **Phone:** 516-472-3750; **Board Cert:** Pediatrics 1979; Pediatric Endocrinology 1983; **Med School:** SUNY Downstate 1973; **Resid:** Pediatric Surgery, LI Jewish Med Ctr 1979; **Fellow:** Pediatric Endocrinology, UCSD Med Ctr 1980; **Fac Appt:** Assoc Prof Ped, Albert Einstein Coll Med

Castro-Magana, Mariano MD (PEn) - **Spec Exp:** Growth/Development Disorders; Adrenal Disorders; Sexual Development Problems; **Hospital:** Winthrop Univ Hosp (page 504); **Address:** Winthrop Univ Hosp, Div Ped Endo, 120 Mineola Blvd, Ste 210, Mineola, NY 11501; **Phone:** 516-663-4600 x2; **Board Cert:** Pediatrics 1983; Pediatric Endocrinology 1983; **Med School:** El Salvador 1974; **Resid:** Pediatrics, Nassau County Med Ctr 1980; **Fellow:** Pediatric Endocrinology, Nassau County Med Ctr 1982; **Fac Appt:** Prof Ped, NYU Sch Med

Frank, Graeme MD (PEn) - **Spec Exp:** Pubertal Disorders; Growth/Development Disorders; Diabetes; Thyroid Disorders; **Hospital:** Steven & Alexandra Cohen Chldn's Med Ctr of NY (page 106); **Address:** 1991 Marcus Ave, Ste M100, Lake Success, NY 11042-2057; **Phone:** 516-472-3750; **Board Cert:** Pediatrics 2005; Pediatric Endocrinology 2010; **Med School:** South Africa 1982; **Resid:** Pediatrics, LIJ-Schneider Chldns Hosp 1991; **Fellow:** Pediatric Endocrinology, Children's Hosp 1994; **Fac Appt:** Assoc Clin Prof Ped, Albert Einstein Coll Med

Kreitzer, Paula MD (PEn) - **Spec Exp:** Diabetes; Growth/Development Disorders; **Hospital:** Steven & Alexandra Cohen Chldn's Med Ctr of NY (page 106), Long Island Jewish Med Ctr (page 106); **Address:** 1991 Marcus Ave, Ste M100, Lake Success, NY 11042-2057; **Phone:** 516-472-3750; **Board Cert:** Pediatrics 1987; Pediatric Endocrinology 2011; **Med School:** Univ NC Sch Med 1982; **Resid:** Pediatrics, LIJ-Schneider Chldns Hosp 1987; Pediatric Endocrinology, LIJ-Schneider Chldns Hosp 1989

Speiser, Phyllis W MD (PEn) - **Spec Exp:** Pubertal Disorders; Growth/Development Disorders; Adrenal Disorders; Thyroid Disorders; **Hospital:** Steven & Alexandra Cohen Chldn's Med Ctr of NY (page 106), N Shore Univ Hosp (page 106); **Address:** 1991 Marcus Ave, Ste M100, Div Ped Endocrinology, 269-01 76th Ave, Lake Success, NY 11042-2057; **Phone:** 516-472-3750; **Board Cert:** Pediatrics 1984; Pediatric Endocrinology 2004; **Med School:** Columbia P&S 1979; **Resid:** Pediatrics, Jacobi Med Ctr 1982; **Fellow:** Pediatric Endocrinology, New York Hosp-Cornell 1984; **Fac Appt:** Prof Ped, NYU Sch Med

Pediatric Gastroenterology

Daum, Fredric MD (PGe) - **Spec Exp:** Inflammatory Bowel Disease; Liver Disease; Incontinence-Fecal; **Hospital:** Winthrop Univ Hosp (page 504); **Address:** 120 Mineola Blvd, Ste 210, Mineola, NY 11501; **Phone:** 516-663-4600; **Board Cert:** Pediatrics 1972; Pediatric Gastroenterology 2005; **Med School:** Tufts Univ 1967; **Resid:** Pediatrics, Jacobi Med Ctr 1969; **Fellow:** Adolescent Medicine, Montefiore Med Ctr 1972

Levine, Jeremiah MD (PGe) - **Spec Exp:** Inflammatory Bowel Disease; Crohn's Disease; Liver Disease; **Hospital:** Steven & Alexandra Cohen Chldn's Med Ctr of NY (page 106); **Address:** 1991 Marcus Ave, Div Pediatric Gastroenterology, Lake Success, NY 11042; **Phone:** 516-472-3650; **Board Cert:** Pediatrics 1985; Pediatric Gastroenterology 2005; **Med School:** Harvard Med Sch 1980; **Resid:** Pediatrics, Albert Einstein Coll Med Ctr 1983; **Fellow:** Pediatric Gastroenterology, Children's Hosp 1985; **Fac Appt:** Prof Ped, Albert Einstein Coll Med

Markowitz, James MD (PGe) - **Spec Exp:** Inflammatory Bowel Disease/Crohn's; Gastroesophageal Reflux Disease (GERD); **Hospital:** Steven & Alexandra Cohen Chldn's Med Ctr of NY (page 106); **Address:** 1991 Marcus Ave, Div Pediatric Gastroenterology, Lake Success, NY 11042; **Phone:** 516-472-3650; **Board Cert:** Pediatrics 1981; Pediatric Gastroenterology 2005; **Med School:** Cornell Univ-Weill Med Coll 1977; **Resid:** Pediatrics, NY Hosp 1980; **Fellow:** Pediatric Gastroenterology, N Shore Univ Hosp 1983; **Fac Appt:** Assoc Prof Ped, NYU Sch Med

Pettei, Michael J MD/PhD (PGe) - **Spec Exp:** Cholesterol/Lipid Disorders; Nutrition; Celiac Disease; **Hospital:** Steven & Alexandra Cohen Chldn's Med Ctr of NY (page 106); **Address:** 1991 Marcus Ave, Div Pediatric Endocrinology, Lake Success, NY 11042; **Phone:** 516-472-3650; **Board Cert:** Pediatrics 1986; Pediatric Gastroenterology 2005; **Med School:** Univ Miami Sch Med 1980; **Resid:** Pediatrics, Mt Sinai Med Ctr 1982; **Fellow:** Pediatric Gastroenterology, Columbia-Presby Med Ctr 1984; **Fac Appt:** Assoc Prof Ped, Albert Einstein Coll Med

Weinstein, Toba MD (PGe) - **Spec Exp:** Inflammatory Bowel Disease/Crohn's; Gastroesophageal Reflux Disease (GERD); Irritable Bowel Syndrome; Constipation; **Hospital:** Steven & Alexandra Cohen Chldn's Med Ctr of NY (page 106); **Address:** 1991 Marcus Ave, Ste M100, Lake Success, NY 11042; **Phone:** 516-472-3650; **Board Cert:** Pediatrics 2007; Pediatric Gastroenterology 2007; **Med School:** Columbia P&S 1986; **Resid:** Pediatrics, Chldn's Hosp Natl Med Ctr 1989; **Fellow:** Pediatric Gastroenterology, Schneider Children's Hosp-LIJ 1991; **Fac Appt:** Assoc Prof Ped, Hofstra N Shore-LIJ Sch Med

Pediatric Hematology-Oncology

Lipton, Jeffrey M MD/PhD (PHO) - **Spec Exp:** Bone Marrow Failure Disorders; Stem Cell Transplant; Bone Marrow Transplant; Bone Marrow Failure Disorders; **Hospital:** Steven & Alexandra Cohen Chldn's Med Ctr of NY (page 106); **Address:** Cohen Children's Medical Center of NY, 269-01 76th Ave, New Hyde Park, NY 11040-1433; **Phone:** 718-470-3460; **Board Cert:** Pediatrics 1981; **Med School:** St Louis Univ 1975; **Resid:** Pediatrics, Boston Chldns Hosp 1977; **Fellow:** Pediatric Hematology-Oncology, Boston Chldns Hosp/Dana Farber Cancer Inst 1979; **Fac Appt:** Prof Ped, Hofstra N Shore-LIJ Sch Med

Redner, Arlene MD (PHO) - **Spec Exp:** Leukemia; Brain Tumors; Solid Tumors; Neuro-Oncology; **Hospital:** Steven & Alexandra Cohen Chldn's Med Ctr of NY (page 106); **Address:** 269-01 76th Ave, rm 255, New Hyde Park, NY 11040-1434; **Phone:** 718-470-3460; **Board Cert:** Pediatrics 1982; Pediatric Hematology-Oncology 1984; **Med School:** Univ Pennsylvania 1977; **Resid:** Pediatrics, Boston Floating Hosp 1980; **Fellow:** Pediatric Hematology-Oncology, Meml Sloan Kettering Hosp 1985; **Fac Appt:** Assoc Clin Prof Ped, Albert Einstein Coll Med

Sabatino, Dominick P MD (PHO) - **Spec Exp:** Cooley's Anemia; Thalassemia; Sickle Cell Disease; **Hospital:** Nassau Univ Med Ctr; **Address:** Nassau Univ Med Ctr, Dept Peds, 2201 Hempstead Tpke, East Meadow, NY 11554; **Phone:** 516-572-6177; **Board Cert:** Pediatrics 1975; Pediatric Hematology-Oncology 1982; **Med School:** Italy 1968; **Resid:** Pediatrics, LI College Hosp 1974; **Fellow:** Pediatric Hematology-Oncology, LI College Hosp 1975; **Fac Appt:** Clin Prof Ped, SUNY Stony Brook

Weinblatt, Mark E MD (PHO) - **Spec Exp:** Leukemia & Lymphoma; Sickle Cell Disease; Bleeding/Coagulation Disorders; Thalassemia; **Hospital:** Winthrop Univ Hosp (page 504); **Address:** 120 Mineola Blvd, Ste 460, Mineola, NY 11501; **Phone:** 516-663-9400; **Board Cert:** Pediatrics 1980; Pediatric Hematology-Oncology 1982; **Med School:** Albert Einstein Coll Med 1976; **Resid:** Pediatrics, Jacobi Med Ctr 1979; **Fellow:** Pediatric Hematology-Oncology, Children's Hosp 1981; **Fac Appt:** Prof Ped, SUNY Stony Brook

Wolfe, Lawrence C MD (PHO) - **Spec Exp:** Palliative Care; Neuroblastoma; Adrenal Cancer; Congenital Hemolytic Anemia; **Hospital:** Steven & Alexandra Cohen Chldn's Med Ctr of NY (page 106); **Address:** Steven & Alexandra Cohen Chldn's Med Ctr, Div Pediatric Hematology/Oncology, 269-01 76th Ave, New Hyde Park, NY 11040; **Phone:** 718-470-3460; **Board Cert:** Pediatrics 1981; Pediatric Hematology-Oncology 1987; Hospice & Palliative Medicine 2011; **Med School:** Harvard Med Sch 1976; **Resid:** Pediatrics, Chldns Hosp 1978; **Fellow:** Pediatric Hematology-Oncology, Chldns Hosp 1991; **Fac Appt:** Prof Ped

Pediatric Infectious Disease

Krilov, Leonard MD (PInf) - **Spec Exp:** Infections-Respiratory; Infections in Int'l Adopted Children; Chronic Fatigue Syndrome; Lyme Disease; **Hospital:** Winthrop Univ Hosp (page 504); **Address:** 120 Mineola Blvd, Ste 210, Mineola, NY 11501; **Phone:** 516-663-4600; **Board Cert:** Pediatrics 1983; Pediatric Infectious Disease 2009; **Med School:** Columbia P&S 1978; **Resid:** Pediatrics, Johns Hopkins Hosp 1981; **Fellow:** Pediatric Infectious Disease, Children's Hosp 1984; **Fac Appt:** Prof Ped, SUNY Stony Brook

Rubin, Lorry MD (PInf) - **Spec Exp:** Kawasaki Disease; Tuberculosis; Fevers of Unknown Origin; **Hospital:** Steven & Alexandra Cohen Chldn's Med Ctr of NY (page 106), N Shore Univ Hosp (page 106); **Address:** 269-01 76th Ave, Div Infectious Disease, New Hyde Park, NY 11040-1433; **Phone:** 718-470-3480; **Board Cert:** Pediatrics 1983; Pediatric Infectious Disease 2009; **Med School:** Rush Med Coll 1978; **Resid:** Pediatrics, Children's Hosp 1980; **Fellow:** Pediatric Infectious Disease, Johns Hopkins Hosp 1982; **Fac Appt:** Prof Ped, Albert Einstein Coll Med

Sood, Sunil K MD (PInf) - **Spec Exp:** Fevers of Unknown Origin; Tuberculosis; Lyme Disease; **Hospital:** Steven & Alexandra Cohen Chldn's Med Ctr of NY (page 106); **Address:** 269-01 76th Ave, New Hyde Park, NY 11040-1433; **Phone:** 718-470-3480; **Board Cert:** Pediatrics 1987; Pediatric Infectious Disease 2009; **Med School:** India 1976; **Resid:** Pediatrics, Baltimore City Hosp 1983; Pediatrics, Georgetown Univ Hosp 1985; **Fellow:** Infectious Disease, Tulane Univ 1988; **Fac Appt:** Assoc Prof Ped, Albert Einstein Coll Med

Pediatric Otolaryngology

Mendelsohn, Michael MD (PO) - **Hospital:** Long Island Jewish Med Ctr (page 106); **Address:** 990 Stewart Ave, Ste 610, Garden City, NY 11530; **Phone:** 516-222-1881; **Board Cert:** Otolaryngology 1999; **Med School:** Boston Univ 1990; **Resid:** Otolaryngology, LI Jewish Med Ctr 1995; **Fellow:** Pediatric Otolaryngology, Univ Virginia Med Ctr 1996; **Fac Appt:** Asst Prof Oto, SUNY Downstate

Smith, Lee P MD (PO) - **Spec Exp:** Airway Disorders; Head & Neck Tumors; Tonsil/Adenoid Disorders; Ear Infections; **Hospital:** Steven & Alexandra Cohen Chldn's Med Ctr of NY (page 106), Long Island Jewish Med Ctr (page 106); **Address:** Steven and Alexandra Cohen Childrens Medical Center, Pediatric Otolaryngology, 430 Lakville Rd, New Hyde Park, NY 11042; **Phone:** 718-470-7550; **Board Cert:** Otolaryngology 2008; **Med School:** NYU Sch Med 2002; **Resid:** Otolaryngology, Univ Miami Hosp 2007; **Fellow:** Pediatric Otolaryngology, Chldns Hosp 2009; **Fac Appt:** Asst Prof Oto, Hofstra N Shore-LIJ Sch Med

Pediatric Pulmonology

Schaeffer, Janis MD (PPul) - **Spec Exp:** Asthma; Cough-Chronic; Lung Disorders-Congenital; **Hospital:** Steven & Alexandra Cohen Chldn's Med Ctr of NY (page 106), N Shore Univ Hosp (page 106); **Address:** 3003 New Hyde Park Rd, Ste 204, New Hyde Park, NY 11042-1214; **Phone:** 516-488-7575; **Board Cert:** Pediatrics 1984; Pediatric Pulmonology 2011; **Med School:** SUNY Downstate 1979; **Resid:** Pediatrics, LI Jewish Med Ctr 1982; **Fellow:** Pediatric Pulmonology, Columbia-Presby Med Ctr 1985; **Fac Appt:** Asst Prof Ped, Albert Einstein Coll Med

Vicencio, Alfin G MD (PPul) - **Spec Exp:** Bronchoscopy; **Hospital:** NS-LIJ Hlth Sys (page 106), Steven & Alexandra Cohen Chldn's Med Ctr of NY (page 106); **Address:** Cohen Children's Med Pul/Cystic, 865 Northern Blvd Ste 103, Great Neck, NY 11021; **Phone:** 516-622-5280; **Board Cert:** Pediatrics 2001; Pediatric Pulmonology 2004; **Med School:** Med Coll OH 1996; **Resid:** Pediatrics, Columbia Presby Med Ctr 1999; **Fellow:** Pediatric Pulmonology, Yale-New Haven Hosp 2002

Pediatric Rheumatology

Gottlieb, Beth S MD (PRhu) - **Spec Exp:** Juvenile Arthritis; Lupus/SLE; Osteoarthritis; Dermato-myositis; **Hospital:** Steven & Alexandra Cohen Chldn's Med Ctr of NY (page 106), NS-LIJ Hlth Sys (page 106); **Address:** 1991 Marcus Ave, Ste M100, Lake Success, NY 11042; **Phone:** 516-472-3700; **Board Cert:** Pediatrics 2010; Pediatric Rheumatology 2006; **Med School:** Israel 1992; **Resid:** Pediatrics, Schneider Children's Hosp 1995; **Fellow:** Pediatric Rheumatology, Schneider Children's Hosp 1998; **Fac Appt:** Asst Prof Ped, Albert Einstein Coll Med

Pediatric Surgery

Coren, Charles V MD (PS) - **Hospital:** Winthrop Univ Hosp (page 504), NY Hosp Queens (page 206); **Address:** 320 Post Ave, Ste 101, Westbury, NY 11590; **Phone:** 516-997-1199; **Board Cert:** Pediatric Surgery 2005; **Med School:** Univ Cincinnati 1978; **Resid:** Surgery, NYU Med Ctr 1983; **Fellow:** Pediatric Surgery, Univ Hosp 1985; **Fac Appt:** Asst Prof S, SUNY Hlth Sci Ctr

Dolgin, Stephen MD (PS) - **Spec Exp:** Neonatal Surgery; Ulcerative Colitis; Inflammatory Bowel Disease/Crohn's; Ovarian Masses in Children/Adolescents; **Hospital:** Steven & Alexandra Cohen Chldn's Med Ctr, Pediatric Surgery, 269-01 76th Ave, Ste 158, New Hyde Park, NY 11040; **Phone:** 718-470-3636; **Board Cert:** Surgery 2011; Pediatric Surgery 2003; Surgical Critical Care 2000; **Med School:** NYU Sch Med 1977; **Resid:** Surgery, Peter Bent Brigham Hosp/Harvard Univ 1982; **Fellow:** Pediatric Surgery, Chldns Meml Hosp/Northwestern Univ 1984; **Fac Appt:** Prof S, Hofstra N Shore-LIJ Sch Med

Hong, Andrew MD (PS) - **Spec Exp:** Neonatal Surgery; Minimally Invasive Surgery; Chest Wall Deformities; **Hospital:** Steven & Alexandra Cohen Chldn's Med Ctr of NY (page 106), N Shore Univ Hosp (page 106); **Address:** Steven & Alexandra Cohen Chldn's Med Ctr, 269-01 76th Ave, Ste 158, New Hyde Park, NY 11040; **Phone:** 718-470-3636; **Board Cert:** Surgery 2002; Pediatric Surgery 2011; **Med School:** Univ Wisc 1985; **Resid:** Surgery, Med Ctr Hosp 1990; **Fellow:** Pediatric Surgery, Montreal Chldns Hosp 1992; **Fac Appt:** Asst Prof S, Albert Einstein Coll Med

Parnell, Vincent MD (PS) - **Spec Exp:** Pediatric Cardiothoracic Surgery; Congenital Heart Disease; **Hospital:** Steven & Alexandra Cohen Chldn's Med Ctr of NY (page 106), N Shore Univ Hosp (page 106); **Address:** Steven & Alexandra Cohen Chldn's Med Ctr, Ped Cardiothoracic Surgery, 269-01 76th Ave, New Hyde Park, NY 11040; **Phone:** 718-470-7350; **Board Cert:** Surgery 2000; Thoracic & Cardiac Surgery 2002; Congenital Cardiac Surgery 2011; **Med School:** SUNY Downstate 1976; **Resid:** Surgery, N Shore Univ Hosp 1981; Thoracic Surgery, Harper Hosp 1983; **Fellow:** Pediatric Cardiac Surgery, Chldns Hosp 1984

Stylianos, Steven MD (PS) - **Spec Exp:** Trauma; Neonatal Surgery; Chest Wall Deformities; Congenital Anomalies; **Hospital:** Steven & Alexandra Cohen Chldn's Med Ctr of NY (page 106); **Address:** 269-01 76th Ave, New Hyde Park, NY 11040; **Phone:** 718-470-3636; **Board Cert:** Surgery 2002; Pediatric Surgery 2003; **Med School:** NYU Sch Med 1983; **Resid:** Surgery, Columbia-Presby Med Ctr 1988; Pediatric Surgery, Chldns Hosp 1992; **Fellow:** Pediatric Trauma, New England Med Ctr 1990; **Fac Appt:** Prof S, FIU Coll Med

Pediatrics

Adesman, Andrew MD (Ped) - **Spec Exp:** Autism; Asperger's Syndrome; Developmental Disorders; Tourette's Syndrome; **Hospital:** Steven & Alexandra Cohen Chldn's Med Ctr of NY (page 106); **Address:** 1983 Marcus Ave Fl 1 - Ste 130, New Hyde Park, NY 11042; **Phone:** 516-802-6100; **Board Cert:** Pediatrics 1987; Neurodevelopmental Disabilities 2001; Developmental-Behavioral Pediatrics 2010; **Med School:** Univ Pennsylvania 1981; **Resid:** Pediatrics, Chldn's Hosp Natl Med Ctr 1984; **Fellow:** Developmental-Behavioral Pediatrics, Chldn's Hosp 1986; **Fac Appt:** Assoc Prof Ped, Albert Einstein Coll Med

Chianese, Maurice J MD (Ped) *PCP* - **Spec Exp:** Pediatric Sports Medicine; Asthma; Behavioral Disorders; **Hospital:** Steven & Alexandra Cohen Chldn's Med Ctr of NY (page 106), N Shore Univ Hosp (page 106); **Address:** ProHealthCare Associates, 7 Vermont Drive, Div of Pediatrics, Lake Success, NY 11042; **Phone:** 516-622-7337; **Board Cert:** Pediatrics 2004; **Med School:** NY Med Coll 1986; **Resid:** Pediatrics, North Shore Univ Hosp 1990; **Fac Appt:** Asst Prof Ped, NYU Sch Med

Cooper, Seymour M MD (Ped) *PCP* - **Hospital:** Winthrop Univ Hosp (page 504), Steven & Alexandra Cohen Chldn's Med Ctr of NY (page 106); **Address:** 1101 Stewart Ave, Ste 306, Garden City, NY 11530; **Phone:** 516-746-2299; **Board Cert:** Pediatrics 1977; **Med School:** NY Med Coll 1972; **Resid:** Pediatrics, Montefiore Hosp Med Ctr 1975

Friedman, Eugene B MD (Ped) *PCP* - **Hospital:** Steven & Alexandra Cohen Chldn's Med Ctr of NY (page 106), Winthrop Univ Hosp (page 504); **Address:** 271 Jericho Tpke, Floral Park, NY 11002; **Phone:** 516-354-7575; **Board Cert:** Pediatrics 1973; **Med School:** NY Med Coll 1968; **Resid:** Pediatrics, Metropolitan Hosp Ctr 1971; **Fac Appt:** Asst Clin Prof Ped, Albert Einstein Coll Med

Galinkin, Lawrence MD (Ped) *PCP* - **Hospital:** N Shore Univ Hosp (page 106), Long Island Jewish Med Ctr (page 106); **Address:** 700 Old Bethpage Rd, Old Bethpage, NY 11804; **Phone:** 516-293-0666; **Board Cert:** Pediatrics 1976; **Med School:** Tulane Univ 1971; **Resid:** Pediatrics, Bronx Muni Hosp 1974

Gerberg, Lynda Frances MD (Ped) *PCP* - **Spec Exp:** Sports Medicine; Obesity; **Hospital:** Long Island Jewish Med Ctr (page 106); **Address:** 200 Middle Neck Rd, Great Neck, NY 11021; **Phone:** 516-466-3311; **Board Cert:** Pediatrics 2009; **Med School:** Mexico 1987; **Resid:** Pediatrics, Schneider Chldns Hosp 1993; **Fellow:** Pediatrics, Children's Hosp 1994; **Fac Appt:** Asst Prof Ped, Albert Einstein Coll Med

Gould, Eric MD (Ped) *PCP* - **Spec Exp:** Developmental Disorders; **Hospital:** Long Island Jewish Med Ctr (page 106), N Shore Univ Hosp (page 106); **Address:** 225 Community Drive, Ste 105, Great Neck, NY 11021-2229; **Phone:** 516-829-9409; **Board Cert:** Pediatrics 1976; **Med School:** NY Med Coll 1970; **Resid:** Pediatrics, Bellevue Hosp Ctr/NYU 1974; **Fellow:** Child Development, Montefiore Med Ctr 1976

Green, Abraham I MD (Ped) *PCP* - **Spec Exp:** Asthma; Nutrition; ADD/ADHD; **Hospital:** Long Island Jewish Med Ctr (page 106), Winthrop Univ Hosp (page 504); **Address:** 115 Franklin Pl, Woodmere, NY 11598; **Phone:** 516-295-1200; **Board Cert:** Pediatrics 2009; **Med School:** Albert Einstein Coll Med 1979; **Resid:** Pediatrics, Jacobi Med Ctr 1983

Grijnsztein, Jacob MD (Ped) *PCP* - **Spec Exp:** Allergy; **Hospital:** Long Island Jewish Med Ctr (page 106), N Shore Univ Hosp (page 106); **Address:** 107 Northern Blvd, Ste 201, Great Neck, NY 11021; **Phone:** 516-487-6565; **Board Cert:** Pediatrics 1979; **Med School:** NYU Sch Med 1973; **Resid:** Pediatrics, Bellevue Hosp 1976

Hankin, Dorie E. MD (Ped) - **Spec Exp:** Developmental Disorders; Behavioral Disorders; **Hospital:** Winthrop Univ Hosp (page 504), Steven & Alexandra Cohen Chldn's Med Ctr of NY (page 106); **Address:** 173 Mineola Blvd, Ste 301B, Mineola, NY 11501; **Phone:** 516-739-1936; **Board Cert:** Pediatrics 1980; Neurodevelopmental Disabilities 2012; Developmental-Behavioral Pediatrics 2010; **Med School:** Albert Einstein Coll Med 1974; **Resid:** Pediatrics, Montefiore Med Ctr 1978; **Fellow:** Child Development, Montefiore-Einstein Med Ctr 1980; **Fac Appt:** Asst Clin Prof Ped, Albert Einstein Coll Med

Leavens-Maurer, Jill MD (Ped) *PCP* - **Hospital:** Winthrop Univ Hosp (page 504); **Address:** Winthrop Pediatrics Assocs, 222 Station Plaza N, Ste 611, Mineola, NY 11501-3893; **Phone:** 516-663-2532; **Board Cert:** Pediatrics 2011; **Med School:** SUNY Upstate Med Univ 1984; **Resid:** Pediatrics, NY Hosp-Cornell Med Ctr 1987

Levy, Morton G MD (Ped) *PCP* - **Hospital:** N Shore Univ Hosp (page 106), Steven & Alexandra Cohen Chldn's Med Ctr of NY (page 106); **Address:** 133 Andover Rd, Roslyn Heights, NY 11577-1009; **Phone:** 516-621-9360; **Board Cert:** Pediatrics 1966; **Med School:** SUNY Downstate 1961; **Resid:** Pediatrics, Mount Sinai 1964; **Fac Appt:** Asst Clin Prof Ped, NYU Sch Med

Marino, Ronald Vincent DO (Ped) *PCP* - **Spec Exp:** Developmental & Behavioral Disorders; **Hospital:** Winthrop Univ Hosp (page 504), Good Samaritan Hosp Med Ctr - West Islip; **Address:** 222 Station Plaza N, Ste 611, Mineola, NY 11501-3808; **Phone:** 516-663-2532; **Board Cert:** Pediatrics 1985; **Med School:** Mich State Univ 1978; **Resid:** Pediatrics, Doctors Hosp 1981; **Fellow:** Behavioral Pediatrics, Univ Maryland Med Ctr 1985; **Fac Appt:** Prof Ped, SUNY Stony Brook

Milanaik, Ruth DO (Ped) *PCP* - **Spec Exp:** Developmental & Behavioral Disorders; Neonatal Care; **Hospital:** NS-LIJ Hlth Sys (page 106); **Address:** 1983 Marcus Ave, Bldg 1 - Fl 1 - Ste 130, Lake Success, NY 11042; **Phone:** 516-802-6100; **Board Cert:** Developmental-Behavioral Pediatrics 2012; Pediatrics 2009; **Med School:** NY Coll Osteo Med 1997; **Resid:** Pediatrics, Winthrop Univ Hosp 2001; **Fellow:** Developmental-Behavioral Pediatrics, North Shore/LI Jewish Med Ctr 2004

Nerwen, Clifford MD (Ped) *PCP* - **Hospital:** Steven & Alexandra Cohen Chldn's Med Ctr of NY (page 106), N Shore Univ Hosp (page 106); **Address:** Steven & Alexandra Cohen Chldn's Med Ctr, 410 Lakeville Rd, Ste 108, Dept Pediatrics, New Hyde Park, NY 11040; **Phone:** 516-465-4377; **Board Cert:** Pediatrics 2010; **Med School:** Univ Conn 1991; **Resid:** Pediatrics, Schneider Chldns Hosp 1994

Rabinowicz, Morris MD (Ped) *PCP* - **Hospital:** Plainview Hosp (page 106), Steven & Alexandra Cohen Chldn's Med Ctr of NY (page 106); **Address:** 995 Old Country Rd, Plainview, NY 11803; **Phone:** 516-935-7333; **Board Cert:** Pediatrics 1985; **Med School:** SUNY Downstate 1978; **Resid:** Surgery, LIJ Med Ctr 1982; Pediatrics, Brookdale Hosp 1983; **Fac Appt:** Asst Prof Ped, Hofstra N Shore-LIJ Sch Med

Resmovits, Marvin MD (Ped) *PCP* - **Hospital:** Steven & Alexandra Cohen Chldn's Med Ctr of NY (page 106), N Shore Univ Hosp (page 106); **Address:** 107 NE Northern Blvd, Fl s, Ste 201, Great Neck, NY 11021-4309; **Phone:** 516-487-6565; **Board Cert:** Pediatrics 1984; **Med School:** SUNY Buffalo 1979; **Resid:** Pediatrics, LI Jewish Hosp 1982

Physical Medicine & Rehabilitation

Lipetz, Jason S MD (PMR) - **Spec Exp:** Spinal Rehabilitation; Pain-Spine; **Hospital:** NS-LIJ Hlth Sys (page 106), N Shore Univ Hosp (page 106); **Address:** LI Spine Rehab Medicine, 801 Merrick Ave, East Meadow, NY 11554; **Phone:** 516-393-8941; **Board Cert:** Physical Medicine & Rehabilitation 2009; Pain Medicine 2012; **Med School:** Columbia P&S 1994; **Resid:** Physical Medicine & Rehabilitation, Kessler Inst-UMDNJ 1998; **Fellow:** Interventional Spine Medicine, Univ Penn Affil Hosp 1999; **Fac Appt:** Asst Prof PMR, Albert Einstein Coll Med

Root, Barry C MD (PMR) - **Spec Exp:** Spinal Cord Injury; Electromyography; Spinal Rehabilitation; **Hospital:** N Shore Univ Hosp (page 106), St. Francis Hosp - The Heart Ctr (page 121); **Address:** Dept Physical Med & Rehab, 101 St Andrews Ln Fl 1 North, Glen Cove, NY 11542-2254; **Phone:** 516-674-7501; **Board Cert:** Physical Medicine & Rehabilitation 1988; Spinal Cord Injury Medicine 2003; **Med School:** Ohio State Univ 1984; **Resid:** Physical Medicine & Rehabilitation, Nassau County Med Ctr 1987; **Fac Appt:** Asst Clin Prof PMR, Cornell Univ-Weill Med Coll

Stein, Adam B MD (PMR) - **Spec Exp:** Spinal Cord Injury; Multiple Sclerosis; Stroke Rehabilitation; **Hospital:** NS-LIJ Hlth Sys (page 106), Glen Cove Hosp (page 106); **Address:** 825 Northern Blvd Fl 1 - Ste 105, Great Neck, NY 11021; **Phone:** 516-465-8609; **Board Cert:** Physical Medicine & Rehabilitation 1992; Spinal Cord Injury Medicine 2003; **Med School:** NYU Sch Med 1987; **Resid:** Physical Medicine & Rehabilitation, Rusk Inst-NYU Med Ctr 1991

Plastic Surgery

Alizadeh, Kaveh MD (PlS) - **Spec Exp:** Breast Cosmetic & Reconstructive Surgery; Facial Plastic & Reconstructive Surgery; Liposuction & Body Contouring; Migraine; **Hospital:** Lenox Hill Hosp (page 106), South Nassau Comm Hosp; **Address:** 1111 Park Ave, New York, NY 10128; **Phone:** 516-742-3404; **Board Cert:** Plastic Surgery 2011; **Med School:** Cornell Univ 1993; **Resid:** Plastic Surgery, Univ Chicago Hosps 1999; **Fellow:** Microsurgery, Meml Sloan Kettering Cancer Ctr 2000; Cosmetic Plastic Surgery, Manhattan EET Hosp 2000

Breitbart, Arnold MD (PlS) - **Spec Exp:** Cosmetic Surgery-Face & Body; Liposuction; Breast Reconstruction; Cosmetic Surgery-Breast; **Hospital:** N Shore Univ Hosp (page 106), NY-Presby/Weill Cornell Med Ctr, NY (page 104); **Address:** 1155 Northern Blvd, Ste 110, Manhasset, NY 11030; **Phone:** 516-365-3511; **Board Cert:** Surgery 2003; Plastic Surgery 2004; **Med School:** NYU Sch Med 1985; **Resid:** Surgery, NYU Med Ctr 1991; Plastic Surgery, NYU Med Ctr 1993; **Fellow:** Craniofacial Surgery, NYU Med Ctr 1994; Microsurgery, Meml Sloan Kettering Cancer Ctr 1995; **Fac Appt:** Asst Prof S, Cornell Univ-Weill Med Coll

DeVita, Gregory MD (PlS) - **Spec Exp:** Rhinoplasty; Rhinoplasty Revision; Cosmetic Surgery-Face; Cosmetic Surgery-Breast; **Hospital:** St. Francis Hosp - The Heart Ctr (page 121), N Shore Univ Hosp (page 106); **Address:** 650 Northern Blvd, Great Neck, NY 11021-5204; **Phone:** 516-466-7000; **Board Cert:** Plastic Surgery 1989; **Med School:** SUNY Downstate 1980; **Resid:** Surgery, St Luke's Hosp 1982; Surgery, Jersey City Med Ctr 1983; **Fellow:** Plastic Surgery, New York Methodist Hosp 1984; Plastic Surgery, SUNY Downstate Med Ctr 1986

DiGregorio, Vincent R MD (PlS) - **Spec Exp:** Rhinoplasty Revision; Cosmetic Surgery-Face; Breast Reconstruction & Augmentation; **Hospital:** Winthrop Univ Hosp (page 504), Mercy Med Ctr - Rockville Centre; **Address:** 999 Franklin Ave, Garden City, NY 11530; **Phone:** 516-742-3404; **Board Cert:** Plastic Surgery 1978; **Med School:** Albany Med Coll 1968; **Resid:** Surgery, Thomas Jefferson Univ Hosp 1974; Plastic Surgery, Nassau County Med Ctr 1976; **Fac Appt:** Assoc Prof PlS, SUNY Stony Brook

Doctor, Naishad MD (PlS) - **Hospital:** Mercy Med Ctr - Rockville Centre, Winthrop Univ Hosp (page 504); **Address:** 2000 N Village Ave, Ste 103, Rockville Centre, NY 11570-1001; **Phone:** 516-678-2517; **Board Cert:** Plastic Surgery 1993; **Med School:** India 1974; **Resid:** Surgery, Univ Hosp 1987; Plastic Surgery, Univ Utah Hosp 1990; **Fellow:** Burn Surgery, Univ Hosp 1988

Dubner, Sanford MD (PlS) - **Spec Exp:** Head & Neck Tumors; Melanoma; Reconstructive Plastic Surgery; **Hospital:** Long Island Jewish Med Ctr (page 106), N Shore Univ Hosp (page 106); **Address:** 410 Lakeville Rd, Ste 310, Lake Success, NY 11042; **Phone:** 516-437-1111; **Board Cert:** Surgery 2006; Plastic Surgery 1992; **Med School:** SUNY Stony Brook 1982; **Resid:** Surgery, Booth Meml Med Ctr 1987; Plastic Surgery, Montefiore Med Ctr 1989; **Fellow:** Head and Neck Surgery, Meml Sloan Kettering Cancer Ctr 1990; **Fac Appt:** Clin Prof S, Hofstra N Shore-LIJ Sch Med

Elkowitz, Marc J MD (PlS) - **Spec Exp:** Cosmetic Surgery; Reconstructive Surgery; **Hospital:** Long Island Jewish Med Ctr (page 106), N Shore Univ Hosp (page 106); **Address:** 107 Northern Blvd, Ste 203, Great Neck, NY 11021; **Phone:** 516-773-9200; **Board Cert:** Surgery 2007; Plastic Surgery 2012; **Med School:** Albany Med Coll 1993; **Resid:** Surgery, NY Med Coll 1998; **Fellow:** Plastic Surgery, Montefiore Med Ctr 2000; **Fac Appt:** Asst Clin Prof PlS, Albert Einstein Coll Med

Feinberg, Joseph MD (PlS) - **Spec Exp:** Cosmetic Surgery-Face & Eyes; Breast Augmentation; Abdominoplasty; **Hospital:** St. Francis Hosp - The Heart Ctr (page 121), N Shore Univ Hosp (page 106); **Address:** 1201 Northern Blvd, Ste 202, Manhasset, NY 11030; **Phone:** 516-869-6200; **Board Cert:** Plastic Surgery 1980; **Med School:** Cornell Univ-Weill Med Coll 1973; **Resid:** Surgery, NY Hosp 1976; Plastic Surgery, NY Hosp 1978; **Fellow:** Facial Plastic & Reconstr Surgery, Meml Sloan Kettering Cancer Ctr; **Fac Appt:** Asst Clin Prof S, Cornell Univ-Weill Med Coll

Funt, David K MD (PlS) - **Spec Exp:** Cosmetic Surgery-Face & Body; Liposuction; Botox Therapy; Facial Rejuvenation; **Hospital:** South Nassau Comm Hosp, N Shore Univ Hosp (page 106); **Address:** 19 Irving Pl, Woodmere, NY 11598; **Phone:** 516-295-0404; **Board Cert:** Plastic Surgery 1987; **Med School:** Geo Wash Univ 1979; **Resid:** Surgery, Montefiore Med Ctr 1983; Plastic Surgery, Montefiore Med Ctr 1985; **Fac Appt:** Asst Clin Prof PlS, Albert Einstein Coll Med

Gallagher, Pamela M MD (PlS) - **Spec Exp:** Abdominoplasty; Body Contouring; Facial Rejuvenation; Breast Augmentation; **Hospital:** Winthrop Univ Hosp (page 504), N Shore Univ Hosp (page 106); **Address:** 190 E Jericho Tpke, Mineola, NY 11501; **Phone:** 516-977-9922; **Board Cert:** Plastic Surgery 1980; **Med School:** Univ Chicago-Pritzker Sch Med 1974; **Resid:** Surgery, NY Hosp 1977; Plastic Surgery, NY Hosp 1979

Gold, Alan H MD (PlS) - **Spec Exp:** Cosmetic Surgery-Face & Eyes; Cosmetic Surgery-Breast; Cosmetic Surgery-Body; Nasal Surgery; **Hospital:** N Shore Univ Hosp (page 106), Long Island Jewish Med Ctr (page 106); **Address:** 833 Northern Blvd, Ste 240, MS 11021, Great Neck, NY 11021-5322; **Phone:** 516-498-2800; **Board Cert:** Plastic Surgery 1979; **Med School:** SUNY Downstate 1971; **Resid:** Surgery, N Shore Univ Hosp 1975; Plastic Surgery, Kings County-Suny Med Ctr 1978; **Fellow:** Hand Surgery, Nassau County Med Ctr 1976

Gotkin, Robert MD (PlS) - **Spec Exp:** Cosmetic Surgery-Face & Breast; Liposuction; Skin Laser Surgery; **Hospital:** NS-LIJ Hlth Sys (page 106); **Address:** 31 Northern Blvd, Greenvale, NY 11548; **Phone:** 516-484-9000; **Board Cert:** Plastic Surgery 1990; **Med School:** Howard Univ 1980; **Resid:** Surgery, SUNY Stony Brook 1985; Plastic Surgery, Georgetown Univ 1988; **Fellow:** Surgical Critical Care, SUNY Stony Brook 1986

Groeger, William E MD (PlS) - **Spec Exp:** Skin Cancer; **Hospital:** Long Beach Med Ctr, South Nassau Comm Hosp; **Address:** 1490 Broadway Fl 2, Hewlett, NY 11557-1645; **Phone:** 516-887-5502; **Board Cert:** Plastic Surgery 1982; **Med School:** SUNY Downstate 1972; **Resid:** Surgery, Beth Israel Hosp 1977; Plastic Surgery, Univ Hosp 1979

Israeli, Ron MD (PlS) - **Spec Exp:** Plastic & Reconstructive Surgery; Breast Reconstruction; Microsurgery; **Hospital:** N Shore Univ Hosp (page 106), St. Francis Hosp - The Heart Ctr (page 121); **Address:** 833 Northern Blvd, Ste 160, Great Neck, NY 11021; **Phone:** 516-498-8400; **Board Cert:** Plastic Surgery 2009; **Med School:** Boston Univ 1990; **Resid:** Surgery, Mt Sinai Hosp 1995; Plastic Surgery, Mass Genl Hosp 1997; **Fellow:** Microsurgery, Mt Sinai Hosp 1992

Kasabian, Armen K MD (PlS) - **Spec Exp:** Hand Reconstruction; Plastic & Reconstructive Surgery; Microsurgery; **Hospital:** NS-LIJ Hlth Sys (page 106); **Address:** Dept of Surgery, 1991 Marcus Ave, Ste 102, Lake Success, NY 11042; **Phone:** 516-233-3659; **Board Cert:** Plastic Surgery 1992; Hand Surgery 2004; **Med School:** Cornell Univ-Weill Med Coll 1982; **Resid:** Surgery, NYU Med Ctr 1987; Plastic Surgery, NYU Med Ctr 1989; **Fellow:** Microsurgery, NYU Med Ctr 1990; **Fac Appt:** Asst Prof PlS, NYU Sch Med

Keller, Alex J MD (PlS) - **Spec Exp:** Breast Reconstruction; Cosmetic Surgery-Face & Breast; Poland Syndrome; **Hospital:** Long Island Jewish Med Ctr (page 106); **Address:** 900 Northern Blvd, Ste 130, Great Neck, NY 11021; **Phone:** 516-482-1100; **Board Cert:** Plastic Surgery 1984; **Med School:** NYU Sch Med 1975; **Resid:** Surgery, NYU Med Ctr 1978; Surgery, LI Jewish Hosp 1980; **Fellow:** Plastic Surgery, NYU Med Ctr 1982; Microsurgery, NYU Med Ctr 1983; **Fac Appt:** Asst Clin Prof PlS, NYU Sch Med

Kessler, Martin E MD (PlS) - **Spec Exp:** Cosmetic Surgery-Face & Body; Reconstructive Surgery-Face; Breast Reconstruction; Hand Surgery; **Hospital:** South Nassau Comm Hosp, N Shore Univ Hosp (page 106); **Address:** 242 Merrick Rd, Ste 302, Rockville Centre, NY 11570-5254; **Phone:** 516-536-5858; **Board Cert:** Plastic Surgery 1987; **Med School:** Cornell Univ-Weill Med Coll 1980; **Resid:** Surgery, NY Hosp 1983; Plastic Surgery, NY Hosp 1985; **Fellow:** Hand Surgery, Cleveland Clinic 1986; Microsurgery, Univ Louisville Hlth Ctr 1986; **Fac Appt:** Assoc Clin Prof PlS, Cornell Univ-Weill Med Coll

Leipziger, Lyle S MD (PlS) - **Spec Exp:** Cosmetic Surgery-Face & Eyes; Cosmetic Surgery-Breast; Breast Reconstruction; Liposuction & Body Contouring; **Hospital:** N Shore Univ Hosp (page 106), Long Island Jewish Med Ctr (page 106); **Address:** 825 Northern Blvd Fl 3, Great Neck, NY 11021; **Phone:** 516-465-8787; **Board Cert:** Plastic Surgery 1994; **Med School:** Cornell Univ-Weill Med Coll 1985; **Resid:** Plastic Surgery, New York Hosp 1990; **Fellow:** Craniofacial Surgery, Johns Hopkins Hosp 1991; **Fac Appt:** Asst Prof S, Albert Einstein Coll Med

Lukash, Frederick MD (PlS) - **Spec Exp:** Pediatric Plastic Surgery; Cosmetic Surgery-Face; Breast Cosmetic & Reconstructive Surgery; Rhinoplasty; **Hospital:** Long Island Jewish Med Ctr (page 106), Steven & Alexandra Cohen Chldn's Med Ctr of NY (page 106); **Address:** 1129 Northern Blvd, Ste 403, Manhasset, NY 11030-3022; **Phone:** 516-365-1040; **Board Cert:** Plastic Surgery 1982; **Med School:** Tulane Univ 1973; **Resid:** Surgery, Emory Univ Hosp 1975; Surgery, Univ Hosp 1980; **Fellow:** Plastic Surgery, Mass Genl Hosp 1981; **Fac Appt:** Asst Prof S, Albert Einstein Coll Med

Silberman, Mark Illan MD (PlS) - **Spec Exp:** Cosmetic Surgery-Face; Breast Cosmetic & Reconstructive Surgery; Facial Rejuvenation; Body Contouring; **Hospital:** N Shore Univ Hosp (page 106), St. Francis Hosp - The Heart Ctr (page 121); **Address:** 650 Northern Blvd, Great Neck, NY 11021-5204; **Phone:** 516-466-7000; **Board Cert:** Plastic Surgery 1988; **Med School:** SUNY Downstate 1980; **Resid:** Surgery, Beth Israel Med Ctr 1983; Plastic Surgery, SUNY Downstate Med Ctr 1985

Simpson, Roger MD (PlS) - **Spec Exp:** Eyelid Surgery; Liposuction & Body Contouring; Cosmetic Surgery-Face & Breast; Burn Care; **Hospital:** Winthrop Univ Hosp (page 504), NS-LIJ Hlth Sys (page 106); **Address:** 999 Franklin Ave, Garden City, NY 11530; **Phone:** 516-742-3404; **Board Cert:** Plastic Surgery 1981; **Med School:** Belgium 1974; **Resid:** Surgery, Nassau Co Med Ctr 1978; Plastic Surgery, Nassau Co Med Ctr 1980; **Fellow:** Hand Surgery, St Luke's-Roosevelt Hosp Ctr 1981; **Fac Appt:** Asst Clin Prof S, SUNY Stony Brook

Psychiatry

Bailine, Samuel MD (Psyc) - **Spec Exp:** Depression; Psychopharmacology; Electroconvulsive Therapy (ECT); **Hospital:** Long Island Jewish Med Ctr (page 106); **Address:** 5 Ridgeway Rd, Port Washington, NY 11050-2729; **Phone:** 516-883-3304; **Board Cert:** Psychiatry 1970; **Med School:** NYU Sch Med 1964; **Resid:** Psychiatry, Tulane Univ Med Ctr 1968; **Fac Appt:** Asst Prof Psyc, Albert Einstein Coll Med

Behr, Raymond MD (Psyc) - **Spec Exp:** Depression; Bipolar/Mood Disorders; Addiction/Substance Abuse; **Hospital:** Long Island Jewish Med Ctr (page 106); **Address:** 81-A Arleigh Rd, Great Neck, NY 11021-1442; **Phone:** 516-482-1980; **Board Cert:** Psychiatry 1981; Child & Adolescent Psychiatry 1982; **Med School:** South Africa 1973; **Resid:** Psychiatry, LI Jewish Med Ctr 1978; **Fellow:** Child & Adolescent Psychiatry, LI Jewish Med Ctr 1980; **Fac Appt:** Asst Clin Prof Psyc, Albert Einstein Coll Med

Benjamin, John MD (Psyc) - **Spec Exp:** Depression; Anxiety Disorders; Schizophrenia; **Hospital:** N Shore Univ Hosp (page 106); **Address:** 1983 Marcus Ave, Ste E132, Lake Success, NY 11042; **Phone:** 516-216-1780; **Board Cert:** Psychiatry 1983; **Med School:** India 1969; **Resid:** Psychiatry, N Shore Univ Hosp 1981; **Fac Appt:** Asst Clin Prof Psyc, NYU Sch Med

Berman, Sheldon S MD (Psyc) - **Spec Exp:** Psychodynamic Psychotherapy; Psychopharmacology; Palliative Care; **Address:** 8 Payne Circle, Hewlett Harbor, NY 11557-2735; **Phone:** 516-374-4417; **Board Cert:** Psychiatry 1979; **Med School:** Ros Franklin Univ/Chicago Med Sch 1969; **Resid:** Psychiatry, Brookdale Hosp 1973; **Fac Appt:** Asst Clin Prof Psyc, SUNY Downstate

Bhatt, Ashok MD (Psyc) - **Spec Exp:** Depression; Psychopharmacology; **Hospital:** Long Beach Med Ctr; **Address:** 871 E Park Ave, Long Beach, NY 11561; **Phone:** 516-889-8844; **Board Cert:** Psychiatry 1985; **Med School:** India 1976; **Resid:** Psychiatry, LI Jewish Med Ctr 1981; **Fellow:** Psychiatry, LI Jewish Med Ctr 1983

Budman, Cathy L MD (Psyc) - **Spec Exp:** Tourette's Syndrome; ADD/ADHD; Obsessive-Compulsive Disorder; Neuro-Psychiatry; **Hospital:** N Shore Univ Hosp (page 106), Long Island Jewish Med Ctr (page 106); **Address:** 400 Community Drive, Dept Psychiatry North Shore-LIJHS, Manhasset, NY 11030; **Phone:** 516-562-3223; **Board Cert:** Psychiatry 1991; **Med School:** SUNY Buffalo 1984; **Resid:** Psychiatry, Langley Porter Psych Inst/UCSF 1986; Psychiatry, N Shore Univ Hosp 1990; **Fellow:** Family Medicine, Sydney Univ-Royal Price Albert Hosp 1988; Neuropsychiatry, N Shore Univ Hosp 1991; **Fac Appt:** Assoc Prof Psyc, Hofstra N Shore-LIJ Sch Med

Crasta, Jovita M MD (Psyc) - **Spec Exp:** Anxiety Disorders; Depression; Bipolar/Mood Disorders; Women's Health-Mental Health; **Hospital:** South Nassau Comm Hosp; **Address:** 2277 Grand Ave, Baldwin, NY 11510-3148; **Phone:** 516-377-5400; **Board Cert:** Psychiatry 1991; **Med School:** India 1981; **Resid:** Psychiatry, Nassau County Med Ctr 1987; **Fac Appt:** Asst Prof Psyc, NY Coll Osteo Med

Gupta, Adarsh MD/PhD (Psyc) - **Spec Exp:** Psychosomatic Disorders; Psychiatry in Physical Illness; Neuro-Psychiatry; **Address:** Great Neck Psychiatry, 1010 Northern Blvd, Ste 208, Great Neck, NY 11021; **Phone:** 516-336-2544; **Board Cert:** Surgery 2007; Psychosomatic Medicine 2005; Sleep Medicine 2011; **Med School:** India 1978; **Resid:** Internal Medicine, St Vincent Hosp 1992; Psychiatry, NYU Med Ctr 1995

Gurevich, Michael I MD (Psyc) - **Spec Exp:** Psychotherapy & Psychopharmacology; Complementary Medicine; Addiction/Substance Abuse; Psychiatry in Physical Illness; **Hospital:** Glen Cove Hosp (page 106); **Address:** 997 Glen Cove Avenue, Glen Head, NY 11545-1584; **Phone:** 516-674-9489; **Board Cert:** Psychiatry 1989; **Med School:** Lithuania 1974; **Resid:** Psychiatry, Elmhurst Hosp Ctr 1987; **Fellow:** Child Psychiatry, Elmhurst Hosp Ctr 1989

Katus, Eli Margrethe MD (Psyc) - **Spec Exp:** Psychopharmacology; Psychotherapy; Child & Adolescent Psychiatry; **Hospital:** N Shore Univ Hosp (page 106), Winthrop Univ Hosp (page 504); **Address:** 1035 Route 106, East Norwich, NY 11732-1005; **Phone:** 516-922-5607; **Board Cert:** Psychiatry 1990; Child & Adolescent Psychiatry 1991; **Med School:** Germany 1982; **Resid:** Psychiatry, N Shore Univ Hosp 1986; **Fellow:** Child & Adolescent Psychiatry, N Shore Univ Hosp 1988

Katz, Jack L MD (Psyc) - **Spec Exp:** Eating Disorders; Mood Disorders; Anxiety Disorders; **Hospital:** N Shore Univ Hosp (page 106), Long Island Jewish Med Ctr (page 106); **Address:** 1010 Northern Blvd, Ste 208, Great Neck, NY 11021; **Phone:** 516-336-2565; **Board Cert:** Psychiatry 1968; **Med School:** Albert Einstein Coll Med 1960; **Resid:** Psychiatry, Montefiore Med Ctr 1966; **Fellow:** Psychiatry, Montefiore Med Ctr-Einstein 1968; **Fac Appt:** Prof Psyc, NYU Sch Med

Sami, Sherif F MD (Psyc) - **Spec Exp:** Depression; Anxiety & Mood Disorders; Geriatric Psychiatry; **Hospital:** Winthrop Univ Hosp (page 504), N Shore Univ Hosp (page 106); **Address:** 7 Bond St, Great Neck, NY 11021; **Phone:** 516-487-9191; **Board Cert:** Psychiatry 1973; **Med School:** Egypt 1961; **Resid:** Psychiatry, Cairo Univ Hosp 1966; Psychiatry, Elmhurst Hosp 1969; **Fellow:** Community Psychiatry, Albert Einstein 1970

Pulmonary Disease

Blum, Alan I MD (Pul) - **Spec Exp:** Cough-Chronic; Asthma; Sleep Disorders; **Hospital:** South Nassau Comm Hosp, Franklin Hosp (page 106); **Address:** 444 Merrick Rd Fl Lower Level 1, Lynbrook, NY 11563-2400; **Phone:** 516-593-9500; **Board Cert:** Internal Medicine 1981; Pulmonary Disease 1984; **Med School:** Mexico 1977; **Resid:** Internal Medicine, Mt Sinai Hosp Ctr 1981; **Fellow:** Pulmonary Disease, Mt Sinai Hosp Ctr 1983

Breidbart, David M MD (Pul) - **Spec Exp:** Asthma; Chronic Obstructive Lung Disease (COPD); Sarcoidosis; **Hospital:** N Shore Univ Hosp (page 106), St. Francis Hosp - The Heart Ctr (page 121); **Address:** 6 Ohio Drive, Ste 201, LSQ Medical Bldg, Lake Success, NY 11042-1129; **Phone:** 516-328-8700; **Board Cert:** Internal Medicine 1982; Pulmonary Disease 1984; **Med School:** SUNY Downstate 1979; **Resid:** Internal Medicine, North Shore Univ Hosp 1982; **Fellow:** Pulmonary Disease, Meml Sloan-Kettering Hosp 1983; Pulmonary Disease, Montefiore-Albert Einstein Med Ctr 1985; **Fac Appt:** Asst Clin Prof Med, NYU Sch Med

Cohen, Michael L MD (Pul) - **Spec Exp:** Asthma; Bronchitis; Emphysema; **Hospital:** N Shore Univ Hosp (page 106); **Address:** N Shore Internal Med Assocs, 560 Northern Blvd, Ste 203, Great Neck, NY 11021-5100; **Phone:** 516-482-0600; **Board Cert:** Internal Medicine 1972; Pulmonary Disease 1974; **Med School:** SUNY Upstate Med Univ 1967; **Resid:** Internal Medicine, Montefiore Hosp Med Ctr 1970; **Fellow:** Pulmonary Disease, Montefiore Hosp Med Ctr 1971; Pulmonary Disease, LI Jewish Med Ctr 1974; **Fac Appt:** Asst Clin Prof Med, NYU Sch Med

Fein, Alan MD (Pul) - **Spec Exp:** Chronic Obstructive Lung Disease (COPD); Asthma; Pneumonia; **Hospital:** N Shore Univ Hosp (page 106), Long Island Jewish Med Ctr (page 106); **Address:** 2800 Marcus Ave, Dept Pulmonary Med, Fl 2 - Ste 202, Lake Success, NY 11042; **Phone:** 516-608-2890; **Board Cert:** Internal Medicine 1976; Pulmonary Disease 1978; Critical Care Medicine 2008; **Med School:** SUNY Downstate 1973; **Resid:** Internal Medicine, Albert Einstein Affil Hosp 1976; **Fellow:** Pulmonary Disease, UC San Francisco Med Ctr 1978

Gordon, Richard Eric MD (Pul) - **Spec Exp:** Emphysema; Sleep Disorders; Asthma; **Hospital:** St. Joseph's Hosp-Nassau, Plainview Hosp (page 106); **Address:** Island Pulmonary Associates, 4271 Hempstead Tpke, Ste 1, Bethpage, NY 11714-5718; **Phone:** 516-796-3700; **Board Cert:** Internal Medicine 1984; Pulmonary Disease 1986; **Med School:** Mount Sinai Sch Med 1980; **Resid:** Internal Medicine, Beth Israel Med Ctr 1983; **Fellow:** Pulmonary Disease, Queens Hosp Ctr 1985

Greenberg, Harly MD (Pul) - **Spec Exp:** Sleep Disorders/Apnea; Lung Disease; Critical Care; **Hospital:** Long Island Jewish Med Ctr (page 106), N Shore Univ Hosp (page 106); **Address:** North Shore LIJ Sleep Disorders Ctr, 410 Lakeville Rd, Ste 107, New Hyde Park, NY 11040; **Phone:** 516-465-3899; **Board Cert:** Internal Medicine 1985; Pulmonary Disease 1988; Sleep Medicine 2011; **Med School:** NYU Sch Med 1982; **Resid:** Internal Medicine, North Shore Univ Hosp 1985; **Fellow:** Pulmonary Disease, NYU-Bellevue Hosp Ctr 1987; **Fac Appt:** Assoc Prof Med, Albert Einstein Coll Med

Leeman, Benjamin J MD (Pul) *PCP* - **Spec Exp:** Asthma; Pneumonia; Chronic Obstructive Lung Disease (COPD); **Hospital:** Franklin Hosp (page 106), South Nassau Comm Hosp; **Address:** 20 W Lincoln Ave, Ste 306, Valley Stream, NY 11580; **Phone:** 516-599-8787; **Board Cert:** Internal Medicine 2006; Pulmonary Disease 2007; **Med School:** SUNY Stony Brook 1988; **Resid:** Internal Medicine, Montefiore Med Ctr-Weiler Div 1991; **Fellow:** Pulmonary Disease, NY Presby-Columbia Med Ctr 1993

Mermelstein, Steve A MD (Pul) - **Spec Exp:** Asthma; Chronic Obstructive Lung Disease (COPD); Cough-Chronic; **Hospital:** South Nassau Comm Hosp, Franklin Hosp (page 106); **Address:** 444 Merrick Rd, Lower Level 1, Lynbrook, NY 11563-2456; **Phone:** 516-593-9500; **Board Cert:** Internal Medicine 1980; Pulmonary Disease 1982; **Med School:** Albert Einstein Coll Med 1977; **Resid:** Internal Medicine, Metropolitan Hosp Ctr 1980; **Fellow:** Pulmonary Disease, St Luke's-Roosevelt Hosp Ctr 1982

Multz, Alan S MD (Pul) - **Spec Exp:** Sepsis; Respiratory Distress Syndrome; Critical Care; **Hospital:** Nassau Univ Med Ctr, N Shore Univ Hosp (page 106); **Address:** 2201 Hemptstead Tpke, East Meadow, NY 11554; **Phone:** 516-572-6501; **Board Cert:** Internal Medicine 1988; Pulmonary Disease 2010; Critical Care Medicine 2000; **Med School:** Boston Univ 1985; **Resid:** Internal Medicine, Montefiore Hosp Med Ctr 1988; **Fellow:** Pulmonary Disease, Montefiore Hosp Med Ctr 1990; Critical Care Medicine, Montefiore Hosp Med Ctr 1991; **Fac Appt:** Assoc Prof Med, Albert Einstein Coll Med

Newmark, Ian H MD (Pul) - **Spec Exp:** Critical Care; Asthma; Lung Cancer; **Hospital:** Plainview Hosp (page 106), Syosset Hosp (page 106); **Address:** 8 Greenfield Rd, Syosset, NY 11791-4831; **Phone:** 516-496-3001; **Board Cert:** Internal Medicine 1982; Pulmonary Disease 1986; Critical Care Medicine 2010; **Med School:** SUNY Hlth Sci Ctr 1979; **Resid:** Internal Medicine, Nassau Co Med Ctr 1982; **Fellow:** Pulmonary Intensive Care, Nassau Co Med Ctr 1984; **Fac Appt:** Asst Clin Prof Med, Hofstra N Shore-LIJ Sch Med

Niederman, Michael S MD (Pul) - **Spec Exp:** Infections-Respiratory; Emphysema; Respiratory Failure; Pneumonia; **Hospital:** Winthrop Univ Hosp (page 504); **Address:** 222 Station Plaza N, Ste 400, Mineola, NY 11501-3893; **Phone:** 516-663-2834; **Board Cert:** Internal Medicine 1980; Pulmonary Disease 1982; Critical Care Medicine 2007; **Med School:** Boston Univ 1977; **Resid:** Internal Medicine, Northwestern Univ Med Ctr 1980; **Fellow:** Pulmonary Disease, Yale-New Haven Hosp 1983; **Fac Appt:** Prof Med, SUNY Stony Brook

Rosen, Mark J MD (Pul) - **Spec Exp:** Cough; Pulmonary Rehabilitation; Sepsis; **Hospital:** Long Island Jewish Med Ctr (page 106), N Shore Univ Hosp (page 106); **Address:** 410 Lakeville Rd, Ste 107, New Hyde Park, NY 11040; **Phone:** 516-465-5400; **Board Cert:** Internal Medicine 1978; Critical Care Medicine 2007; Pulmonary Disease 1980; **Med School:** Brown Univ 1975; **Resid:** Internal Medicine, Mt Sinai Hosp 1978; **Fellow:** Pulmonary Disease, Mt Sinai Hosp 1980; Critical Care Medicine, St Vincent's Med Ctr 1980; **Fac Appt:** Prof Med, Hofstra N Shore-LIJ Sch Med

Schulster, Rita B MD (Pul) - **Spec Exp:** Asthma; Bronchitis; **Hospital:** Long Beach Med Ctr, South Nassau Comm Hosp; **Address:** 442 E Waukena Ave, Oceanside, NY 11572; **Phone:** 516-599-8234; **Board Cert:** Internal Medicine 1977; Pulmonary Disease 1978; **Med School:** Albert Einstein Coll Med 1970; **Resid:** Internal Medicine, Beth Israel Med Ctr 1973; Internal Medicine, Beth Israel Med Ctr 1974; **Fellow:** Pulmonary Disease, LI Jewish Med Ctr 1975; Pulmonary Disease, Beth Israel Med Ctr 1976

Steinberg, Harry MD (Pul) - **Spec Exp:** Asthma; Emphysema; Lung Cancer; Pulmonary Hypertension; **Hospital:** Long Island Jewish Med Ctr (page 106), N Shore Univ Hosp (page 106); **Address:** 410 Lakeville Rd, Ste 107, 270-05 76th Ave, New Hyde Park, NY 11040; **Phone:** 516-465-5400; **Med School:** Temple Univ 1966; **Resid:** Internal Medicine, LI Jewish Med Ctr 1969; Pulmonary Critical Care Medicine, LI Jewish Med Ctr 1970; **Fellow:** Pulmonary Disease, Hosp Univ Penn 1974; **Fac Appt:** Prof Med, Hofstra N Shore-LIJ Sch Med

Wyner, Perry A MD (Pul) - **Spec Exp:** Asthma; Cough-Chronic; Emphysema; Preventive Medicine; **Hospital:** Mercy Med Ctr - Rockville Centre; **Address:** 2 Lincoln Ave, Ste 201, Rockville Centre, NY 11570; **Phone:** 516-536-4960; **Board Cert:** Internal Medicine 1980; Pulmonary Disease 1982; **Med School:** Cornell Univ-Weill Med Coll 1977; **Resid:** Internal Medicine, Med Coll Virginia Hosps 1980; **Fellow:** Pulmonary Disease, Bellevue Hosp 1982

Zupnick, Henry Michael MD (Pul) - **Spec Exp:** Asthma; Bronchitis; Cough; **Hospital:** South Nassau Comm Hosp; **Address:** 158 Hempstead Ave, Lynbrook, NY 11563; **Phone:** 516-593-3541; **Board Cert:** Internal Medicine 1983; Pulmonary Disease 1988; **Med School:** Albert Einstein Coll Med 1980; **Resid:** Internal Medicine, Brookdale Hosp Med Ctr 1983; **Fellow:** Pulmonary Disease, Columbia-Presby Med Ctr 1985; Critical Care Medicine, Mount Sinai Hosp 1987; **Fac Appt:** Asst Clin Prof Med, SUNY Downstate

Radiation Oncology

Bosworth, Jay L MD (RadRO) - **Spec Exp:** Breast Cancer; Prostate Cancer; Lymphoma; **Hospital:** St. Francis Hosp - The Heart Ctr (page 121), N Shore Univ Hosp (page 106); **Address:** 6 Ohio Drive, Lake Success, NY 11042; **Phone:** 516-365-6544; **Board Cert:** Therapeutic Radiology 1974; **Med School:** Albert Einstein Coll Med 1970; **Resid:** Radiation Oncology, Bronx Muni Hosp Ctr 1974

Diamond, Ezriel MD (RadRO) - **Hospital:** Plainview Hosp (page 106), St. Joseph's Hosp-Nassau; **Address:** Advanced Radiation Centers of New York, 688 Old Country Rd, Plainview, NY 11803; **Phone:** 516-932-6007; **Board Cert:** Therapeutic Radiology 1982; **Med School:** NYU Sch Med 1978; **Resid:** Radiation Oncology, NYU Med Ctr 1981; **Fellow:** Radiation Oncology, NY Methodist Hosp 1982

Gewanter, Richard M MD (RadRO) - **Hospital:** Meml Sloan-Kettering Cancer Ctr (page 116); **Address:** MSKCC Long Island, 1000 N Village Ave, Rockville Center, NY 11570; **Phone:** 516-256-3600; **Board Cert:** Radiation Oncology 2002; **Med School:** Albert Einstein Coll Med 1995; **Resid:** Radiation Oncology, NY Presby-Columbia Med Ctr 2002

Haas, Jonathan A MD (RadRO) - **Spec Exp:** Brachytherapy; Prostate Cancer; Lung Cancer; Gynecologic Cancer; **Hospital:** Winthrop Univ Hosp (page 504); **Address:** Winthrop Univ Hosp, Radiation Onc, 264 Old Country Rd, Mineola, NY 11501; **Phone:** 516-663-2501; **Board Cert:** Radiation Oncology 2009; **Med School:** Washington Univ, St Louis 1993; **Resid:** Radiation Oncology, Hosp Univ Penn 1997; **Fac Appt:** Asst Clin Prof RadRO, SUNY Stony Brook

Knisely, Jonathan P S MD (RadRO) - **Spec Exp:** Brain Tumors; Stereotactic Radiosurgery; **Hospital:** NS-LIJ Hlth Sys (page 106); **Address:** North Shore University Hospital, 300 Community Drive, Manhasset, NY 11030; **Phone:** 516-470-7190; **Board Cert:** Internal Medicine 1989; Radiation Oncology 1993; **Med School:** Univ Pennsylvania 1986; **Resid:** Internal Medicine, Michael Reese Hosp 1989; Radiation Oncology, Univ Toronto Med Ctr 1992; **Fac Appt:** Assoc Prof RadRO, Hofstra N Shore-LIJ Sch Med

Marin, Lorraine A MD (RadRO) - **Spec Exp:** Breast Cancer; Gynecologic Cancer; Pediatric Cancers; Lymphoma; **Address:** HealthCare Partners, 501 Franklin Ave, Ste 300, Garden City, NY 11530; **Phone:** 516-746-2200; **Board Cert:** Internal Medicine 1980; Medical Oncology 1983; Therapeutic Radiology 1986; **Med School:** UC Davis 1977; **Resid:** Internal Medicine, Rush Presby/St. Lukes Med Ctr 1978; Internal Medicine, UC Davis Med Ctr 1980; **Fellow:** Medical Oncology, Natl Cancer Inst/NIH 1983; Radiation Oncology, Natl Cancer Inst/NIH 1985; **Fac Appt:** Asst Clin Prof RadRO, Albert Einstein Coll Med

Mullen, Edward E MD (RadRO) - **Spec Exp:** Brain Tumors; Breast Cancer; Stereotactic Radiosurgery; **Hospital:** South Nassau Comm Hosp; **Address:** South Nassau Comm Hosp, One Healthy Way, Dept Radiation Oncology, Oceanside, NY 11572; **Phone:** 516-632-3330; **Board Cert:** Radiation Oncology 1991; **Med School:** Univ VA Sch Med 1986; **Resid:** Radiation Oncology, Columbia-Presby Med Ctr 1990

Pollack, Jed MD (RadRO) - **Spec Exp:** Head & Neck Cancer; Prostate Cancer; Brain Tumors; **Hospital:** N Shore Univ Hosp (page 106), St. Francis Hosp - The Heart Ctr (page 121); **Address:** Long Island Radiation Therapy, 6 Ohio Drive, Ste 103, Lake Success, NY 11042; **Phone:** 516-394-8100; **Board Cert:** Therapeutic Radiology 1985; **Med School:** Univ New Mexico 1981; **Resid:** Therapeutic Radiology, Meml Sloan-Kettering Cancer Ctr 1985; **Fac Appt:** Asst Clin Prof RadRO, Albert Einstein Coll Med

Potters, Louis MD (RadRO) - **Spec Exp:** Prostate Cancer; Intensity Modulated Radiotherapy (IMRT); Brachytherapy; **Hospital:** Long Island Jewish Med Ctr (page 106), N Shore Univ Hosp (page 106); **Address:** N Shore-LIJ, 270-05 76th Ave, New Hyde Park, NY 11040; **Phone:** 718-470-7190; **Board Cert:** Internal Medicine 1988; Radiation Oncology 1999; **Med School:** UMDNJ-NJ Med Sch, Newark 1985; **Resid:** Internal Medicine, Beth Israel Med Ctr 1988; Radiation Oncology, SUNY Downstate Med Ctr 1991; **Fac Appt:** Prof RadRO, Hofstra N Shore-LIJ Sch Med

Reproductive Endocrinology

Brenner, Steven H MD (RE) - **Spec Exp:** Infertility-IVF; Polycystic Ovarian Syndrome; **Hospital:** Long Island Jewish Med Ctr (page 106), John T Mather Meml Hosp; **Address:** 2001 Marcus Ave, Ste N213, Lake Success, NY 11042; **Phone:** 516-358-6363; **Board Cert:** Obstetrics & Gynecology 1985; Reproductive Endocrinology 1987; **Med School:** SUNY Downstate 1978; **Resid:** Obstetrics & Gynecology, Beth Israel Med Ctr 1982; **Fellow:** Reproductive Endocrinology, NYU Med Ctr 1984; **Fac Appt:** Assoc Clin Prof ObG, Hofstra N Shore-LIJ Sch Med

Hershlag, Avner MD (RE) - **Hospital:** N Shore Univ Hosp (page 106); **Address:** 300 Community Drive, Manhasset, NY 11030; **Phone:** 516-562-2229; **Board Cert:** Obstetrics & Gynecology 2011; Reproductive Endocrinology 2011; **Med School:** Israel 1977; **Resid:** Surgery, Hadassah Med 1978; Obstetrics & Gynecology, George Washington Univ Med Ctr 1988; **Fellow:** Reproductive Endocrinology, New Haven Hosp 1990; **Fac Appt:** Assoc Prof ObG, NYU Sch Med

Rosenfeld, David L MD (RE) - **Spec Exp:** Infertility-IVF; Endometriosis; Uterine Fibroids; **Hospital:** N Shore Univ Hosp (page 106); **Address:** Div Human Reproduction, 300 Community Drive Ambulatory Bldg, Manhasset, NY 11030-3816; **Phone:** 516-562-2229; **Board Cert:** Obstetrics & Gynecology 1976; Reproductive Endocrinology 1980; **Med School:** Univ Pennsylvania 1970; **Resid:** Obstetrics & Gynecology, Hosp Univ Penn 1974; **Fellow:** Reproductive Endocrinology, Hosp Univ Penn 1976; **Fac Appt:** Prof ObG, NYU Sch Med

Rheumatology

Belilos, Elise MD (Rhu) - **Spec Exp:** Polymyalgia Rheumatica; Giant Cell Arteritis; Rheumatoid Arthritis; **Hospital:** Winthrop Univ Hosp (page 504); **Address:** Winthrop Univ Hosp, Div Rheum, 120 Mineola Blvd, Ste 410, Mineola, NY 11501; **Phone:** 516-663-2097; **Board Cert:** Internal Medicine 1989; Rheumatology 2004; **Med School:** SUNY Stony Brook 1986; **Resid:** Internal Medicine, Winthrop Univ Hosp 1990; **Fellow:** Rheumatology, Winthrop UnivHosp 1993; **Fac Appt:** Asst Clin Prof Med, SUNY Stony Brook

Blau, Sheldon P MD (Rhu) - **Spec Exp:** Lupus/SLE; Scleroderma; Rheumatoid Arthritis; Osteoporosis; **Hospital:** Winthrop Univ Hosp (page 504); **Address:** 566 Broadway, Massapequa, NY 11758-5017; **Phone:** 516-541-6262; **Board Cert:** Internal Medicine 1969; Rheumatology 1972; **Med School:** Albert Einstein Coll Med 1961; **Resid:** Internal Medicine, Montefiore Med Ctr 1964; **Fellow:** Rheumatology, Albert Einstein Coll Med 1965; **Fac Appt:** Clin Prof Med, SUNY Stony Brook

Carsons, Steven MD (Rhu) - **Spec Exp:** Rheumatoid Arthritis; Sjogren's Syndrome; **Hospital:** Winthrop Univ Hosp (page 504); **Address:** Winthrop Univ Hosp, Div Rhematology, 120 Mineola Blvd, Ste 410, Mineola, NY 11501; **Phone:** 516-663-2097; **Board Cert:** Internal Medicine 1978; Rheumatology 1980; Clinical & Laboratory Immunology 1988; **Med School:** NY Med Coll 1975; **Resid:** Internal Medicine, Maimonides Med Ctr 1978; **Fellow:** Rheumatology, SUNY Brooklyn Med Ctr 1980; **Fac Appt:** Prof Med, SUNY Hlth Sci Ctr

Cohen, Daniel Henry MD (Rhu) - **Spec Exp:** Osteoporosis; Arthritis; **Hospital:** South Nassau Comm Hosp, Franklin Hosp (page 106); **Address:** 1157 Broadway, Hewlett, NY 11557; **Phone:** 516-295-4481; **Board Cert:** Internal Medicine 1981; Rheumatology 1984; **Med School:** NYU Sch Med 1978; **Resid:** Internal Medicine, Columbia-Presby Med Ctr 1981; **Fellow:** Rheumatology, NYU Med Ctr 1983

Furie, Richard A MD (Rhu) - **Spec Exp:** Lupus/SLE; Antiphospholipid Syndrome (APS); Rheumatoid Arthritis; **Hospital:** N Shore Univ Hosp (page 106), Long Island Jewish Med Ctr (page 106); **Address:** 2800 Marcus Ave, Ste 200, Lake Success, NY 11042; **Phone:** 516-708-2550; **Board Cert:** Internal Medicine 1982; Rheumatology 1984; **Med School:** Cornell Univ-Weill Med Coll 1979; **Resid:** Internal Medicine, NY Hosp 1982; **Fellow:** Rheumatology, Hosp Spec Surg 1984; **Fac Appt:** Prof Med, Albert Einstein Coll Med

Greenwald, Robert MD (Rhu) - **Spec Exp:** Rheumatoid Arthritis; Psoriatic Arthritis; Osteoarthritis; **Hospital:** Long Island Jewish Med Ctr (page 106); **Address:** 2 ProHealth Plaza, Lake Success, NY 11042; **Phone:** 516-622-6090; **Board Cert:** Internal Medicine 1973; Rheumatology 1974; **Med School:** Johns Hopkins Univ 1967; **Resid:** Internal Medicine, LI Jewish-Hillside Med Ctr 1970; **Fellow:** Rheumatology, SUNY Brooklyn Med Ctr 1972; **Fac Appt:** Prof Med, Albert Einstein Coll Med

Hoffman, Michael L MD (Rhu) - **Spec Exp:** Lupus/SLE; Rheumatoid Arthritis; Osteoarthritis; Osteoporosis; **Hospital:** Long Island Jewish Med Ctr (page 106), N Shore Univ Hosp (page 106); **Address:** 560 Northern Blvd, Ste 107, Great Neck, NY 11021; **Phone:** 516-498-3500; **Board Cert:** Internal Medicine 1971; **Med School:** SUNY Downstate 1965; **Resid:** Internal Medicine, Maimonides Med Ctr 1967; Internal Medicine, Jacobi Med Ctr 1968; **Fellow:** Rheumatology, Hosp for Special Surg 1970; **Fac Appt:** Assoc Clin Prof Med, Albert Einstein Coll Med

Lipstein-Kresch, Esther MD (Rhu) - **Spec Exp:** Rheumatoid Arthritis; Osteoarthritis; Osteoporosis; Fibromyalgia; **Hospital:** Long Island Jewish Med Ctr (page 106), N Shore Univ Hosp (page 106); **Address:** ProHealth Care Assocs, 2 ProHealth Plaza, Ste 103, Lake Success, NY 11042-1111; **Phone:** 516-622-6090; **Board Cert:** Internal Medicine 1982; Rheumatology 1984; **Med School:** SUNY Hlth Sci Ctr 1979; **Resid:** Internal Medicine, LI Jewish Med Ctr 1982; **Fellow:** Rheumatology, LI Jewish Med Ctr 1984; **Fac Appt:** Asst Prof Med, Mount Sinai Sch Med

Meredith, Gary S MD (Rhu) - **Spec Exp:** Gout; Lupus/SLE; Rheumatoid Arthritis; **Hospital:** St. Francis Hosp - The Heart Ctr (page 121); **Address:** 2 ProHEALTH Plaza, Ste 200, Lake Success, NY 11042; **Phone:** 516-622-6125; **Board Cert:** Internal Medicine 1984; Rheumatology 1986; **Med School:** NYU Sch Med 1981; **Resid:** Internal Medicine, Bellevue Hosp 1984; **Fellow:** Rheumatology, NYU Med Ctr 1986; **Fac Appt:** Asst Clin Prof Med, NYU Sch Med

Porges, Andrew J MD (Rhu) - **Spec Exp:** Osteoporosis; **Hospital:** N Shore Univ Hosp (page 106), Glen Cove Hosp (page 106); **Address:** 1044 Northern Blvd, Ste 104, Roslyn, NY 11576; **Phone:** 516-484-6880; **Board Cert:** Internal Medicine 1989; Rheumatology 2002; **Med School:** Cornell Univ-Weill Med Coll 1986; **Resid:** Internal Medicine, NY Hosp 1989; **Fellow:** Rheumatology, Hosp Special Surg 1992; **Fac Appt:** Asst Prof Med, Cornell Univ-Weill Med Coll

Sullivan, James M MD (Rhu) - **Spec Exp:** Rheumatoid Arthritis; Lupus/SLE; Osteoarthritis; **Hospital:** Winthrop Univ Hosp (page 504); **Address:** 711 Stewart Ave, Garden City, NY 11530; **Phone:** 516-222-8654; **Board Cert:** Internal Medicine 1977; Rheumatology 1980; **Med School:** SUNY Upstate Med Univ 1974; **Resid:** Internal Medicine, Univ Michigan Med Ctr 1977; **Fellow:** Rheumatology, Univ Michigan Med Ctr 1979

Tiger, Louis MD (Rhu) - **Spec Exp:** Rheumatoid Arthritis; Lupus/SLE; Osteoarthritis; **Hospital:** Winthrop Univ Hosp (page 504); **Address:** 566 Broadway, Massapequa, NY 11758-5017; **Phone:** 516-541-6262; **Board Cert:** Internal Medicine 1975; Rheumatology 1976; **Med School:** Univ Louisville Sch Med 1967; **Resid:** Internal Medicine, Maimonides Medical Ctr 1970; **Fellow:** Rheumatology, Albert Einstein Med Ctr 1974; **Fac Appt:** Asst Clin Prof Med, SUNY Stony Brook

Surgery

Auguste, Louis J MD (S) - **Spec Exp:** Breast Disease; Melanoma; Thyroid & Parathyroid Surgery; Hernia; **Hospital:** Long Island Jewish Med Ctr (page 106), N Shore Univ Hosp (page 106); **Address:** 2035 Lakeville Rd, Ste 206, New Hyde Park, NY 11042-1102; **Phone:** 516-775-2070; **Board Cert:** Surgery 2011; **Med School:** Haiti 1973; **Resid:** Surgery, LI Jewish Med Ctr 1980; **Fellow:** Surgical Oncology, Roswell Park Meml Inst 1982; **Fac Appt:** Assoc Clin Prof S, Albert Einstein Coll Med

Bank, Matthew MD (S) - **Spec Exp:** Trauma; **Hospital:** N Shore Univ Hosp (page 106), NS-LIJ Hlth Sys (page 106); **Address:** 1999 Marcus Ave, Lake Success, NY 11030; **Phone:** 516-233-3610; **Board Cert:** Surgical Critical Care 2003; Surgery 2011; **Med School:** NY Med Coll 1995; **Resid:** Surgery, Long Island Jewish Med Ctr 2000; **Fellow:** Surgical Critical Care, Yale-New Haven Hosp 2001

Conte, Charles C MD (S) - **Spec Exp:** Cancer Surgery; Breast Cancer; Pancreatic Cancer; **Hospital:** N Shore Univ Hosp (page 106), Forest Hills Hosp (page 106); **Address:** 600 Northern Blvd, Ste 111, Great Neck, NY 11021; **Phone:** 516-487-9454; **Board Cert:** Surgery 2005; **Med School:** Dartmouth Med Sch 1981; **Resid:** Surgery, Hartford Hosp 1986; **Fellow:** Surgical Oncology, Roswell Park Cancer Inst 1988

Coppa, Gene F MD (S) - **Spec Exp:** Minimally Invasive Surgery; Hepatobiliary Surgery; Gastrointestinal Surgery; Pancreatic Surgery; **Hospital:** N Shore Univ Hosp (page 106); **Address:** N Shore Univ Hosp, 300 Community Drive, Manhasset, NY 11030; **Phone:** 516-562-2870; **Board Cert:** Surgery 2010; **Med School:** NYU Sch Med 1974; **Resid:** Surgery, NYU/Bellevue Med Ctr 1979; **Fac Appt:** Prof S, SUNY Downstate

Datta, Rajiv V MD (S) - **Spec Exp:** Breast Cancer; Colon & Rectal Cancer; Gastrointestinal Cancer; Head & Neck Cancer; **Hospital:** South Nassau Comm Hosp; **Address:** South Nassau Comm Hosp Cancer Center, 1 South Central Ave, Valley Stream, NY 11580; **Phone:** 516-632-3350; **Board Cert:** Surgery 2009; **Med School:** India 1984; **Resid:** Surgery, Maimonides Med Ctr 1998; **Fellow:** Surgical Oncology, Roswell Park Cancer Inst 1999; Head and Neck Surgery, Roswell Park Cancer Inst 2000; **Fac Appt:** Assoc Clin Prof S, NY Coll Osteo Med

Denoto, George MD (S) - **Spec Exp:** Laparoscopic Surgery; Hernia; **Hospital:** St. Francis Hosp - The Heart Ctr (page 121); **Address:** 139 Plandome Rd, Manhasset, NY 11030; **Phone:** 516-627-5262; **Board Cert:** Surgery 2006; **Med School:** SUNY Stony Brook 1988; **Resid:** Surgery, Mt Sinai Hosp 1993

Gecelter, Gary MD (S) - **Spec Exp:** Pancreatic Cancer; Esophageal Surgery; Laparoscopic Surgery; Biliary Surgery; **Hospital:** St. Francis Hosp - The Heart Ctr (page 121); **Address:** 139 Plandome Rd, Manhasset, NY 11030; **Phone:** 516-627-5262; **Med School:** South Africa 1981; **Resid:** Surgery, Johannesburg Hosp 1990; **Fellow:** Gastroenterology, Johannesburg Hosp 1992

Grieco, Michael B MD (S) - **Spec Exp:** Breast Surgery; Laparoscopic Abdominal Surgery; Hernia; Laparoscopic Cholecystectomy; **Hospital:** Glen Cove Hosp (page 106), St. Francis Hosp - The Heart Ctr (page 121); **Address:** 10 Medical Plaza, Glen Cove, NY 11542; **Phone:** 516-676-1060; **Board Cert:** Surgery 2010; Colon & Rectal Surgery 1982; **Med School:** Albany Med Coll 1974; **Resid:** Surgery, N Shore Univ Hosp 1979; **Fellow:** Surgery, Lahey Clinic 1980; Colon & Rectal Surgery, Greater Baltimore Med Ctr 1981; **Fac Appt:** Asst Clin Prof S, SUNY Stony Brook

Khalife, Michael E MD (S) - **Spec Exp:** Laparoscopic Surgery; Breast Surgery; **Hospital:** Winthrop Univ Hosp (page 504), N Shore Univ Hosp (page 106); **Address:** 300 Old Country Rd, Ste 101, Mineola, NY 11501; **Phone:** 516-741-4138; **Board Cert:** Surgery 2003; **Med School:** France 1978; **Resid:** Surgery, Univ Hosp 1984; **Fac Appt:** Asst Clin Prof S, SUNY Stony Brook

Kurtz, Lewis M MD (S) - **Spec Exp:** Breast Surgery; Gallbladder Surgery; Hernia; **Hospital:** St. Francis Hosp - The Heart Ctr (page 121), Long Island Jewish Med Ctr (page 106); **Address:** 310 E Shore Rd, Ste 203, Great Neck, NY 11023; **Phone:** 516-482-8657; **Board Cert:** Surgery 2010; **Med School:** Italy 1972; **Resid:** Surgery, Long Island Jewish-Hillside Med Ctr 1977; **Fellow:** Research, Long Island Jewish-Hillside Med Ctr 1978

Mansouri, Hormoz MD (S) - **Spec Exp:** Varicose Veins; **Hospital:** N Shore Univ Hosp (page 106); **Address:** 175 Jericho Tpke, Ste 201, Syosset, NY 11791; **Phone:** 516-682-4800; **Board Cert:** Surgery 1980; **Med School:** Iran 1964; **Resid:** Surgery, Henry Ford Hosp 1969; Surgery, Nassau Co Med Ctr 1971; **Fac Appt:** Asst Prof S, SUNY Stony Brook

Reed Jr, William P MD (S) - **Spec Exp:** Breast Cancer; Stomach Cancer; **Hospital:** Winthrop Univ Hosp (page 504); **Address:** Winthrop Surgical Assoc, 120 Mineola Blvd, Ste 320, Mineola, NY 11501; **Phone:** 516-663-3300; **Board Cert:** Surgery 2008; **Med School:** Harvard Med Sch 1968; **Resid:** Surgery, Stanford Univ 1976; **Fellow:** Surgical Oncology, Inst Gustave-Roussy 1977; **Fac Appt:** Prof S, SUNY Stony Brook

Reiner, Dan S MD (S) - **Spec Exp:** Laparoscopic Surgery; Hernia; Gastrointestinal Surgery; **Hospital:** N Shore Univ Hosp (page 106), Syosset Hosp (page 106); **Address:** 2800 Marcus Ave, Ste 204, Lake Success, NY 11042-1008; **Phone:** 516-622-6120; **Board Cert:** Surgery 2005; Surgical Critical Care 2007; **Med School:** St Louis Univ 1980; **Resid:** Surgery, St Louis Univ-Group Hosps 1985; **Fellow:** Surgical Critical Care, UMDNJ-NJ Hosp 1986; **Fac Appt:** Assoc Clin Prof S, NYU Sch Med

Romero, Carlos MD (S) - **Spec Exp:** Laparoscopic Surgery; Head & Neck Surgery; Breast Surgery; **Hospital:** Winthrop Univ Hosp (page 504); **Address:** 173 Mineola Blvd, Ste 401, Mineola, NY 11501-2555; **Phone:** 516-741-6464; **Board Cert:** Surgery 2007; **Med School:** Argentina 1969; **Resid:** Surgery, Winthrop Univ Hosp 1975; **Fellow:** Surgical Oncology, Med Coll Virginia 1977; **Fac Appt:** Assoc Prof S, SUNY Stony Brook

Vitale, Gerard F MD (S) - **Spec Exp:** Aneurysm; Carotid Artery Surgery; Varicose Veins; Arterial Bypass Surgery; **Hospital:** Glen Cove Hosp (page 106); **Address:** 10 Medical Plaza, Ste 305, Glen Cove, NY 11542; **Phone:** 516-759-5559; **Board Cert:** Surgery 2010; **Med School:** SUNY Buffalo 1982; **Resid:** Surgery, N Shore Univ Hosp 1987; **Fellow:** Vascular Surgery, St Vincents Hosp 1988

Thoracic & Cardiac Surgery

Andaz, Shahriyour MD (T&CS) - **Spec Exp:** Thoracic Cancers; Lung Cancer; **Hospital:** South Nassau Comm Hosp, Franklin Hosp (page 106); **Address:** 444 Merrick Rd, Ste 380, Lynbrook, NY 11563; **Phone:** 516-255-5010; **Board Cert:** Surgery 2009; Thoracic & Cardiac Surgery 2010; **Med School:** India 1983; **Resid:** Surgery, Bronx Lebanon Hosp; **Fellow:** Thoracic Surgery, SUNY Hlth Sci Ctr

Barrett, Leonard O MD (T&CS) - **Spec Exp:** Chest Trauma; Esophageal Tumors; Critical Care; **Hospital:** Nassau Univ Med Ctr; **Address:** Nassau Univ Med Ctr, 2201 Hempstead Tpke Fl 8, East Meadow, NY 11554; **Phone:** 516-572-6703; **Board Cert:** Surgery 2009; Surgical Critical Care 2001; Thoracic Surgery 2005; **Med School:** SUNY Downstate 1983; **Resid:** Surgery, SUNY Stony Brook Med Ctr 1989; Cardiothoracic Surgery, Beth Israel Med Ctr 1993; **Fellow:** Surgical Critical Care, Winthrop Univ Med Ctr 1990

Esposito, Rick A MD (T&CS) - **Spec Exp:** Cardiac Surgery; Coronary Artery Surgery; Mitral Valve Minimally Invasive Surgery; **Hospital:** N Shore Univ Hosp (page 106); **Address:** N Shore Univ Hospital, Dept Cardiothoracic Surgery, 300 Community Drive, Manhasset, NY 11030; **Phone:** 516-562-4970; **Board Cert:** Thoracic Surgery 2006; **Med School:** Univ Chicago-Pritzker Sch Med 1979; **Resid:** Surgery, NYU Med Ctr 1984; **Fellow:** Thoracic Surgery, NYU Med Ctr 1986; **Fac Appt:** Assoc Clin Prof S, NYU Sch Med

Fernandez, Harold A MD (T&CS) - **Spec Exp:** Cardiac Surgery-High Risk; Minimally Invasive Heart Valve Surgery; Ventricular Assist Device (LVAD); Atrial Fibrillation; **Hospital:** Stony Brook Univ Med Ctr; **Address:** Stony Brook Medicine, HSC Bldg, Ste T19-080, Stony Brook, NY 11794-8191; **Phone:** 631-444-1820; **Board Cert:** Surgery 2003; Thoracic Surgery 2005; **Med School:** Harvard Med Sch 1993; **Resid:** Surgery, NYU Med Ctr 1999; **Fellow:** Thoracic Surgery, NYU Med Ctr 2001; **Fac Appt:** Clin Prof T&CS, SUNY Stony Brook

Glassman, Lawrence R MD (T&CS) - **Spec Exp:** Lung Cancer; Esophageal Cancer; Emphysema; Tracheal Surgery; **Hospital:** N Shore Univ Hosp (page 106); **Address:** 225 Community Drive, Ste 110, Great Neck, NY 11021; **Phone:** 516-918-4388; **Board Cert:** Thoracic Surgery 2000; **Med School:** NYU Sch Med 1981; **Resid:** Surgery, U Minnesota Hosps 1983; Surgery, NYU Med Ctr 1987; **Fellow:** Thoracic Surgery, Meml Sloan Kettering 1988; Thoracic Surgery, NYU Med Ctr 1990

Hartman, Alan R MD (T&CS) - **Spec Exp:** Cardiothoracic Surgery; Minimally Invasive Heart Valve Surgery; Aneurysm-Thoracic Aortic; Coronary Artery Surgery; **Hospital:** N Shore Univ Hosp (page 106), Long Island Jewish Med Ctr (page 106); **Address:** N Shore Univ Hosp, Div Cardiothoracic Surg, 300 Community Drive, Manhasset, NY 11030; **Phone:** 516-562-4970; **Board Cert:** Surgery 2004; Thoracic Surgery 2005; Surgical Critical Care 2000; **Med School:** Mount Sinai Sch Med 1979; **Resid:** Surgery, Bellevue Hosp/NYU Med Ctr 1984; **Fellow:** Cardiothoracic Surgery, Bellevue Hosp/NYU Med Ctr 1986; **Fac Appt:** Assoc Prof S, NYU Sch Med

Kline, Gary M MD (T&CS) - **Spec Exp:** Lung Cancer; Emphysema; Mediastinal Tumors; **Hospital:** Winthrop Univ Hosp (page 504), Holy Name Med Ctr (page 688); **Address:** 332 Summit Ave, Hackensack, NJ 07601; **Phone:** 201-488-6445; **Board Cert:** Surgery 2004; Thoracic Surgery 2005; **Med School:** Wayne State Univ 1986; **Resid:** Surgery, Detroit Med Ctr 1991; **Fellow:** Thoracic Surgery, Hosp Univ Penn 1994; **Fac Appt:** Asst Prof S, Albert Einstein Coll Med

Robinson, Newell B MD (T&CS) - **Spec Exp:** Minimally Invasive Cardiac Surgery; Maze Procedure for Atrial Fibrillation; **Hospital:** St. Francis Hosp - The Heart Ctr (page 121); **Address:** St Francis Hosp-The Heart Ctr, 100 Port Washington Blvd, Ste G01, Roslyn, NY 11576; **Phone:** 516-627-2173; **Board Cert:** Surgery 2005; Thoracic Surgery 2006; **Med School:** Univ Miss 1973; **Resid:** Surgery, NY-Cornell Med Ctr 1984; Surgery, Meml Sloan Kettering Cancer Ctr 1984; **Fellow:** Trauma, Univ Washington Med Ctr 1981; Cardiothoracic Surgery, NY-Cornell Med Ctr 1986

Saha, Chanchal MD (T&CS) - **Spec Exp:** Lung Cancer; Pacemakers; Esophageal Cancer; Mediastinal Tumors; **Hospital:** Plainview Hosp (page 106), St. Joseph's Hosp-Nassau; **Address:** 754 Old Country Rd, Plainview, NY 11804; **Phone:** 516-931-0182; **Board Cert:** Thoracic Surgery 2011; **Med School:** India 1964; **Resid:** Surgery, Hosp for Joint Diseases 1973; Thoracic Surgery, Mt Sinai Hosp 1976; **Fellow:** Cardiothoracic Surgery, Mt Sinai Hosp 1977; **Fac Appt:** Assoc Prof S, Cornell Univ-Weill Med Coll

Schubach, Scott L MD (T&CS) - **Spec Exp:** Cardiac Surgery; Coronary Artery Surgery; Heart Valve Surgery; Minimally Invasive Surgery; **Hospital:** Winthrop Univ Hosp (page 504); **Address:** 120 Mineola Blvd, Ste 300, Mineola, NY 11501; **Phone:** 516-663-4400; **Board Cert:** Surgery 2007; Thoracic Surgery 2010; Surgical Critical Care 2010; **Med School:** Baylor Coll Med 1983; **Resid:** Surgery, Dartmouth Hitchcock Med Ctr Ctr. 1988; Cardiothoracic Surgery, Univ of Pittsburgh Med Ctr 1991

Zeltsman, Vadim MD (T&CS) - **Spec Exp:** Thoracic Cancers; Video Assisted Thoracic Surgery (VATS); **Hospital:** Long Island Jewish Med Ctr (page 106), N Shore Univ Hosp (page 106); **Address:** 225 Community Drive, Ste 110, Great Neck, NY 11021; **Phone:** 516-918-4388; **Board Cert:** Thoracic Surgery 2002; Surgery 2011; **Med School:** Russia 1986; **Resid:** Surgery, Mercy Catholic Med Ctr 1997; **Fellow:** Cardiothoracic Surgery, UMDNJ Affil Hosp 2000; Cardiothoracic Surgery, Univ Pennsylvania 2001

Urology

Ashley, Richard N MD (U) - **Hospital:** N Shore Univ Hosp (page 106); **Address:** 233 7th St, Ste 203, Garden City, NY 11530; **Phone:** 516-294-7666; **Board Cert:** Urology 1980; **Med School:** NY Med Coll 1972; **Resid:** Surgery, St Vincents Hosp 1975; Urology, SUNY Downstate Med Ctr 1978; **Fac Appt:** Asst Clin Prof U, SUNY Stony Brook

Bruno, Anthony MD (U) - **Spec Exp:** Prostate Cancer; Kidney Stones; Voiding Dysfunction; **Hospital:** Winthrop Univ Hosp (page 504); **Address:** 1305 Franklin Ave, Ste 100, Garden City, NY 11530; **Phone:** 516-746-5550; **Board Cert:** Urology 1977; **Med School:** Italy 1968; **Resid:** Surgery, Nassau Hosp 1972; Urology, Bellevue Hosp Ctr 1975; **Fac Appt:** Asst Prof U, SUNY Stony Brook

D'Esposito, Robert F MD (U) - **Hospital:** Winthrop Univ Hosp (page 504); **Address:** 601 Franklin Ave, Ste 300, Garden City, NY 11530-5759; **Phone:** 516-742-3200; **Board Cert:** Urology 1981; **Med School:** Italy 1971; **Resid:** Surgery, Nassau Hosp 1972; Urology, Nassau Hosp 1976; **Fac Appt:** Assoc Clin Prof U, SUNY Stony Brook

Edelman, Robert A MD (U) - **Hospital:** Winthrop Univ Hosp (page 504); **Address:** 601 Franklin Ave, Garden City, NY 11530-5729; **Phone:** 516-742-3200; **Board Cert:** Urology 1981; **Med School:** SUNY Upstate Med Univ 1974; **Resid:** Surgery, Montefiore Med Ctr 1976; Urology, Montefiore Med Ctr 1979; **Fac Appt:** Assoc Clin Prof U, SUNY Stony Brook

Gershbaum, Meyer D MD (U) - **Hospital:** Long Island Jewish Med Ctr (page 106); **Address:** 601 Franklin Ave, Ste 300, 2 Prohealth Plaza, Fl 1, Garden City, NY 11530; **Phone:** 516-742-3200; **Board Cert:** Urology 2005; **Med School:** Albert Einstein Coll Med 1996; **Resid:** Surgery, LI Jewish Med Ctr 1998; Urology, LI Jewish Med Ctr 2002; **Fellow:** Laparoscopic Surgery, VA Med Ctr 2003

Girardi, Sarah K MD (U) - **Spec Exp:** Infertility-Male; Incontinence-Female; **Hospital:** N Shore Univ Hosp (page 106), St. Francis Hosp - The Heart Ctr (page 121); **Address:** 535 Plandome Rd, Ste 3, Manhasset, NY 11030; **Phone:** 516-627-6188; **Board Cert:** Urology 2006; **Med School:** Univ NC Sch Med 1989; **Resid:** Urology, Cornell Univ Med Ctr 1995; **Fellow:** Urology, Yale Univ 1996

Hanna, Moneer K MD (U) - **Spec Exp:** Pediatric Urology; Reconstructive Surgery; Hypospadias; Bladder Surgery; **Hospital:** Steven & Alexandra Cohen Chldn's Med Ctr of NY (page 106), NY-Presby/Weill Cornell Med Ctr, NY (page 104); **Address:** 935 Northern Blvd, Ste 303, Great Neck, NY 11021; **Phone:** 516-466-6950; **Board Cert:** Urology 1978; **Med School:** Egypt 1963; **Resid:** Urology, Univ Affiliated Hosp 1972; Urology, Univ West Ont Affil Hosps 1976; **Fellow:** Pediatric Urology, Hosp For Sick Chldn 1975; **Fac Appt:** Clin Prof U, Cornell Univ-Weill Med Coll

Harris, Steven M MD (U) - **Spec Exp:** Impotence; Prostate Disease; Kidney Stones; **Hospital:** Long Beach Med Ctr, South Nassau Comm Hosp; **Address:** 711 Lincoln Blvd, Long Beach, NY 11561-3241; **Phone:** 516-431-9800; **Board Cert:** Urology 1984; **Med School:** Albert Einstein Coll Med 1976; **Resid:** Urology, Mount Sinai Med Ctr 1981; **Fac Appt:** Asst Prof U, NY Coll Osteo Med

Katz, Aaron E MD (U) - **Spec Exp:** Prostate Cancer-Cryosurgery; Kidney Cancer-Cryosurgery; Complementary Medicine; Nutrition & Cancer Prevention; **Hospital:** Winthrop Univ Hosp (page 504); **Address:** 1401 Franklin Ave, Garden City, NY 11530; **Phone:** 516-535-1900; **Board Cert:** Urology 2006; **Med School:** NY Med Coll 1986; **Resid:** Urology, Maimonides Med Ctr 1992; **Fellow:** Urologic Oncology, Columbia Presby Med Ctr 1993; **Fac Appt:** Assoc Clin Prof U, Columbia P&S

Kavoussi, Louis R MD (U) - **Spec Exp:** Laparoscopic Surgery; Urologic Cancer; Prostate Cancer; Kidney Cancer; **Hospital:** Long Island Jewish Med Ctr (page 106), N Shore Univ Hosp (page 106); **Address:** Arthur Smith Institute for Urology, 450 Lakeville Rd, Ste M-41, New Hyde Park, NY 11042; **Phone:** 516-734-8558; **Board Cert:** Urology 2009; **Med School:** SUNY Buffalo 1983; **Resid:** Surgery, Barnes Jewish Hosp 1985; Urology, Barnes Jewish Hosp 1989; **Fac Appt:** Prof U, Hofstra N Shore-LIJ Sch Med

Layne, Jeffrey MD (U) - **Spec Exp:** Kidney Stones; Incontinence; Impotence; **Hospital:** St. Joseph's Hosp-Nassau, N Shore Univ Hosp (page 106); **Address:** 1181 Old Country Rd, Ste 1, Plainview, NY 11803-5018; **Phone:** 516-933-6060; **Board Cert:** Urology 2007; **Med School:** SUNY Stony Brook 1989; **Resid:** Surgery, New England Med Ctr 1991; Urology, New England Med Ctr 1995

Lieberman, Elliott MD (U) - **Spec Exp:** Urologic Cancer; Interstitial Cystitis; Prostate Disease; **Hospital:** Plainview Hosp (page 106); **Address:** 875 Old Country Road Rd, Ste 301, Plainview, NY 11803-4934; **Phone:** 516-931-1710; **Board Cert:** Urology 1983; **Med School:** SUNY Downstate 1976; **Resid:** Surgery, Mount Sinai 1978; Urology, SUNY-Downstate 1981

Mellinger, Brett MD (U) - **Spec Exp:** Infertility-Male; Impotence; Peyronie's Disease; Andrology; **Hospital:** Winthrop Univ Hosp (page 504), N Shore Univ Hosp (page 106); **Address:** Advanced Urology Ctrs of NY, Garden City East Division, 100 Garden City Plaza, Garden City, NY 11530; **Phone:** 516-873-5353; **Board Cert:** Urology 2010; **Med School:** Indiana Univ 1981; **Resid:** Urology, Downstate Med Ctr 1985; Urology, New York Hosp-Cornell 1986; **Fellow:** Male Infertility, New York Hosp-Cornell 1988; **Fac Appt:** Assoc Clin Prof U, SUNY Stony Brook

Moldwin, Robert MD (U) - **Spec Exp:** Interstitial Cystitis; Prostate Benign Disease; Urinary Tract Infections; **Hospital:** NS-LIJ Hlth Sys (page 106); **Address:** 450 Lakeville Rd, Ste M41, New Hyde Park, NY 11040-1433; **Phone:** 516-734-8500; **Board Cert:** Urology 2012; **Med School:** Univ Chicago-Pritzker Sch Med 1984; **Resid:** Urology, LI Jewish Med Ctr 1990; **Fellow:** Infectious Disease, Thomas Jefferson Univ Hosp 1991; **Fac Appt:** Assoc Clin Prof U, Albert Einstein Coll Med

Paul, Elliot M MD (U) - **Spec Exp:** Prostate Cancer; Kidney Stones; Laparoscopic Surgery; Minimally Invasive Urologic Surery; **Hospital:** Long Island Jewish Med Ctr (page 106), St. Francis Hosp - The Heart Ctr (page 121); **Address:** Advanced Urology Centers of NY, Integrated Medical Professionals, 2001 Marcus Ave, Ste N214, Lake Success, NY 11042; **Phone:** 516-437-4228; **Board Cert:** Urology 2007; **Med School:** Albert Einstein Coll Med 2000; **Resid:** Urology, Long Island Jewish Med Ctr 2005

Richstone, Lee MD (U) - **Hospital:** Long Island Jewish Med Ctr (page 106), NS-LIJ Hlth Sys (page 106); **Address:** 450 Lakeville Rd Ste M41, New Hyde Park, NY 11042; **Phone:** 516-734-8500; **Board Cert:** Urology 2009; **Med School:** Cornell Univ-Weill Med Coll 2000; **Resid:** Urology, Ny Presby Hosp 2006

Shepard, Barry R MD (U) - **Spec Exp:** Kidney Stones; Urologic Cancer; **Hospital:** Winthrop Univ Hosp (page 504), N Shore Univ Hosp (page 106); **Address:** 601 Franklin Ave, Ste 300, Garden City, NY 11530; **Phone:** 516-742-3200; **Board Cert:** Urology 2006; **Med School:** SUNY Downstate 1979; **Resid:** Surgery, LIJ Med Ctr 1981; Urology, Columbia-Presby Med Ctr 1984

Sunshine, Robert D MD (U) - **Spec Exp:** Vasectomy-Scalpelless; Prostate Disease; **Hospital:** St. Joseph's Hosp-Nassau, Plainview Hosp (page 106); **Address:** Advanced Urology Ctrs of NY, 480 Hicksville Rd, Bethpage, NY 11714-5700; **Phone:** 516-796-2222; **Board Cert:** Urology 2005; **Med School:** Mexico 1977; **Resid:** Surgery, Long Island Jewish Hosp 1981; Urology, Mount Sinai Med Ctr 1985

Ziegelbaum, Michael M MD (U) - **Spec Exp:** Incontinence-Male & Female; Prostate Disease; Laparoscopic Surgery; Kidney Stones; **Hospital:** Long Island Jewish Med Ctr (page 106), St. Francis Hosp - The Heart Ctr (page 121); **Address:** 2001 Marcus Ave, Ste N214, Lake Success, NY 11042; **Phone:** 516-437-4228; **Board Cert:** Urology 2010; **Med School:** Cornell Univ-Weill Med Coll 1982; **Resid:** Urology, Cleveland Clinic 1988; **Fellow:** Stone Disease, Univ Hosp 1989; **Fac Appt:** Asst Clin Prof S, Albert Einstein Coll Med

Vascular & Interventional Radiology

Crystal, Kenneth MD (VIR) - **Spec Exp:** Interventional Radiology; Angioplasty; Uterine Fibroid Embolization; **Hospital:** St. Francis Hosp - The Heart Ctr (page 121); **Address:** 100 Port Washington Blvd, Roslyn, NY 11576; **Phone:** 516-562-6509; **Board Cert:** Diagnostic Radiology 1986; **Med School:** Univ Rochester 1981; **Resid:** Internal Medicine, Beth Israel Med Ctr 1982; Diagnostic Radiology, NYU Med Ctr 1986; **Fellow:** Vascular & Interventional Radiology, NYU Med Ctr 1986; **Fac Appt:** Asst Prof Rad, NYU Sch Med

Vascular Surgery

Chaudhry, Saqib S MD (VascS) - **Spec Exp:** Aneurysm-Aortic; Carotid Artery Surgery; Dialysis Access Surgery; Limb Sparing Surgery; **Address:** 2001 Marcus Ave, Ste South-50, Lake Success, NY 11042; **Phone:** 516-328-9800; **Board Cert:** Vascular Surgery 2009; Thoracic & Cardiac Surgery 2011; **Med School:** Iraq 1972; **Resid:** Surgery, Flushing Hosp 1978; Thoracic Surgery, Wayne State Univ Affil Hosps 1980

Faust, Glenn MD (VascS) - **Spec Exp:** Carotid Artery Surgery; Diabetic Leg/Foot; Aneurysm-Abdominal Aortic; Vein Disorders; **Hospital:** Nassau Univ Med Ctr; **Address:** 2201 Hempstead Tpke, East Meadow, NY 11554; **Phone:** 516-572-4848; **Board Cert:** Vascular Surgery 2004; **Med School:** Yale Univ 1986; **Resid:** Surgery, LI Jewish Med Ctr 1991; **Fellow:** Vascular Surgery, LI Jewish Med Ctr 1992; **Fac Appt:** Asst Prof S, Albert Einstein Coll Med

Purtill, William A MD (VascS) - **Spec Exp:** Carotid Artery Surgery; Endovascular Surgery; Lower Limb Arterial Disease; Aneurysm-Aortic; **Hospital:** N Shore Univ Hosp (page 106), St. Francis Hosp - The Heart Ctr (page 121); **Address:** 560 Northern Blvd, Ste 209, Great Neck, NY 11021; **Phone:** 516-466-0485; **Board Cert:** Surgery 2007; Vascular Surgery 2007; **Med School:** Ireland 1989; **Resid:** Surgery, Johns Hopkins Hosp 1993; Surgery, SUNY Stony Brook Med Ctr 1996; **Fellow:** Vascular Surgery, Univ Maryland Med Ctr 1997; **Fac Appt:** Asst Prof S, SUNY Stony Brook

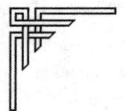

The Best in American Medicine
www.CastleConnolly.com

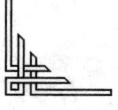
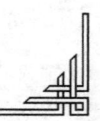

Rockland

Rockland

Allergy & Immunology

Bosso, John MD (A&I) - **Spec Exp:** Asthma; Contact Dermatitis; Food Allergy; Drug Sensitivity; **Hospital:** Nyack Hosp, Valley Hosp (page 689); **Address:** 2 Crosfield Ave, Ste 406, West Nyack, NY 10994-2212; **Phone:** 845-353-9600; **Board Cert:** Internal Medicine 1988; Allergy & Immunology 2011; **Med School:** SUNY Buffalo 1985; **Resid:** Internal Medicine, Staten Island Univ Hosp 1988; **Fellow:** Allergy & Immunology, Scripps Clinic Rsch Fdn 1990

Lo Galbo, Peter MD (A&I) - **Spec Exp:** Asthma; Food Allergy; **Hospital:** Nyack Hosp, Good Samaritan Hosp - Suffern; **Address:** 1 Crossfield Ave, Ste 201, West Nyack, NY 10994; **Phone:** 845-727-1370; **Board Cert:** Pediatrics 1983; Allergy & Immunology 1983; **Med School:** SUNY Stony Brook 1978; **Resid:** Pediatrics, Mount Sinai Med Ctr 1980; **Fellow:** Allergy & Immunology, Duke Univ Med Ctr 1982; **Fac Appt:** Asst Clin Prof Ped, Albert Einstein Coll Med

Cardiovascular Disease

Beniaminovitz, Ainat MD (Cv) - **Spec Exp:** Heart Failure; **Hospital:** Good Samaritan Hosp - Suffern; **Address:** Hudson Heart Associates, 222 Rte 59, Ste 302, Suffern, NY 10901; **Phone:** 845-368-0100; **Board Cert:** Internal Medicine 2003; Cardiovascular Disease 2007; Nuclear Cardiology 2005; **Med School:** Columbia P&S 1990; **Resid:** Internal Medicine, NY-Presby/Columbia Univ Hosp 1994; **Fellow:** Cardiovascular Disease, NY-Presby/Columbia Univ Hosp 1997

Roth, Richard MD (Cv) - **Spec Exp:** Cholesterol/Lipid Disorders; Non-Invasive Cardiology; **Hospital:** Good Samaritan Hosp - Suffern, Nyack Hosp; **Address:** 222 Route 59, Ste 302, Suffern, NY 10901; **Phone:** 845-368-0100; **Board Cert:** Internal Medicine 1978; Cardiovascular Disease 1981; **Med School:** Yale Univ 1975; **Resid:** Internal Medicine, Boston Med Ctr 1978; **Fellow:** Cardiovascular Disease, Boston Med Ctr 1980; **Fac Appt:** Asst Clin Prof Med, Columbia P&S

Southren, David MD (Cv) - **Spec Exp:** Cholesterol/Lipid Disorders; Non-Invasive Cardiology; Preventive Cardiology; **Hospital:** Nyack Hosp, Englewood Hosp & Med Ctr; **Address:** 206 Route 303, Valley Cottage, NY 10989-2019; **Phone:** 845-268-0880; **Board Cert:** Internal Medicine 1984; Cardiovascular Disease 1987; Critical Care Medicine 2011; **Med School:** NY Med Coll 1981; **Resid:** Internal Medicine, Barnes Jewish Hosp 1984; **Fellow:** Cardiovascular Disease, Emory Univ Hosp 1985; Cardiovascular Disease, Westchester Med Ctr 1986

Dermatology

Waldorf, Donald MD (D) - **Spec Exp:** Skin Cancer; Acne; Psoriasis; Cosmetic Dermatology; **Hospital:** Rockland Psych Ctr; **Address:** 57 N Middletown Rd, Nanuet, NY 10954-2312; **Phone:** 845-623-7077; **Board Cert:** Dermatology 1967; **Med School:** Univ Pennsylvania 1962; **Resid:** Dermatology, Hosp Univ Penn 1964; Dermatology, NYU Medical Center 1967; **Fellow:** Dermatology, Natl Cancer Inst 1966

Waldorf, Heidi A MD (D) - **Spec Exp:** Cosmetic Dermatology; Skin Laser Surgery; Skin Cancer; Mohs' Surgery; **Hospital:** Mount Sinai Med Ctr (page 102); **Address:** 57 N Middletown Rd, Nanuet, NY 10954; **Phone:** 845-623-7077; **Board Cert:** Dermatology 2001; **Med School:** Univ Pennsylvania 1990; **Resid:** Internal Medicine, Hosp Univ Penn 1991; Dermatology, Mass Genl Hosp 1994; **Fellow:** Mohs Surgery, Laser & Skin Surg Ctr 1995; **Fac Appt:** Assoc Clin Prof D, Mount Sinai Sch Med

Diagnostic Radiology

Bobroff, Lewis M MD (DR) - **Spec Exp:** Mammography; Nuclear Medicine; PET Imaging; **Hospital:** Good Samaritan Hosp - Suffern; **Address:** 255 Lafayette Ave, Dept Radiology, Suffern, NY 10901-5103; **Phone:** 845-368-5196; **Board Cert:** Diagnostic Radiology 1974; **Med School:** Harvard Med Sch 1969; **Resid:** Diagnostic Radiology, Montefiore Hosp Med Ctr 1973; **Fellow:** Interventional Radiology, Montefiore Hosp Med Ctr 1973

Geller, Mark E MD (DR) - **Spec Exp:** MRI; Ultrasound; Nuclear Medicine; **Hospital:** Nyack Hosp; **Address:** 18 Squadron Blvd, New City, NY 10956; **Phone:** 845-634-9729; **Board Cert:** Diagnostic Radiology 1989; **Med School:** SUNY Downstate 1985; **Resid:** Diagnostic Radiology, Westchester Co Med Ctr 1989; **Fac Appt:** Asst Clin Prof Rad, NY Med Coll

Endocrinology, Diabetes & Metabolism

Cosman, Felicia MD (EDM) - **Spec Exp:** Osteoporosis; Bone Densitometry; **Hospital:** Helen Hayes Hosp, NY-Presby/Columbia Univ Med Ctr, NY (page 104); **Address:** Helen Hayes Hosp, Reg Bone Ctr, Route 9W, West Haverstraw, NY 10993-1195; **Phone:** 845-786-4489; **Board Cert:** Internal Medicine 1986; Endocrinology, Diabetes & Metabolism 1989; **Med School:** SUNY Stony Brook 1983; **Resid:** Internal Medicine, Columbia Presby Med Ctr 1986; **Fellow:** Endocrinology, Columbia Presby Med Ctr 1988; **Fac Appt:** Prof Med, Columbia P&S

Family Medicine

Ibelli, Vincent MD (FMed) *PCP* - **Spec Exp:** Asthma; Hypertension; Osteoporosis; Gastroesophageal Reflux Disease (GERD); **Hospital:** Nyack Hosp; **Address:** 97 Route 303, Tappan, NY 10983-2514; **Phone:** 845-359-5005; **Board Cert:** Family Medicine 2007; **Med School:** Italy 1983; **Resid:** Family Medicine, JFK Med Ctr 1986

Ingrassia, Joseph T MD (FMed) *PCP* - **Hospital:** Good Samaritan Hosp - Suffern, Nyack Hosp; **Address:** 36 College Ave, Nanuet, NY 10954-3093; **Phone:** 845-623-2456; **Board Cert:** Family Medicine 2003; **Med School:** Mexico 1974; **Resid:** Family Medicine, Nassau Co Hosp 1978

Gastroenterology

May, Louis MD (Ge) - **Spec Exp:** Hepatitis; Endoscopy; Pancreatic/Biliary Endoscopy (ERCP); **Hospital:** Good Samaritan Hosp - Suffern, Nyack Hosp; **Address:** 500 New Hempstead Rd, New City, NY 10956; **Phone:** 845-362-3200; **Board Cert:** Internal Medicine 1981; Gastroenterology 1983; **Med School:** Univ Miami Sch Med 1978; **Resid:** Internal Medicine, Univ Utah Med Ctr 1981; **Fellow:** Gastroenterology, Univ Utah Med Ctr 1983

Internal Medicine

Glassman, Charles F MD (IM) *PCP* - **Spec Exp:** Concierge Medicine; Preventive Medicine; Complementary Medicine; **Hospital:** Good Samaritan Hosp - Suffern, Nyack Hosp; **Address:** 7C Medical Park Drive, Pomona, NY 10970; **Phone:** 845-362-1110; **Board Cert:** Internal Medicine 1989; **Med School:** NY Med Coll 1985; **Resid:** Internal Medicine, Westchester Co Med Ctr 1988; **Fac Appt:** Asst Clin Prof Med, NY Med Coll

Handelsman, Richard E DO (IM) - **Spec Exp:** Concierge Medicine; Preventive Medicine; **Hospital:** Nyack Hosp, Good Samaritan Hosp - Suffern; **Address:** 7 Medical Park Drive, Ste C, Pomona, NY 10970-3562; **Phone:** 845-362-1169; **Board Cert:** Internal Medicine 1981; **Med School:** Univ Osteo Med & Hlth Sci, Des Moines 1976; **Resid:** Internal Medicine, UMDNJ Med Ctr 1978; Internal Medicine, Norwalk Hosp 1980; **Fac Appt:** Asst Clin Prof Med, NY Med Coll

Leahy, Mary MD (IM) *PCP* - **Spec Exp:** Preventive Medicine; **Hospital:** Nyack Hosp, Good Samaritan Hosp - Suffern; **Address:** 2 Crosfield Ave, Ste 318, West Nyack, NY 10994; **Phone:** 845-353-5600; **Board Cert:** Internal Medicine 1988; **Med School:** Italy 1983; **Resid:** Internal Medicine, Misericordia Hosp 1986; **Fellow:** Nephrology, Westchester Co Med Ctr 1988

Interventional Cardiology

Innerfield, Michael MD (IC) - **Spec Exp:** Coronary Artery Disease; Preventive Cardiology; **Hospital:** Good Samaritan Hosp - Suffern, Hackensack Univ Med Ctr (page 96); **Address:** 257 Lafayette Ave, Ste 330, Suffern, NY 10901; **Phone:** 845-368-0048; **Board Cert:** Internal Medicine 1984; Cardiovascular Disease 1987; Interventional Cardiology 2009; Nuclear Cardiology 2008; **Med School:** NY Med Coll 1981; **Resid:** Internal Medicine, Bronx Muni Hosp 1984; **Fellow:** Cardiovascular Disease, Montefiore Hosp Med Ctr 1986; Cardiovascular Disease, Cooper Hosp 1987; **Fac Appt:** Asst Prof S, Mount Sinai Sch Med

Medical Oncology

Goldberg, Robert MD (Onc) - **Spec Exp:** Brain Tumors; **Hospital:** Good Samaritan Hosp - Suffern, Nyack Hosp; **Address:** 10 Esquire Rd, Ste 6, New City, NY 10956; **Phone:** 845-634-2727; **Board Cert:** Internal Medicine 1982; Medical Oncology 1985; Hematology 1984; **Med School:** Mount Sinai Sch Med 1979; **Resid:** Internal Medicine, Beth Israel Med Ctr 1982; **Fellow:** Hematology & Oncology, Univ Minnesota Hosp 1985

Lonberg, Mathew MD (Onc) - **Spec Exp:** Lung Cancer; Breast Cancer; Lymphoma; Melanoma; **Hospital:** Nyack Hosp, NY-Presby/Columbia Univ Med Ctr, NY (page 104); **Address:** 255 5th Ave, Nyack, NY 10960; **Phone:** 845-362-1750; **Board Cert:** Internal Medicine 1984; Medical Oncology 1987; Hematology 1988; **Med School:** Univ VA Sch Med 1981; **Resid:** Internal Medicine, Bellevue Hosp Ctr 1982; **Fellow:** Hematology & Oncology, Meml Sloan-Kettering Cancer Ctr 1985; **Fac Appt:** Asst Clin Prof Med, Columbia P&S

Zimmerman, Marc MD (Onc) - **Hospital:** Nyack Hosp, Good Samaritan Hosp - Suffern; **Address:** Pomona Prof Plaza, 974 Rte 45, Ste 1200, Pomona, NY 10970; **Phone:** 845-362-3970; **Board Cert:** Internal Medicine 1980; Medical Oncology 1981; Hematology 1984; **Med School:** Albany Med Coll 1977; **Resid:** Internal Medicine, Albany Med Ctr 1979; **Fellow:** Medical Oncology, Albany Med Ctr 1982

Neonatal-Perinatal Medicine

Mendoza, Glenn MD (NP) - **Hospital:** Good Samaritan Hosp - Suffern, Children's & Women's Phys.of Westchester (page 612); **Address:** Good Samaritan Hosp, Dept Neonatology, 255 Lafayette Ave, Suffern, NY 10901; **Phone:** 845-368-5104; **Board Cert:** Pediatrics 1985; **Med School:** Philippines 1976; **Resid:** Family Medicine, Elyria Meml Hosp 1980; Pediatrics, Brooklyn Jewish Hosp & Med Ctr 1983; **Fellow:** Neonatal-Perinatal Medicine, Mt Sinai Hosp 1985; **Fac Appt:** Asst Prof Ped, Columbia P&S

Nephrology

Kozin, Arthur MD (Nep) - **Spec Exp:** Hypertension; Kidney Failure-Chronic; Diabetic Kidney Disease; **Hospital:** Nyack Hosp, Good Samaritan Hosp - Suffern; **Address:** 2 Crossfield Ave, Ste 312, West Nyack, NY 10994-2212; **Phone:** 845-358-2400; **Board Cert:** Internal Medicine 1985; Nephrology 1988; Critical Care Medicine 2002; **Med School:** Albert Einstein Coll Med 1982; **Resid:** Internal Medicine, Montefiore Hosp Med Ctr 1985; **Fellow:** Nephrology, Bellevue Hosp 1987

Shapiro, Kenneth S MD (Nep) - **Spec Exp:** Hypertension; Diabetic Kidney Disease; Transplant Medicine-Kidney; **Hospital:** Nyack Hosp, Good Samaritan Hosp - Suffern; **Address:** 2 Crosfield Ave, Ste 312, West Nyack, NY 10994-2220; **Phone:** 845-358-2400; **Board Cert:** Internal Medicine 1978; Nephrology 1980; **Med School:** Rush Med Coll 1975; **Resid:** Internal Medicine, Albany Meml Hosp 1978; **Fellow:** Nephrology, New England Med Ctr 1980; **Fac Appt:** Asst Clin Prof Med, NY Med Coll

Yablon, Steven MD (Nep) - **Spec Exp:** Hypertension; Kidney Failure; Dialysis Care; **Hospital:** Nyack Hosp, Good Samaritan Hosp - Suffern; **Address:** 2 Crosfield Ave, Ste 312, West Nyack, NY 10994-2220; **Phone:** 845-358-2400; **Board Cert:** Internal Medicine 1976; Nephrology 1978; **Med School:** UMDNJ-NJ Med Sch, Newark 1973; **Resid:** Internal Medicine, Tufts New England Med Ctr 1975; **Fellow:** Renal Disease, Hosp Univ Penn 1977

Neurological Surgery

Degen, Jeffrey W MD (NS) - **Spec Exp:** Neuro-Endoscopy; Minimally Invasive Spinal Surgery; Brain & Spinal Tumors; **Hospital:** St. Luke's Newburgh, Orange Regl Med Ctr-Horton Campus; **Address:** 222 Route 59, Ste 205, Suffern, NY 10901; **Phone:** 845-368-0286; **Board Cert:** Neurological Surgery 2007; **Med School:** Cornell Univ-Weill Med Coll 1998; **Resid:** Neurological Surgery, Georgetown Univ 2005; **Fac Appt:** Asst Clin Prof NS, NY Med Coll

Oppenheim, Jeffrey S MD (NS) - **Spec Exp:** Spinal Disorders-Degenerative; Brain Tumors; Spinal Surgery; Microsurgery; **Hospital:** Nyack Hosp, Good Samaritan Hosp - Suffern; **Address:** 222 Route 59, Ste 205, Suffern, NY 10901-5206; **Phone:** 845-368-0286; **Board Cert:** Neurological Surgery 1996; **Med School:** Cornell Univ-Weill Med Coll 1988; **Resid:** Neurological Surgery, Mount Sinai Hosp 1994

Spitzer, Daniel MD (NS) - **Spec Exp:** Brain Tumors; Spinal Surgery; Stereotactic Radiosurgery; **Hospital:** Nyack Hosp, Good Samaritan Hosp - Suffern; **Address:** 222 Route 59, Ste 205, Suffern, NY 10901-5206; **Phone:** 845-368-0286; **Board Cert:** Neurological Surgery 1992; **Med School:** NYU Sch Med 1983; **Resid:** Neurological Surgery, Montefiore Med Ctr 1989; **Fac Appt:** Asst Clin Prof NS, Columbia P&S

Neurology

Ober, David T MD (N) - **Spec Exp:** Neuromuscular Disorders; Botox Therapy; Electrodiagnosis; **Hospital:** Nyack Hosp; **Address:** 2 Crosfield Ave, Ste 202, West Nyack, NY 10994; **Phone:** 845-353-4344; **Board Cert:** Neurology 2009; Electrodiagnostic Medicine 2001; **Med School:** Albany Med Coll 1994; **Resid:** Neurology, Mt Sinai Hosp 1998; **Fellow:** Neuroelectrophysiology, St Elizabeth's Med Ctr 1999

Seliger, Glenn MD (N) - **Spec Exp:** Brain Injury; **Hospital:** Helen Hayes Hosp; **Address:** Helen Hayes Hospital, Dept Neurology, Route 9W, MC 51-55, West Haverstraw, NY 10993; **Phone:** 845-786-4459; **Board Cert:** Neurology 1988; **Med School:** SUNY Downstate 1983; **Resid:** Neurology, Neurological Inst 1987; **Fellow:** Neurological Rehabilitation, Braintree Hosp 1988; **Fac Appt:** Assoc Clin Prof N, Columbia P&S

Neuroradiology

Schwartz, Joel M MD (NRad) - **Spec Exp:** Head & Neck Imaging; **Hospital:** Nyack Hosp; **Address:** 18 Squadron Blvd, New City, NY 10956; **Phone:** 845-634-9729; **Board Cert:** Diagnostic Radiology 1990; Neuroradiology 2006; **Med School:** SUNY Upstate Med Univ 1985; **Resid:** Diagnostic Radiology, NYU Med Ctr 1990; **Fellow:** Neuroradiology, NYU Med Ctr 1991

Ophthalmology

Weingarten, Phyllis MD (Oph) - **Spec Exp:** Pediatric Ophthalmology; Strabismus; **Hospital:** Good Samaritan Hosp - Suffern, Beth Israel Med Ctr - Petrie Division (page 94); **Address:** 4A Medical Park Drive, Pomona, NY 10970-3516; **Phone:** 845-354-6225; **Board Cert:** Ophthalmology 1991; **Med School:** NY Med Coll 1986; **Resid:** Ophthalmology, Brookdale Hosp Med Ctr 1990; **Fellow:** Strabismus, Downstate Med Ctr 1991; Pediatric Ophthalmology, Johns Hopkins Hosp 1992

Orthopaedic Surgery

Austin, Kenneth S MD (OrS) - **Spec Exp:** Shoulder Injuries; Knee Injuries; Sports Medicine; **Hospital:** Good Samaritan Hosp - Suffern; **Address:** 327 Route 59, Colonial Square, Airmont, NY 10952; **Phone:** 845-618-1051; **Board Cert:** Orthopaedic Surgery 2007; **Med School:** NYU Sch Med 1988; **Resid:** Orthopaedic Surgery, Bellvue Hosp-NYU Sch Med 1993; **Fellow:** Sports Medicine, Mass Genl Hosp 1994

Kraushaar, Barry S MD (OrS) - **Spec Exp:** Shoulder Arthroscopic Surgery; Rotator Cuff Surgery; Hip & Knee Replacement; Knee Injuries/Ligament Surgery; **Hospital:** Nyack Hosp, Good Samaritan Hosp - Suffern; **Address:** 408 Airport Executive Park, Nanuet, NY 10954; **Phone:** 845-425-0555; **Board Cert:** Orthopaedic Surgery 2009; Orthopaedic Sports Medicine 2007; **Med School:** Albert Einstein Coll Med 1990; **Resid:** Orthopaedic Surgery, Bronx Lebanon Hosp 1995; **Fellow:** Sports Medicine, Arlington Hosp/Georgetown Univ 1996

Medici, Mark MD (OrS) - **Spec Exp:** Sports Medicine; Joint Replacement; Trauma; **Hospital:** Nyack Hosp, Good Samaritan Hosp - Suffern; **Address:** 2 Crosfield Ave, Ste 422, West Nyack, NY 10994; **Phone:** 845-358-1000; **Board Cert:** Orthopaedic Surgery 2012; **Med School:** NY Med Coll 1993; **Resid:** Orthopaedic Surgery, NY Med Coll 1995; Orthopaedic Surgery, Montefiore Med Ctr 1998; **Fellow:** Sports Medicine, Staten Is Ortho & Sports Med 1999

Rubin, Cheryl J MD (OrS) - **Spec Exp:** Shoulder Arthroscopic Surgery; Knee Surgery; **Hospital:** Good Samaritan Hosp - Suffern; **Address:** 327 Route 59, Colonial Square, Airmont, NY 10952; **Phone:** 845-618-1051; **Board Cert:** Orthopaedic Surgery 2003; **Med School:** Mount Sinai Sch Med 1983; **Resid:** Orthopaedic Surgery, Montefiore Med Ctr 1988; **Fellow:** Arthroscopic Surgery, Ortho Research Of Virginia

Pain Medicine

Burns, Paul MD (PM) - **Hospital:** Good Samaritan Hosp - Suffern; **Address:** 100 Route 59, Ste 105, Suffern, NY 10901-5614; **Phone:** 845-357-5745; **Board Cert:** Anesthesiology 1984; Pain Medicine 2007; **Med School:** SUNY Buffalo 1978; **Resid:** Anesthesiology, NY Hosp 1981

Pediatrics

Bernstein, William H MD (Ped) *PCP* - **Hospital:** Nyack Hosp; **Address:** 67 N Main St, New City, NY 10956; **Phone:** 845-634-8911; **Board Cert:** Pediatrics 1966; **Med School:** Vanderbilt Univ 1960; **Resid:** Pediatrics, Bellevue Hosp 1962; Pediatrics, Mt Sinai Hosp 1965; **Fellow:** Neonatology, Mt Sinai Hosp 1966

Diamant, Esther MD (Ped) *PCP* - ; **Address:** Refuah Hlth Ctr, 728 N Main St, Spring Valley, NY 10977-1960; **Phone:** 845-354-9300; **Board Cert:** Pediatrics 2010; **Med School:** Mount Sinai Sch Med 1987; **Resid:** Pediatrics, Mt Sinai Hosp 1991; **Fellow:** Pediatrics, Mt Sinai Hosp 1993

Puder, Douglas R MD (Ped) *PCP* - **Spec Exp:** Asthma; Developmental Disorders; **Hospital:** Nyack Hosp; **Address:** 35 Smith St, Nanuet, NY 10954; **Phone:** 845-623-7100; **Board Cert:** Pediatrics 1987; **Med School:** NYU Sch Med 1982; **Resid:** Pediatrics, NYU/Bellevue Hosp 1985; **Fellow:** Ambulatory Pediatrics, NYU Med Ctr 1987; **Fac Appt:** Assoc Clin Prof Ped, Columbia P&S

Siegal, Elliot MD (Ped) *PCP* - **Spec Exp:** Thyroid Disorders; Growth Disorders; Diabetes; **Hospital:** Nyack Hosp; **Address:** Clarkstown Pediatrics, 200 E Eckerson Rd, New City, NY 10956-7169; **Phone:** 845-352-5511; **Board Cert:** Pediatrics 1973; Pediatric Endocrinology 1978; **Med School:** Univ Pennsylvania 1968; **Resid:** Pediatrics, NY Hosp 1971; **Fellow:** Pediatric Endocrinology, NY Hosp 1972

Physical Medicine & Rehabilitation

Brief, Rochelle MD (PMR) - **Spec Exp:** Electrodiagnosis; **Hospital:** Nyack Hosp; **Address:** 365 Route 304, Bardonia, NY 10954-2042; **Phone:** 845-623-7949; **Board Cert:** Physical Medicine & Rehabilitation 2003; **Med School:** Albert Einstein Coll Med 1987; **Resid:** Physical Medicine & Rehabilitation, Montefiore Med Ctr 1992

Guarracini, Mary MD (PMR) - **Spec Exp:** Amputee Rehabilitation; **Hospital:** Helen Hayes Hosp; **Address:** Helen Hayes Hosp, Route 9W, West Haverstraw, NY 10993; **Phone:** 845-786-4410; **Board Cert:** Physical Medicine & Rehabilitation 1986; **Med School:** St Louis Univ 1982; **Resid:** Physical Medicine & Rehabilitation, Northwestern Univ Med Ctr 1985

Robinson, Michael MD (PMR) - **Spec Exp:** Pain-Neuropathic; Pain-Back & Neck; Musculoskeletal Disorders; **Hospital:** Good Samaritan Hosp - Suffern; **Address:** Rockland Orthopedic & Sports Med, 327 Rte 59, Colonial Square, Airmont, NY 10952; **Phone:** 845-618-1051; **Board Cert:** Physical Medicine & Rehabilitation 2003; Pain Medicine 2000; Electrodiagnostic Medicine 2000; **Med School:** Tufts Univ 1988; **Resid:** Rehabilitation, Walter Reed Army Med Ctr 1992

Psychiatry

Levy, Michael I MD (Psyc) - **Spec Exp:** Psychopharmacology; Geriatric Psychiatry; **Hospital:** Nyack Hosp; **Address:** 160 N Midland Ave, Nyack, NY 10960-2505; **Phone:** 845-348-2116; **Board Cert:** Psychiatry 1982; **Med School:** Albert Einstein Coll Med 1977; **Resid:** Psychiatry, Mount Sinai Hosp 1981; **Fac Appt:** Asst Clin Prof Psyc, NY Med Coll

Schroeder, Karl J MD (Psyc) - **Spec Exp:** Addiction/Substance Abuse; Psychiatry in Physical Illness; Post Traumatic Stress Disorder; **Address:** 104 Montebello Rd, Suffern, NY 10901; **Phone:** 845-357-9367; **Board Cert:** Psychiatry 1980; **Med School:** Columbia P&S 1974; **Resid:** Psychiatry, Columbia-Presby Hosp 1977; **Fac Appt:** Asst Clin Prof Med, Columbia P&S

Pulmonary Disease

Harris, Leon MD (Pul) - **Hospital:** Good Samaritan Hosp - Suffern; **Address:** 2 Crossfield Ave, Ste 318, West Nyack, NY 10994-2212; **Phone:** 845-353-5600; **Board Cert:** Internal Medicine 1979; Pulmonary Disease 1982; Critical Care Medicine 2004; **Med School:** Mount Sinai Sch Med 1976; **Resid:** Internal Medicine, Mt Sinai Hosp 1979; **Fellow:** Pulmonary Disease, Mass Genl Hosp 1981

Hodes, David L MD (Pul) - **Hospital:** Nyack Hosp, Good Samaritan Hosp - Suffern; **Address:** 2 Medical Park Drive, Ste 3, West Nyack, NY 10994; **Phone:** 845-727-7733; **Board Cert:** Internal Medicine 1976; Pulmonary Disease 1978; **Med School:** NYU Sch Med 1973; **Resid:** Internal Medicine, St Luke's Hosp 1976; **Fellow:** Pulmonary Disease, Bellevue Hosp/NYU 1978

Menitove, Stephen MD (Pul) - **Hospital:** Nyack Hosp, Good Samaritan Hosp - Suffern; **Address:** Rockland Pulmonary & Medical Assocs, 2 Crosfield Ave, Ste 318, West Nyack, NY 10994-2212; **Phone:** 845-353-5600; **Board Cert:** Internal Medicine 1980; Pulmonary Disease 1982; **Med School:** Mount Sinai Sch Med 1977; **Resid:** Internal Medicine, Mount Sinai Hospital 1983; **Fellow:** Pulmonary Disease, Bellevue/NYU Med Ctr 1982; **Fac Appt:** Med, Mount Sinai Sch Med

Pellicone, John MD (Pul) - **Spec Exp:** Critical Care; **Hospital:** Helen Hayes Hosp, Nyack Hosp; **Address:** Helen Hayes Hosp, Route 9W, West Haverstraw, NY 10993; **Phone:** 845-786-4410; **Board Cert:** Internal Medicine 1984; Pulmonary Disease 2010; **Med School:** Columbia P&S 1981; **Resid:** Internal Medicine, Montefiore Med Ctr 1984; **Fellow:** Pulmonary Disease, NYU-Bellevue Med Ctr 1986

Rheumatology

Becker, Alfred MD (Rhu) - **Hospital:** Good Samaritan Hosp - Suffern, Nyack Hosp; **Address:** 222 Rte 59, Ste 204, Suffern, NY 10901; **Phone:** 845-357-6464; **Board Cert:** Internal Medicine 1969; Rheumatology 1972; **Med School:** Albert Einstein Coll Med 1962; **Resid:** Internal Medicine, Pittsburgh Hlth Ctr 1967; **Fellow:** Rheumatology, Montefiore Med Ctr 1968; **Fac Appt:** Asst Clin Prof Med, Columbia P&S

Sports Medicine

Berezin, Marc A MD (SM) - **Spec Exp:** Arthroscopic Surgery; Knee Surgery; **Hospital:** Nyack Hosp, Good Samaritan Hosp - Suffern; **Address:** 99 Dutch Hill Rd, Orangeburg, NY 10962-2106; **Phone:** 845-359-1877; **Board Cert:** Orthopaedic Surgery 2012; **Med School:** NY Med Coll 1985; **Resid:** Orthopaedic Surgery, NY Med Coll 1990; **Fellow:** Sports Medicine, Arthoscopy Assoc Ortho 1991

Surgery

Fleischer, Lee S MD (S) - **Spec Exp:** Breast Disease; Laparoscopic Surgery; Gastrointestinal Surgery; **Hospital:** Nyack Hosp; **Address:** 1 Crosfield Ave, Ste 105, West Nyack, NY 10994; **Phone:** 845-535-3362; **Board Cert:** Surgery 2002; **Med School:** McGill Univ 1987; **Resid:** Surgery, Beth Israel Med Ctr 1992

Joseph, Patricia K MD (S) - **Spec Exp:** Breast Cancer; **Hospital:** Nyack Hosp; **Address:** Nyack Breast & Women's Health Ctr, 160 N Midland Ave, Nyack, NY 10960; **Phone:** 845-348-8507; **Board Cert:** Surgery 2005; **Med School:** Univ Fla Coll Med 1979; **Resid:** Surgery, Montefiore Med Ctr 1984

Simon, Lawrence MD (S) - **Spec Exp:** Breast Surgery; Hernia; Gallbladder Surgery; **Hospital:** Nyack Hosp; **Address:** 1 Crosfield Ave, Ste 105, West Nyack, NY 10994; **Phone:** 845-354-2241; **Board Cert:** Surgery 1971; **Med School:** SUNY Upstate Med Univ 1965; **Resid:** Surgery, St Lukes Hosp 1970

Thoracic & Cardiac Surgery

Lundy, Edward MD/PhD (T&CS) - **Spec Exp:** Cardiac Surgery; **Hospital:** Good Samaritan Hosp - Suffern; **Address:** 257 Lafayette Ave, Ste 330, Suffern, NY 10901; **Phone:** 845-368-8800; **Board Cert:** Thoracic Surgery 2009; **Med School:** Univ Mich Med Sch 1981; **Resid:** Surgery, Univ Mich Med Ctr 1987; **Fellow:** Thoracic Surgery, Univ Mich Med Ctr 1989

Urology

Giella, John G MD (U) - **Spec Exp:** Kidney Stones; Prostate Cancer; Prostate Disease; **Hospital:** Nyack Hosp, Good Samaritan Hosp - Suffern; **Address:** 2 Medical Park Drive, Ste 10, West Nyack, NY 10994; **Phone:** 845-354-5000; **Board Cert:** Urology 2002; **Med School:** Harvard Med Sch 1986; **Resid:** Surgery, St Vincent's Hosp 1988; Urology, Columbia-Presby Med Ctr 1992

Suffolk

Suffolk

Allergy & Immunology

Cancellieri, Russell P MD (A&I) - **Spec Exp:** Asthma; **Hospital:** Southampton Hosp; **Address:** 596 Hampton Rd, Southampton, NY 11968; **Phone:** 631-283-3300; **Board Cert:** Pediatrics 1979; Allergy & Immunology 1981; **Med School:** Georgetown Univ 1974; **Resid:** Pediatrics, Georgetown Univ Hosp 1977; Allergy & Immunology, St Luke's-Roosevelt Hosp Ctr 1979

Guida Jr, Louis E MD (A&I) - **Spec Exp:** Allergy; Urticaria; Asthma; Cystic Fibrosis; **Hospital:** Good Samaritan Hosp Med Ctr - West Islip, St. Charles Hosp; **Address:** Bay Shore Allergy & Asthma Specialists, 649 Montauk Hwy, Bay Shore, NY 11706-8542; **Phone:** 631-665-2700; **Board Cert:** Pediatrics 2011; **Med School:** Grenada 1984; **Resid:** Pediatrics, Monmouth Med Ctr 1987; Allergy & Immunology, Nassau Co Med Ctr 1993; **Fellow:** Pediatric Pulmonology, Hahnemann Univ Hosp 1990

Lusman, Paul A MD (A&I) - **Spec Exp:** Asthma; Sinus Disorders; Hives; **Hospital:** John T Mather Meml Hosp, St. Charles Hosp; **Address:** 120 N Country Rd, Port Jefferson, NY 11777; **Phone:** 631-928-4990; **Board Cert:** Pediatrics 1971; Allergy & Immunology 1974; **Med School:** Albert Einstein Coll Med 1965; **Resid:** Pediatrics, Bellevue Hosp 1968; **Fellow:** Allergy & Immunology, Duke Univ Med Ctr 1972; **Fac Appt:** Asst Clin Prof Med, SUNY Stony Brook

Mayer, Daniel L MD (A&I) - **Spec Exp:** Asthma; Allergic Rhinitis; Food Allergy; Sinusitis; **Hospital:** Stony Brook Univ Med Ctr, St. Catherine's of Siena Med Ctr; **Address:** 263 E Main St, Smithtown, NY 11787; **Phone:** 631-366-5252; **Board Cert:** Pediatrics 1983; **Med School:** Italy 1978; **Resid:** Pediatrics, Albany Med Ctr 1985; **Fellow:** Allergy & Immunology, Long Island Hosp 1987; **Fac Appt:** Asst Prof A&I, SUNY Stony Brook

Satnick, Steven MD (A&I) - **Spec Exp:** Asthma; Urticaria; **Hospital:** Stony Brook Univ Med Ctr; **Address:** 900 Main St, Ste 102, Holbrook, NY 11741-1813; **Phone:** 631-588-4486; **Board Cert:** Internal Medicine 1983; Allergy & Immunology 1987; **Med School:** SUNY Downstate 1980; **Resid:** Internal Medicine, Univ Hosp 1984; **Fellow:** Allergy & Immunology, Univ Hosp 1987

Cardiac Electrophysiology

Iwai, Sei MD (CE) - **Spec Exp:** Arrhythmias; Atrial Fibrillation; Radiofrequency Ablation; **Hospital:** Stony Brook Univ Med Ctr; **Address:** 285 Sills Rd, Ste 12-C, East Patchogue, NY 11772; **Phone:** 631-444-3575; **Board Cert:** Internal Medicine 1997; Cardiovascular Disease 2011; Cardiac Electrophysiology 2001; **Med School:** Columbia P&S 1994; **Resid:** Internal Medicine, NY-Presby/Columbia Univ Med Ctr 1997; **Fellow:** Cardiovascular Disease, NY-Presby/Weill Cornell Med Ctr 2000; Cardiac Electrophysiology, NY-Presby/Weill Cornell Med Ctr 2001; **Fac Appt:** Prof Med, SUNY Stony Brook

Rashba, Eric J MD (CE) - **Spec Exp:** Arrhythmias; Pacemakers; Syncope; Atrial Fibrillation; **Hospital:** Stony Brook Univ Med Ctr; **Address:** 101 Nicolls Rd, HSC Bldg Fl 16 - rm 080, Stony Brook, NY 11794-8167; **Phone:** 631-444-3575; **Board Cert:** Internal Medicine 2006; Cardiovascular Disease 2008; Cardiac Electrophysiology 2009; **Med School:** Yale Univ 1992; **Resid:** Internal Medicine, Strong Meml Hosp 1995; **Fellow:** Cardiovascular Disease, New England Med Ctr 1999; Cardiac Electrophysiology, New England Med Ctr 1999; **Fac Appt:** Prof Med, SUNY Stony Brook

Cardiovascular Disease

Altschul, Larry MD (Cv) - **Spec Exp:** Non-Invasive Cardiology; Echocardiography; Nuclear Cardiology; **Hospital:** Good Samaritan Hosp Med Ctr - West Islip, Southside Hosp (page 106); **Address:** 540 Union Blvd, West Islip, NY 11795; **Phone:** 631-669-2555; **Board Cert:** Internal Medicine 1980; Cardiovascular Disease 1983; **Med School:** SUNY Buffalo 1977; **Resid:** Internal Medicine, Nassau County Med Ctr 1980; **Fellow:** Cardiovascular Disease, Nassau County Med Ctr 1982

Borek, Mark G MD (Cv) - **Spec Exp:** Nuclear Cardiology; Echocardiography; Cardiac Catheterization; **Hospital:** Stony Brook Univ Med Ctr; **Address:** Stony Brook Cardiology, 101 Nicholls Rd, HSC Bldg Fl 16 - rm 080, East Setauket, NY 11733; **Phone:** 631-444-1066; **Board Cert:** Internal Medicine 1985; Cardiovascular Disease 1987; **Med School:** SUNY Downstate 1981; **Resid:** Internal Medicine, Nassau Co Med Ctr 1984; **Fellow:** Cardiovascular Disease, Long Island Coll Hosp 1987; **Fac Appt:** Asst Prof Med, SUNY Stony Brook

Brown, David Lloyd MD (Cv) - **Spec Exp:** Heart Valve Disease; Critical Care Medicine; Preventive Cardiology; Coronary Artery Disease; **Hospital:** Stony Brook Univ Med Ctr; **Address:** Division of Cardiology, Stony Brook University School of Medicine, Health Sci Ctr T16-080, Stony Brook, NY 11794; **Phone:** 631-444-3699; **Board Cert:** Internal Medicine 1986; Cardiovascular Disease 2005; **Med School:** Baylor Coll Med 1982; **Resid:** Internal Medicine, Baylor Coll Med 1986; Cardiovascular Disease, UCSF Med Ctr 1990; **Fellow:** Interventional Cardiology, Cleveland Clinic 1993; Hematology, USCF Med Ctr 1988; **Fac Appt:** Prof Med, SUNY Stony Brook

Chengot, Mathew T MD (Cv) - **Spec Exp:** Nuclear Cardiology; Interventional Cardiology; Heart Failure; Echocardiography; **Hospital:** Good Samaritan Hosp Med Ctr - West Islip, St. Joseph's Hosp-Nassau; **Address:** Amityville Heart Ctr, 129 Broadway, Amityville, NY 11701-2729; **Phone:** 631-598-3434; **Board Cert:** Internal Medicine 1980; Cardiovascular Disease 1983; **Med School:** India 1976; **Resid:** Internal Medicine, Lincoln Med Ctr 1982; **Fellow:** Cardiovascular Disease, Mt Sinai Hosp 1984

Dervan, John MD (Cv) - **Spec Exp:** Interventional Cardiology; Cholesterol/Lipid Disorders; Heart Failure; **Hospital:** Stony Brook Univ Med Ctr, St. Charles Hosp; **Address:** Heart Associates of Long Island, 220 Belle Mead Rd, Ste A, East Setauket, NY 11733; **Phone:** 631-941-2273; **Board Cert:** Internal Medicine 1979; Cardiovascular Disease 1985; Interventional Cardiology 2009; **Med School:** St Louis Univ 1976; **Resid:** Internal Medicine, Faulkner Hosp 1980; **Fellow:** Cardiovascular Disease, Beth Israel Hosp 1983; **Fac Appt:** Assoc Clin Prof Med, SUNY Stony Brook

Falco, Thomas MD (Cv) - **Hospital:** Peconic Bay Med Ctr, Eastern Long Island Hosp; **Address:** 1279 E Main St, Riverhead, NY 11901; **Phone:** 631-727-2100; **Board Cert:** Internal Medicine 1985; Cardiovascular Disease 1987; **Med School:** Mexico 1980; **Resid:** Internal Medicine, Winthrop Univ Hosp 1984; Cardiovascular Disease, Winthrop Univ Hosp 1985; **Fellow:** Cardiovascular Disease, Albany Med Ctr 1987

Jeremias, Allen MD (Cv) - **Spec Exp:** Interventional Cardiology; Peripheral Vascular Disease; Percutaneous Vascular Interventions; Vascular Disease; **Hospital:** Stony Brook Univ Med Ctr; **Address:** Stony Brook Univ Med Ctr, Hlth Sci Ctr T16-080, Stony Brook, NY 11794; **Phone:** 631-444-1069; **Board Cert:** Internal Medicine 2002; Cardiovascular Disease 2005; Interventional Cardiology 2006; Vascular Medicine 2006; **Med School:** Germany 1995; **Resid:** Internal Medicine, Cleveland Clinic Hosp 2002; **Fellow:** Cardiovascular Disease, Beth Israel-Deaconess Med Ctr 2004; Interventional Cardiology, Beth Israel-Deaconess Med Ctr 2005; **Fac Appt:** Asst Prof Med, SUNY Stony Brook

Lense, Lloyd MD (Cv) - **Spec Exp:** Cholesterol/Lipid Disorders; Hypertension; Coronary Artery Disease; **Hospital:** Stony Brook Univ Med Ctr; **Address:** Stony Brook Cardiology, 26 Research Way, East Setauket, NY 11733; **Phone:** 631-444-1060; **Board Cert:** Internal Medicine 1980; Cardiovascular Disease 1983; **Med School:** NYU Sch Med 1977; **Resid:** Internal Medicine, Mt Sinai Hosp 1980; **Fellow:** Cardiovascular Disease, Montefiore Med Ctr 1983; **Fac Appt:** Assoc Clin Prof Med, SUNY Stony Brook

Masciello, Michael A MD (Cv) - **Spec Exp:** Coronary Artery Disease; Congestive Heart Failure; **Hospital:** Southside Hosp (page 106), Good Samaritan Hosp Med Ctr - West Islip; **Address:** 540 Union Blvd, West Islip, NY 11795; **Phone:** 631-669-2555; **Board Cert:** Internal Medicine 1983; Cardiovascular Disease 1985; Critical Care Medicine 2003; **Med School:** Univ Miami Sch Med 1980; **Resid:** Cardiovascular Disease, Nassau County Med Ctr 1985

Matilsky, Michael A MD (Cv) - **Spec Exp:** Cholesterol/Lipid Disorders; Hypertension; Coronary Artery Disease; Atrial Fibrillation; **Hospital:** St. Charles Hosp, John T Mather Meml Hosp; **Address:** Three Village Cardiology, 210 Belle Mead Rd, East Setauket, NY 11733-3327; **Phone:** 631-689-1400; **Board Cert:** Internal Medicine 1985; Cardiovascular Disease 1987; **Med School:** SUNY Stony Brook 1982; **Resid:** Internal Medicine, Mt Sinai Hosp 1985; **Fellow:** Cardiovascular Disease, New York Hosp-Cornell 1988; **Fac Appt:** Asst Clin Prof Med, SUNY Stony Brook

Poon, Michael MD (Cv) - **Spec Exp:** Coronary Artery Disease; Pulmonary Hypertension; Cardiac CT Angiography; Cardiac Imaging; **Hospital:** Stony Brook Univ Med Ctr, Mount Sinai Med Ctr (page 102); **Address:** Stony Brook Health Science Ctr, Level 4, rm 120, Stony Brook, NY 11794-8460; **Phone:** 631-444-5400; **Board Cert:** Cardiovascular Disease 2007; **Med School:** Mount Sinai Sch Med 1987; **Resid:** Internal Medicine, Mount Sinai Med Ctr 1991; **Fellow:** Cardiovascular Disease, Mount Sinai Med Ctr 1993; **Fac Appt:** Prof Med, SUNY Stony Brook

Skopicki, Hal A MD/PhD (Cv) - **Spec Exp:** Congestive Heart Failure; **Hospital:** Stony Brook Univ Med Ctr; **Address:** University Physicians at Stony Brook, 3001 Expressway Drive N, Ste 200B, Islandia, NY 11749; **Phone:** 631-444-9600; **Board Cert:** Internal Medicine 2003; Cardiovascular Disease 2007; **Med School:** Ros Franklin Univ/Chicago Med Sch 1990; **Resid:** Internal Medicine, Yale-New Haven Hosp 1993; **Fellow:** Cardiovascular Disease, Mass Genl Hosp 1994; **Fac Appt:** Asst Prof Med, SUNY Stony Brook

Weinberg, Marc MD (Cv) - **Hospital:** Huntington Hosp (page 106); **Address:** West Carver Med Assocs, 200 W Carver St, Ste 8, Huntington, NY 11743-3303; **Phone:** 631-421-0020; **Board Cert:** Internal Medicine 1976; Cardiovascular Disease 1979; Critical Care Medicine 2007; **Med School:** Yale Univ 1973; **Resid:** Internal Medicine, New Haven Hosp 1977; **Fellow:** Cardiovascular Disease, New Haven Hosp 1979

Child & Adolescent Psychiatry

Carlson, Gabrielle A MD (ChAP) - **Spec Exp:** Child Psychiatry; Bipolar/Mood Disorders; ADD/ADHD; **Hospital:** Stony Brook Univ Med Ctr; **Address:** SUNY-Stony Brook, Div Child & Adolescent Psych, Putnam Hall, South Campus, Stony Brook, NY 11794-8790; **Phone:** 631-632-8840; **Board Cert:** Psychiatry 1975; Child & Adolescent Psychiatry 1978; **Med School:** Cornell Univ-Weill Med Coll 1968; **Resid:** Psychiatry, Barnes Hosp-Washington Univ 1970; Psychiatry, Nat Inst Mental Hlth 1972; **Fellow:** Child & Adolescent Psychiatry, UCLA Med Ctr 1978; **Fac Appt:** Prof Psyc, SUNY Stony Brook

Gandhi, Lajpat R MD (ChAP) - **Spec Exp:** Anxiety & Mood Disorders; ADD/ADHD; **Hospital:** Huntington Hosp (page 106); **Address:** 110 E Main St, Ste 5, Huntington, NY 11743; **Phone:** 631-427-6411; **Board Cert:** Psychiatry 1981; Child & Adolescent Psychiatry 1985; **Med School:** India 1975; **Resid:** Psychiatry, Metropolitan Hosp 1979; **Fellow:** Psychiatry, Elmhurst Hosp-Mt Sinai 1980; Child & Adolescent Psychiatry, LI Jewish-Hillside Med Ctr 1981

Pomeroy, John C MD (ChAP) - **Spec Exp:** Autism; Mental Retardation; Developmental Disorders; **Hospital:** Stony Brook Univ Med Ctr; **Address:** The Cody Center for Autism, 37 Research Way, East Setauket, NY 11733; **Phone:** 631-444-4660; **Board Cert:** Psychiatry 1984; Child & Adolescent Psychiatry 1988; **Med School:** England, UK 1973; **Resid:** Psychiatry, St Mary's Hosp 1979; **Fellow:** Child & Adolescent Psychiatry, Univ Iowa Hosps 1981; **Fac Appt:** Assoc Prof Psyc, SUNY Stony Brook

Weisbrot, Deborah M MD (ChAP) - **Spec Exp:** Anxiety & Mood Disorders; Neuro-Psychiatry; **Hospital:** Stony Brook Univ Med Ctr; **Address:** SUNY Stony Brook, Div Child & Adolescent Psych, Putnam Hall, South Campus, Stony Brook, NY 11794-8790; **Phone:** 631-632-8840; **Board Cert:** Psychiatry 1985; Child & Adolescent Psychiatry 1991; **Med School:** SUNY Buffalo 1979; **Resid:** Psychiatry, Yale-New Haven Hosp 1983; **Fellow:** Child Psychiatry, NY Hosp-Payne Whitney Clin 1986; **Fac Appt:** Assoc Clin Prof Psyc, SUNY Stony Brook

Child Neurology

Andriola, Mary R MD (ChiN) - **Spec Exp:** Epilepsy; ADD/ADHD; Headache; Developmental Disorders; **Hospital:** Stony Brook Univ Med Ctr; **Address:** SUNY-Stony Brook, Dept Neurology, 179 Belle Mead Rd, East Setauket, NY 11733; **Phone:** 631-444-2599; **Board Cert:** Pediatrics 1970; Child Neurology 1972; Clinical Neurophysiology 2002; Neurodevelopmental Disabilities 2005; **Med School:** Duke Univ 1965; **Resid:** Pediatrics, Univ Fla Shands Hosp 1967; **Fellow:** Neurology, Univ Fla Shands Hosp 1970; **Fac Appt:** Prof N, SUNY Stony Brook

Clinical Genetics

Hyman, David B MD (CG) - **Spec Exp:** Prenatal Diagnosis; Genetic Disorders; Cancer Risk Assessment; **Hospital:** Stony Brook Univ Med Ctr, St. Catherine's of Siena Med Ctr; **Address:** 48 Route 25-A, Ste 205, Smithtown, NY 11787-1448; **Phone:** 631-862-3620; **Board Cert:** Pediatrics 1983; Clinical Genetics 1984; Clinical Biochemical Genetics 1990; Clinical Molecular Genetics 1990; **Med School:** Univ IL Coll Med 1978; **Resid:** Pediatrics, Yale Univ Sch Med 1980; **Fellow:** Clinical Genetics, Yale Univ Sch Med 1983

McGovern, Margaret MD/PhD (CG) - **Hospital:** Stony Brook Univ Med Ctr; **Address:** Stony Brook Univ Med Ctr, Pediatrics HSC Bldg Fl 11 - rm 020, Nicolls Rd, Stony Brook, NY 11794-8111; **Phone:** 631-444-5437; **Board Cert:** Pediatrics 2005; Clinical Genetics 1990; **Med School:** Mount Sinai Sch Med 1986; **Resid:** Pediatrics, Mt Sinai Hosp 1988; **Fellow:** Genetics, Mt Sinai Hosp 1990; **Fac Appt:** Prof Ped, SUNY Stony Brook

Colon & Rectal Surgery

Leiboff, Arnold R MD (CRS) - **Hospital:** John T Mather Meml Hosp, St. Charles Hosp; **Address:** 3400 Nesconset Hwy, Ste 100, East Setauket, NY 11733; **Phone:** 631-689-2600; **Board Cert:** Surgery 2007; Colon & Rectal Surgery 2001; **Med School:** NY Med Coll 1978; **Resid:** Surgery, SUNY at Stony Brook 1985; **Fellow:** Colon & Rectal Surgery, Carle Foundation Hosp-Univ Ill 1989

Smithy, William B MD (CRS) - **Spec Exp:** Colon & Rectal Cancer; Anorectal Disorders; Colonoscopy; **Hospital:** Stony Brook Univ Med Ctr, St. Catherine's of Siena Med Ctr; **Address:** 222 Middle Country Rd, Ste 209, Smithtown, NY 11787; **Phone:** 631-638-2800; **Board Cert:** Surgery 2009; Colon & Rectal Surgery 1989; **Med School:** Columbia P&S 1981; **Resid:** Surgery, Roosevelt Hosp 1987; **Fellow:** Colon & Rectal Surgery, RWJ Univ Hosp 1988; **Fac Appt:** Asst Clin Prof S, SUNY Stony Brook

Dermatology

Basuk, Pamela MD (D) - **Spec Exp:** Cosmetic Dermatology; Melanoma; Skin Laser Surgery; Skin Cancer; **Hospital:** Southside Hosp (page 106); **Address:** 2011 Union Blvd, Ste 1, Bayshore, NY 11706; **Phone:** 631-666-2900; **Board Cert:** Dermatology 1988; **Med School:** NYU Sch Med 1984; **Resid:** Dermatology, Brown Univ Hosp 1988

Berger, Bernard MD (D) - **Hospital:** Southampton Hosp, Stony Brook Univ Med Ctr; **Address:** 319 Hampton Rd, Southampton, NY 11968-5029; **Phone:** 631-283-7722; **Board Cert:** Dermatology 1975; **Med School:** UC Irvine 1963; **Resid:** Dermatology, Mount Sinai Hosp 1971

Clark, Richard MD (D) - **Spec Exp:** Eczema; Contact Dermatitis; Skin Cancer; **Hospital:** Stony Brook Univ Med Ctr; **Address:** 181 N Belle Meade Rd, Ste 5, East Setauket, NY 11733; **Phone:** 631-444-4200; **Board Cert:** Internal Medicine 1974; Allergy & Immunology 1977; Dermatology 1980; **Med School:** Univ Rochester 1971; **Resid:** Internal Medicine, Strong Meml Hosp 1973; **Fellow:** Allergy & Immunology, Nat Inst Health 1976; Dermatology, Mass Genl Hosp 1980; **Fac Appt:** Prof D, SUNY Stony Brook

Huh, Julie MD (D) - **Spec Exp:** Acne; Skin Cancer; Eczema; **Hospital:** Good Samaritan Hosp Med Ctr - West Islip, Southside Hosp (page 106); **Address:** 332 E Main St, Bayshore, NY 11706-8404; **Phone:** 631-666-0500; **Board Cert:** Dermatology 2005; **Med School:** Columbia P&S 1991; **Resid:** Dermatology, Columbia-Presby Med Ctr 1995

Kristal, Leonard MD (D) - **Spec Exp:** Pediatric Dermatology; **Hospital:** Steven & Alexandra Cohen Chldn's Med Ctr of NY (page 106), Stony Brook Univ Med Ctr; **Address:** 181 N Belle Meade Rd, Ste 5, East Setauket, NY 11733; **Phone:** 631-444-4200; **Board Cert:** Pediatrics 2011; Dermatology 2001; Pediatric Dermatology 2004; **Med School:** Univ Hlth Scis, Chicago Med Sch 1986; **Resid:** Pediatrics, Chldns Hosp 1989; Dermatology, Univ Hosp-SUNY 1993; **Fellow:** Dermatology, Chldns Hosp 1994; **Fac Appt:** Asst Clin Prof Ped, SUNY Stony Brook

Marghoob, Ashfaq A MD (D) - **Spec Exp:** Skin Cancer; Melanoma; **Hospital:** Meml Sloan-Kettering Cancer Ctr (page 116); **Address:** Meml Sloan Kettering Cancer Ctr, 800 Veterans Memorial Hwy, Fl 2, Hauppage, NY 11788; **Phone:** 631-863-5150; **Board Cert:** Dermatology 2005; **Med School:** SUNY Stony Brook 1987; **Resid:** Family Medicine, SUNY Stony Brook Med Ctr 1990; **Fellow:** Dermatology, NYU Med Ctr 1995

Moynihan, Gavan D MD (D) - **Spec Exp:** Melanoma; Skin Cancer; **Hospital:** Good Samaritan Hosp Med Ctr - West Islip, Southside Hosp (page 106); **Address:** 332 E Main St, Bay Shore, NY 11706-8404; **Phone:** 631-666-0500; **Board Cert:** Dermatology 2009; **Med School:** Howard Univ 1973; **Resid:** Dermatology, USPHS Hosp-Staten Island NY & USPHS Hosp 1976; **Fellow:** Dermatology, Columbia-Presby Med Ctr 1977; **Fac Appt:** Asst Prof D, SUNY Stony Brook

Notaro, Antoinette MD (D) - **Spec Exp:** Skin Cancer; Botox Therapy; Psoriasis; Acne; **Hospital:** Eastern Long Island Hosp, Peconic Bay Med Ctr; **Address:** 13405 Main Rd, Box 93, Mattituck, NY 11952-0093; **Phone:** 631-298-1122; **Board Cert:** Dermatology 1982; **Med School:** SUNY Downstate 1978; **Resid:** Dermatology, Montefiore Med Ctr 1982; **Fac Appt:** Asst Clin Prof D, SUNY Stony Brook

Siegel, Daniel M MD (D) - **Spec Exp:** Mohs' Surgery; Dermatologic Surgery; Skin Cancer; **Hospital:** SUNY Downstate Med Ctr (Univ Hosp of Bklyn) (page 419), St. Catherine's of Siena Med Ctr; **Address:** 994 Jericho Tpke, Ste 103, Smithtown, NY 11787; **Phone:** 631-864-6647; **Board Cert:** Dermatology 2009; **Med School:** Albany Med Coll 1981; **Resid:** Dermatology, Parkland Univ Texas SW Med Ctr 1985; **Fellow:** Mohs Surgery, Baylor Coll Med 1986; **Fac Appt:** Clin Prof D, SUNY Downstate

Skrokov, Robert MD (D) - **Spec Exp:** Vascular Malformations/Birthmarks; Psoriasis; Skin Cancer; **Hospital:** Good Samaritan Hosp Med Ctr - West Islip, Southside Hosp (page 106); **Address:** 332 E Main St, Bay Shore, NY 11706-8404; **Phone:** 631-666-0500; **Board Cert:** Dermatology 2009; **Med School:** SUNY Downstate 1982; **Resid:** Dermatology, SUNY-Downstate Med Ctr 1986; **Fac Appt:** Asst Clin Prof D, SUNY Stony Brook

Tom, Jack MD (D) - **Spec Exp:** Acne; Geriatric Dermatology; **Hospital:** Mount Sinai Med Ctr (page 102); **Address:** 207 Hallock Rd, Ste 210, Stony Brook, NY 11790-3076; **Phone:** 631-444-0004; **Board Cert:** Dermatology 1986; **Med School:** NYU Sch Med 1982; **Resid:** Internal Medicine, NYU Med Ctr 1983; Dermatology, Mount Sinai Med Ctr 1986; **Fac Appt:** Asst Clin Prof D, Mount Sinai Sch Med

Wong, Anthony L MD (D) - **Spec Exp:** Mohs' Surgery; Skin Cancer; **Hospital:** NS-LIJ Hlth Sys (page 106); **Address:** Skin Cancer & Dermatologic Surgery, 944 W Jericho Tpke, Ste 103, Smithtown, NY 11787; **Phone:** 631-864-6647; **Board Cert:** Dermatology 2004; **Med School:** SUNY Downstate 2000; **Resid:** Dermatology, SUNY Hlth Sci Ctr 2004; **Fellow:** Mohs Surgery, SUNY Hlth Sci Ctr 2005

Diagnostic Radiology

Brancaccio, William R MD (DR) - **Spec Exp:** Abdominal Imaging; Mammography; **Hospital:** Southampton Hosp, Eastern Long Island Hosp; **Address:** 240 Meeting House Ln, Radiology Dept, Southampton, NY 11968; **Phone:** 631-726-8411; **Board Cert:** Diagnostic Radiology 1981; **Med School:** Geo Wash Univ 1975; **Resid:** Diagnostic Radiology, Univ Hosp 1979; **Fellow:** Diagnostic Radiology, NYU Med Ctr 1980

Kirshy, David MD (DR) - **Spec Exp:** CT Scan; MRI; PET Imaging; **Hospital:** Southampton Hosp; **Address:** 1333 Roanoke Ave, Riverhead, NY 11901; **Phone:** 631-727-2755; **Board Cert:** Diagnostic Radiology 1993; **Med School:** SUNY Downstate 1988; **Resid:** Diagnostic Radiology, SUNY Hlth Sci Ctr 1993

Mankes, Seth MD (DR) - **Hospital:** Stony Brook Univ Med Ctr; **Address:** Radiology Dept, HSC/Level 4/rm 120, Stony Brook, NY 11794-8460; **Phone:** 631-444-7901; **Board Cert:** Diagnostic Radiology 1981; **Med School:** NYU Sch Med 1976; **Resid:** Diagnostic Radiology, NYU Med Ctr 1981; **Fellow:** Ultrasound, NYU Med Ctr 1982

Endocrinology, Diabetes & Metabolism

Balkin, Michael MD (EDM) - **Spec Exp:** Diabetes; Thyroid Disorders; Hirsutism (Excessive Body Hair); Osteoporosis; **Hospital:** Huntington Hosp (page 106), Nassau Univ Med Ctr; **Address:** 191 E Main St, Huntington, NY 11743-2921; **Phone:** 631-549-2525; **Board Cert:** Internal Medicine 1976; Endocrinology 1977; **Med School:** Mount Sinai Sch Med 1972; **Resid:** Internal Medicine, Kings County Med Ctr 1975; **Fellow:** Endocrinology, Diabetes & Metabolism, Mt Sinai Med Ctr 1977; Endocrinology, Diabetes & Metabolism, Meml Sloan Kettering Cancer Ctr 1980; **Fac Appt:** Asst Clin Prof Med, SUNY Stony Brook

Brand, Howard A MD (EDM) - **Spec Exp:** Thyroid Disorders; Pituitary Disorders; Diabetes; Cholesterol/Lipid Disorders; **Hospital:** St. Charles Hosp, John T Mather Meml Hosp; **Address:** 2500 Nesconset Hwy, Bldg 3C, Stony Brook, NY 11790; **Phone:** 631-751-2400; **Board Cert:** Internal Medicine 1987; Endocrinology, Diabetes & Metabolism 2011; **Med School:** UMDNJ-Rutgers Med Sch 1984; **Resid:** Internal Medicine, Mt Sinai Hosp 1987; Internal Medicine, Bronx VA Med Ctr 1988; **Fellow:** Endocrinology, Diabetes & Metabolism, NYU Med Ctr 1990

Carlson, Harold E MD (EDM) - **Spec Exp:** Thyroid Disorders; Pituitary Disorders; Gynecomastia; **Hospital:** Stony Brook Univ Med Ctr; **Address:** Div Endocrinology & Metabolism, 26 Research Way, East Setauket, NY 11733-3453; **Phone:** 631-444-0580; **Board Cert:** Internal Medicine 1974; Endocrinology, Diabetes & Metabolism 1975; **Med School:** Cornell Univ-Weill Med Coll 1968; **Resid:** Internal Medicine, Barnes-Jewish Hosp 1970; Internal Medicine, Natl Inst Hlth 1972; **Fellow:** Endocrinology, Washington Univ 1974; **Fac Appt:** Prof Med, SUNY Stony Brook

Gelato, Marie MD (EDM) - **Spec Exp:** Thyroid Disorders; Pituitary Disorders; Adrenal Disorders; Polycystic Ovarian Syndrome; **Hospital:** Stony Brook Univ Med Ctr; **Address:** 26 Research Way, East Setauket, NY 11733; **Phone:** 631-444-0580; **Board Cert:** Internal Medicine 1982; Endocrinology 1985; **Med School:** Mich State Univ 1979; **Resid:** Internal Medicine, Dartmouth Med Ctr 1982; **Fellow:** Endocrinology, Natl Inst Hlth 1985; **Fac Appt:** Prof Med, SUNY Stony Brook

Gioia, Leonard V MD (EDM) - **Spec Exp:** Diabetes; Thyroid Disorders; **Hospital:** Southside Hosp (page 106), Good Samaritan Hosp Med Ctr - West Islip; **Address:** 53 Brentwood Rd, Ste E, Bay Shore, NY 11706; **Phone:** 631-666-6275; **Board Cert:** Internal Medicine 1979; Endocrinology, Diabetes & Metabolism 1981; **Med School:** SUNY Downstate 1976; **Resid:** Internal Medicine, St Vincent's Hosp & Med Ctr 1979; **Fellow:** Endocrinology, Diabetes & Metabolism, Boston Univ Med Ctr 1981

Goldenberg, Alan MD (EDM) - **Spec Exp:** Diabetes; Thyroid Disorders; Hormonal Disorders; Addison's Disease; **Hospital:** Southampton Hosp, Peconic Bay Med Ctr; **Address:** East End Endocrine Assocs, 189 Main Rd, Riverhead, NY 11901; **Phone:** 631-288-7120; **Board Cert:** Internal Medicine 2008; Endocrinology, Diabetes & Metabolism 2008; **Med School:** SUNY Stony Brook 1993; **Resid:** Internal Medicine, Winthrop Univ Hosp 1996; **Fellow:** Endocrinology, Diabetes & Metabolism, Winthrop Univ Hosp 1998

Weitzman, Steven P MD (EDM) - **Spec Exp:** Hashimoto's Disease; Adrenal Disorders; Thyroid Disorders; **Hospital:** Stony Brook Univ Med Ctr; **Address:** Risk Reduction Disease Mngmt Ctr, 26 Research Way, East Setauket, NY 11733; **Phone:** 631-444-0538; **Board Cert:** Internal Medicine 2005; Endocrinology, Diabetes & Metabolism 2008; **Med School:** SUNY Buffalo 2002; **Resid:** Internal Medicine, Long Island Jewish Med Ctr 2005; **Fellow:** Endocrinology, Diabetes & Metabolism, Univ Hosp- SUNY Stony Brook 2008

Wexler, Craig B MD (EDM) - **Spec Exp:** Diabetes; Thyroid Disorders; Hormonal Disorders; Cholesterol/Lipid Disorders; **Hospital:** Brookhaven Meml Hosp & Med Ctr; **Address:** 285 Sills Rd, Bldg 15 - Ste D, East Patchogue, NY 11772-8810; **Phone:** 631-758-5858; **Board Cert:** Internal Medicine 1981; Endocrinology, Diabetes & Metabolism 1989; **Med School:** Ros Franklin Univ/Chicago Med Sch 1978; **Resid:** Internal Medicine, LIJ-Hillside Med Ctr 1981; **Fellow:** Endocrinology, Diabetes & Metabolism, LIJ-Hillside Med Ctr 1989

Family Medicine

Aponte, Alex M MD (FMed) *PCP* - **Spec Exp:** Preventive Medicine; **Hospital:** Southampton Hosp; **Address:** Westhampton Primary Care, 80 Old Riverhead Rd, Westhampton Beach, NY 11978; **Phone:** 631-288-7746; **Board Cert:** Family Medicine 2009; **Med School:** SUNY Buffalo 1992; **Resid:** Family Medicine, Overlook Hosp 1995

Fishkin, Michael DO (FMed) *PCP* - **Hospital:** John T Mather Meml Hosp, St. Charles Hosp; **Address:** 2500 Nesconset Hwy, Building 7D, Stony Brook, NY 11790-2566; **Phone:** 631-751-3322; **Board Cert:** Family Medicine 2006; **Med School:** Univ Osteo Med & Hlth Sci, Des Moines 1973; **Resid:** Family Medicine, Nassau County Med Ctr 1976; **Fac Appt:** Assoc Prof FMed, SUNY Stony Brook

Giugliano, James E DO (FMed) *PCP* - **Spec Exp:** Lyme Disease; **Hospital:** Southampton Hosp; **Address:** 290 N Sea Rd, Southampton, NY 11968; **Phone:** 631-283-5900; **Board Cert:** Family Medicine 2005; **Med School:** NY Coll Osteo Med 1988; **Resid:** Family Medicine, Southside Hosp 1991; **Fac Appt:** Clin Prof FMed, NY Coll Osteo Med

Greenblatt, Louis DO (FMed) *PCP* - **Spec Exp:** Preventive Medicine; Geriatric Medicine; **Hospital:** St. Catherine's of Siena Med Ctr, Stony Brook Univ Med Ctr; **Address:** 533 Rte 111, Hauppauge, NY 11788; **Phone:** 631-366-1788; **Board Cert:** Family Medicine 2007; Geriatric Medicine 2006; **Med School:** NY Coll Osteo Med 1983; **Resid:** Family Medicine, Univ Hosp 1986; **Fac Appt:** Asst Clin Prof FMed, SUNY Stony Brook

Levites, Kenneth MD (FMed) *PCP* - **Spec Exp:** Asthma; Occupational Medicine; Hypertension; Diabetes; **Hospital:** Southside Hosp (page 106), Good Samaritan Hosp Med Ctr - West Islip; **Address:** 213 Montauk Hwy, West Sayville, NY 11796-1800; **Phone:** 631-563-6205; **Board Cert:** Family Medicine 2003; **Med School:** Albany Med Coll 1974; **Resid:** Family Medicine, Southside Hosp 1977

Schwinn, Hans Dieter MD (FMed) *PCP* - **Hospital:** Southampton Hosp; **Address:** Westhampton Primary Care Center, 80 Old Riverhead Rd, Westhampton Beach, NY 11978-1401; **Phone:** 631-288-7746; **Board Cert:** Family Medicine 2007; **Med School:** Germany 1978; **Resid:** Family Medicine, Community Hosp 1981

Gastroenterology

Cohn, William J MD (Ge) - **Spec Exp:** Liver Disease; **Hospital:** John T Mather Meml Hosp, St. Charles Hosp; **Address:** 3400 Nesconset Hwy, Ste 101, East Setauket, NY 11733-3327; **Phone:** 631-751-8700; **Board Cert:** Internal Medicine 1975; Gastroenterology 1979; **Med School:** Med Coll VA 1972; **Resid:** Internal Medicine, Med Coll Virginia Affil Hosp 1975; **Fellow:** Gastroenterology, Albert Einstein Med Ctr 1978; **Fac Appt:** Asst Clin Prof Med, SUNY Stony Brook

Duva, Joseph M MD (Ge) - **Spec Exp:** Endoscopy & Colonoscopy; Gastroesophageal Reflux Disease (GERD); Irritable Bowel Syndrome; Colonoscopy/Polypectomy; **Hospital:** Peconic Bay Med Ctr; **Address:** 887 Old Country Rd, Ste A, Riverhead, NY 11901-2115; **Phone:** 631-727-6122; **Board Cert:** Internal Medicine 1981; Gastroenterology 2007; **Med School:** Mount Sinai Sch Med 1978; **Resid:** Internal Medicine, Nassau County Med Ctr 1981; **Fellow:** Gastroenterology, Nassau County Med Ctr 1983

Glanzman, Barry MD (Ge) - **Spec Exp:** Colonoscopy; Gastroesophageal Reflux Disease (GERD); Liver Disease; **Hospital:** Huntington Hosp (page 106); **Address:** 152 E Main St, Ste C, Huntington, NY 11743; **Phone:** 631-421-2185; **Board Cert:** Gastroenterology 1989; Internal Medicine 1984; **Med School:** SUNY Downstate 1980; **Resid:** Internal Medicine, LI Jewish hosp 1981; Internal Medicine, LI Jewish Hosp 1983; **Fellow:** Gastroenterology, Med Coll of VA 1986

Harrison, Aaron R MD (Ge) - **Spec Exp:** Gastroesophageal Reflux Disease (GERD); Colon Cancer; Crohn's Disease; **Hospital:** Southside Hosp (page 106), Good Samaritan Hosp Med Ctr - West Islip; **Address:** 375 E Main St, Ste 21, Bay Shore, NY 11706; **Phone:** 631-968-8288; **Board Cert:** Internal Medicine 1977; Gastroenterology 1979; **Med School:** Albert Einstein Coll Med 1974; **Resid:** Internal Medicine, Jacobi Med Ctr 1977; **Fellow:** Gastroenterology, UCLA Med Ctr 1979; **Fac Appt:** Asst Clin Prof Med, SUNY Stony Brook

Lazar, Robert MD (Ge) - **Hospital:** St. Catherine's of Siena Med Ctr; **Address:** 48 Route 25A, Ste 107, Smithtown, NY 11787-1431; **Phone:** 631-862-3680; **Board Cert:** Internal Medicine 1986; Gastroenterology 2011; **Med School:** Mexico 1982; **Resid:** Internal Medicine, Univ Hosp/SUNY Hlth Sci Ctr 1985

Spielberg, Alan MD (Ge) - **Spec Exp:** Inflammatory Bowel Disease; Colitis; Colonoscopy; **Hospital:** St. Catherine's of Siena Med Ctr; **Address:** 48 Route 25A, Ste 203, Smithtown, NY 11787-1448; **Phone:** 631-724-1178; **Board Cert:** Internal Medicine 1977; Gastroenterology 1979; **Med School:** Belgium 1974; **Resid:** Internal Medicine, Albany Med Ctr 1977; **Fellow:** Gastroenterology, Albany Med Ctr 1979

Zinkin, Noah T MD (Ge) - **Spec Exp:** Celiac Disease; Crohn's Disease; Hepatitis; **Hospital:** NS-LIJ Hlth Sys (page 106); **Address:** 755 Park Ave, Ste 225, Huntington, NY 11743; **Phone:** 631-923-1420; **Board Cert:** Internal Medicine 2003; Gastroenterology 2006; **Med School:** Univ Rochester 2000; **Resid:** Internal Medicine, Brigham & Women's Hosp 2003; **Fellow:** Gastroenterology, Beth Israel Deaconess Med Ctr 2004

Geriatric Medicine

Fields, Suzanne D MD (Ger) *PCP* - **Hospital:** Stony Brook Univ Med Ctr; **Address:** 205 N Belle Mead Rd, East Setauket, NY 11733; **Phone:** 631-444-4630; **Board Cert:** Internal Medicine 1982; Geriatric Medicine 2008; **Med School:** Univ Conn 1979; **Resid:** Internal Medicine, Waterbury Hosp 1983; **Fellow:** Internal Medicine, New York Hosp-Cornell 1995; **Fac Appt:** Prof Med, SUNY Stony Brook

Gynecologic Oncology

Pearl, Michael L MD (GO) - **Spec Exp:** Gynecologic Cancer; Gynecologic Surgery-Complex; **Hospital:** Stony Brook Univ Med Ctr; **Address:** 3 Edmund D Pellegrino Rd, Stony Brook, NY 11794-9456; **Phone:** 631-444-2989; **Board Cert:** Obstetrics & Gynecology 2011; Gynecologic Oncology 2011; Hospice & Palliative Medicine 2010; **Med School:** UCSF 1986; **Resid:** Obstetrics & Gynecology, UCSF Med Ctr 1990; **Fellow:** Gynecologic Oncology, Univ Michigan 1994; **Fac Appt:** Prof ObG, SUNY Stony Brook

Hand Surgery

Hurst, Lawrence C MD (HS) - **Spec Exp:** Microvascular Surgery; Nerve Disorders/Surgery; Dupuytren's Contracture; **Hospital:** Stony Brook Univ Med Ctr; **Address:** 14 Technology Drive, Ste 11, E Setauket, NY 11733-3464; **Phone:** 631-444-3145; **Board Cert:** Orthopaedic Surgery 1980; Hand Surgery 2010; **Med School:** Univ VT Coll Med 1973; **Resid:** Orthopaedic Surgery, N Carolina Meml Hosp 1978; **Fellow:** Hand Surgery, Columbia-Presby Med Ctr 1979; **Fac Appt:** Prof OrS, SUNY Stony Brook

Hematology

Avvento, Louis MD (Hem) - **Spec Exp:** Breast Cancer; Lymphoma; **Hospital:** Peconic Bay Med Ctr, Southampton Hosp; **Address:** 1333 E Main St, Riverhead, NY 11901; **Phone:** 631-727-8500; **Board Cert:** Internal Medicine 1985; Medical Oncology 1987; Hematology 2004; **Med School:** Italy 1981; **Resid:** Internal Medicine, Jamaica Med Ctr 1985; **Fellow:** Hematology, Univ Hosp-SUNY 1988

Schulman, Philip MD (Hem) - **Spec Exp:** Leukemia; Lymphoma; Multiple Myeloma; Myelodysplastic Syndromes; **Hospital:** Meml Sloan-Kettering Cancer Ctr (page 116), St. Catherine's of Siena Med Ctr; **Address:** Meml Sloan Kettering at Suffolk, 650 Commack Rd Fl 2, Commack, NY 11725; **Phone:** 631-623-4100; **Board Cert:** Internal Medicine 1977; Medical Oncology 1979; Hematology 1980; **Med School:** SUNY Upstate Med Univ 1974; **Resid:** Internal Medicine, N Shore Univ Hosp 1976; Medical Oncology, Meml Sloan-Kettering 1977; **Fellow:** Medical Oncology, Meml Sloan-Kettering 1978; Hematology, N Shore Univ Hosp 1979; **Fac Appt:** Prof Med, Cornell Univ-Weill Med Coll

Schuster, Michael W MD (Hem) - **Spec Exp:** Bone Marrow Transplant; Hematologic Malignancies; Myelodysplastic Syndromes; Anemia-Aplastic; **Hospital:** Stony Brook Univ Med Ctr; **Address:** HSC T-15, Room 020, Z-8151, Stony Brook University Medical Center, Stony Brook, NY 11794-7909; **Phone:** 631-444-3577; **Board Cert:** Internal Medicine 1984; Hematology 1986; **Med School:** Dartmouth Med Sch 1980; **Resid:** Internal Medicine, Beth Israel Deaconess Med Ctr 1983; **Fellow:** Hematology & Oncology, Beth Israel Deaconess Med Ctr 1987; **Fac Appt:** Prof Hem & Onc, SUNY Stony Brook

Infectious Disease

Nash, Bernard J MD (Inf) - **Hospital:** Good Samaritan Hosp Med Ctr - West Islip, Southside Hosp (page 106); **Address:** 500 Montauk Hwy, Ste S, West Islip, NY 11795; **Phone:** 631-587-7733; **Board Cert:** Internal Medicine 1978; Infectious Disease 1982; **Med School:** Georgetown Univ 1975; **Resid:** Internal Medicine, St Elizabeth Hosp 1978; **Fellow:** Infectious Disease, Boston Univ Med Ctr 1981

Sacks-Berg, Anne C MD (Inf) - **Spec Exp:** Travel Medicine; **Hospital:** Huntington Hosp (page 106); **Address:** 120 New York Ave, Ste 5W, Huntington, NY 11743-2743; **Phone:** 631-423-9809; **Board Cert:** Internal Medicine 1986; Infectious Disease 1988; **Med School:** SUNY Hlth Sci Ctr 1983; **Resid:** Internal Medicine, Winthrop Univ Hosp 1986; **Fellow:** Infectious Disease, Winthrop Univ Hosp 1988

Samuels, Steven MD (Inf) - **Spec Exp:** Lyme Disease; AIDS/HIV; **Hospital:** Good Samaritan Hosp Med Ctr - West Islip, Southside Hosp (page 106); **Address:** 500 Montauk Hwy, Ste S, West Islip, NY 11795; **Phone:** 631-587-7733; **Board Cert:** Internal Medicine 1977; Infectious Disease 1982; **Med School:** NY Med Coll 1974; **Resid:** Internal Medicine, Nassau County Med Ctr 1977; **Fellow:** Immunopathology, UC Irvine Med Ctr 1979; **Fac Appt:** Asst Prof Med, SUNY Stony Brook

Internal Medicine

Balot, Barry DO (IM) *PCP* - **Spec Exp:** Geriatric Medicine; **Hospital:** Good Samaritan Hosp Med Ctr - West Islip, Southside Hosp (page 106); **Address:** 150 E Sunrise Hwy, Ste 101, Lindenhurst, NY 11757; **Phone:** 631-225-6200; **Board Cert:** Internal Medicine 1989; **Med School:** NY Coll Osteo Med 1985; **Resid:** Internal Medicine, Univ Hosp 1987; Internal Medicine, Overlook Hosp 1989

Bernard, Robert MD (IM) *PCP* - **Spec Exp:** Heart Disease; Skin Diseases; **Hospital:** Peconic Bay Med Ctr; **Address:** 6144 Rte 25-A C Bldg - Ste 10, Wading River, NY 11792; **Phone:** 631-929-5900; **Board Cert:** Internal Medicine 1989; **Med School:** Grenada 1986; **Resid:** Internal Medicine, St Joseph's Hosp & Med Ctr 1989

Covey, Alexander J MD (IM) - **Spec Exp:** Aging Skin; **Hospital:** Peconic Bay Med Ctr; **Address:** 445 Main St, Center Moriches, NY 11934; **Phone:** 631-878-9200; **Board Cert:** Internal Medicine 1988; **Med School:** Ros Franklin Univ/Chicago Med Sch 1985; **Resid:** Internal Medicine, Winthrop Univ Hosp 1988

Delman, Michael MD (IM) *PCP* - **Spec Exp:** Addiction/Substance Abuse; Gastroenterology; **Hospital:** Southside Hosp (page 106); **Address:** 301 E Main St, Bay Shore, NY 11706; **Phone:** 631-968-3322; **Board Cert:** Internal Medicine 1972; Gastroenterology 1975; Addiction Medicine 1991; **Med School:** NY Med Coll 1968; **Resid:** Internal Medicine, NY Med-Metro Hosp Ctr 1971; Gastroenterology, NY Med-Metro Hosp Ctr 1972; **Fellow:** Gastroenterology, NY Med-Metro Hosp Ctr 1973; **Fac Appt:** Asst Clin Prof Med, SUNY Stony Brook

Friedling, Steven MD (IM) *PCP* - **Spec Exp:** Preventive Medicine; Chronic Illness; **Hospital:** St. Catherine's of Siena Med Ctr, Stony Brook Univ Med Ctr; **Address:** 267 E Main St A Bldg, Smithtown, NY 11787-2580; **Phone:** 631-724-8348; **Board Cert:** Internal Medicine 1973; Infectious Disease 1980; **Med School:** SUNY Downstate 1968; **Resid:** Medical Oncology, Natl Cancer Inst 1971; Internal Medicine, Barnes Hosp 1973; **Fellow:** Infectious Disease, Barnes Hosp 1974; **Fac Appt:** Asst Prof Med, SUNY Stony Brook

German, Harold MD (IM) *PCP* - **Spec Exp:** Hematology; **Hospital:** Huntington Hosp (page 106); **Address:** 150 Main St, Huntington, NY 11743-6908; **Phone:** 631-271-8700; **Board Cert:** Internal Medicine 1973; Hematology 1978; **Med School:** Columbia P&S 1967; **Resid:** Internal Medicine, Lenox Hill Hosp 1968; Internal Medicine, Columbia Presby Hosp 1972; **Fellow:** Hematology, Columbia Presby Hosp 1973

Hallal Jr, Edward J MD (IM) *PCP* - **Hospital:** Southside Hosp (page 106), Good Samaritan Hosp Med Ctr - West Islip; **Address:** 180 E Main St, Bay Shore, NY 11706; **Phone:** 631-665-0027; **Board Cert:** Internal Medicine 1987; **Med School:** Grenada 1984; **Resid:** Internal Medicine, NY Methodist Hosp 1987

Lalli, Corradino Michael MD (IM) *PCP* - **Spec Exp:** Geriatric Medicine; **Hospital:** St. Catherine's of Siena Med Ctr; **Address:** 59 Southern Blvd, MS 11767, Nesconset, NY 11767; **Phone:** 631-659-1700; **Board Cert:** Internal Medicine 1979; Geriatric Medicine 2008; **Med School:** Albert Einstein Coll Med 1976; **Resid:** Internal Medicine, Nassau County Med Ctr 1979; **Fellow:** Pulmonary Disease, Nassau County Med Ctr 1980; **Fac Appt:** Asst Clin Prof Med, SUNY Stony Brook

Oppenheimer, John MD (IM) *PCP* - **Spec Exp:** Geriatric Medicine; AIDS/HIV; **Hospital:** Southampton Hosp; **Address:** 60 Bay St, Sag Harbor, NY 11963; **Phone:** 631-725-4600; **Board Cert:** Internal Medicine 1984; Geriatric Medicine 2009; **Med School:** Tulane Univ 1981; **Resid:** Internal Medicine, Tulane Univ Hosp 1982; Internal Medicine, Harlem Hosp 1983; **Fac Appt:** Asst Clin Prof Med, SUNY Stony Brook

Romano, Rosario MD (IM) *PCP* - **Spec Exp:** Geriatric Care; Cholesterol/Lipid Disorders; **Hospital:** John T Mather Meml Hosp, St. Charles Hosp; **Address:** 5225-15 Rte 347, Port Jefferson Station, NY 11776-2054; **Phone:** 631-331-1000; **Board Cert:** Internal Medicine 1977; **Med School:** NY Med Coll 1973; **Resid:** Internal Medicine, Lenox Hill Hosp 1977; **Fac Appt:** Asst Clin Prof Med, SUNY Stony Brook

Simon, Lloyd MD (IM) *PCP* - **Spec Exp:** Addiction/Substance Abuse; **Hospital:** Eastern Long Island Hosp; **Address:** 44210C County Rd 48, Box 1341, Southold, NY 11971; **Phone:** 631-765-4150; **Board Cert:** Internal Medicine 1983; **Med School:** SUNY Buffalo 1980; **Resid:** Internal Medicine, Univ Mass Med Ctr 1983

Interventional Cardiology

Ong, Lawrence MD (IC) - **Spec Exp:** Angioplasty & Stent Placement; **Hospital:** Huntington Hosp (page 106), N Shore Univ Hosp (page 106); **Address:** 270 Park Ave, Huntington, NY 11743; **Phone:** 631-351-7948; **Board Cert:** Internal Medicine 1979; Cardiovascular Disease 1981; Interventional Cardiology 2009; **Med School:** UCSF 1976; **Resid:** Internal Medicine, N Shore Univ Hosp 1979; **Fellow:** Cardiovascular Disease, N Shore Univ Hosp 1981; **Fac Appt:** Assoc Prof Med, NYU Sch Med

Medical Oncology

Akhund, Birjis G MD (Onc) - **Spec Exp:** Breast Cancer; Lymphoma; Lung Cancer; **Hospital:** Huntington Hosp (page 106); **Address:** 180 E Pulaski Rd, Huntington Sta, NY 11746; **Phone:** 631-425-2280; **Board Cert:** Internal Medicine 1989; Medical Oncology 2003; Hematology 2004; **Med School:** Lebanon 1986; **Resid:** Internal Medicine, Beth Israel Med Ctr 1990; **Fellow:** Hematology & Oncology, NYU Med Ctr 1992; Hematology Research, NYU Med Ctr 1993

Caruso, Rocco MD (Onc) - **Spec Exp:** Lymphoma; **Hospital:** St. Catherine's of Siena Med Ctr, St. Charles Hosp; **Address:** North Island Hematology Oncology, 2500 Nesconset Hwy 26B Bldg, Stony Brook, NY 11790; **Phone:** 631-751-8305; **Board Cert:** Internal Medicine 1982; Hematology 1984; Medical Oncology 2005; **Med School:** Univ Pennsylvania 1979; **Resid:** Internal Medicine, St Luke's-Roosevelt Hosp Ctr 1982; **Fellow:** Hematology, NYU Med Ctr 1985; Medical Oncology, LI Jewish Med Ctr 1994; **Fac Appt:** Asst Prof Med, SUNY Stony Brook

Fiore, John J MD (Onc) - **Spec Exp:** Lung Cancer; **Hospital:** St. Catherine's of Siena Med Ctr; **Address:** Meml Sloan Kettering at Suffolk, 650 Commack Rd, Commack, NY 11725; **Phone:** 631-623-4100; **Board Cert:** Internal Medicine 1978; Hematology 1982; Medical Oncology 1983; **Med School:** Tufts Univ 1975; **Resid:** Internal Medicine, VA Med Ctr 1979; **Fellow:** Hematology, VA Med Ctr 1981; Medical Oncology, Meml Sloan Kettering Cancer Ctr 1984

Kudelka, Andrzej P MD (Onc) - **Hospital:** Stony Brook Univ Med Ctr; **Address:** 3 Edmund D Pellegrino Rd, Stony Brook, NY 11794; **Phone:** 631-638-1000; **Board Cert:** Internal Medicine 1987; Medical Oncology 1989; Hospice & Palliative Medicine 2010; **Med School:** Poland 1982; **Resid:** Internal Medicine, Coney Island Hosp 1987; **Fellow:** Hematology & Oncology, Stony Brook Univ Hosp 1990

Ostrow, Stanley MD (Onc) - **Spec Exp:** Lymphoma; Breast Cancer; Leukemia; Carcinoid Tumors; **Hospital:** John T Mather Meml Hosp, Brookhaven Meml Hosp & Med Ctr; **Address:** 235 N Belle Mead Rd, East Setauket, NY 11733; **Phone:** 631-751-5151; **Board Cert:** Internal Medicine 1978; Medical Oncology 1979; Hematology 1982; **Med School:** SUNY Downstate 1974; **Resid:** Internal Medicine, Jewish Meml Hosp 1976; **Fellow:** Hematology & Oncology, Natl Cancer Inst 1980; **Fac Appt:** Asst Prof Med, SUNY Stony Brook

Rizvi, Hasan A MD (Onc) - **Hospital:** Good Samaritan Hosp Med Ctr - West Islip, Southside Hosp (page 106); **Address:** 180 E Main St, Bay Shore, NY 11706-8427; **Phone:** 631-666-0262; **Board Cert:** Hematology 2002; **Med School:** Pakistan 1975; **Resid:** Clinical Pathology, Ellis Hosp 1978; Internal Medicine, Mt Sinai Sch Med 1981; **Fellow:** Hematology & Oncology, Winthrop Univ Hosp 1983; Hematology & Oncology, St Elizabeth Hosp 1984

Strauss, Barry MD (Onc) - **Spec Exp:** Lung Cancer; Breast Cancer; Colon Cancer; **Hospital:** Southampton Hosp; **Address:** 353 Meeting House Ln, Southampton, NY 11968-5051; **Phone:** 631-283-6611; **Board Cert:** Internal Medicine 1975; Medical Oncology 1975; **Med School:** Geo Wash Univ 1971; **Resid:** Internal Medicine, Beth Israel Hosp 1973; **Fellow:** Medical Oncology, National Cancer Inst 1975

Neonatal-Perinatal Medicine

Davidson, Dennis MD (NP) - **Spec Exp:** Lung Disease in Newborns; **Hospital:** Stony Brook Univ Med Ctr; **Address:** Stony Brook Long Island Children's Ctr, 101 Nicholls Rd, T-11060, Stony Brook, NY 11794-8111; **Phone:** 631-444-7653; **Board Cert:** Pediatrics 1980; Neonatal-Perinatal Medicine 2009; **Med School:** Loyola Univ-Stritch Sch Med 1974; **Resid:** Pediatrics, Babies Hosp-Columbia Univ 1978; **Fellow:** Neonatal-Perinatal Medicine, Babies Hosp-Columbia Univ 1981; **Fac Appt:** Clin Prof Ped, Albert Einstein Coll Med

Parekh, Aruna MD (NP) - **Hospital:** Stony Brook Univ Med Ctr, SUNY Downstate Med Ctr (Univ Hosp of Bklyn) - LICH (page 420); **Address:** Stony Brook Univ Med Ctr, Dept of Pediatrics, 37 Research Way, MC HSCT-11060, East Setauket, NY 11733; **Phone:** 631-444-5437; **Board Cert:** Pediatrics 1976; Neonatal-Perinatal Medicine 1985; **Med School:** India 1970; **Resid:** Pediatrics, LI Coll Hosp 1975; **Fellow:** Neonatal-Perinatal Medicine, N Shore Univ Hosp 1977

Neurological Surgery

Davis, Raphael P MD (NS) - **Spec Exp:** Acoustic Neuroma; Skull Base Surgery; Spinal Disc Replacement; Brain & Spinal Surgery; **Hospital:** Stony Brook Univ Med Ctr, St. Charles Hosp; **Address:** 24 Research Way, Ste 200, East Setauket, NY 11733; **Phone:** 631-444-1213; **Board Cert:** Neurological Surgery 1990; **Med School:** Mount Sinai Sch Med 1981; **Resid:** Neurological Surgery, Mt Sinai Med Ctr 1987; **Fac Appt:** Prof NS, SUNY Stony Brook

Leon, Steven P MD (NS) - **Spec Exp:** Spinal Surgery; Minimally Invasive Surgery; Spinal Disorders-Degenerative; Spinal Tumors; **Hospital:** St. Charles Hosp; **Address:** Long Island Neuroscience Specialists, 100 Hospital Rd, Ste 216, East Patchoque, NY 11772; **Phone:** 631-475-5511; **Board Cert:** Neurological Surgery 2004; **Med School:** Harvard Med Sch 1994; **Resid:** Neurological Surgery, Brigham & Women's Hosp 2000; **Fellow:** Spinal Surgery, Cleveland Clin 2001; **Fac Appt:** Asst Clin Prof NS, Cornell Univ-Weill Med Coll

Woo, Henry H MD (NS) - **Spec Exp:** Brain Tumors; Aneurysm-Cerebral; Cerebrovascular Surgery; Stroke; **Hospital:** Stony Brook Univ Med Ctr; **Address:** Cerebrovascular Ctr, 24 Research Way, Ste 200, East Setauket, NY 11733; **Phone:** 631-444-1213; **Board Cert:** Neurological Surgery 2008; **Med School:** NYU Sch Med 1995; **Resid:** Neurological Surgery, NYU Med Ctr 2000; **Fellow:** Neuroradiology, NYU Med Ctr; **Fac Appt:** Assoc Prof NS, SUNY Stony Brook

Neurology

Cohen, Daniel H MD/PhD (N) - **Spec Exp:** Stroke; Neuromuscular Disorders; Multiple Sclerosis; Dementia; **Hospital:** Good Samaritan Hosp Med Ctr - West Islip, Southside Hosp (page 106); **Address:** 370 E Main St, Ste 1, Bay Shore, NY 11706; **Phone:** 631-666-4767; **Board Cert:** Neurology 1986; **Med School:** Univ Miami Sch Med 1980; **Resid:** Neurology, Jackson Meml Hosp 1984

Coyle, Patricia K MD (N) - **Spec Exp:** Multiple Sclerosis; Neuro-Immunology; Lyme Disease; Infections-Neurologic; **Hospital:** Stony Brook Univ Med Ctr; **Address:** Dept Neurology, HSC T-12, rm 020, Stonybrook Univ Med Ctr, Stony Brook, NY 11794-8121; **Phone:** 631-444-2599; **Board Cert:** Neurology 2004; **Med School:** Johns Hopkins Univ 1974; **Resid:** Neurology, Johns Hopkins Hosp 1978; **Fellow:** Neurological Immunology, Johns Hopkins Hosp 1980; **Fac Appt:** Prof N, SUNY Stony Brook

Gerber, Oded MD (N) - **Spec Exp:** Stroke; Parkinson's Disease; Neuromuscular Disorders; **Hospital:** Stony Brook Univ Med Ctr; **Address:** SUNY-Stony Brook, Dept Neurology, HSC Bldg Fl T12 - rm 020, Stony Brook, NY 11794-8121; **Phone:** 631-444-2599; **Board Cert:** Neurology 1979; **Med School:** SUNY Downstate 1972; **Resid:** Internal Medicine, Kings County Hosp 1974; Neurology, Mt Sinai Hosp 1977; **Fac Appt:** Asst Clin Prof N, Mount Sinai Sch Med

Moreta, Henry G MD (N) - **Hospital:** Peconic Bay Med Ctr; **Address:** 877 E Main St, Ste 106, Riverhead, NY 11901; **Phone:** 631-727-0660; **Board Cert:** Neurology 1987; **Med School:** Harvard Med Sch 1977; **Resid:** Neurology, New York Hosp 1981

Neuroradiology

Fiorella, David J MD (NRad) - **Spec Exp:** Stroke; Endovascular Surgery; Arteriovenous Malformations; Interventional Neuroradiology; **Hospital:** Stony Brook Univ Med Ctr; **Address:** Stony Brook University Medical Center, Cerebrovascular Center, Hospital Bldg - Fl Level 4 - Ste 430, Stony Brook, NY 11794-7447; **Phone:** 631-444-1213; **Board Cert:** Diagnostic Radiology 2001; Neuroradiology 2004; **Med School:** SUNY Buffalo 1986; **Resid:** Diagnostic Radiology, Duke Univ Med Ctr 2001; **Fellow:** Neurological Radiology, Barrow Neuro Inst 2003; **Fac Appt:** Prof NS, SUNY Stony Brook

Obstetrics & Gynecology

Baker, David A MD (ObG) - **Spec Exp:** Infectious Disease; Premature Labor; Vulvar & Vaginal Disorders; Sexually Transmitted Diseases; **Hospital:** Stony Brook Univ Med Ctr; **Address:** University Assocs in Ob/Gyn, 6 Technology Drive, Nicolls Rd, East Setauket, NY 11733-4079; **Phone:** 631-444-4686; **Board Cert:** Obstetrics & Gynecology 1979; Maternal & Fetal Medicine 1981; **Med School:** SUNY Hlth Sci Ctr 1973; **Resid:** Obstetrics & Gynecology, Hosp Univ Penn 1977; **Fellow:** Maternal & Fetal Medicine, Med Ctr Hosp 1979; **Fac Appt:** Prof ObG, SUNY Stony Brook

Davenport, Deborah M MD (ObG) - **Spec Exp:** Menopause Problems; **Hospital:** Stony Brook Univ Med Ctr; **Address:** 100-16 S Jersey Ave, East Setauket, NY 11733-2036; **Phone:** 631-689-6400; **Board Cert:** Obstetrics & Gynecology 2009; **Med School:** Univ Pennsylvania 1975; **Resid:** Obstetrics & Gynecology, Univ Hosp 1983; **Fac Appt:** Asst Clin Prof ObG, SUNY Stony Brook

Gentilesco, Michael MD (ObG) *PCP* - **Hospital:** St. Catherine's of Siena Med Ctr, Stony Brook Univ Med Ctr; **Address:** 48 Route 25A, Ste 207, Smithtown, NY 11787; **Phone:** 631-862-3800; **Board Cert:** Obstetrics & Gynecology 2011; **Med School:** Albert Einstein Coll Med 1980; **Resid:** Obstetrics & Gynecology, Columbia-Presby Med Ctr 1984

Hirt, Paula MD (ObG) - **Hospital:** Good Samaritan Hosp Med Ctr - West Islip; **Address:** 83 W Main St, East Islip, NY 11730; **Phone:** 631-277-5800; **Board Cert:** Obstetrics & Gynecology 1985; **Med School:** NYU Sch Med 1979; **Resid:** Obstetrics & Gynecology, NYU Med Ctr 1983

Kramer, Mitchell MD (ObG) - **Spec Exp:** Gynecologic Surgery-Complex; Menopause Problems; Minimally Invasive Surgery; Cervical Disease; **Hospital:** Huntington Hosp (page 106), N Shore Univ Hosp (page 106); **Address:** 180 E Pulaski Rd, Huntington Station, NY 11746; **Phone:** 631-425-2218; **Board Cert:** Obstetrics & Gynecology 2011; **Med School:** NY Med Coll 1985; **Resid:** Obstetrics & Gynecology, LI Jewish Med Ctr 1989; **Fac Appt:** Asst Clin Prof ObG, Hofstra N Shore-LIJ Sch Med

Lee, Douglas S MD (ObG) *PCP* - **Spec Exp:** Gynecology Only; Menopause Problems; Cervical Disease; **Hospital:** John T Mather Meml Hosp, St. Charles Hosp; **Address:** 118 N Country Road, Port Jefferson, NY 11777; **Phone:** 631-473-7171; **Board Cert:** Obstetrics & Gynecology 1979; **Med School:** NYU Sch Med 1973; **Resid:** Obstetrics & Gynecology, Bronx Municipal Hosp 1977; **Fac Appt:** Asst Clin Prof ObG, SUNY Stony Brook

Mann, Charles T MD (ObG) *PCP* - **Hospital:** St. Catherine's of Siena Med Ctr, Stony Brook Univ Med Ctr; **Address:** 48 Route 25-A, Ste 207, Smithtown, NY 11787; **Phone:** 631-862-3800; **Board Cert:** Obstetrics & Gynecology 1979; **Med School:** Creighton Univ 1974; **Resid:** Obstetrics & Gynecology, Barnes Hosp 1977

Matalon, Martin MD (ObG) - **Hospital:** Southside Hosp (page 106), Good Samaritan Hosp Med Ctr - West Islip; **Address:** 375 E Main St, Ste 4, Bay Shore, NY 11706-8418; **Phone:** 631-665-8226; **Board Cert:** Obstetrics & Gynecology 1973; **Med School:** Univ Cincinnati 1966; **Resid:** Obstetrics & Gynecology, Brookdale Univ Med Ctr 1971

Ott, Allen Edwin MD (ObG) - **Spec Exp:** Infertility; Colposcopy; Gynecology Only; **Hospital:** Southampton Hosp; **Address:** 595 Hampton Rd, Southampton, NY 11968-3021; **Phone:** 631-283-0918; **Board Cert:** Obstetrics & Gynecology 1979; **Med School:** Boston Univ 1972; **Resid:** Obstetrics & Gynecology, Hosp Univ Penn 1976

San Roman, Gerardo A MD (ObG) - **Spec Exp:** Minimally Invasive Surgery; **Hospital:** St. Charles Hosp, John T Mather Meml Hosp; **Address:** Suffolk OB/GYN, 118 N Country Rd, Port Jefferson, NY 11777; **Phone:** 631-473-7171; **Board Cert:** Obstetrics & Gynecology 2011; **Med School:** Johns Hopkins Univ 1981; **Resid:** Obstetrics & Gynecology, NY Hosp 1985

Segarra, Pedro R MD (ObG) - **Spec Exp:** Pelvic Organ Prolapse Repair; Breast Disease; Gynecologic Surgery; Vaginal Reconstruction; **Hospital:** Lenox Hill Hosp (page 106); **Address:** 595 Hampton Rd, Southampton, NY 11968; **Phone:** 631-283-0918; **Board Cert:** Obstetrics & Gynecology 2010; **Med School:** NY Med Coll 1983; **Resid:** Obstetrics & Gynecology, Lenox Hill Hosp 1987

Ophthalmology

Aries, Philip MD (Oph) - **Hospital:** Southside Hosp (page 106), Good Samaritan Hosp Med Ctr - West Islip; **Address:** Southern Ophthalmology, 375 E Main St, Ste 24, Bay Shore, NY 11706; **Phone:** 631-665-1330; **Board Cert:** Ophthalmology 1975; **Med School:** NY Med Coll 1967; **Resid:** Ophthalmology, Nassau Co Med Ctr 1973

Cossari Jr, Alfred J MD (Oph) - **Spec Exp:** Pediatric Ophthalmology; Strabismus; **Hospital:** John T Mather Meml Hosp, St. Charles Hosp; **Address:** 311 Barnum Ave, Port Jefferson, NY 11777-1682; **Phone:** 631-928-6400; **Board Cert:** Ophthalmology 1976; **Med School:** Italy 1969; **Resid:** Ophthalmology, Nassau County Med Ctr 1974; **Fellow:** Retina, Johns Hopkins Hosp 1974; Pediatric Ophthalmology, Chldns Natl Med Ctr 1975

Di Leo, Frank MD (Oph) - **Spec Exp:** Oculoplastic Surgery; **Hospital:** Southampton Hosp, St. Luke's - Roosevelt Hosp Ctr - Roosevelt Div (page 94); **Address:** 365 County Road 39A, Ste 2, Southampton, NY 11968-5243; **Phone:** 631-283-3677; **Board Cert:** Ophthalmology 1987; **Med School:** Albert Einstein Coll Med 1981; **Resid:** Ophthalmology, St Luke's-Roosevelt Hosp Ctr 1985

Elbaba, Fadi MD (Oph) - **Spec Exp:** Retina/Vitreous Surgery; Diabetic Eye Disease/Retinopathy; Macular Degeneration; HIV Retinitis; **Hospital:** Stony Brook Univ Med Ctr; **Address:** Stony Brook Ophthalmology, 33 Research Way, Ste 13, East Setauket, NY 11733; **Phone:** 631-444-4090; **Board Cert:** Ophthalmology 2003; **Med School:** Amer Univ Beirut 1982; **Resid:** Ophthalmology, Amer Univ Beirut 1987; Ophthalmology, Doheny Eye Inst/USC Med Ctr 1991; **Fellow:** Eye Pathology, Wilmer Eye Inst/Johns Hopkins 1986; Retina, Oregon Lions Sight & Hearing Inst 1987; **Fac Appt:** Assoc Prof Oph, SUNY Stony Brook

Martin, Jeffrey MD (Oph) - **Spec Exp:** Cataract Surgery; Laser Vision Surgery; **Hospital:** St. Catherine's of Siena Med Ctr, Stony Brook Univ Med Ctr; **Address:** 260 Middle Country Rd, Ste 201, Smithtown, NY 11787; **Phone:** 631-265-8780; **Board Cert:** Ophthalmology 1999; **Med School:** SUNY Stony Brook 1994; **Resid:** Ophthalmology, Nassau Co Med Ctr 1998; **Fac Appt:** Asst Clin Prof Oph, SUNY Stony Brook

Morris, Robert P MD (Oph) - **Hospital:** St. Catherine's of Siena Med Ctr; **Address:** 222 E Main St, Ste 330, Smithtown, NY 11787; **Phone:** 631-724-4488; **Board Cert:** Ophthalmology 1974; **Med School:** SUNY Upstate Med Univ 1966; **Resid:** Ophthalmology, SUNY Downstate Med Ctr 1972

Nattis, Richard J MD (Oph) - **Spec Exp:** Cataract Surgery; Laser Vision Surgery; **Hospital:** Good Samaritan Hosp Med Ctr - West Islip, Southside Hosp (page 106); **Address:** 500 W Main St, Ste 210, Babylon, NY 11702; **Phone:** 631-957-3355; **Board Cert:** Ophthalmology 1985; **Med School:** NY Med Coll 1980; **Resid:** Ophthalmology, St Vincent's Hosp 1984; **Fac Appt:** Asst Clin Prof Oph, NY Coll Osteo Med

O'Malley, Grace M MD (Oph) - **Spec Exp:** Cataract Surgery; LASIK-Refractive Surgery; **Hospital:** Southampton Hosp; **Address:** 186 Old Towne Rd, Southampton, NY 11968; **Phone:** 631-283-3533; **Board Cert:** Ophthalmology 1987; **Med School:** NY Med Coll 1981; **Resid:** Ophthalmology, NY Med Coll 1985

Pizzarello, Louis MD (Oph) - **Spec Exp:** Diabetic Eye Disease/Retinopathy; Oculoplastic Surgery; **Hospital:** Southampton Hosp, Eastern Long Island Hosp; **Address:** 137 Hampton Rd, Southampton, NY 11968; **Phone:** 631-283-5152; **Board Cert:** Ophthalmology 1980; **Med School:** Univ VA Sch Med 1975; **Resid:** Ophthalmology, Columbia-Presby Med Ctr 1979

Romanelli, John MD (Oph) - **Spec Exp:** Cataract Surgery; Glaucoma; **Hospital:** St. Catherine's of Siena Med Ctr, Stony Brook Univ Med Ctr; **Address:** 222 E Main St, Ste 330, Smithtown, NY 11787-2814; **Phone:** 631-724-4488; **Board Cert:** Ophthalmology 2003; **Med School:** Harvard Med Sch 1987; **Resid:** Ophthalmology, Manhattan EET Hosp 1991; **Fac Appt:** Clin Prof Oph, SUNY Stony Brook

Rothberg, Charles MD (Oph) - **Spec Exp:** Cataract Surgery; Glaucoma; LASIK-Refractive Surgery; **Hospital:** Brookhaven Meml Hosp & Med Ctr; **Address:** 331 E Main St, Patchogue, NY 11772-3114; **Phone:** 631-758-5300; **Board Cert:** Ophthalmology 1989; **Med School:** SUNY Downstate 1983; **Resid:** Ophthalmology, SUNY Downstate Med Ctr 1987

Schneck, Gideon MD (Oph) - **Spec Exp:** Eyelid Cosmetic Surgery; Thyroid Eye Disease; Orbital Surgery; **Hospital:** Stony Brook Univ Med Ctr, St. Charles Hosp; **Address:** 2500 Nesconset Hwy 17B Bldg, Stony Brook, NY 11790; **Phone:** 631-246-9140; **Board Cert:** Ophthalmology 1991; **Med School:** Boston Univ 1986; **Resid:** Ophthalmology, Northwestern Univ Med Sch 1990; **Fellow:** Oculoplastic Surgery, IL Eye & Ear Infirmary 1991; **Fac Appt:** Asst Clin Prof Oph, SUNY Stony Brook

Sibony, Patrick A MD (Oph) - **Spec Exp:** Neuro-Ophthalmology; Orbital Diseases; **Hospital:** Stony Brook Univ Med Ctr; **Address:** Stony Brook Ophthalmology, 33 Research Way, Ste 13, East Setauket, NY 11733; **Phone:** 631-444-4090; **Board Cert:** Ophthalmology 1982; **Med School:** Boston Univ 1977; **Resid:** Ophthalmology, Boston Univ Med Ctr 1981; **Fellow:** Ophthalmology, Eye & Ear Hosp 1982; **Fac Appt:** Prof Oph, SUNY Stony Brook

Weber, Pamela MD (Oph) - **Spec Exp:** Retinal Disorders; Macular Degeneration; Diabetic Eye Disease/Retinopathy; **Hospital:** Stony Brook Univ Med Ctr, St. Charles Hosp; **Address:** 1500 William Floyd Pkwy, Ste 304, Shirley, NY 11967; **Phone:** 631-924-4300; **Board Cert:** Ophthalmology 1989; **Med School:** Columbia P&S 1984; **Resid:** Ophthalmology, New York Eye & Ear Infirm 1988; **Fellow:** Vitreoretinal Surgery, Retina Assoc 1990; **Fac Appt:** Asst Prof Oph, SUNY Stony Brook

Zweibel, Lawrence MD (Oph) - **Spec Exp:** LASIK-Refractive Surgery; Cataract Surgery; Glaucoma; **Hospital:** St. Catherine's of Siena Med Ctr; **Address:** 260 Middle Country Rd, Ste 201, Smithtown, NY 11787-2982; **Phone:** 631-265-8780; **Board Cert:** Ophthalmology 1977; **Med School:** Albany Med Coll 1972; **Resid:** Ophthalmology, French-Polyclinic Hosp 1976

Orthopaedic Surgery

Dowling Jr, Thomas J MD (OrS) - **Spec Exp:** Spinal Surgery; Spinal Deformity; **Hospital:** St. Catherine's of Siena Med Ctr, Huntington Hosp (page 106); **Address:** 763 Larkfield Rd Fl 2, Commack, NY 11725-2900; **Phone:** 631-462-2225; **Board Cert:** Orthopaedic Surgery 2011; **Med School:** Boston Univ 1981; **Resid:** Surgery, North Shore Univ Hosp 1983; Orthopaedic Surgery, SUNY Univ Hosp 1987; **Fellow:** Spinal Surgery, North Shore Univ Hosp 1983; Spinal Surgery, Univ Toronto 1988

Lewis, Ronald MD (OrS) - **Spec Exp:** Pediatric Orthopaedic Surgery; Arthroscopic Surgery; Sports Medicine; Trauma; **Hospital:** Winthrop Univ Hosp (page 504), Huntington Hosp (page 106); **Address:** Pediatric Orthopaedics of LI, 205 E Main St, Ste 2-6, Huntington, NY 11743; **Phone:** 631-923-2370; **Board Cert:** Orthopaedic Surgery 2012; **Med School:** SUNY Stony Brook 1993; **Resid:** Orthopaedic Surgery, SUNY Stony Brook 1998; **Fellow:** Pediatric Orthopaedic Surgery, Chldns Hosp Med Ctr 1999

Tabershaw, Richard MD (OrS) - **Spec Exp:** Shoulder Surgery; Sports Medicine; Reconstructive Surgery; Arthroscopic Surgery; **Hospital:** Brookhaven Meml Hosp & Med Ctr, St. Joseph's Hosp-Nassau; **Address:** 375 E Main St, Ste 1, Bay Shore, NY 11706-8418; **Phone:** 631-665-8790; **Board Cert:** Orthopaedic Surgery 2009; **Med School:** Georgetown Univ 1980; **Resid:** Surgery, St Vincent Med Ctr 1983; Orthopaedic Surgery, Columbia-Presby Hosp 1986

Otolaryngology

Gargano, Robert M MD (Oto) - **Hospital:** Southside Hosp (page 106), Good Samaritan Hosp Med Ctr - West Islip; **Address:** 375 E Main St, Ste 17, Bay Shore, NY 11706; **Phone:** 631-665-2430; **Board Cert:** Otolaryngology 1989; **Med School:** Tufts Univ 1984; **Resid:** Otolaryngology, New England Med Ctr 1989

Lipinsky, Edward J MD (Oto) - **Spec Exp:** Head & Neck Surgery; **Hospital:** St. Catherine's of Siena Med Ctr; **Address:** 300 E Main St, Apt 1, Smithtown, NY 11787-2900; **Phone:** 631-265-3727; **Board Cert:** Otolaryngology 1976; **Med School:** NYU Sch Med 1972; **Resid:** Otolaryngology, Washington Hosp 1976

Litman, Richard MD (Oto) - **Spec Exp:** Pediatric Otolaryngology; Head & Neck Surgery; Otology; Sinus Surgery; **Hospital:** John T Mather Meml Hosp, St. Charles Hosp; **Address:** 251 E Oakland Ave, Port Jefferson, NY 11777; **Phone:** 631-928-0188; **Board Cert:** Otolaryngology 1976; **Med School:** Wake Forest Univ 1971; **Resid:** Surgery, LIJ Med Ctr 1973; **Fellow:** Otolaryngology, Bronx Muni Hosp 1976; **Fac Appt:** Asst Clin Prof Oto, SUNY Stony Brook

Marotta, James C MD (Oto) - **Spec Exp:** Facial Plastic & Reconstructive Surgery; Cosmetic Surgery-Face; **Hospital:** Stony Brook Univ Med Ctr, St. Catherine's of Siena Med Ctr; **Address:** 267 E Main St, Ste B5, Smithtown, NY 11787; **Phone:** 631-982-2022; **Board Cert:** Otolaryngology 2005; Facial Plastic & Reconstr Surgery 2008; **Med School:** SUNY Stony Brook 1999; **Resid:** Otolaryngology, Yale-New Haven Hosp 2004; **Fellow:** Facial Plastic & Reconstr Surgery, Quatela Ctr for Plastic Surg 2005; **Fac Appt:** Asst Clin Prof Oto, SUNY Stony Brook

Pain Medicine

Gargiulo, Juan MD (PM) - **Spec Exp:** Pain-Chronic; Pain-Back; Pain-Cancer; **Hospital:** Southampton Hosp; **Address:** 365 County Rd 39A, Ste 15-16, Southampton, NY 11968; **Phone:** 631-702-2300; **Board Cert:** Anesthesiology 1993; Pain Medicine 2009; **Med School:** Uruguay 1984; **Resid:** Anesthesiology, Westchester Med Ctr 1991; Pain Medicine, Westchester Med Ctr 1991

Litman, Steven J MD (PM) - **Spec Exp:** Pain-Back & Neck; Pain-after Spinal Intervention; **Hospital:** Good Samaritan Hosp Med Ctr - West Islip, St. Charles Hosp; **Address:** All Island Pain Consultants, 387 E Main St, Ste 104, Bay Shore, NY 11706; **Phone:** 631-665-0075; **Board Cert:** Anesthesiology 2003; Pain Medicine 2007; **Med School:** NY Med Coll 1987; **Resid:** Anesthesiology, Westchester Co Med Ctr 1991; **Fac Appt:** Asst Clin Prof Anes, SUNY Stony Brook

Vaillancourt, Philippe D MD (PM) - **Spec Exp:** Headache; Pain-Chronic; **Hospital:** Southampton Hosp, Peconic Bay Med Ctr; **Address:** 877 E Main St, Ste 106, Riverhead, NY 11901; **Phone:** 631-727-0660; **Board Cert:** Neurology 1986; Pain Medicine 2010; **Med School:** McGill Univ 1978; **Resid:** Neurology, Mount Sinai Med Ctr 1983; **Fac Appt:** Assoc Prof N, SUNY Stony Brook

Pathology

Tornos, Carmen MD (Path) - **Spec Exp:** Gynecologic Cancer; Breast Cancer; Ovarian Cancer; **Hospital:** Stony Brook Univ Med Ctr; **Address:** Stony Brook Univ Hosp, Dept Pathology, Level 2, rm 766, Stony Brook, NY 11794; **Phone:** 631-444-2222; **Board Cert:** Anatomic & Clinical Pathology 1989; **Med School:** Spain 1977; **Resid:** Hematology, Ciudad Sanitaria Valle de Hebron 1982; Anatomic & Clinical Pathology, Univ Texas HSC 1989; **Fellow:** Surgical Pathology, MD Anderson Cancer Ctr 1990; **Fac Appt:** Prof Path, SUNY Stony Brook

Pediatric Cardiology

Biancaniello, Thomas MD (PCd) - **Spec Exp:** Congenital Heart Disease; Fetal Echocardiography; Interventional Cardiology; Cardiac Catheterization; **Hospital:** Morgan Stanley Children's Hosp of NY-Presby, NY (page 104); **Address:** 226 N Belle Mead Rd, East Setauket, NY 11733; **Phone:** 631-265- 3300; **Board Cert:** Pediatrics 1979; Pediatric Cardiology 1981; **Med School:** NY Med Coll 1975; **Resid:** Pediatrics, North Shore Univ Hosp 1977; **Fellow:** Pediatric Cardiology, Cincinnati Chldns Hosp 1980; **Fac Appt:** Prof Ped, Columbia P&S

Pediatric Endocrinology

Wilson, Thomas Allen MD (PEn) - **Spec Exp:** Growth Disorders; Adrenal Disorders; Sexual Differentiation Disorders; Thyroid Disorders; **Hospital:** Stony Brook Univ Med Ctr; **Address:** SUNY Stony Brook, 37 Research Way, E Setauket, NY 11733; **Phone:** 631-444-5437; **Board Cert:** Pediatrics 2009; **Med School:** Univ Pennsylvania 1973; **Resid:** Pediatrics, Chldns Hosp 1976; **Fellow:** Pediatric Endocrinology, Univ Virginia Med Ctr 1982; **Fac Appt:** Prof Ped, SUNY Stony Brook

Pediatric Gastroenterology

Chawla, Anupama MD (PGe) - **Spec Exp:** Gastroesophageal Reflux Disease (GERD); Crohn's Disease; Inflammatory Bowel Disease; **Hospital:** Stony Brook Univ Med Ctr; **Address:** 37 Research Way, East Setauket, NY 11733; **Phone:** 631-444-5437; **Board Cert:** Pediatrics 2008; Pediatric Gastroenterology 2007; **Med School:** India 1980; **Resid:** Pediatrics, Stony Brook Med Ctr 1987; **Fellow:** Pediatric Gastroenterology, N Shore Univ Hosp 1987; **Fac Appt:** Asst Prof Ped, SUNY Stony Brook

Gold, David MD (PGe) - **Spec Exp:** Gastroesophageal Reflux Disease (GERD); Irritable Bowel Syndrome; Ulcerative Colitis/Crohn's; **Hospital:** Good Samaritan Hosp Med Ctr - West Islip; **Address:** 655 Deer Park Ave, Babylon, NY 11702; **Phone:** 631-321-2190; **Board Cert:** Pediatric Gastroenterology 2010; **Med School:** Albert Einstein Coll Med 1987; **Resid:** Pediatrics, LI Jewish Med Ctr 1990; **Fellow:** Pediatric Gastroenterology, LI Jewish Med Ctr 1993

Kessler, Bradley MD (PGe) - **Spec Exp:** Inflammatory Bowel Disease/Crohn's; Liver Disease; Malabsorption; **Hospital:** Good Samaritan Hosp Med Ctr - West Islip, Mercy Med Ctr - Rockville Centre; **Address:** 655 Deer Park Ave, Babylon, NY 11702; **Phone:** 631-321-2190; **Board Cert:** Pediatrics 1988; Pediatric Gastroenterology 2005; **Med School:** SUNY Downstate 1982; **Resid:** Pediatrics, N Shore Univ Hosp 1985; **Fellow:** Pediatric Gastroenterology, Baylor-Tex Chldns Hosp 1987; **Fac Appt:** Assoc Prof Ped, NY Coll Osteo Med

Pediatric Hematology-Oncology

Parker, Robert MD (PHO) - **Spec Exp:** Pediatric Cancers; Bleeding/Coagulation Disorders; Platelet Disorders; Lymphoma; **Hospital:** Stony Brook Univ Med Ctr; **Address:** Stony Brook Univ Hosp, Dept Peds, HSC T-11, Rm 029, Stony Brook, NY 11794-8111; **Phone:** 631-444-7720; **Board Cert:** Pediatrics 1983; Pediatric Hematology-Oncology 1984; **Med School:** Brown Univ 1976; **Resid:** Internal Medicine, Roger Williams Med Ctr 1977; Pediatrics, Rhode Island Hosp 1979; **Fellow:** Pediatric Hematology-Oncology, Natl Cancer Inst 1981; Hematology, Natl Cancer Inst 1984; **Fac Appt:** Prof Ped, SUNY Stony Brook

Pediatric Infectious Disease

Nachman, Sharon MD (PInf) - **Spec Exp:** Lyme Disease; AIDS/HIV; **Hospital:** Stony Brook Univ Med Ctr; **Address:** SUNY at Stony Brook, Dept of Pediatrics, HSC T 11, rm 031, Stony Brook, NY 11794-8111; **Phone:** 631-444-7692; **Board Cert:** Pediatrics 1987; Pediatric Infectious Disease 2009; **Med School:** SUNY Stony Brook 1983; **Resid:** Pediatrics, Schneiders Chldns Hosp 1986; **Fellow:** Pediatric Infectious Disease, NY Med Coll 1987Rockefeller Univ 1989; **Fac Appt:** Prof Ped, SUNY Stony Brook

Pediatric Surgery

Lee, Thomas Kang-Ming MD (PS) - **Spec Exp:** Hernia; Pediatric Cancers; Minimally Invasive Surgery; **Hospital:** Stony Brook Univ Med Ctr; **Address:** 37 Research Way, E Setauket, NY 11733; **Phone:** 631-444-4545; **Board Cert:** Surgery 2005; Pediatric Surgery 2007; **Med School:** Univ Chicago-Pritzker Sch Med 1988; **Resid:** Surgery, NY Hosp-Cornell Med Ctr 1995; **Fellow:** Surgery, Hosps Univ Pittsburgh 1992; Pediatric Surgery, Cardinal Glennon Chldns Hosp/St Louis Univ 1997; **Fac Appt:** Assoc Prof S, SUNY Stony Brook

Scriven, Richard J MD (PS) - **Spec Exp:** Hernia; Minimally Invasive Surgery; **Hospital:** Stony Brook Univ Med Ctr; **Address:** 37 Research Way, East Setauket, NY 11733; **Phone:** 631-444-4545; **Board Cert:** Surgery 1998; Pediatric Surgery 2000; **Med School:** Albert Einstein Coll Med 1990; **Resid:** Surgery, SUNY Hlth Sci Ctr 1997; **Fellow:** Pediatric Surgery, SUNY Hlth Sci Ctr 1999; **Fac Appt:** Assoc Prof S, SUNY Stony Brook

Pediatrics

Bernstein, Harvey E MD (Ped) *PCP* - **Hospital:** St. Catherine's of Siena Med Ctr, Stony Brook Univ Med Ctr; **Address:** 260 Middle Country Rd, Ste 107, Smithtown, NY 11787; **Phone:** 631-979-7222; **Board Cert:** Pediatrics 2009; **Med School:** Univ Pennsylvania 1973; **Resid:** Pediatrics, Bronx Muni Hosp 1976; **Fac Appt:** Assoc Clin Prof Ped, SUNY Stony Brook

Chernobilsky, Lev MD (Ped) *PCP* - **Spec Exp:** Asthma; **Hospital:** Stony Brook Univ Med Ctr, St. Catherine's of Siena Med Ctr; **Address:** 269-D E Main St, Smithtown, NY 11787; **Phone:** 631-361-2121; **Board Cert:** Pediatrics 1987; **Med School:** Russia 1974; **Resid:** Pediatrics, SUNY Med Ctr 1985; **Fac Appt:** Assoc Clin Prof Ped, SUNY Stony Brook

Cusumano, Barbara Jane MD (Ped) *PCP* - **Hospital:** Southampton Hosp; **Address:** 325 Meeting House Ln Bldg 2 - Ste J, Southampton, NY 11968-5087; **Phone:** 631-283-7733; **Board Cert:** Pediatrics 2009; **Med School:** Ros Franklin Univ/Chicago Med Sch 1984; **Resid:** Pediatrics, New York Hosp 1987

Festa, Robert S MD (Ped) *PCP* - **Hospital:** St. Charles Hosp, Stony Brook Univ Med Ctr; **Address:** Pediatric & Adolescent Medicine, 270 Union Ave, Holbrook, NY 11741; **Phone:** 631-588-4442; **Board Cert:** Pediatrics 1978; Pediatric Hematology-Oncology 1980; **Med School:** SUNY Downstate 1972; **Resid:** Pediatrics, Montefiore Med Ctr 1975; **Fellow:** Pediatric Hematology-Oncology, Chldns Hosp 1978

Kaplan, Martin MD (Ped) *PCP* - **Spec Exp:** Asthma; Developmental Disorders; ADD/ADHD; **Hospital:** St. Charles Hosp, Stony Brook Univ Med Ctr; **Address:** Port Jefferson Pediatrics, 12 Medical Drive, Port Jefferson Station, NY 11776-1588; **Phone:** 631-331-1710; **Board Cert:** Pediatrics 1977; **Med School:** NYU Sch Med 1972; **Resid:** Pediatrics, Bellevue Hosp 1974; Pediatrics, Duke Univ Med Ctr 1975; **Fac Appt:** Asst Clin Prof Ped, SUNY Stony Brook

Kolker, Harvey A MD (Ped) *PCP -* **Hospital:** St. Charles Hosp, Stony Brook Univ Med Ctr; **Address:** 111 Sylvan Ave, Miller Place, NY 11764-2420; **Phone:** 631-928-4888; **Board Cert:** Pediatrics 1971; **Med School:** SUNY Downstate 1966; **Resid:** Pediatrics, Madigan Genl Hosp 1969; **Fac Appt:** Assoc Clin Prof Ped, SUNY Stony Brook

Kurfist, Lee A MD (Ped) *PCP -* **Spec Exp:** Adolescent Medicine; **Hospital:** Huntington Hosp (page 106); **Address:** 205 E Main St, Ste 2-8, Huntington, NY 11743; **Phone:** 631-424-1741; **Board Cert:** Pediatrics 2007; **Med School:** Italy 1985; **Resid:** Pediatrics, Nassau County Med Ctr 1988; **Fellow:** Pediatric Gastroenterology, Mt Sinai Hosp 1990

Manners, Richard E MD (Ped) *PCP -* **Hospital:** St. Charles Hosp, Stony Brook Univ Med Ctr; **Address:** Mid-Suffolk Pediatrics, 1770 Motor Pkwy, Islandia, NY 11749; **Phone:** 631-434-1770; **Board Cert:** Pediatrics 1980; **Med School:** Albert Einstein Coll Med 1975; **Resid:** Pediatrics, Univ Minn Med Ctr 1978

McMahon, Donna-Marie DO (Ped) *PCP -* **Hospital:** Good Samaritan Hosp - Suffern, Southside Hosp (page 106); **Address:** Family Health Care Center, 267 Carelton Ave, Central Islip, NY 11722; **Phone:** 631-348-3254; **Board Cert:** Pediatrics 2006; **Med School:** NY Coll Osteo Med 1987; **Resid:** Pediatrics, Winthrop Hosp 1990Chldn's Hosp 1991

Parles, James G MD (Ped) *PCP -* **Hospital:** Stony Brook Univ Med Ctr, St. Catherine's of Siena Med Ctr; **Address:** Smithtown Pediatric Group, 260 Middle Country Rd, Ste 107, Smithtown, NY 11787; **Phone:** 631-979-7222; **Board Cert:** Pediatrics 2009; **Med School:** NYU Sch Med 1985; **Resid:** Pediatrics, Mount Sinai Hospital 1988; **Fac Appt:** Asst Clin Prof Ped, SUNY Upstate Med Univ

Quinn, Joseph B MD (Ped) *PCP -* **Spec Exp:** ADD/ADHD; **Hospital:** Southampton Hosp; **Address:** Southampton Pediatric Assocs, 325 Meetinghouse Ln Bldg 2 - Ste J, Southampton, NY 11968; **Phone:** 631-283-7733; **Board Cert:** Pediatrics 1987; **Med School:** Univ VT Coll Med 1981; **Resid:** Pediatrics, New York Hosp 1984

Sosulski, Richard MD (Ped) *PCP -* **Spec Exp:** Lung Disease in Newborns; Neonatal Critical Care; Neonatology; **Hospital:** Stony Brook Univ Med Ctr, St. Catherine's of Siena Med Ctr; **Address:** 269 E Main St D Bldg, Smithtown, NY 11787-2807; **Phone:** 631-361-2121; **Board Cert:** Pediatrics 1982; Neonatal-Perinatal Medicine 1983; **Med School:** SUNY Downstate 1977; **Resid:** Pediatrics, LI Jewish Med Ctr 1980; **Fellow:** Neonatal-Perinatal Medicine, Chldns Hosp 1982; **Fac Appt:** Assoc Clin Prof Ped, SUNY Stony Brook

Physical Medicine & Rehabilitation

Rosenberg, Craig H MD (PMR) - **Spec Exp:** Pain-Back & Neck; Spasticity Management; **Hospital:** Southside Hosp (page 106), Stony Brook Univ Med Ctr; **Address:** 301 E Main St, Bay Shore, NY 11706; **Phone:** 631-675-4550; **Board Cert:** Physical Medicine & Rehabilitation 1987; **Med School:** Mexico 1981; **Resid:** Physical Medicine & Rehabilitation, NYU Med Ctr/Rusk Inst 1985; **Fac Appt:** Asst Prof PMR, Hofstra N Shore-LIJ Sch Med

Plastic Surgery

Anton, John R MD (PlS) - **Spec Exp:** Cosmetic Surgery-Face; Eyelid Surgery; Liposuction; **Hospital:** Southampton Hosp, Peconic Bay Med Ctr; **Address:** 138 Old Town Rd, Southampton, NY 11968-5011; **Phone:** 631-283-9100; **Board Cert:** Plastic Surgery 1992; **Med School:** Univ VT Coll Med 1981; **Resid:** Surgery, Mass Genl Hosp 1986; Plastic Surgery, Wayne State Univ Med Ctr 1987; **Fellow:** Surgery, Mass Genl Hosp 1986; Plastic Surgery, Nassau County Med Ctr 1988

Dagum, Alexander B MD (PlS) - **Spec Exp:** Reconstructive Plastic Surgery; Cleft Palate/Lip; Hand Surgery; Microsurgery; **Hospital:** Stony Brook Univ Med Ctr; **Address:** 24 Research Way, Ste 100, East Setauket, NY 11733; **Phone:** 631-444-4666; **Board Cert:** Plastic Surgery 2003; Hand Surgery 2004; **Med School:** Canada 1987; **Resid:** Surgery, Univ Ottawa Civic Hosp 1988; Plastic Surgery, Univ Toronto Med Ctr 1993; **Fellow:** Microsurgery, Univ Toronto Med Ctr 1984; Hand Surgery, Stony Brook Univ Hosp 1995; **Fac Appt:** Prof S, SUNY Stony Brook

Duboys, Elliot B MD (PlS) - **Spec Exp:** Cosmetic & Reconstructive Surgery; Pediatric Plastic Surgery; Breast Surgery; Birth Defects; **Hospital:** Plainview Hosp (page 106), Stony Brook Univ Med Ctr; **Address:** Associated Plastic Surgeons/Consultants, 864 W Jericho Tpke, West Hills, NY 11743-6037; **Phone:** 631-423-1000; **Board Cert:** Plastic Surgery 1985; **Med School:** Belgium 1977; **Resid:** Surgery, SUNY - Stony Brook Univ Hosp 1982; Plastic Surgery, Nassau County Med Ctr 1984

Psychiatry

Aronson, Thomas MD (Psyc) - **Spec Exp:** Depression; Bipolar/Mood Disorders; Personality Disorders-Borderline; **Hospital:** St. Catherine's of Siena Med Ctr; **Address:** 2 Brooksite, Ste 220, Smithtown, NY 11787-3400; **Phone:** 631-265-0909; **Board Cert:** Psychiatry 1985; **Med School:** Washington Univ, St Louis 1980; **Resid:** Psychiatry, Hosp Univ Penn 1984; **Fac Appt:** Assoc Clin Prof Psyc, SUNY Stony Brook

Koreen, Amy R MD (Psyc) - ; **Address:** 28 Elm St, Huntington, NY 11743; **Phone:** 631-423-8368; **Board Cert:** Psychiatry 1993; **Med School:** Mount Sinai Sch Med 1988; **Resid:** Psychiatry, Univ Maryland Med Ctr 1991; Psychiatry, LIJ Med Ctr 1992; **Fellow:** Neuropsychopharmacology, LIJ Med Ctr 1993

Lee, Kwang Soo MD (Psyc) - ; **Address:** 221 Broadway, Ste 303, Amityville, NY 11701-2726; **Phone:** 631-789-7448; **Board Cert:** Psychiatry 1979; **Med School:** South Korea 1965; **Resid:** Internal Medicine, Booth Meml Hosp 1967; Psychiatry, Bellevue Hosp 1969; **Fellow:** Psychiatry, Amer Inst Psychoanalysis 1969

Liang, Vera T MD (Psyc) - **Spec Exp:** Women's Health-Mental Health; Depression; Anxiety Disorders; **Hospital:** Long Island Jewish Med Ctr (page 106); **Address:** 221 Broadway, Ste 201, rm A, Amityville, NY 11701-2700; **Phone:** 631-598-7396; **Board Cert:** Psychiatry 1977; Child & Adolescent Psychiatry 1981; **Med School:** Hong Kong 1969; **Resid:** Psychiatry, LI Jewish Med Ctr 1973; **Fellow:** Child & Adolescent Psychiatry, Albert Einstein Coll Med 1975

Nass, Jack MD (Psyc) - **Spec Exp:** Geriatric Rehabilitation; Bipolar/Mood Disorders; Depression; Neuro-Psychiatry; **Hospital:** Good Samaritan Hosp Med Ctr - West Islip; **Address:** 2100 Deer Park Ave, Ste 8, Deer Park, NY 11729; **Phone:** 631-321-7697; **Board Cert:** Psychiatry 1980; **Med School:** Belgium 1975; **Resid:** Psychiatry, LI Jewish Med Ctr 1979

Rosen, Bruce I MD (Psyc) - **Spec Exp:** Depression; Anxiety Disorders; Bipolar/Mood Disorders; Psychopharmacology; **Hospital:** St. Catherine's of Siena Med Ctr, Stony Brook Univ Med Ctr; **Address:** 222 Middle Country Rd, Ste 210, Smithtown, NY 11787-2814; **Phone:** 631-265-6868; **Board Cert:** Psychiatry 1976; **Med School:** Loyola Univ-Stritch Sch Med 1971; **Resid:** Psychiatry, LI Jewish-Hillside Med Ctr 1974; **Fellow:** Psychiatry, LI Jewish-Hillside Med Ctr 1975; **Fac Appt:** Assoc Clin Prof Psyc, SUNY Stony Brook

Schwartz, Michael MD (Psyc) - **Spec Exp:** Forensic Psychiatry; Psychotherapy & Psychophar-macology; Mood Disorders; Anxiety Disorders; **Hospital:** Stony Brook Univ Med Ctr; **Address:** 150 Broadhollow Rd, Ste 204, Melville, NY 11747; **Phone:** 631-385-3313; **Board Cert:** Psychiatry 1984; **Med School:** Univ Miami Sch Med 1977; **Resid:** Internal Medicine, Mount Sinai Hosp 1978; Psychiatry, Mount Sinai Hosp 1981; **Fellow:** Research, Natl Inst Aging 1983; **Fac Appt:** Assoc Prof Psyc, SUNY Stony Brook

Upadhyay, Yogendra MD (Psyc) - **Spec Exp:** Child & Adolescent Psychiatry; Bipolar/Mood Disorders; Depression; **Hospital:** S Oaks Hosp; **Address:** 400 Sunrise Hwy, Amityville, NY 11701-2508; **Phone:** 631-608-5212; **Board Cert:** Pediatrics 1967; Psychiatry 1977; Child & Adolescent Psychiatry 1978; **Med School:** India 1962; **Resid:** Pediatrics, Harlem Hosp Ctr 1965; Psychiatry, Albert Einstein Coll Med 1974; **Fellow:** Child & Adolescent Psychiatry, Johns Hopkins 1972; Child & Adolescent Psychiatry, Albert Einstein Coll Med 1975

Pulmonary Disease

Baram, Daniel MD (Pul) - **Spec Exp:** Critical Care Medicine; Lung Cancer; **Hospital:** John T Mather Meml Hosp; **Address:** 70 North Country Rd, Ste 101, Port Jefferson, NY 11777; **Phone:** 631-473-0037; **Board Cert:** Internal Medicine 2004; Critical Care Medicine 2007; Pulmonary Disease 2008; **Med School:** Jefferson Med Coll 1990; **Resid:** Internal Medicine, New York Hosp 1993; **Fellow:** Critical Care Medicine, Natl Inst of Health 1996; Pulmonary Disease, NYU/Bellevue Hosps 1998

Bernardini, Dennis L MD (Pul) - **Spec Exp:** Chronic Obstructive Lung Disease (COPD); Asthma; Sarcoidosis; Pulmonary Fibrosis; **Hospital:** Huntington Hosp (page 106); **Address:** 175 E Main St, Huntington, NY 11743-2939; **Phone:** 631-424-3787; **Board Cert:** Internal Medicine 1983; Pulmonary Disease 1986; Critical Care Medicine 2002; **Med School:** Johns Hopkins Univ 1980; **Resid:** Internal Medicine, St Luke's Hosp 1983; **Fellow:** Pulmonary Disease, Univ Hospital 1985; Critical Care Medicine, Univ Hospital 1985

Glaser, Morton L MD (Pul) - **Spec Exp:** Emphysema & Asthma; Interstitial Lung Disease; Lung Cancer; Pulmonary Hypertension; **Hospital:** St. Charles Hosp, John T Mather Meml Hosp; **Address:** 60 N Country Rd, Ste 203, Port Jefferson, NY 11777; **Phone:** 631-509-1888; **Board Cert:** Internal Medicine 1980; Pulmonary Disease 1984; Critical Care Medicine 1999; Undersea & Hyperbaric Medicine 2005; **Med School:** Med Coll Wisc 1976; **Resid:** Internal Medicine, Roger Williams Med Ctr 1979; **Fellow:** Pulmonary Disease, Univ Hosp 1981

Sklarek, Howard MD (Pul) - **Spec Exp:** Asthma; Cough; Chronic Obstructive Lung Disease (COPD); Interstitial Lung Disease; **Hospital:** Southampton Hosp; **Address:** Southampton Pulmonary Medicine, 325 Meeting House Ln Bldg 1 - Ste K, Southampton, NY 11968; **Phone:** 631-283-8008; **Board Cert:** Internal Medicine 1984; Pulmonary Disease 1986; Critical Care Medicine 2010; **Med School:** SUNY Buffalo 1981; **Resid:** Internal Medicine, Winthrop Univ Hosp 1984; **Fellow:** Pulmonary Critical Care Medicine, Winthrop Univ Hosp 1986

Walser, Lawrence A MD (Pul) - **Hospital:** Peconic Bay Med Ctr; **Address:** 185 Old Country Rd, Ste 3, Riverhead, NY 11901; **Phone:** 631-727-2523; **Board Cert:** Internal Medicine 1982; Pulmonary Disease 2007; Critical Care Medicine 2007; **Med School:** SUNY Downstate 1979; **Resid:** Internal Medicine, Berkshire Med Ctr 1982; **Fellow:** Pulmonary Disease, SUNY/Univ Hosp 1984

Wohlberg, Gary MD (Pul) - **Spec Exp:** Sleep Disorders/Apnea; Critical Care Medicine; **Hospital:** Southside Hosp (page 106), Good Samaritan Hosp Med Ctr - West Islip; **Address:** 370 E Main St, Ste 5 Bldg, Bay Shore, NY 11706-8405; **Phone:** 631-666-5864; **Board Cert:** Internal Medicine 1985; Pulmonary Disease 1986; Critical Care Medicine 2010; Sleep Medicine 2007; **Med School:** SUNY Hlth Sci Ctr 1981; **Resid:** Internal Medicine, Long Island Hosp 1984; **Fellow:** Pulmonary Disease, Montefiore Hosp Med Ctr 1986

Radiation Oncology

Park, Tae L MD (RadRO) - **Spec Exp:** Prostate Cancer; Breast Cancer; Gynecologic Cancer; **Hospital:** Stony Brook Univ Med Ctr; **Address:** Stony Brook Univ Medical Ctr, Fl Level 2 - rm 664, 100 Nicolls Rd, Stony Brook, NY 11794-7028; **Phone:** 631-444-2210; **Board Cert:** Therapeutic Radiology 1984; **Med School:** South Korea 1976; **Resid:** Radiation Oncology, Kings Co Downstate Med Ctr. 1984; **Fellow:** Radiation Oncology, MD Anderson Cancer Ctr 1985; **Fac Appt:** Assoc Clin Prof RadRO, SUNY Stony Brook

Reproductive Endocrinology

Bronson, Richard A MD (RE) - **Spec Exp:** Infertility-IVF; Pregnancy Loss-Recurrent; Reproductive Immunology; **Hospital:** Stony Brook Univ Med Ctr; **Address:** Department of Obstetrics & Gynecology, Stony Brook University Medical Center, Stony Brook, NY 11794-8091; **Phone:** 631-444-2531; **Board Cert:** Obstetrics & Gynecology 1976; Reproductive Endocrinology 1980; **Med School:** NYU Sch Med 1966; **Resid:** Surgery, NYU Med Ctr 1971; Obstetrics & Gynecology, Hosp Univ Penn 1974; **Fellow:** Reproductive Endocrinology, Pennsylvania Hosp 1976; **Fac Appt:** Prof ObG, SUNY Stony Brook

Kenigsberg, Daniel J MD (RE) - **Spec Exp:** Infertility-IVF; Uterine Fibroids; Endometriosis; Reproductive Surgery; **Hospital:** John T Mather Meml Hosp, Stony Brook Univ Med Ctr; **Address:** 8 Corporate Ctr Drive, Melville, NY 11747; **Phone:** 631-752-0606; **Board Cert:** Obstetrics & Gynecology 1995; Reproductive Endocrinology 1995; **Med School:** NY Med Coll 1978; **Resid:** Obstetrics & Gynecology, Johns Hopkins Hosp 1982; **Fellow:** Reproductive Endocrinology, Natl Inst Hlth 1984; **Fac Appt:** Assoc Clin Prof ObG, SUNY Stony Brook

Lydic, Michael L MD (RE) - **Spec Exp:** Polycystic Ovarian Syndrome; Pregnancy Loss-Recurrent; Infertility; Infertility-IVF; **Hospital:** Stony Brook Univ Med Ctr; **Address:** Reproductive Specialists of NY, 2500 Nesonset Hwy Bldg 23, Stony Brook, NY 11790; **Phone:** 631-246-9100; **Board Cert:** Obstetrics & Gynecology 2011; Reproductive Endocrinology 2011; **Med School:** Hahnemann Univ 1989; **Resid:** Obstetrics & Gynecology, Hahnemann Univ Hosp 1993; **Fellow:** Reproductive Endocrinology, Univ of Cincinnati Hosp 1995; **Fac Appt:** Asst Clin Prof ObG, SUNY Stony Brook

Rheumatology

Hamburger, Max Ira MD (Rhu) - **Spec Exp:** Rheumatoid Arthritis; Gout; Vasculitis; **Hospital:** St. Charles Hosp, John T Mather Meml Hosp; **Address:** 1895 Walt Whitman Rd, Melville, NY 11747; **Phone:** 631-249-9525; **Board Cert:** Internal Medicine 1977; Rheumatology 1980; **Med School:** Albert Einstein Coll Med 1973; **Resid:** Internal Medicine, Bellevue Hosp 1976; **Fellow:** Allergy & Immunology, Nat Inst Health 1979; **Fac Appt:** Asst Clin Prof Med, SUNY Stony Brook

Kaell, Alan T MD (Rhu) - **Spec Exp:** Geriatric Rheumatology; Vasculitis; Connective Tissue Disorders; Osteoporosis; **Hospital:** St. Charles Hosp, John T Mather Meml Hosp; **Address:** 315 Middle Country Rd, Smithtown, NY 11787-2817; **Phone:** 631-360-7778; **Board Cert:** Internal Medicine 1981; Rheumatology 1984; **Med School:** Brown Univ 1978; **Resid:** Internal Medicine, Strong Meml Hosp 1981; **Fellow:** Rheumatology, Hosp For Special Surg 1983; **Fac Appt:** Clin Prof Med, SUNY Stony Brook

Repice, Michael MD (Rhu) - **Spec Exp:** Arthritis; Connective Tissue Disorders; **Hospital:** Huntington Hosp (page 106); **Address:** 5 E Main St, Huntington, NY 11743-2812; **Phone:** 631-271-1640; **Board Cert:** Internal Medicine 1976; Rheumatology 1980; **Med School:** Georgetown Univ 1973; **Resid:** Internal Medicine, Worcester City Hosp 1977; **Fellow:** Rheumatology, Northwestern Univ Hosp 1979; **Fac Appt:** Asst Prof Med, SUNY Stony Brook

Tan, Mark MD (Rhu) - **Spec Exp:** Lupus/SLE; Rheumatoid Arthritis; **Hospital:** St. Catherine's of Siena Med Ctr, St. Charles Hosp; **Address:** 222 Middle Country Rd Fl 3 - Ste 312, Smithtown, NY 11787; **Phone:** 631-724-8900; **Board Cert:** Internal Medicine 1989; Rheumatology 2004; **Med School:** SUNY Buffalo 1983; **Resid:** Internal Medicine, Univ Hosp 1986; **Fellow:** Rheumatology, Johns Hopkins Univ 1989

Sports Medicine

Kottmeier, Stephen A MD (SM) - **Spec Exp:** Trauma; Sports Injuries; **Hospital:** Stony Brook Univ Med Ctr; **Address:** 14 Technology Drive, Ste 11, East Setauket, NY 11733; **Phone:** 631-444-4233; **Board Cert:** Orthopaedic Surgery 2004; **Med School:** SUNY Downstate 1984; **Resid:** Orthopaedic Surgery, SUNY Downstate Med Ctr 1989; **Fellow:** Sports Medicine, Penn State Univ-Hershey Med Ctr 1990; Orthopaedic Trauma Surgery, Southern NJ Regl Trauma Ctr 1991; **Fac Appt:** Asst Prof OrS, SUNY Stony Brook

Putterman, Eric A MD (SM) - **Spec Exp:** Arthroscopic Surgery; **Hospital:** N Shore Univ Hosp (page 106); **Address:** 1800 Walt Whitman Rd, Ste 120, Melville, NY 11747; **Phone:** 631-293-9540; **Board Cert:** Orthopaedic Surgery 2009; **Med School:** Mount Sinai Sch Med 1980; **Resid:** Orthopaedic Surgery, NYU-Bellevue Med Ctr 1985; **Fellow:** Sports Medicine, NYU-Bellevue Med Ctr 1985

Surgery

Busch-Devereaux, Erna MD (S) - **Spec Exp:** Breast Cancer; Breast Surgery; **Hospital:** Huntington Hosp (page 106), N Shore Univ Hosp (page 106); **Address:** 270 Pulaski Rd, Ste A, Greenlawn, NY 11740; **Phone:** 631-423-1414; **Board Cert:** Surgery 2010; **Med School:** UMDNJ-NJ Med Sch, Newark 1985; **Resid:** Surgery, St Vincents Hosp 1990; **Fellow:** Surgical Oncology, Roswell Park Cancer 1993; **Fac Appt:** Asst Prof S, NYU Sch Med

Cohen, Bradley D MD (S) - **Spec Exp:** Breast Disease; Cancer Surgery; Laparoscopic Surgery; Sentinel Node Surgery; **Hospital:** Good Samaritan Hosp Med Ctr - West Islip, Southside Hosp (page 106); **Address:** 15 Park Ave, Bay Shore, NY 11706; **Phone:** 631-581-4400; **Board Cert:** Surgery 2009; **Med School:** Mount Sinai Sch Med 1983; **Resid:** Surgery, Lenox Hill Hosp 1988; **Fellow:** Surgical Oncology, Meml Sloan Kettering Cancer Ctr 1989

Francfort, John MD (S) - **Spec Exp:** Breast Surgery; Gastrointestinal Surgery; Vascular Surgery; Laparoscopic Surgery; **Hospital:** Good Samaritan Hosp Med Ctr - West Islip, Southside Hosp (page 106); **Address:** 580 Union Blvd, West Islip, NY 11795-3105; **Phone:** 631-321-6801; **Board Cert:** Surgery 2005; Vascular Surgery 2006; **Med School:** UMDNJ-NJ Med Sch, Newark 1980; **Resid:** Surgery, Hosp Univ Penn 1986; **Fellow:** Vascular Surgery, Northwesten Univ 1987; **Fac Appt:** Asst Clin Prof S, SUNY Stony Brook

Klausner, Stanley MD (S) - **Spec Exp:** Breast Surgery; **Hospital:** Brookhaven Meml Hosp & Med Ctr; **Address:** 100 Hospital Rd, Ste 106, Patchogue, NY 11772; **Phone:** 631-475-8846; **Board Cert:** Surgery 1975; **Med School:** NYU Sch Med 1967; **Resid:** Surgery, Bronx Muni Hosp 1973

O'Hea, Brian J MD (S) - **Spec Exp:** Breast Cancer; Sentinel Node Surgery; **Hospital:** Stony Brook Univ Med Ctr; **Address:** HSC T-18, Rm 060, Dept of Surgery, Stony Brook, NY 11794-8191; **Phone:** 631-444-1795; **Board Cert:** Surgery 2002; **Med School:** Georgetown Univ 1986; **Resid:** Surgery, St Vincent's Hosp 1991; **Fellow:** Breast Disease, Meml Sloan-Kettering Cancer Ctr 1996; **Fac Appt:** Asst Prof S, SUNY Stony Brook

Sclafani, Lisa MD (S) - **Spec Exp:** Breast Surgery; Breast Cancer; **Hospital:** Meml Sloan-Kettering Cancer Ctr (page 116); **Address:** 650 Commack Rd, Surgical Oncology, Commack, NY 11725; **Phone:** 631-623-4050; **Board Cert:** Surgery 2007; **Med School:** NYU Sch Med 1982; **Resid:** Surgery, Albert Einstein Coll Med 1987; **Fellow:** Surgical Oncology, Meml Sloan Kettering Cancer Ctr 1989; **Fac Appt:** Assoc Clin Prof S, Cornell Univ-Weill Med Coll

Shapiro, Marc MD (S) - **Spec Exp:** Laparoscopic Surgery; Gastrointestinal Surgery; Burn Care; Trauma; **Hospital:** Stony Brook Univ Med Ctr; **Address:** Stony Brook Univ Hosp, 37 Research Way, East Setauket, NY 11733; **Phone:** 631-444-1045; **Board Cert:** Surgery 2004; Surgical Critical Care 2005; **Med School:** Univ Mich Med Sch 1979; **Resid:** Surgery, Henry Ford Hosp 1984; **Fellow:** Critical Care Medicine, Univ Pittsburgh Hosp 1985; **Fac Appt:** Prof S, SUNY Stony Brook

Zingale, Robert MD (S) - **Spec Exp:** Laparoscopic Surgery; Colon & Rectal Cancer; Gastrointestinal Surgery; Breast Disease; **Hospital:** Huntington Hosp (page 106); **Address:** 158 E Main St, Ste 7, Huntington, NY 11743-2988; **Phone:** 631-271-1822; **Board Cert:** Surgery 2007; Surgical Critical Care 1999; **Med School:** SUNY Downstate 1983; **Resid:** Surgery, Maimonides Med Ctr 1988; **Fellow:** Trauma, Coney Island Hosp 1989; **Fac Appt:** Assoc Clin Prof S, NY Med Coll

Thoracic & Cardiac Surgery

Bilfinger, Thomas MD (T&CS) - **Spec Exp:** Cardiac Surgery-Adult; Lung Cancer; **Hospital:** Stony Brook Univ Med Ctr; **Address:** Stony Brook Univ Med Ctr-Surgery, 100 Nichols Rd, HSC Bldg Fl 19 - rm 080, Stony Brook, NY 11794-8191; **Phone:** 631-444-1820; **Board Cert:** Surgery 2006; Thoracic & Cardiac Surgery 2008; Surgical Critical Care 2010; **Med School:** Switzerland 1978; **Resid:** Surgery, Univ Chicago 1982; Surgery, Univ TX Med Branch Hosp 1986; **Fellow:** Thoracic Surgery, Univ TX Med Branch Hosp 1988; **Fac Appt:** Prof T&CS, SUNY Stony Brook

Palatt, Terry MD (T&CS) - **Spec Exp:** Lung Cancer; Video Assisted Thoracic Surgery (VATS); **Hospital:** Good Samaritan Hosp Med Ctr - West Islip, Southside Hosp (page 106); **Address:** 15 Park Ave, Bay Shore, NY 11706; **Phone:** 631-581-4400; **Board Cert:** Thoracic Surgery 2008; **Med School:** Grenada 1981; **Resid:** Surgery, Maimonides Med Ctr 1986; Thoracic Surgery, Maimonides Med Ctr 1988

Rosengart, Todd MD (T&CS) - **Spec Exp:** Transfusion Free Surgery; Gene Therapy-Cardiac Angiogenesis; Minimally Invasive Surgery; Cardiac Surgery; **Hospital:** Stony Brook Univ Med Ctr; **Address:** Stonybrook Univ Hosp, Health Sci Ctr, Cardiothoracic Surgery, HSC-T19, rm 020, Stonybrook, NY 11794-0001; **Phone:** 631-444-7875; **Board Cert:** Surgery 2010; Thoracic Surgery 2001; **Med School:** Northwestern Univ 1983; **Resid:** Surgery, NYU Med Ctr 1985; Surgery, NYU Med Ctr 1989; **Fellow:** Thoracic Surgery, Natl Inst Hlth 1987; Cardiothoracic Surgery, NY-Cornell Med Ctr 1991; **Fac Appt:** Prof S, SUNY Stony Brook

Taylor Jr, James R MD (T&CS) - **Spec Exp:** Thoracic Aortic Surgery; Aneurysm-Aortic; **Hospital:** Stony Brook Univ Med Ctr; **Address:** Stonybrook Univ, Dept Cardiothoracic Surgery, HSC FL 19 rm 080, Stonybrook, NY 11794-8191; **Phone:** 631-444-1820; **Board Cert:** Surgery 2008; Thoracic Surgery 2001; **Med School:** Med Univ SC 1984; **Resid:** Surgery, NY Hosp-Cornell Med Ctr 1989; **Fellow:** Cardiothoracic Surgery, NY Hosp-Cornell Med Ctr 1991

Urology

Beccia, David J MD (U) - **Spec Exp:** Prostate Cancer; Erectile Dysfunction; **Hospital:** Southside Hosp (page 106), Good Samaritan Hosp Med Ctr - West Islip; **Address:** Suffolk Urology, 332 E Main St, Bay Shore, NY 11706-8404; **Phone:** 631-665-3737; **Board Cert:** Urology 1979; **Med School:** NY Med Coll 1970; **Resid:** Surgery, Hartford Hosp 1973; Urology, Boston Univ Med Ctr 1977

Mills, Carl MD (U) - **Spec Exp:** Urologic Cancer; **Hospital:** Brookhaven Meml Hosp & Med Ctr, St. Charles Hosp; **Address:** 250 Yaphank Rd, Ste 15, East Patchogue, NY 11772-4863; **Phone:** 631-475-5051; **Board Cert:** Urology 1984; **Med School:** Geo Wash Univ 1975; **Resid:** Surgery, New York Hosp 1978; Urology, New York Hosp 1982

Wasnick, Robert MD (U) - **Spec Exp:** Undescended Testis; Pediatric Urology; Hydronephrosis; Hypospadias; **Hospital:** Stony Brook Univ Med Ctr, St. Charles Hosp; **Address:** Stony Brook Medical Park, 24 Research Way, Ste 500, East Setauket, NY 11733; **Phone:** 631-444-6270; **Board Cert:** Urology 1982; Pediatric Urology 2008; **Med School:** Jefferson Med Coll 1974; **Resid:** Surgery, St Vincents Hosp Med Ctr 1977; Urology, Downstate Med Ctr 1980; **Fellow:** Pediatric Urology, Alder Hey Chldns Hosp 1981; **Fac Appt:** Clin Prof U, SUNY Stony Brook

Vascular Surgery

Arnold, Thomas E MD (VascS) - **Spec Exp:** Carotid Artery Surgery; Aneurysm-Abdominal Aortic; Varicose Veins; Dialysis Access Surgery; **Hospital:** John T Mather Meml Hosp, St. Charles Hosp; **Address:** 1110 Hallock Ave, Port Jefferson Station, NY 11776; **Phone:** 631-476-9100; **Board Cert:** Surgery 2003; Vascular Surgery 2003; **Med School:** SUNY Downstate 1985; **Resid:** Surgery, Presbyterian Med Ctr/Univ Penn 1987; Surgery, Medical Coll Penn 1991

Pollina, Robert M MD (VascS) - **Spec Exp:** Varicose Veins; Aneurysm; Carotid Artery Surgery; Dialysis Access Surgery; **Hospital:** John T Mather Meml Hosp, St. Charles Hosp; **Address:** 1110 Hallock Ave, Port Jefferson Station, NY 11776; **Phone:** 631-476-9100; **Board Cert:** Vascular Surgery 2007; **Med School:** SUNY Hlth Sci Ctr 1988; **Resid:** Surgery, Kings County Hosp 1993; **Fellow:** Vascular Surgery, Maimonides Medical Ctr 1995

Tassiopoulos, Apostolos K MD (VascS) - **Hospital:** Stony Brook Univ Med Ctr; **Address:** Stony Brook Univ Medical Ctr, HSC Bldg Fl 19 - rm 090, Stony Brook, NY 11794; **Phone:** 631-444-4545; **Board Cert:** Surgery 2010; Vascular Surgery 2002; **Med School:** Greece 1989; **Resid:** Surgery, SUNY Upstate Med Ctr 1999; Vascular Surgery, Loyola Univ Med Ctr 2001; **Fac Appt:** Assoc Prof S, SUNY Stony Brook

The Best in American Medicine
www.CastleConnolly.com

Westchester

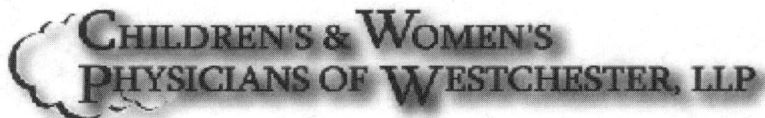

CHILDREN'S & WOMEN'S PHYSICIANS OF WESTCHESTER, LLP

Munger Pavilion, Room 123   Valhalla, New York 10595
Tel: 914-594-4021   Fax: 914-594-4937   www.cwpw.org

GENERAL OVERVIEW

Children's & Women's Physicians of Westchester, LLP (CWPW) is one of the largest physician medical and surgical practices in the Tri-State area, providing a wide-reaching system of primary-care and specialty-care services in both the in-patient and out-patient settings. CWPW is committed to providing comprehensive in-patient and out-patient care to infants, children, adolescents and selected adults throughout the greater New York Metropolitan area, extending from New York City, throughout the Hudson Valley, and into parts of Connecticut. CWPW physicians are world leaders in the diagnosis and treatment of complex illnesses and 41 of our doctors were selected as *Top Doctors* by Castle Connolly.

ACADEMIC AND CLINICAL AFFLIATIONS

CWPW consists of more than 230 practicing physicians who are also faculty at New York Medical College in Valhalla, New York. CWPW pediatricians are also teachers and researchers with access to the most advanced diagnostic and therapeutic approaches and the latest technology in the field of pediatric and adult medicine. CWPW attending physicians are core faculty at the following medical centers: Maria Fareri Children's Hospital at Westchester Medical Center, Sound Shore Medical Center, and Good Samaritan Hospital. CWPW physicians are also on staff at Vassar Brothers Medical Center, Phelps Memorial Hospital, Hudson Valley Hospital, St Luke's Hospital, Putnam Hospital, Norwalk Hospital, Greenwich Hospital and Danbury Hospital. In addition to their academic and clinical affiliations, our physicians also provide an array of primary and specialty-care services in out-patient settings throughout the region.

MEDICAL SPECIALTIES

CWPW physicians are well recognized and renowned in the pediatric medical specialties of: Adolescent and Pediatric Gynecology, Adolescent Medicine, Cardiology, Cardiothoracic Surgery, Critical Care, Developmental Pediatrics, Endocrinology, Gastroenterology, General Pediatrics, Hematology/Oncology/Bone Marrow Transplant, Infectious Disease & Immunology, Medical Genetics, Neonatology, Nephrology, Neurology, Pediatric Surgery, Psychology, Pulmonology, Allergy & Sleep Medicine, Rheumatology and The Medical Home. CWPW physicians are also well recognized in the adult medical specialties of: Gastroenterology, Nephrology and Obstetrics/Gynecology,. CWPW doctors are also leading researchers in all of these disciplines.

PIONEERING, COMPREHENSIVE CARE

CWPW's dedicated and skilled physicians care for low and high risk newborns, as well as mildly to seriously ill children, with a broad range of medical conditions. Our pediatricians and health care professionals make parents feel comfortable when asking about their children's medical problems and treatment options.

CWPW pediatric cardiologists are teaming up with interventional cardiologists to perform 'hybrid' procedures in complex cardiac cases in children. The cardiologists treat cardiac disorders less invasively, but still with outstanding results.

CWPW pediatric oncologists are making new discoveries on how the immune system can be strengthened to counteract neuroblastoma. Their work has helped to develop a procedure where antibodies adhere to the surface of cancer cells, enabling the immune system to target the disease, and eliminate it.

CWPW's Children's Environmental Health Center at Children's is one of only eight such centers in New York State, which treats and studies environmental hazards in the home and in the community.

The goal and philosophy of Children's and Women's Physicians of Westchester is to provide the highest quality medical care in a range of specialties for infants, children and adults every day.

Physician Referral -For a physician referral or more information please contact Children's and Women's Physicians of Westchester at 914-594-4021 or visit www.cwpw.org

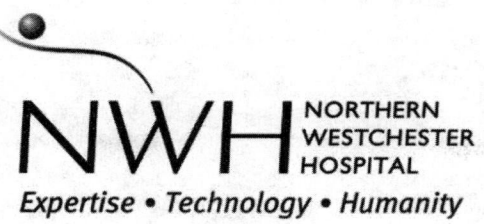

Expertise • Technology • Humanity

<u>Northern Westchester Hospital</u> (NWH) provides quality, patient centered care that is close to home through the right combination of medical expertise, leading edge technology, and a commitment to humanity. Over 750 highly skilled physicians, state-of-the-art technology and professional staff of caregivers are all in place to ensure that you and your family receive treatment in a caring, respectful and nurturing environment.

NWH has established extensive internal quality measurements that surpass the standards defined by the Centers for Medicare & Medicaid Services (CMS) and the Hospital Quality Alliance (HQA) National Hospital Quality Measures. Our high quality standards help to ensure that the treatment you receive at NWH is among the best in the nation. For a complete list of our services, please visit <u>www.nwhc.net</u>.

PHELPS
MEMORIAL HOSPITAL CENTER

701 N. Broadway • Sleepy Hollow, NY 10591 • (914) 366-3000 • www.phelpshospital.org

Sponsorship: Not-for-Profit   Beds: 238
Accreditations: The Joint Commission, College of American Pathologists, the American College of Radiology, and NYS Office of Alcoholism and Substance Abuse Services (OASAS)

A 238-bed acute care community hospital with 475 medical staff members, Phelps Memorial Hospital Center offers a broader range of services than any other community hospital in the region. Its Emergency Department has 32 private rooms. Phelps is the exclusive Westchester location for Memorial Sloan-Kettering Cancer Center. Services include:

Advanced Endoscopy and Gastroenterology: Tertiary-level therapies and groundbreaking techniques to diagnose and treat Barrett's esophagus, intestinal bleeding/ unexplained anemia, abdominal pain, non-cardiac chest pain, swallowing disorders including Zenker's diverticulum, polyps, small pancreatic cancers and other cancerous and precancerous lesions in the digestive tract.

Diabetes and Metabolism Center: Offers adult patients convenient access in one location to a complete range of diabetes and specialty care.

Geriatrics: The Senior Health Consultation Service and Memory Loss Program offer older adults comprehensive health and memory assessments.

Hyperbaric Medicine Center: Therapy for non-healing wounds, post-radiation tissue damage, carbon monoxide poisoning; chronic osteomyelitis, and decompression sickness. The comfortable 12-seat chamber is the largest in the northeast. A hyperbaric nurse or technician accompanies patients and with a primary physician present throughout treatment.

Infusion Center: Patients are administered "biologics," the most advanced class of medications to treat inflammatory diseases and chronic illnesses, including rheumatoid arthritis, psoriatic arthritis, ankylosing spondylitis, juvenile arthritis, psoriasis, and Crohn's disease. One of only a few programs of its kind in the region.

Mental Health:
Inpatient – General psychiatric care is available as well as treatment for mentally ill, chemically addicted adults.
Outpatient – Alcohol and chemical dependency programs, counseling services, continuing day treatment, and supportive case management are offered at the Hospital and in the community.

Orthopedics/Joint Replacement: Over 4,000 total joint replacements performed at Phelps, including the northeast's first anterior approach hip replacement, a minimally invasive operation with less pain and quicker recovery.

Pain Center: Medical specialists from many disciplines use a comprehensive approach to provide diagnostic and therapeutic treatment for acute and chronic pain disorders.

Physical Medicine & Rehabilitation:
Inpatient – Surgical care and acute rehabilitation from a single, integrated team.
Outpatient – physical and occupational therapy with specialists in hand injuries, incontinence, lymphedema, vestibular (dizziness), and aquatherapy in a spacious new facility that includes a therapeutic pool.

Stroke Center: A NYS DOH-designated center. Received the silver performance achievement award from the American Heart Association for outstanding stroke care.

Thoracic Center: Advanced and minimally invasive chest surgery to treat malignant and benign diseases affecting the lungs and other organs inside the chest cavity, except the heart. Quick diagnosis and treatment and full-time care by the Center's director, a renowned cardiothoracic surgeon.

Voice & Swallowing Disorders Institute and the Donald R. Reed Speech & Hearing Center: Comprehensive diagnosis and advanced treatment.

Wound Healing Institute: State-of-the-art outpatient wound care for patients with difficult wounds from diabetes, vascular problems, chronic infections or traumas.

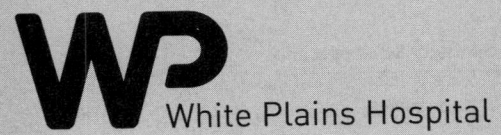

White Plains Hospital

41 East Post Road
White Plains, NY 10601
Tel: (914) 681-0600
www.wphospital.org

Sponsorship: Private, Not-for-Profit
Beds: 292
Accreditation: Joint Commission on Accreditation of Healthcare Organizations, Commission on Cancer of the American College of Surgeons, National Accreditation Program for Breast Centers, College of American Pathologists, American Registry of Radiological Technology, American Society of Radiological Technology, Intersocietal Commission for the Accreditation of Echocardiography Laboratories, American Institute of Ultrasound Medicine, American Academy of Sleep Medicine.

A LEADING COMMUNITY HOSPITAL White Plains Hospital (WPH) is a 292-bed facility that has served Westchester County and the surrounding area since 1893. The Hospital offers much of the technology of large urban specialty teaching hospitals, and combines it with compassionate and personalized care close to home. In addition to a wide range of general acute care services, WPH offers highly sophisticated specialty programs in Oncology, Orthopedics & Joint Replacement, Obstetrics, Neonatal Intensive Care, Radiology, Minimally Invasive & Robotic Surgery, Cardiology, and Stroke Care. An enhanced Emergency Department opened in 2010 and a state-of-the-art Cardiac Catheterization Lab opened in 2008.

The Hospital is a ten-time winner of the Consumer Choice Award for Westchester County, and a 2011 & 2012 winner of the Top 100 Hospitals for Patient Experience. The Hospital received Magnet® recognition from the American Nurses Credentialing Center (ANCC) in 2012. WPH is a member of the NewYork-Presbyterian Healthcare System and the Stellaris Health Network.

AREAS OF DISTINCTION
• **THE RUTH AND JEROME A. SIEGEL STROKE CENTER** The Hospital was the first in Westchester County to receive Stroke Center designation from the New York State Department of Health and the first in the County to receive Gold (Sustained) Award Recognition from the American Stroke Association's Get with the Guidelinessm – Stroke program.

• **WILLIAM & SYLVIA SILBERSTEIN NEONATAL & MATERNITY CENTER** A Labor & Delivery unit, backed up by a Level III Neonatal Intensive Care Unit – the highest designation available to a community hospital – is part of the reason why WPH leads Westchester County in number of deliveries, year after year.

• **DICKSTEIN CANCER TREATMENT CENTER** Part of the Hospital's comprehensive Cancer Program, the Dickstein Center anchors a wide range of services including two linear accelerators for radiation therapy, a state of the art infusion center for chemotherapy and other intravenous treatments, and complementary care programs. Clinical navigation services provide a personal guide for patients at each stage of diagnosis, treatment and follow up care. The Cancer Program has repeatedly received an Outstanding Achievement Award from the American College of Surgeons Commission on Cancer and was recognized by the National Accreditation Program for Breast Centers (NAPBC) in 2012.

• **MINIMALLY INVASIVE & ROBOTIC SURGERY** White Plains Hospital's surgeons perform more minimally invasive surgeries than any other hospital in Westchester. The Hospital was also the first community hospital in the Westchester-Fairfield region to use the da Vinci® Robotic Surgical System for prostate cancer surgery.

• **ORTHOPAEDICS** More hip and knee replacement surgeries – many of them using minimally invasive techniques – have been performed at WPH than at any other hospital in Westchester.

• **CARDIOLOGY** The Hospital's cardiology program includes a new and expansive non-invasive testing center, cardiac catheterization laboratory, and an eight-bed inpatient coronary care unit.

PHYSICIAN REFERRAL:
For a physician referral or more information about our services,
please call (914) 681-1010 or visit www.wphospital.org

Westchester

Addiction Psychiatry

Bisaga, Adam MD (AdP) - **Spec Exp:** Opiate Addiction; Alcohol Abuse; Drug Abuse; **Hospital:** NY-Presby/Columbia Univ Med Ctr, NY (page 104), NY State Psychiatric Inst; **Address:** 547 Saw Mill River Rd, Fl 3, Ste PH, Ardsley, NY 10502; **Phone:** 914-419-8921; **Board Cert:** Psychiatry 2008; Addiction Psychiatry 2011; **Med School:** Poland 1989; **Resid:** Psychiatry, N Shore Univ Hosp 1997; **Fellow:** Addiction Psychiatry, NYSPI-Columbia Univ 1999; **Fac Appt:** Prof Psyc, Columbia P&S

Adolescent Medicine

Browner-Elhanan, Karen MD (AM) - **Hospital:** White Plains Hosp (page 615), Montefiore Med Ctr-Einstein Campus, NY (page 100); **Address:** 222 N Westchester Ave, Ste 201, Bridgespan Medicine, White Plains, NY 10604; **Phone:** 914-698-5544; **Board Cert:** Pediatrics 2011; Adolescent Medicine 2005; **Med School:** Israel 1988; **Resid:** Pediatrics, Maimonides Med Ctr 1996; **Fellow:** Adolescent Medicine, Montefiore Med Ctr 2003; **Fac Appt:** Asst Clin Prof Ped, Cornell Univ-Weill Med Coll

Allergy & Immunology

Geraci-Ciardullo, Kira MD (A&I) - **Spec Exp:** Asthma; Sinus Disorders; Food Allergy; Insect Allergies; **Hospital:** White Plains Hosp (page 615); **Address:** 1600 Harrison Ave, Ste 304, Rockledge Plaza, Mamaroneck, NY 10543-3145; **Phone:** 914-777-1179; **Board Cert:** Pediatrics 1984; Allergy & Immunology 2008; **Med School:** Columbia P&S 1980; **Resid:** Pediatrics, NY-Cornell Hosp 1983; **Fellow:** Allergy & Immunology, NY-Cornell Hosp 1985

Goldman, Neil C MD (A&I) - **Spec Exp:** Asthma; Drug Sensitivity; Sinusitis; **Hospital:** Hudson Valley Hosp Ctr, Phelps Meml Hosp Ctr (page 614); **Address:** 35 S Riverside Ave, Ste 106, Croton On Hudson, NY 10520-2653; **Phone:** 914-271-0001; **Board Cert:** Allergy & Immunology 1977; **Med School:** NY Med Coll 1966; **Resid:** Internal Medicine, Beth Israel Hosp 1968; Internal Medicine, Metropolitan Hosp Ctr 1969; **Fellow:** Allergy & Immunology, Jewish Hosp 1970

Maloney, Patrick F MD (A&I) - **Spec Exp:** Food Allergy; **Hospital:** White Plains Hosp (page 615); **Address:** 1699 Harrison Ave, Ste 304, Rockledge Plaza, Mamaroneck, NY 10543-3145; **Phone:** 917-777-1179; **Board Cert:** Internal Medicine 2002; Allergy & Immunology 2005; **Med School:** SUNY Stony Brook 1999; **Resid:** Internal Medicine, Stony Brook Univ Hosp 2002; **Fellow:** Allergy & Immunology, Stony Brook Univ Hosp 2004

Mechanic, Laura MD (A&I) - **Spec Exp:** Allergic Rhinitis; Eczema; Eye Allergy; Hives; **Hospital:** White Plains Hosp (page 615); **Address:** Westchester Med Grp, 210 Westchester Ave, White Plains, NY 10604; **Phone:** 914-831-6850; **Board Cert:** Internal Medicine 2002; Allergy & Immunology 2005; **Med School:** NYU Sch Med 1989; **Resid:** Internal Medicine, Mt Sinai Med Ctr 1992; **Fellow:** Allergy & Immunology, Mt Sinai Med Ctr 1995; Allergy & Immunology, White Plains Hosp 2006

Osleeb, Craig MD (A&I) - **Hospital:** Northern Westchester Hosp (page 613); **Address:** Mount Kisco Medical Grp, 34 S Bedford Rd, Mt Kisco, NY 10549; **Phone:** 914-242-1580; **Board Cert:** Allergy & Immunology 2003; Pediatrics 2006; **Med School:** Univ Wisc 1988; **Resid:** Pediatrics, UConn Med Ctr 1991; **Fellow:** Allergy & Immunology, Chldns Natl Med Ctr 1993

Pollowitz, James Allen MD (A&I) - **Spec Exp:** Asthma; Food Allergy; Hives; Drug Sensitivity; **Hospital:** White Plains Hosp (page 615), Lawrence Hosp Ctr; **Address:** 281 Garth Rd, Ste A, Scarsdale, NY 10583-4034; **Phone:** 914-472-3833; **Board Cert:** Pediatrics 1978; Allergy & Immunology 1979; **Med School:** NYU Sch Med 1973; **Resid:** Pediatrics, Bronx Muni Hosp Ctr 1976; **Fellow:** Allergy & Immunology, St Vincent Med Ctr 1978; **Fac Appt:** Asst Clin Prof Ped, NY Med Coll

Tuerk-Mendelsohn, Lois MD (A&I) - **Spec Exp:** Asthma; Hay Fever; Food Allergy; Eczema; **Hospital:** Northern Westchester Hosp (page 613); **Address:** 103 S Bedford Rd, Ste 208, Mt Kisco, NY 10549; **Phone:** 914-666-7171; **Board Cert:** Internal Medicine 1989; **Med School:** NY Med Coll 1986; **Resid:** Internal Medicine, Lenox Hill Hosp 1989; **Fellow:** Allergy & Immunology, Mt Sinai Hosp 1991

Cardiac Electrophysiology

Cohen, Martin B MD (CE) - **Spec Exp:** Arrhythmias; Pacemakers; Defibrillators; Coronary Angioplasty/Stents; **Hospital:** Westchester Med Ctr, White Plains Hosp (page 615); **Address:** Westchester Heart & Vascular, 19 Bradhurst Ave Fl 3 - Ste 3850 South, Hawthorne, NY 10532-2140; **Phone:** 914-909-6900; **Board Cert:** Internal Medicine 1983; Cardiovascular Disease 1985; Cardiac Electrophysiology 2006; Interventional Cardiology 2004; **Med School:** SUNY Downstate 1980; **Resid:** Internal Medicine, Univ Hosp 1983; **Fellow:** Cardiovascular Disease, Univ Hosp 1985; Interventional Cardiology, Westchester Co Med Ctr 1986; **Fac Appt:** Assoc Clin Prof Med, NY Med Coll

Rubin, David A MD (CE) - **Spec Exp:** Arrhythmias; Radiofrequency Ablation; Pacemakers/Defibrillators; **Hospital:** NY-Presby/Columbia Univ Med Ctr, NY (page 104), White Plains Hosp (page 615); **Address:** 222 Westchester Ave, White Plains, NY 10604-2906; **Phone:** 914-428-3888; **Board Cert:** Internal Medicine 1978; Cardiovascular Disease 1981; Cardiac Electrophysiology 2002; **Med School:** Columbia P&S 1975; **Resid:** Internal Medicine, Columbia-Presby Hosp 1978; **Fellow:** Cardiovascular Disease, Mount Sinai Hosp 1980; **Fac Appt:** Clin Prof Med, Columbia P&S

Sorbera, Carmine A MD (CE) - **Spec Exp:** Arrhythmias; Cardiac Catheterization; **Hospital:** Westchester Med Ctr; **Address:** 19 Bradhurst Ave, Ste 700, Hawthorne, NY 10532; **Phone:** 914-593-7823; **Board Cert:** Internal Medicine 1987; Cardiovascular Disease 1989; Cardiac Electrophysiology 2004; **Med School:** NY Med Coll 1983; **Resid:** Internal Medicine, Westchester Med Ctr 1987; **Fellow:** Cardiovascular Disease, Westchester Med Ctr 1989; Interventional Cardiology, Westchester Med Ctr 1990

Cardiovascular Disease

Bleiberg, Melvyn S MD (Cv) - **Hospital:** Saint Joseph's Med Ctr - Yonkers; **Address:** 127 S Broadway Fl 4th - Ste 409, Yonkers, NY 10701; **Phone:** 914-378-7583; **Board Cert:** Internal Medicine 1978; Cardiovascular Disease 1981; **Med School:** Albert Einstein Coll Med 1974; **Resid:** Internal Medicine, Brookdale Hosp 1977; **Fellow:** Cardiovascular Disease, Brookdale Hosp 1979

Cappucci, Roger Vincent MD (Cv) - **Spec Exp:** Echocardiography; Cardiac Stress Testing; **Hospital:** White Plains Hosp (page 615); **Address:** Scarsdale Med Grp, 600 Mamaroneck Ave, Ste 200, Harrison, NY 10528; **Phone:** 914-723-8100; **Board Cert:** Internal Medicine 2003; Cardiovascular Disease 2005; **Med School:** Cornell Univ-Weill Med Coll 1989; **Resid:** Internal Medicine, NY-Presby/Weill Cornell Med Ctr 1992; **Fellow:** Cardiovascular Disease, Montefiore Med Ctr 1995

Catanese, James W MD (Cv) - **Spec Exp:** Coronary Artery Disease; Congestive Heart Failure; Heart Valve Disease; **Hospital:** Northern Westchester Hosp (page 613), Westchester Med Ctr; **Address:** Westchester Health- Cardiology, 105 S Bedford Rd, Ste 320, Mt Kisco, NY 10549; **Phone:** 914-242-9400; **Board Cert:** Cardiovascular Disease 2005; **Med School:** Albany Med Coll 1988; **Resid:** Internal Medicine, Montefiore Med Ctr 1991; **Fellow:** Cardiovascular Disease, Montefiore Med Ctr 1992

Charney, Richard MD (Cv) - **Spec Exp:** Interventional Cardiology; Heart Valve Disease; Coronary Artery Disease; Peripheral Vascular Disease; **Hospital:** Sound Shore Med Ctr - Westchester, NY-Presby/Weill Cornell Med Ctr, NY (page 104); **Address:** Sound Shore Cardiology Assocs, 175 Memorial Hwy, Ste 1-1, New Rochelle, NY 10801; **Phone:** 914-235-3535; **Board Cert:** Internal Medicine 1989; Cardiovascular Disease 2011; Interventional Cardiology 2010; **Med School:** Mount Sinai Sch Med 1986; **Resid:** Internal Medicine, Mt Sinai Hosp 1989; **Fellow:** Cardiovascular Disease, Montefiore Med Ctr 1992; Interventional Cardiology, Montefiore Med Ctr 1993; **Fac Appt:** Asst Prof Med, Cornell Univ-Weill Med Coll

Cooper, Jerome MD (Cv) - **Spec Exp:** Coronary Artery Disease; Hypertension; Heart Valve Disease; **Hospital:** Sound Shore Med Ctr - Westchester, NY-Presby/Columbia Univ Med Ctr, NY (page 104); **Address:** Westchester Heart Assocs, 150 Lockwood Ave, Ste 28, New Rochelle, NY 10801; **Phone:** 914-633-7870; **Board Cert:** Internal Medicine 1968; Cardiovascular Disease 1973; **Med School:** SUNY Hlth Sci Ctr 1961; **Resid:** Internal Medicine, Baltimore City Hosps 1963; Cardiovascular Disease, Montefiore Hosp Med Ctr 1964; **Fellow:** Cardiovascular Disease, Johns Hopkins Univ Hosp 1966; Cardiovascular Disease, Johns Hopkins Univ Hosp 1967; **Fac Appt:** Assoc Clin Prof Med, Columbia P&S

Cziner, David MD (Cv) - **Hospital:** White Plains Hosp (page 615), Greenwich Hosp (page 892); **Address:** 210 Westchester Ave, White Plains, NY 10604; **Phone:** 914-305-2700; **Board Cert:** Internal Medicine 1989; Cardiovascular Disease 2011; Neurotology 2003; **Med School:** NYU Sch Med 1986; **Resid:** Internal Medicine, Bellevue/NYU Med Ctr 1989; **Fellow:** Cardiovascular Disease, Bellevue/NYU Med Ctr 1992

Fass, Arthur MD (Cv) - **Spec Exp:** Preventive Cardiology; Coronary Artery Disease; Hypertension; Cholesterol/Lipid Disorders; **Hospital:** Phelps Meml Hosp Ctr (page 614), Westchester Med Ctr; **Address:** 465 N State Rd, Briarcliff Manor, NY 10510; **Phone:** 914-762-5810; **Board Cert:** Internal Medicine 1979; Cardiovascular Disease 1981; **Med School:** NY Med Coll 1976; **Resid:** Internal Medicine, Metropolitan Hosp 1979; **Fellow:** Cardiovascular Disease, Westchester Med Ctr 1981; **Fac Appt:** Assoc Clin Prof Med, NY Med Coll

Feld, Michael MD (Cv) - **Spec Exp:** Pacemakers; Coronary Artery Disease; Congestive Heart Failure; **Hospital:** Phelps Meml Hosp Ctr (page 614), Comm Hosp - Dobbs Ferry; **Address:** 200 S Broadway, Tarrytown, NY 10591-4500; **Phone:** 914-631-2895; **Board Cert:** Internal Medicine 1980; Cardiovascular Disease 1983; **Med School:** Penn State Coll Med 1977; **Resid:** Internal Medicine, Montefiore Med Ctr 1981; **Fellow:** Cardiovascular Disease, Montefiore Med Ctr 1983; **Fac Appt:** Asst Clin Prof Med, Albert Einstein Coll Med

Fishbach, Mitchell MD (Cv) - **Spec Exp:** Non-Invasive Cardiology; Sports Medicine; **Hospital:** Lawrence Hosp Ctr, NY-Presby/Columbia Univ Med Ctr, NY (page 104); **Address:** 73 Market St, Yonkers, NY 10710; **Phone:** 914-631-6880; **Board Cert:** Internal Medicine 1980; Cardiovascular Disease 1983; **Med School:** Albert Einstein Coll Med 1977; **Resid:** Internal Medicine, Montefiore Hosp Med Ctr 1980; **Fellow:** Cardiovascular Disease, Montefiore Hosp Med Ctr 1982

Frishman, William MD (Cv) - **Spec Exp:** Coronary Artery Disease; Preventive Cardiology; Hypertension; Heart Failure; **Hospital:** Westchester Med Ctr; **Address:** NY Med Coll, Dept Med, Munger Pavilion, rm 263, Valhalla, NY 10595; **Phone:** 914-594-4383; **Board Cert:** Internal Medicine 1997; Cardiovascular Disease 1997; Geriatric Medicine 2002; **Med School:** Boston Univ 1969; **Resid:** Internal Medicine, Montefiore Med Ctr 1971; Internal Medicine, Bronx Muni Hosp 1972; **Fellow:** Cardiovascular Disease, NY Hosp 1974; **Fac Appt:** Prof Med, NY Med Coll

Gabelman, Gary S MD (Cv) - **Spec Exp:** Non-Invasive Cardiology; Echocardiography; Nuclear Cardiology; Preventive Cardiology; **Hospital:** Lawrence Hosp Ctr, NY-Presby/Columbia Univ Med Ctr, NY (page 104); **Address:** 73 Market St, Yonkers, NY 10710; **Phone:** 914-831-6880; **Board Cert:** Internal Medicine 1988; Cardiovascular Disease 2001; **Med School:** Mount Sinai Sch Med 1985; **Resid:** Internal Medicine, Montefiore Med Ctr 1989; **Fellow:** Cardiovascular Disease, Montefiore Med Ctr 1991; **Fac Appt:** Assoc Clin Prof Med, Columbia P&S

Gass, Alan MD (Cv) - **Spec Exp:** Heart Failure; Transplant Medicine-Heart; **Hospital:** Westchester Med Ctr; **Address:** E westchester medical center 95 grasslands Rd, Hawthorne, NY 10595-2140; **Phone:** 914-909-6900; **Board Cert:** Cardiovascular Disease 2002; **Med School:** Italy 1984; **Resid:** Internal Medicine, LIJ Med Ctr 1987; **Fellow:** Cardiovascular Disease, Beth Israel Med Ctr 1988; Transplant Medicine, Stanford Univ Med Ctr 1989; **Fac Appt:** Assoc Prof Med, NY Med Coll

Gitler, Bernard MD (Cv) - **Spec Exp:** Hypertension; Cholesterol/Lipid Disorders; Coronary Artery Disease; Heart Valve Disease; **Hospital:** Sound Shore Med Ctr - Westchester, NY-Presby/Columbia Univ Med Ctr, NY (page 104); **Address:** Westchester Heart Specialists, 150 Lockwood Ave, Ste 28, New Rochelle, NY 10801-4913; **Phone:** 914-633-7870; **Board Cert:** Internal Medicine 2009; Cardiovascular Disease 2009; Critical Care Medicine 2010; Echocardiography 2009; **Med School:** Cornell Univ-Weill Med Coll 1976; **Resid:** Internal Medicine, Jacobi Med Ctr 1979; **Fellow:** Cardiovascular Disease, Montefiore Med Ctr 1981; **Fac Appt:** Assoc Clin Prof Med, Albert Einstein Coll Med

Greif, Richard H MD (Cv) - **Hospital:** Saint Joseph's Med Ctr - Yonkers; **Address:** 127 S Broadway Fl 4th - Ste 409, Yonkers, NY 10701; **Phone:** 914-378-7583; **Board Cert:** Internal Medicine 1978; Cardiovascular Disease 1981; **Med School:** NY Med Coll 1975; **Resid:** Internal Medicine, Metropolitan Hosp 1978; **Fellow:** Cardiovascular Disease, St Vincents Hosp 1981; **Fac Appt:** Assoc Clin Prof Med, NY Med Coll

Kaplan, Kenneth C MD (Cv) - **Hospital:** Phelps Meml Hosp Ctr (page 614); **Address:** 160 N State Rd, Briarcliff Manor, NY 10510; **Phone:** 914-762-3821; **Board Cert:** Internal Medicine 1970; Cardiovascular Disease 1975; Echocardiography 1996; **Med School:** NYU Sch Med 1962; **Resid:** Internal Medicine, Bellevue Hosp 1966; **Fellow:** Cardiovascular Disease, Bellevue Hosp/NYU 1969; **Fac Appt:** Asst Clin Prof Med, NY Med Coll

Kay, Richard H MD (Cv) - **Spec Exp:** Preventive Cardiology; Congestive Heart Failure; Non-Invasive Cardiology; **Hospital:** White Plains Hosp (page 615), NY-Presby/Columbia Univ Med Ctr, NY (page 104); **Address:** Columbia Doctors Medical Group, 19 Bradhurst Ave, Ste 700, Hawthorne, NY 10532-2140; **Phone:** 914-593-7800; **Board Cert:** Internal Medicine 1979; Cardiovascular Disease 1981; **Med School:** Johns Hopkins Univ 1976; **Resid:** Internal Medicine, Columbia-Presby Med Ctr 1979; **Fellow:** Cardiovascular Disease, Mount Sinai Hosp 1981; **Fac Appt:** Assoc Prof Med, NY Med Coll

Keltz, Theodore MD (Cv) - **Spec Exp:** Echocardiography; Nuclear Cardiology; Coronary Artery Disease; Preventive Cardiology; **Hospital:** Sound Shore Med Ctr - Westchester, NY-Presby/Columbia Univ Med Ctr, NY (page 104); **Address:** Westchester Heart Assocs, 150 Lockwood Ave, Ste 28, New Rochelle, NY 10801-4913; **Phone:** 914-633-7870; **Board Cert:** Internal Medicine 1983; Cardiovascular Disease 1985; Echocardiography 2006; Nuclear Cardiology 1996; **Med School:** Albany Med Coll 1980; **Resid:** Internal Medicine, Mt Sinai Med Ctr 1983; **Fellow:** Cardiovascular Disease, Montefiore Med Ctr 1985; **Fac Appt:** Assoc Clin Prof Med, Albert Einstein Coll Med

Kupersmith, Andrew C MD (Cv) - **Hospital:** Westchester Med Ctr, White Plains Hosp (page 615); **Address:** Columbia Doctors Medical Group, 19 Bradhurst Ave, Ste 700, Hawthorne, NY 10532; **Phone:** 914-593-7800; **Board Cert:** Cardiovascular Disease 2002; **Med School:** Univ MD Sch Med 1995; **Resid:** Internal Medicine, LIJ Med Ctr 1998; **Fellow:** Cardiovascular Disease, Wesctchester Med Ctr 2000; **Fac Appt:** Asst Prof Med, NY Med Coll

Leonard, Daniel MD (Cv) - **Hospital:** Northern Westchester Hosp (page 613), Westchester Med Ctr; **Address:** Mt Kisco Med Grp, 110 S Bedford Rd Bldg 110, Mt Kisco, NY 10549-3433; **Phone:** 914-241-1050; **Board Cert:** Internal Medicine 1984; Cardiovascular Disease 1987; **Med School:** Univ Cincinnati 1981; **Resid:** Internal Medicine, NY-Presby/Weil Cornell Med Ctr 1984; **Fellow:** Cardiovascular Disease, Albert Einstein Coll Med 1986; **Fac Appt:** Assoc Clin Prof Med, NY Med Coll

Levine, Evan MD (Cv) - **Spec Exp:** Cardiac Stress Testing; **Hospital:** Montefiore Med Ctr-Moses Campus, NY (page 100), St. John's Riverside Hosp-Andrus Pavil; **Address:** Riverside Cardiology, 955 Yonkers Ave, Ste 200, Yonkers, NY 10704; **Phone:** 914-237-1332; **Board Cert:** Internal Medicine 1988; Cardiovascular Disease 2011; **Med School:** Mount Sinai Sch Med 1985; **Resid:** Internal Medicine, Montefiore Med Ctr 1988; **Fellow:** Cardiovascular Disease, Montefiore Med Ctr 1990; **Fac Appt:** Asst Clin Prof Med, Albert Einstein Coll Med

Lieb, Mark MD (Cv) - **Hospital:** Northern Westchester Hosp (page 613); **Address:** 110 S Bedford Rd, Fl 2, Mt Kisco, NY 10549-3412; **Phone:** 914-241-1050; **Board Cert:** Cardiovascular Disease 2006; **Med School:** Boston Univ 1988; **Resid:** Internal Medicine, Mt Sinai Med Ctr 1991; **Fellow:** Cardiovascular Disease, Mt Sinai Med Ctr 1995

Matos, Marshall MD (Cv) - **Spec Exp:** Coronary Artery Disease; Preventive Cardiology; Arrhythmias; Cholesterol/Lipid Disorders; **Hospital:** Sound Shore Med Ctr - Westchester, Lenox Hill Hosp (page 106); **Address:** 140 Lockwood Ave, Ste 310, New Rochelle, NY 10801-4909; **Phone:** 914-576-7171; **Board Cert:** Internal Medicine 1980; Cardiovascular Disease 1985; **Med School:** Albert Einstein Coll Med 1977; **Resid:** Internal Medicine, Bronx Muni Hosp 1981; **Fellow:** Cardiovascular Disease, Albert Einstein Coll Med 1983; **Fac Appt:** Asst Prof Med, NYU Sch Med

McClung, John Arthur MD (Cv) - **Spec Exp:** Echocardiography; **Hospital:** Westchester Med Ctr; **Address:** 19 Bradhurst Ave, Ste 3850 South, Hawthorne, NY 10532; **Phone:** 914-909-6900; **Board Cert:** Internal Medicine 1980; Cardiovascular Disease 1983; **Med School:** NY Med Coll 1975; **Resid:** Internal Medicine, Lincoln Med Ctr 1979; **Fellow:** Cardiovascular Disease, Westchester Med Ctr 1982; **Fac Appt:** Prof Med, NY Med Coll

Medina, Emma MD (Cv) - **Spec Exp:** Non-Invasive Cardiology; **Hospital:** Sound Shore Med Ctr - Westchester, Montefiore Med Ctr-Einstein Campus, NY (page 100); **Address:** 140 Lockwood Ave, Ste 310, New Rochelle, NY 10801-4909; **Phone:** 914-632-1600; **Board Cert:** Internal Medicine 1982; Cardiovascular Disease 1985; **Med School:** NYU Sch Med 1979; **Resid:** Internal Medicine, Jacobi Med Ctr 1982; **Fellow:** Cardiovascular Disease, Jacobi Med Ctr 1984; **Fac Appt:** Asst Clin Prof Med, Albert Einstein Coll Med

Mercando, Anthony MD (Cv) - **Spec Exp:** Cholesterol/Lipid Disorders; Pacemakers/Defibrillators; Preventive Cardiology; **Hospital:** Lawrence Hosp Ctr, NY-Presby/Columbia Univ Med Ctr, NY (page 104); **Address:** Westmed Ridge Hill, 73 Market St, Ste 215, Yonkers, NY 10710; **Phone:** 914-831-6880; **Board Cert:** Internal Medicine 1983; Cardiovascular Disease 1987; **Med School:** Harvard Med Sch 1980; **Resid:** Internal Medicine, Montefiore Med Ctr 1984; **Fellow:** Cardiovascular Disease, Montefiore Med Ctr 1986; **Fac Appt:** Clin Prof Med, Albert Einstein Coll Med

Perry-Bottinger, Lynne V MD (Cv) - **Spec Exp:** Cardiac Catheterization; Coronary Angioplasty/Stents; Heart Disease in Women; Heart Disease in African Americans; **Hospital:** NY-Presby/Columbia Univ Med Ctr, NY (page 104), Sound Shore Med Ctr - Westchester; **Address:** Clinical & Interventional Cardiology, 140A Lockwood Ave, New Rochelle, NY 10801; **Phone:** 914-576-7577; **Med School:** Yale Univ 1986; **Resid:** Internal Medicine, Yale-New Haven Hosp 1990; **Fellow:** Cardiovascular Disease, Johns Hopkins Hosp 1993; Interventional Cardiology, Johns Hopkins Hosp 1994; **Fac Appt:** Asst Clin Prof Med, Columbia P&S

Price Jr, Thomas J MD (Cv) - **Hospital:** Mount Vernon Hosp, Sound Shore Med Ctr - Westchester; **Address:** 105 Stevens Ave, Ste 603, Mt Vernon, NY 10550; **Phone:** 914-664-4052; **Board Cert:** Internal Medicine 1984; Cardiovascular Disease 1987; **Med School:** Univ Cincinnati 1975; **Resid:** Internal Medicine, Harlem Hosp 1979; **Fellow:** Cardiovascular Disease, Harlem Hosp 1983; **Fac Appt:** Asst Clin Prof Med, Columbia P&S

Pucillo, Anthony MD (Cv) - **Spec Exp:** Coronary Angioplasty/Stents; Peripheral Vascular Disease; Cardiac Catheterization; Interventional Cardiology; **Hospital:** Westchester Med Ctr; **Address:** 19 Bradhurst Ave, Ste 700, Hawthorne, NY 10532; **Phone:** 914-593-7800; **Board Cert:** Internal Medicine 1981; Cardiovascular Disease 1983; **Med School:** Mount Sinai Sch Med 1978; **Resid:** Internal Medicine, Columbia-Presby Med Ctr 1981; **Fellow:** Cardiovascular Disease, Columbia-Presby Med Ctr 1984; **Fac Appt:** Assoc Prof Med, NY Med Coll

Sheikh, Shahid MD (Cv) - **Hospital:** St. John's Riverside Hosp-Andrus Pavil, Montefiore Med Ctr-Wakefield Campus, NY (page 100); **Address:** 970 N Broadway, Ste 210, Yonkers, NY 10701-1311; **Phone:** 914-963-0111; **Board Cert:** Internal Medicine 1977; Cardiovascular Disease 1979; **Med School:** Pakistan 1971; **Resid:** Internal Medicine, Our Lady of Mercy Med Ctr 1976

Silver, Michael M MD (Cv) - **Spec Exp:** Hypertension; Cholesterol/Lipid Disorders; Coronary Artery Disease; **Hospital:** White Plains Hosp (page 615), Greenwich Hosp (page 892); **Address:** Westchester Medical Group, 210 Westchester Ave, White Plains, NY 10604; **Phone:** 914-305-2700 x2; **Board Cert:** Internal Medicine 1980; Cardiovascular Disease 1983; **Med School:** SUNY Downstate 1977; **Resid:** Internal Medicine, Thomas Jefferson Univ Hosp 1980; **Fellow:** Cardiovascular Disease, Presby-Hosp Univ Penn 1982

Tartaglia, Joseph J MD (Cv) - **Spec Exp:** Angina; Congestive Heart Failure; Arrhythmias; **Hospital:** White Plains Hosp (page 615), Greenwich Hosp (page 892); **Address:** 311 North St, Ste 402, White Plains, NY 10605-2232; **Phone:** 914-946-3388; **Board Cert:** Internal Medicine 1988; Cardiovascular Disease 2011; Geriatric Medicine 2004; **Med School:** Italy 1984; **Resid:** Internal Medicine, Our Lady of Mercy Med Ctr 1988; **Fellow:** Cardiovascular Disease, N Shore Univ Hosp 1990; **Fac Appt:** Asst Clin Prof Med, NY Med Coll

Weissman, Ronald MD (Cv) - **Spec Exp:** Coronary Artery Disease; Congestive Heart Failure; Arrhythmias; Hypertrophic Cardiomyopathy; **Hospital:** White Plains Hosp (page 615), Westchester Med Ctr; **Address:** 15 N Broadway Fl 2, White Plains, NY 10601; **Phone:** 914-428-6000; **Board Cert:** Internal Medicine 1980; Cardiovascular Disease 1983; **Med School:** NY Med Coll 1977; **Resid:** Internal Medicine, LI Jewish Hosp 1980; **Fellow:** Cardiovascular Disease, LI Jewish Hosp 1982; **Fac Appt:** Assoc Clin Prof Med, NY Med Coll

Zimmerman, Franklin MD (Cv) - **Spec Exp:** Preventive Cardiology; Sports Medicine-Cardiology; Cholesterol/Lipid Disorders; Hypertension; **Hospital:** Phelps Meml Hosp Ctr (page 614), Westchester Med Ctr; **Address:** 465 N State Rd, Briarcliff Manor, NY 10510-1468; **Phone:** 914-762-5810; **Board Cert:** Internal Medicine 1983; Cardiovascular Disease 1987; Critical Care Medicine 2006; **Med School:** Brown Univ 1980; **Resid:** Internal Medicine, St Lukes-Roosevelt Hosp Ctr 1983; **Fellow:** Cardiovascular Disease, St Lukes-Roosevelt Hosp Ctr 1988; **Fac Appt:** Asst Prof Med, Columbia P&S

Child & Adolescent Psychiatry

Cohen, Lee Steven MD (ChAP) - **Spec Exp:** Anxiety & Mood Disorders; Psychopharmacology; ADD/ADHD; Autism; **Hospital:** NY-Presby/Columbia Univ Med Ctr, NY (page 104), St. Luke's - Roosevelt Hosp Ctr - Roosevelt Div (page 94); **Address:** 623 Warburton Ave, Hastings On Hudson, NY 10706-1523; **Phone:** 914-478-1330; **Board Cert:** Psychiatry 1987; Child & Adolescent Psychiatry 1988; **Med School:** SUNY Stony Brook 1982; **Resid:** Psychiatry, Mt Sinai Med Ctr 1985; **Fellow:** Child & Adolescent Psychiatry, Columbia-Presby Med Ctr 1987; **Fac Appt:** Asst Clin Prof Psyc, Columbia P&S

Hyler, Irene MD (ChAP) - **Spec Exp:** Psychotherapy; Psychoanalysis; **Hospital:** NY-Presby/Weill Cornell Med Ctr, NY (page 104); **Address:** 2A Berkeley Rd, Scarsdale, NY 10583-1102; **Phone:** 914-472-8447; **Board Cert:** Psychiatry 1984; Child & Adolescent Psychiatry 1986; **Med School:** Albert Einstein Coll Med 1979; **Resid:** Psychiatry, Bronx Muni Hosp 1982; **Fellow:** Child & Adolescent Psychiatry, Albert Einstein Coll Med 1984; **Fac Appt:** Asst Clin Prof Psyc, Cornell Univ-Weill Med Coll

Kalikow, Kevin T MD (ChAP) - ; **Address:** 83 S Bedford Rd, Mt Kisco, NY 10549; **Phone:** 914-666-3000; **Board Cert:** Psychiatry 1984; Child & Adolescent Psychiatry 1986; **Med School:** Tulane Univ 1979; **Resid:** Psychiatry, NY Hosp-Westchester Div 1983; **Fellow:** Child & Adolescent Psychiatry, NY State Psych Inst 1985; **Fac Appt:** Asst Clin Prof Psyc, NY Med Coll

Rubinstein, Boris MD (ChAP) - **Spec Exp:** Psychopharmacology; Neuro-Psychiatry; Anxiety & Mood Disorders; Developmental Disorders; **Hospital:** Morgan Stanley Children's Hosp of NY-Presby, NY (page 104); **Address:** 623 Warburton Ave, Hastings On Hudson, NY 10706; **Phone:** 914-478-1330; **Board Cert:** Pediatrics 1976; Psychiatry 1979; Child & Adolescent Psychiatry 1981; **Med School:** Mexico 1970; **Resid:** Pediatrics, Chldns Hosp 1974; Psychiatry, Jacobi Med Ctr 1976; **Fellow:** Child & Adolescent Psychiatry, Jacobi Med Ctr 1978; Public Health & Genl Preventive Med, Harvard Sch Pub Hlth 1974; **Fac Appt:** ChAP, Columbia P&S

Schreiber, Klaus MD (ChAP) - **Spec Exp:** Developmental Disorders; **Address:** 1 Neperan Rd, Tarrytown, NY 10591; **Phone:** 914-332-0270; **Board Cert:** Psychiatry 1976; Child & Adolescent Psychiatry 1986; **Med School:** Germany 1966; **Resid:** Psychiatry, Elmhurst City Hosp Ctr 1971; Psychiatry, Westchester Med Ctr 1972; **Fellow:** Child & Adolescent Psychiatry, Westchester Med Ctr 1973; Child & Adolescent Psychiatry, Albert Einstein Coll Med 1982; **Fac Appt:** Asst Prof Psyc, NY Med Coll

Seaver, Robert MD (ChAP) - **Spec Exp:** Forensic Psychiatry; Art & Creativity; Psychopharmacology; **Address:** 83 S Bedford Ave Fl 2nd, Mt Kisco, NY 10549; **Phone:** 914-241-8979; **Board Cert:** Pediatrics 1978; Psychiatry 1984; Child & Adolescent Psychiatry 1986; **Med School:** Mount Sinai Sch Med 1973; **Resid:** Pediatrics, Mt Sinai Hosp 1975; Pediatrics, St Luke's-Roosevelt Hosp 1976; **Fellow:** Psychiatry, NY Hosp-Westchester Div 1984; Child & Adolescent Psychiatry, Jacobi Med Ctr 1985

Silva, Raul R MD (ChAP) - **Spec Exp:** Autism; ADD/ADHD; Depression; Psychopharmacology; **Address:** 2975 Westchester Ave, Ste 308, Purchase, NY 10577; **Phone:** 201-218-1380; **Board Cert:** Psychiatry 1991; Child & Adolescent Psychiatry 1992; **Med School:** Mexico 1983; **Resid:** Psychiatry, St Vincent's Medical Ctr 1988; **Fellow:** Child & Adolescent Psychiatry, St Luke's Hosp 1990; Research, NYU Med Ctr 1992

Silverman, Amy MD (ChAP) - **Spec Exp:** Anxiety & Depression; Anxiety & Mood Disorders; **Hospital:** NY-Presby/Westchester Div, NY (page 104); **Address:** 600 Mamaroneck Ave, Ste 400, Harrison, NY 10528; **Phone:** 914-301-9465; **Board Cert:** Psychiatry 2003; Child & Adolescent Psychiatry 2004; **Med School:** Mount Sinai Sch Med 1998; **Resid:** Psychiatry, Brigham and Women's Hosp 2001; **Fellow:** Child Psychiatry, NY Presby/Cornell Med Ctr 2003; **Fac Appt:** Asst Clin Prof Psyc, Cornell Univ

Slater, Jonathan Allen MD (ChAP) - **Spec Exp:** Psychopharmacology; Psychiatry in Physical Illness; **Hospital:** Morgan Stanley Children's Hosp of NY-Presby, NY (page 104); **Address:** 1 Bridge St, Ste 24 Bldg, Irvington, NY 10533; **Phone:** 914-591-4040; **Board Cert:** Psychiatry 1991; Child & Adolescent Psychiatry 1993; Psychosomatic Medicine 2006; **Med School:** Columbia P&S 1985; **Resid:** Psychiatry, NY State Psych Inst 1990; **Fellow:** Research, Columbia Univ 1986; Child & Adolescent Psychiatry, Columbia Univ 1992; **Fac Appt:** Clin Prof Psyc, Columbia P&S

Walker, Audrey MD (ChAP) - **Hospital:** Montefiore Med Ctr-Moses Campus, NY (page 100); **Address:** 2005 Palmer Ave, Larchmont, NY 10538; **Phone:** 914-834-2214; **Board Cert:** Psychiatry 1992; Child & Adolescent Psychiatry 1994; Psychosomatic Medicine 2005; **Med School:** Albert Einstein Coll Med 1985; **Resid:** Psychiatry, NY Presby-Columbia Med Ctr 1990

Child Neurology

Jacobson, Ronald I MD (ChiN) - **Spec Exp:** Epilepsy; Headache; ADD/ADHD; Autism; **Hospital:** Westchester Med Ctr, Children's & Women's Phys.of Westchester (page 612); **Address:** Pediatric Neurology Associates, 755 N Broadway, Medical Services Bldg, Ste 540, Sleepy Hollow, NY 10591; **Phone:** 914-358-0190; **Board Cert:** Pediatrics 1981; Child Neurology 1984; **Med School:** Albert Einstein Coll Med 1975; **Resid:** Pediatrics, Yale-New Haven Hosp 1978; **Fellow:** Neurological Immunology, Yale Univ School of Med 1979; Pediatric Neurology, Univ Minn Med Ctr 1982; **Fac Appt:** Assoc Clin Prof N, NY Med Coll

Kang, Harriet MD (ChiN) - **Spec Exp:** Epilepsy/Seizure Disorders; **Hospital:** Beth Israel Med Ctr - Petrie Division (page 94); **Address:** 141 S Central Park Ave, Hartsdale, NY 10530; **Phone:** 914-428-0529; **Board Cert:** Pediatrics 1979; Child Neurology 1981; Clinical Neurophysiology 2006; **Med School:** Johns Hopkins Univ 1974; **Resid:** Pediatrics, Johns Hopkins Hosp 1976; Child Neurology, Univ Minn Med Ctr 1979; **Fellow:** Clinical Neurophysiology, Univ Minn Med Ctr 1980; **Fac Appt:** Assoc Prof N, Albert Einstein Coll Med

Kutscher, Martin MD (ChiN) - **Spec Exp:** ADD/ADHD; Asperger's Syndrome; Autism; **Hospital:** Westchester Med Ctr; **Address:** 800 Westchester Ave, Ste N641, Rye Brook, NY 10573; **Phone:** 914-232-1810; **Board Cert:** Pediatrics 1986; Child Neurology 1989; **Med School:** Columbia P&S 1981; **Resid:** Pediatrics, St Christopher's Hosp 1984; Neurology, Montefiore Med Ctr 1987; **Fellow:** Child Neurology, Montefiore Med Ctr 1989; **Fac Appt:** Asst Clin Prof Ped, NY Med Coll

Roseman, Bruce MD (ChiN) - **Spec Exp:** Asperger's Syndrome; **Hospital:** Westchester Med Ctr; **Address:** 125 S Broadway, White Plains, NY 10605-1405; **Phone:** 914-997-2032; **Board Cert:** Pediatrics 1978; Child Neurology 1982; **Med School:** Georgetown Univ 1973; **Resid:** Pediatrics, Johns Hopkins Hosp 1976; **Fellow:** Child Neurology, NY-Presby/Columbia Univ Med Ctr 1979

Sweeney, Tanya-Marie MD (ChiN) - **Spec Exp:** Neurodevelopmental Disabilities; **Hospital:** Northern Westchester Hosp (page 613); **Address:** 110 S Beford Rd, Mount Kisco, NY 10549-3412; **Phone:** 914-241-1050; **Board Cert:** Pediatrics 2005; Child Neurology 2008; **Med School:** SUNY Stony Brook 2002; **Resid:** Pediatrics, Winthrop Univ Hosp 2005; **Fellow:** Child Neurology, N Shore-LIJ Hlth System 2008

Clinical Genetics

Kronn, David F MD (CG) - **Spec Exp:** Bone Disorders-Metabolic; Bone Disorders-Inherited; **Hospital:** Westchester Med Ctr, Children's & Women's Phys.of Westchester (page 612); **Address:** Regional Medical Genetics, 503 Grasslands Rd, Ste 200, Valhalla, NY 10595; **Phone:** 914-304-5300; **Board Cert:** Clinical Genetics 2007; Pediatrics 2002; Clinical Biochemical Genetics 1999; **Med School:** Ireland 1989; **Resid:** Pediatrics, NYU Med Ctr 1996; **Fellow:** Clinical Genetics, NYU Med Ctr 1996; **Fac Appt:** CG, NY Med Coll

Shapiro, Lawrence R MD (CG) - **Spec Exp:** Dysmorphology; Prenatal Diagnosis; Hereditary Cancer; **Hospital:** Westchester Med Ctr; **Address:** Regional Medical Genetics, 503 Grasslands Rd, Ste 200, Valhalla, NY 10595; **Phone:** 914-304-5300; **Board Cert:** Pediatrics 1967; Clinical Genetics 1982; Clinical Cytogenetics 1982; **Med School:** NYU Sch Med 1962; **Resid:** Pediatrics, Chldns Hosp 1964; Pediatrics, Bellevue Hosp 1965; **Fellow:** Clinical Genetics, Mount Sinai Med Ctr 1968; **Fac Appt:** Prof Ped, NY Med Coll

Colon & Rectal Surgery

Krakovitz, Evan K MD (CRS) - **Spec Exp:** Colon & Rectal Cancer & Surgery; Hemorrhoids; Laparoscopic Surgery; Hernia; **Hospital:** Greenwich Hosp (page 892), Lawrence Hosp Ctr; **Address:** Westmed Medical Group, 210 Westchester Ave, Ste 106, White Plains, NY 10604; **Phone:** 914-682-6557; **Board Cert:** Surgery 2005; Colon & Rectal Surgery 2007; **Med School:** Hahnemann Univ 1989; **Resid:** Surgery, Graduate Hospital 1994; **Fellow:** Colon & Rectal Surgery, RWJ Univ Hosp 1995; **Fac Appt:** Clin Prof CRS, Cornell Univ-Weill Med Coll

Wishner, Jerald D MD (CRS) - **Spec Exp:** Colon & Rectal Cancer; Laparoscopic Surgery; **Hospital:** Northern Westchester Hosp (page 613); **Address:** Mount Kisco Med Grp, 110 S Bedford Rd, Mount Kisco, NY 10549; **Phone:** 914-241-1050; **Board Cert:** Surgery 2004; Colon & Rectal Surgery 2006; **Med School:** Northwestern Univ 1988; **Resid:** Surgery, St Luke's-Roosevelt Hosp Ctr 1993; Colon & Rectal Surgery, Grtr Baltimore Med Ctr 1994; **Fellow:** Minimally Invasive Surgery, Eastern Va Med Sch 1995; **Fac Appt:** Asst Prof S, Columbia P&S

Dermatology

Bank, David MD (D) - **Spec Exp:** Liposuction; Skin Laser Surgery; Botox Therapy; **Hospital:** Northern Westchester Hosp (page 613), NY-Presby/Columbia Univ Med Ctr, NY (page 104); **Address:** 359 E Main St, Ste 4G, Mt Kisco, NY 10549; **Phone:** 914-241-3003; **Board Cert:** Dermatology 1989; **Med School:** Columbia P&S 1985; **Resid:** Dermatology, Columbia-Presby Med Ctr 1989; **Fac Appt:** Assoc Clin Prof D, Columbia P&S

Berkowitz, Rhonda K MD (D) - **Spec Exp:** Melanoma; Skin Cancer; **Hospital:** NY-Presby/Columbia Univ Med Ctr, NY (page 104); **Address:** 325 S Highland Ave, Briarcliff Manor, NY 10510-2031; **Phone:** 914-941-5769; **Board Cert:** Dermatology 1986; **Med School:** NYU Sch Med 1982; **Resid:** Internal Medicine, N Shore Univ Hosp 1983; Dermatology, Columbia-Presby Med Ctr 1986

Bronin, Andrew MD (D) - **Spec Exp:** Melanoma; Skin Cancer; Complex Diagnosis; **Hospital:** Greenwich Hosp (page 892), Yale-New Haven Hosp; **Address:** 4 Rye Ridge Plaza, Rye Brook, NY 10573-2820; **Phone:** 914-253-8080; **Board Cert:** Dermatology 1981; **Med School:** NY Med Coll 1975; **Resid:** Dermatology, New York Hosp 1979; **Fac Appt:** Assoc Clin Prof D, Yale Univ

Davis, Ira C MD (D) - **Spec Exp:** Mohs' Surgery; Skin Cancer; Laser Surgery; Cosmetic Dermatology; **Hospital:** Westchester Med Ctr, Richmond Univ Med Ctr; **Address:** 280 N Central Park Ave, Ste 114, Hartsdale, NY 10530; **Phone:** 914-288-0500; **Board Cert:** Dermatology 1990; **Med School:** NYU Sch Med 1986; **Resid:** Dermatology, Duke Univ Med Ctr 1990; **Fellow:** Dermatologic Pharmacology, NYU Med Ctr 1991; Mohs Surgery, Wake Forest Univ Med Ctr 1994; **Fac Appt:** Asst Clin Prof D, NY Med Coll

Evans, Lydia Marion MD (D) - **Spec Exp:** Rosacea; Psoriasis/Eczema; Skin Cancer & Moles; Photodynamic Therapy; **Address:** 229 King Street, Chappaqua, NY 10514; **Phone:** 914-238-1500; **Board Cert:** Dermatology 2001; Internal Medicine 1982; **Med School:** Penn State Coll Med 1979; **Resid:** Dermatology, NY-Presby/Columbia Univ Med Ctr 1993; Internal Medicine, New York Methodist Hosp 1982; **Fellow:** Medical Oncology, Meml Sloan-Kettering Cancer Ctr 1986

Felsenstein, Jerome M MD (D) - **Hospital:** Phelps Meml Hosp Ctr (page 614), NYU Langone Med Ctr (page 108); **Address:** 100 S Highland Ave, Ossining, NY 10562; **Phone:** 914-941-5770; **Board Cert:** Dermatology 1976; **Med School:** NYU Sch Med 1971; **Resid:** Dermatology, Kings County Hosp 1975

Goldberg, Neil S MD (D) - **Spec Exp:** Pediatric Dermatology; Acne; **Hospital:** Lawrence Hosp Ctr; **Address:** 222 Westchester Ave, Ste 203, White Plains, NY 10604-2926; **Phone:** 914-761-8140; **Board Cert:** Dermatology 1986; **Med School:** Northwestern Univ 1982; **Resid:** Dermatology, Northwestern Meml Hosp 1986

Grossman, Marc E MD (D) - **Spec Exp:** Skin Diseases in Transplants/Cancer; Psoriasis; Rare Skin Disorders; Cutaneous Lymphoma; **Hospital:** NY-Presby/Columbia Univ Med Ctr, NY (page 104), White Plains Hosp (page 615); **Address:** 12 Greenridge Ave, White Plains, NY 10605-1238; **Phone:** 914-946-1101; **Board Cert:** Internal Medicine 1977; Dermatology 2009; **Med School:** Univ Pennsylvania 1974; **Resid:** Internal Medicine, Hosp Univ Penn 1976; **Fellow:** Dermatology, Columbia-Presby Med Ctr 1979; **Fac Appt:** Prof D, Columbia P&S

Howanitz, Nancy C MD (D) - **Spec Exp:** Melanoma; Skin Cancer; Rosacea; Cosmetic Dermatology; **Hospital:** Lawrence Hosp Ctr, White Plains Hosp (page 615); **Address:** 700 White Plains Rd, Scarsdale, NY 10583-5013; **Phone:** 914-725-5150; **Board Cert:** Dermatology 1980; **Med School:** Baylor Coll Med 1975; **Resid:** Anatomic Pathology, Texas Houston Med Ctr 1977; Dermatology, NYU Med Ctr 1980; **Fac Appt:** Asst Clin Prof D, NYU Sch Med

Hurwitz, Diana S MD (D) - **Hospital:** White Plains Hosp (page 615); **Address:** Westchester Medical Group, 1 Theall Rd, Ste 211, Rye, NY 10580; **Phone:** 914-848-8840; **Board Cert:** Dermatology 2005; **Med School:** Mount Sinai Sch Med 1992; **Resid:** Dermatology, Mt Sinai Med Ctr 1996

Kaplan, Sherri Kapel MD (D) - **Hospital:** Comm Hosp - Dobbs Ferry; **Address:** 1055 Saw Mill River Rd, Ste 208, Ardsley, NY 10502-1046; **Phone:** 914-693-7191; **Board Cert:** Dermatology 1987; **Med School:** NY Med Coll 1983; **Resid:** Dermatology, Westchester Co Med Ctr 1987

Kaporis, Athena G MD (D) - **Spec Exp:** Cosmetic Dermatology; Skin Cancer; Laser Surgery; **Hospital:** Northern Westchester Hosp (page 613); **Address:** 185 Kisco Ave, Ste 300, Mt. Kisco, NY 10549; **Phone:** 914-242-2020; **Board Cert:** Dermatology 2006; **Med School:** NYU Sch Med 1994; **Resid:** Dermatology, Downstate Med Ctr 1998

Klar, Tobi MD (D) - **Spec Exp:** Skin Cancer; **Hospital:** Sound Shore Med Ctr - Westchester, Montefiore Med Ctr-Einstein Campus, NY (page 100); **Address:** 150 Lockwood Ave, Ste 20, New Rochelle, NY 10801; **Phone:** 914-636-2039; **Board Cert:** Dermatology 1989; **Med School:** SUNY Downstate 1981; **Resid:** Dermatology, Downstate Med Ctr 1986

Lerman, Jay S MD (D) - **Spec Exp:** Acne; Eczema; **Hospital:** Montefiore Med Ctr-Einstein Campus, NY (page 100), Montefiore Med Ctr-Moses Campus, NY (page 100); **Address:** 280 Dobbs Ferry Rd, Ste 205 Bldg, White Plains, NY 10607-1912; **Phone:** 914-949-9196; **Board Cert:** Dermatology 1974; **Med School:** SUNY Downstate 1969; **Resid:** Dermatology, Jacobi Med Ctr 1973; **Fac Appt:** Asst Clin Prof D, Albert Einstein Coll Med

Levy, Ross MD (D) - **Spec Exp:** Skin Laser Surgery; Dermatologic Surgery; Skin Cancer; **Hospital:** Northern Westchester Hosp (page 613), Montefiore Med Ctr-Moses Campus, NY (page 100); **Address:** Mt Kisco Med Group, 110 S Bedford Rd, Mt Kisco, NY 10549; **Phone:** 914-242-1355; **Board Cert:** Dermatology 1981; **Med School:** Albert Einstein Coll Med 1976; **Resid:** Internal Medicine, Montefiore Med Ctr 1978; **Fellow:** Dermatology, Montefiore Med Ctr 1981; **Fac Appt:** Assoc Clin Prof Med, Albert Einstein Coll Med

Lukash, Barbara MD (D) - **Spec Exp:** Skin Cancer; Acne; Psoriasis; Melanoma; **Hospital:** NY-Presby/Columbia Univ Med Ctr, NY (page 104); **Address:** 14 Lawton St, New Rochelle, NY 10801; **Phone:** 914-712-2800; **Board Cert:** Dermatology 1980; **Med School:** Tulane Univ 1976; **Resid:** Dermatology, Univ Chicago Hosps 1980; **Fellow:** Dermatology, Univ of Chicago Hosps 1980; **Fac Appt:** Assoc Clin Prof D, Columbia P&S

Mackler, Karen MD (D) - **Spec Exp:** Pediatric Dermatology; Skin Cancer; **Hospital:** Sound Shore Med Ctr - Westchester, Montefiore Med Ctr-Moses Campus, NY (page 100); **Address:** 150 Lockwood Ave, Ste 34, New Rochelle, NY 10801-4914; **Phone:** 914-576-7070; **Board Cert:** Pediatrics 1978; Dermatology 1983; **Med School:** NYU Sch Med 1973; **Resid:** Pediatrics, NY Hosp 1976; Dermatology, Montefiore Hosp Med Ctr 1983; **Fac Appt:** Asst Prof D, Albert Einstein Coll Med

Mattison, Timothy D MD (D) - **Hospital:** Northern Westchester Hosp (page 613); **Address:** Mt Kisco Medical Group, 90 S Bedford Rd, Mt Kisco, NY 10549-3412; **Phone:** 914-242-1355; **Board Cert:** Dermatology 1980; **Med School:** Dartmouth Med Sch 1976; **Resid:** Dermatology, NYU Med Ctr 1980

Mermelstein, Harold MD (D) - **Spec Exp:** Cosmetic Dermatology; Aging Skin; Sclerotherapy; Laser Surgery; **Hospital:** NYU Langone Med Ctr (page 108), Lawrence Hosp Ctr; **Address:** 559 Gramatan Ave, Ste 205, Mt Vernon, NY 10552; **Phone:** 914-667-2242; **Board Cert:** Dermatology 1979; **Med School:** NY Med Coll 1975; **Resid:** Dermatology, NYU Med Ctr 1979; **Fellow:** Dermatologic Surgery, NYU Med Ctr 1980; **Fac Appt:** Assoc Clin Prof D, NYU Sch Med

Narins, Rhoda S MD (D) - **Spec Exp:** Liposuction; Cosmetic Dermatology; Botox Therapy; Facial Rejuvenation; **Hospital:** NYU Langone Med Ctr (page 108), White Plains Hosp (page 615); **Address:** 222 Westchester Ave, Ste 300, White Plains, NY 10604-2925; **Phone:** 914-684-1000; **Board Cert:** Dermatology 1970; **Med School:** NYU Sch Med 1965; **Resid:** Dermatology, NYU Med Ctr 1969; **Fac Appt:** Clin Prof D, NYU Sch Med

Newburger, Amy E MD (D) - **Spec Exp:** Contact Dermatitis; Cosmetic Dermatology; **Hospital:** White Plains Hosp (page 615), St. Luke's - Roosevelt Hosp Ctr - Roosevelt Div (page 94); **Address:** 2 Overhill Rd, Ste 330, Scarsdale, NY 10583; **Phone:** 914-725-1800; **Board Cert:** Dermatology 1979; **Med School:** NYU Sch Med 1974; **Resid:** Dermatology, Univ Miami Hosps 1978

Schachne, Jeffrey P MD (D) - **Hospital:** Hudson Valley Hosp Ctr; **Address:** 3630 Hill Blvd, Ste 101, Jefferson Valley, NY 10535; **Phone:** 914-962-6222; **Board Cert:** Dermatology 1988; **Med School:** SUNY Downstate 1984; **Resid:** Dermatology, Einstein Affil Hosp 1988

Schliftman, Alan B MD (D) - **Spec Exp:** Skin Laser Surgery; Skin Cancer; Cosmetic Dermatology; **Hospital:** Westchester Med Ctr, White Plains Hosp (page 615); **Address:** 244 Westchester Ave, Ste 211, White Plains, NY 10604-2926; **Phone:** 914-761-1400; **Board Cert:** Dermatology 1981; **Med School:** Geo Wash Univ 1977; **Resid:** Dermatology, Montefiore Med Ctr 1981; **Fac Appt:** Asst Clin Prof D, NY Med Coll

Stillman, Michael MD (D) - **Spec Exp:** Skin Cancer; Acne; Eczema; **Hospital:** Northern Westchester Hosp (page 613); **Address:** Mt Kisco Medical Group, 111 Bedford Rd, Katonah, NY 10536; **Phone:** 914-232-3135; **Board Cert:** Dermatology 1973; **Med School:** SUNY Downstate 1967; **Resid:** Dermatology, NYU Med Ctr 1973; **Fellow:** Dermatology, Letterman Army Inst Rsch 1970

Sturza, Jeffrey MD (D) - **Spec Exp:** Psoriasis; Laser Surgery; Cosmetic Dermatology; **Hospital:** Phelps Meml Hosp Ctr (page 614), Jacobi Med Ctr; **Address:** 150 White Plains Rd, Ste 210, Tarrytown, NY 10591; **Phone:** 914-631-4666; **Board Cert:** Dermatology 1988; **Med School:** SUNY Hlth Sci Ctr 1984; **Resid:** Dermatology, Cook Co Hosp 1988

Treiber, Ruth K MD (D) - **Spec Exp:** Botox Therapy; Acne; Facial Rejuvenation; Skin Cancer; **Hospital:** NY-Presby/Columbia Univ Med Ctr, NY (page 104); **Address:** 175 Purchase St, Rye, NY 10580; **Phone:** 914-967-2153; **Board Cert:** Dermatology 1983; **Med School:** Cornell Univ-Weill Med Coll 1978; **Resid:** Internal Medicine, New York Hosp 1980; Dermatology, Columbia-Presby Med Ctr 1983; **Fac Appt:** Assoc Clin Prof D, Columbia P&S

Zweibel, Stuart M MD/PhD (D) - **Spec Exp:** Mohs' Surgery; Skin Cancer; Skin Laser Surgery; Cosmetic Dermatology; **Hospital:** Northern Westchester Hosp (page 613); **Address:** 185 Kisco Ave, Ste 300, Mt Kisco, NY 10549; **Phone:** 914-242-2020; **Board Cert:** Dermatology 2009; **Med School:** Mount Sinai Sch Med 1985; **Resid:** Dermatology, Rhode Island Hosp 1989; **Fellow:** Mohs Surgery, Univ Wisconsin 1991

Diagnostic Radiology

Hertz, Marc MD (DR) - **Spec Exp:** CT Scan; MRI; **Address:** Mt Kisco Medical Group, Radiology, 90 S Bedford Rd, Mount Kisco, NY 10549; **Phone:** 914-242-1395; **Board Cert:** Diagnostic Radiology 1985; **Med School:** Howard Univ 1979; **Resid:** Pathology, Lenox Hill Hospital 1981; Diagnostic Radiology, Montefiore Hospital 1984; **Fellow:** Ultrasound/CT, North Shore Univ Hosp 1985

Hibbard, Claire MD (DR) - **Spec Exp:** Women's Imaging; Musculoskeletal Imaging; **Hospital:** Northern Westchester Hosp (page 613); **Address:** Mount Kisco Medical Group, Radiology, 110 S Bedford Rd, Mount Kisco, NY 10549-3412; **Phone:** 914-241-1050; **Board Cert:** Diagnostic Radiology 1989; **Med School:** Columbia P&S 1984; **Resid:** Diagnostic Radiology, Hosp U Penn 1989; **Fellow:** Musculoskeletal ImagingHosp U Penn 1990; **Fac Appt:** Asst Clin Prof Rad, Albert Einstein Coll Med

Khoury, Paul MD (DR) - **Hospital:** White Plains Hosp (page 615); **Address:** White Plains Hosp Ctr, Dept Radiology, 41 E Post Rd, White Plains, NY 10601; **Phone:** 914-681-1219; **Board Cert:** Diagnostic Radiology 1979; Nuclear Radiology 1980; **Med School:** Lebanon 1973; **Resid:** Diagnostic Radiology, Hotel Dieu de France Hosp 1975; Diagnostic Radiology, St Luke's-Roosevelt Hosp Ctr 1978

Kutcher, Rosalyn MD (DR) - **Spec Exp:** Mammography; Ultrasound; Women's Imaging; **Hospital:** White Plains Hosp (page 615); **Address:** 90 S Ridge St, Women's Imaging Ctr, Rye Brook, NY 10573; **Phone:** 914-935-0011; **Board Cert:** Diagnostic Radiology 1975; **Med School:** SUNY Hlth Sci Ctr 1970; **Resid:** Diagnostic Radiology, Montefiore Med Ctr 1974; **Fac Appt:** Prof Rad, Albert Einstein Coll Med

Lefkovitz, Zvi MD (DR) - **Spec Exp:** Chest Radiology; **Hospital:** Westchester Med Ctr; **Address:** WMC Advanced Physician Services, 100 Woods Rd, Valhalla, NY 10595; **Phone:** 914-493-2500; **Board Cert:** Diagnostic Radiology 1986; **Med School:** Ros Franklin Univ/Chicago Med Sch 1982; **Resid:** Diagnostic Radiology, Maimonides Med Ctr 1986; **Fellow:** Interventional Radiology, Univ Hosp 1987; **Fac Appt:** Clin Prof Rad, NY Med Coll

Leslie, Denise MD (DR) - **Spec Exp:** Neuroradiology; **Hospital:** Good Samaritan Hosp - Suffern, St. John's Riverside Hosp-Andrus Pavil; **Address:** 141 S Central Ave, Hartsdale, NY 10530; **Phone:** 914-345-0376; **Board Cert:** Diagnostic Radiology 1985; **Med School:** SUNY Buffalo 1981; **Resid:** Diagnostic Radiology, Westchester Co Med Ctr 1985; **Fellow:** Neuroradiology, Westchester Co Med Ctr 1987

LoRusso, Diane MD (DR) - **Spec Exp:** Breast Imaging; Women's Health; Ultrasound; **Address:** Rye Radiology Assoc, 30 Rye Ridge Plaza, Rye Brook, NY 10573-2830; **Phone:** 914-253-9200; **Board Cert:** Diagnostic Radiology 1974; **Med School:** SUNY Upstate Med Univ 1969; **Resid:** Diagnostic Radiology, Montefiore Med Ctr 1974

Poplausky, Maurice R MD (DR) - **Spec Exp:** Interventional Radiology; **Hospital:** Hudson Valley Hosp Ctr, Westchester Med Ctr; **Address:** Hudson Valley Hospital, Dept Radiology, 1980 Crompound Rd, Cortland Manor, NY 10567; **Phone:** 914-734-3680; **Board Cert:** Diagnostic Radiology 1995; Vascular & Interventional Radiology 2008; **Med School:** SUNY Buffalo 1990; **Resid:** Diagnostic Radiology, SUNY Downstate Med Ctr 1995; **Fellow:** Vascular & Interventional Radiology, Mass Genl Hosp 1996; **Fac Appt:** Assoc Prof Rad, NY Med Coll

Staeger-Hirsch, Christine MD (DR) - **Spec Exp:** Breast Imaging; **Address:** Rye Radiology, 30 Rye Ridge Plaza, Rye Brook, NY 10573-2830; **Phone:** 914-253-9200; **Board Cert:** Diagnostic Radiology 2006; **Med School:** NYU Sch Med 2001; **Resid:** Diagnostic Radiology, St Luke's Roosevelt Med Ctr

Weiss, Jonathan D MD (DR) - **Hospital:** White Plains Hosp (page 615); **Address:** Westmed Medical Group, Radiology, 210 Westchester Ave, White Plains, NY 10601; **Phone:** 914-682-6430; **Board Cert:** Diagnostic Radiology 1987; **Med School:** Tufts Univ 1983; **Resid:** Diagnostic Radiology, SUNY Downstate Med Ctr 1987; **Fellow:** Interventional Radiology, SUNY Downstate Med Ctr 1988

Endocrinology, Diabetes & Metabolism

Albin, Joan MD (EDM) - **Spec Exp:** Diabetes; Thyroid Disorders; Polycystic Ovarian Syndrome; **Hospital:** Sound Shore Med Ctr - Westchester, Lawrence Hosp Ctr; **Address:** 140 Lockwood Ave, Ste 212, New Rochelle, NY 10801-4908; **Phone:** 914-235-8503; **Board Cert:** Internal Medicine 1972; Endocrinology, Diabetes & Metabolism 1973; **Med School:** NY Med Coll 1967; **Resid:** Internal Medicine, Metropolitan Hosp 1969; Internal Medicine, Montefiore Hosp Med Ctr 1970; **Fellow:** Endocrinology, Diabetes & Metabolism, Mount Sinai Hosp 1971; Endocrinology, Diabetes & Metabolism, New York Med Coll 1972; **Fac Appt:** Assoc Clin Prof Med, Albert Einstein Coll Med

Bloomgarden, David K MD (EDM) - **Spec Exp:** Diabetes; Osteoporosis; Thyroid Disorders; **Hospital:** White Plains Hosp (page 615); **Address:** Scarsdale Medical Group, 550 Mamaroneck Ave, Ste 101, Harrison, NY 10528; **Phone:** 914-723-8100 x302; **Board Cert:** Internal Medicine 1980; Endocrinology, Diabetes & Metabolism 1983; **Med School:** NYU Sch Med 1977; **Resid:** Internal Medicine, Jacobi Med Ctr 1980; **Fellow:** Endocrinology, Diabetes & Metabolism, Albert Einstein 1982

Blum, David MD (EDM) - **Spec Exp:** Diabetes; Osteoporosis; Thyroid Disorders; **Hospital:** Sound Shore Med Ctr - Westchester; **Address:** Sound Shore Medical Ctr, Endocrinology, 16 Guion Pl, New Rochelle, NY 10802; **Phone:** 914-633-8680; **Board Cert:** Internal Medicine 1977; Endocrinology, Diabetes & Metabolism 1979; **Med School:** Northwestern Univ 1974; **Resid:** Internal Medicine, Mt Sinai Hosp 1977; **Fellow:** Endocrinology, Mt Sinai Hosp 1979; **Fac Appt:** Asst Clin Prof Med, NY Med Coll

Gitler, Ellen MD (EDM) - **Spec Exp:** Cardiac Rehabilitation; **Hospital:** Burke Rehab Hosp; **Address:** 785 Mamaroneck Ave, White Plains, NY 10605-2523; **Phone:** 914-597-2409; **Board Cert:** Internal Medicine 1980; Endocrinology, Diabetes & Metabolism 1983; **Med School:** Cornell Univ-Weill Med Coll 1977; **Resid:** Internal Medicine, Bronx Muni Hosp 1980; **Fellow:** Endocrinology, Diabetes & Metabolism, Mount Sinai Med Ctr 1982

Hellerman, James MD (EDM) - **Spec Exp:** Thyroid Disorders; Diabetes; Calcium Disorders; **Hospital:** Phelps Meml Hosp Ctr (page 614); **Address:** 200 S Broadway, Ste 100, Tarrytown, NY 10591-4504; **Phone:** 914-631-9300; **Board Cert:** Internal Medicine 1979; Endocrinology 1983; **Med School:** Univ Rochester 1976; **Resid:** Internal Medicine, Montefiore Med Ctr 1980; **Fellow:** Endocrinology, Diabetes & Metabolism, Mass Genl Hosp 1984

Kantor, Alan MD (EDM) - **Spec Exp:** Thyroid Disorders; Osteoporosis; Diabetes; Endocrine Tumors; **Hospital:** Northern Westchester Hosp (page 613); **Address:** 1940 Commerce St, Ste 310, Yorktown Heights, NY 10598; **Phone:** 914-245-1111; **Board Cert:** Internal Medicine 1981; Endocrinology, Diabetes & Metabolism 1983; **Med School:** South Africa 1975; **Resid:** Internal Medicine, La Guardia Hosp 1980; Internal Medicine, LI Jewish-Hillside Med Ctr 1981; **Fellow:** Endocrinology, Diabetes & Metabolism, Meml Sloan Kettering Cancer Ctr 1983; **Fac Appt:** Asst Clin Prof Med, NY Med Coll

Leibowitz, Jonas MD (EDM) - **Spec Exp:** Diabetes; Osteoporosis; Thyroid Disorders; Nutrition; **Hospital:** White Plains Hosp (page 615), Lawrence Hosp Ctr; **Address:** 770 B McLean Ave, Yonkers, NY 10704; **Phone:** 914-237-3636; **Board Cert:** Internal Medicine 2005; Endocrinology, Diabetes & Metabolism 2007; **Med School:** SUNY Downstate 1992; **Resid:** Internal Medicine, Mt Sinai Med Ctr 1995; **Fellow:** Endocrinology, Mt Sinai Med Ctr 1997; **Fac Appt:** Asst Clin Prof Med, NY Med Coll

Powell, Jeffrey S MD (EDM) - **Hospital:** Northern Westchester Hosp (page 613); **Address:** Mount Kisco Med Group, 90 S Bedford Rd, Mount Kisco, NY 10549; **Phone:** 914-241-1050; **Board Cert:** Internal Medicine 2008; Endocrinology, Diabetes & Metabolism 2010; **Med School:** Albert Einstein Coll Med 1995; **Resid:** Internal Medicine, Columbia-Presby Med Ctr 1998; **Fellow:** Endocrinology, Diabetes & Metabolism, Columbia-Presby Med Ctr 2001

Pretto, Zorayda MD (EDM) - **Hospital:** White Plains Hosp (page 615); **Address:** Mid-Westchester Medical Assocs, 210 Westchester Ave, White Plains, NY 10605; **Phone:** 914-948-3630; **Board Cert:** Internal Medicine 2005; Endocrinology, Diabetes & Metabolism 2006; **Med School:** Panama 1986; **Resid:** Internal Medicine, St John's Episcopal Hosp 1991; **Fellow:** Endocrinology, Diabetes & Metabolism, Beth Israel Hosp 1993

Rudin, Eric A MD (EDM) - **Spec Exp:** Diabetes; **Hospital:** Northern Westchester Hosp (page 613); **Address:** Mt Kisco Medical Group, 111 Bedford Rd, Katonah, NY 10549; **Phone:** 914-232-3135; **Board Cert:** Internal Medicine 2003; Endocrinology, Diabetes & Metabolism 2005; **Med School:** Mount Sinai Sch Med 2000; **Resid:** Internal Medicine, Thomas Jefferson Univ Hosp` 2003; **Fellow:** Endocrinology, Diabetes & Metabolism, Montefiore Med Ctr 2005

Weiser, Kenneth R MD (EDM) - **Hospital:** White Plains Hosp (page 615); **Address:** Westchester Med Group-Endocrinolgy, 210 Westchester Ave, White Plains, NY 10604; **Phone:** 914-831-4150; **Board Cert:** Internal Medicine 2003; Endocrinology, Diabetes & Metabolism 2005; **Med School:** Albert Einstein Coll Med 1990; **Resid:** Internal Medicine, Jacobi Med Ctr 1993; **Fellow:** Endocrinology, Diabetes & Metabolism, Mt Sinai Med Ctr 1995

Family Medicine

Annabi, Iyad N MD (FMed) *PCP* - **Hospital:** St. John's Riverside Hosp-Andrus Pavil; **Address:** Westchester Family Medicine Practice, 472 Palmer Rd, Yonkers, NY 10701-5207; **Phone:** 914-375-2300; **Board Cert:** Family Medicine 2008; **Med School:** Mexico 1988; **Resid:** Family Medicine, St Joseph Med Ctr 1993

Apuzzo, Thomas MD (FMed) *PCP* - **Hospital:** Saint Joseph's Med Ctr - Yonkers, St. John's Riverside Hosp-Andrus Pavil; **Address:** 755 Yonkers Ave, Yonkers, NY 10704; **Phone:** 914-237-0994; **Board Cert:** Family Medicine 2002; **Med School:** Italy 1985; **Resid:** Family Medicine, St Joseph's Med Ctr 1989

Gottesfeld, Peter MD (FMed) *PCP* - **Spec Exp:** Preventive Medicine; ADD/ADHD; **Hospital:** Northern Westchester Hosp (page 613), Hudson Valley Hosp Ctr; **Address:** 101 S Bedford Rd, Ste 412, MS 10549, Mt Kisco, NY 10549-3455; **Phone:** 914-241-7800; **Board Cert:** Family Medicine 2003; **Med School:** UMDNJ-RW Johnson Med Sch 1985; **Resid:** Family Medicine, Thomas Jefferson U Hosp 1988; **Fac Appt:** Assoc Clin Prof FMed, NY Med Coll

Merker, Edward L MD (FMed) *PCP* - **Spec Exp:** Geriatric Care; **Hospital:** Phelps Meml Hosp Ctr (page 614); **Address:** 180 Marble Ave, Pleasantville, NY 10570; **Phone:** 914-769-7300 x202; **Board Cert:** Family Medicine 2005; **Med School:** Albert Einstein Coll Med 1981; **Resid:** Family Medicine, Overlook Hosp 1984; **Fac Appt:** Asst Clin Prof FMed, Albert Einstein Coll Med

Miller, Daniel MD (FMed) *PCP* - **Hospital:** St. John's Riverside Hosp-Andrus Pavil, Saint Joseph's Med Ctr - Yonkers; **Address:** Hudson River HealthCare, 503 S Broadway, Yonkers, NY 10703; **Phone:** 914-965-9771; **Board Cert:** Family Medicine 2007; **Med School:** Univ Cincinnati 1984; **Resid:** Family Medicine, Montefiore Hosp Med Ctr 1987; **Fac Appt:** Asst Prof FMed, NY Med Coll

Piccirilli, Dora C MD (FMed) *PCP* - **Hospital:** Phelps Meml Hosp Ctr (page 614); **Address:** 180 Marble Ave, Pleasantville, NY 10570; **Phone:** 914-769-7300; **Board Cert:** Family Medicine 2005; **Med School:** SUNY Hlth Sci Ctr 1988; **Resid:** Family Medicine, Overlook Hosp 1991

Sharpe, Arleen S MD (FMed) *PCP* - **Hospital:** Lawrence Hosp Ctr, White Plains Hosp (page 615); **Address:** West Med Group, 73 Market St, Yonkers, NY 10710; **Phone:** 914-693-1660; **Board Cert:** Family Medicine 2005; **Med School:** SUNY Stony Brook 1988; **Resid:** Family Medicine, Montefiore Med Ctr 1991

Strongwater, Richard F MD (FMed) *PCP* - **Spec Exp:** Travel Medicine; **Hospital:** Phelps Meml Hosp Ctr (page 614); **Address:** North Star Medical, 180 Marble Ave, Pleasantville, NY 10570; **Phone:** 914-769-7300; **Board Cert:** Family Medicine 2005; **Med School:** SUNY Upstate Med Univ 1981; **Resid:** Family Medicine, Overlook Hosp 1984

Sutton, Ira MD (FMed) *PCP* - **Spec Exp:** Preventive Medicine; Skin Diseases; **Hospital:** Sound Shore Med Ctr - Westchester, White Plains Hosp (page 615); **Address:** 2 Overhill Rd, Ste 225, SCARSDALE, NY 10583; **Phone:** 914-636-0077; **Board Cert:** Family Medicine 2008; **Med School:** Albert Einstein Coll Med 1980; **Resid:** Family Medicine, Memorial Hosp 1983

Vaidya, Sudhir P MD (FMed) - **Spec Exp:** Primary Care Sports Medicine; Pain Management; Geriatric Rehabilitation; **Hospital:** Burke Rehab Hosp, St. Joseph's Hosp-Nassau; **Address:** Burke Rehab Hosp, 785 Mamaroneck Ave, White Plains, NY 10605; **Phone:** 914-597-2332; **Board Cert:** Family Medicine 2005; Sports Medicine 2011; **Med School:** India 1979; **Resid:** Physical Medicine & Rehabilitation, NHS Hosps-Leicester, Milton Keynes-Bedford 1995; Family Medicine, St Joseph's Hosp 1998; **Fac Appt:** Asst Prof FMed, Cornell Univ-Weill Med Coll

Yudin, Howard MD (FMed) *PCP* - **Hospital:** Greenwich Hosp (page 892); **Address:** 18 Rye Ridge Plaza, Rye Brook, NY 10573-2820; **Phone:** 914-251-1261; **Board Cert:** Family Medicine 2008; **Med School:** Univ Montreal 1974; **Resid:** Family Medicine, Jewish Genl Hosp 1976

Gastroenterology

Abemayor, Elie M MD (Ge) - **Spec Exp:** Inflammatory Bowel Disease; Endoscopy; Irritable Bowel Syndrome; **Hospital:** Northern Westchester Hosp (page 613), NYU Langone Med Ctr (page 108); **Address:** 91 Smith Ave, Mt Kisco, NY 10549-2810; **Phone:** 914-241-9026; **Board Cert:** Internal Medicine 1988; Gastroenterology 2005; **Med School:** SUNY Stony Brook 1985; **Resid:** Internal Medicine, NYU-Bellevue Med Ctr 1988; **Fellow:** Gastroenterology, NYU/Manhattan VA Med Ctr 1990; **Fac Appt:** Asst Clin Prof Med, NYU Sch Med

Antonelle, Robert MD (Ge) - **Spec Exp:** Gastroesophageal Reflux Disease (GERD); Liver & Biliary Disease; Colonoscopy; **Hospital:** White Plains Hosp (page 615); **Address:** 311 North St, rm 403, White Plains, NY 10605-2232; **Phone:** 914-949-7171; **Board Cert:** Gastroenterology 2006; **Med School:** NY Med Coll 1989; **Resid:** Internal Medicine, Westchester Med Ctr 1990; **Fellow:** Gastroenterology, Westchester Med Ctr 1994; **Fac Appt:** Asst Clin Prof Med, NY Med Coll

Auerbach, Mitchell E MD (Ge) - **Spec Exp:** Colonoscopy; Crohn's Disease; Ulcerative Colitis; **Hospital:** Saint Joseph's Med Ctr - Yonkers, St. John's Riverside Hosp-Andrus Pavil; **Address:** Westchester Digestive Disease Group, 469 N Broadway, Yonkers, NY 10701-1923; **Phone:** 914-969-1115; **Board Cert:** Gastroenterology 2008; **Med School:** Tufts Univ 1991; **Resid:** Internal Medicine, Mt Sinai Hosp 1994; **Fellow:** Gastroenterology, Mt Sinai Hosp 1996

Byfield, Floyd MD (Ge) - **Hospital:** Phelps Meml Hosp Ctr (page 614); **Address:** Westchester Gastroenterology Assocs, 777 N Broadway, Ste 305, North Tarrytown, NY 10591; **Phone:** 914-366-6120; **Board Cert:** Internal Medicine 2006; Gastroenterology 2009; **Med School:** Mount Sinai Sch Med 1993; **Resid:** Internal Medicine, Ny Presby-Cornell Med Ctr 1996; **Fellow:** Gastroenterology, NY Presby-Cornell Med Ctr 1998

Chinitz, Marvin MD (Ge) - **Spec Exp:** Colonoscopy; Inflammatory Bowel Disease; Liver Disease; Gastroesophageal Reflux Disease (GERD); **Hospital:** Northern Westchester Hosp (page 613); **Address:** Mt Kisco Medical Group, 90 S Bedford Rd, Mt Kisco, NY 10549-3422; **Phone:** 914-241-1050; **Board Cert:** Internal Medicine 1981; Gastroenterology 1985; **Med School:** Boston Univ 1978; **Resid:** Internal Medicine, Boston Med Ctr 1981; **Fellow:** Gastroenterology, Montefiore Med Ctr 1984; **Fac Appt:** Assoc Prof Med, Albert Einstein Coll Med

Dworkin, Brad M MD (Ge) - **Spec Exp:** Gastrointestinal Motility Disorders; Nutrition; Inflammatory Bowel Disease; **Hospital:** Westchester Med Ctr; **Address:** New York Medical College, Munger Pavilion, Ste 206, Valhalla, NY 10595; **Phone:** 914-493-7337; **Board Cert:** Internal Medicine 1979; Gastroenterology 1981; **Med School:** Jefferson Med Coll 1976; **Resid:** Internal Medicine, New York Hosp 1979; **Fellow:** Gastroenterology, Meml Sloan Kettering Cancer Ctr 1981; **Fac Appt:** Prof Med, NY Med Coll

Ehrlich, James B MD (Ge) - **Spec Exp:** Ulcerative Colitis; Colonoscopy; Gastroesophageal Reflux Disease (GERD); Gastroscopy; **Hospital:** Lawrence Hosp Ctr; **Address:** 73 Market St, Ste 219, Yonkers, NY 10710; **Phone:** 914-831-6820; **Board Cert:** Internal Medicine 1983; Gastroenterology 1985; **Med School:** Univ Hlth Scis, Chicago Med Sch 1980; **Resid:** Internal Medicine, Univ Illinois Med Ctr 1983; **Fellow:** Gastroenterology, Michael Reese Med Ctr 1985

Field, Barry E MD (Ge) - **Spec Exp:** Ulcerative Colitis; Crohn's Disease; **Hospital:** Phelps Meml Hosp Ctr (page 614); **Address:** Westchester Gastroenterology, 777 N Broadway Fl 3 - Ste 305, Sleepy Hollow, NY 10591-1040; **Phone:** 914-366-6120; **Board Cert:** Internal Medicine 1976; Gastroenterology 1979; **Med School:** Albert Einstein Coll Med 1972; **Resid:** Internal Medicine, Metropolitan Hosp Ctr 1976; **Fellow:** Gastroenterology, Harbor Genl Hosp 1978

Finegold, Jonathan MD (Ge) - **Spec Exp:** Barrett's Esophagus; Colon Cancer; Inflammatory Bowel Disease/Crohn's; **Hospital:** Lawrence Hosp Ctr; **Address:** WestMed Med Grp, Ridge Hill, 73 Market St, Ste 219, Yonkers, NY 10710; **Phone:** 914-831-6820; **Board Cert:** Internal Medicine 2005; Gastroenterology 2007; **Med School:** Univ Miami Sch Med 1991; **Resid:** Internal Medicine, NY-Presby/Columbia Med Ctr 1994; **Fellow:** Gastroenterology, NY-Presby/Columbia Med Ctr 1997

Geders, Jane MD/PhD (Ge) - **Spec Exp:** Hepatitis C; Nutrition; Colon Cancer Screening; **Hospital:** Northern Westchester Hosp (page 613); **Address:** 90 S Bedford Rd, Mt Kisco, NY 10549; **Phone:** 914-242-1307; **Board Cert:** Gastroenterology 2003; **Med School:** Univ S Fla Coll Med 1987; **Resid:** Internal Medicine, Meml Sloan Kettering Cancer Ctr 1988; Internal Medicine, N Shore Univ Hosp 1990; **Fellow:** Gastroenterology, Mt Sinai Med Ctr 1992; Hepatology, Mt Sinai Med Ctr 1993; **Fac Appt:** Asst Prof Med, NYU Sch Med

Gendler, Seth MD (Ge) - **Spec Exp:** Pancreatic/Biliary Endoscopy (ERCP); Biliary Disease; Pancreatic Disease; **Hospital:** Sound Shore Med Ctr - Westchester, Westchester Med Ctr; **Address:** 140 Lockwood Ave, Ste 104, New Rochelle, NY 10801-4907; **Phone:** 914-235-9333; **Board Cert:** Internal Medicine 1986; Gastroenterology 2011; **Med School:** Rush Med Coll 1983; **Resid:** Internal Medicine, St Lukes Hosp 1986; **Fellow:** Gastroenterology, St Lukes Hosp 1988; Endoscopy, Univ Hosp 1989; **Fac Appt:** Assoc Prof Med, NY Med Coll

Genn, David A MD (Ge) - **Spec Exp:** Colon Cancer Screening; Biliary Disease; Gastroesophageal Reflux Disease (GERD); Barrett's Esophagus; **Hospital:** Hudson Valley Hosp Ctr; **Address:** 1985 Crompond Road, Bldg D, Cortlandt Manor, NY 10567-4146; **Phone:** 914-739-2400; **Board Cert:** Gastroenterology 2003; **Med School:** Boston Univ 1988; **Resid:** Internal Medicine, Montefiore Med Ctr 1991; **Fellow:** Gastroenterology, Westchester Med Ctr 1993

Goldblatt, Robert MD (Ge) - **Spec Exp:** Liver Disease; Biliary Disease; Endoscopy; Inflammatory Bowel Disease; **Hospital:** White Plains Hosp (page 615), Greenwich Hosp (page 892); **Address:** 18 Rye Ridge Plaza, Rye Brook, NY 10573-2820; **Phone:** 914-253-9252; **Board Cert:** Internal Medicine 1978; Gastroenterology 1979; **Med School:** Geo Wash Univ 1974; **Resid:** Internal Medicine, Univ FL-Shands Hosp 1977; **Fellow:** Gastroenterology, Yale-New Haven Hosp 1979; **Fac Appt:** Asst Prof Med, Cornell Univ-Weill Med Coll

Gould, Richard B MD (Ge) - **Spec Exp:** Colonoscopy; Gastroscopy; **Hospital:** Lawrence Hosp Ctr, Montefiore Med Ctr-Einstein Campus, NY (page 100); **Address:** 1 Pondfield Rd W, Ste 1R, Bronxville, NY 10708; **Phone:** 914-779-6200; **Board Cert:** Internal Medicine 1975; Gastroenterology 1977; **Med School:** SUNY Upstate Med Univ 1972; **Resid:** Internal Medicine, Montefiore Hosp Med Ctr 1975; **Fellow:** Gastroenterology, Montefiore Hosp Med Ctr 1977; **Fac Appt:** Assoc Clin Prof Med, Columbia P&S

Heier, Stephen K MD (Ge) - **Spec Exp:** Colonoscopy/Polypectomy; Gastric & Esophageal Disorders; Pancreatic/Biliary Endoscopy (ERCP); **Hospital:** Phelps Meml Hosp Ctr (page 614); **Address:** Phelps Memorial Hosp, Advanced Endoscopy & Gastroenterology, 755 N Broadway, Ste 530, Sleepy Hollow, NY 10591; **Phone:** 914-366-1190; **Board Cert:** Internal Medicine 1979; Gastroenterology 1981; **Med School:** Albany Med Coll 1976; **Resid:** Internal Medicine, Metro Hosp Ctr 1979; **Fellow:** Gastroenterology, Tufts Univ 1981; **Fac Appt:** Clin Prof Med, NY Med Coll

Jaffe, Alan H MD (Ge) - **Hospital:** White Plains Hosp (page 615); **Address:** Westchester Medical Group, 210 Westchester Ave Fl 2 - Ste 205, White Plains, NY 10604; **Phone:** 914-682-6466; **Board Cert:** Internal Medicine 1977; Gastroenterology 1979; **Med School:** Cornell Univ-Weill Med Coll 1974; **Resid:** Internal Medicine, N Shore U Med Ctr 1977; **Fellow:** Gastroenterology, St Raphael Hosp 1979

Kahn, Oren MD (Ge) - **Spec Exp:** Colon Cancer; Inflammatory Bowel Disease; Peptic Ulcer Disease; Gastroesophageal Reflux Disease (GERD); **Hospital:** Northern Westchester Hosp (page 613); **Address:** 90 S Bedford Rd, Mount Kisco, NY 10549; **Phone:** 914-241-1050; **Board Cert:** Internal Medicine 2004; Gastroenterology 2007; **Med School:** Albert Einstein Coll Med 1990; **Resid:** Internal Medicine, Mt Sinai Med Ctr 1994; **Fellow:** Gastroenterology, Mt Sinai Med Ctr 1996; **Fac Appt:** Assoc Clin Prof Med, Mount Sinai Sch Med

Katz, Henry J MD (Ge) - **Hospital:** Montefiore Med Ctr-Moses Campus, NY (page 100), St. John's Riverside Hosp-Andrus Pavil; **Address:** 1234 Central Park Ave, Yonkers, NY 10704-1068; **Phone:** 914-793-1600; **Board Cert:** Internal Medicine 1983; Gastroenterology 1985; **Med School:** Albany Med Coll 1980; **Resid:** Internal Medicine, Bellevue Hosp 1983; **Fellow:** Gastroenterology, Montefiore Med Ctr 1985

Kozicky, Orest J MD (Ge) - **Spec Exp:** Colitis; Peptic Ulcer Disease; Gastroesophageal Reflux Disease (GERD); **Hospital:** St. John's Riverside Hosp-Andrus Pavil; **Address:** Westchester Digestive Disease Grp, 469 N Broadway, Yonkers, NY 10701-1923; **Phone:** 914-969-1115; **Board Cert:** Internal Medicine 1985; Gastroenterology 1987; **Med School:** NY Med Coll 1981; **Resid:** Internal Medicine, Jacobi Med Ctr 1985; **Fellow:** Gastroenterology, Montefiore Hosp Med Ctr 1987; **Fac Appt:** Asst Clin Prof Med, Albert Einstein Coll Med

Kressner, Michael MD (Ge) - **Spec Exp:** Colon Cancer; Inflammatory Bowel Disease; Biliary Disease; **Hospital:** Sound Shore Med Ctr - Westchester, Mount Vernon Hosp; **Address:** 140 Lockwood Ave, Ste 110, New Rochelle, NY 10801-4907; **Phone:** 914-636-5222; **Board Cert:** Internal Medicine 1980; Gastroenterology 1983; **Med School:** SUNY Buffalo 1977; **Resid:** Internal Medicine, Montefiore Med Ctr 1980; **Fellow:** Gastroenterology, Montefiore Med Ctr 1982; **Fac Appt:** Asst Clin Prof Med, NY Med Coll

Landau, Steven R MD (Ge) - **Spec Exp:** Inflammatory Bowel Disease; Colon Cancer; **Hospital:** White Plains Hosp (page 615); **Address:** 30 Greenridge Ave, White Plains, NY 10605; **Phone:** 914-328-8555; **Board Cert:** Internal Medicine 1984; Gastroenterology 1987; **Med School:** NYU Sch Med 1981; **Resid:** Internal Medicine, Jacobi Med Ctr 1982; Internal Medicine, Montefiore Med Ctr 1984; **Fellow:** Gastroenterology, Mount Sinai Hosp 1986; **Fac Appt:** Asst Prof Med, Albert Einstein Coll Med

Lebovics, Edward MD (Ge) - **Spec Exp:** Hepatitis B & C; Pancreatic/Biliary Endoscopy (ERCP); Crohn's Disease; Liver Disease; **Hospital:** Westchester Med Ctr; **Address:** NY Med College-Div Gastroenterology, Munger Pavilion, Ste 206, Valhalla, NY 10595; **Phone:** 914-493-7337; **Board Cert:** Internal Medicine 1983; Gastroenterology 1985; **Med School:** NYU Sch Med 1980; **Resid:** Internal Medicine, Jewish Hosp 1983; **Fellow:** Hepatology, Mt Sinai Hosp 1984; Gastroenterology, NY Med Coll 1986; **Fac Appt:** Prof Med, NY Med Coll

Liss, Mark MD (Ge) - **Spec Exp:** Endoscopy; Peptic Acid Disorders; Inflammatory Bowel Disease; **Hospital:** Sound Shore Med Ctr - Westchester, Montefiore Med Ctr-Moses Campus, NY (page 100); **Address:** 140 Lockwood Ave, Ste 318, New Rochelle, NY 10801; **Phone:** 914-633-0888; **Board Cert:** Internal Medicine 1980; Gastroenterology 1983; **Med School:** Mount Sinai Sch Med 1977; **Resid:** Internal Medicine, Mt Sinai Hosp 1980; **Fellow:** Gastroenterology, Montefiore Med Ctr 1982; **Fac Appt:** Asst Clin Prof Med, Albert Einstein Coll Med

Martin, Christopher MD (Ge) - **Hospital:** Phelps Meml Hosp Ctr (page 614); **Address:** 777 N Broadway, Ste 305, Sleepy Hollow, NY 10591; **Phone:** 914-366-6120; **Board Cert:** Internal Medicine 2002; Gastroenterology 2005; **Med School:** Cornell Univ-Weill Med Coll 1999; **Resid:** Internal Medicine, NY Presby Hosp-Cornell 2002; **Fellow:** Gastroenterology, St Luke's-Roosevelt Hosp Ctr 2005

Rosemarin, Jack MD (Ge) - **Spec Exp:** Colonoscopy; Peptic Acid Disorders; Nutrition; **Hospital:** White Plains Hosp (page 615); **Address:** 2 Gannett Drive, White Plains, NY 10604; **Phone:** 914-683-1555; **Board Cert:** Internal Medicine 1982; Gastroenterology 1983; **Med School:** NY Med Coll 1978; **Resid:** Internal Medicine, NY Med Coll 1981; **Fellow:** Gastroenterology, Yale Affil Hosps 1983

Roston, Alfred MD (Ge) - **Spec Exp:** Pancreatic/Biliary Endoscopy (ERCP); Barrett's Esophagus; Gastroesophageal Reflux Disease (GERD); Inflammatory Bowel Disease; **Hospital:** White Plains Hosp (page 615); **Address:** 2 Gannett Drive, White Plains, NY 10604; **Phone:** 914-683-1555; **Board Cert:** Gastroenterology 2005; **Med School:** NYU Sch Med 1989; **Resid:** Internal Medicine, Mt Sinai Hosp 1992; **Fellow:** Gastroenterology, NY Hosp-Cornell Univ Med 1994; Endoscopy, Brigham & Women's Hospital 1995

Sgouros, Anthony MD (Ge) - **Spec Exp:** Inflammatory Bowel Disease; Gastrointestinal Cancer; **Hospital:** Northern Westchester Hosp (page 613); **Address:** Westchester Health, 60 Goldens Bridge Rd, Katonah, NY 10536; **Phone:** 914-269-9632; **Board Cert:** Internal Medicine 2003; Gastroenterology 2005; **Med School:** Mount Sinai Sch Med 1990; **Resid:** Internal Medicine, NY-Presby/Columbia Univ Med Ctr 1993; **Fellow:** Gastroenterology, Montefiore Med Ctr 1995

Shapiro, Neil H MD (Ge) - **Spec Exp:** Endoscopy; Liver Disease; Inflammatory Bowel Disease; **Hospital:** White Plains Hosp (page 615), Greenwich Hosp (page 892); **Address:** 18 Rye Ridge Plaza, Rye Brook, NY 10573-2820; **Phone:** 914-253-9252; **Board Cert:** Internal Medicine 1978; Gastroenterology 1981; **Med School:** Wayne State Univ 1975; **Resid:** Internal Medicine, Beth Israel Hosp 1978; Gastroenterology, Montefiore Med Ctr 1980; **Fac Appt:** Asst Clin Prof Med, Cornell Univ-Weill Med Coll

Taffet, Sanford L MD (Ge) - **Spec Exp:** Inflammatory Bowel Disease; Colon Cancer; Liver Disease; **Hospital:** Sound Shore Med Ctr - Westchester, Mount Vernon Hosp; **Address:** 140 Lockwood Ave, Ste 110, New Rochelle, NY 10801-4907; **Phone:** 914-636-5222; **Board Cert:** Internal Medicine 1980; Gastroenterology 1981; **Med School:** NY Med Coll 1976; **Resid:** Internal Medicine, Maimonides Med Ctr 1979; **Fellow:** Gastroenterology, Albert Einstein Med Ctr 1981; **Fac Appt:** Assoc Clin Prof Med, NY Med Coll

Torman, Julie MD (Ge) - **Spec Exp:** Colon Cancer Screening; Swallowing Disorders; **Hospital:** Phelps Meml Hosp Ctr (page 614); **Address:** 2005 Albany Post Rd, Ste 15, Croton-on-Hudson, NY 10520; **Phone:** 914-271-4212; **Board Cert:** Internal Medicine 1983; Gastroenterology 1989; **Med School:** Univ Nevada 1980; **Resid:** Internal Medicine, Brigham & Womens Hosp 1983; **Fellow:** Gastroenterology, Stanford Univ Med Ctr 1985

Wayne, Peter MD (Ge) - **Spec Exp:** Hepatitis; Pancreatic/Biliary Endoscopy (ERCP); Colonoscopy; **Hospital:** Saint Joseph's Med Ctr - Yonkers, St. John's Riverside Hosp-Andrus Pavil; **Address:** 469 N Broadway, Yonkers, NY 10701-1923; **Phone:** 914-969-1115; **Board Cert:** Internal Medicine 1979; Gastroenterology 1981; **Med School:** Albert Einstein Coll Med 1976; **Resid:** Internal Medicine, Montefiore Hosp Med Ctr 1979; **Fellow:** Gastroenterology, Mount Sinai Hosp 1981

Wolf, David C MD (Ge) - **Spec Exp:** Liver Failure; Transplant Medicine-Liver; Liver Disease; Endoscopy; **Hospital:** Westchester Med Ctr; **Address:** 100 Woods Rd, A Wing, Lower Level, Valhalla, NY 10595; **Phone:** 914-493-8916; **Board Cert:** Internal Medicine 1988; Gastroenterology 2011; Transplant Hepatology 2006; **Med School:** Columbia P&S 1985; **Resid:** Internal Medicine, NY Presby Hosp 1988; **Fellow:** Gastroenterology, Montefiore Med Ctr 1991; **Fac Appt:** Clin Prof Med, NY Med Coll

Geriatric Medicine

Banc, Tobe E MD (Ger) - **Hospital:** Phelps Meml Hosp Ctr (page 614); **Address:** 755 N Broadway, Sleepy Hollow, NY 10510; **Phone:** 914-366-3677; **Board Cert:** Internal Medicine 2010; **Med School:** NYU Sch Med 1993; **Resid:** Internal Medicine, Hartford Hosp 1996; **Fellow:** Geriatric Medicine, Mt Sinai Med Ctr 1998

Devons, Cathryn A MD (Ger) - **Spec Exp:** Alzheimer's Disease; Memory Disorders; **Hospital:** Phelps Meml Hosp Ctr (page 614); **Address:** 755 N Broadway, Sleepy Hollow, NY 10591; **Phone:** 914-366-3669; **Board Cert:** Geriatric Medicine 2004; **Med School:** Israel 1988; **Resid:** Internal Medicine, Montefiore Med Ctr 1991; **Fellow:** Geriatric Medicine, Mt Sinai Med Ctr 1993; **Fac Appt:** Asst Prof Med, Mount Sinai Sch Med

Escher, Jeffrey MD (Ger) - **Spec Exp:** Geriatric Care; **Hospital:** Saint Joseph's Med Ctr - Yonkers; **Address:** Geriatric Services, 69 S Broadway, Yonkers, NY 10701; **Phone:** 914-376-5555 x314-376-52; **Med School:** Belgium 1980; **Resid:** Internal Medicine, New Britain Gen Hosp 1983; **Fellow:** Geriatric Medicine, NYU Med Ctr 1985

Kalchthaler, Thomas DO (Ger) *PCP* - **Hospital:** Saint Joseph's Med Ctr - Yonkers; **Address:** 69 S Broadway, Yonkers, NY 10701-4004; **Phone:** 914-376-5555; **Board Cert:** Internal Medicine 1976; **Med School:** Chicago Coll Osteo Med 1971; **Resid:** Internal Medicine, Elmhurst Hosp 1975; **Fellow:** Geriatric Medicine, Elmhurst Hosp 1974; **Fac Appt:** Asst Prof Med, NY Med Coll

Martimucci, William A MD (Ger) *PCP* - **Spec Exp:** Geriatric Care; **Hospital:** White Plains Hosp (page 615); **Address:** Westchester Medical Group, 1 Theall Rd, Rye, NY 10580; **Phone:** 914-848-8700; **Board Cert:** Internal Medicine 1989; **Med School:** Grenada 1985; **Resid:** Internal Medicine, Caledonian Hosp 1988; **Fellow:** Geriatric Medicine, Mt Sinai Med Ctr 1990

Schor, Joshua D MD (Ger) - **Spec Exp:** Alzheimer's Disease; Stroke; Spinal Cord Injury; **Address:** 65 Circle Drive, Hastings-on-Hudson, NY 10706; **Phone:** 877-209-2041; **Board Cert:** Internal Medicine 1988; Geriatric Medicine 2011; **Med School:** Yale Univ 1985; **Resid:** Internal Medicine, Mass General Hosp 1988; **Fellow:** Geriatric Medicine, Beth Israel Med Ctr 1990

Vaughan, Margaret E MD (Ger) - **Hospital:** Northern Westchester Hosp (page 613); **Address:** 111 Bedford Rd, Katonah, NY 10536; **Phone:** 914-232-3135; **Board Cert:** Internal Medicine 2002; Geriatric Medicine 2003; **Med School:** SUNY Upstate Med Univ 1994; **Resid:** Anesthesiology, NY Presby-Cornell Med Ctr 1998; Internal Medicine, St Vincent's Catholic Med Ctr 2001; **Fellow:** Geriatric Medicine, St Vincent's Catholic Med Ctr 2002

Gynecologic Oncology

Chuang, Linus T MD (GO) - **Spec Exp:** Laparoscopic Surgery; Ovarian Cancer; Uterine Cancer; Cervical Cancer; **Hospital:** White Plains Hosp (page 615), Mount Sinai Med Ctr (page 102); **Address:** 15 N Broadway, Ste G, White Plains, NY 10601; **Phone:** 914-761-8901; **Board Cert:** Obstetrics & Gynecology 2009; Gynecologic Oncology 2097; **Med School:** Taiwan 1981; **Resid:** Obstetrics & Gynecology, Flushing Hosp 1990; **Fellow:** Gynecologic Oncology, MD Anderson Cancer Ctr 1994; **Fac Appt:** Assoc Prof ObG, Mount Sinai Sch Med

Gretz, Herbert F MD (GO) - **Spec Exp:** Gynecologic Cancer; Minimally Invasive Surgery; Robotic Surgery; **Hospital:** White Plains Hosp (page 615), Greenwich Hosp (page 892); **Address:** 2 Longview Ave, Ste 302, White Plains, NY 10601; **Phone:** 914-305-2730; **Board Cert:** Obstetrics & Gynecology 2010; Gynecologic Oncology 2010; **Med School:** NY Med Coll 1986; **Resid:** Obstetrics & Gynecology, NYU Med Ctr 1990; **Fellow:** Gynecologic Oncology, Univ Michigan 1993; **Fac Appt:** Assoc Prof ObG, Mount Sinai Sch Med

Hand Surgery

Fragner, Paul D MD (HS) - **Spec Exp:** Hand & Wrist Surgery; Elbow Surgery; **Hospital:** White Plains Hosp (page 615); **Address:** 7 Reservoir Rd, N White Plains, NY 10603; **Phone:** 914-684-0300; **Board Cert:** Orthopaedic Surgery 2006; Hand Surgery 2006; **Med School:** SUNY Upstate Med Univ 1986; **Resid:** Orthopaedic Surgery, SUNY Downstate Med Ctr 1991; **Fellow:** Hand Surgery, Hosp Univ Penn 1992

Magill Jr, Richard M MD (HS) - **Spec Exp:** Hand & Upper Extremity Surgery; Microvascular Surgery; Shoulder Surgery; **Hospital:** Westchester Med Ctr, Phelps Meml Hosp Ctr (page 614); **Address:** University Orthopaedics, 19 Bradhurst Ave, Ste 1300-N, Hawthorne, NY 10532; **Phone:** 914-789-2733; **Board Cert:** Orthopaedic Surgery 2006; Hand Surgery 2006; **Med School:** Temple Univ 1983; **Resid:** Surgery, Temple Univ Hosp 1985; Orthopaedic Surgery, Maimonides Med Ctr 1992; **Fellow:** Hand Surgery, Duke Univ Med Ctr 1993

Schefer, Alan MD (HS) - **Spec Exp:** Hand & Upper Extremity Surgery; **Hospital:** Northern Westchester Hosp (page 613); **Address:** Mt Kisco Medical Group, 90 S Bedford Rd, Mount Kisco, NY 10549; **Phone:** 914-241-1050; **Board Cert:** Orthopaedic Surgery 2009; Hand Surgery 2009; **Med School:** Hahnemann Univ 1990; **Resid:** Orthopaedic Surgery, Mt Sinai Med Ctr 1995; **Fellow:** Hand Surgery, Stony Brook Univ Hosp-SUNY 1996

Hematology

Lester, Thomas J MD (Hem) - **Spec Exp:** Lymphoma; Breast Cancer; **Hospital:** Northern Westchester Hosp (page 613); **Address:** Mt Kisco Medical Group, 90 S Bedford Rd, Mt Kisco, NY 10549; **Phone:** 914-242-2991; **Board Cert:** Internal Medicine 1982; Hematology 1984; Medical Oncology 1987; **Med School:** UMDNJ-Rutgers Med Sch 1979; **Resid:** Internal Medicine, Mt Sinai Hosp 1982; **Fellow:** Hematology, Mt Sinai Hosp 1984; Medical Oncology, Meml Sloan Kettering Cancer Ctr 1986

Nelson, John C MD (Hem) - **Hospital:** Westchester Med Ctr; **Address:** Westchester Hem/Onc Group, 19 Bradhurst Ave, Ste 2100, Hawthorne, NY 10532; **Phone:** 914-493-8353; **Board Cert:** Internal Medicine 1974; Hematology 1976; **Med School:** Harvard Med Sch 1971; **Resid:** Internal Medicine, Mt Sinai Med Ctr 1974; **Fellow:** Hematology, Westchester Med Ctr 1976; **Fac Appt:** Assoc Prof Med, NY Med Coll

Infectious Disease

Berkey, Peter MD (Inf) - **Spec Exp:** Immune Deficiency; Tick-borne Diseases; Travel Medicine; **Hospital:** St. John's Riverside Hosp-Andrus Pavil, Saint Joseph's Med Ctr - Yonkers; **Address:** 970 N Broadway, Ste 212, Yonkers, NY 10701-1311; **Phone:** 914-376-1543; **Board Cert:** Internal Medicine 1985; Infectious Disease 1988; **Med School:** Univ Puerto Rico 1980; **Resid:** Internal Medicine, Westchester Med Ctr 1984; **Fellow:** Infectious Disease, MD Anderson Cancer Ctr 1988

Kesh, Sandra MD (Inf) - **Hospital:** White Plains Hosp (page 615); **Address:** 210 Westchester Ave, WestMed Medical Group, White Plains, NY 10604; **Phone:** 914-682-6511; **Board Cert:** Internal Medicine 2003; Infectious Disease 2007; **Med School:** Cornell Univ-Weill Med Coll 2000; **Resid:** Internal Medicine, NY Presby-Cornell Med Ctr 2003; **Fellow:** Infectious Disease, NY Presby-Cornell Med Ctr 2007

Lederman, Jeffrey A MD (Inf) - **Spec Exp:** Travel Medicine; **Hospital:** Sound Shore Med Ctr - Westchester; **Address:** Sound Shore Medical Ctr, 16 Guion Pl Fl 2, New Rochelle, NY 10802; **Phone:** 914-637-1657; **Board Cert:** Internal Medicine 2000; Infectious Disease 2000; **Med School:** Jefferson Med Coll 1988; **Resid:** Internal Medicine, Mt Sinai Hosp 1991; **Fellow:** Infectious Disease, Montefiore Med Ctr 1995

Moorjani, Harish MD (Inf) - **Spec Exp:** Lyme Disease; AIDS/HIV; **Hospital:** Phelps Meml Hosp Ctr (page 614); **Address:** 127 Woodside Ave, Briarcliff Manor, NY 10510; **Phone:** 914-762-2276; **Board Cert:** Internal Medicine 1992; Infectious Disease 1994; **Med School:** India 1986; **Resid:** Internal Medicine, UMDNJ Med Ctr 1992; **Fellow:** Infectious Disease, Stony Brook Univ Med Ctr 1994

Nadelman, Robert MD (Inf) - **Spec Exp:** Tick-borne Diseases; Lyme Disease; **Hospital:** Westchester Med Ctr; **Address:** NY Med Coll, Div Infectious Disease, Munger Pavillion, rm 245, Valhalla, NY 10595; **Phone:** 914-493-8865; **Board Cert:** Internal Medicine 1983; Infectious Disease 1988; **Med School:** Albert Einstein Coll Med 1980; **Resid:** Internal Medicine, Beth Israel Hosp 1983; **Fellow:** Infectious Disease, Beth Israel Hosp 1985; **Fac Appt:** Prof Med, NY Med Coll

Raffalli, John T MD (Inf) - **Spec Exp:** Lyme Disease; Tick-borne Diseases; **Hospital:** Northern Westchester Hosp (page 613); **Address:** Mt Kisco Medical Group, 90 S Bedford Rd, Mount Kisco, NY 10549; **Phone:** 914-241-1050; **Board Cert:** Internal Medicine 2005; Infectious Disease 2005; **Med School:** SUNY Downstate 1989; **Resid:** Internal Medicine, NYU Med Ctr 1992; **Fellow:** Infectious Disease, Meml Sloan Kettering Cancer Ctr 1992; **Fac Appt:** Assoc Clin Prof Med, NY Med Coll

Rush, Thomas MD (Inf) - **Spec Exp:** AIDS/HIV; Lyme Disease; Travel Medicine; **Hospital:** Phelps Meml Hosp Ctr (page 614), Putnam Hosp Ctr; **Address:** 127 State Woodside Ave, Briarcliff Manor, NY 10510; **Phone:** 914-762-2276; **Board Cert:** Internal Medicine 1981; Infectious Disease 1984; **Med School:** Rush Med Coll 1978; **Resid:** Internal Medicine, Genesee Hosp 1981; **Fellow:** Infectious Disease, Strong Meml Hosp 1983; **Fac Appt:** Asst Clin Prof Med, NY Med Coll

Spicehandler, Debra MD (Inf) - **Hospital:** Northern Westchester Hosp (page 613); **Address:** 16 Bessel Ln, Chappaqua, NY 10514; **Phone:** 914-238-6330; **Board Cert:** Internal Medicine 1983; Infectious Disease 2007; **Med School:** Univ Cincinnati 1980; **Resid:** Internal Medicine, NYU Med Ctr 1983; **Fellow:** Infectious Disease, NYU Med Ctr 1985

Wormser, Gary P MD (Inf) - **Spec Exp:** Lyme Disease; AIDS/HIV; Diagnostic Problems; **Hospital:** Westchester Med Ctr; **Address:** New York Medical College, Munger Pavilion, rm 245, Valhalla, NY 10595; **Phone:** 914-493-8865; **Board Cert:** Internal Medicine 1978; Infectious Disease 1982; **Med School:** Johns Hopkins Univ 1972; **Resid:** Internal Medicine, Mt Sinai Hosp 1975; **Fellow:** Infectious Disease, Mt Sinai Hosp 1977; **Fac Appt:** Prof Med, NY Med Coll

Internal Medicine

Abenavoli, Tancredi J MD (IM) *PCP* - **Hospital:** White Plains Hosp (page 615); **Address:** 446 Westchester Ave, Port Chester, NY 10573; **Phone:** 914-939-1573; **Board Cert:** Internal Medicine 1979; Cardiovascular Disease 1981; **Med School:** NYU Sch Med 1976; **Resid:** Internal Medicine, VA Hosp/NYU Med Ctr 1979; **Fellow:** Cardiovascular Disease, VA Hosp/NYU Med Ctr 1981

Ades, Joseph R MD (IM) *PCP* - **Hospital:** Phelps Meml Hosp Ctr (page 614); **Address:** 150 White Plains Rd, Ste 207, Tarrytown, NY 10591; **Phone:** 914-631-2480; **Board Cert:** Internal Medicine 1985; **Med School:** Albert Einstein Coll Med 1982; **Resid:** Internal Medicine, LAC-USC Med Ctr 1986

Alpert, Barbara MD (IM) *PCP* - **Spec Exp:** Osteoporosis; Lyme Disease; **Hospital:** Northern Westchester Hosp (page 613); **Address:** 90 S Bedford Rd, Mt Kisco, NY 10549; **Phone:** 914-241-1050; **Board Cert:** Internal Medicine 1987; **Med School:** Univ Pennsylvania 1984; **Resid:** Internal Medicine, NY-Cornell Hosp 1987

Altholz, Jeffrey D MD (IM) *PCP* - **Spec Exp:** Occupational Medicine; Addiction/Substance Abuse; **Hospital:** Phelps Meml Hosp Ctr (page 614); **Address:** Westchester Medical Care, 160 S Central Ave, Elmsford, NY 10523; **Phone:** 914-345-3135; **Board Cert:** Internal Medicine 2003; **Med School:** Albert Einstein Coll Med 1986; **Resid:** Internal Medicine, St Vincents Hosp 1989; **Fellow:** Internal Medicine, St Vincents Hosp 1990

Beran, Nancy R MD (IM) *PCP* - **Spec Exp:** Women's Health; **Hospital:** Northern Westchester Hosp (page 613); **Address:** Internal Medicine for Women, 645 Marble Ave, Thornwood, NY 10594; **Phone:** 914-769-1600; **Board Cert:** Internal Medicine 2009; **Med School:** Thomas Jefferson Univ 1995; **Resid:** Internal Medicine, Parkland Meml Hosp 1998

Carosella, Christine MD (IM) *PCP* - **Spec Exp:** Hypertension; Asthma; Cholesterol/Lipid Disorders; **Hospital:** Westchester Med Ctr; **Address:** 19 Bradhurst Ave, Ste 3090 North, Hawthorne, NY 10532; **Phone:** 914-592-2400; **Board Cert:** Internal Medicine 2005; **Med School:** NY Med Coll 1992; **Resid:** Internal Medicine, Westchester Med Ctr 1995; **Fac Appt:** Asst Prof Med, NY Med Coll

Colangelo, Daniel MD (IM) *PCP* - **Hospital:** White Plains Hosp (page 615); **Address:** 1600 Harrison Ave, Ste G 105, Mamaroneck, NY 10543-3149; **Phone:** 914-698-4466; **Board Cert:** Internal Medicine 2004; **Med School:** NYU Sch Med 1980; **Resid:** Internal Medicine, Lenox Hill Hosp 1983

Croen, Kenneth MD (IM) *PCP* - **Spec Exp:** Infectious Disease; Herpes Simplex; **Hospital:** White Plains Hosp (page 615); **Address:** 600 Mamaroneck Ave, Ste 200, Harrison, NY 10583; **Phone:** 914-723-8100; **Board Cert:** Internal Medicine 1984; Infectious Disease 1988; **Med School:** Albert Einstein Coll Med 1980; **Resid:** Internal Medicine, Columbia-Presby Hosp 1983; Internal Medicine, Presby Hosp 1984; **Fellow:** Infectious Disease, Natl Inst Hlth 1989

Dennett, Ronald MD (IM) *PCP* - **Hospital:** Lawrence Hosp Ctr, Montefiore Med Ctr-Moses Campus, NY (page 100); **Address:** 73 Market St, Yonkers, NY 10710; **Phone:** 914-831-6840; **Board Cert:** Internal Medicine 1980; **Med School:** Univ VT Coll Med 1977; **Resid:** Internal Medicine, Univ Colorado Hosp 1980; **Fac Appt:** Asst Clin Prof Med, Albert Einstein Coll Med

Engelhardt III, Martin B DO (IM) *PCP* - **Hospital:** Sound Shore Med Ctr - Westchester; **Address:** North Ridge Medical Group, 77 Quaker Ridge Rd, New Rochelle, NY 10804; **Phone:** 914-235-8224; **Board Cert:** Internal Medicine 2009; **Med School:** Philadelphia Coll Osteo Med 1993; **Resid:** Internal Medicine, Montefiore Med Ctr 1998

Ennis, David T MD (IM) *PCP* - **Hospital:** Northern Westchester Hosp (page 613); **Address:** Westchester Health Assocs, 1838 Commerce St, Yorktown Heights, NY 10598-4400; **Phone:** 914-962-3500; **Board Cert:** Internal Medicine 1986; **Med School:** NY Med Coll 1983; **Resid:** Internal Medicine, Westchester Co Med Ctr 1986

Fazio, Nelson M MD (IM) *PCP* - **Spec Exp:** Skin Diseases; Hypertension; Obesity; Infectious Disease; **Hospital:** Lawrence Hosp Ctr; **Address:** 133 Montgomery Ave, Scarsdale, NY 10583; **Phone:** 914-713-8517; **Board Cert:** Internal Medicine 1986; **Med School:** NY Med Coll 1981; **Resid:** Internal Medicine, Westchester Co Med Ctr 1984; **Fellow:** Infectious Disease, Montefiore Hosp Med Ctr 1994

Fenster, Mitchell MD (IM) *PCP* - **Hospital:** White Plains Hosp (page 615); **Address:** 401 Columbus Ave, Valhalla, NY 10595; **Phone:** 914-769-0268; **Board Cert:** Internal Medicine 1987; **Med School:** Mount Sinai Sch Med 1981; **Resid:** Internal Medicine, Bellevue Med Ctr 1984

Fiorentino, Thomas MD (IM) - **Spec Exp:** Palliative Care; **Hospital:** St. John's Riverside Hosp-Andrus Pavil, Mount Sinai Med Ctr (page 102); **Address:** 984 N Broadway, Ste 303, Yonkers, NY 10701; **Phone:** 914-969-0770; **Board Cert:** Internal Medicine 1975; Hospice & Palliative Medicine 2008; **Med School:** NY Med Coll 1972; **Resid:** Internal Medicine, Metropolitan Hosp 1976

Goldman, Jack S MD (IM) *PCP* - **Spec Exp:** Colonoscopy/Polypectomy; Liver Disease; Endoscopy; **Hospital:** Saint Joseph's Med Ctr - Yonkers, Montefiore Med Ctr-Moses Campus, NY (page 100); **Address:** 750 McLean Ave, Yonkers, NY 10704; **Phone:** 914-237-8686; **Board Cert:** Internal Medicine 1975; Gastroenterology 1979; **Med School:** Albert Einstein Coll Med 1961; **Resid:** Internal Medicine, Bronx Lebanon Hosp 1963; Internal Medicine, VA Med Ctr 1966; **Fellow:** Gastroenterology, VA Med Ctr 1965

Gross, Jeffrey D MD (IM) *PCP* - **Hospital:** Northern Westchester Hosp (page 613); **Address:** Mt Kisco Medical Group, 90 S Bedford Rd, Mt Kisco, NY 10549; **Phone:** 914-241-1050; **Board Cert:** Internal Medicine 2005; **Med School:** SUNY Hlth Sci Ctr 1992; **Resid:** Internal Medicine, Montefiore Med Ctr 1996

Herzog, David A MD (IM) *PCP* - **Spec Exp:** Cholesterol/Lipid Disorders; Preventive Medicine; **Hospital:** White Plains Hosp (page 615), Sound Shore Med Ctr - Westchester; **Address:** 1 Theall Rd, Ste 204, Rye, NY 10580; **Phone:** 914-848-8700; **Board Cert:** Internal Medicine 1984; **Med School:** Mount Sinai Sch Med 1981; **Resid:** Internal Medicine, St Luke's Hosp 1984; **Fac Appt:** Asst Clin Prof Med, NY Med Coll

Higgins, William J MD (IM) *PCP* - **Spec Exp:** Alzheimer's Disease; Geriatric Medicine; **Hospital:** Hudson Valley Hosp Ctr; **Address:** Westchester Medical Practice, 2050 Saw Mill River Rd, Ste 1, Yorktown Heights, NY 10598; **Phone:** 914-962-5533; **Board Cert:** Internal Medicine 2002; **Med School:** Geo Wash Univ 1986; **Resid:** Internal Medicine, Lenox Hill Hosp 1989; **Fellow:** Pulmonary Disease, Lenox Hill Hosp 1991; **Fac Appt:** Assoc Clin Prof Med, NY Med Coll

Hopkins, Arthur MD (IM) *PCP* - **Hospital:** Montefiore Med Ctr-Moses Campus, NY (page 100); **Address:** 1010 Central Park Ave, Yonkers, NY 10704; **Phone:** 914-964-4183; **Board Cert:** Internal Medicine 1986; **Med School:** Univ Pennsylvania 1983; **Resid:** Internal Medicine, Hosp Univ Penn 1986; **Fac Appt:** Asst Prof Med, Albert Einstein Coll Med

Isaacs, Ellen S MD (IM) *PCP* - **Spec Exp:** Hypertension; Heart Disease; **Hospital:** St. John's Riverside Hosp-Andrus Pavil, Saint Joseph's Med Ctr - Yonkers; **Address:** 1019 Yonkers Ave, Yonkers, NY 10704; **Phone:** 914-963-9493; **Board Cert:** Internal Medicine 1972; Cardiovascular Disease 1981; **Med School:** NYU Sch Med 1969; **Resid:** Internal Medicine, Bellevue Hosp 1972; **Fellow:** Cardiovascular Disease, St Vincents Hosp Med Ctr 1974; **Fac Appt:** Asst Prof Med, NY Med Coll

Kapoor, Satish MD (IM) *PCP* - **Spec Exp:** Asthma; Emphysema; Preventive Medicine; **Hospital:** Phelps Meml Hosp Ctr (page 614); **Address:** 362 N Broadway Fl 2, Sleepy Hollow, NY 10591-1040; **Phone:** 914-631-2070; **Board Cert:** Internal Medicine 1979; **Med School:** India 1972; **Resid:** Internal Medicine, Kingsbrook Jewish MC 1979; **Fellow:** Pulmonary Disease, Queens Hosp 1981

Karmen, Carol L MD (IM) *PCP* - **Spec Exp:** Preventive Medicine; **Hospital:** Westchester Med Ctr; **Address:** 19 Bradhurst Ave, Ste 3090 North, Hawthorne, NY 10532; **Phone:** 914-592-2400; **Board Cert:** Internal Medicine 2007; **Med School:** Albert Einstein Coll Med 1986; **Resid:** Internal Medicine, Westchester Med Ctr 1990; **Fac Appt:** Assoc Prof Med, NY Med Coll

Krieger, Sharon MD (IM) *PCP* - **Hospital:** Northern Westchester Hosp (page 613); **Address:** Mt Kisco Medical Group, 90 S Bedford Rd, Mt Kisco, NY 10549-3422; **Phone:** 914-241-1050; **Board Cert:** Internal Medicine 2004; **Med School:** Louisiana State U, New Orleans 1991; **Resid:** Internal Medicine, NY Presby-Cornell Med Ctr 1994

Kubersky, Steven MD (IM) *PCP* - **Hospital:** Lawrence Hosp Ctr; **Address:** WestMed Med Grp, Ridge Hill, 73 Market St Fl 2, Yonkers, NY 10710; **Phone:** 914-831-6860; **Board Cert:** Internal Medicine 2002; **Med School:** NYU Sch Med 1988; **Resid:** Internal Medicine, Mount Sinai Med Ctr 1992

Lebofsky, Martin MD (IM) - **Spec Exp:** Kidney Disease; Hypertension; Dialysis Care; **Hospital:** Lawrence Hosp Ctr, Saint Joseph's Med Ctr - Yonkers; **Address:** 1 Stone Pl, Bronxville, NY 10708-3406; **Phone:** 914-337-9004; **Board Cert:** Internal Medicine 1975; Nephrology 1978; **Med School:** Albert Einstein Coll Med 1972; **Resid:** Internal Medicine, Harlem Hosp 1975; **Fellow:** Nephrology, Montefiore Med Ctr 1978

Lechner, Michael MD (IM) *PCP* - **Spec Exp:** Geriatric Medicine; Geriatric Rehabilitation; **Hospital:** Phelps Meml Hosp Ctr (page 614); **Address:** 14 Church St, Ste 208, Ossining, NY 10562-4831; **Phone:** 914-762-0722; **Board Cert:** Internal Medicine 1980; **Med School:** Albert Einstein Coll Med 1961; **Resid:** Internal Medicine, Westchester Med Ctr 1964; **Fellow:** Hematology, LI Jewish Med Ctr 1965

Margulis, Steven M MD (IM) *PCP* - **Hospital:** Northern Westchester Hosp (page 613); **Address:** Mt Kisco Med Grp, 90 S Bedford Rd, Mt Kisco, NY 10549; **Phone:** 914-241-1050; **Board Cert:** Internal Medicine 2010; **Med School:** Albert Einstein Coll Med 1997; **Resid:** Internal Medicine, Mt Sinai Med Ctr 2000

Melman, Martin MD (IM) *PCP* - **Spec Exp:** Hypertension; Asthma; Geriatric Medicine; **Hospital:** Phelps Meml Hosp Ctr (page 614); **Address:** 87 Grand St, Croton On Hudson, NY 10520-2518; **Phone:** 914-271-4845; **Board Cert:** Internal Medicine 1977; **Med School:** NY Med Coll 1974; **Resid:** Internal Medicine, Metropolitan Hosp Ctr 1977; Internal Medicine, Westchester Med Ctr 1978; **Fac Appt:** Asst Clin Prof Med, NY Med Coll

Pappas, Steven MD (IM) *PCP* - **Spec Exp:** Occupational Medicine; Preventive Medicine; **Hospital:** Sound Shore Med Ctr - Westchester; **Address:** 266 White Plains Rd, Ste 1A, Eastchester, NY 10709; **Phone:** 914-793-1115; **Board Cert:** Internal Medicine 1982; **Med School:** Albert Einstein Coll Med 1978; **Resid:** Internal Medicine, St Luke's Roosevelt Hosp Ctr 1981

Peterson, Stephen J MD (IM) *PCP* - **Spec Exp:** Weight Management; **Hospital:** Westchester Med Ctr; **Address:** NY Med College, Munger Pavilion 256, 95 Grasslands Rd, Valhalla, NY 10595; **Phone:** 914-493-8370; **Board Cert:** Internal Medicine 1985; **Med School:** Philippines 1982; **Resid:** Internal Medicine, Metropolitan Hosp Ctr 1986; **Fac Appt:** Prof Med, NY Med Coll

Pomerantz, Daniel MD (IM) *PCP* - **Spec Exp:** Palliative Care; Ethics; **Hospital:** Sound Shore Med Ctr - Westchester; **Address:** 16 Guion Pl, Goldstein Ambulatory Care Center, New Rochelle, NY 10802; **Phone:** 914-365-3615; **Board Cert:** Internal Medicine 2003; Hospice & Palliative Medicine 2010; **Med School:** Harvard Med Sch 1990; **Resid:** Internal Medicine, NYU Med Ctr 1994; **Fac Appt:** Asst Clin Prof Med, NY Med Coll

Ridge, Gerald A MD (IM) *PCP* - **Spec Exp:** Geriatric Medicine; **Hospital:** Lawrence Hosp Ctr, NY-Presby/Columbia Univ Med Ctr, NY (page 104); **Address:** Lawrence Medical Assocs, 685 White Plains Rd, Eastchester, NY 10709; **Phone:** 914-787-4100; **Board Cert:** Internal Medicine 2008; Geriatric Medicine 2008; **Med School:** UCSF 1979; **Resid:** Internal Medicine, Bronx Muni Hosp Ctr 1981; Neurology, Columbia-Presby Med Ctr 1982; **Fellow:** Internal Medicine, New York Hosp 1983; **Fac Appt:** Clin Prof Med, Columbia P&S

Rosch, Elliott MD (IM) *PCP* - **Spec Exp:** Preventive Medicine; Cholesterol/Lipid Disorders; Hypertension; Weight Management; **Hospital:** St. John's Riverside Hosp-Andrus Pavil, Mount Sinai Med Ctr (page 102); **Address:** 1010 N Broadway, Yonkers, NY 10701-1303; **Phone:** 914-965-4424; **Board Cert:** Internal Medicine 1981; **Med School:** Univ Pennsylvania 1978; **Resid:** Internal Medicine, Pennsylvania Hosp 1981; **Fac Appt:** Asst Prof Med, Mount Sinai Sch Med

Saltzman-Gabelman, Lori MD (IM) *PCP* - **Hospital:** White Plains Hosp (page 615), Greenwich Hosp (page 892); **Address:** 210 Westchester Ave Fl 2, White Plains, NY 10604-2914; **Phone:** 914-682-0700; **Board Cert:** Internal Medicine 1989; **Med School:** NY Med Coll 1986; **Resid:** Internal Medicine, Westchester Med Ctr 1989; **Fac Appt:** , NY Med Coll

Soltren, Rafael MD (IM) *PCP* - **Spec Exp:** Diabetes; Hypertension; **Hospital:** Phelps Meml Hosp Ctr (page 614); **Address:** 100 S Highland Ave, Ossining, NY 10562; **Phone:** 914-941-1277; **Board Cert:** Internal Medicine 1985; **Med School:** Cornell Univ-Weill Med Coll 1981; **Resid:** Internal Medicine, Montefiore Med Ctr 1984

Starke, Charles L MD (IM) *PCP* - **Hospital:** Phelps Meml Hosp Ctr (page 614), Westchester Med Ctr; **Address:** 302 W Chappaqua Rd, Briarcliff Manor, NY 10510-1526; **Phone:** 914-762-4460; **Board Cert:** Internal Medicine 1978; **Med School:** Albert Einstein Coll Med 1975; **Resid:** Internal Medicine, Georgetown Univ Hosp 1978; **Fac Appt:** Prof Med, Columbia P&S

Tang, David J MD (IM) *PCP* - **Hospital:** St. John's Riverside Hosp-Andrus Pavil, Mount Sinai Med Ctr (page 102); **Address:** Mount Sinai Riverside Group, 750 Kimball Ave, Yonkers, NY 10704; **Phone:** 914-237-6763; **Board Cert:** Internal Medicine 2005; **Med School:** Meharry Med Coll 2002; **Resid:** Internal Medicine, LIJ Med Ctr 2005

Turro, James J MD (IM) *PCP* - **Hospital:** Northern Westchester Hosp (page 613); **Address:** 90 S Bedford Rd, Mt Kisco, NY 10549; **Phone:** 914-241-1050; **Board Cert:** Internal Medicine 1985; **Med School:** Cornell Univ-Weill Med Coll 1982; **Resid:** Internal Medicine, Bronx Muni Hosp 1986

Warshafsky, Stephen MD (IM) *PCP* - **Spec Exp:** Lyme Disease; Cholesterol/Lipid Disorders; Preventive Cardiology; Preventive Medicine; **Hospital:** Westchester Med Ctr; **Address:** 1055 Saw Mill River Rd, Ste 206, Ardsley, NY 10502; **Phone:** 914-591-0733; **Board Cert:** Internal Medicine 2004; **Med School:** NY Med Coll 1989; **Resid:** Internal Medicine, Westchester Med Ctr/NY Med Coll 1992; **Fac Appt:** Assoc Clin Prof Med, NY Med Coll

Wolfe, Mary J MD (IM) *PCP* - **Hospital:** Phelps Meml Hosp Ctr (page 614); **Address:** 14 Church St, Ossining, NY 10562; **Phone:** 914-941-1334; **Board Cert:** Internal Medicine 1980; **Med School:** Penn State Coll Med 1976; **Resid:** Internal Medicine, Westchester Med Ctr 1979

Wolfson, Robert A MD (IM) *PCP* - **Hospital:** Northern Westchester Hosp (page 613); **Address:** 90 S Bedford Rd, Mount Kisco, NY 10549; **Phone:** 914-241-1050; **Board Cert:** Internal Medicine 1980; **Med School:** SUNY Downstate 1977; **Resid:** Internal Medicine, Kings Co Hosp 1981

Zarowitz, William MD (IM) *PCP* - **Spec Exp:** Occupational Medicine; Preventive Medicine; **Hospital:** White Plains Hosp (page 615); **Address:** 143 Maple Ave, White Plains, NY 10601; **Phone:** 914-683-8610; **Board Cert:** Internal Medicine 1981; **Med School:** NY Med Coll 1978; **Resid:** Internal Medicine, Montefiore Med Ctr 1981; **Fac Appt:** Assoc Clin Prof Med, NY Med Coll

Interventional Cardiology

Hjemdahl-Monsen, Craig MD (IC) - **Hospital:** NY-Presby/Columbia Univ Med Ctr, NY (page 104); **Address:** 19 Bradhurst Ave, Ste 700, Hawthorne, NY 10532; **Phone:** 914-593-7800; **Board Cert:** Internal Medicine 1983; Cardiovascular Disease 1985; Interventional Cardiology 2009; **Med School:** Johns Hopkins Univ 1980; **Resid:** Internal Medicine, Univ Hosp 1983; **Fellow:** Cardiovascular Disease, Mount Sinai Med Ctr 1985; Interventional Cardiology, Mount Sinai Med Ctr 1987; **Fac Appt:** Asst Clin Prof Med, Columbia P&S

Messinger, David MD (IC) - **Spec Exp:** Coronary Angioplasty/Stents; **Hospital:** NY-Presby/Weill Cornell Med Ctr, NY (page 104), Sound Shore Med Ctr - Westchester; **Address:** Sound-shore Cardiology Associates, 175 Memorial Hwy, New Rochelle, NY 10801; **Phone:** 914-235-3535; **Board Cert:** Cardiovascular Disease 2005; Interventional Cardiology 2009; **Med School:** Cornell Univ-Weill Med Coll 1987; **Resid:** Internal Medicine, NY-Presby/Weill Cornell Med Ctr 1990; **Fellow:** Cardiovascular Disease, NY-Presby/Weill Cornell Med Ctr 1993; Interventional Cardiology, NY-Presby/Weill Cornell Med Ctr 1994

Weiss, Melvin MD (IC) - **Spec Exp:** Cardiac Imaging; Congestive Heart Failure; Diabetes & Heart Disease; Coronary Artery Disease; **Hospital:** NY-Presby/Columbia Univ Med Ctr, NY (page 104), White Plains Hosp (page 615); **Address:** Columbia Doctors Medical Group, 19 Bradhurst Ave, Ste 700, Hawthorne, NY 10532-2140; **Phone:** 914-593-7800; **Board Cert:** Internal Medicine 1972; Cardiovascular Disease 1975; **Med School:** SUNY Hlth Sci Ctr 1967; **Resid:** Internal Medicine, NY Hosp 1971; **Fellow:** Cardiovascular Disease, NY Presby Med Ctr 1972; **Fac Appt:** Prof Med, NY Med Coll

Maternal & Fetal Medicine

Berck, David J MD (MF) - **Spec Exp:** Ultrasound; Pregnancy-High Risk; **Hospital:** Northern Westchester Hosp (page 613); **Address:** Mount Kisco Medical Group, 90 S Bedford Rd, Mount Kisco, NY 10549; **Phone:** 914-241-1050; **Board Cert:** Obstetrics & Gynecology 1999; Maternal & Fetal Medicine 2001; **Med School:** Harvard Med Sch 1991; **Resid:** Obstetrics & Gynecology, Mass Genl Hosp 1995; **Fellow:** Maternal & Fetal Medicine, Columbia Presby Med Ctr 1998

Devine, Patricia Ann MD (MF) - **Spec Exp:** Pregnancy-High Risk; Prenatal Diagnosis; Diabetes in Pregnancy; Premature Labor; **Hospital:** Sound Shore Med Ctr - Westchester; **Address:** Sound Shore Antenatal Testing Lab, 16 Guion Place Fl 4, New Rochelle, NY 10802; **Phone:** 914-365-4263; **Board Cert:** Obstetrics & Gynecology 2010; Maternal & Fetal Medicine 2010; **Med School:** Mount Sinai Sch Med 1987; **Resid:** Obstetrics & Gynecology, Beth Israel Med Ctr 1991; **Fellow:** Maternal & Fetal Medicine, Westchester Co Med Ctr 1993; **Fac Appt:** Assoc Clin Prof ObG, NY Med Coll

Lescale, Keith B MD (MF) - **Spec Exp:** Pregnancy-High Risk; Prenatal Diagnosis; Fetal Ultrasound/Obstetrical Imaging; **Hospital:** White Plains Hosp (page 615), Phelps Meml Hosp Ctr (page 614); **Address:** Hudson Valley Perinatal Consulting, 600 Mamaroneck Ave, Ste 110, Harrison, NY 10528-1647; **Phone:** 914-670-0500; **Board Cert:** Obstetrics & Gynecology 2008; Maternal & Fetal Medicine 2008; **Med School:** Louisiana State U, New Orleans 1987; **Resid:** Obstetrics & Gynecology, New Orleans/LSU Med Ctr 1991; **Fellow:** Maternal & Fetal Medicine, NY Hosp-Cornell Med Ctr 1994

Mootabar, Hamid MD (MF) - **Spec Exp:** Pregnancy-High Risk; **Hospital:** Lawrence Hosp Ctr, NY-Presby/Columbia Univ Med Ctr, NY (page 104); **Address:** Amniocentesis & Genetics Ctr, 77 Pondfield Rd, Bronxville, NY 10708; **Phone:** 914-337-2102; **Board Cert:** Obstetrics & Gynecology 1975; Maternal & Fetal Medicine 1983; **Med School:** Iran 1966; **Resid:** Obstetrics & Gynecology, Roosevelt Hosp 1973; **Fellow:** Maternal & Fetal Medicine, Roosevelt Hosp 1979; **Fac Appt:** Assoc Clin Prof ObG, Columbia P&S

Medical Oncology

Ahmed, Tauseef MD (Onc) - **Spec Exp:** Bone Marrow Transplant; Lymphoma; Brain Tumors; Genitourinary Cancer; **Hospital:** Westchester Med Ctr; **Address:** 19 Bradhurst Ave, Ste 2100, Hawthorne, NY 10532; **Phone:** 914-493-8353; **Board Cert:** Internal Medicine 1980; Hematology 1982; Medical Oncology 1983; **Med School:** Pakistan 1976; **Resid:** Internal Medicine, Mt Sinai Hosp 1980; **Fellow:** Medical Oncology, Meml Sloan Kettering Cancer Ctr 1983; **Fac Appt:** Prof Med, NY Med Coll

Bernhardt, Bernard MD (Onc) - **Spec Exp:** Lung Cancer; Lymphoma; Leukemia-Chronic Lymphocytic; Anemias & Red Cell Disorders; **Hospital:** Sound Shore Med Ctr - Westchester, Montefiore Med Ctr-Einstein Campus, NY (page 100); **Address:** Advanced Oncology Assocs, 50 Guion Pl, Ste 32, New Rochelle, NY 10801-5512; **Phone:** 914-632-5397; **Board Cert:** Internal Medicine 1968; Hematology 1972; Medical Oncology 1973; **Med School:** Northwestern Univ 1961; **Resid:** Internal Medicine, DC Genl Hosp 1963; Internal Medicine, NY Med Coll 1966; **Fellow:** Hematology, Montefiore Hosp Med Ctr 1968; **Fac Appt:** Clin Prof Med, NY Med Coll

Caron, Philip C MD/PhD (Onc) - **Spec Exp:** Lymphoma; Gastrointestinal Cancer; **Hospital:** Meml Sloan-Kettering Cancer Ctr (page 116), Phelps Meml Hosp Ctr (page 614); **Address:** Meml Sloan Kettering at Phelps Meml Hosp, 777 N Broadway, Ste 102, Sleepy Hollow, NY 10591; **Phone:** 914-366-0664; **Board Cert:** Internal Medicine 1989; Medical Oncology 2003; Hematology 2007; **Med School:** NY Med Coll 1986; **Resid:** Internal Medicine, Mt Sinai Hosp 1989; **Fellow:** Hematology & Oncology, Meml Sloan Kettering Cancer Ctr 1992

Feldman, Stuart P MD (Onc) - **Spec Exp:** Breast Cancer; Lymphoma; **Hospital:** White Plains Hosp (page 615), Greenwich Hosp (page 892); **Address:** 210 Westchester Ave, White Plains, NY 10604-2901; **Phone:** 914-681-5200; **Board Cert:** Internal Medicine 1980; Hematology 1982; Medical Oncology 1985; **Med School:** Geo Wash Univ 1977; **Resid:** Internal Medicine, New York Hosp-Cornell 1980; **Fellow:** Hematology & Oncology, Meml Sloan Kettering Cancer Ctr 1983; **Fac Appt:** Asst Clin Prof Med, Cornell Univ-Weill Med Coll

Fialk, Mark A MD (Onc) - **Hospital:** White Plains Hosp (page 615), Westchester Med Ctr; **Address:** 600 Mamaroneck Ave, Harrison, NY 10528; **Phone:** 914-723-8100; **Board Cert:** Internal Medicine 1976; Medical Oncology 1977; Hematology 1978; **Med School:** Tufts Univ 1973; **Resid:** Internal Medicine, NY Hosp-Cornell Med Ctr 1975; Internal Medicine, Meml Sloan-Kettering Cancer Ctr 1976; **Fellow:** Hematology & Oncology, NY Hosp-Cornell Med Ctr 1978; Infectious Disease, Meml Sloan-Kettering Cancer Ctr 1979; **Fac Appt:** Asst Clin Prof Med, NY Med Coll

Goldberg, Jonathan S MD (Onc) - **Spec Exp:** Breast Cancer; Lymphoma; Gastrointestinal Cancer; Lung Cancer; **Hospital:** Northern Westchester Hosp (page 613), Putnam Hosp Ctr; **Address:** Mount Kisco Medical Group, 400 E Main St, Mount Kisco, NY 10549; **Phone:** 914-242-2991; **Board Cert:** Internal Medicine 2007; Hematology 2011; Medical Oncology 2011; **Med School:** Mount Sinai Sch Med 1994; **Resid:** Internal Medicine, NY Presby Med Ctr 1997; **Fellow:** Hematology & Oncology, NY Presby Med Ctr 1999

Halaas, Jeffrey L MD (Onc) - **Hospital:** Northern Westchester Hosp (page 613), Putnam Hosp Ctr; **Address:** Mt Kisco Medical Group, 90 S Bedford Rd, Mt Kisco, NY 10549; **Phone:** 914-241-1050; **Board Cert:** Internal Medicine 2002; Medical Oncology 2005; Hematology 2005; **Med School:** Cornell Univ-Weill Med Coll 1999; **Resid:** Internal Medicine, NY Presby Hosp 2001; **Fellow:** Hematology & Oncology, Meml Sloan Kettering Cancer Ctr 2005

Liu, DeLong MD/PhD (Onc) - **Spec Exp:** Lung Cancer; Leukemia; Bone Marrow Transplant; Lymphoma; **Hospital:** Westchester Med Ctr; **Address:** 19 Bradhurst Ave, Hawthorne, NY 10532; **Phone:** 914-493-8374; **Board Cert:** Internal Medicine 2006; Medical Oncology 2011; Hematology 2002; **Med School:** China 1984; **Resid:** Internal Medicine, Montefiore Med Ctr 1996; **Fellow:** Hematology & Oncology, Meml Sloan Kettering Cancer Ctr 1998; **Fac Appt:** Prof Med, NY Med Coll

Mills, Nancy Ellyn MD (Onc) - **Spec Exp:** Breast Cancer; Gynecologic Cancer; **Hospital:** Phelps Meml Hosp Ctr (page 614), Meml Sloan-Kettering Cancer Ctr (page 116); **Address:** Meml Sloan Kettering @ Sleepy Hollow, 777 N Broadway, Ste 102, Sleepy Hollow, NY 10591; **Phone:** 914-366-0664; **Board Cert:** Internal Medicine 2000; Medical Oncology 2003; Hematology 2004; **Med School:** Mount Sinai Sch Med 1987; **Resid:** Internal Medicine, Mt Sinai Med Ctr 1990; **Fellow:** Hematology & Oncology, NYU Med Ctr 1993; **Fac Appt:** Asst Clin Prof Med, Cornell Univ-Weill Med Coll

Phillips, Elizabeth MD (Onc) - **Spec Exp:** Breast Cancer; Hematology; Lymphoma; Leukemia; **Hospital:** Sound Shore Med Ctr - Westchester, Montefiore Med Ctr-Moses Campus, NY (page 100); **Address:** Advanced Oncology Assocs, 50 Guion Pl, Ste 32, New Rochelle, NY 10801-4914; **Phone:** 914-632-5397; **Board Cert:** Internal Medicine 1974; Hematology 1976; Medical Oncology 1977; **Med School:** Univ Wash 1969; **Resid:** Internal Medicine, Harlem Hosp 1972; Hematology, Montefiore Med Ctr 1973; **Fellow:** Hematology & Oncology, Mem Sloan Kettering Canc Ctr 1976; **Fac Appt:** Assoc Clin Prof Med, NY Med Coll

Provenzano, Anthony F MD (Onc) - **Spec Exp:** Lung Cancer; Breast Cancer; Cancer Genetics; Gastrointestinal Cancer; **Hospital:** Lawrence Hosp Ctr, Mount Vernon Hosp; **Address:** 1 Pondfield Rd W, Ste 1, Bronxville, NY 10708-2635; **Phone:** 914-961-3421; **Board Cert:** Internal Medicine 1979; Medical Oncology 1981; **Med School:** Cornell Univ-Weill Med Coll 1976; **Resid:** Internal Medicine, Lenox Hill Hosp 1978; **Fellow:** Medical Oncology, St Vincents Hosp 1979; Medical Oncology, Lenox Hill Hosp 1981; **Fac Appt:** Asst Clin Prof Med, NY Med Coll

Puccio, Carmelo A MD (Onc) - **Spec Exp:** Breast Cancer; Lung Cancer; Solid Tumors; Gynecologic Cancer; **Hospital:** Westchester Med Ctr, Sound Shore Med Ctr - Westchester; **Address:** 19 Bradhurst Ave, Ste 2100, Hawthorne, NY 10532; **Phone:** 914-493-8353; **Board Cert:** Internal Medicine 1984; Medical Oncology 1989; **Med School:** Mexico 1979; **Resid:** Internal Medicine, Maimonides Med Ctr 1984; **Fellow:** Medical Oncology, Westchester Co Med Ctr 1985; **Fac Appt:** Asst Prof Med, NY Med Coll

Rosen, Norman MD (Onc) - **Spec Exp:** Lung Cancer; Breast Cancer; **Hospital:** St. John's Riverside Hosp-Andrus Pavil; **Address:** 984 N Broadway, Ste 311, Yonkers, NY 10701-1308; **Phone:** 914-965-2060; **Board Cert:** Internal Medicine 1975; Medical Oncology 1977; **Med School:** Tufts Univ 1972; **Resid:** Internal Medicine, Montefiore Med Ctr 1975; **Fellow:** Hematology & Oncology, Montefiore Med Ctr 1977; **Fac Appt:** Asst Clin Prof Med, Albert Einstein Coll Med

Sadan, Sara MD (Onc) - **Spec Exp:** Hematology; **Hospital:** White Plains Hosp (page 615); **Address:** 244 Westchester Ave, Ste 411, White Plains, NY 10604; **Phone:** 914-684-8100; **Board Cert:** Internal Medicine 2002; Medical Oncology 2005; **Med School:** Israel 1984; **Resid:** Internal Medicine, St Luke's-Roosevelt Hosp Ctr 1991; **Fellow:** Hematology & Oncology, Meml Sloan Kettering Cancer Ctr 1994

Saponara, Eduardo M MD (Onc) - **Spec Exp:** Breast Cancer; Hematology; Lymphoma; Multiple Myeloma; **Hospital:** Lawrence Hosp Ctr, Mount Sinai Med Ctr (page 102); **Address:** 77 Pondfield Rd, Bronxville, NY 10708-3809; **Phone:** 914-793-1500; **Board Cert:** Internal Medicine 1977; Hematology 1978; Medical Oncology 1979; **Med School:** Peru 1973; **Resid:** Internal Medicine, Westchester Med Ctr 1976; **Fellow:** Hematology & Oncology, Flower Fifth Ave Hospital/NY Med Coll 1978; Oncology, Mount Sinai Hosp 1979; **Fac Appt:** Asst Clin Prof Onc, NY Med Coll

Schneider, Robert Jay MD (Onc) - **Spec Exp:** Breast Cancer; Genitourinary Cancer; **Hospital:** Northern Westchester Hosp (page 613), Westchester Med Ctr; **Address:** 101 S Bedford, Ste 202A, Mt Kisco, NY 10549-3456; **Phone:** 914-666-8976; **Board Cert:** Internal Medicine 1979; Medical Oncology 1985; **Med School:** Albert Einstein Coll Med 1975; **Resid:** Internal Medicine, Jacobi Med Ctr 1978; **Fellow:** Medical Oncology, Meml Sloan Kettering Cancer Ctr 1980

Seiter, Karen MD (Onc) - **Spec Exp:** Hematologic Malignancies; Leukemia; Myelodysplastic Syndromes; **Hospital:** Westchester Med Ctr; **Address:** 19 Bradhurst Ave, Ste 2100, Hawthorne, NY 10532; **Phone:** 914-493-8353; **Board Cert:** Internal Medicine 1988; Medical Oncology 2011; Hematology 2002; **Med School:** NY Med Coll 1985; **Resid:** Internal Medicine, Albert Einstein Hosp 1988; **Fellow:** Hematology & Oncology, Meml Sloan Kettering Cancer Ctr 1991; **Fac Appt:** Prof Med, NY Med Coll

Wasserheit, Carolyn MD (Onc) - **Spec Exp:** Solid Tumors; Breast Cancer; Gynecologic Cancer; **Hospital:** Meml Sloan-Kettering Cancer Ctr (page 116); **Address:** Memorial Sloan Kettering @ Sleepy Hollow, 777 N Broadway, Ste 102, Sleepy Hollow, NY 10591; **Phone:** 914-366-0664; **Board Cert:** Internal Medicine 1988; Medical Oncology 2011; **Med School:** Mount Sinai Sch Med 1985; **Resid:** Internal Medicine, Mount Sinai Med Ctr 1988; **Fellow:** Hematology, Mount Sinai Med Ctr 1990; Medical Oncology, Meml Sloan-Kettering Cancer Ctr 1992

Neonatal-Perinatal Medicine

Golombek, Sergio G MD (NP) - **Spec Exp:** Prematurity/Low Birth Weight Infants; Lung Disease in Newborns; **Hospital:** Westchester Med Ctr, Children's & Women's Phys.of Westchester (page 612); **Address:** Westchester Med Center-NEO, 100 Woods Rd Ste 2211, Valhalla, NY 10595; **Phone:** 914-493-8558; **Board Cert:** Neonatal-Perinatal Medicine 2005; Pediatrics 2008; **Med School:** Argentina 1983; **Resid:** Pediatrics, Dr Ignacio Pirovano Hosp 1987; Pediatrics, Raymond Blank Meml Hosp Chldn 1991; **Fellow:** Neonatal-Perinatal Medicine, Chldns Mercy Hosp 1996; **Fac Appt:** Prof Ped, NY Med Coll

Jaile-Marti, Jesus MD (NP) - **Spec Exp:** Lung Disease in Newborns; Neonatal Nutrition; **Hospital:** White Plains Hosp (page 615), Morgan Stanley Children's Hosp of NY-Presby, NY (page 104); **Address:** White Plains Hosp Ctr, Div Neonatology, Davis Ave at East Post Rd, White Plains, NY 10601; **Phone:** 914-681-2282; **Board Cert:** Pediatrics 2005; Neonatal-Perinatal Medicine 2003; **Med School:** Columbia P&S 1987; **Resid:** Pediatrics, Columbia-Presby Med Ctr 1990; **Fellow:** Neonatology, Columbia-Presby Med Ctr 1993

La Gamma, Edmund F MD (NP) - **Spec Exp:** Neonatal Infections; Prematurity/Low Birth Weight Infants; Necrotizing Enterocolitis; **Hospital:** Westchester Med Ctr, Children's & Women's Phys.of Westchester (page 612); **Address:** Maria Fareri Chldns Hosp, 100 Woods Rd, rm 2215, Valhalla, NY 10595; **Phone:** 914-493-8558; **Board Cert:** Pediatrics 1981; Neonatal-Perinatal Medicine 1981; **Med School:** NY Med Coll 1976; **Resid:** Pediatrics, NY Hosp-Cornell Med Ctr 1978; **Fellow:** Neonatal-Perinatal Medicine, NY Hosp-Cornell Med Ctr 1980; Cardiovascular Disease, UCSF Med Ctr 1981; **Fac Appt:** Prof Ped, NY Med Coll

Stafford Jr, John R MD (NP) - **Hospital:** Northern Westchester Hosp (page 613); **Address:** 400 E Main St Fl 3, Mt Kisco, NY 10549-3446; **Phone:** 914-666-1272; **Board Cert:** Pediatrics 2008; Neonatal-Perinatal Medicine 2008; **Med School:** SUNY Downstate 1986; **Resid:** Pediatrics, Columbia-Presby Med Ctr 1989; **Fellow:** Neonatology, Columbia-Presby Med Ctr 1992; **Fac Appt:** Clin Prof Ped, Columbia P&S

Nephrology

Adler, Stephen MD (Nep) - **Spec Exp:** Kidney Failure; Glomerulonephritis; Hypertension; Dialysis Care; **Hospital:** Westchester Med Ctr, White Plains Hosp (page 615); **Address:** 19 Bradhurst Ave, Ste 200N, Hawthorne, NY 10532-2169; **Phone:** 914-493-7701; **Board Cert:** Internal Medicine 1979; Nephrology 1982; **Med School:** NYU Sch Med 1976; **Resid:** Internal Medicine, Mt Sinai Hosp 1979; **Fellow:** Nephrology, Boston Univ Med Ctr 1982; **Fac Appt:** Prof Med, NY Med Coll

Buzzeo, Louis MD (Nep) - **Spec Exp:** Hypertension; Kidney Disease; **Hospital:** Phelps Meml Hosp Ctr (page 614); **Address:** 777 N Broadway, Ste 203, Sleepy Hollow, NY 10591-1019; **Phone:** 914-332-9100; **Board Cert:** Internal Medicine 1975; Nephrology 1978; **Med School:** Tufts Univ 1972; **Resid:** Internal Medicine, St Vincent's Hosp & Med Ctr 1975; **Fellow:** Nephrology, NYU Med Ctr 1977

Delaney, Veronica MD/PhD (Nep) - **Spec Exp:** Transplant Medicine-Kidney; Kidney Failure; **Hospital:** Westchester Med Ctr; **Address:** 19 Bradhurst Ave, Ste 200N, Hawthorne, NY 10532; **Phone:** 914-493-7701; **Board Cert:** Internal Medicine 1981; Nephrology 1982; **Med School:** England, UK 1973; **Resid:** Internal Medicine, Dublin Univ Hosps; **Fellow:** Nephrology, Univ Pittsburgh Med Ctr 1983; **Fac Appt:** Assoc Prof Med, NY Med Coll

Garrick, Renee MD (Nep) - **Spec Exp:** Hypertension; Dialysis Care; **Hospital:** Westchester Med Ctr; **Address:** Nephrology Assocs of Westchester, 19 Bradhurst Ave, Ste 200N, Hawthorne, NY 10532; **Phone:** 914-493-7701; **Board Cert:** Internal Medicine 1981; Nephrology 1984; **Med School:** Rush Med Coll 1978; **Resid:** Internal Medicine, Jacobi Med Ctr 1981; **Fellow:** Nephrology, Hosp Univ Penn 1984; **Fac Appt:** Clin Prof Med, NY Med Coll

Reda, Dominick MD (Nep) - **Spec Exp:** Hypertension; Kidney Disease; **Hospital:** Saint Joseph's Med Ctr - Yonkers; **Address:** 136 S Broadway, Yonkers, NY 10701; **Phone:** 914-965-0621; **Board Cert:** Internal Medicine 1987; Nephrology 2010; **Med School:** Italy 1983; **Resid:** Internal Medicine, Our Lady of Mercy 1987; **Fellow:** Nephrology, Lincoln Med Ctr 1989

Rie, Jonathan MD (Nep) - **Spec Exp:** Hypertension; Kidney Stones; **Hospital:** White Plains Hosp (page 615); **Address:** 33 Davis Ave, White Plains, NY 10605; **Phone:** 914-831-2900; **Board Cert:** Internal Medicine 1988; Nephrology 2010; **Med School:** NY Med Coll 1985; **Resid:** Internal Medicine, Montefiore Hosp Med Ctr 1988; **Fellow:** Nephrology, Montefiore Hosp Med Ctr 1990

Rosen, Michael A MD (Nep) - **Spec Exp:** Kidney Disease-Pediatric & Adult; **Hospital:** Northern Westchester Hosp (page 613); **Address:** Mt Kisco Medical Group, 90 S Bedford Rd, Mt Kisco, NY 10549; **Phone:** 914-241-1050; **Board Cert:** Internal Medicine 2004; Nephrology 2007; **Med School:** Indiana Univ 2000; **Resid:** Internal Medicine & Pediatrics, Mt Sinai Med Ctr 2004; **Fellow:** Nephrology, Nt Sinai Med Ctr 2008

Saltzman, Martin MD (Nep) - **Spec Exp:** Kidney Disease; Hypertension; **Hospital:** Northern Westchester Hosp (page 613), Putnam Hosp Ctr; **Address:** 90 S Bedford Rd, Mt Kisco, NY 10549; **Phone:** 914-241-1050; **Board Cert:** Internal Medicine 1977; Nephrology 1978; **Med School:** SUNY Downstate 1972; **Resid:** Internal Medicine, Kings County Hosp 1973; Internal Medicine, Harlem Hosp 1974; **Fellow:** Nephrology, Univ Hosp 1976

Neurological Surgery

Abrahams, John M MD (NS) - **Spec Exp:** Skull Base Surgery; Aneurysm-Cerebral; **Hospital:** White Plains Hosp (page 615), Northern Westchester Hosp (page 613); **Address:** Brain & Spine Surgeons of NY, 244 Westchester Ave, Ste 310, White Plains, NY 10604; **Phone:** 914-948-6688; **Board Cert:** Neurological Surgery 2004; **Med School:** NY Med Coll 1995; **Resid:** Neurological Surgery, Univ Penn Hosp 2002; **Fellow:** Spinal Surgery, Univ Penn Hosp; **Fac Appt:** Assoc Prof NS, NY Med Coll

Benzil, Deborah L MD (NS) - **Spec Exp:** Brain Tumors; Peripheral Nerve Surgery; **Hospital:** Westchester Med Ctr, Northern Westchester Hosp (page 613); **Address:** Mount Kisco Medical Group, 90 S Bedford Rd, Mount Kisco, NY 10530; **Phone:** 914-241-1050; **Board Cert:** Neurological Surgery 1997; **Med School:** Univ MD Sch Med 1985; **Resid:** Neurological Surgery, Rhode Island Hosp 1993; **Fac Appt:** Assoc Prof NS, NY Med Coll

De Lotbiniere, Alain MD (NS) - **Spec Exp:** Movement Disorders; Brain Tumors; Pituitary Tumors; Deep Brain Stimulation; **Hospital:** Northern Westchester Hosp (page 613), White Plains Hosp (page 615); **Address:** Brain & Spine Surgeons of New York, 244 Westchester Ave, Ste 310, White Plains, NY 10604; **Phone:** 914-948-6688; **Board Cert:** Neurological Surgery 1994; **Med School:** McGill Univ 1981; **Resid:** Surgery, Royal Victoria Hosp 1983; Neurological Surgery, Royal Victoria Hosp 1988; **Fellow:** Neurological Surgery, Univ Cambridge 1989

Kornel, Ezriel MD (NS) - **Spec Exp:** Spinal Surgery-Minimally Invasive; Brain Tumors; Spinal Cord Tumors; **Hospital:** Northern Westchester Hosp (page 613), White Plains Hosp (page 615); **Address:** Brain & Spine Surgeons of New York, 244 Westchester Ave, Ste 310, White Plains, NY 10604; **Phone:** 914-948-0444; **Board Cert:** Neurological Surgery 1987; **Med School:** Rush Med Coll 1978; **Resid:** Surgery, Washington Hosp Ctr 1979; Neurological Surgery, Geo Wash Univ Hosp 1984; **Fac Appt:** Asst Clin Prof NS, Columbia P&S

Lee, Thomas T MD (NS) - **Spec Exp:** Spinal Surgery; Minimally Invasive Spinal Surgery; Stereotactic Radiosurgery; **Hospital:** St. John's Riverside Hosp-Andrus Pavil, Mount Sinai Med Ctr (page 102); **Address:** 150 White Plains Rd, Ste 110, Tarrytown, NY 10591; **Phone:** 914-631-9207; **Board Cert:** Neurological Surgery 2012; **Med School:** UCLA 1993; **Resid:** Neurological Surgery, Jackson Meml Med Ctr 1999; **Fac Appt:** Asst Clin Prof NS, Mount Sinai Sch Med

Murali, Raj MD (NS) - **Spec Exp:** Trigeminal Neuralgia; Skull Base Surgery; Aneurysm-Cerebral; Pituitary Tumors; **Hospital:** Westchester Med Ctr; **Address:** Westchester Med Ctr, Dept Neurosurgery, Munger Pavilion, Ste 329, Valhalla, NY 10595; **Phone:** 914-493-8392; **Board Cert:** Neurological Surgery 1982; **Med School:** India 1968; **Resid:** Neurological Surgery, Royal Infirm-Univ Edinburgh 1974; Neurological Surgery, NYU Med Ctr 1979; **Fac Appt:** Prof NS, NY Med Coll

Rosner, Saran S MD (NS) - **Spec Exp:** Spinal Surgery; Brain & Spinal Cord Tumors; **Hospital:** Phelps Meml Hosp Ctr (page 614), Hudson Valley Hosp Ctr; **Address:** 245 Saw Mill River Rd, Hawthorne, NY 10532; **Phone:** 914-741-2666; **Board Cert:** Neurological Surgery 1986; **Med School:** Columbia P&S 1976; **Resid:** Surgery, Johns Hopkins Hosp 1978; Neurological Surgery, Columbia-Presby Med Ctr 1983

Neurology

Ahluwalia, Brij M Singh MD (N) - **Spec Exp:** Dementia; Cerebrovascular Disease; Multiple Sclerosis; **Hospital:** Westchester Med Ctr; **Address:** 19 Bradhurst Ave, Ste 2850, Hawthorne, NY 10532; **Phone:** 914-345-1313; **Board Cert:** Neurology 1974; **Med School:** India 1961; **Resid:** Internal Medicine, Beekman Downtown Hosp 1969; Neurology, Metropolitan Hosp 1972; **Fac Appt:** Prof N, NY Med Coll

Dickoff, David J MD (N) - **Spec Exp:** Epilepsy/Seizure Disorders; Neuromuscular Disorders; Parkinson's Disease; Trigeminal Neuralgia; **Hospital:** St. John's Riverside Hosp-Andrus Pavil, Mount Sinai Med Ctr (page 102); **Address:** 984 N Broadway, Ste 509, Yonkers, NY 10701-1308; **Phone:** 914-968-0620; **Board Cert:** Neurology 1987; Electrodiagnostic Medicine 1989; **Med School:** Albany Med Coll 1982; **Resid:** Neurology, Mt Sinai Hosp 1986; **Fellow:** Neuromuscular Disease, Columbia-Presby Med Ctr 1987; **Fac Appt:** Asst Clin Prof N, Mount Sinai Sch Med

Duncan, David B MD (N) - **Spec Exp:** Multiple Sclerosis; Neurodegenerative Disorders; **Hospital:** Northern Westchester Hosp (page 613); **Address:** Mt Kisco Medical Group, 90 S Bedford Rd, Mt Kisco, NY 10549; **Phone:** 914-241-1050; **Board Cert:** Neurology 2008; **Med School:** Indiana Univ 1988; **Resid:** Neurology, Univ Kentucky Med Ctr 1992

Gross, Elliott George MD (N) - **Spec Exp:** Alzheimer's Disease; Parkinson's Disease; Headache; Pain-Back & Neck; **Hospital:** Montefiore Med Ctr-Moses Campus, NY (page 100); **Address:** 16 Rye Ridge Plaza, Rye Brook, NY 10573-2826; **Phone:** 914-251-1010; **Board Cert:** Neurology 1969; **Med School:** Albert Einstein Coll Med 1962; **Resid:** Neurology, Jacobi Med Ctr 1966; **Fellow:** Neurology, Albert Einstein Med Coll 1970; **Fac Appt:** Asst Clin Prof N, Columbia P&S

Jordan, Barry D MD (N) - **Spec Exp:** Brain Injury; Sports Neurology; Concussion; Memory Disorders; **Hospital:** Burke Rehab Hosp; **Address:** Burke Rehabilitation Hosp, 785 Mamaroneck Ave, White Plains, NY 10605; **Phone:** 914-597-2332; **Board Cert:** Neurology 1989; **Med School:** Harvard Med Sch 1981; **Resid:** Neurology, New York Hosp 1986; **Fellow:** Hosp Spec Surgery 1987UCLA Med Ctr 1998; **Fac Appt:** Assoc Prof N, Cornell Univ-Weill Med Coll

Kranzler, L Stephan MD (N) - **Hospital:** White Plains Hosp (page 615); **Address:** 244 Westchester Ave, Ste 315, White Plains, NY 10604; **Phone:** 914-946-9444; **Board Cert:** Neurology 1990; **Med School:** Univ Pennsylvania 1985; **Resid:** Neurology, Neuro Inst/Columbia-Presby Med Ctr 1989

Laban-Grant, Olgica MD (N) - **Spec Exp:** Epilepsy; Epilepsy in Women; **Hospital:** White Plains Hosp (page 615); **Address:** NE Regional Epilepsy Group, 333 Westchester Ave, Ste E104, White Plains, NY 10604; **Phone:** 914-428-9213; **Board Cert:** Neurology 2003; Clinical Neurophysiology 2005; **Med School:** Yugoslavia 1991; **Resid:** Neurology, NYU Med Ctr 2002; **Fellow:** Clinical Neurophysiology, NYU Med Ctr 2003

Marks, Stephen J MD (N) - **Spec Exp:** Stroke; Alzheimer's Disease; Dementia; **Hospital:** Westchester Med Ctr; **Address:** 19 Bradhurst Ave, Ste 2850, Hawthorne, NY 10532; **Phone:** 914-345-1313; **Board Cert:** Neurology 1985; Vascular Neurology 2006; **Med School:** NY Med Coll 1980; **Resid:** Neurology, Mt Sinai Hosp 1984; **Fellow:** Stroke, Duke Univ Med Ctr 1985; **Fac Appt:** Prof N, NY Med Coll

Morris, James R MD/PhD (N) - **Spec Exp:** Stroke; Headache; Epilepsy; Parkinson's Disease; **Hospital:** Greenwich Hosp (page 892); **Address:** Neurologic Care, 3020 Westchester Ave, Ste 305, Purchase, NY 10577; **Phone:** 203-629-8029; **Board Cert:** Neurology 2006; **Med School:** Indiana Univ 1990; **Resid:** Neurology, Columbia-Presby Med Ctr 1994; **Fellow:** Clinical Neurophysiology, Columbia-Presby Med Ctr 1995

Reding, Michael MD (N) - **Spec Exp:** Neuro-Rehabilitation; **Hospital:** Burke Rehab Hosp; **Address:** 785 Mamaroneck Ave, White Plains, NY 10605-2523; **Phone:** 914-597-2470; **Board Cert:** Internal Medicine 1976; Neurology 1981; **Med School:** Univ Kansas 1973; **Resid:** Internal Medicine, Univ Nebraska Med Ctr 1976; Neurology, Univ Nebraska Med Ctr 1979; **Fellow:** Neurology, NY Hosp/Cornell 1980; **Fac Appt:** Assoc Prof N, Cornell Univ-Weill Med Coll

Rosenkilde, Carl E MD/PhD (N) - **Hospital:** Northern Westchester Hosp (page 613); **Address:** 91 Smith Ave, Neurology Associates, Mt Kisco, NY 10549-2815; **Phone:** 914-241-1717; **Board Cert:** Neurology 1992; **Med School:** Albert Einstein Coll Med 1985; **Resid:** Neurology, Yale-New Haven Hosp 1989; **Fellow:** Neurology, UCLA Med Ctr 1979

Selman, Jay E MD (N) - **Spec Exp:** Pediatric Neurology; Epilepsy/Seizure Disorders; Headache; Tourette's Syndrome; **Hospital:** Blythedale Children's Hosp, Bronx Lebanon Hosp Ctr; **Address:** Blythedale Chldns Hosp, 95 Bradhurst Ave, Valhalla, NY 10595; **Phone:** 914-592-7555 x71513; **Board Cert:** Pediatrics 1978; Child Neurology 1980; Sleep Medicine 2007; Neurodevelopmental Disabilities 2012; **Med School:** Univ Tex SW, Dallas 1973; **Resid:** Pediatrics, Jacobi Med Ctr 1975; Neurology, Jacobi Med Ctr 1978; **Fellow:** Child Neurology, Jacobi Med Ctr 1977; **Fac Appt:** Assoc Clin Prof N, Columbia P&S

Singh, Avtar MD (N) - **Spec Exp:** Stroke; Epilepsy; Headache; **Hospital:** White Plains Hosp (page 615), Westchester Med Ctr; **Address:** 244 Westchester Ave, Ste 315, White Plains, NY 10604; **Phone:** 914-946-9444; **Board Cert:** Neurology 1978; **Med School:** India 1967; **Resid:** Neurology, Metropolitan Hosp Ctr 1976; **Fac Appt:** Assoc Clin Prof N, NY Med Coll

Szabo, Albert MD (N) - **Hospital:** Northern Westchester Hosp (page 613); **Address:** Mt Kisco Medical Group, 90 S Bedford Rd, Mount Kisco, NY 10549; **Phone:** 914-241-1050; **Board Cert:** Neurology 2007; **Med School:** Hungary 1989; **Resid:** Neurology, Mount Sinai Sch Med 1994; **Fellow:** Clinical Neurophysiology, Thomas Jefferson U Hosp 1996; Clinical Neurophysiology, SUNY Hlth Sci Ctr 1997

Tolunsky, Eugene MD (N) - **Hospital:** Northern Westchester Hosp (page 613); **Address:** Mt Kisco Medical Group, 90 S Bedford Rd, Mt Kisco, NY 10549; **Phone:** 914-241-1050; **Board Cert:** Neurology 2002; Clinical Neurophysiology 2003; **Med School:** Univ Pennsylvania 1997; **Resid:** Neurology, Mtr Sinai Hosp 2001; **Fellow:** Neurological Physiology, Mt Sinai Hosp 2002

Weintraub, Michael MD (N) - **Spec Exp:** Carpal Tunnel Syndrome; Peripheral Neuropathy; Pain-Back & Neck; Diabetic Neuropathy; **Hospital:** Phelps Meml Hosp Ctr (page 614), Putnam Hosp Ctr; **Address:** 325 S Highland Ave, Briarcliff Manor, NY 10510-2093; **Phone:** 914-941-0788; **Board Cert:** Neurology 1972; Clinical Neurophysiology 1977; **Med School:** SUNY Buffalo 1966; **Resid:** Neurology, EJ Meyer Meml Hosp 1968; **Fellow:** Neurology, Yale-New Haven Hosp 1970; **Fac Appt:** Clin Prof N, NY Med Coll

Neuroradiology

Tenner, Michael MD (NRad) - **Spec Exp:** Stroke; Brain & Spinal Tumors; Carotid Artery Stent Placement; **Hospital:** Westchester Med Ctr; **Address:** NY Med Coll, Dept Radiology, 100 Woods Rd, Valhalla, NY 10595; **Phone:** 914-493-6692; **Board Cert:** Diagnostic Radiology 1967; Neuroradiology 2007; **Med School:** Univ MD Sch Med 1960; **Resid:** Diagnostic Radiology, Univ Maryland Hosp 1962; Diagnostic Radiology, Univ Maryland Hosp 1966; **Fellow:** Neuroradiology, Neurological Inst-Columbia Presby 1968; **Fac Appt:** Prof Rad, NY Med Coll

Nuclear Medicine

Gerard, Perry S MD (NuM) - **Spec Exp:** PET Imaging; CT Scan; Nuclear Imaging; Nuclear Oncology; **Hospital:** Westchester Med Ctr; **Address:** 100 Woods Rd, Valhalla, NY 10595; **Phone:** 914-493-8260; **Board Cert:** Diagnostic Radiology 1987; Nuclear Radiology 1989; Nuclear Cardiology 2008; **Med School:** Dominica 1980; **Resid:** Diagnostic Radiology, Maimonides Med Ctr 1984; **Fellow:** Diagnostic Imaging, Maimonides Med Ctr 1985; **Fac Appt:** Asst Clin Prof Rad, Mount Sinai Sch Med

Obstetrics & Gynecology

Armbruster, Robert MD (ObG) - **Spec Exp:** Colposcopy; Pregnancy-High Risk; **Hospital:** Lawrence Hosp Ctr; **Address:** 73 Market St, Ste 212, Yonkers, NY 10710; **Phone:** 914-337-3229; **Board Cert:** Obstetrics & Gynecology 1984; **Med School:** Washington Univ, St Louis 1977; **Resid:** Obstetrics & Gynecology, UCLA Med Ctr 1979; Obstetrics & Gynecology, NY-Cornell Hosp 1981

Burns, Elisa MD (ObG) - **Spec Exp:** Minimally Invasive Surgery; Robotic Surgery; Colposcopy; **Hospital:** Northern Westchester Hosp (page 613); **Address:** 90 S Bedford Rd, Mt Kisco Medical Group, Mt Kisco, NY 10549-3433; **Phone:** 914-241-1050; **Board Cert:** Obstetrics & Gynecology 2012; **Med School:** Columbia P&S 1982; **Resid:** Obstetrics & Gynecology, Columbia-Presby Hosp 1986

Eilen, Bonnie MD (ObG) *PCP* - **Hospital:** White Plains Hosp (page 615); **Address:** 170 Maple Ave Fl 3 - rm 309, White Plains, NY 10601; **Phone:** 914-831-6800; **Board Cert:** Obstetrics & Gynecology 2011; **Med School:** Albert Einstein Coll Med 1977; **Resid:** Obstetrics & Gynecology, Bronx Municipal Hosp 1981; **Fac Appt:** Asst Clin Prof ObG, Albert Einstein Coll Med

Florio, Philip L MD (ObG) *PCP* - **Spec Exp:** Pregnancy-High Risk; Laparoscopic Surgery; Gynecologic Cancer; Colposcopy; **Hospital:** St. John's Riverside Hosp-Andrus Pavil; **Address:** 1022 N Broadway, Yonkers, NY 10701-1303; **Phone:** 914-963-0284; **Board Cert:** Obstetrics & Gynecology 1981; **Med School:** SUNY Upstate Med Univ 1974; **Resid:** Obstetrics & Gynecology, St Barnabas Med Ctr 1978

Giuffrida, Regina MD (ObG) *PCP* - **Spec Exp:** Menopause Problems; Gynecologic Surgery; Gynecology Only; **Hospital:** Northern Westchester Hosp (page 613); **Address:** Mt Kisco Med Grp, 90 S Bedford Rd, Mt Kisco, NY 10549; **Phone:** 914-241-1050; **Board Cert:** Obstetrics & Gynecology 2011; **Med School:** NY Med Coll 1980; **Resid:** Obstetrics & Gynecology, UCSD Med Ctr 1984

Grano, Vanessa MD (ObG) - **Spec Exp:** Laparoscopic Surgery; Pap Smear Abnormalities; Colposcopy; **Hospital:** Greenwich Hosp (page 892); **Address:** Westchester Medical Grp, 1 Theall Rd, Rye, NY 10580; **Phone:** 914-253-4912; **Board Cert:** Obstetrics & Gynecology 2010; **Med School:** SUNY Downstate 1988; **Resid:** Obstetrics & Gynecology, Columbia-Presby Hosp 1993

Hayworth, Scott D MD (ObG) - **Spec Exp:** Minimally Invasive Surgery; Endometriosis; Menopause Problems; **Hospital:** Northern Westchester Hosp (page 613); **Address:** 90 S Bedford Rd, Mt Kisco, NY 10549-3412; **Phone:** 914-241-1050; **Board Cert:** Obstetrics & Gynecology 2011; **Med School:** Cornell Univ-Weill Med Coll 1984; **Resid:** Obstetrics & Gynecology, Mount Sinai Med Ctr 1988; **Fac Appt:** Asst Clin Prof ObG, Mount Sinai Sch Med

Keller, Adina H MD (ObG) - **Spec Exp:** Adolescent Gynecology; Robotic Surgery; Minimally Invasive Surgery; Menopause Problems; **Hospital:** Northern Westchester Hosp (page 613); **Address:** 90 S Bedford Rd, Mount Kisco, NY 10549; **Phone:** 914-241-1050; **Board Cert:** Obstetrics & Gynecology 2011; **Med School:** Mount Sinai Sch Med 1993; **Resid:** Obstetrics & Gynecology, Mount Sinai Med Ctr 1997

Maloney, Romelle J MD (ObG) - **Hospital:** Greenwich Hosp (page 892); **Address:** 145 Huguenot St, Ste 215, New Rochelle, NY 10801; **Phone:** 914-235-6060; **Board Cert:** Obstetrics & Gynecology 2000; **Med School:** E Tenn State Univ 1986; **Resid:** Obstetrics & Gynecology, Westchester Med Ctr 1990; **Fac Appt:** Asst Clin Prof ObG, NY Med Coll

McGovern, Catherine A MD (ObG) - **Hospital:** White Plains Hosp (page 615); **Address:** 170 Maple Ave Fl 3 - Ste 309, White Plains, NY 10605; **Phone:** 914-831-6800; **Board Cert:** Obstetrics & Gynecology 2011; **Med School:** Albany Med Coll 1985; **Resid:** Obstetrics & Gynecology, Albany Med Ctr 1989

Meacham, Kevin MD (ObG) - **Spec Exp:** Pregnancy-High Risk; Laparoscopic Surgery; Gynecologic Surgery; **Hospital:** Sound Shore Med Ctr - Westchester; **Address:** 2071 Boston Post Rd, Larchmont, NY 10538-3701; **Phone:** 914-833-1000; **Board Cert:** Obstetrics & Gynecology 2011; **Med School:** NY Med Coll 1986; **Resid:** Obstetrics & Gynecology, LIJ Med Ctr 1990

Mendelowitz, Lawrence G MD (ObG) - **Spec Exp:** Pelvic Reconstruction; Laparoscopic Hysterectomy; Gynecologic Surgery; Pregnancy-High Risk; **Hospital:** Phelps Meml Hosp Ctr (page 614), Westchester Med Ctr; **Address:** 755 N Broadway, Ste 560, Sleepy Hollow, NY 10591; **Phone:** 914-631-0337; **Board Cert:** Obstetrics & Gynecology 2010; **Med School:** NYU Sch Med 1976; **Resid:** Obstetrics & Gynecology, Bellevue Hosp-NYU 1980

Mieszerski, Laura E MD (ObG) - **Spec Exp:** Adolescent Gynecology; Pregnancy-High Risk; **Hospital:** Hudson Valley Hosp Ctr; **Address:** The Westchester Medical Practice, 2241 Crompond Rd, Cortlandt Manor, NY 10567; **Phone:** 914-736-6180; **Board Cert:** Obstetrics & Gynecology 2009; **Med School:** Albany Med Coll 1992; **Resid:** Obstetrics & Gynecology, UTSA Affil Hosp 1996

Nelson, William S MD (ObG) - **Spec Exp:** Menopause Problems; **Hospital:** Greenwich Hosp (page 892); **Address:** Westchester Medical Group, 1 Theall Rd, Rye, NY 10580; **Phone:** 914-253-4912; **Board Cert:** Obstetrics & Gynecology 1981; **Med School:** Albert Einstein Coll Med 1960; **Resid:** Obstetrics & Gynecology, Maimonides Med Ctr 1965; **Fac Appt:** Asst Clin Prof ObG, Albert Einstein Coll Med

Regard, Monique M MD (ObG) - **Spec Exp:** Pediatric Gynecology Only; Birth Defects-Vaginal; Ovarian Masses in Children/Adolescents; **Hospital:** Westchester Med Ctr, Children's & Women's Phys.of Westchester (page 612); **Address:** Children's/Women's Physicians of Westchester, 503 Grasslands Rd, Ste 200, Valhalla, NY 10595; **Phone:** 914-304-5300; **Board Cert:** Obstetrics & Gynecology 2010; **Med School:** Baylor Coll Med 1989; **Resid:** Obstetrics & Gynecology, Univ Minn Med Ctr 1993; **Fac Appt:** Asst Clin Prof Ped, NY Med Coll

Ullman, Joel MD (ObG) - **Spec Exp:** Laparoscopic Surgery-Complex; Uro-Gynecology; Vulvar Disease; Vaginal Surgery; **Hospital:** Sound Shore Med Ctr - Westchester; **Address:** 2071 Boston Post Rd, Larchmont, NY 10538-3701; **Phone:** 914-833-1000; **Board Cert:** Obstetrics & Gynecology 1978; **Med School:** NY Med Coll 1963; **Resid:** Obstetrics & Gynecology, Beth Israel Med Ctr 1969; **Fac Appt:** Asst Clin Prof ObG, Albert Einstein Coll Med

Wysoki, Randee S MD (ObG) - **Hospital:** White Plains Hosp (page 615); **Address:** Westchester Gynecologists, 170 Maple Ave, Ste 309, White Plains, NY 10601; **Phone:** 914-831-6800; **Board Cert:** Obstetrics & Gynecology 2012; **Med School:** Georgetown Univ 1982; **Resid:** Obstetrics & Gynecology, Emory Univ Med Ctr 1986

Ophthalmology

Bansal, Rajendra K MD (Oph) - **Spec Exp:** Glaucoma; **Hospital:** Mount Vernon Hosp; **Address:** 202 Stevens Ave, Mt Vernon, NY 10550-2534; **Phone:** 914-664-3168; **Board Cert:** Ophthalmology 1977; **Med School:** India 1967; **Resid:** Ophthalmology, Univ Delhi Hosp 1973; **Fellow:** Glaucoma, Columbia Presby Med Ctr 1979; **Fac Appt:** Asst Clin Prof Oph, Columbia P&S

Biser, Seth A MD (Oph) - **Spec Exp:** Corneal Disease & Surgery; Cataract Surgery; Refractive Surgery; **Hospital:** Lawrence Hosp Ctr; **Address:** 654 Gramatan Ave, Fleetwood, NY 10552; **Phone:** 914-664-2300; **Board Cert:** Ophthalmology 2003; **Med School:** Univ Pennsylvania 1997; **Resid:** Ophthalmology, Wilmer Eye Inst 2001; **Fellow:** Refractive Surgery, North Shore Hosp 2002

Brustein, Harris MD (Oph) - **Hospital:** Sound Shore Med Ctr - Westchester; **Address:** 77 Quaker Ridge Rd, Ste 203, New Rochelle, NY 10804-2821; **Phone:** 914-235-0022; **Board Cert:** Ophthalmology 1976; **Med School:** Albert Einstein Coll Med 1970; **Resid:** Ophthalmology, Montefiore Med Ctr 1974; **Fellow:** Pediatric Ophthalmology, Chldns Hosp 1975

Dieck, William MD (Oph) - **Spec Exp:** Cataract Surgery; Glaucoma; Lens Implants-Multifocal; Dry Eye Syndrome; **Hospital:** Northern Westchester Hosp (page 613); **Address:** 185 Kisco Ave, Ste 500, Mt Kisco, NY 10549; **Phone:** 914-666-4939; **Board Cert:** Ophthalmology 1990; **Med School:** NY Med Coll 1983; **Resid:** Internal Medicine, Westchester Co Med Ctr 1985; Ophthalmology, Westchester Co Med Ctr 1988

Fleischman, Jay MD (Oph) - **Spec Exp:** Diabetic Eye Disease/Retinopathy; Macular Degeneration; **Hospital:** Montefiore Med Ctr-Moses Campus, NY (page 100); **Address:** 600 Mamaroneck Ave, Ste 103, Harrison, NY 10528-1613; **Phone:** 914-315-5111; **Board Cert:** Ophthalmology 1980; **Med School:** Columbia P&S 1975; **Resid:** Ophthalmology, Johns Hopkins Hosp 1979; **Fac Appt:** Assoc Prof Oph, Albert Einstein Coll Med

Forman, Scott MD (Oph) - **Spec Exp:** Botox Therapy; Eye Muscle Disorders; Neuro-Ophthalmology; **Hospital:** Westchester Med Ctr; **Address:** Westchester Med Ctr, Dept Ophthalmology, 95 Grasslands Rd, Valhalla, NY 10595; **Phone:** 914-493-7666; **Board Cert:** Ophthalmology 1989; **Med School:** UMDNJ-RW Johnson Med Sch 1981; **Resid:** Ophthalmology, New York Med Coll 1986; **Fellow:** Neuro-Ophthalmology, Columbia-Presby Med Ctr 1987; **Fac Appt:** Assoc Prof Oph, NY Med Coll

Glassman, Morris MD (Oph) - **Spec Exp:** Cataract Surgery; Glaucoma; **Hospital:** Northern Westchester Hosp (page 613), Westchester Med Ctr; **Address:** 1940 Commerce St, Yorktown Heights, NY 10598; **Phone:** 914-962-5506; **Board Cert:** Ophthalmology 1975; **Med School:** NYU Sch Med 1968; **Resid:** Ophthalmology, Montefiore Med Ctr 1974; **Fac Appt:** Assoc Clin Prof Oph, Albert Einstein Coll Med

Gordon, James R MD (Oph) - **Spec Exp:** Oculoplastic Surgery; Eyelid Cosmetic & Reconstructive Surgery; **Hospital:** White Plains Hosp (page 615); **Address:** Westchester Eye Assocs, 170 Maple Ave, Ste 402, White Plains, NY 10601; **Phone:** 914-949-9200; **Board Cert:** Ophthalmology 2004; **Med School:** Israel 1996; **Resid:** Ophthalmology, St Vincent's Hosp & Med Ctr 2000

Greenbaum, Allen MD (Oph) - **Spec Exp:** Laser Refractive Surgery; Cataract Surgery; **Hospital:** White Plains Hosp (page 615); **Address:** 170 Maple Ave, Ste 402, White Plains, NY 10601; **Phone:** 914-949-9200; **Board Cert:** Ophthalmology 1985; **Med School:** Mount Sinai Sch Med 1979; **Resid:** Ophthalmology, Mount Sinai Hosp 1983

Greenberg, Steven C MD (Oph) - **Spec Exp:** Pediatric Ophthalmology; **Hospital:** Putnam Hosp Ctr; **Address:** 1 Theall Rd, Rye, NY 10580; **Phone:** 914-848-8999; **Board Cert:** Ophthalmology 1987; **Med School:** Univ Conn 1982; **Resid:** Ophthalmology, NYU Med Ctr 1986; **Fellow:** Pediatric Ophthalmology, Manhattan EET Hosp 1987

Horowitz, Marc A MD (Oph) - **Spec Exp:** Pediatric Ophthalmology; Strabismus; Retinopathy of Prematurity; **Hospital:** Westchester Med Ctr, White Plains Hosp (page 615); **Address:** 14 Harwood Ct, Ste 209, Scarsdale, NY 10583; **Phone:** 914-723-5511; **Board Cert:** Ophthalmology 1983; **Med School:** Mount Sinai Sch Med 1978; **Resid:** Ophthalmology, St Luke's Roosevelt Hosp Ctr 1982; **Fellow:** Pediatric Ophthalmology, Chldns Hosp 1983; **Fac Appt:** Clin Prof Oph, NY Med Coll

Lederman, Martin E MD (Oph) - **Spec Exp:** Pediatric Ophthalmology; Eye Muscle Disorders; Diagnostic Problems; **Hospital:** White Plains Hosp (page 615), NY-Presby/Columbia Univ Med Ctr, NY (page 104); **Address:** 3020 Westchester Ave, Ste 402, Purchase, NY 10577; **Phone:** 914-417-6441; **Board Cert:** Ophthalmology 2005; **Med School:** Albert Einstein Coll Med 1964; **Resid:** Ophthalmology, Albert Einstein Affil Hosp 1968; **Fellow:** Pediatric Ophthalmology, Chldns Hosp 1970; **Fac Appt:** Assoc Clin Prof Oph, Columbia P&S

Lippman, Jay MD (Oph) - **Spec Exp:** Cataract Surgery; LASIK-Refractive Surgery; Cornea Transplant; **Hospital:** New York Eye & Ear Infirm (page 117); **Address:** 828 Pelhamdale Ave, New Rochelle, NY 10801; **Phone:** 914-636-3600; **Board Cert:** Ophthalmology 1972; **Med School:** Ros Franklin Univ/Chicago Med Sch 1964; **Resid:** Ophthalmology, Montefiore Med Ctr 1970; **Fac Appt:** Clin Prof Oph, NY Med Coll

McKee, Heather MD (Oph) - **Spec Exp:** Cataract Surgery; Glaucoma; **Hospital:** Comm Hosp - Dobbs Ferry; **Address:** 200 S Broadway, Ste 202, Tarrytown, NY 10591-4504; **Phone:** 914-631-7300; **Board Cert:** Ophthalmology 1981; **Med School:** Duke Univ 1976; **Resid:** Ophthalmology, Strong Meml Hosp 1980; **Fac Appt:** Asst Clin Prof Oph, NY Med Coll

Mignone, Biagio MD (Oph) - **Spec Exp:** Cataract Surgery; Glaucoma; **Hospital:** Mount Vernon Hosp, Montefiore Med Ctr-Wakefield Campus, NY (page 100); **Address:** 202 Stevens Ave, Mt Vernon, NY 10550-2534; **Phone:** 914-664-6001; **Board Cert:** Ophthalmology 1980; **Med School:** NY Med Coll 1975; **Resid:** Ophthalmology, UMDNJ Med Ctr 1979; **Fac Appt:** Asst Clin Prof Oph, NY Med Coll

Morello, Robert F MD (Oph) - **Spec Exp:** Geriatric Ophthalmology; **Hospital:** Sound Shore Med Ctr - Westchester; **Address:** Westchester Eye MDs, 120 Warren St, New Rochelle, NY 10801; **Phone:** 914-633-7214; **Board Cert:** Ophthalmology 1985; **Med School:** Mexico 1976; **Resid:** Ophthalmology, Bronx Lebanon Hosp 1981

Most, Richard W MD (Oph) - **Spec Exp:** Pediatric Ophthalmology; Strabismus-Adult & Pediatric; Tear Duct Problems; Retinopathy of Prematurity; **Hospital:** Northern Westchester Hosp (page 613), Mount Sinai Med Ctr (page 102); **Address:** 101 S Bedford Rd, Bldg 400 - Ste 401, MS 10549, Mt Kisco, NY 10549; **Phone:** 914-241-2206; **Board Cert:** Ophthalmology 1977; Pediatric Ophthalmology 1978; **Med School:** Italy 1971; **Resid:** Pathology, Maimonides Med Ctr 1973; Ophthalmology, Lenox Hill Hosp 1976; **Fellow:** Pediatric Ophthalmology, NYU Med Ctr/Bellevue Hosp 1977; Pediatric Ophthalmology, Chldns Hosp Natl Med Ctr 1978; **Fac Appt:** Assoc Prof Oph, Mount Sinai Sch Med

Phillips, Howard P MD (Oph) - **Spec Exp:** LASIK-Refractive Surgery; Corneal Disease; **Hospital:** Phelps Meml Hosp Ctr (page 614); **Address:** 24 Saw Mill River Rd, Hawthorne, NY 10532; **Phone:** 914-345-3937; **Board Cert:** Ophthalmology 1982; **Med School:** NYU Sch Med 1977; **Resid:** Ophthalmology, NYU Med Ctr 1981; **Fellow:** Retina, NYU Med Ctr 1982

Ray, Audell MD (Oph) - **Spec Exp:** Cataract Surgery; Glaucoma; **Hospital:** Lawrence Hosp Ctr; **Address:** Bronxville Eye Associates, 77 Pondfield Rd, Bronxville, NY 10708-3809; **Phone:** 914-337-8844; **Board Cert:** Ophthalmology 1979; **Med School:** Columbia P&S 1974; **Resid:** Ophthalmology, Manhattan EET Hosp 1978

Salzman, Jacqueline G MD (Oph) - **Spec Exp:** Cataract Surgery; Diabetic Eye Disease; Glaucoma; Laser Surgery; **Hospital:** Phelps Meml Hosp Ctr (page 614); **Address:** 200 S Broadway, Ste 211, Tarrytown, NY 10591-4504; **Phone:** 914-332-5394; **Board Cert:** Ophthalmology 1985; **Med School:** NYU Sch Med 1979; **Resid:** Ophthalmology, Bellevue Hosp 1983; **Fellow:** Retina, Bellevue Hosp 1984

Solomon, Ira MD (Oph) - **Spec Exp:** Glaucoma; Laser Surgery; Microsurgery; **Hospital:** Lawrence Hosp Ctr, Lenox Hill Hosp (page 106); **Address:** 700 White Plains Rd, Ste 343, Scarsdale, NY 10583; **Phone:** 914-725-5400; **Board Cert:** Ophthalmology 1989; **Med School:** Jefferson Med Coll 1982; **Resid:** Ophthalmology, Montefiore Med Ctr 1986; **Fellow:** Glaucoma, New York E&E Infirm 1987; **Fac Appt:** Asst Clin Prof Oph, Albert Einstein Coll Med

Solomon, Sherry MD (Oph) - **Spec Exp:** Diabetic Eye Disease/Retinopathy; Macular Degeneration; Retinitis Pigmentosa; **Hospital:** Lawrence Hosp Ctr, Sound Shore Med Ctr - Westchester; **Address:** 700 White Plains Rd, Ste 343, Scarsdale, NY 10583; **Phone:** 914-725-5400; **Board Cert:** Ophthalmology 1991; **Med School:** Albert Einstein Coll Med 1986; **Resid:** Ophthalmology, Montefiore Hosp Med Ctr 1990; **Fellow:** Retina, NYU Med Ctr 1991; **Fac Appt:** Asst Clin Prof Oph, Albert Einstein Coll Med

Stein, Mitchell B MD (Oph) - **Spec Exp:** Cataract Surgery; Cornea & External Eye Disease; **Hospital:** Northern Westchester Hosp (page 613); **Address:** 69 S Moger Ave, Mount Kisco, NY 10549-2217; **Phone:** 914-666-2961; **Board Cert:** Internal Medicine 1982; Ophthalmology 2005; **Med School:** Albert Einstein Coll Med 1979; **Resid:** Internal Medicine, Bronx Muni Hosp 1982; Ophthalmology, SUNY-Downstate Med Ctr 1986; **Fellow:** Cornea, Mt Sinai Hosp/Beth Israel Hosp 1987; **Fac Appt:** Asst Clin Prof Med, Albert Einstein Coll Med

Tostanoski, Jean R MD (Oph) - **Hospital:** Phelps Meml Hosp Ctr (page 614); **Address:** 24 Saw Mill River Rd, Ste 202, Hawthorne, NY 10532; **Phone:** 914-345-3937; **Board Cert:** Ophthalmology 2006; **Med School:** Albert Einstein Coll Med 1989; **Resid:** Ophthalmology, Bronx Lebanon Hosp Ctr 1993; Ophthalmology, Manhattan EE&T Hosp 1994

Zaidman, Gerald MD (Oph) - **Spec Exp:** Laser Vision Surgery; Cornea Transplant; Cataract Surgery; Corneal Disease-Pediatric; **Hospital:** Westchester Med Ctr, Montefiore Med Ctr-Wakefield Campus, NY (page 100); **Address:** Westchester Med Ctr, Dept Ophthalmology, Macy Pavilion, rm 1100, Valhalla, NY 10595; **Phone:** 914-493-1599; **Board Cert:** Ophthalmology 1981; **Med School:** Albert Einstein Coll Med 1975; **Resid:** Ophthalmology, Beth Abraham Hosp 1977; Ophthalmology, Lenox Hill Hosp 1980; **Fellow:** Cornea & Ext Eye Disease, Univ Pittsburgh 1982; **Fac Appt:** Assoc Prof Oph, NY Med Coll

Orthopaedic Surgery

Asprinio, David E MD (OrS) - **Spec Exp:** Trauma; **Hospital:** Westchester Med Ctr; **Address:** University Orthopaedics, 19 Bradhurst Ave, Ste 1300-N, Hawthorne, NY 10595; **Phone:** 914-789-2734; **Board Cert:** Orthopaedic Surgery 2008; **Med School:** Univ VT Coll Med 1986; **Resid:** Surgery, Rhode Island Hosp 1989; Orthopaedic Surgery, Rhode Island Hosp 1992; **Fellow:** Trauma, Hosp for Special Surg 1993

Burak, George MD (OrS) - **Spec Exp:** Sports Injuries; Arthritis; **Hospital:** Phelps Meml Hosp Ctr (page 614); **Address:** Hudson Valley Bone & Joint Surgeons, 24 Saw Mill River Rd, Ste 206, Hawthorne, NY 10532-1541; **Phone:** 914-631-7777; **Board Cert:** Orthopaedic Surgery 1971; **Med School:** SUNY Upstate Med Univ 1964; **Resid:** Orthopaedic Surgery, Kings County Hosp 1969; **Fac Appt:** Asst Prof OrS, SUNY Downstate

Cristofaro, Robert MD (OrS) - **Spec Exp:** Pediatric Orthopaedic Surgery; Pediatric Sports Medicine; Foot & Hip Disorders-Complex Pediatric; **Hospital:** Westchester Med Ctr, Greenwich Hosp (page 892); **Address:** 3010 Westchester Ave, Ste 104, Purchase, NY 10577; **Phone:** 914-967-8708; **Board Cert:** Orthopaedic Surgery 1978; **Med School:** SUNY Downstate 1971; **Resid:** Surgery, Montefiore Hosp 1973; Orthopaedic Surgery, Montefiore Hosp 1976; **Fellow:** Pediatric Orthopaedic Surgery, Rancho Los Amigos Med Ctr 1977; **Fac Appt:** Assoc Clin Prof OrS, NY Med Coll

Edelson, Charles MD (OrS) - **Spec Exp:** Reconstructive Surgery; Sports Medicine; Joint Replacement; Knee Replacement; **Hospital:** St. John's Riverside Hosp-Andrus Pavil, Saint Joseph's Med Ctr - Yonkers; **Address:** S Westchester Ortho & Sports Med Assocs, 970 N Broadway, Ste 204, Yonkers, NY 10701-1310; **Phone:** 914-476-4343; **Board Cert:** Orthopaedic Surgery 1979; **Med School:** NY Med Coll 1973; **Resid:** Surgery, Montefiore Med Ctr 1975; Orthopaedic Surgery, Montefiore Med Ctr 1978

Gundy, Edward MD (OrS) - **Spec Exp:** Geriatric Orthopaedic Surgery; Sports Medicine; **Hospital:** White Plains Hosp (page 615), Greenwich Hosp (page 892); **Address:** 1 Theall Rd, Rye, NY 10580; **Phone:** 914-682-6540; **Board Cert:** Orthopaedic Surgery 1983; **Med School:** Cornell Univ-Weill Med Coll 1976; **Resid:** Surgery, Roosevelt Hosp 1978; Orthopaedic Surgery, Hosp Special Surg 1981

Haig, Scott V MD (OrS) - **Spec Exp:** Hip & Knee Surgery; Hip Replacement; Knee Replacement; Arthritis-Hip & Knee; **Hospital:** Lawrence Hosp Ctr; **Address:** 700 White Plains Rd, Ste 10, Scarsdale, NY 10583; **Phone:** 914-723-4244; **Board Cert:** Orthopaedic Surgery 2003; **Med School:** Yale Univ 1984; **Resid:** Surgery, Brigham & Womens Hosp 1986; Orthopaedic Surgery, Columbia-Presby Hosp 1989

Holder, Jonathan L MD (OrS) - **Spec Exp:** Sports Medicine; Foot & Ankle Surgery; Joint Replacement; **Hospital:** White Plains Hosp (page 615), Westchester Med Ctr; **Address:** 170 Maple Ave, Ste 109, White Plains, NY 10601; **Phone:** 914-421-0600; **Board Cert:** Orthopaedic Surgery 2012; **Med School:** NY Med Coll 1985; **Resid:** Orthopaedic Surgery, Metropolitan Hosp Ctr 1990; **Fac Appt:** Asst Clin Prof OrS, NY Med Coll

Karas, Evan H MD (OrS) - **Spec Exp:** Shoulder Surgery; Sports Medicine; **Hospital:** Northern Westchester Hosp (page 613); **Address:** 90 S Bedford Rd, Mt Kisco, NY 10549; **Phone:** 914-241-1050; **Board Cert:** Orthopaedic Surgery 2010; **Med School:** NYU Sch Med 1991; **Resid:** Orthopaedic Surgery, Mt Sinai Hosp 1996; **Fellow:** Sports Medicine, Univ Penn 1997

Khabie, Victor MD (OrS) - **Spec Exp:** Sports Medicine; Shoulder Surgery; Elbow Surgery; Knee Surgery; **Hospital:** Northern Westchester Hosp (page 613), Putnam Hosp Ctr; **Address:** 657 E Main St, Mt Kisco, NY 10549; **Phone:** 914-666-5550; **Board Cert:** Orthopaedic Surgery 2010; Orthopaedic Sports Medicine 2008; **Med School:** Harvard Med Sch 1991; **Resid:** Orthopaedic Surgery, Hosp for Joint Dis 1996; **Fellow:** Sports Medicine, Keral-Jobe Ortho Clinic 1997; **Fac Appt:** Asst Clin Prof OrS, NYU Sch Med

Maddalo, Anthony Vincent MD (OrS) - **Spec Exp:** Sports Medicine; Shoulder & Knee Injuries; Rotator Cuff Surgery; **Hospital:** Phelps Meml Hosp Ctr (page 614), Comm Hosp - Dobbs Ferry; **Address:** 24 Saw Mill River Rd, Ste 206, Hawthorne, NY 10532; **Phone:** 914-631-7777; **Board Cert:** Orthopaedic Surgery 2009; **Med School:** NY Med Coll 1981; **Resid:** Orthopaedic Surgery, Lenox Hill Hosp 1986

Mann, Ronald L MD (OrS) - **Spec Exp:** Pediatric Orthopaedic Surgery; Joint Replacement; Sports Medicine; **Hospital:** Northern Westchester Hosp (page 613); **Address:** 1888 Commerce St, Yorktown Heights, NY 10598-4431; **Phone:** 914-962-7712; **Board Cert:** Orthopaedic Surgery 2009; **Med School:** Univ Pennsylvania 1980; **Resid:** Surgery, Mount Sinai Hosp 1982; Orthopaedic Surgery, Mount Sinai Hosp 1985; **Fellow:** Pediatric Orthopaedic Surgery, Hosp for Special Surgery 1986

Nelson Jr, John M MD (OrS) - **Spec Exp:** Pediatric Orthopaedic Surgery; Joint Replacement; Sports Medicine; **Hospital:** Sound Shore Med Ctr - Westchester, Westchester Med Ctr; **Address:** 3010 Westchester Ave, Ste 104, Lower Level, rm 7, Purchase, NY 10577; **Phone:** 914-632-4420; **Board Cert:** Orthopaedic Surgery 2008; **Med School:** Mount Sinai Sch Med 1979; **Resid:** Orthopaedic Surgery, Hosp for Joint Diseases 1984; **Fellow:** Pediatric Orthopaedic Surgery, Scottish Rite Chldn's Hosp 1985

Oh, Young Don MD (OrS) - **Spec Exp:** Sports Medicine; **Hospital:** White Plains Hosp (page 615), Greenwich Hosp (page 892); **Address:** Westchester Medical Group, 210 Westchester Ave, White Plains, NY 10604; **Phone:** 914-682-6540; **Board Cert:** Orthopaedic Surgery 2012; **Med School:** NYU Sch Med 1993; **Resid:** Surgery, LIJ Med Ctr 1994; Orthopaedic Surgery, LIJ Med Ctr 1998; **Fellow:** Orthopaedic Sports Medicine, UCLA Med Ctr 1999

Pianka, George MD (OrS) - **Spec Exp:** Hand Surgery; Wrist Surgery; Upper Extremity Surgery; Arthroscopic Surgery; **Hospital:** Lenox Hill Hosp (page 106), Phelps Meml Hosp Ctr (page 614); **Address:** 24 Saw Mill River Rd, Ste 206, Hawthorne, NY 10532; **Phone:** 914-631-7777; **Board Cert:** Orthopaedic Surgery 2003; Hand Surgery 2003; **Med School:** Univ Conn 1984; **Resid:** Orthopaedic Surgery, Lenox Hill Hosp 1989; **Fellow:** Hand Surgery, Hosp For Joint Diseases 1990

Pidoriano, Arthur J MD (OrS) - **Spec Exp:** Sports Medicine; Arthroscopic Surgery; Rotator Cuff Surgery; Knee Ligament Reconstruction; **Hospital:** Hudson Valley Hosp Ctr; **Address:** Community Orthopaedic Assocs, 1985 Crompond Rd, Cortlandt Manor, NY 10567; **Phone:** 914-739-2121; **Board Cert:** Orthopaedic Surgery 2008; **Med School:** NY Med Coll 1989; **Resid:** Orthopaedic Surgery, Westchester Med Ctr 1994; **Fellow:** Sports Medicine, Univ Conn 1996

Schlesinger, Iris E MD (OrS) - **Spec Exp:** Pediatric Orthopaedic Surgery; **Hospital:** Westchester Med Ctr, Phelps Meml Hosp Ctr (page 614); **Address:** 19 Bradhurst Ave, Ste 1300N, Hawthorne, NY 10532; **Phone:** 914-789-2731; **Board Cert:** Orthopaedic Surgery 2002; **Med School:** Albany Med Coll 1983; **Resid:** Orthopaedic Surgery, NYU Med Ctr 1988; **Fellow:** Pediatric Orthopaedic Surgery, Hosp Sick Children 1989; **Fac Appt:** Assoc Prof OrS, NY Med Coll

Seebacher, J Robert MD (OrS) - **Spec Exp:** Hip Replacement; Knee Replacement; **Hospital:** Phelps Meml Hosp Ctr (page 614); **Address:** Hudson Valley Bone & Joint Surgeons, 24 Saw Mill River Rd, Ste 206, Hawthorne, NY 10532; **Phone:** 914-631-7777; **Board Cert:** Orthopaedic Surgery 1984; **Med School:** Georgetown Univ 1976; **Resid:** Surgery, Mount Sinai Hosp 1978; Orthopaedic Surgery, Hosp for Special Surgery 1981; **Fellow:** Pediatric Orthopaedic Surgery, Hosp for Sick Children 1982

Voellmicke, Kurt V MD (OrS) - **Spec Exp:** Foot & Ankle Surgery; **Hospital:** Northern Westchester Hosp (page 613), Hosp For Special Surgery (page 115); **Address:** 90 S Bedford Rd, Mount Kisco, NY 10549; **Phone:** 914-241-1050; **Board Cert:** Orthopaedic Surgery 2004; **Med School:** Cornell Univ-Weill Med Coll 1996; **Resid:** Orthopaedic Surgery, Hosp for Special Surgery 2001; **Fellow:** Foot & Ankle Surgery, Hosp for Special Surgery 2002

Weinstein, Richard N MD (OrS) - **Spec Exp:** Shoulder Surgery; Rotator Cuff Surgery; Sports Medicine; **Hospital:** White Plains Hosp (page 615); **Address:** 7 Reservoir Rd, North White Plains, NY 10603; **Phone:** 914-684-0300; **Board Cert:** Orthopaedic Surgery 2010; Orthopaedic Sports Medicine 2007; **Med School:** NYU Sch Med 1991; **Resid:** Orthopaedic Surgery, Bronx Lebanon Hosp 1996; **Fellow:** Sports Medicine, Univ Conn Hlth Syst 1997; **Fac Appt:** , Albert Einstein Coll Med

Yasgur, David MD (OrS) - **Spec Exp:** Knee Replacement; **Hospital:** Northern Westchester Hosp (page 613); **Address:** Mount Kisco Medical Group, 111 Bedford Rd, Katonah, NY 10536; **Phone:** 914-232-3135; **Board Cert:** Orthopaedic Surgery 2010; **Med School:** Cornell Univ 1991; **Resid:** Orthopaedic Surgery, Hosp Joint Diseases 1996; **Fellow:** Beth Israel North Med Ctr 1997

Zelicof, Steven B MD/PhD (OrS) - **Spec Exp:** Joint Reconstruction; Arthritis; Sports Medicine; Hip & Knee Replacement; **Hospital:** Sound Shore Med Ctr - Westchester, Westchester Med Ctr; **Address:** Specialty Orthopedics, 600 Mamaroneck Ave, Ste 101, Harrison, NY 10528; **Phone:** 914-686-0111; **Board Cert:** Orthopaedic Surgery 2003; **Med School:** Univ Pennsylvania 1983; **Resid:** Surgery, Lenox Hill Hosp 1985; Orthopaedic Surgery, Hosp Special Surg 1989; **Fellow:** Orthopaedic Surgery, Brigham & Women's Hosp 1990; **Fac Appt:** Clin Prof OrS, NY Med Coll

Otolaryngology

Fox, Mark L MD (Oto) - **Spec Exp:** Thyroid Surgery; Salivary Gland Surgery; Head & Neck Cancer; Sinus Surgery; **Hospital:** Lawrence Hosp Ctr; **Address:** ENT & Allergy Assocs, 1 Elm St, Ste 2A, Tuckahoe, NY 10707; **Phone:** 914-961-2515; **Board Cert:** Otolaryngology 1979; **Med School:** NY Med Coll 1973; **Resid:** Surgery, Metropolitan Hosp Ctr 1974; Otolaryngology, Manhattan EET Hosp 1979; **Fac Appt:** Asst Clin Prof Oto, Columbia P&S

Kase, Steven B MD (Oto) - **Spec Exp:** Sinus Disorders; Pediatric Otolaryngology; **Hospital:** White Plains Hosp (page 615), Mount Sinai Med Ctr (page 102); **Address:** 75 S Broadway Fl 3, White Plains, NY 10601; **Phone:** 914-681-0300; **Board Cert:** Otolaryngology 1981; **Med School:** Loyola Univ-Stritch Sch Med 1976; **Resid:** Surgery, St Francis Hosp 1977; Otolaryngology, NY E&E Infirmary 1980

Kates, Matthew J MD (Oto) - **Spec Exp:** Sinus Disorders/Surgery; Sleep Disorders/Apnea; Balance Disorders; **Hospital:** Sound Shore Med Ctr - Westchester, Lawrence Hosp Ctr; **Address:** 26 Burling Ln, New Rochelle, NY 10801-4914; **Phone:** 914-235-1888; **Board Cert:** Otolaryngology 1992; **Med School:** Cornell Univ-Weill Med Coll 1986; **Resid:** Surgery, St Vincent's Hosp 1988; Otolaryngology, Manhattan EET Hosp 1991

Meiteles, Lawrence MD (Oto) - **Spec Exp:** Cochlear Implants; Skull Base Surgery; Otology & Neuro-Otology; Balance Disorders; **Hospital:** Westchester Med Ctr; **Address:** The Balance Ctr, 480 Bedford Rd, Mount Kisco, NY 10514; **Phone:** 914-242-8111; **Board Cert:** Otolaryngology 1992; **Med School:** Albert Einstein Coll Med 1986; **Resid:** Surgery, Montefiore Hosp Med Ctr 1987; Otolaryngology, New York Eye & Ear 1991; **Fellow:** Univ Michigan Med Ctr 1993; **Fac Appt:** Asst Prof Oto, NY Med Coll

Ryback, Hyman MD (Oto) - **Spec Exp:** Endoscopic Sinus Surgery; Laryngeal Disorders; Snoring/Sleep Apnea; Reconstructive Surgery; **Hospital:** White Plains Hosp (page 615); **Address:** 75 S Broadway Fl 3, White Plains, NY 10601; **Phone:** 914-949-3888; **Board Cert:** Otolaryngology 1977; **Med School:** McGill Univ 1970; **Resid:** Surgery, Jewish Genl Hosp 1973; Otolaryngology, Mount Sinai Hosp 1977

Scott, John C MD (Oto) - **Spec Exp:** Head & Neck Surgery; Facial Plastic Surgery; Thyroid Surgery; **Hospital:** Northern Westchester Hosp (page 613); **Address:** Mt Kisco Medical Group, 110 S Bedford Rd, Mt Kisco, NY 10549; **Phone:** 914-242-1355; **Board Cert:** Otolaryngology 1994; Facial Plastic & Reconstr Surgery 1997; **Med School:** Univ Mich Med Sch 1988; **Resid:** Otolaryngology, Johns Hopkins Hosp 1993; **Fellow:** Facial Plastic Surgery, Mount Sinai Hosp 1994

Shapiro, Barry M MD (Oto) - **Spec Exp:** Endoscopic Sinus Surgery; Sleep Disorders/Apnea; **Hospital:** Phelps Meml Hosp Ctr (page 614), St. John's Riverside Hosp-Andrus Pavil; **Address:** West Med Medical Group, Ridge Hill, 73 Market St, Yonkers, NY 10510-1469; **Phone:** 914-945-0505; **Board Cert:** Otolaryngology 1983; **Med School:** Mount Sinai Sch Med 1978; **Resid:** Surgery, Mount Sinai Med Ctr 1979; Otolaryngology, Mount Sinai Med Ctr 1982; **Fac Appt:** Asst Clin Prof Oto, Mount Sinai Sch Med

Stidham, Katrina Ruth MD (Oto) - **Spec Exp:** Cochlear Implants; Balance Disorders; Hearing Loss; Ear Disorders; **Hospital:** Westchester Med Ctr, New York Eye & Ear Infirm (page 117); **Address:** 19 Bradhurst Ave, Ste 3600S, Hawthorne, NY 10532; **Phone:** 914-909-4578; **Board Cert:** Otolaryngology 1999; **Med School:** Duke Univ 1993; **Resid:** Otolaryngology, Stanford Univ Hosp 1998; **Fellow:** Neurotology, CA Inst 2000; **Fac Appt:** Assoc Prof Oto, NY Med Coll

Zalvan, Craig H MD (Oto) - **Spec Exp:** Voice Disorders; Swallowing Disorders; Airway Disorders; Vocal Cord Disorders; **Hospital:** Phelps Meml Hosp Ctr (page 614), Westchester Med Ctr; **Address:** Inst Voice & Swallowing Disorders, Phelps Meml Hosp Ctr, 777 N Broadway, Ste 303, North Tarrytown, NY 10591; **Phone:** 914-366-3636; **Board Cert:** Otolaryngology 2002; **Med School:** Albert Einstein Coll Med 1995; **Resid:** Otolaryngology, Manhattan EE&T 1999; Otolaryngology, Ny Presby Columbia Presbyterian Med Ctr 2001; **Fellow:** Laryngology, St Luke's Roosevelt Med Ctr 2002; **Fac Appt:** Assoc Prof Oto, NY Med Coll

Pain Medicine

Kizelshteyn, Grigory MD (PM) - **Spec Exp:** Pain-Back & Neck; Pain-Spine; **Hospital:** St. John's Riverside Hosp-Andrus Pavil; **Address:** Pain Medicine Wellness Ctr of New York, 220 Westchester Ave, White Plains, NY 10604; **Phone:** 914-289-1507; **Board Cert:** Anesthesiology 1991; Pain Medicine 2004; **Med School:** Russia 1977; **Resid:** Anesthesiology, Westchester Med Ctr 1980; **Fellow:** Pain Medicine, Westchester Med Ctr 1987

Lu, Gabriel P MD (PM) - **Spec Exp:** Acupuncture; Pain-Back & Neck; **Address:** 112 Penn Rd, Scarsdale, NY 10583; **Phone:** 914-725-4240; **Board Cert:** Anesthesiology 1984; Pain Medicine 1997; **Med School:** China 1968; **Resid:** Surgery, St Lukes Hospital 1976; Anesthesiology, Montefiore Med Ctr 1978; **Fellow:** Anesthesiology, Montefiore Med Ctr 1979; **Fac Appt:** Prof Anes, Albert Einstein Coll Med

Malits, Bella M MD (PM) - **Spec Exp:** Pain-Chronic; Reflex Sympathetic Dystrophy (RSD); **Hospital:** Northern Westchester Hosp (page 613); **Address:** Mt Kisco Med Grp, 34 S Bedford Rd Bldg 34, Mt Kisco, NY 10549; **Phone:** 914-242-4400; **Board Cert:** Anesthesiology 1995; Pain Medicine 2007; **Med School:** NY Med Coll 1990; **Resid:** Anesthesiology, Mt Sinai Med Ctr 1995; **Fellow:** Pain Management, Mt Sinai Med Ctr 1996

Pediatric Cardiology

Bierman, Fredrick MD (PCd) - **Spec Exp:** Fetal Echocardiography; Kawasaki Disease; Congenital Heart Disease; Echocardiography; **Hospital:** Westchester Med Ctr; **Address:** Munger Bldg, Ste 618, Ave, rm 139, Valhalla, NY 10595; **Phone:** 914-594-4370; **Board Cert:** Pediatrics 1978; Pediatric Cardiology 1981; **Med School:** SUNY Downstate 1973; **Resid:** Pediatrics, Mount Sinai Med Ctr 1976; **Fellow:** Pediatric Cardiology, Harvard Chldns Hosp 1979; **Fac Appt:** Prof Ped, Albert Einstein Coll Med

Fish, Bernard G MD (PCd) - **Spec Exp:** Cardiac Imaging; Fetal Echocardiography; **Hospital:** Westchester Med Ctr, Children's & Women's Phys.of Westchester (page 612); **Address:** NY Med Coll, Ped Cardiology, 19 Bradhurst Ave, Hawthorne, NY 10595; **Phone:** 914-594-4370; **Board Cert:** Pediatrics 1974; Pediatric Cardiology 1975; **Med School:** Univ Chicago-Pritzker Sch Med 1969; **Resid:** Pediatrics, Montefiore Hosp Med Ctr 1971; Pediatric Cardiology, Montefiore Hosp Med Ctr 1973; **Fellow:** Pediatric Cardiology, Yale-New Haven Hosp 1975; **Fac Appt:** Assoc Prof Ped, NY Med Coll

Friedman, Deborah M MD (PCd) - **Spec Exp:** Fetal Cardiology; Echocardiography; Fetal Echocardiography; Congenital Heart Disease; **Hospital:** Westchester Med Ctr, Children's & Women's Phys.of Westchester (page 612); **Address:** New York Med College, Munger Pavillion, rm 509, Valhalla, NY 10595; **Phone:** 914-594-4370; **Board Cert:** Pediatrics 1982; Pediatric Cardiology 1983; Pediatric Critical Care Medicine 2007; **Med School:** Univ Chicago-Pritzker Sch Med 1977; **Resid:** Pediatrics, Bronx Muni Hosp Ctr 1980; **Fellow:** Pediatric Cardiology, NYU Med Ctr 1983; **Fac Appt:** Prof Ped, NY Med Coll

Gewitz, Michael MD (PCd) - **Spec Exp:** Neonatal Cardiology; Kawasaki Disease; Echocardiography; Heart Failure; **Hospital:** Westchester Med Ctr, Children's & Women's Phys.of Westchester (page 612); **Address:** Maria Fareri Children's Hospital, Munger Pavillion, Ste 618, Valhalla, NY 10595; **Phone:** 914-594-4370; **Board Cert:** Pediatrics 1979; Pediatric Cardiology 1981; **Med School:** Hahnemann Univ 1974; **Resid:** Pediatrics, Chldns Hosp 1976; Pediatrics, Hosp Sick Chldn 1977; **Fellow:** Pediatric Cardiology, Yale-New Haven Hosp 1979; **Fac Appt:** Prof Ped, NY Med Coll

Issenberg, Henry J MD (PCd) - **Spec Exp:** Fetal Echocardiography; Congenital Heart Disease-Adult & Child; Kawasaki Disease; Arrhythmias-Fetal; **Hospital:** Westchester Med Ctr, Children's & Women's Phys.of Westchester (page 612); **Address:** NY Med College, Dept Ped Cardiology, Munger Pavilion, rm 618, Valhalla, NY 10595; **Phone:** 914-594-4370; **Board Cert:** Pediatrics 1979; Pediatric Cardiology 1979; **Med School:** Emory Univ 1974; **Resid:** Pediatrics, Jacobi Med Ctr 1977; **Fellow:** Pediatric Cardiology, Childrens Med Ctr 1980; **Fac Appt:** Assoc Prof Ped, NY Med Coll

Pediatric Critical Care Medicine

Goltzman, Carey MD (PCCM) - **Spec Exp:** Respiratory Failure; Sepsis & Septic Shock; **Hospital:** Westchester Med Ctr, Children's & Women's Phys.of Westchester (page 612); **Address:** NY Med Coll, Chldns Physicians of Westchester, Maria Fareri Chlds Hosp, PCCM, rm 2237, Valhalla, NY 10595; **Phone:** 914-493-7513; **Board Cert:** Pediatrics 2007; **Med School:** Mexico 1981; **Resid:** Pediatrics, Westchester Med Ctr 1987; **Fellow:** Pediatric Critical Care Medicine, Henry Ford Hosp 1989; **Fac Appt:** Asst Prof Ped, NY Med Coll

Pediatric Endocrinology

Handelsman, Dan MD (PEn) - **Hospital:** Phelps Meml Hosp Ctr (page 614), Children's & Women's Phys.of Westchester (page 612); **Address:** 755 N Broadway, Ste 500, Sleepy Hollow, NY 10591; **Phone:** 914-366-0015; **Board Cert:** Pediatrics 1973; **Med School:** Albert Einstein Coll Med 1968; **Resid:** Pediatrics, Montefiore Hosp 1971; **Fellow:** Genetics and Metabolism, Montefiore Hosp 1973; **Fac Appt:** Assoc Clin Prof Ped, NY Med Coll

Noto, Richard MD (PEn) - **Spec Exp:** Growth/Development Disorders; Diabetes; Lead Poisoning; Thyroid Disorders; **Hospital:** Westchester Med Ctr, Children's & Women's Phys.of Westchester (page 612); **Address:** 755 N Broadway, Fl 4, Ste 400, Sleepy Hollow, NY 10591; **Phone:** 914-366-3400; **Board Cert:** Pediatrics 1981; Pediatric Endocrinology 1983; **Med School:** Mount Sinai Sch Med 1976; **Resid:** Pediatrics, Beth Israel Med Ctr 1978; **Fellow:** Pediatric Endocrinology, NY-Presby/Weill Cornell Med Ctr 1979; Pediatric Endocrinology, N Shore Univ Hosp 1981; **Fac Appt:** Asst Prof Ped, NY Med Coll

Romano, Alicia MD (PEn) - **Spec Exp:** Growth/Development Disorders; Diabetes; **Hospital:** Westchester Med Ctr, Children's & Women's Phys.of Westchester (page 612); **Address:** Children's Physicians of Westchester, 701 N Broadway, Ste 400, Sleepy Hollow, NY 10591; **Phone:** 914-366-3400; **Board Cert:** Pediatric Endocrinology 2006; **Med School:** SUNY Stony Brook 1985; **Resid:** Pediatrics, Schneider Chldns Hosp 1988; **Fellow:** Pediatric Endocrinology, Schneider Chldns Hosp 1991; **Fac Appt:** Asst Prof Ped, NY Med Coll

Saenger, Paul MD (PEn) - **Spec Exp:** Short Stature in Children; Turner Syndrome; Sexual Differentiation Disorders; **Hospital:** Winthrop Univ Hosp (page 504); **Address:** 150 Lockwood Ave, Ste 34, New Rochelle, NY 10801; **Phone:** 914-636-5924; **Board Cert:** Pediatrics 1973; Pediatric Endocrinology 1978; **Med School:** Germany 1967; **Resid:** Pediatrics, Montefiore Hosp Med Ctr 1970; Pediatrics, Albert Einstein Coll Med 1971; **Fellow:** Pediatric Endocrinology, Cornell Univ Med Ctr 1975; **Fac Appt:** Prof Ped, Albert Einstein Coll Med

Pediatric Gastroenterology

Berezin, Stuart MD (PGe) - **Hospital:** Westchester Med Ctr, Children's & Women's Phys.of Westchester (page 612); **Address:** Chldns & Womens/Pediatric Gastroent, 503 Grasslands Rd, Valhalla, NY 10595; **Phone:** 914-367-0000; **Board Cert:** Pediatrics 1980; Pediatric Gastroenterology 1990; **Med School:** Hahnemann Univ 1976; **Resid:** Pediatrics, Metrohealth Med Ctr 1980; **Fellow:** Gastroenterology, Children's Hosp 1982; **Fac Appt:** Assoc Prof Ped, NY Med Coll

Birnbaum, Audrey MD (PGe) - **Spec Exp:** Food Allergy; Inflammatory Bowel Disease/Crohn's; **Hospital:** Northern Westchester Hosp (page 613); **Address:** 110 S Bedford Rd, Mount Kisco, NY 10549; **Phone:** 914-241-1050; **Board Cert:** Pediatric Gastroenterology 2007; **Med School:** NYU Sch Med 1986; **Resid:** Pediatrics, Mt Sinai Hosp 1989; **Fellow:** Pediatric Gastroenterology, Mt Sinai Hosp 1991

Halata, Michael MD (PGe) - **Spec Exp:** Inflammatory Bowel Disease; Functional Bowel Disorders; Gastroesophageal Reflux Disease (GERD); **Hospital:** Westchester Med Ctr, Children's & Women's Phys.of Westchester (page 612); **Address:** 503 Grasslands Rd, Ste 201, Valhalla, NY 10595; **Phone:** 914-367-0000; **Board Cert:** Pediatrics 1980; Pediatric Gastroenterology 2005; **Med School:** UMDNJ-NJ Med Sch, Newark 1974; **Resid:** Pediatrics, Westchester Med Ctr 1977; **Fellow:** Pediatric Gastroenterology, Westchester Med Ctr 1979; **Fac Appt:** Assoc Clin Prof Ped, NY Med Coll

Newman, Leonard MD (PGe) - **Spec Exp:** Inflammatory Bowel Disease; Celiac Disease; **Hospital:** Westchester Med Ctr, Children's & Women's Phys.of Westchester (page 612); **Address:** 503 Grasslands Rd, Ste 201, Valhalla, NY 10595; **Phone:** 914-367-0000; **Board Cert:** Pediatrics 1975; Pediatric Gastroenterology 2005; **Med School:** NY Med Coll 1970; **Resid:** Pediatrics, UCSD Med Ctr 1972; Pediatrics, NY Med Coll 1973; **Fellow:** Gastroenterology, Bronx Lebanon Hosp/Einstein 1974; **Fac Appt:** Prof Ped, NY Med Coll

Pediatric Hematology-Oncology

Cairo, Mitchell S MD (PHO) - **Spec Exp:** Bone Marrow Transplant; Stem Cell Transplant; Leukemia; Lymphoma; **Hospital:** Westchester Med Ctr, Children's & Women's Phys.of Westchester (page 612); **Address:** New York Medical College, Munger Pavilion, rm 110, Valhalla, NY 10595; **Phone:** 914-594-3650; **Board Cert:** Pediatrics 1980; Pediatric Hematology-Oncology 1982; **Med School:** UCSF 1976; **Resid:** Pediatrics, UCLA Med Ctr 1979; **Fellow:** Pediatric Hematology-Oncology, Indiana Univ Med Ctr 1981; **Fac Appt:** Prof Ped, NY Med Coll

Ozkaynak, Mehmet Fevzi MD (PHO) - **Spec Exp:** Bone Marrow Transplant; **Hospital:** Westchester Med Ctr, Children's & Women's Phys.of Westchester (page 612); **Address:** Westchester Medical Ctr, Munger Pavilion, Ste 180, Valhalla, NY 10595; **Phone:** 914-493-7997; **Board Cert:** Pediatric Hematology-Oncology 2007; **Med School:** Turkey 1978; **Resid:** Pediatrics, Hacettepe Chldn's Hosp 1982; Pediatrics, Chldn's Hosp 1991; **Fellow:** Hematology & Oncology, Chldn's Hosp 1989; **Fac Appt:** Prof Ped, NY Med Coll

Sandoval, Claudio MD (PHO) - **Hospital:** Westchester Med Ctr, Children's & Women's Phys.of Westchester (page 612); **Address:** NY Med Coll, Munger Pavillion, rm 180, Valhalla, NY 10595; **Phone:** 914-493-7997; **Board Cert:** Pediatric Hematology-Oncology 2009; **Med School:** NY Med Coll 1987; **Resid:** Pediatrics, Schneider Chldns Hosp 1990; **Fellow:** Pediatric Hematology-Oncology, St Jude Chldns Rsch Hosp 1991

Tugal, Oya L MD (PHO) - **Spec Exp:** Leukemia & Lymphoma; Brain Tumors; Langerhans Cell Histiocytoma; **Hospital:** Westchester Med Ctr, Children's & Women's Phys.of Westchester (page 612); **Address:** NY Med Coll, Munger Pavilion, rm 180, Valhalla, NY 10595; **Phone:** 914-493-7997; **Board Cert:** Pediatrics 1986; Pediatric Hematology-Oncology 1987; **Med School:** Turkey 1974; **Resid:** Pediatrics, Hacettepe Med Ctr 1977; Pediatrics, Westchester Med Ctr 1985; **Fellow:** Allergy & Immunology, Hacettepe Med Ctr 1978; Pediatric Hematology-Oncology, Mount Sinai Hosp 1987; **Fac Appt:** Prof Ped, NY Med Coll

Pediatric Nephrology

Weiss, Robert Allen MD (PNep) - **Spec Exp:** Kidney Failure; Nephrotic Syndrome; **Hospital:** Westchester Med Ctr, Children's & Women's Phys.of Westchester (page 612); **Address:** Pediatric Nephrology, 19 Bradhurst Ave Fl 1 - rm 1400, Hawthorne, NY 10595; **Phone:** 914-493-7583; **Board Cert:** Pediatrics 1976; Pediatric Nephrology 1979; **Med School:** Georgetown Univ 1971; **Resid:** Pediatrics, Bellevue Hosp Ctr 1974; **Fellow:** Pediatric Nephrology, Montefiore Med Ctr 1978; **Fac Appt:** Prof Ped, NY Med Coll

Pediatric Otolaryngology

De Serres, Lianne M MD (PO) - **Spec Exp:** Airway Disorders; Sinus Disorders; Ear Infections; Sleep Apnea; **Hospital:** Westchester Med Ctr; **Address:** ENT Faculty Practice, 1055 Saw Mill River Rd, Ste 101, Ardsley, NY 10502; **Phone:** 914-693-7636; **Board Cert:** Otolaryngology 1997; **Med School:** Univ NC Sch Med 1990; **Resid:** Otolaryngology, Univ Wash Med Ctr 1996; **Fellow:** Pediatric Otolaryngology, Univ Wash Med Ctr 1998

Keller, Jeffrey L MD (PO) - **Spec Exp:** Otitis Media; Sinusitis; Sleep Disorders/Apnea; **Hospital:** Northern Westchester Hosp (page 613), Mount Sinai Med Ctr (page 102); **Address:** 110 S Bedford Rd, Mount Kisco, NY 10549; **Phone:** 914-242-1355; **Board Cert:** Otolaryngology 1996; **Med School:** Stanford Univ 1990; **Resid:** Otolaryngology, Mt Sinai Hosp 1995; **Fellow:** Pediatric Otolaryngology, Chldns Hosp 1996; **Fac Appt:** Asst Prof Oto, Mount Sinai Sch Med

Merer, David M MD (PO) - **Hospital:** Westchester Med Ctr; **Address:** 1055 Saw Mill River Rd, Ste 101, Ardsley, NY 10502; **Phone:** 914-693-7636; **Board Cert:** Otolaryngology 1996; **Med School:** Albert Einstein Coll Med 1990; **Resid:** Otolaryngology, Montefiore Med Ctr 1995; **Fellow:** Pediatric Otolaryngology, Montefiore Med Ctr 1996; **Fac Appt:** Assoc Prof Oto, NY Med Coll

Pediatric Pulmonology

Amin, Nikhil S MD (PPul) - **Spec Exp:** Cystic Fibrosis; Asthma; Lung Disorders-Congenital; Primary Ciliary Dyskinesia; **Hospital:** Westchester Med Ctr, Children's & Women's Phys.of Westchester (page 612); **Address:** Munger Pavilion, rm 106, Dept Ped Div Pul, Valhalla, NY 10595; **Phone:** 914-493-7585; **Board Cert:** Pediatric Pulmonology 2009; **Med School:** India 1980; **Resid:** Pediatrics, Baroda Med Coll 1984; Pediatrics, NY Med Coll 1988; **Fellow:** Pediatric Pulmonology, NY Med Coll 1994; **Fac Appt:** Assoc Prof Ped, NY Med Coll

Boyer, Joseph MD (PPul) - **Spec Exp:** Asthma; Cystic Fibrosis; **Hospital:** Westchester Med Ctr, Children's & Women's Phys.of Westchester (page 612); **Address:** New York Med Coll, Pediatric Pulmonology, Munger Pavilion, rm 106, Valhalla, NY 10595; **Phone:** 914-493-7585; **Board Cert:** Therapeutic Radiology 2006; **Med School:** SUNY Downstate 1988; **Resid:** Pediatrics, Westchester Co Med Ctr 1991; **Fellow:** Pediatric Pulmonology, Westchester Co Med Ctr 1995

Dozor, Allen J MD (PPul) - **Spec Exp:** Asthma; Cystic Fibrosis; **Hospital:** Westchester Med Ctr, Children's & Women's Phys.of Westchester (page 612); **Address:** NY Med College, Munger Pavilion, Pediatric Pulmonology, Ste 106, Valhalla, NY 10595-1600; **Phone:** 914-493-7585; **Board Cert:** Pediatrics 1981; Pediatric Pulmonology 2003; **Med School:** Penn State Coll Med 1977; **Resid:** Pediatrics, St Vincent's Hosp & Med Ctr 1980; **Fellow:** Pediatric Pulmonology, Chldns Hosp 1982; **Fac Appt:** Prof Ped, NY Med Coll

Kass, Lewis MD (PPul) - **Spec Exp:** Sleep Disorders/Apnea; **Hospital:** Northern Westchester Hosp (page 613), Norwalk Hosp; **Address:** 103 S Bedford Rd, Ste 111, Mount Kisco, NY 10549; **Phone:** 914-242-0445; **Board Cert:** Pediatrics 2010; Pediatric Pulmonology 2012; Sleep Medicine 2007; **Med School:** SUNY Downstate 1991; **Resid:** Pediatrics, SUNY-Chldren's Med Ctr 1995; **Fellow:** Pediatric Pulmonology, Yale New Haven Children's Hosp 1997

Lowenthal, Diana MD (PPul) - **Spec Exp:** Asthma; Cystic Fibrosis; Cough; Bronchoscopy; **Hospital:** Westchester Med Ctr, Children's & Women's Phys.of Westchester (page 612); **Address:** NY Med Coll, Pediatric Pulmology, Munger Pavilion, rm 106, Valhalla, NY 10595; **Phone:** 914-493-7585; **Board Cert:** Pediatric Pulmonology 2007; **Med School:** Albert Einstein Coll Med 1986; **Resid:** Pediatrics, Albert Einstein Coll Med 1989; **Fellow:** Pulmonary Disease, Mount Sinai Hosp 1992; **Fac Appt:** Asst Prof Ped, NY Med Coll

Quittell, Lynne M MD (PPul) - **Spec Exp:** Cystic Fibrosis; Asthma; **Hospital:** Morgan Stanley Children's Hosp of NY-Presby, NY (page 104), NY-Presby/Columbia Univ Med Ctr, NY (page 104); **Address:** Morgan Stanley Children's Hosp of NY, 3959 Broadway, CHONY Bldg - Fl 7, New York, NY 10032; **Phone:** 212-305-5122; **Board Cert:** Pediatrics 1986; Pediatric Pulmonology 2011; **Med School:** Israel 1981; **Resid:** Pediatrics, Schneider Chldns Hosp 1984; **Fellow:** Pediatric Pulmonology, St Christopher's Hosp 1988; **Fac Appt:** Assoc Prof Ped, Columbia P&S

Pediatric Rheumatology

Chao, Chun MD (PRhu) - **Spec Exp:** Juvenile Arthritis; Lupus/SLE; **Hospital:** Westchester Med Ctr, Children's & Women's Phys.of Westchester (page 612); **Address:** Westchester Medical Ctr, Munger Pavilion, rm 119, Valhalla, NY 10595; **Phone:** 914-594-4835; **Board Cert:** Pediatric Rheumatology 2009; **Med School:** Philippines 1982; **Resid:** Pediatrics, Duke Univ Med Ctr 1990; **Fellow:** Pediatric Rheumatology, Univ Tennessee Med Ctr 1993; **Fac Appt:** Asst Prof Ped, NY Med Coll

Pediatric Surgery

McBride, Whitney J MD (PS) - **Spec Exp:** Neonatal Surgery; Laparoscopic Surgery; **Hospital:** Westchester Med Ctr, Children's & Women's Phys.of Westchester (page 612); **Address:** Maria Fereri Children's Hosp, 321 Munger Pavilion, Valhalla, NY 10595; **Phone:** 914-493-7620; **Board Cert:** Surgery 2011; **Med School:** Univ VT Coll Med 1992; **Resid:** Surgery, Fletcher Allen Hlthcare/Univ VT 1998

Stringel, Gustavo MD (PS) - **Spec Exp:** Minimally Invasive Surgery; Cancer Surgery; Neonatal Surgery; **Hospital:** Westchester Med Ctr; **Address:** New York Med College, Div Ped Surgery, 19 Bradhurst Ave, Ste 1400, Hawthorne, NY 10532; **Phone:** 914-493-7620; **Board Cert:** Surgery 2007; Pediatric Surgery 2005; Surgical Critical Care 2007; **Med School:** Mexico 1971; **Resid:** Surgery, Univ Toronto 1977; **Fellow:** Pediatric Surgery, Hosp Sick Chldn 1979; **Fac Appt:** Prof S, NY Med Coll

Zitsman, Jeffrey MD (PS) - **Spec Exp:** Minimally Invasive Surgery; Chest Wall Deformities; Obesity/Bariatric Surgery; **Hospital:** Morgan Stanley Children's Hosp of NY-Presby, NY (page 104), White Plains Hosp (page 615); **Address:** 688 White Plains Rd, Ste 223, Scarsdale, NY 10583-5015; **Phone:** 914-722-6737; **Board Cert:** Surgery 2001; Pediatric Surgery 2005; **Med School:** Tufts Univ 1976; **Resid:** Surgery, New England Med Ctr 1981; **Fellow:** Pediatric Surgery, Babies Hosp/Columbia Presby Med Ctr 1985; **Fac Appt:** Assoc Clin Prof S, Columbia P&S

Pediatrics

Acker, Peter J MD (Ped) *PCP* - **Spec Exp:** Pediatric Dermatology; Adolescent Medicine; Learning Disorders; **Hospital:** Greenwich Hosp (page 892), Westchester Med Ctr; **Address:** Pediatric Associates, 26 Rye Ridge Plaza, Rye Brook, NY 10573; **Phone:** 914-251-1100; **Board Cert:** Pediatrics 2009; **Med School:** Israel 1982; **Resid:** Pediatrics, NYU-Bellevue Hosp 1985; **Fellow:** Ambulatory Pediatrics, NYU-Bellevue Hosp 1987

Altman, Robin MD (Ped) *PCP* - **Spec Exp:** Child Abuse; **Hospital:** Westchester Med Ctr, Children's & Women's Phys.of Westchester (page 612); **Address:** 19 Bradhurst Ave, Ste 2400, Hawthorne, NY 10532; **Phone:** 914-593-8850; **Board Cert:** Pediatrics 1987; **Med School:** UMDNJ-RW Johnson Med Sch 1983; **Resid:** Pediatrics, Colum-Presby Med Ctr 1986; **Fac Appt:** Asst Prof Ped, NY Med Coll

Amler, David H MD (Ped) *PCP* - **Spec Exp:** Adolescent Medicine; **Hospital:** White Plains Hosp (page 615); **Address:** 15 N Broadway, Ste F, White Plains, NY 10601-2214; **Phone:** 914-948-4422; **Board Cert:** Pediatrics 1982; **Med School:** SUNY Buffalo 1969; **Resid:** Pediatrics, NYU Med Ctr 1972

Bailey, Michele L MD (Ped) *PCP* - **Spec Exp:** Asthma; **Hospital:** Montefiore Med Ctr-Wakefield Campus, NY (page 100), Lawrence Hosp Ctr; **Address:** 16 North Broadway, Ste LMG, White Plains, NY 10601; **Phone:** 914-686-1848; **Board Cert:** Pediatrics 2009; **Med School:** West Indies 1989; **Resid:** Pediatrics, Lincoln Med Ctr 1994; **Fac Appt:** Asst Clin Prof Ped, NY Med Coll

Baskind, Lawrence J MD (Ped) *PCP* - **Hospital:** Hudson Valley Hosp Ctr; **Address:** 35 S Riverside Ave, Ste 101, Croton-On-Hudson, NY 10520; **Phone:** 914-271-2424; **Board Cert:** Pediatrics 2010; **Med School:** UMDNJ-NJ Med Sch, Newark 1983; **Resid:** Pediatrics, Univ Hosp 1987

Berkowitz, Norman MD (Ped) *PCP* - **Hospital:** Greenwich Hosp (page 892), Westchester Med Ctr; **Address:** 26 Rye Ridge Plaza, Rye Brook, NY 10573-2820; **Phone:** 914-251-1100; **Board Cert:** Pediatrics 1972; **Med School:** SUNY Buffalo 1967; **Resid:** Pediatrics, Mount Sinai Med Ctr 1970; **Fellow:** Pediatrics, St Christopher Hosp Chldn 1973

Bomback, Fredric MD (Ped) *PCP* - **Spec Exp:** Infectious Disease; Complex Diagnosis; **Hospital:** White Plains Hosp (page 615), NY-Presby/Columbia Univ Med Ctr, NY (page 104); **Address:** Westchester Pediatrics, 99 Fieldstone Drive, Hartsdale, NY 10530; **Phone:** 914-428-2120; **Board Cert:** Pediatrics 1984; **Med School:** NYU Sch Med 1969; **Resid:** Pediatrics, Bronx Muni Hosp 1972; **Fellow:** Genetics and Metabolism, Albert Einstein Coll Med 1976; **Fac Appt:** Clin Prof Ped, Columbia P&S

Bookner, Scott D MD (Ped) *PCP* - **Hospital:** White Plains Hosp (page 615); **Address:** Scarsdale Pediatric Assocs, 7 Popham Rd, Ste 301, Scarsdale, NY 10583; **Phone:** 914-725-0800; **Board Cert:** Pediatrics 2007; **Med School:** SUNY Buffalo 1989; **Resid:** Pediatrics, Chldns Hosp 1992; **Fac Appt:** Asst Clin Prof Ped, NY Med Coll

Coven, Barbara MD (Ped) *PCP* - **Hospital:** Greenwich Hosp (page 892), White Plains Hosp (page 615); **Address:** Westchester Med Grp, Dept Pediatrics, 210 Westchester Ave Fl 2, White Plains, NY 10604; **Phone:** 914-682-0731; **Board Cert:** Pediatrics 1986; **Med School:** Boston Univ 1980; **Resid:** Pediatrics, Boston City Hosp 1983; **Fellow:** Psychosomatic Medicine, Chldns Hosp Med Ctr 1983

Easton, Lon MD (Ped) *PCP* - **Spec Exp:** Sports Medicine; **Hospital:** Montefiore Med Ctr-Moses Campus, NY (page 100), Montefiore Med Ctr-Einstein Campus, NY (page 100); **Address:** 171 Huguenot St, New Rochelle, NY 10801; **Phone:** 718-863-1050; **Board Cert:** Pediatrics 1983; **Med School:** NY Med Coll 1978; **Resid:** Pediatrics, Metropolitan Hosp 1981; **Fac Appt:** Asst Clin Prof Ped, Albert Einstein Coll Med

Edis, Gloria MD (Ped) *PCP* - **Hospital:** White Plains Hosp (page 615); **Address:** 7 Popham Rd, Ste 301, Scarsdale, NY 10583; **Phone:** 914-725-0800; **Board Cert:** Pediatrics 1970; **Med School:** NYU Sch Med 1963; **Resid:** Pediatrics, Montefiore Hosp Med Ctr 1964; Pediatrics, Columbia-Presby 1968; **Fac Appt:** Assoc Clin Prof Ped, Cornell Univ-Weill Med Coll

Hartz, Cindi MD (Ped) *PCP* - **Hospital:** Sound Shore Med Ctr - Westchester; **Address:** 1415 Boston Post Rd, Larchmont, NY 10538; **Phone:** 914-833-1502; **Board Cert:** Pediatrics 2011; **Med School:** Mount Sinai Sch Med 1983; **Resid:** Pediatrics, Mt Sinai Hosp 1986; **Fellow:** Hematology & Oncology, Mt Sinai Hosp 1987

Levitt, Miriam MD (Ped) *PCP* - **Spec Exp:** Travel Medicine; **Hospital:** Lawrence Hosp Ctr, Montefiore Med Ctr-Moses Campus, NY (page 100); **Address:** 1 Pondfield Rd, Ste 303, Bronxville, NY 10708-3706; **Phone:** 914-961-3604; **Board Cert:** Pediatrics 1975; **Med School:** Albert Einstein Coll Med 1971; **Resid:** Pediatrics, Montefiore Hosp Med Ctr 1973; **Fac Appt:** Asst Clin Prof Ped, Albert Einstein Coll Med

London, Ronald MD (Ped) *PCP* - **Hospital:** Montefiore Med Ctr-Moses Campus, NY (page 100), Montefiore Med Ctr-Einstein Campus, NY (page 100); **Address:** Westmed Medical Group, 171 Huguenot St, New Rochelle, NY 10801; **Phone:** 718-863-1050; **Board Cert:** Pediatrics 2003; **Med School:** Israel 1984; **Resid:** Pediatrics, Montefiore Hosp Med Ctr 1987; **Fellow:** Child Development, Albert Einstein 1988

Lubell, Harry R MD (Ped) *PCP* - **Hospital:** Phelps Meml Hosp Ctr (page 614), Westchester Med Ctr; **Address:** 150 White Plains Rd, Ste 101, Tarrytown, NY 10591-2657; **Phone:** 914-332-4141; **Board Cert:** Pediatrics 1969; **Med School:** Ros Franklin Univ/Chicago Med Sch 1964; **Resid:** Pediatrics, Montefiore Hosp Med Ctr 1967; **Fellow:** Pediatric Hematology-Oncology, Babies Hosp-Columbia Preby 1970; **Fac Appt:** Assoc Clin Prof Ped, NY Med Coll

Meisler, Susan MD (Ped) *PCP* - **Spec Exp:** Adolescent Medicine; **Hospital:** Montefiore Med Ctr-Einstein Campus, NY (page 100), Sound Shore Med Ctr - Westchester; **Address:** 145 Hugenot St, Ste 200, New Rochelle, NY 10801-5011; **Phone:** 914-235-1400; **Board Cert:** Pediatrics 2004; **Med School:** SUNY Downstate 1984; **Resid:** Pediatrics, Schneider Chldn's Hosp 1987

Proskin, Wendy MD (Ped) *PCP* - **Hospital:** White Plains Hosp (page 615), Greenwich Hosp (page 892); **Address:** 210 Westchester Ave, White Plains, NY 10604; **Phone:** 914-682-0731; **Board Cert:** Pediatrics 2002; **Med School:** SUNY Downstate 1999; **Resid:** Pediatrics, Montefiore Med Ctr 2002

Richel, Peter MD (Ped) *PCP* - **Hospital:** Northern Westchester Hosp (page 613); **Address:** 36 Smith Ave, Mt Kisco, NY 10549; **Phone:** 914-666-6655; **Board Cert:** Pediatrics 2008; **Med School:** Dominican Republic 1983; **Resid:** Pediatrics, Albany Med Ctr 1987; **Fellow:** Ambulatory Pediatrics, St Luke's-Roosevelt Hosp Ctr 1988; **Fac Appt:** Asst Clin Prof Ped, Albert Einstein Coll Med

Versfelt, Mary MD (Ped) *PCP* - **Spec Exp:** Chronic Illness; Neonatal Care; Adolescent Medicine; **Hospital:** Greenwich Hosp (page 892), Westchester Med Ctr; **Address:** 26 Rye Ridge Plaza, Rye Brook, NY 10573-2820; **Phone:** 914-251-1100; **Board Cert:** Pediatrics 1983; **Med School:** Columbia P&S 1978; **Resid:** Pediatrics, Columbia Presby Med Ctr 1981; **Fac Appt:** Assoc Clin Prof Ped, Columbia P&S

Wager, Marc D MD (Ped) *PCP* - **Spec Exp:** Adolescent Medicine; **Hospital:** Sound Shore Med Ctr - Westchester; **Address:** Pediatric Group of New Rochelle, 140 Lockwood Ave, Ste 115, New Rochelle, NY 10801-4907; **Phone:** 914-235-3800; **Board Cert:** Pediatrics 1986; **Med School:** Albert Einstein Coll Med 1981; **Resid:** Pediatrics, Jacobi Med Ctr 1984; **Fellow:** Adolescent Medicine, Montefiore Med Ctr 1986; **Fac Appt:** Asst Clin Prof Ped, Albert Einstein Coll Med

Weissbrot, Jay M MD (Ped) *PCP* - **Spec Exp:** Adolescent Medicine; **Hospital:** White Plains Hosp (page 615); **Address:** 410 N Broadway, White Plains, NY 10603-3312; **Phone:** 914-948-0353; **Board Cert:** Pediatrics 1986; **Med School:** SUNY Downstate 1980; **Resid:** Pediatrics, Brookdale Univ Hosp 1983; **Fellow:** Adolescent Medicine, Brookdale Univ Hosp 1984

Physical Medicine & Rehabilitation

Pechman, Karen M MD (PMR) - **Spec Exp:** Electrodiagnosis; Musculoskeletal Disorders; Amputee Rehabilitation; Pain Management; **Hospital:** Burke Rehab Hosp, White Plains Hosp (page 615); **Address:** 170 Maple Ave, Ste 510, White Plains, NY 10601; **Phone:** 914-683-0020; **Board Cert:** Physical Medicine & Rehabilitation 1987; Electrodiagnostic Medicine 1989; **Med School:** Boston Univ 1980; **Resid:** Physical Medicine & Rehabilitation, Montefiore-Weiler Einstein Div 1986; **Fellow:** Research, NYU Sch Med 1982; **Fac Appt:** Asst Clin Prof PMR, Cornell Univ-Weill Med Coll

Pici, Ralph A MD (PMR) - **Spec Exp:** Musculoskeletal Disorders; **Hospital:** Lawrence Hosp Ctr; **Address:** Lawrence Hospital, Physical Med & Rehab, 55 Palmer Ave Fl 2, Bronxville, NY 10708; **Phone:** 914-787-3374; **Board Cert:** Physical Medicine & Rehabilitation 1974; **Med School:** Italy 1965; **Resid:** Pediatrics, Grasslands Hosp 1967; Physical Medicine & Rehabilitation, Montefiore-Weiler Einstein Div 1972

Randolph, Audrey L MD (PMR) - **Spec Exp:** Musculoskeletal Disorders; Pain-Back & Neck; **Hospital:** Westchester Med Ctr; **Address:** 19 Bradhurst Ave, Ste 2450N, Hawthorne, NY 10532; **Phone:** 914-909-4168; **Board Cert:** Physical Medicine & Rehabilitation 1970; **Med School:** Med Coll PA Hahnemann 1964; **Resid:** Physical Medicine & Rehabilitation, NYU Med Ctr 1968; **Fac Appt:** Prof PMR, NY Med Coll

Plastic Surgery

Beran, Samuel J MD (PlS) - **Spec Exp:** Reconstructive Surgery; Liposuction; **Hospital:** White Plains Hosp (page 615); **Address:** 440 Mamaroneck Ave, Ste 412, Harrison, NY 10528; **Phone:** 914-761-8667; **Board Cert:** Plastic Surgery 2009; **Med School:** Albany Med Coll 1990; **Resid:** Surgery, T Jefferson Univ Hosp 1995; Plastic Surgery, Univ Tex-SW Med Ctr 1997

Bernard, Robert W MD (PlS) - **Spec Exp:** Cosmetic Surgery-Face; Cosmetic Surgery-Body; Breast Reconstruction; **Hospital:** White Plains Hosp (page 615), Northern Westchester Hosp (page 613); **Address:** 440 Mamaroneck Ave, Ste 412, Harrison, NY 10528; **Phone:** 914-761-8667; **Board Cert:** Surgery 1973; Plastic Surgery 1975; **Med School:** Univ VT Coll Med 1967; **Resid:** Surgery, NYU Med Ctr 1972; Plastic Surgery, NYU Med Ctr 1974

Chin, Simon H MD (PlS) - **Spec Exp:** Hand Surgery; Cosmetic Surgery; Plastic & Reconstructive Surgery; **Hospital:** Putnam Hosp Ctr, Northern Westchester Hosp (page 613); **Address:** Mt Kisco Medical Group, 111 Bedford Rd, Katonah, NY 10536; **Phone:** 914-232-3135; **Board Cert:** Plastic Surgery 2009; Hand Surgery 2010; **Med School:** Vanderbilt Univ 2000; **Resid:** Surgery, Yale-New Haven Hosp 2003; Plastic Surgery, Yale-New Haven Hosp 2006; **Fellow:** Hand Surgery, Univ Washington Med Ctr 2007; Cosmetic Plastic Surgery, NYU Med Ctr 2008

Greenwald, Joshua Adam MD (PlS) - **Spec Exp:** Breast Augmentation; Rhinoplasty; Liposuction & Body Contouring; **Hospital:** White Plains Hosp (page 615); **Address:** 440 Mamaroneck Ave, Ste 412, Harrison, NY 10528; **Phone:** 914-421-0113; **Board Cert:** Plastic Surgery 2005; **Med School:** NYU Sch Med 1995; **Resid:** Surgery, NYU Med Ctr 2001; **Fellow:** Plastic Surgery, Emory Univ Hosp 2004

Khoury, F Frederic MD (PlS) - **Spec Exp:** Pediatric Plastic Surgery; Cosmetic Surgery-Breast; Cosmetic Surgery-Face; **Hospital:** White Plains Hosp (page 615), Greenwich Hosp (page 892); **Address:** 22 Rye Ridge Plaza, Rye Brook, NY 10573-2820; **Phone:** 914-253-9300; **Board Cert:** Plastic Surgery 2004; **Med School:** Lebanon 1971; **Resid:** Surgery, St Luke's-Roosevelt Hosp Ctr 1976; Plastic Surgery, St Luke's-Roosevelt Hosp Ctr 1979; **Fellow:** Plastic Surgery, St Louis Hosp 1977

Kim, Tae Ho MD (PlS) - **Spec Exp:** Craniofacial Surgery; Pediatric Craniofacial Surgery; **Hospital:** Westchester Med Ctr; **Address:** 155 White Plains Rd, Ste 109, Tarrytown, NY 10591; **Phone:** 914-366-6139; **Board Cert:** Plastic Surgery 2003; **Med School:** Univ Pittsburgh 1991; **Resid:** Surgery, UC Irvine Med Ctr 1993; Plastic Surgery, Univ Mass Med Ctr 1999

Kleinman, Andrew MD (PlS) - **Spec Exp:** Cosmetic Surgery; Breast Augmentation; Eyelid Surgery; **Hospital:** Sound Shore Med Ctr - Westchester; **Address:** 800 Westchester Ave, Ste S-512, Rye Brook, NY 10573; **Phone:** 914-253-0700; **Board Cert:** Plastic Surgery 1989; **Med School:** Univ Rochester 1979; **Resid:** Surgery, Harvard Surg Svcs 1982; **Fellow:** Plastic Surgery, Baylor Coll Med 1985

Newman, Scott E MD (PlS) - **Spec Exp:** Breast Reconstruction & Augmentation; Cosmetic Surgery-Breast; Cosmetic Surgery-Body; Abdominoplasty; **Hospital:** St. John's Riverside Hosp-Andrus Pavil, Montefiore Med Ctr-Einstein Campus, NY (page 100); **Address:** 1 Odell Plaza, Yonkers, NY 10701; **Phone:** 914-423-9000; **Board Cert:** Plastic Surgery 2004; **Med School:** NY Med Coll 1985; **Resid:** Surgery, Westchester Med Ctr 1990; Plastic Surgery, Mt Sinai Hosp 1993; **Fac Appt:** Asst Clin Prof PlS, Albert Einstein Coll Med

Palaia, David A MD (PlS) - **Spec Exp:** Cosmetic Surgery-Face; Breast Reconstruction; Rhinoplasty; Reconstructive Surgery; **Hospital:** Northern Westchester Hosp (page 613); **Address:** 400 E Main St, North Bldg, Fl 2, Mt Kisco, NY 10549; **Phone:** 914-242-7610; **Board Cert:** Plastic Surgery 1993; **Med School:** UMDNJ-NJ Med Sch, Newark 1985; **Resid:** Surgery, Montefiore-Weiler Einstein Div 1989; Plastic Surgery, Montefiore-Weiler Einstein Div 1991

Reiffel, Robert S MD (PlS) - **Spec Exp:** Cosmetic & Reconstructive Surgery; Hand Surgery; **Hospital:** White Plains Hosp (page 615); **Address:** 12 Greenridge Ave, Ste Ste 203, White Plains, NY 10605-1238; **Phone:** 914-683-1400; **Board Cert:** Plastic Surgery 1981; **Med School:** Columbia P&S 1972; **Resid:** Surgery, Roosevelt Hosp 1977; Plastic Surgery, NYU Med Ctr 1979; **Fellow:** Hand Surgery, NYU Med Ctr 1980

Rosenberg, Michael H MD (PlS) - **Spec Exp:** Breast Surgery; **Hospital:** Northern Westchester Hosp (page 613), Westchester Med Ctr; **Address:** Northern Westchester Surgical Services, 400 E Main St, Fl 2, Ste North, Mount Kisco, NY 10549; **Phone:** 914-242-7610; **Board Cert:** Surgery 2006; Plastic Surgery 2008; **Med School:** Columbia P&S 1987; **Resid:** Surgery, Columbia Presby Med Ctr 1992; Plastic/Reconstructive Surgery, Columbia Presby Med Ctr 1994; **Fac Appt:** Asst Clin Prof PlS, NY Med Coll

Roth, Douglas A MD (PlS) - **Spec Exp:** Cosmetic Surgery-Face; Cosmetic Surgery-Breast; Facial Plastic & Reconstructive Surgery; Skin Cancer; **Hospital:** Northern Westchester Hosp (page 613), Lenox Hill Hosp (Manh Eye, Ear & Throat Hosp) (page 106); **Address:** Mount Kisco Medical Grp, Dept Plastic Surgery, 110 S Bedford Rd, Mount Kisco, NY 10549; **Phone:** 914-242-5647; **Board Cert:** Surgery 1997; Plastic Surgery 2000; **Med School:** NYU Sch Med 1990; **Resid:** Surgery, NYU Med Ctr 1996; Plastic Surgery, NYU Med Ctr 1998; **Fellow:** Microvascular Surgery, NYU Med Ctr 1999; **Fac Appt:** Asst Clin Prof S, Mount Sinai Sch Med

Suzman, Michael S MD (PlS) - **Spec Exp:** Rhinoplasty; Facial Plastic & Reconstructive Surgery; Breast Surgery; **Hospital:** Greenwich Hosp (page 892), White Plains Hosp (page 615); **Address:** 1 Theall Rd, Ste 211, Rye, NY 10580-1404; **Phone:** 914-848-8880; **Board Cert:** Plastic Surgery 2003; **Med School:** Cornell Univ 1996; **Resid:** Surgery, NY Presby Hosp 2000; Surgical Oncology, Sloan Kettering Cancer Ctr 2000; **Fellow:** Plastic Surgery, NY Presby Hosp 2002

Psychiatry

Addonizio, Gerard C MD (Psyc) - **Spec Exp:** Psychotherapy; Psychopharmacology; Depression; Anxiety Disorders; **Hospital:** NY-Presby/Westchester Div, NY (page 104); **Address:** 21 Bloomingdale Rd, White Plains, NY 10605-1504; **Phone:** 914-997-5864; **Board Cert:** Psychiatry 1983; **Med School:** Columbia P&S 1978; **Resid:** Psychiatry, New Haven Hosp 1982; **Fac Appt:** Prof Psyc, Cornell Univ-Weill Med Coll

Badikian, Arthur V MD (Psyc) - **Spec Exp:** Mood Disorders; Aging; Women's Health-Mental Health; Psychiatry in Cancer; **Hospital:** St. Vincent Cath Med Ctrs - Westchester; **Address:** 600 Mamaroneck Ave, Ste 106, Harrison, NY 10528; **Phone:** 914-948-4277; **Board Cert:** Psychiatry 1981; **Med School:** Univ Fla Coll Med 1976; **Resid:** Psychiatry, NY Med Coll Affil Hosp 1980; **Fac Appt:** Assoc Prof Psyc, NY Med Coll

Bauman, Jonathan H MD (Psyc) - **Spec Exp:** Mood Disorders; Anxiety Disorders; Personality Disorders; **Hospital:** Four Winds Hosp; **Address:** 800 Cross River Rd, Katonah, NY 10536-3549; **Phone:** 914-763-8151; **Board Cert:** Psychiatry 1978; **Med School:** Georgetown Univ 1974; **Resid:** Psychiatry, Univ Va Med Ctr 1975; Psychiatry, Georgetown Univ Med Ctr 1977; **Fac Appt:** Asst Prof Psyc, Albert Einstein Coll Med

Bogen, Steven MD (Psyc) - **Spec Exp:** Addiction/Substance Abuse; **Hospital:** Phelps Meml Hosp Ctr (page 614); **Address:** Phelps Meml Hosp, Dept Psychiatry, 701 N Broadway, Sleepy Hollow, NY 10591; **Phone:** 914-366-3024; **Board Cert:** Psychiatry 2005; Addiction Psychiatry 2006; **Med School:** SUNY Downstate 1988; **Resid:** Psychiatry, Montefiore Med Ctr 1992

Dulit, Rebecca A MD (Psyc) - **Spec Exp:** Personality Disorders-Borderline; Special Needs-Parental Therapy; Anxiety Disorders; Depression; **Hospital:** NY-Presby/Westchester Div, NY (page 104); **Address:** 45 Popham Rd, Ste D, Scarsdale, NY 10583; **Phone:** 914-722-0608; **Board Cert:** Psychiatry 1991; **Med School:** Mount Sinai Sch Med 1985; **Resid:** Psychiatry, Payne Whitney Clinic-Cornell 1989; **Fellow:** Research, Payne Whitney Clinic-Cornell 1992; **Fac Appt:** Assoc Clin Prof Psyc, Cornell Univ-Weill Med Coll

Gabel, Richard MD (Psyc) - **Spec Exp:** Psychopharmacology; Psychotherapy; **Hospital:** White Plains Hosp (page 615); **Address:** 12 Greenridge Ave, White Plains, NY 10605; **Phone:** 914-681-0202; **Board Cert:** Psychiatry 1982; **Med School:** NYU Sch Med 1976; **Resid:** Psychiatry, Mass Genl Hosp 1980

Harlam, Dean MD (Psyc) - **Spec Exp:** Depression; Bipolar/Mood Disorders; Psychopharmacology; Schizophrenia; **Hospital:** Saint Joseph's Med Ctr - Yonkers; **Address:** St Vincent's Hospital, 275 North St, Harrison, NY 10528; **Phone:** 914-925-5490; **Board Cert:** Psychiatry 1979; **Med School:** Albert Einstein Coll Med 1972; **Resid:** Psychiatry, Bronx Municipal Hosp/Einstein 1976; **Fellow:** Psychiatry, NY Hosp-Cornell Med Ctr 1977; **Fac Appt:** Assoc Prof Psyc, NY Med Coll

Kahn, Jeffrey P MD (Psyc) - **Spec Exp:** Anxiety & Depression; Psychotherapy; Work Problems; Psychopharmacology; **Hospital:** NY-Presby/Weill Cornell Med Ctr, NY (page 104), NY-Presby/Westchester Div, NY (page 104); **Address:** 45 Popham Rd, Ste 1F, Scarsdale, NY 10583; **Phone:** 914-725-6303; **Board Cert:** Psychiatry 1986; **Med School:** Columbia P&S 1979; **Resid:** Psychiatry, NY Presby/NY State Psych Inst 1983; **Fellow:** Research, NY Presby/Columbia Med Ctr 1985; **Fac Appt:** Assoc Clin Prof Psyc, Cornell Univ-Weill Med Coll

Klagsbrun, Samuel C MD (Psyc) - **Spec Exp:** Psychiatry in Cancer; Psychiatry in Terminal Illness; **Hospital:** Four Winds Hosp; **Address:** 800 Cross River Rd, Katonah, NY 10536; **Phone:** 914-763-8151 x2222; **Board Cert:** Psychiatry 1977; **Med School:** Ros Franklin Univ/Chicago Med Sch 1962; **Resid:** Psychiatry, Yale-New Haven Hosp 1966; **Fac Appt:** Clin Prof Psyc, Albert Einstein Coll Med

Levin, Andrew P MD (Psyc) - **Spec Exp:** Post Traumatic Stress Disorder; Forensic Psychiatry; Psychopharmacology; Cognitive Psychotherapy; **Hospital:** NY-Presby/Columbia Univ Med Ctr, NY (page 104); **Address:** 141 N Central Ave, Hartsdale, NY 10530-1912; **Phone:** 914-949-7699 x376; **Board Cert:** Psychiatry 1985; Forensic Psychiatry 2006; **Med School:** Univ Pennsylvania 1980; **Resid:** Psychiatry, NYS Psych Inst 1984; **Fellow:** Anxiety Disorder, NYS Psych Inst 1986; **Fac Appt:** Asst Clin Prof Psyc, Columbia P&S

Lew, Arthur MD (Psyc) - **Spec Exp:** Psychoanalysis; Child & Adolescent Psychiatry; Psychotherapy; **Address:** 225 Lyncroft Rd, New Rochelle, NY 10804-4120; **Phone:** 914-632-9679; **Board Cert:** Psychiatry 1974; Child & Adolescent Psychiatry 1979; **Med School:** SUNY Downstate 1968; **Resid:** Psychiatry, SUNY Downstate Med Ctr 1972; **Fellow:** Child & Adolescent Psychiatry, SUNY Downstate Med Ctr 1975; **Fac Appt:** Clin Prof Psyc, NYU Sch Med

Meyers, Barnett MD (Psyc) - **Spec Exp:** Depression; Geriatric Psychiatry; Psychopharmacology; Psychotherapy; **Hospital:** NY-Presby/Westchester Div, NY (page 104); **Address:** 21 Bloomingdale Rd, White Plains, NY 10605-1504; **Phone:** 914-997-5721; **Board Cert:** Psychiatry 1975; Geriatric Psychiatry 2010; **Med School:** NYU Sch Med 1966; **Resid:** Psychiatry, Bronx Muni Hosp 1972; **Fac Appt:** Prof Psyc, Cornell Univ-Weill Med Coll

Milone, Richard MD (Psyc) - **Spec Exp:** Depression; Psychopharmacology; **Hospital:** Saint Joseph's Med Ctr - Yonkers; **Address:** 275 North St, Harrison, NY 10528; **Phone:** 914-925-5311; **Board Cert:** Psychiatry 1970; **Med School:** Creighton Univ 1963; **Resid:** Psychiatry, St Vincent's Hosp & Med Ctr 1967; **Fac Appt:** Assoc Clin Prof Psyc, NY Med Coll

Neschis, Ronald MD (Psyc) - **Spec Exp:** Geriatric Psychiatry; **Hospital:** Saint Joseph's Med Ctr - Yonkers, Rye Hosp Ctr; **Address:** 18 Linden Ave, Larchmont, NY 10538-4139; **Phone:** 914-834-3470; **Board Cert:** Psychiatry 1972; **Med School:** SUNY Downstate 1963; **Resid:** Psychiatry, Montefiore Hosp Med Ctr 1969

Opler, Lewis A MD (Psyc) - **Spec Exp:** Psychopharmacology; Psychotherapy; **Hospital:** NY-Presby/Columbia Univ Med Ctr, NY (page 104); **Address:** 765 Gramatan Ave, Mount Vernon, NY 10552-1043; **Phone:** 914-668-4799; **Board Cert:** Psychiatry 1983; **Med School:** Albert Einstein Coll Med 1976; **Resid:** Psychiatry, Jacobi Med Ctr 1979; **Fac Appt:** Prof Psyc, Columbia P&S

Perlman, Barry B MD (Psyc) - **Hospital:** Saint Joseph's Med Ctr - Yonkers; **Address:** St Joseph's Med Ctr-Dept of Psychiatry, 127 S Broadway, Yonkers, NY 10701-4006; **Phone:** 914-378-7342; **Board Cert:** Psychiatry 1977; **Med School:** Yale Univ 1971; **Resid:** Psychiatry, Mount Sinai Hosp 1975; **Fac Appt:** Assoc Clin Prof Psyc, NY Med Coll

Perry, Bradford MD (Psyc) - **Spec Exp:** Anxiety & Mood Disorders; Psychopharmacology; **Hospital:** NY-Presby/Westchester Div, NY (page 104), White Plains Hosp (page 615); **Address:** 455 Central Park Ave, Ste 214, Scarsdale, NY 10583-1034; **Phone:** 914-472-2167; **Board Cert:** Psychiatry 1989; **Med School:** Univ Miami Sch Med 1984; **Resid:** Psychiatry, NY Hosp 1988; **Fellow:** Psychiatry, Columbia-Presby Med Ctr 1989; **Fac Appt:** Assoc Clin Prof Psyc, Cornell Univ-Weill Med Coll

Russakoff, L Mark MD (Psyc) - **Spec Exp:** Mood Disorders; Anxiety Disorders; **Hospital:** Phelps Meml Hosp Ctr (page 614); **Address:** Phelps Memorial Hospital, 701 N Broadway, Sleepy Hollow, NY 10591-1020; **Phone:** 914-366-3604; **Board Cert:** Psychiatry 1976; **Med School:** SUNY Downstate 1971; **Resid:** Psychiatry, Yale-New Haven Hosp 1975

Sullivan, Timothy B MD (Psyc) - **Spec Exp:** Bipolar/Mood Disorders; Psychotherapy & Psychopharmacology; Schizophrenia; Psychiatry in Physical Illness; **Hospital:** Staten Island Univ Hosp - North (page 106), St. Vincent Cath Med Ctrs - Westchester; **Address:** 30 Glenn St, Ste 305, White Plains, NY 10603; **Phone:** 347-328-2201; **Board Cert:** Internal Medicine 1981; Psychiatry 1986; **Med School:** Dartmouth Med Sch 1977; **Resid:** Internal Medicine, St Vincent's Hosp 1980; Psychiatry, NY Presby Hosp-Westch Div 1984; **Fellow:** Hematology & Oncology, St Vincents Hosp 1981; **Fac Appt:** Assoc Prof Psyc, NY Med Coll

Zolkind, Neil A MD (Psyc) - **Spec Exp:** Depression; Anxiety Disorders; **Hospital:** Westchester Med Ctr; **Address:** Westchester Med Ctr, Behavioral Hlth Ctr, 95 Grasslands Rd, Valhalla, NY 10595; **Phone:** 914-493-1818; **Board Cert:** Psychiatry 1981; **Med School:** Geo Wash Univ 1976; **Resid:** Psychiatry, UCLA Neuropsych Hosp 1980; **Fac Appt:** Asst Prof Psyc, NY Med Coll

Pulmonary Disease

Binder, Ralph E MD (Pul) - **Spec Exp:** Asthma; Chronic Obstructive Lung Disease (COPD); Interstitial Lung Disease; **Hospital:** Lawrence Hosp Ctr; **Address:** 329 Whiteplains Rd, Ste 100, Eastchester, NY 10709; **Phone:** 914-337-1610; **Board Cert:** Internal Medicine 1978; Pulmonary Disease 1980; **Med School:** Yale Univ 1975; **Resid:** Internal Medicine, Bronx Muni Hosp 1978; **Fellow:** Pulmonary Disease, Boston Med Ctr 1980; **Fac Appt:** Asst Prof Med, Columbia P&S

Brill, Joseph J MD (Pul) - **Spec Exp:** Sarcoidosis; Chronic Obstructive Lung Disease (COPD); Asthma; **Hospital:** St. John's Riverside Hosp-Andrus Pavil, Saint Joseph's Med Ctr - Yonkers; **Address:** 102 Park Ave, Yonkers, NY 10703; **Phone:** 914-968-1611; **Board Cert:** Internal Medicine 1988; Pulmonary Disease 2002; **Med School:** Mexico 1981; **Resid:** Internal Medicine, Elmhurst City Hosp 1986; **Fellow:** Pulmonary Disease, Mt Sinai 1988

Bures, Sergio MD (Pul) - **Hospital:** Northern Westchester Hosp (page 613); **Address:** 111 Bedford Rd, Katonah, NY 10536; **Phone:** 914-232-3135; **Board Cert:** Internal Medicine 2010; Pulmonary Disease 2005; Critical Care Medicine 2006; **Med School:** Albany Med Coll 1994; **Resid:** Internal Medicine, Tripler Army Med Ctr 1997; **Fellow:** Pulmonary Critical Care Medicine, Meml Sloan Kettering Cancer Ctr

Casino, Joseph E MD (Pul) - **Spec Exp:** Asthma; Sleep Disorders; **Hospital:** Sound Shore Med Ctr - Westchester; **Address:** 2365 Boston Post Rd, Ste 103, Larchmont, NY 10538; **Phone:** 914-833-2020; **Board Cert:** Internal Medicine 1989; Pulmonary Disease 2010; Critical Care Medicine 2011; **Med School:** Italy 1984; **Resid:** Internal Medicine, New Rochelle Med Ctr 1988; **Fellow:** Pulmonary Critical Care Medicine, RW Johnson Univ Hosp 1991; **Fac Appt:** Asst Clin Prof Med, NY Med Coll

De Matteo, Robert E MD (Pul) - **Spec Exp:** Asthma; Emphysema; Lung Cancer-Early Detection; **Hospital:** St. John's Riverside Hosp-Andrus Pavil, Saint Joseph's Med Ctr - Yonkers; **Address:** 970 N Broadway, Ste 209, Yonkers, NY 10701; **Phone:** 914-965-3366; **Board Cert:** Internal Medicine 1988; Pulmonary Disease 2010; **Med School:** Mexico 1982; **Resid:** Internal Medicine, Mount Sinai/Bronx VA Hosp 1985; **Fellow:** Pulmonary Disease, Westchester Med Ctr 1988

Delorenzo, Lawrence MD (Pul) - **Spec Exp:** Asthma; Emphysema; **Hospital:** Westchester Med Ctr; **Address:** Westchester Med Ctr, Pulmonary Lab - Macy Pavillion, 100 Woods Rd, Valhalla, NY 10595; **Phone:** 914-493-7518; **Board Cert:** Internal Medicine 1979; Pulmonary Disease 1982; Critical Care Medicine 2009; **Med School:** NY Med Coll 1976; **Resid:** Internal Medicine, Metropolitan Hosp Ctr 1979; **Fellow:** Pulmonary Disease, Metropolitan Hosp Ctr 1981; **Fac Appt:** Assoc Clin Prof Med, NY Med Coll

DiCosmo, Bruno F MD (Pul) - **Spec Exp:** Pulmonary Fibrosis; Bronchoscopy; Lung Cancer; Sleep Disorders; **Hospital:** White Plains Hosp (page 615), Greenwich Hosp (page 892); **Address:** 1 Theall Rd, Rye, NY 10580; **Phone:** 914-848-8777; **Board Cert:** Internal Medicine 2011; Pulmonary Disease 2004; Critical Care Medicine 2005; Sleep Medicine 2011; **Med School:** Univ Conn 1988; **Resid:** Internal Medicine, Univ Conn Hlth Ctr 1991; **Fellow:** Pulmonary Disease, Yale-New Haven Hosp 1994; Critical Care Medicine, Yale-New Haven Hosp 1994; **Fac Appt:** Asst Clin Prof Med, Cornell Univ-Weill Med Coll

Frimer, Richard MD (Pul) - **Hospital:** White Plains Hosp (page 615); **Address:** 170 Maple Ave, Ste G1, White Plains, NY 10601-4710; **Phone:** 914-328-0932; **Board Cert:** Internal Medicine 1983; Pulmonary Disease 1986; Critical Care Medicine 2010; **Med School:** SUNY Buffalo 1980; **Resid:** Internal Medicine, Montefiore Med Ctr 1983; **Fellow:** Pulmonary Disease, NYU Med Ctr 1985

Jacobowitz, Marilyn MD (Pul) - **Spec Exp:** Asthma; Cough; **Hospital:** Northern Westchester Hosp (page 613); **Address:** 90 S Bedford Rd, Mt Kisco, NY 10549-3412; **Phone:** 914-241-1050; **Board Cert:** Internal Medicine 2002; Pulmonary Disease 2004; Critical Care Medicine 2005; **Med School:** NYU Sch Med 1989; **Resid:** Internal Medicine, Mt Sinai Hosp 1992; **Fellow:** Pulmonary Disease, Mt Sinai Hosp 1995

Klares, Scott M MD (Pul) - **Spec Exp:** Critical Care; Asthma; Cough; **Hospital:** Northern Westchester Hosp (page 613); **Address:** Mt Kisco Medical Group, 90 S Bedford Rd, Mt Kisco, NY 10549; **Phone:** 914-241-1050; **Board Cert:** Internal Medicine 2006; Pulmonary Disease 2007; Critical Care Medicine 2008; **Med School:** NY Med Coll 1992; **Resid:** Internal Medicine, New Engl Deaconess Hosp 1995; **Fellow:** Pulmonary Critical Care Medicine, Boston Med Ctr 1998

Lehrman, Gary R MD (Pul) - **Spec Exp:** Sleep Disorders; **Hospital:** Phelps Meml Hosp Ctr (page 614); **Address:** 160 N State Rd, Briarcliff Manor, NY 10510-1443; **Phone:** 914-762-8383; **Board Cert:** Internal Medicine 1982; Pulmonary Disease 1986; Critical Care Medicine 2004; Sleep Medicine 2007; **Med School:** NYU Sch Med 1979; **Resid:** Internal Medicine, LI Jewish Med Ctr 1984; **Fellow:** Pulmonary Disease, LIJ Med Ctr/Queens Hosp Affil 1985

Lehrman, Stuart MD (Pul) - **Spec Exp:** Lung Cancer; Asthma; **Hospital:** Westchester Med Ctr; **Address:** Westchester Med Ctr, Macys Pavilon-Pulmonary Lab, 100 Woods Rd, Valhalla, NY 10595; **Phone:** 914-493-7518; **Board Cert:** Internal Medicine 1981; Pulmonary Disease 1984; Critical Care Medicine 2007; Sleep Medicine 2007; **Med School:** SUNY Hlth Sci Ctr 1978; **Resid:** Internal Medicine, Cedars-Sinai Med Ctr 1981; **Fellow:** Pulmonary Disease, Cedars-Sinai Med Ctr 1983; **Fac Appt:** Assoc Clin Prof Med, NY Med Coll

Mandel, Michael MD (Pul) - **Spec Exp:** Sleep Disorders/Apnea; Chronic Obstructive Lung Disease (COPD); Asthma; **Hospital:** Sound Shore Med Ctr - Westchester; **Address:** 2365 Boston Post Rd, Ste 103, Larchmont, NY 10538; **Phone:** 914-833-2020; **Board Cert:** Internal Medicine 1986; Pulmonary Disease 2010; Critical Care Medicine 2011; Sleep Medicine 2009; **Med School:** Columbia P&S 1983; **Resid:** Internal Medicine, St Lukes Roosevelt Hosp 1987; **Fellow:** Pulmonary Critical Care Medicine, UMDNJ Med Ctr 1989; **Fac Appt:** Asst Prof Med, NY Med Coll

Meixler, Steven M MD (Pul) - **Spec Exp:** Asthma; Emphysema; Cough-Chronic; **Hospital:** White Plains Hosp (page 615), Greenwich Hosp (page 892); **Address:** 210 Westchester Ave, White Plains, NY 10604; **Phone:** 914-682-0700; **Board Cert:** Internal Medicine 1987; Pulmonary Disease 2010; Critical Care Medicine 2011; **Med School:** Boston Univ 1984; **Resid:** Internal Medicine, VA Med Ctr 1988; **Fellow:** Pulmonary Disease, Bellevue Hosp/NYU 1990

Novitch, Richard MD (Pul) - **Spec Exp:** Pulmonary Rehabilitation; **Hospital:** Burke Rehab Hosp; **Address:** 785 Mamaroneck Ave, White Plains, NY 10605; **Phone:** 914-597-2226; **Board Cert:** Internal Medicine 1987; **Med School:** Mexico 1983; **Resid:** Internal Medicine, UMDNJ Med Ctr 1987; **Fellow:** Pulmonary Disease, UMDNJ Med Ctr 1989; **Fac Appt:** Asst Clin Prof Med, Cornell Univ-Weill Med Coll

Schreiber, Michael E MD (Pul) - **Spec Exp:** Asthma; Emphysema; **Hospital:** St. John's Riverside Hosp-Andrus Pavil, Saint Joseph's Med Ctr - Yonkers; **Address:** 970 N Broadway, Ste 209, Yonkers, NY 10701; **Phone:** 914-423-8517; **Board Cert:** Internal Medicine 1976; Pulmonary Disease 1978; Sleep Medicine 2011; **Med School:** Univ Ariz Coll Med 1973; **Resid:** Internal Medicine, Montefiore Med Ctr 1976; **Fellow:** Pulmonary Disease, NYU Med Ctr 1978; **Fac Appt:** Asst Clin Prof Med, NY Med Coll

Sherling, Bruce E MD (Pul) - **Hospital:** White Plains Hosp (page 615), Greenwich Hosp (page 892); **Address:** Westchester Medical Group, 1 Theall Rd, Rye, NY 10580; **Phone:** 914-848-8777; **Board Cert:** Internal Medicine 1976; Pulmonary Disease 1978; **Med School:** NY Med Coll 1973; **Resid:** Internal Medicine, Metropolitan Hosp Ctr 1974; **Fellow:** Pulmonary Disease, Metropolitan Hosp Ctr 1977; Pulmonary Disease, Lenox Hill Hosp 1978

Volcovici, Guido MD (Pul) - **Spec Exp:** Asthma; Emphysema; **Hospital:** Saint Joseph's Med Ctr - Yonkers; **Address:** 127 S Broadway, Ste 406, Yonkers, NY 10701; **Phone:** 212-567-2323; **Board Cert:** Internal Medicine 1985; Pulmonary Disease 1988; **Med School:** Romania 1962; **Resid:** Internal Medicine, Jewish Hosp 1974; **Fellow:** Pulmonary Disease, VA Med Ctr 1976

Weinberg, Harlan MD (Pul) - **Spec Exp:** Asthma; Critical Care Medicine; **Hospital:** Northern Westchester Hosp (page 613); **Address:** 83 S Bedford Rd, Mt Kisco, NY 10549; **Phone:** 914-241-8356; **Board Cert:** Internal Medicine 1984; Pulmonary Disease 1986; Critical Care Medicine 2002; **Med School:** Univ Conn 1981; **Resid:** Internal Medicine, McGaw Med Ctr-Northwestern 1984; **Fellow:** Pulmonary Disease, Cedars-Sinai Med Ctr 1986

Radiation Oncology

Fass, Daniel E MD (RadRO) - **Spec Exp:** Prostate Cancer; Breast Cancer; Head & Neck Cancer; **Address:** 1 Theall Rd, Ste 107, Rye, NY 10580; **Phone:** 914-848-8950; **Board Cert:** Radiation Oncology 1987; **Med School:** Howard Univ 1983; **Resid:** Radiation Oncology, NYU Med Ctr 1986; **Fellow:** Brachytherapy, Meml Sloan Kettering Cancer Ctr 1987; **Fac Appt:** Asst Prof RadRO, Cornell Univ-Weill Med Coll

Moorthy, Chitti MD (RadRO) - **Spec Exp:** Prostate Cancer; Breast Cancer; Brain Tumors; Mycosis Fungoides; **Hospital:** Westchester Med Ctr; **Address:** Westchester Med Ctr, 100 Woods Rd, rm 1297, Valhalla, NY 10595; **Phone:** 914-493-8561; **Board Cert:** Radiation Oncology 1979; **Med School:** India 1974; **Resid:** Surgery, Michael Reese Hosp 1976; Radiation Oncology, Michael Reese Hosp 1979; **Fellow:** Brachytherapy, Meml Sloan Kettering Cancer Ctr 1980; **Fac Appt:** Prof RadRO, NY Med Coll

Tinger, Alfred MD (RadRO) - **Spec Exp:** Prostate Cancer; Breast Cancer; Brain Tumors; **Hospital:** Northern Westchester Hosp (page 613); **Address:** 21st Century Oncology, 970 N Broadway, Yonkers, NY 10701; **Phone:** 914-969-1600; **Board Cert:** Radiation Oncology 2008; **Med School:** SUNY Downstate 1992; **Resid:** Radiation Oncology, Washington Univ Med Ctr 1997

Reproductive Endocrinology

Klein, Jeffrey MD (RE) - **Spec Exp:** Infertility-IVF; Infertility; Polycystic Ovarian Syndrome; Endometriosis; **Hospital:** White Plains Hosp (page 615); **Address:** Reproductive Medical Assocs of New York, 15 N Broadway, Garden Level, Ste G, White Plains, NY 10601; **Phone:** 914-997-6200; **Board Cert:** Obstetrics & Gynecology 2006; Reproductive Endocrinology 2006; **Med School:** Albert Einstein Coll Med 1995; **Resid:** Obstetrics & Gynecology, Geo Wash Univ Med Ctr 1999; **Fellow:** Reproductive Endocrinology, Columbia-Presby Med Ctr 2001

Stangel, John MD (RE) - **Spec Exp:** Infertility-IVF; Endometriosis; Miscarriage-Recurrent; **Hospital:** Northern Westchester Hosp (page 613), Phelps Meml Hosp Ctr (page 614); **Address:** Reproductive Medicine Assocs of NY, 15 N Broadway, Lower Level, rm G, White Plains, NY 10601; **Phone:** 914-967-6200; **Board Cert:** Obstetrics & Gynecology 1976; Reproductive Endocrinology 1981; **Med School:** NY Med Coll 1969; **Resid:** Obstetrics & Gynecology, Mount Sinai Med Ctr 1974; **Fellow:** Reproductive Endocrinology, Metropolitan Hosp Ctr 1976

Rheumatology

Barone, Richard P MD (Rhu) - **Spec Exp:** Rheumatoid Arthritis; Lupus/SLE; Psoriatic Arthritis; **Hospital:** Sound Shore Med Ctr - Westchester; **Address:** 421 Huguenot St Fl 4 - Ste 44, New Rochelle, NY 10801-7004; **Phone:** 914-235-3065; **Med School:** Italy 1971; **Resid:** Internal Medicine, Brooklyn Jewish Hosp & Med Ctr 1974; **Fellow:** Rheumatology, Brooklyn Jewish Hosp & Med Ctr 1976; **Fac Appt:** Assoc Clin Prof Med, NY Med Coll

Berger, Jack MD (Rhu) - **Spec Exp:** Rheumatoid Arthritis; Psoriatic Arthritis; Spondylitis; Gout; **Hospital:** White Plains Hosp (page 615); **Address:** 210 Westchester Ave, White Plains, NY 10604; **Phone:** 914-682-6532; **Board Cert:** Internal Medicine 1979; Rheumatology 1982; **Med School:** Albert Einstein Coll Med 1976; **Resid:** Rheumatology, Bellevue Hosp 1979; **Fellow:** Rheumatology, Bellevue Hosp 1981

Burns, Mark R MD (Rhu) - **Spec Exp:** Lupus Nephritis; Rheumatoid Arthritis; **Hospital:** Sound Shore Med Ctr - Westchester; **Address:** 421 Huguenot St, rm 44, New Rochelle, NY 10801-7021; **Phone:** 914-235-3065; **Board Cert:** Internal Medicine 1980; Rheumatology 1984; **Med School:** UCSF 1977; **Resid:** Internal Medicine, Montefiore Med Ctr 1980; **Fellow:** Rheumatology, Montefiore Med Ctr 1983; **Fac Appt:** Asst Clin Prof Med, Albert Einstein Coll Med

Lans, David DO (Rhu) - **Spec Exp:** Rheumatoid Arthritis; Lupus/SLE; Asthma; Osteoporosis; **Hospital:** Lawrence Hosp Ctr, Sound Shore Med Ctr - Westchester; **Address:** 838 Pelhamdale Ave, New Rochelle, NY 10801-1032; **Phone:** 914-235-5577; **Board Cert:** Internal Medicine 1984; Allergy & Immunology 1987; Rheumatology 1988; **Med School:** Univ Osteo Med & Hlth Sci, Des Moines 1981; **Resid:** Internal Medicine, Downstate Univ Hosp 1985; **Fellow:** Allergy & Immunology, New Eng Med Ctr 1987; Rheumatology, Hosp For Special Surgery 1989; **Fac Appt:** Asst Clin Prof Med, NY Med Coll

Lenci, Margaret MD (Rhu) - **Hospital:** Northern Westchester Hosp (page 613); **Address:** 90 S Bedford Rd, Mt Kisco, NY 10549-3433; **Phone:** 914-241-1050; **Board Cert:** Internal Medicine 1983; Rheumatology 1988; **Med School:** SUNY Downstate 1980; **Resid:** Internal Medicine, Montefiore Med Ctr 1983; **Fellow:** Rheumatology, Montefiore Med Ctr 1988

Mascarenhas, Bento MD (Rhu) - **Spec Exp:** Arthritis; Lupus/SLE; Osteoporosis; **Hospital:** Burke Rehab Hosp, Hosp For Special Surgery (page 115); **Address:** 785 Mamaroneck Ave, White Plains, NY 10605-2523; **Phone:** 914-337-5879; **Board Cert:** Internal Medicine 1972; Rheumatology 1974; **Med School:** India 1961; **Resid:** Internal Medicine, Westchester Med Ctr 1967; **Fellow:** Internal Medicine, Cornell Univ Med Ctr 1970; Rheumatology, Hosp for Special Surg 1970; **Fac Appt:** Clin Prof Med, NY Med Coll

Reinitz, Elizabeth MD (Rhu) - **Spec Exp:** Rheumatoid Arthritis; Lupus/SLE; Osteoarthritis; Gout; **Hospital:** White Plains Hosp (page 615); **Address:** Scarsdale Medical Group, 600 Mamaroneck Ave, Ste 200, Harrison, NY 10528; **Phone:** 914-723-8100; **Board Cert:** Internal Medicine 1979; Rheumatology 1982; **Med School:** Albert Einstein Coll Med 1976; **Resid:** Internal Medicine, Boston City Hosp 1979; **Fellow:** Rheumatology, Montefiore Med Ctr 1981

Sloane, Lori E MD (Rhu) - **Spec Exp:** Rheumatoid Arthritis; **Hospital:** Northern Westchester Hosp (page 613); **Address:** Westchester Hlth Assocs, 322 Underhill Ave, Yorktown Heights, NY 10598; **Phone:** 914-962-5501; **Board Cert:** Internal Medicine 1989; **Med School:** SUNY Downstate 1986; **Resid:** Internal Medicine, Jacobi Med Ctr 1989; **Fellow:** Rheumatology, Montefiore Hosp Med Ctr 1991; **Fac Appt:** Asst Clin Prof Med, Albert Einstein Coll Med

Yegudin-Ash, Julia MD (Rhu) - **Spec Exp:** Lupus/SLE; Rheumatoid Arthritis; Psoriatic Arthritis; Scleroderma; **Hospital:** Westchester Med Ctr; **Address:** MRA Physicians, 19 Bradhurst, Ste 3070N, Hawthorne, NY 10532; **Phone:** 914-594-4444; **Board Cert:** Rheumatology 2006; **Med School:** SUNY Stony Brook 1987; **Resid:** Internal Medicine, Winthrop Univ Hosp 1990; **Fellow:** Rheumatology, Mass Genl Hosp 1992; Rheumatology, Hosp Joint Diseases 1993; **Fac Appt:** Asst Prof Med, NY Med Coll

Sports Medicine

Cavaliere, Gregg MD (SM) - **Spec Exp:** Rotator Cuff Surgery; Knee Injuries/Ligament Surgery; Shoulder Instability; Arthroscopic Surgery; **Hospital:** Phelps Meml Hosp Ctr (page 614), Lenox Hill Hosp (page 106); **Address:** 24 Saw Mill River Rd, Ste 2, Hawthorne, NY 10532; **Phone:** 914-631-7777; **Board Cert:** Orthopaedic Surgery 2006; **Med School:** NY Med Coll 1987; **Resid:** Orthopaedic Surgery, Lenox Hill Hosp 1992; **Fellow:** Sports Medicine, NYU Med Ctr 1993

Luks, Howard J MD (SM) - **Hospital:** Westchester Med Ctr; **Address:** 19 Bradhurst Ave, Ste 1300N, Hawthorne, NY 10532; **Phone:** 914-789-2735; **Board Cert:** Orthopaedic Surgery 2010; **Med School:** NY Med Coll 1991; **Resid:** Orthopaedic Surgery, LI Jewish Med Ctr 1996; **Fellow:** Orthopaedic Sports Medicine, Hosp for Joint Diseases 1997

Shifrin, Seth P MD (SM) - **Spec Exp:** Primary Care Sports Medicine; **Hospital:** Northern Westchester Hosp (page 613); **Address:** Mount Kisco Medical Group, 110 S Bedord Rd, Mount Kisco, NY 10549; **Phone:** 914-241-1050; **Board Cert:** Internal Medicine 2004; Sports Medicine 2005; Pediatrics 2005; **Med School:** Univ Chicago-Pritzker Sch Med 2000; **Resid:** Internal Medicine & Pediatrics, Mass General/Boston Children's Hosp 2004; **Fellow:** Sports Medicine, MacNeal Meml Hosp 2005

Small, Eric W MD (SM) - **Spec Exp:** Primary Care Sports Medicine; Reflex Sympathetic Dystrophy (RSD); Concussion; Compartment Syndrome; **Hospital:** Northern Westchester Hosp (page 613); **Address:** Family Sports Medicine & Fitness, 666 Lexington Ave, Ste 210, Mt Kisco, NY 10549; **Phone:** 914-666-7900; **Board Cert:** Pediatrics 2002; Sports Medicine 2008; **Med School:** UMDNJ-NJ Med Sch, Newark 1989; **Resid:** Pediatrics, Mentefiore-Weiler Einstein Med Ctr 1992; **Fellow:** Pediatric Sports Medicine, McMaster Univ/Hamilton 1994; Sports Medicine, Boston Children's Hosp 1995; **Fac Appt:** Asst Clin Prof Ped, Mount Sinai Sch Med

Surgery

Ashikari, Andrew Y MD (S) - **Spec Exp:** Breast Cancer; Breast Disease; **Hospital:** Comm Hosp - Dobbs Ferry, St. John's Riverside Hosp-Andrus Pavil; **Address:** Ashikari Comprehensive Breast Ctr, Community Hospital, 128 Ashford Ave, Dobbs Ferry, NY 10522; **Phone:** 914-693-5025; **Board Cert:** Surgery 2006; **Med School:** Univ Pittsburgh 1991; **Resid:** Surgery, Montefiore Med Ctr 1996; **Fellow:** Surgical Oncology, Univ Chicago Hosps 1999; **Fac Appt:** Assoc Prof S, NY Med Coll

Cahan, Anthony C MD (S) - **Spec Exp:** Breast Surgery; Breast Cancer; **Hospital:** Northern Westchester Hosp (page 613); **Address:** 3010 Westchester Ave, Ste 201, Purchase, NY 10577; **Phone:** 914-517-8220; **Board Cert:** Surgery 2008; **Med School:** Cornell Univ-Weill Med Coll 1982; **Resid:** Surgery, New York Hosp 1987; **Fac Appt:** Asst Clin Prof Med, NY Med Coll

Charny, Caleb K MD/PhD (S) - **Hospital:** Greenwich Hosp (page 892); **Address:** WESTMED Medical Grp, 210 Westchester Ave Fl 3, White Plains, NY 10604; **Phone:** 914-682-6557; **Board Cert:** Surgery 2011; **Med School:** NYU Sch Med 1995; **Resid:** Surgery, New York Hosp 2000

Cleary, Joseph B MD (S) - **Spec Exp:** Breast Surgery; Cancer Surgery; **Hospital:** Westchester Med Ctr; **Address:** New York Med College, 50 Oval Plaza, Munger Pavilion, rm 149, Valhalla, NY 10595; **Phone:** 914-493-0133; **Board Cert:** Surgery 2009; **Med School:** NY Med Coll 1973; **Resid:** Surgery, NY Med Coll Affil Hosps 1978; Hand Surgery, St Luke's Roosevelt Hosp Ctr 1979; **Fellow:** Surgical Oncology, NY Med Coll Affil Hosps 1976; Plastic Surgery, Columbia Presby Med Ctr 1980; **Fac Appt:** Asst Clin Prof S, NY Med Coll

Fou, Adora C MD (S) - **Spec Exp:** Breast Cancer; Breast Disease; **Hospital:** White Plains Hosp (page 615), Greenwich Hosp (page 892); **Address:** Westchester Medical Group, 1 Theall Rd, Rye, NY 10580; **Phone:** 914-848-8960; **Board Cert:** Surgery 2007; **Med School:** Univ Ottawa 2000; **Resid:** Surgery, NY Presby Hosp-Weill Cornell 2005

Gordon, Mark S MD (S) - **Spec Exp:** Breast Cancer; Melanoma; Pancreatic Cancer; Colon Cancer; **Hospital:** White Plains Hosp (page 615), Westchester Med Ctr; **Address:** Dickstein Cancer Ctr, 2 Longview Ave, Ste 302, White Plains, NY 10601-5012; **Phone:** 914-684-5884; **Board Cert:** Surgery 2006; **Med School:** Northwestern Univ 1982; **Resid:** Surgery, New York Hosp 1987; **Fellow:** Surgical Oncology, Meml Sloan Kettering Cancer Ctr 1989; **Fac Appt:** Asst Clin Prof S, NY Med Coll

Josephson, Lynn G MD (S) - **Spec Exp:** Breast Cancer & Surgery; **Hospital:** White Plains Hosp (page 615); **Address:** Westchester Medical Group, 1 Theall Rd, Rye, NY 10580; **Phone:** 914-848-8960; **Board Cert:** Surgery 2002; **Med School:** Mount Sinai Sch Med 1977; **Resid:** Surgery, Columbia-Presby Med Ctr 1981

Kaul, Ashutosh MD (S) - **Spec Exp:** Obesity/Bariatric Surgery; Minimally Invasive Surgery; **Hospital:** Westchester Med Ctr; **Address:** 19 Bradhurst Ave, Hawthorne, NY 10532; **Phone:** 914-347-0162; **Board Cert:** Surgery 2010; **Med School:** India 1988; **Resid:** Surgery, Bronx Lebanon Hosp 1998; Surgery, St Barnabas Med Ctr 2000; **Fac Appt:** Asst Prof S, NY Med Coll

Lau, Har Chi MD (S) - **Spec Exp:** Laparoscopic Surgery; **Hospital:** Phelps Meml Hosp Ctr (page 614); **Address:** Hudson Valley Surgical Group, 777 N Broadway, Ste 204, Sleepy Hollow, NY 10591; **Phone:** 914-631-3660; **Board Cert:** Surgery 2007; **Med School:** Univ Pennsylvania 1992; **Resid:** Surgery, Allegheny Univ Hosps 1998

Lemercier, Maud L MD (S) - **Spec Exp:** Breast Cancer; **Hospital:** Northern Westchester Hosp (page 613); **Address:** Mt Kisco Medical Group, 111 Bedford Rd, Katonah, NY 10536; **Phone:** 914-232-3135; **Board Cert:** Surgery 2006; **Med School:** Temple Univ 1999; **Resid:** Surgery, Univ Conn 2005

Rajdeo, Heena MD (S) - **Spec Exp:** Dialysis Access Surgery; Thyroid & Parathyroid Surgery; Trauma; Laparoscopic Surgery; **Hospital:** Westchester Med Ctr; **Address:** Taylor Pavilion E1, rm E 130, 100 Woods Road, Valhalla, NY 10595; **Phone:** 914-372-7196; **Board Cert:** Surgery 2002; **Med School:** India 1969; **Resid:** Surgery, KEM Hosp 1972; Surgery, Westchester Med Ctr 1982; **Fac Appt:** Asst Prof S, NY Med Coll

Rangraj, Madhu S MD (S) - **Spec Exp:** Laparoscopic Surgery; Obesity/Bariatric Surgery; Hernia; **Hospital:** Sound Shore Med Ctr - Westchester; **Address:** 110 Lockwood Ave, Ste 300, New Rochelle, NY 10801; **Phone:** 914-632-9650; **Board Cert:** Surgery 2009; **Med School:** India 1972; **Resid:** Surgery, New Rochelle Hosp 1978; Surgery, VA Med Ctr 1980

Raniolo, Robert MD (S) - **Spec Exp:** Breast Surgery; Gastrointestinal Surgery; Hernia; **Hospital:** Phelps Meml Hosp Ctr (page 614); **Address:** Hudson Valley Surgical Group, 777 N Broadway, Ste 204, Sleepy Hollow, NY 10591-1019; **Phone:** 914-631-3660; **Board Cert:** Surgery 2007; **Med School:** Mexico 1981; **Resid:** Surgery, Lincoln Hosp 1988

San Filippo, J Anthony MD (S) - **Spec Exp:** Pediatric Surgery; Neonatal Surgery; Hernia; **Hospital:** Westchester Med Ctr, Phelps Meml Hosp Ctr (page 614); **Address:** 19 Bradhurst Ave, Ste 2550, Hawthorne, NY 10532; **Phone:** 914-761-5437; **Board Cert:** Surgery 1973; **Med School:** Georgetown Univ 1965; **Resid:** Surgery, Bellevue Hosp 1967; Surgery, N Shore Univ Hosp 1970; **Fellow:** Pediatric Surgery, Children's Hosp 1972; **Fac Appt:** Prof S, NY Med Coll

Wertkin, Martin G MD (S) - **Spec Exp:** Breast Cancer; Breast Surgery; **Hospital:** St. John's Riverside Hosp-Andrus Pavil, Phelps Meml Hosp Ctr (page 614); **Address:** 1034 N Broadway, Yonkers, NY 10701; **Phone:** 914-965-2026; **Board Cert:** Surgery 2009; **Med School:** SUNY Hlth Sci Ctr 1972; **Resid:** Surgery, Mt Sinai Med Ctr 1978; **Fac Appt:** Asst Clin Prof S, Mount Sinai Sch Med

Thoracic & Cardiac Surgery

Lafaro, Rocco J MD (T&CS) - **Spec Exp:** Minimally Invasive Cardiac Surgery; **Hospital:** Westchester Med Ctr; **Address:** 100 Woods Rd, Macy 114W, Valhalla, NY 10595; **Phone:** 914-493-7676; **Board Cert:** Thoracic Surgery 2011; **Med School:** NY Med Coll 1982; **Resid:** Surgery, Metropolitan Hosp Ctr 1984; Surgery, Westchester Med Ctr 1986; **Fellow:** Thoracic Surgery, Bronx Muni Hosp Ctr 1991; Thoracic Surgery, Montefiore Med Ctr 1993

Lansman, Steven L MD/PhD (T&CS) - **Spec Exp:** Coronary Artery Surgery; Heart Valve Surgery; Ventricular Assist Device (LVAD); Transplant-Heart; **Hospital:** Westchester Med Ctr; **Address:** Westchester Medical Ctr, 100 Woods Rd, Macy Pavilion, rm 114W, Valhalla, NY 10595; **Phone:** 914-493-8793; **Board Cert:** Thoracic Surgery 2004; **Med School:** SUNY Hlth Sci Ctr 1977; **Resid:** Surgery, Montefiore Med Ctr 1982; **Fellow:** Thoracic Surgery, Univ Hosp 1984; **Fac Appt:** Prof S, NY Med Coll

Merav, Avraham D MD (T&CS) - **Spec Exp:** Minimally Invasive Thoracic Surgery; Lung Surgery; Esophageal Surgery; Cardiothoracic Surgery; **Hospital:** Phelps Meml Hosp Ctr (page 614), Westchester Med Ctr; **Address:** 755 N Broadway, Sleepy Hollow, NY 10591; **Phone:** 914-366-2333; **Board Cert:** Surgery 1974; Thoracic Surgery 2004; **Med School:** Switzerland 1964; **Resid:** Surgery, Montefiore Hosp Med Ctr 1973; **Fellow:** Cardiothoracic Surgery, Montefiore Hosp Med Ctr 1975; **Fac Appt:** Assoc Clin Prof TS, Albert Einstein Coll Med

Sett, Suvro S MD (T&CS) - **Spec Exp:** Pediatric Cardiac Surgery; Congenital Heart Disease; Congenital Heart Disease-Adult; **Hospital:** Westchester Med Ctr; **Address:** Munger pav Bldg - Fl 6th - Ste 618, MS 10595, 155 Grasslands Rd, Valhalla, NY 10595; **Phone:** 914-594-3322; **Med School:** Canada 1983; **Resid:** Surgery, Univ of Saskatchewan 1988; Cardiovascular Surgery, Univ of British Columbia 1991; **Fellow:** Pediatric Cardiac Surgery, The Hosp for Sick Chld 1993

Spielvogel, David MD (T&CS) - **Spec Exp:** Aneurysm-Aortic; Transplant-Heart; Coronary Artery Surgery; Heart Valve Surgery; **Hospital:** Westchester Med Ctr; **Address:** 100 Woods Rd, Macy 114W, Valhalla, NY 10595; **Phone:** 914-493-8793; **Board Cert:** Thoracic Surgery 2009; **Med School:** SUNY Downstate 1990; **Resid:** Surgery, SUNY Hlth Sci Ctr 1995; Thoracic Surgery, Mt Sinai Med Ctr 1998; **Fellow:** Cardiac Surgery, Harefield Hosp 1999; **Fac Appt:** Prof S, NY Med Coll

Weiser, Todd MD (T&CS) - **Spec Exp:** Lung Cancer; Esophageal Cancer; Minimally Invasive Surgery; Mediastinal Tumors; **Hospital:** White Plains Hosp (page 615); **Address:** Dickstein Cancer Center, White Plains Hospital Center, 2 Longview Ave, Ste 301, White Plains, NY 10601; **Phone:** 914-681-2750; **Board Cert:** Surgery 2004; Thoracic Surgery 2007; **Med School:** Jefferson Med Coll 1996; **Resid:** Surgery, St Vincent's Hosp & Med Ctr 2003; **Fellow:** Surgical Oncology, Natl Cancer Inst 2000; Thoracic & Cardiac Surgery, Mass Genl Hosp 2005

Urology

Axelrod, Sheldon L MD (U) - **Spec Exp:** Prostate Cancer; Prostate Disease; Robotic Surgery; **Hospital:** Northern Westchester Hosp (page 613); **Address:** Mt Kisco Medical Group, 111 Bedford Rd, Katonah, NY 10536-2190; **Phone:** 914-232-3135; **Board Cert:** Urology 2003; **Med School:** Albert Einstein Coll Med 1982; **Resid:** Surgery, Montefiore Med Ctr 1984; Urology, NY Presby-Columbia Med Ctr 1988

Blair, Bryan P MD (U) - **Hospital:** White Plains Hosp (page 615); **Address:** Westchester Med Grp, 210 Westchester Ave, White Plains, NY 10604; **Phone:** 914-682-6470; **Board Cert:** Urology 2004; **Med School:** Tulane Univ 1994; **Resid:** Urology, Natl Naval Med Ctr 2001

Boczko, Judd MD (U) - **Spec Exp:** Prostate Cancer/Robotic Surgery; Robotic Urologic Surgery; **Hospital:** Greenwich Hosp (page 892); **Address:** 210 Westchester Ave, White Plains, NY 10604; **Phone:** 914-682-6470; **Board Cert:** Urology 2008; **Med School:** Albert Einstein Coll Med 1999; **Resid:** Surgery, Montefiore Med Ctr 2001; Urology, Montefiore Med Ctr 2005; **Fellow:** Urologic Surgery, Strong Meml Hosp 2006; **Fac Appt:** Asst Prof U, NY Med Coll

Breslin, David S MD (U) - **Spec Exp:** Urology-Female; Voiding Dysfunction; Prostate Disease; **Hospital:** Phelps Meml Hosp Ctr (page 614); **Address:** Mount Kisco Medical Group, 1978 Crompond Rd, Cortlandt Manor, NY 10567; **Phone:** 914-737-8675; **Board Cert:** Urology 2007; **Med School:** Mount Sinai Sch Med 1987; **Resid:** Surgery, Mt Sinai Hosp 1989; Urology, Lenox Hill Hosp 1994; **Fellow:** Female Urology, Beth Israel Hosp 1995; **Fac Appt:** Asst Clin Prof U, NY Med Coll

Choudhury, Muhammad MD (U) - **Spec Exp:** Prostate Cancer; Bladder Cancer; Kidney Cancer; Testicular Cancer; **Hospital:** Westchester Med Ctr, Sound Shore Med Ctr - Westchester; **Address:** 19 Bradhurst Ave, Ste 1900, Hawthorne, NY 10532-2144; **Phone:** 914-347-1900; **Board Cert:** Urology 1982; **Med School:** Bangladesh 1972; **Resid:** Urology, Columbia-Presby Med Ctr 1978; Urology, NY Med Coll 1980; **Fellow:** Urologic Oncology, Roswell Park Cancer Inst 1981; **Fac Appt:** Prof U, NY Med Coll

Eshghi, A Majid MD (U) - **Spec Exp:** Kidney Stones; Laparoscopic Surgery; **Hospital:** Westchester Med Ctr, Sound Shore Med Ctr - Westchester; **Address:** 19 Bradhurst Ave, Ste 1900, Hawthorne, NY 10532; **Phone:** 914-347-1900; **Board Cert:** Urology 2005; **Med School:** Iran 1976; **Resid:** Surgery, St Barnabas Med Ctr 1981; Urology, LI Jewish Med Ctr 1985; **Fac Appt:** Prof U, NY Med Coll

Glassman, Charles N MD (U) - **Spec Exp:** Prostate Cancer; Incontinence; Pediatric Urology; Sexual Dysfunction; **Hospital:** White Plains Hosp (page 615); **Address:** 170 Maple Ave, Ste 104, White Plains, NY 10601-4707; **Phone:** 914-949-7556; **Board Cert:** Urology 1980; **Med School:** Tufts Univ 1973; **Resid:** Surgery, UCSF Med Ctr 1975; Urology, UCSF Med Ctr 1978; **Fellow:** Pediatric Urology, Mayo Clinic 1979

Housman, Arno D MD (U) - **Spec Exp:** Kidney Stones; Prostate Cancer; Incontinence; **Hospital:** Phelps Meml Hosp Ctr (page 614); **Address:** 325 S Highland Ave, Briarcliff Manor, NY 10510-2093; **Phone:** 914-631-6382; **Board Cert:** Urology 2009; **Med School:** SUNY Downstate 1980; **Resid:** Surgery, SUNY-Kings Co Hosp Ctr 1983; Urology, Yale-New Haven Hosp 1986

Lerner, Seth E MD (U) - **Spec Exp:** Prostate Cancer/Robotic Surgery; Robotic Urologic Surgery; **Hospital:** White Plains Hosp (page 615); **Address:** 170 Maple Ave, Ste 104, White Plains, NY 10601; **Phone:** 914-949-7556; **Board Cert:** Urology 2005; **Med School:** SUNY Downstate 1988; **Resid:** Surgery, Montefiore-Weiler Einstein Div 1990; Urology, Montefiore-Weler Einstein Div 1994; **Fellow:** Urologic Oncology, Mayo Clinic 1995; **Fac Appt:** Asst Prof U, Albert Einstein Coll Med

Matthews, Gerald J MD (U) - **Spec Exp:** Infertility-Male; Impotence; **Hospital:** Westchester Med Ctr, Montefiore Med Ctr-Wakefield Campus, NY (page 100); **Address:** 19 Bradhurst Ave, Ste 1900, Hawthorne, NY 10532-2144; **Phone:** 914-347-1900; **Board Cert:** Urology 2006; **Med School:** NY Med Coll 1986; **Resid:** Urology, Lenox Hill Hosp 1993; Surgery, St Francis Hosp Med Ctr 1989; **Fellow:** Urology, NY Hosp-Cornell Med Ctr 1995; Urology, Rockefeller Univ Hosp 1995; **Fac Appt:** Assoc Prof U, NY Med Coll

Owens, George F MD (U) - **Spec Exp:** Prostate Disease; Erectile Dysfunction; Incontinence; Minimally Invasive Surgery; **Hospital:** White Plains Hosp (page 615), Westchester Med Ctr; **Address:** 311 North St, Ste 406, White Plains, NY 10605-2232; **Phone:** 914-946-1406; **Board Cert:** Urology 2005; **Med School:** NY Med Coll 1979; **Resid:** Surgery, Montefiore Hosp Med Ctr 1981; Urology, Montefiore Hosp Med Ctr 1984; **Fellow:** Urology, NY Med Coll 1985; **Fac Appt:** Assoc Clin Prof U, NY Med Coll

Putignano, Joseph D MD (U) - **Spec Exp:** Bladder Surgery; Laser Surgery; Kidney Stones; Prostate Surgery; **Hospital:** Lawrence Hosp Ctr, Westchester Med Ctr; **Address:** 26 Pondfield Rd W, Bronxville, NY 10708; **Phone:** 914-793-1200; **Board Cert:** Urology 1975; **Med School:** Canada 1965; **Resid:** Urology, St Lukes-Roosevelt Hosp Ctr 1971; **Fac Appt:** Assoc Prof U, NY Med Coll

Reda, Edward F MD (U) - **Spec Exp:** Pediatric Urology; **Hospital:** Westchester Med Ctr; **Address:** Pediatric Urology Assocs, 150 White Plains Rd, Ste 306, Tarrytown, NY 10591; **Phone:** 914-493-8628; **Board Cert:** Urology 1984; **Med School:** Mexico 1976; **Resid:** Surgery, Bronx Lebanon Hosp 1979; Urology, Montefiore Med Ctr 1982; **Fellow:** Pediatric Urology, Chldns Hosp 1984; **Fac Appt:** Assoc Prof U, NY Med Coll

Riechers, Roger MD (U) - **Spec Exp:** Incontinence-Female; Prostate Cancer; **Hospital:** Northern Westchester Hosp (page 613); **Address:** 110 S Bedford Rd Fl 3, Mt Kisco, NY 10549; **Phone:** 914-242-1520; **Board Cert:** Urology 1976; **Med School:** NYU Sch Med 1968; **Resid:** Urology, Mount Sinai Med Ctr 1973

Roberts, Larry P MD (U) - **Spec Exp:** Infertility-Male; Erectile Dysfunction; Incontinence; **Hospital:** Sound Shore Med Ctr - Westchester, Lawrence Hosp Ctr; **Address:** 175 Memorial Hwy, Ste 3-2, New Rochelle, NY 10801-5641; **Phone:** 914-235-2929; **Board Cert:** Urology 1981; **Med School:** Univ Miami Sch Med 1974; **Resid:** Surgery, Univ Miami Hosps 1976; Urology, Montefiore Hosp 1979; **Fac Appt:** Asst Clin Prof U, Albert Einstein Coll Med

Schrager, Alan MD (U) - **Spec Exp:** Prostate Disease; Urology-Female; Urologic Cancer; Voiding Dysfunction; **Hospital:** Greenwich Hosp (page 892), Sound Shore Med Ctr - Westchester; **Address:** 1600 Harrison Ave, Ste 102-G, Mamaroneck, NY 10543-3124; **Phone:** 914-698-8106; **Board Cert:** Urology 1975; **Med School:** Ros Franklin Univ/Chicago Med Sch 1966; **Resid:** Surgery, Maimonides Med Ctr 1970; Urology, SUNY Downstate Med Ctr 1973

Siegel, Judy F MD (U) - **Spec Exp:** Voiding Dysfunction-Female; Voiding Dysfunction-Pediatric; **Hospital:** St. John's Riverside Hosp-Andrus Pavil, Phelps Meml Hosp Ctr (page 614); **Address:** Family Urology, 623 Warburton Ave, Hastings-on-Hudson, NY 10706; **Phone:** 914-478-3001; **Board Cert:** Urology 2009; **Med School:** Univ VT Coll Med 1988; **Resid:** Surgery, LI Jewish Med Ctr 1990; Urology, LI Jewish Med Ctr 1994; **Fellow:** Pediatric Urology, Schneider Chldns Hosp 1996

Trauzzi, Stephen MD (U) - **Spec Exp:** Prostate Disease; **Hospital:** Sound Shore Med Ctr - Westchester; **Address:** Advanced Urology Centers of NY, 120 Warren St, New Rochelle, NY 10801; **Phone:** 914-636-2121; **Board Cert:** Urology 2006; **Med School:** Georgetown Univ 1988; **Resid:** Urology, St Luke's Hosp 1994

Weinberg, Jerry MD (U) - **Spec Exp:** Robotic Surgery; Minimally Invasive Surgery; **Hospital:** Northern Westchester Hosp (page 613); **Address:** 666 Lexington Ave, Ste 100, Mt Kisco, NY 10549-3632; **Phone:** 914-666-4346; **Board Cert:** Urology 2010; **Med School:** SUNY Downstate 1983; **Resid:** Surgery, LIJ Jewish Med Ctr 1985; **Fellow:** Urology, LIJ Jewish Med Ctr 1989

Werner, Michael A MD (U) - **Spec Exp:** Infertility-Male; Sexual Dysfunction; **Hospital:** White Plains Hosp (page 615); **Address:** 2975 Westchester Ave, Purchase, NY 10577; **Phone:** 914-997-4100; **Board Cert:** Urology 2005; **Med School:** UCSF 1986; **Resid:** Surgery, Beth Israel Med Ctr 1989; Urology, Mt Sinai Med Ctr 1993; **Fellow:** Male Infertility, Boston Univ Med Ctr 1994

Vascular & Interventional Radiology

Hamet, Marc R MD (VIR) - **Spec Exp:** Osteoporosis Spine-Vertebroplasty; Uterine Fibroid Embolization; Endovascular Surgery; Carotid Artery Stent Placement; **Hospital:** White Plains Hosp (page 615), Lawrence Hosp Ctr; **Address:** White Plains Radiology, Davis & Post Roads, White Plains, NY 10601; **Phone:** 914-681-1273; **Board Cert:** Diagnostic Radiology 1995; Vascular & Interventional Radiology 2009; Neuroradiology 2010; **Med School:** Univ MD Sch Med 1991; **Resid:** Diagnostic Radiology, Univ Maryland Med Sys 1995; **Fellow:** Neuroradiology, Univ Maryland Med Sys 1996; Interventional Radiology, Johns Hopkins Hosp 1998

Vascular Surgery

Babu, Sateesh C MD (VascS) - **Spec Exp:** Carotid Artery Surgery; Aneurysm-Abdominal Aortic; Lower Limb Arterial Disease; Vein Disorders; **Hospital:** Westchester Med Ctr, Northern Westchester Hosp (page 613); **Address:** Westchester Heart & Vascular, 19 Bradhurst Ave, Ste 3750 South, Hawthorne, NY 10532-2140; **Phone:** 914-909-6900; **Board Cert:** Vascular Surgery 2001; **Med School:** India 1969; **Resid:** Surgery, Jewish Memorial Hosp 1972; Surgery, Metropolitan Hosp 1975; **Fellow:** Vascular Surgery, Metropolitan Hosp 1977; **Fac Appt:** Clin Prof S, NY Med Coll

Fishman, Eric MD (VascS) - **Hospital:** White Plains Hosp (page 615), Greenwich Hosp (page 892); **Address:** 1 Theall Rd, Rye, NY 10580; **Phone:** 914-723-7737; **Board Cert:** Surgery 2005; Vascular Surgery 2012; **Med School:** Mount Sinai Sch Med 1997; **Resid:** Surgery, Mount Sinai Med Ctr 2005; Vascular Surgery, Mount Sinai Med Ctr 2011

Goyal, Arun MD (VascS) - **Spec Exp:** Endovascular Surgery; Vein Disorders; Aneurysm; **Hospital:** Westchester Med Ctr; **Address:** 19 Bradhurst Ave, Ste 3750 S, Hawthorne, NY 10532; **Phone:** 914-593-1200; **Board Cert:** Surgery 2006; Vascular Surgery 2008; **Med School:** NY Med Coll 1990; **Resid:** Surgery, Mt Sinai Med Ctr 1995; Vascular Surgery, Mt Sinai Med Ctr 1996; **Fac Appt:** Asst Prof S, NY Med Coll

Karanfilian, Richard MD (VascS) - **Spec Exp:** Varicose Veins; Carotid Artery Surgery; Endovascular Surgery; **Hospital:** Sound Shore Med Ctr - Westchester; **Address:** 150 Lockwood Ave, Ste 14, New Rochelle, NY 10801-4912; **Phone:** 914-636-1700; **Board Cert:** Surgery 2002; Vascular Surgery 2006; **Med School:** Italy 1977; **Resid:** Surgery, UMDNJ-NJ Med Sch 1983; **Fellow:** Vascular Surgery, UMDNJ-NJ Med Sch 1985; **Fac Appt:** Assoc Clin Prof S, NY Med Coll

Schwartz, Kenneth S MD (VascS) - **Spec Exp:** Arterial Disease; Dialysis Access Surgery; **Hospital:** White Plains Hosp (page 615), Greenwich Hosp (page 892); **Address:** 1 Theall Rd, Rye, NY 10580; **Phone:** 914-723-7737; **Board Cert:** Surgery 2001; **Med School:** Albert Einstein Coll Med 1977; **Resid:** Surgery, Montefiore Hosp Med Ctr 1981; **Fellow:** Peripheral Vascular Surgery, USC Med Ctr 1982; **Fac Appt:** Asst Clin Prof S, NY Med Coll

Suggs, William D MD (VascS) - **Spec Exp:** Vein Disorders; Wound Healing/Care; Carotid Artery Surgery; **Hospital:** White Plains Hosp (page 615); **Address:** Vascular Associates, 4 Lyon Pl, Lobby Level, Ste 2, White Plains, NY 10601; **Phone:** 914-948-6633; **Board Cert:** Vascular Surgery 2002; **Med School:** Wake Forest Univ 1983; **Resid:** Surgery, Geo Wash Univ Med Ctr 1989; **Fellow:** Vascular Surgery, Emory Univ Hosp 1991; **Fac Appt:** Assoc Prof VascS, Albert Einstein Coll Med

Sun, Lucy MD (VascS) - **Hospital:** Northern Westchester Hosp (page 613); **Address:** 110 S Bedford Rd, Mt Kisco, NY 10549-3412; **Phone:** 914-241-1050; **Board Cert:** Vascular Surgery 2007; **Med School:** SUNY Downstate 1993; **Resid:** Surgery, Univ Iowa Hosps & Clin 1998; Surgery, UCSF Med Ctr 2001; **Fellow:** Vascular Surgery, UMDNJ-RW Johnson Med Ctr 2003

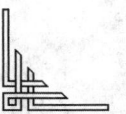
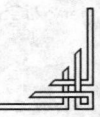

The Best in American Medicine
www.CastleConnolly.com

The State of
New Jersey

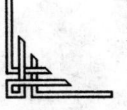
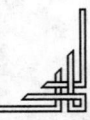

The Best in American Medicine
www.CastleConnolly.com

Bergen

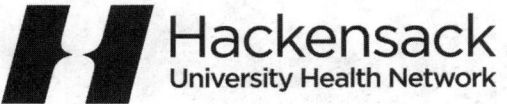

Hackensack
University Health Network

30 Prospect Avenue, Hackensack, NJ, 07601 • 551-996-2000
www.HackensackUHN.org

HackensackUMC *(Hackensack University Medical Center)*
HackensackUMC at Pascack Valley
HackensackUMC Mountainside

Year Founded: 2010
Number of beds: 1,140
Number of employees: 8,265
2011 Admissions: 50,693
Number of Hospitals in System: 3
Nursing: Magnet® Recognized for Nursing Excellence

Academic Affiliations: Saint George's University, Stevens Institute of Technology, University of Medicine and Dentistry of New Jersey - New Jersey Medical School.

Clinical Affiliations: Hackettstown Regional Medical Center, Saint Clare's Health System, Palisades Medical Center and NYU Langone Medical Center's Division of Pediatric Surgery, MinuteClinic

Strategic Alliance: North Shore-LIJ Health System

Hackensack University Health Network (HackensackUHN) is the non-profit, New Jersey-based parent company of HackensackUMC, the HackensackUMC Foundation, Hackensack University HealthPartners Medical Group, and corporate joint venture partners with LHP Hospital Group (Dallas, TX) in ownership of two hospitals: HackensackUMC at Pascack Valley and HackensackUMC Mountainside.

The Network has current clinical collaborations and affiliations with: Hackettstown Regional Medical Center, NYU Langone Medical Center's Division of Pediatric Surgery, Palisades Medical Center, and Saint Clare's Health System. It also formed a strategic alliance with the North Shore-LIJ Health System, and a clinical affiliation with MinuteClinic, the retail healthcare division of CVS Caremark.

• **Health Partners:** Hackensack University Health Network enjoys partnerships with various physician practices throughout the region.

• **Accountable Care Organization (ACO):** In April 2012, Hackensack Physician-Hospital Alliance ACO, LLC, announced it was one of 27 ACOs selected to participate in the Medicare Shared Savings Program (Shared Savings Program) ACO, a multifaceted program sponsored by the Centers for Medicare and Medicaid Services (CMS).

• **United Surgical Partners International:** Hackensack University Health Network entered into a joint venture partnership with community physicians and United Surgical Partners International (USPI) in the acquisition and operation of two ambulatory surgery centers in Bergen County.

For more information, please visit www.HackensackUHN.org.

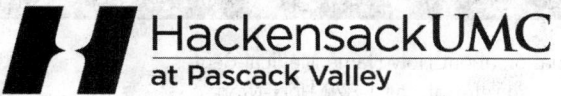

HackensackUMC
at Pascack Valley

250 Old Hook Road, Westwood, NJ 07675 • 201-880-2700
www.hackensackumcpv.com

OPENING SPRING 2013

Number of beds: 128 (in 2013)
Number of employees: Forecasted 350 by spring 2013
2011 Admissions: N/A

Since 2007, Hackensack University Medical Center, a premier healthcare provider ranked among the 50 best hospitals in the nation, has taken a leadership role in serving the needs of Pascack and Northern Valley residents by operating a Satellite Emergency Department at the hospital site.

In 2013, HackensackUMC's commitment to the region will culminate with the opening of HackensackUMC at Pascack Valley, a completely renovated, full-service, state-of-the-art facility. The new world-class, 128-bed community hospital, a joint venture of the Hackensack University Health Network and the LHP Hospital Group Inc., one of the country's leading private hospital management companies, will feature all private rooms and convenient access to the medical services most needed by local residents, including:

- Adult & Pediatric Emergency Care *(currently available)*
- Cardiology & a Catheterization Lab
- Gastroenterology
- Intensive/Critical Care
- Obstetrics and Women's Health Services
- Oncology/Cancer Care
- Outpatient and Inpatient Physical Therapy
- Outpatient Radiology Tests & Procedures *(currently available)*
- Same-Day and Inpatient Surgery
- Sleep Lab
- Urology

The hospital will improve critical travel times for ambulances and mobile intensive care units in the region, times that have more than doubled in recent years due to the absence of a strategically located hospital. It will also promote the establishment of more local medical offices and create residency opportunities in key specialties such as emergency medicine, family medicine, internal medicine, OB/GYN and general surgery at a time when nationwide physician shortages are anticipated. Updates about the opening of HackensackUMC at Pascack Valley are posted regularly on the hospital website.

For more information, please call 201-880-2700 or visit www.HackensackUMCPV.com.

For more information about Holy Name Medical Center
or for a physician referral, call 1-877-HOLY-NAME.
Please mention "Castle Connolly Guide."

Holy Name Medical Center

718 Teaneck Road
Teaneck, NJ 07666
1-877-HOLY-NAME
(1-877-465-9626)
www.holyname.org

THE HOLY NAME HEALING TRADITION

Holy Name Medical Center (HNMC) is a fully accredited, not-for-profit healthcare facility based in Teaneck, New Jersey, with off-site locations throughout Bergen County, and in Hudson and Passaic counties. Founded and sponsored by the Sisters of St. Joseph of Peace in 1925, the comprehensive 361-bed medical center offers leading-edge medical practice and technology administered in an environment rooted in a tradition of compassion and respect for every patient.

COMPREHENSIVE PROGRAMS AND SERVICES

HNMC provides high-quality health care across a continuum that encompasses education, prevention, early intervention, comprehensive treatment options, rehabilitation and wellness maintenance—from pre-conception through end-of-life.

In addition to patient care, HNMC's School of Nursing is renowned for the education of registered nurses and licensed practical nurses.

PERFORMANCE RECOGNITION

- **Top Performer on Key Quality Measures**
  THE JOINT COMMISSION
- **Best Regional Hospitals**
  US News & World Report
- **Distinguished Hospital Award for Clinical Excellence**
  HEALTHGRADES®
- **Magnet Recognition**
  AMERICAN NURSES CREDENTIALING ASSOCIATION
- **Beacon Award**
  AMERICAN ASSOCIATION OF CRITICAL-CARE NURSES
- **Stroke Care Excellence Award™**
  HEALTHGRADES®
- **Community Value Five-Star™ Designation**
  CLEVERLEY + ASSOCIATES
- **Best in Value™ Award**
  DATA ADVANTAGE, LLC
- **Distinguished Hospital Award for Service Excellence**
  MULTIPLE CLINICAL AREAS
  J.D. POWER AND ASSOCIATES
- **Primary Stroke Care Center**
  THE JOINT COMMISSION
- **Accredited Chest Pain Center**
  THE SOCIETY FOR CHEST PAIN CENTERS
- **"An Outstanding Emergency Experience"**
  J.D. POWER AND ASSOCIATES
- **"Best Places to Work in Healthcare"**
  MODERN HEALTHCARE MAGAZINE
- **"Best Places to Work in New Jersey"**
  NJ BIZ MAGAZINE

Centers of Excellence

- Bone and Joint Center
- Cardiovascular Services
- Emergency Care Center
- Interventional Institute
- Maternal/Child Health
- Regional Cancer Center

Robotic and Minimally
Invasive Surgery

Breast Services

Center for Healthy Living

Center for Sleep Medicine

Institute for Clinical Research

Culturally Sensitive Health Care:
– Korean Medical Program
– Hispanic Outreach Program
– Jewish Patient Services

Center for Physical Rehabilitation

HNH Fitness

Home Health Care

Hospice and Palliative Services, and
Villa Marie Claire residential hospice

MS Center

THE VALLEY HOSPITAL

223 North Van Dien Avenue, Ridgewood, NJ 07450
Phone: 201-447-8000 • www.valleyhealth.com
www.facebook.com/valleyhospital • www.twitter.com/valleyhospital

Sponsorship: Voluntary Not-for-Profit   **Beds:** 451 Acute Care Beds
Accredited by The Joint Commission

■ PROFILE

The Valley Hospital is affiliated with the New York-Presbyterian Healthcare System. Valley has been recognized nine consecutive times under the J.D. Power and Associates Distinguished Hospital Program and is a two-time recipient of the Magnet Award for Nursing Excellence.

Valley has been named one of Americas 100 Best Hospitals for Cardiac Care, Cardiac Surgery, Coronary Intervention, Gastrointestinal Care, Joint Replacement, and Orthopedic Surgery by HealthGrades, and has been recognized for clinical excellence in cardiology and cardiac surgery, maternity care, neuroscience and stroke, obstetrics, oncology, orthopedic surgery, and joint replacement.

Valley has earned an impressive 11 Disease-Specific Care Certifications for healthcare quality from the Joint Commission: acute myocardial infarction, heart failure, knee replacement, hip replacement, stroke, colorectal cancer, lung cancer, breast cancer, pancreatic cancer, prostate cancer, and uterine-ovarian cancer. Recognized by HealthGrades as one of America's 100 Best Hospitals for Cardiac Care, Cardiac Surgery, Coronary Intervention and General Surgery.

■ MEDICAL STAFF

The Valley Hospital has more than 1,000 physicians on its Active Medical Staff, 93 percent of whom are board certified.

■ CARDIOLOGY

The Valley Heart and Vascular Institute is a leader in the field of cardiology services, including cardiac surgery; coronary angioplasty and other interventional procedures; electrophysiology studies; and cardiac care research. Valley's cardiac surgery program consistently receives a 3-star rating—the highest designation of quality and clinical excellence—from The Society of Thoracic Surgeons, and is ranked #1 in New Jersey for overall cardiac services by HealthGrades.

■ SURGERY

The Valley Hospital is also known for its comprehensive surgical program, including pioneering advances in surgical oncology, gynecologic oncology, thoracic surgery, and its Center for Minimally Invasive and Robotic Surgery. The hospital has also been designated as a Bariatric Surgery Center of Excellence.

■ ONCOLOGY

Valley is known for its centers specializing in the diagnosis, care and treatment of prostate and lung cancer; as well as its surgical oncology, neuro-oncology, and gynecologic oncology programs; its comprehensive oncology clinical trials program and its Department of Radiation Oncology, including Tomotherapy. In 2011, Valley was the first hospital in northern New Jersey to offer Gamma Knife radiosurgery, a noninvasive tool designed to treat cancer and neurological conditions in the brain

■ OBSTETRICS

The hospital is well known for its maternity services including Maternal-Fetal Medicine, an enhanced Neonatal Intensive Care Unit, a maternal & child health home care program, as well as The Kireker Center for Child Development that offers a full spectrum of services.

Physician Referral: Information on physicians affiliated with The Valley Hospital is available by phone at 1-800-VALLEY 1 (1-800-825-5391) or by visiting **www.valleymedicalstaff.com.**

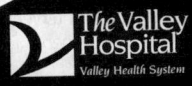

Allergy & Immunology

Falk, Theodore MD (A&I) - **Spec Exp:** Asthma; Immune Deficiency; Chronic Fatigue Syndrome; Pediatric Allergy & Immunology; **Hospital:** Holy Name Med Ctr (page 688), Englewood Hosp & Med Ctr; **Address:** 63 Grand Ave, Ste 100, River Edge, NJ 07661-1930; **Phone:** 201-487-2900; **Board Cert:** Pediatrics 1982; **Med School:** Belgium 1977; **Resid:** Pediatrics, Long Island Jewish Med Ctr 1980; **Fellow:** Allergy & Immunology, Nassau Co Med Ctr 1982

From, Stuart MD (A&I) - **Spec Exp:** Asthma & Allergy; Eczema; Skin Allergies; **Hospital:** Englewood Hosp & Med Ctr, Holy Name Med Ctr (page 688); **Address:** 309 Engle St, Ste 2, Englewood, NJ 07631; **Phone:** 201-568-1480; **Board Cert:** Allergy & Immunology 2003; **Med School:** NY Med Coll 1987; **Resid:** Internal Medicine, Montefiore Med Ctr 1990; **Fellow:** Allergy & Immunology, NY Presby-Cornell Med Ctr 1992

Goodstein, Carolyn E MD (A&I) - **Spec Exp:** Asthma; Rhinitis; Urticaria; Sinusitis; **Hospital:** Englewood Hosp & Med Ctr, Hackensack Univ Med Ctr (page 96); **Address:** 180 N Dean St, Englewood, NJ 07631-2534; **Phone:** 201-871-4755; **Board Cert:** Internal Medicine 1974; Allergy & Immunology 1980; **Med School:** SUNY Downstate 1964; **Resid:** Internal Medicine, Montefiore Med Ctr 1967; Allergy & Immunology, Roosevelt Hosp 1971

Harish, Ziv MD (A&I) - **Spec Exp:** Asthma & Sinusitis; Hay Fever; Urticaria; Hives; **Hospital:** Englewood Hosp & Med Ctr, Hackensack Univ Med Ctr (page 96); **Address:** 200 Engle St, Ste 18, Englewood, NJ 07631; **Phone:** 201-871-7475; **Board Cert:** Allergy & Immunology 2012; **Med School:** Israel 1983; **Resid:** Pediatrics, Montefiore Med Ctr 1989; **Fellow:** Allergy & Immunology, Montefiore Med Ctr 1991; **Fac Appt:** Asst Clin Prof Med, Albert Einstein Coll Med

Michelis, Mary Ann MD (A&I) - **Spec Exp:** Asthma; Immune Deficiency; **Hospital:** Hackensack Univ Med Ctr (page 96); **Address:** Hackensack Univ Med Ctr, 30 Prospect Ave, rm 3674, Hackensack, NJ 07601-1915; **Phone:** 201-996-2065; **Board Cert:** Internal Medicine 1978; Allergy & Immunology 1981; **Med School:** Univ Pittsburgh 1975; **Resid:** Internal Medicine, Lenox Hill Hosp 1978; **Fellow:** Allergy & Immunology, NY Hosp-Cornell Med Ctr 1978; **Fac Appt:** Assoc Clin Prof Med, UMDNJ-NJ Med Sch, Newark

Minikes, Neil I MD (A&I) - **Spec Exp:** Eczema; Food Allergy; Hay Fever; Asthma; **Hospital:** Englewood Hosp & Med Ctr, Hackensack Univ Med Ctr (page 96); **Address:** Allergy & Asthma Ctr Northern NJ, 500 Piermont Rd, Ste 304, Closter, NJ 07624; **Phone:** 201-564-7777; **Board Cert:** Pediatrics 1986; Allergy & Immunology 2011; **Med School:** Columbia P&S 1980; **Resid:** Pediatrics, Columbia-Presby Med Ctr 1983; **Fellow:** Allergy & Immunology, LI Jewish Med Ctr 1990; **Fac Appt:** Asst Clin Prof Ped, Columbia P&S

Perin, Patrick MD (A&I) - **Spec Exp:** Allergy; Asthma; Pediatric Allergy & Immunology; **Hospital:** Holy Name Med Ctr (page 688); **Address:** Advanced Asthma Allergy Care, 185 Cedar Ln, Ste L2, Teaneck, NJ 07666; **Phone:** 201-836-6400; **Board Cert:** Allergy & Immunology 2003; **Med School:** UC Davis 1987; **Resid:** Pediatrics, Univ Hosp-UMDNJ 1990; **Fellow:** Allergy & Immunology, Thomas Jefferson Univ 1992

Cardiac Electrophysiology

Preminger, Mark W MD (CE) - **Spec Exp:** Arrhythmias; **Hospital:** Valley Hosp (page 689), St. Luke's - Roosevelt Hosp Ctr - St Luke's Hosp (page 94); **Address:** The Valley Hospital, 223 N Van Dien Ave, Ridgewood, NJ 07450; **Phone:** 201-432-7837; **Board Cert:** Internal Medicine 1989; Cardiovascular Disease 2001; Cardiac Electrophysiology 2002; **Med School:** Hahnemann Univ 1985; **Resid:** Internal Medicine, N Shore Univ Hosp/Cornell 1988; **Fellow:** Cardiovascular Disease, NY Hosp-Cornell Med Ctr 1991; Cardiac Electrophysiology, Phildelphia Heart Inst 1992; **Fac Appt:** Assoc Prof Med

Cardiovascular Disease

Adibi, Baback MD (Cv) - **Spec Exp:** Cardiac CT Angiography; Coronary Angioplasty/Stents; Cardiac Cathetherization; **Hospital:** Hackensack Univ Med Ctr (page 96); **Address:** Bergen Cardiology Assocs, 400 Frank W. Burr Blvd, Ste 22, Teaneck, NJ 07666; **Phone:** 201-907-0442; **Board Cert:** Internal Medicine 2002; Cardiovascular Disease 2005; **Med School:** Univ Pittsburgh 1999; **Resid:** Internal Medicine, Thomas Jefferson Univ Hosp 2002; **Fellow:** Cardiovascular Disease, Thomas Jefferson Univ Hosp 2005

Blood, David K MD (Cv) - **Spec Exp:** Nuclear Cardiology; Transplant Medicine-Heart; **Hospital:** Englewood Hosp & Med Ctr, NY-Presby/Columbia Univ Med Ctr, NY (page 104); **Address:** 163 Engle St, Bldg 1C, Englewood, NJ 07631; **Phone:** 201-569-3313; **Board Cert:** Internal Medicine 1972; Cardiovascular Disease 1975; **Med School:** Columbia P&S 1966; **Resid:** Internal Medicine, Bellevue Hosp 1968; Internal Medicine, Harlem Hosp 1972; **Fellow:** Cardiovascular Disease, Columbia-Presby Med Ctr 1974; **Fac Appt:** Assoc Clin Prof Med, Columbia P&S

Conroy Jr, Daniel P MD (Cv) - **Spec Exp:** Non-Invasive Cardiology; Hypertension; Cholesterol/Lipid Disorders; Diabetes & Heart Disease; **Hospital:** St. Mary's Hosp - Passaic, Hackensack Univ Med Ctr (page 96); **Address:** 358 Valley Brook Ave, Lyndhurst, NJ 07071; **Phone:** 201-460-0142; **Board Cert:** Internal Medicine 1979; Cardiovascular Disease 1981; **Med School:** Mexico 1975; **Resid:** Internal Medicine, St Michaels Med Ctr 1978; **Fellow:** Cardiovascular Disease, St Michaels Med Ctr 1980

Eichman, Gerard MD (Cv) - **Spec Exp:** Coronary Angioplasty/Stents; Cardiac Cathetherization; Heart Valve Disease; **Hospital:** Holy Name Med Ctr (page 688), Hackensack Univ Med Ctr (page 96); **Address:** Cardiovascular Assocs of Teaneck, 954 Teaneck Rd, Teaneck, NJ 07666-4243; **Phone:** 201-833-2300; **Board Cert:** Cardiovascular Disease 2005; **Med School:** Dominica 1988; **Resid:** Internal Medicine, Monmouth Med Ctr 1991; **Fellow:** Cardiovascular Disease, Seton Hall 1992

Eisenberg, Sheldon B MD (Cv) - **Spec Exp:** Nuclear Cardiology; Preventive Cardiology; Coronary Artery Disease; **Hospital:** Valley Hosp (page 689), Hackensack Univ Med Ctr (page 96); **Address:** 333 Old Hook Rd, Ste 200, Westwood, NJ 07675-3200; **Phone:** 201-664-0201; **Board Cert:** Internal Medicine 1979; Cardiovascular Disease 1981; **Med School:** Cornell Univ-Weill Med Coll 1976; **Resid:** Internal Medicine, N Shore Univ Hosp 1979; **Fellow:** Cardiovascular Disease, N Shore Univ Hosp 1981

Gardin, Julius M MD (Cv) - **Spec Exp:** Echocardiography; Geriatric Cardiology; Preventive Cardiology; Cholesterol/Lipid Disorders; **Hospital:** Hackensack Univ Med Ctr (page 96); **Address:** Hackensack Univ Med Ctr, Dept Medicine, 30 Prospect Ave, 1 Main, Ste 1647, Hackensack, NJ 07601; **Phone:** 551-996-3500; **Board Cert:** Internal Medicine 1975; Cardiovascular Disease 1977; **Med School:** Univ Mich Med Sch 1972; **Resid:** Internal Medicine, Univ Mich Hosp 1975; **Fellow:** Cardiovascular Disease, Georgetown Univ Hosp 1977; **Fac Appt:** Prof Med, UMDNJ-Univ Med Dent NJ

Goldschmidt, Howard Z MD (Cv) - **Spec Exp:** Heart Valve Disease; Pacemakers; Cardiomyopathy; Atrial Fibrillation; **Hospital:** Valley Hosp (page 689); **Address:** 1200 E Ridgewood Ave, Ridgewood, NJ 07450; **Phone:** 201-670-8660; **Board Cert:** Internal Medicine 1986; Cardiovascular Disease 1989; **Med School:** Columbia P&S 1983; **Resid:** Internal Medicine, Mt Sinai Hosp 1986; **Fellow:** Cardiovascular Disease, Mt Sinai Hosp 1988

Goldweit, Richard S MD (Cv) - **Spec Exp:** Interventional Cardiology; Sleep Disorders/Cardiac Risk; Peripheral Vascular Disease; Cardiac Catheterization; **Hospital:** Englewood Hosp & Med Ctr; **Address:** 177 N Dean St Fl 1, Englewood, NJ 07631; **Phone:** 201-569-4901; **Board Cert:** Internal Medicine 1985; Cardiovascular Disease 1987; Interventional Cardiology 2009; **Med School:** Cornell Univ-Weill Med Coll 1982; **Resid:** Internal Medicine, NY Hosp-Cornell Med Ctr 1985; **Fellow:** Cardiovascular Disease, NY Hosp-Cornell Med Ctr 1987

Haft, Jacob I MD (Cv) - **Spec Exp:** Coronary Artery Disease; Arrhythmias; Heart Failure; **Hospital:** Saint Michael's Med Ctr, Hackensack Univ Med Ctr (page 96); **Address:** 20 Prospect Ave, Ste 719, Hackensack, NJ 07601; **Phone:** 201-343-8505; **Board Cert:** Internal Medicine 1968; Cardiovascular Disease 1973; **Med School:** Columbia P&S 1962; **Resid:** Internal Medicine, Beth Israel Hosp 1964; Internal Medicine, Bellevue-Columbia P&S 1968; **Fellow:** Cardiovascular Disease, Mt Sinai Hosp 1965; Cardiovascular Disease, Peter Bent Brigham Hosp 1969; **Fac Appt:** Prof Med, Seton Hall Univ Sch Hlth & Med Scis

Hodges, David MD (Cv) - **Spec Exp:** Stress Management; **Hospital:** Englewood Hosp & Med Ctr; **Address:** 200 Grand Ave, Ste 202, Engelwood, NJ 07631; **Phone:** 201-816-9266; **Board Cert:** Internal Medicine 1987; Cardiovascular Disease 2003; **Med School:** NYU Sch Med 1984; **Resid:** Internal Medicine, Boston Med Ctr 1987; Internal Medicine, Beth Israel Deaconess Med Ctr 1989; **Fellow:** Cardiopulmonary Disease, Brigham and Women's Hosp 1991; **Fac Appt:** Asst Prof Med, Columbia P&S

Jacowitz, Joel MD (Cv) - **Spec Exp:** Echocardiography; Interventional Cardiology; **Hospital:** Valley Hosp (page 689); **Address:** Old Hook Medical Assocs, 452 Old Hook Rd, Emerson, NJ 07630; **Phone:** 201-666-3900; **Board Cert:** Internal Medicine 1981; Cardiovascular Disease 1985; Echocardiography 1993; **Med School:** SUNY Downstate 1977; **Resid:** Internal Medicine, Metropolitan Hosp 1980; Internal Medicine, Harlem Hosp 1982; **Fellow:** Cardiovascular Disease, Harlem Hosp 1985; Interventional Cardiology, Dartmouth-Hitchcock Med Ctr 1993; **Fac Appt:** Assoc Clin Prof Med, Seton Hall Univ Sch Hlth & Med Scis

Landers, David B MD (Cv) - **Spec Exp:** Cardiac Catheterization; Coronary Angioplasty/Stents; Angioplasty; Interventional Cardiology; **Hospital:** Hackensack Univ Med Ctr (page 96), Holy Name Med Ctr (page 688); **Address:** 400 Frank Burr Blvd, Teaneck, NJ 07666; **Phone:** 201-907-0442; **Board Cert:** Internal Medicine 1983; Cardiovascular Disease 1987; Interventional Cardiology 2010; **Med School:** Georgetown Univ 1979; **Resid:** Internal Medicine, St Vincents Hosp 1982; **Fellow:** Cardiovascular Disease, Westchester Co Med Ctr 1985; **Fac Appt:** Asst Clin Prof Med, UMDNJ-NJ Med Sch, Newark

Landzberg, Joel S MD (Cv) - **Spec Exp:** Preventive Cardiology; Coronary Artery Disease; Heart Failure; Heart Valve Disease; **Hospital:** Hackensack Univ Med Ctr (page 96), Valley Hosp (page 689); **Address:** 333 Old Hook Rd, Ste 200, Westwood, NJ 07675-3200; **Phone:** 201-664-0201; **Board Cert:** Internal Medicine 1986; Cardiovascular Disease 1989; Interventional Cardiology 2002; **Med School:** Columbia P&S 1983; **Resid:** Internal Medicine, Vanderbilt Univ Hosp 1986; **Fellow:** Cardiology Research, Moffit Hosp 1987; Cardiovascular Disease, Brigham & Womens Hosp 1991; **Fac Appt:** Assoc Clin Prof Med, UMDNJ-NJ Med Sch, Newark

Lichtstein, Elliott S MD (Cv) - **Spec Exp:** Heart Attack; Congestive Heart Failure; Heart Valve Disease; Heart Failure; **Hospital:** Hackensack Univ Med Ctr (page 96), Valley Hosp (page 689); **Address:** Westwood Cardiology, 333 Old Hook Rd, Ste 200, Westwood, NJ 07675; **Phone:** 201-664-0201; **Board Cert:** Internal Medicine 1984; Cardiovascular Disease 1987; **Med School:** Temple Univ 1981; **Resid:** Internal Medicine, Albany Med Ctr Hosp 1984; **Fellow:** Cardiovascular Disease, LI Jewish Med Ctr 1986

Pumill, Rick MD (Cv) - **Spec Exp:** Coronary Artery Disease; Hypertension; Congestive Heart Failure; **Hospital:** Hackensack Univ Med Ctr (page 96); **Address:** 103 River Rd Fl 2, Edgewater, NJ 07020-1002; **Phone:** 201-941-8100; **Board Cert:** Internal Medicine 1988; Cardiovascular Disease 2001; **Med School:** Dominica 1984; **Resid:** Internal Medicine, Jersey City Med Ctr 1988; **Fellow:** Cardiovascular Disease, Jersey City Med Ctr 1990

Reison, Dennis S MD (Cv) - **Spec Exp:** Interventional Cardiology; **Hospital:** Valley Hosp (page 689); **Address:** 1200 E Ridgewood Ave, Ridgewood, NJ 07450; **Phone:** 201-670-8660; **Board Cert:** Internal Medicine 1978; Cardiovascular Disease 1981; **Med School:** Stanford Univ 1975; **Resid:** Internal Medicine, Columbia Presby Hosp 1978; **Fellow:** Cardiovascular Disease, Mt Sinai Hosp 1979; Cardiovascular Disease, Columbia Presby Hosp 1981; **Fac Appt:** Asst Clin Prof Med, Columbia P&S

Rossakis, Constantine MD (Cv) - **Spec Exp:** Interventional Cardiology; Nuclear Cardiology; **Hospital:** Hackensack Univ Med Ctr (page 96); **Address:** 357 Prospect Ave, Hackensack, NJ 07601-2505; **Phone:** 201-489-3440; **Board Cert:** Internal Medicine 1986; Cardiovascular Disease 1989; Nuclear Cardiology 2009; **Med School:** NYU Sch Med 1983; **Resid:** Internal Medicine, NY Hosp 1986; **Fellow:** Cardiovascular Disease, NY Hosp-Cornell 1989; **Fac Appt:** Asst Clin Prof Med, Cornell Univ-Weill Med Coll

Rothman, Howard C MD (Cv) - **Spec Exp:** Cholesterol/Lipid Disorders; Angina; Women's Health; **Hospital:** Englewood Hosp & Med Ctr, Holy Name Med Ctr (page 688); **Address:** Advanced Cardiology Inst, 2200 Fletcher Ave, Fort Lee, NJ 07024-5005; **Phone:** 201-461-6200; **Board Cert:** Internal Medicine 1975; Cardiovascular Disease 1979; **Med School:** Univ Cincinnati 1970; **Resid:** Internal Medicine, NY Hosp-Cornell Med Ctr 1975; **Fellow:** Cardiovascular Disease, NY Hosp-Cornell Med Ctr 1976; **Fac Appt:** Asst Clin Prof Med, Columbia P&S

Salerno, William D MD (Cv) - **Spec Exp:** Vein Disorders; **Hospital:** Hackensack Univ Med Ctr (page 96); **Address:** Heartcare Ctr, 38 Mayhill St, Saddle Brook, NJ 07663-5307; **Phone:** 201-843-1019; **Board Cert:** Internal Medicine 1987; Cardiovascular Disease 1989; Critical Care Medicine 2011; **Med School:** Mexico 1982; **Resid:** Internal Medicine, Hackensack Med Ctr 1986; Critical Care Medicine, Norwalk Hosp 1987; **Fellow:** Cardiovascular Disease, Hackensack Med Ctr 1989; Interventional Cardiology, Hackensack Med Ctr 1990; **Fac Appt:** Assoc Clin Prof Med, UMDNJ-NJ Med Sch, Newark

Sotsky, Gerald MD (Cv) - **Hospital:** Valley Hosp (page 689); **Address:** 1200 E Ridgewood Ave, Ridgewood, NJ 07450; **Phone:** 201-670-8660; **Board Cert:** Internal Medicine 1984; Cardiovascular Disease 1987; **Med School:** Mount Sinai Sch Med 1981; **Resid:** Internal Medicine, Mt Sinai Med Ctr 1984; **Fellow:** Cardiovascular Disease, Mt Sinai Med Ctr 1986

Teichholz, Louis E MD (Cv) - **Spec Exp:** Mitral Valve Disease; Complementary Medicine; Echocardiography; Cholesterol/Lipid Disorders; **Hospital:** Hackensack Univ Med Ctr (page 96); **Address:** Hackensack Univ Med Ctr, 30 Prospect Ave, 4-Main, Ste 4655, Hackensack, NJ 07601; **Phone:** 201-996-2314; **Board Cert:** Internal Medicine 1972; Cardiovascular Disease 1975; **Med School:** Harvard Med Sch 1966; **Resid:** Internal Medicine, Peter Bent Brigham Hosp 1968; **Fellow:** Cardiovascular Disease, Peter Bent Brigham Hosp 1972; **Fac Appt:** Prof Med, UMDNJ-NJ Med Sch, Newark

Wild, David MD (Cv) - **Hospital:** Holy Name Med Ctr (page 688), Hackensack Univ Med Ctr (page 96); **Address:** 954 Teaneck Rd, Teaneck, NJ 07666; **Phone:** 201-833-2300; **Board Cert:** Cardiovascular Disease 2008; Internal Medicine 2005; **Med School:** UMDNJ-RW Johnson Med Sch 2002; **Resid:** Internal Medicine, Montefiore Med Ctr 2005; **Fellow:** Cardiovascular Disease, St Lukes-Roosevelt Hosp Ctr 2008

Williams, Marcus L MD (Cv) - **Spec Exp:** Cholesterol/Lipid Disorders; Hypertension; Atrial Fibrillation; Coronary Artery Disease; **Hospital:** Valley Hosp (page 689), Chilton Hosp; **Address:** 43 Yawpo Ave, Oakland, NJ 07436; **Phone:** 201-337-0066; **Board Cert:** Internal Medicine 1985; Cardiovascular Disease 1989; **Med School:** Geo Wash Univ 1982; **Resid:** Internal Medicine, Memorial Hosp/Univ NC 1985; **Fellow:** Cardiovascular Disease, Memorial Hosp/Univ NC 1988

Child & Adolescent Psychiatry

Kotler, Lisa A MD (ChAP) - **Spec Exp:** Eating Disorders; ADD/ADHD; Depression; Anxiety Disorders; **Hospital:** NYU Langone Med Ctr (page 108); **Address:** NYU Child Study Ctr-Hackensack, 411 Hackensack Ave Fl 7, Hackensack, NJ 07601; **Phone:** 201-465-8111; **Board Cert:** Psychiatry 2008; Child & Adolescent Psychiatry 2009; **Med School:** Yale Univ 1993; **Resid:** Psychiatry, Mt Sinai Med Ctr 1996; **Fellow:** Child & Adolescent Psychiatry, Columbia-Presby Med Ctr 1998; Eating Disorders Research, NY State Psyc Inst-Columbia Presby MC 1999; **Fac Appt:** Asst Prof Psyc

Pincus, Emile I MD (ChAP) - **Spec Exp:** Substance Abuse; Suicide; **Hospital:** St. Clare's Hosp - Denville; **Address:** 912 Kinderkamack Rd Fl 2, River Edge, NJ 07661; **Phone:** 201-615-1352; **Board Cert:** Psychiatry 1986; Child & Adolescent Psychiatry 2004; **Med School:** Mount Sinai Sch Med 1978; **Resid:** Psychiatry, St Lukes Hosp Ctr 1979; Psychiatry, Mt Sinai Med Ctr 1982; **Fellow:** Child & Adolescent Psychiatry, New York Hosp-Cornell Med Ctr 1984

Colon & Rectal Surgery

Helbraun, Mark E MD (CRS) - **Spec Exp:** Colonoscopy; Rectal Cancer; **Hospital:** Hackensack Univ Med Ctr (page 96); **Address:** 20 Prospect Ave, Ste 811, Hackensack, NJ 07601; **Phone:** 201-525-1660; **Board Cert:** Colon & Rectal Surgery 1978; **Med School:** Wayne State Univ 1972; **Resid:** Surgery, New York Hosp-Cornell 1977; **Fellow:** Colon & Rectal Surgery, Lahey Clin 1978

Nizin, Joel S MD (CRS) - **Spec Exp:** Colon Cancer; Inflammatory Bowel Disease; **Hospital:** Valley Hosp (page 689), Chilton Hosp; **Address:** 140 Chestnut St, Ste 301, Ridgewood, NJ 07450; **Phone:** 201-689-9100; **Board Cert:** Colon & Rectal Surgery 1987; Surgery 2008; **Med School:** Howard Univ 1978; **Resid:** Surgery, St Luke's Hosp 1983; **Fellow:** Colon & Rectal Surgery, Univ Minn Med Ctr 1984

Waxenbaum, Steven I MD (CRS) - **Spec Exp:** Laparoscopic Surgery; Hemorrhoids; Colon Cancer; **Hospital:** Valley Hosp (page 689), Englewood Hosp & Med Ctr; **Address:** 216 Engle St, Englewood, NJ 07631; **Phone:** 201-567-7615; **Board Cert:** Surgery 2003; Colon & Rectal Surgery 2006; **Med School:** UMDNJ-RW Johnson Med Sch 1988; **Resid:** Surgery, Westchester Med Ctr 1993; **Fellow:** Colon & Rectal Surgery, Lehigh Valley Hosp 1994

White, Ronald A MD (CRS) - **Spec Exp:** Hemorrhoids; Colon & Rectal Cancer; Colonoscopy; **Hospital:** Englewood Hosp & Med Ctr, Valley Hosp (page 689); **Address:** 216 Engle St, Ste 203, Englewood, NJ 07631-2428; **Phone:** 201-567-7615; **Board Cert:** Colon & Rectal Surgery 1988; **Med School:** Boston Univ 1981; **Resid:** Surgery, Montefiore Hosp 1986; **Fellow:** Colon & Rectal Surgery, RW Johnson Med Sch 1987

Critical Care Medicine

Cornell, James S MD/PhD (CCM) - **Spec Exp:** Respiratory Distress Syndrome; Lung Cancer; Chronic Obstructive Lung Disease (COPD); **Hospital:** Valley Hosp (page 689); **Address:** 31-00 Broadway Fl 2, Fair Lawn, NJ 07410-2305; **Phone:** 201-796-2255; **Board Cert:** Internal Medicine 2002; **Med School:** Cornell Univ-Weill Med Coll 1988; **Resid:** Internal Medicine, New York Hosp-Cornell 1991; Pulmonary Disease, Meml Sloan Kettering Cancer Ctr 1991; **Fellow:** Pulmonary Critical Care Medicine, New York Hosp-Cornell 1994

Dermatology

Andrews, Alan D MD (D) - **Spec Exp:** Skin Cancer; Phototherapy; **Hospital:** NY-Presby/Columbia Univ Med Ctr, NY (page 104), Holy Name Med Ctr (page 688); **Address:** 500 Piermont Rd, Ste 101, Closter, NJ 07624; **Phone:** 201-767-0501; **Board Cert:** Dermatology 1979; **Med School:** Univ VA Sch Med 1972; **Resid:** Dermatology, NCI Affil Hosp 1975; **Fellow:** Dermatology, Columbia P&S 1979

Ashinoff, Robin MD (D) - **Spec Exp:** Mohs' Surgery; Laser Surgery; Cosmetic Dermatology; Melanoma; **Hospital:** Hackensack Univ Med Ctr (page 96), NYU Langone Med Ctr (page 108); **Address:** 360 Essex St, Ste 201, Hackensack, NJ 07601; **Phone:** 201-336-8660; **Board Cert:** Dermatology 2009; **Med School:** NYU Sch Med 1985; **Resid:** Dermatology, NYU Med Ctr 1989; **Fellow:** Mohs Surgery, NYU Med Ctr 1991; Laser Surgery, NYU Med Ctr 1991; **Fac Appt:** Assoc Clin Prof D, NYU Sch Med

Brauner, Gary J MD (D) - **Spec Exp:** Skin Laser Surgery; Black/Asian Skin Care; Cosmetic Dermatology; Hair Removal-Laser; **Hospital:** Englewood Hosp & Med Ctr, Mount Sinai Med Ctr (page 102); **Address:** 1625 Anderson Ave, Fort Lee, NJ 07024; **Phone:** 201-461-5522; **Board Cert:** Dermatology 1972; Dermatopathology 1978; **Med School:** Harvard Med Sch 1967; **Resid:** Dermatology, Jewish Hosp 1968; Dermatology, Mass Genl Hosp 1971; **Fac Appt:** Assoc Clin Prof D, Mount Sinai Sch Med

Corey, Timothy MD (D) - **Spec Exp:** Psoriasis; Skin Cancer; **Hospital:** Valley Hosp (page 689), NY-Presby/Columbia Univ Med Ctr, NY (page 104); **Address:** 400 Rt 17 S, Ridgewood, NJ 07450; **Phone:** 201-652-4536; **Board Cert:** Dermatology 1979; **Med School:** Columbia P&S 1975; **Resid:** Dermatology, Columbia Presby Med Ctr 1979; **Fac Appt:** Asst Clin Prof D, Columbia P&S

Fishman, Miriam MD (D) - **Spec Exp:** Pediatric Dermatology; Skin Cancer; **Hospital:** Englewood Hosp & Med Ctr; **Address:** 216 Engle St, Ste 104, Englewood, NJ 07631-2428; **Phone:** 201-569-5678; **Board Cert:** Dermatology 2009; **Med School:** NYU Sch Med 1978; **Resid:** Pediatrics, Montefiore Med Ctr 1981; Dermatology, Montefiore Med Ctr 1984

Fried, Sharon MD (D) - **Spec Exp:** Skin Cancer; Acne; Psoriasis; **Hospital:** Englewood Hosp & Med Ctr; **Address:** 180 N Dean St, Ste 2 South, Englewood, NJ 07631-2534; **Phone:** 201-569-9800; **Board Cert:** Internal Medicine 1983; Dermatology 2009; **Med School:** NYU Sch Med 1980; **Resid:** Internal Medicine, NYU Med Ctr 1983; Dermatology, SUNY Downstate HSC 1985

Giardina-Beckett, MarieAnn MD (D) - **Spec Exp:** Acne; Botox Therapy; **Hospital:** Meadowlands Hosp Med Ctr, St. Mary's Hosp - Passaic; **Address:** 71 Union Ave, Rutherford, NJ 07070; **Phone:** 201-804-8900; **Board Cert:** Dermatology 2009; **Med School:** NY Med Coll 1986; **Resid:** Dermatology, New York Med Coll 1990

Grodberg, Michele MD (D) - **Spec Exp:** Cosmetic Dermatology; Hair Removal-Laser; Botox Therapy; Facial Rejuvenation; **Hospital:** Englewood Hosp & Med Ctr; **Address:** 106 Grand Ave Fl 3, Englewood, NJ 07631-3574; **Phone:** 201-567-8884; **Board Cert:** Dermatology 2009; **Med School:** NYU Sch Med 1987; **Resid:** Dermatology, NYU Med Ctr 1991

Heldman, Jay MD (D) - **Spec Exp:** Dermatologic Surgery; **Hospital:** Valley Hosp (page 689); **Address:** 23-00 Route 208 S, Fair Lawn, NJ 07410-1559; **Phone:** 201-797-7770; **Board Cert:** Dermatology 1981; **Med School:** Columbia P&S 1977; **Resid:** Internal Medicine, Columbia-Presby Med Ctr 1978; Dermatology, Mt Sinai Med Ctr 1981

Morman, Manuel R MD/PhD (D) - **Spec Exp:** Mohs' Surgery; Skin Cancer; Reconstructive Surgery; **Hospital:** St. Mary's Hosp - Passaic; **Address:** 47 Orient Way, Rutherford, NJ 07070-2040; **Phone:** 201-460-0280; **Board Cert:** Dermatology 2009; **Med School:** Jefferson Med Coll 1976; **Resid:** Dermatology, Hosp Univ Penn 1979; **Fellow:** Chemosurgery, Cleveland Clinic 1980

Possick, Paul MD (D) - **Spec Exp:** Skin Cancer; Contact Dermatitis; Eczema; Psoriasis; **Hospital:** NYU Langone Med Ctr (page 108); **Address:** 390 Old Hook Rd Fl 2, Westwood, NJ 07675-2616; **Phone:** 201-666-9550; **Board Cert:** Dermatology 2009; **Med School:** Tufts Univ 1964; **Resid:** Internal Medicine, Montefiore Hosp 1966; Dermatology, Univ Hosp 1968; **Fac Appt:** Asst Prof D, NYU Sch Med

Rapaport, Jeffrey A MD (D) - **Spec Exp:** Cosmetic Dermatology; Scar Revision; Laser Surgery; Skin Laser Surgery; **Hospital:** Holy Name Med Ctr (page 688), Englewood Hosp & Med Ctr; **Address:** 333 Sylvan Ave Fl 2 - Ste 207, Englewood Cliffs, NJ 07632; **Phone:** 201-227-1555; **Board Cert:** Dermatology 1983; **Med School:** Emory Univ 1979; **Resid:** Dermatology, Jefferson Univ Hosp 1982

Scherl, Sharon MD (D) - **Spec Exp:** Acne; Cosmetic Dermatology; Photodynamic Therapy; Tattoo Removal; **Hospital:** Englewood Hosp & Med Ctr; **Address:** 45 Central Ave, Tenafly, NJ 07670; **Phone:** 201-568-8400; **Board Cert:** Dermatology 2010; **Med School:** NY Med Coll 1988; **Resid:** Dermatology, Metropolitian Hosp Ctr 1992

Sweeney, Eugene W MD (D) - **Spec Exp:** Skin Cancer; Pediatric Dermatology; Acne; **Hospital:** Holy Name Med Ctr (page 688), Englewood Hosp & Med Ctr; **Address:** 757 N Teaneck Rd, Teaneck, NJ 07666-4241; **Phone:** 201-837-3939; **Board Cert:** Dermatology 1967; **Med School:** NY Med Coll 1960; **Resid:** Dermatology, Columbia-Presby Med Ctr 1966; **Fac Appt:** Assoc Prof D, Columbia P&S

Weiss, Darryl S MD (D) - **Spec Exp:** Hair Restoration/Transplant; Cosmetic Dermatology; Skin Laser Surgery; **Hospital:** Valley Hosp (page 689); **Address:** 23-00 Route 208 S, Fairlawn, NJ 07410; **Phone:** 201-797-7770; **Board Cert:** Dermatology 1990; **Med School:** Med Coll VA 1986; **Resid:** Dermatology, Jackson Meml Hosp 1990

Diagnostic Radiology

Budin, Joel A MD (DR) - **Spec Exp:** Neuroradiology; **Hospital:** Hackensack Univ Med Ctr (page 96); **Address:** 30 S Newman St, Hackensack, NJ 07601; **Phone:** 201-488-1188; **Board Cert:** Diagnostic Radiology 1975; **Med School:** Columbia P&S 1969; **Resid:** Diagnostic Radiology, Columbia-Presby Med Ctr 1975

Calem-Grunat, Jaclyn A MD (DR) - **Spec Exp:** Breast Imaging; Ultrasound; **Hospital:** Valley Hosp (page 689); **Address:** Radiology Assocs of Ridgewood, 20 Franklin Tpke, Waldwick, NJ 07463; **Phone:** 201-445-8822; **Board Cert:** Diagnostic Radiology 1994; **Med School:** Mount Sinai Sch Med 1988; **Resid:** Internal Medicine, Beeth Israel Med Ctr 1990; Diagnostic Radiology, Harbor-UCLA Med Ctr 1994; **Fellow:** Breast Imaging, UCLA Med Ctr 1995

Goldfischer, Mindy A MD (DR) - **Spec Exp:** Breast Imaging; Ultrasound; **Hospital:** Englewood Hosp & Med Ctr; **Address:** 350 Engle St, Englewood, NJ 07631; **Phone:** 201-894-3480; **Board Cert:** Diagnostic Radiology 1986; **Med School:** NYU Sch Med 1982; **Resid:** Diagnostic Radiology, Montefiore Med Ctr 1986; **Fellow:** Diagnostic Radiology, Thomas Jefferson Univ Hosp 1987

Gross, Joshua david MD (DR) - **Spec Exp:** Breast Imaging; Breast Cancer; **Hospital:** Holy Name Med Ctr (page 688); **Address:** Holy Name Hosp, Breast Imaging, 718 Teaneck Rd, Teaneck, NJ 07666; **Phone:** 201-833-7100; **Board Cert:** Diagnostic Radiology 1984; **Med School:** Albert Einstein Coll Med 1980; **Resid:** Diagnostic Radiology, Einstein/Jacobi Hosp 1984

Krinsky, Glenn MD (DR) - **Spec Exp:** MRI; Musculoskeletal Imaging; Gastrointestinal Imaging; **Hospital:** Valley Hosp (page 689); **Address:** Radiology Assocs of Ridgewood, 20 Franklin Tpke, Waldwick, NJ 07463; **Phone:** 201-445-8822; **Board Cert:** Diagnostic Radiology 1994; **Med School:** NYU Sch Med 1988; **Resid:** Surgical Pathology, Bellevue Hosp 1990; Diagnostic Radiology, Bellevue Hosp 1993; **Fellow:** Magnetic Resonance Imaging, NYU/Bellevue Hosp 1994

Levy, Lauren S MD (DR) - **Spec Exp:** Mammography; Breast MRI; Breast Imaging; **Hospital:** Valley Hosp (page 689); **Address:** Radiology Assocs of Ridgewood, 20 Franklin Tpke, Waldwick, NJ 07463; **Phone:** 201-445-8822; **Board Cert:** Diagnostic Radiology 1996; **Med School:** SUNY Downstate 1991; **Resid:** Diagnostic Radiology, NYU-Bellevue Hosp 1996; **Fellow:** Mammography, NYU-Bellevue Hosp 1997

Liebling, Melissa S MD (DR) - **Spec Exp:** Pediatric Radiology; **Hospital:** Hackensack Univ Med Ctr (page 96); **Address:** Hackensack Univ Med Ctr, Dept Radiology, 30 Prospect Ave, rm 1861, Hackensack, NJ 07601; **Phone:** 201-996-2200; **Board Cert:** Diagnostic Radiology 1992; Pediatric Radiology 2006; **Med School:** Albany Med Coll 1987; **Resid:** Diagnostic Radiology, Columbia-Presby Med Ctr 1992; **Fellow:** Pediatric Radiology, Columbia-Presby/Babies Hosp 1994

Lubat, Edward MD (DR) - **Spec Exp:** Abdominal Imaging; Thoracic Radiology; Musculoskeletal Imaging; Nuclear Medicine; **Hospital:** Valley Hosp (page 689); **Address:** Radiology Assocs, 20 Franklin Tpke, Waldwick, NJ 07463-1749; **Phone:** 201-445-8822; **Board Cert:** Diagnostic Radiology 1989; Nuclear Medicine 1989; **Med School:** Jefferson Med Coll 1982; **Resid:** Diagnostic Radiology, NYU Med Ctr 1988; **Fellow:** Nuclear Medicine, NYU Med Ctr 1985

Rakow, Joel MD (DR) - **Spec Exp:** Ultrasound; **Hospital:** Hackensack Univ Med Ctr (page 96); **Address:** Hackensack Univ Med Ctr, Dept Radiology, 30 Prospect Ave, Hackensack, NJ 07601; **Phone:** 201-996-2194; **Board Cert:** Diagnostic Radiology 1986; **Med School:** Albert Einstein Coll Med 1982; **Resid:** Diagnostic Radiology, Montefiore Med Ctr 1986; **Fellow:** Ultrasound, Thomas Jefferson Med Ctr 1987

Rambler, Louis MD (DR) - **Spec Exp:** Ultrasound; **Hospital:** Valley Hosp (page 689); **Address:** Radiology Assocs of Ridgewood, 20 Franklin Tpke, Waldwick, NJ 07463-1749; **Phone:** 201-445-8822; **Board Cert:** Diagnostic Radiology 1977; **Med School:** Cornell Univ-Weill Med Coll 1971; **Resid:** Diagnostic Radiology, Columbia-Presby Med Ctr 1977

Sorabella, Philip MD (DR) - **Spec Exp:** Nuclear Medicine; Breast Imaging; **Hospital:** Valley Hosp (page 689); **Address:** Radiology Assocs of Ridgewood, 20 Franklin Tpke, Waldwick, NJ 07463-1749; **Phone:** 201-445-8822; **Board Cert:** Diagnostic Radiology 1974; Nuclear Medicine 1974; **Med School:** Columbia P&S 1968; **Resid:** Diagnostic Radiology, Columbia-Presby 1974

Toth, Patrick J MD (DR) - **Spec Exp:** Abdominal Imaging; Thoracic Imaging; Interventional Radiology; Nuclear Radiology; **Hospital:** Hackensack Univ Med Ctr (page 96); **Address:** Hackensack Univ Med Ctr, Dept Radiology, 30 Prospect Ave, Hackensack, NJ 07601; **Phone:** 201-996-2194; **Board Cert:** Diagnostic Radiology 1988; **Med School:** Yale Univ 1982; **Resid:** Surgery, Yale-New Haven Hosp 1984; Diagnostic Radiology, NYU Med Ctr 1987; **Fellow:** Abdominal Imaging, NYU Med Ctr 1988; Interventional Radiology, NYU Med Ctr 1989; **Fac Appt:** Asst Clin Prof Rad, NYU Sch Med

Endocrinology, Diabetes & Metabolism

Cobin, Rhoda H MD (EDM) - **Spec Exp:** Thyroid Disorders; Diabetes; Pituitary Disorders; **Hospital:** Valley Hosp (page 689), Mount Sinai Med Ctr (page 102); **Address:** 75 N Maple Ave, Ste 202, Ridgewood, NJ 07450; **Phone:** 201-444-5552; **Board Cert:** Internal Medicine 1972; Endocrinology, Diabetes & Metabolism 1975; **Med School:** Univ Puerto Rico 1969; **Resid:** Internal Medicine, Beth Israel Med Ctr 1972; **Fellow:** Endocrinology, Diabetes & Metabolism, Mt Sinai Hosp 1974; **Fac Appt:** Clin Prof Med, Mount Sinai Sch Med

Daud-Ahmad, Sameera MD (EDM) - **Spec Exp:** Polycystic Ovarian Syndrome; Metabolic Syndrome; Hypogonadism; **Hospital:** Hackensack Univ Med Ctr (page 96), Valley Hosp (page 689); **Address:** Old Hook Medical Assocs, 452 Old Hook Rd, Emerson, NJ 07630; **Phone:** 201-666-3900; **Board Cert:** Internal Medicine 2007; Endocrinology, Diabetes & Metabolism 2009; **Med School:** Pakistan 2002; **Resid:** Internal Medicine, Loma Linda Univ Med Ctr 2006; Internal Medicine, Overlook Hosp 2007; **Fellow:** Endocrinology, Cleveland Clin 2009

Goldman, Michael MD (EDM) - **Spec Exp:** Thyroid Disorders; Diabetes; Pituitary Disorders; Cholesterol/Lipid Disorders; **Hospital:** Englewood Hosp & Med Ctr; **Address:** 600 E Palisade Ave, Ste 1, Englewood Cliffs, NJ 07632-1826; **Phone:** 201-568-1108; **Board Cert:** Internal Medicine 1980; Endocrinology, Diabetes & Metabolism 1981; **Med School:** NY Med Coll 1973; **Resid:** Internal Medicine, Englewood Hosp 1978; **Fellow:** Endocrinology, Diabetes & Metabolism, Columbia-Presby Med Ctr 1980; **Fac Appt:** Asst Prof Med, Mount Sinai Sch Med

Hochstein, Martin MD (EDM) - **Spec Exp:** Thyroid Disorders; Thyroid Cancer; Diabetes; Osteoporosis; **Hospital:** Valley Hosp (page 689); **Address:** 1 W Ridgewood Ave, Ste 301, Paramus, NJ 07652; **Phone:** 201-261-2560; **Board Cert:** Internal Medicine 1973; Endocrinology, Diabetes & Metabolism 1975; **Med School:** Univ Louisville Sch Med 1969; **Resid:** Internal Medicine, Maimoides Med Ctr 1971; Internal Medicine, Jacobi Med Ctr 1972; **Fellow:** Endocrinology, Diabetes & Metabolism, Johns Hopkins Med Ctr 1975; **Fac Appt:** Assoc Clin Prof Med, UMDNJ-RW Johnson Med Sch

Schwartz, Joseph J MD (EDM) - **Hospital:** Holy Name Med Ctr (page 688), Englewood Hosp & Med Ctr; **Address:** 229 Engle St, Englewood, NJ 07631; **Phone:** 201-567-3674; **Board Cert:** Internal Medicine 2001; Endocrinology, Diabetes & Metabolism 2003; **Med School:** Albert Einstein Coll Med 1998; **Resid:** Internal Medicine, LIJ Med Ctr 2001; **Fellow:** Endocrinology, Diabetes & Metabolism, Mt Sinai Med Ctr 2003

Tohme, Jack MD (EDM) - **Spec Exp:** Osteoporosis; Thyroid Disorders; Diabetes; **Hospital:** Valley Hosp (page 689); **Address:** 265 Ackerman Ave, Ste 101, Ridgewood, NJ 07450-4203; **Phone:** 201-444-4363; **Board Cert:** Internal Medicine 1978; Endocrinology, Diabetes & Metabolism 1979; **Med School:** Amer Univ Beirut 1974; **Resid:** Internal Medicine, American Univ Hosp 1976; **Fellow:** Endocrinology, Diabetes & Metabolism, Columbia-Presby Med Ctr 1977; Endocrinology, Diabetes & Metabolism, Barnes Hosp/Wash Univ 1978; **Fac Appt:** Assoc Clin Prof Med, Columbia P&S

Wehmann, Robert MD/PhD (EDM) - **Spec Exp:** Diabetes; Thyroid Disorders; Pituitary Disorders; **Hospital:** Valley Hosp (page 689), Hackensack Univ Med Ctr (page 96); **Address:** 54 Orchard St, Hillsdale, NJ 07642; **Phone:** 201-666-1400; **Board Cert:** Internal Medicine 1977; Endocrinology 1979; **Med School:** Albany Med Coll 1974; **Resid:** Internal Medicine, VA Med Ctr 1976; **Fellow:** Endocrinology, Natl Inst Hlth 1979

Wiesen, Mark MD (EDM) - **Spec Exp:** Diabetes; Thyroid Disorders; Osteoporosis; **Hospital:** Hackensack Univ Med Ctr (page 96), Holy Name Med Ctr (page 688); **Address:** 870 Palisade Ave, Ste 203, Teaneck, NJ 07666; **Phone:** 201-836-5655; **Board Cert:** Internal Medicine 1978; Endocrinology, Diabetes & Metabolism 1981; **Med School:** Columbia P&S 1975; **Resid:** Internal Medicine, Brookdale Hosp 1978; **Fellow:** Endocrinology, Diabetes & Metabolism, Mt Sinai Hosp 1981; **Fac Appt:** Asst Clin Prof Med, UMDNJ-NJ Med Sch, Newark

Family Medicine

Bello, Mary R MD (FMed) *PCP* - **Spec Exp:** Geriatric Care; **Hospital:** Valley Hosp (page 689); **Address:** 400 Franklin Tpke, Ste 106, Mahwah, NJ 07430-3517; **Phone:** 201-327-3333; **Board Cert:** Family Medicine 2010; **Med School:** West Indies 1984; **Resid:** Family Medicine, St Joseph's Hosp 1987; **Fac Appt:** Asst Clin Prof FMed, UMDNJ-NJ Med Sch, Newark

Dombrowski, Mark MD (FMed) *PCP* - **Hospital:** Hackensack Univ Med Ctr (page 96), St. Joseph's Regl Med Ctr - Paterson; **Address:** Old Hook Medical Assocs, 452 Old Hook Rd, Emerson, NJ 07630; **Phone:** 201-666-3900; **Board Cert:** Family Medicine 2004; **Med School:** Italy 1988; **Resid:** Family Medicine, Seton Hall Univ Med Ctr 2002

Gross, Harvey MD (FMed) *PCP* - **Spec Exp:** Geriatric Medicine; Dementia; Myasthenia Gravis; **Hospital:** Englewood Hosp & Med Ctr, Holy Name Med Ctr (page 688); **Address:** 370 Grand Ave, Ste 102, Englewood, NJ 07631; **Phone:** 201-567-3370; **Board Cert:** Family Medicine 2005; Geriatric Medicine 2010; **Med School:** Boston Univ 1970; **Resid:** Family Medicine, Southside Hosp 1974; **Fac Appt:** Asst Clin Prof Med, Mount Sinai Sch Med

Karatoprak, Ohan MD (FMed) *PCP* - **Spec Exp:** Nutrition; Asthma; Obesity; Geriatric Medicine; **Hospital:** Holy Name Med Ctr (page 688); **Address:** 420 Deerwood Rd, Fort Lee, NJ 07024-1643; **Phone:** 201-886-8877; **Board Cert:** Family Medicine 2005; Geriatric Medicine 2003; **Med School:** Turkey 1977; **Resid:** Surgery, Brookdale Univ Hosp 1983; Family Medicine, Southside Hosp 1986; **Fac Appt:** Asst Clin Prof FMed, UMDNJ-NJ Med Sch, Newark

Leipsner, George MD (FMed) *PCP* - **Hospital:** Hackensack Univ Med Ctr (page 96); **Address:** 57 W Pleasant Ave, Maywood, NJ 07607-1334; **Phone:** 201-488-2111; **Board Cert:** Family Medicine 2001; **Med School:** Italy 1966; **Resid:** Family Medicine, Hackensack Hosp 1968; **Fac Appt:** Asst Clin Prof FMed, UMDNJ-Rutgers Med Sch

Gastroenterology

Broussard, Crystal N MD (Ge) - **Spec Exp:** Liver Disease; Hepatitis; **Hospital:** Valley Hosp (page 689); **Address:** Bergen Gastroenterology, 466 Old Hook Rd, Ste 1, Emerson, NJ 07630; **Phone:** 201-967-8221; **Board Cert:** Internal Medicine 2008; Gastroenterology 2009; **Med School:** Case West Res Univ 1992; **Resid:** Internal Medicine, Johns Hopkins Bayview Med Ctr 1995; **Fellow:** Gastroenterology, Cleveland Clinic 1997

Chessler, Richard K MD (Ge) - **Spec Exp:** Pancreatic Cancer; Endoscopy; Pancreatic/Biliary Endoscopy (ERCP); Colonoscopy; **Hospital:** Englewood Hosp & Med Ctr, Hackensack Univ Med Ctr (page 96); **Address:** 140 Sylvan Ave, Fl 1, Ste 101, rm 1, Englewood Cliffs, NJ 07632-2554; **Phone:** 201-945-6564 x320; **Board Cert:** Internal Medicine 1972; Gastroenterology 1975; **Med School:** Ros Franklin Univ/Chicago Med Sch 1969; **Resid:** Internal Medicine, NY Med Coll/Flower-Fifth Ave Hosp 1972; **Fellow:** Gastroenterology, NY Med Coll/Flower-Fifth Ave Hosp 1974; **Fac Appt:** Asst Clin Prof Med, Mount Sinai Sch Med

Fried, Harry A MD (Ge) - **Hospital:** Englewood Hosp & Med Ctr; **Address:** 333 Old Hook Rd, Ste 101, Westwood, NJ 07675; **Phone:** 201-594-0535; **Board Cert:** Internal Medicine 1989; Gastroenterology 2005; **Med School:** SUNY Downstate 1986; **Resid:** Internal Medicine, St Lukes Hosp 1989; **Fellow:** Gastroenterology, Cooper Hosp 1995

Friedrich, Ivan MD (Ge) - **Spec Exp:** Colonoscopy; Inflammatory Bowel Disease; Constipation; Diarrheal Diseases; **Hospital:** Englewood Hosp & Med Ctr, Holy Name Med Ctr (page 688); **Address:** 420 Grand Ave, Englewood, NJ 07631-4152; **Phone:** 201-569-7044; **Board Cert:** Internal Medicine 1979; Gastroenterology 1981; **Med School:** Albany Med Coll 1976; **Resid:** Internal Medicine, Montefiore Med Ctr 1979; **Fellow:** Gastroenterology, Mt Sinai Med Ctr 1982; **Fac Appt:** Asst Clin Prof Med, Mount Sinai Sch Med

Goldfarb, Joel A MD (Ge) - **Spec Exp:** Colonoscopy/Polypectomy; Colon Cancer; Hepatitis; Liver Disease; **Hospital:** Holy Name Med Ctr (page 688), Englewood Hosp & Med Ctr; **Address:** 1086 Teaneck Rd, Ste 4C, Teaneck, NJ 07666; **Phone:** 201-837-9449; **Board Cert:** Internal Medicine 1978; Gastroenterology 1981; **Med School:** NYU Sch Med 1975; **Resid:** Internal Medicine, NYU Med Ctr 1978; Hepatology, Yale-New Haven Hosp 1979; **Fellow:** Gastroenterology, Columbia-Presby Med Ctr 1981; **Fac Appt:** Asst Clin Prof Med, Mount Sinai Sch Med

Klein, Walter A MD (Ge) - **Spec Exp:** Esophageal Disorders; Gastroesophageal Reflux Disease (GERD); Colon Polyps & Cancer; **Hospital:** Englewood Hosp & Med Ctr; **Address:** The Park Medical Group, 274 County Rd, Ste A, Tenafly, NJ 07670; **Phone:** 201-568-0493; **Board Cert:** Internal Medicine 2010; Gastroenterology 2000; **Med School:** Cornell Univ-Weill Med Coll 1987; **Resid:** Internal Medicine, NY Hosp-Cornell Med Ctr 1990; **Fellow:** Gastroenterology, Temple Univ Hosp 1992; **Fac Appt:** Asst Clin Prof Med, Mount Sinai Sch Med

Margulis, Stephen MD (Ge) - **Spec Exp:** Hepatitis; Colonoscopy/Polypectomy; Peptic Ulcer Disease; Inflammatory Bowel Disease; **Hospital:** Valley Hosp (page 689); **Address:** 466 Old Hook Rd, Ste 1, Emerson, NJ 07630-1368; **Phone:** 201-967-8221; **Board Cert:** Internal Medicine 1984; Gastroenterology 1987; **Med School:** Brown Univ 1981; **Resid:** Internal Medicine, New York Hosp-Cornell 1984; **Fellow:** Gastroenterology, New York Hosp-Cornell 1987

Nikias, George A MD (Ge) - **Spec Exp:** Hepatitis; Liver Disease; **Hospital:** Hackensack Univ Med Ctr (page 96); **Address:** 130 Kinderkamack Rd, Ste 301, River Edge, NJ 07661; **Phone:** 201-489-7772; **Board Cert:** Internal Medicine 2002; Gastroenterology 2005; **Med School:** NY Med Coll 1989; **Resid:** Internal Medicine, North Shore Univ Hosp 1992; **Fellow:** Gastroenterology, Meml Sloan-Kettering Cancer Ctr 1995; Hepatology, Mayo Clin 1993; **Fac Appt:** Asst Clin Prof Med, UMDNJ-NJ Med Sch, Newark

Panella, Vincent S MD (Ge) - **Spec Exp:** Colon & Rectal Cancer; Hepatitis C; Inflammatory Bowel Disease; Endoscopy; **Hospital:** Englewood Hosp & Med Ctr, Holy Name Med Ctr (page 688); **Address:** Englewood Endoscopic Associates, 420 Grand Ave, Englewood, NJ 07631-4141; **Phone:** 201-569-7044; **Board Cert:** Internal Medicine 1985; Gastroenterology 1987; **Med School:** NY Med Coll 1982; **Resid:** Internal Medicine, North Shore Univ Hosp 1985; **Fellow:** Gastroenterology, Mem Sloan-Kettering Cancer Cntr 1987; **Fac Appt:** Asst Clin Prof Med, Mount Sinai Sch Med

Rahmin, Michael G MD (Ge) - **Spec Exp:** Endoscopy; Hepatitis; **Hospital:** Valley Hosp (page 689); **Address:** 140 Chestnut St, Ste 300, Ridgewood, NJ 07452; **Phone:** 201-444-2600; **Board Cert:** Internal Medicine 2002; Gastroenterology 2005; **Med School:** NYU Sch Med 1989; **Resid:** Internal Medicine, Mt Sinai Hosp 1992; **Fellow:** Gastroenterology, New York Hosp 1995; Hepatology, Mt Sinai Hosp 1995

Roth, Joseph MD (Ge) - **Spec Exp:** Endoscopy; Inflammatory Bowel Disease; **Hospital:** St. Mary's Hosp - Passaic, St. Joseph's Regl Med Ctr - Paterson; **Address:** 71 Union Ave, Rutherford, NJ 07070-1272; **Phone:** 201-842-0020; **Board Cert:** Internal Medicine 1984; Gastroenterology 1987; **Med School:** Univ Pittsburgh 1981; **Resid:** Internal Medicine, Lenox Hill Hosp 1984; **Fellow:** Gastroenterology, Univ Conn Hlth Ctr 1986

Rubin, Kenneth MD (Ge) - **Spec Exp:** Gastroesophageal Reflux Disease (GERD); Endoscopy; Inflammatory Bowel Disease; Colon Cancer; **Hospital:** Englewood Hosp & Med Ctr, Mount Sinai Med Ctr (page 102); **Address:** 420 Grand Ave, Englewood, NJ 07631-4152; **Phone:** 201-569-7044; **Board Cert:** Internal Medicine 1978; Gastroenterology 1981; **Med School:** UMDNJ-NJ Med Sch, Newark 1975; **Resid:** Internal Medicine, Bronx Muni Hosp 1979; **Fellow:** Gastroenterology, Mount Sinai Hosp 1981; **Fac Appt:** Asst Clin Prof Med, Mount Sinai Sch Med

Rubinoff, Mitchell J MD (Ge) - **Spec Exp:** Hepatitis; Gastroesophageal Reflux Disease (GERD); **Hospital:** Valley Hosp (page 689); **Address:** 140 Chestnut St, Ste 300, Ridgewood, NJ 07450-2536; **Phone:** 201-444-2600; **Board Cert:** Internal Medicine 1982; Gastroenterology 1985; **Med School:** Mount Sinai Sch Med 1979; **Resid:** Internal Medicine, Columbia-Presby Med Ctr 1982; **Fellow:** Gastroenterology, Columbia-Presby Med Ctr 1985

Zingler, Barry M MD (Ge) - **Spec Exp:** Colon Cancer; Hepatitis; Gastroesophageal Reflux Disease (GERD); **Hospital:** Englewood Hosp & Med Ctr, Holy Name Med Ctr (page 688); **Address:** 140 Sylvan Ave, Englewood Cliffs, NJ 07632; **Phone:** 201-945-6564; **Board Cert:** Internal Medicine 1988; Gastroenterology 2011; **Med School:** UMDNJ-Rutgers Med Sch 1985; **Resid:** Internal Medicine, NYU Med Ctr 1988; **Fellow:** Gastroenterology, NYU Med Ctr 1990

Zucker, Ira I MD (Ge) - **Spec Exp:** Colon Cancer; Gastroesophageal Reflux Disease (GERD); Ulcerative Colitis/Crohn's; Hepatitis; **Hospital:** Valley Hosp (page 689), Hackensack Univ Med Ctr (page 96); **Address:** 452 Old Hook Rd, Emerson, NJ 07630; **Phone:** 201-666-3900; **Board Cert:** Internal Medicine 1984; Gastroenterology 1987; **Med School:** Ros Franklin Univ/Chicago Med Sch 1981; **Resid:** Internal Medicine, St Vincents Hosp 1984; **Fellow:** Gastroenterology, St Vincents Hosp 1986

Geriatric Medicine

Chavez, Laura M DO (Ger) - **Spec Exp:** Alzheimer's Disease; **Hospital:** Holy Name Med Ctr (page 688), Hackensack Univ Med Ctr (page 96); **Address:** IMA of Bergen County, 15 Anderson St, Hackensack, NJ 07601; **Phone:** 201-487-3355; **Board Cert:** Internal Medicine 2011; Geriatric Medicine 2004; **Med School:** NY Coll Osteo Med 1998; **Resid:** Internal Medicine, UMDNJ Univ Hosp 2001; **Fellow:** Geriatric Medicine, UMDNJ Univ Hosp 2002

Leifer, Bennett MD (Ger) *PCP* - **Spec Exp:** Dementia; Alzheimer's Disease; **Hospital:** Valley Hosp (page 689); **Address:** 301 Godwin Ave, Midland Park, NJ 07432-1544; **Phone:** 201-444-4526; **Board Cert:** Internal Medicine 2011; Geriatric Medicine 2000; **Med School:** SUNY Upstate Med Univ 1986; **Resid:** Internal Medicine, Hartford Hosp 1989; **Fellow:** Geriatric Medicine, Mt Sinai Hosp 1991

Tank, Lisa K MD (Ger) *PCP* - **Spec Exp:** Cancer in the Elderly; **Hospital:** Hackensack Univ Med Ctr (page 96); **Address:** HUMC Div Geriatric Med, 360 Essex St, Ste 401, Hackensack, NJ 07601; **Phone:** 551-996-1140; **Board Cert:** Internal Medicine 2011; Geriatric Medicine 2003; **Med School:** India 1996; **Resid:** Internal Medicine, NY Methodist Hosp 2001; **Fellow:** Geriatric Medicine, Hackensack Univ Med Ctr 2003

Villongco, Raymond M MD (Ger) - **Spec Exp:** Diabetes; Hypertension; **Hospital:** Mount Sinai Med Ctr (page 102), Holy Name Med Ctr (page 688); **Address:** Salus Medical, 121 Cedar Ln, Ste 2B, Teaneck, NJ 07666; **Phone:** 201-836-4228; **Board Cert:** Internal Medicine 2004; **Med School:** Philippines 1989; **Resid:** Internal Medicine, Jersey City Med Ctr 1994; **Fellow:** Geriatric Medicine, Mt Sinai Med Ctr 1996; **Fac Appt:** Asst Clin Prof Hospice & Palliative Med, Mount Sinai Sch Med

Gynecologic Oncology

Sommers, Gara M MD (GO) - **Spec Exp:** Gynecologic Cancer; **Hospital:** Holy Name Med Ctr (page 688), Newark Beth Israel Med Ctr; **Address:** Holy Name Hosp, Clinical Research Dept, 718 Teaneck Rd, Teaneck, NJ 07666; **Phone:** 201-792-9011; **Board Cert:** Obstetrics & Gynecology 2011; Gynecologic Oncology 2011; **Med School:** NYU Sch Med 1981; **Resid:** Obstetrics & Gynecology, NYU Med Ctr 1985; **Fellow:** Gynecologic Oncology, Barnes Jewish Hosp 1988; Research, Beckman Inst-City of Hope 1988; **Fac Appt:** Asst Clin Prof ObG, Albert Einstein Coll Med

Hand Surgery

Fakharzadeh, Frederick F MD (HS) - **Hospital:** Hackensack Univ Med Ctr (page 96), Valley Hosp (page 689); **Address:** 22 Madison Ave, FL 3, Paramus, NJ 07652-2721; **Phone:** 201-587-7767; **Board Cert:** Orthopaedic Surgery 2009; Hand Surgery 2009; **Med School:** Columbia P&S 1980; **Resid:** Surgery, Roosevelt Hosp 1982; Orthopaedic Surgery, Columbia-Presby Med Ctr 1985; **Fellow:** Hand Surgery, Thomas Jefferson Univ Hosp 1986

Gurland, Mark MD (HS) - **Spec Exp:** Carpal Tunnel Syndrome; Wrist/Hand Injuries; Arthritis Hand Surgery; **Hospital:** Hackensack Univ Med Ctr (page 96), Englewood Hosp & Med Ctr; **Address:** 216 Engle St, Englewood, NJ 07631-2448; **Phone:** 201-568-4066; **Board Cert:** Orthopaedic Surgery 2009; Hand Surgery 2009; **Med School:** NYU Sch Med 1979; **Resid:** Surgery, Hosp Univ Penn 1980; Orthopaedic Surgery, Hosp for Joint Diseases 1984; **Fellow:** Hand Surgery, Thomas Jefferson Univ Hosp

Miller-Breslow, Anne J MD (HS) - **Spec Exp:** Rheumatoid Arthritis; Wrist/Hand Injuries; Arthroscopic Surgery; Fractures; **Hospital:** Englewood Hosp & Med Ctr; **Address:** 401 S Van Brunt St Fl 3, Englewood, NJ 07631-2904; **Phone:** 201-569-2770; **Board Cert:** Orthopaedic Surgery 2012; Hand Surgery 2012; **Med School:** Harvard Med Sch 1983; **Resid:** Orthopaedic Surgery, Montefiore Med Ctr 1988; **Fellow:** Hand Surgery, New England Med Ctr 1989

Rosenstein, Roger G MD (HS) - **Spec Exp:** Arthritis Hand Surgery; Nerve Compression; Carpal Tunnel Syndrome; **Hospital:** Valley Hosp (page 689), Hackensack Univ Med Ctr (page 96); **Address:** 22 Madison Ave, Ste 301, Paramus, NJ 07652-5474; **Phone:** 201-587-7767; **Board Cert:** Orthopaedic Surgery 1984; Hand Surgery 2010; **Med School:** Columbia P&S 1975; **Resid:** Surgery, St Luke's Roosevelt Hosp Ctr 1977; Orthopaedic Surgery, Columbia-Presby Med Ctr 1980; **Fellow:** Hand Surgery, Thomas Jefferson Univ Hosp 1981; **Fac Appt:** Assoc Clin Prof OrS, UMDNJ-NJ Med Sch, Newark

Hematology

Fernbach, Barry R MD (Hem) - **Hospital:** Valley Hosp (page 689); **Address:** 1 Valley Health Plaza, Paramus, NJ 07652; **Phone:** 201-634-5353; **Board Cert:** Internal Medicine 1974; Medical Oncology 1977; Hematology 1982; **Med School:** Harvard Med Sch 1971; **Resid:** Internal Medicine, Mt Sinai Hosp 1973; Hematology, Mt Sinai Hosp 1976; **Fellow:** Neoplastic Diseases, Mt Sinai Hosp 1977

Israel, Alan M MD (Hem) - **Hospital:** Valley Hosp (page 689); **Address:** 270 Old Hook Rd, Westwood, NJ 07675-3102; **Phone:** 201-666-4949; **Board Cert:** Internal Medicine 1982; Medical Oncology 1985; Hematology 1986; **Med School:** NYU Sch Med 1979; **Resid:** Internal Medicine, Mt Sinai Hosp 1982; **Fellow:** Hematology & Oncology, Meml Sloan Kettering Cancer Ctr 1984; Hematology, LI Jewish Hosp 1985

Rowley, Scott D MD (Hem) - **Spec Exp:** Stem Cell Transplant; Bone Marrow Transplant; Graft vs Host Disease; **Hospital:** Hackensack Univ Med Ctr (page 96); **Address:** 92 2nd St, Ste 230, Hackensack, NJ 07601; **Phone:** 201-336-8289 x8291; **Board Cert:** Internal Medicine 1981; Medical Oncology 1983; Hematology 1984; **Med School:** Univ Mass Sch Med 1978; **Resid:** Internal Medicine, Rhode Island Hosp 1981; **Fellow:** Hematology & Oncology, Rhode Island Hosp 1984; **Fac Appt:** Assoc Prof Med, UMDNJ-NJ Med Sch, Newark

Vesole, David H MD/PhD (Hem) - **Spec Exp:** Multiple Myeloma; Stem Cell Transplant; Amyloidosis; Waldenstrom's Macroglobulinemia; **Hospital:** Hackensack Univ Med Ctr (page 96); **Address:** 92 Second St, Hackensack, NJ 07601; **Phone:** 551-996-8704; **Board Cert:** Internal Medicine 1987; Hematology 2000; **Med School:** Northwestern Univ 1984; **Resid:** Internal Medicine, Univ Iowa Hosp 1987; **Fellow:** Hematology & Oncology, Univ Iowa Hosp 1990; **Fac Appt:** Prof Med, UMDNJ-NJ Med Sch, Newark

Infectious Disease

Birch, Thomas MD (Inf) - **Spec Exp:** AIDS/HIV; Lyme Disease; West Nile Virus; Antibiotic Resistance; **Hospital:** Holy Name Med Ctr (page 688), Englewood Hosp & Med Ctr; **Address:** Birch Tree Med Assocs, 718 Teaneck Rd, Teaneck, NJ 07666; **Phone:** 201-833-7274; **Board Cert:** Internal Medicine 1986; Infectious Disease 2004; **Med School:** Univ Wisc 1983; **Resid:** Internal Medicine, Montefiore Med Ctr 1986; **Fellow:** Infectious Disease, Montefiore Med Ctr 1993

Cicogna, Cristina E MD (Inf) - **Spec Exp:** Infections in Immunocompromised Patients; Hospital Acquired Infections; **Hospital:** Hackensack Univ Med Ctr (page 96); **Address:** 20 Prospect Ave Fl 5 - Ste 507, Hackensack, NJ 07601; **Phone:** 201-487-4088; **Board Cert:** Internal Medicine 2002; Infectious Disease 2004; **Med School:** Switzerland 1986; **Resid:** Internal Medicine, St Luke's-Roosevelt Hosp 1989; **Fellow:** Infectious Disease, Meml Sloan-Kettering Cancer Ctr 1991; **Fac Appt:** Asst Prof Med, UMDNJ-RW Johnson Med Sch

Desai, Amita J MD (Inf) - **Spec Exp:** Infections in Transplant Patients; Tropical Diseases; Tuberculosis; **Hospital:** Holy Name Med Ctr (page 688); **Address:** Birch Tree Med/Inst for Clin Rsch, 718 Teaneck Rd, Teaneck, NJ 07666; **Phone:** 201-541-6315; **Board Cert:** Internal Medicine 1987; Infectious Disease 2004; **Med School:** NY Med Coll 1983; **Resid:** Internal Medicine, Montefiore Med Ctr 1986; **Fellow:** Infectious Disease, Mount Sinai Med Ctr 1994

Knackmuhs, Gary G MD (Inf) - **Spec Exp:** Travel Medicine; **Hospital:** Valley Hosp (page 689); **Address:** 947 Lynwood Ave, Ste 2E, Ridgewood, NJ 07450-4407; **Phone:** 201-447-6468; **Board Cert:** Internal Medicine 1979; Infectious Disease 1982; **Med School:** NY Med Coll 1976; **Resid:** Internal Medicine, Mt Sinai Hosp 1979; **Fellow:** Infectious Disease, Montefiore Med Ctr 1981

Kocher, Jeffrey MD (Inf) - **Spec Exp:** Hepatitis B & C; AIDS/HIV; Fungal Infections; Lyme Disease; **Hospital:** Englewood Hosp & Med Ctr; **Address:** 25 Rockwood Pl, Ste 120, Englewood, NJ 07631-4957; **Phone:** 201-568-3335; **Board Cert:** Internal Medicine 1983; Infectious Disease 1986; **Med School:** Cornell Univ-Weill Med Coll 1980; **Resid:** Internal Medicine, New York Hosp 1983; Internal Medicine, St Barnabas Hosp 1984; **Fellow:** Infectious Disease, New York Hosp 1986; **Fac Appt:** Assoc Clin Prof Med, Mount Sinai Sch Med

Weisholtz, Steven J MD (Inf) - **Spec Exp:** AIDS/HIV; Antibiotic Resistance; Travel Medicine; **Hospital:** Englewood Hosp & Med Ctr; **Address:** 25 Rockwood Pl, Ste 120, Englewood, NJ 07631-4957; **Phone:** 201-568-3335; **Board Cert:** Internal Medicine 1981; Infectious Disease 1984; **Med School:** Univ Pennsylvania 1978; **Resid:** Internal Medicine, New York Hosp 1981; **Fellow:** Infectious Disease, New York Hosp 1983; **Fac Appt:** Asst Clin Prof Med, Mount Sinai Sch Med

Internal Medicine

Brunnquell, Stephen MD (IM) *PCP* - **Hospital:** Englewood Hosp & Med Ctr; **Address:** 24 Elm St, Harrington Park, NJ 07640-1902; **Phone:** 201-784-0123; **Board Cert:** Internal Medicine 2002; **Med School:** UMDNJ-NJ Med Sch, Newark 1989; **Resid:** Internal Medicine, Montefiore Med Ctr 1992; **Fac Appt:** Asst Clin Prof Med, Mount Sinai Sch Med

Cacciola, Thomas A MD (IM) *PCP* - **Spec Exp:** Preventive Medicine; Complementary Medicine; **Hospital:** Hackensack Univ Med Ctr (page 96); **Address:** 403 N Farview Ave, Paramus, NJ 07652-4618; **Phone:** 201-261-8386; **Board Cert:** Internal Medicine 1988; **Med School:** Jefferson Med Coll 1983; **Resid:** Internal Medicine, Hackensack Med Ctr 1986; **Fellow:** US Public Hlth Svc 1988

Kushner, Evan G MD (IM) *PCP* - **Spec Exp:** Geriatric Medicine; **Hospital:** Hackensack Univ Med Ctr (page 96), Valley Hosp (page 689); **Address:** Forest Hlthcare Assocs, 277 Forest Ave, Ste 200, Paramus, NJ 07652; **Phone:** 201-986-1881; **Board Cert:** Internal Medicine 1989; Geriatric Medicine 2005; **Med School:** SUNY Upstate Med Univ 1986; **Resid:** Internal Medicine, Univ Hosp 1989

Lan, Vivian E MD (IM) *PCP* - **Spec Exp:** Women's Health; Eating Disorders; **Hospital:** Valley Hosp (page 689); **Address:** 466 Old Hook Rd, Ste 1, Emerson, NJ 07630; **Phone:** 201-967-8221; **Board Cert:** Internal Medicine 2007; **Med School:** Mount Sinai Sch Med 1994; **Resid:** Internal Medicine, Mt Sinai Med Ctr 1997

Lauricella, Joseph MD (IM) *PCP* - **Spec Exp:** Coronary Artery Disease; **Hospital:** Holy Name Med Ctr (page 688); **Address:** 292 Columbia Ave, Fort Lee, NJ 07024-4124; **Phone:** 201-224-0050; **Board Cert:** Internal Medicine 1985; **Med School:** Mexico 1978; **Resid:** Internal Medicine, Rutgers Univ Med Ctr 1985

Miguel, Eduardo E MD (IM) *PCP* - **Spec Exp:** Rheumatoid Arthritis; **Hospital:** Englewood Hosp & Med Ctr; **Address:** 200 Grand Ave, Ste 202, Englewood, NJ 07631; **Phone:** 201-871-3280; **Board Cert:** Internal Medicine 1982; **Med School:** Paraguay 1966; **Resid:** Internal Medicine, VA Med Ctr 1969; Internal Medicine, NY Polyclinic Hosp 1972; **Fellow:** Rheumatology, Albert Einstein Med Ctr 1973

Pelavin, Martin MD (IM) *PCP* - **Hospital:** Valley Hosp (page 689), Englewood Hosp & Med Ctr; **Address:** 215 Old Tappan Rd, Old Tappan, NJ 07675-7428; **Phone:** 201-666-1000; **Board Cert:** Internal Medicine 1976; **Med School:** NYU Sch Med 1973; **Resid:** Internal Medicine, Montefiore Hosp Med Ctr 1976

Schuster, Joseph C MD (IM) *PCP* - **Hospital:** Holy Name Med Ctr (page 688), Hackensack Univ Med Ctr (page 96); **Address:** 175 Cedar Ln, Teaneck, NJ 07666-4315; **Phone:** 201-692-7766; **Board Cert:** Internal Medicine 1984; **Med School:** Albany Med Coll 1981; **Resid:** Internal Medicine, St Luke's-Roosevelt Hosp Ctr 1982; Internal Medicine, Kings County Hosp 1984

Scibetta, Maria MD (IM) *PCP* - **Hospital:** Valley Hosp (page 689); **Address:** 470 N Franklin Tpke, Ramsey, NJ 07446-2034; **Phone:** 201-327-8765; **Board Cert:** Internal Medicine 2003; **Med School:** UMDNJ-RW Johnson Med Sch 1990; **Resid:** Internal Medicine, Mount Sinai Hosp 1993

Valinoti, Anne Marie MD (IM) - **Spec Exp:** Women's Health; **Hospital:** Valley Hosp (page 689); **Address:** 301 Godwin Avenue, Midland Park, NJ 07432; **Phone:** 201-444-4526; **Board Cert:** Internal Medicine 2004; **Med School:** Columbia P&S 1991; **Resid:** Internal Medicine, New York Hosp 1994

Volpe, Anthony P MD (IM) *PCP* - **Spec Exp:** Hypertension; **Hospital:** Valley Hosp (page 689); **Address:** 466 Old Hook Rd, Ste 14, Emerson, NJ 07630-1368; **Phone:** 201-262-6485; **Board Cert:** Internal Medicine 2005; **Med School:** Mexico 1981; **Resid:** Internal Medicine, Texas Tech Hlth Scis Ctr 1986

Wasserman, Kenneth H MD (IM) *PCP* - **Hospital:** Englewood Hosp & Med Ctr, Holy Name Med Ctr (page 688); **Address:** 177 N Dean St Fl 1, Englewood, NJ 07631; **Phone:** 201-567-1140 x10; **Board Cert:** Internal Medicine 1982; **Med School:** Albert Einstein Coll Med 1979; **Resid:** Internal Medicine, Lenox Hill Hosp 1982

Interventional Cardiology

Angeli, Stephen J MD (IC) - **Spec Exp:** Angioplasty & Stent Placement; Cardiac Catheterization; Coronary Artery Disease; **Hospital:** Holy Name Med Ctr (page 688); **Address:** Cardiovascular Assocs of Teaneck, 954 Teaneck Rd, Teaneck, NJ 07666; **Phone:** 201-833-2300; **Board Cert:** Internal Medicine 1984; Cardiovascular Disease 1987; Interventional Cardiology 2009; **Med School:** SUNY Downstate 1981; **Resid:** Internal Medicine, Kings Co Hosp 1984; **Fellow:** Cardiovascular Disease, St Michael Med Ctr 1986

Syed, Tariqshah M MD (IC) - **Spec Exp:** Cardiac Cathetherization; Angiography-Coronary; Angioplasty & Stent Placement; **Hospital:** Hackensack Univ Med Ctr (page 96), Holy Name Med Ctr (page 688); **Address:** Cardiovascular Assocs of Teaneck, 954 Teaneck Rd, Teaneck, NJ 07666; **Phone:** 201-833-2300; **Board Cert:** Internal Medicine 2004; Cardiovascular Disease 2007; Interventional Cardiology 2008; **Med School:** Pakistan 1999; **Resid:** Internal Medicine, St. Luke's Roosevelt Hosp Ctr 2004; **Fellow:** Cardiovascular Disease, Mt. Sinai Hosp 2007; Interventional Cardiology, St. Luke's Roosevelt Hosp Ctr 2008

Maternal & Fetal Medicine

Alvarez, Manuel MD (MF) - **Spec Exp:** Multiple Gestation; Pregnancy-High Risk; **Hospital:** Hackensack Univ Med Ctr (page 96), NYU Langone Med Ctr (page 108); **Address:** 20 Prospect Ave, Ste 601, Hackensack, NJ 07601; **Phone:** 201-996-2765; **Board Cert:** Obstetrics & Gynecology 2011; Maternal & Fetal Medicine 2011; **Med School:** Dominican Republic 1981; **Resid:** Obstetrics & Gynecology, St Joseph Hosp 1987; **Fellow:** Maternal & Fetal Medicine, Mount Sinai Med Ctr 1989; Critical Care Obstetrics, Mount Sinai Med Ctr 1990

Frieden, Faith MD (MF) - **Spec Exp:** Prenatal Ultrasound; Prenatal Diagnosis; **Hospital:** Englewood Hosp & Med Ctr; **Address:** 350 Engle St, Englewood, NJ 07631-1808; **Phone:** 201-894-3669; **Board Cert:** Obstetrics & Gynecology 2011; Maternal & Fetal Medicine 2011; **Med School:** Mount Sinai Sch Med 1984; **Resid:** Obstetrics & Gynecology, Beth Israel Med Ctr 1988; **Fellow:** Maternal & Fetal Medicine, Bellevue Hosp 1990; **Fac Appt:** Asst Clin Prof ObG, Mount Sinai Sch Med

Principe, David L MD (MF) - **Spec Exp:** Pregnancy-High Risk; **Hospital:** St. Joseph's Regl Med Ctr - Paterson, Palisades Med Ctr; **Address:** St Joseph's Perinatal Ctr, 1 Broadway, Ste 203, Elmwood Park, NJ 07407; **Phone:** 973-569-6264; **Board Cert:** Obstetrics & Gynecology 2011; Maternal & Fetal Medicine 2011; **Med School:** Grenada 1991; **Resid:** Obstetrics & Gynecology, St Joseph Hosp 1995; **Fellow:** Maternal & Fetal Medicine, Univ Chicago/Chicago Lying in Hosp 1997; Maternal & Fetal Medicine, Yale New Haven Hosp 1998

Medical Oncology

Attas, Lewis MD (Onc) - **Spec Exp:** Breast Cancer; Lymphoma; Bleeding/Coagulation Disorders; Gaucher Disease; **Hospital:** Englewood Hosp & Med Ctr, Holy Name Med Ctr (page 688); **Address:** 350 Engle St, Englewood, NJ 07631; **Phone:** 201-568-5250; **Board Cert:** Internal Medicine 1985; Medical Oncology 1987; Hematology 1988; **Med School:** Mount Sinai Sch Med 1982; **Resid:** Internal Medicine, Montefiore Hosp Med Ctr 1985; **Fellow:** Hematology & Oncology, North Shore Univ Hosp 1988; **Fac Appt:** Assoc Clin Prof Med, Mount Sinai Sch Med

Condemi, Giuseppe MD (Onc) - **Spec Exp:** Breast Cancer; Prostate Cancer; Colon Cancer; **Address:** Regi Cancer Ctr, 718 Teaneck Rd, Teaneck, NJ 07666; **Phone:** 201-227-6008; **Board Cert:** Internal Medicine 2003; Medical Oncology 2005; **Med School:** Dominica 1998; **Resid:** Internal Medicine, Mt. Sinai Sch Med 2001; **Fellow:** Hematology & Oncology, A Einstein Coll Med 2004

Forte, Francis A MD (Onc) - **Spec Exp:** Breast Cancer; Hematologic Malignancies; Coagulation/Bleeding Disorders; Solid Tumors; **Hospital:** Englewood Hosp & Med Ctr, Holy Name Med Ctr (page 688); **Address:** 350 Engle St Berrie Bldg Fl 1, Englewood, NJ 07631; **Phone:** 201-568-5250; **Board Cert:** Internal Medicine 1971; Hematology 1972; Medical Oncology 1973; **Med School:** Albert Einstein Coll Med 1964; **Resid:** Internal Medicine, Mount Sinai Hosp 1968; **Fellow:** Hematology, Mount Sinai Hosp 1969; **Fac Appt:** Asst Prof Med, Mount Sinai Sch Med

Goldberg, Stuart L MD (Onc) - **Spec Exp:** Leukemia; Stem Cell Transplant; Myelodysplastic Syndromes; **Hospital:** Hackensack Univ Med Ctr (page 96); **Address:** John Theurer Cancer Ctr, HUMC, 92 Second St, Hackensack, NJ 07601; **Phone:** 201-996-5900; **Board Cert:** Internal Medicine 1989; **Med School:** Penn State Coll Med 1986; **Resid:** Internal Medicine, G Washington Univ Hosp 1989; **Fellow:** Hematology & Oncology, G Washington Univ Hosp 1991; Bone Marrow Transplant, Mayo Clin 1992; **Fac Appt:** Assoc Clin Prof Med, UMDNJ-NJ Med Sch, Newark

Goy, Andre MD (Onc) - **Spec Exp:** Lymphoma; Hodgkin's Lymphoma; **Hospital:** Hackensack Univ Med Ctr (page 96); **Address:** 92 2nd St, Hackensack, NJ 07601; **Phone:** 201-996-5900; **Med School:** France 1988; **Resid:** Internal Medicine, Grenoble Univ Med Ctr 1992; **Fellow:** Hematology & Oncology, Grenoble Univ Med Ctr 1993

Harper, Harry MD (Onc) - **Spec Exp:** Lung Cancer; **Hospital:** Hackensack Univ Med Ctr (page 96), Holy Name Med Ctr (page 688); **Address:** John Theurer Cancer Ctr, HUMC, 92 Second St, Hackensack, NJ 07601; **Phone:** 201-996-5900; **Board Cert:** Internal Medicine 1980; Hematology 1982; Medical Oncology 1983; **Med School:** Baylor Coll Med 1977; **Resid:** Internal Medicine, NY-Cornell Med Ctr 1980; **Fellow:** Hematology & Oncology, Meml Sloan-Kettering Cancer Ctr 1983

Jennis, Andrew MD (Onc) - **Spec Exp:** Gastrointestinal Cancer; **Hospital:** Hackensack Univ Med Ctr (page 96); **Address:** John Theurer Cancer Ctr, HUMC, 92 Second St, Hackensack, NJ 07601; **Phone:** 201-996-5900; **Board Cert:** Internal Medicine 1988; Hematology 2002; Medical Oncology 2011; **Med School:** Columbia P&S 1985; **Resid:** Internal Medicine, Mount Sinai Hosp 1988; **Fellow:** Hematology & Oncology, Beth Israel Hosp 1992

Krutchik, Allan MD (Onc) - **Spec Exp:** Breast Cancer; **Hospital:** St. Joseph's Wayne Hosp, Chilton Hosp; **Address:** John Theurer Cancer Ctr, Bldg C, 795 Franklin Ave, Franklin Lakes, NJ 07417; **Phone:** 201-848-8791; **Board Cert:** Internal Medicine 1976; Medical Oncology 2001; **Med School:** Ros Franklin Univ/Chicago Med Sch 1973; **Resid:** Internal Medicine, Beth Israel Hosp 1976; **Fellow:** Medical Oncology, MD Anderson Cancer Ctr 1978; **Fac Appt:** Asst Clin Prof Med, UMDNJ-NJ Med Sch, Newark

Ligresti, Louise G MD (Onc) - **Spec Exp:** Breast Cancer; **Hospital:** Valley Hosp (page 689), Chilton Hosp; **Address:** One Valley Hlth Plaza, Paramus, NJ 07652; **Phone:** 201-634-5353; **Board Cert:** Medical Oncology 2008; Hematology 2008; **Med School:** SUNY Upstate Med Univ 1991; **Resid:** Internal Medicine, NY Hosp-Cornell Med Ctr 1994; **Fellow:** Hematology & Oncology, Meml Sloan Kettering Cancer Ctr 1995

Pascal, Mark MD (Onc) - **Spec Exp:** Lung Cancer; Breast Cancer; Neuro-Oncology; **Hospital:** Hackensack Univ Med Ctr (page 96), Holy Name Med Ctr (page 688); **Address:** John Theurer Cancer Ctr, HUMC, 92 Second St, Hackensack, NJ 07601; **Phone:** 201-996-5266; **Board Cert:** Internal Medicine 1977; Medical Oncology 1979; **Med School:** Jefferson Med Coll 1973; **Resid:** Pathology, NY Hosp-Cornell Univ Med Ctr 1976; Internal Medicine, NY Hosp-Cornell Univ Med Ctr 1977; **Fellow:** Hematology & Oncology, Meml Sloan-Kettering Cancer Ctr 1979

Pecora, Andrew L MD (Onc) - **Spec Exp:** Stem Cell Transplant; Myelodysplastic Syndromes; Melanoma; Immunotherapy; **Hospital:** Hackensack Univ Med Ctr (page 96); **Address:** The Cancer Ctr-Hackensack Univ Med Ctr, 92 2nd St, Hackensack, NJ 07601; **Phone:** 201-996-5814; **Board Cert:** Internal Medicine 1986; Hematology 1988; Medical Oncology 1989; **Med School:** UMDNJ-NJ Med Sch, Newark 1983; **Resid:** Internal Medicine, New York Hosp 1986; **Fellow:** Hematology & Oncology, Meml Sloan Kettering Cancer Ctr 1988; **Fac Appt:** Prof Med, UMDNJ-NJ Med Sch, Newark

Pieczara, Beata K MD (Onc) - **Hospital:** Holy Name Med Ctr (page 688); **Address:** Regional Cancer Ctr at Holy Name, 718 Teaneck Rd, Teaneck, NJ 07666; **Phone:** 201-227-6008; **Board Cert:** Internal Medicine 1999; Medical Oncology 2002; Hematology 2003; **Med School:** Poland 1993; **Resid:** Internal Medicine, Bronx Lebanon Hosp 1999; **Fellow:** Hematology & Oncology, Westchester Med Ctr 1999

Rakowski, Thomas MD (Onc) - **Spec Exp:** Breast Cancer; Lung Cancer; Colon Cancer; **Hospital:** Valley Hosp (page 689); **Address:** One Valley Health Plaza, Paramus, NJ 07652; **Phone:** 201-634-5578; **Board Cert:** Internal Medicine 1979; Medical Oncology 1981; **Med School:** SUNY Upstate Med Univ 1976; **Resid:** Internal Medicine, SUNY Hlth Sci Ctr 1979; Hematology & Oncology, NY Presby Hosp-Columbia Campus 1981

Rivera, Yadyra MD (Onc) - **Spec Exp:** Breast Cancer; Colon Cancer; Lung Cancer; **Hospital:** Holy Name Med Ctr (page 688); **Address:** Regional Cancer Ctr at Holy Name, 718 Teaneck Rd, Teaneck, NJ 07666; **Phone:** 201-227-6008; **Board Cert:** Internal Medicine 2005; Medical Oncology 1998; Hematology 1999; **Med School:** Univ del Caribe Escuela Med 1992; **Resid:** Internal Medicine, Cabrini Med Ctr 1995; **Fellow:** Hematology, Cabrini Med Ctr 1997

Schleider, Michael MD (Onc) - **Spec Exp:** Breast Cancer; Colon Cancer; Bleeding/Coagulation Disorders; **Hospital:** Englewood Hosp & Med Ctr, Holy Name Med Ctr (page 688); **Address:** 350 Engle St Berrie Bldg Fl 1, Englewood, NJ 07631; **Phone:** 201-568-5250; **Board Cert:** Internal Medicine 1974; Hematology 1976; Medical Oncology 1977; **Med School:** Univ Pennsylvania 1969; **Resid:** Internal Medicine, New York Hosp 1974; **Fellow:** Hematology & Oncology, New York Hosp 1977

Waintraub, Stanley E MD (Onc) - **Spec Exp:** Breast Cancer; Bleeding/Coagulation Disorders; **Hospital:** Hackensack Univ Med Ctr (page 96); **Address:** Regional Cancer Care Associates, 92 Second St, Fl 4, Hackensack, NJ 07601; **Phone:** 201-996-5864; **Board Cert:** Internal Medicine 1980; Hematology 1982; Medical Oncology 1983; **Med School:** NY Med Coll 1977; **Resid:** Internal Medicine, Metropolitan Hosp Ctr 1980; **Fellow:** Hematology, Montefiore Hosp Med Ctr 1982; Medical Oncology, Meml Sloan Kettering Cancer Ctr 1983

Neonatal-Perinatal Medicine

Carlin, Elizabeth B MD (NP) - **Spec Exp:** Nutrition; **Hospital:** Englewood Hosp & Med Ctr, Mount Sinai Med Ctr (page 102); **Address:** Englewood Hosp & Med Ctr, 350 Engle St, Englewood, NJ 07631-1808; **Phone:** 201-894-3472; **Board Cert:** Neonatal-Perinatal Medicine 2006; **Med School:** Boston Univ 1990; **Resid:** Pediatrics, Boston City Hosp 1993; **Fellow:** Neonatal-Perinatal Medicine, Mt Sinai Med Ctr 1996; **Fac Appt:** Asst Clin Prof Ped, Mount Sinai Sch Med

Giuliano, Michael A MD (NP) - **Hospital:** Hackensack Univ Med Ctr (page 96); **Address:** Hackensack Univ Med Ctr, 30 Prospect Ave Imus Bldg - rm 217, Hackensack, NJ 07601; **Phone:** 551-996-5362; **Board Cert:** Pediatrics 2010; Neonatal-Perinatal Medicine 2010; **Med School:** SUNY Downstate 1981; **Resid:** Pediatrics, New York Hosp 1984; **Fellow:** Neonatal-Perinatal Medicine, New York Hosp/Cornell 1986

Manginello, Frank P MD (NP) - **Spec Exp:** Prematurity/Low Birth Weight Infants; Lung Disease in Newborns; Developmental Disorders; **Hospital:** Valley Hosp (page 689); **Address:** The Valley Hosp, 223 N Van Dien Ave, Ridgewood, NJ 07450-2736; **Phone:** 201-447-8388; **Board Cert:** Pediatrics 1978; Neonatal-Perinatal Medicine 1979; **Med School:** Georgetown Univ 1973; **Resid:** Pediatrics, Georgetown Univ Hosp 1974; Pediatrics, Georgetown Univ Hosp 1975; **Fellow:** Perinatal Medicine, NY Hosp-Cornell Med Ctr 1977; **Fac Appt:** Asst Prof Ped, Columbia P&S

Perl, Harold MD (NP) - **Spec Exp:** Pulmonary Disease; Jaundice & Bilirubin Metabolism; Sudden Infant Death Syndrome (SIDS); **Hospital:** Hackensack Univ Med Ctr (page 96); **Address:** Hackensack Univ Med Ctr, Dept Pediatrics, 30 Prospect Ave, Imus Bldg, rm 220, Hackensack, NJ 07601-1914; **Phone:** 551-996-5362; **Board Cert:** Pediatrics 1980; Neonatal-Perinatal Medicine 2010; **Med School:** Albert Einstein Coll Med 1975; **Resid:** Pediatrics, Montefiore Med Ctr 1978; **Fellow:** Neonatal-Perinatal Medicine, Montefiore Med Ctr 1980; **Fac Appt:** Asst Clin Prof Ped, UMDNJ-NJ Med Sch, Newark

Nephrology

Fein, Deborah A MD (Nep) - **Spec Exp:** Hypertension; Kidney Disease; Transplant Medicine-Kidney; Lupus Nephritis; **Hospital:** Englewood Hosp & Med Ctr, Holy Name Med Ctr (page 688); **Address:** 177 N Dean St, Ste 207, Englewood, NJ 07631; **Phone:** 201-567-0446; **Board Cert:** Internal Medicine 1983; Nephrology 2004; **Med School:** Tufts Univ 1980; **Resid:** Internal Medicine, Roosevelt Hosp 1983; **Fellow:** Nephrology, NY Hosp 1986

Kozlowski, Jeffrey MD (Nep) - **Spec Exp:** Hypertension; Dialysis Care; Diabetic Kidney Disease; **Hospital:** Valley Hosp (page 689), Hackensack Univ Med Ctr (page 96); **Address:** 44 Godwin Ave, Ste 301, Midland Park, NJ 07432; **Phone:** 201-447-0013; **Board Cert:** Internal Medicine 1981; Nephrology 1984; **Med School:** NYU Sch Med 1978; **Resid:** Internal Medicine, VA Med Ctr 1981; **Fellow:** Nephrology, NYU Med Ctr 1984

Levin, David N MD (Nep) - **Spec Exp:** Hypertension; Dialysis Care; **Hospital:** Holy Name Med Ctr (page 688), Hackensack Univ Med Ctr (page 96); **Address:** 870 Palisade Ave, Ste 202, Teaneck, NJ 07666-3419; **Phone:** 201-836-0897; **Board Cert:** Internal Medicine 1979; Nephrology 1982; **Med School:** UMDNJ-NJ Med Sch, Newark 1976; **Resid:** Internal Medicine, Jacobi Med Ctr 1979; **Fellow:** Nephrology, Albert Einstein Coll Med 1981

Pattner, Austin M MD (Nep) - **Spec Exp:** Hypertension; Dialysis Care; Kidney Disease; **Hospital:** Englewood Hosp & Med Ctr, Hackensack Univ Med Ctr (page 96); **Address:** 177 N Dean St, Ste 207, Englewood, NJ 07631; **Phone:** 201-567-0446; **Board Cert:** Internal Medicine 1974; Nephrology 1976; **Med School:** SUNY Upstate Med Univ 1966; **Resid:** Internal Medicine, Roosevelt Hosp 1969; Internal Medicine, Columbia-Presby Med Ctr 1970; **Fellow:** Nephrology, Columbia-Presby Med Ctr 1972; **Fac Appt:** Asst Prof Med, Mount Sinai Sch Med

Rigolosi, Robert S MD (Nep) - **Spec Exp:** Kidney Disease; Hypertension; Dialysis Care; **Hospital:** Holy Name Med Ctr (page 688), Valley Hosp (page 689); **Address:** Holy Name Med Ctr, 718 Teaneck Rd, Teaneck, NJ 07666-4281; **Phone:** 201-833-3223; **Med School:** Italy 1963; **Resid:** Internal Medicine, Bronx VA Hosp 1967; **Fellow:** Renal Disease, Georgetown Univ Hosp 1969

Salazer, Thomas L MD (Nep) - **Hospital:** Hackensack Univ Med Ctr (page 96), Holy Name Med Ctr (page 688); **Address:** 870 Palisade Ave, Ste 202, Teaneck, NJ 07666; **Phone:** 201-836-0897; **Board Cert:** Internal Medicine 2002; Nephrology 2004; **Med School:** SUNY Stony Brook 1989; **Resid:** Internal Medicine, Mayo Clinic 1992; **Fellow:** Nephrology, Mayo Clinic 1994

Tartini, Albert MD (Nep) - **Spec Exp:** Kidney Disease; Hypertension; Dialysis Care; Anemia; **Hospital:** Valley Hosp (page 689), Holy Name Med Ctr (page 688); **Address:** Holy Name Hosp, 718 Teaneck Rd, Hemodialysis Dept, Teaneck, NJ 07607; **Phone:** 201-833-3223; **Board Cert:** Internal Medicine 1988; Nephrology 2010; **Med School:** Grenada 1984; **Resid:** Internal Medicine, St Joseph Hosp Med Ctr 1988; **Fellow:** Nephrology, Univ Vermont Med Ctr 1990

Weizman, Howard B MD (Nep) - **Spec Exp:** Dialysis Care; Hypertension; **Hospital:** Hackensack Univ Med Ctr (page 96), Valley Hosp (page 689); **Address:** 44 Godwin Ave, Ste 301, Midland Park, NJ 07432-1976; **Phone:** 201-447-0013; **Board Cert:** Internal Medicine 1985; Nephrology 2002; **Med School:** Albert Einstein Coll Med 1982; **Resid:** Internal Medicine, Bronx Muni Hosp 1985; **Fellow:** Nephrology, Mount Sinai Med Ctr 1987

Neurological Surgery

Carpenter, Duncan MD (NS) - **Spec Exp:** Spinal Surgery; Spinal Reconstructive Surgery; **Hospital:** Valley Hosp (page 689); **Address:** 225 Dayton St, Ridgewood, NJ 07450-4407; **Phone:** 201-612-0020; **Board Cert:** Neurological Surgery 1987; **Med School:** Columbia P&S 1978; **Resid:** Surgery, St Lukes Hosp 1980; Neurological Surgery, NY Neuro Inst-Columbia 1985

Fried, Arno H MD (NS) - **Spec Exp:** Epilepsy; Brain Tumors; Head Injury; Pediatric Neuro-surgery; **Hospital:** Hackensack Univ Med Ctr (page 96), St. Peter's Univ Hosp; **Address:** 20 Prospect Ave, Ste 905, Hackensack, NJ 07601; **Phone:** 201-996-5251; **Board Cert:** Neurological Surgery 1990; Pediatric Neurological Surgery 2007; **Med School:** Meharry Med Coll 1980; **Resid:** Neurological Surgery, Albert Einstein Coll Med 1986; Neurological Surgery, Univ Utah 1987; **Fellow:** Pediatric Surgery, Chldns Hosp 1987; **Fac Appt:** Assoc Prof NS, NY Med Coll

Moore, Frank M MD (NS) - **Spec Exp:** Aneurysm-Cerebral; Brain Tumors; Spinal Cord Tumors; Spinal Surgery; **Hospital:** Englewood Hosp & Med Ctr, Mount Sinai Med Ctr (page 102); **Address:** Metropolitan Neurosurgery Assocs, 309 Engle St, Ste 6, Englewood, NJ 07631; **Phone:** 201-569-7737; **Board Cert:** Neurological Surgery 1992; **Med School:** France 1983; **Resid:** Neurological Surgery, Mt Sinai Hosp 1988; **Fac Appt:** Assoc Prof NS, Mount Sinai Sch Med

Roth, Patrick A MD (NS) - **Spec Exp:** Spinal Surgery; Brain Tumors; **Hospital:** Hackensack Univ Med Ctr (page 96), Valley Hosp (page 689); **Address:** 680 Kinderkamack Rd, Ste 300, Oradell, NJ 07649; **Phone:** 201-342-2550; **Board Cert:** Neurological Surgery 1997; **Med School:** Albert Einstein Coll Med 1987; **Resid:** Neurological Surgery, New England Med Ctr 1994; **Fac Appt:** Clin Prof NS, UMDNJ-NJ Med Sch, Newark

Steinberger, Alfred A MD (NS) - **Spec Exp:** Spinal Cord Tumors; Aneurysm; Brain Tumors; Spinal Surgery; **Hospital:** Mount Sinai Med Ctr (page 102), Englewood Hosp & Med Ctr; **Address:** 309 Engle St, Englewood, NJ 07631; **Phone:** 212-410-6990; **Board Cert:** Neurological Surgery 1985; **Med School:** Columbia P&S 1976; **Resid:** Neurological Surgery, Neuro Inst-Columbia-Presby 1982; **Fac Appt:** Asst Clin Prof NS, Mount Sinai Sch Med

Vingan, Roy D MD (NS) - **Spec Exp:** Brain Surgery; Spinal Surgery; **Hospital:** Hackensack Univ Med Ctr (page 96), Valley Hosp (page 689); **Address:** 680 Kinderkamack Rd, Ste 300, Oradell, NJ 07649; **Phone:** 201-342-2550; **Board Cert:** Neurological Surgery 1995; **Med School:** SUNY Downstate 1985; **Resid:** Neurological Surgery, SUNY Hlth Sci Ctr 1992; **Fac Appt:** Asst Clin Prof NS, UMDNJ-NJ Med Sch, Newark

Neurology

Alweiss, Gary S MD (N) - **Spec Exp:** Electromyography; Carpal Tunnel Syndrome; Headache; **Hospital:** Englewood Hosp & Med Ctr; **Address:** 25 Rockwood Pl, Ste 110, Englewood, NJ 07631; **Phone:** 201-894-5805; **Board Cert:** Neurology 1993; **Med School:** Mount Sinai Sch Med 1988; **Resid:** Neurology, Mount Sinai Med Ctr 1992; **Fellow:** Neuromuscular Disease, Columbia-Presby Med Ctr 1993

Effron, Charles MD (N) - **Spec Exp:** Peripheral Neuropathy; **Hospital:** Mount Sinai Med Ctr (page 102); **Address:** 365 W Passaic St, Rochelle Park, NJ 07662; **Phone:** 201-845-6500; **Board Cert:** Neurology 1989; **Med School:** Brown Univ 1983; **Resid:** Neurology, Mt Sinai Hosp 1987

Klein, Patricia MD (N) - **Spec Exp:** Headache; Dizziness; Stroke; **Address:** 680 Kinderka-mack Rd, Ste 302, Oradell, NJ 07649; **Phone:** 201-261-6222; **Board Cert:** Neurology 1980; **Med School:** UMDNJ-NJ Med Sch, Newark 1976; **Resid:** Neurology, UMDNJ 1979; **Fac Appt:** Asst Clin Prof N, UMDNJ-NJ Med Sch, Newark

Levin, Kenneth A MD (N) - **Spec Exp:** Stroke; Alzheimer's Disease; Parkinson's Disease; Epilepsy; **Hospital:** Valley Hosp (page 689); **Address:** 1200 E Ridgewood Ave Fl 2 E Wing, Ridge-wood, NJ 07450; **Phone:** 201-444-0868; **Board Cert:** Neurology 1987; **Med School:** Indiana Univ 1982; **Resid:** Neurology, Indiana Univ Med Ctr 1986

Perron, Reed C MD (N) - **Hospital:** Valley Hosp (page 689); **Address:** 1200 E Ridgewood Ave Fl 2 E Wing, Ridgewood, NJ 07450; **Phone:** 201-444-0868; **Board Cert:** Neurology 1974; **Med School:** Univ Rochester 1966; **Resid:** Internal Medicine, Cleveland Clinic 1970; Neurology, Albert Einstein Coll Med 1973

Rabin, Aaron MD/PhD (N) - **Spec Exp:** Parkinson's Disease; Dementia; Peripheral Neuropathy; **Hospital:** Englewood Hosp & Med Ctr; **Address:** 700 E Palisade Ave, Englewood Cliffs, NJ 07632; **Phone:** 201-568-3412; **Board Cert:** Neurology 1981; **Med School:** Albert Einstein Coll Med 1976; **Resid:** Neurology, Albert Einstein Coll Med Affil Hosps 1980; **Fellow:** Neuroelectrophysiology, Neur Inst-Columbia Presby 1981; **Fac Appt:** Asst Clin Prof Med, Mount Sinai Sch Med

Van Engel, Daniel R MD (N) - **Spec Exp:** Electromyography; **Hospital:** Valley Hosp (page 689); **Address:** 1200 E Ridgewood Ave Fl 2 E Wing, Ridgewood, NJ 07450-3957; **Phone:** 201-444-0868; **Board Cert:** Neurology 1980; **Med School:** SUNY Upstate Med Univ 1973; **Resid:** Internal Medicine, North Shore Univ Hosp 1975; Neurology, Bronx Muni Hosp 1978

Van Slooten, David D MD (N) - **Spec Exp:** Electromyography; Headache; Dementia; Brain & Spinal Imaging; **Hospital:** Holy Name Med Ctr (page 688), Valley Hosp (page 689); **Address:** 680 Kinderkamack Rd, Ste 302, Oradell, NJ 07649-1500; **Phone:** 201-261-6222; **Board Cert:** Neurology 1989; Clinical Neurophysiology 2004; **Med School:** UMDNJ-NJ Med Sch, Newark 1984; **Resid:** Neurology, UMDNJ Univ Hosp 1988; **Fellow:** Clinical Neurophysiology, VA Med Ctr 1989

Willner, Joseph H MD (N) - **Spec Exp:** Multiple Sclerosis; Myasthenia Gravis; Peripheral Neuropathy; **Hospital:** Englewood Hosp & Med Ctr; **Address:** 25 Rockwood Pl, Ste 110, Englewood, NJ 07631-4363; **Phone:** 201-894-5805; **Board Cert:** Neurology 1978; **Med School:** NYU Sch Med 1970; **Resid:** Neurology, Columbia-Presby Hosp 1977; **Fac Appt:** Assoc Clin Prof N, Columbia P&S

Neuroradiology

Lerner, Elliot J MD (NRad) - **Spec Exp:** Brain & Spinal Imaging; Head & Neck Imaging; **Hospital:** Valley Hosp (page 689); **Address:** Radiology Assocs of Ridgewood, 20 Franklin Tpke, Waldwick, NJ 07463-1749; **Phone:** 201-445-8822; **Board Cert:** Diagnostic Radiology 1990; Neuroradiology 2004; **Med School:** Brown Univ 1985; **Resid:** Diagnostic Radiology, Hosp Univ Penn 1989; **Fellow:** Neuroradiology, Hosp Univ Penn 1991

Nuclear Medicine

Agress Jr, Harry MD (NuM) - **Spec Exp:** PET Imaging; Cancer Detection & Staging; Nuclear Oncology; CT Scan; **Hospital:** Hackensack Univ Med Ctr (page 96); **Address:** Hackensack University Medical Center, 30 Prospect Ave, Hackensack, NJ 07601; **Phone:** 201-996-2196; **Board Cert:** Nuclear Medicine 1976; Diagnostic Radiology 1978; **Med School:** Tufts Univ 1972; **Resid:** Radiology, Columbia- Presby Med Ctr 1978; **Fellow:** Nuclear Medicine, Natl Inst Hlth 1975; **Fac Appt:** Clin Prof Rad, Columbia P&S

Brunetti, Jacqueline C MD (NuM) - **Spec Exp:** PET Imaging; CT Scan; Prostate Cancer-MR Spectroscopy (MRSI); **Hospital:** Holy Name Med Ctr (page 688); **Address:** Holy Name Medical Center, 718 Teaneck Rd, Teaneck, NJ 07666-4281; **Phone:** 201-833-3445; **Board Cert:** Diagnostic Radiology 1979; Nuclear Medicine 1980; Nuclear Radiology 1980; **Med School:** SUNY Downstate 1975; **Resid:** Diagnostic Radiology, St Vincents Hosp 1979; Nuclear Radiology, St Vincents Hosp 1980; **Fellow:** Nuclear Medicine, St Vincents Hosp 1980; **Fac Appt:** Assoc Clin Prof, Columbia P&S

Obstetrics & Gynecology

Butler, David G MD (ObG) *PCP* - **Spec Exp:** Gynecologic Surgery; Menopause Problems; **Hospital:** Holy Name Med Ctr (page 688), Englewood Hosp & Med Ctr; **Address:** 420 Grand Ave, Ste 201, Englewood, NJ 07631-4152; **Phone:** 201-871-4040; **Board Cert:** Obstetrics & Gynecology 1972; **Med School:** SUNY Downstate 1965; **Resid:** Obstetrics & Gynecology, St Vincents Hosp 1970

Cavallaro, Barbara MD (ObG) - **Hospital:** Hackensack Univ Med Ctr (page 96); **Address:** 170 Prospect Ave, Bldg 2, Ste 4, Hackensack, NJ 07601-2255; **Phone:** 201-488-2288; **Board Cert:** Obstetrics & Gynecology 2011; **Med School:** NYU Sch Med 1986; **Resid:** Obstetrics & Gynecology, Mt Sinai Med Ctr 1990

Coven, Roger MD (ObG) - **Spec Exp:** Pregnancy-High Risk; **Hospital:** Valley Hosp (page 689); **Address:** 581 N Franklin Tpke, Ramsey, NJ 07446; **Phone:** 201-447-2200; **Board Cert:** Obstetrics & Gynecology 2011; **Med School:** UMDNJ-NJ Med Sch, Newark 1980; **Resid:** Obstetrics & Gynecology, Thomas Jefferson Univ Hosp 1984

Englert, Christopher A MD (ObG) - **Spec Exp:** Gynecologic Surgery; Laparoscopic Surgery; Robotic Surgery; Vulvar & Vaginal Disorders; **Hospital:** Holy Name Med Ctr (page 688); **Address:** 420 Grand Ave, Ste 201, Englewood, NJ 07631-4141; **Phone:** 201-871-4040; **Board Cert:** Obstetrics & Gynecology 2011; **Med School:** Univ Cincinnati 1985; **Resid:** Obstetrics & Gynecology, Thomas Jefferson Univ Hosp 1989

Faust, Michael G MD (ObG) - **Spec Exp:** Gynecologic Surgery; Menopause Problems; Minimally Invasive Surgery; **Hospital:** Valley Hosp (page 689); **Address:** Valley Ctr for Womens Health, 581 N Franklin Tpke, Ramsey, NJ 07446; **Phone:** 201-236-2100; **Board Cert:** Obstetrics & Gynecology 2011; **Med School:** Univ Pittsburgh 1983; **Resid:** Obstetrics & Gynecology, Thos Jefferson Univ Hosp 1987

Fernandez, Jacinto J MD (ObG) - **Spec Exp:** Women's Health; **Hospital:** Holy Name Med Ctr (page 688); **Address:** 870 Palisade Ave, Apt 301, Teaneck, NJ 07666-3446; **Phone:** 201-907-0900; **Board Cert:** Obstetrics & Gynecology 1976; **Med School:** Spain 1967; **Resid:** Obstetrics & Gynecology, St. Joseph's Hosp 1972; **Fellow:** Obstetrics & Gynecology, St. Joseph's Hosp 1974

Hurst, Wendy R MD (ObG) - **Spec Exp:** Gynecology Only; Laparoscopic Surgery; Menopause Problems; Adolescent Gynecology; **Hospital:** Englewood Hosp & Med Ctr; **Address:** 370 Grand Ave, Ste 202, Englewood, NJ 07631-4109; **Phone:** 201-894-9599; **Board Cert:** Obstetrics & Gynecology 2011; **Med School:** Tufts Univ 1986; **Resid:** Obstetrics & Gynecology, Hosp Univ Penn 1990

Meyer, Monica L MD (ObG) *PCP* - **Spec Exp:** Adolescent Gynecology; Gynecology Only; Menopause Problems; **Hospital:** Valley Hosp (page 689); **Address:** The Women's Group of Ridgewood, 1 W Ridgewood Ave, Ste 211, Paramus, NJ 07652; **Phone:** 201-251-2323; **Board Cert:** Obstetrics & Gynecology 2011; **Med School:** SUNY Downstate 1991; **Resid:** Obstetrics & Gynecology, Lenox Hill Hosp 1995

Rezvani, Fred F MD (ObG) - **Spec Exp:** Pregnancy-High Risk; Minimally Invasive Surgery; Congenital Anomalies-Gynecologic; **Hospital:** Valley Hosp (page 689); **Address:** 119 Prospect St, Ridgewood, NJ 07450; **Phone:** 201-444-1600; **Board Cert:** Obstetrics & Gynecology 2007; **Med School:** West Indies 1983; **Resid:** Obstetrics & Gynecology, Lincoln Hosp 1988

Rubenstein, Andrew F MD (ObG) - **Hospital:** Hackensack Univ Med Ctr (page 96); **Address:** 82 E Allendale Rd, Ste 1A, Saddle River, NJ 07458; **Phone:** 201-934-5050; **Board Cert:** Obstetrics & Gynecology 2011; **Med School:** Hahnemann Univ 1980; **Resid:** Obstetrics & Gynecology, Mt Sinai Med Ctr 1994; **Fac Appt:** Asst Clin Prof ObG, UMDNJ-NJ Med Sch, Newark

Ophthalmology

Brown, Andrew C MD (Oph) - **Spec Exp:** LASIK-Refractive Surgery; Cataract Surgery; Macular Degeneration; **Hospital:** Hackensack Univ Med Ctr (page 96); **Address:** Brown Eye Care Assocs, 751 Teaneck Rd, Ste B, Teaneck, NJ 07666; **Phone:** 201-833-0006; **Board Cert:** Ophthalmology 2009; **Med School:** Boston Univ 2002; **Resid:** Ophthalmology, NY Eye & Ear Infirm 2006

Brown, Christopher D MD (Oph) - **Spec Exp:** Corneal Disease; Diabetic Eye Disease/Retinopathy; LASIK-Refractive Surgery; **Hospital:** Englewood Hosp & Med Ctr, Holy Name Med Ctr (page 688); **Address:** Brown Eye Care Assocs, 751 Teaneck Rd, Teaneck, NJ 07666; **Phone:** 201-833-0006; **Board Cert:** Ophthalmology 2012; **Med School:** Boston Univ 1996; **Resid:** Ophthalmology, Wills Eye Hosp 2000; **Fellow:** Refractive Surgery, Vision Correction Ctr 2001

Burke, Patricia A MD (Oph) - **Spec Exp:** Corneal Disease; Cataract Surgery; **Hospital:** Holy Name Med Ctr (page 688); **Address:** One Sears Drive, Paramus, NJ 07652; **Phone:** 201-599-0123; **Board Cert:** Ophthalmology 1991; **Med School:** UMDNJ-NJ Med Sch, Newark 1986; **Resid:** Ophthalmology, Columbia-Presby Med Ctr 1990; **Fellow:** Cornea, Manhattan EET Hosp 1991

Chin, Patrick K MD (Oph) - **Spec Exp:** Laser Vision Surgery; Cataract Surgery; Refractive Surgery; **Hospital:** Valley Hosp (page 689); **Address:** Westwood Ophthalmology Assocs, 300 Fairview Ave, Westwood, NJ 07675; **Phone:** 201-666-4014; **Board Cert:** Ophthalmology 2007; **Med School:** UMDNJ-NJ Med Sch, Newark 1989; **Resid:** Ophthalmology, NYU Med Ctr 1994; **Fellow:** Ophthalmology, Gimbel Eye Ctr 1995

DeLuca, Joseph A MD (Oph) - **Spec Exp:** Cataract Surgery; Laser Refractive Surgery; Anterior Segment Surgery; Trauma; **Hospital:** Clara Maass Med Ctr; **Address:** 20 Park Ave Fl 1, Lyndhurst, NJ 07071-1012; **Phone:** 201-896-0096; **Board Cert:** Ophthalmology 1991; **Med School:** UMDNJ-Rutgers Med Sch 1985; **Resid:** Ophthalmology, United Hosp Med Ctr 1990; **Fac Appt:** Asst Clin Prof Oph, UMDNJ-NJ Med Sch, Newark

Hersh, Peter MD (Oph) - **Spec Exp:** LASIK-Refractive Surgery; Cornea Transplant; Keratoconus; **Hospital:** Univ Hosp-UMDNJ—Newark; **Address:** The Cornea & Laser Eye Institute, Glenpointe Center East, 300 Frank W Burr Blvd, Ste 71, Teaneck, NJ 07666-6704; **Phone:** 201-883-0505; **Board Cert:** Ophthalmology 1987; **Med School:** Johns Hopkins Univ 1982; **Resid:** Internal Medicine, Lenox Hill Hosp 1983; Ophthalmology, Mass Eye & Ear Infirm 1986; **Fellow:** Cornea & Ext Eye Disease, Mass Eye & Ear Infirm 1987; **Fac Appt:** Prof Oph, UMDNJ-NJ Med Sch, Newark

Liva, Douglas MD (Oph) - **Spec Exp:** LASIK-Refractive Surgery; Cataract Surgery; Glaucoma; **Hospital:** Valley Hosp (page 689); **Address:** 1 W Ridgewood Ave, Ste 101, Paramus, NJ 07652-2350; **Phone:** 201-444-7770; **Board Cert:** Ophthalmology 1987; **Med School:** Univ Miami Sch Med 1981; **Resid:** Ophthalmology, UMDNJ Affil Hosps 1986

Silbert, Glenn MD (Oph) - **Spec Exp:** Cataract Surgery; Lens Implants; **Hospital:** Hackensack Univ Med Ctr (page 96), New York Eye & Ear Infirm (page 117); **Address:** 316 State St, Hackensack, NJ 07601-5529; **Phone:** 201-342-8115; **Board Cert:** Ophthalmology 1985; **Med School:** Columbia P&S 1979; **Resid:** Ophthalmology, NYU Med Ctr 1983; **Fac Appt:** Assoc Prof Oph, NY Med Coll

Solomon, Edward MD (Oph) - **Spec Exp:** Cataract Surgery; Laser Surgery; **Hospital:** Valley Hosp (page 689); **Address:** 85 S Maple Ave, Ridgewood, NJ 07450-4500; **Phone:** 201-444-3010; **Board Cert:** Ophthalmology 1976; **Med School:** Tufts Univ 1968; **Resid:** Ophthalmology, NYU Med Ctr 1974

Stabile, John R MD (Oph) - **Spec Exp:** Cataract Surgery; Oculoplastic Surgery; LASIK-Refractive Surgery; **Hospital:** Englewood Hosp & Med Ctr, Holy Name Med Ctr (page 688); **Address:** 111 Dean Drive, Tenafly, NJ 07670-2764; **Phone:** 201-567-5995; **Board Cert:** Ophthalmology 1981; **Med School:** NY Med Coll 1976; **Resid:** Ophthalmology, St Luke's-Roosevelt Hosp Ctr 1980; **Fellow:** Oculoplastic Surgery, Columbia-Presby Med Ctr 1981; **Fac Appt:** Clin Prof Oph, Columbia P&S

Topilow, Harvey MD (Oph) - **Spec Exp:** Retinal Disorders; Macular Degeneration; Retinopathy of Prematurity; **Hospital:** New York Eye & Ear Infirm (page 117); **Address:** 301 Bridge Plaza N, Fort Lee, NJ 07024; **Phone:** 212-288-3860; **Board Cert:** Ophthalmology 1980; **Med School:** Columbia P&S 1975; **Resid:** Ophthalmology, Albert Einstein 1979; **Fellow:** Vitreoretinal Surgery, Mass Eye & Ear Infirmary 1981; **Fac Appt:** Assoc Clin Prof Oph, Albert Einstein Coll Med

Weinberg, Martin R MD (Oph) - **Spec Exp:** Neuro-Ophthalmology; Glaucoma; **Hospital:** Englewood Hosp & Med Ctr, Hackensack Univ Med Ctr (page 96); **Address:** 405 Cedar Ln, Ste 5, Teaneck, NJ 07666-1715; **Phone:** 201-836-8333; **Board Cert:** Ophthalmology 1989; **Med School:** Eastern VA Med Sch 1979; **Resid:** Surgery, Albany Memorial Hosp 1981; Ophthalmology, Kings County Hosp 1986; **Fellow:** Ocular Pathology, Scheie Eye Inst-Univ Penn 1983; Ocular Oncology, Manhattan EET Hosp 1987

Orthopaedic Surgery

Altman, Wayne MD (OrS) - **Spec Exp:** Carpal Tunnel Syndrome; Knee Injuries; Hand & Wrist Injuries; Shoulder Injuries; **Hospital:** Meadowlands Hosp Med Ctr, Hackensack UMC-Mountainside (page 736); **Address:** 85 Orient Way, FL 1, Rutherford, NJ 07070-2045; **Phone:** 201-438-5888; **Board Cert:** Orthopaedic Surgery 2009; **Med School:** UMDNJ-NJ Med Sch, Newark 1978; **Resid:** Orthopaedic Surgery, UMDNJ-Newark 1983; **Fellow:** Hand Surgery, Thomas Jefferson Univ Hosp 1984

Berman, Mark MD (OrS) - **Spec Exp:** Knee Surgery; Shoulder Surgery; Rotator Cuff Surgery; Sports Medicine; **Hospital:** Hackensack Univ Med Ctr (page 96), Holy Name Med Ctr (page 688); **Address:** 920 Main St Fl 2, Hackensack, NJ 07601-3246; **Phone:** 201-489-8250; **Board Cert:** Orthopaedic Surgery 2010; **Med School:** Mount Sinai Sch Med 1981; **Resid:** Surgery, Mount Sinai Hosp 1983; Orthopaedic Surgery, Univ Hosp 1986; **Fellow:** Sports Medicine, Lenox Hill Hosp 1987

Cahill, James W MD (OrS) - **Spec Exp:** Arthroscopic Surgery-Knee; Joint Replacement; Shoulder Arthroscopic Surgery; Cartilage Damage; **Hospital:** Hackensack Univ Med Ctr (page 96), Holy Name Med Ctr (page 688); **Address:** 87 Summit Ave, Hackensack, NJ 07601; **Phone:** 201-489-0022; **Board Cert:** Orthopaedic Surgery 2010; **Med School:** Columbia P&S 1990; **Resid:** Orthopaedic Surgery, Montefiore Med Ctr 1995; **Fellow:** Sports Medicine, Hosp for Joint Diseases 1996

Doidge, Robert DO (OrS) - **Spec Exp:** Knee Surgery; Shoulder Surgery; Sports Medicine; **Hospital:** Englewood Hosp & Med Ctr; **Address:** 370 Grand Ave, Ste 100, Englewood, NJ 07631-4109; **Phone:** 201-567-5700; **Med School:** Philadelphia Coll Osteo Med 1986; **Resid:** Orthopaedic Surgery, Oakland Genl Hosp 1991; **Fellow:** Sports Medicine, Michigan State Univ 1992

Esformes, Ira MD (OrS) - **Spec Exp:** Sports Medicine; Arthroscopic Surgery; Joint Replacement; **Hospital:** Valley Hosp (page 689), Hackensack Univ Med Ctr (page 96); **Address:** 440 Old Hook Rd Fl 2, Emerson, NJ 07630-1325; **Phone:** 201-261-3333; **Board Cert:** Orthopaedic Surgery 1985; Orthopaedic Sports Medicine 2009; **Med School:** Albany Med Coll 1977; **Resid:** Surgery, North Shore Univ Hosp 1979; Orthopaedic Surgery, Hosp For Joint Diseases 1983

Gennace, Ronald MD (OrS) - **Hospital:** Clara Maass Med Ctr, Saint Michael's Med Ctr; **Address:** 312 Belleville Tpke, Ste 2A, North Arlington, NJ 07031; **Phone:** 201-997-8777; **Board Cert:** Orthopaedic Surgery 1982; **Med School:** UMDNJ-NJ Med Sch, Newark 1976; **Resid:** Orthopaedic Surgery, St Joseph's Hosp & Med Ctr 1980

Hartzband, Mark A MD (OrS) - **Spec Exp:** Knee Replacement; Hip Replacement; **Hospital:** Hackensack Univ Med Ctr (page 96), Holy Name Med Ctr (page 688); **Address:** 10 Forest Ave, Paramus, NJ 07652; **Phone:** 201-291-4040; **Board Cert:** Orthopaedic Surgery 2007; **Med School:** McGill Univ 1978; **Resid:** Surgery, Montefiore Med Ctr 1981; Orthopaedic Surgery, Montefiore Med Ctr 1984

Kelly, Michael A MD (OrS) - **Spec Exp:** Knee Surgery; Knee Replacement; Arthroscopic Surgery; **Hospital:** Hackensack Univ Med Ctr (page 96), Lenox Hill Hosp (page 106); **Address:** 360 Essex St, Ste 303, Hackensack, NJ 07601; **Phone:** 201-336-8861; **Board Cert:** Orthopaedic Surgery 2009; **Med School:** Georgetown Univ 1979; **Resid:** Surgery, St Vincents Hosp 1981; Orthopaedic Surgery, Columbia-Presby Hosp 1984; **Fellow:** Knee Surgery, Hosp for Special Surgery 1985

McIlveen, Stephen J MD (OrS) - **Spec Exp:** Joint Replacement; Sports Medicine; Shoulder Surgery; Knee Surgery; **Hospital:** Valley Hosp (page 689), Hackensack Univ Med Ctr (page 96); **Address:** 1 W Ridgewood Ave, Ste 307, Paramus, NJ 07652; **Phone:** 201-670-6702; **Board Cert:** Orthopaedic Surgery 1983; **Med School:** NYU Sch Med 1973; **Resid:** Surgery, Columbia Presby Med Ctr 1975; Orthopaedic Surgery, Columbia Presby Med Ctr 1978; **Fellow:** Joint Replacement Surgery, Columbia Presby Med Ctr 1979; Elbow & Shoulder Surgery, Columbia Presby Med Ctr 1979; **Fac Appt:** Asst Prof OrS, Columbia P&S

Pizzurro, Joseph MD (OrS) - **Spec Exp:** Hip & Knee Replacement; Joint Replacement; **Hospital:** Valley Hosp (page 689); **Address:** 85 S Maple Ave Fl 2, Ridgewood, NJ 07450-4561; **Phone:** 201-445-2830; **Board Cert:** Orthopaedic Surgery 1972; **Med School:** St Louis Univ 1963; **Resid:** Surgery, Bronx VA Hosp 1968; Orthopaedic Surgery, Bellevue Hosp Ctr/NYU 1971; **Fellow:** Orthopaedic Surgery, Amer Acad Ortho Surg 1975

Pollock, Roger G MD (OrS) - **Spec Exp:** Rotator Cuff Surgery; Shoulder Arthroscopic Surgery; Shoulder Injuries; **Hospital:** NY-Presby/Columbia Univ Med Ctr, NY (page 104), Valley Hosp (page 689); **Address:** 1 W Ridgewood Ave, Ste 202, Paramus, NJ 07625; **Phone:** 201-612-9774; **Board Cert:** Orthopaedic Surgery 2005; **Med School:** Columbia P&S 1985; **Resid:** Surgery, St Luke's-Roosevelt 1987; Orthopaedic Surgery, Columbia-Presby Med Ctr 1991; **Fellow:** Shoulder Surgery, Columbia-Presby Med Ctr 1992; **Fac Appt:** Asst Prof OrS, Columbia P&S

Salzer Jr, Richard L MD (OrS) - **Spec Exp:** Hip & Knee Replacement; Knee Surgery; Joint Replacement; Minimally Invasive Surgery; **Hospital:** Englewood Hosp & Med Ctr, Palisades Med Ctr; **Address:** 401 S Van Brunt St Fl 3rd, Englewood, NJ 07631-4800; **Phone:** 201-569-2770; **Board Cert:** Orthopaedic Surgery 1979; **Med School:** Tufts Univ 1973; **Resid:** Surgery, St Paul's Hosp 1975; Orthopaedic Surgery, Hosp Special Surg 1978

Otolaryngology

Henick, David H MD (Oto) - **Spec Exp:** Nasal & Sinus Surgery; Endoscopic Sinus Surgery; Head & Neck Surgery; **Hospital:** Englewood Hosp & Med Ctr, Hackensack Univ Med Ctr (page 96); **Address:** 301 Bridge Plaza N Fl 3, Fort Lee, NJ 07024-5059; **Phone:** 201-592-8200; **Board Cert:** Otolaryngology 1993; **Med School:** SUNY Buffalo 1987; **Resid:** Otolaryngology, Montefiore Med Ctr 1992; **Fellow:** Head and Neck Surgery, Montefiore Med Ctr 1993; Rhinoplasty & Sinus Surgery, Hosp Univ Penn 1994; **Fac Appt:** Asst Clin Prof Oto, UMDNJ-NJ Med Sch, Newark

Ho, Bryan MD (Oto) - **Spec Exp:** Sinus Surgery; Thyroid & Parathyroid Surgery; **Hospital:** Englewood Hosp & Med Ctr, Holy Name Med Ctr (page 688); **Address:** 216 Engle St, Ste 101, Englewood, NJ 07631-2428; **Phone:** 201-816-9800; **Board Cert:** Otolaryngology 1995; **Med School:** Mount Sinai Sch Med 1989; **Resid:** Surgery, Mount Sinai Med Ctr 1991; Otolaryngology, Mount Sinai Med Ctr 1994

Katz, Harry MD (Oto) - **Spec Exp:** Sinus Disorders; **Hospital:** Valley Hosp (page 689); **Address:** 44 Godwin Ave, Ste 300, Midland Park, NJ 07432-1959; **Phone:** 201-445-2900; **Board Cert:** Otolaryngology 1982; **Med School:** NYU Sch Med 1977; **Resid:** Otolaryngology, NYU Med Ctr-Bellevue 1981

Low, Ronald B MD (Oto) - **Spec Exp:** Head & Neck Surgery; Rhinoplasty; Sinus Surgery; **Hospital:** Hackensack Univ Med Ctr (page 96); **Address:** 20 Prospect Ave, Ste 909, Hackensack, NJ 07601-5013; **Phone:** 201-489-6520; **Board Cert:** Otolaryngology 1974; **Med School:** UMDNJ-NJ Med Sch, Newark 1969; **Resid:** Surgery, Montefiore Hosp 1971; Otolaryngology, NYU-Bellevue Hosp Ctr 1974; **Fac Appt:** Asst Clin Prof Oto

Milgrim, Laurence M MD (Oto) - **Spec Exp:** Facial Plastic Surgery; **Hospital:** Holy Name Med Ctr (page 688), Valley Hosp (page 689); **Address:** 1 Degraw Ave, Teaneck, NJ 07666; **Phone:** 201-837-2174; **Board Cert:** Otolaryngology 1995; Facial Plastic & Reconstr Surgery 2000; **Med School:** UMDNJ-Rutgers Med Sch 1989; **Resid:** Otolaryngology, Montefiore Med Ctr 1995; **Fellow:** Facial Plastic & Reconstr Surgery, Mt Sinai Med Ctr 1995

Rosen, Arie MD (Oto) - **Spec Exp:** Head & Neck Tumors; Sinus Disorders; Facial Plastic Surgery; Ear Surgery; **Hospital:** Hackensack Univ Med Ctr (page 96), Englewood Hosp & Med Ctr; **Address:** 2 S Summit Ave, Hackensack, NJ 07601-1117; **Phone:** 201-996-9200; **Board Cert:** Otolaryngology 1995; **Med School:** Israel 1982; **Resid:** Otolaryngology, Univ Chicago-Pritzker Sch Med Hosp 1994; **Fellow:** Otolaryngology, Lenox Hill Hosp 1989

Scherl, Michael MD (Oto) - **Spec Exp:** Hearing Loss/Tinnitus; Nasal & Sinus Disorders; **Hospital:** Englewood Hosp & Med Ctr; **Address:** 3541 Old Hook Rd, Westwood, NJ 07675; **Phone:** 201-666-8787; **Board Cert:** Otolaryngology 1987; **Med School:** Albany Med Coll 1982; **Resid:** Surgery, Mount Sinai Med Ctr 1984; Otolaryngology, Mount Sinai Med Ctr 1987; **Fac Appt:** , Mount Sinai Sch Med

Surow, Jason B MD (Oto) - **Spec Exp:** Pediatric Otolaryngology; Sinus Disorders; Voice Disorders; **Hospital:** Valley Hosp (page 689), Good Samaritan Hosp - Suffern; **Address:** 690 Kinderkamack Rd, Ste 101, Oradell, NJ 07649; **Phone:** 201-722-9850; **Board Cert:** Otolaryngology 1987; **Med School:** Univ Pennsylvania 1982; **Resid:** Surgery, Hosp Univ Penn 1984; Otolaryngology, Hosp Univ Penn 1987

Tobias, Geoffrey W MD (Oto) - **Spec Exp:** Rhinoplasty Revision; Nasal Surgery; Nasal Reconstruction; **Hospital:** Englewood Hosp & Med Ctr, Mount Sinai Med Ctr (page 102); **Address:** 214 Engle St, Ste 22, Englewood, NJ 07631; **Phone:** 201-567-6770; **Board Cert:** Otolaryngology 1978; **Med School:** Tufts Univ 1973; **Resid:** Otolaryngology, Mt Sinai Med Ctr 1978

Pain Medicine

Datta, Samyadev MD (PM) - **Spec Exp:** Complex Regional Pain Syndromes; Pain-Cancer; Pain-Back; **Hospital:** Holy Name Med Ctr (page 688); **Address:** Ctr for Pain Mngmt, 294 State St, Ste 1, Hackensack, NJ 07601; **Phone:** 201-488-7246; **Board Cert:** Anesthesiology 1996; Pain Medicine 2009; **Med School:** India 1979; **Resid:** Anesthesiology, NY Presby Hosp 1994

Park, Kenneth H DO (PM) - **Spec Exp:** Pain-Chronic; Pain-Back; Pain-Neuropathic; Pain-Cancer; **Hospital:** Holy Name Med Ctr (page 688); **Address:** 680 Kinderkamach Rd, Ste 207, Oradell, NJ 07649; **Phone:** 201-487-7246; **Board Cert:** Anesthesiology 2007; Pain Medicine 2007; **Med School:** NY Coll Osteo Med 2002; **Resid:** Anesthesiology, Brigham & Women's Hosp 2006; **Fellow:** Pain Medicine, Brigham & Women's Hosp 2007

Ragukonis, Thomas P MD (PM) - ; **Address:** Bergen Pain Management, 37 W Century Rd, Ste 101, Paramus, NJ 07652; **Phone:** 201-634-9000; **Board Cert:** Anesthesiology 1999; Pain Medicine 2000; **Med School:** UMDNJ-NJ Med Sch, Newark 1991; **Resid:** Anesthesiology, Columbia Presby Med Ctr 1995; **Fac Appt:** Asst Clin Prof Anes, UMDNJ-NJ Med Sch, Newark

Pathology

Sanchez, Miguel A MD (Path) - **Spec Exp:** Breast Cancer; Thyroid Cancer; **Hospital:** Englewood Hosp & Med Ctr; **Address:** 350 Engle St, Dean Bldg - Fl LL1, Englewood, NJ 07631-1898; **Phone:** 201-894-3423; **Board Cert:** Anatomic Pathology 1975; Clinical Pathology 1979; Cytopathology 1991; **Med School:** Spain 1969; **Resid:** Pathology, Englewood Hosp 1972; Pathology, Temple Univ 1973; **Fellow:** Pathology, Meml Sloan Kettering Cancer Ctr 1974; Clinical Pathology, St Vincents Hosp 1975; **Fac Appt:** Assoc Prof Path, Mount Sinai Sch Med

Pediatric Allergy & Immunology

Colenda, Maryann MD (PA&I) - **Spec Exp:** Asthma-Adult & Pediatric; Allergy; **Hospital:** Englewood Hosp & Med Ctr, Meadowlands Hosp Med Ctr; **Address:** 811 Abbott Blvd, Fort Lee, NJ 07024-4116; **Phone:** 201-224-2256; **Board Cert:** Pediatrics 1976; Allergy & Immunology 1979; **Med School:** NY Med Coll 1971; **Resid:** Pediatrics, Columbia-Presby Med Ctr 1974; **Fellow:** Allergy & Immunology, Columbia-Presby Med Ctr 1978; **Fac Appt:** Assoc Clin Prof Ped, Columbia P&S

Hicks, Patricia MD (PA&I) - **Spec Exp:** Asthma & Sinusitis; Asthma in Pregnancy; **Hospital:** Valley Hosp (page 689); **Address:** 119 1st St, Ste 5, Hohokus, NJ 07423-1575; **Phone:** 201-444-5277; **Board Cert:** Pediatrics 1978; Allergy & Immunology 2001; **Med School:** Penn State Coll Med 1973; **Resid:** Pediatrics, Columbia-Presby Med Ctr 1976; **Fellow:** Allergy & Immunology, Columbia-Presby Med Ctr 1981

Pediatric Cardiology

Messina, John J MD (PCd) - **Spec Exp:** Critical Care; Interventional Cardiology; Congenital Heart Disease; **Hospital:** St. Joseph's Regl Med Ctr - Paterson; **Address:** 1 Broadway, Ste 203, Elmwood Park, NJ 07407-1844; **Phone:** 973-569-6250; **Board Cert:** Pediatrics 2009; Pediatric Cardiology 2009; **Med School:** West Indies 1986; **Resid:** Pediatrics, St Joseph's Hosp 1989; **Fellow:** Pediatric Cardiology, NY Hosp 1992; **Fac Appt:** Asst Prof Ped, Columbia P&S

Tozzi, Robert J MD (PCd) - **Spec Exp:** Hypertrophic Cardiomyopathy; Fetal Echocardiography; Sports Medicine; **Hospital:** Hackensack Univ Med Ctr (page 96); **Address:** 155 Polifly Rd, Fl 1, Ste 106, Hackensack, NJ 07601; **Phone:** 201-487-7617; **Board Cert:** Pediatrics 1987; Pediatric Cardiology 2006; **Med School:** UMDNJ-NJ Med Sch, Newark 1983; **Resid:** Pediatrics, Univ Hosp-UMDNJ 1987; **Fellow:** Pediatric Cardiology, NYU Med Ctr 1988

Pediatric Endocrinology

Aisenberg, Javier E MD (PEn) - **Spec Exp:** Diabetes; Growth Disorders; **Hospital:** Hackensack Univ Med Ctr (page 96); **Address:** 30 prospect Ave, wfan Bldg - Fl 2nd - Ste 251, Hackensack, NJ 07601; **Phone:** 551-996-5329; **Board Cert:** Pediatrics 2008; Pediatric Endocrinology 2010; **Med School:** Argentina 1987; **Resid:** Pediatrics, Bellevue Hosp Ctr 1991; **Fellow:** Pediatric Endocrinology, NY Presby/Cornell Med Ctr 1995

Pediatric Hematology-Oncology

Diamond, Steven MD (PHO) - **Spec Exp:** Pediatric Cancers; Sickle Cell Disease; Hemophilia; **Hospital:** Hackensack Univ Med Ctr (page 96); **Address:** Hackensack Univ Med Ctr, Div Ped Hem/Onc, 30 Prospect Ave, Hackensack, NJ 07601-1914; **Phone:** 201-996-5437; **Board Cert:** Pediatrics 1979; Pediatric Hematology-Oncology 1980; **Med School:** Univ Pennsylvania 1974; **Resid:** Pediatrics, Mount Sinai Hosp 1977; **Fellow:** Pediatric Hematology-Oncology, Beth Israel Hosp 1979; **Fac Appt:** Asst Clin Prof Ped, UMDNJ-NJ Med Sch, Newark

Flug, Frances MD (PHO) - **Spec Exp:** Bleeding/Coagulation Disorders; Sickle Cell Disease; Pediatric Cancers; **Hospital:** Hackensack Univ Med Ctr (page 96), Saint Michael's Med Ctr; **Address:** 30 Prospect Ave, Hackensack, NJ 07601-2129; **Phone:** 201-996-5437; **Board Cert:** Pediatrics 1984; Pediatric Hematology-Oncology 1984; **Med School:** SUNY Downstate 1979; **Resid:** Pediatrics, Bellevue/NYU Med Ctr 1982; **Fellow:** Pediatric Hematology-Oncology, Bellevue/NYU Med Ctr 1984; **Fac Appt:** Assoc Prof Ped, UMDNJ-NJ Med Sch, Newark

Halpern, Steven L MD (PHO) - **Spec Exp:** Leukemia & Lymphoma; Brain Tumors; Hodgkin's Lymphoma; Hemophilia; **Hospital:** Morristown Med Ctr (page 92), Overlook Med Ctr (page 92); **Address:** 100 Madison Ave, Morristown, NJ 07960; **Phone:** 973-971-6720; **Board Cert:** Pediatrics 1981; Pediatric Hematology-Oncology 1982; **Med School:** Ros Franklin Univ/Chicago Med Sch 1976; **Resid:** Pediatrics, St Christophers Hosp for Children 1979; **Fellow:** Pediatric Hematology-Oncology, Childrens Hosp 1982; **Fac Appt:** Asst Prof Ped, UMDNJ-NJ Med Sch, Newark

Harris, Michael B MD (PHO) - **Spec Exp:** Leukemia & Lymphoma; Bone Tumors; Cancer Survivors-Late Effects of Therapy; **Hospital:** Hackensack Univ Med Ctr (page 96); **Address:** Tomorrows Chldns Inst, JM Sanzari Chldns Hosp, 30 Prospect Ave, Imus 1-TCI, rm PC116, Hackensack, NJ 07601; **Phone:** 201-996-5437; **Board Cert:** Pediatrics 1974; Pediatric Hematology-Oncology 1974; **Med School:** Albert Einstein Coll Med 1969; **Resid:** Pediatrics, Chldns Hosp 1971; **Fellow:** Pediatric Hematology-Oncology, Chldns Hosp 1974; **Fac Appt:** Prof Ped, UMDNJ-NJ Med Sch, Newark

Pediatric Infectious Disease

Boscamp, Jeffrey R MD (PInf) - **Spec Exp:** Fevers of Unknown Origin; Lyme Disease; **Hospital:** Hackensack Univ Med Ctr (page 96); **Address:** 30 Prospect Ave, WFAN Pediatric Center, Hackensack Univ Med Ctr PC 360, Hackensack, NJ 07601; **Phone:** 551-996-5308; **Board Cert:** Pediatrics 1986; Pediatric Infectious Disease 2009; **Med School:** NY Med Coll 1981; **Resid:** Pediatrics, Columbia-Presby Med Ctr 1984; Internal Medicine, Greenwich Hosp 1985; **Fellow:** Infectious Disease, Montefiore Med Ctr 1987; **Fac Appt:** Assoc Prof Ped, UMDNJ-Univ Med Dent NJ

Piwoz, Julia A MD (PInf) - **Spec Exp:** AIDS/HIV; Congenital Infections; Infections in Transplant Patients; **Hospital:** Hackensack Univ Med Ctr (page 96); **Address:** Joseph M. Sanzari Children's Hosp, 30 Prospect Ave, Don Imus Pediatric Ctr PC360 Bldg, Hackensack, NJ 07601; **Phone:** 201-996-5308; **Board Cert:** Pediatrics 2009; Pediatric Infectious Disease 2007; **Med School:** Hahnemann Univ 1991; **Resid:** Pediatrics, Mt Sinai Med Ctr 1994; **Fellow:** Pediatric Infectious Disease, Mt Sinai Med Ctr 1995; **Fac Appt:** Asst Prof Ped, UMDNJ-NJ Med Sch, Newark

Slavin, Kevin A MD (PInf) - **Spec Exp:** Antibiotic Resistance; Travel Medicine; Infection Control; **Hospital:** Hackensack Univ Med Ctr (page 96); **Address:** Joseph M. Sanzari Children's Hosp, 30 Prospect Ave, Don Imus Pediatric Ctr PC360 Bldg, Hackensack, NJ 07601; **Phone:** 201-996-5308; **Board Cert:** Pediatrics 2012; Pediatric Infectious Disease 2007; **Med School:** UCLA 1993; **Resid:** Pediatrics, UCSF Med Ctr 1996; **Fellow:** Clinical Pharmacology, UCSF Med Ctr 1997; Pediatric Infectious Disease, UCSF Med Ctr 1999; **Fac Appt:** Asst Prof Ped, UMDNJ-NJ Med Sch, Newark

Pediatric Nephrology

Lieberman, Kenneth V MD (PNep) - **Spec Exp:** Nephrotic Syndrome; Glomerulonephritis; Kidney Failure-Chronic; Hypertension; **Hospital:** Hackensack Univ Med Ctr (page 96); **Address:** 30 Prospect Ave, Hackensack, NJ 07601; **Phone:** 551-996-8228; **Board Cert:** Pediatrics 1981; Pediatric Nephrology 1982; **Med School:** Albert Einstein Coll Med 1977; **Resid:** Pediatrics, Mount Sinai Hosp 1979; **Fellow:** Nephrology, New York Hosp-Cornell 1981; **Fac Appt:** Prof Ped, UMDNJ-NJ Med Sch, Newark

Pediatric Otolaryngology

Respler, Don MD (PO) - **Spec Exp:** Airway Disorders; Sinus Disorders; Head & Neck Tumors; Sleep Disorders/Apnea; **Hospital:** Hackensack Univ Med Ctr (page 96), Valley Hosp (page 689); **Address:** 2 S Summit Ave, Hackensack, NJ 07601-1117; **Phone:** 201-996-9200; **Board Cert:** Otolaryngology 1986; **Med School:** Mount Sinai Sch Med 1981; **Resid:** Surgery, Beth Israel Med Ctr 1983; Otolaryngology, Univ Hosp-UMDNJ 1986; **Fellow:** Pediatric Otolaryngology, Chldns Hosp 1988; **Fac Appt:** Asst Clin Prof S, UMDNJ-NJ Med Sch, Newark

Samadi, Sharyar D MD (PO) - **Spec Exp:** Ear Infections; Sinusitis; Tonsil/Adenoid Disorders; Sleep Apnea; **Hospital:** Hackensack Univ Med Ctr (page 96); **Address:** 20 Prospect Ave, Ste 903, Hackensack, NJ 07601; **Phone:** 201-996-1505; **Board Cert:** Otolaryngology 2012; **Med School:** Johns Hopkins Univ 1996; **Resid:** Otolaryngology, Univ Penn Med Ctr 2001; **Fellow:** Pediatric Otolaryngology, Univ Penn Med Ctr 2003

Pediatric Pulmonology

Kanengiser, Steven MD (PPul) - **Spec Exp:** Asthma; Cough-Chronic; Pneumonia; **Hospital:** Valley Hosp (page 689), St. Joseph's Regl Med Ctr - Paterson; **Address:** 505 Goffle Rd, Ridgewood, NJ 07450-4027; **Phone:** 201-447-8026; **Board Cert:** Pediatrics 2003; Pediatric Pulmonology 2009; **Med School:** UCSF 1984; **Resid:** Pediatrics, Children's Hosp 1987; **Fellow:** Pediatric Pulmonology, Westchester Med Ctr 1994; **Fac Appt:** Asst Clin Prof Ped, Columbia P&S

Ngai, Pakkay MD (PPul) - **Spec Exp:** Asthma; Sleep Disorders; **Hospital:** Hackensack Univ Med Ctr (page 96); **Address:** 30 Prospect Ave WFAN Bldg Fl 3, Hackensack, NJ 07601; **Phone:** 201-996-5207; **Board Cert:** Pediatrics 2007; Pediatric Pulmonology 2010; Sleep Medicine 2007; **Med School:** NYU Sch Med 1995; **Resid:** Pediatrics, NY Presby/Columbia Med Ctr 1998; **Fellow:** Pediatric Pulmonology, NY Presby/Columbia Med Ctr 2002

Pediatric Rheumatology

Haines, Kathleen A MD (PRhu) - **Spec Exp:** Juvenile Arthritis; Lupus/SLE; Immune Deficiency; Scleroderma; **Hospital:** Hackensack Univ Med Ctr (page 96), NYU Langone Med Ctr (page 108); **Address:** 30 Prospect Ave Fl 3, Pediatric Ctr, Hackensack, NJ 07601; **Phone:** 551-996-5306; **Board Cert:** Pediatrics 1980; Allergy & Immunology 1981; Pediatric Rheumatology 2007; **Med School:** Albert Einstein Coll Med 1975; **Resid:** Pediatrics, New York Hosp 1977; **Fellow:** Allergy & Immunology, New York Hosp 1980; Rheumatology, NYU Med Sch 1982; **Fac Appt:** Assoc Prof Ped, UMDNJ-NJ Med Sch, Newark

Kimura, Yukiko MD (PRhu) - **Spec Exp:** Juvenile Arthritis; Lupus/SLE; Dermatomyositis; Vasculitis; **Hospital:** Hackensack Univ Med Ctr (page 96); **Address:** HUMC, Div Ped Rheumatology, 30 Prospect Ave WFAN Bldg - rm PC360, Hackensack, NJ 07601; **Phone:** 201-996-5306; **Board Cert:** Pediatrics 1987; Pediatric Rheumatology 2007; **Med School:** Albert Einstein Coll Med 1982; **Resid:** Pediatrics, Babies Hosp/Columbia Presby 1985; **Fellow:** Pediatric Rheumatology, Babies Hosp/Columbia Presby 1991; **Fac Appt:** Assoc Prof Ped, UMDNJ-NJ Med Sch, Newark

Pediatric Surgery

Alexander, Frederick MD (PS) - **Spec Exp:** Inflammatory Bowel Disease; Solid Tumors; Congenital Anomalies-Gastrointestinal; **Hospital:** Hackensack Univ Med Ctr (page 96); **Address:** 30 W Century Rd Fl 2 - Ste 235, Paramas, NJ 07652; **Phone:** 201-225-9440; **Board Cert:** Pediatric Surgery 1999; **Med School:** Columbia P&S 1977; **Resid:** Surgery, Brigham-Womens Hosp 1984; **Fellow:** Pediatric Surgery, Chldns Hosp 1986; **Fac Appt:** Clin Prof S

Friedman, David L MD (PS) - **Spec Exp:** Neonatal Surgery; Gastroesophageal Reflux Disease (GERD); Laparoscopic Surgery; **Hospital:** Valley Hosp (page 689), Hackensack Univ Med Ctr (page 96); **Address:** 30 W Century Rd, Ste 235, Paramus, NJ 07652-1433; **Phone:** 201-225-9440; **Board Cert:** Pediatric Surgery 2009; **Med School:** SUNY Downstate 1971; **Resid:** Surgery, Univ Hosp 1976; **Fellow:** Pediatric Surgery, Univ Hosp 1977; **Fac Appt:** Asst Prof S, Columbia P&S

Gandhi, Rajinder MD (PS) - **Spec Exp:** Gastrointestinal Surgery; Laparoscopic Surgery; Chest Wall Deformities; **Hospital:** Valley Hosp (page 689); **Address:** 30 W Century Rd, Ste 235, Paramus, NJ 07652; **Phone:** 201-225-9440; **Board Cert:** Surgery 1975; Pediatric Surgery 2007; **Med School:** Burma 1966; **Resid:** Surgery, Montefiore Med Ctr-Einstein Div 1974; Pediatric Surgery, Columbia-Presby Med Ctr 1977; **Fellow:** Gastroenterology, Columbia-Presby Med Ctr 1975; **Fac Appt:** Assoc Clin Prof S, Columbia P&S

Valda, Victor MD (PS) - **Spec Exp:** Congenital Anomalies; Cancer Surgery; **Hospital:** Hackensack Univ Med Ctr (page 96); **Address:** 30 W Century Rd, Ste 235, Paramus, NJ 07652; **Phone:** 201-225-9440; **Board Cert:** Surgery 1974; Pediatric Surgery 2007; **Med School:** Bolivia 1962; **Resid:** Surgery, Mt Zion Hosp 1968; Surgery, Maricopa Med Ctr 1972; **Fellow:** Pediatric Surgery, St Christopher's Hosp 1974

Pediatrics

Asnes, Russell MD (Ped) *PCP* - **Spec Exp:** Diagnostic Problems; **Hospital:** Englewood Hosp & Med Ctr, Hackensack Univ Med Ctr (page 96); **Address:** Tenafly Pediatrics, 32 Franklin St, Tenafly, NJ 07670; **Phone:** 201-569-2400; **Board Cert:** Pediatrics 2010; **Med School:** Tufts Univ 1963; **Resid:** Pediatrics, Johns Hopkins Hosp 1966; Pediatrics, Johns Hopkins Hosp 1969; **Fellow:** Neonatology, Babies Hosp/Columbia Univ 1970; **Fac Appt:** Clin Prof Ped, Columbia P&S

Buchalter, Maury MD (Ped) *PCP* - **Spec Exp:** Asthma; Infectious Disease; ADD/ADHD; **Hospital:** Hackensack Univ Med Ctr (page 96), Englewood Hosp & Med Ctr; **Address:** 301 Bridge Plaza N, Fort Lee, NJ 07670; **Phone:** 201-592-8787; **Board Cert:** Pediatrics 2010; **Med School:** Mount Sinai Sch Med 1984; **Resid:** Pediatrics, Mt Sinai Hosp 1987; **Fellow:** Infectious Disease, Chldns Hosp 1988

Hages, Harry A MD (Ped) *PCP* - **Hospital:** Englewood Hosp & Med Ctr, Valley Hosp (page 689); **Address:** 215 Old Tappan Rd, Old Tappan, NJ 07675-7000; **Phone:** 201-666-1001; **Board Cert:** Pediatrics 1973; **Med School:** Univ Pittsburgh 1966; **Resid:** Pediatrics, Chldns Hosp 1968; Pediatrics, New York Hosp 1969

Harlow, Paul J MD (Ped) *PCP* - **Spec Exp:** Anemia; Bleeding/Coagulation Disorders; **Hospital:** Hackensack Univ Med Ctr (page 96), Valley Hosp (page 689); **Address:** 90 Prospect Ave, Ste 1A, Hackensack, NJ 07601; **Phone:** 201-342-4001 x107; **Board Cert:** Pediatrics 1979; Pediatric Hematology-Oncology 1980; **Med School:** SUNY Hlth Sci Ctr 1974; **Resid:** Pediatrics, Jacobi Med Ctr 1977; **Fellow:** Pediatric Hematology-Oncology, Children's Hosp 1979

Hyatt, Alexander C MD (Ped) *PCP* - **Hospital:** Englewood Hosp & Med Ctr, Mount Sinai Med Ctr (page 102); **Address:** Englewood Hosp, Dept Peds, 350 Engle St, Englewood, NJ 07631; **Phone:** 201-894-3158; **Board Cert:** Pediatrics 1980; Infectious Disease 2009; **Med School:** Mount Sinai Sch Med 1975; **Resid:** Pediatrics, Johns Hopkins Hosp 1978; **Fellow:** Infectious Disease, Mount Sinai Med Ctr 1979; Pediatric Pulmonology, Johns Hopkins Hosp 1980; **Fac Appt:** Assoc Prof Ped, Mount Sinai Sch Med

Kanter, Alan MD (Ped) *PCP* - **Spec Exp:** ADD/ADHD; Autism; **Hospital:** Englewood Hosp & Med Ctr, Morgan Stanley Children's Hosp of NY-Presby, NY (page 104); **Address:** 704 Palisade Ave, Teaneck, NJ 07666-3198; **Phone:** 201-836-4301; **Board Cert:** Pediatrics 1977; **Med School:** Albert Einstein Coll Med 1970; **Resid:** Pediatrics, St Christopher's Hosp 1971; Pediatrics, Montefiore Med Ctr 1975; **Fac Appt:** Assoc Clin Prof Ped, Columbia P&S

Kolsky, Neil MD (Ped) *PCP* - **Hospital:** Holy Name Med Ctr (page 688), Hackensack Univ Med Ctr (page 96); **Address:** 870 Palisade Ave, Teaneck, NJ 07666-3419; **Phone:** 201-692-1661; **Board Cert:** Pediatrics 1972; **Med School:** UMDNJ-NJ Med Sch, Newark 1966; **Resid:** Pediatrics, Johns Hopkins Hosp 1969

Kushner, Susan C MD (Ped) *PCP* - **Spec Exp:** Atopic Dermatitis; Allergic Rhinitis; Asthma; Otitis Media; **Hospital:** Hackensack Univ Med Ctr (page 96), Valley Hosp (page 689); **Address:** Forrest Pediatrics, 299 Forrest Ave Fl 3, Paramus, NJ 07652; **Phone:** 201-267-0888; **Board Cert:** Pediatrics 2011; **Med School:** SUNY Upstate Med Univ 1986; **Resid:** Pediatrics, LI Jewish Med Ctr 1989

Namerow, David MD (Ped) *PCP* - **Spec Exp:** Behavioral Disorders; Adolescent Medicine; **Hospital:** Valley Hosp (page 689), St. Joseph's Regl Med Ctr - Paterson; **Address:** 2020 Fair Lawn Ave, Fair Lawn, NJ 07410-2319; **Phone:** 201-791-4545; **Board Cert:** Pediatrics 1977; **Med School:** Univ Louisville Sch Med 1972; **Resid:** Pediatrics, Children's Hosp 1975; **Fellow:** Adolescent Medicine, Univ MD Hosp 1977; **Fac Appt:** Asst Clin Prof Ped, NY Med Coll

O'Brien, Daryl H MD (Ped) *PCP* - **Hospital:** Valley Hosp (page 689); **Address:** Broadway Pediatric Assocs, 336 Center Ave, Westwood, NJ 07675; **Phone:** 201-664-7444; **Board Cert:** Pediatrics 1986; **Med School:** Dartmouth Med Sch 1979; **Resid:** Pediatrics, Duke Univ Med Ctr 1982

Schuss, Steven A MD (Ped) *PCP* - **Hospital:** Englewood Hosp & Med Ctr, Hackensack Univ Med Ctr (page 96); **Address:** 197 Cedar Ln, Teaneck, NJ 07666-4301; **Phone:** 201-836-7171; **Board Cert:** Pediatrics 1986; **Med School:** Albert Einstein Coll Med 1979; **Resid:** Pediatrics, Montefiore Med Ctr 1983; **Fac Appt:** Asst Clin Prof Ped, Albert Einstein Coll Med

Sugarman, Lynn B MD (Ped) *PCP* - **Hospital:** Englewood Hosp & Med Ctr, Hackensack Univ Med Ctr (page 96); **Address:** Tenafly Pediatrics, 32 Franklin St, Tenafly, NJ 07670-2005; **Phone:** 201-569-2400; **Board Cert:** Pediatrics 2010; **Med School:** Harvard Med Sch 1977; **Resid:** Pediatrics, Bronx Muni Hos 1981; **Fellow:** Pediatric Critical Care Medicine, Bronx Muni Hosp 1983; **Fac Appt:** Assoc Clin Prof Ped, Columbia P&S

Weiss, Christopher A DO (Ped) - **Hospital:** Hackensack Univ Med Ctr (page 96), Englewood Hosp & Med Ctr; **Address:** Washington Ave Pediatrics, 95 N Washington Ave, Bergenfield, NJ 07621; **Phone:** 201-384-0300; **Board Cert:** Pediatrics 2008; **Med School:** Nova SE Univ, Coll Osteo Med 1996; **Resid:** Pediatrics, Long Island Jewish Med Ctr 2001

Wisotsky, David H MD (Ped) *PCP* - **Hospital:** Englewood Hosp & Med Ctr, Hackensack Univ Med Ctr (page 96); **Address:** Tenafly Pediatrics, 32 Franklin St, Tenafly, NJ 07670; **Phone:** 201-569-2400; **Board Cert:** Pediatrics 2010; **Med School:** Albert Einstein Coll Med 1974; **Resid:** Pediatrics, Bronx Muni Hosp 1978; **Fac Appt:** Asst Clin Prof Ped, Columbia P&S

Physical Medicine & Rehabilitation

Averill, Allison MD (PMR) - **Spec Exp:** Neuro-Rehabilitation; Brain Injury Rehabilitation; Stroke Rehabilitation; **Hospital:** Kessler Inst for Rehab - Saddle Brook; **Address:** Kessler Institute for Rehab, Saddle Brook Campus, 300 Market St, Saddle Brook, NJ 07663; **Phone:** 201-368-6000; **Board Cert:** Physical Medicine & Rehabilitation 2003; **Med School:** UMDNJ-RW Johnson Med Sch 1988; **Resid:** Physical Medicine & Rehabilitation, Univ Penn Hosp 1992; **Fac Appt:** Asst Prof PMR, UMDNJ-NJ Med Sch, Newark

Liss, Donald MD (PMR) - **Spec Exp:** Pain-Back; Sports Medicine; Osteoarthritis; **Hospital:** NY-Presby/Columbia Univ Med Ctr, NY (page 104), Englewood Hosp & Med Ctr; **Address:** 500 Grand Ave, Englewood, NJ 07631-2920; **Phone:** 201-567-2277; **Board Cert:** Physical Medicine & Rehabilitation 1984; **Med School:** Wayne State Univ 1979; **Resid:** Physical Medicine & Rehabilitation, Columbia-Presby Med Ctr 1982; **Fac Appt:** Assoc Clin Prof PMR, Columbia P&S

Liss, Howard MD (PMR) - **Hospital:** NY-Presby/Columbia Univ Med Ctr, NY (page 104), Englewood Hosp & Med Ctr; **Address:** Physical Medicine & Rehabilitation Ctr, 500 Grand Ave Fl 1, Englewood, NJ 07631-2920; **Phone:** 201-567-2277; **Board Cert:** Physical Medicine & Rehabilitation 1982; **Med School:** Wayne State Univ 1977; **Resid:** Physical Medicine & Rehabilitation, NY-Presby/Columbia Univ Med Ctr 1981; **Fac Appt:** Asst Clin Prof PMR, Columbia P&S

Zimmerman, Jerald R MD (PMR) - **Spec Exp:** Post Polio Syndrome/Rehabilitation; Musculoskeletal Disorders; Pain Management; **Hospital:** Englewood Hosp & Med Ctr, Holy Name Med Ctr (page 688); **Address:** 370 Grand Ave, Ste 102, Englewood, NJ 07631; **Phone:** 201-567-3370; **Board Cert:** Physical Medicine & Rehabilitation 1989; **Med School:** Univ IL Coll Med 1982; **Resid:** Orthopaedic Surgery, Univ Minn Med Ctr 1985; **Fellow:** Physical Medicine & Rehabilitation, Columbia-Presby Med Ctr 1988; **Fac Appt:** Assoc Prof PMR, UMDNJ-NJ Med Sch, Newark

Plastic Surgery

Bikoff, David J MD (PlS) - **Spec Exp:** Cosmetic Surgery-Breast; Breast Reconstruction; Eyelid Surgery; Hand Surgery; **Hospital:** Hackensack Univ Med Ctr (page 96); **Address:** 146 Rte 17 N, Fl 3, Hackensack, NJ 07601; **Phone:** 201-488-8584; **Board Cert:** Plastic Surgery 1980; **Med School:** SUNY Downstate 1973; **Resid:** Surgery, Kings Co Hosp 1977; Plastic Surgery, Kings Co Hosp 1979; **Fellow:** Hand Surgery, Kings Co Hosp 1980

Boss Jr, William K MD (PlS) - **Spec Exp:** Cosmetic & Reconstructive Surgery; **Hospital:** Hackensack Univ Med Ctr (page 96); **Address:** Cosmetic Surgery & Rejuvenation Ctr, 385 Prospect Ave Fl 2, Hackensack, NJ 07601; **Phone:** 201-488-1035; **Board Cert:** Plastic Surgery 1984; **Med School:** UMDNJ-NJ Med Sch, Newark 1975; **Resid:** Surgery, UMDNJ Med Ctr 1980; Plastic Surgery, Yale-New Haven Hosp 1982; **Fellow:** Hand & Microvascular Surgery, RK Davies Med Ctr 1983; **Fac Appt:** Asst Clin Prof PlS, UMDNJ-Univ Med Dent NJ

D'Amico, Richard A MD (PlS) - **Spec Exp:** Cosmetic Surgery-Face; Liposuction & Body Contouring; Breast Augmentation; Facial Rejuvenation; **Hospital:** Englewood Hosp & Med Ctr, Holy Name Med Ctr (page 688); **Address:** 180 N Dean St, Ste 3N, Englewood, NJ 07631-2534; **Phone:** 201-567-9595; **Board Cert:** Plastic Surgery 1986; **Med School:** NYU Sch Med 1976; **Resid:** Surgery, Tulsa Med Ctr 1979; Surgery, Strong Meml Hosp 1981; **Fellow:** Plastic/Reconstructive Surgery, Columbia-Presby Med Ctr 1983; **Fac Appt:** Asst Clin Prof PlS, Mount Sinai Sch Med

Lipson, David E MD (PlS) - **Spec Exp:** Breast Augmentation; Body Contouring; Facial Rejuvenation; **Hospital:** Valley Hosp (page 689); **Address:** 2300 Route 208 South, Fair Lawn, NJ 07410; **Phone:** 201-797-7770; **Board Cert:** Plastic Surgery 1981; **Med School:** Albert Einstein Coll Med 1971; **Resid:** Surgery, Bellevue/NYU Med Ctr 1976; Plastic Surgery, Bellevue/NYU Med Ctr 1978

Ponamgi, Suri MD (PlS) - **Spec Exp:** Cosmetic & Reconstructive Surgery; **Hospital:** Palisades Med Ctr, Holy Name Med Ctr (page 688); **Address:** 1101 Palisades Ave, Fort Lee, NJ 07024-6329; **Phone:** 201-224-8831; **Board Cert:** Plastic Surgery 1984; **Med School:** India 1970; **Resid:** Surgery, Bronx Lebonon Hosp 1979; Plastic Surgery, NY Methodist Hosp 1982; **Fellow:** Surgery, Bronx Lebonon Hosp 1980

Sternschein, Michael J MD (PlS) - **Spec Exp:** Cosmetic Surgery-Face & Breast; Liposuction & Body Contouring; Laser Surgery; **Hospital:** Hackensack Univ Med Ctr (page 96), Valley Hosp (page 689); **Address:** 1200 E Ridgewood Ave, Fl 2 W Wing, Ridgewood, NJ 07450; **Phone:** 201-444-1188; **Board Cert:** Plastic Surgery 1985; **Med School:** Columbia P&S 1976; **Resid:** Surgery, Columbia-Presby Med Ctr 1980; Plastic Surgery, Columbia-Presby Med Ctr 1982; **Fellow:** Microsurgery, Columbia-Presby Med Ctr 1982

Zubowski, Robert I MD (PlS) - **Spec Exp:** Breast Augmentation; Liposuction & Body Contouring; Cosmetic Surgery-Face; **Hospital:** Valley Hosp (page 689); **Address:** 1 Sears Drive, Paramus, NJ 07652; **Phone:** 201-261-7550; **Board Cert:** Plastic Surgery 2003; **Med School:** Mexico 1983; **Resid:** Surgery, Westchester Co Med Ctr 1991; **Fellow:** Plastic Surgery, Cleveland Clinic 1994; **Fac Appt:** Asst Clin Prof S, NY Med Coll

Psychiatry

Chertoff, Harvey R MD (Psyc) - **Spec Exp:** Anxiety & Mood Disorders; Psychoanalysis; **Hospital:** Englewood Hosp & Med Ctr, NY-Presby/Columbia Univ Med Ctr, NY (page 104); **Address:** 205 Engle St, Englewood, NJ 07631-2409; **Phone:** 201-567-4970; **Board Cert:** Psychiatry 1978; **Med School:** Albert Einstein Coll Med 1966; **Resid:** Psychiatry, Columbia-Presby Med Ctr 1970; **Fellow:** Psychoanalysis, Columbia-Psychoanalytic Ctr 1976; **Fac Appt:** Asst Clin Prof Psyc, Columbia P&S

Farkas, Edward MD (Psyc) - **Spec Exp:** Depression in the Elderly; Psychotherapy-Men's Issues; Panic Disorder; **Hospital:** Holy Name Med Ctr (page 688); **Address:** 175 Cedar Ln, Ste A, Teaneck, NJ 07666-4315; **Phone:** 201-692-8354; **Board Cert:** Psychiatry 1988; **Med School:** Italy 1979; **Resid:** Psychiatry, Bronx Lebanon Hosp 1981; Psychiatry, St Luke's-Roosevelt Hosp Ctr 1983; **Fellow:** Psychiatry, William Allison White Inst 1983

Gurland, Frances Effron MD (Psyc) - **Spec Exp:** Eating Disorders; ADD/ADHD; **Address:** 216 Engle St, Englewood, NJ 07631; **Phone:** 201-568-4066; **Board Cert:** Psychiatry 2005; **Med School:** SUNY Hlth Sci Ctr 1989; **Resid:** Psychiatry, St Lukes-Roosevelt Hosp Ctr 1991; **Fellow:** Child & Adolescent Psychiatry, Mount Sinai Hosp 1994; **Fac Appt:** Asst Clin Prof Psyc, Mount Sinai Sch Med

Narula, Amarjot S MD (Psyc) - **Spec Exp:** Geriatric Psychiatry; Mood Disorders; **Hospital:** Valley Hosp (page 689), Bergen Regl Med Ctr; **Address:** 65 N Maple Ave, Ridgewood, NJ 07450-1600; **Phone:** 201-670-4423; **Board Cert:** Psychiatry 1992; Geriatric Psychiatry 2007; **Med School:** India 1979; **Resid:** Psychiatry, Middletown Psychiatric Ctr 1988; **Fellow:** Psychiatry, Metropolitan Hosp 1989

Rosenfeld, David N MD (Psyc) - **Spec Exp:** Mood Disorders; Anxiety Disorders; Personality Disorders; Geriatric Psychiatry; **Hospital:** Valley Hosp (page 689); **Address:** 265 Ackerman Ave, Ste 202, Ridgewood, NJ 07450-4200; **Phone:** 201-447-5630; **Board Cert:** Psychiatry 2005; **Med School:** UMDNJ-RW Johnson Med Sch 1988; **Resid:** Psychiatry, Mount Sinai Sch Med 1990; Psychiatry, Bergen Pines Co 1994

Samuels, Steven MD (Psyc) - **Spec Exp:** Dementia; Depression; Geriatric Psychiatry; **Hospital:** Englewood Hosp & Med Ctr; **Address:** Psyc Med Consultants New Jersey, 60 W Ridgefield Ave Fl 3, Ridgefield, NJ 07451; **Phone:** 201-681-2915; **Board Cert:** Psychiatry 2004; Geriatric Psychiatry 2006; **Med School:** SUNY Buffalo 1989; **Resid:** Psychiatry, St Vincent's Hosp & Med Ctr 1993; **Fellow:** Geriatric Psychiatry, Hosp Univ Penn 1995; **Fac Appt:** Asst Prof Psyc, Mount Sinai Sch Med

Shah, Pritesh J MD (Psyc) - **Spec Exp:** Geriatric Psychiatry; **Hospital:** Holy Name Med Ctr (page 688); **Address:** 354 Old Hook Rd, Ste 102, Westwood, NJ 07675; **Phone:** 201-358-0400; **Board Cert:** Psychiatry 2004; **Med School:** India 1985; **Resid:** Psychiatry, Bergen Regl Med Ctr 1991; **Fellow:** Psychiatry, Bergen Regl Med Ctr 1998

Wagle, Sharad MD (Psyc) - **Spec Exp:** Anxiety Disorders; Forensic Psychiatry; Geriatric Psychiatry; **Hospital:** Holy Name Med Ctr (page 688); **Address:** 718 Teaneck Rd, Teaneck, NJ 07666; **Phone:** 201-833-3291; **Board Cert:** Psychiatry 2006; **Med School:** India 1971; **Resid:** Psychiatry, Hackensack Univ Med Ctr 1976; Psychiatry, Albert Einstein Coll Med 1978; **Fellow:** Child & Adolescent Psychiatry, Psychoanalytic Inst 1978

Zaidi, Syed A R MD (Psyc) - **Spec Exp:** Addiction Psychiatry; **Hospital:** Holy Name Med Ctr (page 688); **Address:** 294 State St, Ste 2, Hackensack, NJ 07601; **Phone:** 201-342-4004; **Board Cert:** Psychiatry 2009; **Med School:** Pakistan 1984; **Resid:** Psychiatry, Temple Univ Hosp 1996; **Fellow:** Geriatric Psychiatry, Mount Sinai Med Ctr 1997

Pulmonary Disease

Benoff, Brian A MD (Pul) - **Hospital:** Englewood Hosp & Med Ctr; **Address:** Bergen Pulmonary & Sleep Specialists, 180 N Dean St, Ste 2N, Englewood, NJ 07631; **Phone:** 201-871-8366; **Board Cert:** Internal Medicine 2007; Pulmonary Disease 2009; Critical Care Medicine 2010; Sleep Medicine 2011; **Med School:** Albert Einstein Coll Med 1994; **Resid:** Internal Medicine, Long Island Jewish Med Ctr 1997; **Fellow:** Pulmonary Critical Care Medicine, Long Island Jewish Med Ctr 2000; **Fac Appt:** Asst Prof Med, Albert Einstein Coll Med

Brauntuch, Glenn R MD (Pul) - **Spec Exp:** Chronic Obstructive Lung Disease (COPD); Asthma; Lung Cancer; **Hospital:** Englewood Hosp & Med Ctr, Holy Name Med Ctr (page 688); **Address:** 180 Engle St, Englewood, NJ 07631-2507; **Phone:** 201-568-8010; **Board Cert:** Internal Medicine 1981; Pulmonary Disease 1984; **Med School:** Columbia P&S 1978; **Resid:** Internal Medicine, St Lukes-Roosevelt Hosp 1981; **Fellow:** Pulmonary Disease, NYU Med Ctr 1984

Bromberg, Assia MD (Pul) - **Spec Exp:** Asthma; Emphysema; Women's Health; **Hospital:** Valley Hosp (page 689); **Address:** 19-20 Fair Lawn Ave, Fairlawn, NJ 07410; **Phone:** 201-794-1963; **Board Cert:** Internal Medicine 1989; Pulmonary Disease 2004; **Med School:** Israel 1974; **Resid:** Anesthesiology, Chaim Sheba Med Ctr 1981; Internal Medicine, Englewood Hosp 1989; **Fellow:** Pulmonary Disease, Bellevue-NYU Med Ctr 1992; **Fac Appt:** Asst Prof Med, UMDNJ-Univ Med Dent NJ

Cole, Randolph P MD (Pul) - **Spec Exp:** Critical Care; **Hospital:** Holy Name Med Ctr (page 688); **Address:** 718 Teaneck Rd, Teaneck, NJ 07666; **Phone:** 201-833-3342; **Board Cert:** Internal Medicine 1976; Pulmonary Disease 1978; Critical Care Medicine 2007; **Med School:** SUNY Downstate 1973; **Resid:** Internal Medicine, Kings Co Hosp 1975; **Fellow:** Pulmonary Disease, Columbia-Presby Med Ctr 1979

Engler, Mitchell S MD (Pul) - **Spec Exp:** Pulmonary Disease; Critical Care; Sleep Disorders; **Hospital:** Holy Name Med Ctr (page 688), Englewood Hosp & Med Ctr; **Address:** 180 Engle St, Englewood, NJ 07631-2507; **Phone:** 201-568-8010; **Board Cert:** Internal Medicine 1981; Pulmonary Disease 1988; Sleep Medicine 2003; **Med School:** Boston Univ 1978; **Resid:** Internal Medicine, St Lukes Hosp 1981; **Fellow:** Pulmonary Disease, St Lukes Hosp 1983

Levine, Selwyn E MD (Pul) - **Spec Exp:** Chronic Obstructive Lung Disease (COPD); Lung Cancer; Asthma; Pneumonia; **Hospital:** Holy Name Med Ctr (page 688), Englewood Hosp & Med Ctr; **Address:** Pulmonary Assocs of Northern NJ, 200 Grand Ave, Ste 102, Englewood, NJ 07631; **Phone:** 201-871-3636; **Board Cert:** Internal Medicine 1985; Pulmonary Disease 1988; **Med School:** NYU Sch Med 1982; **Resid:** Internal Medicine, Bellevue Hosp/NYU Med Ctr 1985; **Fellow:** Pulmonary Disease, Albert Einstein Coll Med 1987

Malovany, Robert MD (Pul) - **Spec Exp:** Exercise Physiology; Interventional Pulmonology; **Hospital:** Englewood Hosp & Med Ctr; **Address:** 180 Engle St, Englewood, NJ 07631-2507; **Phone:** 201-568-8010; **Board Cert:** Internal Medicine 1973; Pulmonary Disease 1976; **Med School:** Jefferson Med Coll 1970; **Resid:** Internal Medicine, Montefiore Med Ctr 1973; **Fellow:** Pulmonary Disease, Montefiore Med Ctr 1975; **Fac Appt:** Asst Clin Prof Med, Mount Sinai Sch Med

Polkow, Melvin MD (Pul) - **Spec Exp:** Asthma; Sarcoidosis; Pulmonary Fibrosis; Lung Cancer; **Hospital:** Hackensack Univ Med Ctr (page 96); **Address:** 211 Essex St, Ste 302, Hackensack, NJ 07601; **Phone:** 201-498-1311; **Board Cert:** Internal Medicine 1980; Pulmonary Disease 1982; Critical Care Medicine 2007; **Med School:** SUNY Downstate 1977; **Resid:** Internal Medicine, Lenox Hill Hosp 1980; **Fellow:** Pulmonary Critical Care Medicine, Univ Hosp 1982; **Fac Appt:** Asst Clin Prof Med, UMDNJ-NJ Med Sch, Newark

Simon, Clifford J MD (Pul) - **Spec Exp:** Asthma; Lung Cancer; **Hospital:** Englewood Hosp & Med Ctr, Holy Name Med Ctr (page 688); **Address:** 180 Engle St, Englewood, NJ 07631-2507; **Phone:** 201-567-2050; **Board Cert:** Internal Medicine 1976; Pulmonary Disease 1980; **Med School:** Cornell Univ-Weill Med Coll 1973; **Resid:** Internal Medicine, Dartmouth Affil Hosps 1975; **Fellow:** Pulmonary Disease, Bellevue Hosp 1977

Radiation Oncology

Dubin, David MD (RadRO) - **Spec Exp:** Breast Cancer; Brachytherapy; Prostate Cancer; **Hospital:** Englewood Hosp & Med Ctr; **Address:** Englewood Hosp, Dept Radiation Oncology, 350 Engle St, Englewood, NJ 07631-1808; **Phone:** 201-894-3125; **Board Cert:** Radiation Oncology 1991; **Med School:** Albert Einstein Coll Med 1986; **Resid:** Radiation Oncology, St Barnabas Hosp 1990

Gejerman, Glen MD (RadRO) - **Spec Exp:** Prostate Cancer; Intensity Modulated Radiotherapy (IMRT); Brachytherapy; Urologic Cancer; **Hospital:** Hackensack Univ Med Ctr (page 96); **Address:** Hackensack University Medical Center, 92 Second St, Hackensack, NJ 07601; **Phone:** 201-996-2464; **Board Cert:** Radiation Oncology 2006; **Med School:** UMDNJ-NJ Med Sch, Newark 1990; **Resid:** Radiation Oncology, Montefiore Med Ctr 1995; **Fac Appt:** Asst Clin Prof RadRO, Albert Einstein Coll Med

Ingenito, Anthony C MD (RadRO) - **Spec Exp:** Brain Tumors; Head & Neck Cancer; Lymphoma; Gastrointestinal Cancer; **Hospital:** Hackensack Univ Med Ctr (page 96); **Address:** Dept Radiation Oncology, 92 Second St, Hackensack, NJ 07601; **Phone:** 201-996-2210; **Board Cert:** Radiation Oncology 2008; **Med School:** UMDNJ-NJ Med Sch, Newark 1991; **Resid:** Radiation Oncology, NY-Presby Hosp 1996

Vialotti, Charles P MD (RadRO) - **Spec Exp:** Lung Cancer; **Hospital:** Holy Name Med Ctr (page 688), St. Mary's Hosp - Passaic; **Address:** Holy Name Med Ctr, Regl Cancer Ctr, Rad Onc Dept, 718 Teaneck Rd, Teaneck, NJ 07666; **Phone:** 201-541-5900; **Board Cert:** Therapeutic Radiology 1975; **Med School:** NY Med Coll 1971; **Resid:** Radiology, NYU Med Ctr 1974; **Fellow:** Therapeutic Radiology, NY Med Ctr 1975

Reproductive Endocrinology

Lesorgen, Philip R MD (RE) - **Spec Exp:** Infertility; Infertility-IVF; **Hospital:** Englewood Hosp & Med Ctr, Holy Name Med Ctr (page 688); **Address:** 106 Grand Ave, Ste 400, Englewood, NJ 07631-3570; **Phone:** 201-569-6979; **Board Cert:** Obstetrics & Gynecology 1984; **Med School:** Boston Univ 1977; **Resid:** Obstetrics & Gynecology, LI Jewish Med Ctr 1981; **Fellow:** Reproductive Endocrinology, Thomas Jefferson Univ Hosp 1983; **Fac Appt:** Asst Clin Prof ObG, Seton Hall Univ Sch Hlth & Med Scis

McGovern, Peter G MD (RE) - **Spec Exp:** Infertility-IVF; Fertility Preservation in Cancer; **Hospital:** Univ Hosp-UMDNJ—Newark, Hackensack Univ Med Ctr (page 96); **Address:** University Reproductive Assocs, 214 Terrace Ave, Hasbrouck Heights, NJ 07604; **Phone:** 201-288-6330; **Board Cert:** Obstetrics & Gynecology 2011; Reproductive Endocrinology/Infertility 2011; **Med School:** NYU Sch Med 1986; **Resid:** Obstetrics & Gynecology, NYU-Bellevue Hosp Ctr 1990; **Fellow:** Reproductive Endocrinology, UMDNJ-Newark 1992; **Fac Appt:** Assoc Prof ObG, UMDNJ-NJ Med Sch, Newark

Miller, Jane E MD (RE) - **Spec Exp:** Infertility-IVF; Laparoscopic Surgery; Hysteroscopic Surgery; **Hospital:** Holy Name Med Ctr (page 688); **Address:** North Hudson IVF Ctr, 385 Sylvan Ave, Englewood Cliffs, NJ 07632; **Phone:** 201-871-1999; **Board Cert:** Obstetrics & Gynecology 2011; Reproductive Endocrinology/Infertility 2011; **Med School:** SUNY Downstate 1978; **Resid:** Obstetrics & Gynecology, Havard Univ Affil Hosp 1983; Obstetrics & Gynecology, Univ Tennessee Med Ctr 1984; **Fellow:** Reproductive Endocrinology, SUNY Downstate Med Ctr 1989

Navot, Daniel MD (RE) - **Spec Exp:** Infertility-IVF; **Hospital:** Englewood Hosp & Med Ctr, Valley Hosp (page 689); **Address:** 400 Old Hook Rd, Fl 2nd, rm 2-3, Westwood, NJ 07675-2732; **Phone:** 201-666-4200; **Board Cert:** Obstetrics & Gynecology 2011; Reproductive Endocrinology 2011; **Med School:** Israel 1978; **Resid:** Obstetrics & Gynecology, Hassadah Hosp 1983; **Fellow:** Reproductive Endocrinology, Jones Inst 1987; **Fac Appt:** Prof ObG, NY Med Coll

Weiss, Gerson MD (RE) - **Spec Exp:** Infertility; Menopause Problems; **Hospital:** Hackensack Univ Med Ctr (page 96), Univ Hosp-UMDNJ—Newark; **Address:** 214 Terrace Ave, Hasbrouck Heights, NJ 07604-1815; **Phone:** 201-288-6330; **Board Cert:** Obstetrics & Gynecology 2011; Reproductive Endocrinology 2011; **Med School:** NYU Sch Med 1964; **Resid:** Obstetrics & Gynecology, Bellevue Hosp Ctr 1969; **Fellow:** Reproductive Endocrinology, Univ Pittsburgh 1973; **Fac Appt:** Prof ObG, UMDNJ-NJ Med Sch, Newark

Rheumatology

Gonter, Neil J MD (Rhu) - **Spec Exp:** Rheumatoid Arthritis; Gout; Osteoporosis; **Hospital:** Hackensack Univ Med Ctr (page 96), Holy Name Med Ctr (page 688); **Address:** Rheumatology Associates of North Jersey, 1415 Queen Anne Rd, Teaneck, NJ 07666; **Phone:** 201-837-7788; **Board Cert:** Rheumatology 2003; **Med School:** SUNY Upstate Med Univ 1998; **Resid:** Internal Medicine, UMDNJ Univ Hosp 2001; **Fellow:** Rheumatology, SUNY Downstate Med Ctr 2003; **Fac Appt:** Asst Prof Med, Columbia P&S

Guma, Michael DO (Rhu) - **Spec Exp:** Arthritis; Autoimmune Disease; Inflammatory Muscle Disease; Osteoporosis; **Hospital:** Saint Michael's Med Ctr; **Address:** North Jersey Rheumatology Assocs, 312 Belleville Tpke, Ste 3A, North Arlington, NJ 07031; **Phone:** 201-998-2800; **Board Cert:** Internal Medicine 2003; Rheumatology 2004; **Med School:** Kirksville Coll Osteo Med 1989; **Resid:** Internal Medicine, St Michaels Med Ctr 1992; **Fellow:** Rheumatology, St Michaels Med Ctr 1994; **Fac Appt:** Asst Clin Prof Med, Univ New Eng Coll Osteo Med

Kopelman, Rima G MD (Rhu) - **Spec Exp:** Rheumatoid Arthritis; Lupus/SLE; Vasculitis; **Hospital:** Valley Hosp (page 689), NY-Presby/Columbia Univ Med Ctr, NY (page 104); **Address:** 301 Godwin Ave, Midland Park, NJ 07432-1544; **Phone:** 201-444-4526; **Board Cert:** Internal Medicine 1980; Rheumatology 1984; **Med School:** Columbia P&S 1977; **Resid:** Internal Medicine, Columbia-Presby Med Ctr 1981; **Fellow:** Rheumatology, Columbia-Presby Med Ctr 1983; **Fac Appt:** Asst Prof Med, Columbia P&S

Leibowitz, Evan H MD (Rhu) - **Spec Exp:** Rheumatoid Arthritis; Gout; Lupus/SLE; **Hospital:** Valley Hosp (page 689); **Address:** Prospect Medical Office, 301 Godwin Ave, Midland Park, NJ 07432; **Phone:** 201-444-4526; **Board Cert:** Rheumatology 2011; **Med School:** UMDNJ-NJ Med Sch, Newark 1996; **Resid:** Internal Medicine, New York Hosp 1999; **Fellow:** Rheumatology, Hosp for Special Surg 2001

Marcus, Ralph E MD (Rhu) - **Spec Exp:** Rheumatoid Arthritis; Osteoporosis; Lupus/SLE; Scleroderma; **Hospital:** Holy Name Med Ctr (page 688), Hackensack Univ Med Ctr (page 96); **Address:** 1415 Queen Anne Rd, Ste 102, Teaneck, NJ 07666-3521; **Phone:** 201-837-7788; **Board Cert:** Internal Medicine 1975; Rheumatology 1976; **Med School:** Albert Einstein Coll Med 1969; **Resid:** Internal Medicine, Mount Sinai Hosp 1974; **Fellow:** Rheumatology, Natl Inst Hlth 1972; Rheumatology, Hosp Special Surg 1976; **Fac Appt:** Assoc Clin Prof Med, UMDNJ-RW Johnson Med Sch

Salem, Noel MD (Rhu) - **Hospital:** Englewood Hosp & Med Ctr; **Address:** 285 Engle St, Englewood, NJ 07631-2406; **Phone:** 201-871-0223; **Board Cert:** Internal Medicine 1976; Rheumatology 1998; Geriatric Medicine 2004; **Med School:** SUNY Buffalo 1972; **Resid:** Internal Medicine, US Public Hlth Svc Hosp 1974; **Fellow:** Rheumatology, Columbia-Presby 1976; **Fac Appt:** Asst Prof Med, Mount Sinai Sch Med

Zalkowitz, Alan MD (Rhu) - **Spec Exp:** Rheumatoid Arthritis; Gout; Collagen Vascular Disorders; **Hospital:** Valley Hosp (page 689); **Address:** 31-00 Broadway, Fl 2nd, Fair Lawn, NJ 07410-2331; **Phone:** 201-796-2255; **Board Cert:** Internal Medicine 1977; Rheumatology 1982; **Med School:** Belgium 1970; **Resid:** Internal Medicine, Yale New Haven Hosp 1971; Internal Medicine, Stamford Hosp 1972; **Fellow:** Rheumatology, Mount Sinai Hosp 1974

Sports Medicine

Gross, Michael L MD (SM) - **Spec Exp:** Shoulder & Knee Injuries; **Hospital:** Hackensack Univ Med Ctr (page 96); **Address:** 25 Prospect Ave, Hackensack, NJ 07601; **Phone:** 201-343-2277; **Board Cert:** Orthopaedic Surgery 2012; Orthopaedic Sports Medicine 2012; **Med School:** NYU Sch Med 1983; **Resid:** Orthopaedic Surgery, Montefiore Med Ctr 1988; **Fellow:** Sports Medicine, UCLA Med Ctr 1989

Savatsky, Gary MD (SM) - **Spec Exp:** Shoulder & Knee Injuries; **Hospital:** Hackensack Univ Med Ctr (page 96); **Address:** 2 Forest Ave, Paramus, NJ 07652; **Phone:** 201-587-1111; **Board Cert:** Orthopaedic Surgery 2007; **Med School:** Columbia P&S 1975; **Resid:** Surgery, St Luke's-Roosevelt Hosp Ctr 1978; Orthopaedic Surgery, Hosp for Special Surg 1983; **Fellow:** Orthopaedic Surgery, Hosp for Special Surg 1979

Surgery

Ahlborn, Thomas N MD (S) - **Spec Exp:** Breast Surgery; Gastrointestinal Surgery; Hernia; Biliary Surgery; **Hospital:** Valley Hosp (page 689); **Address:** 385 S Maple Ave, Glen Rock, NJ 07452; **Phone:** 201-444-5757; **Board Cert:** Surgery 2005; **Med School:** Columbia P&S 1980; **Resid:** Surgery, Columbia-Presby Hosp 1985; **Fellow:** Vascular Surgery, Columbia-Presby Hosp 1986

Bufalini, Bruno MD (S) - **Spec Exp:** Laparoscopic Surgery; Minimally Invasive Surgery; **Hospital:** Englewood Hosp & Med Ctr; **Address:** 200 Grand Ave, Englewood, NJ 07631-4371; **Phone:** 201-871-0303; **Med School:** Italy 1971; **Resid:** Surgery, Englewood Hosp 1976

Christoudias, George MD (S) - **Spec Exp:** Hernia; Laparoscopic Cholecystectomy; Cancer Surgery; **Hospital:** Holy Name Med Ctr (page 688); **Address:** 741 Teaneck Rd, Teaneck, NJ 07666; **Phone:** 201-833-2888; **Med School:** Greece 1969; **Resid:** Surgery, Downstate-Kings Co Med Ctr 1975; **Fellow:** Surgical Oncology, Downstate-Kings Co Med Ctr 1976

Fried, Kenneth S MD (S) - **Spec Exp:** Carotid Artery Surgery; Laparoscopic Surgery; **Hospital:** Englewood Hosp & Med Ctr, Holy Name Med Ctr (page 688); **Address:** 180 N Dean St, Ste 2 South, Englewood, NJ 07631-2541; **Phone:** 201-568-8666; **Board Cert:** Surgery 2004; **Med School:** NYU Sch Med 1978; **Resid:** Surgery, NYU Med Ctr 1983; **Fellow:** Vascular Surgery, NYU Med Ctr 1984; **Fac Appt:** Asst Clin Prof S, Mount Sinai Sch Med

Kagan, Peter E MD (S) - **Spec Exp:** Gastrointestinal Surgery; Laparoscopic Surgery; Obesity/Bariatric Surgery; **Hospital:** Hackensack Univ Med Ctr (page 96), Holy Name Med Ctr (page 688); **Address:** North Jersey Surgical Specialists, 83 Summit Ave, Hackensack, NJ 07601; **Phone:** 201-646-0010; **Board Cert:** Surgery 2011; Vascular Surgery 2006; **Med School:** Grenada 1997; **Resid:** Surgery, UMDNJ-Univ Hospital 2002; **Fellow:** Vascular Surgery, Newark Beth Israel Med Ctr 2004

Licata Jr, Joseph J MD (S) - **Spec Exp:** Laparoscopic Surgery; Breast Surgery; **Hospital:** Valley Hosp (page 689); **Address:** 245 E Main St, Ramsey, NJ 07446-1942; **Phone:** 201-327-0220; **Board Cert:** Surgery 2002; **Med School:** Mexico 1984; **Resid:** Surgery, Westchester Co Med Ctr 1991

McCain, Donald MD/PhD (S) - **Spec Exp:** Cancer Surgery; Breast Cancer; Gastrointestinal Cancer; Melanoma; **Hospital:** Hackensack Univ Med Ctr (page 96); **Address:** 20 Prospect Ave, Ste 603, Hackensack, NJ 07601; **Phone:** 201-342-1010; **Board Cert:** Surgery 2010; **Med School:** Albert Einstein Coll Med 1991; **Resid:** Surgery, Mt Sinai Med Ctr 1996; **Fellow:** Surgical Oncology, Meml Sloan-Kettering Cancer Ctr 1998; **Fac Appt:** Asst Clin Prof S, UMDNJ-NJ Med Sch, Newark

Pereira, Stephen MD (S) - **Spec Exp:** Laparoscopic Abdominal Surgery; **Hospital:** Hackensack Univ Med Ctr (page 96); **Address:** 90 Prospect Ave, Ste 1D, Hackensack, NJ 07601-1918; **Phone:** 201-343-3433; **Board Cert:** Surgery 2007; **Med School:** UMDNJ-RW Johnson Med Sch 1991; **Resid:** Surgery, Northwestern Meml Hosp 1996; **Fellow:** Laparoscopic Surgery, Hackensack Univ Med Ctr 1999; **Fac Appt:** Asst Clin Prof S, UMDNJ-NJ Med Sch, Newark

Poole, John W MD (S) - **Hospital:** Holy Name Med Ctr (page 688); **Address:** 83 Summit Ave, Hackensack, NJ 07601; **Phone:** 201-801-0030; **Board Cert:** Surgery 2008; **Med School:** Univ VA Sch Med 1982; **Resid:** Surgery, Montefiore Med Ctr 1987

Schmidt, Hans J MD (S) - **Spec Exp:** Obesity/Bariatric Surgery; Laparoscopic Abdominal Surgery; **Hospital:** Hackensack Univ Med Ctr (page 96); **Address:** 81 Route 4 W, Ste 401, Paramus, NJ 07652; **Phone:** 201-646-1121; **Board Cert:** Surgery 2008; **Med School:** UMDNJ-NJ Med Sch, Newark 1991; **Resid:** Surgery, Univ Hosp-UMDNJ 1997

Shapiro, Michael E MD (S) - **Spec Exp:** Transplant-Kidney; Transplant-Pancreas; Parathyroid Surgery; Dialysis Access Surgery; **Hospital:** Hackensack Univ Med Ctr (page 96); **Address:** Hackensack Univ Med Ctr, Dept Surg, 30 Prospect Ave, Hackensack, NJ 07601-1914; **Phone:** 201-996-2608; **Board Cert:** Surgery 2005; **Med School:** Univ Rochester 1977; **Resid:** Surgery, Beth Israel Med Ctr 1983; **Fac Appt:** Prof S, UMDNJ-NJ Med Sch, Newark

Sussman, Barry MD (S) - **Spec Exp:** Laparoscopic Surgery; **Hospital:** Englewood Hosp & Med Ctr; **Address:** 375 Engle St, Englewood, NJ 07631-1823; **Phone:** 201-894-0400; **Board Cert:** Surgery 2008; **Med School:** NYU Sch Med 1973; **Resid:** Surgery, NYU Med Ctr 1978; **Fellow:** Vascular Surgery, Englewood Hosp 1979; **Fac Appt:** Asst Clin Prof S, Mount Sinai Sch Med

Yang, Hee K MD (S) - **Spec Exp:** Laparoscopic Surgery; Vascular Surgery; **Hospital:** Holy Name Med Ctr (page 688); **Address:** 464 Hudson Terr, Ste 101, Englewood Cliff, NJ 07632; **Phone:** 201-567-7747; **Board Cert:** Surgery 2006; **Med School:** Rush Med Coll 1989; **Resid:** Surgery, Lenox Hill Hosp 1995

Yiengpruksawan, Anusak MD (S) - **Spec Exp:** Liver & Biliary Surgery; Endoscopic Ultrasound; Robotic Surgery; Minimally Invasive Surgery; **Hospital:** Valley Hosp (page 689), Chilton Hosp; **Address:** 1 Valley Health Plaza, Paramus, NJ 07652; **Phone:** 201-493-1005; **Board Cert:** Surgery 2011; **Med School:** Japan 1978; **Resid:** Surgery, Harlem Hosp 1989; **Fellow:** Surgical Oncology, Meml Sloan Kettering Cancer Ctr 1991

Thoracic & Cardiac Surgery

Elmann, Elie M MD (T&CS) - **Spec Exp:** Robotic Cardiac Surgery; Minimally Invasive Cardiac Surgery; Heart Valve Surgery; Atrial Fibrillation; **Hospital:** Hackensack Univ Med Ctr (page 96), Englewood Hosp & Med Ctr; **Address:** 20 Prospect Ave, Ste 900, Hackensack, NJ 07601; **Phone:** 201-996-2261; **Board Cert:** Surgery 2004; Thoracic Surgery 2005; **Med School:** NY Med Coll 1987; **Resid:** Surgery, Cabrini Med Ctr/NY Med Coll 1992; **Fellow:** Cardiothoracic Surgery, SUNY Downstate Med Ctr 1995; **Fac Appt:** Asst Prof S, UMDNJ-NJ Med Sch, Newark

Park, Bernard J MD (T&CS) - **Spec Exp:** Lung Cancer; Esophageal Cancer; Mediastinal Tumors; Robotic Surgery; **Hospital:** Hackensack Univ Med Ctr (page 96); **Address:** 30 Prospect Ave, Ste 5640, Hackensack, NJ 07601; **Phone:** 551-996-4218; **Board Cert:** Surgery 2011; Thoracic Surgery 2003; **Med School:** Univ Pennsylvania 1993; **Resid:** Surgery, New York Hosp 1996; Surgery, New York Hosp 2000; **Fellow:** Cardiothoracic Surgery, NY Presby/Cornell 2002; Thoracic Surgery, Meml Sloan Kettering Cancer Ctr 2002; **Fac Appt:** Asst Clin Prof TS, UMDNJ-NJ Med Sch, Newark

Zairis, Ignatios MD (T&CS) - **Spec Exp:** Endovascular Surgery; Minimally Invasive Thoracic Surgery; **Hospital:** Englewood Hosp & Med Ctr, Holy Name Med Ctr (page 688); **Address:** 741 Teaneck Rd, Teaneck, NJ 07666-4243; **Phone:** 201-837-8282; **Board Cert:** Surgery 2011; **Med School:** Greece 1973; **Resid:** Surgery, Kings Co Hosp 1984; Thoracic Surgery, SUNY Hlth Sci Ctr 1983; **Fellow:** Cardiothoracic Surgery, SUNY Hlth Sci Ctr 1984

Zapolanski, Alex MD (T&CS) - **Spec Exp:** Minimally Invasive Heart Valve Surgery; Aortic Surgery; Coronary Artery Surgery; **Hospital:** Valley Hosp (page 689); **Address:** Valley Hospital, 223 N Van Dien Ave, Ridgewood, NJ 07450; **Phone:** 201-447-8377; **Board Cert:** Thoracic Surgery 2004; **Med School:** Argentina 1973; **Resid:** Surgery, Cleveland Clinic 1979; Cardiothoracic Surgery, Toronto Genl Hosp 1981

Urology

Basralian, Kevin R MD (U) - **Spec Exp:** Infertility-Male; Prostate Benign Disease; Minimally Invasive Surgery; **Hospital:** Hackensack Univ Med Ctr (page 96), Holy Name Med Ctr (page 688); **Address:** 20 Prospect Ave, Ste 719, Hackensack, NJ 07601; **Phone:** 201-343-0082; **Board Cert:** Urology 2010; **Med School:** Mexico 1979; **Resid:** Surgery, Lenox Hill Hosp 1982; Urology, Lenox Hill Hosp 1985; **Fellow:** Urology, Univ Edinburgh 1986

Berdini, Jeffrey L MD (U) - **Spec Exp:** Kidney Stones; Prostate Cancer; Vasectomy Reversal; **Hospital:** Valley Hosp (page 689); **Address:** 555 Kinderkamack Rd, Oradell, NJ 07649; **Phone:** 201-834-1890; **Board Cert:** Urology 1980; **Med School:** UMDNJ-NJ Med Sch, Newark 1973; **Resid:** Urology, UNDMJ Affil Hosps 1978

Chun, Thomas MD (U) - **Spec Exp:** Prostate Cancer; Kidney Stones; Erectile Dysfunction; **Hospital:** SUNY Downstate Med Ctr (Univ Hosp of Bklyn) - LICH (page 420); **Address:** 300 Grand Ave, Ste 202, Englewood, NJ 07631; **Phone:** 201-816-1900; **Board Cert:** Urology 2008; **Med School:** Geo Wash Univ 1991; **Resid:** Surgery, NYU Langone Med Ctr 1993; **Fellow:** Urology, NYU Langone Med Ctr 1997

Esposito, Michael P MD (U) - **Spec Exp:** Laparoscopic Kidney Surgery; Prostate Cancer/Robotic Surgery; Minimally Invasive Urologic Surgery; Adrenal Surgery; **Hospital:** Hackensack Univ Med Ctr (page 96), Monmouth Med Ctr; **Address:** 255 W Spring Valley Ave, Ste 101, Maywood, NJ 07607; **Phone:** 201-487-8866; **Board Cert:** Urology 2012; **Med School:** UMDNJ-NJ Med Sch, Newark 1994; **Resid:** Urology, UMDNJ Med Ctr 2000; **Fellow:** Urologic Laparoscopic Surg-Endourology, Royal Infirmary/Western Genl Hosp 2001; **Fac Appt:** Asst Clin Prof S, UMDNJ-NJ Med Sch, Newark

Frey, Howard L MD (U) - **Spec Exp:** Prostate Cancer; Bladder Cancer; Kidney Cancer; **Hospital:** Valley Hosp (page 689); **Address:** 4 Godwin Ave, Midland Park, NJ 07432-1980; **Phone:** 201-444-7070; **Board Cert:** Urology 2003; **Med School:** Johns Hopkins Univ 1977; **Resid:** Surgery, Johns Hopkins Hosp 1979; Urology, UCLA Med Ctr 1983

Hajjar, John H MD (U) - **Spec Exp:** Laparoscopic Surgery; Prostate Surgery; **Hospital:** Valley Hosp (page 689); **Address:** 14-01 Broadway, Route 4 West, Fair Lawn, NJ 07410-6001; **Phone:** 201-791-4544; **Board Cert:** Urology 2011; **Med School:** Georgetown Univ 1981; **Resid:** Surgery, NYU Med Ctr 1983; Urology, NYU-Bellevue/Sloan Ketterin 1987; **Fellow:** Research, NYU Med Ctr 1988

Katz, Steven A MD (U) - **Spec Exp:** Transfusion Free Surgery; Prostate Cancer; Laparoscopic Surgery; **Hospital:** Englewood Hosp & Med Ctr; **Address:** 300 Grand Ave, Ste 202, Englewood, NJ 07631; **Phone:** 201-816-1900; **Board Cert:** Urology 1978; **Med School:** SUNY Buffalo 1969; **Resid:** Urology, Metropolitan Hosp Ctr 1976

Lanteri, Vincent J MD (U) - **Spec Exp:** Prostate Cancer/Robotic Surgery; Urologic Cancer; Minimally Invasive Urologic Surgery; **Hospital:** Hackensack Univ Med Ctr (page 96); **Address:** 255 W Spring Valley Ave, Ste 101, Maywood, NJ 07607; **Phone:** 201-487-8866; **Board Cert:** Urology 1982; **Med School:** Mexico 1974; **Resid:** Surgery, UMDNJ Med Ctr 1977; Urology, UMDNJ Med Ctr 1980; **Fellow:** Urologic Oncology, Roswell Park Cancer Inst 1981

Margolis, Eric J MD (U) - **Spec Exp:** Urologic Cancer; Prostate Disease; **Hospital:** Englewood Hosp & Med Ctr; **Address:** 300 Grand Ave, Ste 202, Englewood, NJ 07631; **Phone:** 201-816-1900; **Board Cert:** Urology 2008; **Med School:** SUNY Upstate Med Univ 1990; **Resid:** Urologic Surgery, Mount Sinai Hosp 1996

Munver, Ravi MD (U) - **Spec Exp:** Robotic Surgery; Urologic Cancer; Minimally Invasive Urologic Surgery; Kidney Stones; **Hospital:** Hackensack Univ Med Ctr (page 96); **Address:** Hackensack University Medical Center, 360 Essex St, Ste 403, Hackensack, NJ 07601; **Phone:** 551-996-8090; **Board Cert:** Urology 2005; **Med School:** Cornell Univ-Weill Med Coll 1996; **Resid:** Urology, Duke Univ Med Ctr 2002; **Fellow:** Robotic Surgery, New York Hosp-Cornell Med Ctr 2003; **Fac Appt:** Assoc Prof U, UMDNJ-Univ Med Dent NJ

Rosenberg, Gene S MD (U) - **Spec Exp:** Minimally Invasive Surgery; Prostate Cancer-Cryosurgery; Kidney Cancer-Cryosurgery; **Hospital:** Hackensack Univ Med Ctr (page 96), Holy Name Med Ctr (page 688); **Address:** 20 Prospect Ave, Ste 719, Hackensack, NJ 07601; **Phone:** 201-343-0082; **Board Cert:** Urology 1982; **Med School:** NYU Sch Med 1974; **Resid:** Pathology, Kings Co Hosp 1976; Urology, Bellevue/NYU Med Ctr 1980

Sadeghi-Nejad, Hossein MD (U) - **Spec Exp:** Erectile Dysfunction; Peyronie's Disease; Prostate Disease; Infertility-Male; **Hospital:** Hackensack Univ Med Ctr (page 96), Univ Hosp-UMDNJ—Newark; **Address:** 20 Prospect Ave, rm 711, Hackensack, NJ 07601; **Phone:** 201-342-7977 x214; **Board Cert:** Urology 2009; **Med School:** McGill Univ 1989; **Resid:** Surgery, UCSF Med Ctr 1991; Urology, Boston Univ Med Ctr 1996; **Fellow:** Microsurgery, Boston Univ Med Ctr 1997; Reproductive Medicine, Boston Univ Med Ctr 1997; **Fac Appt:** Prof U, UMDNJ-NJ Med Sch, Newark

Sawczuk, Ihor S MD (U) - **Spec Exp:** Bladder Cancer; Kidney Cancer; Prostate Cancer/Robotic Surgery; Bladder Reconstruction; **Hospital:** Hackensack Univ Med Ctr (page 96), NY-Presby/Columbia Univ Med Ctr, NY (page 104); **Address:** Hackensack Univ Med Ctr, 360 Essex St, Ste 403, Hackensack, NJ 07601; **Phone:** 551-996-8090; **Board Cert:** Urology 2005; **Med School:** Med Coll PA Hahnemann 1979; **Resid:** Surgery, St Vincents Hosp 1981; Urology, Columbia-Presby Med Ctr 1984; **Fellow:** Urologic Oncology, Columbia-Presby Med Ctr 1986; **Fac Appt:** Prof U, Columbia P&S

Tennenbaum, Steven Y MD (U) - **Hospital:** Holy Name Med Ctr (page 688), Valley Hosp (page 689); **Address:** 699 Teaneck Rd, Ste 103, Teaneck, NJ 07666; **Phone:** 201-692-9550; **Board Cert:** Urology 2003; **Med School:** Albert Einstein Coll Med 1984; **Resid:** Surgery, Montefiore Med Ctr 1986; Urology, Montefiore Med Ctr 1990; **Fellow:** Pediatric Urology, San Diego Chldns Hosp 1991; **Fac Appt:** Asst Prof U, Columbia P&S

Vitenson, Jack MD (U) - **Spec Exp:** Prostate Cancer; Bladder Cancer; Erectile Dysfunction; **Hospital:** Hackensack Univ Med Ctr (page 96); **Address:** 277 Forest Ave, Ste 206, Paramus, NJ 07652; **Phone:** 201-489-8900; **Board Cert:** Urology 1974; **Med School:** NY Med Coll 1965; **Resid:** Surgery, VA Med Ctr 1967; Urology, Metropolitan Hosp Ctr 1970; **Fac Appt:** Assoc Clin Prof U, UMDNJ-NJ Med Sch, Newark

Wasserman, Gary D MD (U) - **Spec Exp:** Kidney Stones; Incontinence; Voiding Dysfunction; **Hospital:** Englewood Hosp & Med Ctr, Holy Name Med Ctr (page 688); **Address:** 300 Grand Ave, Ste 202, Englewood, NJ 07631; **Phone:** 201-816-1900; **Board Cert:** Urology 2012; **Med School:** Tulane Univ 1985; **Resid:** Surgery, G Washington Univ Med Ctr 1987; Urology, Tulane Univ Med Ctr 1991

Vascular & Interventional Radiology

Rundback, John H MD (VIR) - **Spec Exp:** Angioplasty; Chemoembolization & Tumor Ablation; Peripheral Vascular Disease; **Hospital:** Holy Name Med Ctr (page 688); **Address:** Holy Name Hosp, Dept Radiology, 718 Teaneck Rd, Teaneck, NJ 07666; **Phone:** 201-833-7268; **Board Cert:** Diagnostic Radiology 1992; Vascular & Interventional Radiology 2006; **Med School:** SUNY Downstate 1987; **Resid:** Diagnostic Radiology, Beth Israel Med Ctr 1992; **Fellow:** Interventional Radiology, Washington Hosp Ctr 1993

Vascular Surgery

Elias, Steven M MD (VascS) - **Spec Exp:** Vein Disorders; Wound Healing/Care; Minimally Invasive Surgery; Varicose Veins; **Hospital:** Englewood Hosp & Med Ctr, NY-Presby/Columbia Univ Med Ctr, NY (page 104); **Address:** Englewood Hosp & Med Ctr, Ctr Vein Disease, 350 Engle St, Englewood, NJ 07631-2541; **Phone:** 201-894-3252; **Board Cert:** Surgery 2007; **Med School:** SUNY Buffalo 1979; **Resid:** Surgery, Millard Filmore Hosp 1981; **Fellow:** Peripheral Vascular Surgery, Englewood Hosp 1985; **Fac Appt:** Asst Prof S, Columbia P&S

Geuder, James W MD (VascS) - **Spec Exp:** Vein Disorders; Carotid Artery Surgery; Aneurysm-Aortic; Endovascular Surgery; **Hospital:** Hackensack Univ Med Ctr (page 96); **Address:** 680 Kinderkamack Rd, Ste 306, Oradell, NJ 07649; **Phone:** 201-262-8346; **Board Cert:** Surgery 2007; Vascular Surgery 2009; **Med School:** Med Coll Wisc 1981; **Resid:** Surgery, Univ Hosp-UMDNJ 1986; **Fellow:** Vascular Surgery, NYU Med Ctr 1988

Manno, Joseph MD (VascS) - **Spec Exp:** Arterial Disease; Angioplasty; Limb Sparing Surgery; **Hospital:** Holy Name Med Ctr (page 688), Hackensack Univ Med Ctr (page 96); **Address:** 83 Summit Ave, Hackensack, NJ 07601-1262; **Phone:** 201-646-0010; **Board Cert:** Surgery 2009; Vascular Surgery 2002; **Med School:** Oral Roberts Sch Med 1982; **Resid:** Surgery, Univ Hosp-UMDNJ 1987; **Fellow:** Vascular Surgery, Univ Hosp-UMDNJ 1989

Wolodiger, Fred A MD (VascS) - **Spec Exp:** Arterial Bypass Surgery-Leg; Carotid Artery Surgery; Laparoscopic Surgery; **Hospital:** Englewood Hosp & Med Ctr; **Address:** 375 Engle St, Englewood, NJ 07631; **Phone:** 201-894-0400; **Board Cert:** Surgery 2004; Vascular Surgery 2008; **Med School:** SUNY Hlth Sci Ctr 1980; **Resid:** Surgery, North Shore Univ Hosp 1985; **Fellow:** Vascular Surgery, Englewood Hosp 1987

Essex

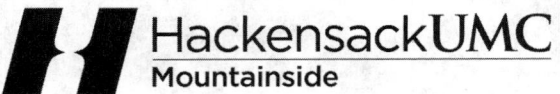

HackensackUMC
Mountainside

1 Bay Avenue, Montclair, NJ 07042 • 973-429-6000
www.mountainsidehosp.com

Number of beds: 365
Number of employees: 1,628
2011 Admissions: 10,793

July 1, 2012 marked the start of a new era for HackensackUMC Mountainside. Our prestigious new affiliation with the Hackensack University Health Network has enhanced the hospital's reputation and paved the way for convenient local access to a larger array of specialized services and medical innovations. This pivotal turning point ensures our ability to grow and uphold our 121-year tradition of service.

With 365 beds and 820,000 square feet, HackensackUMC Mountainside provides a caliber of care within its community hospital setting that rivals the nation's largest and most prestigious facilities. Patients have immediate access to state-of-the-art diagnostic technologies, including high-speed, 3D CT imaging. Innovative and effective treatment alternatives for an array of diverse conditions are available at specialized centers dedicated to: women's health; cancer care; cardiology; surgery; stroke; chronic kidney disease; wound care; and sleep disorders.

Our surgical center is equipped with the most current generation da Vinci robotics, and more than 200 skilled surgeons successfully perform thousands of procedures at HackensackUMC Mountainside each year. The HackensackUMC Mountainside Center for Advanced Bariatric Surgery, which offers a comprehensive range of laparoscopic options, is a recognized Center of Excellence by the American Society of Metabolic and Bariatric Surgery, and our Breast Health Program was recently awarded Breast Center of Excellence status by the American College of Radiology.

Other distinguished programs include the HackensackUMC Mountainside Cancer Center, which is accredited with commendation by the American College of Surgeons, a distinction awarded to only about one-fourth of all hospital cancer centers nationwide.

• American Society for Metabolic and Bariatric Surgery Center of Excellence
• Joint Commission National Quality Approval
• American College of Radiology for Radiation Oncology and Mammography
• American Heart Association/American Stroke Association Get with the Guidelines Gold Plus Achievement Award
• New Jersey Department of Health and Senior Services-designated Primary Stroke Center
• Federal Drug Administration's Mammography Quality Standards Act for Mammography Services
• American College of Surgeons for the Cancer Center
• College of American Pathologists for laboratory services
• National League for Nursing Accrediting Commission for the Mountainside Nursing School
• Intersocietal Commission for the Accreditation of Echocardiography Laboratories

For more information, please call 973-429-6000 or visit Mountainsidehosp.com.

Adolescent Medicine

Johnson, Robert L MD (AM) - **Spec Exp:** AIDS/HIV; Abuse/Neglect; Behavioral Disorders; **Hospital:** Univ Hosp-UMDNJ—Newark; **Address:** 185 S Orange Ave, rm C671, Newark, NJ 07101-1709; **Phone:** 973-972-5277; **Board Cert:** Pediatrics 1977; **Med School:** UMDNJ-NJ Med Sch, Newark 1972; **Resid:** Pediatrics, Martland Hosp 1974; **Fellow:** Adolescent Medicine, NYU Med Ctr 1976; **Fac Appt:** Prof Ped, UMDNJ-NJ Med Sch, Newark

Neal, Wendy P MD (AM) - **Spec Exp:** Nutrition; Eating Disorders; **Hospital:** Newark Beth Israel Med Ctr; **Address:** 166 Lyons Ave, Newark, NJ 07112; **Phone:** 973-926-2676; **Board Cert:** Pediatrics 2010; Adolescent Medicine 2011; **Med School:** Tulane Univ 1991; **Resid:** Pediatrics, Montefiore Med Ctr 1994; **Fellow:** Adolescent Medicine, Montefiore Med Ctr 1997

Stanford, Paulette D MD (AM) - **Spec Exp:** AIDS/HIV in Adolescents; Adolescent Gynecology; Adolescent Behavior-High Risk; **Hospital:** Univ Hosp-UMDNJ—Newark; **Address:** UMDNJ - Dept Pediatrics, Adolescent Med, 90 Bergen St, Ste 4300, Newark, NJ 07103; **Phone:** 973-972-2100; **Board Cert:** Pediatrics 1984; Adolescent Medicine 2009; **Med School:** UMDNJ-NJ Med Sch, Newark 1975; **Resid:** Pediatrics, UMDNJ-Univ Hosp 1977; **Fellow:** Adolescent Medicine, UMDNJ-Univ Hosp 1979; **Fac Appt:** Prof Ped, UMDNJ-NJ Med Sch, Newark

Allergy & Immunology

Perlman, Donald B MD (A&I) - **Spec Exp:** Asthma; Urticaria; Drug Sensitivity; **Hospital:** Saint Barnabas Med Ctr, Newark Beth Israel Med Ctr; **Address:** 741 Northfield Ave, Ste 104, West Orange, NJ 07052-1023; **Phone:** 973-736-7722; **Board Cert:** Pediatrics 1978; Allergy & Immunology 1979; **Med School:** Mount Sinai Sch Med 1973; **Resid:** Pediatrics, Mt Sinai Hosp 1976; **Fellow:** Allergy & Immunology, Duke Univ Med Ctr 1978; **Fac Appt:** Asst Clin Prof Ped, UMDNJ-NJ Med Sch, Newark

Weiss, Steven J MD (A&I) - **Spec Exp:** Asthma; Sinus Disorders; **Hospital:** Saint Barnabas Med Ctr; **Address:** 209 S Livingston Ave, Ste 6, Livingston, NJ 07039-4042; **Phone:** 973-992-4171; **Board Cert:** Internal Medicine 1985; Allergy & Immunology 1987; **Med School:** Ros Franklin Univ/Chicago Med Sch 1982; **Resid:** Internal Medicine, St Lukes Roosevelt Hosp 1985; **Fellow:** Allergy & Immunology, St Lukes Roosevelt Hosp 1987; **Fac Appt:** Asst Clin Prof Med, Mount Sinai Sch Med

Cardiac Electrophysiology

Correia, Joaquim J MD (CE) - **Spec Exp:** Arrhythmias; Pacemakers; Defibrillators; Syncope; **Hospital:** Saint Michael's Med Ctr, Univ Hosp-UMDNJ—Newark; **Address:** 243 Chestnut St, Ste 2L, Newark, NJ 07105; **Phone:** 973-589-8668; **Board Cert:** Internal Medicine 1989; Cardiac Electrophysiology 2004; **Med School:** NYU Sch Med 1986; **Resid:** Internal Medicine, Columbia-Presby Med Ctr 1989; **Fellow:** Cardiovascular Disease, Columbia-Presby Med Ctr 1992; Cardiac Electrophysiology, Columbia-Presby Med Ctr 1993; **Fac Appt:** Asst Prof Med, UMDNJ-NJ Med Sch, Newark

Costeas, Constantinos A MD (CE) - **Spec Exp:** Arrhythmias; Radiofrequency Ablation; Pacemakers; **Hospital:** Saint Michael's Med Ctr, Saint Barnabas Med Ctr; **Address:** NJ Cardiology Assocs, 375 Mount Pleasant Ave Fl 2, West Orange, NJ 07052; **Phone:** 973-731-9598; **Board Cert:** Cardiac Electrophysiology 2008; Cardiovascular Disease 2008; **Med School:** SUNY Stony Brook 1989; **Resid:** Internal Medicine, Univ Hosp 1992; **Fellow:** Cardiovascular Disease, St Vincents Hosp 1996; Cardiac Electrophysiology, Columbia-Presby Med Ctr 1998

Roelke, Marc MD (CE) - **Hospital:** Newark Beth Israel Med Ctr, Saint Barnabas Med Ctr; **Address:** Diagnostic & Clinical Cardiology, 375 Mount Pleasant Ave Fl 2, West Orange, NJ 07052; **Phone:** 973-731-9598; **Board Cert:** Cardiovascular Disease 2003; Cardiac Electrophysiology 2006; **Med School:** Columbia P&S 1987; **Resid:** Internal Medicine, Univ Chicago 1990; **Fellow:** Cardiovascular Disease, Mass Genl Hosp 1993; Cardiac Electrophysiology, Mass Genl Hosp 1994

Sauberman, Roy B MD (CE) - **Spec Exp:** Electrophysiologic Testing; Arrhythmias; Radiofrequency Ablation; Pacemakers/Defibrillators; **Hospital:** Saint Barnabas Med Ctr; **Address:** The Heart Group, 161 Millburn Ave, Millburn, NJ 07041; **Phone:** 973-467-4220; **Board Cert:** Cardiovascular Disease 2008; Cardiac Electrophysiology 2008; **Med School:** Yale Univ 1990; **Resid:** Internal Medicine, NY-Presby/Weill Cornell Med Ctr 1993; **Fellow:** Cardiovascular Disease, NY-Presby/Columbia Univ Med Ctr 1996; Cardiac Electrophysiology, Beth Israel Med Ctr 1998

Cardiovascular Disease

Goldstein, Jonathan E MD (Cv) - **Spec Exp:** Interventional Cardiology; Cardiac Catheterization; **Hospital:** Saint Michael's Med Ctr, Christ Hosp - Jersey City; **Address:** Saint Michaels Med Ctr, 111 Central Ave Fl 5, Newark, NJ 07102; **Phone:** 973-877-5430; **Board Cert:** Internal Medicine 1978; Cardiovascular Disease 1981; **Med School:** UMDNJ-NJ Med Sch, Newark 1973; **Resid:** Internal Medicine, Jackson Meml Hosp 1976; **Fellow:** Cardiovascular Disease, Boston Med Ctr 1978; **Fac Appt:** Assoc Prof Med, Seton Hall Univ Sch Hlth & Med Scis

Klapholz, Marc MD (Cv) - **Spec Exp:** Congestive Heart Failure; Angioplasty; Interventional Cardiology; Pulmonary Hypertension; **Hospital:** Univ Hosp-UMDNJ—Newark; **Address:** 90 Bergen St, Ste 3500, I-538, Newark, NJ 07103-2757; **Phone:** 973-972-4731; **Board Cert:** Internal Medicine 1989; Cardiovascular Disease 2002; Interventional Cardiology 1999; Echocardiography 1997; **Med School:** Albert Einstein Coll Med 1986; **Resid:** Internal Medicine, Bronx Muni Hosp 1989; **Fellow:** Cardiovascular Disease, Bronx Muni Hosp 1992; Interventional Cardiology, Montefiore Med Ctr 1995; **Fac Appt:** Prof Med, UMDNJ-NJ Med Sch, Newark

Rogal, Gary J MD (Cv) - **Spec Exp:** Echocardiography; Coronary Artery Disease; Heart Valve Disease; **Hospital:** Saint Barnabas Med Ctr, Newark Beth Israel Med Ctr; **Address:** New Jersey Cardiology Assocs, 375 Mount Pleasant Ave, W Orange, NJ 07052; **Phone:** 973-731-9442; **Board Cert:** Internal Medicine 1981; Cardiovascular Disease 1983; **Med School:** Geo Wash Univ 1978; **Resid:** Internal Medicine, LI Jewish Med Ctr 1981; **Fellow:** Cardiovascular Disease, Strong Meml Hosp 1984

Saroff, Alan L MD (Cv) - **Spec Exp:** Heart Valve Disease; Cholesterol/Lipid Disorders; Arrhythmias; Preventive Cardiology; **Hospital:** Hackensack UMC-Mountainside (page 736), NY-Presby/Columbia Univ Med Ctr, NY (page 104); **Address:** Montclair Cardiology Group, 123 Highland Ave, Ste 302, Glen Ridge, NJ 07028-1522; **Phone:** 973-748-9555; **Board Cert:** Internal Medicine 1972; Cardiovascular Disease 1975; **Med School:** SUNY Upstate Med Univ 1965; **Resid:** Internal Medicine, SUNY-Syracuse Med Ctr 1967; Internal Medicine, NY Hosp 1970; **Fellow:** Cardiovascular Disease, Columbia Presby Med Ctr 1972; Cardiac Electrophysiology, Columbia Presby Med Ctr 1973; **Fac Appt:** Assoc Clin Prof Med, Columbia P&S

Shamoon, Fayez E MD (Cv) - **Spec Exp:** Interventional Cardiology; Coronary Artery Disease; Nuclear Cardiology; Angioplasty & Stent Placement; **Hospital:** Saint Michael's Med Ctr, Clara Maass Med Ctr; **Address:** Saint Michaels Med Ctr - Cardiology, 111 Central Ave, Newark, NJ 07102; **Phone:** 973-877-5160; **Board Cert:** Internal Medicine 2006; Cardiovascular Disease 2006; Interventional Cardiology 2009; **Med School:** Jordan 1981; **Resid:** Internal Medicine, Jordan Univ Hosp 1985; Internal Medicine, St Michael's Med Ctr 1992; **Fellow:** Cardiovascular Disease, St Michael's Med Ctr 1995; Interventional Cardiology, St Michael's Med Ctr 1996; **Fac Appt:** Assoc Prof Med, Seton Hall Univ Sch Hlth & Med Scis

Wangenheim, Paul M MD (Cv) - **Spec Exp:** Echocardiography; **Hospital:** Saint Barnabas Med Ctr, Morristown Med Ctr (page 92); **Address:** 741 Northfield Ave, Ste 205, West Orange, NJ 07052; **Phone:** 973-467-1544; **Board Cert:** Internal Medicine 1985; Cardiovascular Disease 1987; Echocardiography ; **Med School:** UMDNJ-NJ Med Sch, Newark 1982; **Resid:** Internal Medicine, UMDNJ-Univ Hosp 1985; **Fellow:** Cardiovascular Disease, Newark Beth Israel Med Ctr 1987

Wu, Chia F MD (Cv) - **Hospital:** Saint Barnabas Med Ctr; **Address:** 35 Park Ave, West Orange, NJ 07052-5526; **Phone:** 973-325-3445; **Board Cert:** Internal Medicine 1972; Cardiovascular Disease 1975; **Med School:** Taiwan 1969; **Resid:** Internal Medicine, Martland Hosp 1972; **Fellow:** Cardiovascular Disease, Martland Hosp 1974; **Fac Appt:** Asst Clin Prof Med, UMDNJ-NJ Med Sch, Newark

Zucker, Mark J MD (Cv) - **Spec Exp:** Transplant Medicine-Heart; Heart Failure; Pulmonary Hypertension; Amyloid Heart Disease; **Hospital:** Newark Beth Israel Med Ctr, Saint Barnabas Med Ctr; **Address:** Heart Failure Trmt & Transplant Program, 201 Lyons Ave, Ste L4, Newark, NJ 07112-2027; **Phone:** 973-926-7205; **Board Cert:** Internal Medicine 1984; Cardiovascular Disease 1987; Advanced Heart Failure & Transplant Cardiology 2010; **Med School:** Northwestern Univ 1981; **Resid:** Internal Medicine, Northwestern Meml Hosp 1984; **Fellow:** Cardiovascular Disease, Northwestern Meml Hosp 1987; **Fac Appt:** Clin Prof Med, UMDNJ-NJ Med Sch, Newark

Child & Adolescent Psychiatry

Bartlett, Jacqueline MD (ChAP) - **Spec Exp:** Stress Management; ADD/ADHD; Mood Disorders; **Hospital:** Univ Hosp-UMDNJ—Newark; **Address:** 183 S Orange Ave, BHSB -rmE1547, Newark, NJ 07103; **Phone:** 973-972-2977; **Board Cert:** Psychiatry 1983; **Med School:** Univ Cincinnati 1971; **Resid:** Pediatrics, Montefiore Hospital 1976; Psychiatry, Columbia-Presby Med Ctr 1981; **Fellow:** Child & Adolescent Psychiatry, Columbia-Presby Med Ctr 1979; **Fac Appt:** Assoc Prof Ped, UMDNJ-NJ Med Sch, Newark

Child Neurology

Pak, Jayoung MD (ChiN) - **Spec Exp:** Epilepsy/Seizure Disorders; **Hospital:** Univ Hosp-UMDNJ—Newark; **Address:** 90 Bergen St, rm 8100, Newark, NJ 07103-2406; **Phone:** 973-972-2922; **Board Cert:** Child Neurology 1993; **Med School:** South Korea 1978; **Resid:** Pediatrics, Ewha Women's Univ 1983; Pediatrics, UMDNJ-Univ Hosp 1988; **Fellow:** Child Neurology, UMDNJ-Univ Hosp 1991; Epilepsy, Columbia-Presby Med Ctr 1993; **Fac Appt:** Assoc Prof N, UMDNJ-NJ Med Sch, Newark

Clinical Genetics

Desposito, Franklin MD (CG) - **Spec Exp:** Birth Defects; Genetic Disorders; **Hospital:** Univ Hosp-UMDNJ—Newark, Saint Barnabas Med Ctr; **Address:** 90 Bergen St, Ste 5400, Newark, NJ 07103; **Phone:** 973-972-3300; **Board Cert:** Pediatrics 1986; Clinical Genetics 1982; Clinical Cytogenetics 1990; Clinical Molecular Genetics 2010; **Med School:** Ros Franklin Univ/Chicago Med Sch 1957; **Resid:** Pediatrics, Long Island Jewish Hosp 1961; **Fellow:** Hematology, Univ Wisc Sch Med 1963; **Fac Appt:** Prof Ped, UMDNJ-NJ Med Sch, Newark

Colon & Rectal Surgery

Gilder, Mark E MD (CRS) - **Hospital:** Saint Barnabas Med Ctr, Morristown Med Ctr (page 92); **Address:** Assocs in Colon & Rectal Diseases, 231 Millburn Ave, Millburn, NJ 07041-1718; **Phone:** 973-467-2277; **Board Cert:** Colon & Rectal Surgery 2006; **Med School:** NY Med Coll 1987; **Resid:** Surgery, North Shore Univ Hosp 1992; **Fellow:** Colon & Rectal Surgery, St Francis Hosp 1993

Rothberg, Robert M MD (CRS) - **Spec Exp:** Colon & Rectal Cancer; Colonoscopy; Diverticulitis; **Hospital:** Hackensack UMC-Mountainside (page 736), Saint Barnabas Med Ctr; **Address:** 39 S Fullerton Ave, Montclair, NJ 07042-6303; **Phone:** 973-744-0550; **Board Cert:** Colon & Rectal Surgery 1978; **Med School:** NYU Sch Med 1972; **Resid:** Surgery, Hackensack Hosp 1977; Colon & Rectal Surgery, Muhlenberg Hosp 1978

Dermatology

Connolly, Adrian L MD (D) - **Spec Exp:** Mohs' Surgery; Skin Cancer; **Hospital:** Saint Barnabas Med Ctr; **Address:** 101 Old Short Hills Rd, Ste 503, West Orange, NJ 07052-1023; **Phone:** 973-731-9131; **Board Cert:** Dermatology 2009; **Med School:** UMDNJ-NJ Med Sch, Newark 1975; **Resid:** Dermatology, NYU Med Ctr 1979; **Fellow:** Mohs Surgery, NYU Med Ctr 1980; **Fac Appt:** Asst Clin Prof D, UMDNJ-NJ Med Sch, Newark

Downie, Jeanine B MD (D) - **Spec Exp:** Cosmetic Dermatology; Botox Therapy; Black/Asian Skin Care; Skin Laser Surgery; **Hospital:** Overlook Med Ctr (page 92), Hackensack UMC-Mountainside (page 736); **Address:** 51 Park St, Montclair, NJ 07042; **Phone:** 973-509-6900; **Board Cert:** Dermatology 2006; **Med School:** SUNY Downstate 1992; **Resid:** Pediatrics, New York Hosp 1994; Dermatology, Mt Sinai Med Ctr 1997

Liftin, Alan J MD (D) - **Spec Exp:** Cosmetic Dermatology; Botox Therapy; Facial Rejuvenation; Acne & Rosacea; **Hospital:** Saint Barnabas Med Ctr; **Address:** 22 Old Short Hills Rd, Ste 103, Livingston, NJ 07039-5605; **Phone:** 973-535-5800; **Board Cert:** Dermatology 2009; Anatomic Pathology 1987; Dermatopathology 1989; **Med School:** Mount Sinai Sch Med 1982; **Resid:** Pathology, Mt Sinai Hosp 1985; Dermatology, Mt Sinai Hosp 1990; **Fellow:** Dermatopathology, Hosp Univ Penn 1986

Machler, Brian C MD (D) - **Spec Exp:** Contact Dermatitis; Laser Surgery; Skin Cancer; **Hospital:** Saint Barnabas Med Ctr; **Address:** Center for Dermatology, 101 Old Short Hills Rd, Atkins Kent Bldg, Ste 401, West Orange, NJ 07052; **Phone:** 973-736-9535; **Board Cert:** Dermatology 2004; **Med School:** UMDNJ-NJ Med Sch, Newark 1991; **Resid:** Dermatology, Jackson Meml Hosp 1995; **Fac Appt:** Asst Prof D, NYU Sch Med

Rozanski, Reuben MD (D) - **Spec Exp:** Cosmetic Dermatology; Acne; Rosacea; **Hospital:** Hackensack UMC-Mountainside (page 736); **Address:** 200 Highland Ave, Glen Ridge, NJ 07028-1528; **Phone:** 973-748-9474; **Board Cert:** Dermatology 1979; Internal Medicine 1974; **Med School:** Boston Univ 1970; **Resid:** Internal Medicine, Montefiore Med Ctr 1974; Dermatology, Albert Einstein Coll Med 1976

Schwartz, Robert A MD (D) - **Spec Exp:** Skin Cancer; Atopic Dermatitis; Tuberous Sclerosis; Rare Skin Disorders; **Hospital:** Univ Hosp-UMDNJ—Newark; **Address:** 90 Bergen St, Ste 4400, Newark, NJ 07101; **Phone:** 973-972-1880; **Board Cert:** Dermatology 1978; Clinical & Laboratory Dematologic Immunology 1985; **Med School:** NY Med Coll 1974; **Resid:** Dermatology, Univ Hosp 1977; Dermatology, Roswell Park Meml Inst 1978; **Fellow:** Dermatopathology, NJ Med Sch Affil Hosps 1990; **Fac Appt:** Prof D, UMDNJ-NJ Med Sch, Newark

Siegel, Eric S MD (D) - **Spec Exp:** Cosmetic Dermatology; Skin Laser Surgery; **Hospital:** Saint Barnabas Med Ctr, Overlook Med Ctr (page 92); **Address:** Millburn Laser Center, 12 E Willow St, Millburn, NJ 07041; **Phone:** 973-376-8500; **Board Cert:** Dermatology 2007; **Med School:** SUNY Downstate 1993; **Resid:** Internal Medicine, Staten Island Univ Hosp 1996; Dermatology, Downstate Med Ctr 1999; **Fac Appt:** Assoc Clin Prof D, SUNY Downstate

Diagnostic Radiology

Byk, Cheryl MD (DR) - **Spec Exp:** Mammography; Nuclear Medicine; **Address:** 61 Main St, Ste 61 A, West Orange, NJ 07052; **Phone:** 973-669-1989; **Board Cert:** Diagnostic Radiology 1976; Nuclear Radiology 1977; **Med School:** UMDNJ-NJ Med Sch, Newark 1972; **Resid:** Diagnostic Radiology, St Vincent's Hosp 1976; **Fellow:** Nuclear Medicine, St Vincent's Hosp 1977; **Fac Appt:** Asst Clin Prof, Mount Sinai Sch Med

Lee, Huey-Jen MD (DR) - **Spec Exp:** Brain Imaging; Head & Neck Imaging; Spine Neuroradiologic Diagnosis; Brain Tumors; **Hospital:** Univ Hosp-UMDNJ—Newark; **Address:** 150 Bergen St, Ste C320, Dept of Radiology, Newark, NJ 07103; **Phone:** 973-972-6900; **Board Cert:** Diagnostic Radiology 1990; Neuroradiology 2004; **Med School:** Taiwan 1976; **Resid:** Pediatrics, Taipei Jen-Ai Hosp 1979; Diagnostic Radiology, Beth Israel Med Ctr 1988; **Fellow:** Neuroradiology, NY Med Coll 1989; **Fac Appt:** Prof Rad, UMDNJ-NJ Med Sch, Newark

Sanders, Linda M MD (DR) - **Spec Exp:** Breast Imaging; **Hospital:** Saint Barnabas Med Ctr; **Address:** St Barnabas Breast Center, 200 S Orange Ave, Livingston, NJ 07039; **Phone:** 973-322-7800; **Board Cert:** Diagnostic Radiology 1986; **Med School:** Univ Pennsylvania 1982; **Resid:** Diagnostic Radiology, Columbia-Presby Med Ctr 1986; **Fellow:** Mammography, Meml Sloan-Kettering Cancer Ctr 1987

Endocrinology, Diabetes & Metabolism

Baranetsky, Nicholas G MD (EDM) - **Spec Exp:** Thyroid Disorders; Pituitary Disorders; Adrenal Disorders; **Hospital:** Saint Michael's Med Ctr, Clara Maass Med Ctr; **Address:** St Michaels Med Ctr - Endocrinology, 306 Dr Martin Luther King Blvd, Newark, NJ 07102; **Phone:** 973-877-5185; **Board Cert:** Internal Medicine 1977; Endocrinology, Diabetes & Metabolism 1981; **Med School:** NY Med Coll 1974; **Resid:** Internal Medicine, Stamford Hosp 1977; **Fellow:** Endocrinology, Diabetes & Metabolism, VA Med Ctr-Wadsworth 1979; **Fac Appt:** Prof Med, Seton Hall Univ Sch Hlth & Med Scis

Bleich, David MD (EDM) - **Spec Exp:** Diabetes; Metabolic Disorders; Thyroid Disorders; **Hospital:** Univ Hosp-UMDNJ—Newark; **Address:** UMDNJ Div Endocrinology, 90 Bergen St, DOC 4500, Newark, NJ 07103; **Phone:** 973-972-2500; **Board Cert:** Internal Medicine 1986; Endocrinology, Diabetes & Metabolism 1989; **Med School:** NY Med Coll 1983; **Resid:** Internal Medicine, Maimonides Med Ctr 1986; **Fellow:** Endocrinology, Diabetes & Metabolism, Peter Bent Brigham Hosp 1990; Research, Joslin Diabetes Ctr 1992; **Fac Appt:** Assoc Prof Med, UMDNJ-NJ Med Sch, Newark

Dower, Samuel M MD (EDM) - **Hospital:** Saint Barnabas Med Ctr; **Address:** 200 S Orange Ave, Ste 219, Livingston, NJ 07039; **Phone:** 973-322-7200; **Board Cert:** Internal Medicine 1984; Endocrinology 1987; **Med School:** NYU Sch Med 1981; **Resid:** Internal Medicine, Bronx Muni Hosp 1984; **Fellow:** Endocrinology, Mount Sinai Hosp 1985

Gewirtz, George P MD (EDM) - **Spec Exp:** Diabetes; Thyroid Disorders; Osteoporosis; **Hospital:** Saint Barnabas Med Ctr; **Address:** 200 S Orange Ave, Ste 219, Livingston, NJ 07039; **Phone:** 973-322-7200; **Board Cert:** Internal Medicine 1972; Endocrinology 1975; **Med School:** Harvard Med Sch 1965; **Resid:** Internal Medicine, Bellevue Hosp Ctr 1967; Internal Medicine, Columbia-Presby Med Ctr 1971; **Fellow:** Endocrinology, Diabetes & Metabolism, Mt Sinai Hosp 1973

Sherry, Stephen H MD (EDM) - **Spec Exp:** Thyroid Disorders; Diabetes; Osteoporosis; **Hospital:** Hackensack UMC-Mountainside (page 736); **Address:** 119 Grove St, Montclair, NJ 07042-2629; **Phone:** 973-744-3733; **Board Cert:** Internal Medicine 1979; Endocrinology, Diabetes & Metabolism 1981; **Med School:** Univ Conn 1976; **Resid:** Internal Medicine, New Eng Deaconess 1979; **Fellow:** Endocrinology, Diabetes & Metabolism, New Eng Deaconess 1981; **Fac Appt:** Asst Clin Prof Med, UMDNJ-NJ Med Sch, Newark

Family Medicine

Cirello, Richard MD (FMed) *PCP* - **Hospital:** Hackensack UMC-Mountainside (page 736); **Address:** Town Medical Associates, 271 Grove Ave, Verona, NJ 07044-1730; **Phone:** 973-239-2600; **Board Cert:** Family Medicine 2004; **Med School:** Mexico 1975; **Resid:** Family Medicine, Mountainside Hosp 1979; **Fac Appt:** Asst Clin Prof FMed, UMDNJ-Rutgers Med Sch

Gorman, Robert T MD (FMed) *PCP* - **Hospital:** Hackensack UMC-Mountainside (page 736), Saint Barnabas Med Ctr; **Address:** Town Medical Assocs, 271 Grove Ave, Verona, NJ 07044; **Phone:** 973-239-2600; **Board Cert:** Family Medicine 2005; **Med School:** UMDNJ-NJ Med Sch, Newark 1982; **Resid:** Family Medicine, Mountainside Hosp 1985; **Fac Appt:** Asst Clin Prof FMed, UMDNJ-NJ Med Sch, Newark

Schlam, Everett W MD (FMed) *PCP* - **Spec Exp:** Travel Medicine; **Hospital:** Hackensack UMC-Mountainside (page 736); **Address:** Mountainside Family Practice Assocs, 799 Bloomfield Ave, Verona, NJ 07044; **Phone:** 973-746-7050; **Board Cert:** Family Medicine 2007; Sports Medicine 1999; Adolescent Medicine 2001; **Med School:** UMDNJ-RW Johnson Med Sch 1986; **Resid:** Family Medicine, Mountainside Hosp 1989

Gastroenterology

Finkelstein, Warren MD (Ge) - **Spec Exp:** Crohn's Disease; Ulcerative Colitis; Inflammatory Bowel Disease; **Hospital:** Hackensack UMC-Mountainside (page 736); **Address:** The Gastroenterology Group of New Jersey, 123 Highland Ave, Ste 103, Glen Ridge, NJ 07028; **Phone:** 973-429-8800; **Board Cert:** Internal Medicine 1975; Gastroenterology 1983; **Med School:** Med Coll VA 1972; **Resid:** Internal Medicine, Boston City Hosp 1974; Internal Medicine, Boston VA Med Ctr 1975; **Fellow:** Gastroenterology, Mass Genl Hosp 1977; **Fac Appt:** Assoc Clin Prof Med, UMDNJ-NJ Med Sch, Newark

Fiske, Steven C MD (Ge) - **Spec Exp:** Colon Cancer Screening; Colonoscopy; Peptic Acid Disorders; Gastroesophageal Reflux Disease (GERD); **Hospital:** Saint Barnabas Med Ctr, Clara Maass Med Ctr; **Address:** 1500 Pleasant Valley Way, Ste 306, West Orange, NJ 07052-1104; **Phone:** 973-325-5775; **Board Cert:** Internal Medicine 1977; Gastroenterology 1979; **Med School:** NYU Sch Med 1974; **Resid:** Internal Medicine, NYU-Bellevue Hosp Ctr 1976; **Fellow:** Gastroenterology, Harvard /Brigham & Womens Hosp 1978; **Fac Appt:** Assoc Prof Med, Seton Hall Univ Sch Hlth & Med Scis

Kenny, Raymond MD (Ge) - **Spec Exp:** Liver Disease; Hepatitis B & C; Inflammatory Bowel Disease/Crohn's; Ulcerative Colitis; **Hospital:** Hackensack UMC-Mountainside (page 736); **Address:** The Gastroenterology Group of New Jersey, 123 Highland Ave, Ste 103, Glen Ridge, NJ 07028; **Phone:** 973-429-8800; **Board Cert:** Internal Medicine 1984; Gastroenterology 1987; **Med School:** SUNY Stony Brook 1981; **Resid:** Internal Medicine, Mayo Clinic 1984; **Fellow:** Gastroenterology, Univ Penn Med Ctr 1986; **Fac Appt:** Asst Clin Prof Med, UMDNJ-NJ Med Sch, Newark

Mogan, Glen MD (Ge) - **Spec Exp:** Inflammatory Bowel Disease; Peptic Ulcer Disease; Gastroesophageal Reflux Disease (GERD); **Hospital:** Saint Barnabas Med Ctr; **Address:** 741 N Field Ave, Ste 204, West Orange, NJ 07052-1104; **Phone:** 973-731-8686; **Board Cert:** Internal Medicine 1978; Gastroenterology 1981; **Med School:** SUNY Upstate Med Univ 1975; **Resid:** Internal Medicine, Mount Sinai Hosp 1978; **Fellow:** Gastroenterology, Mount Sinai Hosp 1980; **Fac Appt:** Assoc Clin Prof Med, UMDNJ-Rutgers Med Sch

Spira, Robert S MD (Ge) - **Spec Exp:** Liver Disease; Inflammatory Bowel Disease; Endoscopy; **Hospital:** Saint Michael's Med Ctr, Clara Maass Med Ctr; **Address:** 5 Franklin Ave, Ste 109, Claremont Professional Bldg, Belleville, NJ 07109; **Phone:** 973-759-7240; **Board Cert:** Internal Medicine 1978; Gastroenterology 1981; **Med School:** NYU Sch Med 1975; **Resid:** Internal Medicine, Bellevue Hosp/NYU Med Ctr 1978; **Fellow:** Gastroenterology, VA Med Ctr 1981

Geriatric Medicine

Arunachalam, Muthu R MD (Ger) - **Spec Exp:** Palliative Care; **Hospital:** Newark Beth Israel Med Ctr, Hackensack UMC-Mountainside (page 736); **Address:** 22 Old Short Hills Rd, Ste 110, Livingston, NJ 07039; **Phone:** 973-994-0899; **Board Cert:** Internal Medicine 2000; Geriatric Medicine 2004; **Med School:** India 1993; **Resid:** Internal Medicine, Flushing Hosp Med Ctr 1999; **Fellow:** Geriatric Medicine, Flushing Hosp Med Ctr 2000

Gynecologic Oncology

Anderson, Patrick S MD (GO) - **Spec Exp:** Gynecologic Cancer; Robotic Surgery; **Hospital:** Holy Name Med Ctr (page 688), Montefiore Med Ctr-Moses Campus, NY (page 100); **Address:** Ctr for Gyn Oncology & Women's Hlth, 120 Irvington Ave, South Orange, NJ 07079; **Phone:** 973-762-7270; **Board Cert:** Obstetrics & Gynecology 2011; Gynecologic Oncology 2011; **Med School:** UMDNJ-NJ Med Sch, Newark 1988; **Resid:** Obstetrics & Gynecology, Montefiore Med Ctr 1995; **Fellow:** Gynecologic Oncology, Montefiore Med Ctr 1998; **Fac Appt:** Asst Clin Prof ObG, Albert Einstein Coll Med

Cracchiolo, Bernadette M MD (GO) - **Hospital:** Univ Hosp-UMDNJ—Newark; **Address:** UMDNJ-New Jersey Med Sch, Dept OB/Gyn, 185 S Orange Ave, rm E 506, ACC Level C, Newark, NJ 07101; **Phone:** 973-972-5055; **Board Cert:** Obstetrics & Gynecology 2011; Gynecologic Oncology 2011; Hospice & Palliative Medicine 2008; **Med School:** Univ Hlth Scis, Chicago Med Sch 1991; **Resid:** Obstetrics & Gynecology, Columbia Presby Hosp 1995; **Fellow:** Obstetrics & Gynecology, Yale-New Haven Hosp 1997; **Fac Appt:** Asst Prof ObG, UMDNJ-NJ Med Sch, Newark

Denehy, Thad R. MD (GO) - **Spec Exp:** Robotic Surgery; Ovarian Cancer; Gynecologic Surgery-Complex; Laparoscopic Surgery; **Hospital:** Saint Barnabas Med Ctr, Overlook Med Ctr (page 92); **Address:** Gyn Cancer & Pelvic Surgery, LLC, 101 Old Short Hills Rd, Ste 400, West Orange, NJ 07052; **Phone:** 973-243-9300; **Board Cert:** Gynecologic Oncology 2011; Obstetrics & Gynecology 2011; **Med School:** Wake Forest Univ 1984; **Resid:** Obstetrics & Gynecology, St Barnabas Med Ctr 1988; **Fellow:** Gynecologic Oncology, Strong Meml Hosp 1990

Taylor, Robert R MD (GO) - **Spec Exp:** Pelvic Reconstruction; Gynecologic Cancer; Laparoscopic Surgery; Robotic Surgery; **Hospital:** Saint Barnabas Med Ctr; **Address:** Gynecologic Cancer & Pelvic Surgery, 101 Old Short Hills Rd, Ste 400, West Orange, NJ 07052; **Phone:** 973-243-9300; **Board Cert:** Obstetrics & Gynecology 2011; Gynecologic Oncology 2011; **Med School:** Uniformed Srvs Univ, Bethesda 1985; **Resid:** Obstetrics & Gynecology, United Naval Med Ctr 1989; **Fellow:** Gynecologic Oncology, Walter Reed Army Med Ctr 1994; **Fac Appt:** Assoc Prof ObG, Uniformed Srvs Univ, Bethesda

Hand Surgery

Tan, Virak MD (HS) - **Spec Exp:** Hand & Upper Extremity Surgery; Microvascular Surgery; Nerve Disorders/Surgery; **Hospital:** Univ Hosp-UMDNJ—Newark, Overlook Med Ctr (page 92); **Address:** 90 Bergen St, Ste 1200, Newark, NJ 07103; **Phone:** 973-972-0763; **Board Cert:** Orthopaedic Surgery 2003; Hand Surgery 2004; **Med School:** Univ Pennsylvania 1994; **Resid:** Orthopaedic Surgery, Hosp U Penn 2000; **Fellow:** Hand Surgery, Hosp for Special Surgery 2001; Microvascular Surgery, Chang Gung Meml Hosp 2001; **Fac Appt:** Prof OrS, UMDNJ-NJ Med Sch, Newark

Hematology

Cohen, Alice J MD (Hem) - **Spec Exp:** Bleeding/Coagulation Disorders; **Hospital:** Newark Beth Israel Med Ctr, Saint Barnabas Med Ctr; **Address:** Newark Beth Israel Med Ctr, Div Hem, 201 Lyons Ave, Newark, NJ 07112; **Phone:** 973-926-7230; **Board Cert:** Internal Medicine 1984; Hematology 1986; Medical Oncology 2011; **Med School:** Ros Franklin Univ/Chicago Med Sch 1981; **Resid:** Internal Medicine, NYU-Man VA Med Ctr 1984; **Fellow:** Hematology & Oncology, Geo Wash Univ Med Ctr 1986; Hematology & Oncology, Columbia Presby Med Ctr 1987; **Fac Appt:** Assoc Clin Prof Med, Columbia P&S

Sabnani, Indu MD (Hem) - **Spec Exp:** Lymphoma; **Hospital:** Newark Beth Israel Med Ctr; **Address:** Newark Beth Israel Med Ctr, 2130 Milburn Ave, Ste C11, Maplewood, NJ 07040; **Phone:** 973-762-7676; **Board Cert:** Internal Medicine 1987; Medical Oncology 1989; **Med School:** India 1980; **Resid:** Internal Medicine, United Hosp 1987; **Fellow:** Hematology & Oncology, UMDNJ-Newark 1990

Zager, Robert MD (Hem) - **Hospital:** Hackensack UMC-Mountainside (page 736); **Address:** Richard F Harries Ambulatory Care Pav, 1 Bay Ave Fl 2nd - Ste 1, Montclair, NJ 07042; **Phone:** 973-259-3555; **Board Cert:** Internal Medicine 1973; Hematology 1974; Medical Oncology 1975; **Med School:** Cornell Univ-Weill Med Coll 1968; **Resid:** Internal Medicine, New York Hosp 1970; Medical Oncology, Natl Cancer Inst-NIH 1972; **Fellow:** Hematology & Oncology, New York Hosp 1974; **Fac Appt:** Asst Clin Prof Med, UMDNJ-NJ Med Sch, Newark

Zauber, N Peter MD (Hem) - **Hospital:** Saint Barnabas Med Ctr; **Address:** 22 Old Short Hills Rd, Ste 108, Livingston, NJ 07039; **Phone:** 973-533-9299; **Board Cert:** Internal Medicine 1976; Hematology 1978; **Med School:** Johns Hopkins Univ 1971; **Resid:** Internal Medicine, New York Hosp 1973; Internal Medicine, Baltimore City Hosp 1976; **Fellow:** Hematology & Oncology, Univ Pittsburgh 1978

Infectious Disease

Slim, Jihad G MD (Inf) - **Spec Exp:** AIDS/HIV; Hepatitis C; Hospital Acquired Infections; Osteomyelitis; **Hospital:** Saint Michael's Med Ctr, Newark Beth Israel Med Ctr; **Address:** Saint Michaels Med Ctr, 111 Central Ave, Newark, NJ 07102; **Phone:** 973-877-5644; **Board Cert:** Internal Medicine 1986; Infectious Disease 1988; **Med School:** Lebanon 1980; **Resid:** Internal Medicine, Broussais Hosp 1983; Internal Medicine, Saint Michael's Med Ctr 1986; **Fellow:** Infectious Disease, Saint Michaels Med Ctr 1988; **Fac Appt:** Asst Prof Med, Seton Hall Univ Sch Hlth & Med Scis

Smith, Leon G MD (Inf) - **Spec Exp:** Fevers of Unknown Origin; Bone/Joint Infections; Hepatitis; Chronic Fatigue Syndrome; **Hospital:** Saint Barnabas Med Ctr; **Address:** 189 Engle St, Roseland, NJ 07068; **Phone:** 973-226-3359; **Board Cert:** Internal Medicine 1963; Infectious Disease 1974; **Med School:** Georgetown Univ 1956; **Resid:** Infectious Disease, Nat Inst Hlth 1959; Internal Medicine, Yale-New Haven Hosp 1962; **Fellow:** Infectious Disease, Yale-New Haven Hosp 1960; **Fac Appt:** Prof Med, UMDNJ-NJ Med Sch, Newark

Smith, Stephen M MD (Inf) - **Spec Exp:** AIDS/HIV; Diagnostic Problems; Hepatitis; Sexually Transmitted Diseases; **Hospital:** Saint Barnabas Med Ctr, Saint Michael's Med Ctr; **Address:** 189 Eagle Rock Ave, Roseland, NJ 07068; **Phone:** 973-226-3359; **Board Cert:** Infectious Disease 2004; **Med School:** Yale Univ 1989; **Resid:** Internal Medicine, Univ Virginia Med Ctr 1991; **Fellow:** Infectious Disease, Natl Inst Allergy & Inf Dis 1993; **Fac Appt:** Asst Prof Med, Seton Hall Univ Sch Hlth & Med Scis

Soroko, Theresa A MD (Inf) - **Spec Exp:** AIDS/HIV; Lyme Disease; Skin/Soft Tissue Infections; **Hospital:** Hackensack UMC-Mountainside (page 736), Clara Maass Med Ctr; **Address:** 199 Broad St, Ste 2A, Bloomfield, NJ 07003-2635; **Phone:** 973-748-4583; **Board Cert:** Internal Medicine 1988; Infectious Disease 2002; **Med School:** Grenada 1985; **Resid:** Internal Medicine, St Michael's Med Ctr 1988; **Fellow:** Infectious Disease, St Michael's Med Ctr 1990; **Fac Appt:** Asst Clin Prof Med, UMDNJ-NJ Med Sch, Newark

Youssef-Bessler, Manal F MD (Inf) - **Spec Exp:** AIDS/HIV; Fevers of Unknown Origin; Staphylococcal infections; **Hospital:** Morristown Med Ctr (page 92), Saint Barnabas Med Ctr; **Address:** 22 Old Short Hills Rd, Ste 106, Livingston, NJ 07039; **Phone:** 973-243-8819; **Board Cert:** Internal Medicine 2003; Infectious Disease 2005; **Med School:** Egypt 1992; **Resid:** Internal Medicine, UMDNJ-Univ Hosp 2003; **Fellow:** Infectious Disease, UMDNJ-Univ Hosp 2005

Internal Medicine

Bains, Yatinder MD (IM) *PCP* - **Spec Exp:** Liver Disease; Inflammatory Bowel Disease; Gastroesophageal Reflux Disease (GERD); **Hospital:** Clara Maass Med Ctr, Jersey City Med Ctr; **Address:** 116 Millburn Ave, Ste 102, Millburn, NJ 07041; **Phone:** 973-376-2121; **Board Cert:** Internal Medicine 2002; Gastroenterology 2003; **Med School:** UMDNJ-NJ Med Sch, Newark 1987; **Resid:** Internal Medicine, Univ Hosp-UMDNJ 1990; **Fellow:** Gastroenterology, Univ Hosp-UMDNJ 1992

Chrisanderson, Donna A MD (IM) - **Spec Exp:** Nutrition; **Hospital:** Saint Barnabas Med Ctr; **Address:** 2040 Millburn Ave, Ste 402, Maplewood, NJ 07040; **Phone:** 973-378-9070; **Board Cert:** Internal Medicine 2004; **Med School:** Med Coll GA 1988; **Resid:** Internal Medicine, Greenwich Hosp 1991; **Fellow:** Internal Medicine, Univ Alabama 1993

De Cosimo, Diana R MD (IM) *PCP* - **Spec Exp:** Women's Health; Geriatric Care; Preventive Medicine; **Hospital:** Univ Hosp-UMDNJ—Newark; **Address:** 140 Bergen St, F-Level, Newark, NJ 07103; **Phone:** 973-972-1880; **Board Cert:** Internal Medicine 1977; Cardiovascular Disease 1979; **Med School:** Boston Univ 1974; **Resid:** Internal Medicine, Worcester City Hosp 1977; **Fellow:** Cardiovascular Disease, Univ Mass Med Ctr 1979; **Fac Appt:** Assoc Prof Med, UMDNJ-NJ Med Sch, Newark

Fortunato, Franklin D MD (IM) *PCP* - **Spec Exp:** Asthma; **Hospital:** Hackensack UMC-Mountainside (page 736), Clara Maass Med Ctr; **Address:** 127 Pine St, Montclair, NJ 07042-4835; **Phone:** 973-744-4075; **Board Cert:** Internal Medicine 1978; Pulmonary Disease 1980; **Med School:** UMDNJ-NJ Med Sch, Newark 1975; **Resid:** Internal Medicine, St Michael's Med Ctr 1977; **Fellow:** Pulmonary Disease, St Michael's Med Ctr 1979

Gribbon, John MD (IM) *PCP* - **Spec Exp:** Hypertension; Diabetes; **Hospital:** Hackensack UMC-Mountainside (page 736); **Address:** 62 S Fullerton Ave, Montclair, NJ 07042-2686; **Phone:** 973-744-3382; **Board Cert:** Internal Medicine 1980; **Med School:** UMDNJ-NJ Med Sch, Newark 1977; **Resid:** Internal Medicine, UMDNJ-NJ Med Schl 1980; **Fac Appt:** Asst Clin Prof Med, UMDNJ-NJ Med Sch, Newark

Rommer, James A MD (IM) *PCP* - **Spec Exp:** Preventive Medicine; **Hospital:** Saint Barnabas Med Ctr; **Address:** 349 E Northfield Rd, Ste 110, Livingston, NJ 07039-4807; **Phone:** 973-992-2227; **Board Cert:** Internal Medicine 1981; **Med School:** Cornell Univ-Weill Med Coll 1978; **Resid:** Internal Medicine, NY Hosp-Cornell Med Ctr 1981; **Fellow:** Internal Medicine, Johns Hopkins Med Sch 1982; **Fac Appt:** Asst Clin Prof Med, Mount Sinai Sch Med

Russo, John A MD (IM) *PCP* - **Hospital:** Saint Barnabas Med Ctr; **Address:** 1500 Pleasant Valley Way, Ste 302, West Orange, NJ 07052; **Phone:** 973-736-8119; **Board Cert:** Internal Medicine 1988; **Med School:** Mexico 1981; **Resid:** Internal Medicine & Pediatrics, UMDNJ Affil Hosp 1987

Interventional Cardiology

Cohen, Marc MD (IC) - **Hospital:** Newark Beth Israel Med Ctr; **Address:** Newark Beth Israel Med Ctr, 201 Lyons Ave, Ste C2, Newark, NJ 07112; **Phone:** 973-926-7852; **Board Cert:** Internal Medicine 1980; Cardiovascular Disease 1983; Interventional Cardiology 2009; **Med School:** NYU Sch Med 1977; **Resid:** Internal Medicine, Mt Sinai Hosp 1980; **Fellow:** Cardiovascular Disease, Mt Sinai Hosp 1982; **Fac Appt:** Prof Med, Mount Sinai Sch Med

Miller, Kenneth P MD (IC) - **Spec Exp:** Interventional Cardiology; **Hospital:** Hackensack UMC-Mountainside (page 736), Saint Barnabas Med Ctr; **Address:** 62 S Fullerton Ave, Montclair, NJ 07042-2629; **Phone:** 973-746-8585; **Board Cert:** Internal Medicine 1985; Cardiovascular Disease 1989; Interventional Cardiology 2002; **Med School:** NYU Sch Med 1982; **Resid:** Internal Medicine, Bronx Muni Hosp 1986; **Fellow:** Cardiovascular Disease, Columbia Presby Med Ctr 1989

Maternal & Fetal Medicine

Gimovsky, Martin MD (MF) - **Spec Exp:** Pregnancy-High Risk; **Hospital:** Newark Beth Israel Med Ctr; **Address:** OB/GYN Ultrasound, 201 Lyons Ave, Newark, NJ 07112; **Phone:** 973-926-4882; **Board Cert:** Obstetrics & Gynecology 2010; Maternal & Fetal Medicine 2010; **Med School:** NYU Sch Med 1976; **Resid:** Obstetrics & Gynecology, Sloane Hosp/Columbia Presby hop 1980; **Fellow:** Maternal & Fetal Medicine, USC Med Ctr 1982; **Fac Appt:** Prof ObG, Mount Sinai Sch Med

Smith Jr, Leon G MD (MF) - **Spec Exp:** Ultrasound; Prenatal Diagnosis; Perinatal Infections; Amniocentesis; **Hospital:** Saint Barnabas Med Ctr, Holy Name Med Ctr (page 688); **Address:** NJ Perinatal Associates, 94 Old Short Hills Rd, East Wing, Ste 402, Livingston, NJ 07039-5672; **Phone:** 973-322-5287; **Board Cert:** Obstetrics & Gynecology 2011; Maternal & Fetal Medicine 2011; **Med School:** Georgetown Univ 1985; **Resid:** Obstetrics & Gynecology, Tulane Univ Hosp 1989; **Fellow:** Maternal & Fetal Medicine, Baylor Univ Hosp 1991

Warren, Wendy B MD (MF) - **Spec Exp:** Pregnancy-High Risk; **Hospital:** Saint Barnabas Med Ctr; **Address:** NJ Perinatal Associates, 94 Old Short Hills Rd, East Wing, Ste 402, Livingston, NJ 07039; **Phone:** 973-322-5287; **Board Cert:** Obstetrics & Gynecology 2501; Maternal & Fetal Medicine 2011; **Med School:** Cornell Univ 1982; **Resid:** Obstetrics & Gynecology, T Jefferson Univ Hosp 1986; **Fellow:** Maternal & Fetal Medicine, Columbia Presby Hosp 1991

Medical Oncology

Leitner, Stuart P MD (Onc) - **Spec Exp:** Urologic Cancer; Breast Cancer; **Hospital:** Saint Barnabas Med Ctr; **Address:** Medical Oncology Assocs, 94 Old Short Hills Rd, East Wing, Cancer Ctr, Livington, NJ 07039; **Phone:** 973-322-5200; **Board Cert:** Internal Medicine 1982; Medical Oncology 1985; **Med School:** Mount Sinai Sch Med 1979; **Resid:** Internal Medicine, Univ Tex SW Med Ctr 1982; **Fellow:** Medical Oncology, Meml Sloan Kettering Cancer Ctr 1985

Lippman, Alan MD (Onc) - **Hospital:** Clara Maass Med Ctr, Saint Barnabas Med Ctr; **Address:** 36 Newark Ave, Ste 304, Belleville, NJ 07109; **Phone:** 973-751-8880; **Board Cert:** Internal Medicine 1973; Medical Oncology 1975; **Med School:** Hahnemann Univ 1965; **Resid:** Internal Medicine, Newark Beth Israel Med Ctr 1970; **Fellow:** Medical Oncology, Meml Sloan-Kettering Cancer Ctr 1972; **Fac Appt:** Assoc Clin Prof Med, UMDNJ-NJ Med Sch, Newark

Michaelson, Richard MD (Onc) - **Spec Exp:** Breast Cancer; **Hospital:** Saint Barnabas Med Ctr; **Address:** Medical Oncology Assocs, 94 Old Short Hills Rd, East Wing, Cancer Center, Livingston, NJ 07039; **Phone:** 973-322-5200; **Board Cert:** Internal Medicine 1979; Medical Oncology 1981; **Med School:** Univ Pennsylvania 1976; **Resid:** Internal Medicine, Hosp Univ Penn 1979; **Fellow:** Medical Oncology, Meml Sloan Kettering Cancer Ctr 1981

Sagorin, Charles Elliot MD (Onc) - **Hospital:** Hackensack UMC-Mountainside (page 736); **Address:** 70 Park St, Ste 310, Montclair, NJ 07042-2960; **Phone:** 973-783-3300; **Board Cert:** Internal Medicine 1981; Medical Oncology 1983; Hematology 1986; **Med School:** SUNY Downstate 1971; **Resid:** Internal Medicine, Bronx Municipal Hosp 1973; **Fellow:** Hematology, Montefiore Med Ctr 1974; Medical Oncology, Montefiore Med Ctr 1978

Scoppetuolo, Michael MD (Onc) - **Spec Exp:** Sarcoma; Palliative Care; Hematologic Malignancies; Lung Cancer; **Hospital:** Saint Barnabas Med Ctr; **Address:** Medical Oncology Assocs, 94 Old Short Hills Rd, East Wing, Cancer Center, Livingston, NJ 07039; **Phone:** 973-322-5200; **Board Cert:** Internal Medicine 1982; Medical Oncology 1985; **Med School:** Univ Hlth Scis, Chicago Med Sch 1979; **Resid:** Internal Medicine, Univ Hosp 1982; **Fellow:** Hematology & Oncology, Meml Sloan Kettering Cancer Ctr 1984

Neonatal-Perinatal Medicine

Sun, Shyan-chu MD (NP) - **Spec Exp:** Prematurity/Low Birth Weight Infants; Breathing Disorders; Respiratory Distress Syndrome; **Hospital:** Saint Barnabas Med Ctr; **Address:** Dept Neonatology, 94 Old Short Hills Rd, Livingston, NJ 07039; **Phone:** 973-322-5437; **Board Cert:** Pediatrics 1969; Neonatal-Perinatal Medicine 1975; **Med School:** Taiwan 1961; **Resid:** Pediatrics, Univ London 1967; Pediatrics, Harlem Hosp 1970; **Fellow:** Neonatology, LI Jewish Med Ctr 1972; **Fac Appt:** Clin Prof Ped, UMDNJ-NJ Med Sch, Newark

Nephrology

Byrd, Lawrence H MD (Nep) - **Spec Exp:** Hypertension; Pheochromocytoma; Kidney Tumors; Dialysis Care; **Hospital:** Saint Barnabas Med Ctr, Bayonne Med Ctr; **Address:** 22 Old Short Hills Rd, Ste 212, Livingston, NJ 07039-5605; **Phone:** 973-994-4550; **Board Cert:** Internal Medicine 1977; Nephrology 1978; **Med School:** Med Coll PA 1973; **Resid:** Internal Medicine, Univ Hosp 1976; **Fellow:** Nephrology, New York Hosp-Cornell 1978; **Fac Appt:** Asst Clin Prof Med, UMDNJ-NJ Med Sch, Newark

Grasso, Michael MD (Nep) - **Spec Exp:** Kidney Disease; Hypertension; Dialysis Care; Transplant Medicine-Kidney; **Hospital:** Newark Beth Israel Med Ctr, Saint Barnabas Med Ctr; **Address:** 111 Northfield Ave, Ste 311, West Orange, NJ 07052-4703; **Phone:** 973-325-2103; **Board Cert:** Internal Medicine 1974; Nephrology 1976; **Med School:** Univ MD Sch Med 1970; **Resid:** Internal Medicine, Univ MD Hosp 1974; **Fellow:** Nephrology, Newark Beth Israel Hosp 1976

Mulgaonkar, Shamkant MD (Nep) - **Spec Exp:** Transplant Medicine-Kidney; **Hospital:** Saint Barnabas Med Ctr, Newark Beth Israel Med Ctr; **Address:** St Barnabas Med Ctr, 94 Old Short Hills Rd, Ste 303, Livingston, NJ 07039; **Phone:** 973-322-8216; **Board Cert:** Internal Medicine 1981; Nephrology 1982; **Med School:** India 1975; **Resid:** Internal Medicine, Morristown Meml Hosp 1980; **Fellow:** Nephrology, St Barnabas Med Ctr 1982; **Fac Appt:** Assoc Prof Med, UMDNJ-NJ Med Sch, Newark

Sipzner, Robert J MD (Nep) - **Spec Exp:** Hypertension; Kidney Failure; **Hospital:** Bayonne Med Ctr, Saint Barnabas Med Ctr; **Address:** 22 Old Short Hills Rd, Ste 212, Livingston, NJ 07039; **Phone:** 973-994-4550; **Board Cert:** Internal Medicine 1985; Nephrology 1988; **Med School:** NYU Sch Med 1982; **Resid:** Internal Medicine, SUNY Downstate Med Ctr 1985; **Fellow:** Nephrology, Univ Tenn Hlth Sci Ctr 1987

Neurological Surgery

Heary, Robert F MD (NS) - **Spec Exp:** Spinal Surgery; Spinal Cord Injury; Spinal Deformity; **Hospital:** Univ Hosp-UMDNJ—Newark, Overlook Med Ctr (page 92); **Address:** UMDNJ-NJ Med Sch, Div Neurosurg, 90 Bergen St, Ste 8100, Newark, NJ 07101; **Phone:** 973-972-2323; **Board Cert:** Neurological Surgery 2010; **Med School:** Univ Pittsburgh 1986; **Resid:** Surgery, UMDNJ Univ Hosp 1989; Neurological Surgery, UMDNJ Univ Hosp 1994; **Fellow:** Orthopaedic Surgery, Thomas Jefferson Univ Hosp 1995; **Fac Appt:** Prof NS, UMDNJ-NJ Med Sch, Newark

Hubschmann, Otakar R MD (NS) - **Spec Exp:** Spinal Surgery-Complex; Cerebrovascular Neurosurgery; Chiari's Deformity; Brain Tumors; **Hospital:** Saint Barnabas Med Ctr; **Address:** 101 Old Short Hills Rd, Ste 409, West Orange, NJ 07052; **Phone:** 973-322-6732; **Board Cert:** Neurological Surgery 1978; **Med School:** Czech Republic 1967; **Resid:** Surgery, Montefiore Med Ctr 1970; Neurological Surgery, Montefiore Med Ctr 1976; **Fac Appt:** Clin Prof NS, NY Coll Osteo Med

Neurology

Blady, David MD (N) - **Spec Exp:** Parkinson's Disease; Dementia; Multiple Sclerosis; Stroke; **Hospital:** Hackensack UMC-Mountainside (page 736), Clara Maass Med Ctr; **Address:** 230 Sherman Ave, Ste K, 1100 Clifton Ave, Glen Ridge, NJ 07028-1520; **Phone:** 973-743-9555; **Board Cert:** Neurology 1990; **Med School:** SUNY Downstate 1983; **Resid:** Neurology, Bellevue Hosp/NYU Med Ctr 1987

Cook, Stuart D MD (N) - **Spec Exp:** Multiple Sclerosis; Infectious & Demyelinating Diseases; **Hospital:** Univ Hosp-UMDNJ—Newark; **Address:** 65 Bergen St, rm 1435, Newark, NJ 07101-1709; **Phone:** 973-972-9181; **Board Cert:** Neurology 1970; **Med School:** Univ VT Coll Med 1962; **Resid:** Neurology, Albert Einstein Coll Med 1968; **Fac Appt:** Prof N, UMDNJ-NJ Med Sch, Newark

Geller, Eric B MD (N) - **Spec Exp:** Epilepsy; **Hospital:** Saint Barnabas Med Ctr; **Address:** St Barnabas Inst Neurolgy/Neurosurgery, 200 S Orange Ave, Ste 101, Livingston, NJ 07039; **Phone:** 973-322-7580; **Board Cert:** Neurology 2005; Clinical Neurophysiology 2006; **Med School:** Brown Univ 1989; **Resid:** Neurology, Harvard Med Sch Prog 1993; **Fellow:** Clinical Neurophysiology, Cleveland Clinic 1995

Marks, David A MD (N) - **Spec Exp:** Epilepsy/Seizure Disorders; Headache; Migraine; **Hospital:** Univ Hosp-UMDNJ—Newark; **Address:** 90 Bergen St Fl 8th - Ste 8100, Newark, NJ 07103; **Phone:** 973-972-2550; **Board Cert:** Neurology 1989; **Med School:** South Africa 1983; **Resid:** Neurology, Boston Med Ctr 1988; **Fellow:** Neurological Physiology, New England Med Ctr 1989; Epilepsy, Yale-New Haven Hosp 1991; **Fac Appt:** Assoc Prof Med, UMDNJ-NJ Med Sch, Newark

Ruderman, Marvin MD (N) - **Spec Exp:** Neuromuscular Disorders; Peripheral Neuropathy; Myasthenia Gravis; Demyelinating Neuropathy; **Hospital:** Saint Barnabas Med Ctr; **Address:** 1099 Bloomfield Ave, West Caldwell, NJ 07006-7129; **Phone:** 973-439-7000; **Board Cert:** Neurology 1981; **Med School:** Columbia P&S 1976; **Resid:** Neurology, Barnes Hosp 1980; **Fellow:** Neuromuscular Disease, Neuro Inst 1981; **Fac Appt:** Asst Clin Prof N, UMDNJ-NJ Med Sch, Newark

Nuclear Medicine

Lutzker, Letty G MD (NuM) - **Hospital:** Saint Barnabas Med Ctr; **Address:** St Barnabas Med Ctr, Dept Radiology, 94 Old Short Hills Rd, Livingston, NJ 07039-5672; **Phone:** 973-322-5957; **Board Cert:** Diagnostic Radiology 1973; Nuclear Medicine 1974; Nuclear Radiology 1977; **Med School:** Albert Einstein Coll Med 1968; **Resid:** Diagnostic Radiology, Montefiore Med Ctr 1972; **Fac Appt:** Assoc Clin Prof NuM, Albert Einstein Coll Med

Obstetrics & Gynecology

Apuzzio, Joseph MD (ObG) - **Spec Exp:** Prenatal Diagnosis; Pregnancy-High Risk; Infectious Disease; **Hospital:** Univ Hosp-UMDNJ—Newark, Columbus Hosp; **Address:** UMDNJ Medical School, Dept OB/GYN & Women's Health, 185 S Orange Ave, MSB-rm E506, Newark, NJ 07103-2714; **Phone:** 973-972-5557; **Board Cert:** Obstetrics & Gynecology 2011; Maternal & Fetal Medicine 2011; **Med School:** UMDNJ-NJ Med Sch, Newark 1973; **Resid:** Obstetrics & Gynecology, UMDNJ-Univ Hosp 1976; **Fellow:** Maternal & Fetal Medicine, UMDNJ-Univ Hosp 1982; **Fac Appt:** Prof ObG, UMDNJ-NJ Med Sch, Newark

Cooperman, Alan S MD (ObG) - **Spec Exp:** Laparoscopic Surgery; Pelvic Surgery; Colposcopy; **Hospital:** Overlook Med Ctr (page 92), Saint Barnabas Med Ctr; **Address:** 235 Millburn Ave, Ste 101, Millburn, NJ 07041-1738; **Phone:** 973-467-9440; **Board Cert:** Obstetrics & Gynecology 1979; **Med School:** Italy 1968; **Resid:** Obstetrics & Gynecology, Newark Beth Israel Med Ctr 1973

Crane, Stephen E MD (ObG) - **Hospital:** Saint Barnabas Med Ctr; **Address:** 375 Mount Pleasant Ave, Ste 202, West Orange, NJ 07052; **Phone:** 973-731-7707; **Board Cert:** Obstetrics & Gynecology 2011; **Med School:** UMDNJ-NJ Med Sch, Newark 1986; **Resid:** Obstetrics & Gynecology, St Barnabas Med Ctr 1990

Luciani, Richard L MD (ObG) - **Spec Exp:** Laparoscopic Surgery; Pregnancy-High Risk; Endometriosis; **Hospital:** Overlook Med Ctr (page 92), Saint Barnabas Med Ctr; **Address:** 235 Millburn Ave, Ste 101, Millburn, NJ 07041; **Phone:** 973-467-9440; **Board Cert:** Obstetrics & Gynecology 1982; **Med School:** UMDNJ-NJ Med Sch, Newark 1976; **Resid:** Obstetrics & Gynecology, St Barnabas Hosp 1980

Quartell, Anthony C MD (ObG) - **Spec Exp:** Laparoscopic Surgery-Complex; Pelvic Reconstruction; Robotic Surgery; **Hospital:** Saint Barnabas Med Ctr; **Address:** 316 Eisenhower Pkwy, Ste 202, Livingston, NJ 07039-1718; **Phone:** 973-716-9600; **Board Cert:** Obstetrics & Gynecology 1978; **Med School:** UMDNJ-NJ Med Sch, Newark 1969; **Resid:** Surgery, Univ Hosp 1971; Obstetrics & Gynecology, St Barnabas Med Ctr 1976; **Fac Appt:** Asst Clin Prof ObG, Mount Sinai Sch Med

Ophthalmology

Bhagat, Neelakshi MD (Oph) - **Spec Exp:** Retinal Detachment; Trauma; Diabetic Eye Disease/Retinopathy; Macular Degeneration; **Hospital:** Univ Hosp-UMDNJ—Newark; **Address:** NJ Med Sch Dept Ophthalmology, 90 Bergen St, DOC Bldg - Fl 6th, Newark, NJ 07103; **Phone:** 973-972-2032; **Board Cert:** Ophthalmology 2010; **Med School:** SUNY Stony Brook 1994; **Resid:** Ophthalmology, UMDNJ-NJ Med School 1998; **Fellow:** Retina, Doheny Eye Inst- USC 2000; **Fac Appt:** Assoc Prof Oph, UMDNJ-NJ Med Sch, Newark

Cangemi, Francis E MD (Oph) - **Spec Exp:** Diabetic Eye Disease/Retinopathy; Macular Degeneration; Retinal Detachment; Retinopathy of Prematurity; **Hospital:** Clara Maass Med Ctr, Valley Hosp (page 689); **Address:** 36 Newark Ave, Ste 212, Belleville, NJ 07109-4121; **Phone:** 973-751-8808; **Board Cert:** Ophthalmology 1976; **Med School:** NY Med Coll 1969; **Resid:** Internal Medicine, Mayo Clinic 1971; Ophthalmology, NY EE Infirm 1975; **Fellow:** Retina/Vitreous, Mass EE Infirm 1972; Vitreoretinal Surgery, Mass EE Infirm 1976; **Fac Appt:** Assoc Clin Prof Oph, UMDNJ-NJ Med Sch, Newark

Caputo, Anthony R MD (Oph) - **Spec Exp:** Pediatric Ophthalmology; Strabismus; **Hospital:** Clara Maass Med Ctr; **Address:** 556 Eagle Rock Ave, Ste 203, Roseland, NJ 07068-1500; **Phone:** 973-228-3111; **Board Cert:** Ophthalmology 1976; **Med School:** Italy 1969; **Resid:** Ophthalmology, UMDNJ-Univ Hosp 1974; **Fellow:** Ophthalmology, Wills Eye Hosp 1975; **Fac Appt:** Prof Oph, UMDNJ-NJ Med Sch, Newark

Davidson, Lawrence M MD (Oph) - **Spec Exp:** LASIK-Refractive Surgery; Cataract Surgery; Glaucoma; **Hospital:** Hackensack UMC-Mountainside (page 736), Saint Barnabas Med Ctr; **Address:** 825 Bloomfield Ave Fl 1, Verona, NJ 07044-1300; **Phone:** 973-239-4000; **Board Cert:** Ophthalmology 1975; **Med School:** SUNY Downstate 1969; **Resid:** Ophthalmology, Manhattan EE&T Hosp 1973

Eichler, Joel D MD (Oph) - **Spec Exp:** Diabetic Eye Disease/Retinopathy; Macular Degeneration; Retinal Disorders; **Hospital:** Clara Maass Med Ctr; **Address:** Eye Institute of Essex, 5 Franklin Ave, Ste 209, Belleville, NJ 07109; **Phone:** 973-751-6060; **Board Cert:** Ophthalmology 2004; **Med School:** Geo Wash Univ 1988; **Resid:** Ophthalmology, UMDNJ Affil Hosp 1992; **Fellow:** Vitreoretinal Surgery, Touro Infirm-Touro Hosp 1993

Frohman, Larry P MD (Oph) - **Spec Exp:** Neuro-Ophthalmology; Sarcoidosis; Vision Loss-Unexplained Loss; **Hospital:** Univ Hosp-UMDNJ—Newark; **Address:** 90 Bergen St, Ste 6174, Newark, NJ 07103; **Phone:** 973-972-2065; **Board Cert:** Ophthalmology 1985; **Med School:** Univ Pennsylvania 1980; **Resid:** Ophthalmology, Bellevue Hosp 1984; **Fellow:** Neuro-Ophthalmology, Bellevue Hosp/NYU 1985; **Fac Appt:** Prof Oph, UMDNJ-NJ Med Sch, Newark

Glatt, Herbert L MD (Oph) - **Spec Exp:** Cataract Surgery-Lens Implant; LASIK-Refractive Surgery; **Hospital:** Hackensack UMC-Mountainside (page 736), Clara Maass Med Ctr; **Address:** 1025 Broad St, Bloomfield, NJ 07003-2844; **Phone:** 973-338-1001; **Board Cert:** Ophthalmology 1991; **Med School:** Mexico 1979; **Resid:** Ophthalmology, UMDNJ-NJ Med Sch 1983; **Fac Appt:** Asst Clin Prof Oph, UMDNJ-NJ Med Sch, Newark

Langer, Paul MD (Oph) - **Spec Exp:** Trauma; Orbital Tumors/Cancer; Thyroid Eye Disease; **Hospital:** Univ Hosp-UMDNJ—Newark; **Address:** 90 Bergen St Fl 6 - Ste 6100, Newark, NJ 07103; **Phone:** 973-972-2065; **Board Cert:** Ophthalmology 2005; **Med School:** Johns Hopkins Univ 1989; **Resid:** Ophthalmology, UCSF Med Ctr 1993; **Fellow:** Ophthalmic Plastic Surgery, Univ Utah Affil Hosp 1995; Orbital Surgery, Moorfields Eye Hosp 1995; **Fac Appt:** Assoc Prof Oph, UMDNJ-NJ Med Sch, Newark

Turbin, Roger E MD (Oph) - **Spec Exp:** Neuro-Ophthalmology; Orbital Tumors/Cancer; Oculo-plastic & Orbital Surgery; **Hospital:** Univ Hosp-UMDNJ—Newark, Saint Barnabas Med Ctr; **Address:** 90 Bergen St, Fl 6, Ste 6100, Newark, NJ 07103; **Phone:** 973-972-1244; **Board Cert:** Ophthalmology 2010; **Med School:** Washington Univ, St Louis 1993; **Resid:** Ophthalmology, NYU Med Ctr 1997; **Fellow:** Neuro-Ophthalmology, NYU/NY Eye & Ear/Beth Israel 1998; Oculoplastic Surgery, Allegheny Genl Hosp 1999

Wagner, Rudolph S MD (Oph) - **Spec Exp:** Strabismus; Eye Disorders-Congenital; Botox Therapy; Strabismus; **Hospital:** Clara Maass Med Ctr, Saint Barnabas Med Ctr; **Address:** Childrens Eye Care Ctr New Jersey, 1 Clara Maass Drive, Belleville, NJ 07109; **Phone:** 973-751-1702; **Board Cert:** Ophthalmology 1983; **Med School:** UMDNJ-NJ Med Sch, Newark 1978; **Resid:** Ophthalmology, NJ Med Sch Affil Hosp 1982; **Fellow:** Pediatric Ophthalmology, Wills Eye Hosp 1983; **Fac Appt:** Clin Prof Oph, UMDNJ-NJ Med Sch, Newark

Zarbin, Marco A MD/PhD (Oph) - **Spec Exp:** Macular Degeneration; Diabetic Eye Disease/Retinopathy; Eye Trauma; Retinal Detachment; **Hospital:** Univ Hosp-UMDNJ—Newark, Saint Barnabas Med Ctr; **Address:** 90 Bergen St,, DOC Bldg, Ste 6156, Newark, NJ 07103-2499; **Phone:** 973-972-2065; **Board Cert:** Ophthalmology 1989; **Med School:** Johns Hopkins Univ 1984; **Resid:** Ophthalmology, Johns Hopkins Hosp 1988; **Fellow:** Vitreoretinal Surgery, Johns Hopkins Hosp 1990; **Fac Appt:** Prof Oph, UMDNJ-NJ Med Sch, Newark

Orthopaedic Surgery

Benevenia, Joseph MD (OrS) - **Spec Exp:** Limb Sparing Surgery; Bone Cancer; Sarcoma-Soft Tissue; **Hospital:** Univ Hosp-UMDNJ—Newark; **Address:** 140 Bergen St, Ste ACC1610, Newark, NJ 07103; **Phone:** 973-972-2153; **Board Cert:** Orthopaedic Surgery 2012; **Med School:** UMDNJ-NJ Med Sch, Newark 1984; **Resid:** Orthopaedic Surgery, UMDNJ-NJ Med Sch Hosp 1988; **Fellow:** Orthopaedic Oncology, Case Western Reserve Univ 1991; **Fac Appt:** Prof OrS, UMDNJ-NJ Med Sch, Newark

Berberian, Wayne S MD (OrS) - **Spec Exp:** Joint Infections; Foot & Ankle Deformities; Foot & Ankle Surgery-Complex; **Hospital:** Hackensack Univ Med Ctr (page 96), Univ Hosp-UMDNJ—Newark; **Address:** 90 Bergen St, DOC Bldg, Ste 1200, Newark, NJ 07103; **Phone:** 973-972-8464; **Board Cert:** Orthopaedic Surgery 2012; **Med School:** Univ Pennsylvania 1991; **Resid:** Surgery, St Lukes Roosevelt Hosp 1992; Orthopaedic Surgery, UMDNJ Univ Hosp 1998; **Fac Appt:** Assoc Prof OrS, UMDNJ-NJ Med Sch, Newark

Chase, Mark MD (OrS) - **Spec Exp:** Sports Medicine; **Hospital:** Hackensack UMC-Mountainside (page 736); **Address:** Montclair Orthopaedic Group, 200 Highland Ave, Glen Ridge, NJ 07028-1521; **Phone:** 973-746-2200; **Board Cert:** Orthopaedic Surgery 2012; **Med School:** Boston Univ 1983; **Resid:** Orthopaedic Surgery, Boston Univ Affil Hosps 1988

Decter, Edward MD (OrS) - **Spec Exp:** Knee Reconstruction; Shoulder Reconstruction; Sports Medicine; **Hospital:** Saint Barnabas Med Ctr; **Address:** Center for Orthopaedics, 1500 Pleasant Valley Way, Ste 101, West Orange, NJ 07052; **Phone:** 973-669-5600; **Board Cert:** Orthopaedic Surgery 1982; **Med School:** Creighton Univ 1975; **Resid:** Orthopaedic Surgery, Hosp Joint Diseases 1980

Mendes, John MD (OrS) - **Spec Exp:** Hip & Knee Replacement; Foot & Ankle Surgery; Spinal Disorders; **Hospital:** Hackensack UMC-Mountainside (page 736), Clara Maass Med Ctr; **Address:** Montclair Orthopaedic Group, 200 Highland Ave, Glen Ridge, NJ 07028-1521; **Phone:** 973-746-2200; **Board Cert:** Orthopaedic Surgery 1984; **Med School:** Cornell Univ-Weill Med Coll 1976; **Resid:** Surgery, Bryn Mawr Hosp 1978; Orthopaedic Surgery, Hosp Special Surg 1981; **Fellow:** Penn Hosp 1982

Patterson, Francis MD (OrS) - **Spec Exp:** Musculoskeletal Tumors; Bone Cancer; Limb Sparing Surgery; **Hospital:** Univ Hosp-UMDNJ—Newark; **Address:** 90 Bergen St, Ste 1200, Newark, NJ 07103; **Phone:** 973-972-1993; **Board Cert:** Orthopaedic Surgery 2012; **Med School:** SUNY Buffalo 1993; **Resid:** Orthopaedic Surgery, SUNY Health Sci Ctr 1998; **Fellow:** Musculoskeletal Oncology, Univ Chicago Hosps 1999; **Fac Appt:** Assoc Prof OrS, UMDNJ-NJ Med Sch, Newark

Sabharwal, Sanjeev MD (OrS) - **Spec Exp:** Pediatric Orthopaedic Surgery; Limb Lengthening (Ilizarov Procedure); Limb Deformities; **Hospital:** Univ Hosp-UMDNJ—Newark, Overlook Med Ctr (page 92); **Address:** 90 Bergen St, Ste 1200, Newark, NJ 07103; **Phone:** 973-972-0246; **Board Cert:** Orthopaedic Surgery 2010; **Med School:** India 1986; **Resid:** Surgery, St Elizabeth Hosp 1988; Orthopaedic Surgery, Univ British Columbia 1994; **Fellow:** Pediatric Orthopaedic Surgery, Chldns Hosp/Shriners Hosp 1996; Reconstructive Surgery, Md Ctr for Limb Lengthening & Reconstruction 1996; **Fac Appt:** Prof OrS, UMDNJ-NJ Med Sch, Newark

Schob, Clifford J MD (OrS) - **Spec Exp:** Sports Medicine; Shoulder & Knee Surgery; **Hospital:** Overlook Med Ctr (page 92), Saint Barnabas Med Ctr; **Address:** 235 Millburn Ave, Millburn, NJ 07041; **Phone:** 973-258-1177; **Board Cert:** Orthopaedic Surgery 2003; **Med School:** UMDNJ-RW Johnson Med Sch 1982; **Resid:** Surgery, LIJ Med Ctr 1984; Orthopaedic Surgery, LIJ Med Ctr 1988; **Fellow:** Sports Medicine, Am Sports Med Inst 1990

Seidenstein, Michael K MD (OrS) - **Spec Exp:** Arthroscopic Surgery; Joint Replacement; **Hospital:** Newark Beth Israel Med Ctr; **Address:** 61-C Main St, West Orange, NJ 07052-5338; **Phone:** 973-736-8080; **Board Cert:** Orthopaedic Surgery 1977; **Med School:** NY Med Coll 1970; **Resid:** Orthopaedic Surgery, Hosp for Joint Diseases 1975; **Fellow:** Hip Surgery, Wrightington Hosp Ctr 1975A-O Fellowship 1978; **Fac Appt:** Asst Prof OrS, UMDNJ-NJ Med Sch, Newark

Otolaryngology

Morrow, Todd A MD (Oto) - **Spec Exp:** Cosmetic Surgery-Face; Rhinoplasty; Laser Surgery; Botox Therapy; **Hospital:** Saint Barnabas Med Ctr, Newark Beth Israel Med Ctr; **Address:** 741 Northfield Ave, Ste 104, West Orange, NJ 07052; **Phone:** 973-243-1823; **Board Cert:** Otolaryngology 1992; Facial Plastic & Reconstr Surgery 1995; **Med School:** Jefferson Med Coll 1986; **Resid:** Otolaryngology, UMDNJ-Univ Hosp 1991; **Fellow:** Facial Plastic & Reconstr Surgery, Univ Toronto Med Ctr 1992; **Fac Appt:** Asst Clin Prof Oto, UMDNJ-NJ Med Sch, Newark

Zbar, Lloyd I.S. MD (Oto) - **Spec Exp:** Hearing & Balance Disorders; Nasal & Sinus Disorders; Voice Disorders; **Hospital:** Hackensack UMC-Mountainside (page 736), Overlook Med Ctr (page 92); **Address:** 200 Highland Ave, Ste 250, Glen Ridge, NJ 07028-1528; **Phone:** 973-744-2424; **Board Cert:** Otolaryngology 1970; **Med School:** Queens Univ 1964; **Resid:** Surgery, Beth Israel Hosp 1966; Otolaryngology, NYU-Bellevue Hosp Ctr 1969; **Fellow:** Otolaryngology, NYU-Bellevue Hosp Ctr 1970; **Fac Appt:** Assoc Clin Prof Oto, NYU Sch Med

Pain Medicine

Kaufman, Andrew G MD (PM) - **Spec Exp:** Complex Regional Pain Syndromes; Pain-Back & Neck; Pain-Cancer; Pain-Neuropathic; **Hospital:** Univ Hosp-UMDNJ—Newark, Overlook Med Ctr (page 92); **Address:** 90 Bergen St, Ste 3400, Newark, NJ 07103; **Phone:** 973-972-2085; **Board Cert:** Anesthesiology 1993; Pain Medicine 2005; **Med School:** Univ VA Sch Med 1988; **Resid:** Anesthesiology, Columbia Presby Med Ctr 1992; **Fellow:** Pain Medicine, Beth Israel Hosp/Brigham & Women's/Chldn's Hosp 1993; **Fac Appt:** Assoc Prof Anes, UMDNJ-NJ Med Sch, Newark

Pathology

Heller, Debra S MD (Path) - **Spec Exp:** Gynecologic Pathology; Pediatric Pathology; Perinatal Pathology; **Hospital:** Univ Hosp-UMDNJ—Newark; **Address:** UMDNJ-NJ Med Sch Dept Pathology, 185 S Orange Ave, UH/E158, Newark, NJ 07101; **Phone:** 973-972-0751; **Board Cert:** Anatomic Pathology 1988; Obstetrics & Gynecology 2011; Pediatric Pathology 1999; **Med School:** NY Med Coll 1977; **Resid:** Obstetrics & Gynecology, Beth Israel Med Ctr 1981; Anatomic Pathology, Mt Sinai Med Ctr 1988; **Fellow:** Pediatric Pathology, Mt Sinai Med Ctr 1987; Gynecologic Pathology, Mt Sinai Med Ctr 1989; **Fac Appt:** Prof Path, UMDNJ-NJ Med Sch, Newark

Lara, Jonathan F MD (Path) - **Spec Exp:** Breast Cancer; **Hospital:** Saint Barnabas Med Ctr; **Address:** St Barnabas Medical Ctr, Dept Pathology, 94 Old Short Hills Rd, Livingston, NJ 07039-5672; **Phone:** 973-322-5762; **Board Cert:** Anatomic & Clinical Pathology 1988; Cytopathology 1997; **Med School:** Philippines 1984; **Resid:** Pathology, St Barnabas Med Ctr 1988; **Fellow:** Surgical Pathology, Meml Sloan Kettering Cancer Ctr 1989; **Fac Appt:** Asst Clin Prof Path, UMDNJ-NJ Med Sch, Newark

Pediatric Allergy & Immunology

Fost, Arthur MD (PA&I) - **Spec Exp:** Asthma; Sinusitis; Urticaria; **Hospital:** Clara Maass Med Ctr; **Address:** 197 Bloomfield Ave, Verona, NJ 07044-2702; **Phone:** 973-857-0330; **Board Cert:** Pediatrics 1968; Allergy & Immunology 1972; **Med School:** Jefferson Med Coll 1963; **Resid:** Pediatrics, Chldns Hosp 1965; Pediatrics, Hosp Univ Penn 1966; **Fellow:** Allergy & Immunology, St Vincent's Hosp 1968; **Fac Appt:** Assoc Clin Prof Ped, UMDNJ-NJ Med Sch, Newark

Morrison, Susan MD (PA&I) - **Spec Exp:** Infectious Disease; Travel Medicine; **Hospital:** Clara Maass Med Ctr; **Address:** 36 Newark Ave, Ste 322, Belleville, NJ 07109; **Phone:** 973-450-0100; **Board Cert:** Pediatrics 1986; Allergy & Immunology 2008; Pediatric Infectious Disease 2009; **Med School:** UMDNJ-NJ Med Sch, Newark 1981; **Resid:** Pediatrics, Univ Hosp-UMDNJ 1985; **Fellow:** Pediatric Allergy & Immunology, Univ Hosp-UMDNJ 1988; Pediatric Infectious Disease, Univ Hosp-UMDNJ 1988; **Fac Appt:** Prof Ped, UMDNJ-NJ Med Sch, Newark

Torre, Arthur J MD (PA&I) - **Spec Exp:** Asthma; Diving Medicine; Rhinitis; Sinusitis; **Hospital:** St. Joseph's Regl Med Ctr - Paterson; **Address:** 25 Hollywood Ave, Fairfield, NJ 07004-1113; **Phone:** 973-882-0880; **Board Cert:** Pediatrics 1975; **Med School:** UMDNJ-NJ Med Sch, Newark 1970; **Resid:** Pediatrics, Martland Hosp 1972; **Fellow:** Pediatric Allergy & Immunology, Martland Hosp 1973; **Fac Appt:** Assoc Clin Prof Ped, UMDNJ-NJ Med Sch, Newark

Pediatric Cardiology

Connor, Thomas M MD (PCd) - **Hospital:** Saint Barnabas Med Ctr; **Address:** 101 Old Short Hills Rd, Ste 104, West Orange, NJ 07052; **Phone:** 973-731-5550; **Board Cert:** Pediatrics 1973; Pediatric Cardiology 1977; **Med School:** Italy 1966; **Resid:** Pediatrics, Grasslands Hosp 1970; **Fellow:** Pediatric Cardiology, Yale-New Haven Hosp 1972; **Fac Appt:** Assoc Prof Ped, Columbia P&S

Fernandes, John MD (PCd) - **Spec Exp:** Congenital Heart Disease; Fetal Cardiology; **Hospital:** Saint Barnabas Med Ctr, Morgan Stanley Children's Hosp of NY-Presby, NY (page 104); **Address:** 349 E Northfield Rd, Ste 201, Livingston, NJ 07039-4086; **Phone:** 973-533-1031; **Board Cert:** Pediatric Cardiology 2006; **Med School:** India 1983; **Resid:** Pediatrics, Hahnemann Univ Med Ctr 1988; **Fellow:** Pediatric Cardiology, NYU Med Ctr 1991; Pediatric Cardiology, Johns Hopkins Hosp 1990; **Fac Appt:** Assoc Clin Prof Ped, Columbia P&S

Langsner, Alan MD (PCd) - **Spec Exp:** Fetal Echocardiography; Congenital Heart Disease-Adult & Child; Preventive Cardiology; **Hospital:** NYU Langone Med Ctr (page 108); **Address:** 160 E 32nd St, Fl 3rd, New York, NY 10016; **Phone:** 212-263-5490; **Board Cert:** Pediatrics 1983; Pediatric Cardiology 2010; **Med School:** Mexico 1977; **Resid:** Pediatrics, Metropolitan Hosp Ctr 1981; **Fellow:** Pediatric Cardiology, NYU Med Ctr 1983; **Fac Appt:** Asst Prof Ped, NYU Sch Med

O'Connor, Brian K MD (PCd) - **Hospital:** Newark Beth Israel Med Ctr, Chldns Hosp NJ at Newark; **Address:** Chldns Heart Ctr at Newark Beth Israel, 201 Lyons Ave, Ste L-5, Newark, NJ 07112; **Phone:** 973-926-3500; **Board Cert:** Pediatric Cardiology 2010; **Med School:** Georgetown Univ 1985; **Resid:** Pediatrics, New England Med Ctr 1988; **Fellow:** Pediatric Cardiology, Mott Chldns Hosp 1991; Pediatric Cardiology, Chldns Hosp Univ SC 1995

Putman, Donald C MD (PCd) - **Hospital:** Saint Barnabas Med Ctr, Hackensack UMC-Mountainside (page 736); **Address:** MetroPediatric Cardiology Assocs, 349 E Northfield Rd, Ste 105, Livingston, NJ 07039; **Phone:** 973-597-3333; **Board Cert:** Pediatric Cardiology 2011; **Med School:** Grenada 1989; **Resid:** Pediatrics, NYU/Bellevue Hosp 1992; **Fellow:** Pediatric Cardiology, NYU/Bellevue Hosp 1995

Verma, Rajiv MD (PCd) - **Spec Exp:** Congenital Heart Disease-Adult & Child; Kawasaki Disease; **Hospital:** Newark Beth Israel Med Ctr; **Address:** 201 Lyons Ave, Ste L5, Newark, NJ 07112; **Phone:** 973-926-3500; **Board Cert:** Pediatric Cardiology 2009; **Med School:** Zambia 1984; **Resid:** Pediatrics, NYU Langone Med Ctr 1991; **Fellow:** Pediatric Cardiology, NYU Langone Med Ctr 1994; Interventional Cardiology, Boston Chldns Hosp 1996; **Fac Appt:** Asst Clin Prof Ped, NYU Sch Med

Pediatric Critical Care Medicine

Yeh, Timothy S MD (PCCM) - **Hospital:** Saint Barnabas Med Ctr, Monmouth Med Ctr; **Address:** St Barnabas Med Ctr, 94 Old Short Hills Rd, Fl 4th, rm 4134A, Livingston, NJ 07039; **Phone:** 973-322-5691; **Board Cert:** Pediatrics 1982; Pediatric Critical Care Medicine 2012; **Med School:** UC Davis 1976; **Resid:** Pediatrics, UC Davis Med Ctr 1979; **Fellow:** Pediatric Critical Care Medicine, Chldns Hosp Natl Med Ctr 1981; **Fac Appt:** Clin Prof Ped, UMDNJ-NJ Med Sch, Newark

Pediatric Endocrinology

Brenner, Dennis J MD (PEn) - **Spec Exp:** Growth Disorders; Pubertal Disorders; Diabetes; Turner Syndrome; **Hospital:** Saint Barnabas Med Ctr, Newark Beth Israel Med Ctr; **Address:** 200 S Orange Ave Fl 2 - Ste 225, Pediatric Specialty Center, Livingston, NJ 07039; **Phone:** 973-322-7600; **Board Cert:** Pediatric Endocrinology 2011; **Med School:** SUNY Downstate 1997; **Resid:** Pediatrics, Schneider Chldns Hosp 2000; **Fellow:** Pediatric Endocrinology, Schneider Chldns Hosp 2003; **Fac Appt:** Asst Clin Prof Ped, SUNY Downstate

Sivitz, Jennifer N MD (PEn) - **Spec Exp:** Diabetes; Obesity; **Hospital:** Hackensack Univ Med Ctr (page 96), Newark Beth Israel Med Ctr; **Address:** 30 Prospect Ave WFAN Bldg - rm 251, Hackensack, NJ 07601; **Phone:** 551-996-5329; **Board Cert:** Pediatrics 2005; Pediatric Endocrinology 2009; **Med School:** NY Med Coll 2002; **Resid:** Pediatrics, North Shore LI Jewish Hlth System 2005; **Fellow:** Pediatric Endocrinology, Mass Gen Hosp 2008

Pediatric Gastroenterology

Sunaryo, Francis MD (PGe) - **Spec Exp:** Inflammatory Bowel Disease; Gastroesophageal Reflux Disease (GERD); **Hospital:** Newark Beth Israel Med Ctr, Saint Barnabas Med Ctr; **Address:** 201 Lyons Ave, Newark, NJ 07112; **Phone:** 973-926-7280; **Board Cert:** Pediatrics 1982; Pediatric Gastroenterology 2005; **Med School:** Indonesia 1973; **Resid:** Pediatrics, North Shore Univ Hosp 1979; **Fellow:** Pediatric Gastroenterology, Chldns Hosp 1982; **Fac Appt:** Asst Prof Ped, UMDNJ-Univ Med Dent NJ

Pediatric Hematology-Oncology

Kamalakar, Peri MD (PHO) - **Spec Exp:** Sickle Cell Disease; Thalassemia; Leukemia; Solid Tumors; **Hospital:** Newark Beth Israel Med Ctr, Monmouth Med Ctr; **Address:** Valerie Fund Children's Ctr, 201 Lyons Ave, Ste L5, Newark, NJ 07112-2027; **Phone:** 973-926-7161; **Board Cert:** Pediatrics 1975; Pediatric Hematology-Oncology 1997; **Med School:** India 1967; **Resid:** Pediatrics, Beth Israel Med Ctr 1973; **Fellow:** Pediatric Hematology-Oncology, Childrens Hosp 1976; **Fac Appt:** Asst Clin Prof Ped, UMDNJ-NJ Med Sch, Newark

Pediatric Infectious Disease

Oleske, James M MD (PInf) - **Spec Exp:** AIDS/HIV; Pediatric Allergy & Immunology; Pain Management; Palliative Care; **Hospital:** Univ Hosp-UMDNJ—Newark; **Address:** UMDNJ Dept Ped, MSB-F 572, 570 S Orange Ave, Newark, NJ 07103; **Phone:** 973-972-5066; **Board Cert:** Pediatrics 1976; Allergy & Immunology 1977; Diagnostic Lab Immunology 1986; Hospice & Palliative Medicine 2007; **Med School:** UMDNJ-NJ Med Sch, Newark 1971; **Resid:** Pediatrics, Martland Hosp 1974; **Fellow:** Pediatric Infectious Disease, Grady Meml Hosp 1976; **Fac Appt:** Prof Ped, UMDNJ-NJ Med Sch, Newark

Pediatric Nephrology

Roberti, M Isabel MD/PhD (PNep) - **Spec Exp:** Transplant Medicine-Kidney; Kidney Failure; Hypertension; Kidney Stones; **Hospital:** Saint Barnabas Med Ctr; **Address:** SBMC - Pediatric Nephrology, 94 Old Short Hills Rd, Ste 304, Livingston, NJ 07039; **Phone:** 973-322-5264; **Board Cert:** Pediatrics 2010; Pediatric Nephrology 2005; **Med School:** Brazil 1983; **Resid:** Pediatrics, Hosp Sao Paulo 1986; **Fellow:** Pediatric Nephrology, Hosp Sao Paulo 1989; Pediatric Nephrology, Mount Sinai Hosp 1995; **Fac Appt:** Assoc Clin Prof Ped, Mount Sinai Sch Med

Pediatric Pulmonology

Aguila, Helen MD (PPul) - **Spec Exp:** Asthma; Tuberculosis; **Hospital:** Univ Hosp-UMDNJ—Newark, Columbus Hosp; **Address:** UMDNJ-Univ Hosp-Newark, 90 Bergen St Fl 5th - rm 5100, Dept Ped Pulmonology, Newark, NJ 07103; **Phone:** 973-972-5779; **Board Cert:** Pediatrics 1983; Pediatric Pulmonology 2004; **Med School:** Philippines 1974; **Resid:** Pediatrics, Staten Island Hosp 1979; Pediatrics, Kings Co Hosp/Downstate Med Ctr 1980; **Fellow:** Pediatric Pulmonology, Chldns Hosp Michigan 1983; **Fac Appt:** Asst Prof Ped, UMDNJ-NJ Med Sch, Newark

Bisberg, Dorothy S MD (PPul) - **Spec Exp:** Asthma; Cystic Fibrosis; **Hospital:** Saint Barnabas Med Ctr, Newark Beth Israel Med Ctr; **Address:** 200 S Orange Ave Fl 2 - Ste 225, Pediatric Specialty Center, Livingston, NJ 07039; **Phone:** 973-322-7600 x6; **Board Cert:** Pediatrics 1977; Pediatric Pulmonology 2007; **Med School:** Cornell Univ-Weill Med Coll 1972; **Resid:** Pediatrics, Montefiore Hosp Med Ctr 1974; Pediatrics, Bronx Lebanon Hosp 1975; **Fac Appt:** Asst Prof Ped, UMDNJ-NJ Med Sch, Newark

Kottler, William MD (PPul) - **Spec Exp:** Asthma; Cystic Fibrosis; **Hospital:** Saint Barnabas Med Ctr, Overlook Med Ctr (page 92); **Address:** 48 Essex St, Millburn, NJ 07041; **Phone:** 973-218-0900; **Board Cert:** Pediatric Pulmonology 2009; **Med School:** Dominica 1987; **Resid:** Pediatrics, Overlook Hosp 1990; **Fellow:** Pediatric Pulmonology, Newark Beth Israel Hosp 1991; Pediatric Pulmonology, Univ Florida 1993; **Fac Appt:** Asst Clin Prof Ped, UMDNJ-NJ Med Sch, Newark

Mikkilineni, Sushmita MD (PPul) - **Spec Exp:** Critical Care; Sleep Medicine; **Hospital:** Chldns Hosp NJ at Newark; **Address:** 201 Lyons Ave, Ste L-5, Newark, NJ 07112; **Phone:** 973-926-4273; **Board Cert:** Pediatrics 2009; Pediatric Pulmonology 2007; Pediatric Critical Care Medicine 2010; Sleep Medicine 2007; **Med School:** India 1981; **Resid:** Pediatrics, RW Johnson Univ Hosp 1987; **Fellow:** Pediatric Pulmonary & Critical Care, RW Johnson Univ Hosp 1988; Pediatric Pulmonology, NY-Presby/Columbia Univ Med Ctr 1991; **Fac Appt:** Assoc Prof Ped, UMDNJ-RW Johnson Med Sch

Pediatric Rheumatology

Chalom, Elizabeth C MD (PRhu) - **Hospital:** Saint Barnabas Med Ctr; **Address:** St Barnabas Med Ctr, 200 S Orange Ave, Ste 225, Livingston, NJ 07039; **Phone:** 973-322-7600; **Board Cert:** Pediatrics 2009; Pediatric Rheumatology 2006; **Med School:** Columbia P&S 1991; **Resid:** Pediatrics, Chldns Hosp 1994; **Fellow:** Pediatric Rheumatology, Chldns Hosp 1995; **Fac Appt:** Asst Clin Prof S, UMDNJ-NJ Med Sch, Newark

Pediatric Surgery

Bethel, Colin A MD (PS) - **Spec Exp:** Minimally Invasive Surgery; Neonatal Surgery; **Hospital:** Newark Beth Israel Med Ctr, St. Joseph's Regl Med Ctr - Paterson; **Address:** Pediatric Surgery Group, 2130 Millburn Ave, Ste C-1, Maplewood, NJ 07040; **Phone:** 973-313-3115; **Board Cert:** Surgery 2005; Pediatric Surgery 2007; **Med School:** Columbia P&S 1987; **Resid:** Surgery, Yale-New Haven Hosp 1995; **Fellow:** Pediatric Surgery, Chldns Hosp 1997

Pediatrics

Colyer-Aversa, Lori A. MD (Ped) - **Spec Exp:** Developmental Disorders; **Hospital:** Hackensack UMC-Mountainside (page 736); **Address:** 399 Hoover Ave, Ste 5, Bloomfield, NJ 07003; **Phone:** 973-748-9500; **Board Cert:** Pediatrics 2007; **Med School:** UMDNJ-Univ Med Dent NJ 1989; **Resid:** Pediatrics, Columbia-Presby Med Ctr 1992

Gruenwald, Laurence D MD (Ped) *PCP* - **Spec Exp:** Asthma; Behavioral Disorders; **Hospital:** Saint Barnabas Med Ctr; **Address:** 90 Millburn Ave, Ste 101, Millburn, NJ 07041-1933; **Phone:** 973-378-7990; **Board Cert:** Pediatrics 1981; **Med School:** UMDNJ-NJ Med Sch, Newark 1975; **Resid:** Pediatrics, Chldns Hosp Natl Med Ctr 1978

Marcus, Richard W MD (Ped) *PCP* - **Spec Exp:** ADD/ADHD; **Hospital:** Clara Maass Med Ctr; **Address:** 242 Washington Ave, Ste A, Nutley, NJ 07110-1994; **Phone:** 973-667-6676; **Board Cert:** Pediatrics 1988; **Med School:** UMDNJ-NJ Med Sch, Newark 1982; **Resid:** Pediatrics, Univ Hosp-UMDNJ 1985; **Fac Appt:** Asst Prof Ped, UMDNJ-NJ Med Sch, Newark

Rigtrup, Edward MD (Ped) *PCP* - **Hospital:** Hackensack UMC-Mountainside (page 736), Saint Barnabas Med Ctr; **Address:** 73 Park St, Montclair, NJ 07042-2903; **Phone:** 973-746-7375; **Board Cert:** Pediatrics 1980; **Med School:** NY Med Coll 1975; **Resid:** Pediatrics, Chldns Natl Med Ctr 1978; **Fac Appt:** Assoc Clin Prof Ped, NY Med Coll

Physical Medicine & Rehabilitation

Bach, John MD (PMR) - **Spec Exp:** Neuromuscular Disorders; Amyotrophic Lateral Sclerosis (ALS); Post Polio Syndrome/Rehabilitation; **Hospital:** Univ Hosp-UMDNJ—Newark; **Address:** 90 Bergen St Fl 3 - Ste 3100, Newark, NJ 07103; **Phone:** 973-972-7195; **Board Cert:** Physical Medicine & Rehabilitation 1986; **Med School:** UMDNJ-NJ Med Sch, Newark 1976; **Resid:** Physical Medicine & Rehabilitation, NYU Med Ctr 1980; **Fellow:** Neuromuscular Disease, Univ Hosp 1983; **Fac Appt:** Prof PMR, UMDNJ-NJ Med Sch, Newark

Cole, Jeffrey L MD (PMR) - **Spec Exp:** Pain Management; Neuromuscular Disorders; Electromyography; Electrodiagnosis; **Hospital:** Kessler Inst for Rehab - W Orange; **Address:** Kessler Inst for Rehabilitation, 1199 Pleasant Valley Way, West Orange, NJ 07052; **Phone:** 973-243-6943; **Board Cert:** Physical Medicine & Rehabilitation 1983; Pain Medicine 2003; **Med School:** Mexico 1977; **Resid:** Internal Medicine, NY Hosp-Queens Med Ctr 1979; Physical Medicine & Rehabilitation, Montefiore Med Ctr 1982; **Fellow:** Electrodiagnosis, Booth Meml Med Ctr 1983

Francis, Kathleen D MD (PMR) - **Spec Exp:** Lymphedema; **Address:** Lymphedema Physician Services, 200 S Orange Ave, Ste 111, Livingston, NJ 07039; **Phone:** 973-322-7366; **Board Cert:** Physical Medicine & Rehabilitation 2004; **Med School:** UMDNJ-NJ Med Sch, Newark 1989; **Resid:** Physical Medicine & Rehabilitation, UMDNJ-Kessler Inst Rehab 1993; **Fac Appt:** Asst Clin Prof PMR, UMDNJ-NJ Med Sch, Newark

Kirshblum, Steven C MD (PMR) - **Spec Exp:** Spinal Cord Injury; Spasticity Management; **Hospital:** Kessler Inst for Rehab - W Orange, Saint Barnabas Med Ctr; **Address:** Kessler Institute, 1199 Pleasant Valley Way, West Orange, NJ 07052-1424; **Phone:** 973-731-3600 x2258; **Board Cert:** Physical Medicine & Rehabilitation 1991; Spinal Cord Injury Medicine 2008; **Med School:** Univ Hlth Scis, Chicago Med Sch 1986; **Resid:** Physical Medicine & Rehabilitation, Mount Sinai Med Ctr 1990; **Fac Appt:** Prof PMR, UMDNJ-NJ Med Sch, Newark

Shumko, John Z MD/PhD (PMR) - **Hospital:** Saint Barnabas Med Ctr; **Address:** Sports & Physical Medicine Institute, 200 S Orange Ave, Ste 124, Livingston, NJ 07039; **Phone:** 973-322-7909; **Board Cert:** Physical Medicine & Rehabilitation 2007; **Med School:** UMDNJ-NJ Med Sch, Newark 1992; **Resid:** Physical Medicine & Rehabilitation, Univ Hosp-UMDNJ 1997

Plastic Surgery

Ablaza, Valerie J MD (PlS) - **Spec Exp:** Cosmetic Surgery-Breast; Breast Reconstruction; Liposuction & Body Contouring; **Hospital:** Saint Barnabas Med Ctr, Hackensack UMC-Mountainside (page 736); **Address:** The Plastic Surgery Group, 37 N Fullerton Ave, Montclair, NJ 07042; **Phone:** 973-233-1933; **Board Cert:** Plastic Surgery 2010; **Med School:** Med Coll PA Hahnemann 1989; **Resid:** Surgery, Albert Einstein Med Ctr 1994; Plastic Surgery, New York Hosp 1996; **Fellow:** Breast Surgery, Nashville Plastic Surgery

Cooperman, Ross D MD (PlS) - **Spec Exp:** Reconstructive Surgery; Cosmetic Surgery; **Hospital:** Saint Barnabas Med Ctr; **Address:** 22 Old Short Hills Rd, Ste 101, Livingston, NJ 07039; **Phone:** 973-994-2021; **Board Cert:** Surgery 2008; **Med School:** Geo Wash Univ 2003; **Resid:** Surgery, St Barnabas Med Ctr 2008; **Fellow:** Plastic Surgery, Univ Louisville Sch Med 2010

DiBernardo, Barry E MD (PlS) - **Spec Exp:** Laser Surgery; Hair Restoration/Transplant; Cosmetic Surgery-Face & Body; Body Contouring after Weight Loss; **Hospital:** Hackensack UMC-Mountainside (page 736), Clara Maass Med Ctr; **Address:** 29 Park St, Montclair, NJ 07042; **Phone:** 973-509-2000; **Board Cert:** Plastic Surgery 1994; **Med School:** Cornell Univ-Weill Med Coll 1984; **Resid:** Surgery, Mt Sinai Hosp 1989; Plastic Surgery, Montefiore Med Ctr 1991; **Fac Appt:** Assoc Clin Prof PlS, UMDNJ-NJ Med Sch, Newark

Granick, Mark S MD (PIS) - **Spec Exp:** Reconstructive Surgery; Cosmetic Surgery; Skin Cancer; Liposuction & Body Contouring; **Hospital:** Univ Hosp-UMDNJ—Newark, Newark Beth Israel Med Ctr; **Address:** 140 Bergen St, rm E-1620, Newark, NJ 07103; **Phone:** 973-972-8092; **Board Cert:** Otolaryngology 1982; Plastic Surgery 1985; **Med School:** Harvard Med Sch 1977; **Resid:** Otolaryngology, Mass E&E Hosp 1982; Plastic Surgery, Univ Pittsburgh Med Ctr 1984; **Fac Appt:** Prof PIS, UMDNJ-NJ Med Sch, Newark

LoVerme, Paul J MD (PIS) - **Spec Exp:** Cosmetic Surgery-Face; Liposuction & Body Contouring; Breast Reconstruction & Augmentation; **Hospital:** Hackensack UMC-Mountainside (page 736), Saint Barnabas Med Ctr; **Address:** 825 Bloomfield Ave, Ste 205, Verona, NJ 07044; **Phone:** 973-857-9499; **Board Cert:** Plastic Surgery 1987; **Med School:** UMDNJ-NJ Med Sch, Newark 1978; **Resid:** Surgery, UMDNJ Univ Hosp 1983; Plastic Surgery, Med Coll Hosp 1985; **Fellow:** Surgical Oncology, UMDNJ Univ Hosp 1982; **Fac Appt:** Assoc Clin Prof PIS, UMDNJ-NJ Med Sch, Newark

Rosen, Allen D MD (PIS) - **Spec Exp:** Cosmetic Surgery-Face & Breast; Breast Reconstruction; Liposuction & Body Contouring; Eyelid Surgery; **Hospital:** Hackensack UMC-Mountainside (page 736), Saint Barnabas Med Ctr; **Address:** 37 N Fullerton Ave, Montclair, NJ 07042; **Phone:** 973-233-1933; **Board Cert:** Plastic Surgery 1991; **Med School:** SUNY Buffalo 1983; **Resid:** Surgery, Columbia Presby Med Ctr 1986; Plastic Surgery, Columbia Presby Med Ctr 1988; **Fellow:** Hand Surgery, Columbia Presby Med Ctr 1987; **Fac Appt:** Asst Clin Prof PIS, UMDNJ-NJ Med Sch, Newark

Psychiatry

Caracci, Giovanni MD (Psyc) - **Spec Exp:** Geriatric Psychiatry; Psychopharmacology; Psychotherapy; Post Traumatic Stress Disorder; **Hospital:** Univ Hosp-UMDNJ—Newark; **Address:** 183 S Orange Ave, rm F1436, Box 1709, Newark, NJ 07101; **Phone:** 973-972-7117; **Board Cert:** Psychiatry 1990; **Med School:** Italy 1977; **Resid:** Psychiatry, Metropolitan Hosp 1983; **Fellow:** Psychiatry, Metropolitan Hosp 1984; **Fac Appt:** Assoc Prof Psyc, UMDNJ-NJ Med Sch, Newark

Faber, Mark P MD (Psyc) - **Spec Exp:** Child Psychiatry; Anxiety Disorders; Depression; ADD/ADHD; **Hospital:** Saint Barnabas Med Ctr, Hackensack UMC-Mountainside (page 736); **Address:** 594 Valley Rd, Upper Montclair, NJ 07043-1882; **Phone:** 973-746-6711; **Board Cert:** Psychiatry 1993; Child & Adolescent Psychiatry 2005; **Med School:** Dominica 1988; **Resid:** Psychiatry, CT Valley Hosp-Yale 1991; **Fellow:** Child & Adolescent Psychiatry, UMDNJ-RW Johnson Sch Med 1993; Sleep Medicine, UMDNJ-RW Johnson Sch Med 1996

Nucci, Annamaria MD/PhD (Psyc) - **Spec Exp:** Psychopharmacology; Relationship Problems; Depression; **Address:** 5 Westview Ct, Cedar Grove, NJ 07009-1937; **Phone:** 973-857-2609; **Board Cert:** Psychiatry 1978; **Med School:** Italy 1971; **Resid:** Psychiatry, Manhattan VA Hosp-NYU 1973; Psychiatry, Payne Whitney Clinic 1976; **Fellow:** Child & Adolescent Psychiatry, New York Hosp-Cornell 1976; **Fac Appt:** Asst Clin Prof Psyc, NY Med Coll

Schleifer, Steven J MD (Psyc) - **Spec Exp:** Depression; Psychoneuroimmunology; Anxiety Disorders; **Hospital:** Univ Hosp-UMDNJ—Newark; **Address:** 183 S Orange Ave Bldg BHSB F1430, Newark, NJ 07103; **Phone:** 973-972-5023; **Board Cert:** Psychiatry 1980; **Med School:** Mount Sinai Sch Med 1975; **Resid:** Psychiatry, USC Med Ctr 1976; Psychiatry, Mount Sinai Med Ctr 1979; **Fac Appt:** Prof Psyc, UMDNJ-NJ Med Sch, Newark

Zornitzer, Michael R MD (Psyc) - **Spec Exp:** Pyschopharmacology; Depression; Psychotherapy; **Hospital:** Saint Barnabas Med Ctr; **Address:** 2 W Northfield Rd, Ste 305, Livingston, NJ 07039-3789; **Phone:** 973-992-6090; **Board Cert:** Psychiatry 1976; **Med School:** SUNY Downstate 1971; **Resid:** Internal Medicine, NYU Hosps Ctr 1972; Psychiatry, Jacobi Med Ctr 1975; **Fac Appt:** Asst Clin Prof Psyc, NY Coll Osteo Med

Pulmonary Disease

Gagliardi, Anthony MD (Pul) - **Spec Exp:** Asthma; Lung Cancer; Tuberculosis; **Hospital:** Saint Barnabas Med Ctr; **Address:** Saint Barnabas Med Ctr, Dept of Med, 94 Old Short Hills Rd, Livingston, NJ 07039; **Phone:** 973-322-6256; **Board Cert:** Internal Medicine 1984; Pulmonary Disease 1986; **Med School:** UMDNJ-NJ Med Sch, Newark 1981; **Resid:** Internal Medicine, St Vincent's Hosp & Med Ctr 1984; **Fellow:** Pulmonary Disease, Meml Sloan Kettering Cancer Ctr 1986; **Fac Appt:** Asst Clin Prof Med, NY Med Coll

Greenberg, Martin J MD (Pul) - **Spec Exp:** Asthma; Emphysema; **Hospital:** Saint Barnabas Med Ctr; **Address:** 124 East Mt Pleasant Ave, Livingston, NJ 07039; **Phone:** 973-994-4130; **Board Cert:** Internal Medicine 1987; **Med School:** Dominica 1983; **Resid:** Internal Medicine, Univ Hosp UMDNJ 1986; **Fellow:** Pulmonary Disease, Newark Beth Israel 1989

Miller, Richard A MD (Pul) - **Spec Exp:** Sarcoidosis; Asthma; Sleep Medicine; **Hospital:** Saint Michael's Med Ctr; **Address:** St Michaels Medical Center, 111 Central Ave, Newark, NJ 07102; **Phone:** 973-877-5493; **Board Cert:** Internal Medicine 1989; Pulmonary Disease 2003; Critical Care Medicine 2005; **Med School:** NY Med Coll 1983; **Resid:** Internal Medicine, St Michaels Med Ctr 1988; **Fellow:** Pulmonary Critical Care Medicine, St Michaels Med Ctr 1991

Safirstein, Benjamin MD (Pul) - **Spec Exp:** Asthma; Sarcoidosis; **Hospital:** Hackensack UMC-Mountainside (page 736), Saint Michael's Med Ctr; **Address:** 123 Highland Ave, Ste 101, Glen Ridge, NJ 07028; **Phone:** 973-744-9125; **Board Cert:** Internal Medicine 1970; Pulmonary Disease 1974; **Med School:** Ros Franklin Univ/Chicago Med Sch 1965; **Resid:** Internal Medicine, Mount Sinai Hosp 1969; **Fellow:** Pulmonary Disease, Inst Dis Chest 1972

Shah, Smita MD (Pul) - **Spec Exp:** Asthma; Chronic Obstructive Lung Disease (COPD); Lung Cancer; Pulmonary Hypertension; **Hospital:** Saint Barnabas Med Ctr; **Address:** 96 Millburn Ave, Ste 200-A, Millburn, NJ 07040; **Phone:** 973-763-6800; **Board Cert:** Internal Medicine 1986; Pulmonary Disease 2010; Sleep Medicine 2009; **Med School:** India 1980; **Resid:** Internal Medicine, St Marys Hosp 1986; **Fellow:** Pulmonary Critical Care Medicine, Temple Univ Hosp 1988

Radiation Oncology

Wagman, Raquel T MD (RadRO) - **Spec Exp:** Breast Cancer; **Hospital:** Saint Barnabas Med Ctr; **Address:** St Barnabas Med Ctr, 94 Old Short Hills Rd, Livingston, NJ 07039; **Phone:** 973-322-5630; **Board Cert:** Radiation Oncology 2010; **Med School:** Univ Mich Med Sch 1995; **Resid:** Radiation Oncology, Meml Sloan Kettering Cancer Ctr 2000

Reproductive Endocrinology

Chen, Serena H MD (RE) - **Spec Exp:** Infertility; Laparoscopic Surgery; Hysteroscopic Surgery; **Hospital:** Saint Barnabas Med Ctr; **Address:** IRMS at St. Barnabas, 94 Old Short Hills Rd, East Wing, Ste 403, Livingston, NJ 07039; **Phone:** 973-322-8286; **Board Cert:** Obstetrics & Gynecology 2011; Reproductive Endocrinology 2011; **Med School:** Duke Univ 1988; **Resid:** Obstetrics & Gynecology, Johns Hopkins Hosp 1992; **Fellow:** Reproductive Endocrinology, Johns Hopkins Hosp 1994

Rheumatology

Cannarozzi, Nicholas A MD (Rhu) - **Spec Exp:** Rheumatoid Arthritis; Lupus Nephritis; Osteoporosis; Vasculitis; **Hospital:** Hackensack UMC-Mountainside (page 736); **Address:** 127 Pine St, Montclair, NJ 07042-4835; **Phone:** 973-783-6000; **Board Cert:** Internal Medicine 1980; Rheumatology 1972; **Med School:** Hahnemann Univ 1965; **Resid:** Internal Medicine, Philadelphia Genl Hosp 1967; Internal Medicine, St Michaels Med Ctr 1968; **Fellow:** Rheumatology, Yale-New Haven Hosp 1969; Rheumatology, Yale-New Haven Hosp 1972

Lahita, Robert G MD/PhD (Rhu) - **Spec Exp:** Lupus/SLE; Endocrinology & Joint Disorders; Immunodeficiency Disorders; Lupus/SLE; **Hospital:** Newark Beth Israel Med Ctr; **Address:** 201 Lyons Ave Fl 4, Newark, NJ 07112; **Phone:** 973-926-7472; **Board Cert:** Internal Medicine 2004; Rheumatology 2007; **Med School:** Jefferson Med Coll 1973; **Resid:** Internal Medicine, New York Hosp-Cornell 1976; **Fellow:** Rheumatology, Rockefeller Hosp 1978; **Fac Appt:** Prof Med, Mount Sinai Sch Med

Simon, Jonathan M MD (Rhu) - **Hospital:** Hackensack UMC-Mountainside (page 736); **Address:** 1018 Broad St, Bloomfield, NJ 07003-2807; **Phone:** 973-338-3383; **Board Cert:** Internal Medicine 1981; Rheumatology 1984; **Med School:** NYU Sch Med 1978; **Resid:** Internal Medicine, UMDNJ Univ Hosp 1981; **Fellow:** Rheumatology, UMDNJ Univ Hosp 1983

Sports Medicine

Gehrmann, Robin M MD (SM) - **Spec Exp:** Cartilage Damage & Transplant; Knee Ligament Reconstruction; Shoulder Injuries; Arthroscopic Surgery; **Hospital:** Univ Hosp-UMDNJ—Newark; **Address:** North Jersey Orthopaedic Inst, 90 Bergen St, Ste 1200, Newark, NJ 07103; **Phone:** 973-972-8240; **Board Cert:** Orthopaedic Surgery 2004; Orthopaedic Sports Medicine 2007; **Med School:** Hahnemann Univ 1995; **Resid:** Surgery, UMDNJ Med Ctr 1996; Orthopaedic Surgery, UMDNJ Med Ctr 2000; **Fellow:** Orthopaedic Sports Medicine, Pennsylvania Hosp 2001; **Fac Appt:** Asst Prof OrS, UMDNJ-NJ Med Sch, Newark

Levy, Andrew S MD (SM) - **Spec Exp:** Cartilage Damage & Transplant; Ligament Reconstruction; Shoulder Surgery; **Hospital:** Saint Barnabas Med Ctr, Morristown Med Ctr (page 92); **Address:** 90 Milburn Ave, Ste 204A, Milburn, NJ 07041; **Phone:** 908-598-9199; **Board Cert:** Orthopaedic Surgery 2008; **Med School:** Temple Univ 1987; **Resid:** Orthopaedic Surgery, Albert Einstein Med Ctr 1994; **Fellow:** Sports Medicine, Duke Univ Med Ctr 1995; Shoulder Surgery, Duke Univ Med Ctr 1995; **Fac Appt:** Assoc Clin Prof OrS, UMDNJ-NJ Med Sch, Newark

Surgery

Andrei, Valeriu E MD (S) - **Spec Exp:** Obesity/Bariatric Surgery; Laparoscopic Surgery; **Hospital:** Robert Wood Johnson Univ Hosp - New Brunswick, Saint Barnabas Med Ctr; **Address:** 200 S Orange Ave, Ste 123, Livingston, NJ 07039; **Phone:** 973-322-7265; **Board Cert:** Surgery 2009; **Med School:** Romania 1987; **Resid:** Surgery, Methodist Hosp 1988; **Fellow:** Minimally Invasive Surgery, Mt Sinai Med Ctr 1999

Blackwood, M Michele MD (S) - **Spec Exp:** Breast Cancer; Breast Surgery; Sentinel Node Surgery; Breast Cancer-High Risk Women; **Hospital:** Saint Barnabas Med Ctr; **Address:** 200 S Orange Ave, Ste 102, Livingston, NJ 07039; **Phone:** 973-322-7020; **Board Cert:** Surgery 2003; **Med School:** Med Univ SC 1988; **Resid:** Surgery, Stamford Hosp 1993; **Fellow:** Surgical Oncology, Meml Sloan Kettering Cancer Ctr 1994; **Fac Appt:** Asst Clin Prof S, Columbia P&S

Chamberlain, Ronald S MD (S) - **Spec Exp:** Liver & Biliary Surgery; Cancer Surgery; Laparoscopic Surgery; Pancreatic Cancer; **Hospital:** Saint Barnabas Med Ctr; **Address:** St Barnabas Med Ctr, Dept Surgery, 94 Old Short Hills Rd, Livingston, NJ 07039; **Phone:** 973-322-5195; **Board Cert:** Surgery 2009; **Med School:** Geo Wash Univ 1991; **Resid:** Surgery, Geo Wash Univ Med Ctr 1997; **Fellow:** Surgical Oncology, Natl Cancer Inst-NIH 1996; Hepatobiliary Surgery, Meml Sloan-Kettering Canc Ctr 1999; **Fac Appt:** Prof S, UMDNJ-NJ Med Sch, Newark

Deitch, Edwin A MD (S) - **Spec Exp:** Burn Care; Abdominal Wall Reconstruction; Critical Care; **Hospital:** Univ Hosp-UMDNJ—Newark; **Address:** 185 S Orange Ave, MSB, rm G506, Newark, NJ 07103; **Phone:** 973-972-6639; **Board Cert:** Surgery 2009; Surgical Critical Care 2006; **Med School:** Univ MD Sch Med 1973; **Resid:** Surgery, US Public Hlth Svc Hosp 1976; Surgery, US Public Hlth Svc Hosp 1978; **Fac Appt:** Prof S, UMDNJ-NJ Med Sch, Newark

Huston, Jan A MD (S) - **Spec Exp:** Breast Surgery; Breast Disease; **Hospital:** Saint Michael's Med Ctr, Saint Barnabas Med Ctr; **Address:** Summit Breast Care, SMMC-Connie Dwyer Breast Ctr, 1 Bay Ave, Montclair, NJ 07042; **Phone:** 908-918-0001; **Board Cert:** Surgery 2007; **Med School:** Mich State Univ 1982; **Resid:** Surgery, St Barnabas Hosp 1987; **Fellow:** Vascular Surgery, Lehigh Valley Hosp 1988

Maheshwari, Vivek MD (S) - **Spec Exp:** Gastrointestinal Cancer; Endocrine Tumors; Cancer Surgery; Breast Cancer; **Hospital:** Saint Barnabas Med Ctr, Newark Beth Israel Med Ctr; **Address:** 101 Old Short Hills Rd, Ste 206, West Orange, NJ 07052; **Phone:** 973-731-5005; **Board Cert:** Surgery 2003; **Med School:** India 1992; **Resid:** Surgery, Beth Israel Med Ctr 2002; **Fellow:** Surgical Oncology, Univ Pittsburgh 2004

Mansour, E Hani MD (S) - **Spec Exp:** Burn Care; **Hospital:** Saint Barnabas Med Ctr; **Address:** Burn Surgeons of St Barnabas, 94 Old Short Hills Rd, Livingston, NJ 07039; **Phone:** 973-322-5924; **Board Cert:** Surgery 1999; Surgical Critical Care 2010; **Med School:** Lebanon 1973; **Resid:** Surgery, Union Meml Hosp 1979; **Fellow:** Burn Surgery, Brooke Army Med Ctr

Petrone, Sylvia J MD (S) - **Spec Exp:** Burn Care; Critical Care; **Hospital:** Saint Barnabas Med Ctr; **Address:** Burn Surgeons of St Barnabas, 94 Old Short Hills Rd, Livingston, NJ 07039; **Phone:** 973-322-5924; **Board Cert:** Surgery 2011; Surgical Critical Care 2008; **Med School:** Loyola Univ-Stritch Sch Med 1977; **Resid:** Surgery, Boston Univ Med Ctr 1982; **Fellow:** Burn Surgery, New York Hosp-Cornell 1983

Shack, Robert P MD (S) - **Hospital:** Saint Barnabas Med Ctr; **Address:** 745 Northfield Ave, West Orange, NJ 07052; **Phone:** 973-325-7705; **Board Cert:** Surgery 2005; **Med School:** Jefferson Med Coll 1969; **Resid:** Surgery, Mt Sinai Med Ctr 1975

Thoracic & Cardiac Surgery

Burns, Paul G MD (T&CS) - **Spec Exp:** Cardiac Surgery; **Hospital:** Saint Barnabas Med Ctr; **Address:** St Barnabas Hosp, 94 Old Short Hills Rd, rm 2511, Livingston, NJ 07039; **Phone:** 973-322-2200; **Board Cert:** Thoracic Surgery 2010; **Med School:** Columbia P&S 1989; **Resid:** Surgery, Deaconess Hosp/Harvard 1996; **Fellow:** Cardiothoracic Surgery, New York Hosp/Cornell 1998

Camacho, Margarita T MD (T&CS) - **Spec Exp:** Mechanical Assist Devices; Transplant-Heart; Heart Failure; **Hospital:** Newark Beth Israel Med Ctr; **Address:** Newark Beth Israel Med Ctr, Dept Cardiothoracic Surgery, 201 Lyons Ave, Ste G-5, Newark, NJ 07112; **Phone:** 973-926-6938; **Board Cert:** Thoracic Surgery 2008; **Med School:** NY Med Coll 1984; **Resid:** Surgery, Lenox Hill Hosp 1989; Cardiothoracic Surgery, Albert Einstein Affil Hosp 1991; **Fellow:** Pediatric Cardiothoracic Surgery, LI Jewish Med Ctr 1992; Transplantation/Mechanical Assist Devices, Cleveland Clinic 1994; **Fac Appt:** Assoc Clin Prof TS, Albert Einstein Coll Med

Forman, Mark MD (T&CS) - **Spec Exp:** Lung Cancer; Lung Surgery; Vascular Surgery; Video Assisted Thoracic Surgery (VATS); **Hospital:** Saint Barnabas Med Ctr, Overlook Med Ctr (page 92); **Address:** 1500 Pleasant Valley Way, Ste 302, West Orange, NJ 07052; **Phone:** 973-324-0988; **Board Cert:** Thoracic Surgery 2007; **Med School:** Tulane Univ 1976; **Resid:** Surgery, LI Jewish Med Ctr 1981; Thoracic Surgery, Montefiore Hosp Med Ctr 1984; **Fellow:** Thoracic Surgery, Montefiore Hosp Med Ctr 1982

Goldenberg, Bruce MD (T&CS) - **Spec Exp:** Minimally Invasive Thoracic Surgery; Cardiac Surgery-Adult; Pacemakers; Arrhythmias; **Hospital:** St. Clare's Hosp - Denville, Hackensack UMC-Mountainside (page 736); **Address:** 30 Chatham Rd, Ste 377, Short Hills, NJ 07078; **Phone:** 973-467-5550; **Board Cert:** Thoracic & Cardiac Surgery 2003; **Med School:** Northwestern Univ 1976; **Resid:** Surgery, NYU Med Ctr 1981; **Fellow:** Thoracic & Cardiac Surgery, NYU Med Ctr 1983; **Fac Appt:** Asst Clin Prof S, UMDNJ-NJ Med Sch, Newark

Saunders, Craig R MD (T&CS) - **Spec Exp:** Cardiac Surgery; Minimally Invasive Surgery; **Hospital:** Newark Beth Israel Med Ctr, Saint Barnabas Med Ctr; **Address:** 201 Lyons Ave, Ste G5, Newark, NJ 07112; **Phone:** 973-926-6938; **Board Cert:** Thoracic Surgery 2011; **Med School:** Univ Iowa Coll Med 1970; **Resid:** Surgery, Univ Iowa Hosps 1978; Thoracic Surgery, Cleveland Clinic 1980

Urology

Boorjian, Peter C MD (U) - **Spec Exp:** Kidney Stones; Prostate Benign Disease; Urinary Tract Infections; Urologic Cancer; **Hospital:** Hackensack UMC-Mountainside (page 736); **Address:** Montclair Urological Group, 777 Bloomfield Ave, Glen Ridge, NJ 07028; **Phone:** 973-429-0462; **Board Cert:** Urology 1978; **Med School:** SUNY Downstate 1971; **Resid:** Surgery, Med Coll VA 1973; Urology, SUNY Downstate 1976

Ciccone, Patrick N MD (U) - **Spec Exp:** Prostate Cancer; **Hospital:** Clara Maass Med Ctr, Saint Barnabas Med Ctr; **Address:** 36 Newark Ave, Ste 200, Belleville, NJ 07109; **Phone:** 973-759-6180; **Board Cert:** Urology 1975; **Med School:** Georgetown Univ 1967; **Resid:** Surgery, VA Med Ctr 1969; Urology, VA Med Ctr 1972

Jordan, Mark L MD (U) - **Spec Exp:** Urologic Cancer; Kidney Cancer; Transplant-Kidney; Laparoscopic Surgery; **Hospital:** Univ Hosp-UMDNJ—Newark; **Address:** Univ Hosp-UMDNJ, Dept Urol, 140 Bergen St, Ste G-1680, Newark, NJ 07103; **Phone:** 973-972-2888; **Board Cert:** Urology 2003; **Med School:** Canada 1977; **Resid:** Urologic Surgery, Univ Toronto 1983; **Fellow:** Renal Transplant, Cleveland Clinic 1984; Immunology, Univ Minn 1986; **Fac Appt:** Prof U, UMDNJ-NJ Med Sch, Newark

Katz, Jeffrey I MD (U) - **Spec Exp:** Prostate Disease; Kidney Stones; Urologic Cancer; **Hospital:** Saint Barnabas Med Ctr; **Address:** 741 Northfield Ave, Ste 206, West Orange, NJ 07052; **Phone:** 973-325-6100; **Board Cert:** Urology 1978; **Med School:** Italy 1970; **Resid:** Surgery, Mt Sinai Hosp 1973; Urology, Montefiore Med Ctr 1976

Linsenmeyer, Todd A MD (U) - **Spec Exp:** Infertility-Male in Spinal Cord Injury; Voiding Dysfunction/Spinal Cord Injury; Urodynamics in Spinal Cord Injury; **Hospital:** Kessler Inst for Rehab - W Orange; **Address:** Kessler Inst Rehab, 1199 Pleasant Valley Way, West Orange, NJ 07052; **Phone:** 973-731-3900 x2274; **Board Cert:** Urology 2005; Physical Medicine & Rehabilitation 1990; Spinal Cord Injury Medicine 2002; **Med School:** Univ Hawaii JA Burns Sch Med 1979; **Resid:** Urology, Tripler AMC 1984; **Fellow:** Physical Medicine & Rehabilitation, Stanford Univ Hosp 1989; **Fac Appt:** Assoc Prof S, UMDNJ-NJ Med Sch, Newark

Savatta, Domenico J MD (U) - **Spec Exp:** Robotic Urologic Surgery; Prostate Cancer; Kidney Cancer; Bladder Cancer; **Hospital:** Newark Beth Israel Med Ctr, Saint Barnabas Med Ctr; **Address:** 375 Mt. Pleasant Ave, Ste 250, West Orange, NJ 07052; **Phone:** 973-323-1320; **Board Cert:** Urology 2005; **Med School:** SUNY Stony Brook 1997; **Resid:** Surgery, Indiana Univ Med Ctr 1999; Urologic Surgery, Indiana Univ Med Ctr 2003

Stock, Jeffrey A MD (U) - **Spec Exp:** Pediatric Urology; Robotic Surgery-Pediatric; Minimally Invasive Surgery-Pediatric; **Hospital:** Newark Beth Israel Med Ctr, Mount Sinai Med Ctr (page 102); **Address:** 101 Old Short Hills Rd, Ste 203, West Orange, NJ 07052-1023; **Phone:** 973-325-7188; **Board Cert:** Urology 2010; Pediatric Urology 2010; **Med School:** Mount Sinai Sch Med 1988; **Resid:** Surgery, UMDNJ- Univ Hosp 1990; Urology, UMDNJ- Univ Hosp 1993; **Fellow:** Pediatric Urology, UCSD Med Ctr 1994; **Fac Appt:** Clin Prof U, UMDNJ-NJ Med Sch, Newark

Strauss, Bernard S MD (U) - **Spec Exp:** Kidney Stones; Prostate Disease; Sexual Dysfunction; **Hospital:** Saint Barnabas Med Ctr; **Address:** 741 Northfield Ave, Ste 206, West Orange, NJ 07052; **Phone:** 973-325-6100; **Board Cert:** Urology 1973; **Med School:** Albert Einstein Coll Med 1964; **Resid:** Surgery, Marquette Univ Affil Hosp 1966; **Fellow:** Urology, Bronx Municipal Hosp 1969; **Fac Appt:** Asst Clin Prof S, UMDNJ-NJ Med Sch, Newark

Vascular Surgery

Brener, Bruce J MD (VascS) - **Spec Exp:** Endovascular Surgery; Minimally Invasive Vascular Surgery; Carotid Artery Surgery; Aneurysm-Aortic; **Hospital:** Newark Beth Israel Med Ctr, Saint Barnabas Med Ctr; **Address:** 200 S Orange Ave, Ste 109, Livingston, NJ 07039; **Phone:** 973-322-7233; **Board Cert:** Surgery 1972; Vascular Surgery 2005; **Med School:** Harvard Med Sch 1966; **Resid:** Surgery, Chldns Hosp Med Ctr 1968; Surgery, Peter Bent Brigham Hosp 1972; **Fellow:** Vascular Surgery, Mass Genl Hosp 1973; **Fac Appt:** Assoc Clin Prof S, Columbia P&S

Hudson

Hudson

Cardiovascular Disease

Cruz, Merle C MD (Cv) - **Spec Exp:** Heart Disease; **Hospital:** Christ Hosp - Jersey City; **Address:** 201 St Pauls Ave, Ste 1D, Jersey City, NJ 07306; **Phone:** 201-653-7533; **Board Cert:** Internal Medicine 1983; Cardiovascular Disease 1985; **Med School:** Philippines 1976; **Resid:** Internal Medicine, Jersey City Med Ctr 1982; **Fellow:** Cardiovascular Disease, Brookdale Hosp Med Ctr 1984

Elkind, Barry M MD (Cv) - **Spec Exp:** Non-Invasive Cardiology; Preventive Cardiology; **Hospital:** Bayonne Med Ctr, Newark Beth Israel Med Ctr; **Address:** 1061 Avenue C, Bayonne, NJ 07002; **Phone:** 201-858-0800; **Board Cert:** Internal Medicine 1979; Cardiovascular Disease 1981; **Med School:** UMDNJ-NJ Med Sch, Newark 1976; **Resid:** Internal Medicine, Boston City Hosp 1979; **Fellow:** Cardiovascular Disease, New England Med Ctr 1982

Moussa, Ghias M MD (Cv) - **Spec Exp:** Heart Valve Disease; Congestive Heart Failure; **Hospital:** Christ Hosp - Jersey City; **Address:** 1815 Kennedy Blvd, Jersey City, NJ 07305; **Phone:** 201-333-3311; **Board Cert:** Internal Medicine 1989; **Med School:** Syria 1979; **Resid:** Internal Medicine, Jersey City Med Ctr 1989; **Fellow:** Cardiovascular Disease, Jersey City Med Ctr 1991; **Fac Appt:** Assoc Prof Med, UMDNJ-NJ Med Sch, Newark

Dermatology

Blank, Ellen MD (D) - **Spec Exp:** Acne; **Hospital:** Mount Sinai Med Ctr (page 102); **Address:** 333 Avenue C, Bayonne, NJ 07002; **Phone:** 201-858-4800; **Board Cert:** Dermatology 1979; **Med School:** Mount Sinai Sch Med 1975; **Resid:** Dermatology, Mount Sinai Hosp 1979

Kopec, Anna V MD (D) - **Spec Exp:** Cosmetic Dermatology; Hair & Nail Disorders; **Hospital:** Bayonne Med Ctr; **Address:** 730 Kennedy Blvd, Bayonne, NJ 07002-1838; **Phone:** 201-858-4300; **Board Cert:** Dermatology 1980; **Med School:** UMDNJ-NJ Med Sch, Newark 1975; **Resid:** Dermatology, Albert Einstein 1979; **Fac Appt:** Assoc Clin Prof D, Albert Einstein Coll Med

Endocrinology, Diabetes & Metabolism

Cam, Jenny Rose G MD (EDM) - **Spec Exp:** Diabetes; Thyroid Disorders; Osteoporosis; Adrenal Disorders; **Hospital:** Hoboken Univ Med Ctr - Hoboken, Meadowlands Hosp Med Ctr; **Address:** 10 Huron Ave, Ste 1P, Jersey City, NJ 07306; **Phone:** 201-656-6003; **Board Cert:** Internal Medicine 1988; Endocrinology, Diabetes & Metabolism 1989; **Med School:** Philippines 1979; **Resid:** Internal Medicine, Interfaith Med Ctr 1987; **Fellow:** Endocrinology, Diabetes & Metabolism, UMDNJ-Univ Hosp 1989

Family Medicine

Levine, Martin S DO (FMed) *PCP* - **Spec Exp:** Primary Care Sports Medicine; Osteopathic Manipulation; **Hospital:** Christ Hosp - Jersey City, Bayonne Med Ctr; **Address:** 789 Avenue C, Bayonne, NJ 07002; **Phone:** 201-339-2620; **Board Cert:** Family Medicine 2007; Geriatric Medicine 2011; **Med School:** Kirksville Coll Osteo Med 1980; **Resid:** Family Medicine, Kennedy Meml Hosp 1983; **Fac Appt:** Assoc Clin Prof FMed, Seton Hall Univ Sch Hlth & Med Scis

Sklower, Jay A DO (FMed) *PCP* - **Spec Exp:** Geriatric Medicine; Diabetes; Cholesterol/Lipid Disorders; **Hospital:** Christ Hosp - Jersey City; **Address:** 600 Pavonia Ave, 2nd Fl, Jersey City, NJ 07306-2929; **Phone:** 201-216-3040; **Board Cert:** Family Medicine 2005; **Med School:** SUNY Stony Brook 1971; **Resid:** Family Medicine, Union Meml Hosp 1973; **Fac Appt:** Assoc Prof Ped

Gastroenterology

Hahn, John C MD (Ge) - **Spec Exp:** Colonoscopy; Peptic Acid Disorders; **Hospital:** Bayonne Med Ctr; **Address:** 534 Avenue E, Ste 1C, Bayonne, NJ 07002; **Phone:** 201-823-0450; **Board Cert:** Internal Medicine 1988; Gastroenterology 2011; **Med School:** UMDNJ-NJ Med Sch, Newark 1985; **Resid:** Internal Medicine, Univ Hosp 1988; **Fellow:** Gastroenterology, Univ Hosp 1990

Prakash, Anaka MD (Ge) - **Spec Exp:** Pancreatic/Biliary Endoscopy (ERCP); Capsule Endoscopy; **Hospital:** Bayonne Med Ctr, Jersey City Med Ctr; **Address:** 534 Ave E, Ste 1A, Bayonne, NJ 07002; **Phone:** 201-858-8444; **Board Cert:** Internal Medicine 1976; Gastroenterology 1977; **Med School:** India 1973; **Resid:** Internal Medicine, St Joseph's Hosp 1975; **Fellow:** Gastroenterology, CMDNJ-Newark 1977

Geriatric Medicine

Brown, Mitchell Lee MD (Ger) *PCP* - **Spec Exp:** Alzheimer's Disease; **Hospital:** Bayonne Med Ctr, Jersey City Med Ctr; **Address:** 758 Broadway, Bayonne, NJ 07002; **Phone:** 201-339-2220; **Board Cert:** Geriatric Medicine 2002; **Med School:** West Indies 1987; **Resid:** Internal Medicine, St Elizabeth Hosp 1990; **Fellow:** Geriatric Medicine, St Vincent's Hosp & Med Ctr 1992

Reisner, Michelle MD (Ger) *PCP* - **Hospital:** Jersey City Med Ctr; **Address:** 196 Jewitt Ave, Jersey City, NJ 07304; **Phone:** 201-332-3354; **Board Cert:** Internal Medicine 1989; Geriatric Medicine 2005; Hospice & Palliative Medicine 2008; **Med School:** South Africa 1983; **Resid:** Internal Medicine, Jersey City Med Ctr 1989

Internal Medicine

Cardiello, Gary P MD (IM) *PCP* - **Spec Exp:** Diabetes; Hypertension; Hemochromatosis; **Hospital:** Clara Maass Med Ctr, Saint Michael's Med Ctr; **Address:** 744 Broadway, Bayonne, NJ 07002; **Phone:** 201-436-8888; **Board Cert:** Internal Medicine 1986; **Med School:** Italy 1983; **Resid:** Internal Medicine, St Michael's Med Ctr 1986

Condo, Dominick MD (IM) *PCP* - **Spec Exp:** Geriatric Care; **Hospital:** Bayonne Med Ctr, Overlook Med Ctr (page 92); **Address:** 622 Broadway, Bayonne, NJ 07002; **Phone:** 201-436-2800; **Board Cert:** Internal Medicine 1984; **Med School:** Mexico 1980; **Resid:** Internal Medicine, St Michael's Med Ctr 1984

Dedousis, John T MD (IM) *PCP* - **Hospital:** Bayonne Med Ctr; **Address:** 1166 Kennedy Blvd, Bayonne, NJ 07002-3112; **Phone:** 201-339-1133; **Board Cert:** Internal Medicine 2003; **Med School:** Dominica 1985; **Resid:** Internal Medicine, Univ Hosp 1988

Kozel, Joseph M MD (IM) *PCP* - **Spec Exp:** Asthma; Chronic Obstructive Lung Disease (COPD); Lung Cancer; Lung Disease in Pregnancy; **Hospital:** Hoboken Univ Med Ctr - Hoboken, Jersey City Med Ctr; **Address:** 331 Grand St, Fl Ground, Hoboken, NJ 07030; **Phone:** 201-656-3519; **Board Cert:** Internal Medicine 1984; **Med School:** Mexico 1973; **Resid:** Family Medicine, St Mary Hosp 1979; Internal Medicine, St Michaels Med Ctr 1980; **Fellow:** Pulmonary Disease, St Michaels Med Ctr 1982

Mutterperl, Mitchell MD (IM) *PCP* - **Spec Exp:** Hypertension; Cholesterol/Lipid Disorders; Cardiovascular Disease; **Hospital:** Bayonne Med Ctr, Jersey City Med Ctr; **Address:** 19 W 33rd St, Bayonne, NJ 07002-3916; **Phone:** 201-858-0090; **Board Cert:** Internal Medicine 1985; **Med School:** Italy 1981; **Resid:** Internal Medicine, UMDNJ-NJ Med Ctr 1985

Nephrology

Thomsen, Stephen MD (Nep) - **Spec Exp:** Diabetes; Hypertension; Kidney Disease; **Hospital:** Christ Hosp - Jersey City, Hackensack UMC-Mountainside (page 736); **Address:** 510 31st St, Union City, NJ 07087; **Phone:** 201-866-3322; **Board Cert:** Internal Medicine 1981; Nephrology 2006; **Med School:** Italy 1977; **Resid:** Internal Medicine, Mountainside Hosp 1980; **Fellow:** Nephrology, Univ Hosp-UMDNJ 1982

Neurology

Anselmi, Gregory D MD (N) - **Spec Exp:** Migraine; Multiple Sclerosis; Stroke; **Hospital:** Bayonne Med Ctr, Hoboken Univ Med Ctr - Hoboken; **Address:** 1222 Kennedy Blvd, Bayonne, NJ 07002-3822; **Phone:** 201-339-6531; **Board Cert:** Neurology 2009; Vascular Surgery 2009; **Med School:** Italy 1988; **Resid:** Internal Medicine, SUNY/Univ Hosp 1989; **Fellow:** Neurology, St Vincent's Hosp & Med Ctr 1992

Charles, James A MD (N) - **Spec Exp:** Headache; Clinical Neurophysiology; **Hospital:** Bayonne Med Ctr, Holy Name Med Ctr (page 688); **Address:** 956 Kennedy Blvd, Bayonne, NJ 07002; **Phone:** 201-858-2457; **Board Cert:** Neurology 1984; Clinical Neurophysiology 2005; **Med School:** UMDNJ-NJ Med Sch, Newark 1978; **Resid:** Neurology, UMDNJ Med Ctr 1982; **Fac Appt:** Assoc Clin Prof N, UMDNJ-NJ Med Sch, Newark

Fellus, Jonathan L MD (N) - **Spec Exp:** Brain Injury; Neuro-Rehabilitation; Stroke; Dementia; **Hospital:** Meadowlands Hosp Med Ctr; **Address:** Meadowlands Hospital, 55 Meadowlands Pkwy, Secaucus, NJ 07094; **Phone:** 201-392-3524; **Board Cert:** Neurology 2009; **Med School:** UMDNJ-RW Johnson Med Sch 1992; **Resid:** Neurology, Penn Hosp 1996; **Fellow:** Neurological Rehabilitation, Kernan Hosp/Univ MD Med Ctr 1997; **Fac Appt:** Asst Clin Prof N, UMDNJ-NJ Med Sch, Newark

Sadeghi, Hooshang W MD (N) - **Spec Exp:** Parkinson's Disease; Stroke; Multiple Sclerosis; Dystonia-Cervical; **Hospital:** Bayonne Med Ctr, Jersey City Med Ctr; **Address:** 631 Broadway, FL 3, Bayonne, NJ 07002-3846; **Phone:** 201-823-2888; **Board Cert:** Neurology 1977; **Med School:** Iran 1967; **Resid:** Neurology, UMDNJ Med Ctr 1975; **Fac Appt:** Asst Clin Prof N, UMDNJ-NJ Med Sch, Newark

Obstetrics & Gynecology

Banzon, Manuel MD (ObG) - **Spec Exp:** Laparoscopic Surgery; Vaginal Surgery; Incontinence; **Hospital:** Meadowlands Hosp Med Ctr; **Address:** 1265 Paterson Plank Rd, Ste 3D, Secaucus, NJ 07094; **Phone:** 201-864-4442; **Board Cert:** Obstetrics & Gynecology 1979; **Med School:** Philippines 1962; **Resid:** Obstetrics & Gynecology, Jersey City Med Ctr 1969

Masson, Lalitha MD (ObG) - **Spec Exp:** Infertility; **Hospital:** Christ Hosp - Jersey City; **Address:** 634 Newark Ave, Main Fl, Jersey City, NJ 07306; **Phone:** 201-963-8554; **Board Cert:** Obstetrics & Gynecology 1973; **Med School:** India 1964; **Resid:** Obstetrics & Gynecology, Margaret Hogue Hosp 1969; Obstetrics & Gynecology, St Clares Hosp 1970; **Fellow:** Infertility, UMDNJ-NJ Sch Med 1971

Uy, Vena MD (ObG) *PCP* - **Hospital:** Christ Hosp - Jersey City, Meadowlands Hosp Med Ctr; **Address:** 142 Palisade Ave, Ste 102, Jersey City, NJ 07306; **Phone:** 201-653-0506; **Board Cert:** Obstetrics & Gynecology 1977; **Med School:** Philippines 1968; **Resid:** Obstetrics & Gynecology, Jersey Shore Med Ctr 1973; **Fellow:** Gynecologic Pathology, Magee Womens Hosp 1974

Ophthalmology

Benedetto, Dominick A MD (Oph) - **Spec Exp:** LASIK-Refractive Surgery; Cataract Surgery; **Hospital:** Bayonne Med Ctr, Morristown Med Ctr (page 92); **Address:** EyeMD Associates, 124 Avenue B, Bayonne, NJ 07002-2033; **Phone:** 201-436-1150; **Board Cert:** Ophthalmology 1982; **Med School:** Univ Fla Coll Med 1975; **Resid:** Ophthalmology, Wills Eye Hosp 1981

Constad, William H MD (Oph) - **Spec Exp:** Cornea Transplant; Cataract Surgery; Refractive Surgery; **Hospital:** Jersey City Med Ctr; **Address:** 600 Pavonia Ave Fl 6, Jersey City, NJ 07306-2932; **Phone:** 201-963-3937; **Board Cert:** Ophthalmology 1985; **Med School:** Med Coll PA Hahnemann 1980; **Resid:** Ophthalmology, Univ Hosp-UMDNJ 1984; **Fellow:** Cornea, NY Eye & Ear Infirm 1985; **Fac Appt:** Clin Prof Oph, UMDNJ-NJ Med Sch, Newark

Orthopaedic Surgery

Granatir, Charles MD (OrS) - **Hospital:** Clara Maass Med Ctr; **Address:** 586 Kearny Ave, Kearny, NJ 07032; **Phone:** 201-997-7667; **Board Cert:** Orthopaedic Surgery 2010; **Med School:** Hahnemann Univ 1979; **Resid:** Orthopaedic Surgery, Montefiore Med Ctr 1984

Otolaryngology

Garay, Kenneth F MD (Oto) - **Spec Exp:** Nasal & Sinus Disorders; **Hospital:** Jersey City Med Ctr; **Address:** 355 Grand St, Jersey City, NJ 07302; **Phone:** 201-915-2832; **Board Cert:** Otolaryngology 1982; **Med School:** Temple Univ 1978; **Resid:** Surgery, Abington Meml Hosp 1979; Otolaryngology, Columbia-Presby 1982

Pediatrics

Baker, Azzam A MD (Ped) *PCP* - **Hospital:** Hackensack Univ Med Ctr (page 96), Palisades Med Ctr; **Address:** 714 10th St, Secaucus, NJ 07094-2921; **Phone:** 201-863-3346; **Board Cert:** Pediatrics 2011; **Med School:** Egypt 1972; **Resid:** Pediatrics, Jersey City Med Ctr 1978; **Fellow:** Neonatal-Perinatal Medicine, UMDNJ Univ Hosp 1980

Klos, Andrzej E MD (Ped) *PCP* - **Hospital:** Hoboken Univ Med Ctr - Hoboken, Hackensack Univ Med Ctr (page 96); **Address:** 1327 Willow Ave, Hoboken, NJ 07030; **Phone:** 201-963-5633; **Board Cert:** Pediatrics 2010; **Med School:** Poland 1977; **Resid:** Pediatrics, Jersey City Med Ctr 1994; **Fac Appt:** Asst Clin Prof Ped, UMDNJ-NJ Med Sch, Newark

Oko, Piotr MD (Ped) *PCP* - **Hospital:** Christ Hosp - Jersey City, Hoboken Univ Med Ctr - Hoboken; **Address:** Hoboken Pediatrics, 1327 Willow Ave, Hoboken, NJ 07030; **Phone:** 201-963-5633; **Board Cert:** Pediatrics 2010; **Med School:** Poland 1987; **Resid:** Pediatrics, Jersey City Med Ctr 1995

Skripkus, Aldona J MD (Ped) *PCP* - **Hospital:** Clara Maass Med Ctr; **Address:** 381 Kearny Ave, Kearny, NJ 07032-2603; **Phone:** 201-991-4824; **Board Cert:** Pediatrics 1971; **Med School:** Med Coll PA Hahnemann 1966; **Resid:** Pediatrics, Chldns Hosp 1969

Physical Medicine & Rehabilitation

Filippone, Mark A MD (PMR) - **Spec Exp:** Electrodiagnosis; Electromyography; Pain Management; **Hospital:** Christ Hosp - Jersey City, Hoboken Univ Med Ctr - Hoboken; **Address:** 2012 John F Kennedy Blvd W, Jersey City, NJ 07305-1526; **Phone:** 201-332-6855; **Board Cert:** Physical Medicine & Rehabilitation 1980; **Med School:** Georgetown Univ 1974; **Resid:** Pediatrics, St Vincent's Hosp & Med Ctr 1976; Physical Medicine & Rehabilitation, Bronx Muni Hosp-Einstein 1978; **Fac Appt:** Asst Clin Prof PMR, Albert Einstein Coll Med

Psychiatry

Gewolb, Eric B MD (Psyc) - **Spec Exp:** Anxiety Disorders; Dementia; Bipolar/Mood Disorders; **Hospital:** Bayonne Med Ctr; **Address:** 830 Kennedy Blvd, Bayonne, NJ 07002-2872; **Phone:** 201-339-0200; **Board Cert:** Psychiatry 1979; **Med School:** Tulane Univ 1974; **Resid:** Psychiatry, Mount Sinai Hosp 1978

Jacoby, Jacob H MD/PhD (Psyc) - **Spec Exp:** Psychopharmacology; Mood Disorders; **Hospital:** Bayonne Med Ctr, Saint Barnabas Med Ctr; **Address:** 654 Avenue C, Ste 201, Bayonne, NJ 07002-3899; **Phone:** 201-339-0323; **Board Cert:** Psychiatry 1993; **Med School:** SUNY Buffalo 1980; **Resid:** Psychiatry, Univ Pittsburgh Med Ctr 1981; Psychiatry, Western Psychiatric Inst 1983; **Fellow:** Addiction Psychiatry, Albert Einstein 1983; **Fac Appt:** Assoc Clin Prof Psyc, UMDNJ-NJ Med Sch, Newark

Kurani, Devendra MD (Psyc) - **Spec Exp:** Depression; Anxiety Disorders; Panic Disorder; **Hospital:** Saint Barnabas Med Ctr, Christ Hosp - Jersey City; **Address:** 221 Palisade Ave, Jersey City, NJ 07306; **Phone:** 201-656-3116; **Board Cert:** Psychiatry 1986; **Med School:** India 1975; **Resid:** Psychiatry, Warley Hosp 1981; Psychiatry, Harlem Hosp 1983

Moraille, Pascale MD (Psyc) - **Spec Exp:** Autism; Developmental Disorders; ADD/ADHD; **Hospital:** Hoboken Univ Med Ctr - Hoboken; **Address:** CMHC of Hoboken Univ Med Ctr, 506 Third St, Hoboken, NJ 07030; **Phone:** 201-792-8200; **Board Cert:** Psychiatry 1993; **Med School:** Ponce Med Sch 1988; **Resid:** Psychiatry, UMDNJ-NJ Med Sch 1991; **Fellow:** Child & Adolescent Psychiatry, UMDNJ-NJ Med Sch 1993

Pulmonary Disease

Elamir, Mazhar E MD (Pul) - **Spec Exp:** Sleep Disorders; Allergy; Asthma; **Hospital:** Christ Hosp - Jersey City; **Address:** 192 Harrison Ave, Jersey City, NJ 07304; **Phone:** 201-333-5363; **Board Cert:** Internal Medicine 1987; Pulmonary Disease 2004; Sleep Medicine 2011; **Med School:** Egypt 1982; **Resid:** Internal Medicine, Jersey City Med Ctr 1987; **Fellow:** Pulmonary Disease, Interfaith Med Ctr 1991

Radiation Oncology

Goodman, Robert L MD (RadRO) - **Spec Exp:** Breast Cancer; Lymphoma; Prostate Cancer; Brain Tumors; **Hospital:** Saint Barnabas Med Ctr; **Address:** 631 Grand St, Jersey City, NJ 07304; **Phone:** 201-942-3999; **Board Cert:** Internal Medicine 1971; Therapeutic Radiology 1974; Medical Oncology 1975; **Med School:** Columbia P&S 1966; **Resid:** Internal Medicine, Beth Israel Hosp 1970; Radiation Therapy, Harvard Joint Ctr Rad Therapy 1974; **Fellow:** Hematology, NY-Presby Hosp 1969; **Fac Appt:** Prof RadRO, Univ Pennsylvania

Rheumatology

Scarpa, Nicholas P MD (Rhu) - **Spec Exp:** Lupus/SLE in Pregnancy; Rheumatoid Arthritis; Osteoporosis; **Hospital:** Christ Hosp - Jersey City, Univ Hosp-UMDNJ—Newark; **Address:** 600 Pavonia Ave Fl 5 - Ste 1, Jersey City, NJ 07306-2932; **Phone:** 201-216-3050; **Board Cert:** Internal Medicine 1983; Rheumatology 1986; **Med School:** UMDNJ-NJ Med Sch, Newark 1980; **Resid:** Internal Medicine, Hackensack Univ Med Ctr 1983; **Fellow:** Rheumatology, Hosp for Special Surg 1985; **Fac Appt:** Asst Clin Prof Med, UMDNJ-NJ Med Sch, Newark

Surgery

Gildengers, Jaime N MD (S) - **Spec Exp:** Gallbladder Surgery; Colon Surgery; Breast Surgery; **Hospital:** Palisades Med Ctr, Christ Hosp - Jersey City; **Address:** 313 60th St, West New York, NJ 07093; **Phone:** 201-854-0406; **Board Cert:** Surgery 2006; **Med School:** Argentina 1965; **Resid:** Surgery, Mt Sinai Med Ctr 1970; Surgery, St Clares Hosp 1973; **Fellow:** Surgical Research, St Clares Hosp 1974; **Fac Appt:** Asst Clin Prof S, UMDNJ-NJ Med Sch, Newark

McGovern Jr, Patrick J MD (S) - **Spec Exp:** Vascular Surgery; Aneurysm-Aortic; Carotid Artery Surgery; **Hospital:** Christ Hosp - Jersey City, Bayonne Med Ctr; **Address:** 17 Nardone Pl, Jersey City, NJ 07306; **Phone:** 201-656-0646; **Board Cert:** Surgery 2003; Vascular Surgery 2008; **Med School:** UMDNJ-NJ Med Sch, Newark 1978; **Resid:** Surgery, UMDNJ-Univ Hosp 1983; **Fellow:** Vascular Surgery, UMDNJ-RWJ Univ Hosp 1984

Sultan, Ronald H MD (S) - **Spec Exp:** Hernia; Thyroid Cancer; Breast Cancer; **Hospital:** Jersey City Med Ctr, Palisades Med Ctr; **Address:** 2255 John F Kennedy Blvd, Jersey City, NJ 07304-1428; **Phone:** 201-434-3305; **Board Cert:** Surgery 2009; **Med School:** NYU Sch Med 1973; **Resid:** Surgery, Bronx Muni Hosp 1977; Surgery, Albert Einstein Med Ctr 1980

Urology

Katz, Herbert I MD (U) - **Spec Exp:** Urologic Cancer; Erectile Dysfunction; Kidney Stones; Prostate Disease; **Hospital:** Bayonne Med Ctr; **Address:** 534 Ave E, Ste 2A, Bayonne, NJ 07002; **Phone:** 201-823-1303; **Board Cert:** Urology 1981; **Med School:** Temple Univ 1974; **Resid:** Surgery, Abington Meml Hosp 1976; Urology, Monterfiore-Weiler Einstein Med Ctr 1979

Shulman, Yale MD (U) - **Spec Exp:** Urologic Cancer; Kidney Stones; Sexual Dysfunction; Incontinence; **Hospital:** Christ Hosp - Jersey City, Englewood Hosp & Med Ctr; **Address:** 2255 Kennedy Blvd, Jersey City, NJ 07304-1428; **Phone:** 201-433-1057; **Board Cert:** Urology 1984; **Med School:** Albert Einstein Coll Med 1976; **Resid:** Surgery, Montefiore Hosp Med Ctr 1978; Urology, NYU Med Ctr 1982; **Fac Appt:** Assoc Clin Prof U, NYU Sch Med

Steigman, Elliot G MD (U) - **Spec Exp:** Kidney Stones; Prostate Benign Disease; **Hospital:** Christ Hosp - Jersey City; **Address:** 142 Palisade Ave, Ste 211, Jersey City, NJ 07306-1108; **Phone:** 201-435-2244; **Board Cert:** Urology 1982; **Med School:** SUNY Downstate 1975; **Resid:** Surgery, Brookdale Hosp Med Ctr 1977; Urology, SUNY Downstate Med Ctr 1980

Mercer

Mercer

Allergy & Immunology

Ricketti, Anthony J MD (A&I) - **Spec Exp:** Asthma in Pregnancy; Allergic Aspergillosis; Eosinophilic Lung Disorders; **Hospital:** St. Francis Med Ctr - Trenton, Robert Wood Johnson Univ Hosp Hamilton; **Address:** Allergy & Pulmonary Assocs, 1542 Kuser Rd, Ste B7, Trenton, NJ 08619-3829; **Phone:** 609-581-1400; **Board Cert:** Internal Medicine 1981; Allergy & Immunology 1983; Pulmonary Disease 1986; Critical Care Medicine 2009; **Med School:** Hahnemann Univ 1978; **Resid:** Internal Medicine, Cleveland Clin Fdn 1981; Allergy & Immunology, Northwestern Univ 1983; **Fellow:** Pulmonary Disease, Northwestern Univ 1984; **Fac Appt:** Asst Clin Prof Med, UMDNJ-RW Johnson Med Sch

Winant Jr, John G MD (A&I) - **Spec Exp:** Asthma; **Hospital:** Univ Med Ctr Princeton at Plainsboro; **Address:** 8 Quakerbridge Plaza, Ste E, Mercerville, NJ 08619-1255; **Phone:** 609-890-8782; **Board Cert:** Pediatrics 1980; Allergy & Immunology 1987; **Med School:** Univ Cincinnati 1975; **Resid:** Pediatrics, Chldns Hosp Med Ctr 1978; **Fellow:** Allergy & Immunology, Chldns Hosp Med Ctr 1980

Cardiovascular Disease

Costin, Andrew MD (Cv) - **Hospital:** Univ Med Ctr Princeton at Plainsboro; **Address:** 419 N Harrison St, Princeton, NJ 08540; **Phone:** 609-924-9300; **Board Cert:** Internal Medicine 1989; Cardiovascular Disease 2003; **Med School:** Yale Univ 1986; **Resid:** Internal Medicine, NY Hosp 1989; **Fellow:** Cardiovascular Disease, Hosp Univ Penn 1993

Hagaman, John F MD (Cv) - **Spec Exp:** Heart Failure; **Hospital:** Univ Med Ctr Princeton at Plainsboro; **Address:** 281 Witherspoon St, Ste 210, Princeton, NJ 08540-3210; **Phone:** 609-921-7456; **Board Cert:** Internal Medicine 1977; Cardiovascular Disease 1981; **Med School:** Columbia P&S 1974; **Resid:** Internal Medicine, Univ Mich Hosp 1977; **Fellow:** Cardiovascular Disease, NC Meml Hosp 1980; **Fac Appt:** Asst Clin Prof Med, UMDNJ-RW Johnson Med Sch

Mahalingam, Banu MD (Cv) - **Spec Exp:** Heart Disease in Women; Echocardiography; Preventive Cardiology; **Hospital:** Univ Med Ctr Princeton at Plainsboro, Robert Wood Johnson Univ Hosp - New Brunswick; **Address:** Cardiac Associates of Princeton, 281 Witherspoon St, Ste 210, Princeton, NJ 08542; **Phone:** 609-921-7456; **Board Cert:** Internal Medicine 2008; Cardiovascular Disease 2002; **Med School:** India 1995; **Resid:** Internal Medicine, RW Johnson Med Ctr 1998; **Fellow:** Cardiovascular Disease, RW Johnson Med Ctr 2001

Dermatology

Bagel, Jerry MD (D) - **Spec Exp:** Psoriasis; Atopic Dermatitis; Skin Diseases; Exfoliate Erythroderma; **Hospital:** Univ Med Ctr Princeton at Plainsboro; **Address:** 59 One Mile Rd, Ste G, East Windsor, NJ 08520-2505; **Phone:** 609-443-4500; **Board Cert:** Dermatology 1985; **Med School:** Mount Sinai Sch Med 1981; **Resid:** Dermatology, Columbia-Presby Med Ctr 1985

Notterman, Robyn MD (D) - **Hospital:** Univ Med Ctr Princeton at Plainsboro; **Address:** 800 Bunn Drive, Ste B 201, Princeton, NJ 08540; **Phone:** 609-924-1033; **Board Cert:** Dermatology 2003; **Med School:** Cornell Univ-Weill Med Coll 1983; **Resid:** Dermatology, NYU Med Ctr 1992

Vine, John E MD (D) - **Spec Exp:** Mohs' Surgery; Cosmetic Dermatology; Hyperhidrosis/Axillary Curettage; **Hospital:** Univ Med Ctr Princeton at Plainsboro, Robert Wood Johnson Univ Hosp - New Brunswick; **Address:** 253 Witherspoon St, Ste L, Princeton, NJ 08540; **Phone:** 609-683-0101; **Board Cert:** Dermatology 2005; **Med School:** Brown Univ 1992; **Resid:** Dermatology, Meml Hermann Hosp 1996; **Fellow:** Mohs Surgery, Scripps Clinic 1997

Endocrinology, Diabetes & Metabolism

Shelmet, John J MD (EDM) - **Spec Exp:** Diabetes; Metabolic Disorders; **Hospital:** Univ Med Ctr Princeton at Plainsboro; **Address:** 3131 Princeton Pike, Bldg 2B, Ste 104, Lawrenceville, NJ 08648-2526; **Phone:** 609-896-8050; **Board Cert:** Internal Medicine 1984; **Med School:** UMDNJ-RW Johnson Med Sch 1981; **Resid:** Internal Medicine, Middlesex Genl Hosp/Univ Hosp 1984; **Fellow:** Metabolism, Temple Univ 1986; Diabetes, Temple Univ 1986; **Fac Appt:** Clin Prof Med, UMDNJ-RW Johnson Med Sch

Family Medicine

Lansing, Martha MD (FMed) *PCP* - **Spec Exp:** Chronic Illness; Women's Health; Psychosomatic Disorders; **Hospital:** Capital Health Regl Med Ctr, Capital Health Med Ctr - Hopewell; **Address:** 433 Bellevue Ave, Fl 4th, Trenton, NJ 08618; **Phone:** 609-815-2671; **Board Cert:** Family Medicine 2005; **Med School:** Univ Okla Coll Med 1982; **Resid:** Family Medicine, Univ Tenn 1984; Family Medicine, Williamsport Hosp/Univ Penn 1985; **Fac Appt:** Assoc Prof FMed, UMDNJ-RW Johnson Med Sch

Rednor, Jeffrey DO (FMed) *PCP* - **Spec Exp:** Diabetes; Pain-Back; Preventive Cardiology; **Hospital:** Robert Wood Johnson Univ Hosp Hamilton; **Address:** 1 Washington Blvd, Ste A, Robbinsville, NJ 08691; **Phone:** 609-448-4353; **Board Cert:** Family Medicine 1992; **Med School:** UMDNJ Sch Osteo Med 1989; **Resid:** Family Medicine, Kennedy Meml Hosp 1992

Gastroenterology

Afridi, Shariq A MD (Ge) - **Spec Exp:** Liver Disease; Endoscopy; **Hospital:** Robert Wood Johnson Univ Hosp Hamilton, St. Francis Med Ctr - Trenton; **Address:** 1374 White Horse Square Rd, Yorkshire Bldg - Fl 2, Hamilton, NJ 08690; **Phone:** 609-586-1319; **Board Cert:** Internal Medicine 2002; Gastroenterology 2003; **Med School:** Pakistan 1986; **Resid:** Internal Medicine, Bridgeport Hosp 1991; **Fellow:** Gastroenterology, Bridgeport Hosp 1993

De Antonio, Joseph R MD (Ge) - **Spec Exp:** Liver Disease; **Hospital:** Capital Health Regl Med Ctr; **Address:** 3100 Princeton Pike, Bldg 4 - Ste C, Lawrenceville, NJ 08648; **Phone:** 609-882-2185; **Board Cert:** Internal Medicine 1989; Gastroenterology 2004; **Med School:** St Louis Univ 1982; **Resid:** Internal Medicine, VA Med Ctr 1989; **Fellow:** Gastroenterology, Bellevue Hosp Ctr 1991

Marin, Geobel A MD (Ge) - **Spec Exp:** Peptic Ulcer Disease; Colonoscopy; Inflammatory Bowel Disease; **Hospital:** Capital Health Med Ctr - Hopewell, Robert Wood Johnson Univ Hosp Hamilton; **Address:** 416 Bellevue Ave, Ste 101, Trenton, NJ 08618; **Phone:** 609-394-8844; **Board Cert:** Gastroenterology 1972; Internal Medicine 1977; **Med School:** Columbia P&S 1962; **Resid:** Internal Medicine, Philadelphia Genl Hosp 1966; **Fellow:** Gastroenterology, Philadelphia Genl Hosp 1968

Meirowitz, Robert F MD (Ge) - **Spec Exp:** Inflammatory Bowel Disease; Colon Polyps & Cancer; Colonoscopy; Gastroesophageal Reflux Disease (GERD); **Hospital:** Univ Med Ctr Princeton at Plainsboro; **Address:** 281 Witherspoon St, Ste 230, Princeton, NJ 08542; **Phone:** 609-924-1422; **Board Cert:** Internal Medicine 1987; Gastroenterology 2012; **Med School:** NY Med Coll 1984; **Resid:** Internal Medicine, UMDNJ-RW Johnson Univ Hosp 1988; **Fellow:** Gastroenterology, Univ Maryland 1990; **Fac Appt:** Asst Clin Prof Med

Rosner, Bruce P MD (Ge) - **Spec Exp:** Liver Disease; Gastroesophageal Reflux Disease (GERD); Colon Cancer; **Hospital:** St. Francis Med Ctr - Trenton; **Address:** Gastroenterology Associates, 2275 Whitehorse Mercerville Rd, Ste 2, Trenton, NJ 08619-2643; **Phone:** 609-890-0200; **Board Cert:** Internal Medicine 1979; Gastroenterology 1983; **Med School:** Univ Pennsylvania 1976; **Resid:** Internal Medicine, Penn Hosp 1979; **Fellow:** Gastroenterology, Hahnemann Univ 1981

Rubin, Marc R MD (Ge) - **Hospital:** St. Francis Med Ctr - Trenton; **Address:** Gastroenterology Associates, 2275 Whitehorse Mercerville Rd, Ste 2, Trenton, NJ 08619-2643; **Phone:** 609-890-0200; **Board Cert:** Internal Medicine 1977; Gastroenterology 1979; **Med School:** Albert Einstein Coll Med 1974; **Resid:** Internal Medicine, Penn Hosp 1977; **Fellow:** Gastroenterology, Univ Hosp 1979

Sachs, Jonathan R MD (Ge) - **Spec Exp:** Colon Cancer Screening; Gastroesophageal Reflux Disease (GERD); Inflammatory Bowel Disease; **Hospital:** Univ Med Ctr Princeton at Plainsboro; **Address:** Princeton Gastroenterology, 281 Witherspoon St, Ste 230, Princeton, NJ 08542-3210; **Phone:** 609-924-1422; **Board Cert:** Internal Medicine 1987; Gastroenterology 1989; **Med School:** Med Coll PA Hahnemann 1984; **Resid:** Internal Medicine, Temple Univ Hosp 1987; **Fellow:** Gastroenterology, Graduate Hosp 1989; **Fac Appt:** Clin Prof Med, UMDNJ-RW Johnson Med Sch

Hand Surgery

Ark, Jon Wong Tze-Jen MD (HS) - **Spec Exp:** Hand Surgery; Carpal Tunnel Syndrome; Foot & Ankle Surgery; Arthritis Hand Surgery; **Hospital:** Univ Med Ctr Princeton at Plainsboro; **Address:** 325 Princeton Ave, Princeton, NJ 08540; **Phone:** 609-924-8131; **Board Cert:** Orthopaedic Surgery 2007; Hand Surgery 2007; **Med School:** UMDNJ-RW Johnson Med Sch 1987; **Resid:** Orthopaedic Surgery, Columbia-Presby Med Ctr 1992; **Fellow:** Hand Surgery, Mass Genl Hosp 1993; Foot & Ankle Surgery, Jefferson Hosp 1995

Infectious Disease

Aufiero, Patrick MD (Inf) - **Spec Exp:** AIDS/HIV; Lyme Disease; Osteomyelitis; Skin/Soft Tissue Infections; **Hospital:** Robert Wood Johnson Univ Hosp Hamilton, Capital Health Med Ctr - Hopewell; **Address:** 2085 Klockner Rd, Hamilton, NJ 08690; **Phone:** 609-587-4122; **Board Cert:** Internal Medicine 2005; Infectious Disease 2006; **Med School:** Grenada 1984; **Resid:** Internal Medicine, St Michaels Med Ctr 1989; **Fellow:** Infectious Disease, St Michaels Med Ctr 1991

Cleri, Dennis MD (Inf) - **Spec Exp:** Viral Infections; AIDS/HIV; **Hospital:** St. Francis Med Ctr - Trenton; **Address:** 601 Hamilton Ave, Trenton, NJ 08629; **Phone:** 609-599-5050; **Board Cert:** Internal Medicine 1976; Infectious Disease 1982; **Med School:** Jefferson Med Coll 1972; **Resid:** Internal Medicine, Coney Island Hosp 1975; **Fellow:** Infectious Disease, Kings Co Hosp Ctr 1980

Gekowski, Kathleen MD (Inf) - **Spec Exp:** Travel Medicine; AIDS/HIV; Lyme Disease; **Hospital:** Capital Health Med Ctr - Hopewell, Robert Wood Johnson Univ Hosp Hamilton; **Address:** 1450 Parkside Ave, Ste 4, Ewing, NJ 08638; **Phone:** 609-882-3500; **Board Cert:** Internal Medicine 1979; Infectious Disease 1984; **Med School:** Hahnemann Univ 1976; **Resid:** Internal Medicine, Univ Illinois Hosp 1979; **Fellow:** Infectious Disease, Yale Univ 1982; **Fac Appt:** Assoc Clin Prof Med, UMDNJ-RW Johnson Med Sch

Porwancher, Richard B MD (Inf) - **Spec Exp:** Lyme Disease; AIDS/HIV; Disaster Preparedness; **Hospital:** St. Francis Med Ctr - Trenton, Robert Wood Johnson Univ Hosp Hamilton; **Address:** 1245 Whitehorse-Mercerville Rd, Ste 410-411, Hamilton, NJ 08619-3831; **Phone:** 609-581-2000; **Board Cert:** Internal Medicine 1980; Infectious Disease 1982; **Med School:** Northwestern Univ 1977; **Resid:** Internal Medicine, Med Coll Wisconsin Affil Hosps 1980; **Fellow:** Infectious Disease, VA Med Ctr 1982; **Fac Appt:** Assoc Clin Prof Med

Internal Medicine

Corazza, Douglas P MD (IM) *PCP* - **Hospital:** Univ Med Ctr Princeton at Plainsboro; **Address:** 727 State Road, Princeton, NJ 08540; **Phone:** 609-921-6410; **Board Cert:** Internal Medicine 1988; **Med School:** UMDNJ-Rutgers Med Sch 1985; **Resid:** Internal Medicine, RW Johnson Univ Hosp 1988

Harman, John MD (IM) *PCP* - **Hospital:** Capital Health Med Ctr - Hopewell; **Address:** 2480 Pennington Rd, Ste 108, Pennington, NJ 08534; **Phone:** 609-737-6700; **Board Cert:** Internal Medicine 1972; **Med School:** Univ Pennsylvania 1969; **Resid:** Internal Medicine, Presby Hosp 1972; **Fellow:** Pulmonary Disease, U Penn Hosp 1975

Murray, Simon D MD (IM) *PCP* - **Spec Exp:** Concierge Medicine; Cholesterol/Lipid Disorders; Nutrition; Preventive Medicine; **Hospital:** Univ Med Ctr Princeton at Plainsboro; **Address:** 727 State Rd, Princeton, NJ 08540; **Phone:** 609-921-7444; **Board Cert:** Internal Medicine 1985; **Med School:** Philippines 1980; **Resid:** Internal Medicine, UMDNJ/RWJ Univ Hosp 1984; **Fac Appt:** Asst Clin Prof Med, UMDNJ-RW Johnson Med Sch

Schaeffer, Mark A MD (IM) - **Hospital:** Univ Med Ctr Princeton at Plainsboro; **Address:** 800 Bunn Drive, Ste 302, Princeton, NJ 08540; **Phone:** 609-921-1680; **Board Cert:** Internal Medicine 1989; **Med School:** NY Med Coll 1984; **Resid:** Internal Medicine, RW Johnson Univ Hosp 1989

Warren, Ronald MD (IM) - **Spec Exp:** Pulmonary Disease; **Hospital:** Capital Health Regl Med Ctr; **Address:** Pulmonary & Internal Med, 40 Fuld St, Ste 201, Trenton, NJ 08638-5247; **Phone:** 609-695-4422; **Board Cert:** Internal Medicine 1972; Pulmonary Disease 1976; **Med School:** Univ Pennsylvania 1968; **Resid:** Internal Medicine, Presby Hosp 1970; Internal Medicine, Grady Meml Hosp 1971; **Fellow:** Pulmonary Disease, Emory Hosps 1972

Yamane, Michael H MD (IM) *PCP* - **Hospital:** Capital Health Med Ctr - Hopewell; **Address:** 2480 Pennington Rd, Ste 104, Pennington, NJ 08534-5227; **Phone:** 609-818-1000; **Board Cert:** Internal Medicine 1984; **Med School:** UCSF 1981; **Resid:** Internal Medicine, Univ Hawaii Med Ctr 1984

Interventional Cardiology

Shanahan, Andrew J MD (IC) - **Spec Exp:** Angioplasty; **Hospital:** Univ Med Ctr Princeton at Plainsboro, Robert Wood Johnson Univ Hosp - New Brunswick; **Address:** Cardiology Assocs of Princeton, 281 Witherspoon St, Ste 210, Princeton, NJ 08542; **Phone:** 609-921-7456; **Board Cert:** Internal Medicine 2005; Cardiovascular Disease 2005; Interventional Cardiology 2011; **Med School:** Med Coll Wisc 1989; **Resid:** Internal Medicine, St Lukes-Roosevelt Hosp 1992; **Fellow:** Cardiovascular Disease, St Lukes-Roosevelt Hosp 1995

Medical Oncology

Grossman, Bernard MD (Onc) - **Hospital:** Capital Health Med Ctr - Hopewell, Robert Wood Johnson Univ Hosp Hamilton; **Address:** 2997 Princeton Pike Fl 2, Lawrenceville, NJ 08648; **Phone:** 609-771-0700; **Board Cert:** Internal Medicine 1977; Medical Oncology 1979; Hematology 1980; Hospice & Palliative Medicine 2010; **Med School:** Temple Univ 1974; **Resid:** Internal Medicine, Albany Meml Hosp 1977; **Fellow:** Hematology & Oncology, George Wash Univ Hosp 1979; Oncology, Fox Chase Cancer Ctr 1980

Lerma, Pauline M MD (Onc) - **Spec Exp:** Breast Cancer; Hematologic Malignancies; **Hospital:** Robert Wood Johnson Univ Hosp Hamilton; **Address:** Cancer Inst NJ-Hamilton, 2575 Klockner Rd, Hamilton, NJ 08690; **Phone:** 609-631-6960; **Board Cert:** Internal Medicine 2006; Medical Oncology 2009; Hematology 2010; **Med School:** Philippines 1992; **Resid:** Internal Medicine, Abington Meml Hosp 1996; **Fellow:** Hematology & Oncology, Hahnemann Univ Hosp 1999; Bone Marrow Transplant, Hahnemann Univ Hosp 2000; **Fac Appt:** Asst Prof Med, UMDNJ-RW Johnson Med Sch

Schaebler, David MD (Onc) - **Hospital:** Capital Health Med Ctr - Hopewell, Robert Wood Johnson Univ Hosp Hamilton; **Address:** Mercer Bucks Hem/Onc, 2997 Princeton Pike, Lawrenceville, NJ 08648; **Phone:** 609-771-0700; **Board Cert:** Internal Medicine 2002; Medical Oncology 2003; **Med School:** Jefferson Med Coll 1988; **Resid:** Internal Medicine, Cooper Univ Med Ctr 1991; **Fellow:** Medical Oncology, Fox Chase 1994

Sierocki, John Stanley MD (Onc) - **Spec Exp:** Breast Cancer; Lung Cancer; Lymphoma; Brain Tumors; **Hospital:** Univ Med Ctr Princeton at Plainsboro; **Address:** Princeton Med Grp, 419 N Harrison St, Ste 101, Princeton, NJ 08540-3521; **Phone:** 609-924-9300; **Board Cert:** Internal Medicine 1976; Medical Oncology 1979; **Med School:** Hahnemann Univ 1973; **Resid:** Internal Medicine, Hahnemann Univ Hosp 1976; **Fellow:** Medical Oncology, Meml Sloan-Kettering Cancer Ctr 1978

Yi, Peter I MD (Onc) - **Spec Exp:** Breast Cancer; Lymphoma; Prostate Cancer; Colon Cancer; **Hospital:** Univ Med Ctr Princeton at Plainsboro; **Address:** Princeton HealhCare Center, 419 N Harrison St, Ste 101, Princeton, NJ 08540; **Phone:** 609-924-9300; **Board Cert:** Internal Medicine 1987; Medical Oncology 1989; Hematology 2010; **Med School:** Cornell Univ-Weill Med Coll 1984; **Resid:** Internal Medicine, Brigham & Women's Hosp 1987; **Fellow:** Hematology & Oncology, NY Hosp-Cornell Med Ctr 1990; **Fac Appt:** Asst Clin Prof Med, UMDNJ-RW Johnson Med Sch

Nephrology

Cohen, Barry H MD (Nep) - **Hospital:** Capital Health Med Ctr - Hopewell; **Address:** 40 Fuld St, Ste 401, Trenton, NJ 08638-5247; **Phone:** 609-599-1004; **Board Cert:** Internal Medicine 1971; Nephrology 1974; **Med School:** Hahnemann Univ 1965; **Resid:** Internal Medicine, Hahnemann Univ Hosp 1968; **Fellow:** Nephrology, Hahnemann Univ 1969

Ruddy, Michael MD (Nep) - **Spec Exp:** Hypertension; Renovascular Disease; Diabetic Kidney Disease; Pheochromocytoma; **Hospital:** Univ Med Ctr Princeton at Plainsboro, Robert Wood Johnson Univ Hosp - New Brunswick; **Address:** 88 Princeton-Hightstown Rd, Ste 203, Princeton Junction, NJ 08550-1100; **Phone:** 609-750-7330; **Board Cert:** Internal Medicine 1977; Nephrology 1980; **Med School:** UMDNJ-NJ Med Sch, Newark 1974; **Resid:** Internal Medicine, Rutgers Affil Hosps 1977; **Fellow:** Nephrology, NY Hosp-Cornell Med Ctr 1980; **Fac Appt:** Assoc Clin Prof Med

Sudhakar, Telechery A MD (Nep) - **Spec Exp:** Kidney Disease; **Hospital:** Capital Health Med Ctr - Hopewell, Capital Health Regl Med Ctr; **Address:** 40 Fuld St, Ste 401, Trenton, NJ 08638; **Phone:** 609-599-1004; **Board Cert:** Internal Medicine 1977; Nephrology 1978; **Med School:** India 1971; **Resid:** Internal Medicine, Helene Fuld Med Ctr 1976; **Fellow:** Nephrology, Washington VA Hosp 1978

Wei, Fong MD (Nep) *PCP* - **Spec Exp:** Hypertension; Kidney Stones; **Hospital:** Univ Med Ctr Princeton at Plainsboro; **Address:** 419 N Harrison St, Princeton, NJ 08540; **Phone:** 609-924-9300; **Board Cert:** Internal Medicine 1976; Nephrology 1976; **Med School:** Tufts Univ 1967; **Resid:** Internal Medicine, Boston City Hosp 1969; Internal Medicine, Bronx Municipal Hosp 1970; **Fellow:** Nephrology, Univ NC Hosp 1972; **Fac Appt:** Assoc Clin Prof Med

Neurological Surgery

Chiurco, Anthony A MD (NS) - **Spec Exp:** Aneurysm-Cerebral; Brain Tumors; Spinal Disc Replacement; **Hospital:** Univ Med Ctr Princeton at Plainsboro, Capital Health Med Ctr - Hopewell; **Address:** 3131 Princeton Pike Bldg 4 - Ste 201, Lawrenceville, NJ 08648; **Phone:** 609-895-8898; **Board Cert:** Neurological Surgery 1977; **Med School:** Jefferson Med Coll 1967; **Resid:** Surgery, Univ Iowa Coll Med 1971; Neurological Surgery, Univ Iowa Coll Med 1975; **Fellow:** Neurological Surgery, Penn Hosp 1976; **Fac Appt:** Asst Clin Prof NS

McLaughlin, Mark R MD (NS) - **Spec Exp:** Spinal Surgery-Complex; Spinal Surgery-Minimally Invasive; Trigeminal Neuralgia; **Hospital:** Univ Med Ctr Princeton at Plainsboro, St. Mary Med Ctr - Langhorne, PA; **Address:** Princeton Brain & Spine Care, 731 Alexander Rd, Ste 200, Princeton, NJ 08540; **Phone:** 609-921-9001; **Board Cert:** Neurological Surgery 2004; **Med School:** Med Coll VA 1992; **Resid:** Neurological Surgery, Univ Pittsburgh Med Ctr 1999; **Fellow:** Spinal Surgery, Emory Univ Affil Hosp 2000

Neurology

Kaiser, Paul K MD (N) - **Hospital:** Univ Med Ctr Princeton at Plainsboro, Capital Health Med Ctr - Hopewell; **Address:** 3131 Princeton Pike 3C Bldg - Ste 202, Lawrenceville, NJ 08648-2526; **Phone:** 609-896-1701; **Board Cert:** Neurology 1993; Vascular Neurology 2009; **Med School:** Jefferson Med Coll 1988; **Resid:** Neurology, Temple Univ Hosp 1992; **Fellow:** Clinical Neurophysiology, Temple Univ Hosp 1993

Kososky, Charles S MD (N) - **Hospital:** St. Francis Med Ctr - Trenton; **Address:** St Francis Med Ctr, Neurosci Inst, 601 Hamilton Ave, Trenton, NJ 08629; **Phone:** 609-599-5792; **Board Cert:** Neurology 1981; **Med School:** UMDNJ-NJ Med Sch, Newark 1975; **Resid:** Internal Medicine, Kings Co Hosp 1975; Neurology, UMDNJ-Univ Hosp 1978

Vester, John W MD (N) - **Spec Exp:** Parkinson's Disease; Stroke; Peripheral Neuropathy; Epilepsy/Seizure Disorders; **Hospital:** Univ Med Ctr Princeton at Plainsboro; **Address:** 1000 Herrontown Rd, Princeton, NJ 08540; **Phone:** 609-497-0100; **Board Cert:** Neurology 1979; **Med School:** Georgetown Univ 1973; **Resid:** Internal Medicine, Hartford Hosp 1975; Neurology, Georgetown Univ Hosp 1978

Witte, Arnold S MD (N) - **Spec Exp:** Neuromuscular Disorders; Parkinson's Disease; Electromyography; **Hospital:** Capital Health Med Ctr - Hopewell, Capital Health Regl Med Ctr; **Address:** 2 Princess Rd, Ste 2F, Lawrenceville, NJ 08648; **Phone:** 609-895-9000; **Board Cert:** Internal Medicine 1981; Neurology 1983; **Med School:** Tufts Univ 1977; **Resid:** Internal Medicine, Hosp Univ Penn 1979; Neurology, Hosp Univ Penn 1983

Obstetrics & Gynecology

Brickner, Gary R MD (ObG) *PCP* - **Spec Exp:** Gynecology Only; Menopause Problems; Minimally Invasive Surgery; Weight Management; **Hospital:** Capital Health Med Ctr - Hopewell; **Address:** Brickner-Martell Ctr for Women's Health, Quakerbridge Plaza Building 1A, Hamilton, NJ 08619-1241; **Phone:** 609-689-9991; **Board Cert:** Obstetrics & Gynecology 1981; **Med School:** Univ Pittsburgh 1975; **Resid:** Obstetrics & Gynecology, Pennsylvania Hosp 1979

Friedman, Alan L MD (ObG) - **Spec Exp:** Pregnancy-High Risk; Infertility; **Hospital:** Univ Med Ctr Princeton at Plainsboro; **Address:** 253 Witherspoon St, Ste R, Princeton, NJ 08540; **Phone:** 609-683-9292; **Board Cert:** Obstetrics & Gynecology 2011; **Med School:** Univ Chicago-Pritzker Sch Med 1982; **Resid:** Obstetrics & Gynecology, NYU Medical Ctr 1986

Ophthalmology

Matossian, Cynthia MD (Oph) - **Spec Exp:** Cataract Surgery; Glaucoma; **Hospital:** Capital Health Regl Med Ctr, Doylestown Hosp; **Address:** Two Capital Way, Ste 326, Pennington, NJ 08534; **Phone:** 609-882-8833; **Board Cert:** Ophthalmology 1987; **Med School:** Penn State Coll Med 1981; **Resid:** Ophthalmology, G Washington Univ Hosp 1985

Mulvey, Lauri MD (Oph) - **Spec Exp:** Pediatric Ophthalmology; **Hospital:** Chldns Hosp of Philadelphia; **Address:** CHOP Princeton Specialty Care Ctr, 707 Alexander Rd, Princeton, NJ 08540; **Phone:** 609-520-1717; **Board Cert:** Ophthalmology 1983; **Med School:** Harvard Med Sch 1977; **Resid:** Ophthalmology, Barnes-Jewish Hosp 1981; **Fellow:** Pediatric Ophthalmology, Wills Eye Hosp 1983

Safran, Steven G MD (Oph) - **Spec Exp:** Cataract Surgery; Laser Vision Surgery; Glaucoma; **Hospital:** Capital Health Med Ctr - Hopewell, Robert Wood Johnson Univ Hosp Hamilton; **Address:** 132 Franklin Corner Rd, Ste A-1, Lawrenceville, NJ 08648-2523; **Phone:** 609-896-3931; **Board Cert:** Ophthalmology 2003; **Med School:** SUNY Downstate 1987; **Resid:** Ophthalmology, NYU Med Ctr 1991; **Fellow:** Cornea & Ext Eye Disease, Duke Univ Med Ctr 1992

Wasserman, Barry N MD (Oph) - **Spec Exp:** Pediatric Ophthalmology; LASIK-Refractive Surgery; Eyelid Surgery; Botox Therapy; **Hospital:** St. Peter's Univ Hosp, Univ Med Ctr Princeton at Plainsboro; **Address:** 100 Canal Pointe Blvd, Ste 112, Princeton, NJ 08540; **Phone:** 609-243-8711; **Board Cert:** Ophthalmology 2009; **Med School:** UMDNJ-NJ Med Sch, Newark 1992; **Resid:** Ophthalmology, UMDNJ-Univ Hosp 1996; **Fellow:** Pediatric Ophthalmology, Indiana Univ Med Ctr 1997; Refractive Surgery; **Fac Appt:** Asst Clin Prof Oph, UMDNJ-RW Johnson Med Sch

Wong, Michael Y MD (Oph) - **Spec Exp:** LASIK-Refractive Surgery; Cataract Surgery-Lens Implant; Lens Implants-Multifocal; **Hospital:** Wills Eye Hosp, Univ Med Ctr Princeton at Plainsboro; **Address:** 419 N Harrison St, Ste 104, Princeton, NJ 08540-3521; **Phone:** 609-921-9437; **Board Cert:** Ophthalmology 1983; **Med School:** Albany Med Coll 1978; **Resid:** Ophthalmology, Wills Eye Hosp 1982; **Fac Appt:** Clin Prof Oph, UMDNJ-RW Johnson Med Sch

Wong, Richard H MD (Oph) - **Spec Exp:** Cataract Surgery-Lens Implant; LASIK-Refractive Surgery; **Hospital:** Univ Med Ctr Princeton at Plainsboro; **Address:** 419 N Harrison St, Ste 104, Princeton, NJ 08540-3521; **Phone:** 609-921-9437; **Board Cert:** Internal Medicine 1982; Ophthalmology 1987; **Med School:** UMDNJ-NJ Med Sch, Newark 1979; **Resid:** Internal Medicine, Thomas Jefferson Univ Hosp 1982; Ophthalmology, Wills Eye Hosp 1985

Orthopaedic Surgery

Abrams, Jeffrey S MD (OrS) - **Spec Exp:** Shoulder Surgery; Sports Medicine; Arthroscopic Surgery; Rotator Cuff Surgery; **Hospital:** Univ Med Ctr Princeton at Plainsboro; **Address:** Princeton Orthopaedic Assocs, 325 Princeton Ave, Princeton, NJ 08540-1617; **Phone:** 609-924-8131; **Board Cert:** Orthopaedic Surgery 2009; **Med School:** SUNY Upstate Med Univ 1980; **Resid:** Orthopaedic Surgery, Thomas Jefferson Univ Hosp 1985; **Fellow:** Shoulder Surgery, Univ Western Ontario 1986; Sports Medicine, Hughston Sports Med Hosp 1986; **Fac Appt:** Assoc Clin Prof OrS, Seton Hall Univ Sch Hlth & Med Scis

Costa, Leon N MD (OrS) - **Spec Exp:** Arthroscopic Surgery; Joint Replacement; Sports Medicine; **Hospital:** Univ Med Ctr Princeton at Plainsboro, Capital Health Med Ctr - Hopewell; **Address:** 256 Bunn Dr, Ste 2, Princeton, NJ 08540-2859; **Phone:** 609-924-9229; **Board Cert:** Orthopaedic Surgery 2009; **Med School:** Geo Wash Univ 1980; **Resid:** Surgery, Hosp Univ Penn 1982; Orthopaedic Surgery, NY Ortho Hosp/Colum-Presby 1984; **Fellow:** Sports Medicine, NY Ortho Hosp/Colum-Presby 1985

Gomez, William MD (OrS) - **Spec Exp:** Sports Medicine; Arthroscopic Surgery; Arthritis; **Hospital:** Robert Wood Johnson Univ Hosp Hamilton, St. Francis Med Ctr - Trenton; **Address:** Trenton Orthopaedic Group, 1225 Whitehorse Mercerville Rd, D Bldg - Ste 220, Trenton, NJ 08619-3876; **Phone:** 609-581-2200; **Board Cert:** Orthopaedic Surgery 2011; **Med School:** Columbia P&S 1982; **Resid:** Surgery, St Vincent's Hosp 1984; Orthopaedic Surgery, Columbia-Presby Med Ctr 1987; **Fellow:** Sports Medicine, Univ Pittsburgh Hosp 1988

Grenis, Michael S MD (OrS) - **Spec Exp:** Carpal Tunnel Syndrome; Hand & Wrist Injuries; **Hospital:** Univ Med Ctr Princeton at Plainsboro, Capital Health Med Ctr - Hopewell; **Address:** 256 Bunn Drive, Ste 2, Princeton, NJ 08540; **Phone:** 609-924-9229; **Board Cert:** Orthopaedic Surgery 2012; **Med School:** NY Med Coll 1984; **Resid:** Surgery, NYU-Bellevue Hosp 1985; Orthopaedic Surgery, NYU-Bellevue Hosp 1989; **Fellow:** Hand Surgery, NYU-Bellevue Hosp 1990

Gutowski III, W Thomas MD (OrS) - **Spec Exp:** Hip Replacement; Knee Replacement; Arthroscopic Surgery; Joint Replacement; **Hospital:** Univ Med Ctr Princeton at Plainsboro; **Address:** Princeton Orthopaedic Assocs, 325 Princeton Ave, Princeton, NJ 08540; **Phone:** 609-924-8131; **Board Cert:** Orthopaedic Surgery 2008; **Med School:** Cornell Univ-Weill Med Coll 1980; **Resid:** Orthopaedic Surgery, Yale-New Haven Hosp 1985

Taitsman, James P MD (OrS) - **Spec Exp:** Sports Medicine; **Hospital:** Capital Health Med Ctr - Hopewell, Robert Wood Johnson Univ Hosp Hamilton; **Address:** 123 Franklin Corner Rd, Ste 114, Lawrenceville, NJ 08648-2526; **Phone:** 609-896-0707; **Board Cert:** Orthopaedic Surgery 1977; **Med School:** Univ Rochester 1971; **Resid:** Surgery, Yale-New Haven Hosp 1973; Orthopaedic Surgery, Yale-New Haven Hosp 1976

Otolaryngology

Brunner, Eugenie MD (Oto) - **Spec Exp:** Cosmetic Surgery-Face; Rhinoplasty; Skin Laser Surgery; Blepharoplasty; **Hospital:** Univ Med Ctr Princeton at Plainsboro; **Address:** 256 Bunn Drive, Ste 4, Princeton, NJ 08540-2859; **Phone:** 609-921-9497; **Board Cert:** Otolaryngology 1997; Facial Plastic & Reconstr Surgery 2002; **Med School:** UMDNJ-RW Johnson Med Sch 1990; **Resid:** Surgery, NYU Med Ctr 1992; Otolaryngology, NYU Med Ctr 1996; **Fellow:** Facial Plastic & Reconstr Surgery, Univ Toronto 1997

Pain Medicine

Loren, Gary M MD (PM) - **Spec Exp:** Pain-Back; Reflex Sympathetic Dystrophy (RSD); **Hospital:** St. Francis Med Ctr - Trenton; **Address:** 1666 Hamilton Ave, Ste 2, Hamilton Township, NJ 08629; **Phone:** 609-584-9080; **Board Cert:** Anesthesiology 1988; Pain Medicine 2012; **Med School:** Univ Pittsburgh 1984; **Resid:** Anesthesiology, LI Jewish Med Ctr 1987; **Fellow:** Pediatrics, LI Jewish Med Ctr 1988

Pediatrics

Baiser, Dennis MD (Ped) *PCP* - **Spec Exp:** Developmental Disorders; Asthma; **Hospital:** Capital Health Med Ctr - Hopewell, Robert Wood Johnson Univ Hosp Hamilton; **Address:** Hamilton Pediatrics, 3 Hamilton Health Pl, Ste A, Hamilton, NJ 08690; **Phone:** 609-581-4480; **Board Cert:** Pediatrics 1983; **Med School:** NY Med Coll 1978; **Resid:** Pediatrics, Chldn's Hosp 1981; **Fac Appt:** Ped, Univ Pennsylvania

Boim, Marilynn MD (Ped) *PCP* - **Hospital:** Capital Health Med Ctr - Hopewell, Robert Wood Johnson Univ Hosp Hamilton; **Address:** Hamilton Pediatrics, 3 Hamilton Health Pl, Ste A, Hamilton, NJ 08690; **Phone:** 609-581-4480; **Board Cert:** Pediatrics 2009; **Med School:** Emory Univ 1982; **Resid:** Pediatrics, Mt Sinai Hosp 1986; **Fellow:** Pediatric Endocrinology, Mt Sinai Hosp 2000

Palsky, Glenn S MD (Ped) *PCP* - **Hospital:** Capital Health Med Ctr - Hopewell, Univ Med Ctr Princeton at Plainsboro; **Address:** 132 Franklin Corner Rd, Lawrenceville, NJ 08648-2526; **Phone:** 609-896-4141; **Board Cert:** Pediatrics 1978; **Med School:** Penn State Coll Med 1973; **Resid:** Pediatrics, Albany Med Ctr 1977

Raymond, Gerald M MD (Ped) *PCP* - **Hospital:** Univ Med Ctr Princeton at Plainsboro; **Address:** 196 Princeton Heights Town Rd, West Windsor, NJ 08550; **Phone:** 609-799-5335; **Board Cert:** Pediatrics 1987; **Med School:** Penn State Coll Med 1983; **Resid:** Pediatrics, Columbus Chldns Hosp 1986

Physical Medicine & Rehabilitation

Agri, Robyn F MD (PMR) - **Spec Exp:** Acupuncture; Pain Management; **Hospital:** St. Lawrence Rehab Ctr, Capital Health Med Ctr - Hopewell; **Address:** St Lawrence Rehabilitation Ctr, 2381 Lawrenceville Rd, Lawrenceville, NJ 08648-2024; **Phone:** 609-896-9500; **Board Cert:** Physical Medicine & Rehabilitation 1990; **Med School:** SUNY Upstate Med Univ 1985; **Resid:** Physical Medicine & Rehabilitation, Hosp Univ Penn 1989

Gribbin, Dorota M MD (PMR) - **Spec Exp:** Industrial Injuries; Sports Injuries; Pain Management; **Hospital:** Robert Wood Johnson Univ Hosp Hamilton, Univ Med Ctr Princeton at Plainsboro; **Address:** 2333 Whitehorse-Mercerville Rd, Ste 8, Mercerville, NJ 08619; **Phone:** 609-588-0540; **Board Cert:** Physical Medicine & Rehabilitation 2003; **Med School:** Poland 1984; **Resid:** Internal Medicine, Beth Israel Med Ctr 1989; Physical Medicine & Rehabilitation, New York Hosp 1992; **Fellow:** Internal Medicine, Univ Paris 1985; **Fac Appt:** Asst Clin Prof PMR, Columbia P&S

Plastic Surgery

Drimmer, Marc A MD (PlS) - **Spec Exp:** Cosmetic Surgery; **Hospital:** Univ Med Ctr Princeton at Plainsboro; **Address:** 842 State Rd, Princeton, NJ 08540; **Phone:** 609-924-1026; **Board Cert:** Plastic Surgery 1981; **Med School:** Belgium 1974; **Resid:** Surgery, Beth Israel Med Ctr 1977; Plastic Surgery, Univ Hosp 1979

Leach, Thomas A MD (PlS) - **Spec Exp:** Cosmetic Surgery-Face; Cosmetic Surgery-Breast; Liposuction; **Hospital:** Univ Med Ctr Princeton at Plainsboro, Robert Wood Johnson Univ Hosp - New Brunswick; **Address:** 932 State Rd, Princeton, NJ 08540; **Phone:** 609-921-7161; **Board Cert:** Plastic Surgery 1994; **Med School:** UMDNJ-NJ Med Sch, Newark 1985; **Resid:** Surgery, UMDNJ Med Ctr 1990; **Fellow:** Plastic Surgery, UMDNJ Med Ctr 1992

Smotrich, Gary MD (PlS) - **Hospital:** Capital Health Med Ctr - Hopewell, Robert Wood Johnson Univ Hosp Hamilton; **Address:** Lawrenceville Plastic Surgery, 3131 Princeton Pike, Bldg 5 - Ste 205, Lawrenceville, NJ 08648-2300; **Phone:** 609-896-2525; **Board Cert:** Plastic Surgery 1991; **Med School:** Univ Conn 1982; **Resid:** Surgery, Boston Univ Med Ctr 1987; Plastic Surgery, Univ Louisville Hosp 1989

Psychiatry

Khouri, Philippe J MD (Psyc) - **Spec Exp:** Neuro-Psychiatry; Bipolar/Mood Disorders; Geriatric Psychiatry; **Hospital:** Univ Med Ctr Princeton at Plainsboro, Capital Health Regl Med Ctr; **Address:** 905 Herrontown Rd, Princeton, NJ 08540; **Phone:** 609-497-3300; **Board Cert:** Psychiatry 1977; Geriatric Psychiatry 2005; **Med School:** Lebanon 1972; **Resid:** Psychiatry, Strong Meml Hosp 1973; Psychiatry, Univ Tenn Med Ctr 1975; **Fellow:** Genetics and Metabolism, Nat Inst Mntl Hlth 1977; **Fac Appt:** Prof Psyc

Leifer, Marvin W MD (Psyc) - **Spec Exp:** Psychopharmacology; Anxiety & Mood Disorders; Depression; Bipolar/Mood Disorders; **Hospital:** Univ Med Ctr Princeton at Plainsboro; **Address:** 42 N Tulane St, Princeton, NJ 08542; **Phone:** 609-683-7929; **Board Cert:** Psychiatry 1977; **Med School:** SUNY Downstate 1970; **Resid:** Psychiatry, Albert Einstein 1974; **Fellow:** Psychopharmacology, Albert Einstein 1976

Schneider, Samuel MD (Psyc) - **Spec Exp:** Mood Disorders; Personality Disorders; Addiction/Substance Abuse; **Hospital:** Univ Med Ctr Princeton at Plainsboro; **Address:** 33 State Rd, Ste J, Princeton, NJ 08540-1304; **Phone:** 609-924-3980; **Board Cert:** Psychiatry 1984; Internal Medicine 1978; **Med School:** Penn State Coll Med 1975; **Resid:** Internal Medicine, MS Hershey Med Ctr 1977; Psychiatry, Coll Med NJ 1983

Pulmonary Disease

Seelagy, Marc M MD (Pul) - **Spec Exp:** Sleep Disorders; Lung Disease; Critical Care Medicine; **Hospital:** St. Francis Med Ctr - Trenton, Robert Wood Johnson Univ Hosp Hamilton; **Address:** Allergy & Pulmonary Associates, 1542 Kuser Rd, Ste B7, Trenton, NJ 08619-3829; **Phone:** 609-581-1400; **Board Cert:** Internal Medicine 1989; Pulmonary Disease 2002; Critical Care Medicine 2003; Sleep Medicine 1995; **Med School:** Univ Chicago-Pritzker Sch Med 1986; **Resid:** Internal Medicine, Univ Colorado Hosp 1989; **Fellow:** Pulmonary Disease, Johns Hopkins Hosp 1993; Critical Care Medicine, Johns Hopkins Hosp 1993

Radiation Oncology

McKenna, Michael G MD (RadRO) - **Spec Exp:** Prostate Cancer; Breast Cancer; Head & Neck Cancer; **Hospital:** Robert Wood Johnson Univ Hosp Hamilton; **Address:** Cancer Inst NJ-Radiation Oncology, 2575 Klockner Rd, Hamilton, NJ 08690; **Phone:** 609-584-2800; **Board Cert:** Radiation Oncology 1993; **Med School:** Univ Mass Sch Med 1988; **Resid:** Radiation Oncology, Hosp Univ Penn 1992

Soffen, Edward MD (RadRO) - **Spec Exp:** Prostate Cancer; Breast Cancer; Brachytherapy; **Hospital:** Univ Med Ctr Princeton at Plainsboro, CentraState Med Ctr; **Address:** Med Ctr at Princeton, Dept Rad Onc, 253 Witherspoon St, Princeton, NJ 08540-3298; **Phone:** 609-497-4304; **Board Cert:** Radiation Oncology 1991; **Med School:** Temple Univ 1986; **Resid:** Radiation Oncology, Hosp Univ Penn 1990; **Fac Appt:** Asst Clin Prof RadRO, UMDNJ-RW Johnson Med Sch

Reproductive Endocrinology

O'Shaughnessy, Althea MD (RE) - **Spec Exp:** Infertility; **Hospital:** Capital Health Med Ctr - Hopewell, Univ Med Ctr Princeton at Plainsboro; **Address:** Reproductive Science Ctr of New Jersey, 3131 Princeton Pike, Bldg 6 - Ste 100, Lawrenceville, NJ 08648; **Phone:** 609-895-1114; **Board Cert:** Obstetrics & Gynecology 2011; Reproductive Endocrinology/Infertility 2011; **Med School:** Univ Rochester 1982; **Resid:** Obstetrics & Gynecology, Univ Conn Hlth Ctr 1986; **Fellow:** Reproductive Endocrinology, Downstate Med Ctr 1988

Rheumatology

Carney, Alexander MD (Rhu) - **Hospital:** Univ Med Ctr Princeton at Plainsboro; **Address:** 8 Quakerbridge Plaza, Ste H, Mercerville, NJ 08619; **Phone:** 609-588-9044; **Board Cert:** Internal Medicine 1972; Rheumatology 1978; **Med School:** Cornell Univ-Weill Med Coll 1966; **Resid:** Internal Medicine, Univ Iowa Hosp 1972; **Fellow:** Rheumatology, Univ Iowa Hosp 1974

Gordon, Richard D MD (Rhu) - **Spec Exp:** Rheumatoid Arthritis; Osteoporosis; Osteoarthritis; **Hospital:** Robert Wood Johnson Univ Hosp Hamilton; **Address:** Professional Ctr at Hamilton, 2121 Klockner Rd, Hamilton, NJ 08690; **Phone:** 609-587-9898; **Board Cert:** Internal Medicine 1978; Rheumatology 1980; **Med School:** Jefferson Med Coll 1975; **Resid:** Internal Medicine, Geo Wash Hosp/VA Hosp 1978; **Fellow:** Rheumatology, Georgetown Univ 1979; Rheumatology, St Vincents Hosp 1980

Surgery

Dultz, Rachel P MD (S) - **Spec Exp:** Breast Surgery; Breast Cancer; **Hospital:** Univ Med Ctr Princeton at Plainsboro; **Address:** Princeton Breast Health Ctr, 300-B Princeton-Heightstown Rd, Ste 102, East Windsor, NJ 08520; **Phone:** 609-688-2700; **Board Cert:** Surgery 2006; **Med School:** SUNY Downstate 1991; **Resid:** Surgery, RW Johnson Univ Hosp 1997; **Fellow:** Breast Surgery, Baylor Univ Med Ctr 1998

Gannon, Christopher J MD (S) - **Spec Exp:** Liver & Biliary Surgery; Liver Cancer; Liver Metastases; Reconstructive Surgery; **Hospital:** Capital Health Regl Med Ctr, Capital Health Med Ctr - Hopewell; **Address:** Two Capital Way, Ste 356, Pennington, NJ 08534; **Phone:** 609-537-6000; **Board Cert:** Surgery 2005; **Med School:** Columbia P&S 1998; **Resid:** Surgery, Univ Maryland Med Ctr 2004; **Fellow:** Surgical Oncology, MD Anderson Cancer Ctr 2007

Schell, Harold S MD (S) - **Spec Exp:** Breast Cancer; Thyroid & Parathyroid Surgery; Gastrointestinal Surgery; **Hospital:** Capital Health Med Ctr - Hopewell, Capital Health Regl Med Ctr; **Address:** 850 Bear Tavern Rd, Ste 309, Ewing, NJ 08628; **Phone:** 609-656-8844; **Board Cert:** Surgery 2002; **Med School:** Boston Univ 1970; **Resid:** Surgery, St Vincent's Hosp 1975

Thoracic & Cardiac Surgery

Seinfeld, Fredric I MD (T&CS) - **Spec Exp:** Carotid Artery Surgery; Aneurysm; Esophageal Surgery; Cardiovascular Surgery; **Hospital:** St. Francis Med Ctr - Trenton, Univ Med Ctr Princeton at Plainsboro; **Address:** 601 Hamilton Ave, Trenton, NJ 08629; **Phone:** 609-599-5308; **Board Cert:** Thoracic Surgery 2005; **Med School:** SUNY Buffalo 1976; **Resid:** Surgery, NYU Med Ctr 1981; Thoracic Surgery, Yale-New Haven Hosp 1984

Urology

Rossman, Barry R MD (U) - **Spec Exp:** Kidney Stones; Incontinence-Female; Prostate Cancer; Erectile Dysfunction; **Hospital:** Univ Med Ctr Princeton at Plainsboro, Robert Wood Johnson Univ Hosp - New Brunswick; **Address:** Urology Group of Princeton, 134 Stanhope St, Princeton, NJ 08540; **Phone:** 609-924-6487; **Board Cert:** Urology 2010; **Med School:** Boston Univ 1983; **Resid:** Surgery, Montefiore Med Ctr 1985; Urology, Montefiore Med Ctr 1989; **Fac Appt:** Assoc Clin Prof U, UMDNJ-RW Johnson Med Sch

Vasselli, Anthony J MD (U) - **Hospital:** Univ Med Ctr Princeton at Plainsboro; **Address:** 299 Witherspoon St, Princeton, NJ 08540-3506; **Phone:** 609-252-0575; **Board Cert:** Urology 2006; **Med School:** NY Med Coll 1979; **Resid:** Urology, Albany Meml Hosp 1984

Vukasin, Alexander P MD (U) - **Spec Exp:** Laparoscopic Surgery; Urologic Cancer; Urology-Female; **Hospital:** Univ Med Ctr Princeton at Plainsboro, Robert Wood Johnson Univ Hosp - New Brunswick; **Address:** Urology Group of Princeton, 134 Stanhope St, Princeton, NJ 08540; **Phone:** 609-924-6487; **Board Cert:** Urology 2006; **Med School:** Yale Univ 1989; **Resid:** Urology, New York Hosp 1995; **Fac Appt:** Asst Clin Prof U, UMDNJ-RW Johnson Med Sch

Middlesex

Addiction Psychiatry

Williams, Jill M MD (AdP) - **Spec Exp:** Addiction/Substance Abuse; Alcohol Abuse; Dual Diagnosis; Smoking Cessation; **Hospital:** Robert Wood Johnson Univ Hosp - New Brunswick; **Address:** 671 Hoes Ln, Piscataway, NJ 08855; **Phone:** 732-235-4402; **Board Cert:** Psychiatry 2008; Addiction Psychiatry 2000; **Med School:** UMDNJ-RW Johnson Med Sch 1993; **Resid:** Psychiatry, Duke Univ Med Ctr 1997; **Fellow:** Addiction Psychiatry, UMDNJ-RW Johnson Med Sch 1999; **Fac Appt:** Assoc Prof Psyc, UMDNJ-RW Johnson Med Sch

Adolescent Medicine

Snyder, Barbara K MD (AM) - **Spec Exp:** Eating Disorders; Pediatric Gynecology; **Hospital:** Robert Wood Johnson Univ Hosp - New Brunswick; **Address:** Childrens Health Inst New Jersey, 89 French St, Ste 2230, New Brunswick, NJ 08901; **Phone:** 732-235-7896; **Board Cert:** Pediatrics 1985; Adolescent Medicine 2009; **Med School:** Geo Wash Univ 1979; **Resid:** Pediatrics, Chldns National Med Ctr 1981; Pediatrics, Upstate Med Ctr 1982; **Fellow:** Adolescent Medicine, Univ Rochester 1988; **Fac Appt:** Assoc Prof Ped

Allergy & Immunology

Blum, Jay R MD (A&I) - **Spec Exp:** Rhinitis; Asthma; Hives; Urticaria; **Hospital:** St. Peter's Univ Hosp, Robert Wood Johnson Univ Hosp - New Brunswick; **Address:** 85 Raritan Ave, Highland Park, NJ 08904-2439; **Phone:** 732-846-7861; **Board Cert:** Internal Medicine 1978; Allergy & Immunology 1979; **Med School:** Univ Pennsylvania 1974; **Resid:** Internal Medicine, Beth Israel Hosp 1977; **Fellow:** Allergy & Immunology, New York Hosp 1979

Kesarwala, Hemant MD (A&I) - **Spec Exp:** Food Allergy; Asthma; **Hospital:** St. Peter's Univ Hosp, Robert Wood Johnson Univ Hosp - New Brunswick; **Address:** 3084 State Route 27, Ste 6, Kendall Park, NJ 08824-1657; **Phone:** 732-821-0595; **Board Cert:** Pediatrics 1979; Allergy & Immunology 1979; **Med School:** India 1971; **Resid:** Pediatrics, Lincoln Hosp 1976; **Fellow:** Infectious Disease, UMDNJ-Rutgers Med Sch 1978; Allergy & Immunology, Children's Hosp 1979; **Fac Appt:** Clin Prof Ped, Drexel Univ Coll Med

Leibner, Donald MD (A&I) - **Spec Exp:** Asthma & Allergy; Cough-Chronic; Insect Allergies; Nasal & Sinus Disorders; **Hospital:** Robert Wood Johnson Univ Hosp - New Brunswick, St. Peter's Univ Hosp; **Address:** 579-A Cranbury Rd, Ste 103, East Brunswick, NJ 08816-5426; **Phone:** 732-390-4900; **Board Cert:** Pediatrics 2003; Allergy & Immunology 2005; **Med School:** SUNY Downstate 1981; **Resid:** Pediatrics, UMDNJ-Rutgers 1984; Pediatrics, Beth Israel Med Ctr 1982; **Fellow:** Allergy & Immunology, Long Island Coll Hosp 1986; **Fac Appt:** Asst Clin Prof Ped, Drexel Univ Coll Med

Cardiovascular Disease

Kostis, John B MD (Cv) - **Spec Exp:** Hypertension; Coronary Artery Disease; Cholesterol/Lipid Disorders; **Hospital:** Robert Wood Johnson Univ Hosp - New Brunswick; **Address:** 125 Paterson St, CAB Bldg - Fl 5 - Ste 5200, 1 Robert Wood Johnson Pl, New Brunswick, NJ 08901; **Phone:** 732-235-7685; **Board Cert:** Internal Medicine 1973; Cardiovascular Disease 1973; **Med School:** Greece 1960; **Resid:** Internal Medicine, Evanglismos Hosp 1964; Internal Medicine, Cumberland Med Ctr 1967; **Fellow:** Cardiovascular Disease, Philadelphia Genl Hosp 1969; **Fac Appt:** Prof Med, UMDNJ-RW Johnson Med Sch

Mermelstein, Erwin MD (Cv) - **Spec Exp:** Cholesterol/Lipid Disorders; Cardiac Catheterization; Congestive Heart Failure; Hypertension; **Hospital:** Robert Wood Johnson Univ Hosp - New Brunswick, St. Peter's Univ Hosp; **Address:** Cardiology Assocs New Brunswick, 593 Cranbury Rd, East Brunswick, NJ 08816; **Phone:** 732-390-3333; **Board Cert:** Internal Medicine 1981; Cardiovascular Disease 1983; **Med School:** Cornell Univ 1978; **Resid:** Internal Medicine, New York Hosp 1981; **Fellow:** Cardiovascular Disease, Hosp Univ Penn 1983

Mondrow, Daniel N MD (Cv) - **Spec Exp:** Cardiac Catheterization; Nuclear Stress Testing; Critical Care Medicine; **Hospital:** JFK Med Ctr - Edison, Robert Wood Johnson Univ Hosp - New Brunswick; **Address:** 280 Main St, Metuchen, NJ 08840-2429; **Phone:** 732-494-3177; **Board Cert:** Internal Medicine 1979; Cardiovascular Disease 1985; **Med School:** SUNY Downstate 1976; **Resid:** Internal Medicine, Brookdale Hosp 1979; **Fellow:** Cardiovascular Disease, St Vincents Hosp 1981

Shell, Roger A MD (Cv) - **Spec Exp:** Coronary Artery Disease; Heart Valve Disease; Cholesterol/Lipid Disorders; **Hospital:** Robert Wood Johnson Univ Hosp - New Brunswick, St. Peter's Univ Hosp; **Address:** Cardiology Assocs of New Brunswick, 593 Cranberry Rd, East Brunswick, NJ 08816; **Phone:** 732-390-3333; **Board Cert:** Internal Medicine 1980; Cardiovascular Disease 1983; **Med School:** UMDNJ-Rutgers Med Sch 1977; **Resid:** Internal Medicine, RW Johnson Univ Hosp 1980; **Fellow:** Cardiovascular Disease, Presby Hosp-Univ Penn 1982; **Fac Appt:** Asst Clin Prof Med, UMDNJ-RW Johnson Med Sch

Shindler, Daniel M MD (Cv) - **Spec Exp:** Echocardiography; Echocardiography-Transesophageal; Cardiac Tumors/Cancer; **Hospital:** Robert Wood Johnson Univ Hosp - New Brunswick; **Address:** Univ Med Group, 125 Paterson St, Fl 6th, Ste 6100, New Brunswick, NJ 08901; **Phone:** 732-235-7855; **Board Cert:** Internal Medicine 1987; Cardiovascular Disease 2002; **Med School:** Spain 1979; **Resid:** Internal Medicine, USPHS Hosp 1981; Internal Medicine, RW Johnson Hosp 1984; **Fellow:** Cardiovascular Disease, RW Johnson Hosp 1983; **Fac Appt:** Prof Med, UMDNJ-RW Johnson Med Sch

Child & Adolescent Psychiatry

Shampain, Lawrence R MD (ChAP) - **Spec Exp:** Trauma Psychiatry; Anxiety Disorders; **Hospital:** Somerset Med Ctr, Univ Beh HC-Univ of Med/Dent of NJ; **Address:** 32B Wernik Place, Metuchen, NJ 08840; **Phone:** 732-548-1600; **Board Cert:** Psychiatry 1988; Child & Adolescent Psychiatry 1990; **Med School:** Hahnemann Univ 1982; **Resid:** Psychiatry, Mt Sinai Med Ctr 1985; **Fellow:** Child Psychiatry, UCLA Neuropsych Inst 1987; **Fac Appt:** Assoc Clin Prof Psyc, UMDNJ-RW Johnson Med Sch

Child Neurology

Wollack, Jan B MD (ChiN) - **Spec Exp:** Epilepsy/Seizure Disorders; **Hospital:** Robert Wood Johnson Univ Hosp - New Brunswick; **Address:** 89 French St Fl 2, New Brunswick, NJ 08901; **Phone:** 732-235-7875; **Board Cert:** Pediatrics 1988; Child Neurology 1987; **Med School:** Columbia P&S 1981; **Resid:** Pediatrics, Columbia-Presby Med Ctr 1983; Neurology, Columbia-Presby Med Ctr 1986; **Fac Appt:** Assoc Prof Ped, UMDNJ-RW Johnson Med Sch

Clinical Genetics

Sklower Brooks, Susan MD (CG) - **Spec Exp:** Birth Defects; Inborn Errors of Metabolism; Developmental Disorders; Prenatal Diagnosis; **Hospital:** Robert Wood Johnson Univ Hosp - New Brunswick; **Address:** Child Hlth Inst of NJ, 89 French St, New Brunswick, NJ 08903-2160; **Phone:** 732-235-6230; **Board Cert:** Pediatrics 1979; Clinical Genetics 1982; Clinical Biochemical Genetics 1984; **Med School:** Mount Sinai Sch Med 1975; **Resid:** Pediatrics, Mount Sinai Hosp 1977; **Fellow:** Clinical Genetics, Mount Sinai Hosp 1979; **Fac Appt:** Prof Ped, UMDNJ-RW Johnson Med Sch

Colon & Rectal Surgery

Chinn, Bertram T MD (CRS) - **Spec Exp:** Laparoscopic Surgery; Colon & Rectal Cancer; Inflammatory Bowel Disease; Diverticulitis; **Hospital:** Overlook Med Ctr (page 92), Robert Wood Johnson Univ Hosp - New Brunswick; **Address:** Associated Colon & Rectal Surgeons, 3900 Park Ave, Ste 101, Edison, NJ 08820; **Phone:** 732-494-6640; **Board Cert:** Surgery 2002; Colon & Rectal Surgery 2012; **Med School:** Jefferson Med Coll 1987; **Resid:** Surgery, Thomas Jefferson Univ Hosp 1992; **Fellow:** Colon & Rectal Surgery, UMDNJ-RW Johnson Med Ctr 1993; **Fac Appt:** Asst Clin Prof S, UMDNJ-RW Johnson Med Sch

Eisenstat, Theodore E MD (CRS) - **Spec Exp:** Colon Cancer; Inflammatory Bowel Disease; Anorectal Disorders; Hemorrhoids; **Hospital:** Robert Wood Johnson Univ Hosp - New Brunswick, JFK Med Ctr - Edison; **Address:** 3900 Park Ave, Ste 101, Edison, NJ 08820-3032; **Phone:** 732-494-6640; **Board Cert:** Surgery 1974; Colon & Rectal Surgery 1994; **Med School:** NY Med Coll 1968; **Resid:** Surgery, Thomas Jefferson Univ Hosp 1971; Surgery, Pennsylvania Hosp 1973; **Fellow:** Colon & Rectal Surgery, Muhlenberg Med Ctr 1978; **Fac Appt:** Clin Prof S, UMDNJ-RW Johnson Med Sch

Oliver, Gregory C MD (CRS) - **Spec Exp:** Colon & Rectal Cancer; Incontinence-Fecal; Ulcerative Colitis; Crohn's Disease; **Hospital:** JFK Med Ctr - Edison, Overlook Med Ctr (page 92); **Address:** Assoc Colon & Rectal Surgeons, 3900 Park Ave, Ste 101, Edison, NJ 08820; **Phone:** 732-494-6640; **Board Cert:** Colon & Rectal Surgery 1986; **Med School:** Geo Wash Univ 1976; **Resid:** Surgery, Geo Wash Univ Med Ctr 1983; Surgery, UMDNJ-Rutgers 1985; **Fac Appt:** Assoc Clin Prof S, UMDNJ-RW Johnson Med Sch

Rezac, Craig MD (CRS) - **Spec Exp:** Colon & Rectal Cancer; Inflammatory Bowel Disease; Diverticulitis; Pelvic & Perineal Surgery; **Hospital:** Robert Wood Johnson Univ Hosp - New Brunswick; **Address:** 125 Patterson St, Ste 4100, New Brunswick, NJ 08903; **Phone:** 732-235-7920; **Board Cert:** Surgery 2011; Colon & Rectal Surgery 2012; **Med School:** Italy 1995; **Resid:** Surgery, RW Johnson Medical Ctr 2001; **Fellow:** Colon & Rectal Surgery, RW Johnson Med Ctr 2002; Laparoscopic Surgery, Hackensack Med Ctr 2003; **Fac Appt:** Asst Prof S, UMDNJ-RW Johnson Med Sch

Zinkin, Lewis D MD (CRS) - **Spec Exp:** Colon Cancer; Inflammatory Bowel Disease; **Hospital:** Robert Wood Johnson Univ Hosp - New Brunswick, St. Peter's Univ Hosp; **Address:** 620 Cranbury Rd, Ste 111, East Brunswick, NJ 08816; **Phone:** 732-238-2662; **Board Cert:** Colon & Rectal Surgery 1978; **Med School:** UMDNJ-NJ Med Sch, Newark 1970; **Resid:** Surgery, St Vincents Hosp 1977; Colon & Rectal Surgery, Greater Baltimore Med Ctr 1978; **Fac Appt:** Assoc Clin Prof S

Dermatology

Milgraum, Sandy S MD (D) - **Spec Exp:** Skin Laser Surgery; Tattoo Removal; Cosmetic Dermatology; Pediatric Dermatology; **Hospital:** Robert Wood Johnson Univ Hosp - New Brunswick; **Address:** Academic Dermatology Ctr, 81 Brunswick Woods Drive, East Brunswick, NJ 08816-5601; **Phone:** 732-613-0300; **Board Cert:** Dermatology 1986; Pediatric Dermatology 2006; **Med School:** Australia 1983; **Resid:** Dermatology, Univ Mich Hosp 1986; **Fac Appt:** Assoc Prof D, UMDNJ-RW Johnson Med Sch

Wrone, David A MD (D) - **Spec Exp:** Skin Laser Surgery; Cosmetic Surgery; Mohs' Surgery; Skin Cancer; **Hospital:** Univ Med Ctr Princeton at Plainsboro, Robert Wood Johnson Univ Hosp - New Brunswick; **Address:** 1950 Highway 27, Ste A, North Brunswick, NJ 08902; **Phone:** 609-683-4999; **Board Cert:** Dermatology 2009; **Med School:** Stanford Univ 1996; **Resid:** Dermatology, Univ Wisconsin Med Ctr 1998; Dermatology, Mass Genl Hosp 2001; **Fellow:** Mohs Surgery, UCLA Med Ctr 2002

Diagnostic Radiology

Compito, Gerard A MD (DR) - **Hospital:** Univ Med Ctr Princeton at Plainsboro; **Address:** 3674 Rt 27, Kendall Park, NJ 08824; **Phone:** 732-821-5563; **Board Cert:** Diagnostic Radiology 1990; Neuroradiology 2005; **Med School:** SUNY Upstate Med Univ 1985; **Resid:** Diagnostic Radiology, NY Hosp-Cornell 1990; **Fellow:** Neuroradiology, NY Hosp-Cornell 1992

Epstein, Robert E MD (DR) - **Spec Exp:** MRI; Musculoskeletal Imaging; **Hospital:** Robert Wood Johnson Univ Hosp - New Brunswick; **Address:** University Radiology Group, 579A Cranbury Rd Fl 3, East Brunswick, NJ 08816; **Phone:** 732-390-0040; **Board Cert:** Diagnostic Radiology 1995; **Med School:** Duke Univ 1990; **Resid:** Diagnostic Radiology, Thomas Jefferson Univ Hosp 1995; **Fellow:** Musculoskeletal Imaging, Hosp Univ Penn 1996; **Fac Appt:** Asst Clin Prof Rad, UMDNJ-RW Johnson Med Sch

Ford, Robert R MD (DR) - **Spec Exp:** CT Scan; MRI; Nuclear Medicine; Ultrasound; **Hospital:** Univ Med Ctr Princeton at Plainsboro; **Address:** Princeton Radiology, 3674 Route 27, Kendall Park, NJ 08824; **Phone:** 908-745-9944; **Board Cert:** Diagnostic Radiology 1988; Neuroradiology 2009; **Med School:** UMDNJ-Rutgers Med Sch 1983; **Resid:** Internal Medicine, R W Johnson Univ Hosp 1984; Diagnostic Radiology, NY Hosp-Cornell 1988

Rosenfeld, David L MD (DR) - **Spec Exp:** Pediatric Radiology; **Hospital:** Robert Wood Johnson Univ Hosp - New Brunswick; **Address:** University Radiology Group, 579A Cranbury Rd Fl 3, East Brunswick, NJ 08816; **Phone:** 732-390-0040; **Board Cert:** Diagnostic Radiology 1972; **Med School:** Univ Pittsburgh 1967; **Resid:** Diagnostic Radiology, Montefiore Med Ctr 1971; **Fac Appt:** Clin Prof Rad, UMDNJ-RW Johnson Med Sch

Underberg-Davis, Sharon MD (DR) - **Spec Exp:** Pediatric Radiology; **Hospital:** Robert Wood Johnson Univ Hosp - New Brunswick; **Address:** Univ Radiology Grp, 579A Cranbury Rd Fl 3, East Brunswick, NJ 08816; **Phone:** 732-390-0040; **Board Cert:** Diagnostic Radiology 1993; Pediatric Radiology 2004; **Med School:** Harvard Med Sch 1988; **Resid:** Diagnostic Radiology, Hosp Univ Penn 1993; **Fellow:** Pediatric Radiology, Chldns Hosp 1995

Endocrinology, Diabetes & Metabolism

Agrin, Richard MD (EDM) - Spec Exp: Thyroid Disorders; Parathyroid Disorders; Diabetes; **Hospital:** Robert Wood Johnson Univ Hosp - New Brunswick, Somerset Med Ctr; **Address:** 78 Easton Ave, New Brunswick, NJ 08901; **Phone:** 732-545-1065; **Board Cert:** Internal Medicine 1974; Endocrinology 1977; **Med School:** Univ Pennsylvania 1971; **Resid:** Internal Medicine, USPHS Hosp 1975; **Fellow:** Endocrinology, Boston Univ Hosp 1977; **Fac Appt:** Assoc Clin Prof Med, UMDNJ-RW Johnson Med Sch

Bucholtz, Harvey K MD (EDM) - Spec Exp: Diabetes; Thyroid Disorders; Osteoporosis; **Hospital:** JFK Med Ctr - Edison, Newark Beth Israel Med Ctr; **Address:** 2 Lincoln Hwy, Ste 501, Edison, NJ 08820; **Phone:** 732-549-7470; **Board Cert:** Internal Medicine 1973; Endocrinology 1975; **Med School:** SUNY Hlth Sci Ctr 1968; **Resid:** Internal Medicine, Univ Michigan Med Ctr 1971; **Fellow:** Endocrinology, Duke Univ Med Ctr 1975; **Fac Appt:** Asst Clin Prof Med, UMDNJ-NJ Med Sch, Newark

Maman, Arie MD (EDM) - Spec Exp: Thyroid Disorders; Diabetes; Pituitary Disorders; **Hospital:** Robert Wood Johnson Univ Hosp - New Brunswick, St. Peter's Univ Hosp; **Address:** D3 Brier Hill Ct, East Brunswick, NJ 08816-3335; **Phone:** 732-613-0707; **Board Cert:** Internal Medicine 1977; Endocrinology, Diabetes & Metabolism 1979; **Med School:** France 1974; **Resid:** Internal Medicine, Jewish Hosp 1977; **Fellow:** Endocrinology, Univ Colorado 1979; **Fac Appt:** Assoc Clin Prof Med, UMDNJ-RW Johnson Med Sch

Schneider, Stephen H MD (EDM) - Spec Exp: Diabetes; Nutrition; Cholesterol/Lipid Disorders; **Hospital:** Robert Wood Johnson Univ Hosp - New Brunswick; **Address:** 125 Patterson St, Clinical Academic Bldg Fl 5 - Ste 5100B, New Brunswick, NJ 08901; **Phone:** 732-235-7219; **Board Cert:** Internal Medicine 1975; Endocrinology, Diabetes & Metabolism 1979; **Med School:** Boston Univ 1972; **Resid:** Internal Medicine, Boston Univ Hosp 1974; Internal Medicine, Boston City Hosp 1975; **Fellow:** Endocrinology, Diabetes & Metabolism, Boston City Hosp 1976; **Fac Appt:** Prof Med, UMDNJ-RW Johnson Med Sch

Spiler, Ira MD (EDM) - Spec Exp: Pituitary Disorders; Thyroid Disorders; Calcium Disorders; **Hospital:** Raritan Bay Med Ctr - Perth Amboy, Robert Wood Johnson Univ Hosp - New Brunswick; **Address:** 3 Hospital Plaza, Ste 307, Old Bridge, NJ 08857-3095; **Phone:** 732-360-1122; **Board Cert:** Internal Medicine 1976; Endocrinology, Diabetes & Metabolism 1979; **Med School:** Albert Einstein Coll Med 1971; **Resid:** Internal Medicine, Bronx Municipal Hosp 1973; Internal Medicine, Boston City Hosp 1976; **Fellow:** Endocrinology, Tufts-New England Med Ctr 1978; **Fac Appt:** Assoc Clin Prof Med, UMDNJ-RW Johnson Med Sch

Family Medicine

Metz, John P MD (FMed) *PCP* **- Spec Exp:** Primary Care Sports Medicine; **Hospital:** JFK Med Ctr - Edison; **Address:** 65 James St, Edison, NJ 08818; **Phone:** 732-321-7487; **Board Cert:** Family Medicine 2003; Sports Medicine 2011; **Med School:** Jefferson Med Coll 1994; **Resid:** Family Medicine, Malcolm Grow Med Ctr 1997; **Fellow:** Sports Medicine, Uniformed Srvs U Hlth Scis 2000

Picciano, Anne MD (FMed) *PCP* **- Spec Exp:** Adolescent Medicine; **Hospital:** JFK Med Ctr - Edison; **Address:** 65 James St, Edison, NJ 08818; **Phone:** 732-321-7487; **Board Cert:** Family Medicine 2009; Adolescent Medicine 2003; **Med School:** Univ Pennsylvania 1987; **Resid:** Family Medicine, W Jersey Hlth 1990; **Fac Appt:** Asst Clin Prof FMed, UMDNJ-RW Johnson Med Sch

Swee, David E MD (FMed) *PCP* - **Hospital:** Robert Wood Johnson Univ Hosp - New Brunswick; **Address:** Family Medicine at Monument Square, 317 George St Fl 1 - Ste 100, New Brunswick, NJ 08901; **Phone:** 732-235-8993; **Board Cert:** Family Medicine 2007; **Med School:** Canada 1974; **Resid:** Family Medicine, Somerset Med Ctr 1977; **Fac Appt:** Prof FMed, UMDNJ-RW Johnson Med Sch

Tallia, Alfred F MD (FMed) *PCP* - **Hospital:** Robert Wood Johnson Univ Hosp - New Brunswick; **Address:** Family Med at Monument Square, 317 George St Fl 1 - Ste 100, New Brunswick, NJ 08901-2162; **Phone:** 732-235-8993; **Board Cert:** Family Medicine 2007; **Med School:** UMDNJ-RW Johnson Med Sch 1978; **Resid:** Family Medicine, Jefferson Univ Hosp 1981

Tierney, Peter C MD (FMed) *PCP* - **Hospital:** Univ Med Ctr Princeton at Plainsboro; **Address:** 666 Plainsboro Rd, Ste 1316, Plainsboro, NJ 08536; **Phone:** 609-275-8100; **Board Cert:** Family Medicine 2005; **Med School:** Univ VA Sch Med 1983; **Resid:** Family Medicine, Hunterdon Med Ctr 1986

Winter, Robin O MD (FMed) *PCP* - **Spec Exp:** Geriatric Medicine; **Hospital:** JFK Med Ctr - Edison; **Address:** 65 James St, Edison, NJ 08818; **Phone:** 732-321-7487; **Board Cert:** Family Medicine 2005; Geriatric Medicine 2006; **Med School:** Albert Einstein Coll Med 1978; **Resid:** Family Medicine, Hunterdon Med Ctr 1981; **Fac Appt:** Clin Prof FMed, UMDNJ-RW Johnson Med Sch

Gastroenterology

Hodes, Steven MD (Ge) - **Hospital:** Raritan Bay Med Ctr - Perth Amboy, JFK Med Ctr - Edison; **Address:** 205 May St, Ste 201, Edison, NJ 08837; **Phone:** 732-661-9225; **Board Cert:** Internal Medicine 1977; Gastroenterology 1979; **Med School:** Albert Einstein Coll Med 1974; **Resid:** Internal Medicine, Montefiore Med Ctr 1977; **Fellow:** Gastroenterology, Mt Sinai-Bronx VA Hosps 1979

Pitchumoni, Capecomorin S MD (Ge) - **Spec Exp:** Pancreatic Disease; Gastroesophageal Reflux Disease (GERD); Pancreatic Cancer; Hepatitis C; **Hospital:** St. Peter's Univ Hosp; **Address:** St Peters Univ Hosp, 254 Easton Ave, CARES Bldg Fl 4 - Ste 4013, New Brunswick, NJ 08901; **Phone:** 732-745-7939; **Board Cert:** Gastroenterology 1971; Internal Medicine 1977; **Med School:** India 1960; **Resid:** Internal Medicine, Norwalk Hosp 1968; **Fellow:** Gastroenterology, Yale New Haven Hosp 1969Metropolitan Hosp Ctr 1971; **Fac Appt:** Clin Prof Med

Plumser, Allan B MD (Ge) - **Spec Exp:** Endoscopy; Pancreatic/Biliary Endoscopy (ERCP); Liver Disease; **Hospital:** Robert Wood Johnson Univ Hosp - New Brunswick, St. Peter's Univ Hosp; **Address:** 465 Cranbury Rd, Ste 102, East Brunswick, NJ 08816; **Phone:** 732-390-1995; **Board Cert:** Internal Medicine 1981; Gastroenterology 1983; **Med School:** NY Med Coll 1978; **Resid:** Internal Medicine, SUNY Stonybrook Med Ctr 1981; **Fellow:** Gastroenterology, SUNY Stonybrook Med Ctr 1983

Geriatric Medicine

Bullock, Richard B MD (Ger) *PCP* - **Spec Exp:** Hypertension; Cholesterol/Lipid Disorders; Dementia; **Hospital:** JFK Med Ctr - Edison; **Address:** 225 May St, Ste E, Edison, NJ 08837-3266; **Phone:** 732-661-2020; **Board Cert:** Internal Medicine 1984; Geriatric Medicine 2010; **Med School:** Mount Sinai Sch Med 1981; **Resid:** Internal Medicine, Mt Sinai Hosp 1984; **Fac Appt:** Asst Clin Prof Med

Gynecologic Oncology

Carlson Jr, John A MD (GO) - **Spec Exp:** Gynecologic Cancer; Ovarian Cancer; Gynecologic Surgery-Complex; **Hospital:** St. Peter's Univ Hosp; **Address:** St Peter's Univ Hosp, 254 Easton Ave, Cares Bldg, New Brunswick, NJ 08901; **Phone:** 732-937-6003; **Board Cert:** Obstetrics & Gynecology 1981; Gynecologic Oncology 1982; **Med School:** Georgetown Univ 1974; **Resid:** Obstetrics & Gynecology, Hosp Univ Penn 1978; **Fellow:** Gynecologic Oncology, MD Anderson Cancer Ctr 1980; **Fac Appt:** Prof ObG, Drexel Univ Coll Med

Goldberg, Michael I MD (GO) - **Spec Exp:** Ovarian Cancer; Uterine Cancer; **Hospital:** St. Peter's Univ Hosp; **Address:** 78 Easton Ave, New Brunswick, NJ 08901-1865; **Phone:** 732-828-3300; **Board Cert:** Obstetrics & Gynecology 1977; Gynecologic Oncology 1980; **Med School:** Italy 1970; **Resid:** Obstetrics & Gynecology, Maimonides Med Ctr 1975; **Fellow:** Gynecologic Oncology, Jackson Meml Hosp 1977; **Fac Appt:** Clin Prof ObG, UMDNJ-RW Johnson Med Sch

Rodriguez, Lorna MD/PhD (GO) - **Spec Exp:** Robotic Surgery; Ovarian Cancer; Cervical Cancer; **Hospital:** Robert Wood Johnson Univ Hosp - New Brunswick; **Address:** Cancer Institute of New Jersey, 195 Little Albany St Fl 1 - rm 1100, New Brunswick, NJ 08903; **Phone:** 732-235-7615; **Board Cert:** Obstetrics & Gynecology 2010; Gynecologic Oncology 2010; **Med School:** Puerto Rico 1979; **Resid:** Obstetrics & Gynecology, Cooper Med Ctr 1983; **Fellow:** Gynecologic Oncology, Univ Michigan 1985; **Fac Appt:** Prof ObG, UMDNJ-RW Johnson Med Sch

Hematology

Karp, George I MD (Hem) - **Spec Exp:** Coagulation/Bleeding Disorders; Anemia; Breast Cancer; **Hospital:** Robert Wood Johnson Univ Hosp - New Brunswick, St. Peter's Univ Hosp; **Address:** 205 Easton Ave, New Brunswick, NJ 08901; **Phone:** 732-390-7750; **Board Cert:** Internal Medicine 1979; Medical Oncology 1981; Hematology 1982; **Med School:** Columbia P&S 1976; **Resid:** Internal Medicine, Univ Chicago Hosps 1978; **Fellow:** Hematology & Oncology, Natl Cancer Inst 1979; Hematology & Oncology, Dana Farber Cancer Inst/Beth Israel Hosp 1982; **Fac Appt:** Clin Prof Hem & Onc, UMDNJ-RW Johnson Med Sch

Philipp, Claire S MD (Hem) - **Spec Exp:** Bleeding/Coagulation Disorders; **Hospital:** Robert Wood Johnson Univ Hosp - New Brunswick; **Address:** Robert Wood Johnson Med School, 125 Paterson St, CAB5231, New Brunswick, NJ 08901; **Phone:** 732-235-6531; **Board Cert:** Internal Medicine 1981; Hematology 1984; Medical Oncology 1985; **Med School:** Brown Univ 1978; **Resid:** Internal Medicine, Beth Israel Med Ctr 1981; **Fellow:** Hematology & Oncology, NYU Med Ctr 1984; **Fac Appt:** Prof Med

Strair, Roger MD/PhD (Hem) - **Spec Exp:** Leukemia; Lymphoma; Bone Marrow Transplant; Multiple Myeloma; **Hospital:** Robert Wood Johnson Univ Hosp - New Brunswick; **Address:** Cancer Inst of NJ, 195 Little Albany St, New Brunswick, NJ 08903; **Phone:** 732-235-7464; **Board Cert:** Internal Medicine 1984; Hematology 1986; Medical Oncology 1987; **Med School:** Albert Einstein Coll Med 1981; **Resid:** Internal Medicine, Brigham & Women's Hosp 1984; **Fellow:** Hematology & Oncology, Brigham & Women's Hosp 1988; **Fac Appt:** Assoc Prof Med, UMDNJ-RW Johnson Med Sch

Infectious Disease

Boruchoff, Susan E MD (Inf) - **Spec Exp:** Travel Medicine; AIDS/HIV; Viral Infections; **Hospital:** Robert Wood Johnson Univ Hosp - New Brunswick; **Address:** RWJ Div Infectious Disease/Travel Med, 125 Patterson St Fl 5 - Ste 5100B, New Brunswick, NJ 08901-1928; **Phone:** 732-235-7060; **Board Cert:** Internal Medicine 1985; Infectious Disease 1988; **Med School:** Columbia P&S 1982; **Resid:** Internal Medicine, Geo Wash Univ Hosp 1985; **Fellow:** Infectious Disease, Univ Mass Med Ctr 1988; **Fac Appt:** Prof Med, UMDNJ-RW Johnson Med Sch

Middleton, John R MD (Inf) - **Spec Exp:** AIDS/HIV; Osteomyelitis; **Hospital:** Raritan Bay Med Ctr - Perth Amboy; **Address:** ID Care, 3 Hospital Plaza, Ste 208, Old Bridge, NJ 08857-3093; **Phone:** 732-360-2700; **Board Cert:** Internal Medicine 1973; Infectious Disease 1980; **Med School:** UMDNJ-NJ Med Sch, Newark 1970; **Resid:** Internal Medicine, NY Hosp-Cornell Med Ctr 1973; **Fellow:** Infectious Disease, RWJ Univ Hosp 1977; **Fac Appt:** Assoc Clin Prof Med, UMDNJ-Rutgers Med Sch

Sensakovic, John W MD/PhD (Inf) - **Spec Exp:** Lyme Disease; Fevers of Unknown Origin; Bone Infections; **Hospital:** Saint Michael's Med Ctr, JFK Med Ctr - Edison; **Address:** 113 James St, Edison, NJ 08820; **Phone:** 732-549-3449; **Board Cert:** Internal Medicine 1982; Infectious Disease 1984; **Med School:** UMDNJ-NJ Med Sch, Newark 1977; **Resid:** Internal Medicine, St Michaels Med Ctr 1980; **Fellow:** Infectious Disease, St Michaels Med Ctr 1982; **Fac Appt:** Prof Med, Seton Hall Univ Sch Hlth & Med Scis

Weinstein, Melvin P MD (Inf) - **Spec Exp:** Bone/Joint Infections; Infective Endocarditis; Mycobacterial Infections; **Hospital:** Robert Wood Johnson Univ Hosp - New Brunswick; **Address:** 125 Patterson St, Fl 5, New Brunswick, NJ 08901-1928; **Phone:** 732-235-7713; **Board Cert:** Internal Medicine 1975; Infectious Disease 1978; Medical Microbiology 1983; **Med School:** Geo Wash Univ 1970; **Resid:** Internal Medicine, Hartford Hosp 1975; **Fellow:** Infectious Disease, Univ Colo Hosp 1977; **Fac Appt:** Prof Med, UMDNJ-RW Johnson Med Sch

Internal Medicine

Carson, Jeffrey L MD (IM) *PCP* - **Hospital:** Robert Wood Johnson Univ Hosp - New Brunswick; **Address:** 125 Paterson St, Ste 5100, New Brunswick, NJ 08901; **Phone:** 732-235-6968; **Board Cert:** Internal Medicine 1980; **Med School:** Hahnemann Univ 1977; **Resid:** Internal Medicine, Hahnemann Univ Hosp 1980; **Fellow:** Internal Medicine, Univ Penn 1982; **Fac Appt:** Prof Med, UMDNJ-RW Johnson Med Sch

Cassidy, Brian MD (IM) *PCP* - **Hospital:** JFK Med Ctr - Edison; **Address:** 3910 Park Ave, Ste 8, Edison, NJ 08820; **Phone:** 732-767-3130; **Board Cert:** Internal Medicine 1988; **Med School:** Grenada 1985; **Resid:** Internal Medicine, Muhlenberg Med Ctr 1988

DeSilva Jr, Derrick M MD (IM) *PCP* - **Spec Exp:** Complementary Medicine; **Hospital:** Raritan Bay Med Ctr - Perth Amboy; **Address:** 629 Amboy Ave, Fl 2, Edison, NJ 08837; **Phone:** 732-738-8801; **Med School:** Dominican Republic 1982; **Resid:** Internal Medicine, Raritan Bay Med Ctr-Perth Amboy Div 1988

Gil, Constante MD (IM) *PCP* - **Spec Exp:** Hypertension; Stroke; Heart Failure; Diabetes; **Hospital:** Raritan Bay Med Ctr - Perth Amboy; **Address:** 86 New Brunswick Ave, Hopelawn, NJ 08861; **Phone:** 732-826-1609; **Med School:** Dominican Republic 1981; **Resid:** Internal Medicine, Raritan Bay Med Ctr-Perth Amboy Div 1989; **Fac Appt:** Assoc Clin Prof Med, UMDNJ-RW Johnson Med Sch

Guillen, Gregorio MD (IM) *PCP* - **Spec Exp:** Geriatric Medicine; **Hospital:** Raritan Bay Med Ctr - Perth Amboy, JFK Med Ctr - Edison; **Address:** 400 State St, Ste 2, Perth Amboy, NJ 08861; **Phone:** 732-442-6020; **Med School:** Dominican Republic 1982; **Resid:** Internal Medicine, Raritan Bay Med Ctr 1990; **Fellow:** Geriatric Medicine, Univ Florida 1992

Schaer, Teresa M MD (IM) *PCP* - **Spec Exp:** Concierge Medicine; Geriatric Medicine; **Hospital:** St. Peter's Univ Hosp, Robert Wood Johnson Univ Hosp - New Brunswick; **Address:** 12 Stults Rd, Ste 123, Dayton, NJ 08810; **Phone:** 732-230-3272; **Board Cert:** Internal Medicine 1984; Geriatric Medicine 2010; **Med School:** UCSD 1981; **Resid:** Internal Medicine, Bellevue Hosp Ctr 1984; **Fellow:** Geriatric Medicine, Geo Wash Univ Med Ctr 1986; **Fac Appt:** Assoc Clin Prof Med

Interventional Cardiology

Altmann, Dory B MD (IC) - **Spec Exp:** Coronary Artery Disease; Heart Valve Disease; **Hospital:** Robert Wood Johnson Univ Hosp - New Brunswick, St. Peter's Univ Hosp; **Address:** Cardiology Assocs of New Brunswick, 593 Cranbury Rd, East Brunswick, NJ 08816; **Phone:** 732-390-3333; **Board Cert:** Internal Medicine 1989; Cardiovascular Disease 2011; Interventional Cardiology 2009; **Med School:** Yale Univ 1986; **Resid:** Internal Medicine, New England Med Ctr 1989; **Fellow:** Cardiovascular Disease, Mt Sinai Hosp 1992; Interventional Cardiology, Washington Hosp Ctr 1993; **Fac Appt:** Asst Clin Prof Med, UMDNJ-RW Johnson Med Sch

Maternal & Fetal Medicine

MacMillan, William E MD (MF) - **Spec Exp:** Fetal Diagnosis & Therapy; Diabetes in Pregnancy; Reproductive Genetics; Multiple Gestation; **Hospital:** Robert Wood Johnson Univ Hosp - New Brunswick; **Address:** RWJ Med Group, Dept Ob/Gyn, 125 Paterson St, Ste 4200, New Brunswick, NJ 08901; **Phone:** 732-235-6600; **Board Cert:** Obstetrics & Gynecology 2011; Maternal & Fetal Medicine 2011; **Med School:** Univ Wisc 1985; **Resid:** Obstetrics & Gynecology, Univ Wisc Affil Hosp 1989; **Fellow:** Maternal & Fetal Medicine, SUNY Stony Brook 1991; **Fac Appt:** Asst Prof ObG, UMDNJ-RW Johnson Med Sch

Medical Oncology

Aisner, Joseph MD (Onc) - **Spec Exp:** Lung Cancer; Solid Tumors; Thymoma; Mesothelioma; **Hospital:** Robert Wood Johnson Univ Hosp - New Brunswick; **Address:** Cancer Inst of New Jersey, 195 Little Albany St, rm 2006, New Brunswick, NJ 08903-2681; **Phone:** 732-235-6777; **Board Cert:** Internal Medicine 1973; Medical Oncology 1975; **Med School:** Wayne State Univ 1970; **Resid:** Internal Medicine, Georgetown Univ Hosp 1972; **Fellow:** Medical Oncology, Natl Cancer Inst 1975; **Fac Appt:** Prof Med, UMDNJ-RW Johnson Med Sch

DiPaola, Robert S MD (Onc) - **Spec Exp:** Genitourinary Cancer; Prostate Cancer; Urologic Cancer; **Hospital:** Robert Wood Johnson Univ Hosp - New Brunswick; **Address:** Cancer Inst of New Jersey, 195 Little Albany St, New Brunswick, NJ 08903-2681; **Phone:** 732-235-6777; **Board Cert:** Internal Medicine 2011; Medical Oncology 2005; **Med School:** Univ Utah 1988; **Resid:** Internal Medicine, Duke Univ Med Ctr 1991; **Fellow:** Hematology & Oncology, Univ Penn Hosp 1994; **Fac Appt:** Assoc Prof Med, UMDNJ-RW Johnson Med Sch

Eleff, Michael MD (Onc) - **Spec Exp:** Lung Cancer; Melanoma; **Hospital:** Robert Wood Johnson Univ Hosp - New Brunswick; **Address:** Cancer Institute of New Jersey, 195 Little Ablanty St, New Brunswick, NJ 08901; **Phone:** 732-235-6777; **Board Cert:** Internal Medicine 1982; Medical Oncology 1985; **Med School:** Case West Res Univ 1979; **Resid:** Internal Medicine, Med Coll Va Hosp 1982; **Fellow:** Medical Oncology, Med Coll Va Hosp 1984

Fang, Bruno S MD (Onc) - Spec Exp: Lung Cancer; Head & Neck Cancer; Breast Cancer; Colon Cancer; **Hospital:** Univ Med Ctr Princeton at Plainsboro, St. Peter's Univ Hosp; **Address:** Central Jersey Oncology Ctr, 205 Easton Ave, New Brunswick, NJ 08901; **Phone:** 732-390-7750; **Board Cert:** Internal Medicine 2006; Hematology 2010; Medical Oncology 2010; **Med School:** Brazil 1991; **Resid:** Internal Medicine, Jackson Meml Hosp 1996; Internal Medicine, VA Med Ctr 1997; **Fellow:** Hematology & Oncology, Natl Cancer Inst/NIH 2000

Nissenblatt, Michael J MD (Onc) - Spec Exp: Breast Cancer; Colon Cancer; Lung Cancer; Hereditary Cancer; **Hospital:** Robert Wood Johnson Univ Hosp - New Brunswick, St. Peter's Univ Hosp; **Address:** 205 Easton Ave, New Brunswick, NJ 08901-1722; **Phone:** 732-390-7750; **Board Cert:** Internal Medicine 1976; Medical Oncology 1979; **Med School:** Columbia P&S 1973; **Resid:** Internal Medicine, Johns Hopkins Hosp 1976; **Fellow:** Medical Oncology, Johns Hopkins Hosp 1978; **Fac Appt:** Clin Prof Med, UMDNJ-RW Johnson Med Sch

Salwitz, James C MD (Onc) - Spec Exp: Colon Cancer; Breast Cancer; Lung Cancer; Leukemia & Lymphoma; **Hospital:** Robert Wood Johnson Univ Hosp - New Brunswick, St. Peter's Univ Hosp; **Address:** Central Jersey Oncology Ctr, 205 Easton Ave, New Brunswick, NJ 08901; **Phone:** 732-390-7750; **Board Cert:** Internal Medicine 1984; Medical Oncology 1987; **Med School:** UMDNJ-Rutgers Med Sch 1981; **Resid:** Internal Medicine, Northwestern Univ/McGaw Med Ctr 1984; **Fellow:** Medical Oncology, NIH-Natl Canc Inst 1987

Shypula, Gregory J MD (Onc) - Spec Exp: Hematology; **Hospital:** Raritan Bay Med Ctr - Perth Amboy, JFK Med Ctr - Edison; **Address:** 1030 St Georges Ave, Ste 307, Avenel, NJ 07001-1330; **Phone:** 732-750-1200; **Board Cert:** Internal Medicine 1989; Medical Oncology 2011; Hematology 2007; **Med School:** Poland 1981; **Resid:** Internal Medicine, T Marciniak Univ 1984; Internal Medicine, Raritan Bay Med Ctr-Perth Amboy Div 1988; **Fellow:** Hematology & Oncology, St Luke's-Roosevelt Hosp Ctr 1992; **Fac Appt:** Assoc Clin Prof Med, Columbia P&S

Toppmeyer, Deborah L MD (Onc) - Spec Exp: Breast Cancer; Hereditary Cancer; **Hospital:** Robert Wood Johnson Univ Hosp - New Brunswick; **Address:** Cancer Inst of New Jersey, 195 Little Albany St, New Brunswick, NJ 08903; **Phone:** 732-235-9692; **Board Cert:** Internal Medicine 1988; Medical Oncology 2006; **Med School:** Albany Med Coll 1985; **Resid:** Internal Medicine, Univ Pittsburgh Hlth Ctr Hosp 1988; **Fellow:** Medical Oncology, Dana Farber Cancer Inst 1993; **Fac Appt:** Assoc Prof Med

Neonatal-Perinatal Medicine

Hiatt, I Mark MD (NP) - Spec Exp: Respiratory Failure; Prematurity/Low Birth Weight Infants; Ethics; **Hospital:** St. Peter's Univ Hosp; **Address:** St Peter's Univ Hosp, Div Neonatal Med, 254 Easton Ave, New Brunswick, NJ 08902; **Phone:** 732-745-8523; **Board Cert:** Pediatrics 1978; Neonatal-Perinatal Medicine 1979; **Med School:** Cornell Univ-Weill Med Coll 1972; **Resid:** Pediatrics, NY Hosp-Cornell Med Ctr 1975; **Fellow:** Neonatal-Perinatal Medicine, Babies Hosp-Columbia Univ 1977; **Fac Appt:** Prof Ped, Drexel Univ Coll Med

Mehta, Rajeev MD (NP) - Spec Exp: Neonatal Critical Care; **Hospital:** Robert Wood Johnson Univ Hosp - New Brunswick; **Address:** RW Johnson Med School, 1 RW Johnson Pl, MEB 238, Dept Pediatrics, New Brunswick, NJ 08903-1766; **Phone:** 732-235-7036; **Board Cert:** Neonatal-Perinatal Medicine 2008; **Med School:** India 1979; **Resid:** Pediatrics, Queens Park/St Mary's/Dudley Rd Hosps 1985; Pediatrics, Univ Hosp 1990; **Fellow:** Neonatology, Bradford Royal Infirmary 1989; Neonatology, North Shore Univ Hosp 1993; **Fac Appt:** Prof Ped, UMDNJ-RW Johnson Med Sch

Nephrology

Covit, Andrew B MD (Nep) - **Spec Exp:** Hypertension; Kidney Failure; Renovascular Disease; **Hospital:** Robert Wood Johnson Univ Hosp - New Brunswick, St. Peter's Univ Hosp; **Address:** 8 Old Bridge Tpke, South River, NJ 08882; **Phone:** 732-390-4888; **Board Cert:** Internal Medicine 1982; Nephrology 1986; **Med School:** SUNY Downstate 1979; **Resid:** Internal Medicine, NY Hosp 1982; **Fellow:** Nephrology, NY Hosp 1984; **Fac Appt:** Clin Prof Med, UMDNJ-RW Johnson Med Sch

Sherman, Richard A MD (Nep) - **Spec Exp:** Dialysis Care; Electrolyte Disorders; **Hospital:** Robert Wood Johnson Univ Hosp - New Brunswick; **Address:** RWJ Div Nephrology, 125 Patterson St, Ste 5100, New Brunswick, NJ 08901; **Phone:** 732-235-6512; **Board Cert:** Internal Medicine 1978; Nephrology 1980; **Med School:** Albert Einstein Coll Med 1975; **Resid:** Internal Medicine, Metropolitan Hosp 1977; **Fellow:** Nephrology, Albert Einstein 1979; **Fac Appt:** Prof Med, UMDNJ-RW Johnson Med Sch

Neurological Surgery

Lee, Sun H MD/PhD (NS) - **Spec Exp:** Spinal Surgery-Complex; Brain Tumors; Minimally Invasive Surgery; Pituitary Tumors; **Hospital:** Robert Wood Johnson Univ Hosp - New Brunswick; **Address:** University Neuro Assocs, 125 Patterson St, CAB 2100 Bldg Fl 4 - Ste 4011, New Brunswick, NJ 08901; **Phone:** 732-235-7756; **Board Cert:** Neurological Surgery 2012; **Med School:** Korea 1979; **Resid:** Neurological Surgery, Seoul National Univ Hosp 1984; Neurological Surgery, Thos Jefferson Univ Hosp 1998; **Fellow:** Neurological Surgery, Univ Pittsburgh Med Ctr 1999; **Fac Appt:** Assoc Prof NS, UMDNJ-RW Johnson Med Sch

Nosko, Michael G MD/PhD (NS) - **Spec Exp:** Aneurysm-Cerebral; Brain Tumors; Pituitary Tumors; Cerebrovascular Neurosurgery; **Hospital:** Robert Wood Johnson Univ Hosp - New Brunswick, Univ Med Ctr Princeton at Plainsboro; **Address:** University Neuro Assocs, 125 Paterson St, Bldg 2100 Fl 4 - Ste 4011, New Brunswick, NJ 08901-1962; **Phone:** 732-235-7756; **Board Cert:** Neurological Surgery 1993; **Med School:** Univ Toronto 1982; **Resid:** Neurological Surgery, Univ Alberta Affil Hosp 1991; **Fellow:** Research, Alberta Heritage Fdn Med Rsch 1986; **Fac Appt:** Assoc Prof NS, UMDNJ-RW Johnson Med Sch

Przybylski, Gregory J MD (NS) - **Spec Exp:** Spinal Surgery; Multiple Sclerosis; Vascular Neurosurgery; Spinal Cord Tumors; **Hospital:** JFK Med Ctr - Edison, Jersey Shore Univ Med Ctr; **Address:** NJ Neuroscience Inst, 65 James St Fl 1st, Edison, NJ 08820; **Phone:** 732-321-7010; **Board Cert:** Neurological Surgery 2011; **Med School:** Jefferson Med Coll 1987; **Resid:** Neurological Surgery, Univ Pittsburgh 1994; **Fellow:** Spinal Surgery, Hosp St Vincent de Paul/Hosp St Roch 1995; Spinal Surgery, Med Coll Wisc 1996; **Fac Appt:** Prof NS, Seton Hall Univ Sch Hlth & Med Scis

Neurology

Belsh, Jerry M MD (N) - **Spec Exp:** Neuromuscular Disorders; Amyotrophic Lateral Sclerosis (ALS); **Hospital:** Robert Wood Johnson Univ Hosp - New Brunswick; **Address:** 125 Paterson St, New Brunswick, NJ 08901; **Phone:** 732-235-7340; **Board Cert:** Neurology 1981; **Med School:** Jefferson Med Coll 1975; **Resid:** Neurology, Hahnemann Univ Hosp 1977; Neurology, SUNY-Dwnst Med Ctr 1979; **Fellow:** Neuromuscular Medicine, Mt Sinai Hosp 1980; **Fac Appt:** Prof N, UMDNJ-RW Johnson Med Sch

Gizzi, Martin S MD/PhD (N) - **Spec Exp:** Neuro-Ophthalmology; Stroke; Progressive Supranuclear Palsy (PSP); Stroke; **Hospital:** JFK Med Ctr - Edison; **Address:** 65 James St, NJ Neuroscience Institute, Edison, NJ 08820-3947; **Phone:** 732-321-7010; **Board Cert:** Neurology 1990; Vascular Neurology 2008; **Med School:** Univ Miami Sch Med 1985; **Resid:** Neurology, Mount Sinai Hosp 1989; **Fellow:** Neuro-Ophthalmology, Mount Sinai Hosp 1991; **Fac Appt:** Prof N, Seton Hall Univ Sch Hlth & Med Scis

Golbe, Lawrence I MD (N) - **Spec Exp:** Parkinson's Disease; Progressive Supranuclear Palsy (PSP); Movement Disorders; **Hospital:** Robert Wood Johnson Univ Hosp - New Brunswick; **Address:** 125 Paterson St Fl 6 - rm 6100, New Brunswick, NJ 08901-2160; **Phone:** 732-235-7733; **Board Cert:** Neurology 1984; **Med School:** NYU Sch Med 1978; **Resid:** Internal Medicine, Hahnemann Univ Hosp 1980; Neurology, Bellevue Hosp 1983; **Fac Appt:** Prof N, UMDNJ-RW Johnson Med Sch

Lazar, Mark H MD (N) - **Spec Exp:** Headache; Pain Management; Acupuncture; Sarcoidosis; **Hospital:** Robert Wood Johnson Univ Hosp - New Brunswick; **Address:** 573 Cranbury Rd, Ste A5, East Brunswick, NJ 08816-4026; **Phone:** 732-254-5101; **Board Cert:** Neurology 1982; **Med School:** NYU Sch Med 1977; **Resid:** Neurology, NYU Med Ctr 1981; **Fellow:** Neurology, NY-Cornell Med Ctr 1982; Clinical Neurophysiology, Columbia-Presby Med Ctr 1983; **Fac Appt:** Assoc Clin Prof N, UMDNJ-RW Johnson Med Sch

Lepore, Frederick E MD (N) - **Spec Exp:** Neuro-Ophthalmology; Botox for Blepharospasm; Migraine; Pseudomotor Cerebri; **Hospital:** Robert Wood Johnson Univ Hosp - New Brunswick; **Address:** Dept Neurology, 125 Paterson St, rm 6210, New Brunswick, NJ 08901-2160; **Phone:** 732-235-7729; **Board Cert:** Neurology 1981; **Med School:** Univ Rochester 1975; **Resid:** Internal Medicine, Univ Michigan Med Ctr 1976; Neurology, Univ Virginia Hlth Sci Ctr 1979; **Fellow:** Neuro-Ophthalmology, Bascom Palmer Eye Inst 1980; **Fac Appt:** Prof N, UMDNJ-RW Johnson Med Sch

Oh, Youn K MD (N) - **Spec Exp:** Headache; Stroke; Seizure Disorders; Parkinson's Disease; **Hospital:** JFK Med Ctr - Edison, Robert Wood Johnson Univ Hosp at Rahway; **Address:** 34-36 Progress St, Ste B, Edison, NJ 08820-1197; **Phone:** 908-757-6633; **Board Cert:** Neurology 1979; Psychiatry 1981; **Med School:** South Korea 1964; **Resid:** Psychiatry, Harvard Psy Svc/Boston City Hosp 1973; Neurology, UMDNJ-NJ Med Sch 1975; **Fac Appt:** Assoc Clin Prof N, UMDNJ-RW Johnson Med Sch

Rosenberg, Michael L MD (N) - **Spec Exp:** Neuro-Ophthalmology; Neuro-Otology; Balance Disorders; **Hospital:** JFK Med Ctr - Edison; **Address:** New Jersey Neuroscience Institute, 65 James St, Edison, NJ 08818; **Phone:** 732-321-7010; **Board Cert:** Neurology 1983; **Med School:** Baylor Coll Med 1976; **Resid:** Neurology, Letterman AMC 1981; **Fellow:** Neuro-Ophthalmology, Bascom-Palmer Eye Inst 1981; **Fac Appt:** Prof N, Seton Hall Univ Sch Hlth & Med Scis

Sage, Jacob MD (N) - **Spec Exp:** Parkinson's Disease; **Hospital:** Robert Wood Johnson Univ Hosp - New Brunswick; **Address:** UMDNJ, Dept Neurology, 125 Paterson St Fl 6 - Ste 6100, New Brunswick, NJ 08901-2160; **Phone:** 732-235-7733; **Board Cert:** Neurology 1979; **Med School:** Univ Pittsburgh 1972; **Resid:** Neurology, Univ Pittsburgh Hosps 1978; **Fellow:** Neurological Chemistry, NY Hosp-Cornell 1980; **Fac Appt:** Prof N, UMDNJ-RW Johnson Med Sch

Neuroradiology

Keller, Irwin MD (NRad) - **Spec Exp:** Brain & Spinal Imaging; Interventional Neuroradiology; Aneurysm-Cerebral; **Hospital:** Robert Wood Johnson Univ Hosp - New Brunswick; **Address:** 579A Cranbury Rd, East Brunswick, NJ 08816-5405; **Phone:** 732-390-0040; **Board Cert:** Diagnostic Radiology 1984; Neuroradiology 2005; **Med School:** NY Med Coll 1980; **Resid:** Diagnostic Radiology, Montefiore Hosp Med Ctr 1984; **Fellow:** Neuroradiology, NYU Med Ctr 1986; **Fac Appt:** Assoc Prof Rad, UMDNJ-RW Johnson Med Sch

Roychowdhury, Sudipta MD (NRad) - **Spec Exp:** Interventional Neuroradiology; Pediatric Radiology; **Hospital:** Robert Wood Johnson Univ Hosp - New Brunswick; **Address:** University Radiology Group, 579A Cranbury Rd, East Brunswick, NJ 08816; **Phone:** 732-390-0040; **Board Cert:** Diagnostic Radiology 1997; Neuroradiology 2010; **Med School:** Northwestern Univ 1992; **Resid:** Diagnostic Radiology, Northwestern Univ Hosp 1997; **Fellow:** Neuroradiology, Univ Penn 1999; **Fac Appt:** Asst Clin Prof Rad, UMDNJ-RW Johnson Med Sch

Schonfeld, Steven MD (NRad) - **Spec Exp:** Spine Imaging & Intervention; Interventional Neuroradiology; **Hospital:** Robert Wood Johnson Univ Hosp - New Brunswick; **Address:** University Radiology Group, 579A Cranbury Rd Fl 3, East Brunswick, NJ 08816; **Phone:** 732-390-0040; **Board Cert:** Diagnostic Radiology 1982; Neuroradiology 2005; **Med School:** Mount Sinai Sch Med 1978; **Resid:** Diagnostic Radiology, Montefiore Hosp Med Ctr 1982; **Fellow:** Neuroradiology, NYU Med Ctr 1984; **Fac Appt:** Assoc Clin Prof Rad, UMDNJ-RW Johnson Med Sch

Obstetrics & Gynecology

Bachmann, Gloria A MD (ObG) - **Spec Exp:** Menopause Problems; Sexual Dysfunction; Pelvic Surgery; Uterine Fibroids; **Hospital:** Robert Wood Johnson Univ Hosp - New Brunswick; **Address:** Womens Health Institute, 125 Paterson St, Ste 2104, New Brunswick, NJ 08901-1962; **Phone:** 732-235-7633; **Board Cert:** Obstetrics & Gynecology 1981; **Med School:** Univ Pennsylvania 1974; **Resid:** Obstetrics & Gynecology, Hosp Univ Penn 1978; **Fac Appt:** Prof ObG, UMDNJ-RW Johnson Med Sch

Bochner, Ronnie Z MD (ObG) - **Spec Exp:** Gynecologic Surgery; Laparoscopic Surgery; Uterine Fibroids; Menopause Problems; **Hospital:** Robert Wood Johnson Univ Hosp - New Brunswick; **Address:** 3270 Rt 27, Ste 2200, MS 08824, Kendall Park, NJ 08824-1458; **Phone:** 732-422-8989; **Board Cert:** Obstetrics & Gynecology 2012; **Med School:** Mount Sinai Sch Med 1981; **Resid:** Obstetrics & Gynecology, LI Jewish Med Ctr 1985; **Fac Appt:** Asst Clin Prof ObG, UMDNJ-RW Johnson Med Sch

Davis, Nicole D MD (ObG) - **Spec Exp:** Gynecology Only; **Hospital:** St. Peter's Univ Hosp; **Address:** 620 Cranbury Rd, Ste LL90, East Brunswick, NJ 08816; **Phone:** 732-257-0081; **Board Cert:** Obstetrics & Gynecology 2011; **Med School:** Yale Univ 1988; **Resid:** Obstetrics & Gynecology, New York Hosp 1992

Rathauser, Robert H MD (ObG) - **Hospital:** Robert Wood Johnson Univ Hosp - New Brunswick; **Address:** RWJ OB/GYN Assocs, 3270 Route 27, Ste 2200, Kendall Park, NJ 08824; **Phone:** 732-422-8989; **Board Cert:** Obstetrics & Gynecology 2011; **Med School:** NYU Sch Med 1979; **Resid:** Obstetrics & Gynecology, LI Jewish Med Ctr 1983; **Fac Appt:** Assoc Prof ObG, UMDNJ-RW Johnson Med Sch

Occupational Medicine

Gochfeld, Michael MD/PhD (OM) - **Spec Exp:** Environmental Medicine; Mercury Toxic Exposure; Chemical Exposure; **Hospital:** Robert Wood Johnson Univ Hosp - New Brunswick; **Address:** Enviro & Occupational Health-EOHSI, 170 Frelinghuysen Rd, Ste 200, Piscataway, NJ 08854; **Phone:** 848-445-0123; **Board Cert:** Occupational Medicine 1983; **Med School:** Albert Einstein Coll Med 1965; **Resid:** Behavioral Medicine, Rockefeller Univ 1977; **Fac Appt:** Prof OM, UMDNJ-RW Johnson Med Sch

Kipen, Howard M MD (OM) - **Spec Exp:** Environmental Medicine; Occupational Lung Disease; **Hospital:** Robert Wood Johnson Univ Hosp - New Brunswick; **Address:** UMDNJ-RWJ Med Sch, EOHSI, 170 Frelinghuysen Rd, Ste 200, Piscataway, NJ 08854; **Phone:** 848-445-0123; **Board Cert:** Internal Medicine 1982; Occupational Medicine 1986; **Med School:** UCSF 1979; **Resid:** Internal Medicine, Columbia Presby Med Ctr 1982; Occupational Medicine, Mt Sinai Hosp 1984; **Fac Appt:** Prof Med, UMDNJ-RW Johnson Med Sch

Ophthalmology

Blondo, Dennis L MD (Oph) - **Hospital:** Raritan Bay Med Ctr - Old Bridge Div; **Address:** 28 Throckmorton Ln, Old Bridge, NJ 08857-2558; **Phone:** 732-679-6100; **Board Cert:** Ophthalmology 1979; **Med School:** Med Coll VA 1973; **Resid:** Ophthalmology, NYU Med Ctr 1977

Engel, J Mark MD (Oph) - **Spec Exp:** Pediatric Ophthalmology; **Hospital:** Robert Wood Johnson Univ Hosp - New Brunswick, St. Peter's Univ Hosp; **Address:** University Childrens Eye Ctr, 4 Cornwall Ct, East Brunswick, NJ 08816; **Phone:** 732-613-9191; **Board Cert:** Ophthalmology 2003; **Med School:** Loyola Univ-Stritch Sch Med 1986; **Resid:** Internal Medicine, Evanston Hosp 1988; Ophthalmology, Interfaith Med Ctr 1991; **Fellow:** Pediatric Ophthalmology, Childrens Meml Hosp 1992; **Fac Appt:** Assoc Clin Prof Oph, UMDNJ-NJ Med Sch, Newark

Grabowski, Wayne M MD (Oph) - **Spec Exp:** Diabetic Eye Disease; Laser Vision Surgery; **Hospital:** Univ Med Ctr Princeton at Plainsboro; **Address:** 5 Centre Drive, Ste 1B, Monroe Township, NJ 08831; **Phone:** 609-409-2777; **Board Cert:** Ophthalmology 1982; **Med School:** Albany Med Coll 1977; **Resid:** Ophthalmology, Albany Med Ctr 1981; **Fellow:** Vitreoretinal Surgery, Wills Eye Hosp 1983

Milite, James MD (Oph) - **Spec Exp:** Oculoplastic Surgery; Eyelid Cosmetic Surgery; Eyelid Tumors/Cancer; Thyroid Eye Disease; **Hospital:** New York Eye & Ear Infirm (page 117); **Address:** 485 Route 1 S, A Bldg, Iselin, NJ 08830; **Phone:** 732-750-0400; **Board Cert:** Ophthalmology 2006; **Med School:** NYU Sch Med 1990; **Resid:** Ophthalmology, NY Eye & Ear Infirm 1994; **Fellow:** Ocular Pathology, NY Eye & Ear Infirm 1995; Ophthalmic Plastic Surgery, NY Eye & Ear Infirm 1996; **Fac Appt:** Asst Prof Oph, NY Med Coll

Napolitano, Joseph D MD (Oph) - **Spec Exp:** Pediatric Ophthalmology; Strabismus; Eye Muscle Disorders; **Hospital:** Robert Wood Johnson Univ Hosp - New Brunswick; **Address:** OMNI Eye Services, 485 Route 1 South, A Bldg - Ste 140, Iselin, NJ 08830; **Phone:** 732-750-0400; **Board Cert:** Ophthalmology 2008; **Med School:** UMDNJ-RW Johnson Med Sch 1987; **Resid:** Ophthalmology, Univ Hosp 1992; **Fellow:** Pediatric Ophthalmology, Childrens Hosp 1993

Santamaria II, Jaime MD (Oph) - **Spec Exp:** Cataract Surgery; LASIK-Refractive Surgery; **Hospital:** Raritan Bay Med Ctr - Perth Amboy, NY-Presby/Columbia Univ Med Ctr, NY (page 104); **Address:** 104 Market St, Santamaria Eye Center, Perth Amboy, NJ 08861-4412; **Phone:** 732-826-5159; **Board Cert:** Ophthalmology 1979; **Med School:** Columbia P&S 1973; **Resid:** Ophthalmology, Columbia-Presby Med Ctr 1978; **Fellow:** Research, Columbia Physicians & Surgeons 1975; **Fac Appt:** Asst Clin Prof Oph, Columbia P&S

Orthopaedic Surgery

Garfinkel, Matthew J MD (OrS) - **Spec Exp:** Shoulder & Knee Surgery; Arthroscopic Surgery; Sports Medicine; **Hospital:** JFK Med Ctr - Edison; **Address:** Edison-Metuchen Orthopaedic Group, 10 Parsonage Rd, Ste 500, Edison, NJ 08837-2429; **Phone:** 732-494-6226; **Board Cert:** Orthopaedic Surgery 2005; **Med School:** Cornell Univ-Weill Med Coll 1986; **Resid:** Orthopaedic Surgery, Montefiore/Weiler Einsten Med Ctr 1991; **Fellow:** Sports Medicine, Lankenau Hosp 1992

Lombardi, Joseph S MD (OrS) - **Spec Exp:** Spinal Surgery; Spinal Disc Replacement; **Hospital:** JFK Med Ctr - Edison; **Address:** Edison-Metuchen Orthopaedic Group, 10 Parsonage Rd, Ste 500, Edison, NJ 08837-2475; **Phone:** 732-494-6226; **Board Cert:** Orthopaedic Surgery 2008; **Med School:** UMDNJ-RW Johnson Med Sch 1978; **Resid:** Orthopaedic Surgery, UMDNJ-Univ Hosp 1983; **Fellow:** Spinal Surgery, Long Beach Mem Med Ctr 1984

Piskun, Andrew MD (OrS) - **Spec Exp:** Trauma; Sports Injuries; Arthroscopic Surgery; **Hospital:** Robert Wood Johnson Univ Hosp - New Brunswick, St. Peter's Univ Hosp; **Address:** 1132 S Washington Ave, Piscataway, NJ 08854-3335; **Phone:** 732-752-8484; **Board Cert:** Orthopaedic Surgery 1984; **Med School:** UMDNJ-RW Johnson Med Sch 1977; **Resid:** Orthopaedic Surgery, UMDNJ-RW Johnson Univ Hosp 1982; **Fac Appt:** Asst Clin Prof OrS, UMDNJ-RW Johnson Med Sch

Reich, Steven MD (OrS) - **Spec Exp:** Spinal Surgery; Spinal Disorders; **Hospital:** Robert Wood Johnson Univ Hosp - New Brunswick, St. Peter's Univ Hosp; **Address:** Affiliated Orthopaedic Specialists, 2186 Route 27, Ste 1A, North Brunswick, NJ 08902; **Phone:** 732-422-1222; **Board Cert:** Orthopaedic Surgery 2005; **Med School:** Albert Einstein Coll Med 1986; **Resid:** Orthopaedic Surgery, Hosp for Joint Diseases 1991; **Fellow:** Spinal Surgery, Pennsylvania Hosp 1992; Spinal Surgery, Thomas Jefferson Univ Hosp 1992

Otolaryngology

Edelman, Bruce MD (Oto) - **Spec Exp:** Ear Disorders; Sinusitis; **Hospital:** St. Peter's Univ Hosp; **Address:** B3 Cornwall Drive, East Brunswick, NJ 08816; **Phone:** 732-238-0300; **Board Cert:** Otolaryngology 1990; **Med School:** NYU Sch Med 1984; **Resid:** Surgery, Albert Einstein 1986; Otolaryngology, NYU Med Ctr 1990; **Fellow:** Pediatric Otolaryngology, Children's Hosp 1991

Kay, Scott MD (Oto) - **Spec Exp:** Facial Nerve Disorders; Otology; Hearing Loss; Sinus Surgery; **Hospital:** Univ Med Ctr Princeton at Plainsboro; **Address:** 7 Schalks Crossing Rd, Ste 324, Plainsboro, NJ 08536; **Phone:** 609-897-0203; **Board Cert:** Otolaryngology 1993; **Med School:** Univ Pennsylvania 1986; **Resid:** Surgery, Mt Sinai Hosp 1988; Otolaryngology, Columbia-Presby Med Ctr 1992; **Fellow:** Facial Plastic Surgery, Shadyside Hosp 1993; **Fac Appt:** Prof S

Li, Ronald MD (Oto) - **Spec Exp:** Cosmetic Surgery-Face; Sinus Disorders; Voice Disorders; **Hospital:** Univ Med Ctr Princeton at Plainsboro; **Address:** 2650 US Hwy 130 & Day Rd, Ste B, Cranbury, NJ 08512; **Phone:** 609-655-3000; **Board Cert:** Otolaryngology 1990; **Med School:** Mount Sinai Sch Med 1984; **Resid:** Otolaryngology, Montefiore Med Ctr 1989

Mazzara, Carl A MD (Oto) - **Spec Exp:** Rhinoplasty; Eyelid Surgery; Cancer Reconstruction; Facial Plastic & Reconstructive Surgery; **Hospital:** JFK Med Ctr - Edison, Overlook Med Ctr (page 92); **Address:** Mazzara Aesthetics, 5 Lincoln Hwy, Ste 4, Edison, NJ 08820; **Phone:** 732-635-1800; **Board Cert:** Otolaryngology 1994; Facial Plastic & Reconstr Surgery 1995; **Med School:** Mount Sinai Sch Med 1988; **Resid:** Otolaryngology, UMDNJ- Univ Hosp 1992; **Fellow:** Facial Plastic & Reconstr Surgery, Inst Facial Plastic Surg 1993

Miller, Andrew J MD (Oto) - **Spec Exp:** Cosmetic Surgery-Face; **Hospital:** JFK Med Ctr - Edison; **Address:** Associates in Plastic Surgery, 1150 Amboy Ave, Edison, NJ 08837; **Phone:** 732-548-3200; **Board Cert:** Otolaryngology 2000; Facial Plastic & Reconstr Surgery 2002; **Med School:** Baylor Coll Med 1994; **Resid:** Otolaryngology, Tulane Univ Med Ctr 1999

Rosenbaum, Jeffrey M MD (Oto) - **Spec Exp:** Head & Neck Surgery; Cosmetic Surgery-Face; Salivary Gland Surgery; Thyroid & Parathyroid Surgery; **Hospital:** St. Peter's Univ Hosp; **Address:** B3 Cornwall Drive, East Brunswick, NJ 08816; **Phone:** 732-238-0300; **Board Cert:** Otolaryngology 1978; **Med School:** Albany Med Coll 1973; **Resid:** Surgery, Hartford Hosp 1975; Otolaryngology, NYU Med Ctr 1978; **Fellow:** Plastic Surgery, Wayne Co Genl Hosp 1979; **Fac Appt:** Assoc Prof Oto, NYU Sch Med

Pain Medicine

Grubb, William R MD (PM) - **Spec Exp:** Complex Regional Pain Syndromes; Pain-Cancer; **Hospital:** Robert Wood Johnson Univ Hosp - New Brunswick; **Address:** New Jersey Pain Institute, 125 Patterson St Fl 5 - Ste 5100, New Brunswick, NJ 08901; **Phone:** 732-235-7246; **Board Cert:** Anesthesiology 1990; Pain Medicine 2007; **Med School:** Geo Wash Univ 1985; **Resid:** Anesthesiology, G Washington Univ Med Ctr 1989; **Fellow:** Cardiac Anesthesiology, Univ S Florida 1994; **Fac Appt:** Asst Prof Anes, UMDNJ-RW Johnson Med Sch

Levin, Alexander MD (PM) - **Spec Exp:** Pain-Chronic; **Hospital:** Robert Wood Johnson Univ Hosp - New Brunswick; **Address:** 561 Cranbury Road Fl Ground, East Brunswick, NJ 08816-5400; **Phone:** 732-651-1300; **Board Cert:** Anesthesiology 1990; Pain Medicine 2007; **Med School:** Russia 1978; **Resid:** Anesthesiology, Westchester Med Ctr 1986; **Fellow:** Pain Medicine, Univ Cincinnati 1987

Pathology

Barnard, Nicola J MD (Path) - **Spec Exp:** Breast Pathology; Surgical Pathology; **Hospital:** Robert Wood Johnson Univ Hosp - New Brunswick; **Address:** RJW Dept Surgical Pathology, 1 Robert Wood Johnson Pl, New Brunswick, NJ 08901; **Phone:** 732-937-8592; **Board Cert:** Anatomic Pathology 1981; **Med School:** England, UK 1975; **Resid:** Anatomic Pathology, Yale-New Haven Hosp 1980; Anatomic Pathology, Beth Israel Deaconess Hosp 1982; **Fellow:** Clinical Pathology, Harvard Univ 1982; **Fac Appt:** Assoc Prof Path, UMDNJ-RW Johnson Med Sch

Pediatric Cardiology

Agarwal, Kishan C MD (PCd) - **Spec Exp:** Echocardiography; Heart Disease in Adolescents; Arrhythmias; **Hospital:** JFK Med Ctr - Edison, Children's Specialized Hosp; **Address:** 450 Plainfield Rd, Edison, NJ 08820-2628; **Phone:** 732-494-9500; **Board Cert:** Pediatrics 1990; Pediatric Cardiology 1990; **Med School:** India 1969; **Resid:** Pediatrics, St John's Episcopal Hosp 1977; Pediatrics, SUNY Downstate Med Ctr 1979; **Fellow:** Pediatric Cardiology, Mayo Clinic 1981; **Fac Appt:** Clin Prof Ped, UMDNJ-RW Johnson Med Sch

Gaffney, Joseph W MD (PCd) - **Spec Exp:** Echocardiography; Fetal Echocardiography; Critical Care; **Hospital:** Robert Wood Johnson Univ Hosp - New Brunswick, Morgan Stanley Children's Hosp of NY-Presby, NY (page 104); **Address:** Clin Academic Bldg, 125 Paterson St Fl 6 - Ste 6100, New Brunswick, NJ 08901; **Phone:** 732-235-7905; **Board Cert:** Pediatric Cardiology 2006; **Med School:** NY Med Coll 1981; **Resid:** Pediatrics, Brookdale Hosp Med Ctr 1984; **Fellow:** Pediatric Cardiology, Babies Hosp/Columbia-Presby 1987; **Fac Appt:** Assoc Prof Ped, UMDNJ-RW Johnson Med Sch

Kurer, Cheryl C MD (PCd) - **Spec Exp:** Arrhythmias; Congenital Heart Disease & Acquired; **Hospital:** Chldns Hosp of Philadelphia, St. Peter's Univ Hosp; **Address:** CHOP Cardiac Ctr at St Peter's Univ Hosp, 254 Easton Ave, New Brunswick, NJ 08901-1766; **Phone:** 732-846-2855; **Board Cert:** Pediatrics 1987; Pediatric Cardiology 2006; **Med School:** Mount Sinai Sch Med 1983; **Resid:** Pediatrics, Mt Sinai Hosp 1986; **Fellow:** Pediatric Cardiology, Chldns Hosp 1989; **Fac Appt:** Assoc Clin Prof Ped, Univ Pennsylvania

Pediatric Critical Care Medicine

Anene, Okechukwu P MD (PCCM) - **Hospital:** JFK Med Ctr - Edison; **Address:** Children's Service Dept, JFK Medical Ctr, 65 James St, Edison, NJ 08820; **Phone:** 732-321-7010; **Board Cert:** Pediatric Critical Care Medicine 2011; Pediatrics 2009; **Med School:** Nigeria 1983; **Resid:** Pediatrics, UMDNJ-New Jersey Med Sch 1991; Pediatric Critical Care Medicine, Wayne St Univ-Detroit Med Ctr 1995; **Fellow:** Pediatric Critical Care Medicine, Chldn's Hosp of Michigan 1995; **Fac Appt:** Assoc Prof Ped, Seton Hall Univ Sch Hlth & Med Scis

Jonna, Siva P MD (PCCM) - **Hospital:** St. Peter's Univ Hosp; **Address:** 254 Easton Ave, rm 5094, New Brunswick, NJ 08901; **Phone:** 732-745-8600 x8152; **Board Cert:** Pediatrics 2010; Pediatric Critical Care Medicine 2006; **Med School:** India 1981; **Resid:** Pediatrics, Howard Univ Hosp 1995; **Fellow:** Pediatric Critical Care Medicine, Georgetown Univ Hosp 1995

Pediatric Endocrinology

Marshall, Ian MD (PEn) - **Spec Exp:** Adrenal Disorders; Growth Disorders; Pubertal Disorders; **Hospital:** Robert Wood Johnson Univ Hosp - New Brunswick; **Address:** UMDNJ-RWJ Medical School, Div Pediatric Endocrinology, 89 French St Fl 2 - Ste 2300, New Brunswick, NJ 08901; **Phone:** 732-235-6230; **Board Cert:** Pediatric Endocrinology 2003; **Med School:** South Africa 1991; **Resid:** Pediatrics, Schneider Chldns Hosp 1998; **Fellow:** Pediatric Endocrinology, NY Presby Hosp 2002; **Fac Appt:** Asst Prof Ped

Salas, Max MD (PEn) - **Spec Exp:** Growth Disorders; Pubertal Disorders; Diabetes; **Hospital:** St. Peter's Univ Hosp; **Address:** St Peter's Univ Hosp-Ped Endocrinology, 254 Easton Ave Fl 3, New Brunswick, NJ 08901-1766; **Phone:** 732-745-8574; **Board Cert:** Pediatrics 1968; Pediatric Endocrinology 1986; **Med School:** Mexico 1964; **Resid:** Pediatrics, Children's Hosp 1967; Pediatrics, Children's Hosp 1968; **Fellow:** Pediatric Endocrinology, Children's Hosp 1979; Pediatric Endocrinology, N Shore Univ Hosp 1980; **Fac Appt:** Assoc Prof Ped, Drexel Univ Coll Med

Skuza, Kathryn MD (PEn) - **Spec Exp:** Diabetes; Thyroid Disorders; **Hospital:** St. Peter's Univ Hosp; **Address:** St Peter's Univ Hosp-Ped Endocrinology, 254 Easton Ave Fl 3, New Brunswick, NJ 08901-1766; **Phone:** 732-745-8574; **Board Cert:** Pediatrics 1987; Pediatric Endocrinology 2011; **Med School:** Poland 1982; **Resid:** Pediatrics, UMDNJ-Chldns Hosp 1985; **Fellow:** Endocrinology, Diabetes & Metabolism, UMDNJ-Chldns Hosp 1988; **Fac Appt:** Asst Prof Ped, UMDNJ-NJ Med Sch, Newark

Pediatric Gastroenterology

Koniaris, Soula MD (PGe) - **Spec Exp:** Nutrition; **Hospital:** Robert Wood Johnson Univ Hosp - New Brunswick; **Address:** Child Health Institute NJ, 89 French St, rm 2226, New Brunswick, NJ 08901; **Phone:** 732-235-7885; **Board Cert:** Pediatric Gastroenterology 2005; **Med School:** Univ Tenn Coll Med 1988; **Resid:** Pediatrics, Montefiore Hosp Med Ctr 1991; **Fellow:** Pediatric Gastroenterology, North Shore Univ Hosp 1994; **Fac Appt:** Asst Prof Ped, UMDNJ-RW Johnson Med Sch

Pediatric Hematology-Oncology

Drachtman, Richard A MD (PHO) - **Spec Exp:** Pediatric Cancers; Sickle Cell Disease; **Hospital:** Robert Wood Johnson Univ Hosp - New Brunswick, Jersey Shore Univ Med Ctr; **Address:** Cancer Inst of New Jersey, 195 Little Albany St, rm 3507, New Brunswick, NJ 08903; **Phone:** 732-235-5437; **Board Cert:** Pediatric Hematology-Oncology 2007; **Med School:** Ros Franklin Univ/Chicago Med Sch 1984; **Resid:** Pediatrics, N Shore Univ Hosp 1988; **Fellow:** Pediatric Hematology-Oncology, Mount Sinai Hosp 1991; **Fac Appt:** Prof Ped, UMDNJ-RW Johnson Med Sch

Pediatric Infectious Disease

Tolan Jr, Robert W MD (PInf) - **Spec Exp:** Lyme Disease; Cytomegalovirus; Staphylococcal Infections; Toxic Shock Syndrome; **Hospital:** St. Peter's Univ Hosp, Capital Health Regl Med Ctr; **Address:** Childrens Hosp at St Peters Univ Hosp, 254 Easton Ave, MOB 3110, New Brunswick, NJ 08901; **Phone:** 732-339-7841; **Board Cert:** Pediatrics 2005; Pediatric Infectious Disease 2009; **Med School:** Washington Univ, St Louis 1987; **Resid:** Pediatrics, Riley Childrens Hosp 1990; **Fellow:** Infectious Disease, Childrens Hosp/Barnes Jewish 1994; **Fac Appt:** Assoc Clin Prof Ped, Drexel Univ Coll Med

Whitley-Williams, Patricia N MD (PInf) - **Spec Exp:** AIDS/HIV; Lyme Disease; Neonatal Infections; Travel Medicine; **Hospital:** Robert Wood Johnson Univ Hosp - New Brunswick; **Address:** RWJ Div Pediatric Infectious Disease, 89 French St, New Brunswick, NJ 08903; **Phone:** 732-235-7894; **Board Cert:** Pediatrics 1980; Pediatric Infectious Disease 2005; **Med School:** Johns Hopkins Univ 1975; **Resid:** Pediatrics, Chldns Hosp Med Ctr 1978; **Fellow:** Pediatric Infectious Disease, Boston City Hosp 1980; **Fac Appt:** Prof Ped, UMDNJ-RW Johnson Med Sch

Pediatric Nephrology

Singh, Anup MD (PNep) - **Spec Exp:** Nephrotic Syndrome; Lupus/SLE; Hypertension in Children; Kidney Stones; **Hospital:** St. Peter's Univ Hosp, Staten Island Univ Hosp - South (page 106); **Address:** St Peter's Univ Hospital, 254 Easton Ave MOB-3, New Brunswick, NJ 08901; **Phone:** 732-565-5489; **Board Cert:** Pediatrics 2007; Pediatric Nephrology 2003; **Med School:** Philippines 1985; **Resid:** Pediatrics, SUNY-Downstate Med Ctr 1991; **Fellow:** Pediatric Nephrology, SUNY-Downstate Med Ctr 1994; **Fac Appt:** Assoc Prof Ped, Drexel Univ Coll Med

Weiss, Lynne MD (PNep) - **Spec Exp:** Hypertension; Kidney Disease; Kidney Failure-Chronic; **Hospital:** Robert Wood Johnson Univ Hosp - New Brunswick; **Address:** Robert Wood Johnson Univ Hosp, Pediatric Nephrology, 89 French St Fl 2, New Brunswick, NJ 08901; **Phone:** 732-235-7880; **Board Cert:** Pediatrics 1979; Pediatric Nephrology 1982; **Med School:** Hahnemann Univ 1974; **Resid:** Pediatrics, Michael Reese Hosp 1977; **Fellow:** Pediatric Nephrology, Michael Reese Hosp 1979; **Fac Appt:** Prof Ped, UMDNJ-RW Johnson Med Sch

Pediatric Otolaryngology

Traquina, Diana N MD (PO) - **Spec Exp:** Airway Disorders; Ear Disorders; Sinus Disorders; **Hospital:** Robert Wood Johnson Univ Hosp - New Brunswick; **Address:** University Otolaryngology Assocs, 181 Somerset St Fl 2, New Brunswick, NJ 08901; **Phone:** 732-247-2401; **Board Cert:** Otolaryngology 1989; **Med School:** Yale Univ 1984; **Resid:** Surgery, Yale-New Haven Hosp 1986; Otolaryngology, Yale-New Haven Hosp 1989; **Fellow:** Pediatric Otolaryngology, Montefiore-Weiler Enstein Hosp 1990; **Fac Appt:** Assoc Prof Ped, UMDNJ-RW Johnson Med Sch

Pediatric Surgery

Gallucci, John MD (PS) - **Hospital:** St. Peter's Univ Hosp; **Address:** St Peter's Univ Hosp, 254 Easton Ave, MOB4, New Brunswick, NJ 08901; **Phone:** 732-565-5482; **Board Cert:** Pediatric Surgery 2009; **Med School:** UMDNJ-RW Johnson Med Sch 1990; **Resid:** Surgery, Cooper Univ Hosp 1997; **Fellow:** Pediatric Surgery, McGill Univ Chldn's Hosp 2000

Pediatrics

Chefitz, Dalya L MD (Ped) - **Spec Exp:** Developmental Disorders; **Hospital:** Robert Wood Johnson Univ Hosp - New Brunswick; **Address:** RWJ Dept Pediatrics, 125 Patterson St, MEB 348, New Brunswick, NJ 08901; **Phone:** 732-235-7044; **Board Cert:** Pediatrics 2008; **Med School:** UMDNJ-RW Johnson Med Sch 1990; **Resid:** Pediatrics, RW Johnson Univ Hosp 1994; **Fac Appt:** Asst Clin Prof Ped, UMDNJ-RW Johnson Med Sch

McAbee, Gary N DO (Ped) - **Spec Exp:** Autism; Epilepsy; Headache; **Hospital:** JFK Med Ctr - Edison; **Address:** 65 James St, Edison, NJ 08818; **Phone:** 732-321-7010; **Board Cert:** Pediatrics 1988; Child Neurology 1988; **Med School:** Univ Osteo Med & Hlth Sci, Des Moines 1980; **Resid:** Pediatrics, NY Med Coll 1982; **Fellow:** Child Neurology, St Louis Chldns Hosp 1985; **Fac Appt:** Prof Ped, UMDNJ-RW Johnson Med Sch

Yalamanchi, Krishan MD (Ped) - **Spec Exp:** Neurodevelopmental Disabilities; Brain Injury; Pediatric Rehabilitation; **Hospital:** Children's Specialized Hosp, Robert Wood Johnson Univ Hosp - New Brunswick; **Address:** 200 Somerset St, New Brunswick, NJ 08901; **Phone:** 732-258-7065; **Board Cert:** Pediatrics 2011; Neurodevelopmental Disabilities 2004; **Med School:** India 1981; **Fac Appt:** Asst Clin Prof Ped, UMDNJ-RW Johnson Med Sch

Physical Medicine & Rehabilitation

Brown, David P DO (PMR) - **Spec Exp:** Sports Medicine; Electrodiagnosis; Electromyography; **Hospital:** JFK Med Ctr - Edison; **Address:** JFK Johnson Rehabilitation Inst, 65 James St, Edison, NJ 08820; **Phone:** 732-321-7070; **Board Cert:** Physical Medicine & Rehabilitation 1990; Sports Medicine 2007; **Med School:** Philadelphia Coll Osteo Med 1985; **Resid:** Physical Medicine & Rehabilitation, Walter Reed AMC 1989; **Fac Appt:** Assoc Clin Prof PMR, Seton Hall Univ Sch Hlth & Med Scis

Fantasia, Michele E MD (PMR) - **Spec Exp:** Pediatric Rehabilitation; Spinal Cord Injury-Pediatric; Cerebral Palsy; Neuromuscular Disorders; **Hospital:** Children's Specialized Hosp, Robert Wood Johnson Univ Hosp - New Brunswick; **Address:** Pediatric Phys Med & Rehab, 200 Somerset St, New Brunswick, NJ 08901; **Phone:** 732-258-7065; **Board Cert:** Pediatrics 2007; Physical Medicine & Rehabilitation 2010; Spinal Cord Injury Medicine 2002; Pediatric Rehabilitation Medicine 2004; **Med School:** UMDNJ-NJ Med Sch, Newark 1993; **Resid:** Pediatrics, Univ Hosp-UMDNJ 1996; Physical Medicine & Rehabilitation, Univ Hosp-UMDNJ 1999; **Fac Appt:** Asst Prof PMR, UMDNJ-NJ Med Sch, Newark

Plastic Surgery

Borah, Gregory L MD (PlS) - **Spec Exp:** Cosmetic Surgery-Face; Cosmetic Surgery-Breast; Hand Surgery; **Hospital:** Robert Wood Johnson Univ Hosp - New Brunswick, St. Peter's Univ Hosp; **Address:** RWJUH Div Plastic Surgery, 1 Robert Wood Johnson MEB 506, Box 19, New Brunswick, NJ 08901-1928; **Phone:** 732-235-7865; **Board Cert:** Plastic Surgery 2008; **Med School:** Harvard Med Sch 1978; **Resid:** Surgery, Mass Genl Hosp 1983; Plastic Surgery, Yale-New Haven Hosp 1985; **Fac Appt:** Prof PlS, UMDNJ-RW Johnson Med Sch

Cuber, Shain A MD (PlS) - **Spec Exp:** Cosmetic Surgery-Body; Breast Reconstruction; Cosmetic Surgery-Breast; Liposuction & Body Contouring; **Hospital:** JFK Med Ctr - Edison; **Address:** Assoc in Plastic Surgery, 1150 Amboy Ave, Edison, NJ 08837; **Phone:** 732-548-3200; **Board Cert:** Plastic Surgery 2002; **Med School:** NY Med Coll 1990; **Resid:** Surgery, Univ Texas Hlth Sci Ctr 1994; Plastic/Reconstructive Surgery, Univ Texas Hlth Sci Ctr 1997; **Fellow:** Hand & Microvascular Surgery, UMDNJ Med Ctr 1998

Herbstman, Robert A MD (PlS) - **Spec Exp:** Breast Cosmetic & Reconstructive Surgery; Liposuction & Body Contouring; Facial Rejuvenation; Minimally Invasive Surgery; **Hospital:** Robert Wood Johnson Univ Hosp - New Brunswick, Riverview Med Ctr; **Address:** 579A Cranbury Rd, Ste 202, East Brunswick, NJ 08816; **Phone:** 732-254-1919; **Board Cert:** Plastic Surgery 1992; **Med School:** Univ Rochester 1982; **Resid:** Surgery, RW Johnson Univ Hosp 1987; Plastic Surgery, Univ Hosp 1989; **Fac Appt:** Asst Clin Prof S, UMDNJ-RW Johnson Med Sch

Kaufman, Matthew R MD (PlS) - **Spec Exp:** Rhinoplasty; Rhinoplasty Revision; Cosmetic Surgery-Breast; Peripheral Nerve Surgery; **Hospital:** Somerset Med Ctr, Jersey Shore Univ Med Ctr; **Address:** 30 Rehill Ave, Ste 3400, Somerville, NJ 08876; **Phone:** 908-927-8993; **Board Cert:** Plastic Surgery 2007; Otolaryngology 2004; **Med School:** SUNY Upstate Med Univ 1998; **Resid:** Surgery, Mount Sinai Med Ctr 1999; Otolaryngology, Mount Sinai Med Ctr 2003; **Fellow:** Plastic Surgery, UCLA Med Ctr 2005; **Fac Appt:** Asst Clin Prof S, Drexel Univ Coll Med

Nini, Kevin T MD (PlS) - **Spec Exp:** Cosmetic Surgery-Face; Cosmetic Surgery-Breast; Liposuction & Body Contouring; **Hospital:** St. Peter's Univ Hosp, Robert Wood Johnson Univ Hosp - New Brunswick; **Address:** 78 Easton Ave Fl 2, New Brunswick, NJ 08901-5400; **Phone:** 732-418-0709; **Board Cert:** Plastic Surgery 1994; **Med School:** UMDNJ-RW Johnson Med Sch 1984; **Resid:** Surgery, Pennsylvania Hosp 1989; Plastic Surgery, Shands Hosp-Univ Fla 1991; **Fellow:** Plastic Surgery, Univ Miami Hosps 1992

Wey, Philip D MD (PlS) - **Spec Exp:** Cosmetic Surgery-Face; Breast Cosmetic & Reconstructive Surgery; Liposuction & Body Contouring; **Hospital:** Robert Wood Johnson Univ Hosp - New Brunswick, St. Peter's Univ Hosp; **Address:** 78 Easton Ave, Fl 2, New Brunswick, NJ 08901-1838; **Phone:** 732-418-0709; **Board Cert:** Plastic Surgery 2007; **Med School:** Brown Univ 1986; **Resid:** Surgery, Northwestern Meml Hosp 1990; Plastic Surgery, New York Hosp 1992; **Fellow:** Breast Surgery, NYU/Meml Sloan-Kettering Cancer Ctr 1993; **Fac Appt:** Assoc Clin Prof S, UMDNJ-RW Johnson Med Sch

Psychiatry

Jones Jr, Frank A MD (Psyc) - **Spec Exp:** Depression; Anxiety Disorders; Mood Disorders; **Address:** 2186 Route 27, Ste 2A, North Brunswick, NJ 08902; **Phone:** 732-422-0800; **Board Cert:** Psychiatry 1977; **Med School:** Case West Res Univ 1972; **Resid:** Psychiatry, Boston State Hosp 1973; Psychiatry, Worcester State Hosp 1975; **Fac Appt:** Clin Prof Psyc, UMDNJ-RW Johnson Med Sch

Menza, Matthew A MD (Psyc) - **Spec Exp:** Psychopharmacology; Depression; Anxiety Disorders; **Hospital:** Robert Wood Johnson Univ Hosp - New Brunswick; **Address:** 671 Hoes Ln, Fl 3, Piscataway, NJ 08854; **Phone:** 732-235-7647; **Board Cert:** Psychiatry 1985; **Med School:** Temple Univ 1980; **Resid:** Psychiatry, NYU -Bellevue Hosp 1984; **Fellow:** Psychiatry, Harvard Med Sch 1985; **Fac Appt:** Prof Psyc, UMDNJ-RW Johnson Med Sch

Pulmonary Disease

Goldberg, Jory MD (Pul) - **Spec Exp:** Lung Disease; Asthma; **Hospital:** Univ Med Ctr Princeton at Plainsboro; **Address:** 18 Centre Drive, Ste 103, Monroe Township, NJ 08831-1564; **Phone:** 609-655-1700; **Board Cert:** Internal Medicine 1981; Pulmonary Disease 1984; Critical Care Medicine 2007; **Med School:** Mexico 1976; **Resid:** Internal Medicine, City Hosp Ctr Elmhurst 1979; Internal Medicine, Monmouth Hosp 1980; **Fellow:** Pulmonary Disease, Bergen County Hosp 1982

Goldblatt, Kenneth H MD (Pul) - **Spec Exp:** Asthma; Emphysema; Sarcoidosis; **Hospital:** Univ Med Ctr Princeton at Plainsboro; **Address:** Princeton Healthcare Med Assoc, 5 Plainsboro Rd Fl 3, Plainsboro, NJ 08536; **Phone:** 609-853-7272; **Board Cert:** Internal Medicine 1975; Pulmonary Disease 1978; **Med School:** NY Med Coll 1972; **Resid:** Internal Medicine, CMDNJ-Rutgers Affil Hosp 1975; **Fellow:** Pulmonary Disease, CMDNJ-Rutgers 1977; **Fac Appt:** Assoc Prof Med, UMDNJ-RW Johnson Med Sch

Harangozo, Andrea M MD (Pul) - **Hospital:** Robert Wood Johnson Univ Hosp - New Brunswick, St. Peter's Univ Hosp; **Address:** Pulmonary/Intensive Care Specialists NJ, 593 Cranbury Rd, Ste 1-A, East Brunswick, NJ 08816-4029; **Phone:** 732-613-8880; **Board Cert:** Internal Medicine 1989; Pulmonary Disease 2005; Critical Care Medicine 2005; **Med School:** NYU Sch Med 1984; **Resid:** Internal Medicine, RW Johnson Univ Hosp 1987; **Fellow:** Pulmonary Critical Care Medicine, RW Johnson Univ Hosp 1990; **Fac Appt:** Asst Clin Prof Med, UMDNJ-RW Johnson Med Sch

Melillo, Nicholas MD (Pul) - **Spec Exp:** Chronic Obstructive Lung Disease (COPD); Lung Cancer; Asthma; Chronic Obstructive Lung Disease(COPD); **Hospital:** JFK Med Ctr - Edison; **Address:** 106 James St, Edison, NJ 08820-3945; **Phone:** 732-906-0091; **Board Cert:** Internal Medicine 1983; Pulmonary Disease 1986; Critical Care Medicine 2007; **Med School:** UMDNJ-NJ Med Sch, Newark 1979; **Resid:** Internal Medicine, St Michael's Med Ctr 1983; **Fellow:** Pulmonary Disease, St Michael's Med Ctr 1985; Critical Care Medicine, St Michael's Med Ctr 1986; **Fac Appt:** Assoc Clin Prof Med, Seton Hall Univ Sch Hlth & Med Scis

Riley, David J MD (Pul) - **Spec Exp:** Pulmonary Fibrosis; Interstitial Lung Disease; **Hospital:** Robert Wood Johnson Univ Hosp - New Brunswick; **Address:** RWJ Pulmonary/Critical Care, 125 Patterson St, Ste 5100, New Brunswick, NJ 08901; **Phone:** 732-235-7840; **Board Cert:** Internal Medicine 1980; Pulmonary Disease 1974; **Med School:** Univ MD Sch Med 1968; **Resid:** Internal Medicine, Baltimore City Hosps 1970; Internal Medicine, Johns Hopkins Hosp 1973; **Fellow:** Pulmonary Disease, Hosp Univ Penn 1972; **Fac Appt:** Prof Med, UMDNJ-RW Johnson Med Sch

Radiation Oncology

Baumann, John MD (RadRO) - **Spec Exp:** Breast Cancer; Cervical Cancer; Prostate Cancer; **Hospital:** Univ Med Ctr Princeton at Plainsboro, Hunterdon Med Ctr; **Address:** Edward & Marie Matthews Ctr for Cancer Care, One Plainsboro Rd, Plainsboro, NJ 08536; **Phone:** 609-497-4304; **Board Cert:** Radiation Oncology 1981; **Med School:** Harvard Med Sch 1977; **Resid:** Internal Medicine, Walter Reed AMC 1978; Radiation Oncology, Harvard Joint Program 1981; **Fellow:** Radiation Oncology, Harvard Joint Program

Haas, Alexander MD (RadRO) - **Spec Exp:** Breast Cancer; Prostate Cancer; **Hospital:** St. Peter's Univ Hosp, Robert Wood Johnson Univ Hosp - New Brunswick; **Address:** 254 Easton Ave, New Brunswick, NJ 08901; **Phone:** 732-745-8590; **Board Cert:** Radiation Oncology 1972; **Med School:** Croatia 1962; **Resid:** Diagnostic Radiology, Univ WA Med Ctr 1968; Radiation Oncology, Univ WA Med Ctr 1972; **Fellow:** Neoplastic Diseases, Thomas Jefferson Univ Hosp 1973; **Fac Appt:** Assoc Clin Prof, UMDNJ-RW Johnson Med Sch

Haffty, Bruce MD (RadRO) - **Spec Exp:** Breast Cancer; Head & Neck Cancer; **Hospital:** Robert Wood Johnson Univ Hosp - New Brunswick; **Address:** The Cancer Institute of New Jersey, 195 Little Albany St, rm 2038, New Brunswick, NJ 08903; **Phone:** 732-253-3939; **Board Cert:** Radiation Oncology 1988; **Med School:** Yale Univ 1984; **Resid:** Radiation Oncology, Yale-New Haven Hosp 1988; **Fac Appt:** Prof RadRO, UMDNJ-RW Johnson Med Sch

Macher, Mark MD (RadRO) - **Hospital:** JFK Med Ctr - Edison; **Address:** JFK Med Ctr, Mid-State Rad Oncology, 65 James St, Edison, NJ 08818; **Phone:** 732-321-7167; **Board Cert:** Radiation Oncology 1986; **Med School:** Howard Univ 1982; **Resid:** Diagnostic Radiology, New York Univ Med Ctr 1985; **Fellow:** Diagnostic Radiology, Univ Hosp 1986

Rheumatology

Lichtbroun, Alan S MD (Rhu) - **Spec Exp:** Rheumatoid Arthritis; Sjogren's Syndrome; Fibromyalgia; **Hospital:** Robert Wood Johnson Univ Hosp - New Brunswick, St. Peter's Univ Hosp; **Address:** 63 Brunswick Woods Dr, East Brunswick, NJ 08816-5601; **Phone:** 732-613-1900; **Board Cert:** Internal Medicine 1980; Rheumatology 1984; **Med School:** SUNY Downstate 1977; **Resid:** Internal Medicine, LI Jewish-Hillside Med Ctr 1980; **Fellow:** Rheumatology, Mt Sinai Hosp 1982; **Fac Appt:** Asst Clin Prof Med, UMDNJ-RW Johnson Med Sch

Surgery

August, David MD (S) - **Spec Exp:** Pancreatic Cancer; Esophageal Cancer; Stomach Cancer; Sarcoma-Soft Tissue; **Hospital:** Robert Wood Johnson Univ Hosp - New Brunswick; **Address:** CINJ-195 Little Albany St, New Brunswick, NJ 08903; **Phone:** 732-235-7701; **Board Cert:** Surgery 2005; **Med School:** Yale Univ 1980; **Resid:** Surgery, Yale-New Haven Hosp 1986; **Fellow:** Surgical Oncology, Natl Cancer Inst 1984; **Fac Appt:** Prof S, UMDNJ-RW Johnson Med Sch

Chung-Loy, Harold E MD (S) - **Spec Exp:** Laparoscopic Surgery; Breast Surgery; Vascular Surgery; **Hospital:** JFK Med Ctr - Edison, Robert Wood Johnson Univ Hosp at Rahway; **Address:** 98 James St, Ste 202, Edison, NJ 08820-3902; **Phone:** 732-548-1000; **Board Cert:** Surgery 2007; **Med School:** Howard Univ 1980; **Resid:** Surgery, Mount Sinai Hosp 1985; **Fellow:** Renal Transplant, Mount Sinai Hosp 1983

Dasmahapatra, Kumar MD (S) - **Spec Exp:** Cancer Surgery; Breast Surgery; Laparoscopic Surgery; Pancreatic Surgery; **Hospital:** Raritan Bay Med Ctr - Perth Amboy, JFK Med Ctr - Edison; **Address:** Comprehensive Surgical Assocs, 225 May St, Ste A, Edison, NJ 08837; **Phone:** 732-346-5400; **Board Cert:** Surgery 2009; **Med School:** India 1973; **Resid:** Surgery, Grace Hosp 1979; **Fellow:** Surgical Oncology, Roswell Park Meml Inst 1982; **Fac Appt:** Assoc Clin Prof S, UMDNJ-NJ Med Sch, Newark

Davidson, J Thomas MD (S) - **Spec Exp:** Vascular Surgery; **Hospital:** Univ Med Ctr Princeton at Plainsboro; **Address:** Princeton Surgical Assocs, 5 Plainsboro Rd, Ste 400, Plainsboro, NJ 08536; **Phone:** 609-921-7223; **Board Cert:** Surgery 1974; **Med School:** Cornell Univ-Weill Med Coll 1966; **Resid:** Surgery, NYU Hosp-Bellevue Hosp 1973; **Fellow:** Vascular Surgery, NYU Hosp-Bellevue Hosp 1974; **Fac Appt:** Assoc Clin Prof S, UMDNJ-RW Johnson Med Sch

Goydos, James S MD (S) - **Spec Exp:** Cancer Surgery; Melanoma; Skin Cancer; **Hospital:** Robert Wood Johnson Univ Hosp - New Brunswick, St. Peter's Univ Hosp; **Address:** Cancer Inst of NJ, 195 Little Albany St, rm 3000, New Brunswick, NJ 08901; **Phone:** 732-235-7563; **Board Cert:** Surgery 2006; **Med School:** UMDNJ-RW Johnson Med Sch 1988; **Resid:** Surgery, New Britain Gen Hosp 1993; **Fellow:** Surgical Oncology, Univ Pittsburgh 1995; **Fac Appt:** Assoc Prof S, UMDNJ-RW Johnson Med Sch

Jordan, Lawrence J MD (S) - **Spec Exp:** Laparoscopic Surgery; Biliary Surgery; Cancer Surgery; **Hospital:** Univ Med Ctr Princeton at Plainsboro; **Address:** Princeton Surgical Assocs, 5 Plainsboro Rd, Ste 400, Princeton, NJ 08536; **Phone:** 609-936-9100; **Board Cert:** Surgery 2009; **Med School:** Cornell Univ-Weill Med Coll 1983; **Resid:** Surgery, Columbia-Presby Med Ctr 1988

Kearney, Thomas J MD (S) - **Spec Exp:** Breast Cancer; **Hospital:** Robert Wood Johnson Univ Hosp - New Brunswick, St. Peter's Univ Hosp; **Address:** Cancer Institute New Jersey, 195 Little Albany St, Ste 3000, New Brunswick, NJ 08901; **Phone:** 732-235-8524; **Board Cert:** Surgery 2000; **Med School:** Georgetown Univ 1984; **Resid:** Surgery, Cedars Sinai Med Ctr 1992; **Fellow:** Surgical Oncology, Univ Chicago 1995; **Fac Appt:** Assoc Prof S, UMDNJ-RW Johnson Med Sch

Thoracic & Cardiac Surgery

Heim, John A MD (T&CS) - **Spec Exp:** Cardiothoracic Surgery; **Hospital:** Univ Med Ctr Princeton at Plainsboro; **Address:** Univ Med Ctr at Princeton, 5 Plainsboro Rd, Ste 260, Plainsboro, NJ 08536; **Phone:** 609-853-7200; **Board Cert:** Surgery 2002; Thoracic Surgery 2002; **Med School:** UMDNJ-RW Johnson Med Sch 1985; **Resid:** Surgery, Hartford Hosp 1991; **Fellow:** Thoracic Oncology, Meml Sloan Kettering Cancer Ctr 1992; Cardiothoracic Surgery, Rush Presby-St Lukes Med Ctr 1994; **Fac Appt:** Prof S

Lee, Leonard Y MD (T&CS) - **Spec Exp:** Coronary Artery Surgery; Minimally Invasive Cardiac Surgery; Heart Failure; Gene Therapy-Cardiac Angiogenesis; **Hospital:** Robert Wood Johnson Univ Hosp - New Brunswick; **Address:** UMDNJ-RWJMS, 1 Robert Wood Johnson Pl, MEB 508, Box 19, New Brunswick, NJ 08903; **Phone:** 732-235-8725; **Board Cert:** Surgery 2011; Thoracic & Cardiac Surgery 2002; **Med School:** UMDNJ-RW Johnson Med Sch 1992; **Resid:** Surgery, St Vincent's Hosp 1997; **Fellow:** Thoracic & Cardiac Surgery, NY-Presby/Weill Cornell Med Ctr 2001; **Fac Appt:** Assoc Prof T&CS, UMDNJ-RW Johnson Med Sch

Urology

Fleisher, Michael H MD (U) - **Spec Exp:** Pediatric Urology; **Hospital:** St. Peter's Univ Hosp, Jersey Shore Univ Med Ctr; **Address:** Pediatric Urology Assocs, 557 Cranbury Rd, Ste 4, East Brunswick, NJ 08816-5400; **Phone:** 732-613-9144; **Board Cert:** Urology 1984; Pediatric Urology 2009; **Med School:** SUNY Downstate 1977; **Resid:** Urology, SUNY Downstate Med Ctr 1982; **Fellow:** Transplant Medicine, Montefiore Hosp Med Ctr 1979; Pediatric Urology, Hosp Sick Chldn 1983; **Fac Appt:** Assoc Clin Prof U

Richards, Steven L MD (U) - **Spec Exp:** Kidney Stones; Erectile Dysfunction; **Hospital:** Robert Wood Johnson Univ Hosp - New Brunswick, St. Peter's Univ Hosp; **Address:** 333 Forestgate Drive, Ste 202, Jamesburg, NJ 08831-1567; **Phone:** 732-561-2058; **Board Cert:** Urology 2009; **Med School:** Albert Einstein Coll Med 1993; **Resid:** Surgery, Montefiore Med Ctr 1995; Urology, Montefiore Med Ctr 1999

Solomon, Michael J MD (U) - **Hospital:** St. Peter's Univ Hosp, Robert Wood Johnson Univ Hosp - New Brunswick; **Address:** 579A Cranbury Rd, Ste 104, East Brunswick, NJ 08816-4026; **Phone:** 732-390-8700; **Board Cert:** Urology 1981; **Med School:** Univ Pennsylvania 1973; **Resid:** Surgery, New England Med Ctr 1976; Urology, Lahey Clinic 1979; **Fellow:** Pediatric Urology, Mass Genl Hosp 1981; **Fac Appt:** Assoc Clin Prof U, UMDNJ-RW Johnson Med Sch

Vates III, Thomas S MD (U) - **Spec Exp:** Pediatric Urology; **Hospital:** Robert Wood Johnson Univ Hosp - New Brunswick, Monmouth Med Ctr; **Address:** Pediatric Urology Assocs, 557 Cranbury Rd, Ste 4, East Brunswick, NJ 08816; **Phone:** 732-613-9144; **Board Cert:** Urology 2009; Pediatric Urology 2009; **Med School:** Georgetown Univ 1989; **Resid:** Surgery, RW Johnson Univ Hosp 1991; Urology, RW Johnson Univ Hosp 1995; **Fellow:** Pediatric Urology, Chldns Hosp Michigan 1997

Weiss, Robert E MD (U) - **Spec Exp:** Bladder Cancer; Kidney Cancer; Testicular Cancer; Robotic Surgery; **Hospital:** Robert Wood Johnson Univ Hosp - New Brunswick, Univ Med Ctr Princeton at Plainsboro; **Address:** 1 Robert Wood Johnson Pl Ste MB588, Dept Urology, New Brunswick, NJ 08901-1928; **Phone:** 732-235-7960; **Board Cert:** Urology 2004; **Med School:** NYU Sch Med 1985; **Resid:** Surgery, Mount Sinai Med Ctr 1987; Urology, Mount Sinai Med Ctr 1991; **Fellow:** Urologic Oncology, Meml Sloan Kettering Cancer Ctr 1994; **Fac Appt:** Assoc Prof U, UMDNJ-RW Johnson Med Sch

Vascular & Interventional Radiology

Denny, Donald F MD (VIR) - **Spec Exp:** Dialysis Access; Uterine Fibroids; **Hospital:** Univ Med Ctr Princeton at Plainsboro; **Address:** Princeton Radiology Assocs, 1 Plainsboro Rd, Plainsboro, NJ 08536; **Phone:** 609-497-4310; **Board Cert:** Diagnostic Radiology 1982; Vascular & Interventional Radiology 2005; **Med School:** Hahnemann Univ 1978; **Resid:** Diagnostic Radiology, Yale-New Haven Hosp 1982; **Fellow:** Diagnostic Radiology, Brigham & Womens Hosp 1983; **Fac Appt:** Assoc Clin Prof Rad, Yale Univ

Nosher, John L MD (VIR) - **Spec Exp:** Endovascular Surgery; Uterine Fibroid Embolization; Interventional Oncology; Liver Cancer; **Hospital:** Robert Wood Johnson Univ Hosp - New Brunswick; **Address:** UMDNJ-RW Johnson Med Sch, Dept Radiology, MEB 404, Box 19, New Brunswick, NJ 08903-0019; **Phone:** 732-390-0040; **Board Cert:** Diagnostic Radiology 1975; Vascular & Interventional Radiology 2005; **Med School:** Jefferson Med Coll 1970; **Resid:** Diagnostic Radiology, Columbia Presby Med Ctr 1975; **Fac Appt:** Clin Prof Rad, UMDNJ-RW Johnson Med Sch

Siegel, Randall L MD (VIR) - **Spec Exp:** Endovascular Surgery; Dialysis Access; Pediatric Interventional Radiology; **Hospital:** Robert Wood Johnson Univ Hosp - New Brunswick; **Address:** University Radiology Group, 579A Cranbury Rd, East Brunswick, NJ 08816-5426; **Phone:** 732-390-0040; **Board Cert:** Diagnostic Radiology 1991; Vascular & Interventional Radiology 2005; **Med School:** Univ Pennsylvania 1986; **Resid:** Diagnostic Radiology, RWJ Univ Hosp 1991; **Fellow:** Vascular & Interventional Radiology, RWJ Univ Hosp 1992; **Fac Appt:** Asst Clin Prof Rad, UMDNJ-RW Johnson Med Sch

Vascular Surgery

Goldman, Kenneth A MD (VascS) - **Spec Exp:** Carotid Artery Surgery; Aneurysm-Aortic; Varicose Veins; Endovascular Surgery; **Hospital:** Univ Med Ctr Princeton at Plainsboro; **Address:** Princeton Surgical Assocs, 5 Plainsboro Rd, Ste 400, Princeton, NJ 08536; **Phone:** 609-921-7223; **Board Cert:** Surgery 2003; Vascular Surgery 2004; **Med School:** NYU Sch Med 1988; **Resid:** Surgery, Bellevue Hosp 1993; **Fellow:** Vascular Surgery, NYU Med Ctr 1994

Graham, Alan M MD (VascS) - **Spec Exp:** Endovascular Surgery; Aneurysm-Abdominal & Thoracic Aortic; Carotid Artery Surgery; Peripheral Vascular Disease; **Hospital:** Robert Wood Johnson Univ Hosp - New Brunswick; **Address:** RWJ Vascular Surgery, 125 Paterson St, New Brunswick, NJ 08901; **Phone:** 732-235-8770; **Board Cert:** Vascular Surgery 2006; **Med School:** Canada 1979; **Resid:** Surgery, McGill Univ Med Ctr 1984; **Fellow:** Vascular Surgery, Univ Chicago Hosps 1985; **Fac Appt:** Prof S, UMDNJ-RW Johnson Med Sch

Monmouth

Monmouth

Allergy & Immunology

Gross, Gary L MD (A&I) - **Spec Exp:** Asthma; Cough-Chronic; Sinus Disorders; Atopic Dermatitis; **Hospital:** Jersey Shore Univ Med Ctr, Monmouth Med Ctr; **Address:** 802 W Park Ave, Ste 213, Ocean Township, NJ 07712-4556; **Phone:** 732-695-2555; **Board Cert:** Allergy & Immunology 1987; Pediatrics 1986; **Med School:** NYU Sch Med 1981; **Resid:** Pediatrics, Chldns Hosp 1984; **Fellow:** Allergy & Immunology, Chldns Hosp 1986; **Fac Appt:** Assoc Clin Prof Ped, UMDNJ-RW Johnson Med Sch

Hirsch, Andrew C MD (A&I) - **Spec Exp:** Asthma; Sinusitis; Allergic Rhinitis; Eczema; **Hospital:** Riverview Med Ctr, Monmouth Med Ctr; **Address:** 258 Broad Steet, Red Bank, NJ 07701-5623; **Phone:** 732-741-8900; **Board Cert:** Allergy & Immunology 2005; **Med School:** Temple Univ 1988; **Resid:** Pediatrics, New York Hosp 1991; **Fellow:** Allergy & Immunology, Thomas Jefferson Univ Hosp 1993

Picone, Frank J MD (A&I) - **Spec Exp:** Asthma; Sinus Disorders; Allergy; **Hospital:** Riverview Med Ctr, Monmouth Med Ctr; **Address:** 709 Sycamore Ave, Tinton Falls, NJ 07701; **Phone:** 732-747-8188; **Board Cert:** Pediatrics 1973; Allergy & Immunology 1975; **Med School:** UMDNJ-NJ Med Sch, Newark 1967; **Resid:** Pediatrics, Jackson Meml Hosp 1970; **Fellow:** Allergy & Immunology, Chldns Hosp Med Ctr 1974; **Fac Appt:** Asst Clin Prof Ped, Drexel Univ Coll Med

Sher, Ellen R MD (A&I) - **Spec Exp:** Asthma & Sinusitis; Nasal Allergies; Insect Allergies; Immune Deficiency; **Hospital:** Monmouth Med Ctr, Jersey Shore Univ Med Ctr; **Address:** Atlantic Allergy, Asthma & Immunology, 802 W Park Ave, Ste 213, Ocean Township, NJ 07712; **Phone:** 732-695-2555; **Board Cert:** Internal Medicine 1989; Allergy & Immunology 2003; **Med School:** Georgetown Univ 1986; **Resid:** Internal Medicine, Thomas Jefferson Univ Hosp 1989; **Fellow:** Pulmonary Disease, Thomas Jefferson Univ Hosp 1990; Allergy & Immunology, Natl Jewish Ctr Resp Dis 1992; **Fac Appt:** Asst Clin Prof Med, Drexel Univ Coll Med

Cardiovascular Disease

Beauregard, Lou-Anne M MD (Cv) - **Spec Exp:** Arrhythmias; Heart Disease in Women; Pacemakers; **Hospital:** CentraState Med Ctr; **Address:** Heart Specialists of Central Jersey, 901 W Main St, Ste 205, Freehold, NJ 07728; **Phone:** 732-866-0800; **Board Cert:** Internal Medicine 1983; Cardiovascular Disease 1985; Cardiac Electrophysiology 2002; Nuclear Cardiology 2005; **Med School:** Med Coll PA 1980; **Resid:** Internal Medicine, Temple Univ Hosp 1983; **Fellow:** Cardiovascular Disease, Med Coll Penn 1985; Cardiac Electrophysiology, Cooper Hosp 1986; **Fac Appt:** Assoc Clin Prof Med

Daniels, Jeffrey S MD (Cv) - **Hospital:** Monmouth Med Ctr, Jersey Shore Univ Med Ctr; **Address:** 215 Brighton Ave, Long Branch, NJ 07740; **Phone:** 732-222-5143; **Board Cert:** Internal Medicine 1983; Cardiovascular Disease 1985; **Med School:** Albany Med Coll 1980; **Resid:** Internal Medicine, Mt Sinai Hosp 1983; **Fellow:** Cardiovascular Disease, Mt Sinai Hosp 1985; **Fac Appt:** Asst Clin Prof Med, Drexel Univ Coll Med

Child Neurology

Barabas, Ronald MD (ChiN) - **Spec Exp:** Pediatric Neurology; Developmental Disorders; Neurogenetics; Metabolic Disorders; **Hospital:** Monmouth Med Ctr; **Address:** Child Neurology Associates, 3350 Highway 138W, Ste 117, Wall, NJ 07719; **Phone:** 732-556-0200; **Board Cert:** Child Neurology 2007; Clinical Genetics 2010; Neurodevelopmental Disabilities 2007; **Med School:** UMDNJ-Rutgers Med Sch 1986; **Resid:** Pediatrics, Buffalo Chldns Hosp 1988; **Fellow:** Pediatric Neurology, Chldns Hosp of Pittsburgh 1991; Pediatric Metabolism, Chldns Hosp of Philadelphia 1993; **Fac Appt:** Asst Clin Prof Ped, Drexel Univ Coll Med

Colon & Rectal Surgery

Arvanitis, Michael L MD (CRS) - **Spec Exp:** Laparoscopic Surgery; Colon & Rectal Cancer; Ulcerative Colitis; **Hospital:** Monmouth Med Ctr, Riverview Med Ctr; **Address:** Specialty Surgical Assoc, 10 Industrial Way E, Ste 104, Eatontown, NJ 07724; **Phone:** 732-389-1331; **Board Cert:** Sports Medicine 2008; Colon & Rectal Surgery 2008; **Med School:** Hahnemann Univ 1982; **Resid:** Surgery, St Vincent's Hosp 1987; **Fellow:** Colon & Rectal Surgery, Cleveland Clinic 1988; **Fac Appt:** Assoc Prof S, Hahnemann Univ

Ross, Howard M MD (CRS) - **Spec Exp:** Laparoscopic Surgery; Colon & Rectal Cancer; Inflammatory Bowel Disease; **Hospital:** Riverview Med Ctr; **Address:** Riverview Surgical Assocs, 241 Monmouth Rd, West Longbranch, NJ 07764; **Phone:** 732-403-2075; **Board Cert:** Surgery 2009; Colon & Rectal Surgery 2010; **Med School:** Univ Rochester 1992; **Resid:** Surgery, Univ Conn Hlth Ctr 1994; **Fellow:** Colon & Rectal Surgery, Meml Sloan Kettering Cancer Ctr 1996; Colon & Rectal Surgery, Lahey Clinic 2000; **Fac Appt:** Asst Prof S, Univ Pennsylvania

Dermatology

Grossman, Kenneth A MD (D) - **Spec Exp:** Psoriasis; Skin Cancer; Cutaneous Lymphoma; Cosmetic Dermatology; **Hospital:** Riverview Med Ctr; **Address:** 180 White Rd, Ste 103, Little Silver, NJ 07739-1166; **Phone:** 732-842-5222; **Board Cert:** Internal Medicine 1980; Dermatology 1983; **Med School:** SUNY Hlth Sci Ctr 1977; **Resid:** Internal Medicine, Nassau County Med Ctr 1980; Dermatology, Montefiore Med Ctr 1983

Hametz, Irwin MD (D) - **Hospital:** CentraState Med Ctr; **Address:** 77-55 Schanck Rd, Ste B-3, Freehold, NJ 07728; **Phone:** 732-462-9800; **Board Cert:** Dermatology 1978; **Med School:** NY Med Coll 1973; **Resid:** Pediatrics, Long Island Jewish-Hillside Med Ctr 1975; Dermatology, Brown Univ Affil Hosps 1978; **Fac Appt:** Asst Clin Prof Med, UMDNJ-RW Johnson Med Sch

Orsini, William J MD (D) - **Hospital:** Monmouth Med Ctr; **Address:** 223 Monmouth Rd, W Long Branch, NJ 07764; **Phone:** 732-870-2992; **Board Cert:** Internal Medicine 1975; Dermatology 1977; **Med School:** UMDNJ-NJ Med Sch, Newark 1972; **Resid:** Internal Medicine, Monmouth Med Ctr 1975; Dermatology, Albany Med Ctr 1977

Diagnostic Radiology

Chalal, Jeffrey MD (DR) - **Hospital:** CentraState Med Ctr; **Address:** Freehold Radiology Grp, 901 W Main St, Ground Fl, Freehold, NJ 07728; **Phone:** 732-462-4844; **Board Cert:** Diagnostic Radiology 1982; **Med School:** Univ Pennsylvania 1977; **Resid:** Diagnostic Radiology, Columbia-Presby Med Ctr 1981; **Fellow:** Cross Sectional Imaging, Columbia-Presby Med Ctr 1982

Endocrinology, Diabetes & Metabolism

Nassberg, Barton MD (EDM) - **Spec Exp:** Thyroid Disorders; Diabetes; **Hospital:** Bayshore Community Hosp; **Address:** 723 N Beers St, Ste 2G, Holmdel, NJ 07733-1512; **Phone:** 732-739-0200; **Board Cert:** Internal Medicine 1982; Endocrinology, Diabetes & Metabolism 1985; **Med School:** Belgium 1979; **Resid:** Internal Medicine, Mountainside Hosp 1982; **Fellow:** Endocrinology, Diabetes & Metabolism, MS Hershey Med Ctr 1984

Family Medicine

Bernardo, Salvatore MD (FMed) *PCP* - **Hospital:** CentraState Med Ctr; **Address:** 4255 Rte 9 N, Ste B, Freehold, NJ 07728; **Phone:** 732-683-9897; **Board Cert:** Family Medicine 2009; **Med School:** UMDNJ-NJ Med Sch, Newark 1993; **Resid:** Family Medicine, Somerset Med Ctr 1996

Catanese, Vincent J MD (FMed) *PCP* - **Spec Exp:** Hypertension; Diabetes; Functional Bowel Disorders; **Address:** 733 N Beers St, Ste U3, Holmdel, NJ 07733; **Phone:** 732-264-8484; **Board Cert:** Family Medicine 2005; **Med School:** Penn State Coll Med 1978; **Resid:** Family Medicine, Conemaugh Valley Meml Hosp 1981

Gastroenterology

Binns, Joseph MD (Ge) - **Spec Exp:** Colonoscopy; **Hospital:** Riverview Med Ctr; **Address:** Red Bank Gastroenterology Assocs, 365 Broad St, Ste 1-E, Red Bank, NJ 07701; **Phone:** 732-842-4294; **Board Cert:** Gastroenterology 2003; **Med School:** UMDNJ-RW Johnson Med Sch 1987; **Resid:** Internal Medicine, Pennsylvania Hosp 1990; **Fellow:** Gastroenterology, Graduate Hosp 1992

Fiest, Thomas DO (Ge) - **Spec Exp:** Colitis; Liver Disease; **Hospital:** Monmouth Med Ctr, Jersey Shore Univ Med Ctr; **Address:** Monmouth Gastroenterology, 142 Highway 35, Ste 103, Eatontown, NJ 07724; **Phone:** 732-389-5004; **Board Cert:** Internal Medicine 1989; Gastroenterology 2005; **Med School:** Philadelphia Coll Osteo Med 1985; **Resid:** Internal Medicine, Monmouth Med Ctr 1990; **Fellow:** Gastroenterology, Jersey City Med Ctr 1993

Ludwig, Shelly L MD (Ge) - **Spec Exp:** Inflammatory Bowel Disease; Hepatitis C; Gastroesophageal Reflux Disease (GERD); Endoscopy; **Hospital:** CentraState Med Ctr; **Address:** 535 Iron Bridge Rd, Ste 12, Freehold, NJ 07728; **Phone:** 732-780-4224; **Board Cert:** Internal Medicine 1977; Gastroenterology 1979; **Med School:** Albert Einstein Coll Med 1974; **Resid:** Internal Medicine, LAC-Harbor UCLA Med Ctr 1977; **Fellow:** Gastroenterology, Wadsworth VA Hosp/UCLA 1979; **Fac Appt:** Assoc Clin Prof Med, UMDNJ-RW Johnson Med Sch

Turtel, Penny S MD (Ge) - **Spec Exp:** Inflammatory Bowel Disease; Celiac Disease; Colon Polyps & Cancer; **Hospital:** Monmouth Med Ctr, Jersey Shore Univ Med Ctr; **Address:** Shore Gastroenterology, 1907 Route 35, Ste 1, Oakhurst, NJ 07755-2760; **Phone:** 732-517-0060; **Board Cert:** Internal Medicine 1989; Gastroenterology 2011; **Med School:** Cornell Univ-Weill Med Coll 1986; **Resid:** Internal Medicine, Mount Sinai Hosp 1989; **Fellow:** Gastroenterology, Mount Sinai Hosp 1991

Geriatric Medicine

Israel, Jessica L MD (Ger) - **Spec Exp:** Palliative Care; **Hospital:** Monmouth Med Ctr; **Address:** Monmouth Med Ctr, Dept Geriatrics, 300 Second Ave, Long Branch, NJ 07740; **Phone:** 732-923-7550; **Board Cert:** Geriatric Medicine 2006; **Med School:** Mount Sinai Sch Med 1995; **Resid:** Internal Medicine, Mt Sinai Med Ctr 1998; **Fellow:** Geriatric Medicine, Mt Sinai Med Ctr 2000

Hand Surgery

Lisser, Steven P MD (HS) - **Spec Exp:** Shoulder Surgery; Wrist/Hand Injuries; Ligament Reconstruction; Sports Medicine; **Hospital:** Riverview Med Ctr, Monmouth Med Ctr; **Address:** Orthopaedic, Sports Med & Rehab Ctr, 80 Oak Hill Rd, Red Bank, NJ 07701; **Phone:** 732-741-2313; **Board Cert:** Orthopaedic Surgery 2007; Hand Surgery 2007; Orthopaedic Sports Medicine 2007; **Med School:** Mount Sinai Sch Med 1987; **Resid:** Orthopaedic Surgery, Mt Sinai Med Ctr 1992; **Fellow:** Hand & Microvascular Surgery, Thom Jefferson Univ 1993; Sports Medicine & Shoulder Surgery, Univ Pennsylvania 1994

Hematology

Lerner, William A MD (Hem) - **Spec Exp:** Palliative Care; **Hospital:** Jersey Shore Univ Med Ctr, Ocean Med Ctr; **Address:** 1707 Atlantic Ave, Manasquan, NJ 08736-1147; **Phone:** 732-528-0760; **Board Cert:** Internal Medicine 1980; Hematology 1982; Medical Oncology 1983; Hospice & Palliative Medicine 2008; **Med School:** Belgium 1977; **Resid:** Internal Medicine, Albert Einstein Med Ctr 1980; **Fellow:** Hematology & Oncology, NYU Med Ctr 1983

Topilow, Arthur A MD (Hem) - **Spec Exp:** Lymphoma; Multiple Myeloma; **Hospital:** Jersey Shore Univ Med Ctr, Ocean Med Ctr; **Address:** 1707 Atlantic Ave, Manasquan, NJ 08736-1147; **Phone:** 732-528-0760; **Board Cert:** Internal Medicine 1971; Hematology 1972; Medical Oncology 1981; **Med School:** NY Med Coll 1967; **Resid:** Internal Medicine, Flower/NY Metro Hosp 1970; **Fellow:** Hematology, Flower/NY Metro Hosp 1972; **Fac Appt:** Assoc Clin Prof Med, UMDNJ-NJ Med Sch, Newark

Infectious Disease

Eng, Margaret H MD (Inf) - **Spec Exp:** AIDS/HIV; **Hospital:** Monmouth Med Ctr; **Address:** Monmouth Family Hlth Ctr, 270 Broadway, Long Branch, NJ 07740; **Phone:** 732-923-7139; **Board Cert:** Internal Medicine 1983; Infectious Disease 2010; **Med School:** Albert Einstein Coll Med 1980; **Resid:** Internal Medicine, Kings Co Hosp 1984; **Fellow:** Infectious Disease, Univ Maryland Med Ctr 1986

Internal Medicine

Courtney, Barbara E MD (IM) *PCP* - **Spec Exp:** Geriatric Medicine; **Hospital:** Monmouth Med Ctr; **Address:** Monmouth Med Grp, 370 Highway 35, Red Bank, NJ 07701; **Phone:** 732-842-0290; **Board Cert:** Internal Medicine 1980; Geriatric Medicine 2002; **Med School:** Hahnemann Univ 1977; **Resid:** Internal Medicine, Monmouth Med Ctr 1980; **Fac Appt:** Med

Glowacki, Jan S MD (IM) *PCP* - **Spec Exp:** Preventive Medicine; Diagnostic Problems; **Hospital:** Riverview Med Ctr, Monmouth Med Ctr; **Address:** Fair Haven Internal Medicine, 569 River Rd, Fair Haven, NJ 07704-3262; **Phone:** 732-530-0100; **Board Cert:** Internal Medicine 1980; **Med School:** Jefferson Med Coll 1977; **Resid:** Internal Medicine, Monmouth Med Ctr 1980

Granet, Kenneth M MD (IM) *PCP* - **Hospital:** Monmouth Med Ctr; **Address:** 166 Morris Ave, Long Branch, NJ 07740; **Phone:** 732-229-2020; **Board Cert:** Internal Medicine 1987; **Med School:** SUNY Downstate 1984; **Resid:** Internal Medicine, N Shore Univ Hosp 1987; **Fac Appt:** Asst Clin Prof Med, Drexel Univ Coll Med

Masterson, Raymond M MD (IM) *PCP* - **Spec Exp:** Hypertension; Diabetes; Cholesterol/Lipid Disorders; Peripheral Vascular Disease; **Hospital:** Jersey Shore Univ Med Ctr; **Address:** 700 Highway 71, Ste 9, Sea Girt, NJ 08750-2804; **Phone:** 732-974-0340; **Board Cert:** Internal Medicine 1986; **Med School:** Philippines 1978; **Resid:** Internal Medicine, St Michaels Med Ctr 1982

Maternal & Fetal Medicine

Gonzalez, David MD (MF) - **Spec Exp:** Pregnancy-High Risk; **Hospital:** Monmouth Med Ctr; **Address:** Monmouth Med Group, 73 S Bath Ave, Long Branch, NJ 07740; **Phone:** 732-870-3600; **Board Cert:** Obstetrics & Gynecology 2011; Maternal & Fetal Medicine 2011; **Med School:** Temple Univ 1990; **Resid:** Obstetrics & Gynecology, Univ Hosp-UMDNJ 1994; **Fellow:** Maternal & Fetal Medicine, Univ Hosp-UMDNJ 1996

Medical Oncology

Fitzgerald, Denis B MD (Onc) - **Spec Exp:** Breast Cancer; Lung Cancer; Colon Cancer; Lymphoma, Non-Hodgkin's; **Hospital:** Riverview Med Ctr; **Address:** 180 White Rd, Ste 101, Little Silver, NJ 07739; **Phone:** 732-530-8666; **Board Cert:** Internal Medicine 1981; Medical Oncology 1985; Hematology 1986; **Med School:** SUNY Downstate 1978; **Resid:** Internal Medicine, St Vincents Hosp Med Ctr 1982; **Fellow:** Hematology & Oncology, Univ Rochester 1985

Greenberg, Susan N MD (Onc) - **Spec Exp:** Breast Cancer; Lung Cancer; Palliative Care; **Hospital:** Jersey Shore Univ Med Ctr, Monmouth Med Ctr; **Address:** 39 Sycamore Ave, Little Silver, NJ 07739-1208; **Phone:** 732-576-8610; **Board Cert:** Internal Medicine 1981; Medical Oncology 1983; **Med School:** Med Coll PA Hahnemann 1978; **Resid:** Internal Medicine, Hosp Med Coll Penn 1981; **Fellow:** Hematology & Oncology, Columbia-Presby Med Ctr 1983

Sharon, David J MD (Onc) - **Spec Exp:** Breast Cancer; Lung Cancer; Gastrointestinal Cancer; Hematologic Malignancies; **Hospital:** Monmouth Med Ctr, CentraState Med Ctr; **Address:** The Cancer Ctr - Monmouth Med Ctr, 100 State Highway 36, Ste 1B, West Long Branch, NJ 07764-6205; **Phone:** 732-222-1711; **Board Cert:** Internal Medicine 1980; Medical Oncology 1983; **Med School:** NY Med Coll 1977; **Resid:** Internal Medicine, Beth Israel Med Ctr 1980; **Fellow:** Medical Oncology, Mount Sinai Med Ctr 1982

Walsh, Christina M MD (Onc) - **Spec Exp:** Cancer Genetics; Breast Cancer; **Hospital:** Riverview Med Ctr; **Address:** 180 White Rd, Ste 101, Little Silver, NJ 07739; **Phone:** 732-530-8666; **Board Cert:** Internal Medicine 1980; Hematology 1982; Medical Oncology 1985; **Med School:** Georgetown Univ 1977; **Resid:** Internal Medicine, Georgetown Univ Hosp 1980; **Fellow:** Hematology, Georgetown Univ Hosp 1981; Hematology & Oncology, NYU Med Ctr 1984

Neonatal-Perinatal Medicine

Graff, Michael MD (NP) - **Spec Exp:** Neonatology; **Hospital:** Jersey Shore Univ Med Ctr, Ocean Med Ctr; **Address:** Jersey Shore Univ Med Ctr, Dept Peds, 1945 State Rte 33, Neptune, NJ 07754; **Phone:** 732-776-4283; **Board Cert:** Pediatrics 1981; Neonatal-Perinatal Medicine 1983; **Med School:** Italy 1977; **Resid:** Pediatrics, NYU Med Ctr 1980; **Fellow:** Neonatology, Columbia-Presby Med Ctr 1982; **Fac Appt:** Assoc Clin Prof Ped, UMDNJ-RW Johnson Med Sch

Nephrology

Flis, Raymond S DO (Nep) - **Spec Exp:** Hypertension; Kidney Disease; **Hospital:** Riverview Med Ctr, Monmouth Med Ctr; **Address:** Hypertension & Nephrology Assocs, 6 Industrial Way W, Ste B, Eatontown, NJ 07724-2268; **Phone:** 732-460-1200; **Board Cert:** Internal Medicine 1974; Nephrology 1976; **Med School:** Kirksville Coll Osteo Med 1971; **Resid:** Internal Medicine, Cooper Hosp 1974; **Fellow:** Nephrology, Thomas Jefferson Univ Hosp 1975; Nephrology, Temple Univ Hosp 1976; **Fac Appt:** Assoc Clin Prof Med, Drexel Univ Coll Med

Manning, Eric C MD/PhD (Nep) - **Spec Exp:** Hypertension; Kidney Disease; Dialysis Care; **Hospital:** Robert Wood Johnson Univ Hosp - New Brunswick, Somerset Med Ctr; **Address:** 719 Route 206, Ste 100, Hillsborough, NJ 08844; **Phone:** 908-904-9055; **Board Cert:** Internal Medicine 1989; Nephrology 2002; **Med School:** UC Davis 1985; **Resid:** Internal Medicine, Boston Univ Hosp 1988; **Fellow:** Nephrology, Boston Univ Hosp 1992

Neurological Surgery

Rosenblum, Bruce R MD (NS) - **Spec Exp:** Spinal Surgery; Brain Tumors; Pain-Back & Neck; Chiari's Deformity; **Hospital:** Riverview Med Ctr, Bayshore Community Hosp; **Address:** 160 Ave at the Commons, Ste 2, Shrewsbury, NJ 07702; **Phone:** 732-460-1522; **Board Cert:** Neurological Surgery 1991; **Med School:** Mount Sinai Sch Med 1982; **Resid:** Neurological Surgery, Mount Sinai Med Ctr 1988; **Fellow:** Stroke, Natl Inst Health 1986

Neurology

Gainey, Patrick J MD (N) - **Hospital:** Robert Wood Johnson Univ Hosp - New Brunswick; **Address:** 23 Kilmer Drive Bldg 1 - Ste E, Morganville, NJ 07751; **Phone:** 732-617-0808; **Board Cert:** Neurology 1993; **Med School:** UMDNJ-RW Johnson Med Sch 1988; **Resid:** Neurology, UMDNJ Med Ctr 1990; **Fellow:** Neurology, UMDNJ Med Ctr 1993

Gilson, Noah R MD (N) - **Spec Exp:** Multiple Sclerosis; Headache; Parkinson's Disease; **Hospital:** Monmouth Med Ctr, Riverview Med Ctr; **Address:** Neurology Specialists of Monmouth County, 107 Monmouth Rd, Ste 110, West Long Branch, NJ 07764; **Phone:** 732-935-1850; **Board Cert:** Neurology 1987; Vascular Neurology 2009; **Med School:** Loyola Univ-Stritch Sch Med 1982; **Resid:** Neurology, Mount Sinai Hosp 1986

Herman, Martin MD (N) - **Spec Exp:** Epilepsy; Stroke; **Hospital:** Monmouth Med Ctr, Riverview Med Ctr; **Address:** Neurology Specialists of Monmouth County, 107 Monmouth Rd, Ste 110, West Long Branch, NJ 07764-1000; **Phone:** 732-935-1850; **Board Cert:** Neurology 1973; **Med School:** Northwestern Univ 1964; **Resid:** Psychiatry, Strong Meml Hosp 1965; Neurology, Univ VA Hlth Sci Ctr 1970; **Fellow:** Clinical Neurophysiology, Columbia-Presby Hosp 1971; **Fac Appt:** Assoc Clin Prof N, Drexel Univ Coll Med

Holland, Neil R MD (N) - **Spec Exp:** Neuromuscular Disorders; Peripheral Neuropathy; Electrodiagnosis; Migraine; **Hospital:** Monmouth Med Ctr, Riverview Med Ctr; **Address:** 107 Monmouth Rd, Ste 110, West Long Branch, NJ 07764; **Phone:** 732-935-1850; **Board Cert:** Neurology 2010; Clinical Neurophysiology 2011; Vascular Neurology 2009; Neuromuscular Medicine 2008; **Med School:** England, UK 1991; **Resid:** Neurology, Johns Hopkins Univ Hosp 1996; **Fellow:** Clinical Neurophysiology, Johns Hopkins Univ Hosp 1997; **Fac Appt:** Assoc Prof N, Drexel Univ Coll Med

Silbert, Paul J MD (N) - **Spec Exp:** Parkinson's Disease; Migraine; Carpal Tunnel Syndrome; **Hospital:** Jersey Shore Univ Med Ctr; **Address:** 2100 Corlies Ave, Ste 5, Neptune, NJ 07753-6116; **Phone:** 732-776-8866; **Board Cert:** Neurology 1980; **Med School:** Jefferson Med Coll 1971; **Resid:** Neurology, Columbia-Presby Med Ctr 1975; **Fac Appt:** Asst Clin Prof N

Neuroradiology

Lu, Stanley MD (NRad) - **Hospital:** Monmouth Med Ctr; **Address:** Monmouth Med Ctr-Neuroradiology, 300 Second Ave, Long Branch, NJ 07740; **Phone:** 732-923-6806; **Board Cert:** Diagnostic Radiology 2004; Neuroradiology 2006; **Med School:** NYU Sch Med 1999; **Resid:** Dermatopathology, NYU Med Ctr 2004; **Fellow:** Neurological Radiology, Stanford Univ Med Ctr 2005

Obstetrics & Gynecology

Goldstein, Steven A MD (ObG) - **Spec Exp:** Ultrasound; Menopause Problems; Laparoscopic Hysterectomy; Minimally Invasive Surgery; **Hospital:** CentraState Med Ctr, Monmouth Med Ctr; **Address:** 501 Iron Bridge Rd, Ste 4, Freehold, NJ 07728; **Phone:** 732-431-1807; **Board Cert:** Obstetrics & Gynecology 2011; **Med School:** SUNY Downstate 1985; **Resid:** Obstetrics & Gynecology, RW Johnson Univ Hosp 1989

Martens, Mark G MD (ObG) - **Spec Exp:** Infections in Pregnancy; Vulvar & Vaginal Disorders; Menopause Problems; Viral Infections; **Hospital:** Jersey Shore Univ Med Ctr; **Address:** Jersey Shore Univ Med Ctr, Dept Ob/Gyn, 1945 Rte 33, Neptune, NJ 07753; **Phone:** 732-776-3790; **Board Cert:** Obstetrics & Gynecology 2011; **Med School:** Geo Wash Univ 1982; **Resid:** Obstetrics & Gynecology, Hartford Hosp 1986; **Fellow:** Ob/Gyn Infectious Diseases, Baylor Coll Med 1987; **Fac Appt:** Prof ObG, Univ Okla Coll Med

Seigel, Mark J MD (ObG) - **Spec Exp:** Adolescent Gynecology; Minimally Invasive Surgery; Menopause Problems; **Hospital:** CentraState Med Ctr, Monmouth Med Ctr; **Address:** 501 Iron Bridge Rd, Ste 4, Freehold, NJ 07728-5305; **Phone:** 732-431-1807; **Board Cert:** Obstetrics & Gynecology 2011; **Med School:** Geo Wash Univ 1980; **Resid:** Obstetrics & Gynecology, Columbia-Presby Med Ctr 1984

Ophthalmology

Engel, Mark L MD (Oph) - **Spec Exp:** Cataract Surgery; Glaucoma; **Hospital:** Bayshore Community Hosp, Riverview Med Ctr; **Address:** 733 N Beers St, Ste U4, Holmdel, NJ 07733-1528; **Phone:** 732-739-0707; **Board Cert:** Ophthalmology 1977; **Med School:** SUNY Downstate 1971; **Resid:** Ophthalmology, SUNY Downstate 1975

Goldberg, Daniel B MD (Oph) - **Spec Exp:** LASIK-Refractive Surgery; Cornea Transplant; Cataract Surgery; Lens Implants; **Address:** Atlantic Laser Vision Center, 180 White Rd, Ste 202, Little Silver, NJ 07739-1166; **Phone:** 732-219-9220; **Board Cert:** Ophthalmology 1979; **Med School:** SUNY Downstate 1974; **Resid:** Ophthalmology, SUNY Downstate 1978; **Fellow:** Cornea, Eye & Ear Hosp 1979; **Fac Appt:** Assoc Clin Prof Oph, Drexel Univ Coll Med

Talansky, Marvin MD (Oph) - **Spec Exp:** Cataract Surgery; Diabetic Eye Disease; LASIK-Refractive Surgery; Eyelid Cosmetic Surgery; **Hospital:** Jersey Shore Univ Med Ctr, Monmouth Med Ctr; **Address:** 3333 Fairmont Ave, Asbury Park, NJ 07712; **Phone:** 732-988-4000; **Board Cert:** Ophthalmology 1978; **Med School:** Med Univ SC 1973; **Resid:** Ophthalmology, Storm Eye Inst 1978; **Fellow:** Retina, Storm Eye Inst 1986

Turtel, Lawrence S MD (Oph) - **Spec Exp:** Pediatric Ophthalmology; Strabismus; **Hospital:** Jersey Shore Univ Med Ctr, Monmouth Med Ctr; **Address:** 3333 Fairmont Ave, Asbury Park, NJ 07712; **Phone:** 732-988-4000; **Board Cert:** Ophthalmology 2003; **Med School:** Columbia P&S 1986; **Resid:** Ophthalmology, St Vincents Hosp 1990; **Fellow:** Pediatric Ophthalmology, Manhattan EE&T Hosp 1991

Orthopaedic Surgery

Bade III, Harry A MD (OrS) - **Spec Exp:** Joint Replacement; Shoulder Arthroscopic Surgery; Hand Surgery; Arthroscopic Surgery-Knee; **Hospital:** Monmouth Med Ctr, Riverview Med Ctr; **Address:** Professional Orthopedics Assoc, 776 Shrewsbury Ave, Ste 201, Tinton Falls, NJ 07724-3006; **Phone:** 732-530-4949 x218; **Board Cert:** Orthopaedic Surgery 1984; Orthopaedic Sports Medicine 2007; **Med School:** Jefferson Med Coll 1976; **Resid:** Surgery, Roosevelt Hosp 1978; Orthopaedic Surgery, Hosp for Special Surg 1981; **Fellow:** Shoulder Surgery, Hosp for Special Surg 1982; Hand Surgery, Roosevelt Hosp 1982

Grossman, Robert B MD (OrS) - **Spec Exp:** Knee Surgery; **Hospital:** Monmouth Med Ctr, Riverview Med Ctr; **Address:** Shore Orth Group, 35 Gilbert St S, Tinton Falls, NJ 07701-4917; **Phone:** 732-530-1515; **Board Cert:** Orthopaedic Surgery 1978; **Med School:** Univ MD Sch Med 1972; **Resid:** Orthopaedic Surgery, Univ Vermont Med Ctr 1976; **Fellow:** Sports Medicine, Lenox Hill Hosp 1977; **Fac Appt:** Assoc Prof OrS, Hahnemann Univ

Otolaryngology

Rossos, Apostolos AP MD (Oto) - **Spec Exp:** Pediatric Otolaryngology; Sinus Disorders; Hearing Disorders; **Hospital:** CentraState Med Ctr, Robert Wood Johnson Univ Hosp Hamilton; **Address:** 501 Iron Bridge Rd, Ste 11, Freehold, NJ 07728-5305; **Phone:** 732-409-2500; **Board Cert:** Otolaryngology 1988; **Med School:** Grenada 1981; **Resid:** Surgery, Univ Hosp-UMDNJ 1983; Otolaryngology, Univ Hosp-UMDNJ 1986

Scaccia, Frank J MD (Oto) - **Spec Exp:** Cosmetic Surgery-Face; Rhinoplasty; Nasal & Sinus Surgery; Reconstructive Surgery; **Hospital:** Riverview Med Ctr, Bayshore Community Hosp; **Address:** Riverside Plastic Surgery & Sinus Ctr, 70 E Front St Fl 3, Red Bank, NJ 07701; **Phone:** 732-747-5300; **Board Cert:** Otolaryngology 1993; Facial Plastic & Reconstr Surgery 1995; **Med School:** Wake Forest Univ 1985; **Resid:** Surgery, Monmouth Med Ctr 1988; Otolaryngology, Univ Hosp 1992

Shah, Darsit K MD (Oto) - **Spec Exp:** Head & Neck Cancer & Surgery; Thyroid & Parathyroid Surgery; Parotid Gland Tumors; Neuro-Otology; **Hospital:** Monmouth Med Ctr; **Address:** Central Jersey Otolaryngology, 1131 Broad St, Ste 103, Shrewsbury, NJ 07702; **Phone:** 732-389-3388; **Board Cert:** Otolaryngology 1997; **Med School:** Med Coll PA 1991; **Resid:** Surgery, Mt Sinai Hosp 1992; Otolaryngology, Mt Sinai Hosp 1996; **Fellow:** Neurotology, Michigan Ear Inst; **Fac Appt:** Asst Clin Prof Oto, Drexel Univ Coll Med

Pain Medicine

Bram, Harris MD (PM) - **Spec Exp:** Pain-Back & Neck; Complex Regional Pain Syndromes; **Hospital:** Monmouth Med Ctr, CentraState Med Ctr; **Address:** NJ Pain Care Specialists, 166 Morris Ave Fl 2, Long Branch, NJ 07740; **Phone:** 732-720-0247; **Board Cert:** Anesthesiology 1993; Pain Medicine 2004; **Med School:** Univ Ark 1988; **Resid:** Anesthesiology, Hahnemann Unin Hosp 1992; **Fellow:** Pain Medicine, TJefferson Univ Hosp 1993

Metzger, Scott E MD (PM) - **Spec Exp:** Pain-Back & Neck; **Hospital:** Riverview Med Ctr; **Address:** Premier Pain Centers, 160 Avenue at the Common, Ste 1, Shrewsbury, NJ 07702; **Phone:** 732-380-0200; **Board Cert:** Anesthesiology 1997; Pain Medicine 2009; **Med School:** Boston Univ 1992; **Resid:** Anesthesiology, Johns Hopkins Hosp 1996; **Fellow:** Pain Medicine, Johns Hopkins Hosp 1997

Staats, Peter MD (PM) - **Spec Exp:** Pain-Cancer; Pain-Back; **Hospital:** Riverview Med Ctr, CentraState Med Ctr; **Address:** Premier Pain Centers, 160 Avenue at the Commons, Ste 1, Shrewsbury, NJ 07702; **Phone:** 732-380-0200; **Board Cert:** Anesthesiology 1994; Pain Medicine 2005; **Med School:** Univ Mich Med Sch 1989; **Resid:** Anesthesiology, Johns Hopkins Hosp 1993; **Fellow:** Pain Medicine, Johns Hopkins Hosp 1994

Pediatric Endocrinology

Meyers-Seifer, Cynthia H MD (PEn) - **Spec Exp:** Diabetes; Thyroid Disorders; Growth Disorders; **Hospital:** Jersey Shore Univ Med Ctr, Riverview Med Ctr; **Address:** Meridian Pediatric Assocs, 61 Davis Ave, Ste 1, Neptune, NJ 07753; **Phone:** 732-776-4860; **Board Cert:** Pediatrics 2012; Pediatric Endocrinology 2010; **Med School:** Stanford Univ 1984; **Resid:** Pediatrics, Stanford Univ Hosp 1986; Pediatrics, Univ Hosp 1987; **Fellow:** Anatomic Pathology, Univ Hosp-SUNY 1989; Pediatric Endocrinology, Yale Sch Med 1993

Pediatric Infectious Disease

Fisher, Margaret C MD (PInf) - **Spec Exp:** Pediatric Infections; **Hospital:** Monmouth Med Ctr; **Address:** The Children's Hosp at Monmouth Med Ctr, 300 Second Ave, rm Stanley209, Long Branch, NJ 07740; **Phone:** 732-222-4474; **Board Cert:** Pediatrics 1980; Pediatric Infectious Disease 2009; **Med School:** UCLA 1975; **Resid:** Pediatrics, St Chris Hosp Chldn 1978; **Fellow:** Pediatric Infectious Disease, St Chris Hosp Chldn 1980; **Fac Appt:** Prof Ped, Drexel Univ Coll Med

Pediatric Otolaryngology

Tavill, Michael A MD (PO) - **Hospital:** Monmouth Med Ctr; **Address:** Central Jersey Otolaryngology, 1131 Broad St, Ste 103, Shrewsbury, NJ 07702; **Phone:** 732-389-3388; **Board Cert:** Otolaryngology 1997; **Med School:** Case West Res Univ 1991; **Resid:** Otolaryngology, Hosp Univ Penn 1996; **Fellow:** Pediatric Otolaryngology, Childrens Hosp 1997

Pediatrics

Murphy, Robert D MD (Ped) *PCP* - **Spec Exp:** ADD/ADHD; Asthma; Vaccines; Infectious Disease; **Hospital:** Monmouth Med Ctr; **Address:** Pediatric & Adolescent Med, 223 Monmouth Rd, Ste 2, West Long Branch, NJ 07764; **Phone:** 732-229-4540; **Board Cert:** Pediatrics 1982; **Med School:** Vanderbilt Univ 1977; **Resid:** Pediatrics, Yale-New Haven Hosp 1980

Plastic Surgery

Chidyllo, Stephen A MD/DDS (PlS) - **Spec Exp:** Cosmetic Surgery-Face; Cosmetic Surgery-Breast; Body Contouring; Breast Reconstruction; **Hospital:** Jersey Shore Univ Med Ctr, Southern Ocean Med Ctr; **Address:** Central Jersey Plastic Surgery, 107 Monmouth Rd, Ste 106, West Long Branch, NJ 07764; **Phone:** 732-460-9566; **Board Cert:** Plastic Surgery 2003; **Med School:** Hahnemann Univ 1987; **Resid:** Surgery, NY Infirm-Beekman Downtown Hosp 1990; Plastic Surgery, Univ Illinois Med Ctr 1992; **Fellow:** Craniofacial Surgery, Eastern Va Med Sch 1993; **Fac Appt:** Assoc Clin Prof S, Drexel Univ Coll Med

Dudick, Stephen T MD (PlS) - **Spec Exp:** Breast Reconstruction & Augmentation; Cosmetic Surgery; Cleft Palate/Lip; Body Contouring after Weight Loss; **Hospital:** Jersey Shore Univ Med Ctr, Monmouth Med Ctr; **Address:** 252 Broad St, Red Bank, NJ 07701; **Phone:** 732-741-1303; **Board Cert:** Plastic Surgery 1993; **Med School:** Mexico 1975; **Resid:** Surgery, St Vincents Hosp 1981; Plastic Surgery, Indiana Univ Med Ctr 1983

Glicksman, Caroline A MD (PlS) - **Spec Exp:** Breast Reconstruction & Augmentation; Cosmetic Surgery-Breast; Liposuction & Body Contouring; Rhinoplasty; **Hospital:** Jersey Shore Univ Med Ctr; **Address:** 2164 Hwy 35, Bldg A, Sea Girt, NJ 08750; **Phone:** 732-974-2424; **Board Cert:** Plastic Surgery 1994; **Med School:** SUNY Downstate 1985; **Resid:** Surgery, Mt Sinai Hosp 1988; Plastic Surgery, NY Hosp-Cornell Med Ctr 1991; **Fellow:** Cosmetic Plastic Surgery, Mass Genl Hosp-Newton Wellesley Hosp 1992

Hetzler, Peter T MD (PlS) - **Spec Exp:** Breast Cosmetic & Reconstructive Surgery; Liposuction & Body Contouring; Melanoma; **Hospital:** Riverview Med Ctr, Monmouth Med Ctr; **Address:** 200 White Rd, Ste 211, Little Silver, NJ 07739-1162; **Phone:** 732-219-0447; **Board Cert:** Plastic Surgery 1991; **Med School:** Univ Mich Med Sch 1981; **Resid:** Surgery, MS Hershey Med Ctr 1986; Plastic/Reconstructive Surgery, MS Hershey Med Ctr 1988; **Fellow:** Microsurgery, York Hosp Trauma Ctr 1988; Cosmetic Plastic Surgery, Manhattan Eye & Ear Hosp 1989

Rose, Michael I MD (PlS) - **Spec Exp:** Body Contouring after Weight Loss; Cosmetic Surgery-Face; Breast Cosmetic & Reconstructive Surgery; Reconstructive Surgery; **Hospital:** Jersey Shore Univ Med Ctr, CentraState Med Ctr; **Address:** The Plastic Surgery Center, 535 Sycamore Ave, Shrewsbury, NJ 07702; **Phone:** 732-741-0970; **Board Cert:** Surgery 2009; Plastic Surgery 2003; **Med School:** NYU Sch Med 1994; **Resid:** Surgery, NYU/Bellevue Med Ctr 2000; **Fellow:** Plastic Surgery, Emory Univ Med Ctr 2002

Samra, Said A MD (PlS) - **Spec Exp:** Reconstructive Surgery; Hand Surgery; Cosmetic Surgery; **Hospital:** Bayshore Community Hosp, Raritan Bay Med Ctr - Perth Amboy; **Address:** 733 N Beers St, Ste U-1, Holmdel, NJ 07733-1528; **Phone:** 732-739-2100; **Board Cert:** Plastic Surgery 1988; **Med School:** Syria 1973; **Resid:** Surgery, UMDNJ-NJ Med Sch 1980; Plastic Surgery, St Barnabas Hosp 1982; **Fellow:** Surgery, UMDNJ-NJ Med Sch 1978

Zaccaria, Alan MD (PlS) - **Spec Exp:** Breast Cosmetic & Reconstructive Surgery; Cosmetic Surgery-Face & Body; Botox Therapy; Wound Healing/Care; **Hospital:** Jersey Shore Univ Med Ctr, Monmouth Med Ctr; **Address:** 180 White Rd, Ste 102, Little Silver, NJ 07739; **Phone:** 732-530-8565; **Board Cert:** Surgery 2001; Plastic Surgery 2005; **Med School:** UMDNJ-RW Johnson Med Sch 1986; **Resid:** Surgery, Monmouth Med Ctr 1991; **Fellow:** Plastic Surgery, Univ Illinois 1993

Psychiatry

Rubin, Kenneth MD (Psyc) - **Spec Exp:** Mood Disorders; Anxiety Disorders; Dementia; **Hospital:** Monmouth Med Ctr; **Address:** 170 Morris Ave, Ste D, Long Branch, NJ 07740-6660; **Phone:** 732-870-3535; **Board Cert:** Psychiatry 1979; **Med School:** SUNY Downstate 1974; **Resid:** Psychiatry, Kings County Hosp 1977; **Fac Appt:** Assoc Clin Prof Psyc, Drexel Univ Coll Med

Pulmonary Disease

Davis, George C MD (Pul) - **Spec Exp:** Critical Care; Chronic Obstructive Lung Disease (COPD); Sepsis; **Hospital:** Monmouth Med Ctr; **Address:** 279 3rd Ave, Ste 510, Long Branch, NJ 07740; **Phone:** 732-870-0650; **Board Cert:** Internal Medicine 1976; Pulmonary Disease 1980; **Med School:** Hahnemann Univ 1972; **Resid:** Internal Medicine, Monmouth Med Ctr 1977; **Fellow:** Pulmonary Disease, Monmouth Med Ctr 1979

Reproductive Endocrinology

Damien, Miguel MD (RE) - **Hospital:** Riverview Med Ctr, Monmouth Med Ctr; **Address:** 200 White Rd, Ste 214, Little Silver, NJ 07739; **Phone:** 732-758-6511; **Board Cert:** Obstetrics & Gynecology 2011; Reproductive Endocrinology 2011; **Med School:** Dartmouth Med Sch 1982; **Resid:** Obstetrics & Gynecology, Beth Israel Deaconess Hosp 1986; **Fellow:** Reproductive Endocrinology, Harvard Med Sch 1988; Reproductive Endocrinology, Univ Conn 1989

Rheumatology

Schwartzberg, Mori MD (Rhu) - **Spec Exp:** Rheumatoid Arthritis; Spondylitis; Osteoarthritis; **Hospital:** Jersey Shore Univ Med Ctr; **Address:** 3350 Route 138, Wall Township Bldg 1 Fl 2 - Ste 212, Wall Township, NJ 07719; **Phone:** 732-988-5030; **Board Cert:** Internal Medicine 1976; Rheumatology 1978; **Med School:** SUNY Upstate Med Univ 1973; **Resid:** Internal Medicine, Nassau County Med Ctr 1976; **Fellow:** Rheumatology, Albert Einstein Med Ctr 1978; **Fac Appt:** Asst Clin Prof Med, UMDNJ-RW Johnson Med Sch

Wasser, Kenneth B MD (Rhu) - **Spec Exp:** Rheumatoid Arthritis; Lupus Nephritis; Psoriatic Arthritis; **Hospital:** Riverview Med Ctr, Monmouth Med Ctr; **Address:** 43 Gilbert St N, Ste 7, Tinton Falls, NJ 07701; **Phone:** 732-530-7999; **Board Cert:** Internal Medicine 1981; Rheumatology 1982; **Med School:** Case West Res Univ 1977; **Resid:** Internal Medicine, Univ Hosps 1980; Rheumatology, Univ Hosps 1982; **Fac Appt:** Asst Clin Prof Med, Drexel Univ Coll Med

Sports Medicine

Rice, Stephen G MD/PhD (SM) - **Spec Exp:** Primary Care Sports Medicine; Musculoskeletal Injuries; **Hospital:** Jersey Shore Univ Med Ctr; **Address:** Jersey Shore Sports Med Ctr, 51 Davis Ave, Ste S1-02, Neptune, NJ 07753; **Phone:** 732-776-2433; **Board Cert:** Pediatrics 1981; Sports Medicine 2004; **Med School:** NYU Sch Med 1974; **Resid:** Pediatrics, Chldn's Hosp Med Ctr 1977; **Fac Appt:** Clin Prof Ped, UMDNJ-RW Johnson Med Sch

Sclafani, Michael MD (SM) - **Spec Exp:** Knee Injuries/Ligament Surgery; Shoulder Instability; **Hospital:** Jersey Shore Univ Med Ctr; **Address:** Orthopedic Inst, 2315 Route 34 S, Manasquan, NJ 08736; **Phone:** 732-974-0404; **Board Cert:** Orthopaedic Surgery 2007; **Med School:** NYU Sch Med 1988; **Resid:** Orthopaedic Surgery, NYU Med Ctr 1993; **Fellow:** Sports Medicine, American Sports Med Inst 1994

Surgery

Arbour, Robert MD (S) - **Spec Exp:** Breast Surgery; Colon & Rectal Surgery; Biliary Surgery; Hernia; **Hospital:** Bayshore Community Hosp, Riverview Med Ctr; **Address:** 668 N Beers St, Ste 102, Holmdel, NJ 07733; **Phone:** 732-847-3300; **Board Cert:** Surgery 1972; **Med School:** UMDNJ-NJ Med Sch, Newark 1965; **Resid:** Surgery, Georgetown Univ Hosp 1971

Borao, Frank J MD (S) - **Spec Exp:** Laparoscopic Abdominal Surgery; Obesity/Bariatric Surgery; Gastroesophageal Reflux Disease (GERD); Critical Care; **Hospital:** Monmouth Med Ctr; **Address:** Specialty Surgical Assocs, 10 Industrial Way E, Ste 104, Eatontown, NJ 07724; **Phone:** 732-389-1331; **Board Cert:** Surgery 2010; **Med School:** UMDNJ-NJ Med Sch, Newark 1994; **Resid:** Surgery, Monmouth Med Ctr 1999; **Fellow:** Laparoscopic Surgery, White Plains Hosp 2000; **Fac Appt:** Asst Clin Prof S, Hahnemann Univ

Goldfarb, Michael A MD (S) - **Spec Exp:** Breast Surgery; Telemedicine; **Hospital:** Monmouth Med Ctr; **Address:** 166 Morris Ave Fl 2, Long Branch, NJ 07740; **Phone:** 732-870-6060; **Board Cert:** Surgery 1973; **Med School:** NYU Sch Med 1967; **Resid:** Surgery, Beth Israel Med Ctr 1972; **Fac Appt:** Prof S, Drexel Univ Coll Med

Thoracic & Cardiac Surgery

Neibart, Richard M MD (T&CS) - **Spec Exp:** Coronary Artery Surgery; Cardiac Surgery; **Hospital:** Jersey Shore Univ Med Ctr; **Address:** 1944 Route 33, Ste 201, Neptune, NJ 07753-4463; **Phone:** 732-776-4618; **Board Cert:** Thoracic & Cardiac Surgery 2011; **Med School:** Mount Sinai Sch Med 1982; **Resid:** Surgery, St Vincents Med Ctr 1987; **Fellow:** Thoracic Surgery, Jackson Meml Hosp 1989

Urology

Ebani, Jack MD (U) - **Spec Exp:** Prostate Cancer; Incontinence; **Hospital:** Jersey Shore Univ Med Ctr, Ocean Med Ctr; **Address:** 1820 Corlies Ave, Neptune, NJ 07753-4860; **Phone:** 732-774-4551; **Board Cert:** Urology 2006; **Med School:** SUNY Hlth Sci Ctr 1979; **Resid:** Surgery, North Shore Univ Hosp 1981; Urology, NYU Med Ctr 1985

Geltzeiler, Jules MD (U) - **Spec Exp:** Prostate Cancer; Incontinence; **Hospital:** Monmouth Med Ctr, Jersey Shore Univ Med Ctr; **Address:** New Jersey Urologic Inst, 10 Industrial Way E, Ste 101, Eatontown, NJ 07724; **Phone:** 732-963-9091; **Board Cert:** Urology 2004; **Med School:** Hahnemann Univ 1979; **Resid:** Surgery, Monmouth Med Ctr 1981; Urology, Geo Wash Univ Med Ctr 1984; **Fac Appt:** Asst Clin Prof S, Drexel Univ Coll Med

Grebler, Arnold M MD (U) - **Spec Exp:** Urologic Cancer; Kidney Stones; Incontinence; Impotence; **Hospital:** Monmouth Med Ctr, Jersey Shore Univ Med Ctr; **Address:** New Jersey Urologic Inst, 10 Industrial Way E, Ste 101, Long Branch, NJ 07724; **Phone:** 732-963-9091; **Board Cert:** Urology 1982; **Med School:** Italy 1974; **Resid:** Surgery, Maimonides Med Ctr 1976; Urology, Maimonides Med Ctr 1979; **Fac Appt:** Assoc Clin Prof U, Hahnemann Univ

Litvin, Y Samuel MD (U) - **Spec Exp:** Infertility; Prostate Disease; **Hospital:** Monmouth Med Ctr, Riverview Med Ctr; **Address:** New Jersey Urologic Inst, 10 Industrial Way E, Ste 101, Eatontown, NJ 07724; **Phone:** 732-963-9091; **Board Cert:** Urology 2003; **Med School:** UCLA 1986; **Resid:** Surgery, Beth Israel Med Ctr 1988; Urology, Beth Israel Med Ctr 1991

Rose, John G MD (U) - **Hospital:** Riverview Med Ctr, Bayshore Community Hosp; **Address:** Urology Assocs, 70 E Front St, Red Bank, NJ 07701-1851; **Phone:** 732-741-5923; **Board Cert:** Urology 1977; **Med School:** Cornell Univ-Weill Med Coll 1968; **Resid:** Surgery, New York Hosp 1970; Urology, Univ Virginia Med Ctr 1974; **Fellow:** Urology, Univ Virginia

Rotolo, James MD (U) - **Spec Exp:** Prostate Disease; Urologic Cancer; Kidney Stones; **Hospital:** Ocean Med Ctr, Jersey Shore Univ Med Ctr; **Address:** 2401 Highway 35, Manasquan, NJ 08736; **Phone:** 732-223-7877; **Board Cert:** Urology 2010; **Med School:** Georgetown Univ 1984; **Resid:** Surgery, Georgetown Univ Hosp 1986; Urology, Georgetown Univ Hosp 1990

The Best in American Medicine
www.CastleConnolly.com

Morris

Morris

Adolescent Medicine

Rosenfeld, Walter D MD (AM) - **Spec Exp:** Eating Disorders; **Hospital:** Morristown Med Ctr (page 92), Overlook Med Ctr (page 92); **Address:** Adolescent Medicine, 100 Madison Ave, Morristown, NJ 07962; **Phone:** 973-971-5199; **Board Cert:** Pediatrics 1980; Adolescent Medicine 2009; **Med School:** Temple Univ 1975; **Resid:** Pediatrics, Babies Hosp-Columbia Presby Med Ctr 1978; **Fellow:** Adolescent Medicine, Childrens Hosp 1979; **Fac Appt:** Prof Ped, UMDNJ-NJ Med Sch, Newark

Allergy & Immunology

Applebaum, Eric MD (A&I) - **Spec Exp:** Asthma; Food Allergy; Sinus Disorders; Rhinitis; **Hospital:** Morristown Med Ctr (page 92), St. Clare's Hosp - Denville; **Address:** 3799 Route 46 E, Parsippany, NJ 07054-1101; **Phone:** 973-335-1700; **Board Cert:** Allergy & Immunology 2003; **Med School:** Albert Einstein Coll Med 1987; **Resid:** Internal Medicine, LI Jewish Med Ctr 1990; **Fellow:** Allergy & Immunology, LI Jewish Med Ctr 1992

Chernack, William J MD (A&I) - **Spec Exp:** Asthma; Sinus Disorders; Insect Allergies; **Hospital:** Morristown Med Ctr (page 92), Morgan Stanley Children's Hosp of NY-Presby, NY (page 104); **Address:** 28 Franklin Pl, Morristown, NJ 07960-5305; **Phone:** 973-538-7271; **Board Cert:** Pediatrics 1975; Allergy & Immunology 1977; **Med School:** NY Med Coll 1970; **Resid:** Pediatrics, Columbia-Presby Med Ctr 1972; **Fellow:** Allergy & Immunology, Columbia-Presby Med Ctr 1974; **Fac Appt:** Asst Clin Prof Ped, Columbia P&S

Cardiac Electrophysiology

Winters, Stephen L MD (CE) - **Spec Exp:** Pacemakers/Defibrillators; Catheter Ablation; Atrial Fibrillation; Syncope; **Hospital:** Morristown Med Ctr (page 92), Overlook Med Ctr (page 92); **Address:** Morristown Meml Hosp, 100 Madison Ave, Morristown, NJ 07962-1956; **Phone:** 973-971-4261; **Board Cert:** Internal Medicine 1982; Cardiovascular Disease 1985; Cardiac Electrophysiology 2002; **Med School:** Mount Sinai Sch Med 1979; **Resid:** Internal Medicine, Mt Sinai Med Ctr 1982; **Fellow:** Cardiovascular Disease, Mt Sinai Med Ctr 1985; Cardiac Electrophysiology, Mt Sinai Med Ctr 1986; **Fac Appt:** Assoc Prof Med, UMDNJ-NJ Med Sch, Newark

Cardiovascular Disease

Blick, Michael D MD (Cv) - **Spec Exp:** Cardiac Catheterization; **Hospital:** St. Clare's Hosp-Dover, Morristown Med Ctr (page 92); **Address:** Lakeland Cardiology, 765 Route 10 E, Randolph, NJ 07869; **Phone:** 973-989-2566; **Board Cert:** Internal Medicine 1985; Cardiovascular Disease 1987; **Med School:** Geo Wash Univ 1982; **Resid:** Internal Medicine, LI Jewish Med Ctr 1985; **Fellow:** Cardiovascular Disease, Philadelphia Heart Inst 1987

Blum, Mark A MD (Cv) - **Spec Exp:** Interventional Cardiology; Cholesterol/Lipid Disorders; Hypertrophic Cardiomyopathy; Preventive Cardiology; **Hospital:** Morristown Med Ctr (page 92), Saint Barnabas Med Ctr; **Address:** 95 Madison Ave, Morristown, NJ 07960; **Phone:** 973-889-9001; **Board Cert:** Internal Medicine 1986; Cardiovascular Disease 1989; **Med School:** Mount Sinai Sch Med 1983; **Resid:** Internal Medicine, Montefiore Hosp Med Ctr 1985; Internal Medicine, Mt Sinai Hosp 1986; **Fellow:** Cardiovascular Disease, Mt Sinai Hosp 1988; Interventional Cardiology, Newark Beth Israel Hosp 1989; **Fac Appt:** Asst Clin Prof Med, Mount Sinai Sch Med

Fisch, Arthur P MD (Cv) - **Spec Exp:** Echocardiography; Coronary Artery Disease; Heart Valve Disease; **Hospital:** Morristown Med Ctr (page 92); **Address:** Morristown Cardiology Assocs, 435 South St, Ste 100, Morristown, NJ 07960-5350; **Phone:** 973-267-3944; **Board Cert:** Internal Medicine 1972; Cardiovascular Disease 1975; **Med School:** Boston Univ 1969; **Resid:** Internal Medicine, UCLA Med Ctr 1972; **Fellow:** Cardiovascular Disease, Hosp Univ Penn 1974

Lowell, Barry H MD (Cv) - **Spec Exp:** Interventional Cardiology; **Hospital:** St. Clare's Hosp-Dover, Morristown Med Ctr (page 92); **Address:** Morris Heart Assocs, 400 Valley Rd, Ste 102, Mount Arlington, NJ 07856; **Phone:** 973-770-7899; **Board Cert:** Internal Medicine 1986; Cardiovascular Disease 1989; Interventional Cardiology 2010; **Med School:** SUNY Stony Brook 1982; **Resid:** Internal Medicine, St Lukes Hosp 1985; **Fellow:** Cardiovascular Disease, St Lukes Hosp 1989

Raska, Karel MD (Cv) - **Spec Exp:** Preventive Cardiology; Hypertension; Echocardiography; **Hospital:** Morristown Med Ctr (page 92); **Address:** 435 South St, Ste 100, Morristown, NJ 07960-5350; **Phone:** 973-267-3944; **Board Cert:** Cardiovascular Disease 2005; **Med School:** Harvard Med Sch 1989; **Resid:** Internal Medicine, Mass Genl Hosp 1992; **Fellow:** Cardiovascular Disease, Johns Hopkins Hosp 1995

Child Neurology

Bennett, Harvey S MD (ChiN) - **Spec Exp:** Concussion; Tourette's Syndrome; Cerebral Palsy; **Hospital:** Morristown Med Ctr (page 92), Overlook Med Ctr (page 92); **Address:** Goryeb Children's Hospital, 100 Madison Ave, Box 24, Morristown, NJ 07960; **Phone:** 973-971-5700; **Board Cert:** Pediatrics 1979; Child Neurology 1991; Neurodevelopmental Disabilities 2009; **Med School:** Albert Einstein Coll Med 1975; **Resid:** Pediatrics, St Christopher's Hosp Chldn 1977; Child Neurology, Montefiore Med Ctr 1980; **Fac Appt:** Clin Prof N, Mount Sinai Sch Med

Grossman, Elliot A MD (ChiN) - **Spec Exp:** Migraine; ADD/ADHD; Tourette's Syndrome; Epilepsy; **Hospital:** Saint Barnabas Med Ctr, Morristown Med Ctr (page 92); **Address:** 220 Ridgedale Ave, Ste A3, Florham Park, NJ 07932-1349; **Phone:** 973-966-6333; **Board Cert:** Pediatrics 1987; Child Neurology 1990; **Med School:** Meharry Med Coll 1980; **Resid:** Pediatrics, Bellevue Hosp 1982; Pediatrics, Boston City Hosp 1983; **Fellow:** Pediatric Neurology, Boston City Hosp 1986

Colon & Rectal Surgery

Moskowitz, Richard L MD (CRS) - **Spec Exp:** Colon & Rectal Cancer; Anorectal Disorders; Inflammatory Bowel Disease; **Hospital:** Morristown Med Ctr (page 92), St. Clare's Hosp-Dover; **Address:** 111 Madison Ave, Ste 312, Morristown, NJ 07960-6083; **Phone:** 973-267-1225; **Board Cert:** Surgery 2005; Colon & Rectal Surgery 1985; **Med School:** Penn State Coll Med 1978; **Resid:** Surgery, LI Jewish-Hillside Med Ctr 1983; Colon & Rectal Surgery, Greater Baltimore Med Ctr 1984; **Fellow:** Colon & Rectal Surgery, St Marks Hosp 1985

Dermatology

Almeida, Laila N MD (D) - **Spec Exp:** Psoriasis; Acne; Skin Cancer; **Hospital:** St. Clare's Hosp - Denville, NY-Presby/Columbia Univ Med Ctr, NY (page 104); **Address:** Dermatology Associates in Morris, 199 Baldwin Rd, Ste 230, Parsippany, NJ 07054-2043; **Phone:** 973-335-2560; **Board Cert:** Internal Medicine 1986; Dermatology 2009; **Med School:** Univ Mich Med Sch 1983; **Resid:** Internal Medicine, Columbia-Presby Hosp 1986; Dermatology, Columbia-Presby Hosp 1989

Cooper, Lauren M MD (D) - **Spec Exp:** Sclerotherapy; Botox Therapy; Facial Rejuvenation; **Hospital:** Morristown Med Ctr (page 92); **Address:** Affiliated Dermatologists, 182 South St, Ste 1, Morristown, NJ 07960; **Phone:** 973-267-0300; **Board Cert:** Dermatology 1988; **Med School:** NYU Sch Med 1984; **Resid:** Dermatology, Bellevue/NYU Med Ctr 1988

Diagnostic Radiology

Claps, Richard J MD (DR) - **Spec Exp:** Nuclear Medicine; Ultrasound; Mammography; **Hospital:** St. Clare's Hosp - Denville; **Address:** 25 Pocono Rd, Denville, NJ 07834; **Phone:** 973-625-6000; **Board Cert:** Diagnostic Radiology 1973; Nuclear Medicine 1975; Nuclear Radiology 1978; **Med School:** NY Med Coll 1968; **Resid:** Diagnostic Radiology, Metropolitan Hosp 1972

Murphy, Robyn C MD (DR) - **Spec Exp:** Pediatric Radiology; **Hospital:** Morristown Med Ctr (page 92); **Address:** Morristown Meml Hosp, Dept Radiology, 100 Madison Ave, Ste 408, Morristown, NJ 07960; **Phone:** 973-971-5370; **Board Cert:** Diagnostic Radiology 1997; Pediatric Radiology 2010; **Med School:** Med Coll VA 1992; **Resid:** Diagnostic Radiology, Columbia-Presby Med Ctr 1997; **Fellow:** Pediatric Radiology, NY-Presby Hosp 1998

Endocrinology, Diabetes & Metabolism

Nevin, Marie E MD (EDM) - **Hospital:** Morristown Med Ctr (page 92); **Address:** Endocrine Medical Associates, 25 Lindsley Drive, Morristown, NJ 07960; **Phone:** 973-267-9099; **Board Cert:** Internal Medicine 1989; Endocrinology, Diabetes & Metabolism 2002; **Med School:** UMDNJ-NJ Med Sch, Newark 1986; **Resid:** Internal Medicine, Morristown Meml Hosp 1989; **Fellow:** Endocrinology, Mount Sinai Med Ctr 1991

Family Medicine

Holland Jr, Elbridge MD (FMed) *PCP* - **Hospital:** Overlook Med Ctr (page 92); **Address:** 492 Main St, Chatham, NJ 07928; **Phone:** 973-635-2432; **Board Cert:** Family Medicine 2009; Geriatric Medicine 2007; **Med School:** Univ Chicago-Pritzker Sch Med 1975; **Resid:** Family Medicine, Overlook Hosp 1978; **Fac Appt:** Asst Clin Prof FMed, UMDNJ-NJ Med Sch, Newark

Gastroenterology

Dalena, John M MD (Ge) - **Spec Exp:** Colon Cancer Screening; Endoscopy; Gastroesophageal Reflux Disease (GERD); Inflammatory Bowel Disease; **Hospital:** Morristown Med Ctr (page 92); **Address:** 65 Ridgedale Ave, Cedar Knolls, NJ 07927; **Phone:** 973-401-0500; **Board Cert:** Internal Medicine 1988; Gastroenterology 2011; **Med School:** UMDNJ-NJ Med Sch, Newark 1985; **Resid:** Internal Medicine, Mount Sinai Hosp 1988; **Fellow:** Gastroenterology, UMDNJ-Univ Hosp 1990

Krupnick, Matthew MD (Ge) - **Spec Exp:** Colon Cancer; Crohn's Disease; Ulcerative Colitis; Gastroesophageal Reflux Disease (GERD); **Hospital:** St. Clare's Hosp-Dover, St. Clare's Hosp - Denville; **Address:** 369 W Blackwell St, Ste 120, Dover, NJ 07801; **Phone:** 973-361-7660; **Board Cert:** Gastroenterology 2005; **Med School:** Jefferson Med Coll 1990; **Resid:** Internal Medicine, NYU/Bellevue Med Ctr 1993; **Fellow:** Gastroenterology, NYU Med Ctr 1995

Samach, Michael MD (Ge) - **Spec Exp:** Colonoscopy; Gastroesophageal Reflux Disease (GERD); Hepatitis C; **Hospital:** Morristown Med Ctr (page 92); **Address:** 101 Madison Ave, Ste 100, Morristown, NJ 07960; **Phone:** 973-455-0404; **Board Cert:** Internal Medicine 1974; Gastroenterology 1979; **Med School:** NYU Sch Med 1971; **Resid:** Internal Medicine, Montefiore Med Ctr 1974; **Fellow:** Gastroenterology, Montefiore Med Ctr 1978; **Fac Appt:** Asst Clin Prof Med, Mount Sinai Sch Med

Soriano, John G MD (Ge) - **Hospital:** St. Clare's Hosp - Denville, Morristown Med Ctr (page 92); **Address:** 16 Pocono Rd, Ste 201, Denville, NJ 07834; **Phone:** 973-627-4430; **Board Cert:** Internal Medicine 1986; Gastroenterology 2003; **Med School:** Mexico 1981; **Resid:** Internal Medicine, Morristown Meml Hosp 1987; **Fellow:** Gastroenterology, Long Island Coll Hosp 1989

Stein, Lawrence B MD (Ge) - **Spec Exp:** Hepatitis; Gastroesophageal Reflux Disease (GERD); Endoscopy; **Hospital:** Morristown Med Ctr (page 92), Saint Barnabas Med Ctr; **Address:** 101 Madison Ave, Ste 102, Morristown, NJ 07960; **Phone:** 973-410-0960; **Board Cert:** Internal Medicine 1972; Gastroenterology 1973; **Med School:** Univ Minn 1965; **Resid:** Internal Medicine, Montefiore Med Ctr 1969; **Fellow:** Gastroenterology, Montefiore Med Ctr 1971

Gynecologic Oncology

Heller, Paul B MD (GO) - **Spec Exp:** Gynecologic Cancer; **Hospital:** Morristown Med Ctr (page 92), Overlook Med Ctr (page 92); **Address:** Morristown Meml Hosp, Women's Cancer Ctr, 100 Madison Ave, Morristown, NJ 07962; **Phone:** 973-971-5900; **Board Cert:** Obstetrics & Gynecology 1975; Gynecologic Oncology 1982; **Med School:** NY Med Coll 1968; **Resid:** Obstetrics & Gynecology, Metroplitan Hosp 1971; Obstetrics & Gynecology, Beth Israel Med Ctr 1973; **Fellow:** Gynecologic Oncology, Metropolitan Hosp 1977; **Fac Appt:** Clin Prof ObG, Temple Univ

Tobias, Daniel H MD (GO) - **Spec Exp:** Gynecologic Cancer; Uterine Cancer; Laparoscopic Surgery; **Hospital:** Morristown Med Ctr (page 92), Overlook Med Ctr (page 92); **Address:** Morristown Meml Hosp, Women's Cancer Ctr, 100 Madison Ave, Morristown, NJ 07962; **Phone:** 973-971-5900; **Board Cert:** Obstetrics & Gynecology 2010; Gynecologic Oncology 2010; **Med School:** Univ MO-Kansas City 1992; **Resid:** Obstetrics & Gynecology, Bronx Muni Hosp Ctr 1996; **Fellow:** Gynecologic Oncology, Mt Sinai Med Ctr 1999

Hand Surgery

Ende, Leigh MD (HS) - **Spec Exp:** Arthritis; Carpal Tunnel Syndrome; Hand & Upper Extremity Surgery; **Hospital:** St. Clare's Hosp-Dover, Newton Med Ctr (page 92); **Address:** 121 Center Grove Rd, Randolph, NJ 07869; **Phone:** 973-366-5565; **Board Cert:** Orthopaedic Surgery 2010; Hand Surgery 2010; **Med School:** Tulane Univ 1978; **Resid:** Orthopaedic Surgery, UMDNJ-Univ Hosp 1983; **Fellow:** Hand Surgery, Columbia Presby Med Ctr 1984

Miller, Jeffrey K MD (HS) - **Spec Exp:** Carpal Tunnel Syndrome; Dupuytren's Contracture; Wrist/Hand Injuries; Elbow Surgery; **Hospital:** Morristown Med Ctr (page 92), Saint Barnabas Med Ctr; **Address:** 111 Madison Ave, Ste 302, Morristown, NJ 07960; **Phone:** 973-538-5200; **Board Cert:** Orthopaedic Surgery 2010; Hand Surgery 2010; **Med School:** Univ Pittsburgh 1981; **Resid:** Surgery, Geo Wash Univ Med Ctr; Orthopaedic Surgery, Boston Univ Med Ctr 1986; **Fellow:** Hand Surgery, Thomas Jefferson Med Ctr 1987

Hematology

Frank, Martin J MD (Hem) - **Hospital:** Chilton Hosp; **Address:** Collins Pavilion, 97 West Pkwy, Pompton Plains, NJ 07444; **Phone:** 973-831-5451; **Board Cert:** Internal Medicine 1985; Medical Oncology 1989; **Med School:** Geo Wash Univ 1982; **Resid:** Hematology, Montefiore Med Ctr 1986

Infectious Disease

Allegra, Donald T MD (Inf) - **Spec Exp:** Tropical Diseases; AIDS/HIV; International Health; Travel Medicine; **Hospital:** St. Clare's Hosp - Denville, Morristown Med Ctr (page 92); **Address:** 765 Rte 10 E, Randolph, NJ 07869; **Phone:** 973-989-0068; **Board Cert:** Infectious Disease 1982; Internal Medicine 1978; **Med School:** Harvard Med Sch 1974; **Resid:** Internal Medicine, Univ Colorado Affil Hosps 1978; **Fellow:** Infectious Disease, Emory Univ Hosp 1981

Krieger, Richard E MD (Inf) - **Spec Exp:** Lyme Disease; Endocarditis; **Hospital:** Chilton Hosp, St. Joseph's Wayne Hosp; **Address:** 2035 Hamburg Tpke, Ste F, Wayne, NJ 07470-6251; **Phone:** 908-281-0221; **Board Cert:** Internal Medicine 1981; Infectious Disease 1984; **Med School:** UMDNJ-NJ Med Sch, Newark 1978; **Resid:** Internal Medicine, Med Coll Penn Hosp 1981; **Fellow:** Infectious Disease, Med Coll Penn Hosp 1983

McManus, Edward J MD (Inf) - **Spec Exp:** Antibiotic Resistance; Wound Healing/Care; **Hospital:** St. Clare's Hosp - Denville, Morristown Med Ctr (page 92); **Address:** 765 Route 10 E, Randolph, NJ 07869; **Phone:** 973-989-0068; **Board Cert:** Internal Medicine 1985; Infectious Disease 1988; Undersea & Hyperbaric Medicine 2011; **Med School:** UMDNJ-NJ Med Sch, Newark 1982; **Resid:** Internal Medicine, Univ Wisconsin Hosp 1986; **Fellow:** Infectious Disease, Nat Inst Health 1989

Internal Medicine

Collum, Robert G MD (IM) *PCP* - **Hospital:** St. Clare's Hosp - Denville; **Address:** 16 Pocono Rd, Ste 317, Denville, NJ 07834; **Phone:** 973-627-2650; **Board Cert:** Internal Medicine 2005; **Med School:** Columbia P&S 1992; **Resid:** Internal Medicine, NY-Presby/Cornell Med Ctr 1995

Scaduto, Philip MD (IM) *PCP* - **Spec Exp:** Hypertension; Diabetes; Geriatric Medicine; Preventive Medicine; **Hospital:** St. Clare's Hosp - Denville; **Address:** 223 W Main St, Boonton, NJ 07005-1166; **Phone:** 973-335-8656; **Board Cert:** Internal Medicine 1986; **Med School:** UMDNJ-NJ Med Sch, Newark 1983; **Resid:** Internal Medicine, UMDNJ-Univ Hosp 1986

Silva, Waldemar MD (IM) - **Hospital:** Chilton Hosp, St. Joseph's Regl Med Ctr - Paterson; **Address:** 488 Newark Pompton Tpke, Pompton Plains, NJ 07444; **Phone:** 973-835-9100; **Board Cert:** Internal Medicine 1987; **Med School:** Harvard Med Sch 1982; **Resid:** Internal Medicine, Bronx Muni Hosp 1985

Storch, Kenneth J MD/PhD (IM) - **Spec Exp:** Nutrition; Diabetes; Cholesterol/Lipid Disorders; **Hospital:** Morristown Med Ctr (page 92), Overlook Med Ctr (page 92); **Address:** Storch Med Nutrition Ctr, 147 Columbia Tpke, Ste 308, Florham Park, NJ 07932; **Phone:** 973-765-9355; **Board Cert:** Internal Medicine 1982; **Med School:** SUNY Downstate 1979; **Resid:** Internal Medicine, Staten Island Hosp 1982; **Fellow:** Nutrition & Metabolism, MIT 1986; Nutrition & Metabolism, New England Deaconess 1988; **Fac Appt:** Asst Clin Prof Med, UMDNJ-NJ Med Sch, Newark

Weine, Gary R MD (IM) *PCP* - **Spec Exp:** Hypertension; Cholesterol/Lipid Disorders; **Hospital:** Morristown Med Ctr (page 92); **Address:** 95 Madison Ave, Ste 405, Morristown, NJ 07960-7336; **Phone:** 973-829-9998; **Board Cert:** Internal Medicine 1979; **Med School:** Cornell Univ-Weill Med Coll 1976; **Resid:** Internal Medicine, NY Hosp 1979; **Fac Appt:** Asst Clin Prof Med, UMDNJ-NJ Med Sch, Newark

Maternal & Fetal Medicine

Benito, Carlos W MD (MF) - **Spec Exp:** Pregnancy Loss; Prenatal Diagnosis; Premature Labor; **Hospital:** Morristown Med Ctr (page 92), Overlook Med Ctr (page 92); **Address:** 435 South St, Ste 308, Morristown, NJ 07960; **Phone:** 973-971-7080; **Board Cert:** Obstetrics & Gynecology 2010; Maternal & Fetal Medicine 2010; **Med School:** UMDNJ-RW Johnson Med Sch 1993; **Resid:** Obstetrics & Gynecology, UMDNJ-RWJ Med Ctr 1997; **Fellow:** Maternal & Fetal Medicine, UMDNJ-RWJ Med Ctr 1999; **Fac Appt:** Assoc Prof ObG

Medical Oncology

Adler, Kenneth R MD (Onc) - **Spec Exp:** Breast Cancer; Myeloproliferative Disorders; Lymphoma; **Hospital:** Morristown Med Ctr (page 92); **Address:** Carol G Simon Cancer Ctr, 100 Madison Ave, Box 1089, Morristown, NJ 07962-1089; **Phone:** 973-538-5210; **Board Cert:** Internal Medicine 1976; Hematology 1978; **Med School:** Albany Med Coll 1973; **Resid:** Internal Medicine, Albany Med Ctr 1976; **Fellow:** Hematology & Oncology, Albany Med Ctr 1978; **Fac Appt:** Asst Clin Prof Med, UMDNJ-NJ Med Sch, Newark

Farber, Charles M MD/PhD (Onc) - **Spec Exp:** Leukemia & Lymphoma; Breast Cancer; Ovarian Cancer; Multiple Myeloma; **Hospital:** Morristown Med Ctr (page 92); **Address:** Carol G Simon Cancer Center, 100 Madison Ave, Box 1089, Morristown, NJ 07962-1089; **Phone:** 973-538-5210; **Board Cert:** Medical Oncology 2000; **Med School:** NYU Sch Med 1986; **Resid:** Internal Medicine, NY Hosp 1988; **Fellow:** Hematology & Oncology, NY Hosp 1991; **Fac Appt:** Asst Clin Prof Med, UMDNJ-NJ Med Sch, Newark

Gurubhagavatula, Sarada MD (Onc) - **Spec Exp:** Lung Cancer; **Hospital:** Morristown Med Ctr (page 92), St. Clare's Hosp - Denville; **Address:** Hematology-Oncology Associates, 100 Madison Ave, Fl 2, Box 1089, Morristown, NJ 07962; **Phone:** 973-538-5210; **Board Cert:** Medical Oncology 2004; **Med School:** Johns Hopkins Univ 1998; **Resid:** Internal Medicine, Brigham & Women's Hosp 2001; **Fellow:** Hematology & Oncology, Dana Farber Cancer Inst 2004

Papish, Steven W MD (Onc) - **Spec Exp:** Breast Cancer; Lymphoma; Gynecologic Cancer; **Hospital:** Morristown Med Ctr (page 92), St. Clare's Hosp - Boonton Township NO INPT/ER; **Address:** Carol G Simon Cancer Ctr, 100 Madison Ave, Box 1089, Morristown, NJ 07962-1089; **Phone:** 973-538-5210; **Board Cert:** Internal Medicine 1977; Hematology 1980; Medical Oncology 1981; **Med School:** Univ Pennsylvania 1974; **Resid:** Internal Medicine, Geo Wash Univ Med Ctr 1978; **Fellow:** Hematology, New England Med Ctr 1979; Medical Oncology, Dana Farber Canc Inst 1981

Neonatal-Perinatal Medicine

Skolnick, Lawrence MD (NP) - **Spec Exp:** Neonatal Care; **Hospital:** Morristown Med Ctr (page 92), Overlook Med Ctr (page 92); **Address:** 100 Madison Ave, Morristown, NJ 07960-6136; **Phone:** 973-971-5488; **Board Cert:** Pediatrics 1977; Neonatal-Perinatal Medicine 1977; **Med School:** NYU Sch Med 1972; **Resid:** Pediatrics, Albert Einstein 1975; **Fellow:** Neonatal-Perinatal Medicine, Duke Univ Med Ctr 1977; **Fac Appt:** Assoc Clin Prof Ped, UMDNJ-NJ Med Sch, Newark

Nephrology

Fine, Paul L MD (Nep) - **Spec Exp:** Hypertension; Kidney Failure; Dialysis Care; **Hospital:** Morristown Med Ctr (page 92), St. Clare's Hosp - Denville; **Address:** 2 Franklin Pl, Morristown, NJ 07960-5305; **Phone:** 973-267-7673; **Board Cert:** Internal Medicine 1982; Nephrology 1984; **Med School:** Yale Univ 1979; **Resid:** Internal Medicine, New York Hosp 1982; **Fellow:** Nephrology, Kidney Ctr-Cornell Univ Med Ctr 1984; **Fac Appt:** Asst Clin Prof Med, Mount Sinai Sch Med

Lyman, Neil MD (Nep) - **Spec Exp:** Dialysis Care; Kidney Failure; **Hospital:** Saint Barnabas Med Ctr, Clara Maass Med Ctr; **Address:** 83 Hanover Rd, Ste 290, Florham Park, NJ 07932; **Phone:** 973-736-2212; **Board Cert:** Internal Medicine 1976; Nephrology 1980; **Med School:** Albert Einstein Coll Med 1973; **Resid:** Internal Medicine, Mt Sinai Hosp 1976; Nephrology, Mt Sinai Hosp 1979; **Fellow:** Nephrology, Boston Med Ctr 1977; **Fac Appt:** Asst Prof Med, UMDNJ-NJ Med Sch, Newark

Najarian, James MD (Nep) - **Spec Exp:** Hypertension; Kidney Failure; Transplant Medicine-Kidney; Dialysis Care; **Hospital:** Morristown Med Ctr (page 92), St. Clare's Hosp - Denville; **Address:** 121 Center Grove Rd, Ste 1314, Randolph, NJ 07869; **Phone:** 973-361-3737; **Board Cert:** Internal Medicine 1975; Nephrology 2006; **Med School:** Univ Wisc 1972; **Resid:** Internal Medicine, Beth Israel Hosp 1975; **Fellow:** Nephrology, Montefiore Med Ctr 1978

Neurological Surgery

Beyerl, Brian D MD (NS) - **Spec Exp:** Brain Tumors; Stereotactic Radiosurgery; Arteriovenous Malformations; **Hospital:** Morristown Med Ctr (page 92), Overlook Med Ctr (page 92); **Address:** Atlantic Neurosurgical Specialists, 310 Madison Ave, Ste 200, Morristown, NJ 07960; **Phone:** 973-285-7800; **Board Cert:** Neurological Surgery 1990; **Med School:** Johns Hopkins Univ 1980; **Resid:** Surgery, Johns Hopkins Univ Hosp 1981; Neurological Surgery, Mass Genl Hosp 1986; **Fac Appt:** Asst Clin Prof NS, UMDNJ-NJ Med Sch, Newark

Knightly, John J MD (NS) - **Spec Exp:** Spinal Surgery; Stereotactic Radiosurgery; Minimally Invasive Spinal Surgery; Trauma; **Hospital:** Overlook Med Ctr (page 92), Morristown Med Ctr (page 92); **Address:** Atlantic Neurosurgical Specialists, 310 Madison Ave, Ste 300, Morristown, NJ 07960; **Phone:** 973-285-7800; **Board Cert:** Neurological Surgery 1998; **Med School:** UMDNJ-NJ Med Sch, Newark 1985; **Resid:** Neurological Surgery, Bethesda Navval Hosp 1993; **Fellow:** Neurological Surgery, Barrow Neurol Inst 1993

Zampella, Edward J MD (NS) - **Spec Exp:** Stereotactic Radiosurgery; Pain Management; Brain Tumors; **Hospital:** Overlook Med Ctr (page 92), Morristown Med Ctr (page 92); **Address:** Atlantic Neurosurgical Specialists, 310 Madison Ave Fl 2, Morristown, NJ 07960; **Phone:** 973-285-7800; **Board Cert:** Neurological Surgery 1991; Pain Medicine 1997; **Med School:** Univ Alabama 1982; **Resid:** Neurological Surgery, Univ Alabama Hosp 1988; **Fellow:** Neurology, Natl Hosp Nervous Disorders-Queen Square 1985; **Fac Appt:** Assoc Prof NS, UMDNJ-NJ Med Sch, Newark

Obstetrics & Gynecology

Banks, Judy L MD (ObG) - **Hospital:** Morristown Med Ctr (page 92); **Address:** 256 Columbia Tpke, Ste 212 North, Florham Park, NJ 07932; **Phone:** 973-377-3374; **Board Cert:** Obstetrics & Gynecology 2003; **Med School:** Meharry Med Coll 1975; **Resid:** Obstetrics & Gynecology, Univ Hosp-UMDNJ 1980

Culligan, Patrick J MD (ObG) - **Spec Exp:** Uro-Gynecology; **Hospital:** Overlook Med Ctr (page 92), Morristown Med Ctr (page 92); **Address:** 95 Madison Ave, Ste 204, Morristown, NJ 07962; **Phone:** 973-971-7267; **Board Cert:** Obstetrics & Gynecology 2010; **Med School:** Mercer Univ Sch Med 1993; **Resid:** Obstetrics & Gynecology, Greenville Hosp 1997; **Fellow:** Uro-Gynecology, Evanston Hosp 1999; **Fac Appt:** Assoc Clin Prof ObG, UMDNJ-NJ Med Sch, Newark

Dreyfuss, Patricia MD (ObG) - **Hospital:** St. Clare's Hosp - Denville; **Address:** 115 Route 46 West, D Bldg - Ste 27, Mountain Lakes, NJ 07046; **Phone:** 973-334-3345; **Board Cert:** Obstetrics & Gynecology 1985; **Med School:** UMDNJ-Rutgers Med Sch 1979; **Resid:** Obstetrics & Gynecology, St Barnabas Hosp 1983

Gluck, Ian J MD (ObG) *PCP* - **Hospital:** Morristown Med Ctr (page 92); **Address:** 59 Franklin St, Morristown, NJ 07960; **Phone:** 973-538-1515; **Board Cert:** Obstetrics & Gynecology 1985; **Med School:** NY Med Coll 1979; **Resid:** Obstetrics & Gynecology, Grady Meml Hosp 1983; **Fac Appt:** Asst Clin Prof ObG, UMDNJ-NJ Med Sch, Newark

Iammatteo, Matthew D MD (ObG) - **Spec Exp:** Pregnancy-High Risk; Hysteroscopic Surgery; Laparoscopic Surgery; **Hospital:** Morristown Med Ctr (page 92); **Address:** 111 Madison Ave, Ste 311, Morristown, NJ 07960; **Phone:** 973-971-9950; **Board Cert:** Obstetrics & Gynecology 2010; **Med School:** Dominica 1985; **Resid:** Obstetrics & Gynecology, St Michaels Med Ctr 1989

Mohr, Robert F MD (ObG) *PCP* - **Spec Exp:** Gynecologic Surgery; Laparoscopic Surgery; Menopause Problems; **Hospital:** Morristown Med Ctr (page 92), St. Clare's Hosp - Denville; **Address:** 390 Route 10, Randolph, NJ 07869; **Phone:** 973-328-1262; **Board Cert:** Obstetrics & Gynecology 2003; **Med School:** Hahnemann Univ 1977; **Resid:** Obstetrics & Gynecology, Northwestern Meml Hosp 1981; **Fac Appt:** Asst Prof ObG, UMDNJ-Univ Med Dent NJ

Steer, Robert L MD (ObG) - **Spec Exp:** Pregnancy-High Risk; Multiple Gestation; **Hospital:** Morristown Med Ctr (page 92), Overlook Med Ctr (page 92); **Address:** 60 Franklin St, Morristown, NJ 07960-5217; **Phone:** 973-993-1919; **Board Cert:** Obstetrics & Gynecology 2011; **Med School:** Cornell Univ-Weill Med Coll 1986; **Resid:** Obstetrics & Gynecology, New York Hosp 1990; **Fac Appt:** Assoc Clin Prof ObG, Mount Sinai Sch Med

Wallis, Joseph J DO (ObG) - **Spec Exp:** Laparoscopic Surgery; Endoscopy; Infertility; **Hospital:** St. Clare's Hosp - Denville, St. Clare's Hosp-Dover; **Address:** 600 Mt Pleasant Ave, Ste G, Dover, NJ 07801-1629; **Phone:** 973-989-9000; **Board Cert:** Obstetrics & Gynecology 1977; **Med School:** Philadelphia Coll Osteo Med 1970; **Resid:** Internal Medicine, St Michael's Med Ctr 1972; Obstetrics & Gynecology, St Michael's Med Ctr 1975

Ophthalmology

Chen, Lucy L MD (Oph) - **Spec Exp:** Pediatric Ophthalmology; Strabismus; **Hospital:** St. Clare's Hosp-Sussex, Morristown Med Ctr (page 92); **Address:** 95 Madison Ave, Ste 301, Morristown, NJ 07960-6092; **Phone:** 973-540-8814; **Board Cert:** Internal Medicine 1988; Ophthalmology 2004; **Med School:** Boston Univ 1985; **Resid:** Internal Medicine, NY Presby Hosp 1988; **Fellow:** Pediatric Ophthalmology, Wills Eye Hosp 1992

Kazam, Ezra S MD (Oph) - **Spec Exp:** Glaucoma; Cataract Surgery; Refractive Surgery; **Hospital:** Morristown Med Ctr (page 92); **Address:** 2 Washington Pl, Morristown, NJ 07960-4220; **Phone:** 973-267-8755; **Board Cert:** Ophthalmology 1978; **Med School:** SUNY Downstate 1973; **Resid:** Ophthalmology, Montefiore Hosp 1977; **Fac Appt:** Asst Clin Prof Oph, Albert Einstein Coll Med

Pinke, Robert S MD (Oph) - **Spec Exp:** Cataract Surgery; Glaucoma; Laser Refractive Surgery; **Hospital:** St. Clare's Hosp-Dover, St. Clare's Hosp - Denville; **Address:** 66 Sunset Strip, Ste 107, Succasunna, NJ 07876; **Phone:** 973-584-4451; **Board Cert:** Ophthalmology 1989; **Med School:** Mount Sinai Sch Med 1984; **Resid:** Ophthalmology, Methodist Hosp-Baylor Coll Med 1988

Sachs, Ronald MD (Oph) - **Spec Exp:** Macular Degeneration; Diabetic Eye Disease/Retinopathy; Retinal Disorders; Retina/Vitreous Surgery; **Hospital:** Morristown Med Ctr (page 92), St. Clare's Hosp - Denville; **Address:** 8 Saddle Rd, Ste 201, Cedar Knolls, NJ 07927; **Phone:** 973-539-3600; **Board Cert:** Ophthalmology 2004; **Med School:** NYU Sch Med 1988; **Resid:** Ophthalmology, Montefiore Med Ctr 1992; **Fellow:** Retina, Albert Einstein Med Ctr 1993

Silverman, Cary M MD (Oph) - **Spec Exp:** LASIK-Refractive Surgery; Cataract Surgery; **Hospital:** Saint Barnabas Med Ctr; **Address:** EyeCare 20/20, 46 Eagle Rock Ave, East Hanover, NJ 07936; **Phone:** 973-560-1500; **Board Cert:** Ophthalmology 1987; **Med School:** UMDNJ-NJ Med Sch, Newark 1982; **Resid:** Ophthalmology, Hahnemann Univ Hosp 1986; **Fac Appt:** Clin Prof Oph, UMDNJ-RW Johnson Med Sch

Orthopaedic Surgery

Baydin, Jeffrey MD (OrS) - **Hospital:** Morristown Med Ctr (page 92); **Address:** The Orthopedic Group, 50 Cherry Hill Rd, Ste 203, Parsippany, NJ 07054; **Phone:** 973-263-2828; **Board Cert:** Orthopaedic Surgery 1976; **Med School:** Tufts Univ 1969; **Resid:** Surgery, Boston City Hosp-Harvard 1971; Orthopaedic Surgery, Tufts-New England Med Ctr 1975

Dowling, William J MD (OrS) - **Spec Exp:** Joint Replacement; **Hospital:** Morristown Med Ctr (page 92), Overlook Med Ctr (page 92); **Address:** 111 Madison Ave, Ste 400, Morristown, NJ 07960; **Phone:** 973-971-6895; **Board Cert:** Orthopaedic Surgery 1978; **Med School:** UMDNJ-NJ Med Sch, Newark 1971; **Resid:** Orthopaedic Surgery, UMDNJ-Newark 1976

Montgomery, Kenneth MD (OrS) - **Spec Exp:** Hand Surgery; Shoulder Surgery; Knee Surgery; Rotator Cuff Surgery; **Hospital:** Morristown Med Ctr (page 92); **Address:** TriCounty Orthopaedics, PO Box 1446, 160 E Hanover Ave, Morristown, NJ 07962; **Phone:** 973-538-2334; **Board Cert:** Orthopaedic Surgery 2010; Orthopaedic Sports Medicine 2007; **Med School:** UCSF 1990; **Resid:** Orthopaedic Surgery, Hosp Special Surgery 1995; **Fellow:** Sports Medicine, Lenox Hill Hosp 1996; Obstetrics & Anesthesiology, Brigham & Women's Hosp 1997

Rieger, Mark MD (OrS) - **Spec Exp:** Pediatric Orthopaedic Surgery; Scoliosis; Hip Disorders-Pediatric; Adolescent Sports Medicine; **Hospital:** Morristown Med Ctr (page 92), Saint Barnabas Med Ctr; **Address:** Advocare The Orthopedic Center, 218 Ridgedale Ave, Ste 104, Cedar Knolls, NJ 07927-2109; **Phone:** 973-538-7700; **Board Cert:** Orthopaedic Surgery 2012; **Med School:** Univ Conn 1983; **Resid:** Orthopaedic Surgery, LI Jewish Hosp 1988; **Fellow:** Pediatric Orthopaedic Surgery, DuPont Inst 1989; **Fac Appt:** Asst Clin Prof OrS, NYU Sch Med

Spielman, Joel H MD (OrS) - **Spec Exp:** Spinal Surgery; **Hospital:** St. Clare's Hosp-Dover, St. Clare's Hosp - Denville; **Address:** Ortho Assocs of West Jersey, 600 Mount Pleasant Ave, Dover, NJ 07801-1630; **Phone:** 973-989-0888; **Board Cert:** Orthopaedic Surgery 2005; **Med School:** Albert Einstein Coll Med 1986; **Resid:** Orthopaedic Surgery, Montefiore Med Ctr 1991; **Fellow:** Spinal Surgery, Hosp for Special Surg

Taffet, Berton MD (OrS) - **Hospital:** Morristown Med Ctr (page 92); **Address:** 95 Madison Ave, Ste A07, Morristown, NJ 07960; **Phone:** 973-984-0404; **Board Cert:** Orthopaedic Surgery 2011; **Med School:** Albert Einstein Coll Med 1978; **Resid:** Orthopaedic Surgery, Mt Sinai Med Ctr 1983; **Fellow:** Joint Replacement Surgery, Univ Colorado Hosp 1984

Otolaryngology

Fleming, Gregory MD (Oto) - **Spec Exp:** Endoscopic Sinus Surgery; Sleep Disorders/Apnea; **Hospital:** Morristown Med Ctr (page 92), Overlook Med Ctr (page 92); **Address:** Morristown Otolaryngology Group, 26 Madison Ave, Morristown, NJ 07960; **Phone:** 973-267-1850; **Board Cert:** Otolaryngology 1988; **Med School:** Univ Mass Sch Med 1982; **Resid:** Surgery, Univ Mass Med Ctr 1984; Otolaryngology, Mass EE Infirm 1988

Lachman, Reid MD (Oto) - **Hospital:** Morristown Med Ctr (page 92); **Address:** Advocare ENT Specialist of Morristown, 95 Madison Ave, Ste 105, Morristown, NJ 07960-7331; **Phone:** 973-644-0808; **Board Cert:** Otolaryngology 1986; **Med School:** NY Med Coll 1981; **Resid:** Otolaryngology, Albert Einstein Med Ctr 1986

Taylor, Howard MD (Oto) - **Spec Exp:** Hearing Loss; Sinus Surgery; Throat Disorders; Voice Disorders; **Hospital:** Chilton Hosp; **Address:** 51 State Rte 23 S, Riverdale, NJ 07457-1625; **Phone:** 973-831-1220; **Board Cert:** Otolaryngology 1980; **Med School:** Columbia P&S 1976; **Resid:** Otolaryngology, Univ Chicago Hosps 1980; **Fellow:** Facial Plastic Surgery, Hosp Med Coll Penn 1981; **Fac Appt:** Asst Clin Prof Oto, UMDNJ-NJ Med Sch, Newark

Pediatric Cardiology

Donnelly, Christine M MD (PCd) - **Spec Exp:** Fetal Echocardiography; Congenital Heart Disease; Cardiac Catheterization; **Hospital:** Morristown Med Ctr (page 92), Morgan Stanley Children's Hosp of NY-Presby, NY (page 104); **Address:** Goryeb Chldns Hosp-Ped Cardiology, 100 Madison Ave, Morristown, NJ 07962; **Phone:** 973-971-5996; **Board Cert:** Pediatrics 1985; Pediatric Cardiology 1985; **Med School:** Columbia P&S 1978; **Resid:** Pediatrics, Columbia-Presby Med Ctr 1981; **Fellow:** Pediatric Cardiology, Columbia-Presby Med Ctr 1984; **Fac Appt:** Assoc Clin Prof Ped, Columbia P&S

Pediatric Endocrinology

Chin, Daisy MD (PEn) - **Spec Exp:** Thyroid Disorders; Growth Disorders; Pubertal Disorders; Diabetes; **Hospital:** Morristown Med Ctr (page 92), Overlook Med Ctr (page 92); **Address:** Morristown Medical Center- Atlantic Health, 100 Madison Ave, Box 53, Morristown, NJ 07962; **Phone:** 973-971-4340; **Board Cert:** Pediatric Endocrinology 2007; **Med School:** SUNY Downstate 1992; **Resid:** Pediatrics, Columbia Presby Med Ctr 1995; **Fellow:** Pediatric Endocrinology, NYU Med Ctr 1998

Starkman, Harold MD (PEn) - **Spec Exp:** Diabetes; Growth Disorders; **Hospital:** Morristown Med Ctr (page 92); **Address:** 100 Madison Ave, Morristown Meml Hosp-Atlantic Hlth, Morristown, NJ 07962-6136; **Phone:** 973-971-4340; **Board Cert:** Pediatrics 1980; Pediatric Endocrinology 1983; **Med School:** Albert Einstein Coll Med 1976; **Resid:** Pediatrics, Mount Sinai Hosp 1978; Pediatrics, New York Hosp 1979; **Fellow:** Pediatric Endocrinology, New York Hosp 1980; Pediatric Endocrinology, Joslin Diabetes Center 1983; **Fac Appt:** Assoc Prof Ped, UMDNJ-NJ Med Sch, Newark

Pediatric Gastroenterology

Rosh, Joel MD (PGe) - **Spec Exp:** Inflammatory Bowel Disease; Celiac Disease; Liver Disease; **Hospital:** Morristown Med Ctr (page 92), Overlook Med Ctr (page 92); **Address:** Dept Peds Gastroenterology & Nutrition, 100 Madison Ave, Morristown, NJ 07960-6136; **Phone:** 973-971-5676; **Board Cert:** Pediatric Gastroenterology 2007; **Med School:** Albert Einstein Coll Med 1986; **Resid:** Pediatrics, Babies Hosp/Columbia-Presby Med Ctr 1989; **Fellow:** Pediatric Gastroenterology, Mount Sinai Med Ctr 1991; **Fac Appt:** Assoc Prof Ped, UMDNJ-NJ Med Sch, Newark

Pediatric Pulmonology

Atlas, Arthur B MD (PPul) - **Spec Exp:** Asthma; Cystic Fibrosis; Lung Disease; **Hospital:** Morristown Med Ctr (page 92), Overlook Med Ctr (page 92); **Address:** Morristown Meml Hosp, Resp Ctr for Chldn, 100 Madison Ave, Box 107, Morristown, NJ 07962; **Phone:** 973-971-4142; **Board Cert:** Pediatric Pulmonology 2007; **Med School:** Mexico 1982; **Resid:** Pediatrics, St Louis Chldns Hosp 1986; **Fellow:** Allergy & Immunology, St Louis Chldns Hosp 1989; Pediatric Pulmonology, Chldns Hosp/Univ Pittsburgh 1991; **Fac Appt:** Asst Clin Prof Ped, UMDNJ-NJ Med Sch, Newark

Pediatrics

Gotfried, Fern MD (Ped) *PCP* - **Hospital:** Morristown Med Ctr (page 92); **Address:** Franklin Pediatrics, 91 S Jefferson Rd, Ste 200, Whippany, NJ 07981; **Phone:** 973-538-6116; **Board Cert:** Pediatrics 1986; Adolescent Medicine 2009; **Med School:** UMDNJ-Rutgers Med Sch 1980; **Resid:** Pediatrics, Strong Meml Hosp 1983; **Fellow:** Adolescent Medicine, Strong Meml Hosp 1985

Handler, Robert W MD (Ped) *PCP* - **Spec Exp:** Asthma; Allergy; Behavioral Disorders; **Hospital:** Morristown Med Ctr (page 92), St. Clare's Hosp - Denville; **Address:** Advocare Parsippany Pediatrics, 1140 Parsippany Blvd, Ste 102, Parsippany, NJ 07054; **Phone:** 973-263-0066; **Board Cert:** Pediatrics 1980; **Med School:** UMDNJ-NJ Med Sch, Newark 1975; **Resid:** Pediatrics, Chldns Hosp 1978; **Fac Appt:** Asst Clin Prof Ped, UMDNJ-NJ Med Sch, Newark

Suda, Anjuli MD (Ped) *PCP* - **Spec Exp:** Pulmonary Disease; **Hospital:** Chilton Hosp; **Address:** 170 Kinnelon Rd, Ste 28, Kinnelon, NJ 07405; **Phone:** 973-838-0001; **Board Cert:** Pediatrics 1988; **Med School:** India 1976; **Resid:** Pediatrics, St Joseph's Hosp & Med Ctr 1985

Physical Medicine & Rehabilitation

Klecz, Robert J MD (PMR) - **Spec Exp:** Musculoskeletal Disorders; Stroke Rehabilitation; Spasticity Management; Electromyography; **Hospital:** Morristown Med Ctr (page 92); **Address:** Rehab Inst at Morristown Hosp, 95 Mount Kemble Ave, Baud Bldg Fl 4, Morristown, NJ 07960; **Phone:** 973-796-3600; **Board Cert:** Physical Medicine & Rehabilitation 2006; **Med School:** Poland 1990; **Resid:** Internal Medicine, UMDNJ Univ Hosp 1992; Physical Medicine & Rehabilitation, UMDNJ-Kessler Inst 1995; **Fac Appt:** Assoc Clin Prof PMR, UMDNJ-Univ Med Dent NJ

Mulford, Gregory J MD (PMR) - **Spec Exp:** Sports Medicine; Electrodiagnosis; **Hospital:** Morristown Med Ctr (page 92), Overlook Med Ctr (page 92); **Address:** Assoc in Rehab Medicine, 95 Mt Kemble Ave, Thebaud Bldg - Fl 4, Morristown, NJ 07960; **Phone:** 973-267-2293; **Board Cert:** Physical Medicine & Rehabilitation 1990; Sports Medicine 2011; **Med School:** UMDNJ-RW Johnson Med Sch 1985; **Resid:** Physical Medicine & Rehabilitation, Columbia-Presby Hosp 1989; **Fac Appt:** Assoc Clin Prof PMR, UMDNJ-Univ Med Dent NJ

Valenza, Joseph P MD (PMR) - **Spec Exp:** Pain Management; Complex Regional Pain Syndromes; Repetitive Strain Injuries; Spinal Cord Injury; **Hospital:** Kessler Inst for Rehab - Chester; **Address:** Kessler Inst for Rehab, Dept Pain Management, 201 Pleasant Hill Rd, Chester, NJ 07930; **Phone:** 973-252-6402; **Board Cert:** Physical Medicine & Rehabilitation 2007; Pain Medicine 2012; **Med School:** SUNY Downstate 1992; **Resid:** Physical Medicine & Rehabilitation, UMDNJ 1996; **Fac Appt:** Asst Clin Prof PMR, UMDNJ-NJ Med Sch, Newark

Plastic Surgery

Colon, Francisco G MD (PlS) - **Spec Exp:** Cosmetic Surgery-Face & Body; Reconstructive Plastic Surgery; **Hospital:** Saint Barnabas Med Ctr, Morristown Med Ctr (page 92); **Address:** PeerGroup Plastic Surgery Ctr, 124 Columbia Tpke, Florham Park, NJ 07932; **Phone:** 973-822-3000; **Board Cert:** Plastic Surgery 2007; **Med School:** Columbia P&S 1987; **Resid:** Surgery, St Lukes Roosevelt Hosp 1992; Plastic Surgery, Beth Israel Deaconess Hosp 1994

Pyo, Daniel J MD (PlS) - **Spec Exp:** Cosmetic Surgery-Breast; Liposuction & Body Contouring; Facial Rejuvenation; **Hospital:** Morristown Med Ctr (page 92), Saint Barnabas Med Ctr; **Address:** Plastic Surgery Ctr of NJ, 131 Madison Ave, Ste 120, Morristown, NJ 07960; **Phone:** 973-540-9055; **Board Cert:** Surgery 2009; Plastic Surgery 2009; **Med School:** Mount Sinai Sch Med 1990; **Resid:** Surgery, Strong Meml Hosp 1995; **Fellow:** Plastic Surgery, Yale-New Haven Hosp 1997

Rafizadeh, Farhad MD (PlS) - **Spec Exp:** Breast Reconstruction; Cosmetic Surgery-Face; Cosmetic Surgery-Breast; Facial Rejuvenation; **Hospital:** Morristown Med Ctr (page 92), Saint Barnabas Med Ctr; **Address:** 101 Madison Ave, Ste 105, Morristown, NJ 07960; **Phone:** 973-267-0928; **Board Cert:** Plastic Surgery 1986; **Med School:** Switzerland 1975; **Resid:** Surgery, St Barnabas Med Ctr 1981; Surgery, Morristown Meml Hosp 1982; **Fellow:** Plastic Surgery, New York Hosp-Cornell Med Ctr 1984

Starker, Isaac MD (PlS) - **Spec Exp:** Cosmetic Surgery-Face & Body; Cosmetic Surgery-Breast; Breast Reconstruction; **Hospital:** Morristown Med Ctr (page 92), Saint Barnabas Med Ctr; **Address:** 124 Columbia Tpke, Florham Park, NJ 07932; **Phone:** 973-822-3000; **Board Cert:** Plastic Surgery 1992; **Med School:** NYU Sch Med 1981; **Resid:** Surgery, St Lukes-Roosevelt Hosp Ctr 1986; Plastic Surgery, Montefiore Med Ctr 1988; **Fellow:** Hand Surgery, St Lukes-Roosevelt Hosp Ctr 1989

Weinstein, Larry MD (PlS) - **Spec Exp:** Breast Cosmetic & Reconstructive Surgery; Cosmetic Surgery-Face; Liposuction & Body Contouring; Facial Rejuvenation; **Hospital:** Morristown Med Ctr (page 92), Overlook Med Ctr (page 92); **Address:** 385 State Rte 24, Ste 3K, Chester, NJ 07930-2910; **Phone:** 908-879-2222; **Board Cert:** Plastic Surgery 1993; **Med School:** Mexico 1979; **Resid:** Surgery, Univ Hosp/Morristown Meml Hosp 1984; Surgical Oncology, Meml Sloan-Kettering Cancer Ctr 1985; **Fellow:** Plastic Surgery, Univ Pittsburgh 1986; Plastic Surgery, SUNY-Brooklyn Med Ctr 1988

Psychiatry

Sofair, Jane MD (Psyc) - **Spec Exp:** Anxiety & Depression; Women's Health; **Hospital:** Morristown Med Ctr (page 92); **Address:** 35 Airport Rd, Ste 200, Morristown, NJ 07960; **Phone:** 973-292-0960; **Board Cert:** Psychiatry 1986; **Med School:** NYU Sch Med 1980; **Resid:** Psychiatry, NYU Med Ctr 1984

Pulmonary Disease

Benton, Marc L MD (Pul) - **Spec Exp:** Asthma & Emphysema; Sleep Disorders/Apnea; Cough; **Hospital:** Morristown Med Ctr (page 92); **Address:** 300 Madison Ave, Ste 201, Madison, NJ 07940; **Phone:** 973-822-2772; **Board Cert:** Internal Medicine 1985; Pulmonary Disease 1988; Critical Care Medicine 2005; Sleep Medicine 2011; **Med School:** Mount Sinai Sch Med 1982; **Resid:** Internal Medicine, Mt Sinai Hosp 1985; **Fellow:** Pulmonary Disease, NYU Med Ctr 1988; **Fac Appt:** Asst Clin Prof Med, Mount Sinai Sch Med

Fiel, Stanley MD (Pul) - **Spec Exp:** Cystic Fibrosis; Chronic Obstructive Lung Disease (COPD); Asthma; Cystic Fibrosis; **Hospital:** Morristown Med Ctr (page 92), Overlook Med Ctr (page 92); **Address:** 95 Madison Ave, Ste 411, Morristown, NJ 07960; **Phone:** 973-971-7165; **Board Cert:** Internal Medicine 1976; Pulmonary Disease 1978; **Med School:** Med Coll PA 1973; **Resid:** Internal Medicine, Temple Univ Hosp 1976; Pulmonary Disease, Hosp Univ Penn 1978; **Fac Appt:** Prof Med, Mount Sinai Sch Med

O'Donnell, Timothy DO (Pul) - **Spec Exp:** Asthma; Lung Cancer; Interstitial Lung Disease; **Hospital:** Chilton Hosp, Morristown Med Ctr (page 92); **Address:** 63 Beaver Brook Rd, Ste 301, Lincoln Park, NJ 07035; **Phone:** 973-694-1300; **Board Cert:** Internal Medicine 1989; Pulmonary Disease 2002; Critical Care Medicine 2003; **Med School:** UMDNJ Sch Osteo Med 1985; **Resid:** Internal Medicine, Univ Hosp-UMDNJ 1989; **Fellow:** Pulmonary Critical Care Medicine, UMDNJ-Newark Beth Israel Med Ctr 1992

Radiation Oncology

Wong, James R MD (RadRO) - **Spec Exp:** Prostate Cancer; Head & Neck Cancer; Breast Cancer; Pancreatic Cancer; **Hospital:** Morristown Med Ctr (page 92); **Address:** Morristown Medical Center, Radiation Oncology Dept, 100 Madison Ave, Box 9, Morristown, NJ 07960; **Phone:** 973-971-5329; **Board Cert:** Radiation Oncology 1993; **Med School:** Harvard Med Sch 1986; **Resid:** Radiation Oncology, Harvard Jt Ctr for Rad Therapy 1992; **Fellow:** Radiation Oncology, NY-Presby/Weill Cornell Med Ctr 1997; **Fac Appt:** Assoc Clin Prof RadRO, Columbia P&S

Reproductive Endocrinology

Bergh, Paul A MD (RE) - **Spec Exp:** Infertility-IVF; **Hospital:** Morristown Med Ctr (page 92); **Address:** Reproductive Med Assocs of New Jersey, 111 Madison Ave, Ste 100, Morristown, NJ 07960; **Phone:** 973-971-4600; **Board Cert:** Obstetrics & Gynecology 2011; Reproductive Endocrinology 2011; **Med School:** UMDNJ-RW Johnson Med Sch 1983; **Resid:** Obstetrics & Gynecology, St Barnabas Hosp 1989; **Fellow:** Reproductive Endocrinology, Mount Sinai Med Ctr 1991; **Fac Appt:** Asst Clin Prof ObG, UMDNJ-RW Johnson Med Sch

Rheumatology

Pasik, Deborah MD (Rhu) - **Spec Exp:** Rheumatoid Arthritis; Osteoporosis; Lupus/SLE; **Hospital:** Morristown Med Ctr (page 92); **Address:** 8 Saddle Road, Ste 202, Cedar Knolls, NJ 07927; **Phone:** 973-984-9796; **Board Cert:** Internal Medicine 1985; Rheumatology 1988; **Med School:** Mount Sinai Sch Med 1982; **Resid:** Internal Medicine, Beth Israel Hosp 1985; **Fellow:** Rheumatology, NYU Med Ctr 1988

Sports Medicine

Feldman, David J MD (SM) - **Spec Exp:** Sports Medicine; **Hospital:** St. Clare's Hosp - Denville; **Address:** 16 Pocono Rd, Ste 100, Denville, NJ 07834; **Phone:** 973-625-5700; **Board Cert:** Orthopaedic Surgery 1979; Orthopaedic Sports Medicine 2007; **Med School:** Boston Univ 1972; **Resid:** Surgery, Mt Sinai Med Ctr 1974; Orthopaedic Surgery, Mt Sinai Med Ctr 1977; **Fellow:** Pediatric Orthopaedic Surgery, Stanford Univ Med Ctr 1978

Surgery

Carter, Mitchel S MD (S) - **Spec Exp:** Laparoscopic Surgery; Laparoscopic Cholecystectomy; Gastroesophageal Reflux Disease (GERD); **Hospital:** Morristown Med Ctr (page 92); **Address:** Allied Surgical Group, 261 James St, Ste 2G, Morristown, NJ 07960; **Phone:** 973-267-6400; **Board Cert:** Surgery 2003; **Med School:** Univ Hlth Scis, Chicago Med Sch 1979; **Resid:** Surgery, Einstein Affil Hosp 1984

Diehl, William L MD (S) - **Spec Exp:** Breast Cancer; Pancreatic Cancer; Gastrointestinal Cancer; Colon Cancer; **Hospital:** Morristown Med Ctr (page 92), St. Clare's Hosp - Denville; **Address:** Allied Surgical Group, 261 James St, Ste 2G, Morristown, NJ 07960-6348; **Phone:** 973-267-6400; **Board Cert:** Surgery 2009; **Med School:** Mexico 1981; **Resid:** Surgery, Morristown Meml Hosp 1986; **Fellow:** Surgical Oncology, Meml Sloan Kettering Cancer Ctr 1988

Rolandelli, Rolando H MD (S) - **Spec Exp:** Crohn's Disease; Inflammatory Bowel Disease; Gastrointestinal Surgery; **Hospital:** Morristown Med Ctr (page 92), Overlook Med Ctr (page 92); **Address:** 435 South St, Ste 360, Morristown, NJ 07960; **Phone:** 973-971-7200; **Board Cert:** Surgery 2009; **Med School:** Argentina 1977; **Resid:** Surgery, Central Airforce Hosp 1982; Surgery, Grad Hosp 1990; **Fellow:** Metabolism, Univ Penn 1984

Sacco, Margaret M MD (S) - **Spec Exp:** Breast Surgery; Cancer Surgery; **Hospital:** Chilton Hosp, St. Clare's Hosp-Dover; **Address:** 22 Jackson Ave, Pompton Plains, NJ 07444; **Phone:** 973-835-0564; **Board Cert:** Surgery 2011; **Med School:** Hahnemann Univ 1986; **Resid:** Surgery, UMDNJ Univ Hosp 1991; **Fellow:** Surgical Oncology, UMDNJ-NJ Med Sch 1993

Strutin, Millard D MD (S) - **Hospital:** St. Clare's Hosp - Denville, St. Clare's Hosp-Dover; **Address:** NW Surgical Assocs, 121 Center Grove Rd, Randolph, NJ 07869; **Phone:** 973-328-1414; **Board Cert:** Surgery 2008; Surgical Critical Care 2002; **Med School:** Italy 1981; **Resid:** Surgery, UMDNJ Univ Hosp 1986

Whitman, Eric D MD (S) - **Spec Exp:** Melanoma; Endocrine Tumors; Cancer Surgery; Sarcoma; **Hospital:** Morristown Med Ctr (page 92), Overlook Med Ctr (page 92); **Address:** 95 Madison Ave, Ste 307, Morristown, NJ 07960; **Phone:** 973-971-7111; **Board Cert:** Surgery 2002; **Med School:** Penn State Coll Med 1985; **Resid:** Surgery, Hershey Med Ctr 1991; **Fellow:** Surgical Oncology, Natl Inst Hlth 1992

Thoracic & Cardiac Surgery

Brown III, John M MD (T&CS) - **Spec Exp:** Cardiac Surgery-Adult; Thoracic Cancers; Heart Valve Surgery; **Hospital:** Morristown Med Ctr (page 92); **Address:** 100 Madison Ave, Morristown, NJ 07960-1956; **Phone:** 973-971-7300; **Board Cert:** Surgery 2001; Thoracic Surgery 2003; **Med School:** Cornell Univ-Weill Med Coll 1986; **Resid:** Surgery, NY Hosp-Cornell Univ Med Ctr 1991; **Fellow:** Thoracic Surgery, NY Hosp-Meml Sloan Kettering 1993

Widmann, Mark D MD (T&CS) - **Spec Exp:** Minimally Invasive Thoracic Surgery; Video Assisted Thoracic Surgery (VATS); **Hospital:** Morristown Med Ctr (page 92), Overlook Med Ctr (page 92); **Address:** North Jersey Thoracic Surgical Assocs, 100 Madison Ave, Ste 4101, PO Box 1348, Morristown, NJ 07962-1348; **Phone:** 973-644-4844; **Board Cert:** Thoracic Surgery 2007; **Med School:** Yale Univ 1987; **Resid:** Surgery, Yale-New Haven Hosp 1995; **Fellow:** Thoracic Surgery, Univ Iowa Hosps & Clinics 1998

Urology

Chaikin, David C MD (U) - **Spec Exp:** Voiding Dysfunction; Urology-Female; Neuro-Urology; **Hospital:** Morristown Med Ctr (page 92); **Address:** 261 James St, Ste 1a, Morristown, NJ 07960-6348; **Phone:** 973-539-1050; **Board Cert:** Urology 2007; **Med School:** Albert Einstein Coll Med 1992; **Resid:** Urology, Hosp Univ Penn 1997; **Fellow:** Female Urology, NY Hosp-Cornell Med Ctr 1999; **Fac Appt:** Asst Clin Prof U, Cornell Univ-Weill Med Coll

Colton, Marc D MD (U) - **Spec Exp:** Prostate Cancer; Urologic Cancer; Kidney Stones; Robotic Urologic Surgery; **Hospital:** St. Clare's Hosp - Denville, Morristown Med Ctr (page 92); **Address:** 16 Pocono Rd, Ste 205, Denville, NJ 07834-2907; **Phone:** 973-627-0060; **Board Cert:** Urology 2006; **Med School:** Med Coll PA 1989; **Resid:** Surgery, Temple Univ Hosp 1991; Urology, Temple Univ Hosp 1995

Connor, John Patrick MD (U) - **Spec Exp:** Pediatric Urology; **Hospital:** Morristown Med Ctr (page 92), Overlook Med Ctr (page 92); **Address:** Adult & Pediatric Urology Group, 261 James St, Ste 3A, Morristown, NJ 07960; **Phone:** 973-539-0333; **Board Cert:** Urology 2008; Pediatric Urology 2008; **Med School:** Ireland 1983; **Resid:** Surgery, UCLA Med Ctr 1986; Urology, Columbia-Presby Hosp 1990; **Fellow:** Urologic Oncology, Meml Sloan Kettering 1992; Pediatric Urology, Chldns Hosp Mich 1993; **Fac Appt:** Asst Prof U, Columbia P&S

Stone, Chester I MD (U) - **Spec Exp:** Prostate Cancer; **Hospital:** St. Clare's Hosp-Dover, St. Clare's Hosp - Denville; **Address:** 66 Sunset Strip, Ste 300, Succasunna, NJ 07876; **Phone:** 973-927-3388; **Board Cert:** Urology 1978; **Med School:** UMDNJ-NJ Med Sch, Newark 1971; **Resid:** Surgery, Maimonides Med Ctr 1973; Urology, Mount Sinai Med Ctr 1975

Vascular & Interventional Radiology

Calhoun, Sean K DO (VIR) - **Hospital:** Morristown Med Ctr (page 92); **Address:** 100 Madison Ave, Fl Jeff D, Ste Radiology, Box 31, Morristown, NJ 07962; **Phone:** 973-971-5377; **Board Cert:** Diagnostic Radiology 2001; Vascular & Interventional Radiology 2007; **Med School:** UMDNJ Sch Osteo Med 1996; **Resid:** Diagnostic Radiology, Morristown Meml hosp 2001; **Fellow:** Vascular & Interventional Radiology, Montefiore Med Ctr 2002; **Fac Appt:** Assoc Clin Prof Rad, Mount Sinai Sch Med

Vascular Surgery

Patel, Amit V MD (VascS) - **Spec Exp:** Aneurysm-Aortic; Endovascular Surgery; Carotid Artery Surgery; **Hospital:** Morristown Med Ctr (page 92); **Address:** 131 Madison Ave, Fl 2, Morristown, NJ 07960; **Phone:** 973-540-9700; **Board Cert:** Surgery 2004; Vascular Surgery 2006; **Med School:** Albert Einstein Coll Med 1988; **Resid:** Surgery, Montefiore Med Ctr 1993; **Fellow:** Vascular Surgery, Hosp of Univ Penn 1994

The Best in American Medicine
www.CastleConnolly.com

Passaic

Passaic

Allergy & Immunology

Klein, Robert MD (A&I) - **Spec Exp:** Asthma; Sinusitis; Urticaria; Hereditary Angioedema; **Hospital:** Morgan Stanley Children's Hosp of NY-Presby, NY (page 104), St. Mary's Hosp - Passaic; **Address:** 1005 Clifton Ave, Ste 4, Clifton, NJ 07013-3520; **Phone:** 973-773-7400; **Board Cert:** Pediatrics 1981; **Med School:** NY Med Coll 1976; **Resid:** Pediatrics, Beth Israel Hosp 1979; **Fellow:** Allergy & Immunology, Columbia-Presby Med Ctr 1984; **Fac Appt:** Asst Clin Prof Ped, Columbia P&S

Cardiovascular Disease

Julie, Edward MD (Cv) - **Spec Exp:** Interventional Cardiology; **Hospital:** St. Mary's Hosp - Passaic, St. Joseph's Regl Med Ctr - Paterson; **Address:** 1030 Clifton Ave, Clifton, NJ 07013-3500; **Phone:** 973-778-3777; **Board Cert:** Internal Medicine 1983; Cardiovascular Disease 1987; **Med School:** Albert Einstein Coll Med 1980; **Resid:** Internal Medicine, Mt Sinai Hosp 1983; **Fellow:** Cardiovascular Disease, NY Hosp 1986

Salimi, Mostafa MD (Cv) - **Hospital:** St. Joseph's Wayne Hosp, St. Joseph's Regl Med Ctr - Paterson; **Address:** 510 Hamburg Tpke, Ste 201, Wayne, NJ 07470; **Phone:** 973-942-8176; **Board Cert:** Internal Medicine 1973; Cardiovascular Disease 1977; **Med School:** Iran 1964; **Resid:** Internal Medicine, VA Hospital 1970; **Fellow:** Cardiovascular Disease, George Washington Univ Hosp 1972

Siepser, Stuart L MD (Cv) - **Spec Exp:** Coronary Artery Disease; Hypertension; Nuclear Stress Testing; Cholesterol/Lipid Disorders; **Hospital:** Chilton Hosp, Morristown Med Ctr (page 92); **Address:** 1777 Hamburg Tpke, Ste 102, Wayne, NJ 07470-5243; **Phone:** 973-831-7455; **Board Cert:** Internal Medicine 1972; Cardiovascular Disease 1975; Nuclear Cardiology 2000; **Med School:** NYU Sch Med 1968; **Resid:** Internal Medicine, NYU Med Ctr 1970; Cardiovascular Disease, NYU Med Ctr 1972; **Fac Appt:** Asst Clin Prof Med, UMDNJ-NJ Med Sch, Newark

Strobeck, John E MD/PhD (Cv) - **Spec Exp:** Congestive Heart Failure; Nuclear Cardiology; Cardiac Imaging; **Hospital:** Valley Hosp (page 689); **Address:** Cardiac & Endovascular Assoc, 297 Lafayette Ave, Hawthorne, NJ 07506; **Phone:** 973-423-9388; **Board Cert:** Internal Medicine 1979; Cardiovascular Disease 1983; **Med School:** Univ Cincinnati 1974; **Resid:** Internal Medicine, Peter Bent Brigham Hosp 1976; **Fellow:** Cardiovascular Disease, Albert Einstein Coll Med 1978

Weiss, E Michael MD (Cv) - **Spec Exp:** Preventive Cardiology; Hypertension; Coronary Artery Disease; **Hospital:** St. Mary's Hosp - Passaic; **Address:** 842 Clifton Ave, Ste 5, Clifton, NJ 07013-1881; **Phone:** 973-777-2440; **Board Cert:** Internal Medicine 1984; Cardiovascular Disease 2007; **Med School:** Romania 1980; **Resid:** Internal Medicine, Hackensack Med Ctr 1983; **Fellow:** Cardiovascular Disease, Hackensack Med Ctr 1985; **Fac Appt:** Asst Clin Prof Med, UMDNJ-NJ Med Sch, Newark

Dermatology

Gold, Jonathan A MD (D) - **Spec Exp:** Acne & Rosacea; Eczema; **Hospital:** St. Mary's Hosp - Passaic; **Address:** 1033 Clifton Ave, Clifton, NJ 07013; **Phone:** 973-777-6444; **Board Cert:** Dermatology 1987; **Med School:** Canada 1982; **Resid:** Dermatology, McGill Univ Med Ctr 1986; Dermatology, Montefiore Med Ctr 1987; **Fellow:** Dermatologic Pharmacology, NYU Med Ctr 1988

Maier, Herbert MD (D) - **Spec Exp:** Acne; Connective Tissue Disorders; Rosacea; **Hospital:** St. Joseph's Wayne Hosp; **Address:** 220 Hamburg Tpke Fl 2 - Ste 22, Wayne, NJ 07470; **Phone:** 973-595-6338; **Board Cert:** Dermatology 1975; **Med School:** Geo Wash Univ 1967; **Resid:** Dermatology, Mount Sinai Med Ctr 1973

Pollack, Shoshannah S MD (D) - **Hospital:** Chilton Hosp; **Address:** 1777 Hamburg Tpke, Ste 102, Wayne, NJ 07470; **Phone:** 973-835-1823; **Board Cert:** Dermatology 1990; **Med School:** Albert Einstein Coll Med 1986; **Resid:** Dermatology, Montefiore Med Ctr 1990

Tanzer, Floyd R MD (D) - **Spec Exp:** Acne; Eczema; **Hospital:** St. Joseph's Regl Med Ctr - Paterson, Meadowlands Hosp Med Ctr; **Address:** 992 Clifton Ave, Clifton, NJ 07013-3502; **Phone:** 973-365-1800; **Board Cert:** Dermatology 1977; **Med School:** SUNY Downstate 1973; **Resid:** Dermatology, Kings Co Hosp 1977

Endocrinology, Diabetes & Metabolism

Berkowitz, Richard H MD (EDM) - **Spec Exp:** Diabetes; Cholesterol/Lipid Disorders; Thyroid Disorders; **Hospital:** Chilton Hosp; **Address:** 2025 Hamburg Tpke, Ste D, Wayne, NJ 07470-6250; **Phone:** 973-839-5070; **Board Cert:** Internal Medicine 1975; Endocrinology 1977; **Med School:** SUNY Hlth Sci Ctr 1972; **Resid:** Internal Medicine, Montefiore Med Ctr 1974; Internal Medicine, UMDNJ-Univ Hosp 1975; **Fellow:** Endocrinology, Beth Israel Med Ctr 1977

Gastroenterology

Bleicher, Robert MD (Ge) - **Spec Exp:** Inflammatory Bowel Disease; Irritable Bowel Syndrome; Liver Disease; **Hospital:** Chilton Hosp; **Address:** 1825 Route 23 South, Wayne, NJ 07470; **Phone:** 973-633-1484; **Board Cert:** Internal Medicine 1981; Gastroenterology 1983; **Med School:** Columbia P&S 1978; **Resid:** Internal Medicine, Northwestern Meml Hosp 1981; **Fellow:** Gastroenterology, Northwestern Meml Hosp 1983

Farkas, John J MD (Ge) - **Hospital:** St. Joseph's Regl Med Ctr - Paterson, St. Joseph's Wayne Hosp; **Address:** 716 Broad St Fl 1, Clifton, NJ 07013; **Phone:** 973-777-5717; **Board Cert:** Internal Medicine 1989; **Med School:** West Indies 1983; **Resid:** Internal Medicine, St Joseph's Hosp & Med Ctr 1986; **Fellow:** Gastroenterology, St Joseph's Hosp & Med Ctr 1988

Infectious Disease

Najjar, Sessine MD (Inf) - **Spec Exp:** Travel Medicine; **Hospital:** St. Mary's Hosp - Passaic, Valley Hosp (page 689); **Address:** 975 Clifton Ave Fl 2, Clifton, NJ 07013-2722; **Phone:** 973-778-8666; **Board Cert:** Internal Medicine 1979; Infectious Disease 1984; **Med School:** Lebanon 1974; **Resid:** Internal Medicine, Beekman Downtown Hosp 1977; **Fellow:** Infectious Disease, St Michaels Med Ctr 1979

Weiss, Gabriella A MD (Inf) - **Spec Exp:** Chronic Fatigue Syndrome; Lyme Disease; Bone Infections; **Hospital:** St. Mary's Hosp - Passaic; **Address:** 842 Clifton Ave, Clifton, NJ 07013-1800; **Phone:** 973-777-2418; **Board Cert:** Internal Medicine 1985; **Med School:** Romania 1979; **Resid:** Internal Medicine, Hackensack Med Ctr 1984; **Fellow:** Infectious Disease, Hackensack Med Ctr 1985

Internal Medicine

De Giacomo, Frank C MD (IM) *PCP* - **Spec Exp:** Cholesterol/Lipid Disorders; **Hospital:** St. Mary's Hosp - Passaic; **Address:** New Jersey Physicians, 6 Brighton Rd, Clifton, NJ 07012; **Phone:** 973-472-2100; **Board Cert:** Internal Medicine 1972; **Med School:** Harvard Med Sch 1965; **Resid:** Internal Medicine, Bellevue Hosp 1968; **Fellow:** Cardiovascular Disease, VA Hosp 1969

Gajdos, Robert MD (IM) *PCP* - **Hospital:** Hackensack UMC-Mountainside (page 736), St. Mary's Hosp - Passaic; **Address:** 1005 Clifton Ave, Clifton, NJ 07013-3520; **Phone:** 973-777-2005; **Board Cert:** Internal Medicine 1989; **Med School:** Grenada 1985; **Resid:** Internal Medicine, Mountainside Hosp 1989

Gold, Jeffrey L MD (IM) *PCP* - **Hospital:** St. Joseph's Regl Med Ctr - Paterson; **Address:** 1135 Broad St, Ste 205, Clifton, NJ 07013-3346; **Phone:** 973-471-8850; **Board Cert:** Internal Medicine 1983; **Med School:** Mexico 1977; **Resid:** Internal Medicine, St Josephs Hosp 1981; **Fac Appt:** Asst Clin Prof Med, UMDNJ-NJ Med Sch, Newark

Jawetz, Harold I MD (IM) - **Spec Exp:** Chronic Obstructive Lung Disease (COPD); Pulmonary Disease; Asthma; **Hospital:** St. Mary's Hosp - Passaic, St. Joseph's Regl Med Ctr - Paterson; **Address:** New Jersey Physicians, 6 Brighton Rd, Clifton, NJ 07012; **Phone:** 973-472-2100; **Board Cert:** Internal Medicine 1974; **Med School:** Albert Einstein Coll Med 1971; **Resid:** Internal Medicine, Montefiore Med Ctr 1974; **Fellow:** Pulmonary Disease, Montefiore Med Ctr 1978

Maternal & Fetal Medicine

Sullivan, Christopher A MD (MF) - **Spec Exp:** Pregnancy-High Risk; Perinatal Medicine; Diabetes in Pregnancy; Multiple Gestation; **Hospital:** St. Joseph's Regl Med Ctr - Paterson, Holy Name Med Ctr (page 688); **Address:** Totowa Maternal-Fetal Medicine, 535 Union Blvd, Totowa, NJ 07512; **Phone:** 973-904-9778; **Board Cert:** Obstetrics & Gynecology 2010; Maternal & Fetal Medicine 2010; **Med School:** Albany Med Coll 1989; **Resid:** Obstetrics & Gynecology, St Barnabas Med Ctr 1993; **Fellow:** Maternal & Fetal Medicine, Univ of Miss Med Ctr 1995

Medical Oncology

Uhm, Kyudong MD (Onc) - **Hospital:** St. Mary's Hosp - Passaic, St. Joseph's Regl Med Ctr - Paterson; **Address:** 1117 Route 46 East, Ste 205, Clifton, NJ 07013; **Phone:** 973-471-0981; **Board Cert:** Internal Medicine 1978; Medical Oncology 1979; Hematology 1980; **Med School:** South Korea 1969; **Resid:** Internal Medicine, Englewood 1977; Hematology, Montefiore Hosp Med Ctr 1978; **Fellow:** Medical Oncology, Montefiore Hosp Med Ctr 1980

Nephrology

Vitting, Kevin E MD (Nep) - **Spec Exp:** Hypertension; Kidney Failure; **Hospital:** St. Joseph's Regl Med Ctr - Paterson, St. Joseph's Wayne Hosp; **Address:** 342 Hamburg Tpke, Ste 201, Wayne, NJ 07470; **Phone:** 973-389-1119; **Board Cert:** Internal Medicine 1985; Nephrology 1988; **Med School:** UMDNJ-RW Johnson Med Sch 1982; **Resid:** Internal Medicine, Lenox Hill Hosp 1985; **Fellow:** Nephrology, Lenox Hill Hosp 1987; **Fac Appt:** Asst Clin Prof Med, Mount Sinai Sch Med

Neurology

Chodosh, Eliot H MD (N) - **Spec Exp:** Stroke; Multiple Sclerosis; **Hospital:** St. Joseph's Wayne Hosp, Chilton Hosp; **Address:** 220 Hamburg Tpke, Ste 16, Wayne, NJ 07470-2193; **Phone:** 973-942-4778; **Board Cert:** Neurology 1987; **Med School:** Mexico 1981; **Resid:** Neurology, Boston Univ Med Ctr 1986; **Fellow:** Cerebrovascular Disease, Boston Univ Med Ctr 1987

Knep, Stanley MD (N) - **Spec Exp:** Electromyography; Parkinson's Disease; Headache; **Address:** 905 Allwood Rd, Ste 105, Clifton, NJ 07013; **Phone:** 973-471-3680; **Board Cert:** Neurology 1977; **Med School:** South Africa 1965; **Resid:** Internal Medicine, Johannesburg Hosp 1970; Neurology, Albert Einstein 1975; **Fac Appt:** Asst Clin Prof N, Seton Hall Univ Sch Hlth & Med Scis

Obstetrics & Gynecology

Burns, Les A MD (ObG) *PCP* - **Spec Exp:** Menopause Problems; Pap Smear Abnormalities; Hysterectomy Alternatives; Pregnancy After Age 35; **Hospital:** Chilton Hosp, St. Joseph's Regl Med Ctr - Paterson; **Address:** 1784 Hamburg Tpke, Wayne, NJ 07470-4023; **Phone:** 973-831-9925; **Board Cert:** Obstetrics & Gynecology 2012; **Med School:** Hahnemann Univ 1981; **Resid:** Obstetrics & Gynecology, Danbury Hosp 1985

Kierce, Roger P MD (ObG) - **Hospital:** St. Joseph's Regl Med Ctr - Paterson; **Address:** Willowbrook Obstetrics & Gynecology, 57 Willowbrook Blvd Fl 3 - Ste 301, Wayne, NJ 07470-7045; **Phone:** 973-754-4075; **Board Cert:** Obstetrics & Gynecology 2007; **Med School:** UMDNJ-NJ Med Sch, Newark 1986; **Resid:** Obstetrics & Gynecology, St Josephs Hosp 1990

Ophthalmology

Giliberti, Orazio L MD (Oph) - **Spec Exp:** Laser-Refractive Surgery; Cataract Surgery-Lens Implant; Corneal Disease & Surgery; Glaucoma; **Hospital:** Univ Hosp-UMDNJ—Newark, Clara Maass Med Ctr; **Address:** Giliberti Eye and Laser Center, 415 Totowa Rd, Totowa, NJ 07512-2081; **Phone:** 973-595-0011; **Board Cert:** Ophthalmology 1989; **Med School:** Grenada 1982; **Resid:** Ophthalmology, UMDNJ Affil Hosps 1987; **Fellow:** Ophthalmology, Pennsylvania Hosp 1984; Refractive Surgery, Vision Sculpting; **Fac Appt:** Asst Prof Oph, UMDNJ-NJ Med Sch, Newark

Vogel, Mitchell MD (Oph) - **Spec Exp:** Corneal Disease; Refractive Surgery; Uveitis; Cataract Surgery; **Hospital:** St. Mary's Hosp - Passaic, Overlook Med Ctr (page 92); **Address:** 124 Gregory Ave, Ste 104, Passaic, NJ 07055-4856; **Phone:** 973-779-0808; **Board Cert:** Ophthalmology 2010; **Med School:** Temple Univ 1991; **Resid:** Ophthalmology, Nassau Co Med Ctr 1995; **Fellow:** Cornea, Univ Tex SW Med Ctr 1996

Orthopaedic Surgery

Drillings, Gary MD (OrS) - **Spec Exp:** Knee Injuries; Shoulder Injuries; Sports Medicine; **Hospital:** Chilton Hosp; **Address:** 1777 Hamburg Tpke, Ste 305, Wayne, NJ 07470; **Phone:** 973-831-6666; **Board Cert:** Orthopaedic Surgery 2004; **Med School:** SUNY Upstate Med Univ 1985; **Resid:** Orthopaedic Surgery, Northwestern Med Ctr 1990; **Fellow:** Sports Medicine, Lenox Hill Hosp 1991

Emami, Arash MD (OrS) - **Spec Exp:** Spinal Surgery; Scoliosis; Minimally Invasive Spinal Surgery; Spinal Disc Replacement; **Hospital:** St. Joseph's Regl Med Ctr - Paterson, NYU Hosp For Joint Diseases (page 119); **Address:** 504 Valley Rd, Fl 2 - Ste 203, Wayne, NJ 07470; **Phone:** 973-686-0700; **Board Cert:** Orthopaedic Surgery 2012; **Med School:** Univ Chicago-Pritzker Sch Med 1994; **Resid:** Orthopaedic Surgery, Univ Chicago Hosps 1999; **Fellow:** Spinal Surgery, UCSF Med Ctr 2000; **Fac Appt:** Asst Prof OrS, Seton Hall Univ Sch Hlth & Med Scis

Mc Inerney, Vincent MD (OrS) - **Spec Exp:** Hip Replacement; Minimally Invasive Surgery; Knee Replacement; Shoulder Replacement; **Hospital:** St. Joseph's Regl Med Ctr - Paterson; **Address:** 504 Valley Rd, Wayne, NJ 07470; **Phone:** 973-694-2690; **Board Cert:** Orthopaedic Surgery 1984; **Med School:** UMDNJ-NJ Med Sch, Newark 1977; **Resid:** Orthopaedic Surgery, St Josephs Hosp Med Ctr 1981; **Fellow:** Sports Medicine, Mass Genl Hosp 1982

Reicher, Oscar MD (OrS) - **Spec Exp:** Reconstructive Surgery; Sports Medicine; **Hospital:** Chilton Hosp, St. Joseph's Wayne Hosp; **Address:** 2035 Hamburg Tpke, Ste D, Wayne, NJ 07470; **Phone:** 973-616-0200; **Board Cert:** Orthopaedic Surgery 2007; **Med School:** Univ Pittsburgh 1979; **Resid:** Orthopaedic Surgery, Vanderbilt Univ Hosp 1984

Strongwater, Allan M MD (OrS) - **Spec Exp:** Pediatric Orthopaedic Surgery; Cerebral Palsy; Deformity Reconstruction; **Hospital:** St. Joseph's Regl Med Ctr - Paterson, NYU Langone Med Ctr (page 108); **Address:** St Josephs Childrens Hospital, Dept Orthopaedic Surgery, 703 Main St - Xavier 702, Paterson, NJ 07503; **Phone:** 973-754-2414; **Board Cert:** Orthopaedic Surgery 2007; **Med School:** Rush Med Coll 1978; **Resid:** Orthopaedic Surgery, Yale-New Haven Hosp 1983; **Fellow:** Pediatric Orthopaedic Surgery, Hosp Joint Diseases 1984; **Fac Appt:** Clin Prof OrS, NYU Sch Med

Otolaryngology

Cece, John A MD (Oto) - **Spec Exp:** Sinus Surgery; Cosmetic Surgery-Face; Rhinoplasty; **Hospital:** Chilton Hosp, St. Mary's Hosp - Passaic; **Address:** 1211 Hamburg Tpke, Ste 205, Wayne, NJ 07470; **Phone:** 973-633-0808; **Board Cert:** Otolaryngology 1986; Facial Plastic & Reconstr Surgery 1992; **Med School:** UMDNJ-RW Johnson Med Sch 1981; **Resid:** Otolaryngology, Mount Sinai Med Ctr 1986

La Bagnara Jr, James MD (Oto) - **Spec Exp:** Thyroid & Parathyroid Surgery; Pediatric Otolaryngology; **Hospital:** St. Joseph's Regl Med Ctr - Paterson, St. Joseph's Wayne Hosp; **Address:** 311 Lexington Ave, Paterson, NJ 07502-1010; **Phone:** 973-942-1300; **Board Cert:** Otolaryngology 1978; **Med School:** UMDNJ-NJ Med Sch, Newark 1974; **Resid:** Otolaryngology, UMDNJ Affil Hosp 1978; Otolaryngology, Newark EE Hosp 1981; **Fac Appt:** Assoc Clin Prof Oto, UMDNJ-NJ Med Sch, Newark

Mattel, Stephen F MD (Oto) - **Spec Exp:** Pediatric Otolaryngology; **Hospital:** Chilton Hosp, Hackensack UMC-Mountainside (page 736); **Address:** 1211 Hamburg Tpke, Ste 205, Wayne, NJ 07470; **Phone:** 973-633-0808; **Board Cert:** Otolaryngology 1981; **Med School:** NYU Sch Med 1977; **Resid:** Surgery, Mount Sinai Hosp 1978; Otolaryngology, Bellevue Hosp 1981

Pediatric Hematology-Oncology

Bonilla, Mary Ann MD (PHO) - **Hospital:** St. Joseph's Regl Med Ctr - Paterson; **Address:** St Joseph's Chldns Hosp, 703 Main St, Xavier 7, Paterson, NJ 07503; **Phone:** 973-754-3230; **Board Cert:** Pediatrics 1986; Pediatric Hematology-Oncology 2005; **Med School:** Loyola Univ-Stritch Sch Med 1981; **Resid:** Pediatrics, Brookdale Hosp 1984; **Fellow:** Pediatric Hematology-Oncology, Meml Sloan Kettering Canc Ctr 1988; **Fac Appt:** Asst Prof Ped, Columbia P&S

Pediatric Pulmonology

Nachajon, Roberto MD (PPul) - **Spec Exp:** Asthma; Cystic Fibrosis; Sleep Disorders; Bronchoscopy; **Hospital:** St. Joseph's Regl Med Ctr - Paterson, Mount Sinai Med Ctr (page 102); **Address:** 11 Getty Ave, Paterson, NJ 07503; **Phone:** 973-754-2550; **Board Cert:** Pediatric Pulmonology 2011; Sleep Medicine 2007; **Med School:** Uruguay 1985; **Resid:** Pediatrics, Chldns Hosp Uruguay 1990; Pediatrics, Beth Israel Med Ctr 1993; **Fellow:** Pediatric Pulmonology, Childrens Hosp 1996; **Fac Appt:** Asst Clin Prof Ped, Mount Sinai Sch Med

Pediatric Surgery

Bhattacharyya, Nishith MD (PS) - **Hospital:** St. Joseph's Regl Med Ctr - Paterson, Newark Beth Israel Med Ctr; **Address:** 2130 Milburn Ave, Ste C-1, Maplewood, NJ 07470; **Phone:** 973-313-3115; **Board Cert:** Surgery 2004; Pediatric Surgery 2007; **Med School:** India 1984; **Resid:** Surgery, Univ Hawaii Med Ctr 1994; Surgery, Chldns Hosp 1991; **Fellow:** Pediatric Surgery, Chldns Hosp-Ohio 1996; **Fac Appt:** Asst Clin Prof PS, Seton Hall Univ Sch Hlth & Med Scis

Pediatrics

Scofield, Lisa MD (Ped) *PCP* - **Hospital:** St. Joseph's Regl Med Ctr - Paterson, Chilton Hosp; **Address:** 57 Willowbrook Blvd, Ste 421, Wayne, NJ 07470; **Phone:** 973-754-4025; **Board Cert:** Pediatrics 2009; **Med School:** UMDNJ-NJ Med Sch, Newark 1990; **Resid:** Pediatrics, New York Hosp-Cornell 1994

Plastic Surgery

Ganchi, Parham A MD/PhD (PlS) - **Spec Exp:** Cosmetic Surgery-Face & Body; Cosmetic Surgery-Breast; Facial Rejuvenation; Body Contouring; **Hospital:** Chilton Hosp, St. Joseph's Wayne Hosp; **Address:** 342 Hamburg Tpke, Ste 202, Wayne, NJ 07470; **Phone:** 973-942-6600; **Board Cert:** Plastic Surgery 2003; **Med School:** Duke Univ 1994; **Resid:** Surgery, Brigham & Womens Hosp 1999; **Fellow:** Plastic Surgery, Brigham & Womens Hosp 2002

Psychiatry

Hindin, Lee MD (Psyc) - **Spec Exp:** Addiction Psychiatry; **Hospital:** Saint Barnabas Med Ctr; **Address:** Creative Intervention, 1149 Bloomfield Ave, Clifton, NJ 07012; **Phone:** 973-365-2300; **Board Cert:** Psychiatry 1984; **Med School:** UMDNJ-NJ Med Sch, Newark 1977; **Resid:** Psychiatry, UCLA-Neuropsych Inst 1982

Pulmonary Disease

Amoruso, Robert C MD (Pul) - **Spec Exp:** Asthma; Critical Care; **Hospital:** St. Joseph's Regl Med Ctr - Paterson, St. Joseph's Wayne Hosp; **Address:** 999 McBride Ave, Ste 201B, Woodland Park, NJ 07424; **Phone:** 973-256-0287; **Board Cert:** Internal Medicine 1979; Pulmonary Disease 1982; **Med School:** Italy 1975; **Resid:** Internal Medicine, St Joseph's Hosp Med Ctr 1979; **Fellow:** Pulmonary Disease, College Hosp-UMDNJ 1981

Grizzanti, Joseph N DO (Pul) - **Spec Exp:** Lung Cancer; Asthma; Allergy; Immunologic Lung Disease; **Hospital:** Valley Hosp (page 689); **Address:** 297 Lafayette Ave, Hawthorne, NJ 07506; **Phone:** 973-790-4111; **Board Cert:** Internal Medicine 1979; Pulmonary Disease 1982; Allergy & Immunology 1985; **Med School:** Philadelphia Coll Osteo Med 1976; **Resid:** Internal Medicine, Univ Hosp 1979; Allergy & Immunology, Montefiore-Albert Einstein 1984; **Fellow:** Pulmonary Disease, Montefiore-Albert Einstein 1981; **Fac Appt:** Assoc Clin Prof Med, Albert Einstein Coll Med

Radiation Oncology

Cole, Robert J MD (RadRO) - **Spec Exp:** Brachytherapy; Breast Cancer; Prostate Cancer; **Hospital:** St. Mary's Hosp - Passaic, Robert Wood Johnson Univ Hosp - New Brunswick; **Address:** St Mary's Hosp, Dept Oncology, 350 Boulevard, Passaic, NJ 07055; **Phone:** 973-365-5088; **Board Cert:** Therapeutic Radiology 1983; **Med School:** Wake Forest Univ 1979; **Resid:** Therapeutic Radiology, Univ of VA Health Sci Ctr 1983

Reproductive Endocrinology

Ransom, Mark X MD (RE) - **Spec Exp:** Infertility-IVF; **Hospital:** St. Joseph's Wayne Hosp, Hackensack Univ Med Ctr (page 96); **Address:** 57 Willowbrook Blvd, Wayne, NJ 07470; **Phone:** 973-754-4055; **Board Cert:** Obstetrics & Gynecology 2011; Reproductive Endocrinology 2011; **Med School:** UMDNJ-RW Johnson Med Sch 1987; **Resid:** Obstetrics & Gynecology, RWJ Univ Hosp 1991; **Fellow:** Reproductive Endocrinology, RWJ Univ Hosp 1992

Rheumatology

Goldberg, Marc A MD (Rhu) - **Spec Exp:** Rheumatoid Arthritis; Osteoporosis; Osteoarthritis; **Hospital:** St. Mary's Hosp - Passaic; **Address:** 6 Brighton Rd, Clifton, NJ 07012; **Phone:** 973-473-2597; **Board Cert:** Internal Medicine 1972; Rheumatology 1976; **Med School:** Med Coll VA 1969; **Resid:** Internal Medicine, Univ Maryland Hosp 1972; Rheumatology, Johns Hopkins Hosp 1973; **Fellow:** Rheumatology, Hosp Univ Penn 1976

Lewko, Michael P MD (Rhu) - **Spec Exp:** Geriatric Rheumatology; Arthritis; Osteoporosis; Rheumatoid Arthritis; **Hospital:** St. Joseph's Regl Med Ctr - Paterson; **Address:** 871 Allwood Rd, Clifton, NJ 07012; **Phone:** 973-405-5163; **Board Cert:** Internal Medicine 1988; Rheumatology 2002; Geriatric Medicine 2004; **Med School:** UMDNJ-Rutgers Med Sch 1985; **Resid:** Internal Medicine, RW Johnson Univ Hosp 1988; **Fellow:** Geriatric Medicine, Roger Williams Med Ctr 1989; Rheumatology, Hosp Univ Penn 1991; **Fac Appt:** Asst Clin Prof Med, Mount Sinai Sch Med

Surgery

Budd, Daniel C MD (S) - **Spec Exp:** Breast Cancer; Endocrine Surgery; Gastrointestinal Surgery; **Hospital:** Valley Hosp (page 689), Chilton Hosp; **Address:** 707 Broadway, Paterson, NJ 07514; **Phone:** 973-742-3371; **Board Cert:** Surgery 1975; **Med School:** Duke Univ 1969; **Resid:** Surgery, Columbia-Presby Hosp 1974; **Fac Appt:** Assoc Clin Prof S, UMDNJ-NJ Med Sch, Newark

Feigenbaum, Howard MD (S) - **Spec Exp:** Gastrointestinal Surgery; Colon Surgery; Laparoscopic Surgery; Breast Surgery; **Hospital:** Chilton Hosp, St. Joseph's Wayne Hosp; **Address:** 227 Hamburg Tpke, Pompton Lakes, NJ 07442-1838; **Phone:** 973-839-7999; **Board Cert:** Surgery 2009; **Med School:** NYU Sch Med 1971; **Resid:** Surgery, Bellevue Hosp 1977

Thoracic & Cardiac Surgery

Christakos, Manny E MD (T&CS) - **Spec Exp:** Cardiovascular Surgery; **Hospital:** St. Joseph's Regl Med Ctr - Paterson, St. Mary's Hosp - Passaic; **Address:** 871 Allwood Rd Fl 2, Clifton, NJ 07012-1922; **Phone:** 973-779-2270; **Board Cert:** Thoracic Surgery 2002; **Med School:** SUNY Buffalo 1971; **Resid:** Surgery, EJ Meyer Meml Hosp 1976; Thoracic Surgery, UC Irvine Med Ctr 1980

Connolly, Mark W MD (T&CS) - **Spec Exp:** Minimally Invasive Cardiac Surgery; Coronary Artery Surgery; **Hospital:** St. Joseph's Regl Med Ctr - Paterson; **Address:** St Josephs Regional Med Ctr, Dept Surgery, 703 Main St, Paterson, NJ 07503; **Phone:** 973-754-2486; **Board Cert:** Thoracic Surgery 2011; **Med School:** Northwestern Univ 1982; **Resid:** Surgery, NYU Med Ctr 1988; Cardiothoracic Surgery, Emory Univ Hosps 1991; **Fellow:** Surgical Research, Maimonides Med Ctr 1986

Kaushik, Raj R MD (T&CS) - **Spec Exp:** Minimally Invasive Cardiac Surgery; Atrial Fibrillation; Laser Surgery; **Hospital:** St. Mary's Hosp - Passaic, Hackensack UMC-Mountainside (page 736); **Address:** St Mary's Hosp, Div Cardiac Surgery, 350 Boulevard, Ste 130, Passaic, NJ 07055; **Phone:** 973-365-4567; **Board Cert:** Thoracic Surgery 2009; **Med School:** India 1979; **Resid:** Surgery, Bridgeport Hosp 1985; Cardiothoracic Surgery, Newark Beth Israel Med Ctr 1988; **Fellow:** Cardiac Surgery, Baylor Univ 1989; Cardiac Surgery, Univ W Ontario Med Ctr 1990

Syracuse, Donald MD (T&CS) - **Spec Exp:** Pacemakers; Lung Cancer; Carotid Artery Surgery; **Hospital:** Hackensack UMC-Mountainside (page 736), Clara Maass Med Ctr; **Address:** The Cardiovascular Care Group, 1401 Broad St, Clifton, NJ 07013; **Phone:** 973-759-9000; **Board Cert:** Thoracic Surgery 2001; **Med School:** Columbia P&S 1973; **Resid:** Surgery, Columbia Presby Hosp 1979; Thoracic Surgery, Columbia Presby Hosp 1981; **Fellow:** Cardiovascular Surgery, Nat Inst Health 1977; **Fac Appt:** Asst Clin Prof S, UMDNJ-NJ Med Sch, Newark

Urology

Levine, Seth P MD (U) - **Spec Exp:** Prostate Cancer; **Hospital:** Chilton Hosp, Valley Hosp (page 689); **Address:** 1777 Hamburg Tpke, Ste 304, Wayne, NJ 07470; **Phone:** 973-616-8400; **Board Cert:** Urology 1980; **Med School:** Tufts Univ 1971; **Resid:** Surgery, Mount Sinai Hosp 1973; Urology, Mount Sinai Hosp 1978

Somerset

Somerset

Allergy & Immunology

Caucino, Julie A DO (A&I) - **Spec Exp:** Asthma & Allergy; Food Allergy; Urticaria; **Hospital:** Univ Med Ctr Princeton at Plainsboro; **Address:** Princeton Allergy & Asthma Assoc, 24 Vreeland Drive, Skillnan, NJ 08558-2621; **Phone:** 609-921-2202; **Board Cert:** Allergy & Immunology 2003; **Med School:** Kirksville Coll Osteo Med 1987; **Resid:** Internal Medicine, RWJ Univ Hosp 1991; **Fellow:** Allergy & Immunology, Albert Einstein Coll Med 1993

Fox, James A MD (A&I) - **Spec Exp:** Asthma; Urticaria; Food Allergy; Hereditary Angioedema; **Hospital:** Somerset Med Ctr, Hunterdon Med Ctr; **Address:** 3461 US Highway 22 E, D Bldg, Branchburg, NJ 08876-6021; **Phone:** 908-725-4777; **Board Cert:** Pediatrics 1981; Allergy & Immunology 1983; **Med School:** Yale Univ 1977; **Resid:** Pediatrics, Bronx Municipal Hosp Ctr 1980; **Fellow:** Allergy & Immunology, Columbia-Presby Med Ctr 1982

Krol, Kristine MD (A&I) - **Spec Exp:** Insect Allergies; Drug Sensitivity; Food Allergy; Asthma; **Hospital:** Staten Island Univ Hosp - South (page 106), Somerset Med Ctr; **Address:** 177 W High St, Somerville, NJ 08876; **Phone:** 908-725-8666; **Board Cert:** Internal Medicine 1987; Allergy & Immunology 2011; **Med School:** SUNY Downstate 1981; **Resid:** Internal Medicine, Staten Island Hosp 1985; **Fellow:** Allergy & Immunology, Mass Genl Hosp 1987; **Fac Appt:** Asst Clin Prof Med, SUNY Downstate

Pedinoff, Andrew J MD (A&I) - **Spec Exp:** Allergy; Asthma; Hay Fever; **Hospital:** Univ Med Ctr Princeton at Plainsboro, Robert Wood Johnson Univ Hosp - New Brunswick; **Address:** Princeton Allergy & Asthma Assoc, 24 Vreeland Drive, Skilman, NJ 08558; **Phone:** 609-921-2202; **Board Cert:** Allergy & Immunology 2003; **Med School:** Dominican Republic 1984; **Resid:** Pediatrics, Georgetown Univ Hosp 1987; **Fellow:** Allergy & Immunology, Georgetown Univ Hosp 1989; **Fac Appt:** Asst Clin Prof Ped, UMDNJ-RW Johnson Med Sch

Schulhafer, Edwin MD (A&I) - **Spec Exp:** Asthma; Sinus Disorders; Allergy; Migraine; **Hospital:** Somerset Med Ctr, Hunterdon Med Ctr; **Address:** Allergy, Asthma & Sinus Center, 712 Courtyard Drive, Hillsborough, NJ 08844; **Phone:** 908-526-0200; **Board Cert:** Internal Medicine 1988; Allergy & Immunology 2006; **Med School:** UMDNJ-NJ Med Sch, Newark 1983; **Resid:** Internal Medicine, Overlook Hosp 1986; **Fellow:** Allergy & Immunology, Long Island Hosp 1988

Southern, D Loren MD (A&I) - **Spec Exp:** Asthma & Allergy; Urticaria; Hereditary Angioedema; Food Allergy; **Hospital:** Univ Med Ctr Princeton at Plainsboro; **Address:** 24 Vreeland Drive, Skillman, NJ 08558; **Phone:** 609-921-2202; **Board Cert:** Pediatrics 1976; **Med School:** Columbia P&S 1971; **Resid:** Pediatrics, Columbia-Presby Med Ctr 1974; **Fellow:** Allergy & Immunology, Columbia-Presby Med Ctr 1976

Cardiovascular Disease

Kulkarni, Rachana A MD (Cv) - **Spec Exp:** Nuclear Cardiology; Echocardiography-Transesophageal; **Hospital:** Somerset Med Ctr, Robert Wood Johnson Univ Hosp - New Brunswick; **Address:** Medicor Cardiology, 225 Jackson St, Bridgewater, NJ 08807; **Phone:** 908-526-8668; **Board Cert:** Cardiovascular Disease 2010; Nuclear Cardiology ; **Med School:** India 1988; **Resid:** Internal Medicine, RW Johnson Univ Hosp 1995; **Fellow:** Cardiovascular Disease, UMDNJ-RWJ Univ Hosp 1998

Saulino, Patrick F MD (Cv) - **Spec Exp:** Cardiac Catheterization; Invasive Cardiology; Non-Invasive Cardiology; **Hospital:** Somerset Med Ctr, Robert Wood Johnson Univ Hosp - New Brunswick; **Address:** 3322 Route 22 W, Ste 505, Branchburg, NJ 08876; **Phone:** 908-231-0041; **Board Cert:** Internal Medicine 1984; Cardiovascular Disease 1987; **Med School:** Georgetown Univ 1981; **Resid:** Internal Medicine, Georgetown Univ Hosp 1984; Cardiovascular Disease, Georgetown Univ Hosp 1985; **Fellow:** Cardiovascular Disease, RW Johnson Univ Hosp 1987; Cardiovascular Disease, Georgetown Univ Hosp 1988

Stroh, Jack A MD (Cv) - **Spec Exp:** Angioplasty & Stent Placement; Hypertension; Cholesterol/Lipid Disorders; **Hospital:** Robert Wood Johnson Univ Hosp - New Brunswick, St. Peter's Univ Hosp; **Address:** 75 Veronica Ave, Ste 101, Somerset, NJ 08873-5002; **Phone:** 732-247-7444; **Board Cert:** Internal Medicine 1987; Cardiovascular Disease 1989; Interventional Cardiology 2009; **Med School:** Albert Einstein Coll Med 1984; **Resid:** Internal Medicine, Boston Univ Med Ctr 1987; **Fellow:** Cardiovascular Disease, NYU Med Ctr 1990

Dermatology

Fox, Alissa MD (D) - **Spec Exp:** Acne; Psoriasis; **Hospital:** Somerset Med Ctr, Hunterdon Med Ctr; **Address:** 3461 US Highway 22, Somerville, NJ 08876; **Phone:** 908-725-4777; **Board Cert:** Dermatology 1984; **Med School:** NYU Sch Med 1980; **Resid:** Dermatology, New York Hosp 1984

Pappert, Amy S MD (D) - **Spec Exp:** Contact Dermatitis; **Hospital:** Robert Wood Johnson Univ Hosp - New Brunswick; **Address:** RW Johnson Medical Group, Dept Dermatology, 1 World's Fair Drive, Ste 2400, Somerset, NJ 08873; **Phone:** 732-463-7546; **Board Cert:** Dermatology 2001; **Med School:** UMDNJ-RW Johnson Med Sch 1989; **Resid:** Dermatology, Columbia Presby Med Ctr 1994; **Fellow:** Research, Columbia Presby Med Ctr 1991; **Fac Appt:** Asst Prof D, UMDNJ-RW Johnson Med Sch

Diagnostic Radiology

Greer, Jeannete G MD (DR) - **Spec Exp:** Breast Imaging; **Hospital:** Somerset Med Ctr; **Address:** Somerset Med Ctr, Dept Radiology, 110 Rehill Ave, Somerville, NJ 08876; **Phone:** 732-968-5160; **Board Cert:** Diagnostic Radiology 1994; **Med School:** Harvard Med Sch 1989; **Resid:** Diagnostic Radiology, T Jefferson Univ Hosp 1994; **Fellow:** Breast Imaging, T Jefferson Univ Hosp 1995

Melville, Gordon E MD (DR) - **Spec Exp:** Neuroradiology; MRI; **Hospital:** Somerset Med Ctr; **Address:** Somerset Medical Ctr, Dept Radiology, 100 Rehill Ave, Somerville, NJ 08876; **Phone:** 732-968-5160; **Board Cert:** Diagnostic Radiology 1984; Neuroradiology 2006; **Med School:** Univ NC Sch Med 1979; **Resid:** Diagnostic Radiology, G Washington Univ Hosp 1984; **Fellow:** Neuroradiology, Mass Genl Hosp 1985; **Fac Appt:** Asst Clin Prof Rad, UMDNJ-RW Johnson Med Sch

Yang, Roger S MD (DR) - **Spec Exp:** Breast Imaging; Women's Imaging; **Hospital:** Somerset Med Ctr; **Address:** Somerset Med Ctr, Dept Radiology, 110 Rehill Ave, Somerville, NJ 08876; **Phone:** 908-685-2930; **Board Cert:** Diagnostic Radiology 1997; **Med School:** Northwestern Univ 1992; **Resid:** Diagnostic Radiology, Univ Hosp 1997; **Fellow:** Women's Imaging, Univ Hosp/Kings Co Hosp 1998; **Fac Appt:** Asst Clin Prof, SUNY Downstate

Family Medicine

Corson, Richard L MD (FMed) *PCP* - **Hospital:** Somerset Med Ctr; **Address:** 313 Courtyard Drive, Hillsborough, NJ 08844; **Phone:** 908-722-9962; **Board Cert:** Family Medicine 2004; **Med School:** UMDNJ-RW Johnson Med Sch 1983; **Resid:** Family Medicine, Somerset Med Ctr 1986

Frisoli, Anthony MD (FMed) *PCP* - **Spec Exp:** Sports Medicine; Geriatric Care; **Hospital:** Somerset Med Ctr; **Address:** Martinsville Family Practice, 1973 Washington Valley Rd, Martinsville, NJ 08836; **Phone:** 732-560-9225; **Board Cert:** Family Medicine 2005; **Med School:** UMDNJ-Rutgers Med Sch 1983; **Resid:** Family Medicine, Somerset Med Ctr 1986

Ziering, Thomas S MD (FMed) *PCP* - **Spec Exp:** Anxiety & Depression; Gay/Lesbian/Transgender Health; Skin Diseases; Complementary Medicine; **Hospital:** Morristown Med Ctr (page 92); **Address:** 39 Olcott Sq, Bernardsville, NJ 07924-2317; **Phone:** 908-221-1919; **Board Cert:** Family Medicine 2003; **Med School:** UMDNJ-NJ Med Sch, Newark 1987; **Resid:** Family Medicine, Somerset Med Ctr 1990; **Fac Appt:** Assoc Clin Prof FMed

Gastroenterology

Accurso, Charles A MD (Ge) - **Spec Exp:** Colon Cancer Screening; Irritable Bowel Syndrome; Gastroesophageal Reflux Disease (GERD); Endoscopy; **Hospital:** Somerset Med Ctr; **Address:** 511 Courtyard Drive, Bldg 500, Digestive Healthcare Ctr, 56 hillcrest road, Hillsborough, NJ 08844-2017; **Phone:** 908-218-9222; **Board Cert:** Internal Medicine 1987; Gastroenterology 1989; **Med School:** UMDNJ-NJ Med Sch, Newark 1984; **Resid:** Internal Medicine, Univ Hosp 1987; **Fellow:** Gastroenterology, Univ Hosp/NJ Med Sch 1989; **Fac Appt:** Asst Clin Prof Med, UMDNJ-NJ Med Sch, Newark

Ferges, Mitchell L MD (Ge) - **Spec Exp:** Liver Disease; **Hospital:** St. Peter's Univ Hosp, Robert Wood Johnson Univ Hosp - New Brunswick; **Address:** 33 Clyde Rd, Ste 102, Somerset, NJ 08873; **Phone:** 732-873-9200; **Board Cert:** Internal Medicine 1978; Gastroenterology 1981; **Med School:** UMDNJ-RW Johnson Med Sch 1975; **Resid:** Internal Medicine, UMDNJ Rutgers Affil Hosps 1978; **Fellow:** Gastroenterology, UMDNJ Univ Hosp 1980

Hand Surgery

Coyle Jr, Michael P MD (HS) - **Spec Exp:** Arthritis Hand Surgery; Nerve Compression; Dupuytren's Contracture; Sports Injuries; **Hospital:** Robert Wood Johnson Univ Hosp - New Brunswick, St. Peter's Univ Hosp; **Address:** University Orthopaedic Assocs, 2 Worlds Fair Drive, Somerset, NJ 08873; **Phone:** 732-537-0909; **Board Cert:** Orthopaedic Surgery 2005; Hand Surgery 2010; Orthopaedic Sports Medicine 2007; **Med School:** Columbia P&S 1968; **Resid:** Surgery, UCSF-Moffitt Hosp 1970; Orthopaedic Surgery, NY Orth Hosp 1976; **Fellow:** NY Orth Hosp 1973; Hand Surgery, NY Orth Hosp 1977; **Fac Appt:** Clin Prof OrS, UMDNJ-RW Johnson Med Sch

Hematology

Toomey, Kathleen C MD (Hem) - **Spec Exp:** Breast Cancer; **Hospital:** Somerset Med Ctr, St. Peter's Univ Hosp; **Address:** Steepchase Cancer Ctr, 30 Rehill Ave, Ste 2500, Somerville, NJ 08876; **Phone:** 908-927-8700; **Board Cert:** Internal Medicine 1982; Medical Oncology 1987; Hematology 2003; **Med School:** Italy 1978; **Resid:** Internal Medicine, St Peters Med Ctr 1982; **Fellow:** Hematology & Oncology, UMDNJ-Rutgers Med Sch 1985

Infectious Disease

Herman, David J MD (Inf) - **Spec Exp:** Lyme Disease; AIDS/HIV; Travel Medicine; **Hospital:** Univ Med Ctr Princeton at Plainsboro, Somerset Med Ctr; **Address:** 105 Raider Blvd, Ste 101, Hillsborough, NJ 08844; **Phone:** 908-281-0221; **Board Cert:** Internal Medicine 1988; Infectious Disease 2010; **Med School:** Univ MO-Columbia Sch Med 1985; **Resid:** Internal Medicine, Northwestern Univ 1988; **Fellow:** Infectious Disease, Univ Minn 1991; **Fac Appt:** Assoc Clin Prof Med, UMDNJ-RW Johnson Med Sch

Nahass, Ronald MD (Inf) - **Spec Exp:** HIV; Hepatitis B & C; Diagnostic Problems; Bone Infections; **Hospital:** Robert Wood Johnson Univ Hosp - New Brunswick, Univ Med Ctr Princeton at Plainsboro; **Address:** 105 Raider Blvd, Ste 101, Hillsborough, NJ 08844-4254; **Phone:** 908-281-0221; **Board Cert:** Internal Medicine 1985; Infectious Disease 1988; **Med School:** UMDNJ-RW Johnson Med Sch 1982; **Resid:** Internal Medicine, RWJ Univ Hosp 1986; **Fellow:** Infectious Disease, RWJ Univ Hosp 1988

Internal Medicine

Bell, Kevin E MD (IM) *PCP* - **Spec Exp:** Lyme Disease; Hypertension; **Hospital:** Overlook Med Ctr (page 92); **Address:** 10 Mountain Blvd, Warren, NJ 07059-2639; **Phone:** 908-226-9000; **Board Cert:** Internal Medicine 1978; **Med School:** Columbia P&S 1975; **Resid:** Internal Medicine, Univ Wisconsin Med Ctr 1979; **Fac Appt:** Asst Clin Prof Med, Columbia P&S

Bonaventura, Lisa M MD (IM) *PCP* - **Spec Exp:** Concierge Medicine; **Hospital:** Morristown Med Ctr (page 92); **Address:** 2345 Lamington Rd, Ste 104, Bedminster, NJ 07921-2612; **Phone:** 908-781-9661; **Board Cert:** Internal Medicine 1989; **Med School:** Univ Cincinnati 1986; **Resid:** Internal Medicine, Morristown Meml Hosp 1989

Ferrante, Maurice A MD (IM) *PCP* - **Hospital:** Overlook Med Ctr (page 92); **Address:** 8 Mountain Blvd, Warren, NJ 07059; **Phone:** 908-561-8600; **Board Cert:** Internal Medicine 2010; **Med School:** Jefferson Med Coll 1987; **Resid:** Internal Medicine, Univ Maryland Med Ctr 1990

Neiman, Deborah L MD (IM) - **Spec Exp:** Obesity; Weight Management; **Hospital:** Somerset Med Ctr, Morristown Med Ctr (page 92); **Address:** 311 Omni Drive, Hillsborough, NJ 08844; **Phone:** 908-281-0632; **Board Cert:** Internal Medicine 1987; **Med School:** NY Med Coll 1984; **Resid:** Internal Medicine, Morristown Meml Hosp 1987

Sanchez-Catanese, Betty MD (IM) *PCP* - **Hospital:** Somerset Med Ctr; **Address:** 315 E Main St, Somerville, NJ 08876-3109; **Phone:** 908-722-3442; **Board Cert:** Internal Medicine 1987; **Med School:** NY Med Coll 1983; **Resid:** Internal Medicine, Northshore Univ Hosp 1986

Medical Oncology

Hamilton, Audrey M MD (Onc) - **Spec Exp:** Hematologic Malignancies; **Hospital:** Meml Sloan-Kettering Cancer Ctr (page 116); **Address:** Meml Sloan Kettering Cancer Ctr, 136 Mountain View Blvd, Basking Ridge, NJ 07920; **Phone:** 908-542-3000; **Board Cert:** Internal Medicine 1986; Hematology 2004; Medical Oncology 2005; **Med School:** Harvard Med Sch 1983; **Resid:** Internal Medicine, Brigham & Womens Hosp 1986; **Fellow:** Hematology & Oncology, NY Hosp-Cornell Med Ctr 1989

Wu, Hen-Vai MD (Onc) - **Spec Exp:** Colon & Rectal Cancer; Lung Cancer; Lymphoma, Non-Hodgkin's; **Hospital:** Somerset Med Ctr, St. Peter's Univ Hosp; **Address:** Steepchase Cancer Ctr, 30 Rehill Ave, Ste 2500, Somerville, NJ 08876; **Phone:** 908-927-8700; **Board Cert:** Internal Medicine 1977; Hematology 1978; Medical Oncology 1981; **Med School:** Taiwan 1972; **Resid:** Internal Medicine, Mount Vernon Hosp 1974; Internal Medicine, Helene Fuld Med Ctr 1975; **Fellow:** Hematology, CMDNJ-Rutgers 1977; Medical Oncology, CMDNJ-Rutgers 1980; **Fac Appt:** Asst Clin Prof Med, UMDNJ-Univ Med Dent NJ

Nephrology

Kabis, Suzanne M MD (Nep) - **Spec Exp:** Lupus Nephritis; Hypertension; Glomerulonephritis; Kidney Disease in Pregnancy; **Hospital:** Robert Wood Johnson Univ Hosp - New Brunswick, St. Peter's Univ Hosp; **Address:** 1350 Hamilton St, Somerset, NJ 08873; **Phone:** 732-246-2626; **Board Cert:** Internal Medicine 1982; Nephrology 1988; **Med School:** UMDNJ-Rutgers Med Sch 1979; **Resid:** Internal Medicine, NC Meml Hosp 1982; **Fellow:** Nephrology, NC Meml Hosp 1985; **Fac Appt:** Asst Clin Prof Med

Neurology

Friedlander, Devin S MD (N) - **Spec Exp:** Headache; Botox Therapy; **Hospital:** St. Peter's Univ Hosp; **Address:** Princeton & Rutgers Neurology, 77 Veronica Ave, Ste 102, Somerset, NJ 08873-3448; **Phone:** 732-246-1311; **Board Cert:** Neurology 2003; **Med School:** UMDNJ-RW Johnson Med Sch 1989; **Resid:** Neurology, Albert Einstein Coll Med Affil Hosps 1993; **Fellow:** Neurological Physiology, Lyons VA Med Ctr 1994

Neuroradiology

Lee, S Howard MD (NRad) - **Hospital:** Somerset Med Ctr; **Address:** Radiology Dept, 110 Rehill Ave, Somerville, NJ 08876; **Phone:** 908-685-2930; **Board Cert:** Diagnostic Radiology 1971; Neuroradiology 2007; **Med School:** South Korea 1964; **Resid:** Radiology, Jefferson Hosp 1967; Radiology, Graduate Hosp 1970; **Fellow:** Neurological Radiology, Philadelphia Genl Hosp 1972; **Fac Appt:** Clin Prof Rad

Obstetrics & Gynecology

Sanderson, Rhonda A MD (ObG) - **Spec Exp:** Gynecology Only; **Hospital:** Overlook Med Ctr (page 92); **Address:** 8 Mountain Blvd, Warren, NJ 07059; **Phone:** 908-754-5775; **Board Cert:** Obstetrics & Gynecology 2006; **Med School:** Hahnemann Univ 1980; **Resid:** Obstetrics & Gynecology, Womens/Infants Hosp 1984

Ophthalmology

Angrist, Richard C MD (Oph) - **Spec Exp:** Cataract Surgery; Glaucoma; Eyelid/Tear Duct Disorders; Ophthalmic Plastic Surgery; **Hospital:** Robert Wood Johnson Univ Hosp - New Brunswick, Kimball Med Ctr; **Address:** 1527 State Route 27, Ste 2600, Somerset, NJ 08873; **Phone:** 732-246-1050; **Board Cert:** Ophthalmology 1985; **Med School:** Albany Med Coll 1979; **Resid:** Ophthalmology, NY Eye& Ear Infirm 1983; **Fellow:** Ophthalmic Plastic & Reconstructive Surgery, Univ Wisconsin 1984

Salz, Alan G MD (Oph) - **Spec Exp:** LASIK-Refractive Surgery; Cataract Surgery-Lens Implant; **Hospital:** Somerset Med Ctr; **Address:** The Eye Specialists, 31 Monroe St, Bridgewater, NJ 08807; **Phone:** 908-231-1110; **Board Cert:** Ophthalmology 1987; **Med School:** Boston Univ 1981; **Resid:** Ophthalmology, Wills Eye Hosp 1985

Orthopaedic Surgery

Butler, Mark S MD (OrS) - **Spec Exp:** Trauma; Foot & Ankle Surgery; **Hospital:** Robert Wood Johnson Univ Hosp - New Brunswick, St. Peter's Univ Hosp; **Address:** University Orthopaedic Assocs, 2 Worlds Fair Drive, Somerset, NJ 08873; **Phone:** 732-537-0909; **Board Cert:** Orthopaedic Surgery 2004; **Med School:** UMDNJ-RW Johnson Med Sch 1984; **Resid:** Orthopaedic Surgery, RW Johnson Univ Hosp 1989; **Fellow:** Orthopaedic Trauma Surgery, Maryland Inst EMS 1990; Foot & Ankle Surgery, Maryland Inst EMS 1990; **Fac Appt:** Assoc Prof OrS, UMDNJ-RW Johnson Med Sch

D'Agostini Jr, Robert J MD (OrS) - **Spec Exp:** Joint Replacement; Sports Medicine; **Hospital:** Morristown Med Ctr (page 92); **Address:** Bedminster Orthopaedic & Sports Medicine, 1590 Route 206 N, Bedminster, NJ 07921; **Phone:** 908-234-2002; **Board Cert:** Orthopaedic Surgery 2008; Sports Medicine 2009; **Med School:** UMDNJ-RW Johnson Med Sch 1980; **Resid:** Orthopaedic Surgery, Georgetown Univ Hosp 1985

Dwyer, James W MD (OrS) - **Spec Exp:** Spinal Surgery; Minimally Invasive Spinal Surgery; Spinal Disc Replacement; Spinal Reconstructive Surgery; **Hospital:** Somerset Med Ctr, Univ Hosp-UMDNJ—Newark; **Address:** NJ Spine Institute, 1 Robertson Drive, Ste 11, Bedminster, NJ 07921; **Phone:** 908-722-0822; **Board Cert:** Orthopaedic Surgery 2003; **Med School:** UMDNJ-NJ Med Sch, Newark 1982; **Resid:** Orthopaedic Surgery, UMDNJ Affil Hosps 1989; **Fellow:** Spinal Surgery, Seton Med Ctr/St Marys Spine Ctr 1990; **Fac Appt:** Asst Clin Prof OrS, UMDNJ-NJ Med Sch, Newark

Johnson, Albert MD (OrS) - **Spec Exp:** Hand Surgery; Hip & Knee Replacement; **Hospital:** Somerset Med Ctr; **Address:** Somerset Orthopaedic Assocs, 1081 Route 22 West, Bridgewater, NJ 08807; **Phone:** 908-722-0822; **Board Cert:** Orthopaedic Surgery 1977; **Med School:** India 1967; **Resid:** Surgery, Tufts-New England Med Ctr 1972; Orthopaedic Surgery, Tufts-New England Med Ctr 1975; **Fellow:** Hand Surgery, Roosevelt Hosp 1975

Tria Jr, Alfred J MD (OrS) - **Spec Exp:** Knee Surgery; **Hospital:** St. Peter's Univ Hosp, Robert Wood Johnson Univ Hosp - New Brunswick; **Address:** 1527 Route 27, Ste 1300, Somerset, NJ 08873; **Phone:** 732-249-4444; **Board Cert:** Orthopaedic Surgery 1980; **Med School:** Harvard Med Sch 1972; **Resid:** Surgery, Roosevelt Hosp 1975; Orthopaedic Surgery, New York Hosp 1978; **Fellow:** Knee Surgery, Hosp Special Surg 1979; **Fac Appt:** Clin Prof OrS, UMDNJ-RW Johnson Med Sch

Otolaryngology

Lazar, Amy MD (Oto) - **Spec Exp:** Sinus Disorders; Endoscopic Sinus Surgery; **Hospital:** Somerset Med Ctr; **Address:** ENT & Allergy Assocs, 56 Union Ave, Ste 1, Somerville, NJ 08876-2096; **Phone:** 908-722-1022; **Board Cert:** Otolaryngology 1999; **Med School:** Ros Franklin Univ/Chicago Med Sch 1992; **Resid:** Otolaryngology, Manhattan EE&T Hosp 1995; Otolaryngology, Boston Med Ctr 1998

Pain Medicine

Rudman, Michael E MD (PM) - **Spec Exp:** Pain-Back; Pain-Chronic; Complex Regional Pain Syndromes; **Hospital:** Morristown Med Ctr (page 92); **Address:** New Jersey Pain Consultants, 175 Morristown Rd, Basking Ridge, NJ 07920; **Phone:** 908-630-0175; **Board Cert:** Pain Medicine 2007; Anesthesiology 1993; **Med School:** Penn State Coll Med 1988; **Resid:** Anesthesiology, Hosp Univ Penn 1992

Pediatric Pulmonology

Turcios, Nelson L MD (PPul) - **Spec Exp:** Breathing Disorders; Cough-Chronic; Cystic Fibrosis; Ciliary Dyskinesia; **Hospital:** Somerset Med Ctr, St. Peter's Univ Hosp; **Address:** 282 E Main St, Pediatric Pulmonology & Cystic Fibrosis, Somerville, NJ 08876; **Phone:** 908-526-5212; **Board Cert:** Pediatrics 1982; Pediatric Pulmonology 2007; **Med School:** El Salvador 1973; **Resid:** Pediatrics, Univ Mississippi Med Ctr 1978; Pediatrics, Univ Maryland Hosp 1980; **Fellow:** Pediatric Pulmonology, Childrens Hosp 1982; **Fac Appt:** Assoc Prof Ped, UMDNJ-NJ Med Sch, Newark

Pediatrics

Katz, Andrea G MD (Ped) *PCP* - **Spec Exp:** Developmental & Behavioral Disorders; Chronic Illness; Obesity; **Hospital:** Overlook Med Ctr (page 92); **Address:** 76 Stirling Rd, Ste 201, Overlook Hosp-Pediatrics Div, Warren, NJ 07059; **Phone:** 908-755-5437; **Board Cert:** Pediatrics 2006; **Med School:** NY Med Coll 1988; **Resid:** Pediatrics, NY Hosp-Cornell Med Ctr 1991

Yorke, Eric R MD (Ped) *PCP* - **Hospital:** Somerset Med Ctr, Morristown Med Ctr (page 92); **Address:** Somerset Pediatric Group, 2345 Lamington Rd, Ste 101, Bedminster, NJ 07921; **Phone:** 908-470-1124; **Board Cert:** Pediatrics 2009; **Med School:** Columbia P&S 1982; **Resid:** Pediatrics, Babies Hosp-Columbia 1986

Plastic Surgery

Olson, Robert MD (PlS) - **Spec Exp:** Cleft Palate/Lip; Head & Neck Surgery; Wound Healing/Care; **Hospital:** St. Peter's Univ Hosp, Robert Wood Johnson Univ Hosp - New Brunswick; **Address:** 888 Easton Ave, Ste 6, Somerset, NJ 08873-1898; **Phone:** 732-418-1888; **Board Cert:** Plastic Surgery 1982; **Med School:** Univ Pennsylvania 1974; **Resid:** Surgery, Peter Bent Brigham Hosp 1979; Plastic Surgery, Mayo Clinic 1981; **Fac Appt:** Assoc Prof S, UMDNJ-RW Johnson Med Sch

Perry, Arthur W MD (PlS) - **Spec Exp:** Rhinoplasty; Eyelid Surgery; Liposuction; Abdominoplasty; **Hospital:** Robert Wood Johnson Univ Hosp - New Brunswick, Somerset Med Ctr; **Address:** 3055 Route 27, Franklin Park, NJ 08823-1315; **Phone:** 732-422-9600; **Board Cert:** Plastic Surgery 1989; **Med School:** Albany Med Coll 1981; **Resid:** Surgery, Beth Israel Hosp 1984; Plastic Surgery, Univ Chicago Hosps 1987; **Fellow:** Burn Surgery, New York Hosp-Cornell 1985; Cosmetic Plastic Surgery, Univ Miami/Baker-Gordon Assocs 1987; **Fac Appt:** Assoc Prof PlS, Columbia P&S

Psychiatry

Donnellan, Joseph A MD (Psyc) - **Spec Exp:** Eating Disorders; Obsessive-Compulsive Disorder; **Hospital:** Somerset Med Ctr; **Address:** 422 Courtyard Drive, Hillsborough, NJ 08844; **Phone:** 908-725-5595; **Board Cert:** Psychiatry 1991; **Med School:** UMDNJ-NJ Med Sch, Newark 1986; **Resid:** Psychiatry, UMDNJ Affil Hosp 1990; **Fac Appt:** Asst Clin Prof Psyc, UMDNJ-RW Johnson Med Sch

Rochford, Joseph MD (Psyc) - **Spec Exp:** Depression; Anxiety Disorders; Eating Disorders; **Hospital:** Somerset Med Ctr; **Address:** 407 Omni Drive, Hillsborough, NJ 08844; **Phone:** 908-359-2312; **Board Cert:** Psychiatry 1975; **Med School:** Yale Univ 1969; **Resid:** Psychiatry, Hosp Univ Penn 1973; **Fac Appt:** Assoc Clin Prof Psyc, UMDNJ-RW Johnson Med Sch

Pulmonary Disease

Arno, Louis J MD (Pul) - **Spec Exp:** Critical Care; **Hospital:** Somerset Med Ctr; **Address:** RespaCare, 489 Union Ave, Bridgewater, NJ 08807; **Phone:** 732-356-9950; **Board Cert:** Internal Medicine 2002; Pulmonary Disease 2006; Critical Care Medicine 2008; **Med School:** Grenada 1986; **Resid:** Internal Medicine, St Michaels Med Ctr 1990; **Fellow:** Pulmonary Disease, St Michaels Med Ctr 1992; Critical Care Medicine, St Michaels Med Ctr 1993

Gerhard, Harvey MD (Pul) - **Hospital:** Morristown Med Ctr (page 92); **Address:** The Pulmonary Group, 416 Mount Airy Rd, Basking Ridge, NJ 07920-2438; **Phone:** 908-766-6605; **Board Cert:** Internal Medicine 1977; **Med School:** Yale Univ 1974; **Resid:** Internal Medicine, Bellevue Hosp Ctr 1977; **Fellow:** Pulmonary Disease, Yale-New Haven Hosp 1979

Radiation Oncology

Braver, Joel K MD (RadRO) - **Spec Exp:** Prostate Cancer; Stereotactic Radiosurgery; Merkel Cell Carcinoma; **Hospital:** Somerset Med Ctr; **Address:** 30 Rehill Ave, Ste 1100, Steeplechase Cancer Center-Department of Radiation Oncology, Somerville, NJ 08876; **Phone:** 908-927-8777; **Board Cert:** Radiation Oncology 2006; **Med School:** UMDNJ-RW Johnson Med Sch 1991; **Resid:** Radiation Oncology, Montefiore Med Ctr 1996

Reproductive Endocrinology

Scott, Richard T MD (RE) - **Spec Exp:** Infertility; Infertility-IVF; Fertility Preservation in Cancer; **Hospital:** Morristown Med Ctr (page 92); **Address:** 140 Allen Rd, Basking Ridge, NJ 07920; **Phone:** 908-604-7800; **Board Cert:** Obstetrics & Gynecology 2011; Reproductive Endocrinology 2011; **Med School:** Univ VA Sch Med 1983; **Resid:** Obstetrics & Gynecology, Wilford Hall USAF Med Ctr 1987; **Fellow:** Reproductive Endocrinology, Jones Inst Reproductive Med 1989; **Fac Appt:** Clin Prof ObG

Treiser, Susan L MD/PhD (RE) - **Spec Exp:** Infertility; Infertility-IVF; **Hospital:** St. Peter's Univ Hosp; **Address:** IVF NJ Fertility & Gynecology Ctr, 81 Veronica Ave, Somerset, NJ 08873; **Phone:** 732-220-9060; **Board Cert:** Obstetrics & Gynecology 2011; Reproductive Endocrinology 2011; **Med School:** Georgetown Univ 1983; **Resid:** Obstetrics & Gynecology, UMDNJ Med Ctr 1988; **Fellow:** Reproductive Endocrinology, Columbia Presby Med Ctr 1990

Surgery

Drascher, Gary MD (S) - **Spec Exp:** Laparoscopic Surgery-Complex; Aneurysm; Carotid Artery Surgery; **Hospital:** Somerset Med Ctr, Robert Wood Johnson Univ Hosp - New Brunswick; **Address:** 30 Rehill Ave, Ste 3300, Somerville, NJ 08776; **Phone:** 908-927-8994; **Board Cert:** Surgery 2007; **Med School:** Mount Sinai Sch Med 1981; **Resid:** Internal Medicine, St Luke's-Roosevelt Hosp Ctr 1982; Surgery, St Luke's-Roosevelt Hosp Ctr 1987; **Fellow:** Vascular Surgery, Englewood Hosp 1989

Lanfranchi, Angela E MD (S) - **Spec Exp:** Breast Cancer; Breast Surgery; **Hospital:** Somerset Med Ctr; **Address:** Surgical Assocs Central NJ, 30 Rehill Ave, Ste 3300, Somerville, NJ 08776; **Phone:** 908-927-8994; **Board Cert:** Surgery 2003; **Med School:** Georgetown Univ 1975; **Resid:** Family Medicine, Somerset Hosp 1978; Surgery, SUNY-Univ Affil Hosps 1982; **Fellow:** Vascular Surgery, Nassau Hosp 1983

McManus, Susan A MD (S) - **Spec Exp:** Breast Surgery; Cancer Surgery; **Hospital:** St. Peter's Univ Hosp; **Address:** 1553 Highway 27, Ste 3100, Somerset, NJ 08873; **Phone:** 732-846-3300; **Board Cert:** Surgery 2006; **Med School:** Mexico 1979; **Resid:** Surgery, Beth Israel Med Ctr 1985; **Fac Appt:** Asst Clin Prof S, UMDNJ-RW Johnson Med Sch

Thoracic & Cardiac Surgery

Caccavale, Robert J MD (T&CS) - **Spec Exp:** Video Assisted Thoracic Surgery (VATS); **Hospital:** Somerset Med Ctr, CentraState Med Ctr; **Address:** 35 Clyde Rd, Ste 104, Somerset, NJ 08873; **Phone:** 732-247-3002; **Board Cert:** Thoracic Surgery 2008; **Med School:** SUNY Buffalo 1981; **Resid:** Surgery, NYU Med Ctr 1984; Surgery, Booth Meml Med Ctr 1986; **Fellow:** Thoracic Surgery, Downstate Med Ctr 1988; **Fac Appt:** Assoc Clin Prof S, UMDNJ-RW Johnson Med Sch

Urology

Barone, Joseph G MD (U) - **Spec Exp:** Robotic Surgery-Pediatric; Urinary Reconstruction; Incontinence; Hypospadias; **Hospital:** Robert Wood Johnson Univ Hosp - New Brunswick, Univ Med Ctr Princeton at Plainsboro; **Address:** RWJ Dept Urology, 1 Worlds Fair Drive Fl 1, Somerset, NJ 08873; **Phone:** 732-235-7960; **Board Cert:** Urology 2009; Pediatric Urology 2009; **Med School:** UMDNJ-Rutgers Med Sch 1989; **Resid:** Urology, R W Johnson Univ Hosp 1993; **Fellow:** Pediatric Urology, Emory Univ 1994; **Fac Appt:** Assoc Prof U, UMDNJ-RW Johnson Med Sch

Catanese, Anthony J MD (U) - **Spec Exp:** Urologic Cancer; Kidney Cancer; **Hospital:** Somerset Med Ctr, St. Peter's Univ Hosp; **Address:** Partners in Urology, 315 E Main St, Somerville, NJ 08876-3109; **Phone:** 908-722-6900; **Board Cert:** Urology 2009; **Med School:** NY Med Coll 1983; **Resid:** Surgery, NYU Med Ctr 1985; Urology, NYU Med Ctr 1989

The Best in American Medicine
www.CastleConnolly.com

Union

Trinitas Regional Medical Center

225 WILLIAMSON STREET | ELIZABETH, NEW JERSEY 07207
PH 908.994.5000 | WWW.TRINITASRMC.ORG

Caring For You In Every Way

SPONSORSHIP: Trinitas Regional Medical Center is a voluntary not-for-profit Catholic teaching hospital sponsored by the Sisters of Charity of Saint Elizabeth in partnership with Elizabethtown Healthcare Foundation.

BEDS: 556   *Accredited by The Joint Commission*

MEDICAL STAFF

Trinitas Regional Medical Center has nearly 500 physicians and over 40 residents on its medical staff. Trinitas is a major clinical site for the Seton Hall School of Health and Medical Sciences' Internal Medicine Residency Program.

CENTERS OF EXCELLENCE:

Behavioral Health & Psychiatry: Behavioral Health services at Trinitas are among the most comprehensive in New Jersey and include a full range of inpatient and outpatient psychiatric care for seniors, adults, adolescents and children.

Cancer Care: The Trinitas Comprehensive Cancer Center offers the most advanced medical and radiation technology available, including Rapid Arc radiotherapy, to cancer patients. An interdisciplinary team works with each patient to develop a care plan encompassing the latest diagnostic treatment options, medical technology, clinical trials and integrative therapy.

Cardiology: Trinitas maintains a full-service cardiac facility for the intensive care of patients with heart disease, including elective angioplasty, a cardiac care unit, intermediate coronary care unit, cardiac catheterization lab, non-invasive cardiology services, full-service emergency department, and cardiac rehabilitation services.

Maternal & Child Health: Trinitas offers a Level II Intermediate Care Nursery, a 24-hour in-house pediatrician and obstetrician, and midwifery services. Inpatient care for child/adolescent psychiatric patients is also offered.

Renal Care: Trinitas is committed to patients experiencing kidney failure, and initiated the THRIVE early intervention program to reach high-risk patients.

Seniors Services: The Trinitas commitment to seniors takes many forms, most recently the establishment of the Acute Care for the Elderly (ACE) nursing unit. The Seniors First Membership Program offers special gifts and invitations to special events.

School of Nursing: The third largest school of nursing in the United States, the Trinitas School of Nursing, affiliated with Union County College, is known for an outstanding nursing education program that was recently designated a Center of Excellence in Nursing Education by the National League for Nursing.

Sleep Disorders: The Comprehensive Sleep Disorders Center provides monitored, fully-attended diagnostic sleep studies designed to rule out physical, non-stress related symptoms that may prevent restful sleep in adults and children. Two locations are offered, including the first hotel-based sleep center in New Jersey.

Women's Services: In addition to the latest modalities in digital mammography, breast biopsy, breast MRI, bone density screening and ultrasound, women can visit Trinitas for cosmetic and reconstructive surgery and innovative surgical care using the da Vinci® Robotic Surgical System for female incontinence and prolapse.

Wound Healing/Diabetes Management: The Trinitas Center for Wound Healing and Hyperbaric Medicine has one of the highest heal rates in the nation. Specially-trained certified nurses and physicians treat those with chronic, hard-to-heal wounds. Recognized by the American Diabetes Association, the Diabetes Management Center offers a high quality education program for diabetics.

Allergy & Immunology

Bielory, Leonard MD (A&I) - **Spec Exp:** Dry Eye Syndrome; Asthma; Eye Allergy; Autoimmune Occular Disorders; **Hospital:** Saint Barnabas Med Ctr; **Address:** 400 Mountain Ave, Springfield, NJ 07081; **Phone:** 973-912-9817; **Board Cert:** Internal Medicine 1984; Allergy & Immunology 1985; Clinical & Laboratory Immunology 1986; **Med School:** UMDNJ-NJ Med Sch, Newark 1980; **Resid:** Internal Medicine, Univ Md Hosp 1982; Hematology, Natl Inst Hlth 1983; **Fellow:** Allergy & Immunology, Natl Inst Hlth 1985; Diagnostic Lab Immunology, Natl Inst Hlth 1985; **Fac Appt:** Prof A&I, UMDNJ-NJ Med Sch, Newark

Brown, David K MD (A&I) - **Spec Exp:** Asthma; Sinus Disorders; Headache; **Hospital:** Overlook Med Ctr (page 92); **Address:** Allergy Diagnostic & Treatment Center, 33 Overlook Rd, Ste 307, Summit, NJ 07901-3563; **Phone:** 908-522-9696; **Board Cert:** Internal Medicine 1984; Allergy & Immunology 1987; **Med School:** Med Coll OH 1981; **Resid:** Internal Medicine, Overlook Hosp 1984; **Fellow:** Allergy & Immunology, St Luke's-Roosevelt Hosp Ctr 1986

Goodman, Alan J MD (A&I) - **Spec Exp:** Rhinitis; Sinus Disorders; Asthma; **Hospital:** Saint Barnabas Med Ctr; **Address:** 381 Chestnut St, Union, NJ 07083; **Phone:** 908-688-6200; **Board Cert:** Internal Medicine 1985; Allergy & Immunology 2009; **Med School:** SUNY Upstate Med Univ 1982; **Resid:** Internal Medicine, Washington Hosp Ctr 1985; **Fellow:** Allergy & Immunology, St Luke's-Roosevelt Hosp Ctr 1988

Le Benger, Kerry S MD (A&I) - **Spec Exp:** Asthma; Allergy; **Hospital:** Overlook Med Ctr (page 92), Saint Barnabas Med Ctr; **Address:** Summit Medical Group, 1 Diamond Hill Rd, Berkely Heights, NJ 07922; **Phone:** 908-277-8681; **Board Cert:** Internal Medicine 1983; Allergy & Immunology 1985; **Med School:** NY Med Coll 1980; **Resid:** Internal Medicine, Lenox Hill Hosp 1983; **Fellow:** Allergy & Immunology, New York Hosp 1985; **Fac Appt:** Asst Clin Prof Med, Mount Sinai Sch Med

Maccia, Clement MD (A&I) - **Spec Exp:** Rhinitis; Asthma; Urticaria; Eczema; **Hospital:** JFK Med Ctr - Edison, Robert Wood Johnson Univ Hosp - New Brunswick; **Address:** Asthma, Sinus & Allergy Centers, 19 Holly St, Cranford, NJ 07016-2158; **Phone:** 908-276-0666; **Board Cert:** Pediatrics 1980; Allergy & Immunology 1985; **Med School:** Italy 1971; **Resid:** Pediatrics, Muhlenberg Med Ctr 1974; **Fellow:** Allergy & Immunology, Univ Hosp 1976; **Fac Appt:** Clin Prof A&I

Mendelson, Joel S MD (A&I) - **Spec Exp:** Infectious Disease; Food Allergy; Urticaria; Eczema; **Hospital:** Saint Barnabas Med Ctr, Overlook Med Ctr (page 92); **Address:** 1124 Springfield Ave, Mountainside, NJ 07092; **Phone:** 908-233-4477; **Board Cert:** Pediatrics 1987; Allergy & Immunology 2009; Pediatric Infectious Disease 2005; **Med School:** Dominican Republic 1982; **Resid:** Pediatrics, St Luke's-Roosevelt Hosp 1985; **Fellow:** Allergy & Immunology, UMDNJ Med Ctr 1987; Infectious Disease, UMDNJ Med Ctr 1987; **Fac Appt:** Asst Prof Ped, Grenada

Cardiovascular Disease

Kalischer, Alan L MD (Cv) - **Spec Exp:** Echocardiography; Nuclear Cardiology; Coronary Artery Disease; Arrhythmias; **Hospital:** Overlook Med Ctr (page 92), JFK Med Ctr - Edison; **Address:** Fanwood-Westfield Cardiology, 313 South Ave, Ste 202, Fanwood, NJ 07023; **Phone:** 908-889-1900; **Board Cert:** Internal Medicine 1982; Cardiovascular Disease 1985; Echocardiography 2000; Nuclear Cardiology 2001; **Med School:** NY Med Coll 1977; **Resid:** Internal Medicine, Kings County Hosp 1980; **Fellow:** Cardiovascular Disease, Columbia-Presby Med Ctr 1984; **Fac Appt:** Asst Clin Prof Med, UMDNJ-RW Johnson Med Sch

Sachs, R Gregory MD (Cv) - **Spec Exp:** Heart Disease; Heart Valve Disease; Congenital Heart Disease-Adult; **Hospital:** Overlook Med Ctr (page 92), Morristown Med Ctr (page 92); **Address:** Summit Medical Group, 1 Diamond Hill Rd, Berkeley Heights, NJ 07922; **Phone:** 908-277-8713; **Board Cert:** Internal Medicine 1972; Cardiovascular Disease 1976; **Med School:** Georgetown Univ 1966; **Resid:** Internal Medicine, Georgetown Univ Hosp 1968; **Fellow:** Cardiovascular Disease, Emory Hosps 1970; Cardiovascular Disease, National Heart Hosp 1971; **Fac Appt:** Asst Clin Prof Med, Columbia P&S

Sheris, Steven J MD (Cv) - **Spec Exp:** Echocardiography; Cardiac Stress Testing; Nuclear Cardiology; **Hospital:** Overlook Med Ctr (page 92), Morristown Med Ctr (page 92); **Address:** Assocs in Cardiovascular Disease, 29 South St, New Providence, NJ 07974; **Phone:** 908-464-4200; **Board Cert:** Internal Medicine 2003; Cardiovascular Disease 2007; Nuclear Cardiology 2003; **Med School:** UMDNJ-Rutgers Med Sch 1988; **Resid:** Internal Medicine, Natl Naval Med Ctr 1994; **Fellow:** Cardiovascular Disease, Georgetown Univ Med Ctr 1997

Slama, Robert D MD (Cv) - **Spec Exp:** Echocardiography; Preventive Cardiology; Nuclear Cardiology; **Hospital:** Overlook Med Ctr (page 92), Morristown Med Ctr (page 92); **Address:** Summit Med Grp, 1 Diamond Hill Rd, Berkeley Heights, NJ 07922; **Phone:** 908-277-8714; **Board Cert:** Internal Medicine 1974; Cardiovascular Disease 1977; **Med School:** Temple Univ 1971; **Resid:** Internal Medicine, Boston Med Ctr 1973; Internal Medicine, Georgetown Univ Hosp 1974; **Fellow:** Cardiovascular Disease, Boston Univ Med Ctr 1976

Stein, Elliott M MD (Cv) - **Hospital:** Overlook Med Ctr (page 92); **Address:** 211 Mountain Ave, Springfield, NJ 07081; **Phone:** 973-467-0005; **Board Cert:** Internal Medicine 1974; Cardiovascular Disease 1974; **Med School:** Jefferson Med Coll 1964; **Resid:** Internal Medicine, Mt Sinai Hosp 1969; Cardiovascular Disease, Mt Sinai Hosp 1971

Child & Adolescent Psychiatry

Greenberg, Rosalie MD (ChAP) - **Spec Exp:** Bipolar/Mood Disorders; ADD/ADHD; **Hospital:** Overlook Med Ctr (page 92); **Address:** 33 Overlook Rd, Ste 406, Summit, NJ 07901; **Phone:** 908-598-0200; **Board Cert:** Psychiatry 1982; Child & Adolescent Psychiatry 1983; **Med School:** Columbia P&S 1976; **Resid:** Psychiatry, Columbia-Presby Hosp 1979; **Fellow:** Child & Adolescent Psychiatry, Columbia-Presby Hosp 1981; **Fac Appt:** Asst Clin Prof Psyc, Columbia P&S

Child Neurology

Traeger, Eveline C MD (ChiN) - **Spec Exp:** Autism; ADD/ADHD; Learning Disorders; **Hospital:** Children's Specialized Hosp; **Address:** Chldns Specialized Hosp, 150 New Providence Rd, Mountainside, NJ 07092; **Phone:** 908-233-3720; **Board Cert:** Child Neurology 2004; Clinical Genetics 1990; **Med School:** SUNY Buffalo 1984; **Resid:** Child Neurology, Yeshiva Univ 1986; Pediatrics, Jacobi Med Ctr 1988

Colon & Rectal Surgery

Groff, Walter MD (CRS) - **Spec Exp:** Colonoscopy; Rectal Cancer/Sphincter Preservation; **Hospital:** Overlook Med Ctr (page 92), Saint Barnabas Med Ctr; **Address:** 33 Overlook Rd, Ste 412, Summit, NJ 07901-3564; **Phone:** 908-598-0220; **Board Cert:** Colon & Rectal Surgery 1980; **Med School:** Albany Med Coll 1970; **Resid:** Surgery, St Vincent's Hosp 1979; Colon & Rectal Surgery, Muhlenberg Med Ctr 1980; **Fac Appt:** Assoc Prof S, Columbia P&S

Dermatology

Eisenberg, Richard R MD (D) - **Spec Exp:** Skin Cancer; Melanoma; Acne; **Hospital:** Overlook Med Ctr (page 92); **Address:** 40 Stirling Rd, Ste 203, Watchung, NJ 07069; **Phone:** 908-753-4144; **Board Cert:** Internal Medicine 1985; Dermatology 1989; **Med School:** Cornell Univ-Weill Med Coll 1982; **Resid:** Internal Medicine, NY Hosp-Cornell Med Ctr 1985; Dermatology, NY Hosp-Cornell/Meml Sloan Kettering Cancer Ctr 1989

Weinberger, George I MD (D) - **Spec Exp:** Skin Cancer; **Hospital:** Saint Barnabas Med Ctr; **Address:** 190 Greenbrook Rd, North Plainfield, NJ 07060-3903; **Phone:** 908-561-8070; **Board Cert:** Dermatology 1977; **Med School:** UMDNJ-NJ Med Sch, Newark 1973; **Resid:** Dermatology, Henry Ford Hosp 1977

Zirvi, Monib A MD (D) - **Spec Exp:** Cosmetic Dermatology; Skin Cancer; **Hospital:** Morristown Med Ctr (page 92), Overlook Med Ctr (page 92); **Address:** 1 Diamond Hill Rd, Berkeley Heights, NJ 07922; **Phone:** 908-273-4300; **Board Cert:** Dermatology 2004; **Med School:** Cornell Univ 2000; **Resid:** Dermatology, Univ Penn Affil Hosp 2003

Diagnostic Radiology

Grosso, Sue Jane R MD (DR) - **Spec Exp:** Breast Imaging; Nuclear Radiology; CT Body Scan; **Hospital:** Overlook Med Ctr (page 92); **Address:** Summit Med Grp, 1 Diamond Hill Rd, Berkeley Heights, NJ 07922; **Phone:** 908-273-4300; **Board Cert:** Diagnostic Radiology 1991; **Med School:** Harvard Med Sch 1985; **Resid:** Diagnostic Radiology, NYU Med Ctr 1990; **Fellow:** Breast Imaging, NYU Med Ctr 1991; Nuclear Medicine, NYU Med Ctr 1991

Endocrinology, Diabetes & Metabolism

Fuhrman, Robert MD (EDM) - **Spec Exp:** Diabetes; Thyroid Disorders; Osteoporosis; **Hospital:** Overlook Med Ctr (page 92); **Address:** 552 Westfield Ave, Westfield, NJ 07090-3312; **Phone:** 908-654-3377; **Board Cert:** Internal Medicine 1971; Endocrinology, Diabetes & Metabolism 1972; **Med School:** Ros Franklin Univ/Chicago Med Sch 1966; **Resid:** Internal Medicine, Mount Sinai Hosp 1970; Nuclear Medicine, VA Hospital 1970; **Fellow:** Endocrinology, Diabetes & Metabolism, Mount Sinai Hosp 1970; **Fac Appt:** Asst Clin Prof Med, UMDNJ-NJ Med Sch, Newark

Rosenbaum, Robert L MD (EDM) - **Spec Exp:** Thyroid Disorders; Diabetes; Osteoporosis; **Hospital:** Overlook Med Ctr (page 92); **Address:** Summit Med Grp, One Diamond Hill Rd, Berkeley Heights, NJ 07922-2104; **Phone:** 908-277-8667; **Board Cert:** Internal Medicine 1978; Endocrinology, Diabetes & Metabolism 1981; **Med School:** Columbia P&S 1975; **Resid:** Internal Medicine, Montefiore Hosp Med Ctr 1978; **Fellow:** Endocrinology, Diabetes & Metabolism, Montefiore Hosp Med Ctr 1980; **Fac Appt:** Asst Clin Prof Med, Mount Sinai Sch Med

Selinger, Sharon E MD (EDM) - **Spec Exp:** Diabetes; Thyroid Disorders; Pituitary Disorders; Osteoporosis; **Hospital:** Overlook Med Ctr (page 92); **Address:** Summit Endocrinology & Diabetes, 1 Springfield Ave, Ste 1A, Summit, NJ 07901; **Phone:** 908-273-8300; **Board Cert:** Internal Medicine 1984; Endocrinology, Diabetes & Metabolism 1987; **Med School:** Cornell Univ-Weill Med Coll 1981; **Resid:** Internal Medicine, Montefiore Hosp Med Ctr 1984; **Fellow:** Endocrinology, Diabetes & Metabolism, Bellevue Hosp-NYU Med Ctr 1986

Silverman, Mitchell MD (EDM) - **Spec Exp:** Diabetes; Thyroid Disorders; Adrenal Disorders; **Hospital:** Newark Beth Israel Med Ctr, Saint Barnabas Med Ctr; **Address:** 2333 Morris Ave, Ste B-109, Union, NJ 07083; **Phone:** 908-964-5511; **Board Cert:** Internal Medicine 1983; Endocrinology 1987; **Med School:** Duke Univ 1980; **Resid:** Internal Medicine, Emory Univ Hosp 1983; **Fellow:** Endocrinology, Diabetes & Metabolism, NY Hosp-Meml Sloan-Kettering 1988

Family Medicine

Eisenstat, Steven DO (FMed) *PCP* - **Spec Exp:** Osteoporosis; Hypertension; Alzheimer's Disease; **Hospital:** Overlook Med Ctr (page 92); **Address:** 1050 Galloping Hill Rd, Ste 202, Union, NJ 07083-7980; **Phone:** 908-688-4845; **Board Cert:** Family Medicine 1993; Geriatric Medicine 1991; **Med School:** Ohio State Univ 1984; **Resid:** Family Medicine, Union Hosp 1987; **Fac Appt:** Asst Clin Prof FMed, NY Coll Osteo Med

Podell, Richard N MD (FMed) - **Spec Exp:** Complementary Medicine; Nutrition & Disease Prevention/Control; Fibromyalgia; Chronic Fatigue Syndrome; **Hospital:** Overlook Med Ctr (page 92); **Address:** Medical Arts Center, 11 Overlook Rd, Ste 140, Summit, NJ 07901; **Phone:** 908-273-7770; **Board Cert:** Internal Medicine 1980; Family Medicine 2005; **Med School:** Harvard Med Sch 1969; **Resid:** Internal Medicine, Mt Sinai Hosp 1972; **Fellow:** Nutrition, Harvard Sch Pub Hlth 1973; **Fac Appt:** Clin Prof FMed, UMDNJ-RW Johnson Med Sch

Tabachnick, John F MD (FMed) *PCP* - **Hospital:** Overlook Med Ctr (page 92); **Address:** 563 Westfield Ave, Westfield, NJ 07090; **Phone:** 908-232-5858; **Board Cert:** Family Medicine 2007; **Med School:** Mount Sinai Sch Med 1979; **Resid:** Family Medicine, Overlook Hosp 1982; **Fac Appt:** Asst Clin Prof FMed, UMDNJ Sch Osteo Med

Gastroenterology

Barrison, Adam MD (Ge) - **Spec Exp:** Endoscopy; **Hospital:** Overlook Med Ctr (page 92); **Address:** Summit Medical Group, 1 Diamond Hill Rd, Berkeley Heights, NJ 07922; **Phone:** 908-227-8940; **Board Cert:** Gastroenterology 2011; **Med School:** NYU Sch Med 1995; **Resid:** Internal Medicine, Beth Israel Hosp 1998; **Fellow:** Gastroenterology, Boston Univ Med Ctr 1998

Ben-Menachem, Tamir MD (Ge) - **Spec Exp:** Endoscopy; Pancreatic/Biliary Endoscopy (ERCP); Endoscopic Ultrasound; **Hospital:** Overlook Med Ctr (page 92); **Address:** Summit Medical Group, 1 Diamond Hill Rd, Berkeley Heights, NJ 07922; **Phone:** 908-277-8940; **Board Cert:** Internal Medicine 2004; Gastroenterology 2007; **Med School:** Israel 1989; **Resid:** Internal Medicine, Henry Ford Hosp 1994; **Fellow:** Gastroenterology, Henry Ford Hosp 1997; **Fac Appt:** Assoc Prof Med

Feit, David MD (Ge) - **Spec Exp:** Hepatitis; **Hospital:** Hackensack Univ Med Ctr (page 96); **Address:** Hackensack Digestive Diseases Assocs, 385 Prospect Ave, Hackensack, NJ 07061; **Phone:** 201-488-3003; **Board Cert:** Internal Medicine 1984; Gastroenterology 1989; **Med School:** Columbia P&S 1981; **Resid:** Internal Medicine, Columbia-Presby Med Ctr 1984; **Fellow:** Gastroenterology, Columbia-Presby Med Ctr 1987

Goldenberg, David MD (Ge) - **Spec Exp:** Inflammatory Bowel Disease/Crohn's; Biliary Disease; Gastroesophageal Reflux Disease (GERD); **Hospital:** JFK Med Ctr - Edison, Somerset Med Ctr; **Address:** Gastroenterology Associates, 1165 Park Ave, Plainfield, NJ 07060-3010; **Phone:** 908-754-2992; **Board Cert:** Internal Medicine 1977; Gastroenterology 1981; **Med School:** NY Med Coll 1974; **Resid:** Internal Medicine, Metropolitan Hosp 1977; **Fellow:** Gastroenterology, Emory Univ Hosp 1980

Kerner, Michael B MD (Ge) - **Spec Exp:** Colonoscopy; Biliary Disease; Gastroesophageal Reflux Disease (GERD); Inflammatory Bowel Disease; **Hospital:** Overlook Med Ctr (page 92), Morristown Med Ctr (page 92); **Address:** 25 Morris Ave, Springfield, NJ 07081-1406; **Phone:** 973-467-1313; **Board Cert:** Internal Medicine 1975; Gastroenterology 1977; **Med School:** Wake Forest Univ 1971; **Resid:** Internal Medicine, NYU Med Ctr 1974; **Fellow:** Gastroenterology, Manhattan VA-Bellevue Hosp 1976; **Fac Appt:** Asst Clin Prof Med, Mount Sinai Sch Med

Mahal, Pradeep MD (Ge) - **Spec Exp:** Gastrointestinal Cancer; **Hospital:** Overlook Med Ctr (page 92), Trinitas Reg Med Ctr (page 870); **Address:** 1308 Morris Ave, Ste 202, Union, NJ 07083; **Phone:** 908-851-6767; **Board Cert:** Gastroenterology 1981; Internal Medicine 1978; Geriatric Medicine 2002; Medical Oncology 1983; **Med School:** India 1975; **Resid:** Internal Medicine, UMDNJ Univ Hosp 1978; **Fellow:** Medical Oncology, MD Anderson Tumor Inst 1980; Gastroenterology, MD Anderson Tumor Inst 1980

Tempera, Patrick G MD (Ge) - **Spec Exp:** Biliary Disease; Pancreatic Disease; Gastroesophageal Reflux Disease (GERD); **Hospital:** Overlook Med Ctr (page 92), Somerset Med Ctr; **Address:** 1308 Morris Ave, Ste 102, Union, NJ 07083; **Phone:** 908-851-2771; **Board Cert:** Gastroenterology 2004; **Med School:** Grenada 1986; **Resid:** Surgery, Brooklyn Hosp 1987; Internal Medicine, Seton Hall Univ Hosp 1990; **Fellow:** Gastroenterology, Seton Hall Univ Hosp 1992; **Fac Appt:** Assoc Prof Med, Seton Hall Univ Sch Hlth & Med Scis

Geriatric Medicine

Khimani, Karim J MD (Ger) *PCP* - **Hospital:** Trinitas Reg Med Ctr (page 870); **Address:** 240 Williamson St, Ste 306, Elizabeth, NJ 07202; **Phone:** 908-352-5071; **Board Cert:** Internal Medicine 1986; Geriatric Medicine 2003; Hospice & Palliative Medicine 2008; **Med School:** Dominican Republic 1982; **Resid:** Internal Medicine, St Elizabeth Hosp 1985

Solomon, Robert B MD (Ger) *PCP* - **Spec Exp:** Alzheimer's Disease; Osteoporosis; **Hospital:** Trinitas Reg Med Ctr (page 870), Overlook Med Ctr (page 92); **Address:** 744 Galloping Hill Rd, Roselle Park, NJ 07204-1758; **Phone:** 908-241-0044; **Board Cert:** Internal Medicine 1980; Geriatric Medicine 2008; **Med School:** SUNY Hlth Sci Ctr 1977; **Resid:** Internal Medicine, Westchester Med Ctr 1980; **Fellow:** Geriatric Medicine, NY Hosp 1981

Hematology

Kessler, William MD (Hem) - **Hospital:** Trinitas Reg Med Ctr (page 870); **Address:** 225 Williamson St, Elizabeth, NJ 07207; **Phone:** 908-994-8773; **Board Cert:** Internal Medicine 1978; Hematology 1980; **Med School:** Albert Einstein Coll Med 1975; **Resid:** Internal Medicine, UMDNJ-Newark 1978; **Fellow:** Hematology, VA Hosp 1979

Infectious Disease

Farrer, William Eric MD (Inf) - **Spec Exp:** AIDS/HIV; Diabetic Leg/Foot Infections; Travel Medicine; **Hospital:** Trinitas Reg Med Ctr (page 870); **Address:** 240 Williamson St, Ste 502, Elizabeth, NJ 07202; **Phone:** 908-994-5300; **Board Cert:** Internal Medicine 1978; Infectious Disease 1980; **Med School:** Harvard Med Sch 1975; **Resid:** Internal Medicine, Montefiore Med Ctr 1978; **Fellow:** Infectious Disease, Montefiore Med Ctr 1980; **Fac Appt:** Assoc Prof Med, Seton Hall Univ Sch Hlth & Med Scis

Greenman, James L MD (Inf) - **Spec Exp:** AIDS/HIV; Lyme Disease; **Hospital:** Overlook Med Ctr (page 92); **Address:** Medical Diagnostic Associates, 525 Central Ave, Ste C, Westfield, NJ 07090; **Phone:** 908-233-0895; **Board Cert:** Internal Medicine 1985; Infectious Disease 1988; **Med School:** Albert Einstein Coll Med 1982; **Resid:** Internal Medicine, Columbia-Presby Med Ctr 1985; **Fellow:** Infectious Disease, Montefiore Med Ctr 1988

Roland, Robert DO (Inf) - **Spec Exp:** AIDS/HIV; Travel Medicine; Hepatitis C; **Hospital:** Overlook Med Ctr (page 92), Robert Wood Johnson Univ Hosp at Rahway; **Address:** Overlook Hosp Wound Healing Program, 11 Overlook Rd, MAC II, Ste LL 101, Summit, NJ 07901; **Phone:** 908-522-5900; **Board Cert:** Internal Medicine 1990; Infectious Disease 1992; **Med School:** Kirksville Coll Osteo Med 1985; **Resid:** Internal Medicine, Union Hosp 1989; **Fellow:** Infectious Disease, Kennedy Meml Hosp 1991; **Fac Appt:** Asst Clin Prof Med, NY Coll Osteo Med

Internal Medicine

Alterman, Lloyd H MD (IM) - **Spec Exp:** Hypertension; Kidney Disease-Chronic; **Hospital:** Overlook Med Ctr (page 92); **Address:** 1 Diamond Hill Rd, Berkeley Heights, NJ 07922; **Phone:** 908-277-8683; **Board Cert:** Internal Medicine 1980; Nephrology 1982; **Med School:** Wayne State Univ 1977; **Resid:** Internal Medicine, Overlook Hosp 1980; **Fellow:** Nephrology, Montefiore Med Ctr 1982

DiGiacomo, William A MD (IM) *PCP* - **Hospital:** Saint Michael's Med Ctr, Overlook Med Ctr (page 92); **Address:** 2801 Morris Ave, Union, NJ 07083; **Phone:** 908-851-2500; **Board Cert:** Internal Medicine 1978; **Med School:** Mexico 1974; **Resid:** Internal Medicine, St Michaels Med Ctr 1978; **Fac Appt:** Assoc Prof Med, Seton Hall Univ Sch Hlth & Med Scis

Feldman, Jeffrey N MD (IM) - **Spec Exp:** Kidney Disease-Chronic; Cholesterol/Lipid Disorders; Diabetes; Hypertension; **Hospital:** Overlook Med Ctr (page 92); **Address:** 440 Chestnut St, Fl 1, Union, NJ 07083-9306; **Phone:** 908-686-9330; **Board Cert:** Internal Medicine 1979; Nephrology 1982; **Med School:** Hahnemann Univ 1976; **Resid:** Internal Medicine, Bronx Municipal Hosp 1979; **Fellow:** Nephrology, SUNY Hlth Sci Ctr 1981

Goodgold, Abraham MD (IM) *PCP* - **Hospital:** Trinitas Reg Med Ctr (page 870), Robert Wood Johnson Univ Hosp at Rahway; **Address:** Elizabeth Medical Group, 310 W Jersey St, Elizabeth, NJ 07202-1832; **Phone:** 908-351-2222; **Board Cert:** Internal Medicine 1977; **Med School:** NYU Sch Med 1973; **Resid:** Infectious Disease, Montefiore Med Ctr 1976; **Fellow:** Endocrinology, Mt Sinai Med Ctr 1978

Maglaras, Nicholas C MD (IM) - **Hospital:** Trinitas Reg Med Ctr (page 870); **Address:** 236 E Westfield Ave, Ste 5, Roselle Park, NJ 07204; **Phone:** 908-245-8222; **Board Cert:** Internal Medicine 2003; Pulmonary Disease 2006; **Med School:** Grenada 1987; **Resid:** Internal Medicine, Elmhurst Hosp 1990; **Fellow:** Pulmonary Disease, Elmhurst Hosp 1992

Interventional Cardiology

Lux, Michael S MD (IC) - **Hospital:** Overlook Med Ctr (page 92), Morristown Med Ctr (page 92); **Address:** Assocs in Cardiovascular Disease, 211 Mountain Ave, Springfield, NJ 07081-1581; **Phone:** 973-467-0005; **Board Cert:** Internal Medicine 1980; Cardiovascular Disease 1985; Interventional Cardiology 2002; **Med School:** NYU Sch Med 1977; **Resid:** Internal Medicine, Johns Hopkins Hosp 1980; **Fellow:** Cardiovascular Disease, Johns Hopkins Hosp 1983; **Fac Appt:** Asst Prof Med, Columbia P&S

Mich, Robert J MD (IC) - **Spec Exp:** Arrhythmias; **Hospital:** Morristown Med Ctr (page 92), Overlook Med Ctr (page 92); **Address:** Assocs in Cardiovascular Disease, 29 South St Fl 1, New Providence, NJ 07974-1996; **Phone:** 908-464-4200; **Board Cert:** Internal Medicine 1984; Cardiovascular Disease 1985; Interventional Cardiology 2002; **Med School:** Johns Hopkins Univ 1979; **Resid:** Internal Medicine, John Hopkins Hosp 1982; **Fellow:** Cardiovascular Disease, Vanderbilt Univ Hosp 1984; Cardiovascular Disease, Mass Genl Hosp 1986

Medical Oncology

Guerin, Bonni L MD (Onc) - **Spec Exp:** Breast Cancer; **Hospital:** Overlook Med Ctr (page 92); **Address:** Medical Diagnostic Assocs, Overlook Oncology Ctr, 99 Beauvoir Ave Fl 5, Summit, NJ 07902; **Phone:** 908-608-0078; **Board Cert:** Internal Medicine 2005; Medical Oncology 2005; **Med School:** SUNY Stony Brook 1988; **Resid:** Internal Medicine, Vanderbilt Univ Med Ctr 1991; **Fellow:** Medical Oncology, UCSD Cancer Ctr 1993

Lowenthal, Dennis MD (Onc) - **Spec Exp:** Lung Cancer; Lymphoma; Prostate Cancer; Thoracic Cancers; **Hospital:** Overlook Med Ctr (page 92); **Address:** The Cancer Ctr at Overlook Hosp, 99 Beauvoir Ave Fl 5, Summit, NJ 07902; **Phone:** 908-608-0078; **Board Cert:** Internal Medicine 1982; Medical Oncology 1985; Hematology 1986; **Med School:** Boston Univ 1979; **Resid:** Internal Medicine, Montefiore Med Ctr 1982; **Fellow:** Hematology, Montefiore Med Ctr 1983; Medical Oncology, Mem Sloan Kettering Cancer Ctr 1986; **Fac Appt:** Asst Clin Prof Med, Mount Sinai Sch Med

Moriarty, Daniel J MD (Onc) - **Spec Exp:** Gastrointestinal Cancer; **Hospital:** Overlook Med Ctr (page 92); **Address:** Med Diagnostic Assocs, 99 Beauvoir Ave Fl 5, Summit, NJ 07902; **Phone:** 908-608-0078; **Board Cert:** Internal Medicine 1982; Medical Oncology 1987; **Med School:** Univ VT Coll Med 1976; **Resid:** Internal Medicine, Cambridge Hosp 1984; **Fellow:** Hematology & Oncology, St Elizabeth Hosp 1987

Wax, Michael MD (Onc) - **Hospital:** Overlook Med Ctr (page 92); **Address:** 1 Diamond Hill Rd, Berkeley Hieghts, NJ 07922; **Phone:** 908-277-8890; **Board Cert:** Internal Medicine 1980; Medical Oncology 1983; **Med School:** Med Coll PA Hahnemann 1977; **Resid:** Internal Medicine, Hosp Med Coll Penn 1980; **Fellow:** Hematology & Oncology, Univ Wash Med Ctr 1980; **Fac Appt:** Asst Clin Prof Med, Mount Sinai Sch Med

Nephrology

Goldstein, Carl S MD (Nep) - **Spec Exp:** Hypertension; Kidney Stones; Kidney Failure; Metabolic Syndrome; **Hospital:** Overlook Med Ctr (page 92); **Address:** 215 North Ave W, Westfield, NJ 07090-1428; **Phone:** 908-232-4321; **Board Cert:** Internal Medicine 1981; Nephrology 1984; **Med School:** Washington Univ, St Louis 1978; **Resid:** Internal Medicine, Univ Minn Med Ctr 1981; **Fellow:** Nephrology, Hosp Univ Penn 1984; **Fac Appt:** Clin Prof Med, Mount Sinai Sch Med

McAnally, James F MD (Nep) - **Spec Exp:** Kidney Disease; Hypertension; Diabetes; **Hospital:** Trinitas Reg Med Ctr (page 870); **Address:** 240 Williamson St, Ste 307, Elizabeth, NJ 07202-3672; **Phone:** 908-994-9200; **Board Cert:** Internal Medicine 1978; Nephrology 1980; **Med School:** UMDNJ-NJ Med Sch, Newark 1975; **Resid:** Internal Medicine, CMDNJ-Newark Affil Hosp 1978; Internal Medicine, Georgetown Univ Hosp 1980; **Fellow:** Nephrology, Georgetown Univ Hosp 1980; **Fac Appt:** Assoc Clin Prof Med, Seton Hall Univ Sch Hlth & Med Scis

Neurological Surgery

Friedlander, Marvin E MD (NS) - **Spec Exp:** Spinal Surgery; **Hospital:** Trinitas Reg Med Ctr (page 870), Overlook Med Ctr (page 92); **Address:** 700 Rahway Ave, Union, NJ 07083; **Phone:** 908-688-1999; **Board Cert:** Neurological Surgery 1994; **Med School:** SUNY Downstate 1982; **Resid:** Neurological Surgery, Kings Co Hosp 1989; **Fellow:** Metabolism, SUNY Downstate Med Ctr 1984

Hodosh, Richard M MD (NS) - **Spec Exp:** Acoustic Neuroma; Neurovascular Surgery; Spinal Surgery; **Hospital:** Overlook Med Ctr (page 92), Morristown Med Ctr (page 92); **Address:** Atlantic Brain & Spine Institute, 99 Beauvoir Ave, MS 07902, Clinical Office MAC 1, ste 405, Summit, NJ 07901; **Phone:** 908-522-4979; **Board Cert:** Neurological Surgery 1980; **Med School:** Univ Cincinnati 1972; **Resid:** Neurological Surgery, Univ Tex Hlth Scis Ctr 1978; **Fellow:** Neuroradiology, Natl Hosp Neur Dis 1975; Neurological Surgery, Kantonsspital 1976; **Fac Appt:** Clin Prof NS, UMDNJ-NJ Med Sch, Newark

Neurology

Bansil, Shalini M MD (N) - **Spec Exp:** Stroke; **Hospital:** Overlook Med Ctr (page 92); **Address:** Overlook Hospital, Director, Stroke Center, 99 Beauvoir Ave, Summit, NJ 07902; **Phone:** 908-522-5545; **Board Cert:** Neurology 1989; Vascular Neurology 2006; **Med School:** India 1981; **Resid:** Neurology, UMDNJ Med Ctr 1989; **Fellow:** Stroke, Beth Israel Med Ctr

Halperin, John MD (N) - **Spec Exp:** Neuromuscular Disorders; Lyme Disease; Multiple Sclerosis; **Hospital:** Overlook Med Ctr (page 92), Morristown Med Ctr (page 92); **Address:** Overlook Medical Center, 99 Beauvoir Ave, Department of Neurosciences, Summit, NJ 07902; **Phone:** 908-522-2829; **Board Cert:** Internal Medicine 1978; Neurology 1982; Clinical Neurophysiology 2005; **Med School:** Harvard Med Sch 1975; **Resid:** Internal Medicine, Univ Chicago Hosps 1977; Neurology, Mass Genl Hosp 1980; **Fellow:** Neurology, Mass Genl Hosp 1983; **Fac Appt:** Prof N, Mount Sinai Sch Med

Politsky, Jeffrey M MD (N) - **Spec Exp:** Epilepsy/Seizure Disorders; Critical Care; **Hospital:** Overlook Med Ctr (page 92); **Address:** Atlantic Neuroscience Inst, 99 Beauvoir Ave, Summit, NJ 07901; **Phone:** 908-522-6105; **Board Cert:** Neurology 2005; **Med School:** Canada 1994; **Resid:** Neurology, Univ British Columbia 1999; **Fellow:** Epilepsy, Harvard Med Sch-Mass Genl Hosp 2001

Pollock, Jeffrey C MD (N) - **Hospital:** Overlook Med Ctr (page 92); **Address:** 47 Maple St, Ste 104, Summit, NJ 07901; **Phone:** 908-277-2722; **Board Cert:** Neurology 1987; **Med School:** Med Coll GA 1982; **Resid:** Neurology, UMDNJ Med Ctr 1986

Sachs, Stephen M MD (N) - **Spec Exp:** Headache; Stroke; Dementia; Parkinson's Disease; **Hospital:** Robert Wood Johnson Univ Hosp at Rahway, Trinitas Reg Med Ctr (page 870); **Address:** 700 N Broad St, Ste 201, Elizabeth, NJ 07208; **Phone:** 908-354-3994; **Board Cert:** Neurology 1977; **Med School:** Univ Pennsylvania 1971; **Resid:** Internal Medicine, Bellevue Hosp 1973; Neurology, Columbia-Presby Med Ctr 1976

Schanzer, Bernard MD (N) - **Spec Exp:** Stroke; Headache; Multiple Sclerosis; Amyotrophic Lateral Sclerosis (ALS); **Hospital:** Trinitas Reg Med Ctr (page 870), Robert Wood Johnson Univ Hosp at Rahway; **Address:** 700 N Broad St, Ste 201, Elizabeth, NJ 07208; **Phone:** 908-354-3994; **Board Cert:** Neurology 1972; **Med School:** Belgium 1962; **Resid:** Internal Medicine, Maimonides Med Ctr 1965; Neurology, Bronx Muni Med Ctr 1970; **Fac Appt:** Assoc Clin Prof N, UMDNJ-NJ Med Sch, Newark

Neuroradiology

Horner, Neil B MD (NRad) - **Spec Exp:** MRI & CT of Brain & Spine; Spine Imaging & Intervention; Tumor Imaging; Brain Imaging; **Hospital:** Overlook Med Ctr (page 92), Mount Sinai Med Ctr (page 102); **Address:** Overlook Hosp, Dept Radiology, 99 Beauvoir Ave, Summit, NJ 07902; **Phone:** 908-522-2066; **Board Cert:** Diagnostic Radiology 1988; Nuclear Radiology 1989; Neuroradiology 2005; **Med School:** UMDNJ-Rutgers Med Sch 1983; **Resid:** Diagnostic Radiology, NYU Med Ctr 1988; **Fellow:** Neuroradiology, NYU Med Ctr 1989; Nuclear Radiology, NYU Med Ctr 1989; **Fac Appt:** Asst Clin Prof Rad, Mount Sinai Sch Med

Obstetrics & Gynecology

Beim, Robert B MD (ObG) - **Spec Exp:** Laparoscopic Surgery; Minimally Invasive Surgery; Colposcopy; **Hospital:** St. Peter's Univ Hosp, JFK Med Ctr - Edison; **Address:** 190 Greenbrook Rd, N Plainfield, NJ 07060; **Phone:** 908-226-1555; **Board Cert:** Obstetrics & Gynecology 2010; **Med School:** SUNY Upstate Med Univ 1989; **Resid:** Obstetrics & Gynecology, Robert Wood Johnson Med Ctr 1993; **Fac Appt:** Asst Prof ObG, Drexel Univ Coll Med

Margulis, Elynne B MD (ObG) - **Spec Exp:** Infertility; **Hospital:** Overlook Med Ctr (page 92); **Address:** 522 E Broad St, Westfield, NJ 07090; **Phone:** 908-232-4449; **Board Cert:** Obstetrics & Gynecology 1985; **Med School:** Columbia P&S 1978; **Resid:** Obstetrics & Gynecology, Hosp Univ Penn 1982; **Fac Appt:** Asst Clin Prof ObG, Columbia P&S

Soffer, Jeffrey L MD (ObG) - **Hospital:** Overlook Med Ctr (page 92); **Address:** 522 E Broad St, Westfield, NJ 07090; **Phone:** 908-232-4449; **Board Cert:** Obstetrics & Gynecology 1983; **Med School:** Howard Univ 1975; **Resid:** Obstetrics & Gynecology, Hosp Univ Penn 1979

Ophthalmology

Confino, Joel MD (Oph) - **Spec Exp:** Laser Vision Surgery; Cataract Surgery; Corneal Disease & Transplant; **Hospital:** Overlook Med Ctr (page 92); **Address:** 592 Springfield Ave, Westfield, NJ 07090-1002; **Phone:** 908-789-8999; **Board Cert:** Ophthalmology 1985; **Med School:** Albert Einstein Coll Med 1980; **Resid:** Ophthalmology, Mt Sinai Med Ctr 1984; **Fellow:** Cornea & Ext Eye Disease, UCSD Med Ctr 1985

Natale, Benjamin P DO (Oph) - **Spec Exp:** LASIK-Refractive Surgery; Cataract Surgery; **Hospital:** Saint Barnabas Med Ctr; **Address:** 1050 Galloping Hill Rd, Ste 104, Union, NJ 07083-7983; **Phone:** 908-964-7878; **Board Cert:** Ophthalmology 1991; **Med School:** Coll Osteo Med 1980; **Resid:** Family Medicine, Union Hosp 1982; Ophthalmology, UMDNJ Affil Hosp 1985; **Fellow:** Refractive Surgery, Newark Eye & Ear Infirmary 1986

Orthopaedic Surgery

Barmakian, Joseph T MD (OrS) - **Spec Exp:** Carpal Tunnel Syndrome; Nerve & Tendon Reconstruction; Shoulder Reconstruction; **Hospital:** Overlook Med Ctr (page 92); **Address:** 202 Elmer St, Westfield, NJ 07090-3300; **Phone:** 908-232-7797; **Board Cert:** Orthopaedic Surgery 2003; Hand Surgery 2003; **Med School:** UMDNJ-RW Johnson Med Sch 1984; **Resid:** Surgery, Geo Wash Univ Med Ctr 1986; Orthopaedic Surgery, Columbia-Presby Med Ctr 1989; **Fellow:** Hand Surgery, Hosp for Joint Diseases 1990

Botwin, Clifford DO (OrS) - **Spec Exp:** Arthroscopic Surgery; Hip Surgery; Knee Surgery; **Hospital:** Overlook Med Ctr (page 92), Bayonne Med Ctr; **Address:** Associated Orthopaedics, 900 Stuyvesant Ave, Union, NJ 07083-6936; **Phone:** 908-964-6600; **Resid:** Orthopaedic Surgery, Delaware Valley Hosp 1976

Drzala, Mark R MD (OrS) - **Spec Exp:** Spinal Surgery; **Hospital:** Hackensack UMC-Mountainside (page 736), Overlook Med Ctr (page 92); **Address:** 33 Overlook Rd, Ste 305, Summit, NJ 07901; **Phone:** 908-608-9610; **Board Cert:** Orthopaedic Surgery 2012; **Med School:** UMDNJ-NJ Med Sch, Newark 1991; **Resid:** Orthopaedic Surgery, UMDNJ-NJ Med Sch 1997; **Fellow:** Spinal Surgery, San Francisco Orthopeds 1998; **Fac Appt:** Asst Clin Prof OrS, UMDNJ-NJ Med Sch, Newark

Gallick, Gregory MD (OrS) - **Spec Exp:** Sports Medicine; Knee Reconstruction; Shoulder Reconstruction; **Hospital:** Overlook Med Ctr (page 92); **Address:** 2780 Morris Ave, Ste 2C, Union, NJ 07083; **Phone:** 908-686-6665; **Board Cert:** Orthopaedic Surgery 2009; **Med School:** UMDNJ-Rutgers Med Sch 1980; **Resid:** Surgery, UMDNJ Med Ctr 1981; Orthopaedic Surgery, UMDNJ Med Ctr 1985; **Fellow:** Interventional Cardiology, So CA Sports Medicine 1986

Mackessy, Richard P MD (OrS) - **Spec Exp:** Hand Surgery; **Hospital:** Trinitas Reg Med Ctr (page 870), Robert Wood Johnson Univ Hosp at Rahway; **Address:** 210 W St Georges Ave, Linden, NJ 07036; **Phone:** 908-486-1111; **Board Cert:** Orthopaedic Surgery 2007; Hand Surgery 2007; **Med School:** UMDNJ-NJ Med Sch, Newark 1978; **Resid:** Surgery, St Vincents Hosp 1980; Orthopaedic Surgery, St Lukes Hosp 1983; **Fellow:** Hand Surgery, Thomas Jefferson Univ Hosp 1984

Sarokhan, Alan MD (OrS) - **Spec Exp:** Hip Replacement; Knee Replacement; Hand Surgery; **Hospital:** Overlook Med Ctr (page 92), Saint Barnabas Med Ctr; **Address:** Medical Arts Bldg, 33 Overlook Rd, Ste 201, Summit, NJ 07901-3562; **Phone:** 908-522-4555; **Board Cert:** Orthopaedic Surgery 2007; **Med School:** Harvard Med Sch 1977; **Resid:** Surgery, Peter Bent Brigham Hosp 1979; Orthopaedic Surgery, Harvard Affil Hosps 1982; **Fellow:** Hand Surgery, Roosevelt Hosp 1984

Otolaryngology

Carniol, Paul J MD (Oto) - **Spec Exp:** Facial Plastic Surgery; Facial Rejuvenation; Cosmetic Surgery; Skin Cancer; **Hospital:** Overlook Med Ctr (page 92); **Address:** Medical Arts Bldg, 33 Overlook Rd, Ste 401, Summit, NJ 07901; **Phone:** 908-598-1400; **Board Cert:** Otolaryngology 1981; Facial Plastic & Reconstr Surgery 1991; **Med School:** Univ Pennsylvania 1976; **Resid:** Surgery, North Shore Univ Hosp 1978; **Fellow:** Otolaryngology, Mass Eye & Ear Infirm 1981; Plastic/Reconstructive Surgery, Hosp Univ Penn 1983; **Fac Appt:** Clin Prof S, UMDNJ-NJ Med Sch, Newark

Drake III, William MD (Oto) - **Spec Exp:** Endoscopic Sinus Surgery; Head & Neck Surgery; Thyroid & Parathyroid Surgery; Pediatric Otolaryngology; **Hospital:** Overlook Med Ctr (page 92); **Address:** 213 Summit Rd, Mountainside, NJ 07092; **Phone:** 908-233-2111; **Board Cert:** Otolaryngology 1995; **Med School:** UMDNJ-NJ Med Sch, Newark 1989; **Resid:** Otolaryngology, Mt Sinai Med Ctr 1994

Kwartler, Jed A MD (Oto) - **Spec Exp:** Acoustic Neuroma; Balance Disorders; Cochlear Implants; Cholesteatoma; **Hospital:** Overlook Med Ctr (page 92), Hackensack Univ Med Ctr (page 96); **Address:** 1 Diamond Hill Rd, Berkeley Heights, NJ 07922; **Phone:** 908-277-8681; **Board Cert:** Otolaryngology 1988; Neurotology 2010; **Med School:** UMDNJ-NJ Med Sch, Newark 1983; **Resid:** Surgery, UMDNJ/Univ Hosp 1985; Otolaryngology, UMDNJ/Univ Hosp 1988; **Fellow:** Otology & Neurotology, St Vincent's Hosp & Med Ctr 1990; **Fac Appt:** Assoc Clin Prof Oto, UMDNJ-NJ Med Sch, Newark

Scharf, Richard DO (Oto) - **Spec Exp:** Sinus Disorders/Surgery; Cosmetic Surgery-Face; Head & Neck Cancer; **Hospital:** Saint Barnabas Med Ctr, Bayonne Med Ctr; **Address:** 505 Chestnut St, Roselle Park, NJ 07204; **Phone:** 908-241-0200; **Board Cert:** Otolaryngology 1998; **Med School:** Univ Hlth Sci, Coll Osteo Med 1982; **Resid:** Otolaryngology, Flint Hosp 1990; **Fac Appt:** Assoc Clin Prof Oto, NY Coll Osteo Med

Pediatric Cardiology

Leichter, Donald MD (PCd) - **Spec Exp:** Congenital Heart Disease; Fetal Echocardiography; Echocardiography; **Hospital:** Overlook Med Ctr (page 92), Morgan Stanley Children's Hosp of NY-Presby, NY (page 104); **Address:** 47 Maple St, Ste 406, Summit, NJ 07901; **Phone:** 908-522-5566; **Board Cert:** Pediatrics 1988; Pediatric Cardiology 2010; **Med School:** Cornell Univ-Weill Med Coll 1980; **Resid:** Pediatrics, Chldns Hosp Natl Med Ctr 1983; **Fellow:** Pediatric Cardiology, Columbia Presby Med Ctr 1985; **Fac Appt:** Assoc Clin Prof Ped, Columbia P&S

Pediatric Endocrinology

Anhalt, Henry DO (PEn) - **Spec Exp:** Diabetes; Obesity; Growth Disorders; **Address:** 140 Prospect Ave, Ste 2, Hackensack, NJ 07061; **Phone:** 201-996-0777; **Board Cert:** Pediatric Endocrinology 2012; **Med School:** NY Coll Osteo Med 1988; **Resid:** Pediatrics, Winthrop Univ Hosp 1992; **Fellow:** Pediatric Endocrinology, Stanford Univ Med Ctr 1995; **Fac Appt:** Assoc Prof Ped, SUNY Hlth Sci Ctr

Pediatric Gastroenterology

Tyshkov, Michael MD (PGe) - **Spec Exp:** Nutrition; Crohn's Disease; Colitis; **Hospital:** Overlook Med Ctr (page 92), Staten Island Univ Hosp - North (page 106); **Address:** 33 Overlook Rd, Ste 208, Summit, NJ 07901; **Phone:** 908-273-7745; **Board Cert:** Pediatric Gastroenterology 2010; **Med School:** Russia 1977; **Resid:** Pediatrics, Flushing Hosp 1989; **Fellow:** Pediatric Gastroenterology, Westchester Co Med Ctr 1991; **Fac Appt:** Asst Clin Prof Ped, SUNY Downstate

Pediatric Surgery

Bergman, Kerry S MD (PS) - **Hospital:** Overlook Med Ctr (page 92), Morristown Med Ctr (page 92); **Address:** Overlook Hospital, 99 Beauvoir Ave, Box 220, Summit, NJ 07902; **Phone:** 908-522-3523; **Board Cert:** Surgery 2007; Pediatric Surgery 2009; **Med School:** Albany Med Coll 1982; **Resid:** Surgery, New England Med Ctr 1988; Pediatric Surgery, New England Med Ctr 1991; **Fellow:** Pediatric Surgery-ECMO, Hosp for Sick Children 1989

Pediatrics

Ayyanathan, Karpukarasi MD (Ped) *PCP* - **Hospital:** Trinitas Reg Med Ctr (page 870), JFK Med Ctr - Edison; **Address:** Linden Pediatric Grp, 517 Rahway Ave, Elizabeth, NJ 07202-2308; **Phone:** 908-527-1247; **Board Cert:** Pediatrics 1983; **Med School:** India 1975; **Resid:** Pediatrics, St Elizabeth Hosp 1977; Pediatrics, Rahway Hosp 1979

Corbo, Emanuel MD (Ped) *PCP* - **Spec Exp:** Vaccines; Asthma; Otitis Media; Pneumonia; **Hospital:** Overlook Med Ctr (page 92), Trinitas Reg Med Ctr (page 870); **Address:** 443 E Westfield Ave, Roselle Park, NJ 07204-2428; **Phone:** 908-245-2442; **Board Cert:** Pediatrics 2008; **Med School:** Grenada 1985; **Resid:** Pediatrics, Newark Beth Israel Med Ctr 1990; **Fellow:** Pediatrics, Newark Beth Israel Med Ctr 1991

Davis, Kenneth J MD (Ped) *PCP* - **Hospital:** Overlook Med Ctr (page 92), Trinitas Reg Med Ctr (page 870); **Address:** 701 Newark Ave, Ste 212, Elizabeth, NJ 07208-3550; **Phone:** 908-354-9500; **Board Cert:** Pediatrics 1985; **Med School:** Albert Einstein Coll Med 1980; **Resid:** Pediatrics, Bellevue Hosp 1983

Mehta, Uday C MD (Ped) - **Spec Exp:** Autism; ADD/ADHD; Neurodevelopmental Disabilities; **Hospital:** Children's Specialized Hosp, Robert Wood Johnson Univ Hosp - New Brunswick; **Address:** 150 New Providence Rd, Mountainside, NJ 07092; **Phone:** 908-301-5491; **Board Cert:** Pediatrics 1982; Developmental-Behavioral Pediatrics 2012; **Med School:** India 1971; **Resid:** Pediatrics, Overlook Hosp 1980; **Fellow:** Child Development, Chldns Hosp 1981; **Fac Appt:** Asst Clin Prof Ped, UMDNJ-RW Johnson Med Sch

Panza, Robert MD (Ped) - **Hospital:** Overlook Med Ctr (page 92); **Address:** Pediatric Associates of Westfield, 566 Westfield Ave, Westfield, NJ 07090; **Phone:** 908-233-7171; **Board Cert:** Pediatrics 2011; **Med School:** Italy 1985; **Resid:** Pediatrics, Overlook Hosp 1989

Panzner, Elizabeth A MD (Ped) *PCP* - **Spec Exp:** Acne; Allergy; Asthma; **Hospital:** Saint Barnabas Med Ctr, Overlook Med Ctr (page 92); **Address:** Union Pediatric Medical Group, 1050 Galloping Hill Rd, Ste 200, Union, NJ 07083-9417; **Phone:** 908-688-9900; **Board Cert:** Pediatrics 2011; **Med School:** Mexico 1984; **Resid:** Pediatrics, Univ Hosp 1988

Saraiya, Narendra N MD (Ped) *PCP* - **Spec Exp:** Asthma; Anemia; Sickle Cell Disease; **Hospital:** Trinitas Reg Med Ctr (page 870), JFK Med Ctr - Edison; **Address:** 817 Rahway Ave, Elizabeth, NJ 07202; **Phone:** 908-353-5750; **Board Cert:** Pediatrics 1988; **Med School:** India 1971; **Resid:** Pediatrics, NY Methodist Hosp 1980; **Fellow:** Pediatric Hematology-Oncology, Maimonides Med Ctr 1982; Pediatric Hematology-Oncology, Chldns Hosp Buffalo 1984

Physical Medicine & Rehabilitation

Armento, Michael J MD (PMR) - **Spec Exp:** Pediatric Rehabilitation; Cerebral Palsy; Spina Bifida; Spinal Cord Injury-Pediatric; **Hospital:** Children's Specialized Hosp, Newark Beth Israel Med Ctr; **Address:** Chldns Specialized Hosp, 150 New Providence Rd, Mountainside, NJ 07092; **Phone:** 908-301-5502; **Board Cert:** Physical Medicine & Rehabilitation 2003; Spinal Cord Injury Medicine 2002; Pediatric Rehabilitation Medicine 2004; **Med School:** UMDNJ-NJ Med Sch, Newark 1988; **Resid:** Physical Medicine & Rehabilitation, Univ Hosp-UMDNJ 1992; **Fellow:** Pediatric Rehabilitation Medicine, Chldns Specialized Hosp 1994; **Fac Appt:** Assoc Clin Prof Ped, UMDNJ-NJ Med Sch, Newark

Diamond, Martin MD (PMR) - **Spec Exp:** Cerebral Palsy; Neuromuscular Disorders; Electrodiagnosis; **Hospital:** Children's Specialized Hosp, Newark Beth Israel Med Ctr; **Address:** Chldns Specialized Hosp, 150 New Providence Rd, Mountainside, NJ 07092; **Phone:** 908-301-5502; **Board Cert:** Pediatrics 1983; Physical Medicine & Rehabilitation 1982; Pediatric Rehabilitation Medicine 2003; **Med School:** Univ Pittsburgh 1975; **Resid:** Pediatrics, Chldns Hosp Natl Med Ctr 1978; Physical Medicine & Rehabilitation, Sinai Hosp 1980; **Fac Appt:** Assoc Clin Prof PMR, UMDNJ-NJ Med Sch, Newark

Malanga, Gerard A MD (PMR) - **Spec Exp:** Pain-Back & Neck; Sports Injuries; Pain-Low Back; Shoulder Injuries; **Hospital:** Overlook Med Ctr (page 92), Morristown Med Ctr (page 92); **Address:** 11 Overlook Rd, MAC #2, Ste B110, Summit, NJ 07901; **Phone:** 908-522-2808; **Board Cert:** Physical Medicine & Rehabilitation 2003; Pain Medicine 2002; Sports Medicine 2009; **Med School:** UMDNJ-NJ Med Sch, Newark 1982; **Resid:** Physical Medicine & Rehabilitation, UMDNJ Affil Hosp 1992; **Fellow:** Sports Medicine, Mayo Clinic 1993; **Fac Appt:** Assoc Clin Prof PMR, UMDNJ-NJ Med Sch, Newark

Plastic Surgery

Gardner, James N MD (PIS) - **Spec Exp:** Breast Cosmetic & Reconstructive Surgery; Abdominoplasty; **Hospital:** Overlook Med Ctr (page 92); **Address:** 33 Overlook Rd, Ste 310, Summit, NJ 07901; **Phone:** 908-918-1969; **Board Cert:** Plastic Surgery 2005; **Med School:** UMDNJ-RW Johnson Med Sch 1987; **Resid:** Surgery, UMDNJ Univ Hosp 1992; **Fellow:** Plastic Surgery, UMDNJ Univ Hosp 1994

Hyans, Peter MD (PIS) - **Spec Exp:** Cosmetic Surgery-Breast; Breast Reconstruction; Cosmetic Surgery-Face; Liposuction & Body Contouring; **Hospital:** Overlook Med Ctr (page 92), Saint Barnabas Med Ctr; **Address:** Summit Medical Grp, Plastic Surgery Ctr, Lawrence Pavilion, 1 Diamond Hill Rd, Berkeley Heights, NJ 07922; **Phone:** 908-277-8759; **Board Cert:** Plastic Surgery 2003; **Med School:** UMDNJ-RW Johnson Med Sch 1986; **Resid:** Surgery, Thomas Jefferson Univ Hosp 1991; **Fellow:** Plastic Surgery, Univ Cincinnati Hosp 1993

Tepper, Howard N MD (PIS) - **Spec Exp:** Cosmetic Surgery; Breast Surgery; Hand Surgery; **Hospital:** Overlook Med Ctr (page 92); **Address:** 522 E Broad St, Westfield, NJ 07090-2116; **Phone:** 908-654-6540; **Board Cert:** Plastic Surgery 1983; **Med School:** Albert Einstein Coll Med 1975; **Resid:** Surgery, Montefiore Hosp Med Ctr 1979; Plastic Surgery, Montefiore Hosp Med Ctr 1981; **Fellow:** Hand Surgery, St Luke's-Roosevelt Hosp Ctr 1979

Zeitels, Jerrold R MD (PIS) - **Spec Exp:** Liposuction & Body Contouring; Reconstructive Surgery; Hand Surgery; **Hospital:** Overlook Med Ctr (page 92), Robert Wood Johnson Univ Hosp at Rahway; **Address:** 522 E Broad St, Westfield, NJ 07090-2116; **Phone:** 908-654-6540; **Board Cert:** Plastic Surgery 1989; Hand Surgery 2009; **Med School:** Univ Chicago-Pritzker Sch Med 1980; **Resid:** Surgery, Univ Michigan Med Ctr 1985; Plastic Surgery, Hosp Univ Penn 1987

Psychiatry

Kaplan, Gabriel MD (Psyc) - **Spec Exp:** Psychopharmacology; ADD/ADHD; Depression; **Hospital:** Bergen Regl Med Ctr; **Address:** 535 Morris Ave, Springfield, NJ 07081-1426; **Phone:** 973-376-1020; **Board Cert:** Psychiatry 1987; Child & Adolescent Psychiatry 1989; **Med School:** Argentina 1980; **Resid:** Psychiatry, NY Hosp-Cornell 1986; Child Psychiatry, NY Hosp-Cornell 1988; **Fac Appt:** Assoc Prof Psyc, UMDNJ-NJ Med Sch, Newark

Miller, David G MD (Psyc) - **Spec Exp:** Psychopharmacology; Depression; ADD/ADHD; Bipolar/Mood Disorders; **Address:** 28 Milburn Ave, Ste 5, Springfield, NJ 07081; **Phone:** 973-218-1770; **Board Cert:** Psychiatry 1985; **Med School:** Univ Rochester 1980; **Resid:** Psychiatry, Strong Meml Hosp 1984

Richardson, William T MD (Psyc) - **Spec Exp:** Adolescent Psychiatry; Family Therapy; Psychopharmacology; **Hospital:** Overlook Med Ctr (page 92), Morristown Med Ctr (page 92); **Address:** 33 Overlook Rd, Ste 210, Summit, NJ 07901-3570; **Phone:** 908-598-0008; **Board Cert:** Psychiatry 1980; **Med School:** McGill Univ 1967; **Resid:** Psychiatry, Jewish Genl Hosp 1971; Psychiatry, Payne Whitney Clinic 1974

Silver, Bennett MD (Psyc) - **Spec Exp:** Child & Adolescent Psychiatry; ADD/ADHD; Anxiety Disorders; **Hospital:** Bergen Regl Med Ctr; **Address:** 535 Morris Ave, Springfield, NJ 07081; **Phone:** 973-376-1020; **Board Cert:** Psychiatry 1979; **Med School:** SUNY Downstate 1974; **Resid:** Psychiatry, Mount Sinai Hosp 1978; **Fellow:** Child & Adolescent Psychiatry, Mount Sinai Hosp 1980

Villafranca, Manuel V MD (Psyc) - **Spec Exp:** Psychopharmacology; Depression; Anxiety Disorders; **Hospital:** Summit Oaks Hosp, Christ Hosp - Jersey City; **Address:** 220 Lenox Ave, Westfield, NJ 07090; **Phone:** 908-232-9369; **Board Cert:** Psychiatry 1982; **Med School:** Philippines 1971; **Resid:** Psychiatry, St Vincents Hosp 1978; **Fellow:** Child & Adolescent Psychiatry, St Vincents Hosp 1980

Pulmonary Disease

Cerrone, Federico MD (Pul) - **Spec Exp:** Sleep Disorders; Asthma; Chronic Obstructive Lung Disease (COPD); **Hospital:** Overlook Med Ctr (page 92), Morristown Med Ctr (page 92); **Address:** 1 Springfield Ave, Summit, NJ 07901; **Phone:** 908-934-0555; **Board Cert:** Internal Medicine 1989; Pulmonary Disease 2002; Critical Care Medicine 2003; Sleep Medicine 2007; **Med School:** Georgetown Univ 1986; **Resid:** Internal Medicine, Bronx Muni Hosp 1989; **Fellow:** Pulmonary Critical Care Medicine, Georgetown Univ Hosp 1992

Hwang, Cheng-hong DO (Pul) - **Spec Exp:** Critical Care Medicine; **Hospital:** Robert Wood Johnson Univ Hosp at Rahway; **Address:** 1457 Raritan Rd, Ste 101, Clark, NJ 07066; **Phone:** 908-272-2270; **Board Cert:** Internal Medicine 1983; Pulmonary Disease 1984; Critical Care Medicine 2005; **Med School:** Coll Osteo Med 1978; **Resid:** Internal Medicine, USPHS Hosp 1981; **Fellow:** Pulmonary Disease, UMDNJ-Univ Hosp 1983

Sussman, Robert MD (Pul) - **Spec Exp:** Asthma; Chronic Obstructive Lung Disease (COPD); Pulmonary Fibrosis; Lung Cancer; **Hospital:** Overlook Med Ctr (page 92), Morristown Med Ctr (page 92); **Address:** 1 Springfield Ave, Summit, NJ 07901; **Phone:** 908-934-0555; **Board Cert:** Internal Medicine 1984; Pulmonary Disease 1988; **Med School:** Albert Einstein Coll Med 1981; **Resid:** Internal Medicine, Montefiore Med Ctr 1984; **Fellow:** Pulmonary Disease, NYU/Bellevue Hosp 1987

Radiation Oncology

Schwartz, Louis E MD (RadRO) - **Spec Exp:** Stereotactic Radiosurgery; Prostate Cancer; Brain Tumors; **Hospital:** Overlook Med Ctr (page 92); **Address:** Overlook Hosp, Dept Rad Oncology, 33 Overlook Rd, Ste L05, Medical Arts Ctr 1, Summit, NJ 07901-3561; **Phone:** 908-522-2871; **Board Cert:** Therapeutic Radiology 1979; Pediatrics 1981; **Med School:** SUNY Hlth Sci Ctr 1974; **Resid:** Pediatrics, NY Methodist Hosp 1976; Pediatrics, Chldns Hosp Med Ctr 1977; **Fellow:** Therapeutic Radiology, Columbia-Presby Hosp 1979

Rheumatology

Brodman, Richard R MD (Rhu) - **Spec Exp:** Lupus/SLE; Rheumatoid Arthritis; Osteoporosis; Osteoarthritis; **Hospital:** JFK Med Ctr - Edison; **Address:** 345 Somerset St, Ste 107, North Plainfield, NJ 07060-4774; **Phone:** 908-561-7440; **Board Cert:** Internal Medicine 1976; Rheumatology 1982; **Med School:** SUNY Downstate 1973; **Resid:** Internal Medicine, Rhode Island Hosp 1976; **Fellow:** Rheumatology, Brigham & Womens Hosp 1978; **Fac Appt:** Assoc Clin Prof Med, UMDNJ-RW Johnson Med Sch

Kramer, Neil MD (Rhu) - **Spec Exp:** Rheumatoid Arthritis; Lupus/SLE; Sjogren's Syndrome; Vasculitis; **Hospital:** Overlook Med Ctr (page 92); **Address:** 33 Overlook Rd, Ste 211, Summit, NJ 07901; **Phone:** 908-598-7940; **Board Cert:** Internal Medicine 1977; Rheumatology 1980; **Med School:** Univ Pennsylvania 1974; **Resid:** Internal Medicine, Manhattan VA Hosp/NYU Med Ctr 1978; **Fellow:** Rheumatology, NYU Med Ctr 1980; **Fac Appt:** Assoc Clin Prof Med, Mount Sinai Sch Med

Rosenstein, Elliot D MD (Rhu) - **Spec Exp:** Rheumatoid Arthritis; Lupus/SLE; Sjogren's Syndrome; Behcet's Syndrome; **Hospital:** Overlook Med Ctr (page 92), Atl Hlth (page 92); **Address:** 33 Overlook Rd, Ste 211, Summit, NJ 07901; **Phone:** 908-598-7940; **Board Cert:** Internal Medicine 1981; Rheumatology 1984; **Med School:** Mount Sinai Sch Med 1978; **Resid:** Internal Medicine, NYU/Bellevue Hosp 1982; **Fellow:** Rheumatology, NYU/Bellevue Hosp 1984; **Fac Appt:** Assoc Clin Prof Med, Mount Sinai Sch Med

Worth, David MD (Rhu) - **Spec Exp:** Rheumatoid Arthritis; Osteoporosis; **Hospital:** Overlook Med Ctr (page 92); **Address:** 2376 Morris Ave, Union, NJ 07083-5707; **Phone:** 908-686-6616; **Board Cert:** Internal Medicine 1974; Rheumatology 1978; **Med School:** Univ Rochester 1971; **Resid:** Internal Medicine, Montefiore Med Ctr 1974; **Fellow:** Rheumatology, Montefiore Med Ctr 1975; Rheumatology, Montefiore Med Ctr 1978; **Fac Appt:** Asst Clin Prof Med, Mount Sinai Sch Med

Surgery

Colaco, Rodolfo MD (S) - **Spec Exp:** Hernia; Gallbladder Surgery; Laparoscopic Surgery; Breast Surgery; **Hospital:** Trinitas Reg Med Ctr (page 870); **Address:** 431 Elmora Ave, Elizabeth, NJ 07208; **Phone:** 908-353-4177; **Board Cert:** Surgery 2011; **Med School:** India 1974; **Resid:** Surgery, St Vincent Hosp 1980; Surgery, St Elizabeth Hosp 1983

Digioia, Julia M MD (S) - **Spec Exp:** Breast Disease; Breast Cancer; **Hospital:** Overlook Med Ctr (page 92), Jersey City Med Ctr; **Address:** Medical Arts Ctr, 33 Overlook Rd, Ste 205, Summit, NJ 07901; **Phone:** 908-522-3200; **Board Cert:** Surgery 2005; **Med School:** Italy 1979; **Resid:** Surgery, Jersey City Med Ctr 1984; **Fac Appt:** Asst Clin Prof S, UMDNJ-NJ Med Sch, Newark

Feteiha, Muhammad S MD (S) - **Spec Exp:** Minimally Invasive Surgery; Obesity/Bariatric Surgery; **Hospital:** Overlook Med Ctr (page 92), Trinitas Reg Med Ctr (page 870); **Address:** 155 Morris Ave, Fl 2, Springfield, NJ 07081-1225; **Phone:** 973-232-2300; **Board Cert:** Surgery 2009; **Med School:** Tufts Univ 1995; **Resid:** Surgery, Unv New Mexico Hlth Sci Ctr 2000; **Fellow:** Surgery, Columbia Presby Med Ctr 2001

Frost, James Henry MD (S) - **Spec Exp:** Breast Cancer; Colon Cancer; Laparoscopic Surgery; Vascular Surgery; **Hospital:** Overlook Med Ctr (page 92), Trinitas Reg Med Ctr (page 870); **Address:** Advanced Surgical Assocs, 155 Morris Ave Fl 2, Springfield, NJ 07081; **Phone:** 973-232-2300; **Board Cert:** Surgery 2007; **Med School:** Mexico 1982; **Resid:** Surgery, Univ Illinois Med Ctr 1988

Gumbs, Andrew MD (S) - **Spec Exp:** Gastrointestinal Surgery; Minimally Invasive Surgery; Hepatobiliary Surgery; Pancreatic & Biliary Surgery; **Hospital:** Overlook Med Ctr (page 92); **Address:** 1 Diamond Hill Rd Fl 4, Summit Medical Group, Berkeley Heights, NJ 07922; **Phone:** 908-277-8950; **Board Cert:** Surgery 2006; **Med School:** Yale Univ 1998; **Resid:** Surgery, Yale/New Haven Hosp 2005; **Fellow:** Minimally Invasive Surgery, NY Presby Hosp 2006; Hepatopancreatobiliary Surgery, Univ Rene Descartes Affil Hosp 2007; **Fac Appt:** Asst Clin Prof S, Columbia P&S

Lozner, Jerrold S MD (S) - **Spec Exp:** Breast Cancer & Surgery; Breast Surgery; **Hospital:** Overlook Med Ctr (page 92); **Address:** 1 Diamond Hill Rd, MS 0, Berkeley Heights, NJ 07922; **Phone:** 908-277-8850; **Board Cert:** Surgery 2009; Thoracic Surgery 2001; **Med School:** Univ Louisville Sch Med 1971; **Resid:** Surgery, Univ Cincinnati Med Ctr 1976; **Fellow:** Cardiothoracic Surgery, Univ Cincinnati Med Ctr 1978; **Fac Appt:** Assoc Clin Prof S, Columbia P&S

Mandel, Marc S MD (S) - **Spec Exp:** Gastrointestinal Surgery; Breast Cancer & Surgery; Cancer Surgery; Abdominal Wall Reconstruction; **Hospital:** Overlook Med Ctr (page 92); **Address:** 11 Overlook Rd, Ste 160, Summit, NJ 07901; **Phone:** 908-598-0966; **Board Cert:** Surgery 2009; **Med School:** Albert Einstein Coll Med 1985; **Resid:** Surgery, Montefiore Med Ctr 1988; Surgery, Yale New Haven Hosp 1990; **Fac Appt:** Asst Clin Prof S, Columbia P&S

Nitzberg, Richard S MD (S) - **Spec Exp:** Laparoscopic Surgery; Vein Disorders; Hernia; **Hospital:** Overlook Med Ctr (page 92); **Address:** 1 Diamond Hill Rd, Bensley Pavillion Fl 4, Berkeley Heights, NJ 07922; **Phone:** 908-277-8950; **Board Cert:** Surgery 2009; Vascular Surgery 2010; **Med School:** Harvard Med Sch 1983; **Resid:** Surgery, Columbia-Presby Med Ctr 1988; **Fellow:** Vascular Surgery, New England Med Ctr 1990

Starker, Paul MD (S) - **Spec Exp:** Laparoscopic Surgery; **Hospital:** Overlook Med Ctr (page 92); **Address:** 11 Overlook Rd, Ste 160, Summit, NJ 07901-3564; **Phone:** 908-608-9001; **Board Cert:** Surgery 2006; **Med School:** Columbia P&S 1980; **Resid:** Surgery, Columbia-Presby Med Ctr 1986; **Fellow:** Metabolism, Columbia-Presby Med Ctr 1982; **Fac Appt:** Asst Prof S, Columbia P&S

Urology

Lehrhoff, Bernard J MD (U) - **Spec Exp:** Prostate Cancer; Kidney Stones; Sexual Dysfunction; Bladder Cancer; **Hospital:** Overlook Med Ctr (page 92), Saint Michael's Med Ctr; **Address:** 275 Orchard St, Westfield, NJ 07090; **Phone:** 908-654-5100; **Board Cert:** Urology 1984; **Med School:** UMDNJ-NJ Med Sch, Newark 1976; **Resid:** Urology, Bellevue Hosp 1982; **Fac Appt:** Asst Clin Prof U, Columbia P&S

Ring, Kenneth S MD (U) - **Spec Exp:** Pediatric Urology; Urologic Cancer; Kidney Stones; **Hospital:** Overlook Med Ctr (page 92); **Address:** Premiere Urology Group, 275 Orchard St, Westfield, NJ 07090-3133; **Phone:** 908-654-5100; **Board Cert:** Urology 2012; **Med School:** Mount Sinai Sch Med 1985; **Resid:** Surgery, Mount Sinai Hosp 1987; Urology, Columbia-Presby Med Ctr 1991

Seidman, Barry MD (U) - **Spec Exp:** Sexual Dysfunction; Incontinence; Genitourinary Cancer; **Hospital:** Overlook Med Ctr (page 92); **Address:** 33 Overlook Rd, Ste 408, Summit, NJ 07901; **Phone:** 908-219-4479; **Board Cert:** Urology 2004; **Med School:** Mount Sinai Sch Med 1978; **Resid:** Urology, Mt Sinai 1983

Vascular Surgery

Sales, Clifford MD (VascS) - **Spec Exp:** Varicose Veins; Aneurysm-Abdominal Aortic; Peripheral Vascular Disease; Carotid Artery Surgery; **Hospital:** Overlook Med Ctr (page 92); **Address:** 1801 E 2nd St, Scotch Plains, NJ 07076-1749; **Phone:** 908-490-1699; **Board Cert:** Vascular Surgery 2002; **Med School:** Mount Sinai Sch Med 1986; **Resid:** Surgery, Montefiore Med Ctr 1991; **Fellow:** Vascular Surgery, Montefiore Med Ctr 1993; **Fac Appt:** Asst Clin Prof S, Mount Sinai Sch Med

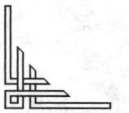

The Best in American Medicine
www.CastleConnolly.com

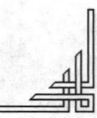

The State of Connecticut

The Best in American Medicine
www.CastleConnolly.com

Fairfield

Greenwich Hospital

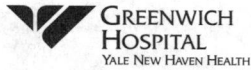
GREENWICH
HOSPITAL
YALE NEW HAVEN HEALTH

GENERAL OVERVIEW

Greenwich Hospital is a progressive, regional medical center and teaching institution with an internal medicine residency, serving lower Fairfield and Westchester counties. Care is provided on a beautiful, modern campus designed to create a healing environment for patients and visitors.

ACADEMIC AND CLINICAL AFFILIATIONS

As a member of the Yale New Haven Health System, Greenwich Hospital is a major affiliate of Yale School of Medicine and maintains affiliations with other leading medical providers. Patients have access to a comprehensive range of medical, surgical, diagnostic, *integrative medicine* and wellness programs. Greenwich Hospital also offers *robotic surgery* and *hyperbaric medicine and wound healing*. It has a State certified and Joint Commission accredited *Stroke Center*, and participates in international clinical trials

OUTSTANDING CLINICAL SERVICES

Specialties include oncology care at the hospital's *Bendheim Cancer Center*; advanced breast care at the *Breast Center*; a comprehensive Maternity program including *Level III NICU* and *fertility services*; a *Pediatric Specialty Center*; a *Weight Loss and Diabetes Center*, expert *neuroscience and spine services* and a wide range of *surgical specialties* including knee, hip and shoulder joint replacment, plus *bariatric surgery*.

SERVICE EXCELLENCE

Greenwich Hospital is renowned for service excellence and has been a five-time recipient of Press Ganey's Summit Award for highest ratings in Patient Satisfaction.

5 Perryridge Road
Greenwich, CT 06830-4697
Tel: 203.863.3000
www.greenwichhospital.org

Physician Referral:
For a prompt, personal Physician Referral please call Greenwich Hospital at 203-863-3627 or *visit us online.*

Sponsorship:
Voluntary,
Not-for-profit

Beds:
206

Accreditation:
The Joint Commission

GREENWICH
HOSPITAL
YALE NEW HAVEN HEALTH

Real Life. Real Care.

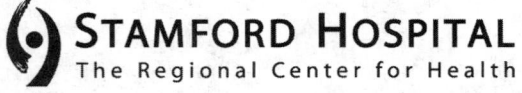

STAMFORD HOSPITAL
The Regional Center for Health

General Overview

Stamford Hospital provides area residents (Fairfield and Westchester Counties) access to the latest technology with a compassionate, patient-centered care approach in keeping with the Planetree philosophy. Stamford is a Level II trauma center with a nationally recognized adult intensive care unit. Our areas of expertise include:

Cancer Care	stamfordhospital.org/cancer
Heart Services	stamfordhospital.org/heart
Orthopedics	stamfordhospital.org/ortho
Women's Health	stamfordhospital.org/womenshealth

Comprehensive Specialty Centers

Bennett Cancer Center provides compassionate, patient-centered care from diagnosis through post-treatment.

Center for Integrative Medicine and Wellness blends conventional and complementary care for patients.

Center for Robotic Surgery using the *da Vinci* Surgical System, enables surgeons to perform even the most complex and delicate procedures through very small incisions with unmatched precision.

Center for Sleep Medicine offers experts in diagnosing and treating pediatric and adult sleep disorders, including snoring, sleep apnea, insomnia, narcolepsy and restless leg syndrome.

Center for Surgical Weight Loss offers the region's only comprehensive weight management program.

CyberKnife Center, located at the first and only hospital in Fairfield and Westchester Counties, provides the technology to destroy tumors with pinpoint accuracy.

Diabetes & Endocrine Center brings together consultative services and complete clinical care, including comprehensive patient education, medical management and treatment.

Women's Breast Center, first in the nation to receive accreditation from the American College of Surgeons for excellence in breast care. The only breast center in the region and among the first in the country, to offer 3-D breast tomosynthesis for breast screeening mammography.

Academic and Clinical Affiliations

Stamford Hospital is an affiliate of the New York–Presbyterian Healthcare System and a major teaching affiliate of the Columbia University College of Physicians & Surgeons.

Accreditation

Joint Commission on Accreditation of Healthcare Organization (JCAHO)

Beds

305

Sponsorship

Voluntary, Not-for-Profit

For a Physician Referral or more information, please call 1.877.233.9355 or visit StamfordHospital.org /doctor.

Stamford Hospital
30 Shelburne Road
Stamford, CT 06902
203.276.1000

StamfordHospital.org

Fairfield

Adolescent Medicine

Schneider, Marcie B MD (AM) - **Spec Exp:** Eating Disorders; Obesity; Menstrual Disorders; **Hospital:** Greenwich Hosp (page 892); **Address:** Greenwich Adolescent Med Srvs, 239 Glenville Rd, Greenwich, CT 06831; **Phone:** 203-532-1919; **Board Cert:** Pediatrics 1987; Adolescent Medicine 2009; **Med School:** Albert Einstein Coll Med 1983; **Resid:** Pediatrics, Montefiore Med Ctr 1986; **Fellow:** Adolescent Medicine, N Shore Univ Hosp 1988; **Fac Appt:** Assoc Clin Prof Ped, Albert Einstein Coll Med

Zolkowski-Wynne, Joanna MD (AM) - **Spec Exp:** Nutrition; Eating Disorders; Parenting Issues; **Hospital:** Bridgeport Hosp; **Address:** Bridgeport Hosp, 267 Grant St, Bridgeport, CT 06610; **Phone:** 203-384-3064; **Board Cert:** Pediatrics 1985; Adolescent Medicine 2009; **Med School:** SUNY Upstate Med Univ 1980; **Resid:** Pediatrics, Rhode Island Hosp 1983; **Fellow:** Adolescent Medicine, New England Bap Hosp 1986; **Fac Appt:** Asst Clin Prof Ped, Yale Univ

Allergy & Immunology

Bell, Jonathan MD (A&I) - **Spec Exp:** Asthma; Insect Allergies; Sinusitis; Hives; **Hospital:** Danbury Hosp; **Address:** 107 Newtown Rd, Ste 1B, Danbury, CT 06810-4156; **Phone:** 203-748-7433; **Board Cert:** Pediatrics 1986; Allergy & Immunology 1987; **Med School:** Georgetown Univ 1980; **Resid:** Pediatrics, St Christopher's Hosp Chldn 1983; **Fellow:** Pediatric Allergy & Immunology, Chldn's Hosp 1987; **Fac Appt:** Asst Clin Prof A&I, NY Med Coll

Hemmers, Philip H DO (A&I) - **Spec Exp:** Pediatric Allergy & Immunology; Food Allergy; **Hospital:** St. Vincent's Med Ctr - Bridgeport, Norwalk Hosp; **Address:** 4675 Main St, Ste 117, Bridgeport, CT 06606-1813; **Phone:** 203-374-6103; **Board Cert:** Pediatrics 2012; Allergy & Immunology 2007; **Med School:** NY Coll Osteo Med 2001; **Resid:** Pediatrics, Mount Sinai Hosp 2004; **Fellow:** Allergy & Immunology, LI College Hosp 2007

Lester, Mitchell R MD (A&I) - **Spec Exp:** Pediatric Allergy & Immunology; Asthma & Allergy; Food Allergy; **Hospital:** Norwalk Hosp, Greenwich Hosp (page 892); **Address:** 148 E Ave, Ste 3G, Norwalk, CT 06851; **Phone:** 203-838-4034; **Board Cert:** Pediatrics 1987; Allergy & Immunology 2003; **Med School:** Brown Univ 1983; **Resid:** Pediatrics, Brown Univ Affil Hosps 1987; **Fellow:** Allergy & Immunology, Natl Jewish Health Ctr 1989

Lindner, Paul S MD (A&I) - **Spec Exp:** Asthma & Sinusitis; Food & Drug Allergy; Immunodeficiency Disorders; Hereditary Angioedema; **Hospital:** Stamford Hosp (page 893); **Address:** 22 Fifth St, Stamford, CT 06905-5030; **Phone:** 203-978-0072; **Board Cert:** Internal Medicine 1989; Allergy & Immunology 2011; **Med School:** SUNY Buffalo 1985; **Resid:** Internal Medicine, Stamford Hosp 1989; **Fellow:** Allergy & Immunology, Nassau Co Med Ctr 1991; **Fac Appt:** Asst Clin Prof Med, Columbia P&S

Litchman, Mark MD (A&I) - **Spec Exp:** Asthma; Immune Deficiency; Lupus/SLE; Vasculitis; **Hospital:** Greenwich Hosp (page 892), Stamford Hosp (page 893); **Address:** 2 1/2 Dearfield Drive, Greenwich, CT 06831-5335; **Phone:** 203-869-2080; **Board Cert:** Internal Medicine 1987; Allergy & Immunology 2011; Rheumatology 1988; **Med School:** Rush Med Coll 1984; **Resid:** Internal Medicine, Greenwich Hosp-Yale Univ 1987; **Fellow:** Allergy & Immunology, Yale-New Haven Hosp 1989; Rheumatology, Yale-New Haven Hosp 1989

Matczuk, Agnieszka MD (A&I) - **Spec Exp:** Pediatric Allergy & Immunology; **Hospital:** Greenwich Hosp (page 892); **Address:** 2 1/2 Deerfield Drive, Greenwich, CT 06831; **Phone:** 203-869-2080; **Board Cert:** Pediatrics 2008; Allergy & Immunology 2003; **Med School:** Poland 1993; **Resid:** Pediatrics, Beth Israel Med Ctr 2000; **Fellow:** Allergy & Immunology, Yale-New Haven Hosp 2002

Santilli, John MD (A&I) - **Spec Exp:** Allergy; Sinusitis; **Hospital:** St. Vincent's Med Ctr - Bridgeport; **Address:** 4675 Main St, Bridgeport, CT 06606-1834; **Phone:** 203-374-6103; **Board Cert:** Pediatrics 1973; Allergy & Immunology 1983; **Med School:** Georgetown Univ 1968; **Resid:** Pediatrics, Georgetown Univ Hosp 1971; **Fellow:** Allergy & Immunology, Georgetown Univ Hosp 1973

Sproviero, Joseph MD/PhD (A&I) - **Hospital:** Norwalk Hosp, Greenwich Hosp (page 892); **Address:** Fairfield Co Allergy & Asthma, 148 East Ave, Ste 3G, Norwalk, CT 06851; **Phone:** 203-838-4034; **Board Cert:** Allergy & Immunology 1991; Internal Medicine 1989; **Med School:** Columbia P&S 1985; **Resid:** Internal Medicine, Yale New Haven Hosp 1988; **Fellow:** Allergy & Immunology, Yale-New Haven Hosp 1989; Rheumatology, Yale-New Haven Hosp 1990; **Fac Appt:** Asst Clin Prof Med, Yale Univ

Cardiac Electrophysiology

Chiravuri, Murali MD (CE) - **Spec Exp:** Arrhythmias; **Hospital:** Danbury Hosp, Bridgeport Hosp; **Address:** Cardiac Specialists, 25 Germantown Rd, Ste 2B, Danbury, CT 06810; **Phone:** 203-794-0090; **Board Cert:** Internal Medicine 2004; Cardiovascular Disease 2007; Cardiac Electrophysiology 2009; **Med School:** Tufts Univ 2001; **Resid:** Internal Medicine, Brigham & Women's Hosp 2003; **Fellow:** Cardiovascular Disease, Mass Genl Hosp 2007; Cardiac Electrophysiology, Brigham & Women's Hosp 2009

McPherson, Craig A MD (CE) - **Spec Exp:** Arrhythmias; Pacemakers/Defibrillators; Atrial Fibrillation; **Hospital:** Bridgeport Hosp, Yale-New Haven Hosp; **Address:** Bridgeport Hosp, Dept Electrophysiology, 267 Grant St Fl 10, Bridgeport, CT 06610; **Phone:** 203-384-3442; **Board Cert:** Internal Medicine 1979; Cardiovascular Disease 1983; Cardiac Electrophysiology 2004; **Med School:** Tufts Univ 1976; **Resid:** Internal Medicine, Tufts-New England Med Ctr 1979; **Fellow:** Cardiovascular Disease, Yale-New Haven Hosp 1982; Cardiac Electrophysiology, Yale-New Haven Hosp 1983; **Fac Appt:** Clin Prof Med, Yale Univ

Winslow, Robert D MD (CE) - **Spec Exp:** Arrhythmias; Atrial Fibrillation; **Hospital:** Bridgeport Hosp; **Address:** Cardiac Specialists, 1305 Post Rd, Fairfield, CT 06824; **Phone:** 203-292-2000; **Board Cert:** Internal Medicine 2002; Cardiovascular Disease 2005; Cardiac Electrophysiology 2007; **Med School:** Northwestern Univ-Feinberg Sch Med 1999; **Resid:** Internal Medicine, Brigham & Women's Hosp 2002; **Fellow:** Cardiovascular Disease, Mount Sinai Hosp 2005; Cardiac Electrophysiology, Brigham & Women's Hosp 2007

Cardiovascular Disease

Augenbraun, Charles B MD (Cv) - **Hospital:** Norwalk Hosp; **Address:** Cardio Assocs Fairfield Co, 40 Cross St, Ste 200, Norwalk, CT 06851-4697; **Phone:** 203-845-2160; **Board Cert:** Internal Medicine 1981; Cardiovascular Disease 1985; **Med School:** Univ Pennsylvania 1978; **Resid:** Internal Medicine, Temple Univ Hosp 1981; Cardiovascular Disease, Hosp Univ Penn 1985

Casale, Linda MD (Cv) - **Spec Exp:** Non-Invasive Cardiology; Women's Health; Echocardiography; **Hospital:** Bridgeport Hosp; **Address:** 1305 Post Rd, Fairfield, CT 06824; **Phone:** 203-292-2000; **Board Cert:** Cardiovascular Disease 2003; **Med School:** NY Med Coll 1986; **Resid:** Internal Medicine, Montefiore Med Ctr 1989; **Fellow:** Cardiovascular Disease, UC San Diego 1992

Copen, David L MD (Cv) - **Spec Exp:** Cardiac Catheterization; Coronary Artery Disease; Congestive Heart Failure; **Hospital:** Danbury Hosp; **Address:** 111 Osborne St Fl 3, Danbury, CT 06810-6099; **Phone:** 203-739-7155; **Board Cert:** Internal Medicine 1972; Cardiovascular Disease 1975; **Med School:** SUNY Downstate 1969; **Resid:** Internal Medicine, Yale-New Haven Hosp 1972; **Fellow:** Cardiovascular Disease, Mass Genl Hosp 1974; **Fac Appt:** Assoc Clin Prof Med, Yale Univ

Fisher, Lawrence I MD (Cv) - **Spec Exp:** Cardiac Catheterization; Pacemakers; Heart Valve Disease; **Hospital:** Danbury Hosp; **Address:** Cardiac Specialists, 25 Germantown Rd, Danbury, CT 06810; **Phone:** 203-794-0090; **Board Cert:** Internal Medicine 1988; Cardiovascular Disease 2011; **Med School:** SUNY Buffalo 1985; **Resid:** Internal Medicine, Bronx Muni Hosp 1988; **Fellow:** Cardiovascular Disease, Albert Einstein Coll Med 1990

Green, Jeffrey A MD (Cv) - **Hospital:** Stamford Hosp (page 893); **Address:** 80 Mill River St, Ste 1300, Stamford, CT 06902; **Phone:** 203-348-7410; **Board Cert:** Cardiovascular Disease 2004; **Med School:** NY Med Coll 1998; **Resid:** Internal Medicine, Montefiore Med Ctr 2001; **Fellow:** Cardiovascular Disease, Montefiore Med Ctr 2004

Heiman, Mark MD (Cv) - **Spec Exp:** Nuclear Cardiology; Cardiac CT Angiography; Clinical Trials; **Hospital:** Stamford Hosp (page 893), St. Vincent's Med Ctr - Bridgeport; **Address:** 177 Summer St, Fl 5, Stamford, CT 06905; **Phone:** 203-353-1133; **Board Cert:** Internal Medicine 1989; Cardiovascular Disease 2011; **Med School:** Albert Einstein Coll Med 1986; **Resid:** Internal Medicine, Montefiore Med Ctr 1989; **Fellow:** Cardiovascular Disease, Montefiore Med Ctr 1991; **Fac Appt:** Assoc Clin Prof Med, Columbia P&S

Horowitz, Steven F MD (Cv) - **Spec Exp:** Nuclear Cardiology; Preventive Cardiology; Complementary Medicine; **Hospital:** Stamford Hosp (page 893); **Address:** Stamford Hospital, Dept Cardiology, 30 Shelburne Rd Fl 2, Stamford, CT 06904-9317; **Phone:** 203-276-7480; **Board Cert:** Internal Medicine 1975; Cardiovascular Disease 1979; **Med School:** NY Med Coll 1972; **Resid:** Internal Medicine, Beth Israel Hosp 1976; **Fellow:** Cardiovascular Disease, Mt Sinai Hosp 1978; Cardiology Research, Mt Sinai Hosp 1979

Keller, Andrew M MD (Cv) - **Spec Exp:** Echocardiography; Cardiac Imaging; **Hospital:** Danbury Hosp; **Address:** Danbury Hospital, Div Cardiology, 111 Osborne St Fl 3, Danbury, CT 06810-6099; **Phone:** 203-739-7155; **Board Cert:** Internal Medicine 1982; Cardiovascular Disease 1985; **Med School:** Ohio State Univ 1979; **Resid:** Internal Medicine, Duke Univ Med Ctr Hosps 1982; **Fellow:** Cardiovascular Disease, Univ Texas-SW Med Ctr 1985; **Fac Appt:** Assoc Clin Prof Med, Columbia P&S

Kosinski, Edward J MD (Cv) - **Spec Exp:** Angioplasty & Stent Placement; **Hospital:** St. Vincent's Med Ctr - Bridgeport, Bridgeport Hosp; **Address:** Cardiology Physicians, 4675 Main St, Bridgeport, CT 06606-4201; **Phone:** 203-683-5100; **Board Cert:** Internal Medicine 1976; Cardiovascular Disease 1979; **Med School:** Wake Forest Univ 1973; **Resid:** Internal Medicine, Columbia-Presby Med Ctr 1976; **Fellow:** Cardiovascular Disease, Peter Bent Brigham Hosp 1978; **Fac Appt:** Assoc Clin Prof Med, Columbia P&S

Kunkes, Steven H MD (Cv) - **Spec Exp:** Cardiovascular Imaging; Diagnostic Problems; **Hospital:** Bridgeport Hosp, Milford Hosp; **Address:** 1305 Post Rd, Cardiac Specialists, Fairfield, CT 06824; **Phone:** 203-292-2000; **Board Cert:** Internal Medicine 1976; Cardiovascular Disease 1979; Geriatric Medicine 2004; **Med School:** Mount Sinai Sch Med 1973; **Resid:** Internal Medicine, Bellevue Hosp Ctr 1976; **Fellow:** Cardiovascular Disease, Mt Sinai Med Ctr 1978; **Fac Appt:** Assoc Clin Prof Med, Yale Univ

Mani, Susan MD (Cv) - **Hospital:** Danbury Hosp; **Address:** Western Med Grp, 111 Osborne St, Med Arts Bldg Fl 3 - Ste 131, Danbury, CT 06810; **Phone:** 203-739-7155; **Board Cert:** Cardiovascular Disease 2005; **Med School:** Johns Hopkins Univ 1998; **Resid:** Internal Medicine, Johns Hopkins Hosp 2001; **Fellow:** Cardiovascular Disease, NY-Presby/Columbia Univ Med Ctr 2005

Marshalko, Stephen MD (Cv) - **Hospital:** Bridgeport Hosp, St. Vincent's Med Ctr - Bridgeport; **Address:** 439 Millhill Ave, Bridgeport, CT 06610; **Phone:** 203-334-2100; **Board Cert:** Internal Medicine 2010; Cardiovascular Disease 2003; Interventional Cardiology 2004; **Med School:** Yale Univ 1996; **Resid:** Internal Medicine, Yale-New Haven Hosp 1999; **Fellow:** Cardiovascular Disease, Yale-New Haven Hosp 2000

Meizlish, Jay Lewis MD (Cv) - **Spec Exp:** Interventional Cardiology; Nuclear Cardiology; Arrhythmias; **Hospital:** Bridgeport Hosp; **Address:** Cardiac Specialists, 1305 Post Rd, Fairfield, CT 06824; **Phone:** 203-292-2000; **Board Cert:** Internal Medicine 1980; Cardiovascular Disease 1983; Nuclear Medicine 1984; Interventional Cardiology 2010; **Med School:** NYU Sch Med 1977; **Resid:** Internal Medicine, Harbor-UCLA Med Ctr 1980; **Fellow:** Cardiovascular Disease, Yale-New Haven Hosp 1983; Nuclear Medicine, Yale-New Haven Hosp

Michaelson, Stephen MD (Cv) - **Spec Exp:** Congestive Heart Failure; Coronary Artery Disease; **Hospital:** Norwalk Hosp; **Address:** Cardio Assocs Fairfield Co, 40 Cross St, Ste 200, Norwalk, CT 06851; **Phone:** 203-845-2160; **Board Cert:** Internal Medicine 1975; Cardiovascular Disease 1977; **Med School:** SUNY Upstate Med Univ 1972; **Resid:** Internal Medicine, Univ VA Hosp 1975; **Fellow:** Cardiovascular Disease, Yale Univ Sch Med 1977

Neeson, Francis J MD (Cv) - **Spec Exp:** Preventive Cardiology; Echocardiography; **Hospital:** Greenwich Hosp (page 892); **Address:** 75 Holly Hill Ln, Greenwich, CT 06830; **Phone:** 203-869-6960; **Board Cert:** Internal Medicine 1988; Cardiovascular Disease 2011; **Med School:** NYU Sch Med 1985; **Resid:** Internal Medicine, Bronx Muni Hosp 1988; **Fellow:** Cardiovascular Disease, Montefiore Med Ctr 1991

Pollack, Brian MD (Cv) - **Spec Exp:** Nuclear Cardiology; **Hospital:** Danbury Hosp; **Address:** 25 Germantown Rd, Ste 2B, Danbury, CT 06810; **Phone:** 203-794-0090; **Board Cert:** Cardiovascular Disease 2000; **Med School:** Mount Sinai Sch Med 1987; **Resid:** Internal Medicine, Mt Sinai Med Ctr 1990; **Fellow:** Cardiovascular Disease, Westchester Med Ctr 1993

Schmierer, Jeffrey A MD (Cv) - **Hospital:** Danbury Hosp; **Address:** 111 Osborne St, Ste 131, Danbury, CT 06810; **Phone:** 203-739-7155; **Board Cert:** Internal Medicine 1982; Cardiovascular Disease 1985; **Med School:** SUNY Downstate 1979; **Resid:** Internal Medicine, NY Hosp/Cornell Med Ctr 1982; **Fellow:** Cardiovascular Disease, Tufts-New Engl Med Ctr 1984

Schuster, Edward MD (Cv) - **Hospital:** Stamford Hosp (page 893); **Address:** 32 Strawberry Hill Ct, Stamford, CT 06902; **Phone:** 203-276-2323; **Board Cert:** Internal Medicine 1980; Cardiovascular Disease 1981; **Med School:** Ros Franklin Univ/Chicago Med Sch 1976; **Resid:** Internal Medicine, Duke Univ Med Ctr 1978; **Fellow:** Cardiovascular Disease, Johns Hopkins Hosp 1980

Taikowski, Richard L MD (Cv) - **Spec Exp:** Echocardiography; Congenital Heart Disease-Adult; Nuclear Cardiology; **Hospital:** Bridgeport Hosp; **Address:** Cardiac Specialists, 1305 Post Rd, Fairfield, CT 06824; **Phone:** 203-292-2000; **Board Cert:** Internal Medicine 1988; Cardiovascular Disease 2002; **Med School:** Boston Univ 1985; **Resid:** Internal Medicine, Boston Univ Med Ctr 1988; **Fellow:** Cardiovascular Disease, Mt Sinai Med Ctr 1991

Tuohy IV, Edward R MD (Cv) - **Spec Exp:** Angioplasty & Stent Placement; Geriatric Cardiology; Cardiac Stress Testing; **Hospital:** Bridgeport Hosp; **Address:** Cardiac Specialists, 999 Silver Ln, Trumbull, CT 06611; **Phone:** 203-385-1111; **Board Cert:** Internal Medicine 2008; Cardiovascular Disease 2011; Interventional Cardiology 2002; **Med School:** NYU Sch Med 1995; **Resid:** Internal Medicine, Yale-New Haven Hosp 1998; **Fellow:** Cardiovascular Disease, Yale-New Haven Hosp 2002

Zarich, Stuart MD (Cv) - **Spec Exp:** Echocardiography; Diabetes & Heart Disease; Cholesterol/Lipid Disorders; **Hospital:** Bridgeport Hosp; **Address:** Bridgeport Hosp, Cardiology Div, 267 Grant St Fl 10, Bridgeport, CT 06605; **Phone:** 203-384-3844; **Board Cert:** Internal Medicine 1984; Cardiovascular Disease 1989; **Med School:** SUNY Upstate Med Univ 1981; **Resid:** Internal Medicine, Beth Israel Deaconess Hosp 1984; **Fellow:** Cardiovascular Disease, Beth Israel Deaconess Hosp/Harvard 1987; **Fac Appt:** Asst Clin Prof Med, Yale Univ

Child & Adolescent Psychiatry

Rosenfeld, Alvin A MD (ChAP) - **Spec Exp:** Psychotherapy; Sexual Development Problems; Overscheduled Children; Family Therapy; **Hospital:** NY-Presby/Weill Cornell Med Ctr, NY (page 104); **Address:** 17 Sherwood Pl, Greenwich, CT 06830; **Phone:** 203-861-0700; **Board Cert:** Psychiatry 1976; Child & Adolescent Psychiatry 1978; **Med School:** Harvard Med Sch 1970; **Resid:** Psychiatry, Mass Mental Hlth Ctr 1973; **Fellow:** Child & Adolescent Psychiatry, Beth Israel Hosp 1975

Colon & Rectal Surgery

Littlejohn, Charles E MD (CRS) - **Spec Exp:** Colon & Rectal Cancer; **Hospital:** Stamford Hosp (page 893), Norwalk Hosp; **Address:** 70 Mill River St, Stamford, CT 06902; **Phone:** 203-323-8989; **Board Cert:** Colon & Rectal Surgery 1985; **Med School:** Dartmouth Med Sch 1978; **Resid:** Surgery, Univ Rochester Affil Hosps 1980; Surgery, UMDNJ Med Ctr 1983; **Fellow:** Colon & Rectal Surgery, UMDNJ Med Ctr 1984; **Fac Appt:** Asst Clin Prof S, Columbia P&S

McClane, Steven J MD (CRS) - **Spec Exp:** Colon & Rectal Cancer & Surgery; Inflammatory Bowel Disease; **Hospital:** Stamford Hosp (page 893); **Address:** 70 Mill River St, Stamford, CT 06902; **Phone:** 203-323-8989; **Board Cert:** Colon & Rectal Surgery 2009; **Med School:** Cornell Univ-Weill Med Coll 1992; **Resid:** Surgery, Hosp Univ Penn 1999; **Fellow:** Colon & Rectal Surgery, Cleveland Clinic 2000; **Fac Appt:** Asst Clin Prof S, Columbia P&S

Thornton, Scott MD (CRS) - **Spec Exp:** Laparoscopic Surgery; Colon & Rectal Cancer; **Hospital:** Bridgeport Hosp; **Address:** 1305 Post Rd, Ste 215, Fairfield, CT 06824; **Phone:** 203-255-7088; **Board Cert:** Colon & Rectal Surgery 2012; Surgery 2011; **Med School:** Univ Pittsburgh 1986; **Resid:** Surgery, Univ Conn Sch Med 1991; Colon & Rectal Surgery, UMDNJ Med Ctr 1992; **Fac Appt:** Clin Prof S, Yale Univ

Dermatology

Connors, Richard C MD (D) - **Spec Exp:** Skin Cancer; **Hospital:** Greenwich Hosp (page 892); **Address:** 1 Perryridge Rd, Greenwich, CT 06830-4607; **Phone:** 203-622-0808; **Board Cert:** Dermatology 1974; Dermatopathology 1976; **Med School:** Cornell Univ-Weill Med Coll 1967; **Resid:** Dermatology, New York Hosp 1974; **Fellow:** Dermatopathology, NYU Med Ctr 1975; **Fac Appt:** Assoc Clin Prof D, NYU Sch Med

Dietz, Stephanie B MD (D) - **Spec Exp:** Sclerotherapy; Laser Hair Removal; **Hospital:** Stamford Hosp (page 893), Yale-New Haven Hosp; **Address:** Dermatology Ctr Stamford, 1290 Summer St, Ste 3600, Stamford, CT 06905; **Phone:** 203-325-3576; **Board Cert:** Dermatology 2008; **Med School:** Univ Pennsylvania 1995; **Resid:** Dermatology, NYU Med Ctr 1999

Drugge, Rhett J MD (D) - **Hospital:** Stamford Hosp (page 893); **Address:** 50 Glenbrook Rd, Ste 1C, Stamford, CT 06902-2949; **Phone:** 203-324-5719; **Board Cert:** Dermatology 2001; **Med School:** NY Med Coll 1988; **Resid:** Dermatology, Univ Michigan Med Ctr 1992

Kolenik III, Steven A MD (D) - **Spec Exp:** Skin Cancer; Mohs' Surgery; **Hospital:** Norwalk Hosp, Yale-New Haven Hosp; **Address:** 761 Main Ave, Ste 102, Norwalk, CT 06851; **Phone:** 203-810-4151; **Board Cert:** Dermatology 2001; **Med School:** Yale Univ 1990; **Resid:** Dermatology, Yale-New Haven Hosp 1994; **Fellow:** Mohs Surgery, Yale-New Haven Hosp 1995; **Fac Appt:** Asst Clin Prof D, Yale Univ

Lipper, Graeme M MD (D) - **Spec Exp:** Pediatric Dermatology; Cosmetic Surgery; Skin Laser Surgery; Botox Therapy; **Hospital:** Danbury Hosp; **Address:** 25 Tamarack Ave, Danbury, CT 06810; **Phone:** 203-797-8990; **Board Cert:** Dermatology 2010; **Med School:** Harvard Med Sch 1997; **Resid:** Dermatology, Mass Genl Hosp 2000; **Fellow:** Cosmetic Surgery, Mass Genl Hosp 2001

Maiocco, Kenneth J MD (D) - **Spec Exp:** Skin Cancer; Dermatologic Surgery; Botox Therapy; **Hospital:** St. Vincent's Med Ctr - Bridgeport, Bridgeport Hosp; **Address:** 4639 Main St, Bridgeport, CT 06606-1873; **Phone:** 203-374-5546; **Board Cert:** Dermatology 1976; **Med School:** Univ Rochester 1967; **Resid:** Surgery, St Vincents Med Ctr 1971; Dermatology, Geisinger Med Ctr 1975

Mayer, Fern E MD (D) - **Spec Exp:** Skin Cancer; Pediatric Dermatology; Immune Deficiency-Skin Disorders; **Hospital:** Stamford Hosp (page 893); **Address:** 132 Morgan St, Stamford, CT 06905; **Phone:** 203-969-0123; **Board Cert:** Dermatology 1990; **Med School:** NYU Sch Med 1986; **Resid:** Dermatology, Downstate Med Ctr 1990

Naidorf, Ellen MD (D) - **Spec Exp:** Skin Cancer; Pediatric Dermatology; **Hospital:** Stamford Hosp (page 893), Yale-New Haven Hosp; **Address:** 22 Long Ridge Rd, Stamford, CT 06905-3812; **Phone:** 203-964-1103; **Board Cert:** Dermatology 2009; Pediatrics 1980; **Med School:** Columbia P&S 1975; **Resid:** Dermatology, NY Presbyterian-Columbia Med Ctr 1978; Pediatrics, Yale-New Haven Hosp 1980

Oestreicher, Mark MD (D) - **Spec Exp:** Hair Loss; Skin Laser Surgery; **Hospital:** Bridgeport Hosp; **Address:** 160 Hawley Ln, Adult & Pediatric Dermatology, Trumbull, CT 06611; **Phone:** 203-377-0639; **Board Cert:** Dermatology 1979; Internal Medicine 1977; **Med School:** Albany Med Coll 1974; **Resid:** Internal Medicine, Albany Med Ctr 1977; Dermatology, UCLA Med Ctr 1979; **Fac Appt:** Asst Prof, Yale Univ

Oshman, Robin G MD/PhD (D) - **Spec Exp:** Skin Cancer; Cosmetic Dermatology; Pediatric Dermatology; **Hospital:** Yale-New Haven Hosp, VA Conn Hlthcre Sys-W Haven Campus; **Address:** 101 Long Lots Rd, Westport, CT 06880-5426; **Phone:** 203-454-0743; **Board Cert:** Dermatology 1990; **Med School:** Brown Univ 1985; **Resid:** Dermatology, Mt Sinai Hosp 1989; **Fac Appt:** Asst Clin Prof D, Yale Univ

Pesce, Joseph R MD (D) - **Hospital:** St. Vincent's Med Ctr - Bridgeport; **Address:** 4699 Main St, Ste 212, Bridgeport, CT 06606-1830; **Phone:** 203-372-8949; **Board Cert:** Dermatology 1972; **Med School:** Belgium 1967; **Resid:** Internal Medicine, Hosp of St Raphael 1968; Dermatology, Dartmouth-Hitchcock Med Ctr 1971

Pruzan-Clain, Debra L MD (D) - **Spec Exp:** Skin Cancer; Cosmetic Dermatology; Pediatric Dermatology; **Hospital:** Stamford Hosp (page 893); **Address:** 1290 Summer St, Ste 3600, Stamford, CT 06905; **Phone:** 203-325-3576; **Board Cert:** Dermatology 1990; **Med School:** Univ Pennsylvania 1986; **Resid:** Dermatology, SUNY Downstate Med Ctr 1990; **Fac Appt:** Asst Prof D, Albert Einstein Coll Med

Sibrack, Laurence A MD (D) - **Spec Exp:** Skin Cancer; Cosmetic Dermatology; **Hospital:** Danbury Hosp, Yale-New Haven Hosp; **Address:** 73 Sand Pit Rd, Ste 207, Danbury, CT 06810; **Phone:** 203-792-4151; **Board Cert:** Dermatology 1978; **Med School:** Univ Mich Med Sch 1974; **Resid:** Dermatology, Yale-New Haven Hosp 1978; **Fac Appt:** Asst Prof D, Yale Univ

Diagnostic Radiology

Cohen, Steven M MD (DR) - **Spec Exp:** Ultrasound; MRI; **Hospital:** Bridgeport Hosp; **Address:** Bridgeport Hosp, Dept Radiology, 267 Grant St, Bridgeport, CT 06610; **Phone:** 203-337-9729; **Board Cert:** Diagnostic Radiology 1987; **Med School:** NY Med Coll 1983; **Resid:** Internal Medicine, Stamford Hosp 1984; Diagnostic Radiology, Montefiore Med Ctr 1987; **Fellow:** Ultrasound/CT/MRI, Thomas Jefferson Univ Hosp 1989; **Fac Appt:** Asst Prof Rad, Columbia P&S

Ehrlich, Conrad MD (DR) - **Spec Exp:** Women's Imaging; Mammography; CT Scan; **Hospital:** Danbury Hosp; **Address:** Housatonic Valley Radiology, 67 Sand Pit Rd, Danbury, CT 06810-4032; **Phone:** 203-797-1770; **Board Cert:** Internal Medicine 1979; Nuclear Medicine 1981; Diagnostic Radiology 1983; **Med School:** Boston Univ 1976; **Resid:** Nuclear Medicine, Beth Israel Deaconess Med Ctr 1981; Diagnostic Radiology, Beth Israel Deaconess Med Ctr 1983; **Fellow:** Ultrasound, Beth Israel Deaconess Med Ctr

Fey, Christopher P MD (DR) - **Hospital:** Greenwich Hosp (page 892); **Address:** Greenwich Radiology Group, 49 Lake Ave, Greenwich, CT 06830; **Phone:** 203-869-6220; **Board Cert:** Diagnostic Radiology 1998; Nuclear Medicine 2009; Nuclear Radiology 1999; **Med School:** Yale Univ 1993; **Resid:** Radiology, Beth Israel Deaconess Med Ctr 1998; **Fellow:** Nuclear Medicine, Harvard Univ Affil Hosp 1999

King, Michael H MD (DR) - **Hospital:** Stamford Hosp (page 893); **Address:** Stamford Hosp, dept Radiology, 30 Shelburne Rd, Stamford, CT 06904; **Phone:** 203-276-7860; **Board Cert:** Diagnostic Radiology 1999; **Med School:** Ros Franklin Univ/Chicago Med Sch 1995; **Resid:** Diagnostic Radiology, Univ Chicago Hosps 1998

Lee, Ronald P MD (DR) - **Spec Exp:** MRI; CT Scan; **Hospital:** Norwalk Hosp; **Address:** Norwalk Radiology, 148 East Ave, Ste 1R, Norwalk, CT 06851; **Phone:** 203-851-5645; **Board Cert:** Diagnostic Radiology 1991; **Med School:** NYU Sch Med 1986; **Resid:** Diagnostic Radiology, Bellevue Hosp/NYU Med Ctr 1991; **Fellow:** Magnetic Resonance Imaging, Johns Hopkins Hosp 1992

Mullen, David MD (DR) - **Hospital:** Greenwich Hosp (page 892); **Address:** 49 Lake Ave, Greenwich, CT 06830-4502; **Phone:** 203-869-6220; **Board Cert:** Diagnostic Radiology 1987; **Med School:** Albert Einstein Coll Med 1983; **Resid:** Diagnostic Radiology, Columbia-Presby Med Ctr 1985; **Fellow:** Abdominal Imaging, Columbia-Presby Med Ctr 1986; **Fac Appt:** Asst Clin Prof, Columbia P&S

Salik, Erez MD (DR) - **Spec Exp:** Interventional Radiology; **Hospital:** Greenwich Hosp (page 892); **Address:** Greenwich Hosp-Dept Radiology, 5 Perryridge Rd, Greenwich, CT 06830; **Phone:** 203-863-3960; **Board Cert:** Diagnostic Radiology 2004; **Med School:** Mount Sinai Sch Med 1999; **Resid:** Radiology, NYU Med Ctr 2004; **Fellow:** Vascular & Interventional Radiology, Yale-New Haven Hosp 2005

Endocrinology, Diabetes & Metabolism

Arden-Cordone, Mary MD (EDM) - **Spec Exp:** Osteoporosis; Thyroid Disorders; **Hospital:** Stamford Hosp (page 893); **Address:** Endocrinology Ctr Stamford, 1275 Summer St, Ste A1, Stamford, CT 06905; **Phone:** 203-359-2444; **Board Cert:** Internal Medicine 1992; Endocrinology, Diabetes & Metabolism 2006; **Med School:** NYU Sch Med 1989; **Resid:** Internal Medicine, NY-Presby/Columbia Univ Med Ctr 1992; **Fellow:** Endocrinology, Diabetes & Metabolism, NY-Presby/Columbia Univ Med Ctr 1995

Goldberg-Berman, Judith C MD/PhD (EDM) - **Spec Exp:** Thyroid Disorders; Osteoporosis; Diabetes; **Hospital:** Greenwich Hosp (page 892); **Address:** 4 Dearfield Drive, Ste 102, Greenwich, CT 06831-5351; **Phone:** 203-622-9160; **Board Cert:** Endocrinology, Diabetes & Metabolism 2000; **Med School:** Cornell Univ-Weill Med Coll 1987; **Resid:** Internal Medicine, NYU/Bellevue Hosp 1990; **Fellow:** Endocrinology, NY CornellHosp/Meml Sloan Kettering 1993

Guoth, Maria S MD (EDM) - **Spec Exp:** Osteoporosis; Thyroid Disorders; Parathyroid Disorders; Diabetes; **Hospital:** Bridgeport Hosp; **Address:** 5520 Park Ave, Ste 306, Trumball, CT 06611; **Phone:** 203-373-7388; **Board Cert:** Endocrinology, Diabetes & Metabolism 2007; **Med School:** Hungary 1980; **Resid:** Internal Medicine, LaGuardia Hosp 1994; **Fellow:** Endocrinology, Diabetes & Metabolism, Yale-New Haven Hosp 1997; **Fac Appt:** Asst Clin Prof Med, Yale Univ

Rennert, Nancy Jill MD (EDM) - **Spec Exp:** Diabetes in Minority Populations; Thyroid Disorders; Endocrine Disorders in Pregnancy; **Hospital:** Norwalk Hosp; **Address:** 120 Connecticut Ave, Norwalk, CT 06856; **Phone:** 203-899-1770; **Board Cert:** Internal Medicine 2003; Endocrinology, Diabetes & Metabolism 2003; **Med School:** Univ Pittsburgh 1987; **Resid:** Internal Medicine, Univ Pitt Hlth Ctr 1990; **Fellow:** Endocrinology, Diabetes & Metabolism, Yale Univ Sch Med 1993; **Fac Appt:** Assoc Clin Prof Med, Yale Univ

Rich, Glenn MD (EDM) - **Spec Exp:** Calcium Disorders; **Hospital:** Bridgeport Hosp; **Address:** Fairfield Co Med Grp, 15 Corporate Drive, Ste 2-1, Trumbull, CT 06611; **Phone:** 203-459-5100; **Board Cert:** Internal Medicine 1989; Endocrinology, Diabetes & Metabolism 2011; **Med School:** Cornell Univ-Weill Med Coll 1986; **Resid:** Internal Medicine, St Lukes Hospital 1989; **Fellow:** Endocrinology, Diabetes & Metabolism, Brigham & Women's Hosp 1992

Rosa, Joseph MD (EDM) - **Spec Exp:** Diabetes; **Hospital:** St. Vincent's Med Ctr - Bridgeport; **Address:** 4699 Main St, Ste 101, Bridgeport, CT 06606; **Phone:** 203-371-7048; **Board Cert:** Internal Medicine 1987; Endocrinology 1989; **Med School:** Mexico 1982; **Resid:** Internal Medicine, St Vincents Med Ctr 1986; **Fellow:** Endocrinology, Diabetes & Metabolism, Univ Conn Med Ctr 1988; **Fac Appt:** Assoc Prof Med, Columbia P&S

Savino, Robert R DO (EDM) - **Spec Exp:** Diabetes; **Hospital:** Danbury Hosp; **Address:** 25 German Town Rd, Danbury, CT 06810; **Phone:** 203-794-5620; **Board Cert:** Internal Medicine 2002; Endocrinology, Diabetes & Metabolism 2005; **Med School:** NY Coll Osteo Med 1988; **Resid:** Internal Medicine, LI Jewish Med Ctr 1992; **Fellow:** Endocrinology, Diabetes & Metabolism, Lahey-Hitchcock Med Ctr 1993; Endocrinology, Diabetes & Metabolism, Joslin Diabetes Ctr 1994; **Fac Appt:** Asst Clin Prof Med, Yale Univ

Family Medicine

Acosta, Rodrigo MD (FMed) *PCP* - **Spec Exp:** Geriatric Care; Preventive Medicine; **Hospital:** Stamford Hosp (page 893); **Address:** Stamford Family Practice, 32 Strawberry Hill Ct Fl 4 - Ste 6, Stamford, CT 06902; **Phone:** 203-977-2566; **Board Cert:** Family Medicine 2008; Geriatric Medicine 2002; **Med School:** Univ Tex SW, Dallas 1984; **Resid:** Family Medicine, St Josephs Med Ctr 1987

Duchen, Douglas MD (FMed) *PCP* - **Hospital:** St. Vincent's Med Ctr - Bridgeport, Bridgeport Hosp; **Address:** 3715 Main St, Ste 200, Bridgeport, CT 06606-3615; **Phone:** 203-372-4065; **Board Cert:** Family Medicine 2004; **Med School:** South Africa 1983; **Resid:** Orthopaedic Surgery, Whittington Hosp 1987; Family Medicine, Brookhaven Meml Hosp 1991

Falkoff, Alan MD (FMed) *PCP* - **Hospital:** Stamford Hosp (page 893); **Address:** High Ridge Family Practice, 30 Buxton Farms Rd, Ste 210, Stamford, CT 06905; **Phone:** 203-322-7070; **Board Cert:** Family Medicine 2007; **Med School:** Grenada 1985; **Resid:** Family Medicine, St Joseph's Med Ctr 1988

Farrell, Matthew M MD (FMed) *PCP* - **Spec Exp:** Primary Care Sports Medicine; Sports Medicine-Aging Athlete; **Hospital:** Danbury Hosp; **Address:** 60 Old New Milford Rd, Ste 2A, Brookfield, CT 06804-2430; **Phone:** 203-775-6365; **Board Cert:** Geriatric Medicine 2006; Family Medicine 2007; Sports Medicine 2003; **Med School:** Columbia P&S 1980; **Resid:** Family Medicine, Somerset Med Ctr 1983; **Fac Appt:** Asst Clin Prof FMed, Univ Conn

Filiberto, Cosmo MD (FMed) *PCP* - **Spec Exp:** Geriatric Care; Cholesterol/Lipid Disorders; Preventive Medicine; **Hospital:** St. Vincent's Med Ctr - Bridgeport, Bridgeport Hosp; **Address:** 3715 Main St, Ste 200, Bridgeport, CT 06606-3611; **Phone:** 203-372-4065; **Board Cert:** Family Medicine 2006; Geriatric Medicine 2000; **Med School:** Italy 1976; **Resid:** Family Medicine, Lutheran Med Ctr 1980; **Fac Appt:** Asst Clin Prof FMed, Univ Conn

Mallozzi, Angelo MD (FMed) *PCP* - **Hospital:** Stamford Hosp (page 893); **Address:** 32 Strawberry Hill Court, Stamford, CT 06902; **Phone:** 203-977-2566; **Board Cert:** Family Medicine 2008; **Med School:** Italy 1978; **Resid:** Family Medicine, St Joseph's Hosp 1982

Sekiguchi, Raymond T MD/PhD (FMed) *PCP* - **Spec Exp:** Pain Management; Pain-Back; **Hospital:** Greenwich Hosp (page 892); **Address:** Greenwich Family Practice & Pain Center, 49 Lake Ave, Greenwich, CT 06830; **Phone:** 203-552-9037; **Board Cert:** Family Medicine 2003; **Med School:** Japan 1988; **Resid:** Family Medicine, N Shore Univ Hosp 1996; **Fellow:** Neuropathology, Univ Washington Med Ctr 1999

Gastroenterology

Barenberg, David MD (Ge) - **Hospital:** Danbury Hosp; **Address:** 111 Osborne St, Ste 121, Danbury, CT 06810; **Phone:** 203-739-7038; **Board Cert:** Internal Medicine 1983; Gastroenterology 1985; **Med School:** SUNY Downstate 1980; **Resid:** Internal Medicine, NY-Presby/Columbia Univ Med Ctr 1983; **Fellow:** Gastroenterology, Brigham & Women's Hosp 1985

Bonheim, Nelson MD (Ge) - **Spec Exp:** Inflammatory Bowel Disease; Hepatitis C; Colon Cancer; **Hospital:** Greenwich Hosp (page 892); **Address:** 500 W Putnam Ave, Ste 100, Greenwich, CT 06830; **Phone:** 203-863-2900; **Board Cert:** Internal Medicine 1973; Gastroenterology 1975; **Med School:** Ros Franklin Univ/Chicago Med Sch 1970; **Resid:** Internal Medicine, Bronx Muni Hosp 1973; **Fellow:** Gastroenterology, NY Hosp-Cornell Med Ctr 1975; **Fac Appt:** Assoc Prof Med, Yale Univ

Dettmer, Robert M MD (Ge) - **Spec Exp:** Endoscopy; Colonoscopy/Polypectomy; **Hospital:** Stamford Hosp (page 893); **Address:** Gastroenterology/Hepatology, 32 Strawberry Hill Ct, Ste 41042, Stamford, CT 06902; **Phone:** 203-348-5355; **Board Cert:** Gastroenterology 2010; **Med School:** Albert Einstein Coll Med 1994; **Resid:** Internal Medicine, Columbia Presby Med Ctr 1998; **Fellow:** Gastroenterology, Columbia Presby Med Ctr 1999

Gardner, Peter W MD (Ge) - **Spec Exp:** Liver Disease; Inflammatory Bowel Disease; **Hospital:** Stamford Hosp (page 893), Greenwich Hosp (page 892); **Address:** 778 Long Ridge Rd, Ste 101, Stamford, CT 06902; **Phone:** 203-967-2100; **Board Cert:** Internal Medicine 1982; Gastroenterology 1987; **Med School:** Georgetown Univ 1979; **Resid:** Internal Medicine, St Vincents Med Ctr 1982; **Fellow:** Gastroenterology, Univ Conn Hlth Ctr 1984; **Fac Appt:** Asst Clin Prof Med, Columbia P&S

Grossman, Edward T MD (Ge) - **Spec Exp:** Inflammatory Bowel Disease; Malabsorption; **Hospital:** St. Vincent's Med Ctr - Bridgeport, Bridgeport Hosp; **Address:** 425 Post Rd, Fl 1, Fairfield, CT 06824; **Phone:** 203-292-9000; **Board Cert:** Internal Medicine 1970; Gastroenterology 1973; **Med School:** Albert Einstein Coll Med 1963; **Resid:** Internal Medicine, Bronx Muni Hosp Ctr 1968; **Fellow:** Gastroenterology, NY Hosp-Cornell Med Ctr 1970; **Fac Appt:** Assoc Clin Prof Med, Univ Conn

Gruss, Claudia B MD (Ge) - **Spec Exp:** Colonoscopy; Gastroesophageal Reflux Disease (GERD); Inflammatory Bowel Disease; Nutrition; **Hospital:** Norwalk Hosp; **Address:** Arbor Med Grp, 73 Redding Rd, Georgetown, CT 06829; **Phone:** 203-544-9517; **Board Cert:** Internal Medicine 1980; Gastroenterology 1983; **Med School:** Brown Univ 1977; **Resid:** Internal Medicine, Rhode Island Hosp 1980; **Fellow:** Gastroenterology, Rhode Island Hosp 1982

Hale, William B MD (Ge) - **Spec Exp:** Liver Disease; **Hospital:** Norwalk Hosp; **Address:** Norwalk Hosp, Dept Gastroenterology, 30 Steven St, Ste D, Norwalk, CT 06850; **Phone:** 203-852-2278; **Board Cert:** Internal Medicine 1983; Gastroenterology 1987; **Med School:** Univ Wisc 1980; **Resid:** Internal Medicine, Boston Med Ctr 1984; **Fellow:** Gastroenterology, Boston Med Ctr 1986

Kapel, Robert C MD (Ge) - **Hospital:** Danbury Hosp; **Address:** 2 Glen Hill Rd, Danbury, CT 06811-4906; **Phone:** 203-748-7460; **Board Cert:** Gastroenterology 2005; **Med School:** Cornell Univ 1989; **Resid:** Internal Medicine, Mount Sinai Med Ctr 1993; **Fellow:** Gastroenterology, Univ Miami/Jackson Memorial Hosp 1995

Khaghan, Neda MD (Ge) - **Spec Exp:** Biliary Disease; Capsule Endoscopy; Pancreatic Cancer; **Hospital:** Greenwich Hosp (page 892); **Address:** Ctr GI Med Fairfield & Westchester, 500 W Putnam Ave, Ste 100, Greenwich, CT 06830; **Phone:** 203-863-2900; **Board Cert:** Internal Medicine 2008; Gastroenterology 2011; **Med School:** Mount Sinai Sch Med 1995; **Resid:** Internal Medicine, Mount Sinai Hosp 1998; **Fellow:** Gastroenterology, St. Luke's-Roosevelt Hosp 2001; **Fac Appt:** Asst Prof Med, NY Med Coll

Landau, Alan MD (Ge) - **Hospital:** St. Vincent's Med Ctr - Bridgeport; **Address:** 888 White Plains Rd, Ste 110, Trumbull, CT 06611; **Phone:** 203-459-4451; **Board Cert:** Internal Medicine 1988; Gastroenterology 2011; **Med School:** Boston Univ 1985; **Resid:** Internal Medicine, St Elizabeths Hosp 1988; **Fellow:** Gastroenterology, VA Med Ctr 1990

Link, Richard J MD (Ge) - **Hospital:** Bridgeport Hosp; **Address:** 4641 Main St, Ste 1, Bridgeport, CT 06606-1827; **Phone:** 203-374-4966; **Board Cert:** Internal Medicine 1974; Gastroenterology 1989; **Med School:** UMDNJ-NJ Med Sch, Newark 1967; **Resid:** Internal Medicine, St Vincent Hosp 1970; **Fellow:** Gastroenterology, Bridgeport Hosp 1972

Mauer, Kenneth MD (Ge) - **Spec Exp:** Endoscopy; Inflammatory Bowel Disease/Crohn's; Capsule Endoscopy; Colonoscopy; **Hospital:** St. Vincent's Med Ctr - Bridgeport, Mount Sinai Med Ctr (page 102); **Address:** 425 Post Rd, Fairfield, CT 06824; **Phone:** 203-292-9000; **Board Cert:** Internal Medicine 1986; Gastroenterology 1989; **Med School:** NYU Sch Med 1983; **Resid:** Internal Medicine, Bronx Muni Hosp Ctr 1987; **Fellow:** Gastroenterology, Mount Sinai Hosp 1989; **Fac Appt:** Assoc Clin Prof Med, Mount Sinai Sch Med

Meighan, Dennis DO (Ge) - **Hospital:** Norwalk Hosp; **Address:** 30 Stevens St, Ste D, Norwalk, CT 06850-3859; **Phone:** 203-852-2278; **Board Cert:** Internal Medicine 1986; Gastroenterology 1989; **Med School:** Univ New Eng Coll Osteo Med 1982; **Resid:** Internal Medicine, Norwalk Hosp 1986; **Fellow:** Gastroenterology, Norwalk Hosp 1987

Nelson, Alan M MD (Ge) - **Hospital:** Bridgeport Hosp; **Address:** 4641 Main St, Ste 1, Bridgeport, CT 06606-1827; **Phone:** 203-374-4966; **Board Cert:** Internal Medicine 1977; Gastroenterology 1979; **Med School:** Georgetown Univ 1974; **Resid:** Internal Medicine, Kings Co Hosp-SUNY Med Ctr 1976; Internal Medicine, Bridgeport Hosp 1977; **Fellow:** Gastroenterology, Yale Univ Affil Hosps 1979

Soloway, Gregory MD (Ge) - **Spec Exp:** Colonoscopy/Polypectomy; **Hospital:** Bridgeport Hosp; **Address:** Gastroenterology Assocs, 2890 Main St Fl 2, Stratford, CT 06614; **Phone:** 203-375-1200; **Board Cert:** Gastroenterology 2004; Internal Medicine 1989; **Med School:** Cornell Univ-Weill Med Coll 1986; **Resid:** Internal Medicine, Montefiore Med Ctr 1990; **Fellow:** Gastroenterology, Montefiore Med Ctr 1992

Spivack, Julie MD (Ge) - **Spec Exp:** Women's Health; Colonoscopy; Gallbladder Disease; **Hospital:** St. Vincent's Med Ctr - Bridgeport; **Address:** Gastroenterology Assocs Fairfield Co, 425 Post Rd, Fairfield, CT 06824; **Phone:** 203-292-9000; **Board Cert:** Gastroenterology 2005; **Med School:** Albert Einstein Coll Med 1990; **Resid:** Internal Medicine, Beth Israel Deaconess Hosp 1993; **Fellow:** Gastroenterology, NY-Presby/Weill Cornell Med Ctr 1994; Hepatobiliary Surgery, Meml Sloan-Kettering Cancer Ctr 1996

Taubin, Howard L MD (Ge) - **Spec Exp:** Colon Cancer Screening; Gastroesophageal Reflux Disease (GERD); Inflammatory Bowel Disease; Liver Disease; **Hospital:** Bridgeport Hosp; **Address:** 2890 Main St Fl 2, Stratford, CT 06614; **Phone:** 203-375-1200; **Board Cert:** Internal Medicine 1972; Gastroenterology 1973; **Med School:** Univ VA Sch Med 1965; **Resid:** Internal Medicine, Montefiore Hosp 1967; Internal Medicine, Yale-New Haven Hosp 1970; **Fellow:** Gastroenterology, Yale-New Haven Hosp 1973; **Fac Appt:** Assoc Clin Prof Med, Yale Univ

Whelan, Thomas Patrick MD (Ge) - **Spec Exp:** Food Allergy; Gastroesophageal Reflux Disease (GERD); Barrett's Esophagus; **Hospital:** Danbury Hosp; **Address:** 2 Elizabeth St, Bethel, CT 06801-2100; **Phone:** 203-791-2221; **Board Cert:** Internal Medicine 1986; Gastroenterology 1989; **Med School:** Univ VT Coll Med 1983; **Resid:** Internal Medicine, Thomas Jefferson Univ Hosp 1986; **Fellow:** Gastroenterology, Temple Univ Hosp 1988

Zwas, Felice R MD (Ge) - **Hospital:** Greenwich Hosp (page 892); **Address:** 500 W Putnam Ave, Ste 100, Greenwich, CT 06831; **Phone:** 203-863-2900; **Board Cert:** Internal Medicine 1983; Gastroenterology 1985; **Med School:** Columbia P&S 1980; **Resid:** Internal Medicine, Columbia-Presby Med Ctr 1983; **Fellow:** Gastroenterology, Beth Israel Deaconess Med Ctr 1985

Geriatric Medicine

Jones, Stephen G MD (Ger) *PCP* - **Spec Exp:** Alzheimer's Disease; **Hospital:** Greenwich Hosp (page 892); **Address:** 5 Perryridge Rd, Greenwich, CT 06830; **Phone:** 203-863-3415; **Board Cert:** Internal Medicine 2002; Geriatric Medicine 2004; **Med School:** SUNY Stony Brook 1985; **Resid:** Geriatric Medicine, SUNY-Stony Brook Hosp 1989; **Fac Appt:** Assoc Clin Prof Med, Yale Univ

Gynecologic Oncology

Wertheim, Iris MD (GO) - **Hospital:** Stamford Hosp (page 893), Northern Westchester Hosp (page 613); **Address:** Tully Hlth Ctr, 32 Strawberry Hill Ct, Ste 41052, Stamford, CT 06902; **Phone:** 203-653-5155; **Board Cert:** Obstetrics & Gynecology 2011; Gynecologic Oncology 2011; **Med School:** Columbia P&S 1989; **Resid:** Obstetrics & Gynecology, Brigham & Women's Hosp 1993; **Fellow:** Gynecologic Oncology, Brigham & Women's Hosp 1996; **Fac Appt:** Asst Prof S, Columbia P&S

Hand Surgery

Backe Jr, Henry A MD (HS) - **Hospital:** St. Vincent's Med Ctr - Bridgeport, Bridgeport Hosp; **Address:** 75 Kings Highway Cutoff, Fairfield, CT 06824; **Phone:** 203-337-2600; **Board Cert:** Orthopaedic Surgery 2006; Hand Surgery 2006; **Med School:** Temple Univ 1986; **Resid:** Orthopaedic Surgery, Temple Univ Hosp 1991; **Fellow:** Hand Surgery, Hosp for Joint Diseases 1992; Joint Reconstruction, Hosp Special Surgery 1993

Brown, Lionel G MD (HS) - **Spec Exp:** Hand Reconstruction; Carpal Tunnel Syndrome; **Hospital:** Danbury Hosp; **Address:** 35 Tamarack Ave, Danbury, CT 06811; **Phone:** 203-792-4263; **Board Cert:** Hand Surgery 2008; **Med School:** UCSF 1964; **Resid:** Surgery, UCSF Med Ctr 1976; **Fellow:** Hand Surgery, UCSF Med Ctr 1975

Kavookjian, Haik G MD (HS) - **Spec Exp:** Hand & Upper Extremity Surgery; **Hospital:** Stamford Hosp (page 893), Norwalk Hosp; **Address:** 555 Newfield Ave, Stamford, CT 06905; **Phone:** 203-358-0661; **Board Cert:** Orthopaedic Surgery 2008; Hand Surgery 2008; **Med School:** NY Med Coll 1985; **Resid:** Orthopaedic Surgery, Boston Univ Med Ctr 1989; **Fellow:** Hand Surgery, NY Presby-Columbia Med Ctr 1999

Lunt, John MD (HS) - **Spec Exp:** Pediatric Hand/Arm Surgery; Sports Injuries; Carpal Tunnel Syndrome; **Hospital:** Danbury Hosp; **Address:** Danbury Orthopedics, 35 Tamarack Ave, Danbury, CT 06811; **Phone:** 203-792-4263; **Board Cert:** Orthopaedic Surgery 2006; Hand Surgery 2006; **Med School:** Columbia P&S 1986; **Resid:** Orthopaedic Surgery, Long Island Jewish Med Ctr 1992; **Fellow:** Surgery, NY-Presby/Columbia Univ Med Ctr 1993

Rago, Thomas A MD (HS) - **Spec Exp:** Hand & Wrist Surgery; **Hospital:** St. Vincent's Med Ctr - Bridgeport; **Address:** 3101 Main St, Bridgeport, CT 06606; **Phone:** 203-374-5892; **Board Cert:** Orthopaedic Surgery 2007; Hand Surgery 2007; **Med School:** Columbia P&S 1977; **Resid:** Surgery, Roosevelt Hosp 1979; Orthopaedic Surgery, Presby Hosp 1982; **Fellow:** Hand Surgery, Columbia-Presby Med Ctr 1983

Hematology

Bar, Michael MD (Hem) - **Spec Exp:** Multiple Myeloma; Leukemia & Lymphoma; Bleeding/Coagulation Disorders; Gaucher Disease; **Hospital:** Stamford Hosp (page 893); **Address:** 34 Shelburne Rd, Stamford, CT 06902; **Phone:** 203-325-2695; **Board Cert:** Internal Medicine 1986; Medical Oncology 1989; Hematology 2010; **Med School:** Columbia P&S 1983; **Resid:** Internal Medicine, Columbia-Presby Med Ctr 1986; **Fellow:** Hematology & Oncology, UCSF Med Ctr 1990; **Fac Appt:** Asst Clin Prof Med, Columbia P&S

Boyd, D Barry MD (Hem) - **Spec Exp:** Hematologic Malignancies; Breast Cancer; Complementary Medicine; **Hospital:** Greenwich Hosp (page 892); **Address:** Boyd Ctr for Integrative Health, 15 Valley Drive Fl 2, Greenwich, CT 06831; **Phone:** 203-869-2111; **Board Cert:** Internal Medicine 1982; Medical Oncology 1987; **Med School:** Cornell Univ-Weill Med Coll 1979; **Resid:** Internal Medicine, NY Hosp-Cornell Med Ctr 1982; **Fellow:** Hematology & Oncology, NY Hosp-Cornell Med Ctr 1986; **Fac Appt:** Asst Clin Prof Med, Yale Univ

Cohen, Neil S MD (Hem) - **Spec Exp:** Leukemia; **Hospital:** Stamford Hosp (page 893); **Address:** Hematology Oncology, 34 Shelburne Rd, Stamford, CT 06902-3658; **Phone:** 203-325-2695; **Board Cert:** Internal Medicine 1983; Medical Oncology 1987; Hematology 1988; **Med School:** NY Med Coll 1980; **Resid:** Internal Medicine, Stamford Hosp 1983; **Fellow:** Hematology & Oncology, U Mass Med Ctr 1987; Hematology & Oncology, N Shore Univ Hosp 1988; **Fac Appt:** Assoc Clin Prof Med, Columbia P&S

Duda, E Andrew MD (Hem) - **Hospital:** St. Vincent's Med Ctr - Bridgeport, Bridgeport Hosp; **Address:** Medical Specialists of Fairfield, 425 Post Rd, Fairfield, CT 06824; **Phone:** 203-255-4545; **Board Cert:** Internal Medicine 1988; Medical Oncology 1989; Hematology 2002; **Med School:** Yale Univ 1984; **Resid:** Internal Medicine, Yale-New Haven Hosp 1987; **Fellow:** Hematology & Oncology, Dana Farber Cancer Ctr 1991; **Fac Appt:** Asst Clin Prof Med, Columbia P&S

Mazur, Eric M MD (Hem) - **Spec Exp:** Bleeding/Coagulation Disorders; Platelet Disorders; **Hospital:** Norwalk Hosp; **Address:** Norwalk Hosp, Div Hematology/Oncology, 34 Maple St, Norwalk, CT 06856; **Phone:** 203-852-2325; **Board Cert:** Hematology 1980; Medical Oncology 1981; Internal Medicine 1978; **Med School:** Johns Hopkins Univ 1975; **Resid:** Internal Medicine, Strong Meml Hosp 1977; Internal Medicine, Yale-New Haven Hosp 1979; **Fellow:** Hematology, Yale Univ Sch Med 1981; **Fac Appt:** Assoc Clin Prof Med, Yale Univ

Infectious Disease

Adler-Klein, Debra MD (Inf) - **Spec Exp:** Lyme Disease; AIDS/HIV; Pneumonia; **Hospital:** Stamford Hosp (page 893); **Address:** Med Assocs Stamford, 1100 Bedford St, Stamford, CT 06905; **Phone:** 203-323-4458; **Board Cert:** Internal Medicine 1988; Infectious Disease 2010; **Med School:** Albert Einstein Coll Med 1984; **Resid:** Internal Medicine, Stamford Hosp 1988; **Fellow:** Infectious Disease, NY-Presby/Columbia Univ Med Ctr 1990; **Fac Appt:** Clin Prof Med, Columbia P&S

Cipriani, Ralph MD (Inf) - **Spec Exp:** Lyme Disease; Fevers of Unknown Origin; **Hospital:** Greenwich Hosp (page 892); **Address:** 5 Perryridge Rd, Ste 108, Greenwich, CT 06830; **Phone:** 203-869-8838; **Board Cert:** Infectious Disease 2011; Internal Medicine 2011; **Med School:** Albert Einstein Coll Med 1996; **Resid:** Internal Medicine, Mt Sinai Hosp 1999; **Fellow:** Infectious Disease, Mt Sinai Hosp 2001; **Fac Appt:** Asst Clin Prof Med, NY Med Coll

Herbin, Joseph T MD (Inf) - **Spec Exp:** Lyme Disease; Infectious Disease in Elderly; **Hospital:** St. Vincent's Med Ctr - Bridgeport; **Address:** 2150 Black Rock Tpke, Ste 201, Fairfield, CT 06825; **Phone:** 203-384-0451; **Board Cert:** Internal Medicine 1972; **Med School:** Switzerland 1965; **Resid:** Internal Medicine, St Vincent's Hosp & Med Ctr 1970; **Fellow:** Infectious Disease, Med Ctr Hosp 1971; **Fac Appt:** Asst Clin Prof Med, Columbia P&S

McLeod, Gavin MD (Inf) - **Spec Exp:** AIDS/HIV; Travel Medicine; Hospital Acquired Infections; Pneumonia; **Hospital:** Stamford Hosp (page 893); **Address:** 166 W Broad St, Ste 202, Stamford, CT 06902; **Phone:** 203-353-1427; **Board Cert:** Internal Medicine 1988; Infectious Disease 2002; **Med School:** Univ Conn 1985; **Resid:** Internal Medicine, North Shore Univ Hosp 1988; **Fellow:** Infectious Disease, New England Deaconess Med Ctr 1992; **Fac Appt:** Assoc Clin Prof Med, Columbia P&S

Sabetta, James MD (Inf) - **Spec Exp:** Lyme Disease; Tropical Diseases; Bone & Joint Infections; Fevers of Unknown Origin; **Hospital:** Greenwich Hosp (page 892); **Address:** 5 Perryridge Rd, Ste 108, Greenwich, CT 06830; **Phone:** 203-869-8838; **Board Cert:** Internal Medicine 1981; Infectious Disease 1984; **Med School:** Brown Univ 1978; **Resid:** Internal Medicine, Rhode Island Hosp 1981; **Fellow:** Infectious Disease, Yale-New Haven Hosp 1984; **Fac Appt:** Assoc Clin Prof Med, Yale Univ

Saul, Zane MD (Inf) - **Spec Exp:** Lyme Disease; AIDS/HIV; **Hospital:** Bridgeport Hosp; **Address:** 3241 Main St, Ste B, Stratford, CT 06614; **Phone:** 203-383-4466; **Board Cert:** Internal Medicine 2011; Infectious Disease 2000; **Med School:** Grenada 1985; **Resid:** Internal Medicine, Brooklyn Hosp 1988; **Fellow:** Infectious Disease, Hackensack Univ Med Ctr 1990

Schleiter, Gary S MD (Inf) - **Hospital:** Danbury Hosp, New Milford Hosp; **Address:** 33 Germantown Rd, Danbury, CT 06810-6148; **Phone:** 203-739-8310; **Board Cert:** Internal Medicine 1983; Infectious Disease 1986; **Med School:** Wake Forest Univ 1980; **Resid:** Internal Medicine, John Dempsey Hosp 1983; **Fellow:** Infectious Disease, Univ Mass Med Ctr 1985; **Fac Appt:** Asst Clin Prof Med, Yale Univ

Yee, Arthur MD (Inf) - **Spec Exp:** Lyme Disease; Infections-Respiratory; Hospital Acquired Infections; **Hospital:** Norwalk Hosp; **Address:** 40 Cross St, Ste 400, Norwalk, CT 06851; **Phone:** 203-845-4838; **Board Cert:** Internal Medicine 1986; Infectious Disease 1988; **Med School:** Univ Conn 1982; **Resid:** Internal Medicine, Columbia-Presby Med Ctr 1985; **Fellow:** Infectious Disease, Hosp Univ Penn 1988; **Fac Appt:** Asst Clin Prof Med, Yale Univ

Internal Medicine

Altbaum, Robert A MD (IM) *PCP* - **Spec Exp:** Hypertension; Asthma; Osteoporosis; **Hospital:** Norwalk Hosp, Bridgeport Hosp; **Address:** 162 Kings Hwy N, Westport, CT 06880-2425; **Phone:** 203-226-0731; **Board Cert:** Internal Medicine 1978; **Med School:** Harvard Med Sch 1975; **Resid:** Internal Medicine, Mass Genl Hosp 1977; Internal Medicine, Yale-New Haven Hosp 1979

Berman, Edward Roy MD (IM) - **Hospital:** Danbury Hosp; **Address:** 30 Prospect St, Ste 500, Ridgefield, CT 06877; **Phone:** 203-438-0364; **Board Cert:** Internal Medicine 1979; Occupational Medicine 1992; **Med School:** Boston Univ 1976; **Resid:** Internal Medicine, Wayne State Univ Affil Hosp 1978; Internal Medicine, Norwalk Hosp 1979

Bivona, James J MD (IM) *PCP* - **Hospital:** Stamford Hosp (page 893); **Address:** Stamford Primary Care, 1275 Summer St, Ste 105, Stamford, CT 06905; **Phone:** 203-325-2667; **Board Cert:** Internal Medicine 2011; **Med School:** Dominica 1997; **Resid:** Internal Medicine, Stamford Hosp 2000

Blumberg, Joel M MD (IM) *PCP* - **Spec Exp:** Preventive Cardiology; Hypertension; Cholesterol/Lipid Disorders; Echocardiography; **Hospital:** Greenwich Hosp (page 892); **Address:** 55 Holly Hill Ln, MS 0, Greenwich, CT 06830; **Phone:** 203-661-4242; **Board Cert:** Internal Medicine 1972; Cardiovascular Disease 1974; **Med School:** NYU Sch Med 1966; **Resid:** Internal Medicine, Bellevue Hosp 1971; **Fellow:** Cardiovascular Disease, New York Hosp 1973

Costanzo, Joseph V MD (IM) *PCP* - **Hospital:** Stamford Hosp (page 893); **Address:** 80 Mill River St, Ste 2400, Stamford, CT 06902; **Phone:** 203-348-9455; **Board Cert:** Internal Medicine 2010; **Med School:** Harvard Med Sch 1987; **Resid:** Internal Medicine, Bronx Muni Hosp 1990

Dreyer, Neil P MD (IM) *PCP* - **Spec Exp:** Hypertension; Preventive Medicine; **Hospital:** Stamford Hosp (page 893); **Address:** 51 Schuyler Ave, Stamford, CT 06902; **Phone:** 203-327-1187; **Board Cert:** Internal Medicine 1980; Nephrology 1974; **Med School:** NYU Sch Med 1967; **Resid:** Internal Medicine, Bronx Municipal Hosp Ctr 1972; **Fellow:** Nephrology, Montefiore Med Ctr 1973; **Fac Appt:** Asst Clin Prof Med, Columbia P&S

Fennell, Gail M MD (IM) *PCP* - **Spec Exp:** Women's Health; Hypertension; Cholesterol/Lipid Disorders; **Hospital:** Greenwich Hosp (page 892); **Address:** Greenwich Medical Group, 75 Holly Hill Ln, Greenwich, CT 06830; **Phone:** 203-413-1130; **Board Cert:** Internal Medicine 2006; **Med School:** Univ Conn 1992; **Resid:** Internal Medicine, Greenwich Hosp 1995

Hoffman, Pamela B MD (IM) *PCP* - **Spec Exp:** Geriatric Care; **Hospital:** St. Vincent's Med Ctr - Bridgeport; **Address:** 2800 Main St, Bridgeport, CT 06606-4201; **Phone:** 203-576-5710; **Board Cert:** Internal Medicine 1983; **Med School:** Univ VA Sch Med 1978; **Resid:** Internal Medicine, St Vincent's Hosp & Med Ctr 1981; **Fellow:** Geriatric Medicine, Jewish Inst Geriatric Care 1983

Israel, Shara MD (IM) *PCP* - **Hospital:** Stamford Hosp (page 893); **Address:** 51 Schuyler Ave, Stamford, CT 06902; **Phone:** 203-327-1187; **Board Cert:** Internal Medicine 2005; **Med School:** Columbia P&S 1992; **Resid:** Internal Medicine, NY-Presby/Weill Cornell Med Ctr 1995

Klein, Neil C MD (IM) - **Spec Exp:** Inflammatory Bowel Disease/Crohn's; Ulcerative Colitis; **Hospital:** Stamford Hosp (page 893); **Address:** 1450 Washington Blvd, Stamford, CT 06902-2451; **Phone:** 203-327-9321; **Board Cert:** Internal Medicine 1974; Gastroenterology 1975; **Med School:** Cornell Univ-Weill Med Coll 1960; **Resid:** Internal Medicine, NY Hosp 1963; Internal Medicine, NY Hosp 1965; **Fellow:** Gastroenterology, NY Hosp 1967; **Fac Appt:** Clin Prof Med, Columbia P&S

Mickley, Diane W MD (IM) - **Spec Exp:** Eating Disorders; **Address:** 7 Riversville Rd Fl 3, Greenwich, CT 06831; **Phone:** 203-531-1909; **Board Cert:** Internal Medicine 1974; **Med School:** Tufts Univ 1971; **Resid:** Internal Medicine, Barnes Jewish Hosp 1973; Internal Medicine, Montefiore Med Ctr 1974; **Fac Appt:** Assoc Clin Prof Med, Yale Univ

Mickley, Steven P MD (IM) *PCP* - **Hospital:** Greenwich Hosp (page 892); **Address:** Glenville Med Assocs, 7 Riversville Rd Fl 1, Greenwich, CT 06831-3697; **Phone:** 203-531-1808; **Board Cert:** Internal Medicine 1974; **Med School:** Harvard Med Sch 1971; **Resid:** Internal Medicine, Barnes Hospital 1973; Internal Medicine, USPHS 1974; **Fac Appt:** Asst Clin Prof Med, Yale Univ

Miner III, Charles MD (IM) - **Hospital:** Stamford Hosp (page 893), Norwalk Hosp; **Address:** 36 Old Kings Hwy S, Darien, CT 06820-4523; **Phone:** 203-655-8749; **Board Cert:** Internal Medicine 1982; **Med School:** Univ Cincinnati 1979; **Resid:** Internal Medicine, Lenox Hill Hosp 1982

Molloy, Edward M MD (IM) *PCP* - **Spec Exp:** Hypertension; Diabetes; Preventive Medicine; **Hospital:** St. Vincent's Med Ctr - Bridgeport; **Address:** 134 Round Hill Rd, Fl 2, Fairfield, CT 06824; **Phone:** 203-255-0695; **Board Cert:** Internal Medicine 1974; **Med School:** UMDNJ-NJ Med Sch, Newark 1966; **Resid:** Internal Medicine, St Vincent's Hosp & Med Ctr 1972

Olin, Craig H MD (IM) *PCP* - **Spec Exp:** Preventive Medicine; Metabolic Disorders; **Hospital:** Stamford Hosp (page 893); **Address:** 5 High Ridge Park, Ste 103, Stamford, CT 06905; **Phone:** 203-276-4644; **Board Cert:** Internal Medicine 2006; **Med School:** NYU Sch Med 1993; **Resid:** Internal Medicine, NY-Presby/Weill Cornell Med Ctr 1996; **Fac Appt:** Asst Clin Prof Med, Columbia P&S

Osnoss, Kenneth MD (IM) *PCP* - **Spec Exp:** Asthma; Lung Disease; **Address:** 79 Sand Pit Rd, Ste 102, Danbury, CT 06810-6099; **Phone:** 203-749-5700; **Board Cert:** Internal Medicine 1978; Pulmonary Disease 1980; **Med School:** Tufts Univ 1975; **Resid:** Internal Medicine, Hosp Univ Penn 1978; **Fellow:** Pulmonary Disease, Hosp Univ Penn 1980

Radin, Alan M MD (IM) *PCP* - **Spec Exp:** Geriatric Medicine; **Hospital:** Norwalk Hosp; **Address:** Arbor Med Grp, 195 Danbury Rd, Whitlock Bldg - Ste 210, Wilton, CT 06897-3003; **Phone:** 203-762-3353; **Board Cert:** Internal Medicine 1977; **Med School:** Penn State Coll Med 1974; **Resid:** Internal Medicine, Univ Vermont Med Ctr 1978

Ralabate, James P MD (IM) _PCP_ - **Hospital:** Bridgeport Hosp; **Address:** 2890 Main St, Ste 2A, Primary Care Assoc, Stratford, CT 08614; **Phone:** 203-378-3696; **Board Cert:** Internal Medicine 1986; Pediatrics 1987; **Med School:** Albany Med Coll 1981; **Resid:** Internal Medicine, Bridgeport Hospital; Pediatrics, Bridgeport Hospital

Skluth, Myra MD/PhD (IM) _PCP_ - **Spec Exp:** Women's Health; Diabetes; Cardiovascular Disease; **Hospital:** Norwalk Hosp; **Address:** 10 Mott Ave, Ste 3A, Norwalk, CT 06850; **Phone:** 203-866-4455; **Board Cert:** Internal Medicine 1989; Geriatric Medicine 2006; **Med School:** Albert Einstein Coll Med 1986; **Resid:** Internal Medicine, Montefiore Med Ctr 1989; **Fac Appt:** Asst Clin Prof Med, Yale Univ

Slogoff, Frederick B MD (IM) _PCP_ - **Spec Exp:** Preventive Medicine; Cardiovascular Disease; Anxiety & Mood Disorders; **Hospital:** Stamford Hosp (page 893); **Address:** 5 High Ridge Park, Ste 104, Stamford, CT 06905; **Phone:** 203-968-9500; **Board Cert:** Internal Medicine 2009; **Med School:** Mount Sinai Sch Med 1996; **Resid:** Internal Medicine, New York Hosp-Cornell Med Ctr 1999; **Fac Appt:** Clin Prof Med, Columbia P&S

Spano, Frank MD (IM) _PCP_ - **Spec Exp:** Preventive Medicine; **Hospital:** Bridgeport Hosp, St. Vincent's Med Ctr - Bridgeport; **Address:** Fairfield County Medical Group, 15 Corporate Drive, Ste 2-1, Trumbull, CT 06611; **Phone:** 203-459-5100; **Board Cert:** Internal Medicine 1987; **Med School:** Albert Einstein Coll Med 1984; **Resid:** Internal Medicine, Jacobi Hosp 1987

Thomas, Byron S MD (IM) _PCP_ - **Spec Exp:** Geriatric Care; **Hospital:** Danbury Hosp; **Address:** 79 Sand Pit Rd, Ste 102, Danbury, CT 06810; **Phone:** 203-749-5700; **Board Cert:** Internal Medicine 1978; Geriatric Medicine 2002; **Med School:** Univ Pittsburgh 1975; **Resid:** Internal Medicine, Mt Sinai Hosp 1978; **Fac Appt:** Asst Clin Prof Med, Yale Univ

Walsh, Francis X MD (IM) _PCP_ - **Spec Exp:** Kidney Disease; Hypertension; Dialysis Care; **Hospital:** Greenwich Hosp (page 892), Stamford Hosp (page 893); **Address:** 31 River Rd, Ste 200, Cos Cob, CT 06830-5694; **Phone:** 203-661-9433; **Board Cert:** Internal Medicine 1972; Nephrology 1974; **Med School:** NY Med Coll 1967; **Resid:** Internal Medicine, Greenwich Hosp 1970; **Fellow:** Nephrology, Duke Univ Med Ctr 1972; **Fac Appt:** Asst Clin Prof Med, Yale Univ

Zucker, Michael MD (IM) _PCP_ - **Hospital:** Stamford Hosp (page 893); **Address:** 555 Newfield Ave, Stamford, CT 06905-3330; **Phone:** 203-359-4444; **Board Cert:** Internal Medicine 1988; **Med School:** NYU Sch Med 1985; **Resid:** Internal Medicine, Stamford Hospital 1988

Interventional Cardiology

Driesman, Mitchell MD (IC) - **Spec Exp:** Cardiac Catheterization; **Hospital:** Bridgeport Hosp; **Address:** Cardiac Specialists, 1305 Post Rd, Fairfield, CT 06824; **Phone:** 203-292-2000; **Board Cert:** Internal Medicine 1980; Cardiovascular Disease 1983; Interventional Cardiology 2009; **Med School:** Brown Univ 1977; **Resid:** Internal Medicine, Tufts-New Eng Med Ctr 1980; **Fellow:** Cardiovascular Disease, Mt Sinai Hosp 1982; **Fac Appt:** Asst Clin Prof Med, Yale Univ

Fishman, Robert MD (IC) - **Spec Exp:** Carotid Artery Stent Placement; Peripheral Vascular Disease; **Hospital:** Bridgeport Hosp; **Address:** Cardiac Specialists, 1305 Post Rd, Fairfield, CT 06824; **Phone:** 203-292-2000; **Board Cert:** Internal Medicine 1988; Cardiovascular Disease 2011; Interventional Cardiology 2009; **Med School:** Boston Univ 1985; **Resid:** Internal Medicine, Beth Israel Hosp 1990; **Fellow:** Cardiovascular Disease, Beth Israel Hosp 1992

Howes, Christopher J MD (IC) - **Hospital:** Greenwich Hosp (page 892), Yale-New Haven Hosp; **Address:** 55 Holly Hill Ln, Ste 240, Cardiology Svcs of Greenwich, Greenwich, CT 06830; **Phone:** 203-863-4210; **Board Cert:** Internal Medicine 2002; Cardiovascular Disease 2007; Interventional Cardiology 2009; Echocardiography 2011; **Med School:** Albert Einstein Coll Med 1989; **Resid:** Internal Medicine, Yale-New Haven Hosp 1992; **Fellow:** Cardiovascular Disease, Yale-New Haven Hosp 1997; **Fac Appt:** Asst Prof Med, Yale Univ

Warshofsky, Mark MD (IC) - **Spec Exp:** Coronary Artery Disease; Heart Valve Disease; **Hospital:** Danbury Hosp, NY-Presby/Columbia Univ Med Ctr, NY (page 104); **Address:** Western CT Med Grp, 24 Hospital Ave Fl 7, Danbury, CT 06810; **Phone:** 203-739-7436; **Board Cert:** Cardiovascular Disease 2007; Interventional Cardiology 2009; **Med School:** Geo Wash Univ 1990; **Resid:** Internal Medicine, Columbia-Presby Med Ctr 1993; **Fellow:** Cardiovascular Disease, Columbia-Presby Med Ctr 1996; Interventional Cardiology, Columbia-Presby Med Ctr 1998; **Fac Appt:** Asst Prof Med, Columbia P&S

Wasserman, Hal S MD (IC) - **Spec Exp:** Coronary Angioplasty/Stents; Heart Valve Disease; Coronary Artery Disease; **Hospital:** Danbury Hosp; **Address:** Western CT Med Grp, 24 Hospital Ave, 7 Tower, Danbury, CT 06810; **Phone:** 203-739-7600; **Board Cert:** Internal Medicine 1985; Cardiovascular Disease 1987; Interventional Cardiology 2009; **Med School:** Columbia P&S 1982; **Resid:** Internal Medicine, NY Presby/Columbia Med Ctr 1985; **Fellow:** Cardiovascular Disease, NY Presby/Columbia Med Ctr 1987; Interventional Cardiology, NY Presby/Columbia Med Ctr 1988; **Fac Appt:** Assoc Clin Prof Med, Columbia P&S

Maternal & Fetal Medicine

Bobby, Paul D MD (MF) - **Spec Exp:** Pregnancy-High Risk; Prenatal Diagnosis; **Hospital:** Stamford Hosp (page 893); **Address:** Stamford Hosp, Dept Maternal/Fetal Med, 30 Shelburne Rd, Stamford, CT 06902; **Phone:** 203-276-7172; **Board Cert:** Obstetrics & Gynecology 2011; Maternal & Fetal Medicine 2011; **Med School:** Boston Univ 1990; **Resid:** Obstetrics & Gynecology, NYU Med Ctr 1994; **Fellow:** Maternal & Fetal Medicine, Montefiore Med Ctr 1996; **Fac Appt:** Assoc Clin Prof ObG, Albert Einstein Coll Med

Bond, Annette L MD (MF) - **Spec Exp:** Pregnancy-High Risk; Multiple Gestation; Prenatal Diagnosis; Hypertension in Pregnancy; **Hospital:** Greenwich Hosp (page 892); **Address:** Greenwich Hospital, 5 Perryridge Rd, rm 1-251, Greenwich, CT 06830; **Phone:** 203-863-3674; **Board Cert:** Obstetrics & Gynecology 2011; Maternal & Fetal Medicine 2011; **Med School:** Harvard Med Sch 1983; **Resid:** Obstetrics & Gynecology, NY Hosp-Cornell Med Ctr 1987; **Fellow:** Perinatal Medicine, NY Hosp-Cornell Med Ctr 1989

Dunston-Boone, Gina A MD (MF) - **Spec Exp:** Amniocentesis; Multiple Gestation; **Hospital:** Bridgeport Hosp; **Address:** 226 Mill Hill Ave, Bridgeport, CT 06610; **Phone:** 203-384-3544; **Board Cert:** Obstetrics & Gynecology 2011; Maternal & Fetal Medicine 2011; **Med School:** Tufts Univ 1985; **Resid:** Obstetrics & Gynecology, NY-Presby/Weill Cornell Med Ctr 1992; **Fellow:** Maternal & Fetal Medicine, Thom Jeff Univ Hosp 1995

Laifer, Steven A MD (MF) - **Spec Exp:** Prenatal Diagnosis; Obesity in Pregnancy; **Hospital:** Bridgeport Hosp, Greenwich Hosp (page 892); **Address:** 267 Grant St Fl 5, Bridgeport, CT 06610; **Phone:** 203-384-3544; **Board Cert:** Obstetrics & Gynecology 2011; Maternal & Fetal Medicine 2011; **Med School:** SUNY Downstate 1982; **Resid:** Obstetrics & Gynecology, Johns Hopkins Hosp 1987; **Fellow:** Maternal & Fetal Medicine, Magee Womens Hosp 1989; **Fac Appt:** Asst Clin Prof ObG, Yale Univ

Shevell, Tracy MD (MF) - **Spec Exp:** Pregnancy-High Risk; Prenatal Diagnosis; **Hospital:** Stamford Hosp (page 893); **Address:** 30 Shelburne Rd, Whittingham Pavilion, Stamford, CT 06904; **Phone:** 203-276-7060; **Board Cert:** Obstetrics & Gynecology 2011; Maternal & Fetal Medicine 2011; **Med School:** Albert Einstein Coll Med 1997; **Resid:** Obstetrics & Gynecology, Mt Sinai Med Ctr 2001; **Fellow:** Maternal & Fetal Medicine, NY Presby-Columbia Univ Med Ctr 2004; **Fac Appt:** Asst Clin Prof ObG, Albert Einstein Coll Med

Stiller, Robert J MD (MF) - **Spec Exp:** Prenatal Diagnosis; Ultrasound; Pregnancy-High Risk; Infectious Disease in Pregnancy; **Hospital:** Bridgeport Hosp, Greenwich Hosp (page 892); **Address:** Bridgeport Hosp, 267 Grant St Fl 5, Bridgeport, CT 06610; **Phone:** 203-384-3544; **Board Cert:** Obstetrics & Gynecology 2011; Maternal & Fetal Medicine 2011; **Med School:** UMDNJ-Rutgers Med Sch 1979; **Resid:** Obstetrics & Gynecology, Univ Conn Med Ctr 1983; **Fellow:** Maternal & Fetal Medicine, Pennsylvania Hosp-UPHS 1985; **Fac Appt:** Assoc Clin Prof ObG, Yale Univ

Medical Oncology

Abrams, Martin MD (Onc) - **Hospital:** Danbury Hosp; **Address:** 95 Locust Ave, Stroock Bldg Fl 1, Danbury, CT 06810; **Phone:** 203-739-7029; **Board Cert:** Internal Medicine 1983; Medical Oncology 1985; **Med School:** Tufts Univ 1980; **Resid:** Internal Medicine, St Elizabeths Hosp 1983; **Fellow:** Hematology & Oncology, Boston Univ Hosp 1985

Delprete, Salvatore A MD (Onc) - **Spec Exp:** Lung Cancer; Ovarian Cancer; Melanoma; Colon Cancer; **Hospital:** Stamford Hosp (page 893); **Address:** Bennett Cancer Ctr, 34 Shelburne Rd, Stamford, CT 06902-3658; **Phone:** 203-325-2695; **Board Cert:** Internal Medicine 1981; Medical Oncology 1985; Hematology 1986; **Med School:** Columbia P&S 1978; **Resid:** Internal Medicine, Dartmouth-Hitchcock Med Ctr 1981; **Fellow:** Pathology, Dartmouth-Hitchcock Med Ctr 1982; Hematology & Oncology, Dartmouth-Hitchcock Med Ctr 1984; **Fac Appt:** Assoc Clin Prof Med, NY Med Coll

Drucker, Beverly J MD/PhD (Onc) - **Spec Exp:** Breast Cancer; Head & Neck Cancer; Colon & Rectal Cancer; Clinical Trials; **Hospital:** Greenwich Hosp (page 892); **Address:** Hematology & Oncology Assocs Greenwich, 77 Lafayette Pl, Ste 260, Greenwich, CT 06830; **Phone:** 203-863-3737; **Board Cert:** Medical Oncology 2009; **Med School:** Columbia P&S 1994; **Resid:** Internal Medicine, Columbia Presby Med Ctr 1997; **Fellow:** Medical Oncology, John Hopkins 1999

Fischbach, Neal A MD (Onc) - **Spec Exp:** Breast Cancer; Lung Cancer; Colon Cancer; **Hospital:** Bridgeport Hosp, St. Vincent's Med Ctr - Bridgeport; **Address:** Oncology Assocs Bridgeport, 111 Beach Rd Fl 3, Fairfield, CT 06824; **Phone:** 203-255-2766; **Board Cert:** Medical Oncology 2002; **Med School:** Harvard Med Sch 1995; **Resid:** Internal Medicine, UCSF Med Ctr 1999; **Fellow:** Hematology & Oncology, UCSF Med Ctr 2002

Folman, Robert S MD (Onc) - **Spec Exp:** Breast Cancer; Lung Cancer; Colon & Rectal Cancer; Genitourinary Cancer; **Hospital:** Bridgeport Hosp, St. Vincent's Med Ctr - Bridgeport; **Address:** 5520 Park Ave, Ste 203, Trumbull, CT 06611-1351; **Phone:** 203-502-8400; **Board Cert:** Internal Medicine 1975; Medical Oncology 1977; **Med School:** SUNY Buffalo 1972; **Resid:** Internal Medicine, Buffalo Gen Hosp 1975; Internal Medicine, Meml Sloan Kettering Cancer Ctr 1976; **Fellow:** Medical Oncology, Meml Sloan Kettering Cancer Ctr 1977; **Fac Appt:** Asst Prof Med, Yale Univ

Frank, Richard C MD (Onc) - **Spec Exp:** Leukemia; Lymphoma; **Hospital:** Norwalk Hosp; **Address:** Whittingham Cancer Ctr, 24 Stevens St, Norwalk, CT 06856; **Phone:** 203-845-4899; **Board Cert:** Medical Oncology 2005; Hematology 2008; **Med School:** SUNY Stony Brook 1985; **Resid:** Internal Medicine, Columbia-Presby Med Ctr 1992; **Fellow:** Hematology & Oncology, Meml Sloan Kettering Cancer Ctr 1996

Hollister Jr, Dickerman MD (Onc) - **Spec Exp:** Breast Cancer; Lung Cancer; Colon Cancer; Leukemia & Lymphoma; **Hospital:** Greenwich Hosp (page 892); **Address:** 77 Lafayette Pl, Ste 260, Greenwich, CT 06830; **Phone:** 203-863-3737; **Board Cert:** Internal Medicine 1978; Hematology 1980; Medical Oncology 1981; **Med School:** Univ VA Sch Med 1975; **Resid:** Internal Medicine, NY Hosp-Cornell Med Ctr 1978; **Fellow:** Hematology & Oncology, NY Hosp-Cornell Med Ctr 1981; **Fac Appt:** Asst Clin Prof Med, Yale Univ

Kloss, Robert MD (Onc) - **Spec Exp:** Breast Cancer; Colon Cancer; Lung Cancer; **Hospital:** Danbury Hosp; **Address:** 95 Locust Ave Fl 1, Danbury, CT 06810-6010; **Phone:** 203-739-7029; **Board Cert:** Internal Medicine 1979; Medical Oncology 1981; Hospice & Palliative Medicine 2008; **Med School:** Jefferson Med Coll 1976; **Resid:** Internal Medicine, Univ Hosp 1979; **Fellow:** Hematology & Oncology, Columbia-Presby Med Ctr 1981

Lo, K M Steve MD (Onc) - **Spec Exp:** Breast Cancer; Lymphoma; **Hospital:** Stamford Hosp (page 893); **Address:** 34 Shelburne Rd, Stamford, CT 06902-3658; **Phone:** 203-325-2695; **Board Cert:** Internal Medicine 1989; Medical Oncology 2011; Hematology 2002; **Med School:** Harvard Med Sch 1985; **Resid:** Internal Medicine, Brigham & Women's Hosp 1988; **Fellow:** Hematology & Oncology, Dana Farber Cancer Inst 1991; Hematology, Dana Farber Cancer Inst 1992; **Fac Appt:** Asst Clin Prof Med, Columbia P&S

Weinstein, Paul MD (Onc) - **Spec Exp:** Breast Cancer; Lung Cancer; Colon Cancer; **Hospital:** Stamford Hosp (page 893); **Address:** 34 Shelburne Rd, Bennett Cancer Ctr, Hematology-Oncology, Stamford, CT 06902-3628; **Phone:** 203-325-2695; **Board Cert:** Internal Medicine 1973; Medical Oncology 1977; Hematology 1978; **Med School:** Ros Franklin Univ/Chicago Med Sch 1970; **Resid:** Internal Medicine, Montefiore Med Ctr 1973; **Fellow:** Hematology & Oncology, Montefiore Med Ctr 1975; **Fac Appt:** Assoc Clin Prof Med, Columbia P&S

Zelkowitz, Richard S MD (Onc) - **Spec Exp:** Breast Cancer; Hematology; Bone Marrow Transplant; **Hospital:** Norwalk Hosp; **Address:** 40 Cross St, Norwalk, CT 06851; **Phone:** 203-845-4890; **Board Cert:** Internal Medicine 1986; Hematology 1988; Medical Oncology 1989; **Med School:** NY Med Coll 1983; **Resid:** Internal Medicine, Westchester Co Med Ctr 1986; **Fellow:** Hematology & Oncology, Brown Univ Hosps 1989; **Fac Appt:** Asst Prof Med, Cornell Univ-Weill Med Coll

Neonatal-Perinatal Medicine

Herzlinger, Robert A MD (NP) - **Spec Exp:** Neonatology; **Hospital:** Bridgeport Hosp, Yale-New Haven Hosp; **Address:** Bridgeport Hosp, 267 Grant St, Ste 6, Bridgeport, CT 06610-2870; **Phone:** 203-384-3486; **Board Cert:** Pediatrics 1974; Neonatal-Perinatal Medicine 1977; **Med School:** NY Med Coll 1969; **Resid:** Pediatrics, Westchester Co Med Ctr 1971; Pediatrics, Columbia-Presby Med Ctr 1972; **Fellow:** Neonatal-Perinatal Medicine, Columbia-Presby Med Ctr 1973; Neonatal-Perinatal Medicine, Montefiore Med Ctr 1976; **Fac Appt:** Assoc Clin Prof Ped, Yale Univ

Rakos, Gerald B MD (NP) - **Hospital:** Stamford Hosp (page 893); **Address:** Stamford Hosp, Dept Pediatrics, 30 Shelburne Rd, Box 9317, Stamford, CT 06904; **Phone:** 203-276-7085; **Board Cert:** Pediatrics 1985; Neonatal-Perinatal Medicine 1985; **Med School:** SUNY Upstate Med Univ 1980; **Resid:** Pediatrics, Univ Mass Medical Ctr 1983; **Fellow:** Neonatology, Montefiore Med Ctr 1985; **Fac Appt:** Asst Clin Prof Ped, Columbia P&S

Theofanidis, Stylianos MD (NP) - **Hospital:** Greenwich Hosp (page 892), Yale-New Haven Hosp; **Address:** 5 Perryridge Rd, Greenwich, CT 06830-4608; **Phone:** 203-863-3515; **Board Cert:** Neonatal-Perinatal Medicine 2004; **Med School:** Greece 1980; **Resid:** Pediatrics, St Lukes Hosp 1985; **Fellow:** Neonatal-Perinatal Medicine, NY Hosp-Cornell Med Ctr 1987; **Fac Appt:** Asst Clin Prof Ped, Yale Univ

Nephrology

Brown, Eric Y MD (Nep) - **Spec Exp:** Kidney Disease; Hypertension; Glomerulonephritis; **Hospital:** Stamford Hosp (page 893); **Address:** 30 Commerce Rd, Stamford, CT 06902-4550; **Phone:** 203-324-7666; **Board Cert:** Internal Medicine 1988; Nephrology 2010; **Med School:** Emory Univ 1985; **Resid:** Internal Medicine, Johns Hopkins Hosp 1988; **Fellow:** Nephrology, Yale-New Haven Hosp 1990; **Fac Appt:** Asst Clin Prof Med, Columbia P&S

Chan, Brenda MD (Nep) - **Spec Exp:** Dialysis Care; Kidney Failure-Chronic; Lupus Nephritis; Glomerulonephritis; **Hospital:** Stamford Hosp (page 893), Greenwich Hosp (page 892); **Address:** Stamford Nephrology, 30 Commerce Rd, Stamford, CT 06902; **Phone:** 203-324-7666; **Board Cert:** Nephrology 2007; **Med School:** Mount Sinai Sch Med 1990; **Resid:** Internal Medicine, Montefiore Med Ctr 1993; **Fellow:** Nephrology, Montefiore Med Ctr 1996

Feintzeig, Irwin D MD (Nep) - **Spec Exp:** Kidney Disease; Hypertension; Dialysis Care; **Hospital:** Bridgeport Hosp, St. Vincent's Med Ctr - Bridgeport; **Address:** 900 Madison Ave, Ste 209, Bridgeport, CT 06606-5534; **Phone:** 203-335-0195; **Board Cert:** Internal Medicine 1982; Nephrology 1984; **Med School:** Univ Chicago-Pritzker Sch Med 1979; **Resid:** Internal Medicine, Temple Univ Hosp 1982; **Fellow:** Nephrology, Boston Univ Med Ctr 1985; **Fac Appt:** Asst Clin Prof Med, Yale Univ

Fogel, Mitchell A MD (Nep) - **Spec Exp:** Kidney Disease-Chronic; Glomerulonephritis; Dialysis Care; **Hospital:** St. Vincent's Med Ctr - Bridgeport, Bridgeport Hosp; **Address:** Nephrology Assocs, 900 Madison Ave, Ste 209, Bridgeport, CT 06606; **Phone:** 203-335-0195; **Board Cert:** Internal Medicine 1986; Nephrology 1988; **Med School:** Univ Pennsylvania 1982; **Resid:** Internal Medicine, Boston Univ Med Ctr 1985; **Fellow:** Nephrology, Boston Univ Med Ctr 1988; **Fac Appt:** Assoc Clin Prof Med, Columbia P&S

Hines, William H MD (Nep) - **Spec Exp:** Dialysis Care; Hypertension; Kidney Disease; **Hospital:** Stamford Hosp (page 893); **Address:** 30 Commerce Rd, Stamford, CT 06902-4550; **Phone:** 203-324-7666; **Board Cert:** Internal Medicine 1984; Nephrology 1986; **Med School:** Cornell Univ-Weill Med Coll 1981; **Resid:** Internal Medicine, Hosp Univ Penn 1984; **Fellow:** Nephrology, Hosp Univ Penn 1988; **Fac Appt:** Asst Clin Prof Med, Columbia P&S

Hunt, William A MD (Nep) - **Spec Exp:** Hypertension; **Hospital:** Bridgeport Hosp; **Address:** 900 Madison Ave, Ste 209, Bridgeport, CT 06606-5534; **Phone:** 203-335-0195; **Board Cert:** Internal Medicine 1984; Nephrology 1986; **Med School:** Yale Univ 1981; **Resid:** Internal Medicine, Univ Hosps Cleveland 1984

Neurological Surgery

Apostolides, Paul J MD (NS) - **Spec Exp:** Minimally Invasive Spinal Surgery; Spinal Surgery; Spinal Disc Replacement; **Hospital:** Greenwich Hosp (page 892), Stamford Hosp (page 893); **Address:** Orthopaedic & Neurosurgery Specialists, 6 Greenwich Office Park, 10 Valley Drive, Greenwich, CT 06831; **Phone:** 203-869-1145; **Board Cert:** Neurological Surgery 2002; **Med School:** Univ Mass Sch Med 1991; **Resid:** Neurological Surgery, Barrow Neuro Inst/St Joseph's Hosp 1998; **Fellow:** Spinal Surgery, Barrow Neuro Inst/St Joseph's 1997

Camel, Mark W MD (NS) - **Spec Exp:** Brain Tumors; Spinal Surgery; Minimally Invasive Spinal Surgery; **Hospital:** Greenwich Hosp (page 892); **Address:** Orthopaedic & Neurosurgery Specialists, 6 Greenwich Office Park, 10 Valley Drive, Greenwich, CT 06831; **Phone:** 203-869-1145 x616; **Board Cert:** Neurological Surgery 1990; **Med School:** Washington Univ, St Louis 1981; **Resid:** Neurological Surgery, Barnes Jewish Hosp 1986; **Fellow:** Neurological Surgery, Barnes Jewish Hosp 1987; **Fac Appt:** Asst Clin Prof S, Columbia P&S

Fiore, Amory J MD (NS) - **Spec Exp:** Minimally Invasive Spinal Surgery; Brain Tumors; **Hospital:** Greenwich Hosp (page 892), Stamford Hosp (page 893); **Address:** 6 Greenwich Office Park, Valley Drive, Orthopaedic & Neurosurgery Specialists, Greenwich, CT 06831; **Phone:** 203-869-1145; **Board Cert:** Neurological Surgery 2006; **Med School:** Columbia P&S 1995; **Resid:** Neurological Surgery, NY-Presby/Columbia Univ Med Ctr 2001; **Fellow:** Spinal Surgery, Emory Clinic 2002

Ghogawala, Zoher MD (NS) - **Spec Exp:** Minimally Invasive Spinal Surgery; Vascular Neurosurgery; Carotid Artery Surgery; Cerebrovascular Neurosurgery; **Hospital:** Greenwich Hosp (page 892), Yale Med Group (page 940); **Address:** CSI-Greenwich Neurosurgery, 25 Valley Drive, Greenwich, CT 06831; **Phone:** 203-661-3333; **Board Cert:** Neurological Surgery 2004; **Med School:** Harvard Med Sch 1991; **Resid:** Neurological Surgery, Mass Genl Hosp 1999; **Fac Appt:** Asst Clin Prof NS, Yale Univ

Lipow, Kenneth MD (NS) - **Spec Exp:** Spinal Surgery; Brain Surgery; **Hospital:** Bridgeport Hosp; **Address:** 267 grant St, Fl 8, Ste shein, 52 Beach Rd, Ste 204B, Bridgeport, CT 06610-2870; **Phone:** 203-384-4500; **Board Cert:** Neurological Surgery 1989; **Med School:** Albert Einstein Coll Med 1978; **Resid:** Neurological Surgery, Montefiore Med Ctr 1984

Mintz, Abraham MD (NS) - **Spec Exp:** Spinal Surgery; **Hospital:** St. Vincent's Med Ctr - Bridgeport, Bridgeport Hosp; **Address:** 5520 Park Ave, Ste 210, Trumbull, CT 06611; **Phone:** 203-372-6460; **Board Cert:** Neurological Surgery 1992; **Med School:** Mexico 1982; **Resid:** Neurological Surgery, Jackson Meml Hosp 1989

Shahid, Syed J MD (NS) - **Spec Exp:** Brain Tumors; Spinal Surgery; Spinal Tumors; **Hospital:** Danbury Hosp, Norwalk Hosp; **Address:** 148 East Ave, Ste 3D, Norwalk, CT 06851; **Phone:** 203-853-0003; **Board Cert:** Neurological Surgery 1983; **Med School:** Pakistan 1972; **Resid:** Surgery, Kings County Hosp 1977; Neurological Surgery, Kings County Hosp 1980

Shear, Perry MD (NS) - **Hospital:** Bridgeport Hosp, St. Vincent's Med Ctr - Bridgeport; **Address:** 75 Kings Hwy Cutoff Fl 2, Fairfield, CT 06824; **Phone:** 203-337-2629; **Board Cert:** Neurological Surgery 1996; **Med School:** Univ Toronto 1984; **Resid:** Neurological Surgery, Toronto Genl Hosp 1991

Simon, Scott L MD (NS) - **Spec Exp:** Spinal Surgery; Scoliosis; Stereotactic Radiosurgery; Minimally Invasive Spinal Surgery; **Hospital:** Stamford Hosp (page 893), Greenwich Hosp (page 892); **Address:** Orthopaedic & Neurosurgery Specialists, 32 Strawberry Hill Ct, Stamford, CT 06902; **Phone:** 203-487-0363; **Board Cert:** Neurological Surgery 2009; **Med School:** UMDNJ-RW Johnson Med Sch 1998; **Resid:** Neurological Surgery, Hosp Univ Penn 2005; **Fellow:** Spinal Surgery, Shriners Hosp for Chldn 2004

Zimmerman, Gary A MD (NS) - **Spec Exp:** Spinal Surgery; **Hospital:** Bridgeport Hosp, St. Vincent's Med Ctr - Bridgeport; **Address:** CT Neurosurgical Specialists, 267 Grant St Fl Shine 8, Bridgeport, CT 06610-2805; **Phone:** 203-384-4500; **Board Cert:** Neurological Surgery 2011; **Med School:** SUNY Downstate 1990; **Resid:** Neurological Surgery, NY-Presby/Weill Cornell Med Ctr 1996; **Fellow:** Cerebrovascular Disease, Univ Hosp 1997

Neurology

Butler, James B MD (N) - **Spec Exp:** Headache; Migraine; **Hospital:** Bridgeport Hosp; **Address:** Neurological Specialists, 4 Corporate Drive, Ste 192, Shelton, CT 06484; **Phone:** 203-924-8664; **Board Cert:** Internal Medicine 1982; Neurology 1987; **Med School:** Belgium 1979; **Resid:** Internal Medicine, Hosp St Raphael 1982; Neurology, Yale-New Haven Hosp 1985; **Fac Appt:** Assoc Clin Prof N, Yale Univ

Cuzzone, Louis J MD (N) - Spec Exp: Migraine; **Hospital:** Norwalk Hosp; **Address:** 637 West Ave, Ste 200, Norwalk, CT 06850; **Phone:** 203-853-5000; **Board Cert:** Neurology 1980; **Med School:** Albert Einstein Coll Med 1975; **Resid:** Neurology, Montefiore Med Ctr 1979; **Fellow:** Electromyography, NYU Med Ctr 1980

Gross, Jeffrey L MD (N) - Spec Exp: Multiple Sclerosis; **Hospital:** St. Vincent's Med Ctr - Bridgeport, Milford Hosp; **Address:** 75 Kings Hwy Cutoff Fl 5, Fairfield, CT 06824; **Phone:** 203-333-1133; **Board Cert:** Neurology 1985; **Med School:** Case West Res Univ 1977; **Resid:** Internal Medicine, Hosp Univ Penn 1980; Neurology, Hosp Univ Penn 1983; **Fellow:** Neuromuscular Disease, Hosp Univ Penn 1984

Litchman, Charisse D MD (N) - Spec Exp: Headache; Migraine; **Hospital:** Stamford Hosp (page 893); **Address:** 1290 Summer St, Ste 5200, Stamford, CT 06905; **Phone:** 203-969-7662; **Board Cert:** Neurology 1993; **Med School:** Yale Univ 1988; **Resid:** Neurology, NY Presby-Cornell Med Ctr 1992; **Fac Appt:** Asst Clin Prof N, Columbia P&S

McAllister, Peter J MD (N) - Spec Exp: Headache; **Hospital:** St. Vincent's Med Ctr - Bridgeport, Bridgeport Hosp; **Address:** Assoc Neurologists of S Connecticut, 75 Kings Hwy Cutoff, Fairfield, CT 06430; **Phone:** 203-333-1133; **Board Cert:** Neurology 2007; **Med School:** Univ Conn 1991; **Resid:** Neurology, Med Coll Virginia 1995; **Fellow:** Neuromuscular Medicine, Med Coll Virginia 1996

Nahm, Frederick K MD/PhD (N) - Spec Exp: Cerebrovascular Disease; Stroke; **Hospital:** Greenwich Hosp (page 892); **Address:** Neurology of Greenwich, 49 Lake Ave, Ste LL3, Greenwich, CT 06830; **Phone:** 203-661-9383; **Board Cert:** Neurology 2003; **Med School:** Univ Mich Med Sch 1996; **Resid:** Neurology, Beth Israel Deaconess Med Ctr 2000; **Fellow:** Clinical Neurophysiology, Mass Genl Hosp 2001

Resor, Louise D MD (N) - Hospital: Stamford Hosp (page 893); **Address:** 166 W Broad St, Ste 203, Stamford, CT 06902; **Phone:** 203-978-0283; **Med School:** Washington Univ, St Louis 1974; **Resid:** Neurology, Ny Presbyterian-Columbia Med Ctr 1978

Rusk, Alice H MD (N) - Spec Exp: Movement Disorders; Parkinson's Disease; Dystonia; **Hospital:** Greenwich Hosp (page 892), Stamford Hosp (page 893); **Address:** Greenwich Neurology, 25 Valley Drive, Greenwich, CT 06831; **Phone:** 203-869-6446; **Board Cert:** Neurology 2006; **Med School:** Univ Conn 1991; **Resid:** Neurology, NY Hosp-Cornell Med Ctr 1995; **Fellow:** Clinical Neurophysiology, Columbia Presby Med Ctr 1996

Sena, Kanaga N MD (N) - Spec Exp: Stroke; Neuro-Rehabilitation; Headache; **Hospital:** Bridgeport Hosp; **Address:** 2590 Main St Fl 2, Stratford, CT 06615-5838; **Phone:** 203-377-5988; **Board Cert:** Neurology 1979; **Med School:** Sri Lanka 1969; **Resid:** Internal Medicine, Bridgeport Hosp 1973; Neurology, Yale-New Haven Hosp 1976; **Fac Appt:** Assoc Clin Prof N, Yale Univ

Siegel, Kenneth C MD (N) - Spec Exp: Parkinson's Disease; Headache; Stroke; Movement Disorders; **Hospital:** St. Vincent's Med Ctr - Bridgeport; **Address:** Assoc Neurologists of S Connecticut, 75 Kings Hwy Cutoff, Fairfield, CT 06824; **Phone:** 203-333-1133; **Board Cert:** Neurology 1975; **Med School:** Meharry Med Coll 1969; **Resid:** Neurology, Bellevue Med Ctr/NYU 1973; **Fac Appt:** Assoc Clin Prof N, Yale Univ

Story, Daryl MD (N) - Spec Exp: Stroke; Vascular Neurology; **Hospital:** Norwalk Hosp; **Address:** 637 West Ave, Ste 200, Neurology Associates of Norwalk, Norwalk, CT 06850; **Phone:** 203-853-5000; **Board Cert:** Neurology 2012; Vascular Neurology 2008; **Med School:** NY Med Coll 1997; **Resid:** Neurology, Yale-New Haven Hosp 2000; **Fellow:** Vascular Neurology, Yale-New Haven Hosp 2002; **Fac Appt:** Asst Clin Prof N, NY Med Coll

Wirz, Diane MD (N) - **Spec Exp:** Headache; Migraine; **Hospital:** Danbury Hosp; **Address:** Associated Neurologists, 69 Sand Pit Rd, Ste 300, Danbury, CT 06810; **Phone:** 203-748-2551; **Board Cert:** Integrative Medicine 1982; Neurology 1986; Headache Medicine ; **Med School:** Albany Med Coll 1979; **Resid:** Internal Medicine, Danbury Hosp 1982; Neurology, John Dempsey Hosp/U Conn 1985

Neuroradiology

Sullivan, Scott J MD (NRad) - **Spec Exp:** Neuroradiology; **Hospital:** Greenwich Hosp (page 892); **Address:** Greenwich Hosp-Dept Radiology, 5 Perryridge Rd, Greenwich, CT 06830; **Phone:** 203-863-3960; **Board Cert:** Diagnostic Radiology 1996; Neuroradiology 2004; **Med School:** Georgetown Univ 1991; **Resid:** Radiology, Yale-New Haven Hosp 1995; **Fellow:** Neuroradiology, Yale-New Haven Hosp 1996

Nuclear Medicine

Johns, William D MD (NuM) - **Hospital:** Danbury Hosp; **Address:** 24 Hospital Ave, Tower 2, Danbury, CT 06810; **Phone:** 203-739-7222; **Board Cert:** Internal Medicine 1986; Nuclear Medicine 1988; **Med School:** Univ Conn 1983; **Resid:** Internal Medicine, Danbury Hosp 1986; Nuclear Medicine, Brigham & Women's Hosp 1988

Obstetrics & Gynecology

Ayoub, Thomas V MD (ObG) - **Spec Exp:** Menopause Problems; **Hospital:** Norwalk Hosp; **Address:** Women's Hlthcare New England, 761 Main Ave, Ste 100, Norwalk, CT 06851; **Phone:** 203-644-1100; **Board Cert:** Obstetrics & Gynecology 2010; **Med School:** NYU Sch Med 1980; **Resid:** Obstetrics & Gynecology, Bellevue Hosp Ctr 1984

Besser, Gary S MD (ObG) - **Spec Exp:** Laparoscopic Surgery-Complex; Uro-Gynecology; Pelvic Surgery; Robotic Surgery; **Hospital:** Stamford Hosp (page 893); **Address:** Whittingham Pavilion, 190 W Broad St, Ste G-401, Stamford, CT 06902-3661; **Phone:** 203-325-4321; **Board Cert:** Obstetrics & Gynecology 2012; **Med School:** SUNY Downstate 1982; **Resid:** Obstetrics & Gynecology, Stamford Hosp 1986; **Fac Appt:** Assoc Prof ObG, Columbia P&S

Blair, Emily DO (ObG) - **Spec Exp:** Pregnancy-High Risk; **Hospital:** Bridgeport Hosp; **Address:** 1735 Post Rd, Fairfield, CT 06824; **Phone:** 203-256-3990; **Board Cert:** Obstetrics & Gynecology 2011; **Med School:** Univ Osteo Med & Hlth Sci, Des Moines 1986; **Resid:** Obstetrics & Gynecology, Bridgeport Hosp 1990; **Fac Appt:** Assoc Prof ObG, Univ Conn

Bruck, Lance MD (ObG) - **Spec Exp:** Minimally Invasive Surgery; Gynecologic Surgery; **Hospital:** Stamford Hosp (page 893); **Address:** Stamford Hosp-Dept Ob/Gyn, 30 Shelburne Rd, Stamford, CT 06902; **Phone:** 203-276-7853; **Board Cert:** Obstetrics & Gynecology 2011; **Med School:** NY Med Coll 1992; **Resid:** Obstetrics & Gynecology, Montefiore Med Ctr 1997; **Fac Appt:** Assoc Clin Prof ObG, Albert Einstein Coll Med

Cuteri, Joseph MD (ObG) - **Spec Exp:** Pregnancy-High Risk; Colposcopy; Ultrasound; **Hospital:** Bridgeport Hosp; **Address:** 4 Corporate Drive, Ste 286, Shelton, CT 06484; **Phone:** 203-929-9000; **Board Cert:** Obstetrics & Gynecology 2011; **Med School:** Mexico 1984; **Resid:** Obstetrics & Gynecology, Brooklyn Hosp 1987; Obstetrics & Gynecology, Bridgeport Hosp 1989; **Fac Appt:** Asst Clin Prof ObG, Yale Univ

Donovan, Leslie MD (ObG) - **Spec Exp:** Adolescent Gynecology; Menopause Problems; Sexually Transmitted Diseases; Gynecology Only; **Hospital:** Greenwich Hosp (page 892); **Address:** Brookside Gynecology, 159 W Putnam Ave, Greenwich, CT 06830; **Phone:** 203-869-7080; **Board Cert:** Obstetrics & Gynecology 2011; **Med School:** Univ Mass Sch Med 1993; **Resid:** Obstetrics & Gynecology, St Joseph's Med Ctr 1999

Ferrucci, Leonard MD (ObG) - **Hospital:** Stamford Hosp (page 893); **Address:** Ferrucci & Ferrucci, 833 Summer St, Ste 1B, Stamford, CT 06901; **Phone:** 203-325-4665; **Board Cert:** Obstetrics & Gynecology 2011; **Med School:** NY Med Coll 1987; **Resid:** Obstetrics & Gynecology, Stamford Hosp 1990

Ferrucci, Vito MD (ObG) - **Hospital:** Stamford Hosp (page 893); **Address:** 833 Summer St, Ste 1B, Stamford, CT 06901; **Phone:** 203-325-4665; **Board Cert:** Obstetrics & Gynecology 2011; **Med School:** NY Med Coll 1985; **Resid:** Obstetrics & Gynecology, Stamford Hosp 1989

Geer-Yan, Lisa MD (ObG) *PCP* - **Hospital:** Norwalk Hosp; **Address:** Avery Ctr for Ob/Gyn, 12 Avery Pl, Westport, CT 06880; **Phone:** 203-227-5125; **Board Cert:** Obstetrics & Gynecology 2007; **Med School:** SUNY Upstate Med Univ 2001; **Resid:** Obstetrics & Gynecology, Thomas Jefferson Univ Hosp 2005

Hines, Brian J MD (ObG) - **Spec Exp:** Uro-Gynecology; Incontinence; Pelvic Organ Prolapse Repair; **Hospital:** Stamford Hosp (page 893), Bridgeport Hosp; **Address:** 1351 Washington Blvd, Ste 201, Stamford, CT 06902; **Phone:** 203-391-6620; **Board Cert:** Obstetrics & Gynecology 2011; **Med School:** Boston Univ 1996; **Resid:** Obstetrics & Gynecology, Mt Sinai Med Ctr 2000; **Fellow:** Uro-Gynecology, NYU Med Ctr 2002; **Fac Appt:** Asst Prof Med, Columbia P&S

Schechter, Michael D MD (ObG) - **Hospital:** Greenwich Hosp (page 892); **Address:** Putnam Gynecology & Obstetrics, 500 W Putnam Ave, Greenwich, CT 06830; **Phone:** 203-622-0303; **Board Cert:** Obstetrics & Gynecology 2009; **Med School:** NYU Sch Med 1988; **Resid:** Obstetrics & Gynecology, St Lukes-Roosevelt Hosp 1992

Szeto, Marjorie MD (ObG) - **Spec Exp:** Pregnancy-High Risk; **Hospital:** Norwalk Hosp; **Address:** Avery Ctr for Ob/Gyn, 12 Avery Pl, Westport, CT 06880; **Phone:** 203-227-5125; **Board Cert:** Obstetrics & Gynecology 2011; **Med School:** NYU Sch Med 1985; **Resid:** Obstetrics & Gynecology, Beth Israel Med Ctr 1989

Ugol, Jay H MD (ObG) - **Hospital:** Norwalk Hosp; **Address:** Women's Hlth Care New England, 761 Main Ave, Norwalk, CT 06851; **Phone:** 203-644-1100; **Board Cert:** Obstetrics & Gynecology 2007; **Med School:** Geo Wash Univ 1982; **Resid:** Obstetrics & Gynecology, Univ Colorado Hosp 1986

Violi, Caterina MD (ObG) - **Spec Exp:** Endometriosis; Pelvic Organ Prolapse Repair; Pregnancy-High Risk; Laparoscopic Surgery-Complex; **Hospital:** Greenwich Hosp (page 892); **Address:** 2 1/2 Dearfield Drive, Ste 101, Greenwich, CT 06831; **Phone:** 203-861-9586; **Board Cert:** Obstetrics & Gynecology 2010; **Med School:** Univ Rochester 1994; **Resid:** Obstetrics & Gynecology, Winthrop Univ Hosp 1998

Weinstein Jr, David B MD (ObG) - **Spec Exp:** Pregnancy-High Risk; **Hospital:** Stamford Hosp (page 893); **Address:** Whittingham Pavilion, 190 W Broad St, Ste G-401, Stamford, CT 06902; **Phone:** 203-325-4321; **Board Cert:** Obstetrics & Gynecology 2011; **Med School:** Univ Chicago-Pritzker Sch Med 1969; **Resid:** Obstetrics & Gynecology, NY-Presby/Weill Cornell Med Ctr 1974; **Fac Appt:** Asst Clin Prof ObG, Cornell Univ-Weill Med Coll

Ophthalmology

Altman, Bruce S MD (Oph) - **Spec Exp:** Glaucoma; **Hospital:** Danbury Hosp; **Address:** 69 Sand Pit Rd, Ste 101, Danbury, CT 06810-4005; **Phone:** 203-791-2020; **Board Cert:** Ophthalmology 2003; **Med School:** Univ Pennsylvania 1986; **Resid:** Ophthalmology, Hahnemann Hosp 1991; **Fellow:** Ophthalmology, Barnes-Jewish W Co Hosp 1992; Ophthalmology, Scheie Eye Inst 1988

DeBroff, Brian MD (Oph) - **Spec Exp:** Refractive Surgery; Cataract Surgery; Cataract-Pediatric; Anterior Segment Surgery; **Hospital:** Yale-New Haven Hosp, Bridgeport Hosp; **Address:** Eye Surgery Associates, 495 Hawley Ln, Stratford, CT 06614; **Phone:** 203-375-5819; **Board Cert:** Ophthalmology 2005; **Med School:** Tufts Univ 1989; **Resid:** Ophthalmology, Univ Pittsburg/Eye & Ear Inst 1993; **Fellow:** Anterior Segment - External Disease, Gimbel Eye Ctr 1994; **Fac Appt:** Assoc Clin Prof Oph, Yale Univ

Doctor, Leslie MD (Oph) - **Spec Exp:** Cataract Surgery; Anterior Segment Surgery; Refractive Surgery; **Hospital:** Yale-New Haven Hosp; **Address:** 129 Kings Hwy N, Westport, CT 06880; **Phone:** 203-227-4113; **Board Cert:** Ophthalmology 2008; **Med School:** Ohio State Univ 1989; **Resid:** Ophthalmology, OH State Univ Med Ctr 1993; **Fellow:** Cornea & Ext Eye Disease, OH State Univ Med Ctr 1994

Finlay, Alexis E MD (Oph) - **Spec Exp:** Refractive Surgery; Cornea & Cataract Surgery; Lens Implants; **Hospital:** Greenwich Hosp (page 892); **Address:** 38 B Grove St, Lower Floor, Ridgefield, CT 06877; **Phone:** 203-403-3375; **Board Cert:** Ophthalmology 1989; **Med School:** Hahnemann Univ 1981; **Resid:** Ophthalmology, NY E&E Informary 1985; **Fellow:** Ophthalmic Pathology, Johns Hopkins Hosp 1986

Gewirtz, Joan MD (Oph) - **Spec Exp:** Cataract Surgery; Glaucoma; Dry Eye Syndrome; **Hospital:** Stamford Hosp (page 893); **Address:** 70 Mill River St, Ste LL3, Stamford, CT 06902; **Phone:** 203-348-0868; **Board Cert:** Ophthalmology 2010; **Med School:** SUNY Downstate 1980; **Resid:** Ophthalmology, Lenox Hill Hosp 1987; **Fellow:** Ophthalmology, NY-Presby/Weill Cornell Med Ctr 1983

Gladstein, Gina F MD (Oph) - **Spec Exp:** Glaucoma; Cataract Surgery; **Hospital:** Greenwich Hosp (page 892); **Address:** Greenwich Ophthalmology Assocs, 4 Dearfield Drive, Greenwich, CT 06831; **Phone:** 203-869-3082; **Board Cert:** Ophthalmology 1989; **Med School:** Albert Einstein Coll Med 1983; **Resid:** Ophthalmology, Manhattan EE&T Hosp 1987; **Fellow:** Ophthalmology, Manhattan EE&T Hosp 1988

Kaplan, Jeffrey N MD (Oph) - **Spec Exp:** Corneal Disease; Cataract Surgery; **Hospital:** Bridgeport Hosp; **Address:** 4699 Main St, Ste 106, Bridgeport, CT 06606; **Phone:** 203-374-8182; **Board Cert:** Ophthalmology 1987; **Med School:** SUNY Stony Brook 1981; **Resid:** Ophthalmology, SUNY Downstate Med Ctr 1985; **Fellow:** Cornea, Dubroff Eye Ctr 1986

Mandava, Suresh MD (Oph) - **Spec Exp:** LASIK-Refractive Surgery; Cataract Surgery; Cornea Transplant; Cornea & External Eye Disease; **Hospital:** Greenwich Hosp (page 892); **Address:** Greenwich Ophthalmology Assocs, 4 Dearfield Drive, Greenwich, CT 06831; **Phone:** 203-869-3082; **Board Cert:** Ophthalmology 2009; **Med School:** Yale Univ 1993; **Resid:** Ophthalmology, Manhattan EE&T 1997; **Fellow:** Cornea & Refractive Surgery, Univ Minnesota Med Ctr 1998

Manjoney, Delia Mary MD (Oph) - **Spec Exp:** Cataract Surgery; Glaucoma; Eyelid Cosmetic Surgery; **Hospital:** St. Vincent's Med Ctr - Bridgeport; **Address:** 2720 Main St, Fl 3rd, Bridgeport, CT 06606; **Phone:** 203-576-6500; **Board Cert:** Pediatrics 1982; Ophthalmology 1988; **Med School:** Univ VT Coll Med 1977; **Resid:** Pediatrics, Parkland Hosp/Chldns Med Ctr 1980; Ophthalmology, Colum Presby Med Ctr/Harkness 1986

Mathias, Stephen Audley MD (Oph) - **Spec Exp:** Pediatric Ophthalmology; Eye Muscle Disorders; **Hospital:** Danbury Hosp; **Address:** 69 Sand Pit Rd, Ste 101, Danbury Eye Physicians, Danbury, CT 06810-4005; **Phone:** 203-791-2020; **Board Cert:** Ophthalmology 1987; **Med School:** Univ Cincinnati 1982; **Resid:** Ophthalmology, Columbia Presby Med Ctr 1986; **Fellow:** Pediatrics, Columbia Presby Med Ctr 1987

Musto, Anthony MD (Oph) - **Spec Exp:** Cataract Surgery-Lens Implant; Eyelid Surgery; **Hospital:** Bridgeport Hosp; **Address:** 495 Hawley Ln, Stratford, CT 06614; **Phone:** 203-375-5819; **Board Cert:** Ophthalmology 1975; **Med School:** Georgetown Univ 1968; **Resid:** Ophthalmology, USPHS 1971; Ophthalmology, Manhattan EE&T Infirm 1973; **Fac Appt:** Asst Clin Prof Oph, Yale Univ

Ostriker, Glenn E MD (Oph) - **Spec Exp:** Cataract Surgery; Glaucoma; **Hospital:** Stamford Hosp (page 893); **Address:** 71 Strawberry Hill Ave, Ste 116, Stamford, CT 06902; **Phone:** 203-348-6300; **Board Cert:** Ophthalmology 1987; **Med School:** NYU Sch Med 1982; **Resid:** Ophthalmology, NYU Med Ctr 1986; **Fellow:** Neurological Physiology, NYU Med Ctr 1983; **Fac Appt:** Assoc Clin Prof Oph, NYU Sch Med

Paul, Matthew D MD (Oph) - **Spec Exp:** Cataract Surgery; **Hospital:** Danbury Hosp; **Address:** Danbury Eye Phys & Surgeons, 69 Sand Pit Rd, Ste 101, Danbury, CT 06810; **Phone:** 203-791-2020; **Board Cert:** Ophthalmology 1985; **Med School:** Columbia P&S 1980; **Resid:** Ophthalmology, NY-Presby/Columbia Univ Med Ctr 1984

Pinke, James MD (Oph) - **Spec Exp:** Cataract Surgery; Glaucoma; Lens Implants; **Hospital:** Griffin Hosp; **Address:** 9 Cots St, Shelton, CT 06484-3866; **Phone:** 203-924-8800; **Board Cert:** Ophthalmology 1983; **Med School:** Tufts Univ 1978; **Resid:** Ophthalmology, Tufts Med Ctr 1982

Potter, William S MD (Oph) - **Spec Exp:** Pediatric Ophthalmology; Strabismus-Adult & Pediatric; Lens Implants; Amblyopia; **Hospital:** Greenwich Hosp (page 892), Stamford Hosp (page 893); **Address:** Greenwich Ophthalmology Assocs, 4 Dearfield Drive, Greenwich, CT 06831; **Phone:** 203-869-3082; **Board Cert:** Ophthalmology 1991; **Med School:** NY Med Coll 1985; **Resid:** Ophthalmology, NY E&E Infirmary 1989; **Fellow:** Strabismus, Wills Eye Hosp 1990

Rabinowitz, Stephen MD (Oph) - **Spec Exp:** Cataract Surgery; Glaucoma; Diabetic Eye Disease/Retinopathy; Lens Implants; **Hospital:** Bridgeport Hosp; **Address:** Ophthalmic Surgeons Grtr Bridgeport, 2371 Black Rock Tpke, Fairfield, CT 06825; **Phone:** 203-371-0141; **Board Cert:** Ophthalmology 1990; **Med School:** NYU Sch Med 1984; **Resid:** Ophthalmology, Lenox Hill Hosp 1988; **Fellow:** Cornea & Ext Eye Disease, Bascom Palmer Eye Inst 1989

Reppucci, Vincent S MD (Oph) - **Spec Exp:** Retinal Disorders; Diabetic Eye Disease; Macular Disease/Degeneration; **Hospital:** Danbury Hosp, New York Eye & Ear Infirm (page 117); **Address:** 65 North St, Danbury, CT 06810; **Phone:** 203-792-6291; **Board Cert:** Ophthalmology 1989; **Med School:** Albert Einstein Coll Med 1983; **Resid:** Ophthalmology, NY-Presby/Columbia Univ Med Ctr 1987; **Fellow:** Vitreoretinal Surgery & Disease, NY-Presby/Weill Cornell Med Ctr 1988; **Fac Appt:** Assoc Prof Oph, Cornell Univ-Weill Med Coll

Robbins, Kim P MD (Oph) - **Spec Exp:** Cataract Surgery; LASIK-Refractive Surgery; **Hospital:** Bridgeport Hosp; **Address:** 4695 Main St, Bridgeport, CT 06606; **Phone:** 203-371-5800; **Board Cert:** Ophthalmology 1985; **Med School:** NY Med Coll 1978; **Resid:** Internal Medicine, Stamford Hosp 1980; Ophthalmology, St Vincents Hosp 1983

Siderides, Elizabeth MD (Oph) - **Spec Exp:** Cataract Surgery; **Hospital:** Stamford Hosp (page 893); **Address:** Stamford Ophthalmology, 1351 Washington Blvd, Ste 101, Stamford, CT 06902-2453; **Phone:** 203-327-5808; **Board Cert:** Ophthalmology 1991; **Med School:** Columbia P&S 1985; **Resid:** Ophthalmology, NYU Med Ctr 1989; **Fellow:** Medical Retina, NYU Med Ctr 1990

Vietorisz, Esteban MD (Oph) - **Spec Exp:** Corneal & External Eye Disease; Cataract Surgery; Glaucoma; **Hospital:** Stamford Hosp (page 893); **Address:** Stamford Ophthalmology, 1351 Washington Blvd, Ste 101, Stamford, CT 06902; **Phone:** 203-327-5808; **Board Cert:** Ophthalmology 2008; **Med School:** Cornell Univ-Weill Med Coll 1991; **Resid:** Ophthalmology, NY-Presby/Weill Cornell Med Ctr 1997; **Fellow:** Cornea, Duke Univ Eye Ctr 1998

Wasserman, Eric L MD (Oph) - **Spec Exp:** Cataract Surgery; Glaucoma; **Hospital:** Stamford Hosp (page 893); **Address:** 1275 Summer St, Ste 200, Stamford, CT 06905-5315; **Phone:** 203-978-0800; **Board Cert:** Ophthalmology 1988; **Med School:** NY Med Coll 1979; **Resid:** Ophthalmology, NY Med Coll 1983; **Fellow:** Anterior Segment - External Disease, John H Sheets Eye Fdn 1984

Weber, Richard B MD (Oph) - **Spec Exp:** Retinal Disorders; **Hospital:** Stamford Hosp (page 893), Greenwich Hosp (page 892); **Address:** 1275 Summer St, Ste 103, Stamford, CT 06905; **Phone:** 203-353-1857; **Board Cert:** Internal Medicine 1979; Ophthalmology 1985; **Med School:** Albert Einstein Coll Med 1976; **Resid:** Internal Medicine, Bronx Muni Hosps 1979; Ophthalmology, Mass E&E Infirm 1984; **Fellow:** Retina, Mass E&E Infirm 1985

Orthopaedic Surgery

Bindelglass, David MD (OrS) - **Spec Exp:** Arthritis; Minimally Invasive Surgery; Hip Replacement; Knee Replacement; **Hospital:** Bridgeport Hosp; **Address:** Orthopaedic Specialty Grp, 75 Kings Hwy Cutoff Fl 2, Fairfield, CT 06824; **Phone:** 203-337-2600; **Board Cert:** Orthopaedic Surgery 2005; **Med School:** Columbia P&S 1985; **Resid:** Surgery, Beth Israel Hosp 1987; Orthopaedic Surgery, Columbia-Presby Med Ctr 1990; **Fellow:** Orthopaedic Surgery, Kerlan-Jobe Ortho Clin 1991

Bomback, David Aaron MD (OrS) - **Spec Exp:** Scoliosis; **Hospital:** Danbury Hosp; **Address:** CT Neck & Back Specialists, 20 Germantown Rd, Ste 2, Danbury, CT 06810-5023; **Phone:** 203-744-9700; **Board Cert:** Orthopaedic Surgery 2007; **Med School:** Columbia P&S 1999; **Resid:** Orthopaedic Surgery, Yale-New Haven Hosp 2004; **Fellow:** Spinal Surgery, Hosp for Special Surgery 2005

Boone, Peter S MD (OrS) - **Spec Exp:** Sports Medicine; Knee Replacement; Hip Replacement; **Hospital:** St. Vincent's Med Ctr - Bridgeport; **Address:** Orthopaedic & Sports Medicine Ctr, 888 White Plains Rd, Trumbull, CT 06611; **Phone:** 203-268-2882; **Board Cert:** Orthopaedic Surgery 2005; **Med School:** Univ Pennsylvania 1985; **Resid:** Surgery, Bellevue/NYU Med Ctr 1986; Orthopaedic Surgery, UMDNJ Med Ctr 1991; **Fellow:** Joint Replacement Surgery, Univ Indiana 1992

Brittis, Dante MD (OrS) - **Spec Exp:** Sports Medicine; Shoulder & Knee Surgery; **Hospital:** Bridgeport Hosp; **Address:** Orthopaedic Specialty Grp, 75 Kings Hwy Cutoff Fl 2, Fairfield, CT 06824; **Phone:** 203-337-2600; **Board Cert:** Orthopaedic Surgery 2008; **Med School:** NY Med Coll 1987; **Resid:** Orthopaedic Surgery, NY-Presby/Columbia Univ Med Ctr 1993; **Fellow:** Sports Medicine, Lenox Hill Hosp 1994

Brown, David B MD (OrS) - **Hospital:** Bridgeport Hosp; **Address:** Orthocare Specialists, 4747 Main St, Bridgeport, CT 06606-1804; **Phone:** 203-372-0649; **Board Cert:** Orthopaedic Surgery 2007; **Med School:** St Louis Univ 1974; **Resid:** Internal Medicine, George Washington Univ Sch Med 1976; Orthopaedic Surgery, Long Island Jewish Med Ctr 1981; **Fellow:** Surgery, Mount Sinai Med Ctr 1978

Clain, Michael R MD (OrS) - **Spec Exp:** Foot & Ankle Surgery; Sports Medicine; **Hospital:** Greenwich Hosp (page 892); **Address:** Orthopaedic & Neurosurgery Specialists, 6 Greenwich Office Park, 10 Valley Drive, Greenwich, CT 06831; **Phone:** 203-869-1145; **Board Cert:** Orthopaedic Surgery 2004; **Med School:** Columbia P&S 1984; **Resid:** Orthopaedic Surgery, Lenox Hill Hosp 1990; **Fellow:** Foot & Ankle Surgery, Baylor Coll Med 1991

Crowe, John F MD (OrS) - **Spec Exp:** Upper Extremity Surgery; Hip & Knee Replacement; Sports Medicine; **Hospital:** Greenwich Hosp (page 892); **Address:** Orthopaedic & Neurosurgery Specialists, 6 Greenwich Office Park, 10 Valley Drive, Greenwich, CT 06831; **Phone:** 203-869-1145 x263; **Board Cert:** Orthopaedic Surgery 1977; **Med School:** Cornell Univ-Weill Med Coll 1971; **Resid:** Surgery, Roosevelt Hosp 1973; Orthopaedic Surgery, Hosp Special Surgery 1976; **Fellow:** Hand Surgery, Roosevelt Hosp 1979

Cunningham, James G MD (OrS) - **Spec Exp:** Arthroscopic Surgery; Shoulder Surgery; Knee Surgery; Sports Medicine; **Hospital:** Greenwich Hosp (page 892); **Address:** Orthopaedic & Neurosurgery Specialists, 6 Greenwich Offfice Park Drive, 10 Valley Drive, Greenwich, CT 06831; **Phone:** 203-869-1145; **Board Cert:** Orthopaedic Surgery 2009; Orthopaedic Sports Medicine 2007; **Med School:** NYU Sch Med 1983; **Resid:** Orthopaedic Surgery, Mt Sinai Med Ctr 1988; Surgery, Mt Sinai Med Ctr 1984; **Fellow:** Sports Medicine, New England Baptist Hosp 1989

D'Amico, Joseph MD (OrS) - **Spec Exp:** Knee Replacement; Hip Replacement; Sports Medicine; **Hospital:** Stamford Hosp (page 893); **Address:** 90 Morgan St, Ste 207, Stamford, CT 06905-5436; **Phone:** 203-325-4087; **Board Cert:** Orthopaedic Surgery 2003; **Med School:** Univ Tenn Coll Med 1982; **Resid:** Orthopaedic Surgery, St Lukes-Roosevelt Med Ctr 1988

Deluca, Jeffrey V MD (OrS) - **Spec Exp:** Arthroscopic Surgery; Knee Replacement; **Hospital:** Norwalk Hosp; **Address:** Coastal Orthopaedics, 40 Cross St, Ste 300, Norwalk, CT 06851-2439; **Phone:** 203-845-2200; **Board Cert:** Orthopaedic Surgery 2005; **Med School:** Temple Univ 1984; **Resid:** Orthopaedic Surgery, Eastern Virginia Med Sch 1991; **Fellow:** Orthopaedic Surgery, Boston Med Ctr 1987; Orthopaedic Surgery, Washington Ortho & Knee Clin 1992

Ennis Jr, Francis A MD (OrS) - **Spec Exp:** Hip & Knee Replacement; Arthroscopic Surgery; **Hospital:** Greenwich Hosp (page 892); **Address:** Orthopaedic & Neurosurgery Specialists, 6 Greenwich Office Park, 10 Valley Drive, Greenwich, CT 06831; **Phone:** 203-869-1145; **Board Cert:** Orthopaedic Surgery 2007; **Med School:** Duke Univ 1999; **Resid:** Orthopaedic Surgery, Yale-New Haven Hosp 2004; **Fellow:** Reconstructive Surgery, New England Baptist Hosp 2005

FitzGibbons, James J MD (OrS) - **Spec Exp:** Arthroscopic Surgery; Joint Replacement; Sports Medicine; **Hospital:** St. Vincent's Med Ctr - Bridgeport; **Address:** Orthopaedic Specialty Grp, 75 Kings Hwy Cutoff Fl 3, Fairfield, CT 06824-5340; **Phone:** 203-337-2600; **Board Cert:** Orthopaedic Surgery 2011; **Med School:** Loyola Univ-Stritch Sch Med 1992; **Resid:** Orthopaedic Surgery, Northwestern Meml Hosp 1997; **Fellow:** Orthopaedic Sports Medicine, Harvard Univ/Mass Genl Hosp 1998

Henshaw, D Ross MD (OrS) - **Spec Exp:** Shoulder Surgery; Rotator Cuff Surgery; Sports Medicine; Knee Surgery; **Hospital:** Danbury Hosp; **Address:** Danbury Orthopaedic Assocs, 73 Sand Pit Rd, Ste 204, Danbury, CT 06810; **Phone:** 203-797-1500; **Board Cert:** Orthopaedic Surgery 2007; Orthopaedic Sports Medicine 2008; **Med School:** Columbia P&S 1998; **Resid:** Orthopaedic Surgery, Ny Presby-Columbia Med Ctr 2003; **Fellow:** Sports Medicine & Shoulder Surgery, Hosp for Special Surgery 2005

Hermele, Herbert I MD (OrS) - **Hospital:** Bridgeport Hosp, St. Vincent's Med Ctr - Bridgeport; **Address:** Orthopaedic Specialty Grp, 75 Kings Hwy Cutoff Fl 2, Fairfield, CT 06824-5340; **Phone:** 203-337-2600; **Board Cert:** Orthopaedic Surgery 1975; **Med School:** Albert Einstein Coll Med 1969; **Resid:** Orthopaedic Surgery, Albert Einstein Affil Hosps 1974

Hindman, Steven MD (OrS) - **Spec Exp:** Sports Injuries; **Hospital:** Greenwich Hosp (page 892); **Address:** Orthopaedic & Neurosurgery Specialists, 6 Greenwich Office Park, 10 Valley Drive, Greenwich, CT 06831-5151; **Phone:** 203-869-1145; **Board Cert:** Orthopaedic Surgery 2010; **Med School:** Albert Einstein Coll Med 1982; **Resid:** Orthopaedic Surgery, Montefiore Med Ctr 1987

Hughes, Peter MD (OrS) - **Spec Exp:** Hip Replacement; Knee Replacement; Sports Medicine; **Hospital:** Stamford Hosp (page 893); **Address:** 90 Morgan St, Ste 207, Stamford, CT 06905; **Phone:** 203-325-4087; **Board Cert:** Orthopaedic Surgery 1978; **Med School:** NY Med Coll 1972; **Resid:** Orthopaedic Surgery, Metropolitan Hosp Ctr 1976; **Fellow:** Surgery, Hosp for Special Surg 1977; **Fac Appt:** Asst Clin Prof OrS, Columbia P&S

Kavanagh, Brian MD (OrS) - **Spec Exp:** Hip Replacement; Knee Replacement; Arthritis; **Hospital:** Greenwich Hosp (page 892); **Address:** 6 Greenwich Office Park, ONS, Greenwich, CT 06831; **Phone:** 203-869-1145; **Board Cert:** Orthopaedic Surgery 2007; **Med School:** Univ Conn 1979; **Resid:** Orthopaedic Surgery, Mayo Clinic 1984; **Fac Appt:** Asst Clin Prof OrS, Yale Univ

Kramer, David Lawrence MD (OrS) - **Hospital:** Danbury Hosp; **Address:** CT Neck & Back Specialists, 20 Germantown Rd Fl 2, Danbury, CT 06810-5023; **Phone:** 203-744-9700; **Board Cert:** Orthopaedic Surgery 2009; **Med School:** Dartmouth Med Sch 1989; **Resid:** Orthopaedic Surgery, Mass Genl Hosp 1994; Orthopaedic Surgery, Beth Israel Hosp 1994; **Fellow:** Orthopaedic Surgery, Inselspital-Maurice E Muller 1995; Orthopaedic Surgery, Thomas Jefferson Univ Hosp 1996

Lynch, Michael MD (OrS) - **Spec Exp:** Arthroscopic Surgery; Sports Medicine; Knee Replacement; **Hospital:** Stamford Hosp (page 893), Norwalk Hosp; **Address:** 40 Cross St, Ste 300, Coastal Orthopaedics, Norwalk, CT 06851-4646; **Phone:** 203-845-2200; **Board Cert:** Orthopaedic Surgery 2005; **Med School:** Dartmouth Med Sch 1984; **Resid:** Orthopaedic Surgery, Mass Genl Hosp 1990; Pediatric Orthopaedic Surgery, Children's Hosp 1991; **Fellow:** Sports Medicine, Union Meml Hosp 1992

Marks, Michael R MD (OrS) - **Hospital:** Norwalk Hosp; **Address:** Norwalk Hosp, 34 Maple St, Norwalk, CT 06856; **Phone:** 203-852-2000; **Board Cert:** Orthopaedic Surgery 2011; **Med School:** Geo Wash Univ 1982; **Resid:** Orthopaedic Surgery, G Washington Univ Hosp 1987; **Fellow:** Spinal Cord Injury Medicine, Cleveland Clinic 1988

McGinniss, George Hoyt MD (OrS) - **Hospital:** Stamford Hosp (page 893); **Address:** Orthopaedic Surgery & Sports, 1290 Summer St Ste 4400, Stamford, CT 06905-5331; **Phone:** 203-323-7331; **Board Cert:** Orthopaedic Surgery 2010; **Med School:** Georgetown Univ 1978; **Resid:** Orthopaedic Surgery, Mount Sinai Med Ctr 1983; **Fellow:** Knee Surgery, Dr. Frank Noyes 1984

Miller, Seth R MD (OrS) - **Spec Exp:** Shoulder Surgery; Rotator Cuff Surgery; Sports Medicine; **Hospital:** Greenwich Hosp (page 892), NYU Hosp For Joint Diseases (page 119); **Address:** Orthopaedic & Neurosurgery Specialists, 6 Greenwich Office Park, 10 Valley Drive, Greenwich, CT 06831; **Phone:** 203-869-1145; **Board Cert:** Orthopaedic Surgery 2012; **Med School:** Mount Sinai Sch Med 1982; **Resid:** Surgery, Mt Sinai Hosp 1985; Orthopaedic Surgery, Columbia-Presby Med Ctr 1988; **Fellow:** Shoulder Surgery, Columbia-Presby Med Ctr 1989; **Fac Appt:** Assoc Prof S, NYU Sch Med

Polifroni, Nicholas V MD (OrS) - **Spec Exp:** Sports Medicine; Joint Replacement; **Hospital:** Norwalk Hosp; **Address:** Coastal Orthopaedics, 40 Cross St, Ste 300, Norwalk, CT 06851; **Phone:** 203-845-2200; **Board Cert:** Orthopaedic Surgery 1984; **Med School:** NY Med Coll 1977; **Resid:** Orthopaedic Surgery, Lenox Hill Hosp 1982

Sethi, Paul MD (OrS) - **Spec Exp:** Sports Medicine; Knee Surgery; Shoulder Surgery; **Hospital:** Greenwich Hosp (page 892); **Address:** Orthopaedic and Neurosurgery Specialists, 6 Greenwich Office Park, 10 Valley Drive, Greenwich, CT 06831; **Phone:** 203-869-1145; **Board Cert:** Orthopaedic Surgery 2005; Orthopaedic Sports Medicine 2007; **Med School:** Mount Sinai Sch Med 1997; **Resid:** Orthopaedic Surgery, Yale-New Haven Hosp 2002; **Fellow:** Sports Medicine, Kerlan Jobe Ortho Clin 2003; Arthroscopic Surgery, Kerlan Jobe Ortho Clin 2004

Spak, James I MD (OrS) - **Spec Exp:** Sports Medicine; **Hospital:** St. Vincent's Med Ctr - Bridgeport; **Address:** Orthopaedic & Sports Med Ctr, 888 White Plains Rd, Trumbull, CT 06611; **Phone:** 203-268-2882; **Board Cert:** Orthopaedic Surgery 2011; Orthopaedic Sports Medicine 2010; **Med School:** Harvard Med Sch 1992; **Resid:** Orthopaedic Surgery, Brigham & Women's Hosp 1997; **Fellow:** Sports Medicine, Tahoe Fracture & Ortho Cl 1998; Trauma, Tahoe Fracture & Ortho Cl 1998

Stovell, Peter B MD (OrS) - **Spec Exp:** Joint Replacement; Sports Medicine; **Hospital:** Norwalk Hosp; **Address:** 40 Cross St, Ste 300, Coastal Orthopaedics, Norwalk, CT 06851-5726; **Phone:** 203-845-2200; **Board Cert:** Orthopaedic Surgery 1976; **Med School:** Columbia P&S 1968; **Resid:** Surgery, St Luke's-Roosevelt Hosp Ctr 1970; Orthopaedic Surgery, Hosp for Special Surgery 1975

Troy, Allen MD (OrS) - **Spec Exp:** Foot & Ankle Surgery; Sports Medicine; **Hospital:** Stamford Hosp (page 893); **Address:** 90 Morgan St Fl 2 - Ste 207, Stamford, CT 06905; **Phone:** 203-325-4087; **Board Cert:** Orthopaedic Surgery 2010; **Med School:** SUNY Downstate 1979; **Resid:** Orthopaedic Surgery, NYU Med Ctr 1984; **Fellow:** Foot & Ankle Surgery, Hosp Joint Disease 1985; **Fac Appt:** Asst Clin Prof OrS, Columbia P&S

Wilchinsky, Mark MD (OrS) - **Spec Exp:** Arthroscopic Surgery; Joint Replacement; **Hospital:** St. Vincent's Med Ctr - Bridgeport, Griffin Hosp; **Address:** Orthopaedic & Sports Medicine Ctr, 888 White Plains Rd, Trumbull, CT 06611; **Phone:** 203-268-2882; **Board Cert:** Orthopaedic Surgery 2007; **Med School:** Tulane Univ 1979; **Resid:** Surgery, Univ Mass Med Ctr 1980; Orthopaedic Surgery, Univ Mass Med Ctr 1984; **Fac Appt:** Asst Prof OrS, Univ Mass Sch Med

Otolaryngology

Aferzon, Mark MD (Oto) - **Spec Exp:** Allergy; Nasal & Sinus Disorders; Snoring/Sleep Apnea; Thyroid & Parathyroid Surgery; **Hospital:** Griffin Hosp; **Address:** 2 Ivy Brook Road, Ste 110, Shelton, CT 06484; **Phone:** 203-954-0019; **Board Cert:** Otolaryngology 2003; **Med School:** Brown Univ 1997; **Resid:** Surgery, SUNY Upstate Med Univ 1999; Otolaryngology, Geisinger Med Ctr 2002

Bard, Michael C MD (Oto) - **Spec Exp:** Head & Neck Surgery; Sleep Disorders/Apnea; Sinus Disorders/Surgery; **Hospital:** Danbury Hosp; **Address:** Advanced Specialty Care, 107 Newton Rd, Ste 2A, Danbury, CT 06810; **Phone:** 203-830-4700; **Board Cert:** Otolaryngology 1993; **Med School:** Mount Sinai Sch Med 1987; **Resid:** Otolaryngology, Mayo Grad Sch Med 1992; **Fellow:** Otolaryngology, Royal Natl Throat,Nose & Ear Hosp 1993

Bianchi, Mark S MD (Oto) - **Spec Exp:** Hearing Disorders; Balance Disorders; **Hospital:** Bridgeport Hosp; **Address:** 2526 Main St, Stratford, CT 06615; **Phone:** 203-459-8330; **Board Cert:** Otolaryngology 1997; Sleep Medicine 2012; **Med School:** Yale Univ 1991; **Resid:** Otolaryngology, Yale-New Haven Hosp 1996

Brauer, Richard J MD (Oto) - **Spec Exp:** Head & Neck Surgery; Thyroid Cancer; **Hospital:** Greenwich Hosp (page 892); **Address:** 49 Lake Ave, Ste 205, Greenwich, CT 06830; **Phone:** 203-869-0177; **Board Cert:** Otolaryngology 1981; **Med School:** Hahnemann Univ 1976; **Resid:** Otolaryngology, Bellevue Hosp Ctr 1980; **Fellow:** Head and Neck Surgery, Montefiore Med Ctr 1982

Breda, Stephen D MD (Oto) - **Spec Exp:** Head & Neck Surgery; **Hospital:** St. Vincent's Med Ctr - Bridgeport; **Address:** 4695 Main St, Ste 1, Bridgeport, CT 06606; **Phone:** 203-371-5166; **Board Cert:** Otolaryngology 1988; **Med School:** NYU Sch Med 1983; **Resid:** Otolaryngology, NYU Med Ctr 1988; **Fellow:** Head and Neck Surgery, NYU Med Ctr 1988

Gordon, Neil A MD (Oto) - **Spec Exp:** Cosmetic Surgery-Face; **Hospital:** Norwalk Hosp, Yale-New Haven Hosp; **Address:** Spilt Rock Surgical Assocs, 539 Danbury Rd, Wilton, CT 06897; **Phone:** 203-661-1715; **Board Cert:** Otolaryngology 1996; Facial Plastic & Reconstr Surgery 1998; **Med School:** Albert Einstein Coll Med 1990; **Resid:** Otolaryngology, Yale-New Haven Hosp 1995; **Fellow:** Facial Plastic Surgery, Tulane Univ Med Ctr 1996

Klarsfeld, Jay MD (Oto) - **Spec Exp:** Sinus Disorders; Thyroid & Parathyroid Surgery; **Hospital:** Danbury Hosp; **Address:** 107 Newtown Rd, Ste 2A, Danbury, CT 06810-4151; **Phone:** 203-830-4700; **Board Cert:** Otolaryngology 1986; **Med School:** Mount Sinai Sch Med 1981; **Resid:** Surgery, Mt Sinai Hosp 1983; Otolaryngology, Mt Sinai Hosp 1986

Klenoff, Bruce MD (Oto) - **Spec Exp:** Ear Disorders/Surgery; Sinus Disorders/Surgery; Pediatric Otolaryngology; **Hospital:** Stamford Hosp (page 893); **Address:** Ear, Nose & Throat Ctr - Tully Hlth Ctr, 32 Strawberry Hill Ct, Fl 4 - Ste 4, Stamford, CT 06902; **Phone:** 203-353-0000; **Board Cert:** Otolaryngology 1976; **Med School:** Tufts Univ 1969; **Resid:** Surgery, St Elizabeth Hosp 1973; Otolaryngology, Mass Eye & Ear Infirm 1976; **Fac Appt:** Asst Clin Prof S, Columbia P&S

Lane, Edward M MD (Oto) - **Hospital:** Bridgeport Hosp, Norwalk Hosp; **Address:** 4675 Main St, Bridgeport, CT 06606-1813; **Phone:** 203-372-0009; **Board Cert:** Otolaryngology 1982; **Med School:** Columbia P&S 1977; **Resid:** Otolaryngology, St Lukes Roosevelt Hosp 1979; Otolaryngology, Columbia-Presby Hosp 1982; **Fellow:** Surgery, UnivTexas MD Anderson Cancer Ctr 1983

Levin, Richard A MD (Oto) - **Spec Exp:** Sinus Disorders; Ear Infections; Facial Plastic & Reconstructive Surgery; **Hospital:** St. Vincent's Med Ctr - Bridgeport, Bridgeport Hosp; **Address:** 1305 Post Rd, Ste 302, Fairfield, CT 06824; **Phone:** 203-259-4700; **Board Cert:** Otolaryngology 1993; **Med School:** Tufts Univ 1987; **Resid:** Otolaryngology, Mount Sinai Hosp 1993; **Fac Appt:** Asst Prof S, Yale Univ

Levine, Steven B MD (Oto) - **Spec Exp:** Sinus Disorders; Allergy & Immunotherapy; Snoring/Sleep Apnea; **Hospital:** Bridgeport Hosp; **Address:** 160 Hawley Ln, Ste 202, Trumbull, CT 06611; **Phone:** 203-380-3707; **Board Cert:** Otolaryngology 1986; **Med School:** Univ Rochester 1981; **Resid:** Surgery, Penn Hosp 1983; Otolaryngology, Hosp Univ Penn 1986; **Fellow:** Otolaryngology, NY Hosp 1986; **Fac Appt:** Asst Clin Prof S, Yale Univ

Salzer, Stephen MD (Oto) - **Spec Exp:** Thyroid & Parathyroid Surgery; Pediatric Otolaryngology; Sinus Disorders/Surgery; Thyroid Cancer; **Hospital:** Greenwich Hosp (page 892), Stamford Hosp (page 893); **Address:** 49 Lake Ave Fl 1, Greenwich, CT 06830-4519; **Phone:** 203-869-2030; **Board Cert:** Otolaryngology 1995; **Med School:** Johns Hopkins Univ 1989; **Resid:** Otolaryngology, Yale-New Haven Hosp 1994; **Fellow:** Otolaryngology, Laennec Hosp 1995

Pain Medicine

Boolbol, Robert MD (PM) - **Hospital:** Bridgeport Hosp, Hartford Hosp; **Address:** CT Pain Care, 5520 Park Ave, Ste 303, Trumball, CT 06611; **Phone:** 203-373-7330; **Board Cert:** Anesthesiology 1994; Pain Medicine 2003; **Med School:** NY Med Coll 1989; **Resid:** Anesthesiology, Univ Chicago Hosps 1992; **Fellow:** Pain Medicine, Univ Chicago Hosps 2002

Pathology

Pinto, Marguerite MD (Path) - **Spec Exp:** Gynecologic Pathology; Breast Pathology; **Hospital:** Bridgeport Hosp; **Address:** Bridgeport Hosp, Yale Pathology, 267 Grant St Fl 2, Bridgeport, CT 06610; **Phone:** 203-384-3157; **Board Cert:** Pathology 1975; Cytopathology 1989; **Med School:** India 1970; **Resid:** Pathology, Bridgeport Hosp; **Fac Appt:** Asst Prof Path, Yale Univ

Pediatric Allergy & Immunology

Burstein, Ora MD (PA&I) - **Hospital:** Stamford Hosp (page 893); **Address:** 22 Fifth St Fl 3, Stamford, CT 06905; **Phone:** 203-978-0072; **Board Cert:** Pediatrics 2005; Allergy & Immunology 2005; **Med School:** Tufts Univ 1984; **Resid:** Pediatrics, Montefiore Med Ctr 1987; **Fellow:** Allergy & Immunology, Montefiore Med Ctr 1989

Pediatric Cardiology

Berkwits, Kieve M MD (PCd) - **Spec Exp:** Congenital Heart Disease; **Hospital:** Bridgeport Hosp, St. Vincent's Med Ctr - Bridgeport; **Address:** Bridgeport Hosp, Dept Peds, 226 Mill Hill Ave, Bridgeport, CT 06610; **Phone:** 203-384-3783; **Board Cert:** Pediatrics 1986; Pediatric Cardiology 2003; **Med School:** Mexico 1979; **Resid:** Pediatrics, Beth Israel Med Ctr 1983; **Fellow:** Pediatric Cardiology, NY Hosp-Cornell Med Ctr 1985; **Fac Appt:** Asst Clin Prof Ped, Yale Univ

Snyder, Michael MD (PCd) - **Spec Exp:** Echocardiography; Fetal Echocardiography; **Hospital:** Stamford Hosp (page 893); **Address:** 1500 Boston Post Rd Fl 2, Darien, CT 06820-5936; **Phone:** 203-662-0313; **Board Cert:** Pediatrics 1984; Pediatric Cardiology 1985; **Med School:** Cornell Univ-Weill Med Coll 1979; **Resid:** Pediatrics, NY Hosp 1982; **Fellow:** Pediatric Cardiology, NY Hosp 1984; **Fac Appt:** Assoc Prof Ped, Columbia P&S

Pediatric Gastroenterology

Glassman, Mark MD (PGe) - **Spec Exp:** Inflammatory Bowel Disease/Crohn's; Gastroesophageal Reflux Disease (GERD); Diarrheal Diseases; Food Allergy; **Hospital:** Norwalk Hosp, Children's & Women's Phys.of Westchester (page 612); **Address:** 149 East Ave, Ste 39, Norwalk, CT 06851; **Phone:** 203-853-7170; **Board Cert:** Pediatrics 1983; Pediatric Gastroenterology 2012; **Med School:** SUNY Buffalo 1978; **Resid:** Pediatrics, Yale-New Haven Hosp 1981; **Fellow:** Gastroenterology, Chldns Hosp 1983; **Fac Appt:** Prof Ped, NY Med Coll

Pediatric Pulmonology

Dworkin, Gregory MD (PPul) - **Spec Exp:** Asthma; Chronic Lung Disease; **Hospital:** Danbury Hosp; **Address:** 79 Sand Pit Rd, Ste 201, Danbury, CT 06810; **Phone:** 203-790-5437; **Board Cert:** Pediatrics 1987; Pediatric Pulmonology 2004; **Med School:** Albany Med Coll 1982; **Resid:** Pediatrics, Mount Sinai 1985; Pediatrics, Mount Sinai 1986; **Fellow:** Pediatric Pulmonology, Mount Sinai 1989; **Fac Appt:** Asst Clin Prof Ped, NY Med Coll

Hen Jr, Jacob MD (PPul) - **Spec Exp:** Asthma; Critical Care; **Hospital:** Bridgeport Hosp; **Address:** Bridgeport Hosp, Dept Peds, 267 Grant St, Box 5000, Bridgeport, CT 06610-2870; **Phone:** 203-384-3711; **Board Cert:** Pediatrics 1980; Pediatric Pulmonology 2006; Pediatric Critical Care Medicine 2009; **Med School:** UMDNJ-NJ Med Sch, Newark 1975; **Resid:** Pediatrics, UMDNJ-Univ Hosp 1977; **Fellow:** Pediatric Pulmonology, Yale-New Haven Hosp 1981; **Fac Appt:** Assoc Clin Prof Ped, Yale Univ

Sadeghi, Hossein MD (PPul) - **Spec Exp:** Asthma; Neonatal Chronic Lung Disease; Cystic Fibrosis; Bronchoscopy; **Hospital:** Stamford Hosp (page 893), Greenwich Hosp (page 892); **Address:** 32 Strawberry Hill Ct, Ste 11, Stamford, CT 06902-2777; **Phone:** 203-276-5949; **Board Cert:** Pediatrics 2010; Pediatric Pulmonology 2006; **Med School:** Australia 1990; **Resid:** Pediatrics, Royal Chldns Hosp 1992; Pediatrics, Med Coll Va Hosp 1995; **Fellow:** Pediatric Pulmonology, Westchester Co Med Ctr 1998; **Fac Appt:** Asst Clin Prof Ped, Columbia P&S

Pediatrics

Chessin, Robert D MD (Ped) *PCP* - **Spec Exp:** Child Development; Developmental Disorders; **Hospital:** Bridgeport Hosp, St. Vincent's Med Ctr - Bridgeport; **Address:** 4699 Main St, Ste 215, Bridgeport, CT 06606-1830; **Phone:** 203-452-8322; **Board Cert:** Pediatrics 1978; Developmental-Behavioral Pediatrics 2004; **Med School:** Johns Hopkins Univ 1973; **Resid:** Pediatrics, Duke Univ Med Ctr 1976; **Fac Appt:** Assoc Clin Prof Ped, Yale Univ

Freedman, Richard M MD (Ped) *PCP* - **Spec Exp:** Neonatology; **Hospital:** Bridgeport Hosp, Yale-New Haven Hosp; **Address:** 4699 Main St, Ste 215, Bridgeport, CT 06606-1830; **Phone:** 203-452-8322; **Board Cert:** Pediatrics 1979; Neonatal-Perinatal Medicine 1981; **Med School:** Boston Univ 1975; **Resid:** Pediatrics, Yale-New Haven Hosp 1978; **Fellow:** Neonatology, Yale-New Haven Hosp 1980; **Fac Appt:** Assoc Clin Prof Ped, Yale Univ

Hedrick, David A MD (Ped) *PCP* - **Hospital:** Greenwich Hosp (page 892); **Address:** Children's Medical Group, 42 Sherwood Pl, Greenwich, CT 06830; **Phone:** 203-661-2440; **Board Cert:** Pediatrics 1981; **Med School:** Univ VA Sch Med 1976; **Resid:** Pediatrics, Children's Hosp of Pittsburgh 1079

Juan, Paul E MD (Ped) *PCP* - **Spec Exp:** Developmental Disorders; Asthma; **Hospital:** Greenwich Hosp (page 892); **Address:** Valley Pediatrics of Greenwich, 25 Valley Drive Fl 2, Greenwich, CT 06830; **Phone:** 203-622-4301; **Board Cert:** Pediatrics 2009; **Med School:** NY Med Coll 1990; **Resid:** Pediatrics, Med Coll of Virginia 1993

Klenk, Rosemary MD (Ped) *PCP* - **Spec Exp:** ADD/ADHD; Eating Disorders; **Hospital:** Stamford Hosp (page 893), NY-Presby/Columbia Univ Med Ctr, NY (page 104); **Address:** New England Pediatrics, 183 Cherry St, Ste 103, New Canaan, CT 06840; **Phone:** 203-972-5232; **Board Cert:** Pediatrics 1987; **Med School:** Cornell Univ-Weill Med Coll 1980; **Resid:** Pediatrics, Columbia-Presby Med Ctr 1983

Korval, Arnold MD (Ped) *PCP* - **Hospital:** Greenwich Hosp (page 892), Stamford Hosp (page 893); **Address:** Greenwich Pediatric Assocs, 8 W End Ave, Old Greenwich, CT 06870-1642; **Phone:** 203-637-0186; **Board Cert:** Pediatrics 2009; **Med School:** St Louis Univ 1974; **Resid:** Pediatrics, Chldn's Hosp-Univ Penn 1977

Levine, Dorothy MD (Ped) *PCP* - **Spec Exp:** Complex Diagnosis; **Hospital:** Stamford Hosp (page 893), NY-Presby/Columbia Univ Med Ctr, NY (page 104); **Address:** 166 W Broad St, Ste 103, Stamford, CT 06902; **Phone:** 203-323-1770; **Board Cert:** Pediatrics 1985; **Med School:** Albert Einstein Coll Med 1980; **Resid:** Pediatrics, Columbia-Presby Med Ctr 1983; **Fac Appt:** Asst Clin Prof Ped, Columbia P&S

Magner, Joan A MD (Ped) - **Hospital:** Danbury Hosp; **Address:** Ctr For Pediatric Med, 107 Newtown Rd, Ste 1D, Danbury, CT 06810-4180; **Phone:** 203-790-0822; **Board Cert:** Pediatrics 1986; **Med School:** Univ Hawaii JA Burns Sch Med 1980; **Resid:** Pediatrics, Ohio State Univ Columbus Chldn's Hosp 1984

Marks, Laura MD (Ped) - **Spec Exp:** Nutrition; Immune Deficiencies-Primary; **Hospital:** Norwalk Hosp; **Address:** 1563 Post Rd E, Willows Pediatric Grp, Westport, CT 06880; **Phone:** 203-319-3939; **Board Cert:** Pediatrics 2010; **Med School:** Yale Univ 1992; **Resid:** Pediatrics, Yale-New Haven Hosp 1995

Mini, Katherine N MD (Ped) *PCP* - **Hospital:** Greenwich Hosp (page 892); **Address:** Chldns Med Grp, 42 Sherwood Pl, Greenwich, CT 06830; **Phone:** 203-661-2440; **Board Cert:** Pediatrics 2005; **Med School:** Albert Einstein Coll Med 1994; **Resid:** Pediatrics, Yale-New Haven Hosp 1997

Mongillo, Nicholas MD (Ped) *PCP* - **Spec Exp:** AIDS/HIV; Sports Medicine; ADD/ADHD; **Hospital:** Bridgeport Hosp; **Address:** 25 Constitution Blvd, Shelton, CT 06484; **Phone:** 203-924-7334; **Board Cert:** Pediatrics 2003; **Med School:** Grenada 1987; **Resid:** Pediatrics, Bridgeport Hosp 1990

Morelli, Alan MD (Ped) *PCP* - **Hospital:** Stamford Hosp (page 893); **Address:** New England Pediatrics, 166 W Broad St, Ste 103, Stamford, CT 06902; **Phone:** 203-323-1770; **Board Cert:** Pediatrics 1987; **Med School:** NY Med Coll 1982; **Resid:** Pediatrics, Yale-New Haven Hosp 1985

Romanowitz, Harry MD (Ped) *PCP* - **Hospital:** Stamford Hosp (page 893), Greenwich Hosp (page 892); **Address:** 35 River Rd, Fl 2, Cos Cob, CT 06807; **Phone:** 203-329-5800; **Board Cert:** Pediatrics 1989; **Med School:** Yale Univ 1973; **Resid:** Pediatrics, Strong Memorial Hosp 1976; **Fac Appt:** Asst Prof Ped, Yale Univ

Schiz, Steven L MD (Ped) *PCP* - **Hospital:** Greenwich Hosp (page 892); **Address:** Children's Medical Group, 42 Sherwood Pl, Greenwich, CT 06830-5633; **Phone:** 203-661-2440; **Board Cert:** Pediatrics 2009; **Med School:** Columbia P&S 1980; **Resid:** Pediatrics, Children's Hosp of Pittsburgh 1983

Physical Medicine & Rehabilitation

Aaronson, Beth MD (PMR) - **Spec Exp:** Acupuncture; Neurologic Rehabilitation; Cancer Rehabilitation; Lymphedema; **Hospital:** Danbury Hosp; **Address:** 235 Main St, Ste 102, Danbury, CT 06810-6606; **Phone:** 203-730-5929; **Board Cert:** Physical Medicine & Rehabilitation 2005; **Med School:** SUNY Stony Brook 1990; **Resid:** Physical Medicine & Rehabilitation, NY-Presby/Columbia Univ Med Ctr 1994

Grant, Linda MD (PMR) - **Spec Exp:** Lymphedema; Acupuncture; **Hospital:** Greenwich Hosp (page 892); **Address:** Greenwich Hosp, Physical Med & Rehab, 5 Perryridge Rd, Greenwich, CT 06830; **Phone:** 203-863-3290; **Board Cert:** Physical Medicine & Rehabilitation 1990; **Med School:** UMDNJ-Rutgers Med Sch 1985; **Resid:** Physical Medicine & Rehabilitation, NYU Med Ctr 1989

Heftler, Jeffrey M MD (PMR) - **Spec Exp:** Pain Management; Spinal Rehabilitation; **Hospital:** Greenwich Hosp (page 892); **Address:** Orthopaedic & Neurosurgery Specialists, 6 Greenwich Office Park, 10 Valley Drive, Greenwich, CT 06831; **Phone:** 203-869-1145; **Board Cert:** Physical Medicine & Rehabilitation 2012; Pain Medicine 2003; **Med School:** UMDNJ-RW Johnson Med Sch 1997; **Resid:** Physical Medicine & Rehabilitation, Thos Jefferson Univ Med Ctr 2001; **Fellow:** Pain Management, Beth Israel Med Ctr 2002

Richter, Edwin MD (PMR) - **Spec Exp:** Neuro-Rehabilitation; Brain Injury Rehabilitation; Amputee Rehabilitation; Lymphedema; **Hospital:** Stamford Hosp (page 893); **Address:** 166 W Broad St, Ste 305, Stamford, CT 06902; **Phone:** 203-316-0610; **Board Cert:** Physical Medicine & Rehabilitation 1992; **Med School:** NYU Sch Med 1987; **Resid:** Physical Medicine & Rehabilitation, NYU Med Ctr 1991; **Fac Appt:** Asst Clin Prof PMR, NYU Sch Med

Snowball, Halina MD (PMR) - **Spec Exp:** Pain Management; Acupuncture; **Hospital:** Greenwich Hosp (page 892); **Address:** 2015 W Main St, Ste 100, Stamford, CT 06902; **Phone:** 203-863-4588; **Board Cert:** Physical Medicine & Rehabilitation 1990; **Med School:** Univ Fla Coll Med 1985; **Resid:** Physical Medicine & Rehabilitation, Stanford Univ Med Ctr 1989

Plastic Surgery

Attkiss, Keith J MD (PlS) - **Spec Exp:** Breast Cosmetic & Reconstructive Surgery; Liposuction & Body Contouring; **Hospital:** Greenwich Hosp (page 892); **Address:** 2 1/2 Dearfield Drive, Ste 203, Greenwich, CT 06831; **Phone:** 203-862-2700; **Board Cert:** Plastic Surgery 2001; **Med School:** Columbia P&S 1992; **Resid:** Surgery, UC Davies Med Ctr 1997; Plastic Surgery, Yale-New Haven Hosp 2000

Gewirtz, Harold S MD (PlS) - **Spec Exp:** Cosmetic Surgery-Face; Breast Cosmetic & Reconstructive Surgery; Liposuction & Body Contouring; Melanoma; **Hospital:** Stamford Hosp (page 893), Greenwich Hosp (page 892); **Address:** 70 Mill River St, Stamford, CT 06902-3725; **Phone:** 203-325-1381; **Board Cert:** Plastic Surgery 1984; **Med School:** Johns Hopkins Univ 1975; **Resid:** Surgery, UCLA Med Ctr 1980; Plastic Surgery, NYU Med Ctr 1982; **Fac Appt:** Assoc Clin Prof PlS, Columbia P&S

Goldenberg, David M MD (PlS) - **Spec Exp:** Cosmetic Surgery; Breast Reconstruction; Wound Healing/Care; **Hospital:** Danbury Hosp; **Address:** 107 Newtown Rd, Ste 2C, Danbury, CT 06810-4151; **Phone:** 203-791-9661; **Board Cert:** Plastic Surgery 1990; **Med School:** NY Med Coll 1982; **Resid:** Surgery, Montefiore Med Ctr-Einstein Div 1986; **Fellow:** Plastic Surgery, Montefiore Med Ctr-Einstein Div 1988; **Fac Appt:** Prof S, NY Med Coll

Newman, Fredric A MD (PlS) - **Spec Exp:** Rhinoplasty; Breast Augmentation; Eyelid Surgery; Abdominoplasty; **Hospital:** Greenwich Hosp (page 892), Stamford Hosp (page 893); **Address:** 722 Post Rd, Ste 200, Darien, CT 06820; **Phone:** 203-656-9999; **Board Cert:** Plastic Surgery 1985; **Med School:** SUNY Downstate 1974; **Resid:** Surgery, Beth Israel Med Ctr 1977; Surgery, SUNY Downstate 1979; **Fellow:** Plastic/Reconstructive Surgery, NYU Med Ctr 1981; Plastic Surgery, Jackson Meml Hosp 1982; **Fac Appt:** Asst Prof PlS, NY Med Coll

O'Connell, Joseph B MD (PlS) - **Spec Exp:** Liposuction & Body Contouring; Cosmetic Surgery-Face; Cosmetic Surgery-Breast; **Hospital:** Bridgeport Hosp; **Address:** 208 Post Rd W, Westport, CT 06880; **Phone:** 203-454-0044; **Board Cert:** Plastic Surgery 2007; **Med School:** Cornell Univ-Weill Med Coll 1981; **Resid:** Surgery, St Vincents Med Ctr 1986; **Fellow:** Plastic Surgery, New York Hosp 1988

Passaretti, David MD (PlS) - **Spec Exp:** Cosmetic Surgery-Face; Breast Cosmetic & Reconstructive Surgery; Body Contouring after Weight Loss; **Hospital:** Greenwich Hosp (page 892); **Address:** 722 Post Rd, Ste 200, Darien, CT 06820; **Phone:** 203-656-9999; **Board Cert:** Plastic Surgery 2005; **Med School:** Tufts Univ 1997; **Resid:** Plastic Surgery, Univ Hosps 2005; **Fellow:** Plastic Surgery, Mass Genl Hosp 2006

Raskin, Elsa M MD (PlS) - **Spec Exp:** Eyelid Cosmetic & Reconstructive Surgery; Cosmetic Surgery-Face; Cosmetic Surgery-Breast; **Hospital:** Greenwich Hosp (page 892), Lenox Hill Hosp (page 106); **Address:** 2 1/2 Dearfield Drive, Ste 102, Greenwich, CT 06831-5335; **Phone:** 203-861-6620; **Board Cert:** Plastic Surgery 2012; **Med School:** Switzerland 1987; **Resid:** Ophthalmology, NY Eye & Ear Infirm 1995; Surgery, NYU Med Ctr 1999; **Fellow:** Plastic Surgery, Univ Pittsburgh Med Ctr 1996; Plastic/Reconstructive Surgery, NY Presby Hosp 2001

Rosenstock, Arthur MD (PlS) - **Spec Exp:** Cosmetic Surgery-Face; Eyelid Surgery; Cosmetic Surgery-Breast; **Hospital:** Stamford Hosp (page 893); **Address:** 1290 Summer St, Ste 3100, Stamford, CT 06905-5326; **Phone:** 203-359-1959; **Board Cert:** Plastic Surgery 1985; **Med School:** Belgium 1976; **Resid:** Surgery, Westchester Co Med Ctr 1981; **Fellow:** Plastic/Reconstructive Surgery, Med Coll Virginia 1983; **Fac Appt:** Asst Clin Prof S, Columbia P&S

Psychiatry

Hart, Sidney MD (Psyc) - **Spec Exp:** Anxiety Disorders; Mood Disorders; Psychotherapy; **Hospital:** Greenwich Hosp (page 892); **Address:** 282 Railroad Ave Fl 2, Greenwich, CT 06830; **Phone:** 203-622-1722; **Board Cert:** Psychiatry 1973; **Med School:** Albert Einstein Coll Med 1964; **Resid:** Psychiatry, Bronx Municipal Hosp 1971; **Fellow:** Liaison Psychiatry, Montefiore Hosp Med Ctr 1973

Kalman, Arlene Diane MD (Psyc) - **Hospital:** Danbury Hosp; **Address:** 54 Arrowhead Rd, Brookfield, CT 06804-1532; **Phone:** 203-775-6100; **Board Cert:** Psychiatry 1985; **Med School:** SUNY Downstate 1980; **Resid:** Psychiatry, Bronx Muni Hosp Ctr 1983; **Fellow:** Child & Adolescent Psychiatry, Albert Einstein Coll Med Bronx Muni Ctr 1985

Lorefice, Laurence S MD (Psyc) - **Spec Exp:** Depression; Bipolar/Mood Disorders; Obsessive-Compulsive Disorder; Anxiety Disorders; **Address:** 1445 E Putnam Ave, Old Greenwich, CT 06870; **Phone:** 203-637-4006; **Board Cert:** Psychiatry 1979; **Med School:** Univ Pennsylvania 1975; **Resid:** Psychiatry, Mass General Hosp 1979

Morgan, Charles J MD (Psyc) - **Spec Exp:** Alcohol Abuse; Mood Disorders; Substance Abuse; **Hospital:** Bridgeport Hosp; **Address:** 267 Grant St Fl 9, Bridgeport, CT 06610; **Phone:** 203-384-3897; **Board Cert:** Psychiatry 1990; **Med School:** Cornell Univ-Weill Med Coll 1983; **Resid:** Psychiatry, Yale-New Haven Hosp 1987

Mueller, F Carl MD (Psyc) - **Spec Exp:** Anxiety & Depression; Obsessive-Compulsive Disorder; Psychopharmacology; **Hospital:** Stamford Hosp (page 893); **Address:** 999 Summer St, Ste 200, Stamford, CT 06905-5513; **Phone:** 203-357-7773; **Board Cert:** Psychiatry 1987; **Med School:** Univ Conn 1982; **Resid:** Psychiatry, Yale-New Haven Hosp 1985; **Fellow:** Psychiatry, Yale-New Haven Hosp 1986; **Fac Appt:** Asst Clin Prof Psyc, Yale Univ

Schechter, Justin MD (Psyc) - **Spec Exp:** Anxiety Disorders; Mood Disorders; Eating Disorders; Forensic Psychiatry; **Hospital:** Stamford Hosp (page 893); **Address:** 22 Fifth St, Fl 3rd, Stamford, CT 06905-5030; **Phone:** 203-323-7760; **Board Cert:** Psychiatry 1986; Forensic Psychiatry 2008; **Med School:** SUNY Stony Brook 1981; **Resid:** Psychiatry, Yale-New Haven Hosp 1985; **Fac Appt:** Asst Clin Prof Psyc, Yale Univ

Shapiro, Bruce MD (Psyc) - **Spec Exp:** Forensic Psychiatry; Psychopharmacology; Anxiety & Depression; Bipolar/Mood Disorders; **Address:** 666 Glenbrook Rd, River Suite, Stamford, CT 06906; **Phone:** 203-327-4144; **Board Cert:** Psychiatry 1976; **Med School:** NY Med Coll 1972; **Resid:** Psychiatry, Metropolitan Hosp Ctr 1975; **Fac Appt:** Clin Prof Psyc, Columbia P&S

Smith, Joann M MD (Psyc) - **Spec Exp:** Mood Disorders; Anxiety Disorders; Women's Health-Mental Health; **Hospital:** St. Vincent's Med Ctr - Bridgeport; **Address:** 160 Hawley Ln, Ste 001, Trumbull, CT 06611-5300; **Phone:** 203-377-0111; **Board Cert:** Psychiatry 1980; **Med School:** SUNY Hlth Sci Ctr 1974; **Resid:** Psychiatry, Georgetown Univ Hosp 1979

Tamerin, John MD (Psyc) - **Spec Exp:** Psychotherapy; Bipolar/Mood Disorders; Substance Abuse; Alcohol Abuse; **Hospital:** NY-Presby/Weill Cornell Med Ctr, NY (page 104), Greenwich Hosp (page 892); **Address:** 27 Stag Ln, Greenwich, CT 06831-3137; **Phone:** 203-661-8282; **Board Cert:** Psychiatry 1970; **Med School:** NYU Sch Med 1963; **Resid:** Psychiatry, Yale-New Haven Hosp 1965; Psychiatry, Mt Sinai Med Ctr 1967; **Fellow:** Child Psychiatry, Mt Sinai Med Ctr 1967; **Fac Appt:** Assoc Clin Prof Psyc, Cornell Univ-Weill Med Coll

Waynik, Mark MD (Psyc) - **Hospital:** St. Vincent's Med Ctr - Bridgeport; **Address:** 52 Beach Rd, Ste 104, Fairfield, CT 06824; **Phone:** 203-254-2000; **Board Cert:** Psychiatry 1987; **Med School:** Mexico 1979; **Resid:** Psychiatry, Inst Living 1984

Pulmonary Disease

Brown, Robert B MD (Pul) - **Spec Exp:** Critical Care; **Hospital:** St. Vincent's Med Ctr - Bridgeport; **Address:** 2800 Main St, Bridgeport, CT 06606; **Phone:** 203-576-5711; **Board Cert:** Internal Medicine 1981; Pulmonary Disease 1984; Critical Care Medicine 2007; **Med School:** SUNY Downstate 1978; **Resid:** Internal Medicine, Westchester Med Ctr 1981; **Fellow:** Pulmonary Disease, NY Med Coll 1984; **Fac Appt:** Asst Prof Med, NY Med Coll

Chronakos, John MD (Pul) - **Spec Exp:** Sleep Disorders; **Hospital:** Danbury Hosp; **Address:** Western CT Med Grp, 24 Hospital Ave, Danbury, CT 06810; **Phone:** 203-739-7070; **Board Cert:** Internal Medicine 2001; Pulmonary Disease 2003; Critical Care Medicine 2005; **Med School:** NYU Sch Med 1998; **Resid:** Internal Medicine, NYU Langone Med Ctr 2001; **Fellow:** Pulmonary Disease, Mt Sinai Med Ctr 2004

Fine, Jonathan MD (Pul) - **Spec Exp:** Asthma; **Hospital:** Norwalk Hosp; **Address:** Norwalk Hosp, Div of Pulmonology, 34 Maple St Fl 3, Norwalk, CT 06856; **Phone:** 203-852-2392; **Board Cert:** Internal Medicine 1984; Pulmonary Disease 1986; Critical Care Medicine 2011; **Med School:** Yale Univ 1981; **Resid:** Internal Medicine, Yale-New Haven Hosp 1984; **Fellow:** Pulmonary Disease, Yale-New Haven Hosp 1985; Pulmonary Critical Care Medicine, UCSF Med Ctr 1988

Krinsley, James MD (Pul) - **Spec Exp:** Asthma; Emphysema; Critical Care; **Hospital:** Stamford Hosp (page 893); **Address:** Pulmonary Associates, 190 W Broad St, Stamford, CT 06902; **Phone:** 203-348-2437; **Board Cert:** Internal Medicine 1983; Pulmonary Disease 1986; Critical Care Medicine 2009; **Med School:** Cornell Univ-Weill Med Coll 1980; **Resid:** Internal Medicine, NYU/VA Med Ctr 1983; **Fellow:** Pulmonary Disease, Yale-New Haven Hosp 1986; **Fac Appt:** Assoc Clin Prof Med, Columbia P&S

Kurtz, Caroline MD (Pul) - **Spec Exp:** Asthma; Emphysema; **Hospital:** Norwalk Hosp; **Address:** 30 Stevens St, Ste C, Norwalk, CT 06850; **Phone:** 203-855-3888; **Board Cert:** Internal Medicine 1988; Pulmonary Disease 2010; **Med School:** NYU Sch Med 1984; **Resid:** Internal Medicine, Mt Sinai Hosp 1987; **Fellow:** Pulmonary Critical Care Medicine, Mt Sinai Hosp 1990

Marino, A Michael MD (Pul) - **Spec Exp:** Asthma; Bronchitis; Emphysema; Lung Cancer; **Hospital:** Greenwich Hosp (page 892); **Address:** 5 Perryridge Rd, Greenwich, CT 06830; **Phone:** 203-661-5379; **Board Cert:** Internal Medicine 1972; Pulmonary Disease 1972; **Med School:** Georgetown Univ 1964; **Resid:** Internal Medicine, VA Med Ctr 1967; **Fellow:** Pulmonary Disease, VA Med Ctr 1969; **Fac Appt:** Assoc Clin Prof Med, Yale Univ

McCalley, Stuart W MD (Pul) - **Spec Exp:** Sleep Disorders; Chronic Obstructive Lung Disease (COPD); Asthma; Pulmonary Fibrosis; **Hospital:** Greenwich Hosp (page 892); **Address:** 75 Holly Hill Ln, Greenwich Medical Group, Greenwich, CT 06830; **Phone:** 203-869-6960; **Board Cert:** Internal Medicine 1972; Pulmonary Disease 1974; Sleep Medicine 2002; **Med School:** Case West Res Univ 1969; **Resid:** Internal Medicine, Univ Conn Hlth Ctr 1971; Internal Medicine, Univ Vermont Med Ctr 1972; **Fellow:** Pulmonary Disease, Bronx Muni Hosp 1974

Rudolph, Daniel J MD (Pul) - **Hospital:** Bridgeport Hosp; **Address:** 15 Corporate Drive, Trumbull, CT 06611; **Phone:** 203-261-3980; **Board Cert:** Internal Medicine 1985; Pulmonary Disease 1988; **Med School:** NYU Sch Med 1982; **Resid:** Internal Medicine, SUNY Stony Brook Med Ctr 1985; **Fellow:** Pulmonary Disease, Montefiore Med Ctr 1986

Sachs, Paul MD (Pul) - **Spec Exp:** Pulmonary Rehabilitation; Asthma; **Hospital:** Stamford Hosp (page 893); **Address:** 190 W Broad St, Stamford, CT 06902-3633; **Phone:** 203-348-2437; **Board Cert:** Internal Medicine 1985; Pulmonary Disease 1988; Critical Care Medicine 2009; **Med School:** NYU Sch Med 1982; **Resid:** Internal Medicine, NY Hosp 1985; **Fellow:** Pulmonary Disease, Montefiore Med Ctr 1987

Turetsky, Arthur S MD (Pul) - **Hospital:** Bridgeport Hosp; **Address:** 15 Corporate Drive, Lower Level, Trumbull, CT 06611; **Phone:** 203-261-3980; **Board Cert:** Internal Medicine 1977; Pulmonary Disease 1980; Sleep Medicine 2009; **Med School:** Albert Einstein Coll Med 1974; **Resid:** Internal Medicine, Einstein Bronx Muncipal Hosp Ctr 1977; Pulmonary Disease, Bronx Municipal Hosp 1979; **Fac Appt:** Asst Clin Prof Med, Albert Einstein Coll Med

Winter, Stephen M MD (Pul) - **Spec Exp:** Respiratory Failure; Sepsis; Critical Care; Ethics; **Hospital:** Norwalk Hosp; **Address:** Norwalk Hosp, Sect Pulm & Crit Care Med, 34 Maple St Fl 3, Norwalk, CT 06856; **Phone:** 203-852-2392; **Board Cert:** Internal Medicine 1984; Pulmonary Disease 1986; Critical Care Medicine 2007; **Med School:** Cornell Univ-Weill Med Coll 1981; **Resid:** Internal Medicine, NY-Presby/Weill Cornell Med Ctr 1984; **Fellow:** Pulmonary Disease, Yale-New Haven Hosp 1987; **Fac Appt:** Clin Prof Med, Yale Univ

Radiation Oncology

Dowling, Sean MD (RadRO) - **Spec Exp:** Breast Cancer; Gynecologic Cancer; **Hospital:** Stamford Hosp (page 893); **Address:** Dept Radiation Oncology, 34 Shelburne Rd, Stamford, CT 06902; **Phone:** 203-276-7886; **Board Cert:** Internal Medicine 1986; Radiation Oncology 1990; **Med School:** Yale Univ 1983; **Resid:** Internal Medicine, Yale-New Haven Hosp 1986; Radiation Oncology, Yale-New Haven Hosp 1989

Fang, Deborah X MD (RadRO) - **Spec Exp:** Breast Cancer; Gastrointestinal Cancer; **Hospital:** St. Vincent's Med Ctr - Bridgeport; **Address:** 2800 Main St, Bridgeport, CT 06606; **Phone:** 203-576-5085; **Board Cert:** Radiation Oncology 2011; **Med School:** China 1987; **Resid:** Radiation Oncology, Mount Sinai Med Ctr 2001

Masino, Frank A MD (RadRO) - **Spec Exp:** Breast Cancer; Prostate Cancer; Brachytherapy; Stereotactic Radiosurgery; **Hospital:** Stamford Hosp (page 893); **Address:** 34 Shelburne Rd, 32 Strawberry Hill Ct, Stamford, CT 06902-3628; **Phone:** 203-276-7886; **Board Cert:** Therapeutic Radiology 1982; **Med School:** Albert Einstein Coll Med 1978; **Resid:** Therapeutic Radiology, Yale-New Haven Hosp 1982

Pathare, Pradip M MD (RadRO) - **Spec Exp:** Breast Cancer; Prostate Cancer; Head & Neck Cancer; Brain Tumors; **Hospital:** Norwalk Hosp; **Address:** Whittingham Cancer Ctr, 24 Stevens St, Norwalk, CT 06856; **Phone:** 203-852-2719; **Board Cert:** Radiology 1980; Therapeutic Radiology 1981; **Med School:** India 1975; **Resid:** Radiology, Misericordia/Lincoln Hosp 1979; Therapeutic Radiology, Yale-New Haven Hosp 1981; **Fac Appt:** Assoc Prof RadRO, Yale Univ

Spera, John A MD (RadRO) - **Spec Exp:** Breast Cancer; Prostate Cancer; Intensity Modulated Radiotherapy (IMRT); **Hospital:** Danbury Hosp; **Address:** Danbury Hosp, Dept Radiation Oncology, 24 Hospital Ave, Danbury, CT 06810-6099; **Phone:** 203-739-7190; **Board Cert:** Radiation Oncology 1987; **Med School:** Georgetown Univ 1979; **Resid:** Surgery, Hosp Univ Penn 1981; Urology, Hosp Univ Penn 1983; **Fellow:** Radiation Oncology, Hosp Univ Penn 1987

Reproductive Endocrinology

Chacho, Karol J MD (RE) - **Hospital:** Bridgeport Hosp, St. Vincent's Med Ctr - Bridgeport; **Address:** 4699 Main St, Ste 210, Bridgeport, CT 06606-1830; **Phone:** 203-372-5282; **Board Cert:** Obstetrics & Gynecology 2011; Reproductive Endocrinology/Infertility 2011; **Med School:** Loyola Univ-Stritch Sch Med 1978; **Resid:** Obstetrics & Gynecology, Michael Reese Hosp Med Ctr 1982; **Fellow:** Reproductive Endocrinology, Michael Reese Hosp Med Ctr 1984

Doyle, Michael B MD (RE) - **Spec Exp:** Infertility-IVF; Endometriosis; **Hospital:** Norwalk Hosp, St. Vincent's Med Ctr - Bridgeport; **Address:** 4920 Main St, Ste 301, Bridgeport, CT 06606-1300; **Phone:** 203-373-1200; **Board Cert:** Obstetrics & Gynecology 2011; **Med School:** UCSF 1985; **Resid:** Obstetrics & Gynecology, Hosp Univ Penn 1989; **Fellow:** Reproductive Endocrinology, Yale-New Haven Hosp 1991

Ginsburg, Frances W MD (RE) - **Spec Exp:** Infertility-IVF; Menopause Problems; Endometriosis; Menstrual Disorders; **Hospital:** Stamford Hosp (page 893); **Address:** Stamford Hosp, 30 Shelburne Rd, Stamford, CT 06904-9317; **Phone:** 203-276-7559; **Board Cert:** Obstetrics & Gynecology 2011; Reproductive Endocrinology 2011; **Med School:** NYU Sch Med 1980; **Resid:** Obstetrics & Gynecology, NYU Med Ctr 1984; **Fellow:** Reproductive Endocrinology, NYU Med Ctr 1986; **Fac Appt:** Asst Clin Prof ObG, Columbia P&S

Richlin, Spencer S MD (RE) - **Spec Exp:** Infertility-IVF; Reproductive Surgery; Fertility Preservation; **Hospital:** Norwalk Hosp, Stamford Hosp (page 893); **Address:** 10 Glover Ave, MS 06850, Norwalk, CT 06850-1202; **Phone:** 203-750-7400; **Board Cert:** Obstetrics & Gynecology 2010; Reproductive Endocrinology/Infertility 2010; **Med School:** USC-Keck School of Medicine 1994; **Resid:** Obstetrics & Gynecology, Stamford Hosp 1999; **Fellow:** Reproductive Endocrinology, Emory Univ Hosp 2002

Witt, Barry R MD (RE) - **Spec Exp:** Infertility-IVF; **Hospital:** Greenwich Hosp (page 892); **Address:** 55 Holly Hill Ln, Ste 270, Greenwich, CT 06830; **Phone:** 203-863-2990; **Board Cert:** Obstetrics & Gynecology 2011; Reproductive Endocrinology 2011; **Med School:** NY Med Coll 1984; **Resid:** Obstetrics & Gynecology, Montefiore-Weiler Einstein Med Ctr 1988; **Fellow:** Reproductive Endocrinology, Tulane Univ Med Ctr 1990; **Fac Appt:** Assoc Prof ObG, NYU Sch Med

Rheumatology

Danehower, Richard L MD (Rhu) - **Spec Exp:** Rheumatoid Arthritis; Temporal Arteritis; Psoriatic Arthritis; Osteoarthritis; **Hospital:** Greenwich Hosp (page 892); **Address:** 49 Lake Ave, Ste 2, Greenwich, CT 06830-4501; **Phone:** 203-869-5715; **Board Cert:** Internal Medicine 1971; Rheumatology 1974; **Med School:** Univ Pennsylvania 1965; **Resid:** Internal Medicine, Univ Michigan Med Ctr 1969; **Fellow:** Rheumatology, Univ Michigan Med Ctr 1970; **Fac Appt:** Asst Clin Prof Med, Yale Univ

Gladstein, Geoffrey S MD (Rhu) - **Hospital:** Bridgeport Hosp; **Address:** 5520 Park Ave, Ste 101, Trumbull, CT 06611; **Phone:** 203-371-5873; **Board Cert:** Internal Medicine 1976; Rheumatology 1978; **Med School:** Geo Wash Univ 1973; **Resid:** Internal Medicine, Albany Med Ctr 1976; **Fellow:** Rheumatology, Albany Med Ctr 1978

Miller, Kenneth A MD (Rhu) - **Spec Exp:** Rheumatoid Arthritis; Osteoporosis; Vasculitis; Lupus/SLE; **Hospital:** Danbury Hosp, New Milford Hosp; **Address:** 27 Hospital Ave, Ste 205, Danbury, CT 06810-5954; **Phone:** 203-794-0599; **Board Cert:** Internal Medicine 1978; Rheumatology 1980; **Med School:** Rush Med Coll 1975; **Resid:** Internal Medicine, GW Univ Hosp 1978; **Fellow:** Rheumatology, Worcester City Hosp 1980

Nascimento, Joao M A MD (Rhu) - **Spec Exp:** Rheumatoid Arthritis; Lupus/SLE; Psoriatic Arthritis; **Hospital:** St. Vincent's Med Ctr - Bridgeport, Bridgeport Hosp; **Address:** 3203 Main St, Bridgeport, CT 06606-4225; **Phone:** 203-371-0009; **Board Cert:** Internal Medicine 1989; Rheumatology 2002; **Med School:** Portugal 1984; **Resid:** Internal Medicine, Bridgeport Hosp 1989; **Fellow:** Rheumatology, Brown Univ Med Ctr 1991; **Fac Appt:** Asst Clin Prof Med, Columbia P&S

Novack, Stuart N MD (Rhu) - **Spec Exp:** Lupus/SLE; Osteoporosis; Rheumatoid Arthritis; **Hospital:** Norwalk Hosp; **Address:** Norwalk Med Grp, 40 Cross St Fl 4, Norwalk, CT 06851; **Phone:** 203-845-4830; **Board Cert:** Internal Medicine 1971; Rheumatology 1972; **Med School:** SUNY Hlth Sci Ctr 1966; **Resid:** Internal Medicine, Maimonides Med Ctr 1968; Internal Medicine, UCLA Med Ctr 1969; **Fellow:** Rheumatology, UCLA Med Ctr 1970; **Fac Appt:** Assoc Clin Prof Med, Yale Univ

Spiegel, Michael MD (Rhu) - **Spec Exp:** Lupus/SLE; Osteoporosis; Rheumatoid Arthritis; **Hospital:** Danbury Hosp; **Address:** Orthopaedics Assocs, 266 White St, Danbury, CT 06810; **Phone:** 203-702-6630; **Board Cert:** Internal Medicine 1987; Rheumatology 2000; **Med School:** SUNY Downstate 1984; **Resid:** Internal Medicine, St. Francis Hosp 1987; **Fellow:** Rheumatology, Roger Williams Hosp 1987

Surgery

Capasse, Jeanne S MD (S) - **Spec Exp:** Breast Surgery; **Hospital:** Norwalk Hosp; **Address:** Surgical Breast Care of Connecticut, 148 East Ave, Ste 2L, Norwalk, CT 06851; **Phone:** 203-846-8885; **Board Cert:** Surgery 2002; **Med School:** Cornell Univ-Weill Med Coll 1987; **Resid:** Surgery, St Lukes-Roosevelt Hosp Ctr 1992

Choi, Laura Hargie MD (S) - **Hospital:** Danbury Hosp; **Address:** Ctr Weight Loss Surgery, 111 Osborne St Fl 2, Danbury, CT 06810-6000; **Phone:** 203-739-7131; **Board Cert:** Surgery 2004; **Med School:** NYU Sch Med 1998; **Resid:** Surgery, St. Luke's-Roosevelt Hosp Ctr 2003

Dong, Xiang Da MD (S) - **Spec Exp:** Gastrointestinal Cancer; Rectal Cancer; Sarcoma; Melanoma; **Hospital:** Stamford Hosp (page 893); **Address:** Fairfield Co Surgical Specialists, 1351 Washington Blvd Fl 6, Stamford, CT 06902; **Phone:** 203-276-5959; **Board Cert:** Surgery 2005; **Med School:** Duke Univ 1999; **Resid:** Surgery, Drexel Univ Med Ctr 2005; **Fellow:** Surgical Oncology, Univ Pittsburgh Med Ctr 2006

Garvey, Richard J MD (S) - **Spec Exp:** Colon & Rectal Surgery; **Hospital:** Bridgeport Hosp; **Address:** 310 Mill Hill Ave, Genl Surgeons Bridgeport, Bridgeport, CT 06610-2863; **Phone:** 203-366-3211; **Board Cert:** Surgery 2009; **Med School:** Georgetown Univ 1974; **Resid:** Surgery, Boston Univ Med Ctr 1979

Kenler, Andrew S MD (S) - **Hospital:** Bridgeport Hosp; **Address:** Park Avenue Surgical Assocs, 5520 Park Ave, Ste 207, Trumbull, CT 06611; **Phone:** 203-373-9015; **Board Cert:** Surgery 2006; **Med School:** Cornell Univ-Weill Med Coll 1988; **Resid:** Orthopaedic Surgery, NE Deaconess Hosp 1991; Surgery, NE Deaconess Hosp 1995

Lazarus, Laura MD (S) - **Spec Exp:** Breast Surgery; Breast Cancer; **Hospital:** Greenwich Hosp (page 892); **Address:** Breast Care Services of Greenwich, 77 Lafayette Pl, Ste 302, Greenwich, CT 06830; **Phone:** 203-863-4250; **Board Cert:** Surgery 2010; **Med School:** Hahnemann Univ 1996; **Resid:** Surgery, LSU Med Ctr 2001; **Fellow:** Breast Surgery, Northwestern Meml Hosp 2002

Marcus, Stuart G MD (S) - **Spec Exp:** Liver Cancer; Pancreatic Surgery; **Hospital:** St. Vincent's Med Ctr - Bridgeport; **Address:** Cancer Ctr, 2800 Main St, Bridgeport, CT 06606; **Phone:** 203-576-6235; **Board Cert:** Surgery 2005; **Med School:** Duke Univ 1987; **Resid:** Surgery, NYU Med Ctr 1995; **Fellow:** Surgical Oncology, NCI-NIH 1992; **Fac Appt:** Assoc Clin Prof S, NYU Sch Med

McWhorter, Philip MD (S) - **Spec Exp:** Cancer Surgery; Gastrointestinal Surgery; **Hospital:** Greenwich Hosp (page 892); **Address:** 77 Lafayette Pl, Ste 301, Greenwich, CT 06830; **Phone:** 203-863-4300; **Board Cert:** Surgery 1997; **Med School:** Cornell Univ-Weill Med Coll 1973; **Resid:** Surgery, New York Hosp 1977

Miller, Kevin D MD (S) - **Spec Exp:** Hepatobiliary Surgery; Trauma; **Hospital:** Stamford Hosp (page 893); **Address:** 1351 Washington Blvd, Ste 601, Stamford, CT 06902; **Phone:** 203-276-5959; **Board Cert:** Surgery 2010; **Med School:** Columbia P&S 1994; **Resid:** Surgery, Beth Israel Deaconess Hosp 1999

Molinelli, Bruce M MD (S) - **Spec Exp:** Minimally Invasive Surgery; Laparoscopic Surgery; Hernia; Obesity/Bariatric Surgery; **Hospital:** Greenwich Hosp (page 892); **Address:** 77 Lafayette Pl, Ste 301, Greenwich, CT 06831; **Phone:** 203-863-4300; **Board Cert:** Surgery 2004; **Med School:** NYU Sch Med 1988; **Resid:** Surgery, St Lukes-Roosevelt Hosp 1993

Pass, Helen A MD (S) - **Spec Exp:** Breast Cancer; Breast Disease; **Hospital:** Stamford Hosp (page 893); **Address:** Women's Breast Center, Fairfield Co Surgical Specialists, 32 Strawberry Hill Court, Stamford, CT 06902; **Phone:** 203-276-4255; **Board Cert:** Surgery 2003; **Med School:** Univ Mich Med Sch 1987; **Resid:** Surgery, Univ Texas Affil Hosp 1989; Surgery, Georgetown Univ Hosp 1994; **Fellow:** Surgical Oncology, NCI/NIH 1992; **Fac Appt:** Asst Clin Prof S, Columbia P&S

Passeri, Daniel J MD (S) - **Spec Exp:** Cancer Surgery; Laparoscopic Surgery; **Hospital:** St. Vincent's Med Ctr - Bridgeport, Bridgeport Hosp; **Address:** 888 White Plains Rd Fl 2 - Ste 206, Trumbull, CT 06611-4552; **Phone:** 203-459-2666; **Board Cert:** Surgery 2011; **Med School:** Yale Univ 1975; **Resid:** Surgery, Yale-New Haven Hosp 1980; **Fac Appt:** Assoc Clin Prof S, NY Med Coll

Sarnelle, James A MD (S) - **Hospital:** Stamford Hosp (page 893); **Address:** 90 Morgan St, Ste 304, Stamford, CT 06905-5436; **Phone:** 203-353-8088; **Board Cert:** Surgery 2006; **Med School:** NYU Sch Med 1981; **Resid:** Surgery, Stamford Hosp 1985; **Fellow:** Surgery, Lehigh Valley Hosp Ctr 1986

Ward, Barbara A MD (S) - **Spec Exp:** Breast Cancer; Breast Surgery; Breast Disease; **Hospital:** Greenwich Hosp (page 892); **Address:** 77 Lafayette Pl, Ste 302, Greenwich, CT 06830-5426; **Phone:** 203-863-4250; **Board Cert:** Surgery 2002; **Med School:** Temple Univ 1983; **Resid:** Surgery, Yale-New Haven Hosp 1990; **Fellow:** Surgical Oncology, Natl Cancer Inst 1987; **Fac Appt:** Assoc Clin Prof S, Yale Univ

Thoracic & Cardiac Surgery

Coady, Michael A MD (T&CS) - **Spec Exp:** Thoracic Aortic Surgery; Heart Valve Surgery; **Hospital:** Stamford Hosp (page 893); **Address:** 32 Strawberry Hill Ct, Fl 2nd, Heart and Vascular Institute, Stamford, CT 06904; **Phone:** 203-276-4415; **Board Cert:** Surgery 2010; Thoracic & Cardiac Surgery 2004; **Med School:** Geo Wash Univ 1993; **Resid:** Surgery, Yale New Haven Hosp 2000; Cardiothoracic Surgery, Stanford Univ Hosp & Clin 2003; **Fac Appt:** Asst Prof T&CS, Columbia P&S

Lettera, James V MD (T&CS) - **Spec Exp:** Minimally Invasive Thoracic Surgery; Aneurysm-Aortic; Vascular Surgery; **Hospital:** Bridgeport Hosp, Norwalk Hosp; **Address:** CT Vascular & Surgical Assocs, 501 Kings Hwy E, Ste 112, Fairfield, CT 06825; **Phone:** 203-382-1900; **Board Cert:** Thoracic Surgery 2003; **Med School:** Georgetown Univ 1977; **Resid:** Surgery, St Vincent's Hosp Med Ctr 1982; Thoracic Surgery, Jackson Meml Hosp 1984; **Fac Appt:** Asst Clin Prof S, NY Med Coll

Squitieri, Rafael P MD (T&CS) - **Spec Exp:** Cardiothoracic Surgery; Aneurysm-Aortic; Maze Procedure for Atrial Fibrillation; Lung Cancer; **Hospital:** St. Vincent's Med Ctr - Bridgeport; **Address:** Dept Thoracic & Cardiac Surgery, 2800 Main St, Bridgeport, CT 06606; **Phone:** 203-576-5708; **Board Cert:** Thoracic Surgery 2002; **Med School:** Mount Sinai Sch Med 1993; **Resid:** Surgery, Morristown Meml Hosp 1998; **Fellow:** Thoracic Surgery, Mt Sinai Med Ctr 2001

Tittle, Shawn L MD (T&CS) - **Spec Exp:** Thoracic Cancers; Lung Cancer; Minimally Invasive Thoracic Surgery; **Hospital:** Danbury Hosp; **Address:** 10 S St, Ste 202, Richfield, CT 06877; **Phone:** 203-403-3490; **Board Cert:** Thoracic Surgery 2006; **Med School:** Wayne State Univ 1997; **Resid:** Surgery, St Mary's Hosp 2003; **Fellow:** Cardiothoracic Surgery, Yale/New Haven Hosp 2005; **Fac Appt:** Asst Prof S, NY Med Coll

Waters, Paul F MD (T&CS) - **Spec Exp:** Lung Cancer; Esophageal Surgery; Thoracic Cancers; **Hospital:** Greenwich Hosp (page 892); **Address:** 77 Lafayette Pl, Ste 302, Greenwich, CT 06830; **Phone:** 203-863-4341; **Board Cert:** Surgery 2004; **Med School:** Univ Toronto 1974; **Resid:** Surgery, Univ Toronto Med Ctr 1979; Thoracic Surgery, Univ Toronto Med Ctr 1980; **Fellow:** Esophageal Surgery, Univ Chicago Hosps 1981

Urology

Andriani, Rudy MD (U) - **Spec Exp:** Urologic Cancer; Kidney Stones; Incontinence; **Hospital:** Stamford Hosp (page 893); **Address:** 166 W Broad St, Ste 404, Stamford, CT 06902-3661; **Phone:** 203-356-9692; **Board Cert:** Urology 2008; **Med School:** NY Med Coll 1981; **Resid:** Surgery, St Vincent's Hosp & Med Ctr 1983; Urology, Duke Univ Med Ctr 1987; **Fac Appt:** Asst Clin Prof U, Columbia P&S

Dodds, Peter MD (U) - **Hospital:** Norwalk Hosp; **Address:** 12 Elmcrest Terr, Urology Associates Of Norwalk, Norwalk, CT 06850-3964; **Phone:** 203-853-4200; **Board Cert:** Urology 2004; **Med School:** Columbia P&S 1977; **Resid:** Surgery, Yale-New Haven Hosp 1980; Urology, Yale-New Haven Hosp 1983

Hennessy, William T MD (U) - **Hospital:** Danbury Hosp; **Address:** Urology Assocs Danbury, 51-53 Kenosia Ave, Danbury, CT 06810; **Phone:** 203-748-0330; **Board Cert:** Urology 1982; **Med School:** Georgetown Univ 1976; **Resid:** Urology, Hosp Univ Penn - UPHS 1980; **Fellow:** Urologic Oncology, Meml Sloan Kettering Cancer Center 1982

Muldoon, Lawrence D MD (U) - **Hospital:** St. Vincent's Med Ctr - Bridgeport, Bridgeport Hosp; **Address:** Greater Bridgeport Urology, 425 Post Rd Fl 2, Fairfield, CT 06824; **Phone:** 203-254-1576; **Board Cert:** Urology 2012; **Med School:** Northwestern Univ 1984; **Resid:** Surgery, Univ Hosps 1987; Urology, Univ Hosps 1990

Ranta, Jeffrey A MD (U) - **Spec Exp:** Prostate Cancer; Bladder Cancer; Kidney Stones; **Hospital:** Greenwich Hosp (page 892); **Address:** 49 Lake Ave, Greenwich Med Bldg, Ste 201, Greenwich, CT 06830-4520; **Phone:** 203-869-1285; **Board Cert:** Urology 2004; **Med School:** Georgetown Univ 1979; **Resid:** Surgery, Georgetown Univ Hosp 1981; Urology, Lahey Clinic 1984

Shield, Dennis MD (U) - **Spec Exp:** Prostate Cancer; **Hospital:** Norwalk Hosp; **Address:** Urology Assocs of Norwalk, 12 Elmcrest Terr, Ste 1, Norwalk, CT 06850; **Phone:** 203-853-4200; **Board Cert:** Urology 1978; **Med School:** Yale Univ 1970; **Resid:** Surgery, Yale-New Haven Hosp 1972; Urology, Yale-New Haven Hosp 1976

Viner, Nicholas MD (U) - **Spec Exp:** Prostate Cancer; Kidney Stones; Bladder Cancer; **Hospital:** Bridgeport Hosp, St. Vincent's Med Ctr - Bridgeport; **Address:** 160 Hawley Ln, Ste 2, Trumbull, CT 06611-6058; **Phone:** 203-375-3456; **Board Cert:** Urology 1977; **Med School:** Vanderbilt Univ 1968; **Resid:** Surgery, Greenwich Hosp 1970; Urology, Vanderbilt Univ Hosp 1974

Waxberg, Jonathan MD (U) - **Spec Exp:** Prostate Cancer; Erectile Dysfunction; Kidney Stones; Incontinence; **Hospital:** Stamford Hosp (page 893), NY-Presby/Columbia Univ Med Ctr, NY (page 104); **Address:** 35 Hoyt St, Stamford, CT 06905-5602; **Phone:** 203-324-2268; **Board Cert:** Urology 2008; **Med School:** Univ Cincinnati 1980; **Resid:** Urology, Maimonides Med Ctr 1986; **Fac Appt:** Clin Prof U, Univ Cincinnati

Zuckerman, Howard L MD (U) - **Spec Exp:** Incontinence; Prostate Cancer; Pediatric Urology; **Hospital:** Bridgeport Hosp, St. Vincent's Med Ctr - Bridgeport; **Address:** 160 Hawley Ln, Ste 2, Trumbull, CT 06611; **Phone:** 203-375-3456; **Board Cert:** Urology 1977; **Med School:** St Louis Univ 1967; **Resid:** Surgery, Med Coll Virginia Hosp 1969; Urology, Albert Einstein Coll Med 1975

Vascular & Interventional Radiology

Hodges, Laura J MD (VIR) - **Spec Exp:** Uterine Fibroid Embolization; **Hospital:** Greenwich Hosp (page 892); **Address:** Greenwich Hospital, Dept Radiology, 49 Lake Ave, Ste LL2, Greenwich, CT 06830; **Phone:** 203-863-3042; **Board Cert:** Diagnostic Radiology 1999; Vascular & Interventional Radiology 2002; **Med School:** Albert Einstein Coll Med 1994; **Resid:** Diagnostic Radiology, Yale-New Haven Hosp 1999; **Fellow:** Vascular & Interventional Radiology, NY-Presby/Cornell Med Ctr 2000

Strauss, Edward B MD (VIR) - **Hospital:** Norwalk Hosp; **Address:** Norwalk Hosp, Radiology, 34 Maple St, Norwalk, CT 06856-3894; **Phone:** 203-852-2715; **Board Cert:** Diagnostic Radiology 1983; Nuclear Medicine 1984; Vascular & Interventional Radiology 2005; **Med School:** Yale Univ 1979; **Resid:** Diagnostic Radiology, Yale-New Haven Hosp 1983; **Fellow:** Nuclear Medicine, Yale-New Haven Hosp 1984

Vascular Surgery

Dietzek, Alan M MD (VascS) - **Spec Exp:** Aneurysm-Aortic; Minimally Invasive Vascular Surgery; Arterial Bypass Surgery-Leg; Carotid Artery Surgery; **Hospital:** Danbury Hosp; **Address:** 41 Germantown Rd, Ste 101, Danbury, CT 06810; **Phone:** 203-794-5680; **Board Cert:** Vascular Surgery 2009; **Med School:** Loyola Univ-Stritch Sch Med 1983; **Resid:** Surgery, LI Jewish Med Ctr 1988; **Fellow:** Vascular Surgery, Montefiore Med Ctr 1990; **Fac Appt:** Asst Clin Prof S, NY Med Coll

Gagne, Paul J MD (VascS) - **Spec Exp:** Endovascular Surgery; Aneurysm-Abdominal Aortic; Carotid Artery Surgery; Vein Disorders; **Hospital:** Norwalk Hosp, Bridgeport Hosp; **Address:** Southern Connecticut Vascular Ctr, 495 Hawley Ln, Ste 2B, Stratford, CT 06614; **Phone:** 203-375-2861; **Board Cert:** Surgery 2001; Vascular Surgery 2005; **Med School:** NYU Sch Med 1986; **Resid:** Surgery, NYU Med Ctr 1991; **Fellow:** Vascular Surgery, UAMS Med Ctr 1995

Huribal, Marsel MD (VascS) - **Spec Exp:** Endovascular Surgery; Aneurysm-Aortic; Varicose Veins; **Hospital:** Bridgeport Hosp, St. Vincent's Med Ctr - Bridgeport; **Address:** Southern CT Vascular Ctr, 495 Hawley Ln, Ste 2A, Stratford, CT 06614; **Phone:** 203-375-2861; **Board Cert:** Vascular Surgery 2008; **Med School:** Amer Univ Caribbean 1987; **Resid:** Surgery, Bridgeport Hosp 1994; **Fellow:** Vascular Surgery, SUNY Buffalo 1996; **Fac Appt:** Asst Clin Prof VascS, Yale Univ

Marsan, Ben U MD (VascS) - **Spec Exp:** Peripheral Vascular Disease; Vein Disorders; Aneurysm-Aortic; Endovascular Surgery; **Hospital:** Norwalk Hosp, Bridgeport Hosp; **Address:** Southern Connecticut Vascular Ctr, 495 Hawley Ln, Ste 2B, Stratford, CT 06614; **Phone:** 203-375-2861; **Board Cert:** Vascular Surgery 2009; **Med School:** Oregon Hlth & Sci Univ 1989; **Resid:** Surgery, Flushing Hosp Med Ctr 1995; **Fellow:** Vascular Surgery, SUNY Buffalo 1997

New Haven

Yale Medical Group

Administrative Offices

300 George Street, 6th Floor, New Haven, CT 06519
Phone 203-785-6592   Fax 203-785-4327
www.yalemedicalgroup.org

GENERAL OVERVIEW

Yale Medical Group is one of the largest academic multispecialty group practices in the United States, providing compassionate, state-of-the-art care in 160 specialties. It has centers of excellence in such areas as cardiac care, organ transplantation, minimally invasive surgery and cancer, and serves as a major referral center for Connecticut and New England.

ACADEMIC AND CLINICAL AFFILIATIONS

Yale Medical Group consists of more than 850 practicing physicians who are full-time faculty at Yale School of Medicine. These clinicians are also teachers and researchers with access to the most advanced diagnostic and therapeutic approaches, and the latest technology. Yale Medical Group physicians are attending physicians at Yale-New Haven Hospital (YNHH), the primary teaching hospital of the Yale School of Medicine. YNHH is a 1,519-bed teaching hospital that includes the Yale-New Haven Children's Hospital and the Yale-New Haven Psychiatric Hospital. Yale Medical Group physicians also provide world-class cancer care at Smilow Cancer Hospital at Yale-New Haven.

INNOVATIVE PHYSICIANS

Many Yale Medical Group physicians have advanced training from the world's most prominent institutions, and have distinguished reputations as national and international leaders in their fields. Some are on the cutting edge of their fields, and attract patients not only from Connecticut and nationwide, but from outside of the U.S. as well. In some cases they are able to provide patients with options that are difficult to find elsewhere, such as an internationally recognized ocular oncologist and new types of Natural Orifice Translumenal Endoscopic Surgery (NOTES), a minimally invasive approach that doesn't require incisions.

PIONEERING, COMPREHENSIVE CARE

Yale Medical Group physicians are clinical pioneers who have made historic contributions to medicine, such as the first X-ray performed in the United States, the first use of chemotherapy to treat cancer and the first working model of an artificial heart. Others continue to perform groundbreaking procedures, such as Connecticut's first appendectomy without an abdominal incision. They often engage in translational research to offer new therapies, such as the development of man-made vascular grafts that have the ability to grow from the patients' own tissue.

The goal and philosophy of Yale Medical Group specialists is to collaborate to provide each patient with a thoughtful and effective multidisciplinary plan of care.

Physician Referral

For a physician referral or for more information, please contact Yale Medical Group at 1-888-YMG4MDS (964-4637) or visit www.yalemedicalgroup.org.

Allergy & Immunology

Adelsberg, Bernard Roy MD (A&I) - **Spec Exp:** Asthma & Allergy; Allergic Rhinitis; Food Allergy; **Hospital:** Yale-New Haven Hosp - St Raphael Campus, Yale-New Haven Hosp; **Address:** Allergy & Pulmonary Assoc, CT Medical Group, 2416 Whitney Ave Fl 3, Hamden, CT 06518; **Phone:** 203-287-9355; **Board Cert:** Internal Medicine 1975; Allergy & Immunology 1979; Diagnostic Lab Immunology 1986; **Med School:** SUNY Downstate 1972; **Resid:** Internal Medicine, Mt Sinai Hosp 1975; **Fellow:** Immunology, Scripps Clinic And Research 1977

Askenase, Philip MD (A&I) - **Spec Exp:** Asthma; Urticaria; Sinusitis; **Hospital:** Yale-New Haven Hosp, Yale Med Group (page 940); **Address:** Yale Allergy & Immunology, 800 Howard Ave Fl 3, New Haven, CT 06520-8013; **Phone:** 203-785-4143; **Board Cert:** Internal Medicine 1973; Allergy & Immunology 1974; **Med School:** Yale Univ 1965; **Resid:** Internal Medicine, Boston City Hosp 1967; **Fellow:** Allergy & Immunology, Yale/ New Haven Hosp 1971; **Fac Appt:** Prof Med, Yale Univ

Kaufman, Richard E MD (A&I) - **Spec Exp:** Asthma; Urticaria; Allergy; **Hospital:** Yale-New Haven Hosp; **Address:** 960 Main St, Branford, CT 06405; **Phone:** 203-488-6358; **Board Cert:** Internal Medicine 1976; Allergy & Immunology 1979; **Med School:** Yale Univ 1971; **Resid:** Internal Medicine, Yale-New Haven Hosp 1976; **Fellow:** Immunology, Yale-New Haven Hosp 1978; **Fac Appt:** Assoc Clin Prof Med, Yale Univ

Cardiac Electrophysiology

Schoenfeld, Mark MD (CE) - **Spec Exp:** Arrhythmias; **Hospital:** Yale-New Haven Hosp - St Raphael Campus; **Address:** 330 Orchard St, Ste 210, New Haven, CT 06511; **Phone:** 203-867-5400; **Board Cert:** Internal Medicine 1982; Cardiovascular Disease 1985; Cardiac Electrophysiology 2002; **Med School:** Harvard Med Sch 1979; **Resid:** Internal Medicine, Mass Genl Hosp 1982; **Fellow:** Cardiovascular Disease, Mass Genl Hosp 1985; Cardiac Electrophysiology, Mass Genl Hosp 1986; **Fac Appt:** Clin Prof Med, Yale Univ

Cardiovascular Disease

Cabin, Henry S MD (Cv) - **Spec Exp:** Interventional Cardiology; Cardiac Catheterization; **Hospital:** Yale-New Haven Hosp, Yale Med Group (page 940); **Address:** 11 Harrison Ave, Branford, CT 06405; **Phone:** 203-483-8300; **Board Cert:** Internal Medicine 1978; Cardiovascular Disease 1983; **Med School:** Yale Univ 1975; **Resid:** Internal Medicine, Yale-New Haven Hosp 1978; **Fellow:** Internal Medicine, Natl Heart Lung and Blood Inst 1981; Cardiovascular Disease, Yale-New Haven Hosp 1982; **Fac Appt:** Prof Med, Yale Univ

Cleman, Michael W MD (Cv) - **Spec Exp:** Interventional Cardiology; Angioplasty; Cardiac Catheterization; **Hospital:** Yale-New Haven Hosp, Yale Med Group (page 940); **Address:** Yale Cardiology, 11 Harrison Ave, Branford, CT 06405; **Phone:** 203-483-8300; **Board Cert:** Internal Medicine 1980; Cardiovascular Disease 1985; Interventional Cardiology 2011; **Med School:** Johns Hopkins Univ 1977; **Resid:** Internal Medicine, Univ Fla-Shands Hosp 1980; **Fellow:** Cardiovascular Disease, Yale-New Haven Hosp 1981; **Fac Appt:** Prof Med, Yale Univ

Freed, Lisa A MD (Cv) - **Spec Exp:** Heart Disease in Women; Mitral Valve Prolapse; **Hospital:** Yale-New Haven Hosp, Yale-New Haven Hosp - St Raphael Campus; **Address:** Cardiology Assocs of New Haven, 40 Temple St, Ste 6A, New Haven, CT 06510; **Phone:** 203-789-2272; **Board Cert:** Cardiovascular Disease 2009; **Med School:** Johns Hopkins Univ 1992; **Resid:** Internal Medicine, NY Hosp-Cornell Med Ctr 1995; **Fellow:** Cardiovascular Disease, Mass Genl Hosp 1998; Cardiovascular Disease, Framingham Heart Study 1999

Child & Adolescent Psychiatry

Gammon, G Davis MD (ChAP) - **Hospital:** Yale-New Haven Hosp; **Address:** 33 Edgehill Terrace, Hamden, CT 06517; **Phone:** 203-865-6540; **Board Cert:** Psychiatry 1981; Child & Adolescent Psychiatry 1992; **Med School:** Temple Univ 1976; **Resid:** Psychiatry, Yale-New Haven Hosp 1980; Child Psychiatry, Yale-New Haven Hosp 1984; **Fellow:** Epidemiology, Yale Univ 1983

Leckman, James F MD (ChAP) - **Spec Exp:** Tourette's Syndrome; Obsessive-Compulsive Disorder; Autism; **Hospital:** Yale-New Haven Hosp, Yale Med Group (page 940); **Address:** Yale Child Study Ctr, 230 S Frontage Rd, Box 207900, New Haven, CT 06520-7900; **Phone:** 203-785-7971; **Board Cert:** Psychiatry 1980; Child & Adolescent Psychiatry 1982; **Med School:** Univ New Mexico 1973; **Resid:** Psychiatry, Yale Univ 1979; Child Psychiatry, Yale Chld Stdy Ctr 1980; **Fellow:** Psychiatry, Natl Inst Mental Hlth 1976; **Fac Appt:** Prof Psyc, Yale Univ

Madigan, Janet A MD (ChAP) - **Spec Exp:** Developmental Disorders; Psychotherapy; Psychoanalysis; Attachment Disorders; **Hospital:** Yale-New Haven Hosp; **Address:** 291 Whitney Ave, Ste 203, New Haven, CT 06511; **Phone:** 203-787-5420; **Board Cert:** Psychiatry 1982; Child & Adolescent Psychiatry 1986; **Med School:** NY Med Coll 1977; **Resid:** Psychiatry, Yale-New Haven Hosp 1981; **Fellow:** Child & Adolescent Psychiatry, Yale-New Haven Hosp 1983; **Fac Appt:** Asst Clin Prof Psyc, Yale Univ

Child Neurology

Levy, Susan Ruth MD (ChiN) - **Spec Exp:** Epilepsy; Neurophysiology; Pediatric Neurology; Headache; **Hospital:** Yale-New Haven Hosp; **Address:** Child Neurology Assoc, 5 Durham Rd, Ste A-7, Guilford, CT 06437-2076; **Phone:** 203-453-2181; **Board Cert:** Pediatrics 1984; Child Neurology 1986; **Med School:** Wake Forest Univ 1978; **Resid:** Pediatrics, N Carolina Baptist Hosp 1981; Pediatric Neurology, Univ Mass Med Ctr 1984; **Fellow:** Neurological Physiology, Mass Genl Hosp 1985; **Fac Appt:** Clin Prof N, Yale Univ

Ment, Laura R MD (ChiN) - **Spec Exp:** Developmental Disorders; Stroke; **Hospital:** Yale-New Haven Hosp, Yale Med Group (page 940); **Address:** Chldns Hosp Yale New Haven, Dept Pediatrics, Sch Med, 333 Cedar St, Ste LMP3089, New Haven, CT 06520; **Phone:** 203-785-5708; **Board Cert:** Pediatrics 1979; Child Neurology 1980; **Med School:** Tufts Univ 1973; **Resid:** Pediatrics, Massachusetts Genl Hosp 1976; Pediatrics, Massachusetts Genl Hosp 1979; **Fellow:** Pediatrics, Hammersmith Hosp 1979

Shaywitz, Bennett A MD (ChiN) - **Spec Exp:** Learning Disorders; Dyslexia; Headache; **Hospital:** Yale-New Haven Hosp, Yale Med Group (page 940); **Address:** Yale Univ Sch Med, Dept Peds, 333 Cedar St, Box 208064, New Haven, CT 06520-8064; **Phone:** 203-785-4641; **Board Cert:** Pediatrics 1968; Child Neurology 1973; **Med School:** Washington Univ, St Louis 1963; **Resid:** Pediatrics, Bronx Muni Hosp Ctr 1967; **Fellow:** Child Neurology, Albert Einstein Coll Med 1970; **Fac Appt:** Prof Ped, Yale Univ

Testa, Francine M MD (ChiN) - **Spec Exp:** Epilepsy; **Hospital:** Yale-New Haven Hosp, Yale Med Group (page 940); **Address:** 5 Durham Rd, Ste A-7, Guilford, CT 06437; **Phone:** 203-453-2181; **Board Cert:** Child Neurology 1994; **Med School:** SUNY Downstate 1986; **Resid:** Pediatrics, Yale-New Haven Hosp 1988; Child Neurology, NY Presby Hosp/Columbia 1991; **Fellow:** Neurological Physiology, Ny Presby Hosp/Columbia 1992; **Fac Appt:** Clin Prof N, Yale Univ

Clinical Genetics

Bale, Allen E MD (CG) - **Spec Exp:** Cancer Genetics; **Hospital:** Yale-New Haven Hosp, Yale Med Group (page 940); **Address:** 333 Cedar St, SHM Bldg - rm I321, New Haven, CT 06519; **Phone:** 203-785-2660; **Board Cert:** Internal Medicine 1983; Clinical Genetics 1987; Clinical Molecular Genetics 2006; **Med School:** Univ Mass Sch Med 1979; **Resid:** Internal Medicine, Western Penn Hosp 1983; **Fellow:** Medical Genetics, Natl Inst of Health 1987; **Fac Appt:** Assoc Prof CG, Yale Univ

Mahoney, Maurice J MD (CG) - **Spec Exp:** Fetal Therapy; Prenatal Diagnosis; **Hospital:** Yale-New Haven Hosp, Yale Med Group (page 940); **Address:** Yale Genetics Consultation Serv, 333 Cedar St, rm WWW330, New Haven, CT 06520-8005; **Phone:** 203-785-2661; **Board Cert:** Pediatrics 1967; Clinical Genetics 1982; Clinical Biochemical Genetics 1982; **Med School:** Univ Pittsburgh 1962; **Resid:** Pediatrics, Johns Hopkins Hosp 1965; Pediatrics, Childrens Hosp 1966; **Fellow:** Clinical Genetics, Yale Univ Sch Med 1970; **Fac Appt:** Prof CG, Yale Univ

Seashore, Margretta MD (CG) - **Spec Exp:** Inherited Metabolic Disorders; **Hospital:** Yale-New Haven Hosp, Yale Med Group (page 940); **Address:** Yale Univ Sch Med, Dept Genetics, 333 Cedar St, rm 305, Box 208005, New Haven, CT 06520-8005; **Phone:** 203-785-2660; **Board Cert:** Pediatrics 1970; Clinical Biochemical Genetics 1982; Clinical Genetics 1982; **Med School:** Yale Univ 1965; **Resid:** Pediatrics, Yale-New Haven Hosp 1968; **Fellow:** Clinical Genetics, Yale-New Haven Hosp 1970; **Fac Appt:** Prof CG, Yale Univ

Colon & Rectal Surgery

Longo, Walter E MD (CRS) - **Spec Exp:** Colon & Rectal Cancer; Gastrointestinal Surgery; Inflammatory Bowel Disease; **Hospital:** Yale-New Haven Hosp, Yale Med Group (page 940); **Address:** Dept Surgery/Gastroenterology, 330 Cedar St, rm LH118, Box 208062, New Haven, CT 06520-8062; **Phone:** 203-785-2616; **Board Cert:** Surgery 2001; Colon & Rectal Surgery 2006; **Med School:** NY Med Coll 1984; **Resid:** Surgery, Yale-New Haven Hosp 1990; **Fellow:** Research, Yale-New Haven Hosp 1988; Colon & Rectal Surgery, Cleveland Clinic 1991; **Fac Appt:** Prof S, Yale Univ

Dermatology

Antaya, Richard J MD (D) - **Spec Exp:** Pediatric Dermatology; Dermatologic Surgery; Laser Surgery; Vascular Malformations/Birthmarks; **Hospital:** Yale-New Haven Hosp; **Address:** Yale Dermatology Assocs, 2 Church St S, Ste 305, New Haven, CT 06519; **Phone:** 203-789-1249; **Board Cert:** Dermatology 2007; Pediatrics 2007; Pediatric Dermatology 2004; **Med School:** Tufts Univ 1989; **Resid:** Pediatrics, Tripler Army Med Ctr 1992; Dermatology, Duke Univ Med Ctr 1998; **Fac Appt:** Prof D, Yale Univ

Bolognia, Jean L MD (D) - **Spec Exp:** Melanoma; Skin Cancer; **Hospital:** Yale-New Haven Hosp, Yale Med Group (page 940); **Address:** 2 Church St S, Ste 305, New Haven, CT 06519; **Phone:** 203-789-1249; **Board Cert:** Dermatology 2009; **Med School:** Yale Univ 1980; **Resid:** Internal Medicine, Yale-New Haven Hosp 1982; Dermatology, Yale-New Haven Hosp 1985; **Fellow:** Dermatology, Yale-New Haven Hosp 1987; **Fac Appt:** Prof D, Yale Univ

Edelson, Richard L MD (D) - **Spec Exp:** Cutaneous Lymphoma; Immune Deficiency-Skin Disorders; **Hospital:** Yale-New Haven Hosp, Yale Med Group (page 940); **Address:** 2 Church St S, Ste 305, New Haven, CT 06519; **Phone:** 203-789-1249; **Board Cert:** Dermatology 1977; **Med School:** Yale Univ 1970; **Resid:** Dermatology, Mass Genl Hosp 1972; Dermatology, Natl Inst Hlth 1975; **Fac Appt:** Prof D, Yale Univ

Leffell, David J MD (D) - **Spec Exp:** Mohs' Surgery; Melanoma; Skin Cancer; Skin Laser Surgery; **Hospital:** Yale-New Haven Hosp, Yale Med Group (page 940); **Address:** 40 Temple St, Ste 5a, New Haven, CT 06510; **Phone:** 203-785-3466; **Board Cert:** Internal Medicine 1984; Dermatology 2009; **Med School:** McGill Univ 1981; **Resid:** Internal Medicine, New York Hosp 1984; Dermatology, Meml Sloan Kettering Cancer Ctr 1986; **Fellow:** Dermatology, Yale Sch Med 1987; Dermatologic Surgery, Univ Michigan Med Ctr 1988; **Fac Appt:** Prof D, Yale Univ

Savin, Ronald MD (D) - **Spec Exp:** Hair loss; Skin Tumors; Psoriasis; **Hospital:** Yale-New Haven Hosp, Yale-New Haven Hosp - St Raphael Campus; **Address:** 134 Park St Fl 3, New Haven, CT 06511-5416; **Phone:** 203-865-6143; **Board Cert:** Dermatology 1968; **Med School:** Univ Fla Coll Med 1961; **Resid:** Dermatology, Yale-New Haven Hosp 1965; **Fellow:** Dermatology, Yale-New Haven Hosp 1965; **Fac Appt:** Clin Prof D, Yale Univ

Diagnostic Radiology

Hammers, Lynwood DO (DR) - **Spec Exp:** Ultrasound; **Address:** Hammers Healthcare Imaging, 2 Church St S, Ste 110, New Haven, CT 06519; **Phone:** 203-773-8959; **Board Cert:** Diagnostic Radiology 1984; **Med School:** Philadelphia Coll Osteo Med 1979; **Resid:** Diagnostic Radiology, SUNY Downstate Med Ctr 1983; **Fellow:** Ultrasound, Yale-New Haven Hosp 1985

McCarthy, Shirley M MD/PhD (DR) - **Spec Exp:** Gynecologic Cancer; Pelvic Imaging; **Hospital:** Yale-New Haven Hosp, Yale Med Group (page 940); **Address:** Yale-New Haven Hosp, 333 Cedar St, Ste TE2, PO Box 208042, New Haven, CT 06520-3206; **Phone:** 203-785-2384; **Board Cert:** Diagnostic Radiology 1983; **Med School:** Yale Univ 1979; **Resid:** Diagnostic Radiology, Yale-New Haven Hosp 1983; **Fellow:** Cross Sectional Imaging, UCSF Med Ctr 1984; **Fac Appt:** Prof Rad, Yale Univ

McClennan, Bruce MD (DR) - **Spec Exp:** Genitourinary Imaging; Abdominal Imaging; **Hospital:** Yale-New Haven Hosp, Yale Med Group (page 940); **Address:** YNHH, Dept Radiology, 20 York St, South Pavilion 2, New Haven, CT 06520-8042; **Phone:** 203-785-2384; **Board Cert:** Diagnostic Radiology 1972; **Med School:** SUNY Upstate Med Univ 1967; **Resid:** Diagnostic Radiology, Mary Imogene Bassett Hosp 1968; **Fellow:** Diagnostic Radiology, Columbia-Presby Med Ctr 1971; **Fac Appt:** Prof Rad, Yale Univ

Weinreb, Jeffrey C MD (DR) - **Spec Exp:** MRI; Breast Cancer; Abdominal Imaging; CT Body Scan; **Hospital:** Yale-New Haven Hosp, Yale Med Group (page 940); **Address:** Yale Univ Sch Medicine, Dept Radiology, 333 Cedar St, rm MRC165, Box 208042, New Haven, CT 06520-8042; **Phone:** 203-785-5913; **Board Cert:** Diagnostic Radiology 1983; **Med School:** Mount Sinai Sch Med 1978; **Resid:** Diagnostic Radiology, LI Jewish Med Ctr 1982; **Fellow:** Ultrasound/CT, Hosp Univ Penn 1983; **Fac Appt:** Prof Rad, Yale Univ

Endocrinology, Diabetes & Metabolism

Inzucchi, Silvio E MD (EDM) - **Spec Exp:** Diabetes; Pituitary Disorders; Growth Hormone Disorder-Adult; Cholesterol/Lipid Disorders; **Hospital:** Yale-New Haven Hosp, Yale Med Group (page 940); **Address:** Yale Diabetes Center, 789 Howard Ave, Dana Clinic Bldg fl 2, New Haven, CT 06520; **Phone:** 203-737-1932; **Board Cert:** Internal Medicine 1988; Endocrinology, Diabetes & Metabolism 2006; **Med School:** Harvard Med Sch 1985; **Resid:** Internal Medicine, Yale-New Haven Hosp 1988; **Fellow:** Endocrinology, Diabetes & Metabolism, Yale-New Haven Hosp 1994; **Fac Appt:** Prof Med, Yale Univ

Wysolmerski, John J MD (EDM) - **Spec Exp:** Bone Disorders-Metabolic; Osteoporosis; Parathyroid Disorders; **Hospital:** Yale-New Haven Hosp, Yale Med Group (page 940); **Address:** Yale Sch Med-Div Endocrinology, Bone Ctr, 789 Howard Ave Fl 2, New Haven, CT 06520-8020; **Phone:** 203-737-1058; **Board Cert:** Internal Medicine 1989; **Med School:** Yale Univ 1986; **Resid:** Internal Medicine, New England Med Ctr 1989; **Fellow:** Endocrinology, Yale Univ Sch Med 1993; **Fac Appt:** Assoc Prof Med, Yale Univ

Gastroenterology

Aslanian, Harry R MD (Ge) - **Spec Exp:** Endoscopic Ultrasound; Esophageal Cancer; Pancreatic Cancer; Rectal Cancer; **Hospital:** Yale-New Haven Hosp; **Address:** 333 Cedar St, Fl 1080 Imp, Box 208019, Department of Internal Medicine, New Haven, CT 06520-8019; **Phone:** 203-200-5083; **Board Cert:** Gastroenterology 2002; **Med School:** Brown Univ 1996; **Resid:** Internal Medicine, Mayo Clin 1999; **Fellow:** Gastroenterology, Yale Univ Affil Hosp 2002; Endoscopy, Yale Univ Affil Hosp 2003; **Fac Appt:** Assoc Prof Med, Yale Univ

Dobbins, John Whitby MD (Ge) - **Spec Exp:** Pancreatic & Biliary Disease; Inflammatory Bowel Disease; **Hospital:** Yale-New Haven Hosp, Yale-New Haven Hosp - St Raphael Campus; **Address:** Connecticut Gastroenterlogy Consultants PC, 40 Temple St, Ste 4A, New Haven, CT 06510; **Phone:** 203-777-0304; **Board Cert:** Internal Medicine 1973; Gastroenterology 2005; **Med School:** Univ Wash 1968; **Resid:** Internal Medicine, George Washington Univ Hosp 1973; **Fellow:** Gastroenterology, Yale/ New Haven Hosp 1976; **Fac Appt:** Prof Med, Yale Univ

Fisher, Rosemarie Louise MD (Ge) - **Spec Exp:** Nutrition; Nutrition in Bowel Disorders; Inflammatory Bowel Disease/Crohn's; Endoscopy; **Hospital:** Yale-New Haven Hosp, St. Mary's Hosp - Waterbury; **Address:** 20 York St, Tompkins Bldg Fl 236, New Haven, CT 06510; **Phone:** 203-688-1449; **Board Cert:** Internal Medicine 1975; Gastroenterology 1977; **Med School:** Tufts Univ 1971; **Resid:** Internal Medicine, Montefiore Med Ctr 1973; **Fellow:** Gastroenterology, Yale-New Haven Hosp 1975; **Fac Appt:** Prof Med, Yale Univ

Jamidar, Priya A MD (Ge) - **Spec Exp:** Gallbladder Disease; Pancreatic Disease; Gastrointestinal Cancer; Pancreatic/Biliary Endoscopy (ERCP); **Hospital:** Yale-New Haven Hosp, Yale Med Group (page 940); **Address:** 20 York Ave Fl 4, New Haven, CT 06510; **Phone:** 203-200-5083; **Board Cert:** Internal Medicine 1988; Gastroenterology 2002; **Med School:** Ireland 1984; **Resid:** Internal Medicine, Univ Conn Hlth Ctr 1988; **Fellow:** Gastroenterology, USC/LAC Med Ctr 1990; Gastroenterology, Indiana Univ Med Ctr 1992; **Fac Appt:** Assoc Prof Med, Yale Univ

Proctor, Deborah D MD (Ge) - **Spec Exp:** Inflammatory Bowel Disease; Colon Cancer Screening; Endoscopy; **Hospital:** Yale-New Haven Hosp, Yale Med Group (page 940); **Address:** 40 Temple St, Ste 1A, New Haven, CT 06519; **Phone:** 203-785-4138; **Board Cert:** Gastroenterology 2003; **Med School:** Univ Cincinnati 1982; **Resid:** Internal Medicine, Beth Israel Hosp 1990; **Fellow:** Gastroenterology, Beth Israel Hosp 1992; **Fac Appt:** Prof Med, Yale Univ

Geriatric Medicine

Cooney Jr, Leo M MD (Ger) - **Spec Exp:** Geriatric Functional Assessment; Rheumatology; Mobility Evaluation & Treatment; **Hospital:** Yale-New Haven Hosp, Yale Med Group (page 940); **Address:** Yale-New Haven Hosp, Adler Geriatric Ctr, 20 York St, New Haven, CT 06510; **Phone:** 203-688-2204; **Board Cert:** Internal Medicine 1974; Rheumatology 1978; **Med School:** Yale Univ 1969; **Resid:** Internal Medicine, Boston City Hosp 1971; Internal Medicine, Boston City Hosp 1974; **Fellow:** Rheumatology, Boston Med Ctr 1975; **Fac Appt:** Prof Med, Yale Univ

Gill, Thomas M MD (Ger) - **Spec Exp:** Geriatric Functional Assessment; **Hospital:** Yale-New Haven Hosp, Yale Med Group (page 940); **Address:** Yale New Haven Hosp, 20 York St, New Haven, CT 06510; **Phone:** 203-688-6361; **Board Cert:** Geriatric Medicine 2000; **Med School:** Univ Chicago-Pritzker Sch Med 1987; **Resid:** Internal Medicine, Univ Wash 1990; **Fellow:** Internal Medicine, Yale-New Haven Hosp 1993; Geriatric Medicine, Yale-New Haven Hosp 1994; **Fac Appt:** Assoc Prof Med, Yale Univ

Tinetti, Mary E MD (Ger) - **Spec Exp:** Falls in the Elderly; Geriatric Functional Assessment; **Hospital:** Yale-New Haven Hosp, Yale Med Group (page 940); **Address:** Yale-New Haven Hosp, Adler Geriatric Ctr, 20 York St, New Haven, CT 06510; **Phone:** 203-688-6361; **Board Cert:** Internal Medicine 1981; **Med School:** Univ Mich Med Sch 1978; **Resid:** Internal Medicine, Univ Minnesota 1981; **Fellow:** Geriatric Medicine, Univ Rochester 1984; **Fac Appt:** Prof Med, Yale Univ

Geriatric Psychiatry

van Dyck, Christopher H MD (GerPsy) - **Spec Exp:** Alzheimer's Disease; **Hospital:** Yale-New Haven Hosp, Yale Med Group (page 940); **Address:** Yake New Haven Hosp, 874 Howard Ave, New Haven, CT 06510; **Phone:** 203-688-6361; **Board Cert:** Psychiatry 1991; Geriatric Psychiatry 2005; **Med School:** Northwestern Univ 1984; **Resid:** Psychiatry, Yale-New Haven Hosp 1988; **Fellow:** Geriatric Psychiatry, Yale-New Haven Hosp 1990; **Fac Appt:** Assoc Prof Psyc, Yale Univ

Gynecologic Oncology

Azodi, Masoud MD (GO) - **Spec Exp:** Laparoscopic Surgery; Ovarian Cancer-Early Detection; Uterine Cancer; **Hospital:** Yale-New Haven Hosp, Yale Med Group (page 940); **Address:** Smilow Cancer Hosp, 25 Park St, Ste B, New Haven, CT 06519; **Phone:** 203-785-4013; **Board Cert:** Gynecologic Oncology 2009; Obstetrics & Gynecology 2009; **Med School:** Wright State Univ 1992; **Resid:** Obstetrics & Gynecology, Aultman Hospital 1996; **Fellow:** Obstetrics & Gynecology, Yale-New Haven Hosp 1999; **Fac Appt:** Assoc Prof ObG, Yale Univ

Rutherford, Thomas J MD (GO) - **Spec Exp:** Ovarian Cancer; Uterine Cancer; Ovarian Cancer-Early Detection; Cervical Cancer; **Hospital:** Yale-New Haven Hosp, Yale Med Group (page 940); **Address:** Smilow Cancer Hosp, 25 Park St Fl 1, New Haven, CT 06519; **Phone:** 203-200-4176; **Board Cert:** Obstetrics & Gynecology 2011; Gynecologic Oncology 2011; **Med School:** Med Coll OH 1989; **Resid:** Obstetrics & Gynecology, Cooper Hosp 1993; **Fellow:** Gynecologic Oncology, Yale-New Haven Hosp 1995; **Fac Appt:** Assoc Prof ObG, Yale Univ

Santin, Alessandro MD (GO) - **Spec Exp:** Immunotherapy; Ovarian Cancer; Vulvar & Vaginal Cancer; **Hospital:** Yale-New Haven Hosp, Yale Med Group (page 940); **Address:** Yale Gynecologic Oncology, 333 Cedar St, PO Box 208063, New Haven, CT 06510; **Phone:** 203-200-4176; **Med School:** Italy 1989; **Resid:** Obstetrics & Gynecology, Univ Brescia Sch Med 1993; **Fellow:** Gynecologic Oncology, UC Irvine 1995; Gynecologic Oncology, UAMS Med Ctr 2000; **Fac Appt:** Prof ObG, Yale Univ

Schwartz, Peter E MD (GO) - **Spec Exp:** Ovarian Cancer; Uterine Cancer; Gynecologic Surgery-Complex; Cervical Cancer; **Hospital:** Yale-New Haven Hosp, Yale Med Group (page 940); **Address:** 20 York St, New Haven, CT 06510-3289; **Phone:** 203-785-4014; **Board Cert:** Obstetrics & Gynecology 1973; Gynecologic Oncology 1979; **Med School:** Albert Einstein Coll Med 1966; **Resid:** Obstetrics & Gynecology, Yale-New Haven Hosp 1970; **Fellow:** Gynecologic Oncology, MD Anderson Cancer Ctr 1975; **Fac Appt:** Prof ObG, Yale Univ

Hand Surgery

Thomson, J Grant MD (HS) - **Spec Exp:** Carpal Tunnel Syndrome; Hand Reconstruction; Microsurgery; Arthritis; **Hospital:** Yale-New Haven Hosp, Yale Med Group (page 940); **Address:** Yale Plastic Surgery, 800 Howard Ave Fl 4, New Haven, CT 06519; **Phone:** 203-737-5130; **Board Cert:** Hand Surgery 2004; Plastic Surgery 2004; **Med School:** McGill Univ 1983; **Resid:** Surgery, Montreal Genl Hosp 1988; Plastic Surgery, Montreal Genl Hosp 1990; **Fellow:** Hand Surgery, Barnes Jewish Hosp 1991; **Fac Appt:** Assoc Prof PlS, Yale Univ

Hematology

Duffy, Thomas P MD (Hem) - **Spec Exp:** Mast Cell Diseases; Leukemia; Lymphoma; Mast Cell Diseases; **Hospital:** Yale-New Haven Hosp, Yale Med Group (page 940); **Address:** Yale Univ, Sect Hematology, 35 Park St Fl 7, New Haven, CT 06520-8021; **Phone:** 203-785-4744; **Board Cert:** Internal Medicine 1972; Hematology 1974; **Med School:** Johns Hopkins Univ 1962; **Resid:** Internal Medicine, Johns Hopkins Hosp 1965; **Fellow:** Hematology, Johns Hopkins Hosp 1970; **Fac Appt:** Prof Med, Yale Univ

Marks, Peter W MD/PhD (Hem) - **Spec Exp:** Leukemia; Platelet Disorders; Bleeding/Coagulation Disorders; Hemophilia; **Hospital:** Yale-New Haven Hosp, Yale Med Group (page 940); **Address:** Yale Hematology, 333 Cedar St, Box 208302, New Haven, CT 06520; **Phone:** 203-200-4363; **Board Cert:** Internal Medicine 2004; Hematology 2007; Medical Oncology 2007; **Med School:** NYU Sch Med 1991; **Resid:** Internal Medicine, Brigham & Women's Hosp 1994; **Fellow:** Hematology & Oncology, Brigham & Women's Hosp 1996; **Fac Appt:** Assoc Prof Med, Yale Univ

Sabbath, Kert David MD (Hem) - **Hospital:** St. Mary's Hosp - Waterbury, Waterbury Hosp; **Address:** 1075 Chase Pkwy, Ste B, Waterbury, CT 06708-2948; **Phone:** 203-755-6311; **Board Cert:** Internal Medicine 1982; Medical Oncology 1985; Hematology 1986; **Med School:** Boston Univ 1979; **Resid:** Internal Medicine, Boston Med Ctr 1982; **Fellow:** Hematology, Mass Genl Hosp 1985

Infectious Disease

Quagliarello, Vincent MD (Inf) - **Spec Exp:** Meningitis; Pneumonia; Endocarditis; **Hospital:** Yale-New Haven Hosp, Yale Med Group (page 940); **Address:** Yale Univ Sch Med, TAC S169A, 300 Cedar St, New Haven, CT 06520-8022; **Phone:** 203-785-4140; **Board Cert:** Internal Medicine 1984; Infectious Disease 1988; **Med School:** Washington Univ, St Louis 1980; **Resid:** Internal Medicine, Yale-New Haven Hosp 1984; **Fellow:** Infectious Disease, Univ VA Hlth Sci Ctr 1987; **Fac Appt:** Prof Med, Yale Univ

Internal Medicine

Eilbott, David J MD (IM) *PCP* - **Hospital:** Yale-New Haven Hosp, Yale-New Haven Hosp - St Raphael Campus; **Address:** 500 E Main St, Ste 212, Branford, CT 06405; **Phone:** 203-481-5665; **Board Cert:** Internal Medicine 1986; **Med School:** Univ Rochester 1981; **Resid:** Internal Medicine, Waterbury Hosp 1985; **Fellow:** Infectious Disease, SUNY Stony Brook 1988; **Fac Appt:** Asst Clin Prof Med, Yale Univ

Ellman, Matthew S MD (IM) *PCP* - **Spec Exp:** Preventive Medicine; **Hospital:** Yale-New Haven Hosp, Yale Med Group (page 940); **Address:** Yale Int Med Assocs, 800 Howard Ave Fl 2, New Haven, CT 06510; **Phone:** 203-785-7411; **Board Cert:** Internal Medicine 2011; **Med School:** Harvard Med Sch 1987; **Resid:** Internal Medicine, Bellevue Hosp-NYU 1990; **Fellow:** Epidemiology, Yale-New Haven Hosp 1993; **Fac Appt:** Asst Prof Med, Yale Univ

Kernan Jr, Walter N MD (IM) *PCP* - **Spec Exp:** Stroke; Hypertension; **Hospital:** Yale-New Haven Hosp, Yale Med Group (page 940); **Address:** 20 York St, New Haven, CT 06520-1744; **Phone:** 203-688-2984; **Board Cert:** Internal Medicine 1987; **Med School:** Dartmouth Med Sch 1984; **Resid:** Internal Medicine, Johns Hopkins Hosp 1987; **Fellow:** Internal Medicine, Yale New Haven Hosp 1989; **Fac Appt:** Prof Med, Yale Univ

O'Connor, Patrick G MD (IM) *PCP* - **Spec Exp:** Addiction/Substance Abuse; **Hospital:** Yale-New Haven Hosp, Yale Med Group (page 940); **Address:** Yale Univ School Medicine, PO Box 208093, 333 Cedar Street, New Haven, CT 06520-8093; **Phone:** 203-688-6532; **Board Cert:** Internal Medicine 1986; Addiction Medicine 2009; **Med School:** Albany Med Coll 1982; **Resid:** Internal Medicine, Univ Rochester Med Ctr 1985; Internal Medicine, Univ Rochester Med Ctr 1986; **Fellow:** Internal Medicine, Yale-New Haven Hosp 1988; **Fac Appt:** Prof Med, Yale Univ

Street, Lynn MD (IM) *PCP* - **Hospital:** Yale-New Haven Hosp; **Address:** University Towers, 100 York St, Ste 2E, New Haven, CT 06511; **Phone:** 203-787-3588; **Med School:** Yale Univ 1987; **Resid:** Internal Medicine, NYU-Bellvue Hosp 1990; **Fellow:** Epidemiology, RWJ Johnson Med Ctr 1992; Geriatric Medicine, Yale-New Haven Hosp 2000

Maternal & Fetal Medicine

Copel, Joshua A MD (MF) - **Spec Exp:** Prenatal Diagnosis; Fetal Echocardiography; Pregnancy-High Risk; Fetal Diagnosis & Therapy; **Hospital:** Yale-New Haven Hosp, Yale Med Group (page 940); **Address:** Yale Maternal/Fetal Medicine, 150 Sargent Drive, New Haven, CT 06511; **Phone:** 203-785-5682; **Board Cert:** Obstetrics & Gynecology 2011; Maternal & Fetal Medicine 2011; **Med School:** Tufts Univ 1979; **Resid:** Obstetrics & Gynecology, Pennsylvania Hosp 1983; **Fellow:** Maternal & Fetal Medicine, Yale-New Haven Hosp 1985; **Fac Appt:** Prof ObG, Yale Univ

Magriples, Urania MD (MF) - **Spec Exp:** Pregnancy-High Risk; **Hospital:** Yale-New Haven Hosp, Yale Med Group (page 940); **Address:** YNHH, Dept Maternal-Fetal Med, 150 Sargent Drive Fl 2, New Haven, CT 06520-8063; **Phone:** 203-785-5682; **Board Cert:** Obstetrics & Gynecology 2011; Maternal & Fetal Medicine 2011; **Med School:** Mount Sinai Sch Med 1987; **Resid:** Obstetrics & Gynecology, Yale-New Haven Hosp 1991; **Fellow:** Perinatal Medicine, Yale-New Haven Hosp 1994; **Fac Appt:** Assoc Prof ObG, Yale Univ

Paidas, Michael J MD (MF) - **Spec Exp:** Pregnancy-High Risk; Clotting Disorders in Pregnancy; Miscarriage-Recurrent; **Hospital:** Yale-New Haven Hosp, Yale Med Group (page 940); **Address:** Yale Maternal/Fetal Medicine, 150 Sargent Drive, New Haven, CT 06511; **Phone:** 203-785-5682; **Board Cert:** Obstetrics & Gynecology 2011; Maternal & Fetal Medicine 2011; **Med School:** Tufts Univ 1987; **Resid:** Obstetrics & Gynecology, Pennsylvania Hosp 1991; **Fellow:** Maternal & Fetal Medicine, Mount Sinai Med Ctr 1993; **Fac Appt:** Assoc Prof ObG, Yale Univ

Medical Oncology

Cooper, Dennis L MD (Onc) - **Spec Exp:** Lymphoma; Stem Cell Transplant; Leukemia; **Hospital:** Yale-New Haven Hosp, Yale Med Group (page 940); **Address:** Yale Univ Sch Med, 333 Cedar St, FMP-122, Box 208032, New Haven, CT 06520-8032; **Phone:** 203-737-5751; **Board Cert:** Internal Medicine 1983; Medical Oncology 1985; **Med School:** Rush Med Coll 1979; **Resid:** Internal Medicine, Yale-New Haven Hosp 1982; Internal Medicine, Presby-Univ Hosp 1983; **Fellow:** Medical Oncology, Yale-New Haven Hosp 1985; **Fac Appt:** Prof Med, Yale Univ

DeVita Jr, Vincent T MD (Onc) - **Spec Exp:** Lymphoma Consultation; Hodgkin's Disease Consultation; **Hospital:** Yale-New Haven Hosp, Yale Med Group (page 940); **Address:** Yale Cancer Ctr, 333 Cedar St, rm FMP117, New Haven, CT 06520-8028; **Phone:** 203-737-1010; **Board Cert:** Internal Medicine 1974; Hematology 1972; Medical Oncology 1973; **Med School:** Geo Wash Univ 1961; **Resid:** Internal Medicine, Geo Wash Hosp 1963; Internal Medicine, Yale-New Haven Hosp 1966; **Fellow:** Medical Oncology, Natl Cancer Inst 1965; **Fac Appt:** Prof Med, Yale Univ

Foss, Francine M MD (Onc) - **Spec Exp:** Lymphoma, Cutaneous T Cell (CTCL); Stem Cell Transplant; Graft vs Host Disease; Multiple Myeloma; **Hospital:** Yale-New Haven Hosp, Yale Med Group (page 940); **Address:** 35 Park St Fl 7, New Haven, CT 06520-8032; **Phone:** 203-200-4363; **Board Cert:** Internal Medicine 1985; Medical Oncology 1987; **Med School:** Univ Mass Sch Med 1982; **Resid:** Internal Medicine, Brigham & Womens Hosp 1985; **Fellow:** Medical Oncology, Natl Cancer Inst 1988; **Fac Appt:** Prof Med, Yale Univ

Herbst, Roy S MD/PhD (Onc) - **Spec Exp:** Lung Cancer; Thoracic Cancers; Drug Development; Clinical Trials; **Hospital:** Yale-New Haven Hosp; **Address:** Smilow Cancer Hosp, Thoracic Cancer Div, 20 York St Fl 4, New Haven, CT 06504; **Phone:** 203-200-5864; **Board Cert:** Medical Oncology 2007; **Med School:** Cornell Univ-Weill Med Coll 1991; **Resid:** Internal Medicine, Brigham & Women's Hosp 1994; **Fellow:** Medical Oncology, Dana Farber Cancer Inst 1996; **Fac Appt:** Assoc Prof Med, Univ Tex, Houston

Hochster, Howard S MD (Onc) - **Spec Exp:** Gastrointestinal Cancer; Gynecologic Cancer; Colon & Rectal Cancer; **Hospital:** Yale-New Haven Hosp, Yale Med Group (page 940); **Address:** Smilow Cancer Center, 333 Cedar St, Box 208028, New Haven, CT 06520-8028; **Phone:** 203-785-4191; **Board Cert:** Internal Medicine 1983; Medical Oncology 1985; Hematology 1986; **Med School:** Yale Univ 1980; **Resid:** Internal Medicine, NYU Med Ctr 1983; **Fellow:** Hematology & Oncology, NYU Med Ctr 1985; Medical Oncology, Jules Bordet Inst 1986; **Fac Appt:** Prof Med, Yale Univ

Lacy, Jill MD (Onc) - **Spec Exp:** Colon & Rectal Cancer; Gastrointestinal Cancer; Brain Tumors; Pancreatic Cancer; **Hospital:** Yale-New Haven Hosp, Yale Med Group (page 940); **Address:** Yale Univ Sch Med-Div Medical Oncology, 333 Cedar St, PO Box 208032, New Haven, CT 06520-8032; **Phone:** 203-785-4191; **Board Cert:** Internal Medicine 1982; Medical Oncology 2005; **Med School:** Yale Univ 1978; **Resid:** Internal Medicine, Yale-New Haven Hosp 1981; **Fellow:** Medical Oncology, Yale-New Haven Hosp 1985; **Fac Appt:** Assoc Prof Onc, Yale Univ

Lundberg, Walter B MD (Onc) - **Spec Exp:** Lymphoma; Colon Cancer; Lung Cancer; **Hospital:** Yale-New Haven Hosp - St Raphael Campus, Yale-New Haven Hosp; **Address:** 1450 Chapel St, Ste A, McGivney Center for Cancer Care, New Haven, CT 06511; **Phone:** 203-867-5420; **Board Cert:** Internal Medicine 1973; Hematology 1974; Blood Banking 1974; Medical Oncology 1975; **Med School:** Columbia P&S 1970; **Resid:** Internal Medicine, Columbia Presby Hosp 1972; Medical Oncology, Yale-New Haven Hosp 1976; **Fellow:** Internal Medicine, Harvard Med Sch 1971; Hematology, NIH 1974; **Fac Appt:** Assoc Clin Prof Med, Yale Univ

Lynch Jr, Thomas J MD (Onc) - **Spec Exp:** Lung Cancer; Thoracic Cancers; **Hospital:** Yale-New Haven Hosp, Yale Med Group (page 940); **Address:** 35 Park St Fl 4, New Haven, CT 06510; **Phone:** 203-688-5864; **Board Cert:** Internal Medicine 1989; Medical Oncology 2003; **Med School:** Yale Univ 1986; **Resid:** Internal Medicine, Mass Genl Hosp 1989; **Fellow:** Medical Oncology, Dana-Farber Cancer Inst 1991; **Fac Appt:** Assoc Prof Med, Yale Univ

Petrylak, Daniel P MD (Onc) - **Spec Exp:** Testicular Cancer; Prostate Cancer; Bladder Cancer; Kidney Cancer; **Hospital:** Yale-New Haven Hosp, Greenwich Hosp (page 892); **Address:** 333 Cedar St, New Haven, CT 06520; **Phone:** 203-200-4822; **Board Cert:** Internal Medicine 2001; Medical Oncology 2003; **Med School:** Case West Res Univ 1985; **Resid:** Internal Medicine, Jacobi Med Ctr 1988; **Fellow:** Oncology, Meml-Sloan Kettering Cancer Ctr 1991; **Fac Appt:** Prof Onc, Yale Univ

Neonatal-Perinatal Medicine

Ehrenkranz, Richard A MD (NP) - **Spec Exp:** Nutrition; Lung Disease in Newborns; **Hospital:** Yale-New Haven Hosp, Yale Med Group (page 940); **Address:** Yale Univ-Dept Ped, 333 Cedar Street, PO Box 208064, New Haven, CT 06520-8064; **Phone:** 203-688-2320; **Board Cert:** Pediatrics 1977; Neonatal-Perinatal Medicine 1979; **Med School:** SUNY Downstate 1972; **Resid:** Pediatrics, Yale-New Haven Hosp 1974; **Fellow:** Neonatal-Perinatal Medicine, Yale-New Haven Hosp 1978; **Fac Appt:** Prof Ped, Yale Univ

Gross, Ian MD (NP) - **Spec Exp:** Breathing Disorders; Critical Care; **Hospital:** Yale-New Haven Hosp, Yale Med Group (page 940); **Address:** Yale Sch Med, Dept Pediatrics, 333 Cedar St, PO Box 208064, New Haven, CT 06520-8064; **Phone:** 203-688-2320; **Board Cert:** Pediatrics 1974; Neonatal-Perinatal Medicine 1977; **Med School:** South Africa 1967; **Resid:** Pediatrics, Univ Witwatersrand Affil Hosps 1971; Pediatrics, Chldns Hosp Med Ctr 1973; **Fellow:** Neonatal-Perinatal Medicine, Yale-New Haven Hosp 1974; **Fac Appt:** Prof Ped, Yale Univ

Nephrology

Bia, Margaret MD (Nep) - **Spec Exp:** Transplant Medicine-Kidney; **Hospital:** Yale-New Haven Hosp, Yale Med Group (page 940); **Address:** YNHH, Dept Organ Transplant Ctr, 800 Howard Ave Fl 4, New Haven, CT 06520; **Phone:** 203-785-2565; **Board Cert:** Internal Medicine 1975; Nephrology 1978; **Med School:** Cornell Univ-Weill Med Coll 1972; **Resid:** Internal Medicine, Univ Hosp Penn 1975; **Fellow:** Renal Disease, Univ Hosp Penn 1976; **Fac Appt:** Prof Med, Yale Univ

Formica Jr, Richard N MD (Nep) - **Spec Exp:** Transplant Medicine-Kidney; **Hospital:** Yale-New Haven Hosp; **Address:** YNHH, Dept Nephrology, 800 Howard Ave Fl 4, New Haven, CT 06520-8029; **Phone:** 203-785-2565; **Board Cert:** Internal Medicine 2007; Nephrology 2009; **Med School:** Boston Univ 1993; **Resid:** Internal Medicine, Boston Univ Hosp 1997; **Fellow:** Nephrology, Yale New-Haven Hosp 1997; **Fac Appt:** Assoc Prof S, Yale Univ

Kliger, Alan MD (Nep) - **Spec Exp:** Kidney Disease; Kidney Disease-Metabolic; **Hospital:** Yale-New Haven Hosp - St Raphael Campus; **Address:** 136 Sherman Ave, New Haven, CT 06511; **Phone:** 203-787-0117 x307; **Board Cert:** Internal Medicine 1973; Nephrology 1976; **Med School:** SUNY Upstate Med Univ 1970; **Resid:** Internal Medicine, SUNY Upstate Med Ctr 1973; **Fellow:** Nephrology, Georgetown Univ Hosp 1975; **Fac Appt:** Clin Prof Med, Yale Univ

Rastegar, Asghar MD (Nep) - **Spec Exp:** Glomerulonephritis; Amyloidosis; Electrolyte Disorders; **Hospital:** Yale-New Haven Hosp, Yale Med Group (page 940); **Address:** YNHH, Dept Nephrology, 800 Howard Ave Fl 4, New Haven, CT 06519; **Phone:** 203-785-2565; **Board Cert:** Internal Medicine 1972; Nephrology 1978; **Med School:** Univ Wisc 1968; **Resid:** Internal Medicine, Hosp Univ Penn 1973; **Fellow:** Nephrology, Hosp Univ Penn 1972; **Fac Appt:** Prof Med, Yale Univ

Neurological Surgery

Duncan, Charles C MD (NS) - **Spec Exp:** Pediatric Neurosurgery; **Hospital:** Yale-New Haven Hosp, Yale Med Group (page 940); **Address:** YNH-Chldns Hosp, 1 Park St Fl 2, New Haven, CT 06520-8082; **Phone:** 203-785-2809; **Board Cert:** Neurological Surgery 1979; Pediatric Neurological Surgery 1996; **Med School:** Duke Univ 1971; **Resid:** Neurological Surgery, Duke Univ Med Ctr 1977; **Fac Appt:** Prof NS, Yale Univ

Piepmeier, Joseph MD (NS) - **Spec Exp:** Neuro-Oncology; Brain & Spinal Cord Tumors; **Hospital:** Yale-New Haven Hosp, Yale Med Group (page 940); **Address:** 35 Park St Fl 8, New Haven, CT 06520; **Phone:** 203-785-2791; **Board Cert:** Neurological Surgery 1984; **Med School:** Univ Tenn Coll Med 1975; **Resid:** Neurological Surgery, Yale-New Haven Hosp 1982; **Fac Appt:** Prof NS, Yale Univ

Spencer, Dennis D MD (NS) - **Spec Exp:** Epilepsy/Seizure Disorders; Brain Tumors; **Hospital:** Yale-New Haven Hosp, Yale Med Group (page 940); **Address:** Yale Univ Sch Med, Dept Neurosurgery, 333 333 Cedar St, PO Box 208082, New Haven, CT 06520; **Phone:** 203-785-4891; **Board Cert:** Neurological Surgery 1980; **Med School:** Washington Univ, St Louis 1971; **Resid:** Surgery, Barnes Hosp 1972; Neurological Surgery, Yale-New Haven Hosp 1976; **Fac Appt:** Prof NS, Yale Univ

Neurology

Duckrow, Robert B MD (N) - **Spec Exp:** Epilepsy; **Hospital:** Yale-New Haven Hosp, Yale Med Group (page 940); **Address:** 800 Howard Ave Fl LL, New Haven, CT 06520; **Phone:** 203-785-4085 x8; **Board Cert:** Neurology 1984; Clinical Neurophysiology 2004; **Med School:** Yale Univ 1975; **Resid:** Neurology, Yale-New Haven Hosp 1979; **Fellow:** Metabolic Neurology, Univ Miami Hosp 1981; **Fac Appt:** Assoc Prof N, Yale Univ

Goldstein, Jonathan M MD (N) - **Spec Exp:** Myasthenia Gravis; Peripheral Neuropathy; **Hospital:** Yale-New Haven Hosp, Yale Med Group (page 940); **Address:** 800 Howard Ave Fl LL, New Haven, CT 06520; **Phone:** 203-785-4085; **Board Cert:** Neurology 1991; Neuromuscular Medicine 2011; **Med School:** Brown Univ 1986; **Resid:** Neurology, Yale-New Haven Hosp 1990; **Fellow:** Clinical Neurophysiology, Yale-New Haven Hosp 1991; Neurological Immunology, Yale-New Haven Hosp 1992; **Fac Appt:** Assoc Prof N, Yale Univ

Greer, David M MD (N) - **Spec Exp:** Stroke; Cerebrovascular Disease; **Hospital:** Yale-New Haven Hosp, Yale Med Group (page 940); **Address:** Yale Univ Sch Medicine, Dept Neurology, 15 York St, PO Box 208018, New Haven, CT 06520-8018; **Phone:** 203-737-1057; **Board Cert:** Neurology 2010; Vascular Neurology 2008; **Med School:** Univ Fla Coll Med 1995; **Resid:** Neurology, Mass General Hosp 1999; **Fellow:** Vascular Neurology, Mass General Hosp 2001

Katz, Amiram MD (N) - **Spec Exp:** Seizure Disorders; Lyme Disease; Diving Medicine; Sleep Medicine; **Hospital:** Norwalk Hosp, Yale-New Haven Hosp; **Address:** 325 Boston Post Rd, Ste 1B, Orange, CT 06477; **Phone:** 203-795-5425; **Board Cert:** Neurology 1993; **Med School:** Israel 1976; **Resid:** Neurology, Sheba Hosp 1980; Neurology, Tel Aviv Med Ctr 1984; **Fellow:** Clinical Neurophysiology, Cleveland Clinic 1988; Epilepsy, Yale Univ 1991; **Fac Appt:** Asst Clin Prof N, Yale Univ

Neuroradiology

Sze, Gordon K MD (NRad) - **Spec Exp:** Brain Tumors; Spinal Cord Tumors; Head & Neck Cancer; MRI; **Hospital:** Yale-New Haven Hosp, Yale Med Group (page 940); **Address:** Yale-New Haven Hospital, Yale Diagnostic Radiology, 20 York St, New Haven, CT 06510; **Phone:** 203-785-3667; **Board Cert:** Diagnostic Radiology 1985; Neuroradiology 2008; **Med School:** Harvard Med Sch 1981; **Resid:** Diagnostic Radiology, UCSF Med Ctr 1985; **Fellow:** Neuroradiology, UCSF Med Ctr 1986; **Fac Appt:** Prof Rad, Yale Univ

Obstetrics & Gynecology

Fine, Emily A MD (ObG) - **Spec Exp:** Menopause Problems; Vulvar Disease; **Hospital:** Yale-New Haven Hosp; **Address:** 60 Washington Ave, Ste 201, Hamden, CT 06518; **Phone:** 203-230-2939; **Board Cert:** Obstetrics & Gynecology 1984; **Med School:** Yale Univ 1978; **Resid:** Obstetrics & Gynecology, Yale-New Haven Hosp 1982; **Fac Appt:** Asst Clin Prof ObG, Yale Univ

Guess, Marsha Kathleen MD (ObG) - **Spec Exp:** Incontinence; Pelvic Organ Prolapse Repair; **Hospital:** Yale-New Haven Hosp; **Address:** Yale Urogyn & Reconstruc Pelvic Surg, 800 Howard Ave, Yale Physicians Bldg, Fl 3, New Haven, CT 06510; **Phone:** 203-785-6927; **Board Cert:** Obstetrics & Gynecology 2011; **Med School:** UCLA 1997; **Resid:** Obstetrics & Gynecology, UCLA Med Ctr 2001; **Fellow:** Reconstructive Pelvic Surgery, Albert Einstein Coll of Med/Montefiore Med Ctr 2004; **Fac Appt:** Asst Prof ObG, Yale Univ

Lynch, Vincent A MD (ObG) - **Spec Exp:** Laparoscopic Surgery; Menopause Problems; Heart Disease in Pregnancy; **Hospital:** Yale-New Haven Hosp, Yale Med Group (page 940); **Address:** 46 Prince St, Ste 207, New Haven, CT 06519; **Phone:** 203-787-2264; **Board Cert:** Obstetrics & Gynecology 1986; **Med School:** NY Med Coll 1967; **Resid:** Obstetrics & Gynecology, Yale-New Haven Hosp 1972; **Fac Appt:** Clin Prof ObG, Yale Univ

Ophthalmology

Lesser, Robert L MD (Oph) - **Spec Exp:** Neuro-Ophthalmology; Myasthenia Gravis; Pseudotumor Cerebri; Temporal Arteritis; **Hospital:** Yale-New Haven Hosp, St. Mary's Hosp - Waterbury; **Address:** The Eye Care Group, 40 Temple St, Ste 5B, New Haven, CT 06510; **Phone:** 203-789-2020; **Board Cert:** Ophthalmology 1975; **Med School:** Cornell Univ-Weill Med Coll 1967; **Resid:** Ophthalmology, Yale-New Haven Hosp 1974; **Fellow:** Neuro-Ophthalmology, Bascom Palmer Eye Inst 1972; **Fac Appt:** Clin Prof Oph, Yale Univ

Tom, David MD (Oph) - **Spec Exp:** Retinal Disorders; **Hospital:** Yale-New Haven Hosp, Greenwich Hosp (page 892); **Address:** 2200 Whitney Ave, Ste 300, Hamden, CT 06518; **Phone:** 203-288-2020; **Board Cert:** Ophthalmology 2008; **Med School:** Geo Wash Univ 1991; **Resid:** Ophthalmology, Yale-New Haven Hosp 1996; **Fellow:** Vitreoretinal Surgery, Manhattan EE & T 1997; **Fac Appt:** Asst Clin Prof Oph, Yale Univ

Tsai, James C MD (Oph) - **Spec Exp:** Glaucoma; **Hospital:** Yale-New Haven Hosp, Yale Med Group (page 940); **Address:** 40 Temple St, New Haven, CT 06520-8061; **Phone:** 203-785-2020; **Board Cert:** Ophthalmology 2006; **Med School:** Stanford Univ 1989; **Resid:** Ophthalmology, Doheny Eye Inst/USC 1993; **Fellow:** Glaucoma, Bascom Palmer Eye Inst 1994; Glaucoma, Moorfields Eye Hosp 1995; **Fac Appt:** Prof Oph, Yale Univ

Orthopaedic Surgery

Baumgaertner, Michael R MD (OrS) - **Spec Exp:** Trauma; Hip & Knee Reconstruction; Fractures-Complex & Non Union; **Hospital:** Yale-New Haven Hosp, Yale Med Group (page 940); **Address:** 800 Howard Ave, Yale Physicians Bldg, Fl 1, New Haven, CT 06520; **Phone:** 203-737-5667; **Board Cert:** Orthopaedic Surgery 2010; **Med School:** UCSD 1982; **Resid:** Orthopaedic Surgery, UCSF Med Ctr 1987; **Fellow:** Plastic Surgery, Univ Mass Med Ctr 1988; Trauma, AO Foundation 1989; **Fac Appt:** Prof OrS, Yale Univ

Friedlaender, Gary E MD (OrS) - **Spec Exp:** Bone & Soft Tissue Tumors; Limb Surgery/Reconstruction; Fractures-Complex & Non Union; Tissue Banking; **Hospital:** Yale-New Haven Hosp, Yale Med Group (page 940); **Address:** 800 Howard Ave, Yale Physicians Building YPB 133 Fl 1, New Haven, CT 06519; **Phone:** 203-737-5660; **Board Cert:** Orthopaedic Surgery 1975; **Med School:** Univ Mich Med Sch 1969; **Resid:** Surgery, Michigan Med Ctr 1971; Orthopaedic Surgery, Yale-New Haven Hosp 1974; **Fellow:** Musculoskeletal Oncology, Mass Genl Hosp 1983; **Fac Appt:** Prof OrS, Yale Univ

Jokl, Peter MD (OrS) - **Spec Exp:** Knee Surgery; Sports Medicine; Shoulder Surgery; **Hospital:** Yale-New Haven Hosp, Yale Med Group (page 940); **Address:** Yale Sports Med, Dept Orthopaedics, 800 Howard Ave, New Haven, CT 06519-1369; **Phone:** 203-785-2579; **Board Cert:** Orthopaedic Surgery 1974; **Med School:** Yale Univ 1968; **Resid:** Orthopaedic Surgery, Yale-New Haven Hosp 1972; **Fac Appt:** Prof OrS, Yale Univ

Marsh, James S MD (OrS) - **Spec Exp:** Pediatric Orthopaedic Surgery; **Hospital:** Yale-New Haven Hosp, Yale-New Haven Hosp - St Raphael Campus; **Address:** 34 York St, Ste 2, Guilford, CT 06437; **Phone:** 203-453-1088; **Med School:** Harvard Med Sch 1981; **Resid:** Orthopaedic Surgery, Stanford Univ 1986; **Fellow:** Pediatric Orthopaedic Surgery, Mass Genl Hosp 1987; **Fac Appt:** Assoc Prof OrS, Yale Univ

Smith, Brian Gerard MD (OrS) - **Spec Exp:** Pediatric Orthopaedic Surgery; Spinal Deformity; Scoliosis; Foot Deformities; **Hospital:** Yale-New Haven Hosp, Yale Med Group (page 940); **Address:** 800 Howard Ave, Yale Physicians Bldg Fl 1, New Haven, CT 06519; **Phone:** 203-737-1616; **Board Cert:** Orthopaedic Surgery 2010; **Med School:** Georgetown Univ 1982; **Resid:** Orthopaedic Surgery, Georgetown Univ Hosp 1987; **Fellow:** Pediatric Orthopaedic Surgery, Children's Hosp 1992; **Fac Appt:** Assoc Prof OrS, Yale Univ

Otolaryngology

Kveton, John F MD (Oto) - **Spec Exp:** Ear Disorders/Surgery; Cochlear Implants; Acoustic Neuroma; Hearing Loss; **Hospital:** Yale-New Haven Hosp; **Address:** ENT Med & Surgical Grp, 46 Prince St, Ste 601, New Haven, CT 06519-1634; **Phone:** 203-752-1726; **Board Cert:** Otolaryngology 1982; Neurotology 2004; **Med School:** St Louis Univ 1978; **Resid:** Otolaryngology, Yale-New Haven Hosp 1982; **Fellow:** Neurotology, The Otology Group 1983; **Fac Appt:** Clin Prof Oto, Yale Univ

Michaelides, Elias M MD (Oto) - **Spec Exp:** Neuro-Otology; Hearing Loss; Balance Disorders; Pediatric Otolaryngology; **Hospital:** Yale-New Haven Hosp, Yale Med Group (page 940); **Address:** 800 Howard Ave, Yale Physicians Bldg, Fl 4, New Haven, CT 06519; **Phone:** 203-785-7656; **Board Cert:** Otolaryngology 1999; Neurotology 2008; **Med School:** SUNY Stony Brook 1993; **Resid:** Otolaryngology, Med Coll Va 1998; **Fellow:** Otology, Michigan Ear Inst 2000; **Fac Appt:** Asst Prof S, Yale Univ

Sasaki, Clarence T MD (Oto) - **Spec Exp:** Head & Neck Cancer; Swallowing Disorders; Zenker Diverticulum; Voice Disorders; **Hospital:** Yale-New Haven Hosp, Yale Med Group (page 940); **Address:** Yale Sch Med, Dept Otolaryngology, 333 Cedar St, Box 208041, New Haven, CT 06520-8041; **Phone:** 203-785-2592; **Board Cert:** Otolaryngology 1973; **Med School:** Yale Univ 1966; **Resid:** Surgery, Mary Hitchcock Hosp 1968; Otolaryngology, Yale-New Haven Hosp 1973; **Fellow:** Head and Neck Surgery, Univ of Milan 1978; Skull Base Surgery, Univ Zurich 1982; **Fac Appt:** Prof Oto, Yale Univ

Vining, Eugenia M MD (Oto) - **Spec Exp:** Sinus Disorders/Surgery; Skull Base Tumors; Sinus Tumors; **Hospital:** Yale-New Haven Hosp; **Address:** ENT Medical & Surgical Grp, 46 Prince St, Ste 601, New Haven, CT 06519; **Phone:** 203-752-1726; **Board Cert:** Otolaryngology 1993; **Med School:** Yale Univ 1987; **Resid:** Otolaryngology, Yale-New Haven Hosp 1991; Otolaryngology, Yale-New Haven Hosp 1992; **Fellow:** Sinus Surgery, Univ Penn 1993

Young, Nwanmegha O MD (Oto) - **Spec Exp:** Voice Disorders; Vocal Cord Disorders; Laryngeal Disorders; Swallowing Disorders; **Hospital:** Yale-New Haven Hosp; **Address:** Yale-New Haven Hosp, Dept Otolaryngology, 333 Cedar St, Box 208041, New Haven, CT 06520-8041; **Phone:** 203-785-2593; **Board Cert:** Otolaryngology 2008; **Med School:** UC Davis 1999; **Resid:** Otolaryngology, Barnes Jewish Hosp 2005; **Fellow:** Neurotology, St Lukes Roosevelt Hosp 2007

Pain Medicine

Saberski, Lloyd MD (PM) - ; **Address:** Adavanced Diagnostic Pain Treatment Ctr, 1 Long Wharf Drive Fl 2 - Ste 212, New Haven, CT 06511; **Phone:** 203-624-4208; **Board Cert:** Internal Medicine 1985; Anesthesiology 1988; Pain Medicine 2004; **Med School:** NY Med Coll 1982; **Resid:** Internal Medicine, Albany Meml Hosp 1985; Anesthesiology, Albany Meml Hosp 1987; **Fellow:** Pain Medicine, Albany Meml Hosp 1988; **Fac Appt:** Asst Prof Anes, Yale Univ

Pathology

Morrow, Jon S MD/PhD (Path) - **Spec Exp:** Kidney Cancer; Colon Cancer; Breast Cancer; Hematopathology; **Hospital:** Yale-New Haven Hosp; **Address:** Yale Pathology, Bady Memorial Laboratory, 310 Cedar St, BML 140, New Haven, CT 06510; **Phone:** 203-785-3624; **Board Cert:** Pathology 1980; **Med School:** Yale Univ 1976; **Resid:** Pathology, Yale-New Haven Hosp 1978; **Fellow:** Pathology, Yale-New Haven Hosp 1980; **Fac Appt:** Prof Path, Yale Univ

Pediatric Cardiology

Friedman, Alan H MD (PCd) - **Spec Exp:** Echocardiography; Fetal Echocardiography; Cardiac Imaging; Sports Medicine; **Hospital:** Yale-New Haven Hosp, Yale Med Group (page 940); **Address:** Yale Univ, Dept Pediatrics, 333 Cedar St, 302 LCI, New Haven, CT 06519; **Phone:** 203-785-2022; **Board Cert:** Pediatric Cardiology 2004; **Med School:** Wayne State Univ 1987; **Resid:** Pediatrics, Chldns Meml Hosp 1991; **Fellow:** Pediatric Cardiology, New Haven Hosp 1994; **Fac Appt:** Prof Ped, Yale Univ

Hellenbrand, William E MD (PCd) - **Spec Exp:** Interventional Cardiology; **Hospital:** Yale-New Haven Hosp; **Address:** 333 cedar St, Box 208064, LLCI Bldg, rm 301, New Haven, CT 06520-8064; **Phone:** 203-785-2022; **Board Cert:** Pediatrics 1975; Pediatric Cardiology 1977; **Med School:** SUNY Downstate 1970; **Resid:** Pediatrics, Yale-New Haven Hosp 1972; **Fellow:** Pediatric Cardiology, Yale-New Haven Hosp 1976; **Fac Appt:** Prof Ped, Columbia P&S

Pediatric Endocrinology

Carpenter, Thomas O MD (PEn) - **Spec Exp:** Calcium Disorders; Bone Disorders-Metabolic; Thyroid Disorders; Parathyroid Disorders; **Hospital:** Yale-New Haven Hosp, Yale Med Group (page 940); **Address:** Yale Sch Med, Dept Pediatrics, 2 Church St S, Ste 511, New Haven, CT 06520-8064; **Phone:** 203-764-9199; **Board Cert:** Pediatrics 1982; Pediatric Endocrinology 1999; **Med School:** Univ Alabama 1977; **Resid:** Pediatrics, Univ Alabama Hosp 1980; **Fellow:** Pediatric Endocrinology, Children's Hosp 1983; **Fac Appt:** Prof Ped, Yale Univ

Tamborlane, William V MD (PEn) - **Spec Exp:** Diabetes; **Hospital:** Yale-New Haven Hosp, Yale Med Group (page 940); **Address:** Yale Pediatric Endocrinology, 333 Cedar St, rm 3091-LMP, New Haven, CT 06519; **Phone:** 203-764-6747; **Board Cert:** Pediatrics 1978; Pediatric Endocrinology 1986; **Med School:** Georgetown Univ 1972; **Resid:** Pediatrics, Georgetown Univ Hosp 1975; **Fellow:** Pediatric Endocrinology, Yale-New Haven Hosp 1977; **Fac Appt:** Prof Ped, Yale Univ

Pediatric Hematology-Oncology

Kadan-Lottick, Nina S MD (PHO) - **Spec Exp:** Cancer Survivors-Late Effects of Therapy; **Hospital:** Yale-New Haven Hosp, Yale Med Group (page 940); **Address:** Yale Pediatric Hematology/Oncology, PO Box 208064, 333 Cedar St, LMP 2073, New Haven, CT 06520; **Phone:** 203-785-4640; **Board Cert:** Pediatrics 2004; Pediatric Hematology-Oncology 2009; **Med School:** Johns Hopkins Univ 1993; **Resid:** Pediatrics, Johns Hopkins Hosp 1996; **Fellow:** Pediatric Hematology-Oncology, Chldns Hosp 1999; Cancer Epidemiology, Univ Minnesota 2000; **Fac Appt:** Asst Prof Ped, Yale Univ

McNamara, Joseph M MD (PHO) - **Hospital:** Yale-New Haven Hosp, Yale Med Group (page 940); **Address:** Pediatric Hematology/Oncology Assocs, 405 Church St, Guilford, CT 06437; **Phone:** 203-453-2013; **Board Cert:** Pediatrics 1987; Pediatric Hematology-Oncology 2005; **Med School:** Italy 1982; **Resid:** Pediatrics, Misericordia Hosp 1985; **Fellow:** Pediatric Hematology-Oncology, Schneider Chldns Hosp 1987

Pediatric Infectious Disease

Andiman, Warren A MD (PInf) - **Spec Exp:** AIDS/HIV; Viral Infections; Lyme Disease; Infectious Mononucleosis; **Hospital:** Yale-New Haven Hosp, Yale Med Group (page 940); **Address:** Yale Univ Sch Med, Dept Pediatrics, 333 Cedar St, Box 208064, New Haven, CT 06520-8064; **Phone:** 203-785-4730; **Board Cert:** Pediatrics 1975; **Med School:** Albert Einstein Coll Med 1969; **Resid:** Pediatrics, Babies Hosp-Columbia Presby 1971; **Fellow:** Pediatric Infectious Disease, Yale Un 1973; **Fac Appt:** Prof Ped, Yale Univ

Baltimore, Robert MD (PInf) - **Spec Exp:** Neonatal Infections; Hospital Acquired Infections; Tuberculosis; **Hospital:** Yale-New Haven Hosp, Yale Med Group (page 940); **Address:** Yale Univ Sch Med, Dept Pediatrics, 333 Cedar St, Box 208064, New Haven, CT 06520-8064; **Phone:** 203-785-4750; **Board Cert:** Pediatrics 1975; Pediatric Infectious Disease 2009; **Med School:** SUNY Buffalo 1968; **Resid:** Pediatrics, Univ Chicago Hosps 1971; **Fellow:** Infectious Disease, Boston City Hosp-Harvard 1976; **Fac Appt:** Prof Ped, Yale Univ

Shapiro, Eugene D MD (PInf) - **Spec Exp:** Lyme Disease; Vaccines; **Hospital:** Yale-New Haven Hosp, Yale Med Group (page 940); **Address:** Yale Univ Sch Med, Dept Pediatrics, 333 Cedar St, Box 208064, New Haven, CT 06520-8064; **Phone:** 203-688-4518; **Board Cert:** Pediatrics 1980; Pediatric Infectious Disease 2009; **Med School:** UCSF 1976; **Resid:** Pediatrics, Chldns Hosp 1979; **Fellow:** Pediatric Infectious Disease, Chldns Hosp 1981; Research, Yale Univ 1983; **Fac Appt:** Prof Ped, Yale Univ

Pediatric Pulmonology

Bazzy-Asaad, Alia MD (PPul) - **Spec Exp:** Asthma; Sleep Disorders; **Hospital:** Yale-New Haven Hosp, Yale Med Group (page 940); **Address:** 333 Cedar St, PO Box 208064, New Haven, CT 06520-8064; **Phone:** 203-785-2480; **Board Cert:** Pediatrics 1987; Pediatric Pulmonology 2009; **Med School:** Amer Univ Beirut 1978; **Resid:** Pediatrics, Amer Univ Beirut 1980; **Fellow:** Pediatric Pulmonology, NY Presby Hosp 1983; **Fac Appt:** Assoc Prof Ped, Yale Univ

Pediatric Rheumatology

McCarthy, Paul L MD (PRhu) - **Spec Exp:** Lupus/SLE; Juvenile Arthritis; Dermatomyositis; Vasculitis; **Hospital:** Yale-New Haven Hosp, Yale Med Group (page 940); **Address:** Yale Sch Med, 333 Cedar St, Box 208064, New Haven, CT 06520-3206; **Phone:** 203-688-2475; **Board Cert:** Pediatrics 1974; Pediatric Rheumatology 2007; **Med School:** Georgetown Univ 1969; **Resid:** Pediatrics, Chldns Hosp 1972; **Fellow:** Pediatrics, Chldns Hosp 1974; **Fac Appt:** Prof Ped, Yale Univ

Pediatric Surgery

Caty, Michael G MD (PS) - **Spec Exp:** Neonatal Surgery; Thoracic Surgery; Gastrointestinal Motility Disorders; Laparoscopic Surgery; **Hospital:** Yale-New Haven Hosp; **Address:** Yale Pediatric Surgery, 330 Cedar St, FMB-131, PO Box 208062, New Haven, CT 06520-8062; **Phone:** 203-785-2701; **Board Cert:** Surgery 2001; Pediatric Surgery 2003; **Med School:** Univ Mass Sch Med 1985; **Resid:** Surgery, Univ Michigan Hosps 1991; Pediatric Surgery, Boston Chldns Hosp 1993; **Fac Appt:** Prof S, Yale Univ

Pediatrics

Angoff, Ronald MD (Ped) *PCP* - **Hospital:** Yale-New Haven Hosp - St Raphael Campus, Yale-New Haven Hosp; **Address:** 200 Orchard St, Ste 108, New Haven, CT 06511; **Phone:** 203-865-3737; **Board Cert:** Pediatrics 1978; **Med School:** Univ Cincinnati 1973; **Resid:** Pediatrics, Yale-New Haven Hosp 1975; **Fellow:** Child Development, Yale-New Haven Hosp 1977; **Fac Appt:** Assoc Prof Ped, Yale Univ

Canny, Christopher R MD (Ped) *PCP* - **Spec Exp:** Behavioral Disorders; Developmental Disorders; **Hospital:** Yale-New Haven Hosp, Yale-New Haven Hosp - St Raphael Campus; **Address:** 9 Washington Ave, Fl 2, Hamden, CT 06518; **Phone:** 203-287-0552; **Board Cert:** Pediatrics 2010; **Med School:** Washington Univ, St Louis 1976; **Resid:** Pediatrics, Yale-New Haven Hosp 1978; **Fellow:** Child Development, Yale Child Study Ctr 1980; **Fac Appt:** Assoc Clin Prof Ped, Yale Univ

Gruskay, Jeffrey MD (Ped) *PCP* - **Hospital:** Milford Hosp, Yale-New Haven Hosp; **Address:** 20 Commerce Park, Milford, CT 06460; **Phone:** 203-882-2066; **Board Cert:** Pediatrics 1985; Neonatal-Perinatal Medicine 1987; **Med School:** Yale Univ 1981; **Resid:** Pediatrics, Childrens Hosp 1984; **Fellow:** Neonatal-Perinatal Medicine, Childrens Hosp 1986; **Fac Appt:** Assoc Clin Prof Ped, Yale Univ

Morgan Jr, James L MD (Ped) *PCP* - **Spec Exp:** Sports Medicine; **Hospital:** Yale-New Haven Hosp, Yale-New Haven Hosp - St Raphael Campus; **Address:** 240 Indian River Rd, Ste B1, Orange, CT 06477; **Phone:** 203-795-6025; **Board Cert:** Pediatrics 1983; **Med School:** Med Coll VA 1978; **Resid:** Pediatrics, Chldn's Hosp 1982

Robert, Marie F MD (Ped) *PCP* - **Hospital:** Yale-New Haven Hosp, Yale Med Group (page 940); **Address:** 240 Indian River Rd, Ste B1, Orange, CT 06477; **Phone:** 203-795-6025; **Board Cert:** Pediatrics 1984; **Med School:** McGill Univ 1976; **Resid:** Pediatrics, Chldn's Hosp 1978; Allergy & Immunology, Yale-New Haven Hosp 1979; **Fellow:** Infectious Disease, Yale Univ 1984

Shaywitz, Sally E MD (Ped) - **Spec Exp:** Learning Disorders; Dyslexia; **Hospital:** Yale-New Haven Hosp, Yale Med Group (page 940); **Address:** Yale Univ Dept Pediatrics, 333 Cedar St, PO Box 208064, New Haven, CT 06520-8064; **Phone:** 203-785-4641; **Board Cert:** Pediatrics 1971; **Med School:** Albert Einstein Coll Med 1966; **Resid:** Pediatrics, Albert Einstein Coll Med 1970; **Fellow:** Pediatrics, Bronx Muni Hosp Ctr 1968; Behavioral Pediatrics, Albert Einstein Coll Med 1970; **Fac Appt:** Prof Ped, Yale Univ

Plastic Surgery

Ariyan, Stephan MD (PlS) - **Spec Exp:** Melanoma; **Hospital:** Yale-New Haven Hosp; **Address:** New Haven Hosp, 60 Temple St, Ste 4B, New Haven, CT 06510-2716; **Phone:** 203-786-3000; **Board Cert:** Plastic Surgery 1978; **Med School:** NY Med Coll 1966; **Resid:** Surgery, Yale-New Haven Hosp 1975; Plastic Surgery, Yale-New Haven Hosp 1976; **Fellow:** Surgical Oncology, Yale-New Haven Hosp 1971; **Fac Appt:** Clin Prof S, Yale Univ

Persing, John A MD (PlS) - **Spec Exp:** Craniofacial Surgery; Vascular Malformations; Cosmetic Surgery; **Hospital:** Yale-New Haven Hosp, Yale Med Group (page 940); **Address:** Yale Plastic Surgery, 330 Cedar St Boardroom Bldg Fl 3, New Haven, CT 06519-3218; **Phone:** 203-785-2570; **Board Cert:** Plastic Surgery 1985; Neurological Surgery 1986; **Med School:** Univ VT Coll Med 1974; **Resid:** Surgery, Univ Arizona Med Ctr 1976; Neurological Surgery, Univ Virginia Med Ctr 1982; **Fellow:** Plastic Surgery, Univ Virginia Med Ctr 1984; **Fac Appt:** Prof PlS, Yale Univ

Price, Gary J MD (PlS) - **Spec Exp:** Cosmetic Surgery-Face; Cosmetic Surgery-Breast; Liposuction & Body Contouring; **Hospital:** Yale-New Haven Hosp; **Address:** 5 Durham Rd, Ste 1-8, Guilford, CT 06437; **Phone:** 203-453-6635; **Board Cert:** Plastic Surgery 1986; **Med School:** Penn State Coll Med 1978; **Resid:** Surgery, Yale New-Haven Hosp 1983; Plastic Surgery, Yale New Haven Hosp 1985; **Fellow:** Adolescent Psychiatry; **Fac Appt:** Assoc Clin Prof PlS, Yale Univ

Restifo, Richard MD (PlS) - **Spec Exp:** Breast Surgery; Abdominoplasty; Liposuction & Body Contouring; **Hospital:** St. Vincent's Med Ctr - Bridgeport, Yale-New Haven Hosp; **Address:** 59 Elm St, Ste 560, New Haven, CT 06510; **Phone:** 203-772-1444; **Board Cert:** Plastic Surgery 2005; **Med School:** Harvard Med Sch 1986; **Resid:** Surgery, Georgetown Univ Hosp 1991; Plastic Surgery, Univ Pittsburgh Med Ctr 1993

Stahl, Richard S MD (PlS) - **Spec Exp:** Abdominal Wall Reconstruction; Chest Wall Reconstruction; Breast Reconstruction; Chest Wall Deformities; **Hospital:** Yale-New Haven Hosp, Yale-New Haven Hosp - St Raphael Campus; **Address:** 5 Durham Rd, Guilford, CT 06437; **Phone:** 203-458-4440; **Board Cert:** Surgery 2001; Plastic Surgery 1984; **Med School:** Vanderbilt Univ 1976; **Resid:** Surgery, Yale New Haven Hosp 1981; **Fellow:** Plastic Surgery, Emory Univ Med Ctr 1983; **Fac Appt:** Clin Prof S, Yale Univ

Psychiatry

Lewis, Dorothy Otnow MD (Psyc) - **Spec Exp:** Dissociative Disorders; Aggression Disorders; **Hospital:** Yale-New Haven Hosp, Bellevue Hosp Ctr; **Address:** 100 York St, 8H, New Haven, CT 06511; **Phone:** 203-624-3933; **Board Cert:** Psychiatry 1972; **Med School:** Yale Univ 1963; **Resid:** Psychiatry, Yale-New Haven Hosp 1967; **Fellow:** Child & Adolescent Psychiatry, Yale-New Haven Hosp 1969; Psychiatric Research, Natl Inst Mental Hlth 1967; **Fac Appt:** Clin Prof Psyc, Yale Univ

Pulmonary Disease

Friedman, Lloyd Neal MD (Pul) - **Spec Exp:** Tuberculosis; **Hospital:** Milford Hosp, Yale-New Haven Hosp; **Address:** Milford Hospital, 300 Seaside Ave, Milford, CT 06460; **Phone:** 203-876-4070; **Board Cert:** Internal Medicine 1983; Pulmonary Disease 1988; Critical Care Medicine 2009; **Med School:** Yale Univ 1979; **Resid:** Internal Medicine, Beth Israel Med Ctr 1980; Internal Medicine, Oregon Hlth Scis Univ 1983; **Fellow:** Pulmonary Intensive Care, Yale-New Haven Hosp 1988; **Fac Appt:** Clin Prof Med, Yale Univ

Redlich, Carrie MD (Pul) - **Spec Exp:** Occupational Lung Disease; **Hospital:** Yale-New Haven Hosp, Yale Med Group (page 940); **Address:** Yale Occupational & Environmental Med, 135 College St Fl 3 - Ste 392, New Haven, CT 06510; **Phone:** 203-785-4197; **Board Cert:** Internal Medicine 1986; Occupational Medicine 1990; Pulmonary Disease 2002; **Med School:** Yale Univ 1982; **Resid:** Internal Medicine, Yale-New Haven Hosp 1986; Occupational Medicine, Yale-New Haven Hosp 1987; **Fellow:** Pulmonary Disease, Univ Washington 1989; **Fac Appt:** Assoc Prof Med, Yale Univ

Rochester, Carolyn L MD (Pul) - **Spec Exp:** Chronic Obstructive Lung Disease (COPD); **Hospital:** VA Conn Hlthcre Sys-W Haven Campus, Yale-New Haven Hosp; **Address:** Yale Univ Sch Med, Pulm & Crit Care Sect, 300 Cedar St, Box 208057, New Haven, CT 06520-8057; **Phone:** 203-785-3207; **Board Cert:** Internal Medicine 1986; Pulmonary Disease 2002; Critical Care Medicine 2006; **Med School:** Columbia P&S 1983; **Resid:** Internal Medicine, Columbia Presby Med Ctr 1986; **Fellow:** Pulmonary Disease, Columbia Presby Med Ctr 1988; **Fac Appt:** Asst Prof Med, Yale Univ

Tanoue, Lynn MD (Pul) - **Spec Exp:** Lung Cancer; **Hospital:** Yale-New Haven Hosp, Yale Med Group (page 940); **Address:** Winchester Chest Clin, 789 Howard Ave, Ste 209FB, New Haven, CT 06519; **Phone:** 203-785-4198; **Board Cert:** Internal Medicine 1985; Pulmonary Disease 1988; Critical Care Medicine 2002; **Med School:** Yale Univ 1982; **Resid:** Internal Medicine, Yale-New Haven Hosp 1985; **Fellow:** Pulmonary Disease, Yale-New Haven Hosp 1988; Critical Care Medicine, Yale-New Haven Hosp 1988; **Fac Appt:** Assoc Prof Med, Yale Univ

Trow, Terence MD (Pul) - **Spec Exp:** Pulmonary Hypertension; Pulmonary Vascular Disease; **Hospital:** Yale-New Haven Hosp, Yale Med Group (page 940); **Address:** Winchester Chest Clinic, 20 York St, Ste 209FB, New Haven, CT 06510; **Phone:** 203-785-4198; **Board Cert:** Internal Medicine 1989; Critical Care Medicine 2003; Pulmonary Disease 2002; **Med School:** Dartmouth Med Sch 1986; **Resid:** Internal Medicine, Hosp Univ Penn-UPHS 1987; Internal Medicine, NY-Presby/Weill Cornell Med Ctr 1989; **Fellow:** Pulmonary Critical Care Medicine, Yale-New Haven Hosp 1993; **Fac Appt:** Asst Clin Prof Med, Yale Univ

Radiation Oncology

Higgins, Susan A MD (RadRO) - **Spec Exp:** Gynecologic Cancer; Vulvar/Vaginal Cancer; Breast Cancer; Gastrointestinal Cancer; **Hospital:** Smilow Cancer Hosp at Yale-New Haven, Yale Med Group (page 940); **Address:** Smilow Cancer Hosp, 35 Park St, Ste LL515, New Haven, CT 06520; **Phone:** 203-785-7033; **Board Cert:** Radiation Oncology 2004; **Med School:** Univ Rochester 1990; **Resid:** Radiology, Yale-New Haven Hosp 1993; **Fac Appt:** Assoc Prof RadRO, Yale Univ

Peschel, Richard E MD (RadRO) - **Spec Exp:** Prostate Cancer; Testicular Cancer; **Hospital:** Yale-New Haven Hosp, Yale Med Group (page 940); **Address:** 35 Park St, rm LL-510, MS 06510, New Haven, CT 06510; **Phone:** 203-785-2958; **Board Cert:** Therapeutic Radiology 1982; **Med School:** Yale Univ 1977; **Resid:** Radiation Oncology, Yale-New Haven Hosp 1981; **Fac Appt:** Prof RadRO, Yale Univ

Roberts, Kenneth MD (RadRO) - **Spec Exp:** Pediatric Cancers; Lymphoma; Hodgkin's Lymphoma; **Hospital:** Yale-New Haven Hosp, Yale Med Group (page 940); **Address:** Yale Univ Sch Med, Dept Radiation Therapy, 15 York St, New Haven, CT 06520-8040; **Phone:** 203-785-2957; **Board Cert:** Internal Medicine 1987; Medical Oncology 1989; Radiation Oncology 1995; **Med School:** Duke Univ 1984; **Resid:** Internal Medicine, Ohio State Univ Hosps 1987; Radiation Oncology, Duke Univ Med Ctr 1992; **Fellow:** Hematology & Oncology, Duke Univ Med Ctr 1989; **Fac Appt:** Assoc Prof Rad, Yale Univ

Weidhaas, Joanne B MD (RadRO) - **Spec Exp:** Breast Cancer; Gynecologic Cancer; **Hospital:** Smilow Cancer Hosp at Yale-New Haven, Yale-New Haven Hosp; **Address:** Smilow Cancer Hosp, 35 Park St, Ste LL515, New Haven, CT 06520; **Phone:** 203-785-7033; **Board Cert:** Radiation Oncology 2005; **Med School:** Tufts Univ 1999; **Resid:** Radiation Oncology, Meml Sloan Kettering Cancer Ctr 2005; **Fac Appt:** Asst Prof RadRO, Yale Univ

Wilson, Lynn D MD (RadRO) - **Spec Exp:** Cutaneous Lymphoma; Lung Cancer; Head & Neck Cancer; **Hospital:** Yale-New Haven Hosp, Yale Med Group (page 940); **Address:** Yale Univ Sch Med, Dept Therapeutic Rad, PO Box 208040, New Haven, CT 06520-8040; **Phone:** 203-737-1202; **Board Cert:** Radiation Oncology 2004; **Med School:** Geo Wash Univ 1990; **Resid:** Therapeutic Radiology, Yale-New Haven Hosp 1994; **Fac Appt:** Prof RadRO, Yale Univ

Reproductive Endocrinology

Patrizio, Pasquale MD (RE) - **Spec Exp:** Infertility-IVF; Fertility Preservation in Cancer; **Hospital:** Yale-New Haven Hosp, Yale Med Group (page 940); **Address:** Yale Fertility Ctr, Dept OB/GYN, 150 Sargent Drive, New Haven, CT 06511; **Phone:** 203-785-4708; **Board Cert:** Obstetrics & Gynecology 2007; Reproductive Endocrinology 2010; **Med School:** Italy 1983; **Resid:** Obstetrics & Gynecology, Univ Naples 1987; Reproductive Endocrinology, Univ Pisa 1990; **Fellow:** Infertility, UC Irvine 1995; **Fac Appt:** Prof ObG, Yale Univ

Taylor, Hugh S MD (RE) - **Spec Exp:** Infertility-IVF; Endometriosis; Menopause Problems; Vaginal/Uterine Abnormalities; **Hospital:** Yale-New Haven Hosp, Yale Med Group (page 940); **Address:** Yale Univ School Med, Dept OB/GYN, 333 Cedar St, New Haven, CT 06520; **Phone:** 203-785-4708; **Board Cert:** Obstetrics & Gynecology 2011; Reproductive Endocrinology 2011; **Med School:** Univ Conn 1988; **Resid:** Obstetrics & Gynecology, Yale-New Haven Hosp 1997; **Fellow:** Reproductive Endocrinology, Yale-New Haven Hosp 1998; **Fac Appt:** Prof ObG, Yale Univ

Rheumatology

Hutchinson, Gordon J MD (Rhu) - **Spec Exp:** Rheumatoid Arthritis; Lyme Disease; Polymyositis; **Hospital:** Yale-New Haven Hosp - St Raphael Campus, Yale-New Haven Hosp; **Address:** 136 Sherman Ave, Ste 104, New Haven, CT 06511; **Phone:** 203-785-0885; **Board Cert:** Internal Medicine 1980; Rheumatology 1982; **Med School:** Switzerland 1976; **Resid:** Internal Medicine, Hosp St Raphael 1980; **Fellow:** Rheumatology, Yale Univ Med Ctr 1982; **Fac Appt:** Assoc Clin Prof Med, Yale Univ

Liebling, Anne MD (Rhu) - **Spec Exp:** Arthritis; Juvenile Arthritis; Fibromyalgia; **Hospital:** Yale-New Haven Hosp, Yale Med Group (page 940); **Address:** 60 Temple St, Ste 6A, New Haven, CT 06510; **Phone:** 203-789-2255; **Board Cert:** Rheumatology 2000; Pediatric Rheumatology 2009; **Med School:** SUNY Downstate 1986; **Resid:** Internal Medicine & Pediatrics, Univ Chicago Hosps 1990; **Fellow:** Rheumatology, Univ Chicago Hosps 1993; Pediatric Rheumatology, Univ Chicago Hosps 1993

Schoen, Robert T MD (Rhu) - **Spec Exp:** Rheumatoid Arthritis; Lyme Disease; Osteoporosis; **Hospital:** Yale-New Haven Hosp; **Address:** 60 Temple St, Ste 6A, New Haven, CT 06510-2716; **Phone:** 203-789-2255; **Board Cert:** Internal Medicine 1979; Rheumatology 1982; **Med School:** Columbia P&S 1976; **Resid:** Internal Medicine, Yale New Haven Hosp 1979; **Fellow:** Rheumatology, Brigham & Womens Hosp 1981; **Fac Appt:** Clin Prof Med, Yale Univ

Surgery

Barcewicz, Paul MD (S) - **Spec Exp:** Cancer Surgery; Laparoscopic Surgery; Soft Tissue Tumors; Endoscopy; **Hospital:** Yale-New Haven Hosp - St Raphael Campus, Yale-New Haven Hosp; **Address:** Surgl Assocs New Haven, 60 Temple St, Ste 5A, New Haven, CT 06510; **Phone:** 203-772-0650 x248; **Board Cert:** Surgery 2002; **Med School:** Univ Rochester 1977; **Resid:** Surgery, Hartford Hosp 1982; **Fellow:** Surgical Oncology, Roswell Park Cancer Ctr 1984; **Fac Appt:** Asst Clin Prof S, Yale Univ

Chagpar, Anees B MD (S) - **Spec Exp:** Breast Cancer & Surgery; Breast Disease; **Hospital:** Yale-New Haven Hosp; **Address:** Yale-New Haven Breast Ctr, Smilow Cancer Hospital, North Pavilion, 20 York St, Fl 1, Ste A, New Haven, CT 06510; **Phone:** 203-200-2328; **Board Cert:** Surgery 2004; **Med School:** Canada 1996; **Resid:** Surgery, Univ Saskatchewan 2002; **Fellow:** Breast Cancer, MD Anderson Cancer Ctr 2003; **Fac Appt:** Assoc Prof Surg & Onc, Yale Univ

Duffy, Andrew J MD (S) - **Spec Exp:** Laparoscopic Surgery; Gastrointestinal Surgery; Diverticulitis; Colon & Rectal Cancer; **Hospital:** Yale-New Haven Hosp; **Address:** Yale GI Surgery, Temple Medical Bldg, 40 Temple St, Ste 7B, New Haven, CT 06510; **Phone:** 203-785-6060; **Board Cert:** Surgery 2004; **Med School:** Univ Mass Sch Med 1996; **Resid:** Surgery, UMass Meml Med Ctr 2003; **Fellow:** Surgery, NY-Presby/Weill Cornell Univ Med Ctr 2004; **Fac Appt:** Assoc Prof S, Yale Univ

Emre, Sukru MD (S) - **Spec Exp:** Transplant-Liver-Adult & Pediatric; Hepatobiliary Surgery; Liver Cancer; Portal Hypertension; **Hospital:** Yale-New Haven Hosp, Yale Med Group (page 940); **Address:** 330 Cedar St, FMB121 Bldg - Fl 1, FMB 121, New Haven, CT 07520-8062; **Phone:** 203-737-2804; **Med School:** Turkey 1977; **Resid:** Surgery, Univ Istanbul 1982; **Fellow:** Hepatobiliary Surgery, Univ Istanbul 1988; Transplant Surgery, Mount Sinai Med Ctr 1994; **Fac Appt:** Prof S, Yale Univ

Kurtzman, Scott H MD (S) - **Spec Exp:** Breast Cancer & Surgery; Sarcoma; **Hospital:** Waterbury Hosp; **Address:** 1625 Straits Tpke, Ste 200, Middlebury, CT 06762; **Phone:** 203-568-2929; · **Board Cert:** Surgery 2009; **Med School:** Albany Med Coll 1981; **Resid:** Surgery, Univ Maryland Hosp 1983; Surgery, UMDNJ Affil Hosp 1988; **Fellow:** Surgical Oncology, Natl Cancer Inst 1985; Surgical Oncology, Meml Sloan Kettering Cancer Ctr 1990; **Fac Appt:** Prof S, Univ Conn

Lannin, Donald R MD (S) - **Spec Exp:** Breast Cancer; Breast Surgery; **Hospital:** Yale-New Haven Hosp, Yale Med Group (page 940); **Address:** Yale-New Haven Breast Ctr, 20 York St, New Haven, CT 06510; **Phone:** 203-785-2328; **Board Cert:** Surgery 2002; **Med School:** Univ Minn 1974; **Resid:** Surgery, Univ Minnesota Med Ctr 1982; **Fac Appt:** Prof S, Yale Univ

Nadzam, Geoffrey S MD (S) - **Spec Exp:** Obesity/Bariatric Surgery; **Hospital:** Yale-New Haven Hosp - St Raphael Campus; **Address:** Orchard Surgical Specialists, 330 Orchard St, Ste 309, New Haven, CT 06511; **Phone:** 203-776-4677; **Board Cert:** Surgery 2004; **Med School:** UMDNJ-NJ Med Sch, Newark 1996; **Resid:** Surgery, Stanford Univ Med Ctr 2002; **Fellow:** Bariatric Surgery, Stanford Univ 2004; Robotic Surgery, Stanford Univ 2004

Salem, Ronald R MD (S) - **Spec Exp:** Cancer Surgery; Liver & Biliary Surgery; Gastrointestinal Cancer; Liver Cancer; **Hospital:** Yale-New Haven Hosp, Yale Med Group (page 940); **Address:** Dept Surgery, 333 Cedar St, FMB 130, New Haven, CT 06520-8062; **Phone:** 203-785-3577; **Board Cert:** Surgery 2011; **Med School:** Zimbabwe 1978; **Resid:** Surgery, Hammersmith Hosp 1985; Surgery, New England Deaconess Hosp 1989; **Fac Appt:** Prof S, Yale Univ

Sosa, Julie A MD (S) - **Spec Exp:** Thyroid Cancer; Parathyroid Cancer; Endocrine Cancers; **Hospital:** Yale-New Haven Hosp; **Address:** 800 Howard Ave, New Haven, CT 06520; **Phone:** 203-785-2314; **Board Cert:** Surgery 2004; **Med School:** Johns Hopkins Univ 1994; **Resid:** Surgery, Johns Hopkins Hosp 2001; **Fellow:** Surgical Oncology, Johns Hoplins Hosp 2002; **Fac Appt:** Assoc Prof S, Yale Univ

Udelsman, Robert MD (S) - **Spec Exp:** Parathyroid Cancer; Adrenal Tumors; Thyroid Cancer; Endocrine Surgery; **Hospital:** Yale-New Haven Hosp, Yale Med Group (page 940); **Address:** Yale-New Haven Hosp, Dept Surgery, 330 Cedar St, Box 208062, New Haven, CT 06520-8062; **Phone:** 203-785-2697; **Board Cert:** Surgery 2009; **Med School:** Geo Wash Univ 1981; **Resid:** Surgery, Natl Inst Hlth 1986; Surgery, Johns Hopkins Hosp 1989; **Fellow:** Gastrointestinal Surgery, Johns Hopkins Hosp 1990; Surgical Oncology, Natl Cancer Inst 1985; **Fac Appt:** Prof S, Yale Univ

Thoracic & Cardiac Surgery

Detterbeck, Frank C MD (T&CS) - **Spec Exp:** Lung Cancer; Mediastinal Tumors; **Hospital:** Yale-New Haven Hosp; **Address:** Yale Sch Medicine - Thoracic Surg, 330 Cedar St, BB205, New Haven, CT 06520-8062; **Phone:** 203-785-4931; **Board Cert:** Thoracic Surgery 2011; **Med School:** Northwestern Univ 1983; **Resid:** Surgery, Virginia Mason Hosp 1988; **Fellow:** Cardiothoracic Surgery, Univ North Carolina Hosps 1991; **Fac Appt:** Prof S, Yale Univ

Elefteriades, John MD (T&CS) - **Spec Exp:** Aneurysm-Thoracic Aortic; Transplant-Heart; Ventricular Assist Device (LVAD); **Hospital:** Yale-New Haven Hosp, Yale Med Group (page 940); **Address:** 333 Cedar St, Boardman 2, Dept Cardiothoracic Surgery, PO Box 208039, New Haven, CT 06520; **Phone:** 203-785-2705; **Board Cert:** Thoracic Surgery 2004; **Med School:** Yale Univ 1976; **Resid:** Surgery, Yale-New Haven Hosp 1981; Cardiothoracic Surgery, Yale-New Haven Hosp 1983; **Fellow:** Cardiothoracic Surgery, Yale-New Haven Hosp 1983; **Fac Appt:** Prof S, Yale Univ

Hashim, Sabet W MD (T&CS) - **Spec Exp:** Mitral Valve Surgery; Heart Valve Surgery; Maze Procedure for Atrial Fibrillation; **Hospital:** Yale-New Haven Hosp, Yale Med Group (page 940); **Address:** Yale Univ Cardiothoracic Surgery, 330 Cedar St, Ste BB204, PO Box 208039, New Haven, CT 06520-8039; **Phone:** 203-785-6214; **Board Cert:** Thoracic Surgery 2001; **Med School:** Lebanon 1975; **Resid:** Surgery, St Lukes Roosevely Hosp 1979; Cardiothoracic Surgery, Yale-New Haven Hosp 1981; **Fac Appt:** Assoc Prof S, Yale Univ

Kopf, Gary S MD (T&CS) - **Spec Exp:** Cardiac Surgery; Pediatric Cardiothoracic Surgery; Congenital Heart Disease; **Hospital:** Yale-New Haven Hosp, Yale Med Group (page 940); **Address:** Yale Univ Sch Med, Dept of Surgery, Box 208039, New Haven, CT 06520-8039; **Phone:** 203-785-2702; **Board Cert:** Thoracic Surgery 2011; **Med School:** Harvard Med Sch 1970; **Resid:** Surgery, Peter Bent Brigham Hosp 1977; Cardiothoracic Surgery, Chldns Hosp Med Ctr 1980; **Fellow:** Cardiothoracic Surgery, Peter Bent Brigham Hosp 1980; **Fac Appt:** Prof S, Yale Univ

Sanchez, Juan A MD (T&CS) - **Spec Exp:** Lung Surgery; Esophageal Surgery; Cardiac Surgery; Thymoma; **Hospital:** St. Mary's Hosp - Waterbury, Bridgeport Hosp; **Address:** 56 Franklin St, Waterbury, CT 06706; **Phone:** 203-709-6315; **Board Cert:** Thoracic Surgery 2004; Surgery 2008; **Med School:** Univ Fla Coll Med 1984; **Resid:** Surgery, Georgetown Univ 1989; Thoracic Surgery, Yale-New Haven Hosp 1993; **Fellow:** Research, Columbia-Presby Med Ctr 1990; Transplant Surgery, Yale-New Haven Hosp 1991; **Fac Appt:** Prof S, Univ Conn

Urology

Colberg, John W MD (U) - **Spec Exp:** Prostate Cancer; Bladder Cancer; Kidney Cancer; Testicular Cancer; **Hospital:** Yale-New Haven Hosp, Yale Med Group (page 940); **Address:** 20 York St, New Haven, CT 06510; **Phone:** 203-785-2815; **Board Cert:** Urology 2001; **Med School:** Washington Univ, St Louis 1985; **Resid:** Surgery, Yale-New Haven Hosp 1987; Urology, Yale-New Haven Hosp 1990; **Fac Appt:** Assoc Prof U, Yale Univ

Flanagan, Michael J MD (U) - **Spec Exp:** Prostate Disease; Incontinence; Incontinence-Fecal; **Hospital:** Waterbury Hosp, St. Mary's Hosp - Waterbury; **Address:** Urology Specialists, 1579 Straits Tpke, Ste 2A, Middlebury, CT 06762; **Phone:** 203-757-8361; **Board Cert:** Urology 2003; **Med School:** UMDNJ-Univ Med Dent NJ 1985; **Resid:** Surgery, Waterbury Hosp 1988; Urology, Temple Univ Hosp 1992

Foster Jr, Harris E MD (U) - **Spec Exp:** Incontinence; Urodynamics; Voiding Dysfunction; Urology-Female; **Hospital:** Yale-New Haven Hosp, Yale Med Group (page 940); **Address:** 35 Park St, New Haven, CT 06520-8062; **Phone:** 203-200-4822; **Board Cert:** Urology 2012; **Med School:** Univ Miami Sch Med 1987; **Resid:** Surgery, Univ Michigan Med Ctr 1989; Urology, Univ Michigan Med Ctr 1992; **Fac Appt:** Prof U, Yale Univ

Passarelli, Marianne MD (U) - **Spec Exp:** Urology-Female; Incontinence; **Hospital:** Yale-New Haven Hosp - St Raphael Campus, Yale-New Haven Hosp; **Address:** 9 Washington Ave, Ste 3A, Hamden, CT 06518; **Phone:** 203-288-4663; **Board Cert:** Urology 2003; **Med School:** Univ VT Coll Med 1986; **Resid:** Surgery, SUNY Hlth Sci Ctr 1988; Urology, SUNY Hlth Sci Ctr 1992

Singh, Dinesh MD (U) - **Spec Exp:** Laparoscopic Surgery; Robotic Surgery; Kidney Cancer; Prostate Cancer; **Hospital:** Yale-New Haven Hosp, Yale Med Group (page 940); **Address:** 35 Park St Fl 4, New Haven, CT 06519; **Phone:** 203-785-2815; **Board Cert:** Urology 2006; **Med School:** Columbia P&S 1997; **Resid:** Surgery, Brigham & Women's Hosp 1999; Urology, Harvard Med Sch Affil Hosp 2003; **Fellow:** Research, Dana Farber Cancer Inst 2001; Laparoscopic Surgery, Cleveland Clin 2004; **Fac Appt:** Asst Prof U, Yale Univ

Weiss, Robert M MD (U) - **Spec Exp:** Pediatric Urology; Testicular Cancer; Penile Cancer; Bladder Cancer; **Hospital:** Yale-New Haven Hosp, Yale Med Group (page 940); **Address:** 1 Long Wharf Drive, New Haven, CT 06511; **Phone:** 203-785-2815; **Board Cert:** Urology 1970; **Med School:** SUNY Downstate 1960; **Resid:** Surgery, Beth Israel Hosp 1962; Urology, Columbia Presby Hosp 1967; **Fellow:** Pharmacology, Columbia Presby Hosp 1965; **Fac Appt:** Prof U, Yale Univ

Vascular & Interventional Radiology

Aruny, John E MD (VIR) - **Spec Exp:** Thrombolytic Therapy; Dialysis Access; Vascular Disease; Vein Disorders; **Hospital:** Yale-New Haven Hosp, Yale Med Group (page 940); **Address:** Yale Univ School of Medicine, 333 Cedar St, New Haven, CT 06520; **Phone:** 203-785-7026; **Board Cert:** Diag Rad with Spec Comp in Nuc Rad 1989; Vascular & Interventional Radiology 2009; **Med School:** Mexico 1983; **Resid:** Diagnostic Radiology, Westch Co Med Ctr 1989; **Fellow:** Interventional Radiology, Brigham & Women's Hosp 1992; **Fac Appt:** Assoc Prof Rad, Yale Univ

White Jr, Robert I MD (VIR) - **Spec Exp:** Uterine Fibroid Embolization; Pelvic Congestion Syndrome; Varicocele Embolization; Hereditary Hemorrhagic Telangiectasia; **Hospital:** Yale-New Haven Hosp, Yale Med Group (page 940); **Address:** Yale Univ Sch Med, Vasc & Interventional Rad, PO Box 208042, New Haven, CT 06520-8042; **Phone:** 203-737-5395; **Board Cert:** Diagnostic Radiology 1970; **Med School:** Baylor Coll Med 1963; **Resid:** Internal Medicine, Johns Hopkins Hosp 1967; Diagnostic Radiology, Johns Hopkins Hosp 1969; **Fellow:** Cardiovascular Disease, Johns Hopkins Hosp 1958; Cardiovascular Radiology, Univ Minn Med Ctr 1971; **Fac Appt:** Prof Rad, Yale Univ

Vascular Surgery

DeNatale, Ralph MD (VascS) - **Hospital:** Yale-New Haven Hosp - St Raphael Campus, Yale-New Haven Hosp; **Address:** Connecticut Vascular Ctr, 280 State St, North Haven, CT 06473; **Phone:** 203-288-2886; **Board Cert:** Vascular Surgery 2009; **Med School:** Italy 1979; **Resid:** Surgery, Hosp St Raphael 1984; Vascular Surgery, Baylor Coll Med 1985; **Fellow:** Cardiovascular Surgery, Baylor Coll Med 1986

Sumpio, Bauer E MD/PhD (VascS) - **Spec Exp:** Diabetic Leg/Foot; Endovascular Surgery; **Hospital:** Yale-New Haven Hosp, Yale Med Group (page 940); **Address:** Yale Univ School Medicine, Dept Surgery, 333 Cedar St, Box 208062, BB 204, New Haven, CT 06520; **Phone:** 203-785-6217; **Board Cert:** Vascular Surgery 2009; Surgery 2009; **Med School:** Cornell Univ-Weill Med Coll 1980; **Resid:** Surgery, Yale-New Haven Hosp 1986; **Fellow:** Vascular Surgery, Univ N Carolina Hosp 1987; **Fac Appt:** Prof S, Yale Univ

Sweeney, Thomas F MD (VascS) - **Spec Exp:** Minimally Invasive Vascular Surgery; Varicose Veins; Vein Disorders; **Hospital:** Yale-New Haven Hosp, Yale-New Haven Hosp - St Raphael Campus; **Address:** 280 State St, North Haven, CT 06473; **Phone:** 203-288-2886; **Board Cert:** Vascular Surgery 2008; **Med School:** Yale Univ 1973; **Resid:** Surgery, Yale-New Haven Hosp 1977; **Fellow:** Vascular Surgery, Yale-New Haven Hosp 1978; **Fac Appt:** Assoc Clin Prof S, Yale Univ

Section Four

Centers of Excellence

Adolescent Medicine

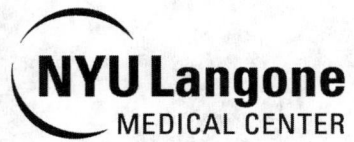
CHILD STUDY CENTER

The Child Study Center is the world's leading institution for transformative science and innovation in the diagnosis and treatment of children with mental illness and learning disabilities. Since 1997, The Child Study Center has treated thousands of children from around the world at its Faculty Group Practices in Manhattan and satellite clinical campuses in New Jersey and Long Island. Through its website, www.AboutOurKids.org, and through professional education programs, parents and practitioners are provided with the tools and knowledge needed to promote children's mental health. The Child Study Center, part of the Hassenfeld Pediatric Center, as well as NYU Langone's Department of Child and Adolescent Psychiatry, provides the following services:

Anxiety and Mood Disorders
The Anita Saltz Institute for Anxiety and Mood Disorders offers the most advanced treatment and evaluation of children, adolescents and young adults. Our psychopharmacologists are experts in understanding the issues of treating children with bipolar disorder and our researchers explore treatments for children with severe temper outbursts and adolescent depression.

Attention Deficit Hyperactivity and Behavior Disorders
The Institute for Attention Deficit Hyperactivity and Behavior Disorders focuses on the treatment of ADHD. Our Parent-Child Interaction Therapy Program (PCIT) offers state-of-the-art treatment for behavioral problems in young children and is the largest program of its kind in the Northeast.

Autism, Asperger's Syndrome and Communication Disorders
The Autism Spectrum programs at the Child Study Center provide extensive evaluations for toddlers and preschoolers with social and communication difficulties. Our Early Social Interaction treatment is a home-based intervention for children identified with symptoms of autism. Center specialists are also experienced at supporting the needs of teens and young adults who have been diagnosed with Asperger's.

Learning Disorders
The Institute for Learning and Academic Achievement evaluates children with suspected learning weaknesses or poor academic achievement using a multidisciplinary team-based approach.

Tics and Tourette Disorder
The Center's Tics and Tourette Clinical and Research programs are dedicated to the evaluation and treatment of individuals with tics, Tourette disorder and related problems. Treatment includes Habit Reversal Therapy (HRT).

Birthing Services

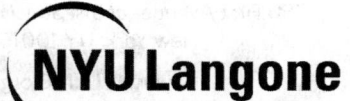

550 First Avenue *(at 31st Street)*
New York, NY 10016
www.NYULMC.org
Physician Referral: **888-7-NYU-MED** *(888-769-8633)*

OBSTETRICS AND GYNECOLOGY

About the Department of Obstetrics and Gynecology
NYU Langone Medical Center provides comprehensive programs and services designed specifically for women, from primary care to highly specialized programs that are supported by sophisticated research and advanced training. We specialize in the following areas:

Fertility-Related Services
NYU Langone offers state-of-the-art programs in egg donation, egg freezing and wellness (acupuncture, mind/body, psychology and yoga). Diagnosis and treatment include ovulation induction, assisted reproductive technologies and surgical options that incorporate the latest endoscopic techniques. The Center also tests for genetic abnormalities, as well as for immunity and infectious diseases.

Gynecologic Oncology
The NCI-designated NYU Cancer Institute's Women's Cancer Program specializes in the treatment of cervical cancer, endometrial cancer, ovarian cancer, uterine cancer, vaginal cancer and vulvar cancer.

Maternal Fetal Medicine
Prenatal care for high-risk pregnancies and detailed consultations before, during and after pregnancy are offered. Special attention is given to multifetal pregnancies and to women who have other medical conditions that may complicate a pregnancy, such as diabetes, heart problems, high blood pressure and lupus.

Obstetrics
We offer a broad range of obstetrical services, including prenatal care that gives equal emphasis to the well-being of the mother and the fetus; fetal monitoring through ultrasound and other techniques; childbirth preparedness and breastfeeding classes; consultation for high-risk pregnancies, including treatment for women who have experienced recurrent pregnancy loss.

Specialty Services
In addition to routine gynecological care, we offer pelvic ultrasound; aspiration of breast cysts; evaluation of infertility (including the special needs of same-sex couples); colposcopy (a diagnostic evaluation of abnormal pap smears); LEEP (a loop electrosurgical procedure used to diagnose and treat cervical cancer); cryotherapy for vaginal warts; and bone density testing.

Urogynecology and Reconstructive Pelvic Surgery
Our urogynecologists treat all forms of incontinence and pelvic disorders; malformations of the reproductive tract found at birth, during childhood or in young adults; and conditions such as overactive bladder, urinary and/or fecal incontinence and pelvic organ prolapse.

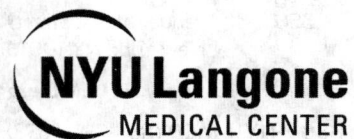

MATERNAL-FETAL MEDICINE

About the Division of Maternal-Fetal Medicine

The Division of Maternal-Fetal Medicine at NYU Langone Medical Center is committed to ensuring that both mother and fetus receive the highly specialized care they need. The Division focuses on multifetal pregnancies, genetic counseling, women who have miscarried, preterm deliveries and other medical complications that can occur during pregnancy. We also specialize in helping women who have other medical conditions that may complicate a pregnancy, such as diabetes, heart problems, high blood pressure, and lupus, among others. The Division offers the latest techniques for in-utero diagnosis and treatment as well as advanced care of complex obstetrical patients. We specialize in the following areas:

Patient Care

The Division of Maternal-Fetal Medicine focuses on ensuring that each patient delivers a healthy baby. Using minimally invasive techniques, doctors at NYU Langone Medical Center are able to repair a number of life-threatening conditions in a child before it is even born, reducing the risks of preterm labor and the need for Cesarean births. Our physicians have developed numerous new treatment protocols for high-risk obstetrics that have been adopted around the world.

Research

The Division of Maternal-Fetal Medicine has generated new treatments for high-risk obstetrics patients and introduced effective new methods of diagnosis and treatment for the fetus.

The Best in American Medicine
www.CastleConnolly.com

Breast Disease

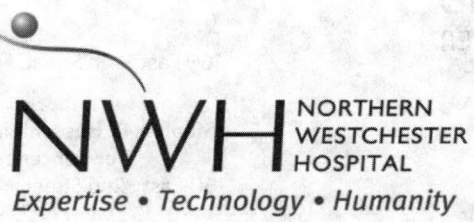

Expertise • Technology • Humanity

<u>The Breast Institute at Northern Westchester</u> Hospital (NWH) provides an environment of compassion, comfort, and expert medical support. Our staff of dedicated professionals includes oncologists, radiologists, and surgeons with specialized training in using the latest techniques for restoring women to the best possible health. The Breast Institute's Care Team treats your needs—physical, emotional, and spiritual—as our top priorities in one convenient hospital-based location, using innovative, leading-edge technologies.

<u>Northern Westchester Hospital (NWH)</u> provides quality, patient centered care that is close to home through the right combination of medical expertise, leading edge technology, and a commitment to humanity. Over 750 highly skilled physicians, state-of-the-art technology and professional staff of caregivers are all in place to ensure that you and your family receive treatment in a caring, respectful and nurturing environment.

NWH has established extensive internal quality measurements that surpass the standards defined by the Centers for Medicare & Medicaid Services (CMS) and the Hospital Quality Alliance (HQA) National Hospital Quality Measures. Our high quality standards help to ensure that the treatment you receive at NWH is among the best in the nation. For a complete list of our services, please visit www.nwhc.net.

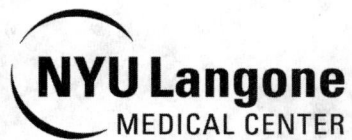

NYU Langone Medical Center
550 First Avenue , New York, NY 10016
www.NYULMC.org

Clinical Cancer Center
160 East 34th Street, New York, NY 10016
www.NYUCI.org

**The Stephen D. Hassenfeld Children's Center
for Cancer and Blood Disorders**
160 East 32nd Street, New York, NY 10016
www.NYUMC.org/Hassenfeld

NYU CANCER INSTITUTE

The NYU Cancer Institute is an NCI-designated cancer center providing personalized patient care that is compassionate and state-of-the-art. The doctors and researchers work together to develop innovative therapies for patients. The Cancer Institute is world-renowned for excellence in cancer-focused research, personalized care, education and community outreach. Its mission is to discover the origins of human cancer and to use that knowledge to eradicate the personal and societal burden of cancer in our community, the nation and the world. For more information about our expert physicians, call 212-731-5000.

Patient-Focused Setting

The Clinical Cancer Center is the principal outpatient facility of The Cancer Institute. The Center and its multidisciplinary team of experts provide access to the latest treatment options and clinical trials, along with a variety of programs in cancer risk reduction/prevention, screening, diagnostics, genetic counseling and supportive services. In addition, the Center emphasizes the importance of a holistic approach involving integrative health, psychosocial support, survivorship and palliative care. Radiology and infusion services are available in Rego Park, NY, as well.

Renowned Expertise

The NYU Cancer Institute brings together experts from a variety of disciplines to create collaborative research endeavors and clinical care teams. It offers a continuum of personalized care, from prevention through diagnosis, treatment and post-treatment support. Additionally, we have created special programs to treat diseases such as breast cancer, brain cancer, melanoma, GI cancer, prostate cancer, hematologic malignancies and lung cancer, as well as translational programs in cancer healthcare disparities, molecularly targeted therapy, and the cell signaling pathways involved in cancer.

A Translational Approach

Our scientists and researchers excel in uncovering how cancer develops at the molecular level, and how we can harness that knowledge to reduce the risk of cancer and treat the disease.

Stephen D. Hassenfeld Children's Center for Cancer and Blood Disorders

The center is a leading pediatric outpatient facility for the treatment of childhood cancers and blood diseases. Its unique interdisciplinary and family-centered approach combines the most advanced medical treatments with psychosocial and emotional support services for young patients and their families.

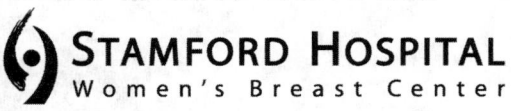

STAMFORD HOSPITAL
Women's Breast Center

Women's Breast Center

Stamford Hospital's Women's Breast Center is the first center in the nation to be recognized as a national Accreditation Program for Breast Centers. Our Center offers women a multi-disciplinary approach to care by focusing on imaging, pathology, medical and radiation oncology, genetic testing, nursing, and surgical care to treat diseases of the breast. Our facility is one of five out of the state's 133 breast imaging centers to have been designated a Breast Imaging Center of Excellence by the American College of Radiology.

Advanced Technology

The only breast center in the region and among the first in the country, to offer 3-D breast tomosynthesis for breast screening mammography. Used in conjunction with a traditional digital mammogram, 3-D breast tomosynthesis presents a clearer more definitive image.

Multi-disciplinary Team Approach

Our expert team is comprised of fellowship-trained female breast surgeons, reconstructive plastic surgeons, breast imaging fellowship-trained radiologists, breast pathologists, medical and radiation oncologists, nurse navigator and genetic counselor. The team meets on a weekly basis to discuss the best possible individualized treatment for each patient.

Personalized Care

In the event a problem is identified, our patients will have immediate follow up testing, see a surgeon within 24–26 hours and have the support of a dedicated nurse navigator to guide them through the process, from diagnosis through treatment and beyond. We work closely with the Integrative Medicine and Wellness team and the Bennett Cancer Center, in providing support services. We offer a warm setting for breast care designed with soft touches to make each and every patient feel as relaxed and comfortable as possible.

Academic and Clinical Affiliations

Stamford Hospital is an affiliate of the New York–Presbyterian Healthcare System and a major teaching affiliate of the Columbia University College of Physicians & Surgeons.

Accreditation

Joint Commission on Accreditation of Healthcare Organization (JCAHO)

Beds

305

Sponsorship

Voluntary, Not-for-Profit

For a Physician Referral or more information, please call 1.877.233.9355 or visit StamfordHospital.org /doctor.

Stamford Hospital
30 Shelburne Road
Stamford, CT 06902
203.276.1000

StamfordHospital.org

Cancer Care

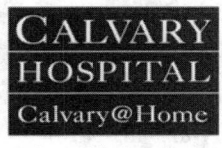

Where Life Continues

CALVARY HOSPITAL
1740 Eastchester Road
Bronx, NY 10461
Tel: (718) 518-2000
www.calvaryhospital.org

PALLIATIVE CARE INSTITUTE
Calvary's Teaching and Research Arm

The mission of the Palliative Care Institute (PCI), which was founded in 1985, is to transmit, through research and education, Calvary's competence in the care of patients with advanced disease. To date, we have welcomed healthcare professionals from more than 30 countries.

Each year, we train more than 800 medical students, residents, and fellows in palliative care. This includes formalized palliative care observership rotations for residency and fellowship programs throughout the New York area, including Memorial Sloan-Kettering Cancer Center, Mount Sinai School of Medicine, and State University of New York Health Science Center at Brooklyn.

A Model for Excellent Care

Calvary earned a reputation for skillful and compassionate control of patients' symptoms long before palliative and hospice care became popular disciplines.

In 2005, the National Cancer Institute designated Calvary an "international center for training in palliative care" and an alliance was formed between the NCI, Calvary Hospital, and the Middle East Cancer Consortium. Through this alliance, physicians and nurses from Israel, Jordan, Cyprus, Turkey, Egypt, and the Palestinian Authority are sent to Calvary to learn palliative care and increase access to palliative care throughout the Middle East.

Wound Care

The PCI directs Calvary Hospital's Center for Curative and Palliative Wound Care, dedicated to the treatment of complex, intractable wounds related to diabetes, cancer, peripheral vascular disease, and other disorders. For more information about our outstanding wound care services, call (718) 518-2577.

Research Initiatives

The PCI conducts research focusing on wound care, the psychological and emotional impact of terminal illness on patients and families, pain management, and ethical issues concerning end-of-life care.

> *For more information about*
> *Calvary's Palliative Care Institute,*
> *please call (718) 518-2147.*

For more information about the Regional Cancer Center, call 1-877-HOLY-NAME. Please mention "Castle Connolly Guide."

718 Teaneck Road
Teaneck, NJ 07666
1-877-HOLY-NAME
(1-877-465-9626)
www.holyname.org

Holy Name Medical Center
Regional Cancer Center

Holy Name Medical Center's Regional Cancer Center offers leading-edge diagnosis, staging and treatment services for people with cancer. Holy Name's outstanding team of board-certified specialists cares for patients in an environment that promotes personalized service and ready access to multiple disciplines. The Regional Cancer Center is accredited by the American College of Radiology, the American Society for Radiation Oncology, and the American College of Surgeons Commission on Cancer as a Comprehensive Community Cancer Program— accreditations that ensure access to a broad spectrum of services, and high-quality patient care, safety and technical standards.

A TEAM APPROACH

Individualized treatment plans are formulated not by a single physician, but with input from medical, radiation and surgical oncologists, pathologists and radiologists; specially trained and certified oncology nurses; and other medical specialists who render care in both outpatient and inpatient settings. State-of-the-art noninvasive technologies, including fusion PET/CT, high-resolution CT, PET, MRI, breast MRI, extremity MRI and low-dose mammography, produce exquisitely detailed images for diagnostic and treatment planning purposes.

PATIENT-CENTERED CARE

Holy Name simplifies the logistics associated with cancer therapy with ready access to services and physicians, minimal waiting, and easy parking. Oncology patients needing emergency care related to their diagnosis are admitted directly to the specialized nursing unit, without the delays associated with first visiting the Emergency Care Center.

The Regional Cancer Center features a one-stop concept with the full range of services located in a single convenient setting. Patients can arrange a consultation with their oncologist, receive radiation treatment or chemotherapy, have imaging procedures, biopsies and other tests, and receive physical rehabilitation. They can meet with the Center's oncology-certified dietitian, take part in a support group or seek the assistance of a social worker. Genetic counselors are available to work with patients and their family members.

**Accurate diagnosis and staging +
Targeted, precision therapy =
Fewer complications, minimal side
effects and improved outcomes**

- PET and fusion PET/CT
- High-resolution CT and MRI
- Breast MRI
- SPECT imaging
- Low-dose digital mammography
- Robotic-assisted surgery
- Intensity-modulated radiation therapy (IMRT)
- Image-guided radiation therapy (IGRT)
- CT-guided prone breast radiation therapy
- Stereotactic body radiotherapy (SBRT)
- High-dose brachytherapy for prostate
- Stereotactic radiosurgery
- Microsphere embolization for liver
- Radiofrequency ablation
- Clinical research trials
- Supportive care, nutrition and pharmacy services, physical rehabilitation, palliative services, and home care
- Genetic counseling

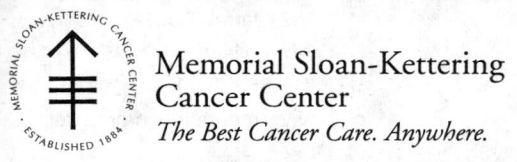

Memorial Sloan-Kettering Cancer Center
The Best Cancer Care. Anywhere.

1275 York Avenue
New York, NY 10065
Make an Appointment: (800) 525-2225
www.mskcc.org

At Memorial Sloan-Kettering Cancer Center, our sole focus is cancer. Our doctors are among the most skilled and experienced in the world in treating all kinds of cancer. The knowledge, talent, and expertise of our medical professionals lead to superb patient care, and often, a significant positive impact on the chances that a patient's cancer will be cured or controlled.

TREATMENT PLANNING BY TEAMS OF SPECIALISTS

Our patients benefit from individualized treatment plans developed by a team of specialists with unsurpassed depth and breadth of experience. The teams include surgeons, medical and radiation oncologists, radiologists, pathologists, nurses, and others who are specialists in a specific type of cancer. They develop treatment plans that reflect their combined expertise, so patients who need several different types of therapy will receive the best combination for them.

RESEARCH EXPANDS TREATMENT OPTIONS

One of Memorial Sloan-Kettering's great strengths is the close relationship between scientists and clinicians. Through the constant collaboration between our doctors and research scientists, new drugs and therapies developed in the laboratory can be quickly translated into improved treatment options for patients.

NURSING AND SUPPORTIVE CARE

Nurses are essential members of the healthcare team. Our specially trained oncology nurses care for patients throughout their treatment, help manage clinical trials, and educate patients about all aspects of their care.

Specialized psychiatrists and psychologists help patients deal with the stress, anxiety, and depression that sometimes accompany cancer and its treatment. Our social workers ensure that patients who need it receive assistance with needs such as housing and transportation. They offer individual and family counseling, as well as support groups for both inpatients and outpatients. After treatment, the Post-Treatment Resource Program offers patients seminars, lectures, support groups, and practical advice on various issues such as insurance and employment.

INTEGRATIVE MEDICINE

Our Integrative Medicine Service offers a full range of complementary therapies, including massage, reflexology, meditation, music therapy, and acupuncture. These do not replace medical care but are used along with clinical treatments to help patients relieve stress, reduce pain and anxiety, manage symptoms, and promote a feeling of well-being.

INSURANCE

Memorial Sloan-Kettering Cancer Center is in-network with most New York–area insurance plans.

A TRADITION OF EXCELLENCE

From its founding in 1884, Memorial Sloan-Kettering Cancer Center has been guided by a clear mission: to offer the best possible care for patients today, and to seek strategies to prevent, control, and ultimately cure cancer in the future. We are proud of our designation as one of the few select National Cancer Institute Comprehensive Cancer Centers and a member of the National Comprehensive Cancer Network.

To see one of our specialized cancer experts, call us at (800) 525-2225.

Sponsorship: Private, Non-Profit

Beds: 470

Accreditation: Awarded Accreditation from the Joint Commission on Accreditation of Healthcare Organizations (JCAHO)

Locations in Manhattan, Westchester, Long Island and New Jersey.

MAKE AN APPOINTMENT: (800) 525-2225

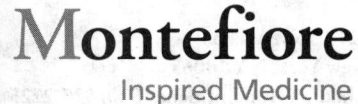

1521 Jarrett Place
Bronx, New York 10461
718-862-8840
www.montefiore.org/cancer

Montefiore Einstein Center for Cancer Care

Montefiore Einstein Center for Cancer Care works closely with its research partner, the National Cancer Institute–designated Albert Einstein Cancer Center, to deliver groundbreaking treatments for patients with common and rare cancers. The Center for Cancer Care's renowned clinicians deliver multidisciplinary care that is supported by cutting-edge technologies and treatments, including the latest da Vinci SI robotic surgical equipment, minimally invasive procedures, GPS-powered image-guided radiation therapy, high-energy focused ultrasound, and targeted immunotherapies that zero in on tumors and protect healthy tissue.

The Center for Cancer Care provides patients with novel drug treatments and delivery systems that are designed with the primary goal of reducing toxicity while increasing effectiveness. **It is the first facility in the Northeast to provide regional perfusion therapy.** This procedure isolates the abdominal cavity or the blood circulatory system in the arms, legs or liver and then delivers concentrated doses of anticancer drugs to the targeted area of the body at levels higher than can be safely given intravenously.

Montefiore is also one of a select number of medical centers offering high-dose interleukin-2 (IL-2) therapy, a complex therapy that achieves complete remission in some patients with advanced-stage melanoma. Physicians at Montefiore are currently conducting clinical trials of a promising group of targeted agents known as B-RAF inhibitors, as well as immunotherapy with anti-CTLA-4.

Patients with liver cancer who are candidates for surgical resection may benefit from **robotic-assisted lobectomy, a recent addition to Montefiore's treatment caché that offers the potential for reduced surgical risk and postoperative discomfort.**

The Center for Cancer Care offers more than 100 clinical trials. These involve orally administered drugs, inhaled drugs for the prevention and treatment of lung cancer, and molecularly targeted and genetically driven therapies. The Center for Cancer Care was also one of five sites recently selected for a $15 million National Institutes of Health grant to study the development of "nanomedicines" to treat patients with pancreatic and ovarian cancer.

The Center for Cancer Care is leading the field in optimizing the patient experience through our Patient Navigator program, which partners patients with staff members who manage their journey through the care process so that patients can focus on getting well.

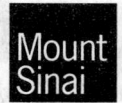
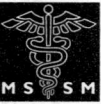

MOUNT SINAI
SCHOOL OF
MEDICINE

THE TISCH CANCER INSTITUTE
AT THE MOUNT SINAI MEDICAL CENTER

One Gustave L. Levy Place
Fifth Avenue and 100th Street
New York, NY 10029-6574
Physician Referral: 1-800-MD-SINAI (637-4624)
www.tischcancerinstitute.org

THE TISCH CANCER INSTITUTE is embedded within a renowned medical center that has world-class research facilities, one of the nation's top-ranked hospitals, and an outstanding medical school. Patients have access to the best possible cancer care across a variety of disciplines, including hematology and medical oncology, surgery, radiation therapy, bone marrow transplantation, radiology, palliative care, psychosocial services, and clinical trials. For fully integrated, multidisciplinary care, our patients are also treated by the best specialists in every field at Mount Sinai and can receive seamless referrals.

Services and Programs – The Tisch Cancer Institute employs a multidisciplinary treatment approach, providing access to clinical breakthroughs, innovative techniques, leading-edge technologies, and a wide range of diagnostic, therapeutic, and support services for all types of cancer. The Institute treats: breast cancer; hematological malignancies (including multiple myeloma, myelodysplastic syndrome, and myeloproliferative disorders); genitourinary cancers (including prostate, bladder, and kidney); head and neck cancers; thoracic cancer (including lung and esophagus); gynecologic cancers; brain tumors; and other diagnoses. In addition to surgical treatment, the Institute provides radiation and medical oncology therapies, as well as bone marrow transplantation. The Dubin Breast Center, consisting of 15,000 square feet, is a recently constructed facility that opened in April 2011 and significantly expands the treatment space for breast cancer patients. In 2012, the Derald H. Ruttenberg Treatment Center will double in size upon its move to the Leon and Norma Hess Center for Science and Medicine at 1470 Madison Avenue (at 101st Street).

THE RUTTENBERG TREATMENT CENTER
The Derald H. Ruttenberg Treatment Center houses the ambulatory cancer program of The Tisch Cancer Institute and is operated by the Mount Sinai Hospital.

THE DUBIN BREAST CARE CENTER
The Dubin Breast Care Center offers the latest, most innovative approaches available for breast health and the treatment of breast cancer.

The Tisch Cancer Institute encourages collaboration with colleagues across the Medical Center, drawing upon the knowledge of a vast network of specialists who are outstanding in their fields. These experts consist of award-winning physicians and surgeons specializing in cardiac care, neurology, urology, pediatrics, digestive diseases, obstetrics and gynecology, and other therapeutic areas. Oncologists, surgeons, radiation oncologists, and specialists from across the medical spectrum work together to provide the highest quality care to all cancer patients. Furthermore, Mount Sinai's nursing staff is an important part of the Medical Center's focus on delivering exceptional patient care, and it has received the prestigious Magnet Award for nursing excellence. Mount Sinai is also renowned for its palliative care program, which provides the highest level of care, focusing on the relief of pain, symptoms, and stress in cancer patients in both an inpatient and outpatient setting.

A Heritage of Breakthroughs – Teams of physicians and scientists at The Tisch Cancer Institute at Mount Sinai work together to rapidly translate laboratory research into new patient treatments. Among the advances pioneered at Mount Sinai are the first successful treatment of tumors of the bladder by transurethral electrocoagulation, the first demonstration of how asbestos can cause cancerous changes in the DNA of cells, and the first development of an ultrasound-guided technique to insert radioactive seeds into the prostate to treat prostate cancer.

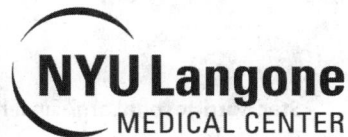

NYU Langone Medical Center
550 First Avenue , New York, NY 10016
www.NYULMC.org

Clinical Cancer Center
160 East 34th Street, New York, NY 10016
www.NYUCI.org

**The Stephen D. Hassenfeld Children's Center
for Cancer and Blood Disorders**
160 East 32nd Street, New York, NY 10016
www.NYUMC.org/Hassenfeld

NYU CANCER INSTITUTE

The NYU Cancer Institute is an NCI-designated cancer center providing personalized patient care that is compassionate and state-of-the-art. The doctors and researchers work together to develop innovative therapies for patients. The Cancer Institute is world-renowned for excellence in cancer-focused research, personalized care, education and community outreach. Its mission is to discover the origins of human cancer and to use that knowledge to eradicate the personal and societal burden of cancer in our community, the nation and the world. For more information about our expert physicians, call 212-731-5000.

Patient-Focused Setting
The Clinical Cancer Center is the principal outpatient facility of The Cancer Institute. The Center and its multidisciplinary team of experts provide access to the latest treatment options and clinical trials, along with a variety of programs in cancer risk reduction/prevention, screening, diagnostics, genetic counseling and supportive services. In addition, the Center emphasizes the importance of a holistic approach involving integrative health, psychosocial support, survivorship and palliative care. Radiology and infusion services are available in Rego Park, NY, as well.

Renowned Expertise
The NYU Cancer Institute brings together experts from a variety of disciplines to create collaborative research endeavors and clinical care teams. It offers a continuum of personalized care, from prevention through diagnosis, treatment and post-treatment support. Additionally, we have created special programs to treat diseases such as breast cancer, brain cancer, melanoma, GI cancer, prostate cancer, hematologic malignancies and lung cancer, as well as translational programs in cancer healthcare disparities, molecularly targeted therapy, and the cell signaling pathways involved in cancer.

A Translational Approach
Our scientists and researchers excel in uncovering how cancer develops at the molecular level, and how we can harness that knowledge to reduce the risk of cancer and treat the disease.

Stephen D. Hassenfeld Children's Center for Cancer and Blood Disorders
The center is a leading pediatric outpatient facility for the treatment of childhood cancers and blood diseases. Its unique interdisciplinary and family-centered approach combines the most advanced medical treatments with psychosocial and emotional support services for young patients and their families.

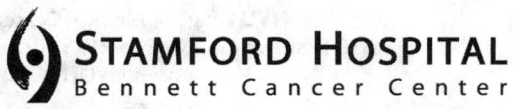

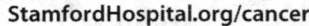

Bennett Cancer Center

Stamford Hospital's Carl & Dorothy Bennett Cancer Center provides compassionate, patient-centered care from diagnosis through post treatment. We are accredited as an Academic Comprehensive Cancer Program and received the outstanding Achievement Award from the American College of Surgeons Commission on Cancer. A multidisciplinary team of physicians, oncology nurses, nurse navigators and radiation therapists, offers advanced surgical, medical and technological services in a warm, caring environment.

Expertise Combined With Comfort

Our physicians' skill, knowledge and expertise are equaled only by their compassion in dealing with our patients. They are represented on the consulting staff of Memorial Sloan-Kettering Cancer Center and teaching faculty of Columbia University College of Physicians and Surgeons. They are also active participants in national research groups. The Center is involved with more clinical trials than any other area hospital.

Genetic Counseling

We offer the only full-time cancer genetic counselor in Fairfield County, ensuring timely delivery of genetic counseling services and superior interaction with other specialists, as well as the most current information in both genetics and oncology.

Treatment Beyond the Disease

We provide chemotherapy and immunotherapy in an outpatient setting, where patients can be treated in private suites with a home-like ambiance or a group room in the company of others. Cancer cases are reviewed by a multidisciplinary team of physicians and staff. This offers patients the benefit of different specialists combining their expertise.

Our Integrative Medicine Program and other support services including the *Transitions: Choices in Recovery* post-treatment survivorship program, offer a wide range of complementary therapies along with stress management, individual, family and group therapy.

Technology That Doesn't Forget Humanity

We are the only hospital in Fairfield and Westchester counties to offer CyberKnife™ stereoatactic radiosurgery to treat tumors with pinpoint accuracy. Additional technology includes simulator and linear accelerator machines with both Intensity Modulated Radiation Therapy and Image-Guided Radiation Therapy. Our diagnostic imaging services include a 64-slice CT scan, ultrasound, nuclear medicine, PET CT and MRI.

Academic and Clinical Affiliations
Stamford Hospital is an affiliate of the New York–Presbyterian Healthcare System and a major teaching affiliate of the Columbia University College of Physicians & Surgeons.

Accreditation
Joint Commission on Accreditation of Healthcare Organization (JCAHO)

Beds
305

Sponsorship
Voluntary, Not-for-Profit

For a Physician Referral or more information, please call 1.877.233.9355 or visit StamfordHospital.org /doctor.

Stamford Hospital
30 Shelburne Road
Stamford, CT 06902
203.276.1000

StamfordHospital.org

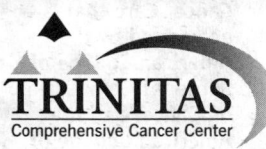

TRINITAS CONTINUES ITS AGGRESSIVE PURSUIT OF EXCELLENCE IN CANCER CARE

As just one of eight healthcare facilities in New Jersey to receive the American College of Surgeons National Accreditation Program for Breast Centers (NAPBC), Trinitas Regional Medical Center has been recognized for its voluntary commitment to providing the best in breast cancer diagnosis and treatment and its compliance with established NAPBC standards. Both the Diagnostic Imaging Center and the Trinitas Comprehensive Cancer Center have received this accreditation for cancer diagnosis and cancer care services.

"When the Trinitas Comprehensive Cancer Center opened its doors in 2005, it did so with the commitment to providing superior, compassionate care to those who use our many services," explains Barry Levinson, MD, Medical Director of the center. "We approach each patient with the utmost of care and direct our attention to giving them not only the best care and treatment but also the best quality of life as they survive cancer. The NAPBC accreditation underscores that commitment and encourages us to maintain the very highest standards for our patients."

Located on the main campus of Trinitas Regional Medical Center in Elizabeth, the Center is the home of the most advanced technology available to cancer patients, including the first Trilogy Linear Accelerator for radiation therapy in New Jersey. The Center is also the site of the state's first AccuBoost breast cancer treatment, and the first RapidArc radiotherapy procedure.

A major quality initiative at the Cancer Center involves a system-wide evaluation of the benefits, risks and efficient management of the increasing number of oral oncology drugs that have become available. These drugs offer a more convenient and less invasive treatment option, but they require a new model for patient education, monitoring, communications and support. Trinitas is well ahead of this curve with the development of in-depth 14-step program that features safeguards, intensive follow-up and a comprehensive system of checks and balances.

Support services include: nutrition/dietician services, genetic counseling, fatigue management, complementary therapies and services, social work, lymphedema management, Look Good – Feel Better, Made for Me boutique, art therapy, pet therapy and pain management.

Trinitas was awarded Comprehensive Cancer Program status by the American College of Surgeons' Commission on Cancer. Further, we are an approved Member of the prestigious Radiation Therapy Oncology Group. Our clinical research program gives many patients access to new treatment approaches that might not otherwise be available.

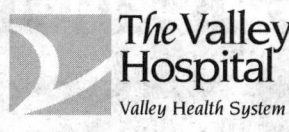

THE VALLEY HOSPITAL

An affiliate of the New York-Presbyterian Healthcare System

223 North Van Dien Avenue, Ridgewood, NJ 07450
Phone: 201-447-8000 • www.valleyhealth.com
www.facebook.com/valleyhospital • www.twitter.com/valleyhospital

The Daniel & Gloria Blumenthal Cancer Center

Our cancer care experts focus on delivering today's most promising therapies with compassion and dignity. Our multidisciplinary team of board-certified medical, surgical, and radiation oncologists; specialty physicians; Magnet-recognized oncology nurses; and award-winning allied health professionals is dedicated to providing personalized care that meets every person's unique needs and expectations. Our growing clinical and translational research programs offer patients access to new therapies and innovative protocols that are unavailable at other area hospitals. Our outreach educational programs and cancer screenings strive to prevent cancer and/or detect it at an early, treatable stage. Our cancer program has earned 6 Disease-Specific Care Certifications for healthcare quality from the Joint Commission for colorectal cancer, lung cancer, breast cancer, pancreatic cancer, prostate cancer, and uterine-ovarian cancer.

Diagnostic Imaging and Testing

Our state-of-the-art capabilities help physicians detect, stage, and monitor cancer. Our technology includes low-dose CT scanning, MRI, PET scanning, endoscopic ultrasound, endobronchial ultrasound, and digital mammography.

Powerful Therapies

Our Radiation Oncology Department and specialized centers provide all of the latest advanced modalities of radiation therapy to treat numerous cancers. Our Centers of Excellence include our Institute for Brain and Spine Surgery, Gamma Knife Center, Lung Cancer Center, Urologic Oncology Center, and Breast Center. Our surgical oncologists and other surgical specialists use the robotic daVinci Surgical System, laparoscopic techniques, and other minimally invasive options to offer patients gentler procedures with quicker recoveries. Our ambulatory Medical Infusion Center provides a comfortable site for receiving outpatient chemotherapy and other infusion therapies. Our hyperthermic intraperitoneal chemotherapy (HIPEC) program is the only one in New Jersey and one of the largest in the metropolitan area.

Patient- and Family-Centered Care

At The Valley Hospital, we espouse patient- and family-centered care, which recognizes the impact a diagnosis of cancer can have on the entire family and offers services, education, and guidance for all. Our holistic nursing care and integrative medicine therapies support healing of the mind, body and spirit. Support services, such as nutrition counseling, genetic counseling, social work services, pastoral care, psychosocial counseling, rehabilitation therapy, support groups, home care, and educational programs assist patients during and after cancer care and help to improve their quality of life.

A Dedication to Research

Our oncology research program endeavors to find answers to the complex questions of how cancer develops, how it behaves, why it mutates, and how it can be stopped or controlled. Included among our research are studies in using microRNA to screen for cancer, immune response to lung cancer, a brain cancer vaccine, and stereotactic radiosurgery outcomes.

Cancer Care that is accredited by the American College of Surgeons Commission on Cancer and the American College of Radiology

■ Infusion Center and chemotherapy, including NJ's only hyperthermic intraperitoneal chemotherapy program

■ Image-guided TomoTherapy

■ Intensity-modulated radiation therapy

■ Gamma Knife Center

■ Stereotactic body radiotherapy

■ High-dose-rate after-loading brachytherapy

■ Lung Cancer, Breast, Urologic Oncology, and Barrett's Esophagus Centers

■ Surgical, gynecologic, urologic, and thoracic oncologists

■ Single-port video-assisted thoracic surgery (VATS)

■ Minimally invasive breast oncoplastics surgery

■ Cancer genetics

■ Integrative healing services

■ Holistic nursing care

■ Home care and hospice

Daniel & Gloria Blumenthal Center, 1-634-5339; www.valleyhealth.com/oncology

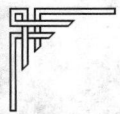

The Best in American Medicine
www.CastleConnolly.com

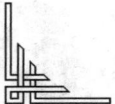
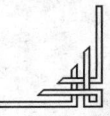

Cardiac Electrophysiology

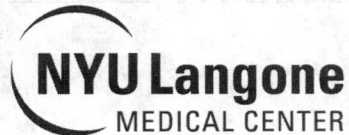

CARDIAC AND VASCULAR INSTITUTE
550 First Avenue *(at 31st Street)*
New York, NY 10016
www.NYULMC.org
Physician Referral: **888-7-NYU-MED** *(888-769-8633)*

ADULT CARDIOVASCULAR SERVICES

The Cardiac and Vascular Institute (CVI) at NYU Langone Medical Center continues to advance new techniques for repairing heart valves, curing heart rhythm disorders, and treating aortic diseases and congestive heart failure. CVI is consistently ranked among the leading heart and heart surgery centers in U.S. News & World Report's annual 'Best Hospitals.'

Cardiac Catheterization
The Cardiac Catheterization Laboratory offers superior catheter-based diagnosis and evaluation of cardiac health. It provides a full range of procedures to evaluate heart muscle, valves, and coronary arteries and recommends appropriate treatment as needed.

Cardiac Rehabilitation and Prevention
The Joan and Joel Smilow Cardiopulmonary Rehabilitation and Prevention focuses on individualized patient care in a state-of-the-art facility.

Cardiac Surgery
The Division of Cardiac Surgery is a nationally recognized leader with a multidisciplinary approach in performing more than 6,000 minimally invasive heart surgery procedures since pioneering the technique in 1996. Moreover it offers over 30 years experience in mitral valve repairs as well as heart valve replacements and aortic aneurysm repairs.

Cardiology
The Leon H. Charney Division of Cardiology is a leader in cardiovascular patient care, biomedical research, and education. Clinicians and researchers are advancing the field of cardiovascular medicine and contributing to the reputation of NYU Langone Medical Center as a comprehensive cardiovascular center of excellence.

Heart Failure
The cardiologists and surgeons at the Heart Failure Center offer advanced echocardiograms, pacemaker/defibrillator implantations, open heart surgeries and ventricular assist devices.

Nuclear Cardiology/Stress
The Nuclear Cardiology/Stress Laboratory performs a range of tests that assist cardiologists in the assessment and diagnosis of heart disease.

Vascular Surgery
The Division of Vascular and Endovascular Surgery has treated thousands of patients for arterial aneurysms, deep vein thrombosis, carotid stenosis and limb salvage, emphasizing minimally invasive diagnostic and treatment approaches.

Cardiovascular Disease

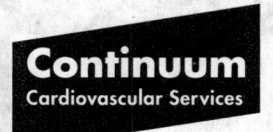

Beth Israel Medical Center
Beth Israel Brooklyn
Roosevelt Hospital
St. Luke's Hospital

Cardiovascular Specialists
Referral Service
800.420.4004

Continuum Cardiovascular Centers of New York
New Cardiac and Vascular Programs of Excellence

The newly conceived Continuum Cardiovascular Centers of New York, led by the internationally renowned Interventional Cardiologist Gary Roubin, MD, PhD, is moving forward to expand the extensive cardiac and vascular services now offered at St. Luke's and Roosevelt Hospitals and Beth Israel Medical Center. By adding preeminent experts and expanding and upgrading facilities, Continuum Cardiovascular Services will provide the most cutting-edge, patient-oriented, compassionate care in the region.

The first expansion milestone has been reached: the opening of the Al-Sabah Arrhythmia Institute in the fall of 2012. This world-class electrophysiology facility is being directed by nationally celebrated physician leaders in management of complex arrhythmias and ablation therapy. Heralding facility upgrades throughout the Continuum Cardiovascular Centers across New York, the new arrhythmia center is equipped with state-of-the-art technology that enhances both outcomes and patient experience.

The driving force behind the development of the Continuum Cardiovascular Centers of New York is our commitment to excellence. A well-developed integrated clinical care system combines the world's most innovative physicians, gifted researchers, educators, and professional staff. We are building our reality upon a foundation of advanced technology and sophisticated facilities to ensure continued superior clinical outcomes and patient satisfaction.

For a referral to one of the expert cardiovascular specialists at the Continuum Cardiovascular Centers of New York, please call 800.420.4004.

Visit us online:
BethIsraelNY.org
StLukesHospitalNYC.org
RooseveltHospitalNYC.org

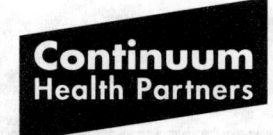

Beth Israel Medical Center
Beth Israel Brooklyn
Roosevelt Hospital
St. Luke's Hospital
NY Eye and Ear Infirmary

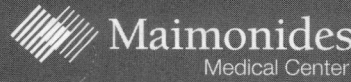
Having pioneered numerous heart care innovations through the years, the Cardiac Institute offers diagnostic studies and therapeutic treatments, procedures and surgeries. It has been ranked by the Centers for Medicare and Medicaid Services among the few hospitals which have achieved excellent ratings in both heart attack and heart failure patient outcomes.

Cardiology
Among the most published and respected in the field, the Maimonides cardiology team continuously sets higher standards for patient care. Edgar Lichstein, MD, Chair of Medicine, has been chief investigator of NIH-sponsored cardiac drug trials, and our Congestive Heart Failure (CHF) Program is among the most effective in the nation.

Interventional Cardiology
Led by Cardiac Institute Chair, Jacob Shani, MD, numerous therapeutic devices have been developed and implemented here. Our Electrophysiology Lab has a superb record of achievement in diagnosing and treating arrhythmias. Close collaboration with the Department of Emergency Medicine ensures that chest pain patients are evaluated immediately and that interventional procedures are used to stop heart attacks in progress whenever necessary.

Cardiothoracic Surgery
The Maimonides Division of Cardiothoracic Surgery has an illustrious history, setting a national standard for advances in cardiothoracic. Under the direction of Greg Ribakove, MD, minimally invasive and robotic heart surgeries, as well as advanced procedures such as LVAD and TAVI, are offered in state-of-the-art facilities, including a hybrid OR. In collaboration with Electrophysiology, Cardiothoracic Surgery has established an Atrial Fibrillation Center of Excellence. Maimonides provides one of the most prestigious cardiothoracic residency programs in the US.

Historic Moments
- In 1967, the first successful human heart transplant in the nation was performed at Maimonides.
- The intra-aortic balloon pump was developed here in 1970.
- Surgical techniques that protect the spine during cardiothoracic surgery were perfected here in 1982.
- Revolutionary cardiac catheterization devices were invented here in 1992 and 1997.
- Maimonides was the first hospital in the US to implement fully automatic external cardiac defibrillators in 2001.

The Centers for Medicare and Medicaid Services, an agency of the federal government, recently published the latest data on 30-day mortality rates for hospitals across the country. Maimonides Medical Center achieved better-than-expected results in all three categories measured – heart attack, heart failure and pneumonia – a distinction only 22 hospitals in the U.S. achieved.

Maimonides Medical Center
Passionate about medicine.
Compassionate about people.

www.maimonidesmed.org/cardiac

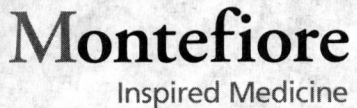
Montefiore Einstein Center for Heart and Vascular Care

Montefiore Einstein Center for Heart and Vascular Care is a national leader in treating patients with cardiovascular disease, offering innovative therapies and exceptional outcomes. **For three consecutive years, the Society of Thoracic Surgeons has recognized the Center's commitment to surgical excellence with its prestigious "three-star" ranking, placing Montefiore in the nation's top 12 percent of participating open-heart surgery programs.**

The Center's comprehensive Heart Valve Repair Program offers the full spectrum of valve repair options. A strong commitment to repair results in risk-adjusted operative mortality rates for mitral valve repair that are among the best in the nation. Valve-sparing aortic repair surgery is offered for individuals with thoracic aortic aneurysms and other conditions such as bicuspid aortic valve disease. **As one of eight U.S. centers selected to participate in the National Institutes of Health/National Heart, Lung, and Blood Institute's Cardiothoracic Surgery Network, Montefiore is advancing mitral valve repair surgery, the use of stem cell therapy for heart failure, and treatments for other cardiac conditions, such as atrial fibrillation.**

Adult and pediatric patients benefit from the Center's Heart Failure Program, which offers the latest ventricular assist devices and surgical interventions—including transplant. **In 2011, Montefiore performed 29 transplants (20 adults, 9 pediatric), with outcomes better than 85 percent of the heart transplant programs in the nation. Over the past two years, the 52 patients who received heart transplants had a one-year survival rate of approximately 100 percent.** The New York State Department of Health has recognized the Center as the leader among the state's transplant/heart failure programs in achieving appropriate treatment measures and one of the lowest mortality rates.

The Center's specialists in the Pediatric Heart Center at The Children's Hospital at Montefiore (CHAM) offer advanced options for children with all forms of cardiac defects and anomalies. In 2011, CHAM expanded its capabilities with a state-of-the-art pediatric hybrid cardiac catheterization lab.

Additionally, the Center for Heart and Vascular Care possesses expertise in catheter-based management of aortic valve replacement and implantation of arrhythmia management devices. The Center also has a growing specialized extracorporeal membrane oxygenation (ECMO) program for both children and adults living with heart failure. This dedicated team boasts a success rate greater than 80 percent, exceeding national benchmarks.

The Center excels in the treatment of patients with peripheral vascular disease and offers surgical, interventional and hybrid revascularization options for these patients. In the area of cardiac interventions, the Center possesses an exceptionally low mortality rate and an expanded team that includes a renowned electrocardiologist and structural interventionalists.

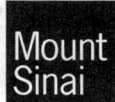
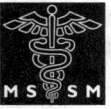

THE MOUNT SINAI MEDICAL CENTER
MOUNT SINAI HEART - CARDIOVASCULAR HEALTH

One Gustave L. Levy Place
Fifth Avenue and 100th Street
New York, NY 10029-6574
Physician Referral: 1-800-MD-SINAI (637-4624)
www.mountsinai.org/heart

At MOUNT SINAI HEART, our integrated system of care brings together the world's most accomplished physicians, research scientists, and educators who share the common goal of preventing and treating cardiovascular disease. **In 2012,** *U.S. News & World Report* **ranked our cardiology and heart surgery service 10th in the nation.**

With access to the latest discoveries and a diversity of the most experienced minds, our doctors ensure that patients receive the best individualized care. The rapid translation of innovative research into prevention, diagnosis, and therapy means that patients receive multidisciplinary treatment of unprecedented quality. Our programs treat patients of all ages – from the unborn fetus well into the advanced elderly years.

We specialize in consultative cardiology, cardiac catheterization, heart and lung transplantation, cardiovascular surgery, heart failure, pulmonary hypertension, lipid management, and hypertension, as well as:

Noninvasive diagnostic imaging – We offer state-of-the-art echocardiography, nuclear cardiology, PET, CT, and MRI technology.

Coronary artery disease – We are ranked as New York State's safest and busiest center for coronary angioplasty and other catheter-based procedures. We lead many innovative device trials in the development phase before getting final approval for commercial use.

Cardiac rhythm disturbances – We manage all aspects of heart rhythm disorders under the auspices of pioneers in the field, including atrial fibrillation (AFib), the most common abnormal heart rhythm, and ventricular tachycardias, the most common cause of sudden cardiac death, as well as implantable devices, such as pacemakers and defibrillators.

Valvular heart disease – We deliver medical and surgical options, including a leading valve-repair program and long-term follow-up care. We are one of the few centers in the country to provide both types of percutaneous non-surgical aortic valves.

Aortic diseases – We pioneer and advance techniques for stent-graft repair of thoracic and abdominal aortic aneurysms and for surgical correction of the most complex aortic pathology.

Congenital heart disease – Our cardiologists offer minimally invasive approaches to the correction of congenital heart defects in children and adults.

Cardiac failure and transplantation – We take a multidisciplinary team approach to comprehensive, compassionate care for patients with the most advanced forms of heart failure and cardiomyopathy.

Comprehensive cardiac disease prevention and rehabilitation –
Our unique synergy provides unparalleled superior patient care and breakthroughs in cardiovascular disease prevention and treatment, while promoting cardiovascular health globally through six projects around the world.

Vascular medicine and surgery – We offer an interdisciplinary approach to disease management, including medical, surgical, catheter-based, and gene therapy techniques for arterial obstruction, limb salvage, venous, and lymphatic diseases. A pioneer in large-artery stenting, Mount Sinai fostered the development of stenting of abdominal aortic aneurysms.

Mount Sinai's Cardiac Catheterization Laboratory – We study the heart with the most precise technologies available, including diagnostic angiography, angioplasty, and biopsy. In a statewide study, our Cath Lab was found to be the safest, with the lowest 30-day risk-adjusted mortality rate for percutaneous coronary intervention (angioplasty), as well as the busiest.

LEADING SURGEONS, INNOVATIVE TREATMENTS
Under the direction of internationally renowned cardiologist Valentin Fuster, MD, PhD, Mount Sinai Heart is recognized worldwide for expert evaluation, management, and prevention of cardiovascular disease through integrated patient care, education, and research. Mount Sinai Heart encompasses the Zena and Michael A. Wiener Cardiovascular Institute and the Marie-Josée and Henry R. Kravis Center for Cardiovascular Health at Mount Sinai, both preeminent resources for the study and treatment of heart and blood vessel diseases.

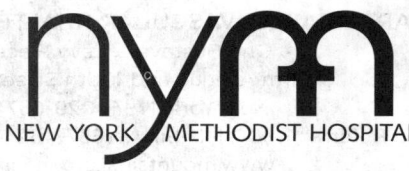
NEW YORK METHODIST HOSPITAL

THE INSTITUTE FOR CARDIOLOGY AND CARDIAC SURGERY

New York Methodist Hospital
506 Sixth Street, Brooklyn, N.Y. 11215
Phone 866 84-HEART (866 844-3278)
http://www.nym.org

SPECIALISTS AND MEDICAL SERVICES

The Institute is the Hospital's program for the prevention, diagnosis and treatment of all types of heart disease. The Institute brings together a panel of specialists and a range of services in all areas related to cardiac disease. These services, which range from screening and diagnostic procedures to emergency and ongoing treatment for heart attacks and chronic heart disease, are provided at the Hospital's specialized laboratories and clinical units, on both an inpatient and outpatient basis. New York Methodist houses state-of-the-art diagnostic and surgical facilities, including three cardiac catheterization laboratories and the most modern cardiac surgery suite in the area. The Institute's staff of physicians includes specialists in all areas of cardiology, electrophysiology, interventional cardiology and cardiac surgery.

PROGRAMS OFFERED

The programs and services offered by the Institute include consultative services, a chest pain emergency center (located in the Emergency Department), diagnostic evaluation (including cardiac MRI) and medical treatment for heart disease, interventional cardiology procedures (angioplasty and stents), electrophysiology (pacemakers, implantable defibrillators, ablation, etc.) and cardiac surgery.

* * *

Referrals to the specialists or to cardiac programs and services can be made through an individual's primary care physician or requested directly through the Institute's referral service. More information (and on-line physician referral) is available at the Hospital's website, http://www.nym.org.

THE NEW YORK METHODIST-CORNELL HEART CENTER

The New York Methodist-Cornell Heart Center is one of only three programs approved to perform cardiac surgery in Brooklyn. It is staffed by physicians from the prestigious Weill Cornell Medical Center of NewYork-Presbyterian Hospital. The Center is located in a state-of-the-art cardiac surgery suite.

Procedures performed at the Center include coronary bypass surgery, off-pump bypass surgery, valve replacement and repair, thoracic aneurysm repair, minimally invasive cardiac surgery and bloodless heart surgery.

⌐ NewYork-Presbyterian
¬ The University Hospital of Columbia and Cornell

Affiliated with Columbia University College of Physicians and Surgeons and Weill Cornell Medical College

NewYork-Presbyterian Hospital	NewYork-Presbyterian Hospital
Columbia University Medical Center	Weill Cornell Medical Center
622 West 168th Street	525 East 68th Street
New York, NY 10032	New York, NY 10065

1-877-NYP-WELL (1-877-697-9355)   www.nyp.org/heart

NewYork-Presbyterian Heart

In 2012-2013, NewYork-Presbyterian Hospital's heart and heart surgery program was ranked 4th in the nation in the annual 'Best Hospitals' survey conducted by *U.S. News & World Report*™. NewYork-Presbyterian has leading clinical programs for patients with coronary artery disease and a wide range of other heart disorders, with particular expertise in the management of:

- Aortic aneurysms, acute dissections, and trauma, with rapid diagnosis and effective medical and surgical interventions
- Heart failure, featuring a robust mechanical circulatory support program. Patients come from all over the world for placement of ventricular assist devices to be used long-term or as a bridge to transplant. NewYork-Presbyterian Hospital/Columbia University Medical Center is one of the world's leading institutions for heart transplantation and is one of the few centers offering patients a total artificial heart
- Adults with congenital heart disorders: echocardiography, interventional cardiac catheterization, interventional electrophysiology, and surgery. NewYork-Presbyterian's adult congenital heart surgeons are among the world's best for complex congenital heart surgery and cardiac transplantation. Related care is provided by specialists in high-risk pregnancy, genetics, fetal echocardiography, GI and liver disease, pulmonary, and hematology
- Cardiac rhythm abnormalities, with experienced electrophysiologists who diagnose and treat atrial fibrillation and other arrhythmias using pacemakers, implantable cardioverter defibrillators, ablation, and novel approaches to restore normal heart rhythm
- Valve disorders: using minimally invasive surgical approaches whenever possible. NewYork-Presbyterian Hospital investigators led the PARTNER Trial, which in 2011 demonstrated that transcatheter aortic valve replacement (TAVR) was as effective as conventional open-heart surgery for reducing mortality among high-risk patients with aortic stenosis. We've performed more TAVR procedures than any other center in the country. In addition, NewYork-Presbyterian Hospital is participating in the EVEREST II clinical trial, evaluating a new device to repair mitral valve leakage
- Heart disorders in the elderly: NewYork-Presbyterian Hospital surgeons have earned a reputation for performing heart surgery on the very elderly (over age 80), achieving excellent outcomes
- Patients who require surgery may receive treatment using a robotic approach, delivered using the Siemens Artis zeego® medical imaging system. This system provides surgeons with exceptional visualization of blood vessels.

A Reputation for Excellence

At NewYork-Presbyterian Hospital, the optimal care of patients with heart disease is achieved by combining an experienced team of clinicians with the latest advances in technology. Basic science and clinical research efforts are aimed at developing more effective ways to prevent, diagnose, and treat cardiac disorders. NewYork-Presbyterian Hospital features renowned cardiac care programs in the following areas:

- Cardiac diagnostics
- Electrophysiology
- Clinical cardiology
- Interventional cardiology
- Cardiac assist devices
- Cardiothoracic surgery, including transplantation
- Mitral valve repair

NewYork-Presbyterian Hospital is designated by the Society of Chest Pain Centers as an Accredited Chest Pain Center, dedicated to reducing heart-related deaths by improving the response time for the diagnosis and treatment of chest pain.

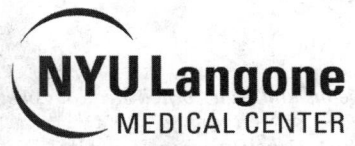

ADULT CARDIOVASCULAR SERVICES

The Cardiac and Vascular Institute (CVI) at NYU Langone Medical Center continues to advance new techniques for repairing heart valves, curing heart rhythm disorders, and treating aortic diseases and congestive heart failure. CVI is consistently ranked among the leading heart and heart surgery centers in U.S. News & World Report's annual 'Best Hospitals.'

Cardiac Catheterization
The Cardiac Catheterization Laboratory offers superior catheter-based diagnosis and evaluation of cardiac health. It provides a full range of procedures to evaluate heart muscle, valves, and coronary arteries and recommends appropriate treatment as needed.

Cardiac Rehabilitation and Prevention
The Joan and Joel Smilow Cardiopulmonary Rehabilitation and Prevention focuses on individualized patient care in a state-of-the-art facility.

Cardiac Surgery
The Division of Cardiac Surgery is a nationally recognized leader with a multidisciplinary approach in performing more than 6,000 minimally invasive heart surgery procedures since pioneering the technique in 1996. Moreover it offers over 30 years experience in mitral valve repairs as well as heart valve replacements and aortic aneurysm repairs.

Cardiology
The Leon H. Charney Division of Cardiology is a leader in cardiovascular patient care, biomedical research, and education. Clinicians and researchers are advancing the field of cardiovascular medicine and contributing to the reputation of NYU Langone Medical Center as a comprehensive cardiovascular center of excellence.

Heart Failure
The cardiologists and surgeons at the Heart Failure Center offer advanced echocardiograms, pacemaker/defibrillator implantations, open heart surgeries and ventricular assist devices.

Nuclear Cardiology/Stress
The Nuclear Cardiology/Stress Laboratory performs a range of tests that assist cardiologists in the assessment and diagnosis of heart disease.

Vascular Surgery
The Division of Vascular and Endovascular Surgery has treated thousands of patients for arterial aneurysms, deep vein thrombosis, carotid stenosis and limb salvage, emphasizing minimally invasive diagnostic and treatment approaches.

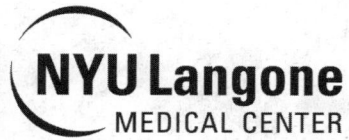

CARDIAC SURGERY

NYU Langone Medical Center is one of the largest cardiac surgery centers in the country, and a nationally recognized leader in advanced treatment for the most complex cases of adult, pediatric and congenital heart disease. World renowned surgeons at the Medical Center pioneered minimally invasive heart surgery and valve repair or replacement, and have since performed over 6,000 minimally invasive procedures. They also perform state-of-the-art surgical procedures for aortic aneurysm disease, coronary artery disease, heart valve disease, and congenital heart disease, while specializing in cardiac surgery for high-risk and elderly patients.

Structural and Valvular Heart Disease Center
Mitral Valve Repair. NYU Langone's heart surgeons introduced mitral valve repair to the U.S. more than 30 years ago, and have since performed more than 4,000 mitral valve repairs, the most in the country.
High Risk Cardiac Surgery. Our cardiac surgery team specializes in the surgical care of high-risk patients, including re-operative surgery in the elderly, coronary bypass surgery, heart valve repair or replacement, surgical repair of the failing heart, and ventricular assist device implantation.
Minimally Invasive Cardiac Surgery. NYU Langone is in the vanguard of minimally invasive cardiac surgery, the benefits of which include reduced pain, lower risk of bleeding and infection, and a faster recovery.

Aortic Disease Center
The Medical Center is committed to a multidisciplinary approach in the treatment of complex aortic disease, and the long-term management of patients with aortic dissection and connective tissue disorders. A wide range of treatment and therapeutic options is offered, including open surgery and stent graft therapy for patients with aortic aneurysms, aortic dissections and genetic diseases of the aorta, like Marfan's syndrome.

Pediatric and Adult Congenital Heart Disease Center
The Division of Pediatric and Adult Congenital Cardiac Surgery treats patients of all ages with inherited and acquired cardiac defects. Our surgeons are experts in reconstructive procedures for complex cardiovascular disorders. The Division maintains a highly experienced team of specialists in pediatric and adult cardiology, neonatal and pediatric cardiac intensive care, pediatric cardiac anesthesiology, nursing, and extracorporeal perfusion.

St. Francis Hospital The Heart Center®

100 Port Washington Blvd.
Roslyn, New York 11576
www.stfrancisheartcenter.com
(516) 562-6000 1-888-HEARTNY

A Leader in Cardiac Care

St. Francis Hospital, The Heart Center® is New York State's only specialty designated cardiac center and is one of the busiest heart centers in the nation. Located in Roslyn, New York, on Long Island's North Shore, St. Francis Hospital has been ranked among the best hospitals in the United States by *U.S. News & World Report* for the six consecutive years. In 2012-13, the Hospital was nationally ranked in cardiology and heart surgery, gastroenterology, geriatrics, and neurology and neurosurgery.

St. Francis Hospital:

• Has a highly experienced team of physicians and surgeons with one of the largest volumes in the nation for cardiac surgery, interventional cardiology and arrhythmia procedures

• Offers innovative approaches to cardiac surgery, including minimally invasive procedures and off-pump coronary artery bypass surgery, designed to minimize trauma and reduce surgical complications

• Performs one of the region's highest volumes of catheter-based techniques to correct congenital heart defects such as atrial septal defects (ASDs) and patent foramen ovale (PFO)

• Operates a nationally recognized Arrhythmia and Pacemaker Center staffed with electrophysiologists with over a decade of experience in radiofrequency ablation, a permanent cure for certain arrhythmias, including atrial fibrillation

• Maintains a high volume center for the implantation of cardiac pacemakers and defibrillators

• Offers a world-class program in cardiac imaging that fully integrates all technologies, including advanced methods in cardiac MRI, coronary CT angiography, PET/CT and three-dimensional echocardiography

• Has received the Magnet Award for excellence in nursing services for the second consecutive three-year approval period

• Is a premier center for clinical trials and studies of the application of image-guided methods of diagnosis and treatment of heart disease, such as CoreValve, eValve, CREST, and Symplicity

St. Francis Hospital has near-perfect patient satisfaction ratings, with over 99 percent of patients saying they would recommend the Hospital to family and friends.

"Our large cardiac caseload and our growing research program put us in an excellent position to introduce new techniques that can benefit thousands of people in need each year."

–Alan D. Guerci, M.D.
President and Chief Executive Officer
St. Francis Hospital, The Heart Center®

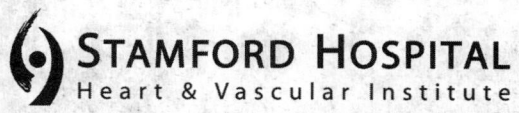

STAMFORD HOSPITAL
Heart & Vascular Institute

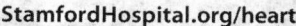

Heart and Vascular Institute

Stamford Hospital's Heart and Vascular Institute is the only comprehensive cardiovascular program to include open heart surgery and elective and primary angioplasty in lower Fairfield County. We offer the finest cardiac services, including cardiovascular screening, diagnostic services, advanced cardiac non-surgical and surgical treatment, cardiac rehabilitation and integrative services and wellness programs.

Nationally Recognized Critical Care Unit

Stamford Hospital's Critical Care Unit has been recognized as one of the best in the country and earned the prestigious, national Codman Award, from the Joint Commission, for development of a life-saving protocol.

Cardiac Catheterization

Our two brand-new, state-of-the-art Cardiac Catheterization Labs, enable diagnosis and treatment of heart conditions, emergency angioplasty to open blocked coronary arteries during heart attacks, electrophysiology procedures that diagnose and treat heart arrhythmias, and the insertion of pacemakers and internal defibrillators. Emergency and elective angioplasty are performed for the treatment of acute myocardial infarction (heart attack) and coronary blockages.

Open Heart Surgery

Our expert team is equipped to handle any emergent and non-emergent surgical issue including CABG, valve repairs and replacements and aneurysm's using state-of-the-art surgical techniques. We have a dedicated team of surgeons, cardiac anesthesiologist, physician assistants, registered nurses and a clinical coordinator who provide patient-centered care.

Cardiac Rehabilitation

Located at the Tully Health Center, we help patients with heart disease recover faster and return to full, productive lives. Together with medical and surgical treatment, cardiac rehab includes exercise, education, counseling and behavioral change strategies that lead to a healthier life.

Integrative Cardiology and Wellness Programs

Offered through our Center for Integrative Medicine and Wellness, this program will offer multiple lifestyle techniques to complement and support the treatment of heart disease. The program is built on the belief that health and wellness involve healing of the spirit, mind and body not solely the treatment of heart disease.

Academic and Clinical Affiliations
Stamford Hospital is an affiliate of the New York–Presbyterian Healthcare System and a major teaching affiliate of the Columbia University College of Physicians & Surgeons.

Accreditation
Joint Commission on Accreditation of Healthcare Organization (JCAHO)

Beds
305

Sponsorship
Voluntary, Not-for-Profit

For a Physician Referral or more information, please call 1.877.233.9355 or visit StamfordHospital.org /doctor.

Stamford Hospital
30 Shelburne Road
Stamford, CT 06902
203.276.1000

StamfordHospital.org

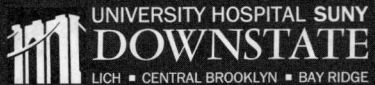
UNIVERSITY HOSPITAL SUNY
DOWNSTATE
LICH ■ CENTRAL BROOKLYN ■ BAY RIDGE

FIND A PHYSICIAN
(888) 270-SUNY
physicians.downstate.edu

Center for Cardiovascular Medicine

Our exceptional team of cardiologists and surgeons works together to provide a full range of state-of-the-art cardiology services, ranging from prevention and diagnosis to evaluation and treatment.

Preventive Cardiology Program
Experts in hypertension, metabolic syndrome, lipid disorders, diabetes, nutrition, psychology and sleep disorders utilize the latest diagnostic techniques to accurately evaluate risks for heart problems in this outpatient service. Patients are given individualized programs of risk modification to prevent heart attacks, strokes and other heart problems. The program may include cardiac rehabilitation, nutritional counseling, weight management, smoking cessation, a cardiac fitness program and medications to reduce risk.

Clinical Cardiology
Consultation and a comprehensive evaluation are followed by determination of the optimal management strategies, potentially including diet, medications, interventional procedures, etc.

Non-invasive Cardiac Testing and Imaging
The most appropriate technique is determined for each individual: echocardiography, CT scan, MRI, EKG, stress testing with EKG, echo or radionuclides, or specialized radioisotope testing (e.g., PET scanning).

Comprehensive Heart Failure Service
A specialized team of doctors and nurses evaluates and monitors patients with heart failure. Treatment is designed to minimize symptoms, reduce the need for hospitalization and maximize survival. In addition to tailored drug and diet therapy, options such as biventricular pacemakers, LVADs and ICDs can improve survival.

Interventional Cardiology
The Interventional Cardiac Catheterization Laboratory excels in diagnosis and non-surgical treatment for patients with coronary artery blockages, heart valve and congenital abnormalities, and hypertrophic obstructive cardiomyopathy.

Cardiac Electrophysiology
Our superb electrophysiology team recently performed the first implantation in NYC of the world's smallest, thinnest defibrillator device (CRT-D). Treatment options include atrial fibrillation "ablation" (pulmonary vein isolation procedure); focal ablation procedures for supraventricular (atrial) and ventricular tachycardia; biventricular pacing for heart failure; tilt table and Microvolt T-wave alternans testing; and laser lead extraction.

Division of Cardiothoracic Surgery
This highly specialized team, consisting of skilled surgeons, critical care physicians, anesthesiologists, physician assistants and nurses equipped with the latest equipment and innovative techniques, provides surgical care for patients with the most complex cardiovascular diseases and at the highest risk. Specialized services include, but are not limited to, off-pump coronary artery by-pass, complete arterial coronary revascularization and and minimally invasive heart surgery and endoscopic leg vein and forearm radial artery harvest. Innovative procedures recently introduced include complex mitral valve repair and endovascular stent-grafting for aortic arch aneurysms. Our cardiac surgical research program is funded by the National Institutes of Health, the only Brooklyn program so recognized.

Cardiac Progressive Care Unit
When patients with arrhythmias, heart failure, or recovering from complicated heart attacks or cardiac surgery do not need intensive care, this unit, staffed only by cardiologists, provides continuous cardiac monitoring and a comprehensive approach to speed recovery and release from the hospital.

The Howard Gilman Institute for Heart Valve Disease www.GilmanHeartValve.us
Institute Director Dr. Jeffrey S. Borer has been a leader in the field of heart valve disease for over three decades. The Institute team has been at the forefront of research, evaluation and treatment of valvular heart disease. Their work has formed the foundation of the best solutions available today for those with valve disease. Our team works hand-in-hand with referring cardiologists and internists, so they can take advantage of cutting-edge research and technology, providing the highest level of patient care. The team also performs ground-breaking research at the fundamental (cellular and molecular) level to increase understanding of heart valve disease and enable new and novel treatments

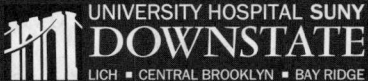

Center for Cardiovascular Medicine

Downstate UHB Central Brooklyn Campus

JEFFREY S. BORER, MD
Chair, Department of Medicine
Chief, Division of Cardiovascular Medicine

ADAM S. BUDZIKOWSKI, MD, PhD
Cardiac Electrophysiology

JOSHUA H. BURACK, MD
Cardiothoracic Surgery

ERDAL CAVUSOGLU, MD
Director, Observation Unit
Interventional Cardiology

ALAN FEIT, MD
Director, Progressive Care Unit
Interventional Cardiology

EDMUND M. HERROLD, MD, PhD
Director, Clinical Cardiology

JOHN KASSOTIS, MD, ENG SCI D
Director, Cardiac Electrophysiology
General Cardiology

JASON M. LAZAR, MD
Director, Non-invasive Cardiac
Testing and Imaging

DANIEL LEE, MD
Cardiothoracic Surgery

JONATHAN D. MARMUR, MD
Director, Interventional Cardiology
Director, Coronary Care Unit

JUDITH E. MITCHELL, MD
Director, Heart Failure Service

CRISTINA MITRE, MD
Clinical Cardiology and Cardiac Electrophysiology

JACEK J. PREIBISZ, MD, PhD
Director, Preventive Cardiology Program

LOUIS SALCICCIOLI, MD
Co-Director, Progressive Care Unit
Non-invasive Imaging

VINAY M. TAK, MD, FRCS
Interim Chief, Division of Cardiothoracic Surgery

PETER TERRY, MD
Cardiothoracic Surgery

Downstate UHB LICH Campus

BALENDU VASAVADA, MD
Chief of Service, LICH
Echocardiography

JOSEPH FRANCIOSA, MD
Director, Heart Failure Program

VLADIMIR FRIDMAN, MD
General Cardiology

NIKI KANTROWITZ, MD
Interventional Cardiology

CARLOS RODRIGUEZ, MD
General Cardiology

CESARE SAPONIERI, MD
Cardiac Electrophysiology

SUDHAKAR PRABHU, MD
General and Non-Invasive Cardiology

FURQUAN TEJANI, MD
General Cardiology

SUNY DOWNSTATE CENTRAL BROOKLYN

University Hospital of Brooklyn
445 Lenox Road, Brooklyn, NY 11203

General Appointments (718) 270-1081
Cardiovascular Medicine (718) 270-1568
Cardiothoracic Surgery (718) 270-1981
Electrophysiology (718) 270-4147
Interventional Cardiology (718) 270-3273
Preventive Cardiology (718) 270-2107

SUNY DOWNSTATE BAY RIDGE

699 92nd Street, Brooklyn, NY 11228

Cardiac Electrophysiology (718) 567-1755 / 270-4147
General Cardiology (718) 567-1755 / (718) 833-2620

SUNY DOWNSTATE LONG ISLAND COLLEGE HOSPITAL

339 Hicks Street, Brooklyn, NY 11201

Interventional Cardiology (718) 780 4626
Cardiac Electrophysiology (718) 780 4841
Echocardiography (718) 780 2944
General Cardiology:
(718) 780- 4841 (Fridman)
(718) 780 1852 (Rodriguez)
(718) 780 4979 (Tejani)

MANHATTAN

635 Madison Avenue, New York, NY 10022

Jeffrey S. Borer, MD, Edmund M. Herrold, MD, PhD
and Jacek J. Preibisz, MD, PhD (212) 289-7777

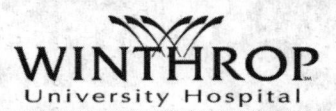

HEART AND VASCULAR INSTITUTE
259 First Street, Mineola, NY 11501
Tel: 1-866-WINTHROP
www.winthrop.org

WINTHROP-UNIVERSITY HOSPITAL offers a unique and comprehensive multifaceted approach to the prevention and treatment of

CARDIOVASCULAR DISEASE.

Made up of several centers of excellence, **the cardiovascular specialists of** Winthrop-University Hospital bring each patient a focused and individualized level of care not accessible elsewhere.

WINTHROP'S highly skilled and experienced cardiologists, cardiothoracic surgeons, specialized nurses, physician assistants, cardiology fellows and cardiovascular technologists provide patients and their primary care physicians with a wide range of sophisticated services; including access to consistently **outstanding interventional cardiology, cardiac surgery, state-of-the-art computerized diagnostic cardiac catheterization procedures and expert drug-eluding stent placement - as well as innovative electrophysiology used to evaluate and treat all types of heart-rhythm disturbances with the latest generation of implantable electronic devices and pacemakers.**

THORACIC AORTIC VASCULAR TREATMENT CENTER

Winthrop recently became one of only 70 centers in the United States to offer the Edwards Sapien Transcathether Heart Valve (TAVR), one of the newest techniques that allows a heart valve to be replaced without open-heart surgery. Surgeons insert a catheter into an artery in the groin, pass a thin wire through the catheter with the new valve attached and install the new valve from the inside. Percutaneous valve replacement has proven especially helpful for elderly patients who are not candidates for open-heart surgery, providing improved quality of life for these patients and their families.

THE PACEMAKER/ARRHYTHMIA CENTER

The Pacemaker/Arrhythmia Center at Winthrop is a state-of-the-art facility that offers cutting-edge services with highly skilled clinical cardiac electrophysiologists who specialize in the entire range of heart rhythm diagnostic and therapeutic procedures. The Center offers both inpatient and outpatient services.

Physicians at Winthrop were the first on Long Island to offer a new therapy for patients with Paroxysmal atrial fibrillation (PAF) – the Arctic Front® Cardiac CryoAblation Catheter system, the first and only cryoballoon in the United States indicated to treat certain cases of PAF. Recently approved by the U.S. Food and Drug Administration, the cryoballoon treatment involves a minimally-invasive procedure that efficiently uses freezing to scar or kill the tissue that is causing the erratic electrical signals that cause the irregular heartbeat.

HYPERTROPHIC CARDIOMYOPATHY TREATMENT CENTER

Winthrop-University Hospital's Hypertrophic Cardiomyopathy (HCM) Treatment Center — one of the nation's handful of comprehensive resources for HCM and the only one on Long Island — treats hundreds of patients and families from the tri-state area and beyond, offering expert, specialized services that address all facets of the disease. The HCM Center is recognized as a national center of excellence by the National Hypertrophic Cardiomyopathy Association.

THE WOMEN'S CARDIOVASCULAR WELLNESS AND PREVENTION CENTER

Winthrop's Women's Cardiovascular Wellness and Prevention Center is a comprehensive prevention, treatment and recovery 'patient-centric' philosophy designed for those women with cardiovascular disease or at risk for such. The Center provides a full complement of cardiac and wellness services for women, including fitness referrals, patient education, medical screening and counseling.

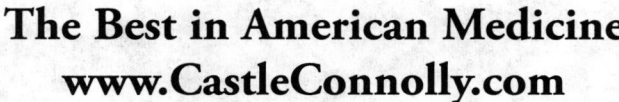

The Best in American Medicine
www.CastleConnolly.com

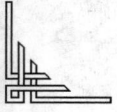
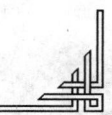

Clinical Genetics

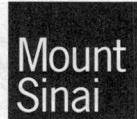 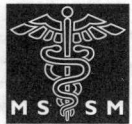

THE MOUNT SINAI MEDICAL CENTER
GENETICS AND GENOMIC SCIENCES
One Gustave L. Levy Place
Fifth Avenue and 100th Street
New York, NY 10029-6574
Physician Referral: 212-241-6947
www.mountsinaimedicalgenetics.org

MOUNT SINAI
SCHOOL OF
MEDICINE

THE DEPARTMENT OF GENETICS AND GENOMIC SCIENCES at The Mount Sinai Medical Center is one of the largest medical genetics centers in the nation, providing expert diagnostic, therapeutic, and counseling services for patients and families with or at risk for genetics disorders or birth defects. The department performs sophisticated diagnostic tests in its state-of-the-art molecular, biochemical, and cytogenetics laboratories, which are New York State and Clinical Laboratory Improvement Amendments (CLIA) licensed, and certified by the College of American Pathologists (CAP).

The department has more than 50 internationally recognized faculty members, including physicians, counselors, and laboratory geneticists who are certified by the American Board of Medical Genetics or the American Board of Genetic Counseling.

Programs and services offered by the department include:

- Clinical Genetic Disorders Program
- Program for Inherited Metabolic Diseases
- Reproductive Genetic Counseling Program
- Cancer Genetic Counseling Program
- Mount Sinai Center for Jewish Genetic Diseases
- International Center for Fabry Disease
- Mount Sinai Comprehensive Gaucher Disease Treatment Center
- Porphyria Comprehensive Diagnostic and Treatment Center
- Congenital Anomalies and Craniofacial Program
- Cardiovascular Genetics Program
- Niemann Pick Disease Center

Advances In Diagnosis And Disease Treatment – In the past several years, Mount Sinai researchers have identified genes responsible for various genetic diseases and developed new treatments for inherited disorders. The following are some examples and results of this important work:

- We have identified genes involved in over a dozen diseases, most recently a debilitating juvenile arthritis, several dystonias, and an inherited form of obesity. The identification of these genes leads to precise diagnosis, understanding disease pathogenesis, and new treatments for these diseases. We have also recently identified a gene linked to prostate cancer.

- Our researchers helped identify eight genes involved in causing Noonan syndrome, a common genetic disorder that causes congenital heart defects. Affected families can now receive early diagnosis and prevention.

- Research pioneered by the Department of Genetics and Genomic Sciences resulted in the development of a safe, effective, FDA-approved treatment for Fabry disease, an inherited metabolic disorder that can cause kidney failure, heart disease, stroke, and premature death.

- Departmental faculty have developed a treatment for Niemann-Pick Type B disease, a hereditary disorder that results in death in childhood or early adulthood.

GROUNDBREAKING RESEARCH AND NEW FORMS OF TREATMENT
There are more than 10,000 known genetic disorders, and current research is identifying the genetic susceptibilities and causative genes for many of these diseases. The faculty of the Department of Genetics and Genomic Sciences at Mount Sinai is performing research to develop new and improved methods for the diagnosis, prevention, and treatment of rare and common diseases. The Human Genome Project, and advances in gene analysis technology and stem cell biology, have accelerated this research.

Colon & Rectal Surgery

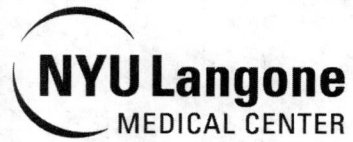

COLON AND RECTAL SURGERY

About the Division of Colon and Rectal Surgery

Colorectal surgeons at NYU Langone perform more than 5,000 outpatient and inpatient procedures each year using laser, laparoscopic, endoscopic and other minimally invasive techniques. Candidates for surgery receive same-day care that includes imaging, radiation and nutritional support. We specialize in cancer, diverticulitis, IBD, anorectal conditions, and bowel disorders.

Adrenalectomies

Our surgeons are skilled at performing adrenalectomies, the surgical removal of one or both of the adrenal glands. This procedure is usually advised for patients with tumors of the adrenal glands, which may be malignant or benign. Adrenalectomy, once performed by conventional (open) surgery, is now routinely done laparoscopically through four very small incisions, which allows patients to usually be discharged within 36 hours.

Colorectal Cancer

We offer the most advanced screening options available for the diagnosis of colon cancer, the second leading cause of cancer death in the U.S. Additionally, we continue to investigate colorectal cancer screenings in special populations such as women, veterans, immigrants, minorities and patients with HIV, and offer the use of virtual colonoscopy for the detection of colorectal polyps and cancer.

Laparoscopic Techniques

Surgeons at NYU Langone use tiny incisions to remove a segment of the colon, which dramatically speeds recovery and reduces the need for pain medication. Laparoscopic techniques are used to treat pancreatic tumors, splenic related conditions, hiatus hernias, small bowel tumors and adrenalectomies.

Liver Lesions

Our surgeons treat liver lesions with painless radiofrequency ablation. Minimally invasive resections and open liver surgery are also routinely performed.

Virtual Colonoscopy

The Medical Center offers the latest developments in colon cancer detection, including virtual colonoscopy. This noninvasive procedure makes use of sophisticated imaging techniques to generate a 3-D reconstruction of the inner surface of the colon, which can then be evaluated for abnormalities by specially trained radiologists.

Dermatology

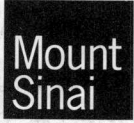 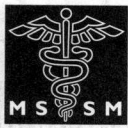

THE MOUNT SINAI DEPARTMENT OF DERMATOLOGY
One Gustave L. Levy Place
Fifth Avenue and 100th Street
New York, NY 10029-6574
Physician Referral: 1-800-MD-SINAI (637-4624)
www.mountsinai.org/dermatology

MOUNT SINAI
SCHOOL OF
MEDICINE

The Mount Sinai Department of Dermatology has one of the most comprehensive programs for skin health and the treatment of skin diseases in the nation. In addition to our offices at Mount Sinai Hospital, the department has satellite offices throughout New York City and in the suburbs.

Skin Cancer
Our department is at the forefront of research in the treatment and prevention of skin cancer. Drs. Hooman Khorasani and David Kriegel perform state-of-the-art surgical treatment and repairs for all types of skin cancer.

Dr. Orit Markowitz uses new imaging techniques for the early diagnosis and prevention of melanoma. We are one of the few dermatology departments with optical coherence tomography (OCT) technology, Molemax technology and Melafind systems. The latter devices are useful for evaluating non-melanoma skin cancers and pigmented lesions and for following and diagnosing melanoma.

Drs. Czernik, Goldenberg, Goldstein, Lamb, Lebwohl, Levitt, Markowitz, Shim-Chang, and Zeichner have expertise in the diagnosis, prevention, and treatment of all skin cancers and have developed many of the treatments currently in use to prevent and treat cancerous and precancerous skin lesions. We also treat one of the largest groups of patients with cutaneous T-cell lymphoma.

General Dermatology
Psoriasis:
Our faculty number among the country's leading experts in psoriasis, including our department chairman, Dr. Mark Lebwohl, and Drs. Norman Goldstein, Gary Goldenberg, Jacob Levitt, Annette Czernik and Angela Lamb. Our center includes a state-of- the-art phototherapy unit, an infusion center for intravenous treatments, and a research center where many new therapies available for psoriasis are tested.

Autoimmune and inflammatory skin diseases:
We have one of the largest centers for inflammatory skin diseases where we treat psoriasis, atopic dermatitis and contact dermatitis. Dr. Emma Guttman is doing clinical research in new targeted therapies for severe atopic dermatitis. Dr. Suhail Hadi is one of the most experienced in the use of the excimer laser for psoriasis and vitiligo. Our faculty also includes three renowned acne experts, Drs. Angela Lamb, Joshua Zeichner, and Susan Bershad.

Our bullous disease center is run by Drs. Jacob Levitt and Annette Czernik. We are one of the few dermatology departments in the nation with its own infusion unit, so patients may be treated either as outpatients in the infusion unit or as inpatients at The Mount Sinai Medical Center.

Pediatric and Adolescent Dermatology
Our faculty treats all ages for skin. Dr. Susan Bershad is a board-certified pediatric and adolescent dermatologist. Dr. Emma Guttman is a trailblazer in research on atopic dermatitis and other forms of eczema.

Cosmetic Dermatology Center
We were one of the first programs in the nation to have a procedural dermatology fellowship, which is run by Drs. David Kriegel and Hooman Khorasani. Along with Drs. Marsha Gordon, Heidi Waldorf, Gary Goldenberg, Joshua Zeichner, and Helen Shim-Chang, our team is renowned for noninvasive skin rejuvenation combining topical regimens, soft tissue fillers, botulinum toxin, photodynamic therapy and laser and radio frequency devices. Members of our faculty perform liposuction, blepharoplasty, microdermabrasion, laser hair removal, sclerotherapy, skin tightening procedures, laser removals of tattoos, and pigmented and vascular lesions as well as laser resurfacing such as fraxel and total Fx.

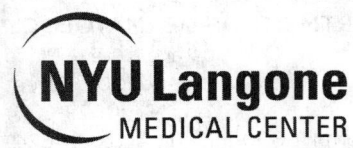

DERMATOLOGY

About the Ronald O. Perelman Department of Dermatology
The Ronald O. Perelman Department of Dermatology is a national and international leader in dermatology, employing the most advanced science and medicine to diagnose and treat skin disorders. The Department provides dermatologic care for more than 100,000 patients each year, as well as conducting research into some of the most significant dermatologic problems. Services include adult and pediatric medical dermatology, dermatologic/skin cancer surgery and cosmetic dermatology. We specialize in the following areas:

Dermatologic / Skin Cancer Surgery and Cosmetic Dermatology
NYU Langone Medical Center's dermatologists provide specialized care for the treatment of malignant and benign skin lesions and offer cutting-edge therapies for aesthetic and cosmetic concerns.

General Dermatology
Dermatologic associates offer multi-subspecialty dermatology care in private office settings for patients with disorders of the skin, hair, and nails, including inflammatory skin diseases such as psoriasis and lupus, cancers and other skin tumors, hair loss, infections and allergic skin diseases such as eczema, contact dermatitis and hives.

Pediatric and Adolescent Dermatology
The Medical Center also boasts a specialized professional practice dedicated to the treatment of diseases affecting the skin, hair, and nails of infants, children and adolescents. These disorders include acne, atopic dermatitis/eczema, hair loss, hemangiomas, moles, birthmarks, vitiligo and genetic disorders affecting the skin.

Charles C. Harris Skin and Cancer Unit / Dermatology Clinical Trials Unit
The Charles C. Harris Skin and Cancer Unit at Tisch Hospital is an outpatient dermatology teaching center combining unique patient care with superior medical education. Resident and attending physicians provide diagnosis and treatment of skin diseases that include acne, eczema and warts as well as complex medical conditions such as connective tissue disorders, pigmented lesions, skin allergies and skin cancers.

Dermatopathology
Highly trained dermatopathologists at the Medical Center examine skin tissues submitted by physicians from biopsies and surgeries to diagnose skin diseases and malignancies. One of the busiest academic skin pathology units in the country, the Dermatopathology section of the Department also provides consultative services for the review of skin pathology specimens performed elsewhere.

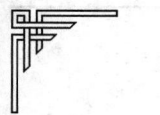

The Best in American Medicine
www.CastleConnolly.com

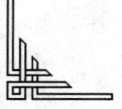
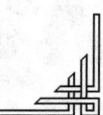

Diabetes Management/ Wound Care

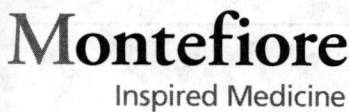

Montefiore
Inspired Medicine

111 East 210th Street
Bronx, New York 10467
1-866-MED-TALK
www.montefiore.org/endocrinology

Clinical Diabetes Center at Montefiore

Montefiore Medical Center's comprehensive approach to diabetes management is nationally recognized and serves as a model for clinical excellence. Approximately 11 percent of adults in the Bronx have diabetes, one of the highest percentages in New York City and in the nation. Every year, more than 4,000 adults visit Montefiore's Clinical Diabetes Center for care and support.

The Center, which is nationally ranked by *U.S. News & World Report*'s 2012–13 "America's Best Hospitals," comprises a multidisciplinary team of experienced endocrinologists, nurse practitioners, clinical nurse specialists, certified diabetes educators and nutritionists who provide care in both inpatient and outpatient settings. The medical faculty of the Center are all full-time members of the Division of Endocrinology of the Departments of Medicine and Pediatrics. This 50-member team provides comprehensive care for adults and children with diabetes (types 1 and 2) and endocrine disease. A distinguishing feature of the Center is its designation by the New York Department of Health as a Diabetes Center of Excellence. As part of this recognition, the Center was awarded a five-year, $500,000 grant to further the care of women with gestational diabetes. Only five sites in the state have received this honor.

The Clinical Diabetes Center emphasizes empowerment through education, teaching patients how to improve their health through diet and medication, use their insulin pumps and monitor their glucose subcutaneously. **Montefiore's diabetes self-management program, the Proactive Managed Information System for Education in Diabetes (PROMISED©), has been twice nationally recognized by the American Diabetes Association for exemplary performance and the consistent achievement of national standards.** Support groups are a mainstay of the Center's activities and serve to help patients maintain lasting health management skills and stabilize their chronic conditions. The Center is active in community outreach and collaborates closely with primary care physicians in the Bronx, Westchester County and surrounding boroughs of New York City.

Faculty of the Clinical Diabetes Center are also members of the Einstein Diabetes Research Center, which has been continually funded by the National Institutes of Health for 35 years. The Diabetes Research Center serves as a major site for many basic and clinical research advancements in the areas of diabetes, obesity and metabolic diseases.

Diagnostic Radiology

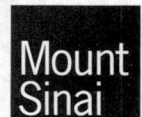
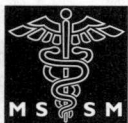

MOUNT SINAI SCHOOL OF MEDICINE

THE MOUNT SINAI MEDICAL CENTER RADIOLOGY

One Gustave L. Levy Place
Fifth Avenue and 100th Street
New York, NY 10029-6574
Physician Referral: 1-800-MD-SINAI (637-4624)
www.mountsinai.org/imaging

THE DEPARTMENT OF RADIOLOGY at Mount Sinai offers patients one of the world's most comprehensive and sophisticated arrays of diagnostic and interventional radiology services. The department uses filmless digital technology that spans magnetic resonance imaging (MRI), multi-slice computed tomography (CT), positron emission tomography CT (PET-CT), single photon emission computed tomography CT (SPECT-CT), advanced ultrasound, conventional radiography, angiography, digital mammography, and state-of-the-art Picture Archiving Communication System (PACS) technology.

Comprehensive Diagnostic Services – Mount Sinai provides the entire range of diagnostic radiology services in a patient-friendly environment. Its nationally renowned radiologic physicians specialize in every area of disease diagnosis, as well as disease prevention and innovative therapeutic approaches. The combination of state-of-the-art imaging equipment with the finest imaging physicians makes Mount Sinai Radiology the place to go for all your imaging needs.

Early Detection Programs – We are committed to special screening approaches for early disease detection. We provide radiological screenings for colon, breast, and lung cancer and atherosclerosis. The early detection programs use a variety of imaging techniques, such as CT and MRI for atherosclerosis, CT for lung and colon cancer, PET for oncology, digital and 3D mammography, MRI, ultrasound, and computer-aided diagnosis for breast cancer.

Minimally Invasive Procedures – Radiology at Mount Sinai has moved beyond diagnosis to the most sophisticated therapeutic interventions. Interventional radiologists at Mount Sinai perform biopsies, vascular therapies, and uterine artery embolization for fibroids—an alternative to hysterectomy—as well as treatments for aneurysms, atherosclerosis, and many types of cancer. In addition, advanced CT and MR angiography techniques are widely utilized to diagnose vascular diseases in a minimally invasive yet highly accurate manner.

Oncology Imaging – Radiologists work closely with surgeons, oncologists, and other caregivers to optimize the diagnosis and treatment of patients with head and neck, liver, lung, breast, and gastrointestinal cancers. State of the art CT, MRI, ultrasound, SPECT and PET CT are utilized to make the most accurate, least invasive and lowest dose diagnosis.

DEVELOPING NEW DIAGNOSTIC TOOLS

Radiology at Mount Sinai is an active center of imaging research and development. Mount Sinai physicians and scientists developed a special form of MRI to diagnose heart disease and atherosclerosis noninvasively and thereby identify patients at greatest risk for stroke and heart attack. We actively collaborate with other disciplines to develop and refine imaging tools that will make prevention and diagnosis increasingly effective. That is the case, for example, in neuroscience, where the imaging innovations impact our understanding of neurodegenerative conditions, such as Parkinson's disease, multiple sclerosis, stroke, brain tumors, and various psychiatric disorders; cardiovascular disease, where studies are under way to predict the risk associated with atherosclerotic plaques and assess new therapies for aortic and cerebral artery aneurysms; and liver disease, where radiologists, transplant surgeons, and hepatologists collaborate closely to develop optimal therapeutic strategies.

Emergency Services

For more information about the Emergency Care Center
or for a physician referral, call 1-877-HOLY-NAME.
Please mention "Castle Connolly Guide."

718 Teaneck Road
Teaneck, NJ 07666
1-877-HOLY-NAME
(1-877-465-9626)
www.holyname.org

Holy Name Medical Center
Emergency Care Center

Holy Name Medical Center's George P. Pitkin MD Emergency Care Center is an ultramodern facility that combines an experienced, specialized staff with today's best practices in health care and the highest industry standards for a superior care experience. Accommodating 55,000 visits per year, Holy Name's emergency division offers a physical space engineered for efficiency, comfort and privacy, and a care delivery system focused on quality and patient satisfaction.

The Center is staffed by board-certified emergency medicine physicians, physician assistants, nurse practitioners and registered nurses with certification in emergency nursing. In the Pediatric Fast Track, on-site board-certified pediatricians and specialized pediatric nurses provide safe, compassionate care, private rooms and a kid-friendly atmosphere to ensure that a visit to Holy Name's ER is as positive an experience as possible.

Designated by the State of New Jersey as a Medical Coordination Center for large-scale emergency preparedness—the only one in Bergen County—Holy Name's Emergency Care Center is able to manage any mass casualty situation, and has special accommodations and procedures in place for decontamination and radiation detection.

EMERGENCY RESPONDERS IN THE COMMUNITY

Holy Name Medical Center (HNMC) provides pre–Medical Center life support services to our surrounding communities. The first Medical Center–based Basic Life Support (BLS) provider in Bergen County, HNMC also supplies Mobile Intensive Care Units staffed by emergency medical technicians and paramedics trained in CPR, cardiac life support, trauma life support, incident command, HAZMAT and CBRNE (chemical, biological, radiological, nuclear and explosive) response.

Holy Name is the only hospital in the area bringing the Hybrid Ambulance to the community, combining advanced life support (ALS) and basic life support (BLS) in a single mobile intensive care unit. The Medical Center's Special Operations unit provides support to mass-gathering events, patient rescue and all-terrain transport, and EMS branch communications. To further its commitment to the community it serves, Holy Name EMS professionals also offer emergency medical training for first responders, EMTs, paramedics and other emergency service personnel.

Awards and Accreditations

- Top Performer on Key Quality Measures—from The Joint Commission for excellence in heart attack, heart failure, pneumonia and surgical care

- Magnet Recognition—from the American Nurses Credentialing Center for excellence in patient care

- J.D. Power and Associates Distinguished Hospital Award—for excellence in emergency service

- Top 10% national ranking for stroke care from HealthGrades®

- Beacon Award for Critical Care Excellence®—from the American Association of Critical-Care Nurses (AACN)

- Primary Stroke Care Certification—from The Joint Commission for excellence in stroke patient care

- Accredited Chest Pain Center—from The Society of Chest Pain Centers for excellence in the ability to diagnose and treat chest pain and acute coronary symptoms

Gastroenterology

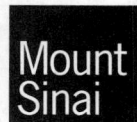 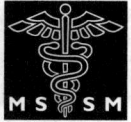

**MOUNT SINAI
SCHOOL OF
MEDICINE**

THE MOUNT SINAI MEDICAL CENTER
GASTROINTESTINAL AND SURGICAL SPECIALTIES
One Gustave L. Levy Place
Fifth Avenue and 100th Street
New York, NY 10029-6574
Physician Referral: 1-800-MD-SINAI (637-4624)
www.mountsinai.org

Mount Sinai's **DIVISIONS OF GASTROENTEROLOGY, COLON AND RECTAL SURGERY, LIVER DISEASES, PEDIATRIC GASTROENTEROLOGY, AND PEDIATRIC HEPATOLOGY** are renowned for their delivery of patient care, research, and education in diseases of the gastrointestinal (GI) tract. In 2000, the National Institutes of Health (NIH) recognized the importance of Mount Sinai as a research center with a grant for GI/Liver fellowship training. Mount Sinai is the only medical school in New York City to earn this prestigious award.

Mount Sinai's Division of Gastroenterology ranks 7th among all institutions in the country, according to the *U.S. News & World Report's* 2012–2013 "Best Hospitals" issue. Successes include breakthroughs in the medical and surgical management of the inflammatory bowel diseases (IBD): ulcerative colitis, and Crohn's disease. Mount Sinai spearheaded novel therapies for treating severe IBD and helped establish the role of colonoscopy in preventing colon cancer by removing precancerous polyps. More recent innovations include employing a tiny camera within a swallowable capsule to capture images in the stomach and intestines. Mount Sinai offers patients advanced comprehensive and interdisciplinary care; newer agents through clinical trials; services of psychologists and nutritionists; and world-class expertise in endoscopic procedures.

Division of Colon and Rectal Surgery — Continuing a long tradition of expertise in gastrointestinal disorders, Mount Sinai surgeons focus on surgical therapies for all diseases involving the colon, rectum, and anus. Highly skilled in the treatment of Crohn's disease (which was first described at Mount Sinai in 1932), ulcerative colitis, colon and rectal cancer, and diverticulitis, they specialize in the most advanced techniques of rectal surgery with an emphasis on colostomy avoidance. They also employ minimally invasive techniques and cutting-edge technologies for the treatment of hemorrhoids, fistulas, rectal tumors, and fecal incontinence.

Division of Liver Diseases — With a program that is among the largest and most successful in the world, Mount Sinai carries out a diverse portfolio of research projects. Featuring both clinical care and scientific investigations, they involve transplantation; diagnosis and treatment of viral hepatitis, including trials for revolutionary new drugs for Hepatitis B and C; treatment of scarring, or fibrosis; management of primary biliary cirrhosis, an autoimmune disease of bile ducts; treatment of liver cancer; and diagnosis and treatment of genetic liver diseases, including Wilson's disease (copper overload) and hemachromatosis (iron overload).

Division of Pediatric Gastroenterology — The division provides consultation and treatment for the full range of children's digestive and nutritional diseases. The Children's IBD Center offers comprehensive, multidisciplinary, family-centered care for pediatric patients with Crohn's disease and ulcerative colitis, and receives referrals from across the country. The division also provides care to families of infants, children, and teens who have the full range of both complex and common digestive disorders, including celiac disease, gastroesophageal reflux disease, and irritable bowel syndrome. Additionally, the division is involved in both basic science and clinical research, allowing physicians to provide state-of-the-art, evidence-based care.

Division of Pediatric Hepatology — The Transplant Program is one of the largest in the nation and was the first program in New York to perform liver transplants and, later, small bowel transplants. The division is active in clinical research in IBD, focusing on issues of genetic factors, psychosocial interactions, and drug trials in liver disease.

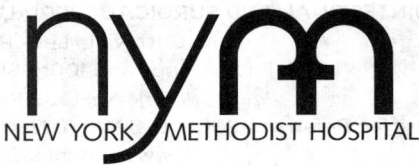

NEW YORK METHODIST HOSPITAL

THE INSTITUTE FOR DIGESTIVE AND LIVER DISORDERS

New York Methodist Hospital
506 Sixth Street, Brooklyn, N.Y. 11215
Phone 866 DIGEST-1 (866 344-3781)
http://www.nym.org

SPECIALISTS AND MEDICAL SERVICES

The Institute's panel of physician specialists includes gastroenterologists, hepatologists, surgeons, laparoscopic surgeons, radiologists, medical and radiation oncologists and pathologists. Nutritionists and psychologists are also members of the team. The latest advances in the diagnosis and treatment of the gastrointestinal tract and the liver are available. These include endoscopic ultrasound, pediatric and adult capsule endoscopy and advanced laparoscopic surgery. In addition, the Endoscopy Suite at New York Methodist Hospital enables physicians to perform highly advanced diagnostic and treatment procedures that can detect and determine disorders of the gastrointestinal tract and bile ducts as well as perform the non-surgical removal of bile duct gallstones.

PROGRAMS OFFERED

Among the programs and services offered by the Institute are a Barrett's esophagus program, colorectal cancer program, heartburn (GERD) program, chronic Hepatitis B & C program, liver transplantation evaluation program, ulcer program, bowel disorders program and pediatric gastroenterology program. Gallbladder and pancreatic conditions are also treated.

* * *

Referrals to the Institute's specialists, programs and services can be made through an individual's primary care physician or requested directly through the Institute's telephone referral service. More information (and on-line physician referral) is available at the Hospital's website, http://www.nym.org.

THE PEDIATRIC GASTROENTEROLOGY PROGRAM

Problems commonly seen by physicians affiliated with the program include regurgitation, colic, constipation, diarrhea, recurrent abdominal pain, jaundice, blood in the stool, failure to thrive and formula intolerances. Children with these disorders present a special challenge because, along with the medical treatment that they receive, they need special care to ensure that their normal growth and development is not disrupted.

Special procedures that can be used to evaluate and diagnose pediatric gastrointestinal disorders include upper and lower endoscopies, liver biopsies and suction rectal biopsies. These procedures are performed by board certified specials in pediatric gastroenterology.

NewYork-Presbyterian
The University Hospital of Columbia and Cornell

Affiliated with Columbia University College of Physicians and Surgeons and Weill Cornell Medical College

NewYork-Presbyterian Hospital
Columbia University Medical Center
622 West 168th Street
New York, NY 10032

Center for Advanced Digestive Care
NewYork-Presbyterian Hospital
Weill Cornell Medical Center
525 East 68th Street
New York, NY 10065

1-877-NYP-WELL (1-877-697-9355)   www.nyp.org/digestive

NewYork-Presbyterian Digestive Disease Services

Since 2010, NewYork-Presbyterian Hospital's gastroenterology program has ranked among the top ten in the nation in the annual 'Best Hospitals' survey conducted by *U.S. News & World Report*™. NewYork-Presbyterian's Digestive Disease Services feature a collaborative team approach, an exceptional track record of routine and advanced procedures, prevention programs, and basic science and clinical research aimed at developing novel therapies.

- Interventional endoscopic procedures to treat disorders such as pancreatic cancer, pancreatitis, biliary and pancreatic stones, Barrett's esophagus, and polyps.
- Endoscopic sewing and radiofrequency ablation for gastroesophageal reflux disease (GERD).
- Minimally invasive surgical approaches, including single-incision, endolumenal, "needlescopic" procedures and combined endoscopic laparoscopic surgery (CELS).
- The Center for Liver Disease and Transplantation achieves extraordinary outcomes in living and deceased liver transplant and features laparoscopic removal of living donor liver tissue for select cases.
- Colorectal surgery is enhanced by the state-of-the-art Siemens Artis zeego® medical imaging system. This system provides real-time, more accurate 3-D images of the body and enables surgeons to transition seamlessly from diagnosis to surgical remedy.

Patients benefit from a range of routine diagnostic tests such as endoscopy, colonoscopy, and flexible sigmoidoscopy, as well as laparoscopy to diagnose and stage digestive cancers. Interventional endoscopic approaches are also available, including:

- Endoscopic retrograde cholangiopancreatography (ERCP) to evaluate the ducts of the gallbladder, pancreas, and liver.
- Endoscopic ultrasound (EUS) to diagnose pancreatic disorders and stage esophageal, gastric, and rectal cancers. NewYork-Presbyterian Hospital is one of only a few centers using EUS for needle aspiration of pancreatic cysts and tumors.
- Cholangioscopy to evaluate stones or strictures in the pancreatic or bile ducts.
- Double-balloon and spiral enteroscopy to investigate possible intestinal bleeding.
- Probe-based confocal laser endomicroscopy to enhance the early detection and treatment of cancers and precancerous conditions.
- Endoscopic stenting to relieve obstructions and improve symptoms.

Comprehensive and Compassionate Care

Patients who come to NewYork-Presbyterian Hospital benefit from a personalized multidisciplinary approach to the care of:

- Cancers of the esophagus, liver, pancreas, colon, stomach, and rectum
- Inflammatory bowel diseases (Crohn's disease and ulcerative colitis)
- Liver disease, including fatty liver and cirrhosis and hepatitis B and C
- Esophageal disorders, such as GERD and Barrett's esophagus
- Disorders of the pancreas, gallbladder, and bile ducts
- Celiac disease
- Polyps, particularly in the colon
- Peptic ulcer and other stomach diseases
- Anal and rectal diseases
- Obesity (through weight loss surgery)
- Type 2 diabetes (through metabolic surgery)

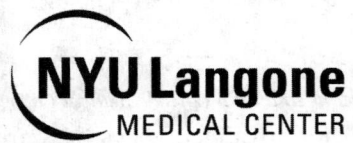

GASTROENTEROLOGY

About the Division of Gastroenterology, Department of Medicine
The Division of Gastroenterology at NYU Langone Medical Center is dedicated to the diagnosis and treatment of patients with diseases of the gastrointestinal tract. Physicians draw on their extensive knowledge and experience in the diagnosis and management of inflammatory bowel disease, peptic ulcer disease, esophageal disorders, gastrointestinal cancer, and liver, biliary and pancreatic diseases. We specialize in the following areas:

Colorectal Cancer
The Medical Center offers the most advanced screening options available for the diagnosis of colon cancer. Additionally, physicians continue to investigate colorectal cancer in special populations such as women, veterans, immigrants, minorities and patients with HIV, and offer the use of virtual colonoscopy for the detection of colorectal polyps and cancer.

Esophageal Diseases
The Esophageal Disease Center offers patients state-of-the-art diagnosis and treatment of esophageal disorders. The Center focuses on gastroesophageal reflux disease, esopha-geal motility disorders, Barrett's esophagus, adenocarcinoma of the esophagus and swal-lowing disorders. It also offers diagnostic studies on esophageal manometry, impedance testing for swallowing, pH catheter and impedance testing for reflux and BRAVO capsule pH testing, as well as such therapies as Barrett's ablation and esophageal dilations.

Gastrointestinal Cancers
Cancer Institute physicians treat patients with all types of gastrointestinal cancers, including those of the esophagus, stomach, colon/rectum, small intestine, liver, pancreas, gallbladder, and biliary tract. They also treat individuals with complex recurring disease, including those origi-nally treated elsewhere. Patients have the opportunity to participate in numerous clinical trials.

Complex Treatments and Diagnosis
Physicians in the Division of Gastroenterology are highly experienced in the use of enter-oscopy and capsule endoscopy for the diagnosis of gastrointestinal bleeding of unknown origin. They have special interest in the diagnosis and treatment of patients with complex pancreatic-biliary disease through the use of ERCP and endoscopic ultrasound.

Virtual Colonoscopy
NYU Langone Medical Center is in the vanguard of advanced colon cancer detection through virtual colonoscopy. The study gives a complete evaluation of the entire surface of the colon and ensures greater accuracy and less patient discomfort.

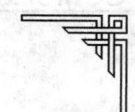
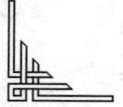
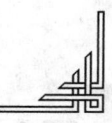

The Best in American Medicine
www.CastleConnolly.com

Geriatric Medicine

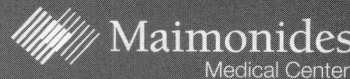
Maimonides serves one of the oldest populations in New York City, with one quarter of our patients over the age of 75. The Geriatrics Program at Maimonides is fully equipped to meet the special needs of this growing segment of the population. Directed by Barbara Paris, MD, the program encompasses inpatient and outpatient services, featuring the Acute Care for Elderly (ACE) Unit and the Safe at Home program. The staff is focused on the continuity, coordination, quality and dignity of care provided.

Patient Evaluation
ACE Unit services focus on acute medical care and account for the complex needs of hospitalized elderly patients. Special attention is given to the assessment of memory loss and understanding the underlying causes of geriatric syndromes that result in falls, incontinence and frailty. Psychosocial issues affecting elderly patients, such as loneliness and end-of-life care, are also addressed.

Wound Care and Hyperbaric Center
Elderly patients can often have wounds that do not heal easily, which is why we have a dedicated wound care team available. Individualized wound treatment is dependent upon the type and severity of the wound. Treatments include conventional and advanced wound dressings, antibiotic therapy, protective footwear, and hyperbaric oxygen therapy.

Safe at Home Program
The Safe at Home program actively manages the care of the frail elderly to keep them in their homes and within their communities. The program is designed to identify patients aged 75 years and older who are at high risk during the transitional period from hospital to home; provide them with coordinated comprehensive care after the transition from hospital to home; actively engage family caregivers and community support networks; increase patient satisfaction with their care during this transitional period; and reduce re-hospitalizations, emergency room visits, and nursing home placements.

Outpatient Geriatric Services
Our geriatric team offers comprehensive assessment and primary care services throughout Southern Brooklyn.

Relying heavily on evidence-based medicine, Maimonides Medical Center has been commended for outstanding services by a number of independent rating organizations. Earlier this year, Maimonides was named a Distinguished Hospital for Clinical Excellence by Healthgrades – one of only three hospitals in the metropolitan area; the American Stroke Association bestowed its Gold Plus Achievement Award on the hospital; and the American Hospital Association once again named it a Most Wired Hospital.

Maimonides Medical Center
Passionate about medicine.
Compassionate about people.

www.maimonidesmed.org/geriatrics

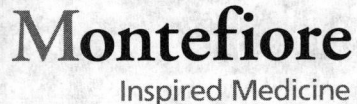
Montefiore
Inspired Medicine

111 East 210th Street
Bronx, New York 10467
1-866-MED-TALK
www.montefiore.org/geriatrics

Geriatrics at Montefiore

Montefiore Medical Center's Division of Geriatrics is widely recognized as a pioneer in the field and a leader in clinical innovation. **The Division provides outstanding primary and consultative care for older adults, and is recognized as high performing by *U.S. News & World Report*'s 2012–13 "America's Best Hospitals."**

Montefiore is committed to developing revolutionary approaches to address the physical and mental challenges associated with the aging process. Leading this charge is Joe Verghese, MD, Chief of the Division of Geriatrics. An internationally respected neurologist, Dr. Verghese brings a unique perspective and strengthens the collaborative ties between the fields of neurology and geriatrics.

The integration of these fields opens the door to new investigative and clinical opportunities. **In collaboration with NIH-funded researchers from Albert Einstein College of Medicine's Institute for Aging Research, our physicians are working to understand the effects of aging and diseases such as Alzheimer's and Parkinson's on cognition and mobility.**

Of special note is the Einstein Aging Study, which focuses on the aging brain and examines both normal aging and the special challenges of Alzheimer's and other dementing disorders. This project has been supported by grants from the National Institute on Aging since 1980. Another effort that has garnered significant attention is the Longevity Genes Project, which is led by Nir Barzilai, MD, and seeks to identify longevity genes that could lead to new drug therapies and ultimately longer, healthier lives.

Montefiore serves the needs of geriatric patients across all points in the care continuum—from outpatient clinics to nursing homes. **All physicians are dual certified in geriatrics and palliative care and are supported by specialists from neurology, geriatric psychiatry, physical medicine and rehabilitation, orthopaedics, nursing, social work and other areas.**

The Division is widely celebrated for its exceptional education programs for physicians and has one of the oldest geriatrics fellowship programs in the nation. Under the leadership of Laurie Jacobs, MD, Vice Chairman of Medicine, **Montefiore was the recipient of a $2 million grant from the Donald W. Reynolds Foundation to establish the GeriEd Program, which aims to improve primary care physicians' skills and knowledge of geriatric medicine, with a special focus on older adults with complex medical and neurologic disease such as dementia, falls and delirium.**

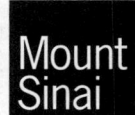
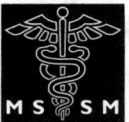

**MOUNT SINAI
SCHOOL OF
MEDICINE**

THE MOUNT SINAI MEDICAL CENTER
THE BROOKDALE DEPARTMENT OF
GERIATRICS AND PALLIATIVE MEDICINE
One Gustave L. Levy Place
Fifth Avenue and 100th Street
New York, NY 10029-6574
Physician Referral: 1-800-MD-SINAI (637-4624)
www.mountsinai.org/geriatrics
www.mountsinai.org/palliative

The Best in Clinical Care

In recognition of the care offered to older patients, The Mount Sinai Medical Center's **BROOKDALE DEPARTMENT OF GERIATRICS AND PALLIATIVE MEDICINE** is cited time and time again among the finest in the nation. In 2012, *U.S. News & World Report* ranked our geriatrics specialty #2 and our medical school program #1 in the United States.

We offer a full spectrum of patient care, including a specialized inpatient care team for the elderly to minimize complications sometimes associated with an older person's hospital stay, a primary care geriatrics practice for older adults living in the community, a hospital-based consultation service for patients throughout Mount Sinai, a number of community-linked programs and partnerships, and a palliative care team dedicated to ensuring the highest quality care and support for patients and families facing serious illnesses.

The Martha Stewart Center for Living, a modern facility designed by renowned architect C.C. Pei, provides clinical care and education for patients and serves as a training ground for physicians. Our newly opened Wiener Family Palliative Care Unit, the only one of its kind in Manhattan, provides inpatient care for patients and families facing serious and life-threatening illness.

Groundbreaking Research—Mount Sinai's researchers continue to advance the understanding, prevention, and treatment of age-related disorders. The extensive research on aging conducted by the Brookdale Department of Geriatrics and Palliative Medicine includes studies on health services, medical decision making and ethical dilemmas, palliative care, the neurobiology of aging, and clinical interventions to promote independence in old age. The department's expertise serves as a renowned educational resource for all Mount Sinai affiliates and other institutions in teaching geriatrics and palliative medicine to medical students, medical residents, geriatrics and palliative care fellows, established physicians, and health profession trainees in other disciplines.

History Of Excellence—The Mount Sinai Medical Center is a pioneer in geriatric medicine. In 1909, a Mount Sinai physician coined the term "geriatrics," and in 1914, he wrote the first textbook on medical care for older adults. Today, the Brookdale Department of Geriatrics and Palliative Medicine continues to break new ground, offering comprehensive care, disease prevention, and the promotion of healthy and productive aging. The department's enhanced expertise in assessing and managing patients with dementia greatly complements its established, interdisciplinary approach to patient care, in which medical staff and social workers address each patient's needs as a team. Our newly opened Wiener Family Palliative Care Unit, the only one of its kind in Manhattan, provides inpatient care for patients and families facing serious and life-threatening illness.

THE FIRST FREESTANDING DEPARTMENT OF GERIATRICS AT A U.S. MEDICAL SCHOOL
Mount Sinai's Brookdale Department of Geriatrics and Palliative Medicine was the first freestanding department of geriatrics established by a U.S. medical school, and it continues to be one of the very best. It offers unparalleled inpatient and outpatient care, as well as numerous treatment programs designed to meet the unique needs of older adults. Mount Sinai is also home to world-class researchers dedicated to advancing our understanding of Alzheimer's disease and other common geriatric conditions. At the department's heart are its patients. The geriatricians of The Mount Sinai Medical Center work hard to improve life and longevity for New York's elderly.

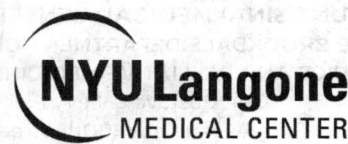

550 First Avenue *(at 31st Street)*
New York, NY 10016
www.NYULMC.org
Physician Referral: **888-7-NYU-MED** *(888-769-8633)*

GERIATRIC MEDICINE

About the Section of Geriatrics, Division of General Internal Medicine, Department of Medicine
NYU Langone Medical Center has a distinguished history as a federally designated research center and leader in the care of geriatrics. We specialize in the following areas:

Inpatient Geriatrics Services
Using a team approach, a senior geriatrician leads nurses, pharmacists, geropsychiatrists, rehabilitation experts and fellowship trainees in caring for geriatric patients with complex conditions. If screening reveals a hospitalized patient is suffering from a geriatric problem (such as cognitive impairment), special consultation is offered to the patient's health care team.

The Healthy Aging Initiative
A fundamental part of the care provided by geriatricians within NYU Langone Medical Center's faculty group practice is assessing and advising older individuals on how to avoid developing problems like cognitive or functional impairment.

The William and Sylvia Silberstein Aging and Dementia Research Center
The Silberstein Aging and Dementia Research Center is a National Institute on Aging-designated Center of Excellence in Alzheimer's treatment. The facility provides comprehensive diagnostic evaluations to determine if memory loss is "normal" or more serious; a memory enhancement program for age-related memory decline; clinical trials for mild memory loss and for Alzheimer's treatment; state-of-the-art brain imaging techniques; methods to minimize disability in Alzheimer's patients; and comprehensive counseling and support groups for patients, caregivers and family members.

The Pearl Barlow Center for Memory Evaluation and Treatment
The Pearl Barlow Center for Memory Evaluation and Treatment is the clinical care and diagnostic unit of the Silberstein Alzheimer's Institute at NYU Langone Medical Center. The Pearl Barlow Center for Memory Evaluation and Treatment is focused on patients with memory impairments caused by neurological, psychological and physical ailments, as well as memory issues resulting from medication side effects, anxiety, depression and the effects of normal aging, including Alzheimer's disease. This multidisciplinary medical approach, integrated with advanced research capabilities, is the first of its kind in New York City for the treatment of memory disorders.

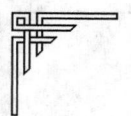

The Best in American Medicine
www.CastleConnolly.com

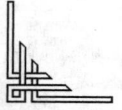
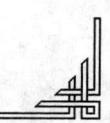

Hand Surgery

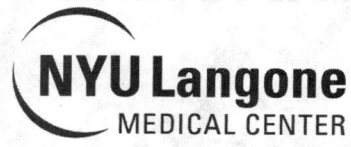

HAND SURGERY

NYU Langone Medical Center's Department of Orthopaedic Surgery provides the full continuum of care for patients with hand and wrist disorders through its specialized Division of Hand Surgery. These include fractures, congenital anomalies, soft tissue and skeletal trauma, degenerative and rheumatoid arthritis, sports-related injuries, vascular disorders, tumors and occupational disorders.

The Hand Division specializes in fractures of the wrist and distal radius and reconstructive hand surgery. Hand surgery experts have particular expertise in post-traumatic injuries, arthritis and congenital, neuromuscular and neoplastic conditions. Offering one of the largest hand programs in the United States, the Division's hand specialists provide extensive care for the many problems that affect the upper extremity, including acute traumatic injuries (fractures, dislocations and tendon, nerve and vascular lacerations), post-traumatic and arthritic deformities, acquired problems (nerve compressions and tumors), congenital deformities and neuromuscular disorders such as cerebral palsy. Board-certified and fellowship-trained orthopaedists perform more than 5,000 procedures on adults and children each year.

After surgery, hand therapy helps surgical patients recover full or partial use of their hands, providing comprehensive rehabilitation for a variety of ailments associated with the hand and upper body. The hand therapy unit, located at NYU Langone's new, state-of-the-art Center for Musculoskeletal Care, specializes in fractures, traumatic injuries, tendonitis, sports injuries, work-related injuries, repetitive stress injuries, carpal tunnel syndrome, tendon and nerve repairs and arthritis. Hand therapy is provided by the expert occupational therapists of Rusk Rehabilitation, who specialize in treatment of the hand and upper extremities.

Research within the Hand Service focuses on a variety of clinical problems including wrist fractures, non-unions of the scaphoid (bone between the hand and the forearm), Kienbock's disease (the death and fracture of bone tissue due to interruption of blood supply), intercarpal subluxations (incomplete or partial dislocation) and neuropathies (disorders of the nerves) of the upper extremities.

Home Health Care

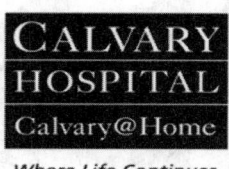

Where Life Continues

CALVARY HOSPITAL
1740 Eastchester Road
Bronx, NY 10461
Tel: (718) 518-2000
www.calvaryhospital.org

CALVARY@HOME
HOME CARE, HOSPICE, AND NURSING HOME HOSPICE

Calvary@Home, the umbrella for our Home Care, Hospice, and Nursing Home Hospice program, brings compassionate care to patients who can be cared for at home. Our inter-disciplinary team includes physicians, nurses, aides, social workers, spiritual care providers, volunteers, bereavement support workers, and other providers as needed. In 2009, The Joint Commission gave Calvary@ Home a Gold Seal of Approval™. Calvary received a 2012 Circle of Life Award® for innovative palliative and end-of-life care. Calvary@Home cares for more than 2,300 patients and families each year.

Certified Home Health Agency
Established in 1985, serves patients with all acute, chronic or life-limiting illnesses. We provide a full range of specialized home healthcare experts to support patients and families. Home care patients approaching the end of life have access to palliative care services such as pain and symptom management, assistance with advance care planning, and psychosocial support. We strive to ensure continuity of care by assigning a core group of caregivers to each patient. Our community health nurses work with the patient's personal physicians to deliver appropriate care. Our home care services are available in Manhattan, the Bronx, Queens, and Westchester.

Hospice
Established in 1998, brings comprehensive care to people at home with all end-stage ill-nesses. Calvary assembles a core group of permanent staff to care for each patient, creating continuity of service for patients and families. Patients who require short-stay inpatient care can be admitted to Calvary in a seamless process. In addition to nurses, physicians and aides, social workers, spiritual counselors, and volunteers make home visits to ensure that physical, psychosocial, emotional and spiritual needs are met. We provide bereavement services for 13 months for families. Staffing exceeds national recommendations. Our hospice services are available in Manhattan, the Bronx, Queens, Brooklyn, as well as Nassau, Westchester and Rockland counties.

Nursing Home Hospice
Brings comprehensive palliative care to nursing home residents suffering from all end-stage illnesses. Provides appropriate care to all dually eligible (Medicare/Medicaid) residents, and bereavement services for loved ones. Through a partnership with Mary Manning Walsh Home in Manhattan, Calvary provides an inpatient level of care for a select number of pa-tients.

Calvary Nursing Home Hospice has contracts with more than 30 facilities in: Manhattan, the Bronx, Queens, Brooklyn, as well as Nassau, Westchester and Rockland Counties.

For information about Calvary@Home, please call 718-518-2465.

Infectious Disease

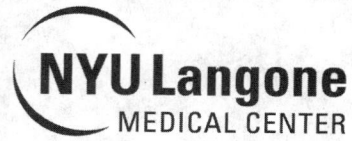

INFECTIOUS DISEASES

About the Division of Infectious Diseases and Immunology

NYU Langone Medical Center has extensive expertise in the diagnosis, treatment and prevention of rare and common acute and chronic infectious diseases. Physicians and fellows within the Division of Infectious Diseases and Immunology are actively involved in the management of complicated bone and joint infections, prevention of infection in cancer and transplant patients and developing strategies for managing hepatitis B and C. They also offer the opportunity for patients with HIV to enroll in clinical trials of new drugs that are not yet widely available. We specialize in the following areas:

HIV Prevention

The Division of Infectious Diseases and Immunology has developed a unique program in HIV prevention that has gained wide recognition and has extended the hospital's expertise from New York City to West and East Africa.

AIDS Clinical Trials

The AIDS Clinical Trials Unit is one of 35 units designated and supported by the National Institute of Allergy and Infectious Diseases, and is a dedicated resource for healthcare providers, researchers and scientists working in the field of HIV/AIDS research. It is one of the most active units in the nation in enrolling adult and pediatric patients in clinical trials supported by the NIH. Data generated by the unit has supported the licensing of several drugs and plays an essential role in defining optimal therapies and preventing complications.

Population Biology of Infectious Diseases

This novel program combines laboratory and clinical studies with epidemiology and genetics to optimize patient outcomes. Researchers in the Division of Infectious Diseases and Immunology are extensively involved in local and international studies into the early diagnosis, treatment and prevention of chronic infections such as tuberculosis and Helicobacter (bacteria associated with stomach ulcers).

Medical and Molecular Parasitology

The Division of Infectious Diseases and Immunology works alongside NYU Langone Medical Center's Department of Medical Parasitology to bring malaria and other parasitic diseases under control.

Internal Medicine

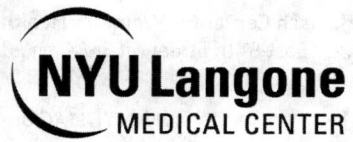
INTERNAL MEDICINE

About the Division of General Internal Medicine, Department of Medicine

Internal medicine physicians at NYU Langone Medical Center are dedicated to treating the whole patient, and not just their disease. Bound by the highest standards of their profession, they address both the physical and psychological aspects of health and disease through clear communication and a fully integrated regimen of care. We specialize in the following areas:

Primary and Specialized Healthcare

The Division of General Internal Medicine offers a multidisciplinary medical approach to treating illnesses involving the heart, lungs, gastrointestinal tract, joints, bones, muscles, endocrine organs and kidneys. A wide range of laboratory, imaging and advanced diagnostic testing, ranging from throat cultures to the complex mapping of the electrical surface of the heart, is available on-site or by referral. Comprehensive women's healthcare, including cancer screening and osteoporosis prevention and treatment, is also available.

Geriatrics

Our geriatric specialists provide comprehensive and multidisciplinary care, consultation and follow-up for elderly patients ranging from prevention and healthy aging to the treatment and care of chronic conditions including dementia, functional impairment and degenerative disorders.

Center for Healthful Behavior Change

The Center for Healthful Behavior Change (CHBC) focuses on developing evidence-based behavioral interventions aimed at improving patient health. CHBC originates, tests and spreads innovative evidence-based behavioral interventions into everyday clinical practice and community settings for patients with high blood pressure and other conditions associated with cardiovascular risk, including obesity and high cholesterol.

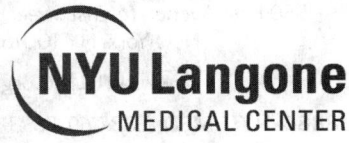

Joan H. Tisch Center for Women's Health
207 East 84th Street *(at 3rd Avenue)*
New York, NY

www.NYULMC.org

646-754-3300

Physician Referral: **888-7-NYU-MED** *(888-769-8633)*

THE JOAN H. TISCH CENTER FOR WOMEN'S HEALTH

About the Joan H. Tisch Center for Women's Health

Because many diseases and conditions impact women differently than men, NYU Langone Medical Center has created the Joan H. Tisch Center for Women's Health. Offering a comprehensive array of primary and specialty care, the Joan H. Tisch Center for Women's Health is New York City's premier destination for healthcare services tailored to the special needs of women. Conveniently located in the heart of Manhattan's Upper East Side, the Center combines NYU Langone's tradition of excellence with a multidisciplinary approach to providing individuals with the best possible medical care. At the Joan H. Tisch Center for Women's Health, the goal is maintaining excellent health and the vehicle is a caring, nurturing environment which understands that women are more than a collection of symptoms and medical conditions.

Expert Staff

Primary and specialty care physicians at the Joan H. Tisch Center for Women's Health have been carefully chosen for their ability to render quality, compassionate care to women. These healthcare professionals are focused on the holistic needs of patients in a state-of-the-art setting that relies heavily on teamwork. As part of a major academic medical institution, the Center is able to draw on additional healthcare resources and innovative research, when the need arises.

Comprehensive Range of Services

The Joan H. Tisch Center for Women's Health offers a wide range of primary and specialty medical care geared to women at a single location. Specialty services include breast health, cardiology, dermatology, endocrinology, ear/nose/throat, gastroenterology, gynecology, internal medicine, mental health, neurology, orthopaedics, plastic surgery, podiatry, pulmonary medicine, rehabilitation medicine, rheumatology, urology, vascular and women's imaging.

Technology Edge

The Joan H. Tisch Center for Women's Health has incorporated sophisticated technology into all levels of the patient experience. This ranges from the Center's informative website to its use of Epic, the Medical Center's up-to-the-minute electronic medical records system. In addition, patients can confidentially view their medical records and test results, as well as make appointment, request prescriptions and communicate with their physicians, through myNYULMC, a secure online service.

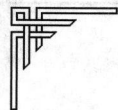

The Best in American Medicine
www.CastleConnolly.com

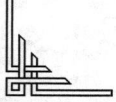
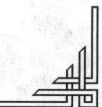

Interventional Cardiology

For more information about the Interventional Institute or for a physician referral, call 1-877-HOLY-NAME. Please mention "Castle Connolly Guide."

Holy Name Medical Center
Interventional Institute

718 Teaneck Road
Teaneck, NJ 07666
1-877-HOLY-NAME
(1-877-465-9626)
www.holyname.org

A REVOLUTIONARY, NONSURGICAL APPROACH

The Interventional Institute at Holy Name Medical Center offers innovative, nonsurgical treatment options for a broad spectrum of illnesses, from vascular conditions and gynecologic health problems to skeletal disease and cancer.

A dynamic field whose treatment techniques are adaptable to many different medical problems, interventional radiology is a rapidly growing medical specialty devoted to advancing patient care through minimally invasive, targeted treatments that are performed with the assistance of imaging guidance.

Under the leadership of John H. Rundback, MD, an internationally recognized specialist in the field of interventional radiology (IR), board-certified interventionalist physicians insert narrow catheters and miniature instruments through tiny incisions, and navigate them directly to the treatment site. Often performed on an outpatient basis, IR carries fewer risks than surgery, with less discomfort and faster recovery. More important, treatment results are comparable to those of traditional approaches.

TREAT A WIDE VARIETY OF MEDICAL PROBLEMS

This revolutionary branch of medicine can shrink uterine fibroid tumors that once necessitated a hysterectomy, clear a life-threatening blood clot in a deep leg vein, eliminate leg pain and amputation risk from plaque buildup in the peripheral arteries, resolve unsightly varicose veins, stabilize painful spine fractures due to osteoporosis, and deliver chemotherapy directly to cancer cells.

Services of the Interventional Institute at Holy Name Medical Center:

- Peripheral artery disease (PAD) treatment
- Limb salvage
- Chemoembolization and transcatheter chemoembolization
- Radiofrequency ablation (RFA)
- Ablation of nonresectable lung cancers
- Uterine fibroid embolization
- Fallopian tube recanalization
- Pelvic congestion syndrome
- Deep vein thrombosis (DVT) treatment
- Endovenous laser treatment for varicose veins
- Kyphoplasty and vertebroplasty for osteoporosis
- Microsphere radioembolization (TheraSphere® and SIR-Sphere® brachytherapy for liver cancer)

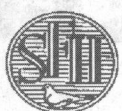

St. Francis Hospital The Heart Center®
100 Port Washington Blvd.
Roslyn, New York 11576
www.stfrancisheartcenter.com
(516) 562-6000   1-888-HEARTNY

Noninvasive Cardiac Imaging

Using the latest in noninvasive cardiac imaging technology, St. Francis Hospital's physicians can evaluate blood flow, heart muscle strength, anatomy, and coronary artery blockages, allowing them to more effectively guide a patient's course of treatment.

Among the most recent advances in St. Francis Hospital's range of services are:

Coronary CT Angiography

St. Francis Hospital was the first hospital on Long Island to offer Multidetector Computed Tomography (MDCT) for noninvasive coronary artery imaging. Now, with installation of more advanced technology, St. Francis can minimize radiation exposure for every patient.

Cardiac MRI

The only center on Long Island with a dedicated Cardiac MRI program and world-class expertise in cardiac MRI, St. Francis Hospital uses MRI to evaluate heart anatomy, function, blood flow, scarring, and inflammation using advanced techniques on two state-of-the-art scanners. Cardiac MRI allows physicians to evaluate effects of heart attack and coronary artery blockages and non-coronary causes of heart failure to determine whether or not patients will benefit from heart surgery or other therapies. World-renowned cardiac MRI authority Nathaniel Reichek, M.D., leads St. Francis Hospital's clinical and research applications with cardiac MRI.

Three-Dimensional Echocardiography

St. Francis Hospital is an internationally recognized leader in three-dimensional echocardiography for quantifying the effects of heart disease and is the leading center in the New York metropolitan area in this field. By creating three-dimensional reconstructions of the heart and blood flow within it, this technology provides diagnostic information that far surpasses that available with conventional echocardiography in many patients.

Nuclear Imaging

Conventional nuclear imaging involves the injection of nuclear isotopes and imaging by a gamma camera that circles the patient's body, improving the accuracy of stress testing. St. Francis Hospital offers the latest advances in nuclear cardiology, such as positron emission tomography of the heart with CT attenuation correction (PET/CT). The nuclear cardiology laboratory at St. Francis Hospital is also a leader in developing new types of computer analysis to improve the value of all forms of cardiac nuclear imaging, and was among the first facilities in the U.S. to receive accreditation from The Intersocietal Commission for the Accreditation of Nuclear Medicine Laboratories.

Noninvasive Imaging at St. Francis Hospital

Noninvasive imaging services at St. Francis Hospital include:

• Multidetector computed tomographic coronary angiography
• Cardiac MRI
• SPECT/CT nuclear Imaging
• Cardiac PET/CT imaging
• Transesophageal echocardiography
• Three-dimensional echocardiography
• Stress testing with nuclear, echocardiographic or MRI imaging.

St. Francis Hospital's leading-edge noninvasive imaging technology is also being applied in its research programs on cardiovascular disease. Drawing on its depth of experience with various imaging modalities, the Hospital has launched a multi-disciplinary effort at its Cardiac Research Institute to improve methods for the diagnosis and treatment of cardiac disease. Past research efforts at the Hospital include The St. Francis Heart Study – a pioneering effort and the largest study of CT calcium scoring to be conducted at any single center – which supported the use of CT calcium scoring for atherosclerotic plaque detection as a tool in cardiac risk evaluation.

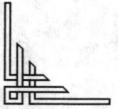
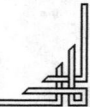

The Best in American Medicine
www.CastleConnolly.com

Medical Oncology

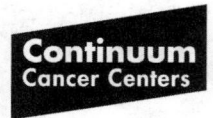

Beth Israel Medical Center
Beth Israel Brooklyn
Roosevelt Hospital
St. Luke's Hospital
NY Eye and Ear Infirmary

Continuum Cancer Centers of New York

Continuum Cancer Centers of New York

212.844.6027

The hospitals of Continuum – Beth Israel Medical Center, Beth Israel Brooklyn, St. Luke's Hospital, Roosevelt Hospital and The New York Eye and Ear Infirmary – are leading providers of cancer care through Continuum Cancer Centers of New York (CCCNY).

We are dedicated to delivering care in ways that are more efficient, more attractive and more convenient for patients. Our cancer patients benefit from system-wide cancer expertise, facilities and resources. Continuum Cancer Centers feature world-renowned cancer specialists, including top-rated surgeons, medical oncologists, radiation oncologists, radiologists, pathologists, and oncology nurses.

Comprehensive diagnostic and treatment services are available for:

- Breast cancer
- Prostate cancer
- Brain cancer
- Thyroid cancer
- Skin cancer
- Lung cancer

- Colorectal cancer
- Gastrointestinal cancer
- Lymphoma/Hodgkin's Disease
- Gynecological cancer
- Head and neck cancer
- Cancer of the central nervous system

Our services also include prevention programs, expert diagnosis, outpatient treatment, inpatient services and home care. In addition, our Research Program offers patients access to investigational protocols through a wide number of clinical trials. Our physicians are leaders in both non-invasive and minimally invasive cancer treatments that focus on maximizing both the cure rate and the quality of life.

Support Services also play an important role at Continuum Cancer Centers. Our nurses, social workers, psychiatrists, chaplains, pharmacists, rehabilitation therapists and nutritionists all have specialized knowledge and expertise in the field of oncology.

In June 2011, CCCNY received a full three-year network accreditation from the American College of Surgeons Commission on Cancer (CoC), with commendation, and is the only hospital system in the metropolitan area to earn this designation.

Minimally Invasive Surgery

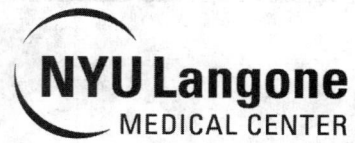

MINIMALLY INVASIVE SURGERY

NYU Langone Medical Center has been at the forefront of minimally invasive surgery for more than 20 years, treating conditions from heart disease and prostate cancer to obesity and fetal abnormalities in utero.

Robotic Surgery

NYU Langone Medical Center was the first hospital in New York City to use the minimally invasive da Vinci Si HD robotic surgical system which allows a 40 percent higher definition view of the surgical field. The Robotic Surgery Center combines world-class experience with the latest technology to treat a number of cardiac, gynecologic, thoracic, and urologic conditions.

Laparoscopic Surgery

Surgeons at NYU Langone Medical Center use laparoscopic techniques to manage kidney cancers, remove adrenal glands, perform renal biopsies, remove renal cysts and perform innovative urinary reconstruction. Kidney donations can also be performed laparoscopically.

Cardiac Surgery

Since 1996, over 6,000 minimally invasive heart surgery procedures have been performed by our cardiac surgeons. Most patients are candidates for minimally invasive procedures.

Thoracic Surgery

We offer a minimally invasive thoracic surgery program, incorporating video-assisted techniques along with the newest methods for post-operative pain relief.

Neurosurgical Technology

NYU Langone Medical Center was the first hospital in the Northeast with the highly advanced Leksell Gamma Knife, allowing neurosurgeons to remove deep-seated tumors, vascular malformations and other disease sites with outstanding results. Assisted by three-dimensional MRI technology, the Leksell Gamma Knife bombards its target with precise doses of radiation, while preserving healthy tissue.

Gynecologic Surgery

Minimally invasive gynecological surgery, including surgery for endometriosis and laparoscopic hysterectomy, are routinely performed at NYU Langone Medical Center.

Varicose Veins

Our physicians pioneered two minimally invasive procedures that do not require surgical incisions to treat varicose veins. They are endovascular closure, which uses radio heat waves to close down inadequate valves, and scope-based varicose vein treatment which allows veins to be removed without an open incision.

Neonatal-Perinatal Medicine

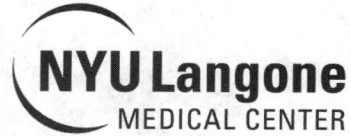

550 First Avenue *(at 31st Street)*
New York, NY 10016
www.NYULMC.org
Children's Services Access Line: **855-NYU-KIDS**

NEONATAL PERINATAL MEDICINE

Neonatal Perinatal Medicine is part of the Hassenfeld Pediatric Center, a full service specialty Children's Hospital, which supports the array of children's health services across the Medical Center where newborns, children, adolescents and young adults receive the most comprehensive and advanced care by a team of pediatricians and pediatric specialists.

The Neonatology Program at NYU Langone Medical Center addresses the unique emotional and developmental needs of infants with a program that combines family-centered care and state-of-the-art technology. We specialize in the following areas:

Neonatal Intensive Care
The Neonatal Intensive Care Unit (NICU) provides the most advanced care in New York City for neonates requiring intensive care and works closely with pediatric general and cardiac surgery, neurosurgery and craniofacial surgery. As a Regional Perinatal Center, the program additionally offers early intervention evaluation services and comprehensive family support and education.

Continuing Care
Because many premature babies may be at an increased risk for problems in growth and development, the Neonatal Comprehensive Continuing Care Program (NCCCP) follows these infants from birth through pre-school, providing evaluation and assessment of problems as soon as they arise.

Hypothermia Program
The Hypothermia Program at NYU Langone Medical Center is a full multidisciplinary service with neonatal transport and inpatient and outpatient follow-up services. The program provides rapid response treatment and assessment of infants who have birth asphyxia.

Infant Apnea and SIDS
The Infant Apnea and SIDS Program at the Bellevue Hospital Center, an affiliate of NYU Langone Medical Center, provides treatment to critically ill infants through its Neonatal Intensive Care Unit, and to other children at risk for apnea, sudden infant death syndrome (SIDS) and other life-threatening events.

Neonatal Transport
As a designated New York State Regional Perinatal Center, the Division of Neonatology cares for over one-fifth of New York City's mothers and infants. As part of that massive effort, it offers an active transport program to bring mothers and/or their newborns to NYU Langone Medical Center's Tisch Hospital for specialized intensive care.

Nephrology

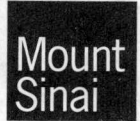 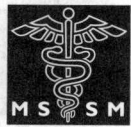

MOUNT SINAI
SCHOOL OF
MEDICINE

THE MOUNT SINAI MEDICAL CENTER
NEPHROLOGY
One Gustave L. Levy Place
Fifth Avenue and 100th Street
New York, NY 10029-6574
Physician Referral: 1-800-MD-SINAI (637-4624)
www.mountsinai.org/kidney

Mount Sinai's Department of Nephrology ranks among the best in the nation, according to the 2012-2013 issue of *U.S. News & World Report's* "Americas Best Hospitals."

We have been an international leader in the treatment of kidney disease since we performed the first hemodialysis in the United States in the 1950s. We established New York State's first dialysis center in 1957. We currently operate the largest home dialysis program in New York City, and our **Geriatric Nephrology Program** is the only one of its kind in the country.

Under the direction of Barbara Murphy, M.D., Acting Chair, Department of Medicine and Division Chief of Nephrology, we are continuing our leadership in patient care, research and education. Proof of our clinical excellence is evident daily in our practice and hospital. Our physicians care for patients referred to us by other nephrologists who recognize the need for our expertise in their most challenging and complex cases.

Our expertise spans numerous kidney diseases and treatments, including:

- Chronic kidney disease
- Polycystic kidney disease
- Geriatric kidney disease
- Diabetes-related kidney disease
- Glomerular disease
- Hypertensive kidney disease
- HIV-associated nephropathy
- Kidney transplantation
- Hemodialysis
- Peritoneal Dialysis

EXPERT PHYSICIANS

Building on the talent and expertise of our physicians, including Jonathan Winston, M.D., Tonia Kim, M.D., Mark Swidler, M.D., Joseph Vassalotti, M.D, Brian Radbill, M.D., and Richard Stein, M.D., along with transplantation specialists, Bernd Schroppel, M.D. and Vinay Nair, M.D., we provide patients with the most advanced and appropriate approach to care. With so much research taking place, we can also offer patients access to experimental treatments often unavailable elsewhere.

Initiated in 1967, our **kidney transplant program** is now one of the largest and most successful in the country, with our physician-scientists actively investigating new and innovative ways to detect, prevent, and treat rejection.

A Strong Focus on Research
With one of the largest National Institutes of Health research budgets of any nephrology division in the country, we conduct and support numerous clinical trials, and our faculty members have achieved international recognition as authorities on the causes and treatments of all forms of kidney diseases and disorders.

Neurological Surgery

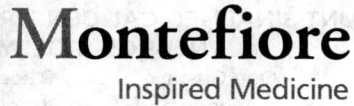

Neurological Surgery at Montefiore

Few neurosurgery programs possess the depth of experience and expertise found in the Department of Neurological Surgery at Montefiore Medical Center. **The Department, which was recognized as high performing in *U.S. News & World Report*'s 2012–13 "America's Best Hospitals," provides advanced surgical treatment for both adults and children with all forms of neurological** conditions.

The Department offers the full spectrum of diagnostic modalities, including intraoperative imaging that provides surgeons with up-to-the-minute information during surgery. Other services include a state-of-the-art intensive care unit, dedicated operating rooms and endovascular procedure rooms. Montefiore's neurosurgeons are experienced and accomplished in all aspects of neurological surgery, and each possesses diverse subspecialty expertise to further enhance patient care. The use of minimally invasive treatment—such as endovascular coiling and stenting, stereotactic-guided radiosurgery and microneurosurgery—is emphasized.

The Cerebrovascular Center offers patients with disorders related to the blood vessels of the brain, including stroke, carotid artery disease, intracranial aneurysms and cerebrovascular malformations, early diagnosis and treatment for patients with these conditions. At Montefiore, nearly half of all aneurysms are treated using catheter techniques that avoid open procedures, while the Department's expertise with angioplasty and stenting has further increased its ability to manage complex disorders. Endovascular and microsurgical management of arteriovenous malformations is also provided.

When performing delicate spine surgery for the common causes of back pain—disk disease and degenerative arthritis—the Department employs the latest technologies, including imaging guidance and neurophysiologic monitoring.

Collaboration across specialty areas is the centerpiece of the Department's approach to patient care. This is evident in its treatment of patients with brain and spine cancers. When planning a patient's course of treatment, neurosurgeons, neuro-oncologists and radiation oncologists work together to identify the best approach. This ensures that patients consistently receive the appropriate diagnostic and treatment interventions for their specific conditions.

At The Children's Hospital at Montefiore, the Department's neurosurgeons expertly manage all aspects of neurological disorders in children, including congenital problems, hydrocephalus and epilepsy. They also excel in the management of rare and difficult problems, treating conjoined twins, spinal cord and skull-base tumors, and birth disorders such as malformations of the face and skull.

Research activities currently under way within the Department focus on outcomes in patients with traumatic brain injury, stroke and Parkinson's disease.

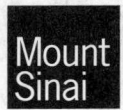
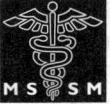

MOUNT SINAI SCHOOL OF MEDICINE

THE MOUNT SINAI MEDICAL CENTER
NEUROSURGERY
One Gustave L. Levy Place
Fifth Avenue and 100th Street
New York, NY 10029-6574
Physician Referral: 1-800-MD-SINAI (637-4624)
www.mountsinai.org/neurosurgery

THE DEPARTMENT OF NEUROSURGERY at Mount Sinai, established in 1920, has earned a distinguished international reputation. Since assuming the position of Chair four years ago, Joshua Bederson, MD, has expanded the department by more than 50 percent through a combination of strategic recruitments, new hospital affiliations, and numerous outreach programs. Neurosurgery is the fastest growing surgical subspecialty at Mount Sinai, performing more than 2,500 procedures a year at The Mount Sinai Hospital. Areas of clinical expertise include the treatment of meningiomas and other skull base tumors, primary and metastatic brain tumors, pituitary adenomas and acoustic neuromas, deep brain stimulation for movement disorders and minimally invasive treatment of spine and spinal cord disorders. The department is a regional leader in endovascular and microsurgical treatment of aneurysms, arteriovenous malformations and stroke, microvascular decompression for trigeminal neuralgia and hemifacial spasm. We are the first medical center in the nation to use the Neurotouch virtual reality brain surgery simulator, which will be used to train our residents, assess skill level and to rehearse upcoming cases.

The Meningioma Program has pioneered endoscopic, minimally invasive surgical approaches for the treatment of meningiomas. Transnasal endoscopic tumor resections and computer-aided navigation help our surgeons achieve even greater precision during surgery. Both tactics reduce risk to the patient and help us avoid critical vascular and intracranial structures. Working with the Minimally Invasive and Endoscopic Skull Base Surgery Program, we unite specialists in neurosurgery, otolaryngology, head and neck cancer, craniofacial surgery, oral and maxillofacial surgery, and microvascular and reconstructive procedures.

The Comprehensive Brain Tumor Program collaborates with The Tisch Cancer Institute and the Departments of Neurology, Radiation Oncology, Radiology, and Pathology to provide comprehensive therapies for primary and metastatic brain tumors. We have pioneered minimally invasive approaches using imaging technology, frameless stereotaxy, awake and asleep brain mapping, and advanced microneurosurgery. Stereotactic radiosurgery, a minimally invasive treatment that does not require open surgery, gene therapy, and clinical trials are also possible options.

The Cerebrovascular Program is composed of an experienced team that provides a complete range of services for the diagnosis and treatment of patients with neurovascular disorders of the brain and spinal cord. Some current treatments include microsurgical treatment of aneurysms and AVMs with clipping and resection, endovascular treatment of aneurysms with coils and/or stents, endovascular treatment of AVMs with liquid acrylics, stereotactic radiosurgical treatment of AVMs, endovascular treatment of stenoses with stents and angioplasty and microsurgical treatment of stenoses and occlusions with bypass. We are the most experienced program in stent-assisted embolization of cerebral aneurysms and stent treatment of carotid artery disease amongst neurovascular centers in New York.

The Neurosurgery Spinal Disorders Program offers treatment for all disorders of the spinal column and spinal cord, including degenerative disorders, trauma, infections, congenital disorders (including scoliosis), and tumors. Our neurosurgeons have pioneered endoscopic, minimally invasive approaches for tumor resection and treatment of degenerative diseases. These approaches reduce pain and hospital stays, and facilitate an early return to normal activity.

The Neuroendocrine Program sees more than 200 new pituitary tumor patients each year, more than 300 follow-up patients annually, and has performed more than 2,500 transphenoidal pituitary operations.

The Center for Neuromodulation, a collaboration between the Departments of Neurology and Neurosurgery, uses the latest technology to precisely target areas of abnormal activity in the brain and spinal cord. Our physicians are focused on developing minimally invasive neurosurgical techniques that either modulate neural function, replace lost neuronal populations, or halt the neurodegenerative process altogether. Currently, deep brain stimulation dominates this field, but many technologies with great potential are on the horizon.

 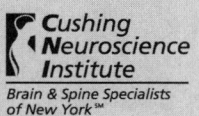

300 Community Drive, 9 Tower
Manhasset, NY 11030
(516) 562-3822
www.neurocni.com
neuro@nshs.edu

North Shore-LIJ's Cushing Neuroscience Institute (CNI) specializes in the diagnosis and treatment of neurological and neurosurgical diseases. Established in 2006, CNI combines clinical programs with advanced medicine and surgical techniques, state-of-the art technology and cutting-edge research to bring patients the best possible care.

Award-Winning Care
Our outcomes and capabilities have led to various designations and acknowledgements, **including *U.S. News & World Report's* ranking of North Shore University Hospital as one of the nation's top 50 hospitals for neurology and neurosurgery.**

In addition, several of our neurosurgeons and neurologists have been named as recipients of the **2011 Patients' Choice Awards**. Only physicians who have received top scores by their patients and pass other quality measures are awarded this honor.

Treatments for a Wide Range of Conditions
Our highly skilled and compassionate team of neurospecialists includes neurologists who diagnose and treat conditions that involve the brain, spine, nerves and muscles, as well as surgeons who provide the latest treatment options while contributing to advances in their field. This multidisciplinary team expertly treats patients for brain aneurysms, stroke, brain tumors, brain injuries, movement disorders, epilepsy, neuromuscular disorders and spinal disease.

We are committed to serve our patients and community with a blend of technical expertise and compassion while maintaining the highest ethical standards, and we continually work to discover new and cutting-edge treatments through clinical research.

Our Neuroscience Centers:

- Brain Aneurysm Center
- Brain Tumor Center
- Chiari Institute
- Comprehensive Epilepsy Care Center
- General Neurology
- Headache Center
- Hyperhidrosis Center
- Hypothalamic Hamartoma Center
- Memory Disorders Center
- Movement Disorders Center
- Moyamoya Center of New York
- Multiple Sclerosis Center
- Nerve Disorders Center
- Neurocritical Care Center
- Normal Pressure Hydrocephalus Center
- Pain Center
- Pediatric Neuroscience Center
- Skull Base Center
- Spine Center
- Stroke Center
- Traumatic Brain Injury Center

To find a doctor: **1-888-321-DOCS** or visit **www.northshorelij.com**

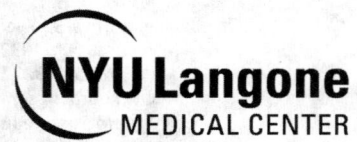
NEUROSURGERY

The Department of Neurosurgery at NYU Langone Medical Center offers some of the nation's most skilled and experienced surgeons in advanced, minimally invasive procedures. Patients also benefit from cutting-edge research and fully integrated approach to medical care.

Brain Tumor
The Department of Neurosurgery specializes in both malignant and benign brain tumors, including skull base tumors. Expertise includes glioblastoma, ependymoma, hemangioblastoma, other gliomas, meningiomas and vestibular schwannomas (acoustic neuromas).

Cerebrovascular Surgery
The Division of Cerebrovascular Surgery is a premier center for brain aneurysms, giant intracranial aneurysms, brain vascular malformations and cavernomas, and stroke.

Epilepsy
The Comprehensive Epilepsy Center is the largest epilepsy center in the U.S. offering patients an array of advanced surgical and medical options.

Spinal Neurosurgery
The Division of Spine Surgery provides treatment for degenerative spinal diseases, spinal tumors, spinal trauma and spinal infections.

Hyperhidrosis
The Department offers expertise in the surgical treatment of primary hyperhidrosis (excessive sweating) including Endoscopic Thoracic Sympathectomy.

Neurosurgical Technology
Our neurosurgeons remove deep-seated tumors, vascular malformations and other disease sites using a highly advanced Leksell Gamma Knife. Aided by 3-D MRI technology, the Gamma Knife bombards its target with precise doses of radiation, while preserving healthy tissue.

We also provide state-of-the-art care and research through the following divisions:
- Facial Pain: provides patients a thorough examination and, if required, nerve injections and minimally invasive surgery.
- Functional Neurosurgery: offers diagnosis and treatment of Parkinson's disease and conditions that involve involuntary muscle contractions.
- Pediatric Neurosurgery: provides treatment to children with brain and spinal cord tumors, congenital and development disorders.
- Peripheral Nerve Surgery: focuses on the diagnosis and treatment of nerve compressions, nerve tremors, Brachial Plexus (nerve fiber) and nerve injuries.

Neuro-Critical Care
Intensive care and treatment of critical neurosurgical illnesses is provided.

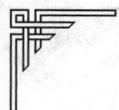

The Best in American Medicine
www.CastleConnolly.com

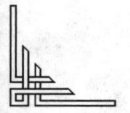
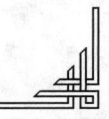

Neurology

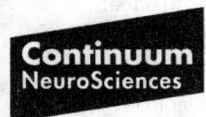

Neurology and Neurosurgery Expertise

800.420.4004

Continuum Health Partners, Inc.

The member hospitals of the Continuum Neurosciences consortium—St. Luke's and Roosevelt Hospitals and Beth Israel Medical Center—are home to many international leaders in neurology, neurosurgery, neuro-radiology and endovascular neurosurgery. Each of the hospitals has clinicians who are nationally and internationally recognized for their accomplishments and attract patients from throughout the United States and other countries who are looking for innovative treatment programs delivered by physicians specializing in both clinical care and research. Our expertise includes treatments for:

- Complex brain tumors, spine and spinal cord; chordomas, meningiomas, acoustic neuromas, trigeminal neuralgia and hemifacial spasms
- Headaches
- Disorders of the brain, spinal cord, peripheral nerves and muscles
- Stroke/cerebrovascular diseases
- Epilepsy and seizures
- Movement disorders (Parkinson's disease, dystonia and essential tremor)
- Neuro-ophthalmologic conditions
- Neuro-oncology-related illnesses
- Neuro-psychiatry/psychology-based conditions
- Many adult and pediatric neurologic conditions

A few of our Centers of Excellence include:

Beth Israel Medical Center

- The Alan and Barbara Mirken Department of Neurology
- Bachmann-Strauss Dystonia Center of Excellence
- National Parkinson Foundation Center of Excellence
- The Betty and Morton Yarmon Stroke Center
- Internationally respected divisions of adult and pediatric epilepsy
- ALS (Lou Gehrig's disease) Center sponsored by the ALS Association
- Adult Neurosurgery
- Pediatric Neurosurgery
- Peripheral Nerve Center

St. Luke's and Roosevelt Hospitals

- The Hyman-Newman Institute for Neurology and Neurosurgery
- Center for Endovascular Surgery
- The Vascular Birthmarks Institute
- Vascular Malformations Center of NY
- New York Brain Tumor Center
- The Headache Institute
- The Stroke Center
- Adult Neurosurgery
- Pediatric Neurosurgery

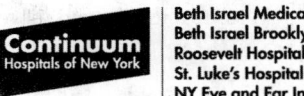

Beth Israel Medical Center
Beth Israel Brooklyn
Roosevelt Hospital
St. Luke's Hospital
NY Eye and Ear Infirmary

www.chpnyc.org

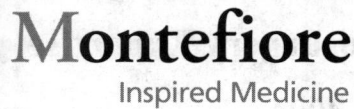

111 East 210th Street
Bronx, New York 10467
718-920-4656
www.montefiore.org/neurology

Neurology at Montefiore

The Department of Neurology at Montefiore Medical Center is among the largest and most respected in the nation. With more than 300 neurological specialists in its larger network, the Department offers state-of-the-art treatments, technological advancements and groundbreaking research for all forms of neurological disease. **The Department, which was recognized as high performing in *U.S. News & World Report*'s 2012–13 "America's Best Hospitals," is a recent recipient of a prestigious National Institutes of Health (NIH)/National Institute of Neurological Disorders and Stroke (NINDS) Einstein-Montefiore Neurological Clinical Trials Network (NeuroNEXT) grant.**

Innovation is a hallmark of the Department and has led to several noteworthy advances over its half-century history. Counted among these is its pioneering Headache Center, founded more than 60 years ago. Its Sleep-Wake Disorders Center, the first of its kind worldwide and accredited by the American Academy of Sleep Medicine, focuses on complex neurological sleep disorders. A primary goal of the Center is to promote wellness and longevity and to prevent neurological diseases by identifying pre-clinical stages of the disease process. The Department also offers a comprehensive and unique program in **neurotoxicology, as well as premier programs in aging and dementia, gait disorders and frailty, stroke, neuro-oncology, multiple sclerosis and allied disorders, neuromuscular disorders, neurological critical care and interventional neuroradiology.** In addition, the Department's world-renowned **Comprehensive Epilepsy Center** includes separate pediatric and adult inpatient epilepsy continuous monitoring units.

Pediatric epilepsy is a strong focus for the Department, and its specialists work with The Children's Hospital at Montefiore (CHAM) to ensure that patients with this condition receive the constant monitoring and treatment they require. In collaboration with CHAM, the Department also offers comprehensive centers devoted to the diagnosis and treatment of patients with autism spectrum disorders, attention deficit and hyperactivity disorders, and Rett syndrome, among others.

Research is pivotal to the advancement of this specialty, and the Department is involved in many NIH- and foundation-sponsored basic, translational and clinical neuroscience research studies focused on autism, neurodegenerative diseases and other neurological disorders. Under the leadership of Chairman Mark F. Mehler, MD, FAAN, the Department is also exploring the reparative potential of neural stem cells present within the brain and the prospective use of epigenetics in healing injured brain tissue through stem cell reprogramming and dynamic tissue remodeling.

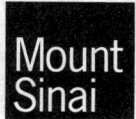
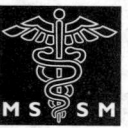

MOUNT SINAI
SCHOOL OF
MEDICINE

THE MOUNT SINAI MEDICAL CENTER
NEUROLOGY

One Gustave L. Levy Place
Fifth Avenue and 100th Street
New York, NY 10029-6574
Physician Referral: 1-800-MD-SINAI (637-4624)
www.mountsinai.org/neurology

THE ESTELLE AND DANIEL MAGGIN DEPARTMENT OF NEUROLOGY at Mount Sinai provides compassionate, state-of-the-art, interdisciplinary care for disorders of the brain and nervous system. *US News World & Report* recently ranked Mount Sinai Neurology and Neurosurgery as a top program nationwide in recognition of our ability to care for patients with complex diseases of the nervous system.

The Robert and John M. Bendheim Parkinson and Movement Disorders Center is one of the world's leading multidisciplinary centers for clinical care and translational research aimed at Parkinson's disease, dystonia, tremor, and a variety of movement disorders. The Center incorporates a world-renowned deep-brain stimulation program, and is at the forefront in clinical trials and experimental therapeutics for movement disorders.

The Corinne Goldsmith Dickinson Center for Multiple Sclerosis is an internationally recognized comprehensive center, uniting the efforts of leading physicians and scientists from many disciplines to understand the causes and consequences of MS. The Center provides services in all aspects of diagnosis, disease management, rehabilitation, and patient support, and the opportunity for patients to participate in potentially groundbreaking clinical trials.

The Clinical Program for Cerebrovascular Disorders comprises an outstanding team of medical experts who specialize in the most advanced approaches in the evaluation, treatment, and rehabilitation of patients with cerebrovascular diseases. Services include the early diagnosis of stroke, a specialized Neurointensive Care Unit, and an advanced inpatient stroke unit. Physicians are available at all times for emergency consultation with referring physicians. The Stroke Center was the first JCAHO-certified primary stroke center in Manhattan.

The NeuroAIDS Program provides diagnosis and treatment for neurological disorders associated with HIV disease. This program is one of the few in the world to treat the various complications of the disease that affect the central and peripheral nervous systems in as many as 70 percent of patients.

The Epilepsy Center provides specific expertise in the diagnosis and treatment of epilepsy and related disorders. The Center encompasses outstanding epileptologists, a new modern inpatient epilepsy monitoring unit, and full outpatient EEG and diagnostic capabilities.

The Center for Headache and Pain Medicine is a multidisciplinary center for the diagnosis and treatment of chronic and acute headaches and other painful disorders of the skull, brain, or face in both adults and children. Specialists in neurology, pain medicine, ENT, ophthalmology, psychiatry, and rehabilitation medicine are available to evaluate and treat individuals with painful disorders.

The Division of Neuromuscular Diseases provides diagnosis, treatment, and compassionate care for patients with disorders in neuromuscular transmission, muscle diseases, peripheral nerve problems, and spasticity resulting from stroke or damage to the central nervous system.

The Center for Cognitive Health provides state-of-the-art diagnosis and treatment for memory disorders, dementias, traumatic brain injury and other cognitive disorders. Our multi-disciplinary team of neurologists, psychiatrists, neuro-psychiatrists, neuro-scientists and patient care managers bridge the brain related specialties to provide individualized comprehensive care.

The Eye Movement and Vestibular Disorder Program provides outstanding diagnosis and treatment for visual problems, balance problems, and motion sickness. Our physicians participate in NASA programs, employing technology used to assess these disorders in space, and studying possible treatment applications on earth.

THE ESTELLE AND DANIEL MAGGIN DEPARTMENT OF NEUROLOGY is renowned for its unique integration of outstanding patient care and cutting-edge research in neurological disease, and can bring the latest advances in treatment to our patients. Our physicians and neuroscientists have made enormous strides in basic and translational research, bringing medical breakthroughs that will change the course of neurological treatment. The department is led by some of the most prominent figures in American neurology, is #3 nationally in the number of academic neurologists trained in our residency program, and receives annual research grants of more than $20 million.

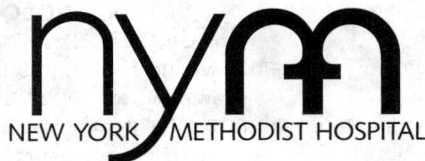

THE INSTITUTE FOR NEUROSCIENCES

New York Methodist Hospital
506 Sixth Street, Brooklyn, N.Y. 11215
Phone: 866 DO-NEURO (866 366-3876)
http://www.nym.org

SPECIALISTS AND MEDICAL SERVICES

The Institute for Neurosciences at New York Methodist Hospital brings together a unique group of specialists and medical services, offering diagnosis and treatment of a broad range of neurological conditions, ranging from frequent headaches to Parkinson's disease to multiple sclerosis.

The Institute's panel of physician specialists includes neurologists, neurosurgeons, psychiatrists, endocrinologists, neuroradiologists, radiation oncologists, physiatrists, geriatricians, psychologists and rehabilitation therapists.

All diagnostic and therapeutic procedures are performed at New York Methodist Hospital or at individual physicians' offices. State-of-the-art equipment to perform computed tomography (CT), magnetic resonance imaging (MRI), and magnetic resonance angiography (MRA) is located in the Hospital's Radiology Department. In addition, equipment and specialists trained to perform neurological diagnostic tests, such as electroencephalography (EEG), electromyography (EMG), and evoked potential examinations are available on the main campus.

The Institute also has a satellite office in Staten Island, located at 1 Harvey Avenue. It can be reached by calling 718 494-4360.

PROGRAMS OFFERED

Special programs and services offered by the Institute include an Alzheimer's disease/memory center, a neuropathy program, pediatric and adult epilepsy programs that offer diagnosis via video EEG, a Parkinson's disease and other movement disorders program, a pituitary program, a multiple sclerosis center, a neuro-oncology service, inpatient and outpatient psychiatry programs, rehabilitation services and a New York State–designated Stroke Center. Neurosurgeons on the Institute's panel perform highly sophisticated procedures, including deep brain stimulation surgery, vascular neurosurgery, skull base surgery and spinal surgery. A stereotactic radiosurgery service is also available at the Hospital's regional radiation oncology center.

***

Referrals to the Institute, its programs and physicians can be made through an individual's primary care physician or requested directly through the Institute's telephone referral service. More information (and on-line physician referral) is available at the Hospital's website, http://www.nym.org.

NYM's CENTER FOR PARKINSON'S DISEASE AND OTHER MOVEMENT DISORDERS

NYM's Center for Parkinson's Disease and Other Movement Disorders is the only such medical center–based program in the New York City area. The Center simplifies the diagnostic and treatment process for patients by consolidating all services.

Treatment for Parkinson's may include medication, surgery and/or specialized therapies. Some patients may be candidates for deep brain stimulation, a neurosurgical procedure that can have dramatic results. NYM is the only Hospital in Brooklyn where this surgery is performed.

The Center has a patient care coordinator to help patients with appointments, treatment regimens, transportation and coordination with insurance companies. For more information, call 718 246-8820.

NewYork-Presbyterian

⌐ The University Hospital of Columbia and Cornell

Affiliated with Columbia University College of Physicians and Surgeons and Weill Cornell Medical College

NewYork-Presbyterian Hospital	NewYork-Presbyterian Hospital
Columbia University Medical Center	Weill Cornell Medical Center
622 West 168th Street	525 East 68th Street
New York, NY 10032	New York, NY 10065

1-877-NYP-WELL (1-877-697-9355) www.nyp.org/neuro

NewYork-Presbyterian Neuroscience

In 2012–2013, NewYork-Presbyterian's neurology and neurosurgery program was ranked 4th in the nation in the annual 'Best Hospitals' survey conducted by *U.S. News & World Report*™. Our Neuroscience Centers offer innovative treatments to improve the quality of life of patients with neurological disorders, including:

- **Stroke:** Our three comprehensive Stroke Center locations are among the few NYS designated primary stroke centers. Round-the-clock surveillance and state-of-the-art brain monitoring in our Neuro-ICU minimizes damage and maximizes the chance for a full recovery.
- **Epilepsy:** Comprehensive Epilepsy Centers use the latest monitoring and imaging tools to locate the source of a patient's seizures and tailor medical and/or surgical treatment.
- **Pediatric neurology/neurosurgery:** Specialists are sensitive to the special needs of children with epilepsy, brain tumors, stroke, craniofacial disorders, vascular anomalies, and movement disorders.
- **Spinal disorders:** Neurosurgeons, rehabilitation medicine physicians, physical therapists, pain management physicians, nurse practitioners, and neurologists personalize a plan of care for patients with neck and back pain and disorders such as scoliosis, disc disease, and compression fractures.
- **Brain and spinal tumors:** Neurosurgeons, neuro-oncologists, radiation oncologists, and others care for patients with brain and spinal tumors. Translational research programs aim to understand the biology of these diseases and develop innovative therapies.
- **Neuro-immune disorders:** Comprehensive care is delivered to patients with multiple sclerosis as well as less common diseases, such as Behcet's disease, sarcoidosis, and vasculitis.
- **Neuro-muscular disorders:** Our multidisciplinary team cares for people with neuromuscular diseases such as ALS (Lou Gehrig's Disease), Guillain-Barre syndrome, muscular dystrophy, myasthenia gravis, myopathy, and neuropathy.
- **Movement disorders:** NewYork-Presbyterian Hospital treats one of the world's largest populations of patients with movement disorders, especially Parkinson's disease. Researchers assess new drugs, imaging techniques, surgical therapies (such as deep brain stimulation), and gene therapy.
- **Memory disorders:** Our programs feature advanced care for patients with Alzheimer's disease or other memory disorders and their families, as well as clinical and laboratory research to better understand these disorders, with the goal of treating them sooner and more effectively.

Highlights:

- Researchers demonstrated that two genes associated with ALS work in tandem to support long-term survival of motor neurons.

- Neurologists, neurosurgeons, and radiologists collaborated to show that intensive medical therapy is more effective than stenting for preventing a second stroke.

- Investigators devised a computer model of the spread of dementia that can be used to predict future disease patterns years before they occur in a patient.

- NewYork-Presbyterian is participating in NeuroNEXT (Network for Excellence in Neuroscience Clinical Trials), an NIH-funded national effort to accelerate the development of therapies for people with neurological diseases.

- Neuro-oncologists are devising innovative approaches, such as the use of microcatheters, to bypass the blood-brain barrier and deliver chemotherapy directly to brain tumors.

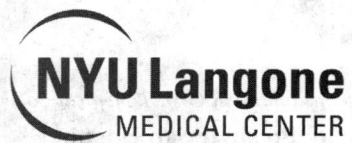

NEUROLOGY

NYU Langone Medical Center evaluates and treats adults and children with a broad spectrum of neurological diseases, including stroke, epilepsy, cerebrovascular diseases, behavioral disorders and dementia, brain tumors, genetic and degenerative diseases, nerve and muscle problems, headache and pain syndromes and movement disorders. We are home to the largest multiple sclerosis (MS) program in New York and were first primary Stroke Center in NYC.

Autonomic Diseases

Our specialized Center evaluates and treats children and adults with familial dysautonomia and other inherited or acquired autonomic nervous system diseases, including orthostatic hypotension and rare forms of hereditary sensory neuropathy.

Epilepsy

The Comprehensive Epilepsy Center offers the most advanced medical and surgical options. Complementary management approaches complete the comprehensive management plan.

Multiple Sclerosis

The Comprehensive MS Care Center provides state-of-the-art diagnostic evaluations and follow-up care as part of a comprehensive program.

Neurogenetics

We focus on inherited diseases of the nervous system. Services include diagnosis and management of inherited diseases, biochemical and molecular testing and genetic counseling.

Neuro-oncology

NYU Cancer Institute includes one of the nation's leading brain and spinal cord tumor programs, with physicians highly experienced in neuro-oncology, neurosurgery and neuroradiology.

Neuromuscular Diseases

We offer multidisciplinary programs for neuromuscular diseases, including acquired peripheral neuropathy, Charcot Marie Tooth neuropathy, myasthenia gravis, amyotrophic lateral sclerosis, spinal muscular atrophy, post-polio syndrome, muscular dystrophy and Lyme neuroborreliosis.

Parkinson's Disease and Movement Disorders

The Parkinson's disease and Movement Disorders Center helps individuals and families achieve the highest possible quality of life.

Stroke Care

The multidisciplinary Comprehensive Stroke Care Center provides rapid diagnosis, effective intervention and early rehabilitation from debilitating stroke.

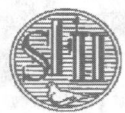

St. Francis Hospital The Heart Center®

100 Port Washington Blvd.
Roslyn, New York 11576
www.stfrancisheartcenter.com
(516) 562-6000   Physician referral: 1-888-HEARTNY
A member of Catholic Health Services of Long Island

Long Island's Highest-Ranked Neurological and Neurosurgical Programs

St. Francis Hospital, The Heart Center® was recognized by *U.S. News & World Report* as one of the nation's best hospitals for neurology and neurosurgery in 2012-13. The Division of Neurology and Neurosurgery at St. Francis provides high quality neurological care to hospital and emergency room patients with acute and chronic neurological issues. Under the leadership of Division Director of Neurology, Anthony Cohen, M.D., and Richard Johnson, M.D., Division Director of Neurosurgery, our team of highly skilled board certified physicians diagnose, treat, and manage patients with various conditions including stroke, neuromuscular disorders, seizure disorders, diagnosis and treatment of brain and spinal tumors, treatment of herniated disks, movement disorders, multiple sclerosis, Alzheimer's disease, and headache. Many of the physicians have subspecialty training in these areas. Combining their knowledge and expertise in the field with advanced technology and diagnostic testing, the staff provides the most comprehensive care available.

An Award-Winning Stroke Center

Under its Director, Paul Wright, M.D., and a team of experienced physicians, mid-level practitioners and nurses, the Stroke Center at St. Francis Hospital has become a leader in the diagnosis, treatment, and support of stroke patients. The Hospital provides advanced treatment in emergency settings, facilitating the diagnosis and expeditious management of stroke victims. The Stroke Center is staffed with neurologically trained and certified nurses, with specific expertise in the management of acute stroke patients. By creating an environment with superior neurological care and compassionate and Magnet Award-winning nursing staff, St. Francis strives to be at the forefront of leading hospitals regionally and nationally.

An Innovative Neurosurgery Program

Dr. Johnson leads a team of Board Certified neurosurgeons who specialize in treating debilitating conditions that affect the brain and spine. The Hospital offers advanced, minimally invasive procedures for patients suffering from lumbar and cervical spinal stenosis. Some other minimally invasive therapies that can decompress and fuse the spine for patients suffering from chronic back pain and herniated disks are also offered at the Hospital. For patients with cervical myelopathy or a compression of the cervical spine, St. Francis surgeons can now operate to remove bone, ligaments or discs that press against the spine. Using pieces of bone or a carbon fiber composite, they can reconstruct and stabilize the spine. St. Francis offers an outstanding intracranial neurosurgical service, having acquired the latest technology and equipment for removal of brain tumors and other intracranial lesions. The Hospital also has state-of-the-art operating rooms and navigational technology to remove extremely small brain tumors. With its Magnet designated nurses, 24-hour ICU intensivists, and dedicated mid-level practitioners, St. Francis consistently provides patients with high quality care.

Conditions Treated

- Stroke
- Headache and facial pain
- Multiple Sclerosis
- Parkinson's disease
- Lou Gehrig's disease
- Epilepsy
- Neck pain
- Back pain
- Coma
- Infections of the nervous system
- Alzheimer's
- Dementia
- Dizziness
- Vertigo
- Brain tumors
- Spinal cord injuries and tumors
- Herniated Disks
- Spinal Stenosis
- Spondylolisthesis
- Hydrocephalus

Key treatments: Pain Management

Under the leadership of Daniel Sajewski, M.D., and Patrick Annello, M.D., the Division of Pain Management has enjoyed dramatic growth in the services it offers and in patient care visits. Trusha Shah, M.D., and Steven Yap, M.D., manage a broad range of medical and invasive therapies which represent the leading edge of pain management.

Comprehensive Spine Care

St. Francis Hospital has acquired the key elements in the diagnosis and treatment of all varieties of spinal pathology. Physicians have the newest MRIs and neuroradiographic equipment. The Cardiac Fitness Center at the DeMatteis Center for Cardiac Research and Education is the ideal place for physical therapy for spinal conditions, especially if patients have cardiac conditions. Up-to-date technology and innovations are available at the facility. Pain management physicians, neurologists, neuroradiologists, orthopedic and neurosurgical spine surgeons meet at the Center to discuss weekly cases and have combined interdisciplinary conferences to discuss the treatment of patients with these complex neurological disorders.

Nuclear Medicine

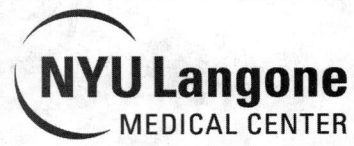

550 First Avenue *(at 31st Street)*
New York, NY 10016
www.NYULMC.org
Physician Referral: **888-7-NYU-MED** *(888-769-8633)*

NUCLEAR MEDICINE

About the Division of Nuclear Medicine, Department of Radiology

Nuclear medicine at NYU Langone Medical Center spans all medical specialties to deliver safe techniques that image body physiology for the diagnosis, monitoring and prevention of disease. In addition to cutting-edge imaging, the Medical Center offers a full spectrum of radioiodine therapy protocols for the treatment of hyperthyroidism and thyroid cancer. Our nuclear medicine physicians are also experts in the field of radioimmunotherapy for lymphoma. We specialize in the following areas:

Advanced Imaging Equipment

NYU Langone Medical Center houses some of the most advanced nuclear medicine equipment in the world, including best-of-breed SPECT, SPECT and PET/CT scanners. Cameras are linked by advanced data management systems to allow rapid, accurate reading and digital report generation. Image data is available to referring physicians over a digital network that allows for timely patient management.

Nuclear Medicine

NYU Langone Medical Center's Tisch Hospital offers a wide range of nuclear medicine services, specializing in a full complement of non-invasive nuclear imaging techniques designed to diagnose and monitor disease of the neurological, cardiovascular, endocrine, gastrointestinal, pulmonary, genitourinary and hepatobiliary systems. Specialized blood volume and lymphedema evaluation protocols are also offered. Advanced dosimetry protocols are used to optimize therapy for patients with thyroid cancer and lymphoma.

PET/CT Scans

PET/CT scans allow for simultaneous imaging of metabolic processes as well as anatomic structures in the body. These advanced scanners have revolutionized the care of cancer patients and are making great strides in the diagnosis and management of neurological and cardiac diseases. NYU Langone Medical Center's nuclear medicine physicians are fellowship-trained experts in the field of PET/CT.

Obstetrics & Gynecology

Maimonides Medical Center
STELLA AND JOSEPH PAYSON BIRTHING CENTER

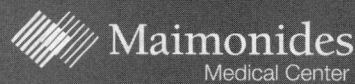
Maimonides
Medical Center

4802 Tenth Avenue • Brooklyn, New York 11219
Phone: 718.283.7048 • Fax: 718.283.7167
www.maimonidesmed.org/obgyn

The Birthing Center features private suites with hardwood floors and a home-like environment. At the same time, physician coverage is provided 24/7 in our advanced Neonatal Intensive Care Unit. Our 36 obstetricians and 26 midwives have found that most families appreciate having the best of both worlds available to them.

Maimonides provides other unique services to its maternity patients. The largest doula program in the metropolitan area can be found at Maimonides. These fully-trained childbirth assistants are available to patients before, during and after delivery at no cost to families. And the maternity units utilize an electronic patient record that sets industry standards for patient safety and hospital efficiency.

This combination of family-centered services and advanced technology continues to have enormous appeal to the women served — over 7,800 of them last year alone. Our highly trained staff includes the finest nurses, physicians, midwives and specialists to ensure the safety and comfort of our patients. Several physicians specialize in high-risk pregnancy, including the Chair of Obstetrics & Gynecology, Howard Minkoff, MD.

Women who give birth at Maimonides also have a variety of other services available to them, including:

- A Perinatal Testing Center, directed by Shoshana Haberman, MD, offering amniocentesis, 3-D ultrasound, fetal echo-cardiograms and other diagnostic exams.

- Neonatologists on-site around-the-clock. The Norma Sutton Center for Neonatology adjoins the Payson Birthing Center and provides the most sophisticated care in a family-friendly environment.

The Stella and Joseph Payson Birthing Center is ranked among the best in the nation for maternity care by HealthGrades, the nation's leading source for independent health care quality information. In recognition of its excellence in obstetrics and pediatrics, Maimonides was designated a Regional Perinatal Center by the New York State Department of Health. More babies are delivered at Maimonides than at any other single-campus hospital in New York State.

Maimonides Medical Center
Passionate about medicine.
Compassionate about people.

www.maimonidesmed.org/obgyn

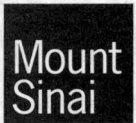 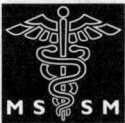

**MOUNT SINAI
SCHOOL OF
MEDICINE**

THE MOUNT SINAI MEDICAL CENTER OBSTETRICS, GYNECOLOGY, AND REPRODUCTIVE SCIENCE

One Gustave L. Levy Place
Fifth Avenue and 100th Street
New York, NY 10029-6574
Physician Referral: 1-800-MD-SINAI (637-4624)
www.mountsinai.org/obgyn

Building on more than a century of leadership in providing health care to women, the **DEPARTMENT OF OBSTETRICS, GYNECOLOGY, AND REPRODUCTIVE SCIENCE** at The Mount Sinai Medical Center offers special expertise in:

General obstetrics – Genetic counseling, prenatal care, labor and delivery management, and postpartum care. In addition to our talented physicians, other health care professionals are integrated into our practice, including genetic counselors, nutritionists, social workers, nurse midwives, childbirth educators, and lactation/breastfeeding specialists.

High-risk obstetrics – Advanced techniques in prenatal diagnosis and consultations in the management of complicated pregnancies. Our ultrasound unit is recognized for its expertise in fetal anatomy ultrasound assessments. The latest technology, including 4D imaging, is employed. Antepartum testing, including amniocentesis, chorionic villus sampling, and fetal blood sampling, are all routinely performed at Mount Sinai.

Reproductive endocrinology and infertility – Diagnosis and treatment of both female and male factor infertility. Treatment options for women include fertility medications, intrauterine insemination, in vitro fertilization, intracytoplasmic sperm injection, and ovum donation.

General gynecology – Cancer screening, management of abnormal Pap smears, family planning, and surgical management of fibroids, endometriosis, and other benign gynecologic conditions.

Gynecologic infectious diseases – Treatment and prevention of sexually transmitted infections and consultations on obstetrical and gynecological infections.

Gynecologic oncology – Care for women with cancers of the ovary, uterus, cervix, vulva, and vagina.

Minimally invasive surgery – For many conditions.

Urogynecology and reconstructive pelvic surgery – Lower urinary tract disorders.

INNOVATIVE APPROACHES TO PRENATAL CARE AND THE TREATMENT OF GYNECOLOGIC CANCERS
Known worldwide for excellence and innovative approaches to prenatal diagnosis and fetal therapy, Mount Sinai's Department of Obstetrics, Gynecology, and Reproductive Science has a long tradition of advancing clinical practice through patient-oriented research. Faculty members are pioneering work in diverse areas, including first- and second-trimester screening for fetal chromosomal abnormalities, vaccines for the prevention of sexually transmitted infections, minimally invasive surgical techniques, and new approaches to the diagnosis and treatment of gender-specific cancers.

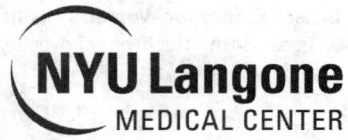
OBSTETRICS AND GYNECOLOGY

About the Department of Obstetrics and Gynecology
NYU Langone Medical Center provides comprehensive programs and services designed specifically for women, from primary care to highly specialized programs that are supported by sophisticated research and advanced training. We specialize in the following areas:

Fertility-Related Services
NYU Langone offers state-of-the-art programs in egg donation, egg freezing and wellness (acupuncture, mind/body, psychology and yoga). Diagnosis and treatment include ovulation induction, assisted reproductive technologies and surgical options that incorporate the latest endoscopic techniques. The Center also tests for genetic abnormalities, as well as for immunity and infectious diseases.

Gynecologic Oncology
The NCI-designated NYU Cancer Institute's Women's Cancer Program specializes in the treatment of cervical cancer, endometrial cancer, ovarian cancer, uterine cancer, vaginal cancer and vulvar cancer.

Maternal Fetal Medicine
Prenatal care for high-risk pregnancies and detailed consultations before, during and after pregnancy are offered. Special attention is given to multifetal pregnancies and to women who have other medical conditions that may complicate a pregnancy, such as diabetes, heart problems, high blood pressure and lupus.

Obstetrics
We offer a broad range of obstetrical services, including prenatal care that gives equal emphasis to the well-being of the mother and the fetus; fetal monitoring through ultrasound and other techniques; childbirth preparedness and breastfeeding classes; consultation for high-risk pregnancies, including treatment for women who have experienced recurrent pregnancy loss.

Specialty Services
In addition to routine gynecological care, we offer pelvic ultrasound; aspiration of breast cysts; evaluation of infertility (including the special needs of same-sex couples); colposcopy (a diagnostic evaluation of abnormal pap smears); LEEP (a loop electrosurgical procedure used to diagnose and treat cervical cancer); cryotherapy for vaginal warts; and bone density testing.

Urogynecology and Reconstructive Pelvic Surgery
Our urogynecologists treat all forms of incontinence and pelvic disorders; malformations of the reproductive tract found at birth, during childhood or in young adults; and conditions such as overactive bladder, urinary and/or fecal incontinence and pelvic organ prolapse.

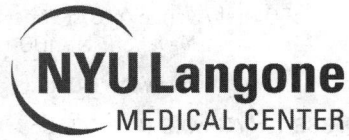

Joan H. Tisch Center for Women's Health
207 East 84th Street *(at 3rd Avenue)*
New York, NY
www.NYULMC.org
646-754-3300
Physician Referral: **888-7-NYU-MED** *(888-769-8633)*

THE JOAN H. TISCH CENTER FOR WOMEN'S HEALTH

About the Joan H. Tisch Center for Women's Health

Because many diseases and conditions impact women differently than men, NYU Langone Medical Center has created the Joan H. Tisch Center for Women's Health. Offering a comprehensive array of primary and specialty care, the Joan H. Tisch Center for Women's Health is New York City's premier destination for healthcare services tailored to the special needs of women. Conveniently located in the heart of Manhattan's Upper East Side, the Center combines NYU Langone's tradition of excellence with a multidisciplinary approach to providing individuals with the best possible medical care. At the Joan H. Tisch Center for Women's Health, the goal is maintaining excellent health and the vehicle is a caring, nurturing environment which understands that women are more than a collection of symptoms and medical conditions.

Expert Staff

Primary and specialty care physicians at the Joan H. Tisch Center for Women's Health have been carefully chosen for their ability to render quality, compassionate care to women. These healthcare professionals are focused on the holistic needs of patients in a state-of-the-art setting that relies heavily on teamwork. As part of a major academic medical institution, the Center is able to draw on additional healthcare resources and innovative research, when the need arises.

Comprehensive Range of Services

The Joan H. Tisch Center for Women's Health offers a wide range of primary and specialty medical care geared to women at a single location. Specialty services include breast health, cardiology, dermatology, endocrinology, ear/nose/throat, gastroenterology, gynecology, internal medicine, mental health, neurology, orthopaedics, plastic surgery, podiatry, pulmonary medicine, rehabilitation medicine, rheumatology, urology, vascular and women's imaging.

Technology Edge

The Joan H. Tisch Center for Women's Health has incorporated sophisticated technology into all levels of the patient experience. This ranges from the Center's informative website to its use of Epic, the Medical Center's up-to-the-minute electronic medical records system. In addition, patients can confidentially view their medical records and test results, as well as make appointment, request prescriptions and communicate with their physicians, through myNYULMC, a secure online service.

The Best in American Medicine
www.CastleConnolly.com

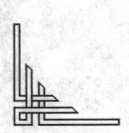
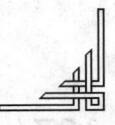

Ophthalmology

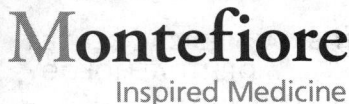

111 East 210th Street
Bronx, New York 10467
718-920-2020
www.montefiore.org/eyes

Ophthalmology and Visual Sciences at Montefiore Medical Center

With more than 30 full-time faculty members and annual patient volumes exceeding 125,000, the Department of Ophthalmology and Visual Sciences at Montefiore Medical Center is among the largest in the country. Here patients with all forms of ophthalmologic conditions receive exceptional care from highly skilled physicians, many of whom are leaders in the field. The Department offers specialty programs in **neuro-ophthalmology, the retina and the cornea, refractive surgery (LASIK), uveitis, glaucoma and ocular pathology as well as a full range of surgical and general ophthalmologic services for children and adults.**

To address the high rates of diabetic blindness and glaucoma among the Bronx's adult population, the Department offers strong treatment programs emphasizing early diagnosis and intervention. **Montefiore's ophthalmologists, led by Department Chairman Roy Chuck, MD, PhD, use the most advanced technology and treatment approaches when caring for patients with these and other vision conditions.** An example of such technology is the Trabectome (NeoMedix), a surgical device co-invented by Dr. Chuck, which is used to extract the meshwork tissue in glaucoma cases.

Meeting the vision needs of the region's vast pediatric population is a particular focus of the Department. **Led by respected congenital glaucoma and corneal transplant expert and Emeritus Trustee of the Foundation of the American Academy of Ophthalmology Norman Medow, MD, FACS, the Department's six pediatric specialists** diagnose and treat patients with such common conditions as refractive error or clogged tear ducts as well as urgent or uncommon conditions including ocular cancers, retinopathy of prematurity, genetic conditions and malformations. Few ophthalmology programs in the nation possess this same depth and volume of pediatric experience.

Through collaboration with Albert Einstein College of Medicine, the Department advances its research mission and aggressively competes for prestigious national grants. The Department's research arm—led by Barrett Katz, MD, MBA—has 14 National Institutes of Health grants and a fully unrestricted grant from Research to Prevent Blindness, Inc. Current research endeavors focus on ocular stem cells, information transfers between retinal cells, resistance to retinal ischemia and cataractogenesis, and surgical technique and instrument development.

The Department's commitment to improving the patient experience has spurred aggressive expansion and recruitment efforts. In addition to building its team of surgeons, optometrists and orthoptists, the Department has offices in eight locations from the Bronx to Scarsdale.

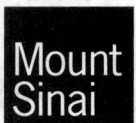 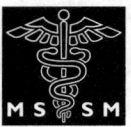

Mount Sinai

M S S M

MOUNT SINAI
SCHOOL OF
MEDICINE

THE MOUNT SINAI MEDICAL CENTER
OPHTHALMOLOGY

One Gustave L. Levy Place
Fifth Avenue and 100th Street
New York, NY 10029-6574
Physician Referral: 1-800-MD-SINAI (637-4624)
www.mountsinai.org/opthalmology

Specializing in the prevention, diagnosis, and treatment of eye disorders, Mount Sinai's **DEPARTMENT OF OPHTHALMOLOGY** features faculty with wide experience in special eye problems, offers comprehensive eye care services, and houses a state-of-the-art optical shop.

Services include:

- Comprehensive ophthalmology, refractive errors, and cataract surgery
- Corneal and external diseases of the eye
- Refractive surgery
- Retinal disorders (diabetic retinopathy, macular degeneration, inherited retinal diseases, retinal detachment)
- Glaucoma
- Pediatric eye care and strabismus
- Uveitis (inflammation of the eye)
- Neuro-ophthalmic disorders
- Oculplastic surgery, including cosmetic surgery, orbital tumors, and thyroid-related eye problems

Specialized treatments and procedures include:

- LASIK and other refractive surgical procedures
- Cataract surgery, including premium intraocular lenses
- Specialists in dry eye management
- Cosmetic lid treatments, including Botox and Restalayne injections
- Laser surgery
- Management of macular degeneration, including Lucentis and Avastin injections
- Advanced management for severe uveitis, including immunosuppressive drug therapy

INTERNATIONAL LEADERS IN THE FIELD OF UVEITIS

Uveitis, a collection of 30 diseases characterized by inflammation inside the eye, is the 5th leading cause of blindness in the United States. Management of severe uveitis often requires the skilled use of systemically-administered, immunosuppressive drugs, resulting in superior outcomes. Mount Sinai ophthalmologists have been pioneers in these treatments and are internationally recognized for their leadership in the field. A team of four uveitis specialists, augmented by the only uveitis training program in New York, offer a comprehensive treatment approach to these diseases.

We offer the full range of sophisticated diagnostic tests for evaluating patient conditions, including spectral domain optical coherence tomography, fluorescein angiography, indocyanine green angiography, autofluorescence, diagnostic ultrasound, electroretinography, visually evoked potential measurements, electro-oculography, corneal topography, confocal microscopy, state-of-the-art perimetry, HRT II imaging, allowing for faster, more accurate diagnosis and help determining the best treatment plan for each patient.

We perform cataract surgery, corneal transplants, refractive, glaucoma, strabismus, laser, ophthalmic plastic and reconstructive surgery, and vitreoretinal surgery for complicated retinal problems. We also offer minimally invasive procedures to treat eye disease, including non-laser refractive surgeries, and small-incision cataract surgery.

LEADERS IN CLINICAL RESEARCH

Mount Sinai ophthalmologists helped pioneer and evaluate new treatments for eye diseases and problems, including glaucoma, uveitis, ocular infections and farsightedness.

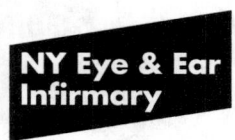

Continuum Health Partners, Inc.

THE NEW YORK EYE AND EAR INFIRMARY

310 East 14th Street
New York, New York 10003
Tel. 212.979.4000   Fax. 212.228.0664
http://www.nyee.edu

PROVIDING EXCEPTIONAL EYE CARE

The Department of Ophthalmology is the region's most comprehensive center for the delivery of primary through tertiary eye care. It is also by far the largest provider of eye care in the metropolitan area—with some 155,000 outpatient visits and 22,000 surgical cases performed each year. 365 board-certified ophthalmologists located throughout New York City and its tri-state area comprise the attending Medical Staff.

IN A HIGHLY SPECIALIZED SETTING

As a specialty hospital, The New York Eye and Ear Infirmary is uniquely qualified to handle the most complicated cases. It serves as a nationwide referral center with a commitment to teaching, research, and high-technology based patient care. Cutting edge ocular imaging instrumentation provides highest resolution to diagnose diseases of the cornea, retina and optic nerve and glaucoma. Highly experienced staff in state-of-the-art facilities have made The New York Eye and Ear Infirmary's 17 operating rooms a national benchmark in efficiency in eye surgery cases.

FOR PATIENTS OF ALL AGES

The New York Eye and Ear Infirmary's Ophthalmology staff are sensitive to the specific needs of patients of all ages. Senior citizens are the vast majority of the NYEE's 12,000 cataract patients each year, as well as individuals receiving treatment for age-related macular degeneration. Young children are now 25 percent of the patient population, with conditions such as strabismus, acquired and congenital cataracts, corneal diseases and ocular trauma. For those rare cases of children who have a disease ordinarily associated with age, the Infirmary runs New York's only Pediatric Glaucoma Service. Active adults of all ages utilize the New York Metropolitan Eye Trauma Center and Oculoplastic and Orbital Surgery Services.

Ophthalmology Clinical Services

Ambulatory Care Services
Comprehensive Eye Care
Cornea & Refractive Surgery
Eye Trauma
Glaucoma
Low Vision
Neuro-Ophthalmology
Ocular Pathology
Ocular Tumor
Oculoplastic &
Orbital Surgery
Pediatric Ophthalmology
& Strabismus
Retinal-Vitreal
Uveitis/Ocular Immunology

Facilities

Ambulatory Surgery Center
Bendheim Family Retina Center
Einhorn Clinical Trials Area
(supporting more than 100 ophthalmology studies a year)
Jorge N. Buxton Microsurgical
Education Center
(for residents, fellows and attending physicians)

About The New York Eye and Ear Infirmary

Founded in 1820, it is the nation's first and foremost, continuously operating specialty hospital. More than 10 million people have sought treatment here since its inception.

**Physician Referral
1.800.449.HOPE (4673)**

Orthopaedic Surgery

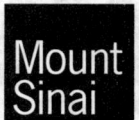 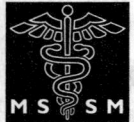

MOUNT SINAI
SCHOOL OF
MEDICINE

**THE MOUNT SINAI MEDICAL CENTER
ORTHOPAEDICS**
One Gustave L. Levy Place
Fifth Avenue and 100th Street
New York, NY 10029-6574
Physician Referral: 1-800-MD-SINAI (637-4624)
www.mountsinai.org/orthopaedics

Beyond its reputation for depth and breadth of expertise, **THE LENI AND PETER W. MAY DEPARTMENT OF ORTHOPAEDICS** at The Mount Sinai Medical Center is known for personalized care. The faculty and staff invest the time to get to know their patients as individuals, ensuring that they receive direct care from superb subspecialty-trained orthopedists. The faculty share expertise in surgery of the foot and ankle, knee, hip, hand, elbow, shoulder, and spine; total joint replacement; microvascular surgery; cancer surgery; and minimally invasive surgery. Taking a whole-patient approach to care, they work in close collaboration with specialists in geriatrics, neurology, oncology, pathology, and rehabilitation medicine.

Investigation and Innovation – Recent years have seen successive refinements in the techniques of orthopedic surgery at Mount Sinai, including joint replacement, minimally invasive fracture repair, and microvascular surgery. Faculty members have been instrumental in the design and perfection of hip and shoulder prostheses. Additionally, Mount Sinai has broadened the applications of arthroscopic surgery—the fiber optic technology that first heralded the arrival of minimally invasive surgery.

Mount Sinai orthopedic bone, spine and tendon scientists are known for their studies of diseases of the skeletal system. Researchers are currently investigating disc degeneration in the spine; rotator cuff degeneration; and the fundamental molecular mechanisms of tendon failure and regeneration.

Use of Cutting-Edge Techniques – Mount Sinai uses innovative, minimally invasive approaches for joint replacement and fracture repair. The Department's Oncology Service is renowned for saving limbs with both bone and joint malignancies.

The Sports Service provides patients with the full spectrum of non-operative and operative treatment including arthroscopic surgery of the hip, shoulder, knee, and elbow. Patients have the ability to return to activities faster and with less pain with this minimally invasive procedure. Our arthroscopists also specialize in cartilage preservation techniques, including cartilage transplantation, allowing patients to preserve their own joints and delaying the need for joint replacement surgery.

GROUNDBREAKING PROCEDURES ENHANCE QUALITY OF LIFE
Today at Mount Sinai, arthroscopy is used to repair not only the knee but virtually every joint. Converting what used to be major open surgery to outpatient procedures has dramatically shortened rehabilitation and return to work times. More significantly, it has allowed many more patients to get help for painful, function-limiting conditions. That is the case for many elderly or frail patients who are physically unable to undergo major surgery. The fact that such procedures are now more widely accessible is enhancing the quality of life for many patients and allowing them to lead more active lives.

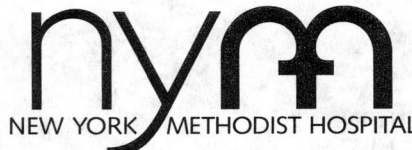

THE INSTITUTE FOR ORTHOPEDIC MEDICINE AND SURGERY

New York Methodist Hospital
506 Sixth Street, Brooklyn, N.Y. 11215
Phone: 866 ORTHO-11 (866 678-4611)
http://www.nym.org.

SPECIALISTS AND MEDICAL SERVICES

The Institute for Orthopedic Medicine and Surgery at New York Methodist Hospital brings together a unique team of specialists, facilities and medical services to provide comprehensive treatment of a broad range of orthopedic disorders.

The Institute's panel of physicians includes specialists in adult and pediatric orthopedic surgery, emergency medicine, rheumatology, podiatric medicine and surgery, endocrinology, sports medicine, pain management, orthopedic oncology and neurosurgery. Other important health care team members include physical and occupational therapists. All diagnostic and therapeutic procedures are performed at New York Methodist Hospital or in the offices of the referred physicians.

PROGRAMS OFFERED

In addition to emergency orthopedic services, programs offered through the Institute include joint replacement, arthroscopic knee surgery and cartilage restoration, medical treatments for arthritis, the geriatric hip fracture program, medical and surgical treatment for hand and shoulder injuries and degenerative conditions, spine surgery, physical therapy and pain management. Podiatric physicians specialize in all foot disorders, including reconstructive foot surgery. In addition, the Institute offers complementary medicine services including chiropractic care, acupuncture and medical massage.

* * *

Referrals to the Institute, its programs and physicians can be made through an individual's primary care physician or requested directly through the Institute's telephone referral service. More information (and on-line physician referral) is available at the Hospital's website, http://www.nym.org.

THE COMPREHENSIVE BACK AND NECK PAIN CENTER

NYM's Comprehensive Back and Neck Pain Center is dedicated to providing patients with the best clinical treatment for disorders of the back and neck. Diagnosis and treatment are centrally coordinated, so that patients avoid duplication of screening and testing procedures, if they need to see more than one specialist.

The Center focuses on conservative treatment, most commonly medication and/or rehabilitation (physical or occupational) therapy. Many other modalities are also available. If surgery is recommended, minimally invasive procedures may be applicable. Treatment decisions are made with consideration for the nature and severity of the condition, as well as the patient's lifestyle and preferences. For information or to make an appointment, call 718 369-BACK (2225).

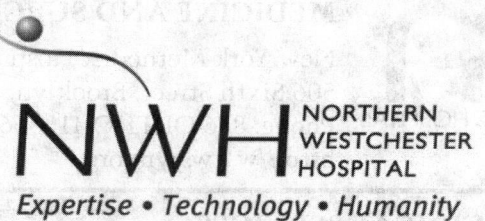

NWH NORTHERN
WESTCHESTER
HOSPITAL

Expertise • Technology • Humanity

The professionals at <u>The Orthopedic and Spine Institute</u> <u>at Northern Westchester Hospital</u> (NWH) provide high-quality, leading edge orthopedic and spine care through the application of <u>the latest minimally invasive and</u> <u>arthroscopic surgical techniques and advanced</u> <u>technologies</u>. Whether you are recovering from an injury or simply wanting to return to a healthier, more active lifestyle, the experts at the Orthopedic and Spine Institute (OSI) can help. <u>The OSI surgeons</u> are highly experienced, board certified, and have trained at the nation's leading medical schools to treat a complete range of orthopedic, spine, and sports medicine conditions.

<u>Northern Westchester Hospital (NWH)</u> provides quality, patient centered care that is close to home through the right combination of medical expertise, leading edge technology, and a commitment to humanity. Over 750 highly skilled physicians, state-of-the-art technology and professional staff of caregivers are all in place to ensure that you and your family receive treatment in a caring, respectful and nurturing environment.

NWH has established extensive internal quality measurements that surpass the standards defined by the Centers for Medicare & Medicaid Services (CMS) and the Hospital Quality Alliance (HQA) National Hospital Quality Measures. Our high quality standards help to ensure that the treatment you receive at NWH is among the best in the nation. For a complete list of our services, please visit <u>www.nwhc.net</u>.

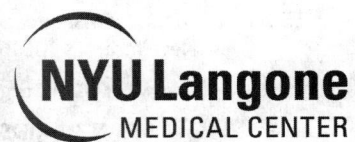

The Center for Musculoskeletal Care
333 East 38th Street *(between First and Second Avenues)*
New York, NY 10016
www.NYULMC.org/CMC
646-501-7070

THE CENTER FOR MUSCULOSKELETAL CARE

The new Center for Musculoskeletal Care (CMC) is the largest, free-standing musculoskeletal center of its kind in the country to bring clinical care, wellness programs, and access to clinical trials together at a single point of service. CMC combines state-of-the-art therapeutic and medical technology with the expertise of NYU Langone physicians, ranked among the country's top 10 in orthopaedics, rheumatology and rehabilitation by *U.S. News & World Report.*

CMC provides the full spectrum of outpatient bone and joint care for a wide range of conditions. The multidisciplinary team approach allows musculoskeletal experts to collaborate across centers and disciplines to provide the most comprehensive and seamless patient care.

Joint Replacement Center/Adult Reconstructive physicians evaluate degenerative conditions of the hip and knee caused by arthritis, injuries, congenital problems and general wear-and-tear to determine the best course of treatment.

Sports Medicine and primary care sports medicine physicians treat sports-related injuries or conditions of the knee, shoulder, elbow and ankle, using joint preservation techniques as well as surgical procedures.

The Spine Center provides conservative orthopaedic care for a broad range of spinal disorders, including problems associated with failed previous surgery, idiopathic disorders, growth disorders, neuromuscular disease, degenerative and congenital conditions, and traumatic deformity.

Rheumatology physicians care for arthritis or autoimmune conditions such as rheumatoid arthritis, osteoarthritis, psoriatic arthritis, lupus, osteoporosis, and Behçet's Syndrome.

The Infusion Center offers biologic agents and medications via infusion therapy, in a comfortable, private environment.

Rehabilitation Services, provided by the world-renowned Rusk Rehabilitation, include rehabilitation medicine (physiatry), physical therapy, occupational therapy, and hand therapy.

The Center for the Study and Treatment of Pain is an American Pain Society-designated Center of Excellence, where specialists partner with a patient's physician to manage pain associated with bone and joint conditions.

The Center for Diagnostic Imaging provides cutting-edge, on-site radiology services to facilitate quick and convenient diagnosis as well as interventional radiology procedures, and is recognized as one of the strongest musculoskeletal radiology departments in the world.

Sports Performance Center specialists assist active individuals in reaching their full potential through a state-of-the-art health and fitness evaluation and personalized athletic training plan.

Biomedical Research is woven into clinical care at CMC, offering patients access to cutting edge musculoskeletal therapies, techniques and devices.

The Outpatient Surgery Center is part of the CMC and offers same-day surgery in a unique, state-of-the art facility for minimally-invasive orthopaedic surgical procedures.

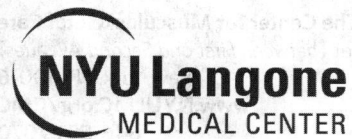

PEDIATRIC ORTHOPAEDICS

Pediatric Orthopaedics is part of the Hassenfeld Pediatric Center, a full service specialty Children's Hospital, which supports the array of children's health services across the Medical Center where newborns, children, adolescents and young adults receive the most comprehensive and advanced care by a team of pediatricians and pediatric specialists.

From common injuries to the most complex congenital disorders, NYU Langone's pediatric orthopaedic service, based at the Hospital for Joint Diseases (HJD), is one of the most extensive orthopaedic programs for children in the country and is a renowned multidisciplinary center featuring a strong collaborative approach to care. Areas of specialization include scoliosis, limb deformities, hip dysplasia, cerebral palsy, congenital insensitivity to pain, arthrogryposis, sports injuries, anterior cruciate ligament injuries, bone tumors, juvenile idiopathic arthritis, Charcot-Marie-Tooth disease, and brachial plexus injuries.

Specialized Orthopaedic Services
The Center for Children at HJD is a full-service pediatric outpatient facility that offers multidisciplinary management of pediatric musculoskeletal and neuromuscular disorders and brings together outstanding board-certified pediatric specialists in orthopaedic surgery, rheumatology, genetics, neurology, rehabilitation and pediatrics.

The Orthopaedic Immediate Care Center (i-Care), New York City's only walk-in orthopaedic clinic, uses state-of-the-art diagnostic equipment to evaluate and treat urgent orthopaedic injuries, such as fractures, dislocation or joint injury, sprains, and bone or joint infection.

The Ambulatory Care Clinic is available for convenient, streamlined treatment of both children and adults. A team of pediatric hospitalists evaluates patients with multiple medical problems prior to surgery, and helps to manage their postoperative care.

Nationally Recognized Surgical Care
The Wallace B. Lehman, MD, Center for Pediatric Orthopaedic Surgery at HJD is at the forefront of specialized surgery and personalized care for children. The Center is proud to be the largest teaching program in the country to offer a pediatric orthopaedic surgical residency, as well as fellowship training. It is also a recognized leader in surgical innovation and advanced technology, which helps ensure that patients receive the best possible care.

Convenient Satellite Sites
Satellite locations in the outlying areas of Westchester, Long Island, Rockland and New Jersey provide added convenience for parents seeking top orthopaedic care for their children within their own communities.

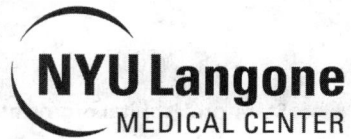

ORTHOPAEDIC PROGRAMS

The **Department of Orthopaedic Surgery** at NYU Langone Medical Center continues to be recognized as a national leader, ranked #6 nationwide in *U.S. News & World Report's* 2012-2013 "Best Hospitals" survey. Expert physicians combine extensive experience with cutting-edge research and technology to address bone and joint problems that affect a patient's ability to function. The department provides care at NYU Langone's premier outpatient facility, The Center for Musculoskeletal Care, as well as at the Hospital for Joint Diseases, our internationally-renowned inpatient musculoskeletal hospital. The clinical expertise of our world-class orthopaedic surgeons represents the full range of subspecialty areas including Adult Reconstructive, Sports Medicine, Spine, Shoulder & Elbow, Foot & Ankle, Hand Surgery, Trauma & Fracture, Orthopaedic Oncology, and Pediatric Orthopaedics; additional areas of focus include minimally-invasive surgery and robotic-assisted joint replacement.

The department also features a number of specialized orthopaedic patient care centers:
The Bone Healing Center evaluates and treats problem fractures and are leaders in technologies and procedures to help patients facing a long and difficult recovery from complex fracture reconstruction or fracture healing problems.
Harkness Center for Dance Injuries offers many subsidized and free services for dancers, including clinics staffed by orthopaedists and dance physical therapists. The Center also offers state-of-the-art rehabilitation technology and free injury prevention screenings and lectures.
The Diabetes Foot and Ankle Center focuses on the prevention and recurrence of foot and ankle problems associated with complications of diabetes.
The Hip Center evaluates and treats developmental, traumatic, and degenerative hip disorders and specializes in the cutting-edge, minimally invasive anterior total hip replacement technique.
The Orthopaedic Immediate Care Center ("i-Care"), New York City's only walk-in orthopaedic clinic, uses state-of-the-art diagnostic equipment to evaluate and treat hand and foot injuries, hip, arm or leg fractures, dislocation or joint injury, sprains, and bone or joint infection.
The Joint Preservation Center (JPC) is dedicated to operative and non-operative treatment of joint problems, aiming to reduce symptoms, restore function and delay the onset of degenerative arthritis and potential need for an eventual joint replacement.
Joint Replacement Center physicians are experts in knee, hip and shoulder replacements, complex joint revisions, and minimally invasive surgeries, conducting 3,000+ procedures annually.
The Occupational and Industrial Orthopaedic Center (OIOC) provides clinical, educational, research and consulting services in the prevention and treatment of musculoskeletal injuries and disorders that arise from work or the work environment.
The Spine Center specializes in spine disorders, including lower back and neck pain, scoliosis, osteoporosis and complex spine problems. The Center performs minimally invasive spinal fusions and was one of the first in the country to successfully perform artificial disc implantation.

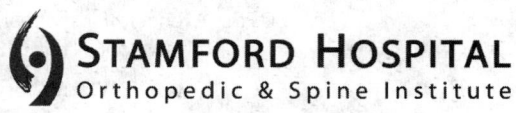
STAMFORD HOSPITAL
Orthopedic & Spine Institute

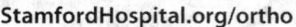

Orthopedic and Spine Institute

Stamford Hospital was the first in the region to earn the Joint Commission certification for our Total Hip and Total Knee Replacement programs in addition to our Spine Fusion Program. We were awarded the Gold Seal of Approval™ for complying with the highest national standards for safety and quality of care. Our doctors and nurses earned this distinction by undergoing a lengthy process of professional review, including on-site evaluations.

Joint Replacements

We provide comprehensive orthopedic services, including prevention, assessment, treatment and rehabilitation. Our fellowship-trained surgeons routinely perform total hip and knee replacements, as well as minimally invasive joint replacements and hip fracture surgeries using leading-edge technology to improve patient care and outcomes.

Spine Center

Experts in total spine care, we perform more complex spine surgeries than any other hospital in the region. From acute neck and back pain to spinal instability and deformity, we provide relief to those who may have previously tried non-surgical options. A team of dedicated orthopedic and neurosurgeons, nurses, anesthesiologists, physical therapists and pain-management specialists, are experienced in treating the most challenging spinal conditions.

Sports Medicine

No matter your age or level of play, amateur or seasoned professional, we can help you stay in the game. We combine hands-on evaluation and appropriate diagnostic testing to determine the best plan of care. We provide the latest surgical techniques and are experienced in performing a wide variety of advanced procedures. Our surgeons are fellowship-trained in sports medicine from some of the top programs in the country.

Academic and Clinical Affiliations

Stamford Hospital is an affiliate of the New York–Presbyterian Healthcare System and a major teaching affiliate of the Columbia University College of Physicians & Surgeons.

Accreditation

Joint Commission on Accreditation of Healthcare Organization (JCAHO)

Beds

305

Sponsorship

Voluntary, Not-for-Profit

For a Physician Referral or more information, please call 1.877.233.9355 or visit StamfordHospital.org /doctor.

Stamford Hospital
30 Shelburne Road
Stamford, CT 06902
203.276.1000

StamfordHospital.org

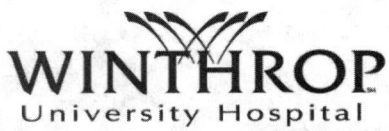

Your Health Means Everything.™

WINTHROP-UNIVERSITY HOSPITAL
is committed to being a leading
center of excellence for

ORTHOPAEDIC SURGERY
on Long Island.

Dedicated to a highly individualized,
multidisciplinary team approach to
address the musculoskeletal needs
of each patient as a whole person,
Winthrop's orthopedic surgeons
address a full range of orthopaedic
conditions, using both surgical and
non-surgical procedures to
relieve pain, discomfort, and
maximize each patient's mobility.

THE WINTHROP ORTHOPAEDIC TEAM
is comprised of specialists who
address several specialty areas of
orthopaedics including: pediatric
orthopaedics, hand and upper
extremity surgery, minimally
invasive surgery, arthroscopy, sports
medicine, trauma and fracture
repair, arthritis treatment, joint
replacement and reconstruction
surgery, spine surgery, and podiatry.

This combination of advanced
treatment options and specialists in
virtually every area of adult and
pediatric orthopaedic medicine places
**Winthrop's program at the
forefront of ORTHOPAEDIC CARE
ON LONG ISLAND.**

ROBOTIC ORTHOPAEDIC SURGERY
A leader in total joint replacement, Winthrop continues to
reach new frontiers in total hip replacement surgery, total
knee replacements and joint replacement revision surgery.
The joint replacement team also specializes in performing
minimally-invasive, bone-sparing, and tissue-conserving
total hip replacements. The department also offers
robotically assisted total knee replacement – a highly
accurate approach to knee replacement surgery only
offered at Winthrop.

SPORTS MEDICINE
Winthrop's comprehensive Sports Medicine Center
features orthopaedic surgeons who focus on every joint in
the body – from ankles and wrists to knees and hips – for
both adults and children. Physicians work with patients
individually to attain the highest levels of achievement
despite any injury they may have.

HAND INJURIES
The hand service treats children and adults with a
variety of bone and soft tissue conditions of the hand and
upper extremity. Some of the more common conditions
include carpal tunnel syndrome, tennis elbow, and trigger
finger. The department also specializes in the treatment of
deformities, reimplantations, metabolic bone disease,
complex fractures, and sports-related injuries.

FOOT AND ANKLE TREATMENT
Winthrop's foot and ankle team specializes in a wide
range of treatments, which can range from bracing and
physical therapy to surgical procedures such as bunion
surgery, ankle arthroscopy, complex ligament and tendon
reconstructions, total ankle replacements,
and osteochondral grafting procedures.

PEDIATRIC CARE
Children's growth plates are delicate and are especially
prone to fracture. Because many childhood fractures
involve growth plates, it is vital for children to be
evaluated quickly when a fracture occurs in order to
determine the best course of treatment and avoid growth
deformity. Winthrop's Division of Pediatric Orthopaedic
Surgery treats pediatric patients from new born to young
adulthood.

WINTHROP's mission is founded upon the basic core value of "YOUR HEALTH MEANS EVERYTHING"
and all of its employees are committed to ensuring
the integrity, comfort and well-being of every individual.

Otolaryngology

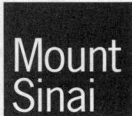
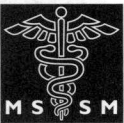

MOUNT SINAI SCHOOL OF MEDICINE

THE MOUNT SINAI MEDICAL CENTER
OTOLARYNGOLOGY – EAR, NOSE, AND THROAT

One Gustave L. Levy Place
Fifth Avenue and 100th Street
New York, NY 10029-6574
Physician Referral: 1-800-MD-SINAI (637-4624)
www.mountsinai.org/ENT

Mount Sinai's **DEPARTMENT OF OTOLARYNGOLOGY – HEAD AND NECK SURGERY** – ranks as one of the finest in the nation. In 2012, *U.S. News & World Report* again placed us among the top 15 in the United States, continuing our impressive history of achievement. Since the early nineteenth century, we have pioneered surgical advances in endoscopy, otology, skull-base surgery, laryngology, rhinology, facial plastic surgery, and head and neck oncology and reconstruction. More recently, we have incorporated advanced technology in robotic and endoscopic surgery, basic science research, and translational science programs.

Robotic Head and Neck Surgery – We are a world leader in robotic head and neck surgery. Our surgeons and researchers have published techniques that have changed the paradigm for management of head and neck cancer, allowing for endoscopic surgery without external incisions, shortening hospital stays, and improving outcomes.

Endoscopic Laser Surgery of the Larynx and Trachea – Our surgeons and scientists have introduced techniques in laryngeal and tracheal surgery, including endoscopic laser surgery, tracheal transplantation, and reconstructive surgery, allowing removal of malignant disease while preserving voice and swallowing functions.

The Grabscheid Voice Center – Our multidisciplinary group provides professional singers and patients in need with cutting-edge treatments, using endoscopic laser and minimally invasive surgery. We pioneered office-based procedures that offer patients the opportunity to undergo therapy without the need for general anesthesia.

Cranial Base Surgery – Techniques in endoscopic trans-nasal surgery have revolutionized the management of skull base tumors and cerebrospinal leaks. We have developed procedures for accessing the cranial base and frontal lobes of the brain through the nose, delivering excellent outcomes with lower complications rates.

Thyroid and Parathyroid Surgery – We are nationally recognized for excellence in clinical care and clinical outcomes research. Our minimally invasive and robotic surgical techniques offer patients surgery through tiny incisions. Cure rates for thyroid cancer using these techniques are higher than 95 percent. Parathyroid surgery is performed using similar techniques and intraoperative parathyroid hormone monitoring.

Otology and Neurotology – Long recognized among the best in the nation, our otologic surgeons have pioneered surgical techniques to manage chronic ear disease and cochlear implantation that have resulted in excellent outcomes.

THE MULTIDISCIPLINARY HEAD AND NECK ONCOLOGY TEAM—Acclaimed as one of the finest in the country, our multidisciplinary team includes 35 physicians, surgeons, and ancillary staff from 12 departments. We offer top-rated courses, training and research fellowships and enjoy national recognition for expertise in head, neck, and skull-base cancer. Our minimally invasive and endoscopic team includes surgeons and oncologists focused on treating tumors of the oral cavity, jaw, and larynx, while preserving each patient's quality of life. Speech and swallowing rehabilitation therapists work with patients to help them recover, all of which keeps Mount Sinai on the cutting edge of head and neck cancer therapy, reconstruction, and rehabilitation.

The Center for Comprehensive Management of Nasal and Sinus Disease – We deliver the most advanced care for patients suffering from allergic and invasive fungal sinusitis, acute and chronic sinusitis, benign and malignant tumors of the sinonasal cavity, cerebrospinal fluid leaks and encephalocele treatment and inflammatory polyp disease.

The Sleep Surgery Center – We offer comprehensive management and treatment of obstructive sleep apnea (OSA) and snoring. Collaboration with the divisions of pulmonary medicine, sleep medicine and endocrinology, provides the collective expertise of a multidisciplinary approach, which is necessary to address all conditions in sleep disordered breathing.

Center for Facial Plastic and Reconstructive Surgery – Our plastic surgeons provide expertise in the areas of facial plastic surgery and complex reconstructive surgery. Our team is expert in the areas of congenital and traumatic deformities, skin cancer, and facial nerve paralysis with reanimation. With expertise, they reverse the signs of aging, remove contour irregularities or deformities, and make the overall appearance of the face more natural and youthful.

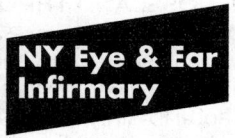

NY Eye & Ear Infirmary

Continuum Health Partners, Inc.

THE NEW YORK EYE AND EAR INFIRMARY

310 East 14th Street
New York, New York 10003
Tel. 212.979.4000   Fax. 212.228.0664
http://www.nyee.edu

PROVIDING EXCEPTIONAL CARE OF THE EAR, NOSE, THROAT, AND HEAD & NECK

Established in 1820 the Department of Otolaryngology/Head & Neck Surgery is the first training program in this specialty in the Western Hemisphere. Over nearly two centuries the department has evolved to be an international referral center for the medical and surgical treatment of diseases of the ear, nose, throat and face.

OUTSTANDING SERVICES:

Ear Institute (Otology – Neuro-otology): Specializing in the care of acute and chronic ear disease including hearing loss, cochlear implantation, dizziness, tinnitus, intra cranial tumors and facial nerve disorders. Our advanced otologic and vestibular diagnostic labs assist physicians in treatment.

Facial Plastic Surgery: Highly specialized and renowned surgeons perform in-office or ambulatory procedures utilizing state-of-the-art technology and techniques to produce outstanding results with minimal incisions, rapid recovery and a natural, youthful appearance.

Facial Paralysis: Comprehensive center treating all causes and offering reconstruction of the paralyzed face.

Head & Neck Oncology: A multi-disciplinary team including board-certified surgeons, medical & radiation oncologists, nutritionists and rehabilitation specialists insure rapid recovery from complex, life-saving surgical procedures and return to daily activities.

Pediatric Otolaryngology: Treating children has long been a priority at the Infirmary. Pediatric care ranges from middle ear infection, tonsil and adenoid disease, and neck masses to complex sinus and airway diseases.

Rhinology and Sinus Surgery: Internationally known specialists utilize minimally invasive techniques to treat disorders from sinusitis to intra cranial tumors.

Thyroid Center: A comprehensive program to streamline the diagnosis and treatment of thyroid diseases and cancers. A highly skilled team of surgeons, endocrinologists and radiologists manage the patient's care.

Voice & Swallowing Institute: Combining the expertise of physicians, speech pathologists and a voice physiologist to diagnose and treat voice problems – not only for performing artists but also for teachers, stockbrokers, receptionists, salespeople – anyone for whom voice is an important part of life.

Otolaryngology Clinical Services

General Otolaryngology *plus*
Facial Plastic & Reconstructive Surgery
Cochlear Implantation
Voice & Vocal Dynamics
Head & Neck Oncology
Laryngology
Otology & Neuro-otology
Pediatric Otolaryngology
Rhinology & Sinus Surgery
Swallowing Disorders
Thyroid Center

Facilities

Academic Faculty Practice,
including multiple locations throughout metropolitan NY
Hearing Aid Dispensary
Vestibular Rehabilitation
Ambulatory Care Services

About The New York Eye and Ear Infirmary

The New York Eye and Ear Infirmary is the nation's first specialty hospital and one of the most experienced in terms of the number of patients it treats and complexity of its cases. Each year the otolaryngology department performs more than 6,000 surgeries and sees more than 70,000 visits from outpatients.

Physician Referral
1.800.449.HOPE (4673)

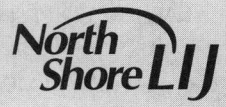 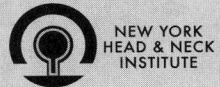

Lenox Hill Hospital (Black Hall)
130 East 77th Street, 10th Floor
(between Lexington & Park Avenues)
New York, NY 10075
(212) 434-4500
www.nyhni.org

New York Head & Neck Institute (NYHNI)

NYHNI, part of North Shore-LIJ Health System, provides seamless, integrated care across several specialty fields for people with disorders of the head and neck.

We are committed to compassionate treatment and trusted doctor–patient relationships. We share all available information with our patients, empowering them as equal partners when it comes to decisions regarding their care. At NYHNI, our patients always come first.

Many Specialists, One Team

NYHNI consists of nine centers, each focusing on a type of disorder or anatomical area of the head and neck, allowing us to treat the entire range of these disorders in adults and children. Each center offers medical therapy and the newest minimally invasive surgical techniques to cure the condition or improve the patient's life.

At NYHNI, we use a minimally invasive approach to all procedures, which ensures a faster, more comfortable recovery for the patient.

The physicians, surgeons (more than 60 — and growing) and professional staff of NYHNI all have regional, national or international reputations within their particular head and neck specialty areas. They bring vast experience and training to effectively diagnose and treat head and neck disorders while providing the most advanced patient-centered care.

We have offices in Manhattan, Staten Island and Long Island.

Our Areas of Expertise:

- Aesthetic Plastic Surgery

- Cranial Base Surgery
  (Skull Base Surgery)

- Facial Reconstruction

- Head and Neck Oncology
  (Head and Neck Cancer)

- Hearing and Balance
  (Diseases of the Ear)

- Allergies, Asthma, Nasal and
  Sinus Disorders

- Sleep Disorders
  (Obstructive Sleep Apnea)

- Thyroid and Parathyroid Surgery

- Voice and Swallowing Disorders

To find a doctor: **1-888-321-DOCS** or visit **www.northshorelij.com**

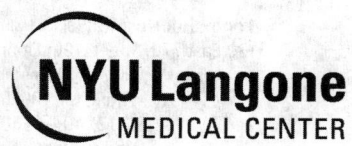
OTOLARYNGOLOGY

About the Department of Otolaryngology
The Department of Otolaryngology at NYU Langone Medical Center provides the highest quality treatment for ear, nose, throat, head and neck disorders, including one of the premier head and neck surgery programs in the country. We specialize in the following areas:

Cochlear Implants
Patients are provided with extensive evaluation, device programming and speech rehabilitation both pre- and post-operatively.

Facial Plastic and Reconstructive Surgery
Care is provided to patients requiring facial reconstructive surgery for a wide variety of facial deformities, and to those seeking facial cosmetic surgery. Specialties include functional and aesthetic rhinoplasty, facial rejuvenation surgery, injectable fillers, Botulinum Toxin (Botox) for facial spasm or wrinkles, and chemical peels and microdermabrasion.

General Otolaryngology and Sleep Surgery
Care is provided to adult patients with voice, sleep, allergy and nasal breathing disorders. Additionally, services for children are provided through our pediatric otolaryngologists.

Head and Neck Surgery and Oncology
Care is provided to patients with cancer of the head and neck, including cancer of the larynx, oral cavity, throat, nasal cavity and sinuses, salivary glands and lymph nodes in the neck.

Neutology/Skull Base Program
The Otolaryngology team provides expert care to patients with hearing loss, facial nerve palsy, vertigo and tinnitus, and treats lesions such as acoustic neuromas and skull base meningiomas. Featured services include facial palsy rehabilitation, auditory brainstem implants, cochlear implants, laser surgery and endoscopic anterior and lateral skull base surgery.

Voice and Swallowing Disorders
We treat voice and swallowing disorders, including sore throat, chronic cough, hoarseness, voice loss, swallowing dysfunction, benign growths and cancerous tumors, vocal cord paralysis, the aging voice, recurrent or chronic laryngitis, gastroesophageal reflux, and injuries from overuse and misuse of the voice.

Audiology treats patients suffering with hearing or balance disorders; Head and Neck Speech Pathology treats voice, speech or swallowing problems; Rhinology treats all diseases of the paranasal sinuses, nose and related structures; Skull Base Surgery offers a minimally invasive and advanced surgical approach to tumors of the anterior and posterior skull base.

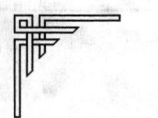

The Best in American Medicine
www.CastleConnolly.com

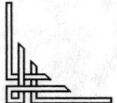

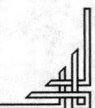

Pediatric Endocrinology

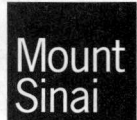
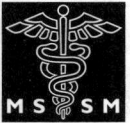

THE MOUNT SINAI MEDICAL CENTER
PEDIATRIC DIABETES AND ENDOCRINOLOGY

One Gustave L. Levy Place
Fifth Avenue and 100th Street
New York, NY 10029-6574
Physician Referral: 1-800-MD-SINAI (637-4624)
www.kravischildrenshospital.org

PEDIATRIC DIABETES AND ENDOCRINOLOGY
INNOVATIVE MEDICINE, FAMILY-CENTERED CARE

The Hall Family Center for Pediatric Endocrinology and Diabetes at Kravis Children's Hospital at Mount Sinai is dedicated to excellence in clinical care, education and research – a fact that has led to our being **named among the top 25 pediatric diabetes and endocrinology services in America,** according to *The U.S. News & World Report's* 2012-2013 ranking of "Best Children's Hospitals."

Under the direction of Robert Rapaport, M.D., Division Chief, we use a team approach, which is patient and family centered, to manage:

- Diabetes (type 1 and type 2, medication-related, monogenic and pre-diabetes)
- Short stature
- Growth disorders, including growth hormone deficiency, growth in children born small for gestational age, and early and late puberty
- Genetic disorders, including Turner Syndrome and Noonan Syndrome
- Congenital and acquired hypothyroidism and hyperthyroidism
- Hyperparathyroidism
- Congenital adrenal hyperplasia/hypoplasia
- Obesity and other nutritional disorders, including Vitamin D deficiency.

Diabetes – We offer the complete spectrum of high level diagnostic and treatment services, including simulation testing, for children and adolescents and bring families into their circle of care. Since education and support are vital to managing diabetes, we offer a variety of programs for patients and their families, including "Toddlers and Grandparents," "College Prep," for teens entering college, and a free one-week day camp in Central Park in conjunction with the Barton Center for Diabetes Education.

We are currently collaborating with four other medical centers on the **R.O.A.D. (Reduce Obesity and Diabetes)** project, to study and educate middle school children in Harlem. By identifying the metabolic factors that lead from obesity to diabetes, we will develop a protocol for detecting which children will most likely develop diabetes, allowing us to streamline interventions and identify where best to allocate resources.

Endocrine Disorders and Growth - With our faculty leading investigations into both international and multi-center trials, we enjoy a stellar reputation for identifying and treating a host of common and complex endocrine disorders, including growth hormone deficiency, growth in children born small for gestational age, and other disorders caused by Turner or Noonan Syndrome, and congenital hypothyroidism. In addition to offering expert consultations, we employ early screening methods and breakthrough growth hormone therapy that enables children to grow and develop normally.

We also excel at diagnosing and treating children with **precocious or delayed puberty** and have developed methods to identify and manage these conditions before they appear clinically obvious.

ANNUAL SYMPOSIUM

Our physician-scientists conduct investigations into the causes and treatments of childhood endocrine conditions, and we are committed to translating research into better methods of clinical care. To that end, we hold an annual symposium each November to update pediatricians practicing within the community on the latest advances in pediatric endocrinology and diabetes.

Pediatric Gastroenterology

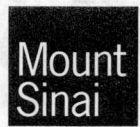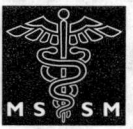

MOUNT SINAI
SCHOOL OF
MEDICINE

THE MOUNT SINAI MEDICAL CENTER
PEDIATRIC GASTROENTEROLOGY
One Gustave L. Levy Place
Fifth Avenue and 100th Street
New York, NY 10029-6574
Physician Referral: 1-800-MD-SINAI (637-4624)
www.mountsinai.org/kravis

PEDIATRIC GASTROENTEROLOGY
Innovative Medicine, Family-Centered Care

In recognition of our tradition of excellence in patient care, research and education, **Mount Sinai's Kravis Children's Hospital was named among the country's best in Pediatric Gastroenterology**, according to *U.S. News and World Report's* 2012-2013 edition of "America's Best Children's Hospitals."

Under the direction of Keith Benkov, M.D., Chief of Pediatric Gastroenterology, we deliver expert consultation and compassionate, evidence-based care to pediatric patients with common and complex digestive disorders, including inflammatory bowel disease, celiac disease, gastroesophageal reflux disease and irritable bowel syndrome.

With a reputation for providing the highest level of innovative and comprehensive care to patients with Crohn's disease and ulcerative colitis, our nationally recognized **Children's IBD Center** receives referrals from across the country. We are currently following over 500 children and have seen over 1700 patients with IBD in the last 10 years. The combination of this extensive experience, our focus on basic science and clinical research, and our collaboration with Mount Sinai's internationally renowned adult IBD program, enables us to deliver a unique approach to IBD care in children.

To optimize outcomes, our entire team of healthcare professionals participates in every patient's circle of care. We address each patient's specific needs, including management, nutrition, growth, body image and coping methods for a chronic illness. The center fosters family participation and encourages patients to gather to share ideas. Lectures, discussions and support groups are open to all families.

In addition, we continually strive to advance our knowledge of IBD and its treatments through research. In conjunction with Department of Pediatric Allergy and Immunology, we are currently investigating the benefits of an herbal medicine developed as a complementary therapy for children with Crohn's disease.

IBD runs the spectrum from mild to severe disease. No matter how seriously a child is affected, our ultimate goal is to help every child who comes to us with IBD lead a normal, productive life and achieve all his or her personal aspirations.

Pediatric Hematology-Oncology

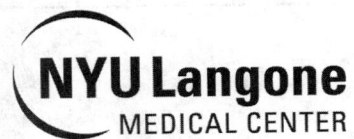
PEDIATRIC HEMATOLOGY/ONCOLOGY

Pediatric Hemaology/Oncology is part of the Hassenfeld Pediatric Center, a full service specialty Children's Hospital, which supports the array of children's health services across the Medical Center where newborns, children, adolescents and young adults receive the most comprehensive and advanced care by a team of pediatricians and pediatric specialists.

We are committed to providing modern, family-centered and highly personalized care to children with cancer and blood disorders. Teams of specialists deliver personalized care in a healing environment promoting physical, emotional and spiritual well-being of children and their families.

Hematologic Malignancies
We offer new treatments for childhood acute lymphoblastic leukemia (ALL) and are a national leader in clinical trials for children with newly diagnosed leukemia and recurrent diseases.

Hematology
We provide treatment for children and adolescents with all types of blood disorders including Sickle Cell Disease, other hemoglobinopathies, bleeding disorders and aplastic anemia.

Pediatric Neuro-Oncology
We provide multidisciplinary comprehensive care for children from infants to young adults with primary central nervous system, slow-growing and malignant tumors assuring the safest and most effective treatments for newly diagnosed or recurrent tumors.

Pediatric Special Hematology Laboratory
NYU Langone offers comprehensive homeostasis and red cell testing incorporating the latest developments in the field.

Psychosocial Services
Our holistic approach to care includes art therapy, relaxation training, play therapy, psychiatric evaluation, neuropsychological assessment, individual/group counseling and patient education.

Sarcoma and Solid Tumor Program
We offer cutting-edge medical, surgical and radiotherapy treatments for bone and soft tissue sarcomas, and all pediatric solid tumors including Wilms' Tumor and neuroblastoma and are developing national trials for the treatment of sarcomas and offer a number of clinical trials.

Stephen D. Hassenfeld Children's Center for Cancer and Blood Disorders
As a member of the NCI-designated NYU Cancer Institute, we are constantly developing new ways to treat childhood cancer. Our unique interdisciplinary and family-centered approach combines the most advanced medical treatments with psychosocial and emotional support.

Pediatric Nephrology

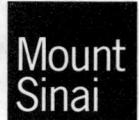 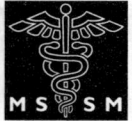

MOUNT SINAI
SCHOOL OF
MEDICINE

THE MOUNT SINAI MEDICAL CENTER
NEPHROLOGY
One Gustave L. Levy Place
Fifth Avenue and 100th Street
New York, NY 10029-6574
Physician Referral: 1-800-MD-SINAI (637-4624)
www.mountsinai.org/kidney

Mount Sinai's Department of Nephrology ranks among the best in the nation, according to the 2012-2013 issue of *U.S. News & World Report's* "Americas Best Hospitals."

We have been an international leader in the treatment of kidney disease since we performed the first hemodialysis in the United States in the 1950s. We established New York State's first dialysis center in 1957. We currently operate the largest home dialysis program in New York City, and our **Geriatric Nephrology Program** is the only one of its kind in the country.

Under the direction of Barbara Murphy, M.D., Acting Chair, Department of Medicine and Division Chief of Nephrology, we are continuing our leadership in patient care, research and education. Proof of our clinical excellence is evident daily in our practice and hospital. Our physicians care for patients referred to us by other nephrologists who recognize the need for our expertise in their most challenging and complex cases.

Our expertise spans numerous kidney diseases and treatments, including:

- Chronic kidney disease
- Polycystic kidney disease
- Geriatric kidney disease
- Diabetes-related kidney disease
- Glomerular disease
- Hypertensive kidney disease
- HIV-associated nephropathy
- Kidney transplantation
- Hemodialysis
- Peritoneal Dialysis

EXPERT PHYSICIANS

Building on the talent and expertise of our physicians, including Jonathan Winston, M.D., Tonia Kim, M.D., Mark Swidler, M.D., Joseph Vassalotti, M.D, Brian Radbill, M.D., and Richard Stein, M.D., along with transplantation specialists, Bernd Schroppel, M.D. and Vinay Nair, M.D., we provide patients with the most advanced and appropriate approach to care. With so much research taking place, we can also offer patients access to experimental treatments often unavailable elsewhere.

Initiated in 1967, our **kidney transplant program** is now one of the largest and most successful in the country, with our physician-scientists actively investigating new and innovative ways to detect, prevent, and treat rejection.

A Strong Focus on Research
With one of the largest National Institutes of Health research budgets of any nephrology division in the country, we conduct and support numerous clinical trials, and our faculty members have achieved international recognition as authorities on the causes and treatments of all forms of kidney diseases and disorders.

Pediatric Pulmonology

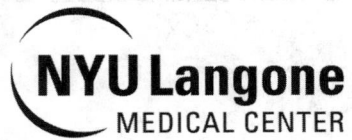

PEDIATRIC PULMONOLOGY

Pediatric Pulmonology is part of the Hassenfeld Pediatric Center, a full service specialty Children's Hospital, which supports the array of children's health services across the Medical Center where newborns, children, adolescents and young adults receive the most comprehensive and advanced care by a team of pediatricians and pediatric specialists.

About Pediatric Pulmonology, Department of Pediatrics

The Division of Pediatric Pulmonology provides comprehensive care to children -- from infancy to adolescence to young adulthood -- with a variety of conditions affecting the respiratory system. Physicians in the Division are committed to providing both family-centered and multidisciplinary care, collaborating with specialists in other divisions throughout NYU Langone Medical Center. For example, physicians in the Division work closely with the Infant Apnea/SIDS Program to follow children discharged from the Neonatal Intensive Care Unit; with the Division of Pediatric Gastroenterology and the Swallowing Center to follow children with feeding difficulties and swallowing dysfunction; with the Division of Pediatric Surgery to follow children with congenital lung lesions through minimally invasive surgery; and with the Division of Orthopaedics to optimize the care of children with neuromuscular disease undergoing spine surgery. We specialize in the following areas:

Pulmonologists in the Division care for children with a wide range of problems, including asthma, bronchopulmonary dysplasia (chronic lung disease of prematurity), cystic fibrosis, chronic respiratory failure and pulmonary complications of neuromuscular disease, congenital lung malformations, chest wall deformities, interstitial lung disease, and obstructive sleep apnea. Consultation for chronic cough, noisy breathing, and exercise intolerance is also provided.

Flexible bronchoscopy

Using specialized pediatric equipment, the airways of even the tiniest infants can be examined in the state-of-the-art endoscopy suite at NYU Langone Medical Center, with multiple specialists often involved in the procedure. Because the equipment is mobile, procedures can also be performed at bedside in the Pediatric Intensive Care Unit.

Pediatric Rheumatology

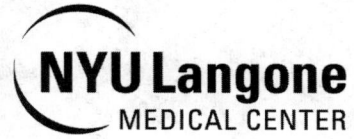
PEDIATRIC RHEUMATOLOGY

Pediatric Rheumatology is part of the Hassenfeld Pediatric Center, a full service specialty Children's Hospital, which supports the array of children's health services across the Medical Center where newborns, children, adolescents and young adults receive the most comprehensive and advanced care by a team of pediatricians and pediatric specialists.

About the Division of Pediatric Rheumatology, Department of Pediatrics

Pediatric rheumatology specialists at the NYU Langone Medical Center are dedicated to the complete care of children with rheumatic disease. In conjunction with our multidisciplinary team of specialists, we treat children with a variety of rheumatologic conditions, including Juvenile Idiopathic Arthritis (JIA), systemic lupus erythematosus, juvenile dermatomyositis, Kawasaki's disease, and others. Through early diagnosis and appropriately intensive treatment we aim to achieve disease quiescence as quickly and safely as possible, with the ultimate goal of returning children to full physical functionality.

In addition to our clinical services, we are committed to the continued formal education of residents, rheumatology fellows and medical students, as well as the general public through our community outreach programs and in collaboration with the adult Rheumatology Division, we have initiated an annual pediatric rheumatology CME course which is well-attended by general physicians and rheumatologists. Our emphasis on providing high-level clinical services and teaching is complemented by the Division's collaboration with national pediatric rheumatology research organizations in several clinical research projects pertaining to drug exposure in children with rheumatic disease. We specialize in the following areas:

Juvenile Idiopathic Arthritis

An umbrella term for several different patterns of arthritis in children, juvenile idiopathic arthritis (JIA) refers to arthritic disorders caused by an autoimmune reaction. Our Pediatric rheumatologists diagnose and treat different types of JIA. The use of methotrexate in combination with newly discovered biologic agents, such as Etanercept and Infliximab, gives even greater reason for optimism. Juvenile arthritis, once a crippler of children, is fast becoming a highly manageable disease.

Pediatric Arthritis

A bacterial joint infection in children, known as septic arthritis, is a painful condition requiring urgent care to prevent the spread of infection and the possibility of permanent damage to the joint. At the first sign of septic arthritis, NYU Langone's Pediatric staff takes quick action to fight the infection at its source.

Pediatric Surgery

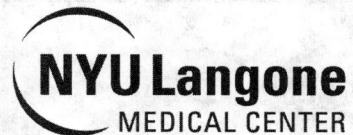

PEDIATRIC SURGERY

Pediatric Surgery is part of the Hassenfeld Pediatric Center, a full service specialty Children's Hospital, which supports the array of children's health services across the Medical Center where newborns, children, adolescents and young adults receive the most comprehensive and advanced care by a team of pediatricians and pediatric specialists.

The Division of Pediatric Surgery at NYU Langone Medical Center provides comprehensive pediatric surgical care for the smallest preterm infant to the adolescent. Our surgeons are experts at minimally invasive procedures (resulting in shorter hospitals stays and faster recoveries), as well as in conventional surgical techniques. In addition to highly-skilled surgeons and surgical nurses, we offer a wide array of Child Life Services to help children and their families become familiar with the hospital environment and lessen fears.

Surgical Expertise
NYU Langone Medical Center is renowned for its achievements in the full spectrum of pediatric surgical specialties, including abdominal and thoracic surgery, neonatal surgery, surgery for all congenital anomalies, cancer surgery, urology, cardiac surgery, neurosurgery, orthopaedics, plastic and reconstructive surgery, repair of cleft lips and palates, ophthalmology, and ENT, among others.

Pediatric Anesthesia
We are proud of our expert team of fellowship-trained pediatric anesthesiologists who serve the pediatric population. These anesthesiologists are involved in preoperative and postoperative care as well as in administering anesthesia, and they have close working relationships with our pediatric surgeons.

Child Life Services
The pediatric unit is home to The Child Life Program which is focused on creating a supportive environment for children undergoing surgery and their families through a total care approach. Child Life personnel meet with parents and their child prior to surgery and provide a continuum of care to the entire family throughout the hospital experience.

Pre-Admission Orientation and Information
Informational packets about what to expect are given to families during the pre-admission testing process. Parents and their children are also encouraged to attend an orientation session.

Facilities
Day surgery facilities include an expansive playroom with computers, games and Child Life personnel to care for the family. A separate recovery room area provides a calming environment for children during their emergence from anesthesia.

Pediatrics

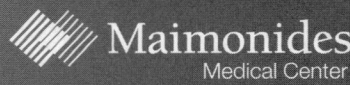
The Maimonides Infants & Children's Hospital is a NACHRI-certified children's hospital-within-a-hospital. Offering over 30 sub-specialty divisions as well as primary care, the Pediatrics program is unrivaled in the region and serves one of the largest pediatric populations in the nation.

Danielle Laraque, MD, Vice President of the Infants & Children's Hospital, leads a family-centered pediatrics program in a state-of-the-art medical environment, where babies, children and adolescents receive the best and most appropriate care. For most children, this involves preventing illness and promoting healthy growth. For those whose problems are more complicated, Maimonides specialists can treat every manner of childhood disorder, no matter how rare or complex. The level and quality of critical care provided is evidenced by the demand for the Maimonides Pediatric Transport Program, through which critically ill children from other hospitals are transferred to Maimonides.

In recognition of its excellence in obstetrics and pediatrics, Maimonides was designated a Regional Perinatal Center by the New York State Department of Health.

Pediatric specialties include:

Allergy	Infectious Disease
Behavioral & Developmental Pediatrics	Neonatology
	Nephrology
Cardiology	Neurology
Critical Care Medicine	Ophthalmology
Dentistry & Dental Surgery	Orthopedic Surgery
Emergency Medicine	Otolaryngology
Endocrinology	Psychiatry/Psychology
Gastroenterology	Pulmonology
Genetics	Rheumatology
Hematology/Oncology	Surgery
Immunology	Urology

Relying heavily on evidence-based medicine, Maimonides Medical Center has been commended for outstanding services by a number of independent rating organizations. Earlier this year, Maimonides was named a Distinguished Hospital for Clinical Excellence by Healthgrades — one of only three hospitals in the metropolitan area; the American Stroke Association bestowed its Gold Plus Achievement Award on the hospital; and the American Hospital Association once again named it a Most Wired Hospital.

Maimonides Medical Center
Passionate about medicine.
Compassionate about people.

www.maimonidesmed.org/pediatrics

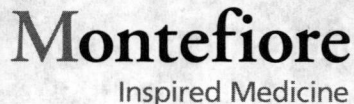

Pediatric Services

The Children's Hospital at Montefiore (CHAM) offers the full spectrum of advanced services for pediatric patients and is a recognized leader in the areas of cardiology, nephrology, oncology, orthopaedics, endocrinology, gastroenterology, neurology and surgery, among others. **CHAM is consistently recognized among the nation's top children's hospitals by *U.S. News & World Report*.**

Children with all forms of cardiac defects and anomalies benefit from the vast resources of CHAM's Pediatric Heart Center, including its state-of-the-art pediatric hybrid cardiac catheterization lab. This lab is one of the first of its kind in the area and boasts a 96 percent success rate in the area of cardiac ablation procedures. Montefiore's experienced cardiologists and cardiothoracic surgeons employ the most advanced therapies and procedures available to treat patients with both common and rare heart conditions.

CHAM's pediatric oncology program specializes in all forms of hematologic malignancies, such as leukemia and lymphoma, sarcomas and neuroblastomas, and treats more than 150 new cases each year. CHAM specialists employ the full range of advanced medical, surgical and radiation treatments, including novel surgical approaches coupled with new chemotherapy agents. **This multidisciplinary approach has helped CHAM achieve a 95 percent cure rate for leukemia.**

CHAM's transplant program is the second busiest in New York State and reports one-year patient survival rates approaching 100 percent for heart, liver and kidney. The program is one of only a few in the nation offering comprehensive intestinal rehabilitation, including intestinal transplantation.

Orthopaedic surgeons at CHAM are highly respected for their ability to expertly treat patients with a wide range of musculoskeletal conditions, including scoliosis, hip dysplasia and developmental extremity malformations as well as bone and soft-tissue tumors. Additionally, CHAM boasts a 95 percent survival rate for babies treated in its NICU and is home to exceptional general, head and neck, plastic and neurosurgery programs.

All of the Hospital's programs are supported by superior family- and patient-centered services. CHAM consistently ranks in the 90th percentile or above on national patient satisfaction surveys, leading its peers in delivering an exceptional experience to children and their families.

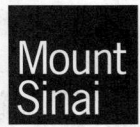 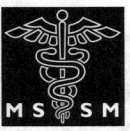

**MOUNT SINAI
SCHOOL OF
MEDICINE**

**THE KRAVIS CHILDREN'S HOSPITAL
AT THE MOUNT SINAI MEDICAL CENTER**
One Gustave L. Levy Place
Fifth Avenue and 100th Street
New York, NY 10029-6574
Physician Referral: 1-800-MD-SINAI (637-4624)
www.mountsinai.org/kravis

THE KRAVIS CHILDREN'S HOSPITAL AT THE MOUNT SINAI MEDICAL CENTER

At the Kravis Children's Hospital at The Mount Sinai Medical Center, we offer the most advanced treatments and technologies available, supported by groundbreaking research, because the health and care of your child is our first priority.

This year the Kravis Children's Hospital saw significant gains in the *U.S. News & World Report* pediatric rankings, which **placed it among the country's best children's hospitals in six of the ten pediatric specialties**, as noted in the 2012-13 edition of the annual "Best Children's Hospitals" report. The six specialties are: gastroenterology (ranked #21 nationally), diabetes and endocrinology (#23), urology (#23), nephrology (#29), cancer (#32), and pulmonology (#34).

The rankings reflect not only double-digit gains within specialties, but also **first-time rankings in two new areas – cancer and urology –** placing these specialties among the best pediatric programs in the United States.

In all of our services, including 31 subspecialty areas of care, we offer advanced treatments, supported by research, community outreach, and advocacy programs. Our ongoing efforts to recruit the finest physicians and scientists have resulted in our ability to provide fundamental insights into the causes of childhood diseases and to deliver breakthrough treatments.

We will soon be opening a new Pediatric Intensive Care Unit (PICU), a 15-bed unit that will wed state-of-the-art medical technology with a family-friendly facility for our most critically ill children. Upon completion of the PICU in the fall of 2012, construction will immediately begin on a new 46-bed Neonatal Intensive Care Unit (NICU).

THE ZONE SPACE AT KRAVIS

An especially unique feature of the Kravis Children's Hospital at Mount Sinai is the Zone - a 3,000 square foot state-of-the-art therapeutic and educational play environment for pediatric patients and their families. **The Zone space at Kravis is the only one of its kind in the northeast region of the United States.**

The area is staffed by the Child Life and Creative Arts Therapy Department, a full-time pediatric medical librarian, and numerous consultants and volunteers who share their talents in art, music, cooking, knitting and more. The facility includes a lounge, theatre, family resource center, teen area, full kitchen and performing space. **The Zone features KidsZone TV (KZTV), the first live, interactive broadcast studio in a children's hospital.** The space is also used as a pediatric television programming training site for hospitals across the country and abroad.

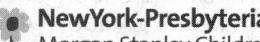

NewYork-Presbyterian

The University Hospital of Columbia and Cornell

Affiliated with Columbia University College of Physicians and Surgeons and Weill Cornell Medical College

NewYork-Presbyterian
Morgan Stanley Children's Hospital
Columbia University Medical Center
3959 Broadway
New York, NY 10032

NewYork-Presbyterian
Phyllis and David Komansky
Center for Children's Health
Weill Cornell Medical Center
525 East 68th Street
New York, NY 10065

1-800-245-KIDS (1-800-245-5437)   www.childrensnyp.org

Accreditation: The Joint Commission

Overview

The pediatric services of NewYork-Presbyterian Hospital are comprised of NewYork-Presbyterian Morgan Stanley Children's Hospital, which is affiliated with Columbia University College of Physicians and Surgeons, and the NewYork-Presbyterian Phyllis and David Komansky Center for Children's Health, which is affiliated with Weill Cornell Medical College. Together, they serve as one of the nation's premier centers for comprehensive pediatric care. Skilled and experienced physicians, surgeons, nurses and other pediatric healthcare professionals manage some of the most complex medical conditions of children at every stage of development. Their expertise includes general pediatric care and the full range of medical and surgical subspecialties:

- Adolescent Medicine
- Allergy and Immunology
- Anesthesiology
- Blood Disorders
- Blood and Marrow Transplantation
- Cancer
- Cardiology and Cardiac Surgery
- Craniofacial and Plastic Surgery
- Critical Care
- Dermatology
- Digestive Disease
- Ear, Nose and Throat
- Emergency Department, including specialized units for burns and trauma injuries
- Endocrinology, Diabetes and Metabolism
- Epilepsy
- Genetics
- Infectious Diseases

- Kidney Disease
- Liver Disease
- Lung Disease
- Maternal Fetal Medicine (high-risk pregnancy)
- Neonatal Medicine
- Neurology and Neurological Surgery
- Nutrition
- Obesity and Bariatric Surgery
- Ophthalmology
- Oral and Maxillofacial Surgery and Pediatric Dentistry
- Organ Transplantation
- Orthopaedic Surgery
- Pain Medicine
- Pediatric Surgery
- Pregnancy and Newborn Services
- Primary Care/General Pediatrics
- Psychiatry
- Radiology
- Rheumatology
- Urology

Highlights at a Glance:

- A national leader in pediatric heart surgery with one of the largest heart transplant programs in the nation.
- A pediatric kidney and liver transplant program, which includes a Living Donor Program and leading edge therapies to help reduce the side effects of anti-rejection drugs.
- Pediatric cardiac surgeons at the forefront of ventricular assist devices for infants and small children as a bridge to recovery or transplantation.
- One of three Level 1-designated Regional Pediatric Trauma Centers in New York State and the only one in New York City.
- Maternal-Fetal Medicine Divison designated a Regional Perinatal Center, the highest hospital classification, able to care for the most complex, highest-risk cases.
- One of the largest Type 1 diabetes programs in New York State.
- Outstanding neonatal intensive care programs setting standards of care nationwide for extremely ill newborns.
- The only program in the New York tri-state area that has active programs in both liver and small bowel transplantation.

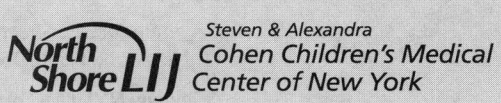 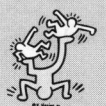
Cohen Children's Medical Center

Steven and Alexandra Cohen Children's Medical Center of New York is the largest provider of pediatric health services in New York State, serving 1.8 million children in Brooklyn, Queens, Nassau and Suffolk counties.

Cohen Children's Medical Center, located on Long Island, is a full-service acute, medical, surgical, dental and psychiatric facility dedicated to providing the highest levels of care to children, from newborns to adolescents. Our expert pediatric specialists screen, diagnose, and treat a wide variety of injuries and illnesses in our 164-bed hospital.

Cohen Children's is ranked by *U.S. News and World Report* as one of the nation's top 50 children's hospitals in cancer care, diabetes/endocrinology, neonatology, neurology/neurosurgery, nephrology, pulmonary and urology. In addition, we're the only hospital on Long Island to offer pediatric open heart surgery and bone marrow transplantation, along with a dedicated Pediatric Trauma Center.

Child-Friendly and Family-Centered Care

Cohen Children's is designed exclusively for children and their families. Caring for children includes providing them with a warm, comforting, homelike setting. That's why every aspect of our spacious open building is child oriented — from the fold-out beds for parents to the fully staffed playrooms on each floor. Our caregivers are dedicated to providing the most skilled and sensitive treatment for all your child's healthcare needs. Our goal is to help children feel comfortable, safe and stress-free.

At Cohen Children's, family-centered care is an essential part of each child's experience. Our family-centered approach to healthcare involves patients, families and healthcare professionals forming a partnership that benefits everyone.

A Growing Network of Care

State-of-the-art care for children's medical, surgical, psychiatric and dental needs are provided in both inpatient and outpatient settings. Outpatient services are available at our main campus in New Hyde Park and at regional consultation centers in Commack, Hewlett, Bensonhurst, Williamsburg and Flushing.

Our Services Include:

- Adolescent Medicine
- Allergy/Immunology
- Asthma
- Cardiology
- Children's Cancer Center
- Children's Heart Center
- Craniofacial and Cleft Palate
- Critical Care
- Cystic Fibrosis
- Developmental/Behavioral Pediatrics
- Emergency Medicine
- Endocrinology/Diabetes
- Epilepsy
- Gastroenterology
- Infectious Diseases
- Neonatology
- Nephrology (Kidney Disease)
- Neurology
- Nutritional Disorders
- Ophthalmology
- Orthopaedics
- Otolaryngology (ENT)
- Pediatric/Adolescent Gynecology
- Pediatric Dental Services
- Pulmonology (Lung Disease)
- Rheumatology
- Sleep Study Center
- Trauma
- Urgent Care
- Urology

To find a doctor: **1-888-321-DOCS** or visit **www.northshorelij.com**

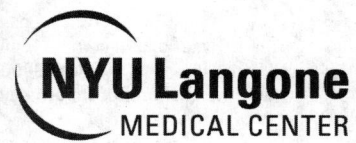

HASSENFELD PEDIATRIC CENTER

The new Hassenfeld Pediatric Center (HPC) is a full-service specialty children's hospital that works as a cohesive team across all children's health services at NYU Langone Medical Center. At HPC, newborns, children, adolescents and young adults receive the most comprehensive and advanced care possible from a team of pediatricians and pediatric specialists across more than 30 medical and surgical disciplines. With more than 150 full-time pediatric specialists, as well as pediatric nurses, child life specialists and social workers, the Hassenfeld Pediatric Center is uniquely equipped to provide innovative pediatric subspecialty care in a highly personalized manner.

About Children's Services at NYU Langone

NYU Langone Medical Center is nationally recognized in many pediatric specialty fields, including craniofacial anomalies, cardiac surgery, orthopaedic surgery, rehabilitation medicine, brain tumors, leukemia, sarcoma, and epilepsy. Our specialists work collaboratively to optimize care for each child, from the operating room and pediatric intensive care unit to the Emergency Department and pediatric inpatient unit.

A Family-Centered Approach

Integral to the care we provide is a myriad of support services for children and their families. We recognize that the best outcomes are achieved when the child's family is actively involved in every step of care. For that reason, our trained specialists address the needs of not just the patient, but of parents and siblings through ongoing education and communication.

The Future Shape of Pediatric Care at HPC

In 2017, a 160,000 square foot pediatric hospital, on the Medical Center's main campus, will become the inpatient centerpiece of the Hassenfeld Pediatric Center. This state-of-the-art facility will enhance the Center's ability to deliver world-class care through all private rooms, a feature that increases patient safety by decreasing exposure to infections, while providing a private, supportive environment for the patients and their families. HPC will be the only pediatric inpatient facility in Manhattan with this amenity, which will also include a "family zone" offering a sleep-in couch, storage, and Web access for each room.

The new pediatric hospital will also include a child-friendly pre-operative unit along with recovery bays where parents can be by the child's bedside during post-operation. Rounding out the new hospital will be a Family Center for orientation activities geared to patients, space for child-life activities and performances, as well as support, education and respite services for families.

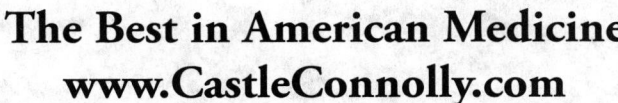

The Best in American Medicine
www.CastleConnolly.com

Physical Medicine & Rehabilitation

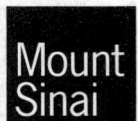
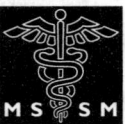

MOUNT SINAI SCHOOL OF MEDICINE

THE MOUNT SINAI MEDICAL CENTER
REHABILITATION MEDICINE

One Gustave L. Levy Place
Fifth Avenue and 100th Street
New York, NY 10029-6574
Faculty Practice: 212-241-6321
Inpatient Admitting: 212-241-541
www.mountsinai.org/rehab

THE DEPARTMENT OF REHABILITATION MEDICINE at Mount Sinai is a Center of Excellence in the delivery of complete care for people with disabilities. A wide range of comprehensive patient care services is available for individuals with spinal cord injuries, brain injuries, and a variety of neuromuscular, musculoskeletal, and chronic conditions. We are accredited by the Commission on Accreditation of Rehabilitation Facilities (CARF) for our inpatient spinal cord injury, amputation and brain injury programs—the only such accredited programs at non-VA hospitals in New York City—as well as for our comprehensive rehabilitation medicine program. Our Amputation Specialty Program was the first such CARF-accredited program in New York State.

Pivotal to successful rehabilitation, the multidisciplinary team approach at Mount Sinai takes advantage of all areas of expertise to provide the highest quality of coordinated care. Our experienced professionals evaluate each patient and meet regularly to develop and implement individualized treatment plans in partnership with patients and their families. Our goal is to make each individual with a disability maximally self-sufficient and mobile, and able to return to community life.

The Mount Sinai Rehabilitation Center team is led by Kristjan T. Ragnarsson, MD, whose leadership and innovative approach to patient care has had a major impact in the field of rehabilitation medicine. The Center includes physicians, primary rehabilitation nurses, nurse practitioners, and professional staff in physical therapy, occupational therapy, speech therapy, nutrition, social work, psychology, therapeutic recreation, and vocational counseling. Special rehabilitation medicine programs include the following:

MODEL SYSTEMS OF CARE

The Department of Rehabilitation Medicine provides comprehensive services that serve as national models of care.

- Consistently ranked among the top rehabilitation centers by *U.S. News & World Report*, currently # 12.

- One of 16 programs designated by NIDRR as a Model System of Care for Traumatic Brain Injury, the only such designated program in New York State.

- The first CDC Injury Control Research Center focusing on traumatic brain injury research.

- **The Spinal Cord Injury Rehabilitation Program** provides comprehensive care to individuals with spinal cord injuries. This includes a full range of innovative medical and rehabilitation services. For example, our "Do It" program is a unique outpatient program that facilitates community integration.

- **The Brain Injury Rehabilitation Program** provides comprehensive care to individuals with brain injuries. It is well recognized that the treatment of individuals with cognitive and behavioral challenges is critical to community integration. Our program contains specialists uniquely qualified to meet these challenges.

- **The Interventional Spine and Sports Medicine Program** provides the highest quality, evidence-based care for spine and musculoskeletal disorders. Our physiatrists combine a thorough examination with the latest high-tech diagnostic procedures to precisely identify and treat each patient. Our treatment options include physical and occupational therapy, medications, bracing, as well as ultrasound and fluoroscopic guided injections.

- **The Amputation Specialty Program** is designed to anticipate and meet the needs of persons with limb loss, as well as to prevent secondary complications and further amputations. Our interdisciplinary team works closely with other departments throughout the Medical Center to provide an integrated approach to our patients' healthcare.

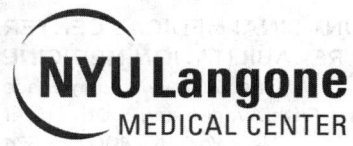

Rusk Rehabilitation
400 East 34th Street *(between 1st Avenue and FDR Drive)*
New York, NY 10016
HJD: 301 East 17th Street *(at 2nd Avenue)*
New York, NY 10003
www.NYULMC.org/RUSK
Children's Services Access Line: **855-NYU-KIDS**

PEDIATRIC REHABILITATION MEDICINE

Pediatric Rehabilitation is part of the Hassenfeld Pediatric Center, a full service special-ty Children's Hospital, which supports the array of children's health services across the Medical Center where newborns, children, adolescents and young adults receive the most comprehensive and advanced care by a team of pediatricians and pediatric specialists.

About the Pediatric Rehabilitation Program
The Pediatric Rehabilitation Medicine Division is a key component Rusk Rehabilitation at NYU Langone (Rusk), providing world-class inpatient and outpatient rehabilitation ser-vices for children, from birth through early adulthood. Rusk has been ranked the best rehabilitation hospital in New York and among the top ten in the country by *U.S. News & World Report* for 23 consecutive years. At Rusk, the focus is on early intervention and a family-centered approach that includes sibling and family support groups and counseling.

Areas of Expertise
The pediatric rehabilitation team is particularly skilled in treating the multiple challenges of children with developmental disorders such as cerebral palsy, spina bifida, muscu-lar dystrophy, reflex sympathetic dystrophy, limb deficiencies, arthrogryposis, and spinal cord injuries. Children with traumatic brain injuries, brain tumors, and oncologic diagno-ses (such as bone tumors or musculoskeletal disease) also benefit from our specialized services, as do youngsters affected by stroke or cerebrovascular accidents, viral infec-tions or inflammatory diseases, and rheumatic disease.

Spanning the Continuum of Care
In addition to inpatient services, we offer extensive outpatient programs for young pa-tients, including physical therapy, occupational therapy, speech therapy, feeding and swallowing, vocational services, psychological services, and other specialized therapies.

Rusk's pediatric services are delivered at Rusk's 34th Street location as well as at the world-renowned Hospital for Joint Diseases. Moreover, specialized rehabilitation care for premature infants is provided by the Medical Center's neonatal intensive care unit.

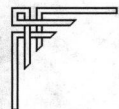

The Best in American Medicine
www.CastleConnolly.com

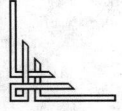
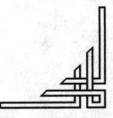

Plastic Surgery

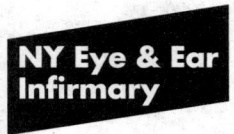

NY Eye & Ear Infirmary

Continuum Health Partners, Inc.

THE NEW YORK EYE AND EAR INFIRMARY

310 East 14th Street
New York, New York 10003
Tel. 212.979.4000   Fax. 212.228.0664
http://www.nyee.edu

PROVIDING EXCEPTIONAL CARE

The Department of Plastic & Reconstructive Surgery is one of the region's most comprehensive centers for surgery which restores the body and spirit. More than 1,500 procedures a year are performed here, and 50 of the most noted board-certified plastic surgeons located throughout New York City and tri-state area comprise the attending medical staff.

IN A HIGHLY SPECIALIZED SETTING

As a specialty hospital, the Infirmary is uniquely qualified to handle the most complicated cases. It serves as a nationwide referral center with a commitment to teaching, research, and high-technology based patient care. Highly experienced staff using state-of-the-art instrumentation have made the Infirmary's 17 operating rooms a national benchmark in efficiency. In addition, private premium patient accommodations are available to assure that the hospital experience is as comfortable and convenient as possible.

FOR PATIENTS OF ALL AGES

The Department treats more than 1,500 patients a year who seek reconstructive surgery of the body as well as facial area as a result of accident, birth defect or cancer, and those who elect cosmetic surgery. It is one of the few hospitals in the region to perform breast reconstruction after mastectomy with microvascular surgery to harvest tissue from patients' lower body to create living, natural, and normal looking breasts, often preferred to artificial implants. State-of-the-art lymph node transfer to cure post-mastectomy lymphedema is also available.

Childhood problems, such as cleft lip and palate and ear deformities also fall under the care of our surgeons.

Innovative cosmetic surgery procedures such as endoscopic and other minimally invasive operations are offered. The Center for Nasal Plastic specializes in closed (no scar) nasal plastic techniques as well as repair of previous nasal surgeries, the secondary nasal plasty. Liposuction using the latest instrumentation and fat grafting by the latest technology is also available as are the latest variants of the abdominoplasty (tummy tuck) operation.

The latest version of a skin tightening Fraxel Re:pair laser enables many patients to avoid a surgical face and eyelid plastic operation.

The hospital has a Post Graduate Cosmetic Surgery Program which offers a year of intensive cosmetic surgery training to surgeons who have completed a formal plastic surgery residency. The program is the largest and most sought-after in the US and also provides a source for affordable cosmetic surgery for the community.

Plastic Surgery Clinical Services

Facial plasty

Eyelid plastic operations

Nasal plastic operations

Breast augmentation
Breast reduction procedures
and suspension

Breast reconstruction using
patient's own tissue
(DIEP, S-GAP, I-GAP and
SIEA flap procedures)

Liposuction

Abdominoplasty

Facial resurfacing and
dermabrasion

Fraxel laser

Botox

About The New York Eye and Ear Infirmary

Founded in 1820, it is the nation's oldest, continuously operating specialty hospital. Throughout its history, the Infirmary has led clinical advances and research in vision, hearing, speech and restoration of the physical appearance.

**Physician Referral
1.800.449.HOPE (4673)**

Psychiatry

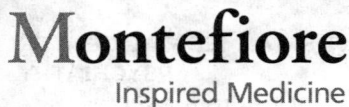

Montefiore
Inspired Medicine

111 East 210th Street
Bronx, New York 10467
1-800-MD-MONTE
www.montefiore.org/psychiatry

Psychiatry and Behavioral Sciences at Montefiore

The Department of Psychiatry and Behavioral Sciences at Montefiore Medical Center, which was recognized as high performing in *U.S. News & World Report*'s 2012–13 "America's Best Hospitals," is among the most established and respected in the country. It specializes in providing quality, compassionate care for patients with complicated medical and neuropsychiatric presentations.

One of the Department's most valuable resources is **its esteemed team of psychiatrists, many of whom have been named "Best Doctors" by *New York* magazine.** These physicians draw upon the latest medical advances to treat the full spectrum of mental health conditions in adults and children, including anxiety and depression, alcohol and substance dependency, autism, obsessive-compulsive disorder, bipolar disorder and schizophrenia. Supporting their efforts is the Department's 22-bed neuropsychiatric unit at the Moses Campus—which offers an intimate setting where patients receive individualized care—and a 33-bed adult unit at the Wakefield Campus.

The Department is home to one of the first child behavioral consultation teams in the nation and has led the way in the creation of both a residency and a fellowship program in child/adolescent psychosomatic medicine. Its child psychiatrists collaborate with experts at The Children's Hospital at Montefiore to treat pediatric patients with such conditions as autism, autism spectrum disorders and obsessive-compulsive disorder. The Department's Dialectical Behavior Therapy (DBT) Program serves as a model for other mental health programs in the United States and addresses the critical needs of at-risk adolescents suffering from anxiety, depression or suicidal tendencies.

Other services offered by the Department include cognitive behavior therapy and family therapy. It is one of only a few in the region to also provide electroconvulsive therapy.

Through its 10-bed medically managed detoxification unit at Montefiore's Wakefield Campus and New Directions Recovery Center, the Department helps individuals maintain a drug-free lifestyle. The Department's Caregiver Support Center meets the emotional needs of individuals who care for a friend or loved one on an ongoing basis. Additionally, construction is currently under way on a new building to accommodate the Department's expanded substance abuse treatment program.

Research is the focus of the Autism and Obsessive-Compulsive Spectrum Program. A collaboration between the Department and Albert Einstein College of Medicine, this program seeks to bridge and translate basic neuroscience discoveries into innovative experimental therapeutics and new clinical treatments. Other research efforts focus on developing more-targeted treatments for disorders such as anxiety and depression.

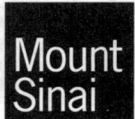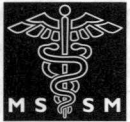

MOUNT SINAI
SCHOOL OF
MEDICINE

THE MOUNT SINAI MEDICAL CENTER PSYCHIATRY

One Gustave L. Levy Place
Fifth Avenue and 100th Street
New York, NY 10029-6574
Physician Referral: 1-800-MD-SINAI (637-4624)
www.mountsinai.org/psychiatry
www.mssm.edu/psychiatry

THE DEPARTMENT OF PSYCHIATRY at Mount Sinai strives to bring breakthrough discoveries from neuroscience research to clinical care today. We provide services for children, adolescents, adults, and seniors, offering mental health evaluation and treatment for autism, attention-deficit hyperactivity disorder (ADHD), behavioral disorders, schizophrenia, Alzheimer's disease, mood and anxiety disorders, obsessive-compulsive disorder (OCD), tics and Tourette's Disorder (TD), substance abuse, post-traumatic stress disorder (PTSD), eating disorders, and personality disorders.

Clinical Services – The Department of Psychiatry is organized around key Centers of Excellence that link academic thought leaders to clinicians throughout the department. We offer a full range of diagnostic and treatment services, including psychotherapy, psychopharmacology, emergency services, electroconvulsive therapy, neuropsychological testing, and management of difficult clinical cases. We also provide mental health services in the Mount Sinai's World Trade Center Medical Monitoring and Treatment Program.

Specialty Programs – The Seaver Autism Center of Excellence offers a comprehensive assessment and treatment program that provides the finest patient care informed by the latest research. Our expert clinical staff is experienced in autism spectrum disorders, specializing in personalized and evidence-based treatment for very young children and high-functioning adults, as well as those individuals considered most difficult to assess and treat. The ADHD Center serves children and adults providing state-of-the-art psychiatric evaluation, psychological testing, behavioral and cognitive-behavioral treatments, and medication management. Our Center for Eating and Weight Disorders serves adults and children, offering innovative and evidence-based treatment for anorexia nervosa, bulimia nervosa, binge eating disorder, and obesity.

The Mood and Anxiety Disorders Program (MAP) is devoted to understanding the causes of mood and anxiety disorders and aims to advance the latest integrative treatment strategies for patients who suffer from major depression, bipolar disorder, PTSD, panic attacks, generalized anxiety disorder, and social phobia. MAP at Mount Sinai uses state-of-the-art brain imaging, and genetic, and clinical trials methods to enhance our understanding of brain processes associated with these disorders.

TRANSLATING KNOWLEDGE INTO NEW SOLUTIONS
Mount Sinai is at the forefront of unlocking the interactions between biological processes and the myriad states of the human mind. Among our major research programs in psychiatry are the Alzheimer's Disease Research Center, which conducts both basic science and clinical research, and The Seaver Autism Center for Research and Treatment, which is dedicated to unraveling the biological causes of this disorder and to developing innovative treatment strategies. In shedding important new light on mental illness, psychiatrists at Mount Sinai are frequently able to offer experimental interventions for treatment-resistant cases of depression, OCD, and other disorders.

The OCD Center of Excellence provides state-of-the-art diagnostic evaluation and specializes in treating severe or treatment-resistant OCD. The Center offers comprehensive evaluations, expert consultations, outpatient services, novel and evidence-based treatments, and research studies. We specialize in biological interventions for patients who have not responded to conventional therapies. In addition, the **Tics and TD Clinical and Research Program** is dedicated to enhancing the understanding, evaluation, and treatment of children, adolescents, and adults with tics, TD, and related problems such as OCD and ADHD.

The Best in American Medicine
www.CastleConnolly.com

Pulmonary Disease

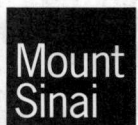
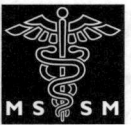

MOUNT SINAI
SCHOOL OF
MEDICINE

THE MOUNT SINAI MEDICAL CENTER
PULMONARY MEDICINE
One Gustave L. Levy Place
Fifth Avenue and 100th Street
New York, NY 10029-6574
Physician Referral: 1-800-MD-SINAI (637-4624)
www.mountsinai.org/pulmonary

The mission of Mount Sinai's **DIVISION OF PULMONARY, CRITICAL CARE, AND SLEEP MEDICINE** is to offer state-of-the-art clinical care to patients with all forms of lung disease and critical illness, cutting-edge research that will translate into improved patient care and outcomes, and hands-on training of future leaders in the field.

To achieve this goal, every faculty member is charged with the success of a specific program. Mount Sinai's Pulmonary Division has a long history of providing specialized care and key research in several disease areas that include sarcoidosis and occupational lung diseases. Mount Sinai's Sarcoidosis Service, the largest of its kind in the world, is a Center of Excellence for sarcoidosis research. It is the only site in the United States that performs the diagnostic Kveim- Siltzbach skin test for sarcoidosis, which eliminates the need for more invasive, uncomfortable, and expensive procedures. Through its Pulmonary Physiology Laboratory, Mount Sinai has been instrumental in establishing normal values for various pulmonary function tests and is currently conducting clinical studies of new tests for obesity, sarcoidosis, asthma, and lung cancer.

Pulmonary specialists at Mount Sinai are investigating asthma and emphysema, lung cancer, collagen vascular diseases, pulmonary infections, and occupational lung diseases. Mount Sinai has the largest screening program for workers and anyone in the general population exposed to polluted air at the World Trade Center catastrophe site. Our critical care physicians are experts in treating liver disease and acute and chronic respiratory failure, using the most modern forms of delivery of intensive care and providing compassionate end-of-life care.

The Asthma Program uses a multidisciplinary team approach, focusing on patient education and skill-building to foster self-management.

The Chronic Obstructive Pulmonary Disease Program offers a screening and a coordinated approach of exercise, treatment, and education that improves symptoms and quality of life, for one of the nation's most underdiagnosed conditions.

The Critical Care Medicine Program features state-of-the-art medical intensive care and respiratory care units.

The Interventional Pulmonary Service performs cutting-edge diagnostic and therapeutic procedures for patients with advanced pulmonary diseases.

The Lung Cancer/Thoracic Oncology Service provides specialized care for lung cancer diagnosis and staging and for coordinating multidisciplinary medical care for lung cancer.

The Occupational Lung Disorders Program specializes in the diagnosis and management of occupational lung disorders, such as occupational asthma and bronchitis, asbestosis, silicosis, and heavy metal lung injury.

The Pulmonary Fibrosis/Interstitial Lung Disease Program treats patients with chronic inflammatory and scarring disorders of the lungs, including idiopathic pulmonary fibrosis and collagen vascular-associated pulmonary diseases.

The Pulmonary Physiology Laboratory, performs the full range of physiological lung function and cardiopulmonary exercise testing for lung disease.

The Pulmonary Rehabilitation Program provides occupational, physical, and cardiopulmonary rehabilitation programs for patients with disabling lung disorders, as well as pre- and post-operative consultation and therapy.

The Thoracic Oncology Service provides multidisciplinary medical care for lung cancer, as a joint effort with the Department of Cardiothoracic Surgery.

The Sarcoidosis Service, which has passed its 20,000 enrollee count, offers standard care as well as the opportunity to participate in new clinical trials to 60 new enrollees per week.

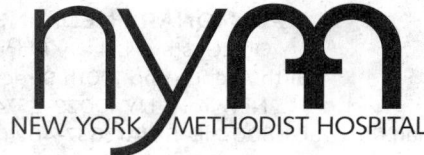

THE INSTITUTE FOR ASTHMA AND OTHER LUNG DISEASES

New York Methodist Hospital
506 Sixth Street, Brooklyn, N.Y. 11215
Phone: 866 ASK-LUNG (866 275-5864)
http://www.nym.org

SPECIALISTS AND MEDICAL SERVICES

The Institute for Asthma and Other Lung Diseases brings together a unique group of specialists and medical services to offer comprehensive diagnosis and treatment of a broad range of lung conditions. The Institute's panel of physician specialists includes both pediatric and adult pulmonologists and allergists. A larger constellation of physicians—medical oncologists, radiologists, radiation oncologists and surgeons—is available as needed. For diagnostic purposes, state-of-the-art specialty facilities— including the interventional bronchoscopy suite, the pulmonary function laboratory, the Pulmonary Hypertension Center and the Sleep Disorders Center— are conveniently located on the Hospital campus. These facilities are used to diagnose and treat a variety of lung disorders and are staffed by registered respiratory therapists, board-certified pulmonary function technologists and exercise physiologists.

PROGRAMS OFFERED

In addition to the treatment of pediatric and adult asthma, physicians affiliated with the Institute diagnose and care for patients with chronic obstructive lung disease (COPD), interstitial lung disease, infectious lung disease, pulmonary hypertension and lung cancer. Highly sophisticated interventional pulmonary services and advanced thoracic surgery procedures are performed at the Hospital, which is a Center of Excellence Epicenter for Robotic Thoracic Surgery.

* * *

Referrals to the Institute, its programs and physicians can be made through an individual's primary care physician or requested directly through the Institute's telephone referral service. More information (and on-line physician referral) is available at the Hospital's website, http://www.nym.org.

COMPREHENSIVE LUNG CANCER CENTER

New York Methodist Hospital's Comprehensive Lung Cancer Center coordinates and consolidates all services related to the treatment of lung cancer. One of the advantages NYM offers patients is a range of minimally invasive screening, diagnostic and treatment techniques that offer a high degree of accuracy while reducing patient discomfort.

Treatment options include surgery (both robotic and traditional), radiation and medical oncology, but even patients who are not eligible for surgery, radiation or chemotherapy may benefit from specialized interventional pulmonology treatments.

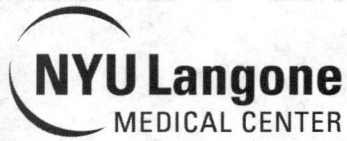
PULMONOLOGY

About the Division of Pulmonary, Critical Care and Sleep Medicine

NYU Langone's Pulmonary, Critical Care and Sleep Medicine Division offers a full range of services for the diagnosis and treatment of inpatient and ambulatory patients. Services include pulmonary function laboratories; specialized medical critical care units at Tisch Hospital and the Hospital for Joint Diseases; and a multidisciplinary interventional bronchoscopy program integrated with thoracic radiology at Tisch Hospital. Research grant support includes the National Institutes of Health and the Centers for Disease Control and Prevention. We specialize in the following areas:

Asthma

The Division of Pulmonary Medicine is experienced in treating all aspects of asthma and airway disorders. The Bellevue Asthma Clinic at Bellevue Hospital Center, an affiliate of NYU Langone Medical Center, offers an active research program dealing exclusively with particulate matter pollution and asthma.

Pulmonary Services

The Division of Pulmonary Medicine provides clinical chest services at Tisch Hospital which care for patients with tuberculosis, lung cancer, asthma and interstitial fibrosis. Hospital consultation services are available for interstitial lung diseases, sarcoidosis, pulmonary hypertension, COPD, lung cancer, occupational lung diseases, bronchiectasis, and myobacterial other than TB.

Interventional Bronchoscopy

The Interventional Bronchoscopy Program at Tisch Hospital employs leading-edge techniques to diagnose and treat tumors and inflammatory conditions of the lung.

Lung Cancer Screening Program

Individuals at high risk for lung cancer may schedule a CT-scan as part of our lung cancer screening program. Eligible patients are also choose to contribute to our research efforts by participating in our lung cancer biomarker screening study.

Sleep Disorders

The Sleep Disorders Center at NYU Langone Medical Center offers clinical and research services for physicians and patients in the diagnosis and treatment of severe or prolonged sleeping difficulties. The Center is also equipped for limited home or in-hospital patient monitoring.

Radiation Oncology

Maimonides Medical Center
MAIMONIDES CANCER CENTER
6300 Eighth Avenue • Brooklyn, New York 11220
Phone: 718.765.2500 • Fax: 718.765.2574
www.maimonidesmed.org/cancer

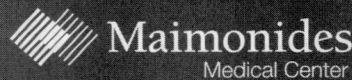
Maimonides
Medical Center

The Maimonides Cancer Center offers a fully integrated, multimodal approach to cancer care that includes prevention, education, screening, diagnostics, treatment, palliative care and clinical research. The Lena Cymbrowitz Pavilion contains the following specialty divisions:

Radiation Oncology: equipped with state-of-the art imaging and treatment delivery technologies; offers patients the most precise treatments available, yet does so in an airy, life-affirming environment.

Medical Oncology: provides comprehensive diagnosis, oral drug therapies, intravenous chemotherapy infusions, and biological and hormonal therapies.

Pediatric Oncology: treats children with cancer and diseases of the blood in a child-friendly environment, and features special areas set aside for parent conferences.

Surgical Oncology: provides a convenient location for minor surgical procedures, as well as innovative surgical techniques such as sentinel node mapping and biopsy, skin/tissue-sparing mastectomy, and nerve-sparing prostatectomy.

Research Center: conducts basic science and genetic research, as well as clinical trials that offer appropriately screened patients, who wish to volunteer, new therapies and medications.

Resource Center: offers access to integrative (complementary) oncology services, dietary advice, as well as psychological and social services.

Located around the block from the Lena Cymbrowitz Pavilion, the newly opened Rivera Pavilion houses the **Maimonides Breast Cancer Center**. With a spa-like decor and life-affirming environment, the Center provides digital mammography, sonography, computerized interpretation, digital stereotactic biopsies, breast-specific gamma imaging, and treatment plans tailored to each patient. A genetics counselor is also on-site.

Clinicians at the Maimonides Cancer Center — Brooklyn's only dedicated cancer center — are talented specialists, recruited specifically for their expertise. Our doctors emphasize multimodal care, which means that multiple methods of treatment are available to patients, sometimes simultaneously. Every week, physicians from radiology, surgery, pathology, radiation oncology, and medical oncology meet to discuss patient treatment at our case management meetings. The patient's needs, as well as the disease, are considered from many angles.

Maimonides Medical Center
Passionate about medicine.
Compassionate about people.
www.maimonidesmed.org/cancer

Rehabilitation Medicine

THE CENTER FOR MUSCULOSKELETAL CARE

The new Center for Musculoskeletal Care (CMC) is the largest, free-standing musculoskeletal center of its kind in the country to bring clinical care, wellness programs, and access to clinical trials together at a single point of service. CMC combines state-of-the-art therapeutic and medical technology with the expertise of NYU Langone physicians, ranked among the country's top 10 in orthopaedics, rheumatology and rehabilitation by *U.S. News & World Report.*

CMC provides the full spectrum of outpatient bone and joint care for a wide range of conditions. The multidisciplinary team approach allows musculoskeletal experts to collaborate across centers and disciplines to provide the most comprehensive and seamless patient care.

Joint Replacement Center/Adult Reconstructive physicians evaluate degenerative conditions of the hip and knee caused by arthritis, injuries, congenital problems and general wear-and-tear to determine the best course of treatment.

Sports Medicine and primary care sports medicine physicians treat sports-related injuries or conditions of the knee, shoulder, elbow and ankle, using joint preservation techniques as well as surgical procedures.

The Spine Center provides conservative orthopaedic care for a broad range of spinal disorders, including problems associated with failed previous surgery, idiopathic disorders, growth disorders, neuromuscular disease, degenerative and congenital conditions, and traumatic deformity.

Rheumatology physicians care for arthritis or autoimmune conditions such as rheumatoid arthritis, osteoarthritis, psoriatic arthritis, lupus, osteoporosis, and Behçet's Syndrome.

The Infusion Center offers biologic agents and medications via infusion therapy, in a comfortable, private environment.

Rehabilitation Services, provided by the world-renowned Rusk Rehabilitation, include rehabilitation medicine (physiatry), physical therapy, occupational therapy, and hand therapy.

The Center for the Study and Treatment of Pain is an American Pain Society-designated Center of Excellence, where specialists partner with a patient's physician to manage pain associated with bone and joint conditions.

The Center for Diagnostic Imaging provides cutting-edge, on-site radiology services to facilitate quick and convenient diagnosis as well as interventional radiology procedures, and is recognized as one of the strongest musculoskeletal radiology departments in the world.

Sports Performance Center specialists assist active individuals in reaching their full potential through a state-of-the-art health and fitness evaluation and personalized athletic training plan.

Biomedical Research is woven into clinical care at CMC, offering patients access to cutting edge musculoskeletal therapies, techniques and devices.

The Outpatient Surgery Center is part of the CMC and offers same-day surgery in a unique, state-of-the art facility for minimally-invasive orthopaedic surgical procedures.

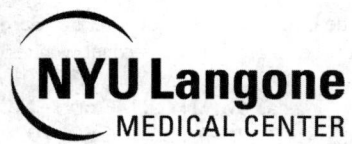

Rusk Rehabilitation
550 First Avenue *(at 31st Street)*
New York, NY 10016
www.NYULMC.org/RUSK
Physician Referral: **888-7-NYU-MED** (888-769-8633)

RUSK INSTITUTE OF REHABILITATION MEDICINE

Rusk Rehabilitation at NYU Langone Medical Center (Rusk) has been ranked the best rehabilitation hospital in New York and among the top ten in the country by *U.S. News & World Report* for 23 consecutive years. Rusk is internationally renowned for the treatment of adults and children with disabilities, providing the full continuum of inpatient and outpatient rehabilitation care at multiple, state-of-the-art NYU Langone facilities and across all specialties: physical, occupational, speech/swallowing and vocational therapy, psychology, music and recreational therapy, nutrition, nursing, and social work.

Rusk's CARF-Accredited Brain Injury Rehabilitation Program is tailored for patients who have medical, physical, cognitive, and behavioral changes as a result of a brain injury or neurological illness.

The Amputee Program provides specialized limb deficiency rehabilitation to patients who have undergone amputations.

The Joan and Joel Smilow Cardiac and Pulmonary Rehabilitation & Prevention Center offers a model of transitional care for patients with cardiac and lung conditions.

Orthopaedic/Musculoskeletal Rehabilitation is offered for patients with back, neck, hip, elbow and shoulder disorders, arthritis-related joint pain, conditions affecting the bones, tendon, ligaments and muscles, and for pre- and post-surgical patients.

The Spinal Cord Injury program offers a comprehensive, patient-centered array of specialized and innovative clinical and educational programs to optimize quality of life.

Sports Injury Rehabilitation addresses the needs of patients with sports-related conditions, including post-operative rehabilitation for patients who require orthopaedic surgery.

Rusk's CARF-Accredited Stroke Program offers an interdisciplinary team with specialized training in the medical, nursing or therapeutic care and treatment of stroke patients.

Vestibular Rehabilitation addresses the evaluation and treatment of patients suffering from dizziness and imbalance.

The Women's Health Program addresses issues that uniquely affect women, including pelvic floor muscle dysfunction/pain, urinary incontinence, cancer rehabilitation and lymphedema, and prenatal and postpartum musculoskeletal conditions.

Chest Physical Therapy cares for individuals with lung congestion, secretion retention or areas of lung collapse.

The Outpatient Rehabilitation Psychology Service provides care to patients with neurological and medical conditions on an outpatient basis.

Speech-Language Pathology & Swallowing is dedicated to patients with communication disorders due to neurological problems as well as diagnosis and management of swallowing and feeding disorders.

Vocational Services provides disabled individuals with the competencies needed to return to school or work and to lead a productive life.

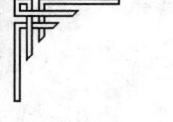

The Best in American Medicine
www.CastleConnolly.com

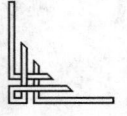
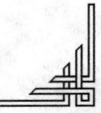

Reproductive Endocrinology

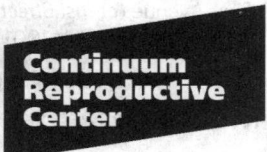

The Continuum Reproductive Center
212.523.7751

The Continuum Reproductive Center (CRC) is one of New York's leading providers of reproductive medicine and fertility care. Our physicians have expertise in many areas of reproductive care including the management of:

- Ovulation Disorders
- Polycystic Ovary Syndrome
- Fallopian Tube Disease
- Fibroid Tumors of the Uterus
- Unexplained Infertility
- Recurrent Pregnancy Loss
- Endometriosis and Pelvic Pain
- Benign Disorders of the Ovaries and Uterus
- Assisted Reproductive Technologies, such as In Vitro Fertilization (IVF)
- Male Factor Infertility

The physicians of the CRC are all double board-certified in both obstetrics and gynecology, and reproductive endocrinology and fertility. Our physicians are well-respected for their clinical and research contributions, have published in peer-review journals, and presented at national and international meetings.

In addition to our physicians, the staff at the CRC is comprised of nurses, medical assistants, and administrators who form an expert, cohesive and professional team with many years of experience in the care of fertility and reproductive endocrinology. Our laboratory is directed by a Ph.D. reproductive physiologist accredited by the American Association of Bioanalysts as a high-complexity laboratory director (HCLD). Our team of embryologists and andrologists possesses a wealth of specialized training and experience in the culture and manipulation of human sperm, eggs and embryos. The result is comprehensive and personalized care with excellent success rates.

We deliver care to patients in the tri-state area, with broader insurance coverage and lower out-of-pocket fees than available from most of our competitors. In addition to our main center in Manhattan, we have a Mount Kisco, NY, office. Please call 914.244.8749 for additional information.

The physicians of the Continuum Reproductive Center are affiliated with St. Luke's and Roosevelt Hospitals, an Academic Affiliate of the Columbia University College of Physicians and Surgeons.

Continuum Reproductive Centers
Manhattan: 425 West 59th Street
Mt. Kisco, NY: 83 South Bedford Road

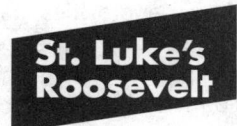

www.ContinuumFertility.com

Continuum Health Partners, Inc.

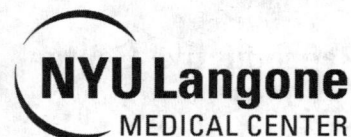

550 First Avenue *(at 31st Street)*
New York, NY 10016
www.NYULMC.org
Physician Referral: **888-7-NYU-MED** *(888-769-8633)*

PROGRAM FOR IVF REPRODUCTIVE SURGERY AND INFERTILITY

About the Division of Reproductive Endocrinology and Infertility, Department of Obstetrics and Gynecology

The Division of Reproductive Endocrinology and Infertility offers the most advanced technology available to help infertile women and men realize their dreams of parenthood. The Division is highly experienced in all aspects of reproductive endocrinology, including the diagnosis and treatment of endometriosis, fibroids, problems with ovulation or sperm function, and recurring pregnancy loss. Its clinical staff includes seasoned technicians and physicians who have pioneered new innovations and been honored for their contributions to the field.

Patient-Centered Care

From the initial diagnosis through all stages of treatment, couples at NYU Langone Medical Center receive state-of-the-art, compassionate care tailored to their specific needs. After a comprehensive evaluation to determine the cause of infertility, couples are counseled on whether assisted reproduction is necessary.

In Vitro Fertilization (IVF)

When medical conditions prevent the sperm from reaching the egg, skilled physicians and laboratory staff at the Fertility Center assist patients with retrieving their eggs, insemination in the lab, and insertion back into the patient's uterus as embryos. Preimplantation Genetic Screening (PGS) at the Fertility Center offers tests for aneuploidy (an abnormal number of chromosomes). Some of the genetic disorders identified with PGS include cystic fibrosis, Down syndrome, hemophilia, Huntington's disease, Marfan's disease, muscular dystrophy and sickle cell anemia. State-of-the-art technology is also used to increase chances of delivery in some women with a history of recurrent miscarriage or previous IVF failures.

Complex Cases

The Center offers the most advanced care available for complex cases of infertility including those which may not have been successful in other centers and may even have been told there is no hope.

IVF for Male Factor Infertility

The Fertility Center provides male patients with experienced urologists who can provide expert fertility treatment. Men receive a complete evaluation, including a fertility history, physical exam, blood testing and semen analysis. Surgical treatment of male infertility is performed on-site at the Center's surgical suites on an outpatient basis and may include testicular biopsy, vasectomy reversal, epididymal tissue repair and varicose vein repair.

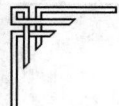

The Best in American Medicine
www.CastleConnolly.com

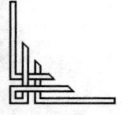

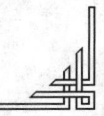

Rheumatology

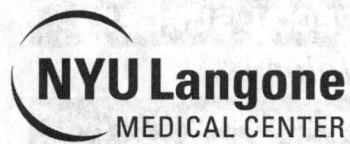
RHEUMATOLOGY

Rheumatologists at NYU Langone Medical Center are dedicated to the diagnosis and treatment of patients with rheumatic illnesses, particularly autoimmune diseases. *U.S. News and World Report* has repeatedly recognized the Division of Rheumatology as one of the best in the country, ranking #7 nationwide in the 2012-2013 "Best Hospitals" survey. The division provides care at NYU Langone's premier outpatient facility, The Center for Musculoskeletal Care; the internationally-renowned, inpatient Hospital for Joint Diseases; and at the medical center's Tisch Hospital.

Arthritis and Autoimmunity: We offer a comprehensive program for the prevention, diagnosis and treatment of all rheumatologic conditions. Patients also have access to complete rheumatologic evaluations, orthopaedic and neurological consultative services, and participation in clinical trials using the most advanced interventional therapies, highly sophisticated diagnostic testing, and complementary medicine.

Behçet's Syndrome: We have the largest North American Behçet's Center for research and the evaluation and treatment of patients with Behçet's Syndrome, a disease that involves inflammation of the blood vessels.

Biological Treatment: Biological treatments for inflammatory arthritis, rheumatoid arthritis, lupus, psoriatic arthritis, vasculitis, and osteoporosis are administered by the Medical Center's infusion centers.

Lupus: The Center for Lupus Care and Research is devoted to the treatment and research of patients with this autoimmune disease. Patients have access to world renowned specialists in lupus, lupus and pregnancy, and related sub-specialties.

Osteoporosis: We offer comprehensive care for the prevention, evaluation and treatment of osteoporosis, including state-of-the art bone densitometers, a range of advanced drug therapies, and programs in balance training and exercise.

Psoriatic Arthritis: Patients at the Psoriatic Arthritis Center, a collaborative effort with the Department of Dermatology, are seen by both a rheumatologist and dermatologist who specialize in psoriasis and psoriatic arthritis.

We are also leaders in rheumatology research, focusing on the study of drugs, drug delivery systems and protocols, and the roles genes play in the development and treatment of rheumatic diseases, positioning us at the forefront of basic science and translational research, personalized medicine and the genetics of rheumatic diseases. The Peter D. Seligman Center for Advanced Therapeutics, renowned for breakthrough research in arthritis and Systematic Lupus Erythematosus, conducts clinical studies using a wide variety of newly developed therapies.

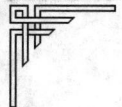

The Best in American Medicine
www.CastleConnolly.com

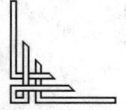
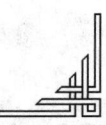

Sleep Disorders

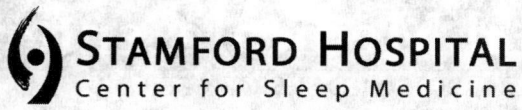

STAMFORD HOSPITAL
Center for Sleep Medicine

Center for Sleep Medicine

Stamford Hospital's Center for Sleep Medicine is Accredited by the American Academy of Sleep Medicine. All of our physicians are board-certified and highly skilled in diagnosing and treating sleep disorders including: snoring, sleep apnea, insomnia, narcolepsy and restless legs syndrome.

In addition, The Center includes one of Fairfield County's few board-certified sleep specialists trained in pediatric sleep medicine, providing special expertise in the treatment of sleep problems in infancy through teenage years.

Personalized Care

We are one of the state's larger sleep centers, and are able to schedule appointments and sleep studies faster than other facilities.

Located in the Hospital, all rooms are private with their own bath with shower. Each hotel-like room is furnished with a queen-size bed, reclining chair and cable television. Our rooms are large enough to accommodate a caregiver, especially important for pediatric patients.

Sleep Study

Some patients require an overnight sleep study. This non-invasive test monitors heart activity, breathing, oxygenation, position, limb movement, snoring and brain activity. During this painless process, a patient will be free to watch television or read until ready to go to sleep. The sleep study will be conducted throughout the night while the patient sleeps. Patients can leave the following morning for work or whatever their normal routine may be. In special circumstances, a home study can be performed.

Treatment Options

There are numerous treatment options available at the Center for Sleep Medicine—behavior modification, medication and in some instances custom made medical devices. Regardless of your sleep disorder, our physicians are experts in their field and will work with you to achieve a good night's sleep.

Academic and Clinical Affiliations

Stamford Hospital is an affiliate of the New York–Presbyterian Healthcare System and a major teaching affiliate of the Columbia University College of Physicians & Surgeons.

Accreditation

Joint Commission on Accreditation of Healthcare Organization (JCAHO)

Beds

305

Sponsorship

Voluntary, Not-for-Profit

For a Physician Referral or more information, please call 1.877.233.9355 or visit StamfordHospital.org /doctor.

Stamford Hospital
30 Shelburne Road
Stamford, CT 06902
203.276.1000

StamfordHospital.org

Trinitas Regional Medical Center

COMPREHENSIVE SLEEP DISORDERS CENTER

210 WILLIAMSON STREET | ELIZABETH, NEW JERSEY 07207
PH 908.994.8694 | WWW.NJSLEEPDISORDERSCENTER.COM

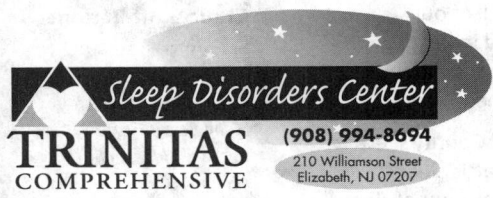

Sleep Disorders Center

TRINITAS
COMPREHENSIVE

(908) 994-8694
210 Williamson Street
Elizabeth, NJ 07207

Accredited by The American Academy of Sleep Medicine

Getting a good night's sleep is an essential part of healthy living, but for the millions of Americans who suffer from sleep disorders, getting enough rest can be difficult, if not impossible. Left untreated, sleep disorders can have harmful, even life-threatening effects on health, well-being and safety.

The Comprehensive Sleep Disorders Center at Trinitas Regional Medical Center provides a monitored, fully attended diagnostic sleep study designed to rule out physical, non-stress related symptoms that may prevent restful sleep. The medical director is board certified in Internal Medicine, Critical Care, Sleep Medicine and Pulmonary Medicine. A team of trained sleep specialists supervises each study and coordinates follow-up care with the patient's physician. These professionals can quickly diagnose any sleep problem and, working closely with each patient's primary physician, provide expert treatment and follow-up.

Located within the main campus of Trinitas Regional Medical Center, the state-of-the-art Comprehensive Sleep Disorders Center is designed to diagnose sleep disorders, including insomnia, sleep apnea, restless leg syndrome, snoring and narcolepsy, among others. The private, comfortable testing is performed in home-like suites with soft designer sheets, pillows and a private shower. Studies are provided for adults and children as young as 18 months. Daytime studies are available to meet patient needs.

In 2010, a second sleep center was unveiled in Homewood Suites by Hilton, Cranford. The site is the first hotel-based sleep center in New Jersey.

Both locations offer state-of-the-art diagnostic sleep studies performed by specially trained sleep pulmonologists, registered poly-somnographers and licensed, credentialed respiratory therapists.

The Trinitas Comprehensive Sleep Disorders Center is a fully staffed center accredited by The American Academy of Sleep Medicine - the "gold standard" accrediting body for sleep centers - offering the benefits of two distinct locations. With one location on the campus of Trinitas Regional Medical Center, a comprehensive, state-of-the-art medical facility and the other at a nearby nationally known hotel chain, patients who have sleep studies performed at Trinitas receive the high level of attention or treatment that is simply not possible to receive at a neighborhood sleep center.

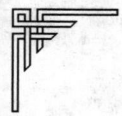

The Best in American Medicine
www.CastleConnolly.com

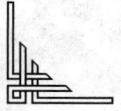
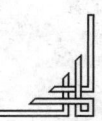

Stroke Care

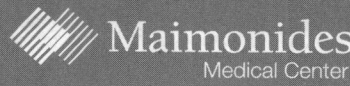

Surgery

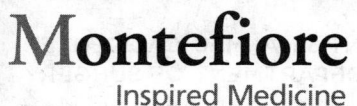

111 East 210th Street
Bronx, New York 10467
718-920-4800
www.montefiore.org/surgery

Surgery at Montefiore

High volumes and exceptional outcomes are distinguishing traits of the Department of Surgery at Montefiore Medical Center. The Department's five divisions collectively perform more than 8,000 procedures on adult and pediatric patients annually. **In 2011, the Department received national recognition for exemplary outcomes by the American College of Surgeons' National Surgical Quality Improvement Program.** Exemplary outcomes were achieved in the categories of overall morbidity, unplanned intubations, ventilator requirement greater than 48 hours and renal failure. This success is attributed largely to the caliber of the Department's surgical team.

The Department's Division of Breast Surgery is widely recognized for its personalized approach to care and extensive surgical offerings for the treatment of patients with breast cancer and other breast disorders. Breast reconstructions are performed by the Division of Plastic and Reconstructive Surgery, which uses state-of-the-art techniques to create replacement breasts that look and feel natural.

The Division of Plastic and Reconstructive Surgery's highly trained experts employ the latest microsurgical techniques when performing delicate cranial/facial, limb and hand reconstruction/reimplantation surgeries in adult and pediatric patients.

Our Division of General Surgery has achieved national prominence in the area of robotic and minimally invasive surgery. These approaches encompass all surgical specialties, including colon, gastrointestinal, stomach, pancreas and weight reduction surgery, and are used as often as possible to the benefit of patients. Of particular note is the Division's recent addition of robotic-assisted liver resection for patients with liver cancer.

Montefiore's Division of Transplant Surgery offers comprehensive treatment for adult and pediatric patients with diseases of the pancreas, kidney and liver—**including solid organ and living donor transplants. The Division's one-year outcomes in all areas exceed state and national averages.**

Cancer patients at Montefiore benefit from a number of sophisticated surgical treatment options that include minimally invasive procedures as well as robotic surgery. Cancer patients can also receive one of the three types of perfusion treatments offered by the Division of General Surgery—hyperthermic intraperitoneal chemotherapy, isolated limb perfusion (for sarcoma or melanoma) and liver perfusion.

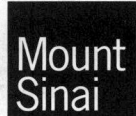 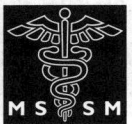

**MOUNT SINAI
SCHOOL OF
MEDICINE**

THE MOUNT SINAI MEDICAL CENTER
DEPARTMENT OF SURGERY
One Gustave L. Levy Place
Fifth Avenue and 100th Street
New York, NY 10029-6574
Physician Referral: 1-800-MD-SINAI (637-4624)
www.mountsinai.org/surgery

THE DEPARTMENT OF SURGERY continues to build upon the legacy of those who have gone before, caring for the very sickest of patients while developing new therapies and training tomorrow's physicians to save and enhance lives. Patients today are experiencing less pain, shorter hospital stays, and faster recovery times than was ever imaginable just 20 years ago.

Bariatric Surgery – The latest minimally invasive techniques are used to perform laparoscopic gastric bypass, lap band placement, duodenal switch, and sleeve gastrectomy.

Colon and Rectal Surgery – Leaders in the treatment of gastrointestinal disorders, our surgeons care for a wide range of diseases, including: inflammatory bowel disease (Crohn's disease and ulcerative colitis), diverticulitis, colon and rectal cancer, and fecal incontinence. We offer many important procedures not commonly available.

General Surgery – The Division of General Surgery specializes in the treatment of abdominal surgical conditions. These include benign and malignant diseases of the gallbladder and gastrointestinal track (stomach, intestine, and colon). Our Comprehensive Hernia Center offers state-of-the-art repair of inguinal, ventral and hiatal hernias. We use minimally invasive and evidence-based surgery to deliver the highest standard of care to our patients.

Laparoscopic and Minimally Invasive Surgery – Mount Sinai surgeons rank as some of the world's most respected and innovative surgeons, performing more laparoscopic procedures than surgeons at any other hospital in New York.

Metabolic, Endocrine and Minimally Invasive Surgery – This division was formed to serve as the backbone for several disease-specific multidisciplinary programs. Ours is a truly novel metabolic surgery program that brings together traditional endocrine, bariatric and laparoscopic techniques to treat diseases of metabolism and the endocrine system.

Pediatric Surgery – Surgeries involving children can be met with even more apprehension than those for adults. Fortunately, Mount Sinai surgeons offer a full range of pediatric surgical procedures in a family-focused, child-sensitive environment.

Plastic and Reconstructive Surgery – Surgical care from aesthetic to complex reconstruction is offered for benign and malignant disease, as well as for deformities that are either congenital or acquired. The aim is to restore function and correct deformities caused by birth defects, aging, accident, or illness.

Surgical Oncology – Our surgeons provide expert care for both minimally invasive and open complex malignancies. Patients are seen promptly and are cared for by a multidisciplinary team of medical and surgical experts, enabling them to benefit from the opinions of dozens of nationally renowned doctors.

Vascular Surgery – Mount Sinai is a recognized world leader in the development of new minimally invasive techniques for the treatment of aortic aneurysms, carotid stenosis for the prevention of stroke and lower extremity ischemia. Mount Sinai performs research in areas ranging from stem cell therapy to specialized vascular devices. Our research serves to advance the field of vascular surgery. A wide array of advanced patient services is available, ensuring that conditions are managed successfully.

TOP-RANKING MINIMALLY INVASIVE SURGEONS
In surveys of leading minimally invasive surgeons in a variety of specialties, Mount Sinai's physicians are consistently at the top of the list in surgery of the colon and rectum, liver and bile ducts, thyroid, hernia, chest, and blood vessels.

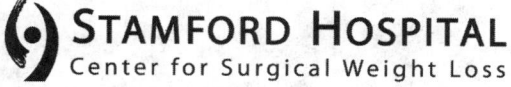

Center for Surgical Weight Loss

At Stamford Hospital's Center for Surgical Weight Loss, patients benefit from a comprehensive program led by an expert team of weight management specialists. Surgeons, physicians, dedicated nurse practitioner, registered dietitian, psychologist and exercise physiologist provide patients with the knowledge and skills needed to achieve the best possible results. In addition to surgical procedures, the Center offers medically supervised weight management for patients who do not qualify for surgery or simply prefer to take a different approach.

Surgical Procedures

The Center offers four types of weight loss surgery: gastric bypass, gastric banding, sleeve gastrectomy and duodenal switch, all of which are performed laparoscopically (tiny incisions) and result in less pain and scarring with a faster recovery.

Integrated Care

We offer an extraordinary breadth of expertise across many medical and support disciplines to guide a patient to success. *Our comprehensive plan includes:*

Surgical Preparatory Program

We offer educational seminars, consultations, complimentary 90-day membership at our Health & Fitness Institute and support groups.

Center for Integrative Medicine and Wellness

Patients learn mind-body, guided imagery techniques to prepare emotionally and physically for surgery as well as to help heal and recover faster and more comfortably. In addition, acupuncture, stress management and nutritional counseling support are offered.

Health & Fitness Institute

An innovative wellness facility, offering medically supervised fitness and lifestyle change, includes a dedicated exercise physiologist on staff who specializes in working with bariatric patients. The use of state-of-the-art exercise equipment, 25-yard lap pool, warm water therapeutic pool and Jacuzzi helps patients achieve weight loss and fitness goals. To take a tour of the facility, and to view the pool and class schedule, visit StamfordHospital.org/HFI.

Academic and Clinical Affiliations

Stamford Hospital is an affiliate of the New York–Presbyterian Healthcare System and a major teaching affiliate of the Columbia University College of Physicians & Surgeons.

Accreditation

Joint Commission on Accreditation of Healthcare Organization (JCAHO)

Beds

305

Sponsorship

Voluntary, Not-for-Profit

For a Physician Referral or more information, please call 1.877.233.9355 or visit StamfordHospital.org /doctor.

Stamford Hospital
30 Shelburne Road
Stamford, CT 06902
203.276.1000

StamfordHospital.org

Thoracic & Cardiac Surgery

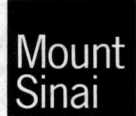
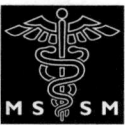

**MOUNT SINAI
SCHOOL OF
MEDICINE**

THE MOUNT SINAI MEDICAL CENTER
CARDIOTHORACIC SURGERY

One Gustave L. Levy Place
Fifth Avenue and 100th Street
New York, NY 10029-6574
Physician Referral: 1-800-MD-SINAI (637-4624)
www.mountsinai.org/heart
www.mitralvalverepair.org

THE DEPARTMENT OF CARDIOTHORACIC SURGERY at Mount Sinai is one of the nation's most prestigious programs. **In 2012, *U.S. News & World Report* ranked our cardiology and heart surgery service 10th in the country.** Cardiothoracic surgical patients benefit from an integrated and personalized care plan designed in coordination with expert cardiologists, anesthesiologists, perfusionists, and intensive care physicians. Mount Sinai is a quaternary referral center, meaning its surgeons often operate on the sickest and most complicated patients.

The Mitral Valve Repair Reference Center is one of the largest and most advanced in the nation. The superiority of mitral valve repair over replacement with a mechanical or bioprosthetic valve is now well established. Directed by David H. Adams, MD, Mount Sinai's Mitral Valve Repair Reference Center offers patients one of the highest percentages of successful valve repair in the world. In patients with mitral valve prolapse, our success rate in avoiding valve replacement approaches 100 percent. Our physicians are experts in mitral valve repair for patients with advanced cardiomyopathy. For patients who have associated atrial fibrillation, we offer the latest in concomitant arrhythmia surgery, including the MAZE procedure. Mitral valve repair with minimally invasive approaches is also performed when appropriate. Learn more about our Reference Center at www.mitralvalverepair.org.

The Cardiac Transplant and Assist Program, one of the largest in the nation, is under the direction of Anelechi Anyanwu, MD. We have been involved in the field of mechanical cardiac assistance from its inception, and have experience with most of the available FDA-approved devices. We have also played an active role in multi-institutional studies exploring permanent mechanical heart support.

Transcatheter Aortic Valve Replacement/Implantation (TAVR/TAVI) Program offers breakthrough treatment. Our physicians have been performing TAVR/TAVI for two years, with patients coming from around the world for this treatment. We were the first institution in the country to implant the Medtronic CoreValve Transcatheter Aortic Valve replacement device, and we are the first hospital in New York State able to implant both the Edwards Sapien Valve and the Medtronic CoreValve. These minimally invasive treatments spare patients from open-heart surgery and offer quicker recovery and return to daily activities. Our TAVR/TAVI program is led by Dr. David Adams, the National Co-Principal Investigator of the United States FDA pivotal trial of the Medtronic CoreValve Transcatheter Aortic Valve replacement device, and Dr. Samin Sharma, Director of Clinical Cardiology and Interventional Cardiology who, according to NYS Department of Health reports, has had the highest angioplasty success rate (lowest mortality less than 0.1 percent) for an interventional cardiologist in the state since 1994.

Pediatric and Congenital Cardiac Surgery Program achieves exceptional results. Led by Dr. Khanh Nguyen, patients from newborns to young adults are cared for in this program, which has achieved outstanding results with challenging problems by incorporating the most advanced techniques available. Part of only three active pediatric heart transplant centers in the state, our program also provides support for very sick hearts in infants and older children, using Extra-Corporeal Membrane Oxygenators (ECMO) or Ventricular Assist Devices (VAD). The care extended to the patient and family is supported by an outstanding multidisciplinary team. Superb post-operative care is provided in a dedicated Pediatric Cardiac Surgical Intensive Care Unit, under the direction of pediatric cardiologists, intensivists, and surgeons.

**LEADING SURGEONS, UNPARALLELED POSSIBILITIES
The Department of Cardiothoracic Surgery at Mount Sinai** is chaired by David H. Adams, MD, the Marie-Josée and Henry R. Kravis Professor. Dr. Adams is a world-renowned mitral repair surgeon. Anelechi Anyanwu, MD, leads one of the largest ventricular assist device and heart transplant centers in the country. He is also an expert in complex and re-operative valve surgery. Paul Stelzer, MD, is a specialist in aortic root surgery whose experience with the Ross procedure is unmatched, exceeding 20 years and 500 cases. These leaders work in concert with other members of Mount Sinai Heart, which is under the direction of world-renowned cardiologist Valentin Fuster, MD, PhD, to deliver unparalleled possibilities for patients with cardiovascular disease.

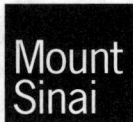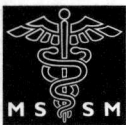

THE MOUNT SINAI MEDICAL CENTER
THORACIC SURGERY

One Gustave L. Levy Place
Fifth Avenue and 100th Street
New York, NY 10029-6574
Physician Referral: 1-800-MD-SINAI (637-4624)
www.mountsinai.org/thoracicsurgery

MOUNT SINAI
SCHOOL OF
MEDICINE

THORACIC SURGERY at The Mount Sinai Medical Center is known for its state-of-the-art surgery, multidisciplinary team approach to treatment, and commitment to compassionate patient care. Protocol-driven therapy ensures that Mount Sinai patients are given access to many clinical trials.

The Division of Thoracic Surgery at Mount Sinai engages in multidisciplinary collaboration, partnering with medical oncology, radiation oncology, pulmonary medicine, diagnostic and interventional radiology, gastroenterology, neurology, and anesthesiology, so patients can benefit from the insights of multiple experts across different specialties. This coordination among teams ensures seamless delivery of high-quality care to patients.

With an integrated approach to clinical care and research, our team of dedicated thoracic surgeons are experts in the treatment of all primary cancers of the chest, lung, esophagus, mediastinum, and airway, and all metastatic tumors of the chest. We also diagnose and treat patients who are affected by benign esophageal disorders such as gastroesophageal reflux disease, achalasia, and motility disorders.

Minimally Invasive Care: Minimally invasive interventions are preferred whenever possible, allowing less tissue damage, faster recovery time, and less scarring than open surgery. Mount Sinai's Division of Thoracic Surgery offers state-of-the-art assessment and treatment approaches, including thoroscopy, rigid and flexible bronchoscopy, and endoscopic laser resection in the diagnosis and management of thoracic conditions. The division has led the national trials for VATS (video-assisted thoracoscopic surgery) lobectomy, a procedure using three small incisions, which is now the surgical approach of choice, particularly for patients with early-stage lung cancer.

Personalized and Targeted Therapy: A unique part of our division is the integration and application of groundbreaking scientific research into the clinical care of our patients. These research efforts are being carried out in the Thoracic Surgery Translational Laboratory. Mount Sinai's thoracic surgeons and physician-scientists are conducting state-of-the-art translational thoracic research, including genomic analysis of tumors to better understand and predict behavior, in order to develop more directed, personalized, therapeutic approaches to treatment with novel targeted therapies.

Lung and Esophageal Cancer: Mount Sinai is New York City's leading center for comprehensive screening for lung and esophageal cancer, including CT scans for early detection, advanced endoscopic techniques, PET scans, and innovative MRI technology with ultrasensitive resolution. Our team is unique in our abilities to screen for cancers in people at risk, treat early cancers less invasively, and provide the most advanced protocol driven treatments available. Our approach to lung cancer care focuses on patients first, providing not only VATS and advanced minimally invasive techniques, but also an ability to treat advanced and challenging cases that require skills and expertise found in few other medical centers.

Mesothelioma: Irving J. Selikoff, MD, was the first to determine the association between mesothelioma and asbestos exposure. His tireless research efforts at Mount Sinai led to the Selikoff Center for Occupational and Environmental Medicine. This tradition of cutting-edge developments continues with Raja M. Flores' work using different modalities in the treatment of mesothelioma, such as the extrapleural pneumonectomy and pleurectomy (decortication) procedures. The Division of Thoracic Surgery is also currently involved in several ongoing studies with the goal of discovering new treatments for mesothelioma.

LEADING SURGEONS, PIONEERING RESEARCH

Led by Raja M. Flores, the Division of Thoracic Surgery is internationally recognized as a leader in thoracic surgery drawing patients from across the globe to seek our expertise.

Dr. Flores is a recognized leader in the treatment of mesothelioma and one of the first physicians in the world to use robotic surgery to treat lung and esophageal cancer. Dr. Flores established VATS lobectomy as the gold standard in the surgical treatment of lung cancer. He is one of the foremost educators of other surgeons about the VATS lobectomy.

Our award-winning physicians have consistently contributed to the evolution of this field through their efforts to bring about new technologies and therapies.

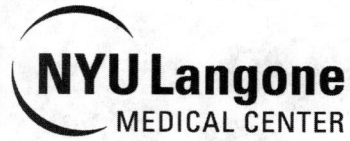

550 First Avenue (*at 31st Street*)
New York, NY 10016
www.NYULMC.org
Physician Referral: **888-7-NYU-MED** (*888-769-8633*)

THORACIC SURGERY

About the Division of Thoracic Surgery

Thoracic Surgeons at NYU Langone Medical Center offer the most advanced diagnosis and treatment options available to patients for either benign or malignant lesions of the lung, esophagus, mediastinum and chest wall. All thoracic attending surgeons at the Medical Center are experts in minimally invasive, video-assisted thoracic surgery which minimizes patient discomfort and shortens recuperation time. We specialize in the following areas:

Airway Stenting

Patients experiencing trouble breathing may require stenting to maintain an open airway (windpipe). Treatment of primary and metastatic lung cancer often requires the use of hollow tubes (stents) to maintain an unobstructed airway. At NYU Langone, stent placement is performed in the operating room by an experienced team that includes a surgeon, anesthesiologist and nursing staff. The procedure can be performed through either rigid or flexible bronchoscopy using temporary (plastic) or more permanent (metal) stents. Post-operative patients are carefully monitored by a multidisciplinary team to ensure their comfort and care.

Minimally Invasive Thoracic Surgery

The Division of Thoracic Surgery offers a minimally invasive surgery program, incorporating both video-assisted and "open chest" techniques along with the newest methods for post-operative pain relief. The use of video-assisted equipment allows for a smaller incision without spreading the rib spaces, leading to greater patient comfort, a shorter recovery time and decreased length of stay for patients. Procedures offered include video-assisted thoracoscopy for biopsy with or without removal of a portion of the lungs, as well as repair of hiatal hernias and minimally invasive esophagectomy.

Pioneering Treatments

NYU Langone Medical Center continues to pioneer new treatments for the early detection of airway malignancies, diagnosis and treatment strategies for endobronchial abnormalities, investigation of non-surgical techniques for destruction of lung cancer nodules, and the use of stents (including replaceable stents) to relieve blockages of the windpipe and esophagus.

Research

NYU Langone is committed to state-of-the-art surgical management and development of novel treatment strategies through clinical trials. We also leverage the resources of the New York Thoracic Surgery Laboratory at Bellevue Hospital Center to search for genes and proteins in malignancies of the chest in order to develop novel targeted therapies.

Transplantation

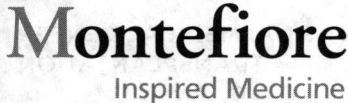
Montefiore
Inspired Medicine

111 East 210th Street
Bronx, New York 10467
Heart: 718-920-6515
Liver: 888-795-4837
Kidney: 877-287-3536
www.montefiore.org/transplant

Montefiore Einstein Center for Transplantation

Montefiore Einstein Center for Transplantation is widely recognized for its excellent outcomes and holistic approach to care. Here, adults and children with end-stage organ disease receive all aspects of treatment and counseling in one convenient location. Additionally, **the Center's one-year survival rates exceed 90 percent in all areas (heart, liver, pancreatic and kidney), surpassing the national average of 75 to 80 percent.** Our Pediatric Transplant Program is the only program in the Bronx and Westchester for patients with type 1 diabetes and severe end-stage renal failure.

Critical to the Center's success is its nationally renowned Kidney Transplant Program, one of the nation's oldest and most respected. The Program maintains a proven track record of success and growth. In addition to its exceptional patient survival rates, the Program achieves superior graft survival rates. The Center's commitment to its pediatric population resulted in the establishment of the first pediatric dialysis center in the United States.

Montefiore Einstein Center for Heart and Vascular Care has the highest transplant survival rates for both children and adults in the region. The Center also identifies alternatives to transplant for heart failure patients, including novel therapies and ventricular assist devices (VADs). In 2011, Montefiore performed a total of 29 heart transplants (20 adult and 9 pediatric), with a one-year survival rate of 100 percent. **The Center's Liver Disease and Transplant Program combines specialty programs in liver transplantation (deceased and living donor), liver cancer, pediatric liver disease, general consultative hepatology and hepatobiliary surgery.** Since the Program's launch, it has accelerated the rate at which patients are placed on the transplant waiting list, added hepatologists to meet the growing needs of the community, and expanded its reach to help serve patients with liver disease. In 2011, our specialists transplanted 25 livers, a figure that includes rare "split-liver" grafts in which an adult donor liver is split and offered to two recipients. In 25 percent of transplants performed at Montefiore, the patients had unresectable liver cancer.

In addition to performing clinical trials for new therapies for hepatitis C, the Center is collaborating with the Marion Bessin Liver Research Center at Albert Einstein College of Medicine to conduct pioneering work in liver stem cells and hepatocyte transplantation for metabolic disease.

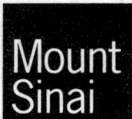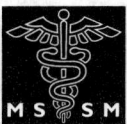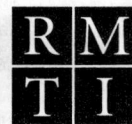

MOUNT SINAI
SCHOOL OF
MEDICINE

THE MOUNT SINAI MEDICAL CENTER TRANSPLANTATION
One Gustave L. Levy Place
Fifth Avenue and 100th Street
New York, NY 10029-6574
Physician Referral: 1-800-MD-SINAI (637-4624)
212-731-RMTI (7684)
www.mountsinai.org/rmti

Scientific breakthroughs, technological advances, and improved clinical therapies make it possible to save more lives through organ transplantation than ever before. The Mount Sinai Medical Center's **RECANATI MILLER/TRANSPLANTATION INSTITUTE (RMTI)** has been a world leader in these advances. The RMTI brings together clinical programs in adult and pediatric liver, kidney, pancreas, and intestinal transplantation. It is one of the largest transplant centers in the United States and performs more than 350 transplant procedures annually. In addition, RMTI surgeons also perform complex hepatobiliary surgical procedures.

History of Achievement – The kidney transplant program was instituted at Mount Sinai in 1967 and is now one of the largest adult and pediatric programs in the nation, having performed more than 2,500 transplants. The first liver transplant to be performed in New York State was in 1988 at Mount Sinai. There have been many other firsts in the program's 22-year history, including the first pediatric liver transplant and the first adult-to-adult living-donor liver transplant in New York State. Our surgeons have successfully performed more than 3,000 liver transplants and over 250 living donor liver transplants.

Tradition of Excellence – Mount Sinai is one of the few hospitals in the country that offers comprehensive, multi-organ transplant services for both children and adults. Our physicians are able to accept and care for the sickest and most complex patients.

Innovative Programs

- **HIV/Protocol Study** – Since 2001, the RMTI has been one of the only transplant centers to participate in a National Institutes of Health study on transplantation for carefully selected patients with HIV.

- **Living Donor Program** – Mount Sinai has an active living-donor program. The newly endowed **Zweig Family Center for Living Donation** is the first multi-organ living donor center where dedicated resources ensure the well-being of these heroes who give one, or a part, of their own organs to save another person's life. We also participate in local and national paired-exchange and donor-chain initiatives.

- **Multi-organ Transplantation and Intestinal Rehabilitation Program** – We have performed many combined transplant procedures. Our rehabilitation program offers patients with intestinal failure the opportunity, when possible, to avoid transplantation through medical and/or surgical interventions.

- **Translational Research** – Our scientists are actively investigating new and innovative ways to detect, prevent and treat rejection. We have nationally-recognized and well-funded transplant, genomic, and proteomic projects.

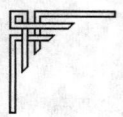

The Best in American Medicine
www.CastleConnolly.com

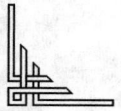
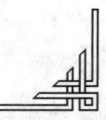

Urology

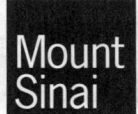
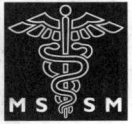

MOUNT SINAI SCHOOL OF MEDICINE

**THE MOUNT SINAI MEDICAL CENTER
UROLOGY**
One Gustave L. Levy Place
Fifth Avenue and 100th Street
New York, NY 10029-6574
Physician Referral: 1-800-MD-SINAI (637-4624)
www.mountsinai.org/urology

UROLOGY

The Milton and Carroll Petrie Department of Urology at The Mount Sinai Medical Center offers the latest technologic advances for the diagnosis and treatment of urologic diseases and conditions while supporting a translational and clinical research program.

Prostate Cancer: The Department of Urology's Barbara and Maurice Deane Health and Research Center is at the forefront of diagnosis, treatment and management of localized and advanced prostate cancer. Our surgeons are among the few trained in open, laparoscopic, and robotic surgery. The Robotics Prostatectomy program is one of the world's busiest, with over 4,000 surgeries to date. For men with low grade cancer, we oversee structured and personalized active surveillance. Our research focus is on multi-modal and novel therapies for advanced cancer; our work led to the approval of *Provenge®*, a cellular immunotherapeutic treatment.

Bladder Cancer: As recognized leaders in the assessment and treatment of all forms of bladder cancer, Mount Sinai urologic oncologists are successfully using tumor markers and new diagnostic techniques. Our surgeons employ robotic and laparoscopic surgery to perform cystectomies (removal of bladder) resulting in minimal impact on quality of life.

Kidney Cancer: Mount Sinai specialists helped pioneer robotic partial nephrectomy for the treatment of small kidney cancers. Other minimally invasive options such as cryoablation (freezing) or radiofrequency ablation (heating) are offered as a means to treat small cancers while preserving maximum kidney function.

Benign Prostatic Hyperplasia (BPH): The Deane Center offers the latest minimally invasive technologies and treatments for BPH, including Holium Laser Enucleation, Greenlight ™ Laser Photoselective Vaporization of the Prostate and bipolar cautery vaporization (Button TURP) in addition to TURP for symptoms of an enlarged prostate. Many of these procedures can be performed on an ambulatory basis.

Reconstructive Urology, Female Urology and Voiding Dysfunction: The Department of Urology provides comprehensive resources for the evaluation and treatment of urinary incontinence, neuro-urologic problems (e.g., spinal cord injury, multiple sclerosis) and pelvic pain syndrome for both men and women. Our specialists are among the few in the country with advanced training in urethral reconstruction. A state-of-the-art continence center provides the convenience of on-site diagnosis and treatment.

Erectile Dysfunction and Infertility: The Mount Sinai Sexual Health Program uses the most advanced techniques available to evaluate the causes of erectile dysfunction. Treatment options are extensive and effective. Importantly, patients and their partners receive the guidance they need to make the appropriate personal decision regarding treatment.

Kidney Stones: Mount Sinai's specialists utilize minimally invasive procedures to treat kidney stones, including laser and ultrasonic lithotripsy techniques. Medical and surgical care is highly customized based on type of stone and stone burden.

Infertility: Mount Sinai's state-of-the-art use of medications, in vitro fertilization techniques and microsurgical repairs have resulted in high success rates.

Pediatric Urology: Mount Sinai excels in treating urologic problems in newborns, infants, children and adolescents, The Division of Pediatric Urology is the only NYC pediatric urology service to be ranked by *U.S. News & World Report* and noted as "superior" for numerous clinical and family services. Minimally invasive procedures are utilized whenever possible, including robotic assisted surgery.

THE BARBARA AND MAURICE DEANE PROSTATE HEALTH AND RESEARCH CENTER offers a multidisciplinary approach for the assessment and treatment of all aspects of prostate disease, including cancer, benign enlargement, and inflammation. The Center strives to empower the patient and his family and help them better understand various prostate conditions so they can choose the most appropriate treatment for lasting benefits.

Mount Sinai offers a comprehensive **Minimally Invasive Urologic Surgery Program** and is a recognized leader in the greater New York area for performing complex and laparoscopic procedures to treat urologic cancers. Areas of focus also include the treatment and management of stone disease and reconstructive procedures for various urologic cancers and anatomic abnormalities.

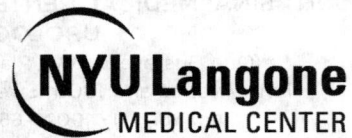

UROLOGY

Urologists at NYU Langone Medical Center continue to pioneer in the surgical and medical treatment of urological disease and are recognized as a top urology program in the country by U.S. News and World Report.

Smilow Comprehensive Prostate Cancer Center
As part of the NCI-designated NYU Cancer Institute, the Center offers care by a team of uro-oncologic surgeons, radiation oncologists, oncologists, naturopathic doctors and radiologists.

Benign Prostatic Diseases
Innovative medical and surgical therapies for benign prostatic disease (as well as for prostatitis (the inflammation of the prostate gland), are offered.

Urological Diseases Center of Excellence
We are focused on discovering novel treatments for bladder and prostate cancer, while exploring how cancer markers can be used to determine how cancer treatments are working.

Female Urology and Incontinence
NYU Langone specializes in urological problems unique to women, including recurrent urinary tract infections, pelvic pain, prolapse and sexual dysfunction.

Latest Minimally Invasive Treatments
The Smilow Comprehensive Prostate Cancer Center, offers advances in prostate imaging and computer biopsy are providing valuable information about tumor location and growth to enable targeted treatment.

Male Sexual Health
Working in collaboration with NYU Langone's Fertility Center, urologists use the latest techniques to enable infertile couples to have children. Treatment is also offered to men suffering from erectile dysfunction and low testosterone.

Pediatric Urology and Reconstructive Surgery
Pediatric urologists focus on urinary system disorders in children from birth to early adults.

Robotic Urological Surgery
The Department's robotic surgery program includes prostate and kidney cancers, as well as female incontinence and urinary tract reconstruction.

Urologic Oncology
Because cancer treatment often requires a collaborative approach, urologists work closely with their colleagues at the NYU Cancer Institute to tailor treatments for each patient.

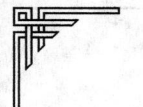

The Best in American Medicine
www.CastleConnolly.com

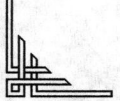
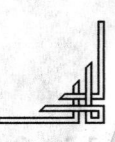

Vascular Surgery

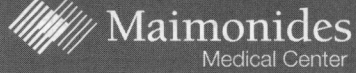

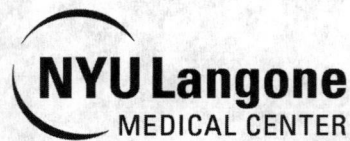

VASCULAR SURGERY

Staffed by one of the largest vascular surgery teams in the country, NYU Langone Medical Center emphasizes both expert patient care and minimally invasive therapies. Physicians have extensive experience performing the most advanced procedures, including stents and angioplasty for carotid artery disease, aortic aneurysm repair and the repair and removal of blockages in arteries throughout the body. In addition to its expertise in arterial disease, NYU Langone is proud to offer one of the few academic Vein Centers in the United States. We specialize in the following areas:

Aortic Pathology
The Medical Center offers minimally invasive surgical solutions as well as treatments for complex aortic problems. Patients usually require no blood transfusions and are able to leave the hospital one or two days after surgery. We are also a training center for endovascular management of abdominal and thoracic aneurysms.

Carotid Artery Disease
NYU Langone remains a leader in both the screening for carotid disease and the prevention of stroke in patients being treated for carotid artery occlusive disease. Our physicians helped pioneer carotid endarterectomy as an open surgical procedure, and played a pivotal role in the development of carotid stenting.

Peripheral Arterial Disease
Vascular surgeons at the Medical Center draw on a wealth of experience in treating peripheral arterial disease (PAD). The team specializes in new and innovative technologies such as laser and "Silverhawk" atherectomy procedures, as well as cryoplasty. Additionally, we offer drug-eluting stents, which are coated with special medicines to prevent scar formation and reocclusion of the stent.

Vascular Screenings
Our physicians are committed to improving public awareness and understanding of vascular disease through preventative screenings. Vascular disease is among the leading causes of death in the U.S., yet is generally asymptomatic until a stroke or aneurysm occurs. Effective screening techniques include ultrasound scans of the aorta, ultrasound scans of the carotid arteries, and advanced blood pressure measurements.

Venous Disease
The Vein Center at NYU Langone is considered an authority in the minimally invasive treatment of venous disease. The Center treats patients with all forms of venous pathology, from venous insufficiency and varicose veins to occlusive disease and deep vein thrombosis.

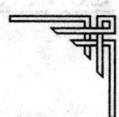

The Best in American Medicine
www.CastleConnolly.com

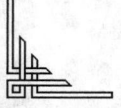
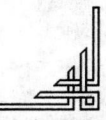

Women's Health

For more information about Women's and Children's Health, call 1-877-Holy-Name. Please mention "Castle Connolly Guide."

Holy Name Medical Center
Women's and Children's Health

718 Teaneck Road
Teaneck, NJ 07666
1-877-Holy-Name
(1-877-465-9626)
www.holyname.org

WOMEN'S AND CHILDREN'S HEALTH DISTINGUISHED FOR SERVICE EXCELLENCE

Recognized for service excellence by both J.D. Power and Associates and HealthGrades®, Holy Name Medical Center's Women's and Children's Health service features superior medical care with a family-centered focus. At the core of Women's and Children's Health is the Medical Center's staff of specialized physicians and mother-baby nurses, whose expertise fosters the highly positive patient and family experience traditionally associated with Holy Name.

A COMPREHENSIVE PROGRAM OF CARE, EDUCATION AND SUPPORT

Holy Name's beautifully designed BirthPlace offers hotel-like accommodations and amenities, supported by advanced monitoring and infant care technology. The BirthPlace is equipped to address emergencies and cesarean sections with round-the-clock anesthesia coverage, and has an intermediate level II special care nursery with board-certified obstetricians, pediatricians, neonatologists and high-risk specialists available 24/7.

Board-certified perinatologists in Maternal-Fetal Medicine work as consultants with obstetricians to treat women who anticipate or are experiencing a complicated or high-risk pregnancy. They advocate a personalized, hands-on approach to patient care, meeting with the patient at every appointment. The medical team includes perinatal sonographers with advanced training and expertise in perinatal ultrasound, and genetic counselors with extensive training in high-risk pregnancy care.

- Private LDRP suites
- On-unit cesarean-section rooms
- Dedicated nursing staff for labor and delivery, postpartum, and special care nursery
- 24-hour access to board-certified anesthesiologists, obstetrician/gynecologists, pediatricians and neonatologists
- Intermediate level II special care nursery
- Maternal-fetal medicine program and perinatal high-risk services
- Genetic counseling
- Central fetal monitoring and maternal monitoring
- Education classes, support groups and infant care hotline
- State-of-the-art electronic security system
- Participant in National Cord Blood Stem Cell Program (umbilical cord blood storage for future lifesaving interventions)

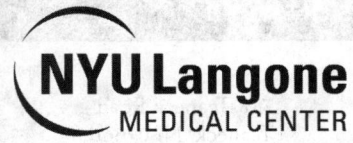

Joan H. Tisch Center for Women's Health
207 East 84th Street *(at 3rd Avenue)*
New York, NY

www.NYULMC.org

646-754-3300

Physician Referral: **888-7-NYU-MED** *(888-769-8633)*

THE JOAN H. TISCH CENTER FOR WOMEN'S HEALTH

About the Joan H. Tisch Center for Women's Health

Because many diseases and conditions impact women differently than men, NYU Langone Medical Center has created the Joan H. Tisch Center for Women's Health. Offering a comprehensive array of primary and specialty care, the Joan H. Tisch Center for Women's Health is New York City's premier destination for healthcare services tailored to the special needs of women. Conveniently located in the heart of Manhattan's Upper East Side, the Center combines NYU Langone's tradition of excellence with a multidisciplinary approach to providing individuals with the best possible medical care. At the Joan H. Tisch Center for Women's Health, the goal is maintaining excellent health and the vehicle is a caring, nurturing environment which understands that women are more than a collection of symptoms and medical conditions.

Expert Staff

Primary and specialty care physicians at the Joan H. Tisch Center for Women's Health have been carefully chosen for their ability to render quality, compassionate care to women. These healthcare professionals are focused on the holistic needs of patients in a state-of-the-art setting that relies heavily on teamwork. As part of a major academic medical institution, the Center is able to draw on additional healthcare resources and innovative research, when the need arises.

Comprehensive Range of Services

The Joan H. Tisch Center for Women's Health offers a wide range of primary and specialty medical care geared to women at a single location. Specialty services include breast health, cardiology, dermatology, endocrinology, ear/nose/throat, gastroenterology, gynecology, internal medicine, mental health, neurology, orthopaedics, plastic surgery, podiatry, pulmonary medicine, rehabilitation medicine, rheumatology, urology, vascular and women's imaging.

Technology Edge

The Joan H. Tisch Center for Women's Health has incorporated sophisticated technology into all levels of the patient experience. This ranges from the Center's informative website to its use of Epic, the Medical Center's up-to-the-minute electronic medical records system. In addition, patients can confidentially view their medical records and test results, as well as make appointment, request prescriptions and communicate with their physicians, through myNYULMC, a secure online service.

Trinitas Regional Medical Center
WOMEN'S SERVICES

225 WILLIAMSON STREET | ELIZABETH, NEW JERSEY 07207
PH 908.994.5138 | WWW.TRINITASRMC.ORG

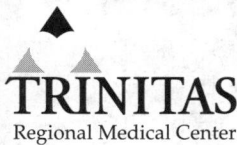

TRINITAS
Regional Medical Center

Trinitas Regional Medical Center offers a number of advanced services just for women that range from the latest in imaging and diagnostic technology, to state-of-the-art, minimally invasive procedures used for hysterectomies and in the treatment of incontinence and prolapse.

WOMEN'S IMAGING CENTER

Our new, technologically advanced, FDA-approved and MQSA (Mammography Quality Standards Act) certified facility provides the services - digital mammography, stereotactic needle biopsy, ultrasound and bone densitometry - that are essential in addressing women's concerns.

The staff in the Women's Imaging Center has had specialized training, and they will work with you and your physician to provide services in a comfortable and professional environment. State-of-the-art digital mammography equipment further enhances the diagnostic quality of the images of the breast tissue and the accuracy of the interpretation of the mammogram. All studies are interpreted by Board Certified Radiologists.

Procedures may be scheduled by calling 908-994-5984.

TREATMENT FOR INCONTINENCE AND PROLAPSE

Trinitas is a pioneer in the latest, minimally invasive procedures for the treatment of female incontinence and vaginal prolapse. A new approach to prolapse includes a single-incision approach that shortens surgical time, minimizes tissue trauma and reduces recovery time. The treatment of incontinence is also accomplished with highly effective, minimally invasive techniques, many

performed for the first time in New Jersey at Trinitas Regional Medical Center. Single-incision techniques involve the placement of an internal supporting sling that is highly effective in eliminating stress incontinence. Procedures are commonly performed on an outpatient basis.

MINIMALLY INVASIVE HYSTERECTOMY

Trinitas Regional Medical Center offers a non-surgical option for women who undergo hysterectomy to treat excessive menstrual or uterine bleeding. Endometrial Ablation involves removing only the lining of a woman's uterus using warmed water.

In the event that surgery is necessary, Trinitas now offers a precise, minimally invasive option for hysterectomy through the use of the da Vinci® Surgical System. The da Vinci system provides surgeons with an alternative to both traditional open surgery and conventional laparoscopy, putting a surgeon's hands at the controls of a state-of-the-art robotic platform. The da Vinci® Surgical System enables surgeons to perform even the most complex and delicate procedures through very small incisions with unmatched precision. Benefits for patients include significantly less pain, less blood loss, less scarring, shorter recovery time, a faster return to normal daily activities and, in many cases, better clinical outcomes.

Wound Care

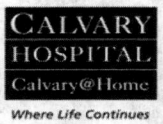
CENTER FOR CURATIVE AND PALLIATIVE WOUND CARE

Founded in 1899, Calvary Hospital is the nation's only acute care specialty hospital dedicated to caring for inpatients with advanced cancer. We serve people of all faith traditions in a restraint-free environment that offers 24/7 visiting hours and extensive bereavement support for families and friends. In addition to inpatient care, we offer outpatient care, home care, hospice, nursing home hospice, and wound care. All Calvary care is guided by our core values of compassion, respect for the dignity of every patient, and non-abandonment of patients and families.

Calvary Wound Care: A Proud Tradition

In the course of caring for people with advanced cancer, Calvary has developed outstanding expertise in the care of complex, intractable wounds. We extend this care to people in the community through our outpatient clinic. In 2004, we established the Center for Curative and Palliative Wound Care, where we treat patients with chronic wounds secondary to diabetes, neuropathy, chronic venous insufficiency, immobility, lymphedema, peripheral vascular disease, cancer, and other inflammatory or hematological disorders that can cause wounds. Since its inception, Calvary's Wound Care Center has recorded more than 36,000 patient visits.

A Personalized Approach

Our personalized approach to wound management goes beyond established curative protocols to address the larger goals of patient care, by seeking to enhance quality of life for patients and families. We strive to relieve the suffering of patients when wounds do not respond to standard interventions, or when demands of treatment are beyond their tolerance or stamina.

The Center for Curative and Palliative Wound Care offers treatment options for chronic wounds such as:

Venous Ulcers	Diabetic Foot Ulcers	Arterial Ulcers
Pressure Ulcers	Inflammatory Wounds	Vasculitic Ulcers
Lymphedema	Sickle Cell Ulcers	Fungating Tumors
Post-op Wounds	Wound Infection	Wounds from Radiation or Chemotherapy

Wound care personnel are available to consult with nursing homes and long-term care facilities on request. Specially trained visiting nurses and therapists provide expert wound care services for patients at home.

We are a community resource for Bronx residents, where the prevalence of Type 2 Diabetes is the highest in New York and among the highest in the country.

Support for Families

Family members often serve as caregivers. Our physicians and nurses strive to build a foundation of trust and open communication with patients and families. We teach family members to clean wounds and change dressings, and we are always available to answer questions or offer guidance about wound care.

Research is integral to the mission of the Center, which is now pursuing a number of protocols focusing on novel treatments for wounds related to diabetes and other disorders.

For information or to refer a patient to the Wound Care Center, please call (718) 518-2577.

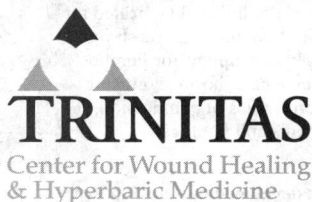

SECTION FIVE

Appendices

Appendix A:
Medical Boards

Intro to ABMS and Osteopathic Specialties

The following pages contain descriptions of the "official" medical specialties, approved by the American Board of Medical Specialists (for M.D.s) or by the American Osteopathic Association (for D.O.s). These are important because they are the only specialties recognized by the official governing boards. There may be physicians who call themselves one kind of specialist or another, but they may not be certified by the "official" boards. There are, in fact, over 100 such "self-designated" boards, some simply groups of physicians interested in a given area of medicine with no qualifications for membership to other groups with very specific qualifications for membership.

It is important for the medical consumer to seek out physicians certified by the ABMS or AOA to assure their doctor has had the appropriate training and passed the board certification exam.

ABMS

The ABMS is an organization of ABMS approved medical specialty boards. The mission of the ABMS is to maintain and improve the quality of medical care by assisting the Member Boards in their efforts to develop and utilize professional and educational standards for the evaluation and certification of physician specialists. The intent of certification of physicians is to provide assurance to the public that a physician specialist certified by a Member Board of the ABMS has successfully completed an approved educational program and evaluation process which includes an examination designed to assess the knowledge, skills, and experience required to provide quality patient care in that specialty. The ABMS serves to coordinate the activities of its Member Boards and to provide information to the public, the government, the profession and its Members concerning issues involving specialization and certification in medicine.

Following is a list of the addresses of the various medical specialty boards approved by the ABMS. Note that there are 24 board organizations for 25 medical specialties. Psychiatry and Neurology share the same board.

Appendix A: Medical Boards

To find out if a physician is certified, consumers can call the individual boards which may charge a fee for the information, or they can contact the ABMS at 866-275-2267 (no fee) or www.abms.org.

American Board of Allergy and Immunology
111 South Independence Mall East
Suite 701
Philadelphia, PA 19106
(215) 592-9466, (866) 264-5568

General Certification in Allergy and Immunology. Certifications awarded since 1989 are valid for 10 years. For those certified prior to 1989 there is no recertification requirement.

American Board of Anesthesiology
4208 Six Forks Rd, Ste 900
Raleigh, NC 27609-5735
(919) 745-2200

General Certification in Anesthesiology; with Special and Added Qualifications in Critical Care Medicine, Hospice & Palliative Medicine, Pain Medicine and Pediatric Anesthesiology. Certifications awarded since 2000 are valid for 10 years.

American Board of Colon and Rectal Surgery
20600 Eureka Road, Suite 600
Taylor, MI 48180
(734) 282-9400

General Certification in Colon and Rectal Surgery. Certifications awarded since 1990 are valid for 10 years.

American Board of Dermatology
Henry Ford Health System
1 Ford Place
Detroit, MI 48202-3450
(313) 874-1088

General Certification in Dermatology; with Special Qualifications in Dermatopathology, and Pediatric Dermatology. Certifications awarded since 1991 are valid for 10 years.

American Board of Emergency Medicine
3000 Coolidge Road
East Lansing, MI 48823-6319
(517) 332-4800

General Certification in Emergency Medicine; with Special and Added Qualifications in Critical Care Medicine, Emergency Medical Services, Hospice & Palliative Medicine, Medical Toxicology, Pediatric Emergency Medicine, Sports Medicine and Undersea and Hyperbaric Medicine. Certifications awarded since 1980 are valid for 10 years.

American Board of Family Practice
1648 McGrathiana Parkway, Suite 550
Lexington, KY 40511
(859) 269-5626, (888) 995-5700

General Certification in Family Practice; with Added Qualifications in Adolescent Medicine, Geriatric Medicine, Hospice & Palliative Medicine, Sleep Medicine and Sports Medicine. Certifications awarded since 1970 are valid for 7 years.

American Board of Internal Medicine
510 Walnut Street, Suite 1700
Philadelphia, PA 19106-3699
(215) 446-3500, (800) 441-ABIM

General Certification in Internal Medicine; with Special Qualifications in Cardiovascular Disease, Endocrinology, Diabetes and Metabolism, Gastroenterology, Hematology, Infectious Disease, Medical Oncology, Nephrology, Pulmonary Disease, and Rheumatology; and Added Qualifications in Adolescent Medicine, Advanced Heart Failure & Transplant Cardiology, Clinical Cardiac Electrophysiology, Critical Care Medicine, Geriatric Medicine, Hospice & Palliative Medicine, Interventional Cardiology, Sleep Medicine, Sports Medicine and Transplant Hepatology. Certifications awarded since 1990 are valid for 10 years.

American Board of Medical Genetics
9650 Rockville Pike
Bethesda, MD 20814-3998
(301) 634-7315

General Certification in Clinical Genetics (MD), Clinical Biochemical Genetics, Clinical Cytogenetics and Clinical Molecular Genetics; with Added Qualifications in Medical Biochemical Genetics, Molecular Genetic Pathology. Certifications awarded since 2002 are valid for 2 years.

Appendix A: Medical Boards

American Board of Neurological Surgery

245 Amity Road, Suite 208
Woodbridge, CT 06525
(713) 441-6015

General Certification in Neurological Surgery. Certifications awarded since 1999 are valid for 10 years.

American Board of Nuclear Medicine

4555 Forest Park Boulevard, Suite 119
St. Louis, MO 63108
(314) 367-2225

General Certification in Nuclear Medicine. Certifications awarded since 1992 are valid for 10 years.

American Board of Obstetrics and Gynecology

2915 Vine Street
Dallas, TX 75204
(214) 871-1619

General Certification in Obstetrics and Gynecology; with Special Qualifications in Gynecologic Oncology, Maternal and Fetal Medicine, Reproductive Endocrinology/Infertility; and Added Qualifications in Female Pelvic Medicine & Reconstructive Surgery, Hospice & Palliative Medicine and Critical Care Medicine. Certifications awarded since 1986 are valid for 6 years.

American Board of Ophthalmology

111 Presidential Boulevard, Suite 241
Bala Cynwyd, PA 19004-1075
(610) 664-1175

General certification in Ophthalmology. Certifications awarded since 1992 are valid for 10 years. For those certified prior to 1992 there is no recertification requirement.

American Board of Orthopaedic Surgery

400 Silver Cedar Court
Chapel Hill, NC 27514
(919) 929-7103

General Certification in Orthopaedic Surgery; with Added Qualification in Hand Surgery and Orthopaedic Sports Medicine. Certifications awarded since 1986 are valid for 10 years.

American Board of Otolaryngology
5615 Kirby Drive, Suite 600
Houston, TX 77005
(713) 850-0399

General Certification in Otolaryngology; with Added Qualifications in Neurotology, Pediatric Otolaryngology, Plastic Surgery within the Head and Neck and Sleep Medicine. Certifications awarded since 2002 are valid for 10 years.

American Board of Pathology
4830 Kennedy Boulevard
Suite 690
Tampa, FL 33609
(813) 286-2444

General Certification in Anatomic and Clinical Pathology, Anatomic Pathology and Clinical Pathology; with Special Qualifications in Blood Banking/Transfusion Medicine, Chemical Pathology, Dermatopathology, Forensic Pathology, Hematology, Medical Microbiology, Molecular Genetic Pathology, Neuropathology and Pediatric Pathology; and Added Qualifications in Clinical Informatics and Cytopathology. Certifications awarded since 1997 are valid for 10 years.

American Board of Pediatrics
111 Silver Cedar Court
Chapel Hill, NC 27514-1651
(919) 929-0461

General Certification in Pediatrics; with Special Qualifications in Adolescent Medicine, Developmental-Behavioral Pediatrics, Neonatal-Perinatal Medicine, Pediatric Cardiology, Pediatric Critical Care Medicine, Pediatric Emergency Medicine, Pediatric Endocrinology, Pediatric Gastroenterology, Pediatric Hematology-Oncology, Pediatric Infectious Diseases, Pediatric Nephrology, Pediatric Pulmonology, and Pediatric Rheumatology; and Added Qualifications in Child Abuse Pediatrics, Hospice & Palliative Medicine, Medical Toxicology, Neurodevelopmental Disabilities, Pediatric Transplant Hepatology, Sleep Medicine and Sports Medicine. Certifications awarded since 1988 valid for 7 years.

Appendix A: Medical Boards

American Board of Physical Medicine and Rehabilitation
3015 Allegro Park Lane, S.W.
Rochester, MN 55902-4139
(507) 282-1776

General Certification in Physical Medicine and Rehabilitation; with Special Qualifications in Pain Medicine, Pediatric Rehabilitation Medicine, and Spinal Cord Injury Medicine; and Added Qualifications in Brain Injury Medicine, Hospice & Palliative Medicine, Neuromuscular Medicine and Sports Medicine. Certifications awarded since 1993 are valid for 10 years.

American Board of Plastic Surgery
Seven Penn Center, Suite 400
1635 Market Street
Philadelphia, PA 19103-2204
(215) 587-9322

General Certification in Plastic Surgery; with Added Qualifications in Hand Surgery and Head & Neck Surgery. Certifications awarded since 1995 are valid for 10-years.

American Board of Preventive Medicine
111 W. Jackson, Suite 1110
Chicago, IL 60604
(312) 939-ABPM [2276]

General Certification in Aerospace Medicine, Occupational Medicine and Public Health and General Preventive Medicine; with Added Qualifications in Clinical Informatics, Medical Toxicology and Undersea and Hyperbaric Medicine. Certifications awarded since 1997 are valid for 10 years.

American Board of Psychiatry and Neurology
2150 E. Lake Cook Road, Suite 900
Buffalo Grove, IL 60089
(847) 229-6500

General Certification in Psychiatry, Neurology and Neurology with Special Qualification in Child Neurology; with Special Qualifications in Child and Adolescent Psychiatry, Epilepsy, Hospice & Palliative Medicine, Pain Medicine and Sleep Medicine; and Added Qualifications in Addiction Psychiatry, Brain Injury Medicine, Clinical Neurophysiology, Epilepsy, Forensic Psychiatry, Geriatric Psychiatry, Hospice & Palliative Medicine, Neurodevelopmental Disabilities, Psychosomatic Medicine and Vascular Neurology. Certifications awarded since 1994 are valid for 10 years.

American Board of Radiology

5441 E. Williams Boulevard, Suite 200
Tucson, AZ 85711
(520) 790-2900

General Certification in Diagnostic Radiology, Medical Physics or Radiation Oncology; with Special Competency in Nuclear Radiology; and Added Qualifications in Hospice & Palliative Medicine, Neuroradiology, Pediatric Radiology and Vascular and Interventional Radiology. Radiological Physics is a non-clinical certification. Certificates are valid for 10 years.

American Board of Surgery

1617 John F. Kennedy Boulevard, Suite 860
Philadelphia, PA 19103-1847
(215) 568-4000

General Certification in Surgery and Vascular Surgery; with Special Qualifications in Pediatric Surgery and Surgery of the Hand; and Added Qualifications in Complex General Surgical Oncology, Hospice & Palliative Medicine and Surgical Critical Care. Certifications awarded since 1976 are valid for 10 years.

American Board of Thoracic Surgery

633 North St. Clair Street, Suite 2320
Chicago, IL 60611
(312) 202-5900

General Certification in Thoracic and Cardiac Surgery; and Added Qualifications in Congenital Cardiac Surgery. Certifications awarded since 1976 are valid for 10 years.

American Board of Urology

600 Peter Jefferson Parkway, Suite 150
Charlottesville, VA 22911
(434) 979-0059

General Certification in Urology; and Added Qualifications in Pediatric Urology. Certifications awarded as of 1985 are valid for 10 years.

Osteopathic

The American Osteopathic Association (AOA) is a member association representing more than 78,000 osteopathic physicians (D.O.s). The AOA serves as the primary certifying body for D.O.s, and is the accrediting agency for all osetopathic medical colleges and healthcare facilities. The AOA's mission is to advance the philosophy and practice of osteopathic medicine by promoting excellence in education, research, and the delivery of quality, cost-effective healthcare within a distinct, unified profession.

American Osteopathic Association
142 E Ontario Street
Chicago, IL 60611

Consumers may call the American Osteopathic Association at (800) 621-1773 or visit the website, www.osteopathic.org, for general certification information.

American Osteopathic Board of Anesthesiology

General certification in Anesthesiology; with Added Qualifications in Critical Care Medicine, and Pain Management. Certifications awarded since 2004 are valid for 10 years. For those certified prior to 2004 there is no recertification requirement.

American Osteopathic Board of Dermatology

General certification in Dermatology; with Added Qualifications in Dermatopathology and Mohs'-Micrographic Surgery. Certifications awarded since 2004 are valid for 10 years.

American Osteopathic Board of Emergency Medicine

General certification in Emergency Medicine; with Added Qualifications in Emergency Medical Services, Medical Toxicology, and Sports Medicine. Certifications awarded since 1994 are valid for 10 years.

American Osteopathic Board of Family Physicians

General certification in Family Practice and Osteopathic Manipulative Treatment (OMT); with Added Qualifications in Geriatric Medicine, Hospice & Palliative Medicine, Sleep Medicine, Sports Medicine and Undersea & Hyperbaric Medicine. Certifications awarded since March 1,1997 are valid for 8 years.

American Osteopathic Board of Internal Medicine

General certification in Internal Medicine; with Special Qualifications in Allergy/Immunology, Cardiology, Endocrinology, Gastroenterology, Hematology, Infectious Disease, Nephrology, Oncology, Pulmonary Disease, Rheumatology; with Added Qualifications in Addiction Medicine, Critical Care Medicine, Clinical Cardiac Electrophysiology, Hospice & Palliative Medicine, Geriatric Medicine, Interventional Cardiology, Sleep Medicine, Sports Medicine and Undersea & Hyperbaric Medicine. Certifications awarded since 1993 are valid for 10 years.

American Osteopathic Board of Neurology and Psychiatry

General certification in Neurology and Psychiatry; with Special Qualifications in Child/Adolescent Psychiatry and Child/Adolescent Neurology; with Added Qualifications in Addiction Medicine, Geriatric Psychiatry, Hospice & Palliative Medicine, Neurophysiology, and Sleep Medicine. Certifications awarded since 1995 are valid for 10 years.

American Osteopathic Board of Neuromusculoskeletal Medicine

General certification in Neuromusculoskelatal Medicine & Osteopathic Manipulative Medicine; with Added qualifications in Sports Medicine.

American Osteopathic Board of Nuclear Medicine

General certification in Nuclear Medicine. Certifications awarded since 1995 are valid for 10 years. This certification is no longer issued.

American Osteopathic Board of Obstetrics and Gynecology

General certification in Obstetrics and Gynecology; with Special Qualifications in Gynecologic Oncology; Maternal and Fetal Medicine and Reproductive Endocrinology. Certifications awarded since June 2002 are valid for 6 years.

American Osteopathic Board of Ophthalmology and Otolaryngology - Head & Neck Surgery

General certification in Ophthalmology, Otolaryngology, Facial Plastic Surgery and Otolaryngology/Facial Plastic Surgery; with Added Qualifications in Otolaryngic Allergy and Sleep Medicine. Certifications awarded in Ophthalmology since 2000 are valid for 10 years. For those certified prior to 2000 there is no recertification requirement. Certifications awarded in Otolaryngology and/or Otolaryngology/Facial Plastic Surgery since 2002 are valid for 10 years.

American Osteopathic Board of Orthopaedic Surgery

General certification in Orthopaedic Surgery; with Added Qualifications in Hand Surgery. Certifications awarded since 1994 are valid for 10 years.

American Osteopathic Board of Pathology

General certification in Laboratory Medicine, Anatomic Pathology and Anatomic Pathology and Laboratory Medicine; with Special Qualifications in Forensic Pathology; and with Added Qualifications in Dermatopathology. Certifications awarded since 1995 are valid for 10 years.

Appendix A: Medical Boards

American Osteopathic Board of Pediatrics

General certification in Pediatrics with Special Qualifications in Adolescent and Young Adult Medicine, Neonatology, Pediatric Allergy/Immunology and Pediatric Endocrinology; with Added Qualifications in Sports Medicine. Certifications awarded since 1995 are valid for 7 years.

American Osteopathic Board of Physical Medicine and Rehabilitation Medicine

General certification in Physical Medicine and Rehabilitation; with Added Qualifications in Hospice & Palliative Medicine and Sports Medicine. Certifications awarded since 2004 are valid
for 10 years.

American Osteopathic Board of Preventive Medicine

General certification in Preventive Medicine/Aerospace Medicine, Preventive Medicine/Occupational-Environmental Medicine and Preventive Medicine/Public Health; with Added Qualifications in Undersea & Hyperbaric Medicine. Certifications awarded since 1994 are valid for 10 years.

American Osteopathic Board of Proctology

General certification in Proctology. Certifications awarded since 2004 are valid for 10 years.

American Osteopathic Board of Radiology

General certification in Diagnostic Radiology and Radiation Oncology; with Added Qualifications in Angiography & Interventional Radiology, Neuroradiology, Pediatric Radiology and Vascular & Interventional Radiology. Certifications awarded since 2002 are valid for 10 years.

American Osteopathic Board of Surgery

General certification in General Vascular Surgery, Surgery, Neurological Surgery, Plastic and Reconstructive Surgery, Thoracic Cardiovascular Surgery, Urological Surgery; with Added Qualifications in Surgical Critical Care. Certifications awarded since 1997 are valid for 10 years.

Appendix B:
Self-Designated Medical Specialties

This list of self-designated medical specialty groups was obtained from the American Board of Medical Specialties. However, it is important to point out that these groups are not recognized by the ABMS, the governing board for the recognized twenty-four medical specialty boards (listed in Appendix A).

The organizations listed below range from highly organized groups that are attempting to formalize training and certification in their field to informal groups interested in a particular aspect of medicine.

If you wish to obtain information from any of these groups you will have to do some detective work. Because so many are informal, the location, phone and mailing addresses change frequently, depending upon the person who is functioning as secretary or administrator.

The best way to track down one of these groups is to consult the doctor listings to find a doctor who has expressed a special interest in that field, and call his or her office. You might also call a nearby academic health center in the area to see if they have a faculty or staff member known to be involved in that particular medical interest. If that fails, take the same approach with your community hospital.

A

Abdominal Surgeons

Acupuncture Medicine

Addiction Medicine

Addictionology

Adolescent Psychiatry

Aesthetic Plastic Surgery

Alcoholism and Other Drug
        Dependencies (AMSAODD)

Algology (Chronic Pain)

Alternative Medicine

Ambulatory Anesthesia

Ambulatory Foot Surgery

Anesthesia

Arthroscopic Surgery

Arthroscopy (Board of North America)

B

Bariatric Medicine

Bionic Psychology

Bloodless Medicine & Surgery

C

Chelation Therapy

Chemical Dependence

Clinical Chemistry

Clinical Ecology

Clinical Medicine and Surgery

Clinical Neurology

Clinical Neurophysiology

Clinical Neurosurgery

Clinical Nutrition

Clinical Orthopaedic Surgery

Clinical Pharmacology

Clinical Polysomnography

Clinical Psychiatry

Clinical Psychology

Clinical Toxicology

Cosmetic Plastic Surgery

Cosmetic Surgery

Council of Non-Board Certified Physicians

Critical Care in Medicine & Surgery

D

Disability Analysis

Disability Evaluating Physicians

E

Electrodiagnostic Medicine

Electroencephalography

Electromyography & Electrodiagnosis

Environmental Medicine

Epidemiology (College)

Eye Surgery

F

Facial Cosmetic Surgery

Facial Plastic & Reconstructive Surgery

Family Practice, Certification

Forensic Examiners

Forensic Psychiatry

Forensic Toxicology

H

Hand Surgery

Head, Facial & Neck Pain & TMJ Orthopaedics

Health Physics

Homeopathic Physicians

Homeotherapeutics

Hypnotic Anesthesiology, National Board for

I

Independent Medical Examiners

Industrial Medicine & Surgery

Insurance Medicine

International Cosmetic & Plastic
        Facial Reconstructive Standards

Interventional Radiology

L

Laser Surgery
Law in Medicine
Longevity Medicine/Surgery

M

Malpractice Physicians
Maxillofacial Surgeons
Medical Accreditation (American Federation for)
Medical Hypnosis
Medical Laboratory Immunology
Medical-Legal Analysis of Medicine & Surgery
Medical Legal & Workers
      Comp. Medicine & Surgery
Medical-Legal Consultants
Medical Management
Medical Microbiology
Medical Preventics (Academy)
Medical Psychotherapists
Medical Toxicology
Microbiology (Medical Microbiology)
Military Medicine
Mohs' Micrographic Surgery &
      Cutaneous Oncology

N

Neuroimaging
Neurologic & Orthopaedic Dental
      Medicine and Surgery
Neurological & Orthopaedic Medicine
Neurological & Orthopaedic Surgery
Neurological Microsurgery
Neurology
Neuromuscular Thermography
Neuro-Orthopaedic Dental Medicine
Neuro-Orthopaedic Electrodiagnosis
Neuro-Orthopaedic Laser Surgery
Neuro-Orthopaedic Psychiatry
Neuro-Orthopaedic Thoracic Medicine
Neurorehabilitation
Nutrition

O

Orthopaedic Medicine
Orthopaedic Microneurosurgery
Otorhinolaryngology

P

Pain Management (American Academy of)
Pain Management Specialties
Pain Medicine
Palliative Medicine
Percutaneous Diskectomy
Plastic Esthetic Surgeons
Prison Medicine
Professional Disability Consultants
Psychiatric Medicine
Psychiatry (American National Board of)
Psychoanalysis (American Examining
      Board in)
Psychological Medicine (International)

Q

Quality Assurance & Utilization Review

R

Radiology & Medical Imaging
Rheumatologic Surgery
Rheumatological & Reconstructive Medicine
Ringside Medicine & Surgery

S

Skin Specialists
Sleep Medicine (Polysomnography)
Spinal Cord Injury
Spinal Surgery
Sports Medicine
Sports Medicine/Surgery

T

Toxicology
Trauma Surgery
Traumatologic Medicine & Surgery
Tropical Medicine

U

Ultrasound Technology
Urologic Allied Health Professionals
Urological Surgery

W

Weight Reduction Medicine

APPENDIX C:
Hospital Listings

The following is an alphabetical listing of all hospitals that have at least one Castle Connolly Top Doctor in this guide. Institutions listed in **Bold** are profiled in this Guide in association with Castle Connolly's Partnership for Excellence program. The abbreviations as they appear in the listings are in italics below. Due to the many changes taking place in the hospital industry, the names on this list may have changed subsequent to publication of this guide.

Bayonne Medical Center		(201) 858-5000
Bayonne Med Ctr		
29 E 29th St	Bayonne, NJ 07002	HUDSON

Bayshore Community Hospital		(732) 739-5900
Bayshore Community Hosp		
727 North Beers Street	Holmdel, NJ 07733	MONMOUTH

Bellevue Hospital Center		(212) 562-1000
Bellevue Hosp Ctr		
462 First Avenue	New York, NY 10016	NEW YORK

Bergen Regional Medical Center		(201) 967-4000
Bergen Regl Med Ctr		
230 East Ridgewood Avenue	Paramus, NJ 07652	BERGEN

Beth Israel Medical Center - Kings Highway Division		(718) 252-3000
Beth Israel Med Ctr- Kings Hwy Div		
3201 Kings Highway	Brooklyn, NY 11234	KINGS

Beth Israel Medical Center - Milton & Caroll Petrie Division		(212) 420-2000
Beth Israel Med Ctr - Petrie Division		
First Avenue at 16th Street	New York, NY 10003	NEW YORK

Blythedale Children's Hospital		(914) 592-7555
Blythedale Children's Hosp		
95 Bradhurst Avenue	Valhalla, NY 10595	WESTCHESTER

Bridgeport Hospital		(203) 384-3000
Bridgeport Hosp		
267 Grant St	Bridgeport, CT 06610	FAIRFIELD

Bronx Children's Psychiatric Center | (718) 239-3600
Bronx Children's Psych Ctr
1000 Waters Place | Bronx, NY 10461 | BRONX

Bronx Lebanon Hospital Center | (718) 590-1800
Bronx Lebanon Hosp Ctr
1276 Fulton Ave | Bronx, NY 10457 | BRONX

Bronx Psychiatric Center | (718) 931-0600
Bronx Psych Ctr
1500 Waters Place | Bronx, NY 10461 | BRONX

Brookdale University Hospital Medical Center | (718) 240-5000
Brookdale Univ Hosp Med Ctr
One Brookdale Plaza | Brooklyn, NY 11212 | KINGS

Brookhaven Memorial Hospital & Medical Center | (631) 654-7100
Brookhaven Meml Hosp & Med Ctr
101 Hospital Road | Patchogue, NY 11772 | SUFFOLK

Brooklyn Hospital Center-Downtown | (718) 250-8000
Brooklyn Hosp Ctr-Downtown
121 DeKalb Avenue | Brooklyn, NY 11201 | KINGS

Burke Rehabilitation Hospital | (914) 597-2500
Burke Rehab Hosp
785 Mamaroneck Avenue | White Plains, NY 10605 | WESTCHESTER

Calvary Hospital | (718) 518-2000
Calvary Hosp
1740 Eastchester Road | Bronx, NY 10461 | BRONX

Capital Health Medical Center - Hopewell | (609) 303-4000
Capital Health Med Ctr - Hopewell
One Capital Way | Pennington, NJ 08534 | MERCER

Capital Health Regional Medical Center | (609) 394-6000
Capital Health Regl Med Ctr
750 Brunswick Avenue | Trenton, NJ 08638-4174 | MERCER

CentraState Medical Center | (732) 431-2000
CentraState Med Ctr
901 West Main Street | Freehold, NJ 07728 | MONMOUTH

Children's Hospital of NJ at Newark | (973) 926-7000
Chldns Hosp NJ at Newark
201 Lyons Ave N New Jersey | Newark, NJ 07112 | ESSEX

Children's Hospital of Philadelphia   (215) 590-1000
Chldns Hosp of Philadelphia
34th St & Civic Center Blvd   Philadelphia, PA 19104   PHILADELPHIA

Children's Specialized Hospital   (908) 233-3720
Children's Specialized Hosp
150 New Providence Rd   Mountainside, NJ 07092   UNION

Chilton Hospital   (973) 831-5000
Chilton Hosp
97 West Parkway   Pompton Plains, NJ 07444   MORRIS

Christ Hospital - Jersey City   (201) 795-8200
Christ Hosp - Jersey City
176 Palisade Avenue   Jersey City, NJ 07306   HUDSON

Clara Maass Medical Center   (973) 450-2000
Clara Maass Med Ctr
One Clara Maass Drive   Belleville, NJ 07109   ESSEX

Community Hospital - Dobbs Ferry   (914) 693-0700
Comm Hosp - Dobbs Ferry
128 Ashford Ave   Dobbs Ferry, NY 10522-1924   WESTCHESTER

Coney Island Hospital   (718) 616-3000
Coney Island Hosp
2601 Ocean Parkway   Brooklyn, NY 11235   KINGS

Danbury Hospital   (203) 739-7000
Danbury Hosp
24 Hospital Avenue   Danbury, CT 06810   FAIRFIELD

Eastern Long Island Hospital   (631) 477-1000
Eastern Long Island Hosp
201 Manor Place   Greenport, NY 11944   SUFFOLK

Elmhurst Hospital Center   (718) 334-4000
Elmhurst Hosp Ctr
79-01 Broadway   Elmhurst, NY 11373   QUEENS

Englewood Hospital & Medical Center   (201) 894-3000
Englewood Hosp & Med Ctr
350 Engle Street   Englewood, NJ 07631   BERGEN

Flushing Hospital Medical Center   (718) 670-5000
Flushing Hosp Med Ctr
4500 Parsons Blvd   Flushing, NY 11355   QUEENS

Forest Hills Hospital (718) 830-4000
Forest Hills Hosp
102-01 66th Rd   Forest Hills, NY 11375   QUEENS

Four Winds Hospital (914) 763-8151
Four Winds Hosp
800 Cross River Road   Katonah, NY 10536   WESTCHESTER

Franklin Hospital (516) 256-6000
Franklin Hosp
900 Franklin Avenue   Valley Stream, NY 11580   NASSAU

Glen Cove Hospital (516) 674-7300
Glen Cove Hosp
101 St Andrew's Ln   Glen Cove, NY 11542   NASSAU

Good Samaritan Hospital - Suffern (845) 368-5000
Good Samaritan Hosp - Suffern
255 Lafayette Ave   Suffern, NY 10901   ROCKLAND

Good Samaritan Hospital Medical Center - West Islip (631) 376-4444
Good Samaritan Hosp Med Ctr - West Islip
1000 Montauk Highway   West Islip, NY 11795   SUFFOLK

Gracie Square Hospital (212) 988-4400
Gracie Square Hosp
420 E 76th St   New York, NY 10021   NEW YORK

Greenwich Hospital (203) 863-3000
Greenwich Hosp
Five Perryridge Road   Greenwich, CT 06830   FAIRFIELD

Griffin Hospital (203) 735-7421
Griffin Hosp
130 Division St   Derby, CT 06418-1377   NEW HAVEN

Hackensack University Medical Center (551) 996-2000
Hackensack Univ Med Ctr
30 Prospect Avenue   Hackensack, NJ 07601   BERGEN

Hackensack University Medical Center-Mountainside (973) 429-6000
Hackensack UMC-Mountainside
1 Bay Ave   Montclair, NJ 07042   ESSEX

Harlem Hospital Center (212) 939-1000
Harlem Hosp Ctr
506 Lenox Avenue   New York, NY 10037   NEW YORK

Helen Hayes Hospital — (845) 786-4000
Helen Hayes Hosp
51-55 Route 9W North   West Haverstraw, NY 10993   ROCKLAND

Hoboken University Medical Center — (201) 418-1000
Hoboken Univ Med Ctr - Hoboken
308 Willow Ave   Hoboken, NJ 07030   HUDSON

Holy Name Medical Center — (201) 833-3000
Holy Name Med Ctr
718 Teaneck Road   Teaneck, NJ 07666-4281   BERGEN

Hospital for Special Surgery — (212) 606-1000
Hosp For Special Surgery
535 East 70th Street   New York, NY 10021   NEW YORK

Hudson Valley Hospital Center — (914) 737-9000
Hudson Valley Hosp Ctr
1980 Crompond Road   Cortland Manor, NY 10567   WESTCHESTER

Huntington Hospital — (631) 351-2000
Huntington Hosp
270 Park Avenue   Huntington, NY 11743   SUFFOLK

Interfaith Medical Center — (718) 613-4000
Interfaith Med Ctr
1545 Atlantic Avenue   Brooklyn, NY 11213   KINGS

Jacobi Medical Center — (718) 918-5000
Jacobi Med Ctr
1400 Pelham Parkway South   Bronx, NY 10461   BRONX

Jamaica Hospital Medical Center — (718) 206-6000
Jamaica Hosp Med Ctr
8900 Van Wyck Expressway   Jamaica, NY 11418   QUEENS

James J. Peters VA Medical Center-Bronx — (718) 584-9000
James J. Peters VA Med Ctr-Bronx
130 W Kingsbridge Rd   Bronx, NY 10468   BRONX

Jersey City Medical Center — (201) 915-2000
Jersey City Med Ctr
355 Grand Street   Jersey City, NJ 07302   HUDSON

Jersey Shore University Medical Center — (732) 775-5500
Jersey Shore Univ Med Ctr
1945 Route 33   Neptune, NJ 07753   MONMOUTH

JFK Medical Center - Edison   (732) 321-7000
JFK Med Ctr - Edison
65 James St   Edison, NJ 08820   MIDDLESEX

John T Mather Memorial Hospital   (631) 473-1320
John T Mather Meml Hosp
75 N Country Rd   Port Jefferson, NY 11777   SUFFOLK

Kessler Institute for Rehabiitation - Saddle Brook   (201) 368-6000
Kessler Inst for Rehab - Saddle Brook
300 Market St   Saddle Brook, NJ 07663   BERGEN

Kessler Institute for Rehabilitation - Chester   (973) 252-6300
Kessler Inst for Rehab - Chester
201 Pleasant Hill Rd   Chester, NJ 07930   MORRIS

Kessler Institute for Rehabilitation - West Orange   (973) 731-3600
Kessler Inst for Rehab - W Orange
1199 Pleasant Valley Way   West Orange, NJ 07052-1499   ESSEX

Kings County Hospital Center   (718) 245-3131
Kings County Hosp Ctr
451 Clarkson Avenue   Brooklyn, NY 11203   KINGS

Kingsbrook Jewish Medical Center   (718) 604-5000
Kingsbrook Jewish Med Ctr
585 Schenectady Avenue   Brooklyn, NY 11203   KINGS

Lawrence Hospital Center   (914) 787-1000
Lawrence Hosp Ctr
55 Palmer Avenue   Bronxville, NY 10708   WESTCHESTER

Lenox Hill Hospital   (212) 434-2000
Lenox Hill Hosp
100 East 77th Street   New York, NY 10021   NEW YORK

Lenox Hill Hospital (Manhattan Eye, Ear & Throat Hosp)   (212) 838-9200
Lenox Hill Hosp (Manh Eye, Ear & Throat Hosp)
210 East 64th Street   New York, NY 10021   NEW YORK

Lincoln Medical & Mental Health Center   (718) 579-5000
Lincoln Med & Mental Hlth Ctr
234 East 149th St.   Bronx, NY 10451   BRONX

Long Beach Medical Center   (516) 897-1000
Long Beach Med Ctr
455 East Bay Drive   Long Beach, NY 11561   NASSAU

Long Island Jewish Medical Center   (718) 470-7000
Long Island Jewish Med Ctr
270-05 76th Avenue   New Hyde Park, NY 11040   NASSAU

Lutheran Medical Center - Brooklyn   (718) 630-7000
Lutheran Med Ctr - Brooklyn
150 55th Street   Brooklyn, NY 11220   KINGS

Maimonides Medical Center   (718) 283-6000
Maimonides Med Ctr
4802 Tenth Avenue   Brooklyn, NY 11219   KINGS

Meadowlands Hospital Medical Center   (201) 392-3100
Meadowlands Hosp Med Ctr
55 Meadowland Parkway   Secaucus, NJ 07094   HUDSON

Memorial Sloan-Kettering Cancer Center   (212) 639-2000
Meml Sloan-Kettering Cancer Ctr
1275 York Avenue   New York, NY 10021   NEW YORK

Mercy Medical Center - Rockville Centre   (516) 705-2525
Mercy Med Ctr - Rockville Centre
1000 North Village Avenue   Rockville Centre, NY 11570   NASSAU

Metropolitan Hospital Center - NY   (212) 423-6262
Metropolitan Hosp Ctr - NY
1901 First Avenue   New York, NY 10029   NEW YORK

Milford Hospital   (203) 876-4000
Milford Hosp
300 Seaside Ave   Milford, CT 06460   NEW HAVEN

Monmouth Medical Center   (732) 222-5200
Monmouth Med Ctr
300 2nd Ave   Long Branch, NJ 07740-6300   MONMOUTH

Montefiore Medical Center-Einstein Campus, NY   (718) 904-2000
Montefiore Med Ctr-Einstein Campus, NY
1825 Eastchester Road   Bronx, NY 10461   BRONX

Montefiore Medical Center-Moses Campus, NY   (718) 920-4321
Montefiore Med Ctr-Moses Campus, NY
111 East 210 Street   Bronx, NY 10467   BRONX

Montefiore Medical Center-Wakefield Campus, NY   (718) 920-9000
Montefiore Med Ctr-Wakefield Campus, NY
600 E 233rd St   Bronx, NY 10466   BRONX

Morgan Stanley Children's Hospital of NewYork-Presbyterian, NY (212) 305-5437
Morgan Stanley Children's Hosp of NY-Presby, NY
3959 Broadway   New York, NY 10032   NEW YORK

Morristown Medical Center   (973) 971-5000
Morristown Med Ctr
100 Madison Avenue   Morristown, NJ 07960-6095   MORRIS

Mount Sinai Hospital of Queens   (718) 932-1000
Mount Sinai Hosp of Queens
25-10 30th Avenue   Long Island City, NY 11102   QUEENS

Mount Sinai Medical Center   (212) 241-6500
Mount Sinai Med Ctr
One Gustave L. Levy Pl   New York, NY 10029   NEW YORK

Mount Vernon Hospital   (914) 664-8000
Mount Vernon Hosp
12 N Seventh Ave   Mount Vernon, NY 10550   WESTCHESTER

Nassau University Medical Center   (516) 572-0123
Nassau Univ Med Ctr
2201 Hempstead Tpke   East Meadow, NY 11554   NASSAU

New York Community Hospital   (718) 692-5300
New York Comm Hosp
2525 Kings Highway   Brooklyn, NY 11229   KINGS

New York Downtown Hospital   (212) 312-5000
NY Downtown Hosp
170 William Street   New York, NY 10038   NEW YORK

New York Eye & Ear Infirmary   (212) 979-4000
New York Eye & Ear Infirm
310 East 14th Street   New York, NY 10003   NEW YORK

New York Hospital Queens   (718) 670-2000
NY Hosp Queens
56-45 Main Street   Flushing, NY 11355   QUEENS

New York Methodist Hospital   (718) 780-3000
New York Methodist Hosp
506 Sixth Street   Brooklyn, NY 11215   KINGS

New York State Psychiatric Institute   (212) 543-5000
NY State Psychiatric Inst
1051 Riverside Dr   New York, NY 10032   NEW YORK

New York Westchester Square Medical Center   (718) 430-7300
NY Westchester Sq Med Ctr
2475 St Raymond Ave   Bronx, NY 10461   BRONX

Newark Beth Israel Medical Center   (973) 926-7000
Newark Beth Israel Med Ctr
201 Lyons Ave   Newark, NJ 07112   ESSEX

NewYork-Presbyterian/Columbia University Medical Center, NY   (212) 305-2500
NY-Presby/Columbia Univ Med Ctr, NY
622 W 168th St   New York, NY 10032   NEW YORK

NewYork-Presbyterian/The Allen Hospital, NY   (212) 932-4000
NY-Presby Hosp/The Allen Hosp
5141 Broadway   New York, NY 10034   NEW YORK

NewYork-Presbyterian/Weill Cornell Medical Center, NY   (212) 746-5454
NY-Presby/Weill Cornell Med Ctr, NY
525 E 68th St   New York, NY 10021   NEW YORK

NewYork-Presbyterian/Westchester Division, NY   (914) 997-5780
NY-Presby/Westchester Div, NY
21 Bloomingdale Rd   White Plains, NY 10605   WESTCHESTER

North Shore University Hospital   (516) 562-0100
N Shore Univ Hosp
300 Community Dr   Manhasset, NY 11030   NASSAU

North Shore-LIJ Health System   (516) 465-2550
NS-LIJ Hlth Sys
125 Community Drive   Great Neck, NY 11021   NASSAU

Northern Westchester Hospital   (914) 666-1200
Northern Westchester Hosp
400 East Main Street   Mount Kisco, NY 10549   WESTCHESTER

Norwalk Hospital   (203) 852-2000
Norwalk Hosp
34 Maple Street   Norwalk, CT 06856   FAIRFIELD

Nyack Hospital   (845) 348-2000
Nyack Hosp
160 North Midland Avenue   Nyack, NY 10960   ROCKLAND

NYU Hospital for Joint Diseases   (212) 598-6000
NYU Hosp For Joint Diseases
301 East 17th Street   New York, NY 10003   NEW YORK

NYU Langone Medical Center   (212) 263-7300
NYU Langone Med Ctr
550 First Avenue   New York, NY 10016   NEW YORK

NYU Rusk Institute   (212) 263-1999
NYU Rusk Inst
400 East 34th Street   New York, NY 10016   NEW YORK

Ocean Medical Center   (732) 840-2200
Ocean Med Ctr
425 Jack Martin Blvd   Brick, NJ 08724   OCEAN

Overlook Medical Center   (908) 522-2000
Overlook Med Ctr
99 Beauvoir Ave   Summit, NJ 07901   UNION

Palisades Medical Center   (201) 854-5000
Palisades Med Ctr
7600 River Road   North Bergen, NJ 07047   HUDSON

Peconic Bay Medical Center   (631) 548-6000
Peconic Bay Med Ctr
1300 Roanoke Avenue   Riverhead, NY 11901   SUFFOLK

Phelps Memorial Hospital Center   (914) 366-3000
Phelps Meml Hosp Ctr
701 N Broadway   Sleepy Hollow, NY 10591   WESTCHESTER

Plainview Hospital   (516) 719-3000
Plainview Hosp
888 Old Country Rd   Plainview, NY 11803   NASSAU

Putnam Hospital Center   (845) 279-5711
Putnam Hosp Ctr
670 Stoneleigh Ave   Carmel, NY 10512   PUTNAM

Queens Hospital Center - Jamaica   (718) 883-3000
Queens Hosp Ctr - Jamaica
82-68 164th Street   Jamaica, NY 11432   QUEENS

Raritan Bay Medical Center - Old Bridge Division   (732) 360-1000
Raritan Bay Med Ctr - Old Bridge Div
One Hospital Plaza   Old Bridge, NJ 08857   MIDDLESEX

Raritan Bay Medical Center - Perth Amboy Division   (732) 442-3700
Raritan Bay Med Ctr - Perth Amboy
530 New Brunswick Avenue   Perth Amboy, NJ 08861-3654   MIDDLESEX

Richmond University Medical Center   (718) 818-1234
Richmond Univ Med Ctr
355 Bard Ave   Staten Island, NY 10310-1699   RICHMOND

Riverview Medical Center   (732) 741-2700
Riverview Med Ctr
1 Riverview Plaza   Red Bank, NJ 07701   MONMOUTH

Robert Wood Johnson University Hospital - Hamilton   (609) 586-7900
Robert Wood Johnson Univ Hosp Hamilton
1 Hamilton Health Pl   Hamilton, NJ 08690   MERCER

Robert Wood Johnson University Hospital - New Brunswick   (732) 828-3000
Robert Wood Johnson Univ Hosp - New Brunswick
1 Robert Wood Johnson Pl   New Brunswick, NJ 08903   MIDDLESEX

Robert Wood Johnson University Hospital at Rahway   (732) 381-4200
Robert Wood Johnson Univ Hosp at Rahway
865 Stone St   Rahway, NJ 07065   UNION

Rockland Psychiatric Center   (845) 359-1000
Rockland Psych Ctr
140 Old Orangeburg Rd   Orangeburg, NY 10962-1196   ROCKLAND

Saint Barnabas Medical Center   (973) 322-5000
Saint Barnabas Med Ctr
94 Old Short Hills Rd   Livingston, NJ 07039-5672   ESSEX

Saint Joseph's Medical Center - Yonkers   (914) 378-7000
Saint Joseph's Med Ctr - Yonkers
127 South Broadway   Yonkers, NY 10701   WESTCHESTER

Saint Michael's Medical Center   (973) 877-5000
Saint Michael's Med Ctr
111 Central Avenue Blvd   Newark, NJ 07102   ESSEX

Saint Vincent Catholic Medical Centers - St. Vincent's Westchester   (914) 967-6500
St. Vincent Cath Med Ctrs - Westchester
275 North Street   Harrison, NY 10528   WESTCHESTER

Silver Hill Hospital   (203) 966-3561
Silver Hill Hosp
208 Valley Rd   New Canaan, CT 06840-3899   FAIRFIELD

Smilow Cancer Hospital at Yale-New Haven   (203) 688-2000
Smilow Cancer Hosp at Yale-New Haven
20 York St   New Haven, CT 06510   FAIRFIELD

Somerset Medical Center   (908) 685-2200
Somerset Med Ctr
110 Rehill Ave   Somerville, NJ 08876   SOMERSET

Sound Shore Medical Center - Westchester   (914) 632-5000
Sound Shore Med Ctr - Westchester
16 Guion Pl   New Rochelle, NY 10801   WESTCHESTER

South Nassau Communities Hospital   (516) 632-3000
South Nassau Comm Hosp
1 Healthy Way   Oceanside, NY 11572   NASSAU

South Oaks Hospital   (631) 264-4000
S Oaks Hosp
400 Sunrise Hwy   Amityville, NY 11701   SUFFOLK

Southampton Hospital   (631) 726-8200
Southampton Hosp
240 Meeting House Ln   Southampton, NY 11968   SUFFOLK

Southside Hospital   (631) 968-3000
Southside Hosp
301 E Main St   Bay Shore, NY 11706   SUFFOLK

St. Barnabas Hospital - Bronx   (718) 960-9000
St. Barnabas Hosp - Bronx
4422 Third Avenue   Bronx, NY 10457   BRONX

St. Catherine's of Siena Medical Center   (631) 862-3000
St. Catherine's of Siena Med Ctr
50 Rt 25A   Smithtown, NY 11787   SUFFOLK

St. Charles Hospital   (631) 474-6000
St. Charles Hosp
200 Belle Terre Rd   Port Jefferson, NY 11777   SUFFOLK

St. Clare's Hospital - Denville   (973) 625-6000
St. Clare's Hosp - Denville
25 Pocono Road   Denville, NJ 07834   MORRIS

St. Clare's Hospital at Sussex   (973) 702-2600
St. Clare's Hosp-Sussex
20 Walnut St   Sussex, NJ 07461   SUSSEX

St. Clare's Hospital-Dover   (973) 989-3000
St. Clare's Hosp-Dover
400 W Blackwell St   Dover, NJ 07801   MORRIS

St. Francis Hospital - The Heart Center   (516) 562-6000
St. Francis Hosp - The Heart Ctr
100 Port Washington Boulevard   Roslyn, NY 11576   NASSAU

St. Francis Medical Center - Trenton   (609) 599-5000
St. Francis Med Ctr - Trenton
601 Hamilton Avenue   Trenton, NJ 08629   MERCER

St. John's Episcopal Hospital - South Shore   (718) 869-7000
St. John's Epis Hosp - S Shore
327 Beach 19th Street   Far Rockaway, NY 11691   QUEENS

St. John's Riverside Hospital-Andrus Pavilion   (914) 964-4444
St. John's Riverside Hosp-Andrus Pavil
967 N Broadway   Yonkers, NY 10701   WESTCHESTER

St. Joseph's Hospital-Nassau   (516) 579-6000
St. Joseph's Hosp-Nassau
4295 Hempstead Turnpike   Bethpage, NY 11714   NASSAU

St. Joseph's Regional Medical Center - Paterson   (973) 754-2000
St. Joseph's Regl Med Ctr - Paterson
703 Main St   Paterson, NJ 07503   PASSAIC

St. Joseph's Wayne Hospital   (973) 942-6900
St. Joseph's Wayne Hosp
224 Hamburg Turnpike   Wayne, NJ 07470   PASSAIC

St. Lawrence Rehabilitation Center   (609) 896-9500
St. Lawrence Rehab Ctr
2381 Lawrencville Rd   Lawrencville, NJ 08648   MERCER

St. Luke's - Roosevelt Hospital Center - Roosevelt Division   (212) 523-4000
St. Luke's - Roosevelt Hosp Ctr - Roosevelt Div
1000 Tenth Avenue   New York, NY 10019   NEW YORK

St. Luke's - Roosevelt Hospital Center - St Luke's Hospital   (212) 523-4000
St. Luke's - Roosevelt Hosp Ctr - St Luke's Hosp
1111 Amsterdam Ave   New York, NY 10025   NEW YORK

St. Luke's-Cornwall Hospital of Newburgh   (845) 561-4400
St. Luke's Newburgh
70 Dubois St   Newburgh, NY 12550   ORANGE

St. Mary's Hospital - Passaic   (973) 365-4300
St. Mary's Hosp - Passaic
350 Boulevard   Passaic, NJ 07055   PASSAIC

St. Mary's Hospital - Waterbury   (203) 709-6000
St. Mary's Hosp - Waterbury
56 Franklin St   Waterbury, CT 06706-1200   FAIRFIELD

St. Peter's University Hospital   (732) 745-8600
St. Peter's Univ Hosp
254 Easton Ave   New Brunswick, NJ 08901-1780   MIDDLESEX

St. Vincent's Medical Center - Bridgeport   (203) 576-6000
St. Vincent's Med Ctr - Bridgeport
2800 Main St   Bridgeport, CT 06606   FAIRFIELD

Stamford Hospital   (203) 276-1000
Stamford Hosp
30 Shelburne Rd   Stamford, CT 06902   FAIRFIELD

Staten Island University Hospital - North   (718) 226-9000
Staten Island Univ Hosp - North
475 Seaview Avenue   Staten Island, NY 10305   RICHMOND

Staten Island University Hospital - South   (718) 226-2000
Staten Island Univ Hosp - South
375 Seguine Avenue   Staten Island, NY 10309   RICHMOND

Steven and Alexandra Cohen Children's Medical Center of New York   (718) 470-3000
Steven & Alexandra Cohen Chldn's Med Ctr of NY
269-01 76th Ave   New Hyde Park, NY 11040   NASSAU

Stony Brook University Medical Center   (631) 444-4000
Stony Brook Univ Med Ctr
101 Nicolls Rd   Stony Brook, NY 11794-8410   SUFFOLK

Summit Oaks Hospital   (908) 522-7000
Summit Oaks Hosp
19 Prospect St   Summit, NJ 07902   UNION

SUNY Downstate Medical Center (University Hospital of Brooklyn)   (718) 270-1000
SUNY Downstate Med Ctr (Univ Hosp of Bklyn)
450 Clarkson Ave   Brooklyn, NY 11203   KINGS

SUNY Downstate Medical Center at LongIsland College Hospital   (718) 780-1000
SUNY Downstate Med Ctr at LICH
339 Hicks Street   Brooklyn, NY 11201   KINGS

Syosset Hospital   (516) 496-6500
Syosset Hosp
221 Jericho Tpke   Syosset, NY 11791-4536   NASSAU

Trinitas Regional Medical Center (908) 994-5000
Trinitas Reg Med Ctr
225 Williamson St Elizabeth, NJ 07207 UNION

University Hospital-UMDNJ-Newark (973) 972-4300
Univ Hosp-UMDNJ—Newark
150 Bergen St Newark, NJ 07103-2406 ESSEX

University Medical Center of Princeton at Plainsboro (609) 853-7000
Univ Med Ctr Princeton at Plainsboro
One Plainsboro Rd Plainsboro, NJ 08536 MIDDLESEX

VA Connecticut Healthcare System-West Haven Campus (203) 932-5711
VA Conn Hlthcre Sys-W Haven Campus
950 Campbell Ave West Haven, CT 06516 NEW HAVEN

VA NY Harbor Healthcare System-Brooklyn Campus (718) 630-6600
VA NY Harbor Hlthcr Sys-Brooklyn Campus
800 Poly Pl Bay Ridge, NY 11209 KINGS

VA NY Harbor Healthcare System-Manhattan Campus (212) 686-7500
VA NY Harbor Hlthcare Sys-Manhattan Campus
423 E 23rd St New York, NY 10010 NEW YORK

Valley Hospital (201) 447-8000
Valley Hosp
223 N Van Dien Ave Ridgewood, NJ 07450-2736 BERGEN

Waterbury Hospital (203) 573-6000
Waterbury Hosp
64 Robbins St Waterbury, CT 06721 NEW HAVEN

Westchester Medical Center (914) 493-7000
Westchester Med Ctr
95 Grasslands Road Valhalla, NY 10595 WESTCHESTER

White Plains Hospital (914) 681-0600
White Plains Hosp
Davis Ave at E Post Rd White Plains, NY 10601 WESTCHESTER

Wills Eye Hospital (215) 928-3000
Wills Eye Hosp
840 Walnut St Philadelphia, PA 19107-5598 PHILADELPHIA

Winthrop University Hospital (516) 663-0333
Winthrop Univ Hosp
259 1st St Mineola, NY 11501 NASSAU

Woodhull Medical & Mental Health Center   (718) 963-8000
Woodhull Med & Mental Hlth Ctr
760 Broadway   Brooklyn, NY 11206   KINGS

Wyckoff Heights Medical Center   (718) 963-7272
Wyckoff Heights Med Ctr
374 Stockholm Street   Brooklyn, NY 11237   KINGS

Yale-New Haven Hospital   (203) 688-4242
Yale-New Haven Hosp
20 York St   New Haven, CT 06510   NEW HAVEN

Yale-New Haven Hospital St Raphael Campus   (203) 789-3000
Yale-New Haven Hosp - St Raphael Campus
1450 Chapel Street   New Haven, CT 06511   NEW HAVEN

Zucker Hillside Hospital   (718) 470-8100
Zucker Hillside Hosp
75-59 263rd St   Glen Oaks, NY 11004   QUEENS

Appendix D:
Selected Resources

GENERAL RESOURCES

AMERICAN AMBULANCE ASSOCIATION (AAA)
The American Ambulance Association represents emergency and non-emergency medical transportation providers, advocating high quality pre-hospital care and keeping these providers aware of legislation and news that may affect them.

8400 Westpark Drive
Second Floor
McLean, VA 22102

800-523-4447
703-610-9018
fax 703-610-0210
www.the-aaa.org/

AMERICA'S HEALTH INSURANCE PLANS (AHIP)
America's Health Insurance Plans is a national trade association representing nearly 1,300 member companies providing health benefits to more than 200 million Americans.

601 Pennsylvania Ave, NW
South Building Suite 500
Washington, DC 20004

202-778-3200
fax: 202-331-7487
www.ahip.org/

AMERICAN BOARD OF MEDICAL SPECIALTIES (ABMS)
The ABMS is the authoritative body for the recognition of medical specialties, coordinating 24 medical specialty boards (including 25 medical specialties) and providing information on the board certification of doctors.

222 N LaSalle St, Ste 1500
Chicago, IL 60601

312-436-2600
fax 312-436-2700
www.abms.org

AMERICAN HOSPITAL ASSOCIATION (AHA)
A national health advocacy organization, the AHA represents hospitals and healthcare networks in legislative and regulatory matters. In 1973 the AHA adopted the Patient Bill of Rights to help patients understand their rights and responsibilities.

155 N Wacker Drive
Chicago, IL 60606

800-424-4301 or 312-422-3000
fax 312-422-4796
www.aha.org/

325 7th St. NW
Washington, DC 20004

800-424-4301 or 202-638-1100
fax 202-626-3245

AMERICAN MEDICAL ASSOCIATION (AMA)
The AMA is an association that maintains information on physicians practicing throughout the nation. Healthcare consumers can use their database to check the location, licensing, education and specialty of many doctors in the United States.

515 North State Street
Chicago, IL 60654

800-621-8335
www.ama-assn.org/

CENTER FOR MEDICAL CONSUMERS

Provides volume and outcome data on certain medical procedures performed in New York state.

239 Thompson St.
New York, NY 10012

212-674-7105
fax 212-674-7100

CenterForMedicalConsumers@gmail.com

www.medicalconsumers.org

CENTERS FOR DISEASE CONTROL AND PREVENTION (CDC)

Part of the Department of Health and Human Services, the CDC's mission is to prevent and manage diseases and illnesses. Its website contains information on a range of illnesses and the research being pursued to manage them. It also provides free faxed reports on disease risk and prevention in various parts of the world.

Public Inquiries/MASO
Mailstop E11
1600 Clifton Road
Atlanta, GA 30333

1-800-CDC-INFO

toll free number for international travelers 877 FYI-TRIP or 404-639-3534
fax information service for international travelers 888-232-3299
www.cdc.gov/netinfo.htm

THE CENTERWATCH CLINICAL TRIALS LISTING SERVICE

Profiles centers conducting clinical research by therapeutic area and geographic region, including more than 41,000 international industry and government-sponsored clinical trials and new FDA approved drug therapies, as well as 5,200 clinical trials that are actively recruiting patients.

10 Winthrop Square, Fl 5
Boston, MA 02110

617-948-5100
fax 617-948-5101
www.centerwatch.com

HEALTH CARE CHOICES

Provides information on volume and outcomes of certain medical procedures performed in hospitals in various states throughout the country.

P.O. Box 21039
Columbus Circle Station
New York, NY 10023

212-724-9395
www.healthcarechoices.org

INTERNATIONAL ASSOCIATION FOR MEDICAL ASSISTANCE TO TRAVELLERS (IAMAT)

IAMAT is a non-profit organization that disseminates information on health and sanitary conditions worldwide. Membership is free but donations are appreciated. Members will receive a membership card making them eligible to access English speaking physicians all over the world. The organization also provides information on immunization requirements, malaria, and other tropical diseases, and sanitary and climactic conditions around the world. For information, send request in writing.

1623 Military Road #279
Niagra Falls, NY 14304-1745

716-754-4883
www.iamat.org

JOINT COMMISSION ON ACCREDITATION OF HEALTHCARE ORGANIZATIONS

The Joint Commission (JCAHO) is an independent, not-for-profit organization, which evaluates the quality and safety of care for nearly 17,000 health care organizations. To maintain and earn accreditation, organizations must have an extensive on-site review by a team of JCAHO health care professionals, at least once every three years. JCAHO is governed by a board that includes physicians, nurses, and consumers. JCAHO sets the standards by which health care quality is measured in America and around the world.

One Renaissance Boulevard
Oakbrook Terrace, IL 60181

630-792-5800
fax 630-792-5005
www.jointcommission.org

MEDIC ALERT FOUNDATION

The Medic Alert Foundation (a non-profit organization) provides an "ID tag" engraved with personal medical facts, as well as a 24-hour emergency response center which can release additional personal medical details. Membership is $45/year and members need to purchase the "ID tag" which sells for as low as $35.

2323 Colorado Avenue
Turlock, CA 95382

888-633-4298
Fax 209-669-2450
www.medicalert.org

MEDLINE

One Medline Place
Mundelein, IL 60060

1-800-MEDLINE (800-633-5463)
fax 1-800-351-1512
www.medline.com

A medical database including millions of medical references and abstracts from thousands of scientific and medical journals.

THE NATIONAL CANCER INSTITUTE (NCI)

Part of the NIH, the NCI sponsors cancer clinical trials at more than 100 sites in the United States. Trials are carried out in major medical research centers, such as teaching hospitals, as well as in community hospitals, specialized medical clinics and even in doctors' offices.

Clinical Studies Support Center (CSSC)
6116 Executive Boulevard
Bethesda, MD 20892-8322

800-4-CANCER (800-422-6237)
www.nci.nih.gov
www.cancer.gov
cancergovstaff@mail.nih.gov

NATIONAL CENTER FOR COMPLEMENTARY AND ALTERNATIVE MEDICINE CLEARINGHOUSE (NCCAMC)

The NCCAMC facilitates the evaluation of alternative medical treatment modalities to help determine their effectiveness and bring alternative medicine into mainstream medicine. This agency does not provide referrals.

PO Box 7923
Gaithersburg, MD 20898

888-644-6226
fax 866-464-3616
www.nccam.nih.gov
info@nccam.nih.gov

NATIONAL CONSUMERS LEAGUE (NCL)

NCL is a private, nonprofit consumer advocacy organization. NCL strives to investigate, educate, and advocate on a variety of issues including healthcare. Membership is $35 annually, but individuals can also write to the organization for a list of publications that non-members can purchase.

1701 K Street, NW, Suite 1200
Washington, DC 20006

202-835-3323
fax 202-835-0747
www.nclnet.org
info@nclnet.org

THE NATIONAL INSTITUTES OF HEALTH (NIH)

An organization operated by the U.S. government, the NIH operates its own hospital at which the care provided is usually related to clinical studies its researchers are undertaking. Information about the Warren G. Magnuson Clinical Center is also available.

Patient Recruitment Referral Center
9000 Rockville Pike
Bethesda, MD 20892

800-411-1222 or 301-496-4000
www.nih.gov
www.clinicaltrials.gov
nihinfo@od.nih.gov

NATIONAL INSURANCE INFORMATION INSTITUTE

The National Insurance Information Institute Helpline advises consumers on how to choose an insurance company or broker. It also offers an analysis of life insurance and assists in insurance complaints.

110 William Street
New York, NY 10038

800-942-4242 or 212-346-5500
www.iii.org

THE PATIENT ADVOCATE FOUNDATION

A national non-profit organization that provides consultation, referrals and case management to patients to ensure that they are not denied access to healthcare, insurance coverage, employment and public assistance programs during an illness. In particular, the organization maintains comprehensive information on cancer treatment options that are available to consumers through a separate website: www.oncology.com.

421 Butler Farm Rd
Hampton, VA 23666

800-532-5274
fax 757-873-8999
www.patientadvocate.org/
help@patientadvocate.org

PEOPLE'S MEDICAL SOCIETY

The People's Medical Society, a nonprofit organization, is focused on educating the healthcare consumer about healthcare issues and medical rights. Their website provides information on useful books and publications as well as the latest healthcare developments.

P.O. Box 868
Allentown, PA 18105

610-770-1670
www.peoplesmed.org
cbi@peoplesmed.org

PERSONS UNITED LIMITING SUBSTANDARDS AND ERRORS IN HEALTHCARE (P.U.L.S.E.)

A support group for the survivors of medical malpractice and substandard healthcare, this nonprofit group also advocates patient education and patient-doctor communication.

PO Box 353
Wantagh, NY 11793-0353

800-96-pulse (800-967-8573) or
516-579-4711
fax: 516-520-8105
www.PULSEamerica.org
www.PULSEofNY.org
pulse516@aol.com

Colorado Office

719-250-1286
PULSECOLO@YAHOO.COM

PUBLIC CITIZEN'S HEALTH AND RESEARCH GROUP

A non-profit organization, the Public Citizen's Group acts as a watchdog agency by advocating accountability and the open use of doctors' disciplinary backgrounds.

1600 20th Street NW
Washington, DC 20009

202-588-1000
www.citizen.org/hrg/

VERITAS MEDICINE

An organization that allows individuals to perform confidential, personalized searches of their clinical trials database and to access information on new treatment and drug options. The text is submitted by Harvard-affiliated doctors.

11 Cambridge Center
Cambridge, MA 02142

617-234-1500

Appendix E:
State Agencies

While there is a wealth of information available through these state agencies, much of it is not user-friendly. Complicated contractual agreements and other legal documents contain information that might prove to be valuable, providing a consumer can locate it and then review it with some understanding. Often a department will suggest that a consumer visit the office for guidance in reviewing the documents. However, some of these agencies provide useful information on doctors, hospitals, and HMOs. They may also offer statistical reports and consumer-oriented studies.

CONNECTICUT

DOCTORS

Department of Public Health State of Connecticut
Practitioner Licensing and Investigations Section
410 Capitol Avenue, MS#12MQA
P.O. Box 340308
Hartford, CT 06134-0308
(860) 509-7603
www.dph.state.ct.us
Attn: Physician renewal of verification

Department of Public Health State of Connecticut
Legal Office
410 Capitol Avenue, MS#12LEG
P.O. Box 340308
Hartford, CT 06134-0308
(860) 509-7600

HOSPITALS

Department of Public Health State of Connecticut
Facilities Licensing and Investigations Section
410 Capitol Avenue, MS#12HSR
P.O. Box 340308
Hartford, CT 06134-0308
(860) 509-7400

Appendix E

HMOs

Department of Insurance (Location address)
153 Market Street, 7th Floor
Hartford, CT 06103-0816
(860) 297-3800

Department of Insurance (Mailing address)
P.O. Box 816
Hartford, CT 06142-0816
(860) 297-3800

www.ct.gov/cid/site/default.asp

Office of Health Care Access
410 Capitol Avenue, MS#13HCA
P.O. Box 340308
Hartford, CT 06134-0308
800-797-9688

TDD 860-418-7001

www.ct.gov/ohca/site/default.asp

NEW JERSEY

DOCTORS

New Jersey State Board of Medical Examiners (Location address)
140 East Front Street, 2nd Floor
Trenton, NJ 08608
(609) 826-7100

New Jersey State Board of Medical Examiners (Mailing address)
P.O. Box 360
Trenton, NJ 08625-0360

http://www.state.nj.us/lps/ca/bme/index.html
bme@dca.lps.state.nj.us

HOSPITALS

Department of Health
Division of Health Facilities Evaluation and Licensing
P.O. Box 360
120 S Stockton Street
Trenton, NJ 08625-0360
(609) 292-7837

http://www.nj.gov/health/

HMOs

Department of Health
Division of Health Facilities Evaluation and Licensing
P.O. Box 360
120 S Stockton Street
Trenton, NJ 08625-0360
(609) 292-7837

Department of Health
Office of Managed Care
20 West State St, 11th Fl
P.O. Box 325
Trenton, NJ 08625
(609) 292-5427

http://www.state.nj.us/dobi/managed.htm

Department of Banking & Insurance (Location address)
Division of Insurance, Life and Health Division
Managed Healthcare Bureau
20 West State St
P.O. Box 325
Trenton, NJ 08625
(609) 292-7272

http://www.state.nj.us/dobi/

Department of Banking & Insurance (Mailing address)
Division of Insurance, Life and Health Division
Managed Healthcare Bureau
20 West State St
P.O. Box 325
Trenton, NJ 08625
(609) 292-7272

Office of Managed Care Hotline: 1-888-393-1062
Office of managed Care Fax: (609) 633-0807
Consumer Protection Services Main Line: (609) 292-7272

NEW YORK

DOCTORS

New York State Department of Health
Office of Professional Medical Conduct
433 River Street, Suite 303
Troy, NY 12180
(518) 402-0836
www.health.state.ny.us
opmc@health.state.ny.us

New York State Education Department
Division of Professional Licensing Services
State Education Building - 2nd floor
89 Washington Avenue
Albany, NY 12234
(518) 474-3817
http://www.op.nysed.gov/home.html

op4info@mail.nysed.gov

Hospitals

Office of Health Systems Management
Corning Tower, Fl 14
Empire State Plaza
Albany, NY 12237
(518) 474-7028

New York State Department of Health
Bureau of Biometrics
Corning Tower, Room 2348
Empire State Plaza
Albany, NY 12237
(518) 474-3189

HMOs

New York State Insurance Department
Health Bureau
99 Washington Ave.
Albany, NY 12257
(518) 474-6272

New York State Insurance Department
Life Policy Bureau
1 Commerce Plaza, Suite 1910
Albany, NY 12257
(518) 474-4552

New York State Department of Health
Office of Managed Care
Corning Tower, Room 1911
Albany, NY 12237
(518) 473-4178

New York State Department of Health
Records Access Office
Corning Tower, Room 2364
Empire State Plaza
Albany, NY 12237
(518) 486-9144

Appendix F:
Sources of Quality Data on Hospitals

U.S. NEWS AND WORLD REPORT

U.S. News & World Report has been the nation's leading source of information on hospital rankings since 1990. The Best Hospitals rankings evaluate medical centers on their competence in high-stakes situations. Their annual feature on Best Hospitals has become the standard in the field where rankings are concerned and is heavily anticipated and utilized by consumers and members of the health care profession. Castle Connolly teamed up with *U.S. News & World Report* in July 2011 to bring its listing of Top Doctors online to www.usnews.com/health in conjunction with the Top Hospitals rankings. There, consumers can search the full Castle Connolly database of nearly 30,000 Top Doctors across the nation.

WWW.WHYNOTTHEBEST.ORG

WhyNotTheBest.org was created and is maintained by The Commonwealth Fund, a private foundation working toward a high performance health system. It is a free resource for health care professionals and consumers interested in tracking performance on various measures of health care quality. It enables organizations to compare their performance against that of peer organizations, against a range of benchmarks and over a given period of time. Case studies and improvement tools spotlight successful improvement strategies of the nation's top performers. A regional map shows performance at the county, state and national levels. This site also includes process-of-care measures, patient satisfaction measures, readmission rates, mortality rates and average reimbursement rates. All of these performance measures are publicly reported on the Centers for Medicare and Medicaid Services website, Hospital Compare, and include data from nearly all U.S. hospitals.

THE LEAPFROG GROUP

The Leapfrog Group, http://www.leapfroggroup.org/cp, started in 1998 by a group of large employers. The Leapfrog Hospital Survey compares hospitals' performance on the national standards of safety, quality and efficiency - areas of healthcare that are most relevant to consumers. Hospitals that participate in The Leapfrog Hospital Survey achieve hospital-wide improvements that translate into saving millions of lives and cutting costs for hospitals and consumers. Leapfrog's survey results are later used to inform key employees on purchasing strategies.

HOSPITAL COMPARE

The Hospital Compare website was created through the efforts of the Centers for Medicare & Medicaid Services (CMS), an agency of the U.S. Department of Health and Human Services (DHHS), along with the Hospital Quality Alliance (HQA). The HQA was established to promote reporting on hospital quality of care. The HQA consists of organizations that represent consumers, hospitals, doctors and nurses, employers, accrediting organizations and Federal agencies. The information on this website can be used by patients requiring hospital care. This information helps the consumer and health care providers to compare the quality of care provided in participating hospitals. This information not only helps one to make good decisions about health care, but also encourages hospitals to improve the quality of the care that they provide to their communities. This website can be found at: http://www.hospitalcompare.hhs.gov/hospital-search.aspx or http://bit.ly/jdvCzW

SECTION SIX

Indices

The Best in American Medicine
www.CastleConnolly.com

Subject Index

A

Academic Medical Center 14, 21-22, 71

Alternative medicine 43-45, 51

Alternative therapy 40, 45

American Board of Medical Specialties (ABMS) 4, 14, 16, 18, 41, 75, 77, 81, 82

American Board of Radiology 17, 19

American Medical Association (AMA) 32, 33, 51, 53

American Medical News 25

B

Bachelor of Medicine 8

Baseline tests 32, 34

Board certification 12, 17-19, 23, 41, 53, 73-75, 79, 81

Board eligibility 19

C

Capitation 60, 63, 64

Chiropractors 8

Chronic condition 51

Clinical trials 39, 45-46

Community hospitals 12, 21-22

Compendium of Certified Medical Specialists 16

Continuing Medical Education (CME) 18

Credentialing 14, 20

Cultural sensitivity 26

D

E

F

G

H

Health Maintenance Organization (HMO) 58-67

Hippocratic Oath xiii

Hospital appointment 15, 20-21

Hospital referral services 7

I

Indemnity insurance 14, 32

IPA 60, 62-63

J

J.D. Power and Associates 66

L

LEXIS/NEXIS 54, 58

Licensed nurse practitioners 24

Licensure 14, 17, 24

Louis Harris Associates 66

Lupus 4, 6

Lyme disease 4, 6, 23

M

Malpractice insurance 21

Managed care 4, 6, 20, 32-33, 42, 51, 60-66

Medical history 34-35

Medical records 30, 35, 48, 52-53

Medical school faculty appointment 22

Medical schools 16-17, 21-22, 26

Subject Index

Medical societies 2, 7

MedStat Group 66

Midlevel providers 24-25

Multi-specialty group 24

N

National Practitioner Data Bank 50, 54

New England Journal of Medicine 44

O

Office and practice arrangements 15, 24

P

Physician's assistants 24

Placebo 40, 45

Podiatrists 8

PPO 60-63, 66

Preventive medicine 4, 6

Primary care physicians 3-5

PSO 60, 63

Psychologists 8

Public Citizen Health Research Group 50, 54

Q

Questionable doctors 53

R

S

T

U

W

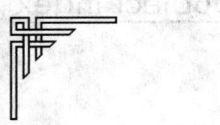

The Best in American Medicine
www.CastleConnolly.com

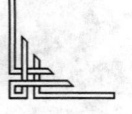

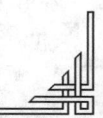

Specialty & Special Expertise Index

This index lists the areas that the physicians listed in the Guide have identified as their "special expertise." They are specific elements of disease, procedures, techniques and treatments for which these physicians are best known and are referred patients. Each doctor's medical specialty is also included.

Spec	Name	St	Pg

A

Abdominal Imaging

Spec	Name	St	Pg
DR	Baer, J	NY	160
DR	Brancaccio, W	NY	588
DR	Lubat, E	NJ	698
DR	McClennan, B	CT	945
DR	Megibow, A	NY	163
DR	Newhouse, J	NY	163
DR	Prince, M	NY	164
DR	Toth, P	NJ	699
DR	Weinreb, J	CT	945
DR	Wolf, E	NY	389

Abdominal Wall Reconstruction

Spec	Name	St	Pg
PlS	Stahl, R	CT	958
PS	Weinberg, G	NY	408
S	Deitch, E	NJ	762
S	Mandel, M	NJ	887

Abdominoplasty

Spec	Name	St	Pg
PlS	Almeyda, E	NY	312
PlS	Feinberg, J	NY	555
PlS	Friedman, D	NY	314
PlS	Gallagher, P	NY	555
PlS	Gardner, J	NJ	884
PlS	Godfrey, P	NY	315
PlS	Goldstein, R	NY	410
PlS	Kolker, A	NY	316
PlS	Lesesne, C	NY	316
PlS	Matarasso, A	NY	316
PlS	Newman, F	CT	929
PlS	Newman, S	NY	668
PlS	Perrotti, J	NY	317
PlS	Perry, A	NJ	865
PlS	Pitman, G	NY	317
PlS	Restifo, R	CT	958
PlS	Wells, S	NY	320

Abuse/Neglect

Spec	Name	St	Pg
AM	Diaz, A	NY	130
AM	Johnson, R	NJ	738
Ger	Lachs, M	NY	182

Acanthamoeba Keratitis

Spec	Name	St	Pg
Oph	Auran, J	NY	248

Achalasia

Spec	Name	St	Pg
Ge	Lambroza, A	NY	176

Acne

Spec	Name	St	Pg
D	Almeida, L	NJ	832
D	Aprile, G	NY	515
D	Aranoff, S	NY	151
D	Berson, D	NY	152
D	Blank, E	NJ	767
D	Bruckstein, R	NY	515
D	Davis, J	NY	153
D	Deitz, M	NY	428
D	Demar, L	NY	153
D	Dolitsky, C	NY	515
D	Eisenberg, R	NJ	874
D	Falcon, R	NY	515
D	Feldman, P	NY	428
D	Fox, A	NJ	860
D	Fried, S	NY	696
D	Giardina-Beckett, M	NJ	696
D	Goldberg, N	NY	626
D	Hefter, H	NY	516
D	Hisler, B	NY	516
D	Huh, J	NY	587
D	Lerman, J	NY	627
D	Lukash, B	NY	627
D	Maier, H	NJ	850
D	Notaro, A	NY	587
D	Rosen, D	NY	387
D	Rozanski, R	NJ	741
D	Scherl, S	NJ	697
D	Seidenberg, R	NY	158
D	Stillman, M	NY	628
D	Sweeney, E	NJ	697
D	Tanzer, F	NJ	850
D	Tom, J	NY	588
D	Treiber, R	NY	628
D	Waldorf, D	NY	573
D	Walther, R	NY	159
D	Wattenberg, D	NY	160
D	Wechsler, A	NY	160
D	Wexler, P	NY	160
Ped	Panzner, E	NJ	883

Acne & Rosacea

Spec	Name	St	Pg
D	Baldwin, H	NY	427
D	Danziger, S	NY	428
D	Felderman, L	NY	153
D	Gold, J	NJ	849
D	Liftin, A	NJ	741

Acoustic Neuroma

Spec	Name	St	Pg
NS	Davis, R	NY	595
NS	Golfinos, J	NY	228
NS	Gutin, P	NY	228
NS	Hodosh, R	NJ	879
NS	Jafar, J	NY	228
NS	Post, K	NY	229
NS	Sisti, M	NY	230
NS	Stieg, P	NY	230
Oto	Chandrasekhar, S	NY	279
Oto	Feghali, J	NY	404
Oto	Kohan, D	NY	281
Oto	Kveton, J	CT	954
Oto	Kwartler, J	NJ	881
Oto	Linstrom, C	NY	283
Oto	Roland, J	NY	284
Oto	Selesnick, S	NY	285
Oto	Storper, I	NY	286

Acupuncture

Spec	Name	St	Pg
FMed	Kligler, B	NY	169
IM	Ehrlich, M	NY	200
IM	Gazzara, P	NY	494
IM	Lu, B	NY	437
IM	Strauss, M	NY	206
N	Lazar, M	NJ	800
PM	Agin, C	NY	545
PM	Lu, G	NY	660
PM	Moqtaderi, F	NY	288
PM	Ngeow, J	NY	288
PMR	Aaronson, B	CT	928
PMR	Agri, R	NJ	783
PMR	Atakent, P	NY	457
PMR	Dillard, J	NY	309
PMR	Grant, L	CT	928
PMR	Snowball, H	CT	929
Rhu	Meed, S	NY	348
SM	Hamner, D	NY	351

Acute Coronary Syndromes

Spec	Name	St	Pg
Cv	Dangas, G	NY	136
Cv	Menegus, M	NY	385

ADD/ADHD

Spec	Name	St	Pg
ChAP	Abright, A	NY	144
ChAP	Bartlett, J	NJ	740
ChAP	Bird, H	NY	145
ChAP	Boorady, R	NY	145
ChAP	Burkes, L	NY	145
ChAP	Carlson, G	NY	585
ChAP	Coffey, B	NY	145
ChAP	Cohen, L	NY	623
ChAP	Gandhi, L	NY	586
ChAP	Greenberg, R	NJ	873
ChAP	Hertzig, M	NY	145
ChAP	Hirsch, G	NY	146
ChAP	Holzer, B	NY	426
ChAP	Kafantaris, V	NY	473

Specialty & Special Expertise Index

Specialty & Special Expertise Index

Specialty & Special Expertise Index

Spec	Name	St	Pg
Management			
VascS	Riles, T	NY	379
Aneurysm-Cerebral			
NRad	Bello, J	NY	401
NRad	Berenstein, A	NY	239
NRad	Keller, I	NJ	800
NRad	Meyers, P	NY	240
NS	Abrahams, J	NY	648
NS	Bederson, J	NY	226
NS	Chiurco, A	NJ	780
NS	Flamm, E	NY	399
NS	Holtzman, R	NY	534
NS	Jafar, J	NY	228
NS	Langer, D	NY	534
NS	Moore, F	NJ	711
NS	Murali, R	NY	649
NS	Nosko, M	NJ	799
NS	Patel, A	NY	229
NS	Riina, H	NY	229
NS	Solomon, R	NY	230
NS	Woo, H	NY	595
Aneurysm-Thoracic Aortic			
T&CS	Abrol, S	NY	465
T&CS	Elefteriades, J	CT	962
T&CS	Hartman, A	NY	566
T&CS	Stelzer, P	NY	366
T&CS	Tranbaugh, R	NY	367
Angina			
Cv	Askanas, A	NY	134
Cv	Lucariello, R	NY	385
Cv	Rothman, H	NJ	694
Cv	Schulman, I	NY	142
Cv	Siskind, S	NY	473
Cv	Sklaroff, H	NY	143
Cv	Tartaglia, J	NY	622
Angiography-Coronary			
Cv	Pappas, T	NY	512
Cv	Zaloom, R	NY	426
IC	Abittan, M	NY	529
IC	Moses, J	NY	208
IC	Syed, T	NJ	706
Angioplasty			
Cv	Cleman, M	CT	942
Cv	Coppola, J	NY	135
Cv	Green, S	NY	510
Cv	Klapholz, M	NJ	739
Cv	Landers, D	NJ	693
Cv	Sherman, W	NY	142
IC	Shanahan, A	NJ	778
VascS	Manno, J	NJ	734
VIR	Crystal, K	NY	569
VIR	Rundback, J	NJ	733

Spec	Name	St	Pg
Angioplasty & Stent Placement			
Cv	Dangas, G	NY	136
Cv	Jauhar, R	NY	511
Cv	Kosinski, E	CT	897
Cv	Shamoon, F	NJ	739
Cv	Stroh, J	NJ	860
Cv	Tuohy, E	CT	898
IC	Angeli, S	NJ	706
IC	Brener, S	NY	438
IC	Kodali, S	NY	207
IC	Lituchy, A	NY	529
IC	Malpeso, J	NY	495
IC	Moses, J	NY	208
IC	Ong, L	NY	594
IC	Shani, J	NY	439
IC	Sharma, S	NY	208
IC	Stone, G	NY	208
IC	Syed, T	NJ	706
Angiosarcoma			
S	Bernik, S	NY	353
Ankle Reconstruction			
OrS	Levine, D	NY	270
Ankle Replacement & Revision			
OrS	Greisberg, J	NY	268
OrS	O'Malley, M	NY	272
OrS	Sands, A	NY	274
Anorectal Disorders			
CRS	Arnell, T	NY	149
CRS	Brandeis, S	NY	149
CRS	Eisenstat, T	NJ	791
CRS	Greenwald, M	NY	514
CRS	Lee, S	NY	150
CRS	Moseson, M	NY	515
CRS	Moskowitz, R	NJ	832
CRS	Procaccino, J	NY	515
CRS	Smithy, W	NY	587
Anorectal Malformations			
PS	Velcek, F	NY	304
Anterior Segment Surgery			
Oph	DeBroff, B	CT	919
Oph	DeLuca, J	NJ	714
Oph	Doctor, L	CT	919
Oph	Sherman, S	NY	449
Anterior Segment Trauma/Reconstruction			
Oph	Florakis, G	NY	252
Antibiotic Resistance			
Inf	Birch, T	NJ	704
Inf	Chapnick, E	NY	435

Spec	Name	St	Pg
Inf	McManus, E	NJ	835
Inf	McMeeking, A	NY	195
Inf	Weisholtz, S	NJ	705
PInf	Slavin, K	NJ	720
Antiphospholipid Syndrome (APS)			
Rhu	Belmont, H	NY	346
Rhu	Furie, R	NY	562
Rhu	Salmon, J	NY	349
Anxiety & Depression			
ChAP	Bird, H	NY	145
ChAP	Silverman, A	NY	624
FMed	Ziering, T	NJ	861
Psyc	Almeleh, J	NY	321
Psyc	Aronoff, M	NY	321
Psyc	Brodie, J	NY	322
Psyc	Bronheim, H	NY	323
Psyc	Goldberg, J	NY	458
Psyc	Kahn, J	NY	670
Psyc	Kranzler, E	NY	326
Psyc	Mellman, L	NY	328
Psyc	Mueller, F	CT	930
Psyc	Muskin, P	NY	328
Psyc	Osei-Tutu, J	NY	411
Psyc	Pfeffer, C	NY	329
Psyc	Sacks, M	NY	330
Psyc	Sadock, V	NY	331
Psyc	Schwartz, B	NY	411
Psyc	Shapiro, B	CT	931
Psyc	Sofair, J	NJ	842
Psyc	Tancredi, L	NY	333
Psyc	Wallack, J	NY	334
Anxiety & Mood Disorders			
AdP	Frances, R	NY	129
ChAP	Boorady, R	NY	145
ChAP	Cohen, L	NY	623
ChAP	Fox, S	NY	145
ChAP	Gandhi, L	NY	586
ChAP	Hirsch, G	NY	146
ChAP	Koplewicz, H	NY	146
ChAP	Moreau, D	NY	146
ChAP	Rubinstein, B	NY	623
ChAP	Shatkin, J	NY	147
ChAP	Silverman, A	NY	624
ChAP	Weisbrot, D	NY	586
IM	Slogoff, F	CT	910
Psyc	Appelbaum, P	NY	321
Psyc	Barbuto, J	NY	322
Psyc	Chertoff, H	NJ	724
Psyc	Friedman, R	NY	324
Psyc	Gorman, L	NY	325
Psyc	Kahn, D	NY	325
Psyc	Leifer, M	NJ	784
Psyc	Lipton, B	NY	327
Psyc	Papp, L	NY	329
Psyc	Perry, B	NY	671
Psyc	Rosenthal, R	NY	330
Psyc	Sami, S	NY	558

Specialty & Special Expertise Index

Specialty & Special Expertise Index

Spec	Name	St	Pg
Ped	Harlow, P	NJ	722
PHO	Bussel, J	NY	297
PHO	Flug, F	NJ	719
PHO	Kulpa, J	NY	454
PHO	Marcus, J	NY	298
PHO	Parker, R	NY	601
PHO	Sadanandan, S	NY	454
PHO	Weinblatt, M	NY	549

Blepharoplasty
Oph	Garber, P	NY	539
Oto	Brunner, E	NJ	782
Oto	Zimbler, M	NY	287
PlS	Silich, R	NY	318

Blistering Diseases
D	Shupack, J	NY	159

Blount's Disease
OrS	Fragomen, A	NY	267

Body Contouring
D	Grossman, M	NY	155
PlS	Chidyllo, S	NJ	824
PlS	Gallagher, P	NY	555
PlS	Ganchi, P	NJ	854
PlS	Jacobs, E	NY	315
PlS	Lipson, D	NJ	724
PlS	Schulman, M	NY	318
PlS	Silberman, M	NY	556
PlS	Verga, M	NY	320
PlS	Zevon, S	NY	320

Body Contouring after Weight Loss
PlS	DiBernardo, B	NJ	758
PlS	Dudick, S	NJ	824
PlS	Kolker, A	NY	316
PlS	Passaretti, D	CT	930
PlS	Razaboni, R	NY	317
PlS	Rose, M	NJ	824

Body Dysmorphic Disorder (BDD)
Psyc	Hollander, E	NY	325

Bone & Joint Infections
Inf	Sabetta, J	CT	907

Bone & Joint Pathology
Path	Schiller, A	NY	291

Bone & Soft Tissue Tumors
HS	Athanasian, E	NY	186
OrS	Friedlaender, G	CT	954
OrS	Lee, F	NY	270

Bone Cancer
DR	Panicek, D	NY	163
OrS	Benevenia, J	NJ	752
OrS	Geller, D	NY	403
OrS	Lane, J	NY	270
OrS	Patterson, F	NJ	753
PHO	Wexler, L	NY	299

Bone Densitometry
DR	Barone, C	NY	161
DR	Berson, B	NY	161
EDM	Cosman, F	NY	574

Bone Disorders-Inherited
CG	Kronn, D	NY	625

Bone Disorders-Metabolic
CG	Kronn, D	NY	625
EDM	Bilezikian, J	NY	166
EDM	Bockman, R	NY	166
EDM	Klyde, B	NY	167
EDM	Mechanick, J	NY	168
EDM	Shane, E	NY	168
EDM	Siris, E	NY	169
EDM	Wysolmerski, J	CT	946
Nep	Stern, L	NY	225
OrS	Lane, J	NY	270
PEn	Carpenter, T	CT	956

Bone Imaging
DR	Brill, P	NY	161
NuM	Scharf, S	NY	242

Bone Infections
Inf	Nahass, R	NJ	862
Inf	Sensakovic, J	NJ	796
Inf	Weiss, G	NJ	850
OrS	Fragomen, A	NY	267

Bone Marrow Failure Disorders
Hem	Castro-Malaspina, H	NY	189
PHO	Lipton, J	NY	549
PHO	Lipton, J	NY	549

Bone Marrow Pathology
Path	Orazi, A	NY	290

Bone Marrow Transplant
Hem	Castro-Malaspina, H	NY	189
Hem	Cook, P	NY	189
Hem	Isola, L	NY	190
Hem	Rowley, S	NJ	704
Hem	Schuster, M	NY	592
Hem	Scigliano, E	NY	191
Hem	Strair, R	NJ	795
Hem	Tallman, M	NY	192
Onc	Abramowitz, A	NY	479

Spec	Name	St	Pg
Onc	Ahmed, T	NY	644
Onc	Jakubowski, A	NY	215
Onc	Liu, D	NY	645
Onc	Moskowitz, C	NY	217
Onc	Zelkowitz, R	CT	913
PHO	Cairo, M	NY	662
PHO	Garvin, J	NY	298
PHO	Kernan, N	NY	298
PHO	Kushner, B	NY	298
PHO	Lipton, J	NY	549
PHO	O'Reilly, R	NY	299
PHO	Ozkaynak, M	NY	662

Bone Pathology
Path	Antonescu, C	NY	289
Path	Kahn, L	NY	546
Path	Vigorita, V	NY	452

Bone Tumors
Onc	Maki, R	NY	216
OrS	Healey, J	NY	269
OrS	Kenan, S	NY	542
OrS	Wittig, J	NY	277
Path	Schiller, A	NY	291
PHO	Aledo, A	NY	297
PHO	Gorlick, R	NY	406
PHO	Harris, M	NJ	719
PHO	Meyers, P	NY	299

Bone Tumors-Benign
OrS	Lee, F	NY	270

Bone Tumors-Metastatic
OrS	Lee, F	NY	270

Bone/Joint Infections
Inf	Brause, B	NY	193
Inf	Helfgott, D	NY	194
Inf	Romagnoli, M	NY	196
Inf	Smith, L	NJ	746
Inf	Weinstein, M	NJ	796

Botox for Blepharospasm
N	Lepore, F	NJ	800

Botox for Muscle Overactivity
N	Kelemen, J	NY	535

Botox Therapy
D	Albom, M	NY	151
D	Avram, M	NY	152
D	Bank, D	NY	625
D	Berry, R	NY	427
D	Brandt, F	NY	152
D	Cooper, L	NJ	833
D	Dolitsky, C	NY	515
D	Downie, J	NJ	741
D	Gendler, E	NY	154

Specialty & Special Expertise Index

Specialty & Special Expertise Index

Spec	Name	St	Pg
PlS	Chidyllo, S	NJ	824
PlS	Choi, M	NY	313
PlS	Cordeiro, P	NY	313
PlS	Cuber, S	NJ	808
PlS	Disa, J	NY	314
PlS	Friedman, D	NY	314
PlS	Goldenberg, D	CT	929
PlS	Grant, R	NY	315
PlS	Hoffman, L	NY	315
PlS	Hyans, P	NJ	884
PlS	Israeli, R	NY	556
PlS	Keller, A	NY	556
PlS	Kessler, M	NY	556
PlS	Kolker, A	NY	316
PlS	Leipziger, L	NY	556
PlS	Levine, J	NY	316
PlS	Mehrara, B	NY	316
PlS	Palaia, D	NY	668
PlS	Rafizadeh, F	NJ	842
PlS	Razaboni, R	NY	317
PlS	Rosen, A	NJ	759
PlS	Sabry, M	NY	317
PlS	Stahl, R	CT	958
PlS	Starker, I	NJ	842
PlS	Sultan, M	NY	319
PlS	Talmor, M	NY	319
PlS	Ting, J	NY	320
S	Osborne, M	NY	358

Breast Reconstruction & Augmentation

Spec	Name	St	Pg
PlS	DiGregorio, V	NY	554
PlS	Dudick, S	NJ	824
PlS	Gayle, L	NY	314
PlS	Glicksman, C	NJ	824
PlS	LoVerme, P	NJ	759
PlS	Newman, S	NY	668

Breast Surgery

Spec	Name	St	Pg
PlS	Broumand, S	NY	313
PlS	Cherofsky, A	NY	499
PlS	Choi, M	NY	313
PlS	Duboys, E	NY	604
PlS	Goldstein, R	NY	410
PlS	Restifo, R	CT	958
PlS	Rosenberg, M	NY	668
PlS	Suzman, M	NY	669
PlS	Tepper, H	NJ	884
PlS	Zevon, S	NY	320
S	Agarwal, N	NY	414
S	Ahlborn, T	NJ	729
S	Arbour, R	NJ	826
S	Blackwood, M	NJ	761
S	Boolbol, S	NY	354
S	Borriello, R	NY	463
S	Busch-Devereaux, E	NY	607
S	Cahan, A	NY	676
S	Capasse, J	CT	934
S	Cassell, L	NY	354
S	Chung-Loy, H	NJ	810
S	Cleary, J	NY	676

Spec	Name	St	Pg
S	Colaco, R	NJ	886
S	Dasmahapatra, K	NJ	810
S	Dresner, L	NY	463
S	Dultz, R	NJ	785
S	Feigenbaum, H	NJ	855
S	Feldman, S	NY	355
S	Fogler, R	NY	463
S	Francfort, J	NY	607
S	Genato, R	NY	463
S	Gildengers, J	NJ	772
S	Goldfarb, M	NJ	826
S	Grieco, M	NY	564
S	Hornyak, S	NY	501
S	Huston, J	NJ	762
S	Khalife, M	NY	564
S	Kimmelstiel, F	NY	357
S	Klausner, S	NY	608
S	Kurtz, L	NY	564
S	Lanfranchi, A	NJ	867
S	Lannin, D	CT	962
S	Lazarus, L	CT	935
S	Licata, J	NJ	730
S	Lozner, J	NJ	886
S	Manasseh, D	NY	464
S	McManus, S	NJ	867
S	Mills, C	NY	357
S	Pace, B	NY	486
S	Rajpal, S	NY	464
S	Raniolo, R	NY	677
S	Romero, C	NY	565
S	Sacco, M	NJ	844
S	Sclafani, L	NY	608
S	Simon, L	NY	580
S	Steiner, H	NY	464
S	Wallack, M	NY	361
S	Ward, B	CT	936
S	Wertkin, M	NY	677

Breathing Disorders

Spec	Name	St	Pg
NP	Gross, I	CT	951
NP	Steele, A	NY	532
NP	Sun, S	NJ	748
PPul	Loughlin, G	NY	302
PPul	Turcios, N	NJ	865

Bronchiolitis Obliterans

Spec	Name	St	Pg
Pul	Stover-Pepe, D	NY	339

Bronchitis

Spec	Name	St	Pg
IM	Feuer, M	NY	200
Ped	Kotin, N	NY	305
Pul	Blair, L	NY	336
Pul	Cohen, M	NY	558
Pul	Kolodny, E	NY	337
Pul	Marino, A	CT	932
Pul	Schulster, R	NY	560
Pul	Stein, S	NY	339
Pul	Zupnick, H	NY	560

Bronchoscopy

Spec	Name	St	Pg
IM	Horovitz, L	NY	202
PPul	Lowenthal, D	NY	664
PPul	Nachajon, R	NJ	854
PPul	Sadeghi, H	CT	927
PPul	Ting, A	NY	302
PPul	Vicencio, A	NY	551
Pul	Addrizzo-Harris, D	NY	335
Pul	DiCosmo, B	NY	672
Pul	Fishman, D	NY	336
Pul	Marino, W	NY	413
Pul	Maxfield, R	NY	337

Brugada Syndrome

Spec	Name	St	Pg
Cv	Kerstein, J	NY	425

Burn Care

Spec	Name	St	Pg
PlS	Greenstein, B	NY	411
PlS	Liebling, R	NY	411
PlS	Simpson, R	NY	556
S	Bessey, P	NY	353
S	Deitch, E	NJ	762
S	Mansour, E	NJ	762
S	Petrone, S	NJ	762
S	Shapiro, M	NY	608
S	Yurt, R	NY	361

Burns-Reconstructive Plastic Surgery

Spec	Name	St	Pg
PlS	Greenstein, B	NY	411
PlS	Rose, E	NY	317

C

Calcium Disorders

Spec	Name	St	Pg
EDM	Bergman, D	NY	165
EDM	Brickman, A	NY	429
EDM	Goldman, J	NY	429
EDM	Hellerman, J	NY	630
EDM	Jacobs, T	NY	167
EDM	Rich, G	CT	902
EDM	Seltzer, T	NY	168
EDM	Silverberg, S	NY	168
EDM	Spiler, I	NJ	793
EDM	Warman, J	NY	430
EDM	Weinerman, S	NY	520
PEn	Agarwal, C	NY	406
PEn	Carey, D	NY	547
PEn	Carpenter, T	CT	956

Cancer Detection & Staging

Spec	Name	St	Pg
NuM	Agress, H	NJ	712

Cancer Genetics

Spec	Name	St	Pg
CG	Bale, A	CT	944

Specialty & Special Expertise Index

Specialty & Special Expertise Index

Spec	Name	St	Pg
Cv	Skopicki, H	NY	585
Cv	Slama, R	NJ	873
Cv	Slater, W	NY	143
Cv	Sokol, S	NY	513
Cv	Sotsky, G	NJ	694
Cv	Southren, D	NY	573
Cv	Spadaro, L	NY	513
Cv	Stein, E	NJ	873
Cv	Stein, R	NY	143
Cv	Steingart, R	NY	143
Cv	Strobeck, J	NJ	849
Cv	Stroh, J	NJ	860
Cv	Taikowski, R	CT	898
Cv	Tartaglia, J	NY	622
Cv	Teichholz, L	NJ	694
Cv	Tenenbaum, J	NY	143
Cv	Tenet, W	NY	513
Cv	Traube, C	NY	425
Cv	Tuohy, E	CT	898
Cv	Tyberg, T	NY	143
Cv	Unger, A	NY	144
Cv	Varriale, P	NY	144
Cv	Vazzana, T	NY	492
Cv	Wangenheim, P	NJ	740
Cv	Weg, I	NY	513
Cv	Wein, P	NY	426
Cv	Weinberg, M	NY	585
Cv	Weintraub, H	NY	144
Cv	Weisenseel, A	NY	144
Cv	Weiss, E	NJ	849
Cv	Weissman, R	NY	622
Cv	Wild, D	NJ	695
Cv	Williams, M	NJ	695
Cv	Winter, S	NY	492
Cv	Wolk, M	NY	144
Cv	Wu, C	NJ	740
Cv	Zaloom, R	NY	426
Cv	Zarich, S	CT	899
Cv	Zeldis, S	NY	513
Cv	Zimmerman, F	NY	623
Cv	Zucker, M	NJ	740
IM	Gambarin, B	NY	437
IM	Legato, M	NY	203
IM	Mutterperl, M	NJ	768
IM	Sherman, F	NY	438
IM	Skluth, M	CT	910
IM	Slogoff, F	CT	910
IM	Zaremski, B	NY	207

Cardiovascular Disease/Young Adult

Cv	Chen, T	NY	509

Cardiovascular Imaging

Cv	Kunkes, S	CT	897
DR	Wolff, S	NY	165

Cardiovascular Surgery

T&CS	Christakos, M	NJ	856
T&CS	Seinfeld, F	NJ	785

Career Related Problems

Psyc	Borbely, A	NY	322

Caribbean Health Care

FMed	Krotowski, M	NY	430

Carotid Artery Medical Management

VascS	Riles, T	NY	379

Carotid Artery Stent Placement

Cv	Cohen, H	NY	135
IC	Fishman, R	CT	910
IC	Petrossian, G	NY	529
IC	Roubin, G	NY	208
NRad	Tenner, M	NY	651
VascS	Karwowski, J	NY	378
VIR	Hamet, M	NY	681

Carotid Artery Surgery

NS	Ghogawala, Z	CT	915
NS	Langer, D	NY	534
NS	Quest, D	NY	229
S	Drascher, G	NJ	867
S	Fried, K	NJ	729
S	McGovern, P	NJ	772
S	Vitale, G	NY	565
T&CS	Seinfeld, F	NJ	785
T&CS	Syracuse, D	NJ	856
VascS	Adelman, M	NY	376
VascS	Arnold, T	NY	609
VascS	Ascher, E	NY	467
VascS	Babu, S	NY	681
VascS	Bernik, T	NY	377
VascS	Brener, B	NJ	764
VascS	Cayne, N	NY	377
VascS	Chaudhry, S	NY	569
VascS	D'Ayala, M	NY	467
VascS	Deitch, J	NY	502
VascS	Dietzek, A	CT	938
VascS	Faries, P	NY	377
VascS	Faust, G	NY	569
VascS	Gagne, P	CT	938
VascS	Geuder, J	NJ	733
VascS	Goldman, K	NJ	812
VascS	Graham, A	NJ	812
VascS	Green, R	NY	377
VascS	Grossi, R	NY	378
VascS	Harrington, E	NY	378
VascS	Harrington, M	NY	378
VascS	Jacobowitz, G	NY	378
VascS	Karanfilian, R	NY	681
VascS	Karwowski, J	NY	378
VascS	Landis, G	NY	487
VascS	Lipsitz, E	NY	416
VascS	McKinsey, J	NY	378
VascS	Morrissey, N	NY	379
VascS	Patel, A	NJ	845
VascS	Pollina, R	NY	609
VascS	Purtill, W	NY	569

VascS	Rockman, C	NY	379
VascS	Sales, C	NJ	887
VascS	Suggs, W	NY	681
VascS	Todd, G	NY	380
VascS	Weiser, R	NY	467
VascS	Wolodiger, F	NJ	734

Carpal Tunnel Syndrome

HS	Ark, J	NJ	777
HS	Botwinick, N	NY	186
HS	Brown, L	CT	906
HS	Ende, L	NJ	834
HS	Gluck, R	NY	524
HS	Gurland, M	NJ	703
HS	Kamler, K	NY	524
HS	King, W	NY	187
HS	Kulick, R	NY	394
HS	Lane, L	NY	524
HS	Lenzo, S	NY	187
HS	Lunt, J	CT	906
HS	Miller, J	NJ	834
HS	Pruzansky, M	NY	187
HS	Raskin, K	NY	187
HS	Rosenstein, R	NJ	703
HS	Rosenwasser, M	NY	188
HS	Teplitz, G	NY	525
HS	Thomson, J	CT	948
N	Alweiss, G	NJ	711
N	Belok, L	NY	231
N	Silbert, P	NJ	821
N	Weintraub, M	NY	651
NS	Zonenshayn, M	NY	443
OrS	Altman, W	NJ	715
OrS	Barmakian, J	NJ	880
OrS	Green, S	NY	267
OrS	Grenis, M	NJ	782

Cartilage Damage

DR	Potter, H	NY	164
OrS	Cahill, J	NJ	715
OrS	Cushner, F	NY	265
OrS	Gladstone, J	NY	267
SM	Rodeo, S	NY	352

Cartilage Damage & Transplant

OrS	Levitz, C	NY	542
OrS	Plancher, K	NY	273
SM	Gehrmann, R	NJ	761
SM	Levy, A	NJ	761
SM	Williams, R	NY	352

Cataract Surgery

Oph	Accardi, F	NY	248
Oph	Angrist, R	NJ	863
Oph	Asbell, P	NY	248
Oph	Auran, J	NY	248
Oph	Benedetto, D	NJ	770
Oph	Biser, S	NY	653
Oph	Braunstein, R	NY	249
Oph	Brown, A	NY	714

Specialty & Special Expertise Index

Specialty & Special Expertise Index

Specialty & Special Expertise Index

Spec	Name	St	Pg
Onc	Dosik, D	NY	440
Onc	Fang, B	NJ	798
Onc	Fischbach, N	CT	912
Onc	Fitzgerald, D	NJ	819
Onc	Friscia, P	NY	495
Onc	Fuks, J	NY	397
Onc	Greenberg, H	NY	479
Onc	Hirschman, R	NY	214
Onc	Hirshaut, Y	NY	214
Onc	Holland, J	NY	215
Onc	Hollister, D	CT	913
Onc	Jarowski, C	NY	215
Onc	Kappel, B	NY	531
Onc	Kemeny, N	NY	216
Onc	Kloss, R	CT	913
Onc	Lundberg, W	CT	950
Onc	Marino, J	NY	531
Onc	Nissenblatt, M	NJ	798
Onc	Rakowski, T	NJ	708
Onc	Rivera, Y	NJ	708
Onc	Salwitz, J	NJ	798
Onc	Schleider, M	NJ	709
Onc	Schwartz, P	NY	531
Onc	Shum, K	NY	479
Onc	Strauss, B	NY	595
Onc	Weinstein, P	CT	913
Onc	Yi, P	NJ	779
Path	Morrow, J	CT	955
S	Diehl, W	NJ	844
S	Edye, M	NY	354
S	Frost, J	NJ	886
S	Gordon, M	NY	677
S	Michelassi, F	NY	357
S	Salky, B	NY	359

Colon Cancer Screening

Spec	Name	St	Pg
Ge	Accurso, C	NJ	861
Ge	Aisenberg, J	NY	170
Ge	Baiocco, P	NY	170
Ge	Bartolomeo, R	NY	520
Ge	Ben-Zvi, J	NY	171
Ge	Bernstein, B	NY	521
Ge	Cerulli, M	NY	521
Ge	Cooper, R	NY	172
Ge	Dalena, J	NJ	833
Ge	Fiske, S	NJ	743
Ge	Geders, J	NY	633
Ge	Genn, D	NY	633
Ge	Gettenberg, G	NY	431
Ge	Goldberg, M	NY	174
Ge	Goldman, I	NY	522
Ge	Grosman, I	NY	431
Ge	Krumholz, M	NY	176
Ge	Nussbaum, M	NY	476
Ge	Proctor, D	CT	946
Ge	Robilotti, J	NY	179
Ge	Sachs, J	NJ	777
Ge	Schneebaum, C	NY	180
Ge	Schwartz, G	NY	523
Ge	Taubin, H	CT	905
Ge	Torman, J	NY	636
Ge	Zimbalist, E	NY	432

Colon Polyps & Cancer

Spec	Name	St	Pg
Ge	Klein, W	NJ	701
Ge	Meirowitz, R	NJ	776
Ge	Turtel, P	NJ	817

Colon Surgery

Spec	Name	St	Pg
S	Adler, H	NY	462
S	Feigenbaum, H	NJ	855
S	Gildengers, J	NJ	772
S	Schwartzman, A	NY	464

Colonoscopy

Spec	Name	St	Pg
CRS	Fleischer, M	NY	427
CRS	Greenwald, M	NY	514
CRS	Groff, W	NJ	873
CRS	Helbraun, M	NJ	695
CRS	Lacqua, F	NY	427
CRS	Rothberg, R	NJ	741
CRS	Smithy, W	NY	587
CRS	White, R	NJ	695
Ge	Ackert, J	NY	170
Ge	Adler, H	NY	170
Ge	Antonelle, R	NY	632
Ge	Antony, M	NY	391
Ge	Auerbach, M	NY	632
Ge	Bartolomeo, R	NY	520
Ge	Bernstein, D	NY	521
Ge	Binns, J	NJ	817
Ge	Bruckstein, A	NY	493
Ge	Chessler, R	NJ	701
Ge	Chinitz, M	NY	632
Ge	Cohen, J	NY	172
Ge	Cohen, S	NY	172
Ge	Ehrlich, J	NY	633
Ge	Fazio, R	NY	493
Ge	Ferran, E	NY	173
Ge	Fiske, S	NJ	743
Ge	Foong, A	NY	173
Ge	Frank, M	NY	173
Ge	Friedlander, C	NY	173
Ge	Friedrich, I	NJ	701
Ge	Gamss, J	NY	431
Ge	Glanzman, B	NY	590
Ge	Goldberg, M	NY	174
Ge	Gould, R	NY	634
Ge	Green, P	NY	174
Ge	Gruss, C	CT	904
Ge	Gutwein, I	NY	392
Ge	Hahn, J	NJ	768
Ge	Hammerman, H	NY	174
Ge	Harooni, R	NY	476
Ge	Iswara, K	NY	431
Ge	Katz, S	NY	522
Ge	Kerner, M	NJ	876
Ge	Krumholz, M	NY	176
Ge	Kummer, B	NY	176
Ge	Lustbader, I	NY	177
Ge	Marin, G	NJ	776
Ge	Marion, J	NY	177
Ge	Mauer, K	CT	904
Ge	Meirowitz, R	NJ	776

Spec	Name	St	Pg
Ge	Rand, J	NY	476
Ge	Rieber, J	NY	179
Ge	Rosemarin, J	NY	635
Ge	Rubin, M	NY	179
Ge	Salik, J	NY	179
Ge	Samach, M	NJ	834
Ge	Schmerin, M	NY	180
Ge	Sherman, H	NY	393
Ge	Spielberg, A	NY	591
Ge	Spivack, J	CT	905
Ge	Talansky, A	NY	523
Ge	Waye, J	NY	181
Ge	Wayne, P	NY	636
IM	Gelberg, B	NY	527

Colonoscopy/Polypectomy

Spec	Name	St	Pg
CRS	Moseson, M	NY	515
Ge	Dettmer, R	CT	903
Ge	Duva, J	NY	590
Ge	Goldfarb, J	NJ	701
Ge	Heier, S	NY	634
Ge	Knapp, A	NY	175
Ge	Margulis, S	NJ	701
Ge	Romeu, J	NY	179
Ge	Soloway, G	CT	905
IM	Goldman, J	NY	640

Colostomy Avoidance

Spec	Name	St	Pg
CRS	Steinhagen, R	NY	150

Colposcopy

Spec	Name	St	Pg
ObG	Armbruster, R	NY	651
ObG	Beim, R	NJ	880
ObG	Blanco, J	NY	242
ObG	Burns, E	NY	651
ObG	Cooperman, A	NJ	750
ObG	Cuteri, J	CT	917
ObG	Florio, P	NY	652
ObG	Grano, V	NY	652
ObG	Ott, A	NY	597
ObG	Reilly, J	NY	497

Coma

Spec	Name	St	Pg
N	Mayer, S	NY	236

Community Medicine

Spec	Name	St	Pg
Ped	Murphy, R	NY	306

Compartment Syndrome

Spec	Name	St	Pg
SM	Small, E	NY	676

Complementary Medicine

Spec	Name	St	Pg
Cv	Goodman, D	NY	137
Cv	Horowitz, S	CT	897
Cv	Teichholz, L	NJ	694
FMed	Kligler, B	NY	169
FMed	Podell, R	NJ	875
FMed	Schiller, R	NY	170

Specialty & Special Expertise Index

Specialty & Special Expertise Index

Spec	Name	St	Pg
DR	Hertz, M	NY	628
DR	Kirshy, D	NY	588
DR	Lee, R	CT	901
DR	Mollin, J	NY	474
DR	Rifkin, M	NY	164
DR	Rozenblit, A	NY	388
DR	Sherman, S	NY	517
DR	Yoon, S	NY	518
NRad	Knopp, E	NY	240
NuM	Agress, H	NJ	712
NuM	Brunetti, J	NJ	712
NuM	Freeman, L	NY	401
NuM	Gerard, P	NY	651
NuM	Scharf, S	NY	242

Cultural Psychiatry

Spec	Name	St	Pg
Psyc	Ferran, E	NY	324

Cushing's Syndrome

Spec	Name	St	Pg
EDM	Young, I	NY	169

Cutaneous Lymphoma

Spec	Name	St	Pg
D	Belsito, D	NY	152
D	Edelson, R	CT	944
D	Grossman, K	NJ	816
D	Grossman, M	NY	626
D	Katz, S	NY	155
D	Lebwohl, M	NY	156
D	Myskowski, P	NY	156
D	Ramsay, D	NY	157
Path	Magro, C	NY	290
RadRO	Wilson, L	CT	960

Cutaneous Lymphoma, T-cell

Spec	Name	St	Pg
Hem	Hymes, K	NY	190

Cystic Fibrosis

Spec	Name	St	Pg
A&I	Guida, L	NY	583
PPul	Amin, N	NY	663
PPul	Atlas, A	NJ	841
PPul	Bisberg, D	NJ	756
PPul	Boyer, J	NY	663
PPul	Dimaio, M	NY	301
PPul	Dozor, A	NY	664
PPul	Giusti, R	NY	455
PPul	Kattan, M	NY	302
PPul	Kottler, W	NJ	757
PPul	Lowenthal, D	NY	664
PPul	Nachajon, R	NJ	854
PPul	Quittell, L	NY	664
PPul	Sadeghi, H	CT	927
PPul	Ting, A	NY	302
PPul	Turcios, N	NJ	865
Pul	Fiel, S	NJ	843
Pul	Fiel, S	NJ	843
Pul	Kaplan, R	NY	336

Cystic Fibrosis Infection

Spec	Name	St	Pg
PInf	Saiman, L	NY	300

Spec	Name	St	Pg

Cytomegalovirus

Spec	Name	St	Pg
PInf	Tolan, R	NJ	806

D

Dance Medicine

Spec	Name	St	Pg
OrS	Hamilton, W	NY	268
OrS	Padgett, D	NY	272

Dance/Ballet Injuries

Spec	Name	St	Pg
OrS	Rose, D	NY	273
SM	Metzl, J	NY	352

Dance/Sports Medicine

Spec	Name	St	Pg
OrS	Bauman, P	NY	263

Deep Brain Stimulation

Spec	Name	St	Pg
NS	De Lotbiniere, A	NY	648
NS	Kaplitt, M	NY	228

Defibrillators

Spec	Name	St	Pg
CE	Biviano, A	NY	132
CE	Chinitz, L	NY	133
CE	Cohen, M	NY	618
CE	Correia, J	NJ	738
CE	Evans, S	NY	133
CE	Jadonath, R	NY	508
CE	Lerman, B	NY	133
CE	Matos, J	NY	133
CE	Turitto, G	NY	423
T&CS	Camunas, J	NY	362

Deformity Reconstruction

Spec	Name	St	Pg
OrS	Helfet, D	NY	269
OrS	Strongwater, A	NJ	853

Dementia

Spec	Name	St	Pg
FMed	Gross, H	NJ	700
Ger	Bloom, P	NY	181
Ger	Bullock, R	NJ	794
Ger	Callahan, E	NY	181
Ger	Chang, C	NY	182
Ger	Chun, A	NY	182
Ger	Gomolin, I	NY	523
Ger	Leifer, B	NJ	702
Ger	Macina, L	NY	523
Ger	Siegler, E	NY	183
Ger	Wolf-Klein, G	NY	524
GerPsy	Greenwald, B	NY	476
GerPsy	Kennedy, G	NY	394
GerPsy	Reisberg, B	NY	183
IM	Bharathan, T	NY	436
IM	Taubman, L	NY	528
N	Ahluwalia, B	NY	649
N	Azhar, S	NY	443

Spec	Name	St	Pg
N	Blady, D	NJ	749
N	Cohen, D	NY	595
N	Crystal, H	NY	443
N	Feinberg, T	NY	232
N	Fellus, J	NJ	769
N	Foo, S	NY	233
N	Gendelman, S	NY	233
N	Gordon, M	NY	535
N	Kay, A	NY	443
N	Kessler, J	NY	536
N	Levine, D	NY	235
N	Marder, K	NY	235
N	Marks, S	NY	650
N	Mayeux, R	NY	236
N	Rabin, A	NJ	712
N	Relkin, N	NY	237
N	Sachs, S	NJ	879
N	Van Slooten, D	NJ	712
N	Yellin, J	NY	445
Psyc	Brenner, R	NY	482
Psyc	Gewolb, E	NJ	771
Psyc	Rubin, K	NJ	825
Psyc	Samuels, S	NJ	725
Psyc	Teusink, J	NY	333

Demyelinating Neuropathy

Spec	Name	St	Pg
N	Ruderman, M	NJ	750

Depression

Spec	Name	St	Pg
ChAP	Gabbay, V	NY	145
ChAP	Kotler, L	NJ	695
ChAP	Silva, R	NY	624
Ger	Chun, A	NY	182
GerPsy	Amin, R	NY	433
GerPsy	Devanand, D	NY	183
GerPsy	Greenwald, B	NY	476
GerPsy	Kennedy, G	NY	394
GerPsy	Reisberg, B	NY	183
GerPsy	Serby, M	NY	183
Psyc	Addonizio, G	NY	669
Psyc	Appelbaum, P	NY	321
Psyc	Aronson, T	NY	604
Psyc	Asnis, G	NY	411
Psyc	Bailine, S	NY	557
Psyc	Behr, R	NY	557
Psyc	Benjamin, J	NY	557
Psyc	Berkowitz, H	NY	457
Psyc	Bhatt, A	NY	557
Psyc	Brenner, R	NY	482
Psyc	Chung, H	NY	323
Psyc	Crasta, J	NY	557
Psyc	Di Buono, M	NY	500
Psyc	Douglas, C	NY	324
Psyc	Dulit, R	NY	669
Psyc	Eitan, N	NY	458
Psyc	Faber, M	NJ	759
Psyc	Friedman, R	NY	324
Psyc	Gelfand, J	NY	411
Psyc	Harlam, D	NY	670
Psyc	Heller, S	NY	325
Psyc	Hoffman, J	NY	325

Specialty & Special Expertise Index

Specialty & Special Expertise Index

Specialty & Special Expertise Index

Specialty & Special Expertise Index

Specialty & Special Expertise Index

Spec	Name	St	Pg
Endocarditis			
Inf	Hartman, B	NY	194
Inf	Krieger, R	NJ	835
Inf	Quagliarello, V	CT	948
Endocrine Cancers			
S	Sosa, J	CT	962
Endocrine Disorders in Pregnancy			
EDM	Rennert, N	CT	902
Endocrine Pathology			
Path	Wenig, B	NY	291
Endocrine Radiology			
NRad	Knopp, E	NY	240
Endocrine Surgery			
S	Budd, D	NJ	855
S	Fahey, T	NY	355
S	Heller, K	NY	356
S	Lee, J	NY	357
S	Udelsman, R	CT	962
S	Zarnegar, R	NY	361
Endocrine Tumors			
EDM	Kantor, A	NY	630
S	Maheshwari, V	NJ	762
S	Whitman, E	NJ	844
Endocrinology			
EDM	Guzman, R	NY	389
IM	Liu, G	NY	204
Endocrinology & Joint Disorders			
Rhu	Lahita, R	NJ	761
Endocrinology, Diabetes & Metabolism			
EDM	Agrin, R	NJ	793
EDM	Albin, J	NY	629
EDM	Aloia, J	NY	518
EDM	Arden-Cordone, M	CT	901
EDM	Balkin, M	NY	588
EDM	Baranetsky, N	NJ	742
EDM	Bergman, D	NY	165
EDM	Berkowitz, R	NJ	850
EDM	Bhatt, A	NY	518
EDM	Bilezikian, J	NY	166
EDM	Bitton, R	NY	518
EDM	Bleich, D	NJ	742
EDM	Bloomgarden, D	NY	630
EDM	Bloomgarden, Z	NY	166
EDM	Blum, C	NY	166
EDM	Blum, D	NY	630
EDM	Bockman, R	NY	166

Spec	Name	St	Pg
EDM	Brand, H	NY	589
EDM	Brett, E	NY	166
EDM	Brickman, A	NY	429
EDM	Brillon, D	NY	166
EDM	Bucholtz, H	NJ	793
EDM	Bukberg, P	NY	166
EDM	Cam, J	NJ	767
EDM	Carlson, H	NY	589
EDM	Cobin, R	NJ	699
EDM	Cohen, C	NY	389
EDM	Cohen, N	NY	493
EDM	Cosman, F	NY	574
EDM	Das, S	NY	493
EDM	Daud-Ahmad, S	NJ	699
EDM	Davies, T	NY	167
EDM	Dower, S	NJ	742
EDM	Friedman, S	NY	518
EDM	Fuhrman, R	NJ	874
EDM	Gelato, M	NY	589
EDM	Gewirtz, G	NJ	742
EDM	Giegerich, E	NY	429
EDM	Gioia, L	NY	589
EDM	Gitler, E	NY	630
EDM	Goland, R	NY	167
EDM	Goldberg-Berman, J	CT	902
EDM	Goldenberg, A	NY	589
EDM	Goldman, J	NY	429
EDM	Goldman, M	NJ	699
EDM	Gordon, J	NY	518
EDM	Grajower, M	NY	389
EDM	Greene, L	NY	167
EDM	Greenfield, M	NY	519
EDM	Guoth, M	CT	902
EDM	Guzman, R	NY	389
EDM	Hellerman, J	NY	630
EDM	Hochstein, M	NJ	699
EDM	Hoffman, R	NY	493
EDM	Hupart, K	NY	519
EDM	Inzucchi, S	CT	945
EDM	Jacobs, T	NY	167
EDM	Kantor, A	NY	630
EDM	Kaplan, J	NY	519
EDM	Kleinberg, D	NY	167
EDM	Klyde, B	NY	167
EDM	Leibowitz, J	NY	630
EDM	Levine, A	NY	167
EDM	Lomasky, S	NY	519
EDM	Lorber, D	NY	474
EDM	Maman, A	NJ	793
EDM	Margulies, P	NY	519
EDM	McConnell, R	NY	168
EDM	Mechanick, J	NY	168
EDM	Nassberg, B	NJ	817
EDM	Nevin, M	NJ	833
EDM	Peck, V	NY	168
EDM	Poretsky, L	NY	168
EDM	Powell, J	NY	630
EDM	Pretto, Z	NY	630
EDM	Rennert, N	CT	902
EDM	Resta, C	NY	429
EDM	Rich, G	CT	902
EDM	Rosa, J	CT	902
EDM	Rosenbaum, R	NJ	874

Spec	Name	St	Pg
EDM	Rosenthal, D	NY	519
EDM	Rosman, L	NY	474
EDM	Rothman, J	NY	493
EDM	Rudin, E	NY	631
EDM	Savino, R	CT	902
EDM	Schneider, S	NJ	793
EDM	Schwartz, J	NJ	699
EDM	Selinger, S	NJ	874
EDM	Seltzer, T	NY	168
EDM	Seplowitz, A	NY	168
EDM	Shamoon, H	NY	389
EDM	Shane, E	NY	168
EDM	Shapiro, L	NY	519
EDM	Shelmet, J	NJ	776
EDM	Sherry, S	NJ	743
EDM	Silverberg, A	NY	429
EDM	Silverberg, S	NY	168
EDM	Silverman, M	NJ	875
EDM	Siris, E	NY	169
EDM	Spiler, I	NJ	793
EDM	Surks, M	NY	389
EDM	Tibaldi, J	NY	475
EDM	Tohme, J	NJ	699
EDM	Tuttle, R	NY	169
EDM	Vaswani, A	NY	519
EDM	Wardlaw, S	NY	169
EDM	Warman, J	NY	430
EDM	Wehmann, R	NJ	700
EDM	Weinerman, S	NY	520
EDM	Weiser, K	NY	631
EDM	Weitzman, S	NY	589
EDM	Wexler, C	NY	589
EDM	Wiesen, M	NJ	700
EDM	Wysolmerski, J	CT	946
EDM	Young, I	NY	169
EDM	Zonszein, J	NY	390
EDM	Zweig, S	NY	169
Endometriosis			
ObG	Goldman, G	NY	244
ObG	Goldstein, M	NY	244
ObG	Hayworth, S	NY	652
ObG	Luciani, R	NJ	750
ObG	Violi, C	CT	918
RE	David, S	NY	343
RE	Doyle, M	CT	933
RE	Fateh, M	NY	343
RE	Ginsburg, F	CT	933
RE	Kenigsberg, D	NY	606
RE	Klein, J	NY	674
RE	Mukherjee, T	NY	344
RE	Quagliarello, J	NY	344
RE	Rosenfeld, D	NY	562
RE	Stangel, J	NY	674
RE	Taylor, H	CT	960
Endoscopic Sinus Surgery			
Oto	Branovan, D	NY	278
Oto	Close, L	NY	279
Oto	Drake, W	NJ	881
Oto	Edelstein, D	NY	279

Specialty & Special Expertise Index

Specialty & Special Expertise Index

Specialty & Special Expertise Index

Spec	Name	St	Pg
Exercise Physiology			
PCd	Arnon, R	NY	292
PCd	Schiller, M	NY	405
Pul	Malovany, R	NJ	726
Exfoliate Erythroderma			
D	Bagel, J	NJ	775
Eye Allergy			
A&I	Bielory, L	NJ	872
A&I	Mechanic, L	NY	617
Eye Disorders-Congenital			
Oph	Derespinis, P	NY	497
Oph	Wagner, R	NJ	752
Eye Infections			
Oph	Eichenbaum, J	NY	251
Oph	Koplin, R	NY	254
Oph	Mayers, M	NY	402
Oph	Newton, M	NY	257
Oph	Ritterband, D	NY	258
Oph	Samson, C	NY	259
Oph	Starr, M	NY	261
Eye Muscle Disorders			
Oph	Campolattaro, B	NY	249
Oph	Derespinis, P	NY	497
Oph	Forman, S	NY	654
Oph	Hall, L	NY	254
Oph	Lederman, M	NY	654
Oph	Mathias, S	CT	920
Oph	Napolitano, J	NJ	802
Oph	Steele, M	NY	261
Oph	Wang, F	NY	261
Oph	Winterkorn, J	NY	481
Oph	Wisnicki, H	NY	262
Eye Trauma			
Oph	Koplin, R	NY	254
Oph	Zarbin, M	NJ	752
Eye Tumors/Cancer			
Oph	Abramson, D	NY	248
Oph	Finger, P	NY	252
Oph	Friedman, A	NY	252
Oph	Rodriguez-Sains, R	NY	259
RadRO	McCormick, B	NY	341
RadRO	Rotman, M	NY	461
Eyelid Cosmetic & Reconstructive Surgery			
Oph	Gordon, J	NY	654
Oph	Lisman, R	NY	255
Oph	Rodgers, I	NY	259
Oph	Rodriguez-Sains, R	NY	259
Oph	Schlessinger, D	NY	541

Spec	Name	St	Pg
PIS	Raskin, E	CT	930
Eyelid Cosmetic Surgery			
Oph	Ackerman, J	NY	446
Oph	Goldberg, L	NY	539
Oph	Manjoney, D	CT	919
Oph	Marks, A	NY	540
Oph	Milite, J	NJ	802
Oph	Relland, M	NY	258
Oph	Schneck, G	NY	599
Oph	Talansky, M	NJ	822
Eyelid Surgery			
Oph	Dweck, M	NY	447
Oph	Musto, A	CT	920
Oph	Wasserman, B	NJ	781
Oto	Mazzara, C	NJ	803
PIS	Anton, J	NY	603
PIS	Bikoff, D	NJ	724
PIS	Broumand, S	NY	313
PIS	Cutolo, L	NY	499
PIS	Imber, G	NY	315
PIS	Kleinman, A	NY	668
PIS	Newman, F	CT	929
PIS	Perry, A	NJ	865
PIS	Rosen, A	NJ	759
PIS	Rosenstock, A	CT	930
PIS	Simpson, R	NY	556
PIS	Tabbal, N	NY	319
Eyelid Surgery/Blepharoplasty			
PIS	Scott, S	NY	318
PIS	Spinelli, H	NY	319
Eyelid Tumors/Cancer			
Oph	Charles, N	NY	250
Oph	Della Rocca, R	NY	251
Oph	Elahi, E	NY	251
Oph	Kazim, M	NY	254
Oph	Milite, J	NJ	802
Oph	Rodriguez-Sains, R	NY	259
Eyelid/Tear Duct Disorders			
Oph	Angrist, R	NJ	863
Oph	Perry, H	NY	540
Oph	Rodgers, I	NY	259
Eyelid/Tear Duct Reconstruction			
Oph	Lisman, R	NY	255
Oph	Moazed, K	NY	257

F

Spec	Name	St	Pg
Fabry's Disease			
N	Kolodny, E	NY	234

Spec	Name	St	Pg
Facial Nerve Disorders			
Oto	Kay, S	NJ	803
Oto	Lalwani, A	NY	282
Oto	Miller, P	NY	283
Oto	Roland, J	NY	284
Facial Paralysis Reconstruction			
PIS	Rose, E	NY	317
Facial Plastic & Reconstructive Surgery			
Oto	Levin, R	CT	925
Oto	Marotta, J	NY	600
Oto	Mazzara, C	NJ	803
Oto	Portnoy, W	NY	284
Oto	Rizk, S	NY	284
Oto	Romo, T	NY	284
Oto	Shikowitz, M	NY	544
Oto	Turk, J	NY	286
PIS	Alizadeh, K	NY	554
PIS	Cordeiro, P	NY	313
PIS	Monasebian, D	NY	317
PIS	Rose, E	NY	317
PIS	Roth, D	NY	669
PIS	Sherman, J	NY	318
PIS	Suzman, M	NY	669
Facial Plastic Surgery			
Oph	Elahi, E	NY	251
Oto	Carniol, P	NJ	881
Oto	Goldstein, S	NY	404
Oto	Milgrim, L	NJ	717
Oto	Rosen, A	NJ	717
Oto	Scott, J	NY	659
Oto	Zimbler, M	NY	287
Facial Rejuvenation			
D	Cooper, L	NJ	833
D	DeLeo, V	NY	153
D	Dolitsky, C	NY	515
D	Felderman, L	NY	153
D	Gendler, E	NY	154
D	Gordon, M	NY	154
D	Green, M	NY	154
D	Grodberg, M	NJ	697
D	Grossman, M	NY	155
D	Liftin, A	NJ	741
D	Narins, R	NY	627
D	Polis, L	NY	157
D	Sklar, J	NY	516
D	Treiber, R	NY	628
D	Wexler, P	NY	160
Oto	Carniol, P	NJ	881
Oto	Constantinides, M	NY	279
Oto	Miller, P	NY	283
PIS	D'Amico, R	NJ	724
PIS	Diktaban, T	NY	314
PIS	Funt, D	NY	555
PIS	Gallagher, P	NY	555
PIS	Ganchi, P	NJ	854

Specialty & Special Expertise Index

Spec	Name	St	Pg
PlS	Herbstman, R	NJ	808
PlS	Hoffman, L	NY	315
PlS	Lipson, D	NJ	724
PlS	Pyo, D	NJ	842
PlS	Rafizadeh, F	NJ	842
PlS	Silberman, M	NY	556
PlS	Weinstein, L	NJ	842

Facial Surgery-Chin & Lip

Spec	Name	St	Pg
PlS	Zide, B	NY	320

Failure to Thrive

Spec	Name	St	Pg
PGe	McFarlane-Ferreira, Y	NY	453

Falls in the Elderly

Spec	Name	St	Pg
Ger	Karp, A	NY	182
Ger	Sherman, F	NY	183
Ger	Tinetti, M	CT	947
Ger	Wolf-Klein, G	NY	524

Family & Couples Therapy

Spec	Name	St	Pg
Psyc	Aronoff, M	NY	321
Psyc	Spitz, H	NY	332

Family Medicine

Spec	Name	St	Pg
FMed	Acosta, R	CT	902
FMed	Annabi, I	NY	631
FMed	Aponte, A	NY	589
FMed	Apuzzo, T	NY	631
FMed	Arcati, A	NY	520
FMed	Arcati, R	NY	520
FMed	Athanail, S	NY	430
FMed	Bello, M	NJ	700
FMed	Bernardo, S	NJ	817
FMed	Biagiotti, W	NY	390
FMed	Calman, N	NY	169
FMed	Capobianco, L	NY	520
FMed	Catanese, V	NJ	817
FMed	Cirello, R	NJ	743
FMed	Coloka-Kump, R	NY	390
FMed	Cordero, E	NY	390
FMed	Corson, R	NJ	860
FMed	Delaney, B	NY	390
FMed	Dombrowski, M	NJ	700
FMed	Duchen, D	CT	902
FMed	Edelstein, M	NY	520
FMed	Eisenstat, S	NJ	875
FMed	Falkoff, A	CT	903
FMed	Farrell, M	CT	903
FMed	Filiberto, C	CT	903
FMed	Fisher, G	NY	475
FMed	Fishkin, M	NY	590
FMed	Franzetti, C	NY	390
FMed	Frisoli, A	NJ	861
FMed	Giugliano, J	NY	590
FMed	Gorman, R	NJ	743
FMed	Gottesfeld, P	NY	631
FMed	Greenblatt, L	NY	590
FMed	Gross, H	NJ	700

Spec	Name	St	Pg
FMed	Holland, E	NJ	833
FMed	Ibelli, V	NY	574
FMed	Ingrassia, J	NY	574
FMed	Istrico, R	NY	475
FMed	Karatoprak, O	NJ	700
FMed	Kligler, B	NY	169
FMed	Krotowski, M	NY	430
FMed	Lansing, M	NJ	776
FMed	Leeds, G	NY	169
FMed	Leipsner, G	NJ	700
FMed	Levine, M	NJ	767
FMed	Levites, K	NY	590
FMed	Levy, A	NY	170
FMed	Lopez, C	NY	430
FMed	Lyon, V	NY	170
FMed	Mallozzi, A	CT	903
FMed	Maselli, F	NY	390
FMed	Merker, E	NY	631
FMed	Metz, J	NJ	793
FMed	Miller, D	NY	631
FMed	Molnar, T	NY	475
FMed	Morrow, R	NY	390
FMed	Moskowitz, G	NY	430
FMed	Moynihan, B	NY	520
FMed	Muraca, G	NY	475
FMed	Nepola, N	NY	493
FMed	Picciano, A	NJ	793
FMed	Piccirilli, D	NY	631
FMed	Podell, R	NJ	875
FMed	Rechter, L	NY	520
FMed	Reddy, M	NY	475
FMed	Rednor, J	NJ	776
FMed	Roth, A	NY	475
FMed	Sadovsky, R	NY	430
FMed	Schiller, R	NY	170
FMed	Schiowitz, E	NY	430
FMed	Schlam, E	NJ	743
FMed	Schwinn, H	NY	590
FMed	Sekiguchi, R	CT	903
FMed	Sharpe, A	NY	631
FMed	Sheridan, B	NY	430
FMed	Sklower, J	NJ	767
FMed	Soloway, B	NY	390
FMed	Soskel, N	NY	520
FMed	Strongwater, R	NY	632
FMed	Sutton, I	NY	632
FMed	Swee, D	NJ	794
FMed	Tabachnick, J	NJ	875
FMed	Tallia, A	NJ	794
FMed	Tierney, P	NJ	794
FMed	Vaidya, S	NY	632
FMed	Vincent, M	NY	430
FMed	Winter, R	NJ	794
FMed	Yudin, H	NY	632
FMed	Ziering, T	NJ	861

Family Therapy

Spec	Name	St	Pg
ChAP	Rosenfeld, A	CT	899
Psyc	Richardson, W	NJ	884

Female Genital Cosmetic

Surgery

Spec	Name	St	Pg
PlS	Hunter, J	NY	315

Fertility Preservation

Spec	Name	St	Pg
RE	Kofinas, G	NY	461
RE	Richlin, S	CT	933

Fertility Preservation in Cancer

Spec	Name	St	Pg
GO	Sonoda, Y	NY	185
RE	Copperman, A	NY	343
RE	Grazi, R	NY	461
RE	Grifo, J	NY	343
RE	Licciardi, F	NY	344
RE	McGovern, P	NJ	727
RE	Noyes, N	NY	344
RE	Patrizio, P	CT	960
RE	Rosenwaks, Z	NY	344
RE	Scott, R	NJ	866
RE	Seifer, D	NY	461
U	Sheinfeld, J	NY	373

Fetal Abnormalities

Spec	Name	St	Pg
MF	Genc, M	NY	209

Fetal Cardiology

Spec	Name	St	Pg
PCd	Fernandes, J	NJ	754
PCd	Friedman, D	NY	660

Fetal Diagnosis & Therapy

Spec	Name	St	Pg
MF	Copel, J	CT	949
MF	MacMillan, W	NJ	797
ObG	Evans, M	NY	243

Fetal Echocardiography

Spec	Name	St	Pg
MF	Copel, J	CT	949
PCd	Better, D	NY	546
PCd	Biancaniello, T	NY	601
PCd	Bierman, F	NY	660
PCd	Borg, M	NY	292
PCd	Brick, D	NY	293
PCd	Donnelly, C	NJ	840
PCd	Fish, B	NY	660
PCd	Friedman, A	CT	955
PCd	Friedman, D	NY	660
PCd	Gaffney, J	NJ	804
PCd	Issenberg, H	NY	661
PCd	Langsner, A	NY	755
PCd	Leichter, D	NJ	882
PCd	Parness, I	NY	293
PCd	Presti, S	NY	452
PCd	Ramaswamy, P	NY	452
PCd	Schiff, R	NY	547
PCd	Shapir, Y	NY	547
PCd	Shenoy, R	NY	405
PCd	Snyder, M	CT	926
PCd	Tozzi, R	NJ	719
PCd	Vallone, A	NY	547

Specialty & Special Expertise Index

Specialty & Special Expertise Index

Specialty & Special Expertise Index

Specialty & Special Expertise Index

Spec	Name	St	Pg
GO	Maiman, M	NY	494
GO	Menzin, A	NY	524
GO	Pearl, M	NY	591
GO	Poynor, E	NY	185
GO	Rahaman, J	NY	185
GO	Rodriguez, L	NJ	795
GO	Rutherford, T	CT	947
GO	Santin, A	CT	947
GO	Schwartz, P	CT	947
GO	Serur, E	NY	434
GO	Smith, H	NY	394
GO	Smotkin, D	NY	394
GO	Sommers, G	NJ	703
GO	Sonoda, Y	NY	185
GO	Taylor, R	NJ	744
GO	Tobias, D	NJ	834
GO	Wallach, R	NY	185
GO	Welshinger, M	NY	477
GO	Wertheim, I	CT	905
GO	Zakashansky, K	NY	186

Gynecologic Pathology

Spec	Name	St	Pg
Path	Heller, D	NJ	754
Path	Pinto, M	CT	926
Path	Soslow, R	NY	291

Gynecologic Surgery

Spec	Name	St	Pg
ObG	Ascher-Walsh, C	NY	242
ObG	Benedict, L	NY	537
ObG	Bochner, R	NJ	801
ObG	Bruck, L	CT	917
ObG	Butler, D	NJ	713
ObG	Cox, K	NY	243
ObG	Englert, C	NJ	713
ObG	Faust, M	NJ	713
ObG	Giuffrida, R	NY	652
ObG	Levine, R	NY	245
ObG	Meacham, K	NY	652
ObG	Mendelowitz, L	NY	652
ObG	Mohr, R	NJ	838
ObG	Rodke, G	NY	246
ObG	Sassoon, R	NY	247
ObG	Schwartz, J	NY	247
ObG	Segarra, P	NY	597
RE	Quagliarello, J	NY	344

Gynecologic Surgery-Complex

Spec	Name	St	Pg
GO	Carlson, J	NJ	795
GO	Chi, D	NY	184
GO	Denehy, T	NJ	744
GO	Pearl, M	NY	591
GO	Poynor, E	NY	185
GO	Schwartz, P	CT	947
ObG	Evanko, J	NY	243
ObG	Kramer, M	NY	597

Gynecologic Ultrasound

Spec	Name	St	Pg
ObG	Goldstein, S	NY	244
ObG	Veloso, M	NY	538

Gynecology Only

Spec	Name	St	Pg
ObG	Barzegar, H	NY	445
ObG	Brickner, G	NJ	780
ObG	Cox, K	NY	243
ObG	Davis, N	NJ	801
ObG	Diamond, S	NY	243
ObG	Donovan, L	CT	918
ObG	Fishbane-Mayer, J	NY	243
ObG	Giuffrida, R	NY	652
ObG	Harris, D	NY	244
ObG	Haselkorn, J	NY	537
ObG	Hurst, W	NJ	713
ObG	Kent, J	NY	245
ObG	Lee, D	NY	597
ObG	Lustig, I	NY	246
ObG	Meyer, M	NJ	713
ObG	Ott, A	NY	597
ObG	Phillips, R	NY	246
ObG	Reizis, I	NY	446
ObG	Sadarangani, B	NY	246
ObG	Sailon, P	NY	246
ObG	Sanderson, R	NJ	863
ObG	Snyder, J	NY	247
ObG	Sullum, S	NY	247
ObG	Veloso, M	NY	538
ObG	Yarberry-Allen, P	NY	247
ObG	Young, C	NY	401

Gynecomastia

Spec	Name	St	Pg
EDM	Carlson, H	NY	589
PlS	Jacobs, E	NY	315

H

Hair & Nail Disorders

Spec	Name	St	Pg
D	Kopec, A	NJ	767

Hair loss

Spec	Name	St	Pg
D	Davis, J	NY	153

Hair Loss

Spec	Name	St	Pg
D	Oestreicher, M	CT	900

Hair loss

Spec	Name	St	Pg
D	Savin, R	CT	945

Hair Loss in Women

Spec	Name	St	Pg
D	Bernstein, R	NY	152

Hair Removal-Laser

Spec	Name	St	Pg
D	Berry, R	NY	427
D	Brauner, G	NJ	696
D	Grodberg, M	NJ	697
D	Rosen, D	NY	387
D	Vogel, L	NY	159

Hair Restoration/Transplant

Spec	Name	St	Pg
D	Avram, M	NY	152
D	Bernstein, R	NY	152
D	Orentreich, D	NY	157
D	Unger, W	NY	159
D	Weiss, D	NJ	697
PlS	DiBernardo, B	NJ	758

Hairy Cell Leukemia

Spec	Name	St	Pg
Hem	Tallman, M	NY	192

Hand & Elbow Nerve Disorders

Spec	Name	St	Pg
HS	Strauch, R	NY	188

Hand & Elbow Surgery

Spec	Name	St	Pg
HS	Polatsch, D	NY	187

Hand & Microvascular Surgery

Spec	Name	St	Pg
PlS	Chiu, D	NY	313

Hand & Upper Extremity Surgery

Spec	Name	St	Pg
HS	Athanasian, E	NY	186
HS	Carlson, M	NY	186
HS	Catalano, L	NY	186
HS	Choueka, J	NY	434
HS	Ende, L	NJ	834
HS	Kavookjian, H	CT	906
HS	Kulick, R	NY	394
HS	Magill, R	NY	637
HS	Schefer, A	NY	637
HS	Tan, V	NJ	745

Hand & Upper Extremity Tumors

Spec	Name	St	Pg
HS	Athanasian, E	NY	186

Hand & Wrist Injuries

Spec	Name	St	Pg
HS	Lenzo, S	NY	187
OrS	Altman, W	NJ	715
OrS	Grenis, M	NJ	782

Hand & Wrist Surgery

Spec	Name	St	Pg
HS	Beldner, S	NY	186
HS	Caligiuri, D	NY	434
HS	Fragner, R	NY	637
HS	Glickel, S	NY	187
HS	Rago, T	CT	906
HS	Strauch, R	NY	188
OrS	Green, S	NY	267

Hand Reconstruction

Spec	Name	St	Pg
HS	Brown, L	CT	906
HS	King, W	NY	187
HS	Lane, L	NY	524
HS	Strauch, R	NY	188
HS	Thomson, J	CT	948

Specialty & Special Expertise Index

Specialty & Special Expertise Index

Specialty & Special Expertise Index

Specialty & Special Expertise Index

Specialty & Special Expertise Index

Specialty & Special Expertise Index

Specialty & Special Expertise Index

Specialty & Special Expertise Index

Specialty & Special Expertise Index

Spec	Name	St	Pg
Knee Reconstruction			
OrS	Cushner, F	NY	265
OrS	Decter, E	NJ	752
OrS	Gallick, G	NJ	881
OrS	Grelsamer, R	NY	268
OrS	Scuderi, G	NY	275
OrS	Zambetti, G	NY	277
Knee Replacement			
OrS	Adler, E	NY	263
OrS	Alexiades, M	NY	263
OrS	Asnis, S	NY	542
OrS	Bindelglass, D	CT	921
OrS	Boone, P	CT	921
OrS	Bostrom, M	NY	264
OrS	Bronson, M	NY	264
OrS	Buly, R	NY	264
OrS	Cobelli, N	NY	403
OrS	D'Amico, J	CT	922
OrS	Deluca, J	CT	922
OrS	Edelson, C	NY	656
OrS	Fealy, S	NY	266
OrS	Gutowski, W	NJ	782
OrS	Haas, S	NY	268
OrS	Haig, S	NY	656
OrS	Hartzband, M	NJ	716
OrS	Hughes, P	CT	923
OrS	Jaffe, F	NY	269
OrS	Kavanagh, B	CT	923
OrS	Kelly, M	NJ	716
OrS	Lynch, M	CT	923
OrS	Macaulay, W	NY	271
OrS	Mani, J	NY	449
OrS	Marx, R	NY	271
OrS	Mc Inerney, V	NJ	853
OrS	Menezes, P	NY	450
OrS	Pellicci, P	NY	273
OrS	Rich, D	NY	543
OrS	Salvati, E	NY	274
OrS	Sarokhan, A	NJ	881
OrS	Scott, W	NY	275
OrS	Scuderi, G	NY	275
OrS	Seebacher, J	NY	658
OrS	Wilson, A	NY	403
OrS	Windsor, R	NY	277
OrS	Yasgur, D	NY	658
OrS	Zuckerman, J	NY	278
SM	Nisonson, B	NY	352
Knee Replacement & Revision			
OrS	Meere, P	NY	271
OrS	Westrich, G	NY	277
Knee Surgery			
OrS	Bauman, P	NY	263
OrS	Berman, M	NJ	715
OrS	Bosco, J	NY	264
OrS	Botwin, C	NJ	881
OrS	Cunningham, J	CT	922
OrS	D'Agostino, R	NY	542

Spec	Name	St	Pg
OrS	Doidge, R	NJ	716
OrS	Figgie, M	NY	266
OrS	Glashow, J	NY	267
OrS	Grossman, R	NJ	822
OrS	Haas, S	NY	268
OrS	Henshaw, D	CT	922
OrS	Jokl, P	CT	954
OrS	Kelly, M	NJ	716
OrS	Khabie, V	NY	657
OrS	Levy, H	NY	270
OrS	Lubliner, J	NY	271
OrS	McIlveen, S	NJ	716
OrS	Montgomery, K	NJ	839
OrS	Rozbruch, J	NY	274
OrS	Rubin, C	NY	577
OrS	Salzer, R	NJ	716
OrS	Schwartz, E	NY	481
OrS	Sethi, P	CT	924
OrS	Tria, A	NJ	864
OrS	Turtel, A	NY	276
SM	Altchek, D	NY	351
SM	Berezin, M	NY	579
SM	Hershman, E	NY	351
SM	Williams, R	NY	352
Knee-Patella Problems			
OrS	Gladstone, J	NY	267
OrS	Grelsamer, R	NY	268

L

Spec	Name	St	Pg
Lacrimal Gland Disorders			
Oph	Gallin, P	NY	253
Oph	Garber, P	NY	539
Oph	Lauer, S	NY	255
Langerhans Cell Histiocytoma			
PHO	Tugal, O	NY	663
Laparoscopic Abdominal Surgery			
S	Borao, F	NJ	826
S	Edye, M	NY	354
S	Grieco, M	NY	564
S	Pereira, S	NJ	730
S	Pomp, A	NY	358
S	Salky, B	NY	359
S	Schmidt, H	NJ	730
S	Vine, A	NY	361
S	Zeitlin, A	NY	486
Laparoscopic Cholecystectomy			
S	Carter, M	NJ	844
S	Christoudias, G	NJ	729
S	Grieco, M	NY	564

Spec	Name	St	Pg
Laparoscopic Hysterectomy			
ObG	Goldstein, S	NJ	821
ObG	Mendelowitz, L	NY	652
Laparoscopic Kidney Surgery			
U	DelPizzo, J	NY	368
U	Esposito, M	NJ	732
Laparoscopic Surgery			
CRS	Arnell, T	NY	149
CRS	Arvanitis, M	NJ	816
CRS	Chessin, D	NY	149
CRS	Chinn, B	NJ	791
CRS	Greenwald, M	NY	514
CRS	Krakovitz, E	NY	625
CRS	Milsom, J	NY	150
CRS	Ross, H	NJ	816
CRS	Sonoda, T	NY	150
CRS	Temple, L	NY	150
CRS	Thornton, S	CT	899
CRS	Waxenbaum, S	NJ	695
CRS	Weiser, M	NY	151
CRS	Whelan, R	NY	151
CRS	Wishner, J	NY	625
GO	Azodi, M	CT	947
GO	Barakat, R	NY	184
GO	Brown, C	NY	184
GO	Chuang, L	NY	637
GO	Curtin, J	NY	184
GO	Denehy, T	NJ	744
GO	Dottino, P	NY	184
GO	Herzog, T	NY	185
GO	Holcomb, K	NY	185
GO	Poynor, E	NY	185
GO	Rahaman, J	NY	185
GO	Serur, E	NY	434
GO	Sonoda, Y	NY	185
GO	Taylor, R	NJ	744
GO	Tobias, D	NJ	834
ObG	Banzon, M	NJ	769
ObG	Beim, R	NJ	880
ObG	Bochner, R	NJ	801
ObG	Brodman, M	NY	242
ObG	Cooperman, A	NJ	750
ObG	Englert, C	NJ	713
ObG	Florio, P	NY	652
ObG	Goldstein, M	NY	244
ObG	Grano, V	NY	652
ObG	Haselkorn, J	NY	537
ObG	Hurst, W	NJ	713
ObG	Iammatteo, M	NJ	838
ObG	Krim, E	NY	538
ObG	Luciani, R	NJ	750
ObG	Lynch, V	CT	953
ObG	Meacham, K	NY	652
ObG	Mohr, R	NJ	838
ObG	Nimaroff, M	NY	538
ObG	Olanescu, A	NY	481
ObG	Reilly, J	NY	497
ObG	Sailon, P	NY	246
ObG	Sassoon, R	NY	247

Specialty & Special Expertise Index

Spec	Name	St	Pg
Oph	Yagoda, A	NY	262
Oph	Zaidman, G	NY	656

Laser-Refractive Surgery

Spec	Name	St	Pg
Oph	D'Aversa, G	NY	539
Oph	Giliberti, O	NJ	852
Oph	Klapper, D	NY	254
Oph	Marks, A	NY	540
Oph	Perry, H	NY	540

LASIK-Refractive Surgery

Spec	Name	St	Pg
Oph	Asbell, P	NY	248
Oph	Benedetto, D	NJ	770
Oph	Braunstein, R	NY	249
Oph	Brown, A	NJ	714
Oph	Brown, C	NJ	714
Oph	Buxton, D	NY	249
Oph	Chaiken, B	NY	249
Oph	Cykiert, R	NY	250
Oph	Davidson, L	NJ	751
Oph	Fishman, A	NY	481
Oph	Fong, R	NY	252
Oph	Fox, M	NY	252
Oph	Glatt, H	NJ	751
Oph	Goldberg, D	NJ	821
Oph	Goldberg, L	NY	539
Oph	Goldstein, M	NY	253
Oph	Guillory, S	NY	253
Oph	Hatsis, A	NY	540
Oph	Hersh, P	NJ	714
Oph	Kelly, S	NY	254
Oph	Klein, N	NY	254
Oph	Lebowitz, M	NY	448
Oph	Lippman, J	NY	654
Oph	Liva, D	NJ	714
Oph	Mackool, R	NY	481
Oph	Mandava, S	CT	919
Oph	Mandel, E	NY	256
Oph	Natale, B	NJ	880
Oph	Nightingale, J	NY	257
Oph	O'Malley, G	NY	598
Oph	Phillips, H	NY	655
Oph	Robbins, K	CT	920
Oph	Rothberg, C	NY	598
Oph	Rudick, A	NY	259
Oph	Salz, A	NJ	864
Oph	Santamaria, J	NJ	802
Oph	Sciortino, P	NY	448
Oph	Shulman, J	NY	260
Oph	Silverman, C	NJ	839
Oph	Stabile, J	NJ	715
Oph	Starr, M	NY	261
Oph	Talansky, M	NJ	822
Oph	Wasserman, B	NJ	781
Oph	Wong, M	NJ	781
Oph	Wong, R	NJ	781
Oph	Zweibel, L	NY	599

Latex Allergy

Spec	Name	St	Pg
A&I	Fine, S	NY	472

Lead Poisoning

Spec	Name	St	Pg
PEn	Noto, R	NY	661

Learning Disorders

Spec	Name	St	Pg
AM	Lopez, R	NY	130
ChiN	De Carlo, R	NY	492
ChiN	Kaufman, D	NY	147
ChiN	Nass, R	NY	148
ChiN	Shaywitz, B	CT	943
ChiN	Traeger, E	NJ	873
Ped	Acker, P	NY	665
Ped	Cross, J	NY	304
Ped	McCarton, C	NY	306
Ped	Shaywitz, S	CT	958
Psyc	Wachtel, A	NY	333

Lens Implants

Spec	Name	St	Pg
Oph	Finlay, A	CT	919
Oph	Goldberg, D	NJ	821
Oph	Pinke, J	CT	920
Oph	Potter, W	CT	920
Oph	Rabinowitz, S	CT	920
Oph	Silbert, G	NJ	715

Lens Implants-Multifocal

Spec	Name	St	Pg
Oph	Dieck, W	NY	653
Oph	Mackool, R	NY	481
Oph	Malik, S	NY	540
Oph	Wong, M	NJ	781

Leukemia

Spec	Name	St	Pg
Hem	Cohen, N	CT	906
Hem	Cook, P	NY	189
Hem	Duffy, T	CT	948
Hem	Halperin, I	NY	190
Hem	Kempin, S	NY	190
Hem	Leonard, J	NY	190
Hem	Marks, P	CT	948
Hem	Maslak, P	NY	191
Hem	Mears, J	NY	191
Hem	Meyer, R	NY	191
Hem	Ossias, A	NY	191
Hem	Rai, K	NY	525
Hem	Raphael, B	NY	191
Hem	Schulman, P	NY	592
Hem	Strair, R	NJ	795
Hem	Tallman, M	NY	192
Hem	Troy, K	NY	192
Hem	Wisch, N	NY	192
Onc	Berman, E	NY	211
Onc	Cooper, D	CT	950
Onc	Feldman, E	NY	212
Onc	Frank, R	CT	912
Onc	Gabrilove, J	NY	213
Onc	Goldberg, S	NJ	707
Onc	Jakubowski, A	NY	215
Onc	Jurcic, J	NY	215
Onc	Klafter, R	NY	216
Onc	Liu, D	NY	645
Onc	Ostrow, S	NY	594

Spec	Name	St	Pg
Onc	Phillips, E	NY	645
Onc	Raza, A	NY	219
Onc	Roboz, G	NY	219
Onc	Scheinberg, D	NY	220
Onc	Seiter, K	NY	646
PHO	Aledo, A	NY	297
PHO	Cairo, M	NY	662
PHO	Carroll, W	NY	297
PHO	Guarini, L	NJ	453
PHO	Kamalakar, P	NJ	756
PHO	Kernan, N	NY	298
PHO	Kulpa, J	NY	454
PHO	Marcus, J	NY	298
PHO	Redner, A	NY	549
PHO	Sundaram, R	NY	454
PHO	Weiner, M	NY	299

Leukemia & Lymphoma

Spec	Name	St	Pg
Hem	Allen, S	NY	525
Hem	Bar, M	CT	906
Hem	Dosik, H	NY	434
Hem	Hymes, K	NY	190
Hem	Kolitz, J	NY	525
Hem	Vogel, J	NY	192
Onc	Coleman, M	NY	212
Onc	Decter, J	NY	212
Onc	Farber, C	NJ	836
Onc	Hollister, D	CT	913
Onc	Salwitz, J	NJ	798
Onc	Silverman, L	NY	221
PHO	Halpern, S	NJ	719
PHO	Harris, M	NJ	719
PHO	Steinherz, P	NY	299
PHO	Tugal, O	NY	663
PHO	Weinblatt, M	NY	549

Leukemia-Chronic Lymphocytic

Spec	Name	St	Pg
Onc	Bernhardt, B	NY	644

Liaison Psychiatry

Spec	Name	St	Pg
Psyc	Heisman, A	NY	458
Psyc	Kalash, G	NY	483
Psyc	Shapiro, P	NY	331
Psyc	Vivek, S	NY	483

Ligament Reconstruction

Spec	Name	St	Pg
HS	Lee, S	NY	187
HS	Lisser, S	NJ	818
OrS	Hannafin, J	NY	268
OrS	Hubbard, C	NY	269
SM	Hershman, E	NY	351
SM	Levy, A	NJ	761

Limb Deformities

Spec	Name	St	Pg
OrS	Feldman, D	NY	266
OrS	Fragomen, A	NY	267
OrS	Rozbruch, S	NY	274
OrS	Sabharwal, S	NJ	753
OrS	Widmann, R	NY	277

Specialty & Special Expertise Index

Spec	Name	St	Pg
Limb Lengthening			
OrS	Fragomen, A	NY	267
OrS	Rozbruch, S	NY	274
OrS	Widmann, R	NY	277
Limb Lengthening (Ilizarov Procedure)			
OrS	Egol, K	NY	266
OrS	Sabharwal, S	NJ	753
OrS	Vitale, M	NY	276
Limb Sparing Surgery			
OrS	Benevenia, J	NJ	752
OrS	Patterson, F	NJ	753
VascS	Ascher, E	NY	467
VascS	Chaudhry, S	NY	569
VascS	Lipsitz, E	NY	416
VascS	Manno, J	NJ	734
VascS	Marin, M	NY	378
VascS	Mendes, D	NY	379
Limb Surgery/Reconstruction			
OrS	Friedlaender, G	CT	954
OrS	Rozbruch, S	NY	274
Liposuction			
D	Bank, D	NY	625
D	Kenet, B	NY	156
D	Narins, R	NY	627
D	Orentreich, D	NY	157
D	Sobel, H	NY	159
D	Urbanek, R	NY	492
D	Wexler, P	NY	160
PlS	Almeyda, E	NJ	312
PlS	Anton, J	NY	603
PlS	Beran, S	NY	667
PlS	Breitbart, A	NY	554
PlS	Cutolo, L	NY	499
PlS	Funt, D	NY	555
PlS	Gotkin, R	NY	555
PlS	Karpinski, R	NY	316
PlS	Leach, T	NJ	783
PlS	Matarasso, A	NY	316
PlS	Perry, A	NJ	865
PlS	Pitman, G	NY	317
PlS	Schulman, M	NY	318
PlS	Schulman, M	NY	318
PlS	Verga, M	NY	320
PlS	Zevon, S	NY	320
Liposuction & Body Contouring			
D	Katz, B	NY	155
PlS	Ablaza, V	NJ	758
PlS	Alizadeh, K	NY	554
PlS	Aston, S	NY	312
PlS	Attkiss, K	CT	929
PlS	Broumand, S	NY	313
PlS	Colen, H	NY	313
PlS	Cuber, S	NJ	808

Spec	Name	St	Pg
PlS	D'Amico, R	NJ	724
PlS	Diktaban, T	NY	314
PlS	Friedman, D	NY	314
PlS	Gewirtz, H	CT	929
PlS	Glicksman, C	NJ	824
PlS	Godfrey, P	NY	315
PlS	Granick, M	NJ	759
PlS	Greenwald, J	NY	668
PlS	Herbstman, R	NJ	808
PlS	Hetzler, P	NJ	824
PlS	Hoffman, L	NY	315
PlS	Hyans, P	NJ	884
PlS	Karp, N	NY	316
PlS	Leipziger, L	NY	556
PlS	LoVerme, P	NJ	759
PlS	Nini, K	NJ	808
PlS	O'Connell, J	CT	929
PlS	Perrotti, J	NY	317
PlS	Price, G	CT	958
PlS	Pyo, D	NJ	842
PlS	Restifo, R	CT	958
PlS	Romita, M	NY	317
PlS	Rosen, A	NJ	759
PlS	Sherman, J	NY	318
PlS	Simpson, R	NY	556
PlS	Skolnik, R	NY	318
PlS	Sternschein, M	NJ	724
PlS	Sultan, M	NY	319
PlS	Weinstein, L	NJ	842
PlS	Wey, P	NJ	808
PlS	Zeitels, J	NJ	884
PlS	Zubowski, R	NJ	724
Liver & Biliary Cancer			
S	Emond, J	NY	355
S	Fong, Y	NY	355
S	Kinkhabwala, M	NY	414
S	Newman, E	NY	358
Liver & Biliary Disease			
Ge	Antonelle, R	NY	632
Ge	Jacobson, I	NY	175
Ge	Tobias, H	NY	180
Liver & Biliary Surgery			
S	Chabot, J	NY	354
S	Chamberlain, R	NJ	762
S	Gannon, C	NJ	785
S	Kinkhabwala, M	NY	414
S	Salem, R	CT	962
S	Yiengpruksawan, A	NJ	730
Liver Cancer			
Onc	Grace, W	NY	213
Onc	Holcombe, R	NY	214
Onc	Kemeny, N	NY	216
Onc	O'Reilly, E	NY	218
PS	La Quaglia, M	NY	303
S	Cherqui, D	NY	354
S	Emond, J	NY	355

Spec	Name	St	Pg
S	Emre, S	CT	961
S	Gannon, C	NJ	785
S	Hiotis, S	NY	356
S	Jarnagin, W	NY	356
S	Karpeh, M	NY	357
S	Kemeny, M	NY	485
S	Labow, D	NY	357
S	Libutti, S	NY	414
S	Marcus, S	CT	935
S	Salem, R	CT	962
S	Schwartz, M	NY	359
S	Teperman, L	NY	360
VIR	Brown, K	NY	375
VIR	Cynamon, J	NY	416
VIR	Nosher, J	NJ	812
VIR	Solomon, S	NY	376
Liver Disease			
DR	Rozenblit, A	NY	388
Ge	Afridi, S	NJ	776
Ge	Antony, M	NY	391
Ge	Bernstein, D	NY	521
Ge	Bleicher, R	NJ	850
Ge	Borcich, A	NY	171
Ge	Broussard, C	NJ	700
Ge	Brown, R	NY	171
Ge	Cantor, M	NY	171
Ge	Chinitz, M	NY	632
Ge	Cohn, W	NY	590
Ge	De Antonio, J	NJ	776
Ge	Dieterich, D	NY	172
Ge	Ferges, M	NJ	861
Ge	Ferran, E	NY	173
Ge	Fiest, T	NJ	817
Ge	Gaglio, P	NY	391
Ge	Gardner, P	CT	903
Ge	Glanzman, B	NY	590
Ge	Goldblatt, R	NY	633
Ge	Goldfarb, J	NJ	701
Ge	Goldin, H	NY	174
Ge	Grendell, J	NY	522
Ge	Grosman, I	NY	431
Ge	Gupta, S	NY	391
Ge	Hale, W	CT	904
Ge	Hammerman, H	NY	174
Ge	Kenny, R	NJ	743
Ge	Kim-Schluger, H	NY	175
Ge	Knapp, A	NY	175
Ge	Korsten, M	NY	392
Ge	Lax, J	NY	176
Ge	Lebovics, E	NY	635
Ge	Lucak, S	NY	177
Ge	Maizel, B	NY	432
Ge	Marsh, F	NY	178
Ge	Min, A	NY	178
Ge	Miskovitz, P	NY	178
Ge	Nikias, G	NJ	701
Ge	Plumser, A	NJ	794
Ge	Remy, P	NY	392
Ge	Rosner, B	NJ	777
Ge	Salik, J	NY	179
Ge	Schiano, T	NY	180

Specialty & Special Expertise Index

Specialty & Special Expertise Index

Medications in the Elderly

Specialty & Special Expertise Index

Specialty & Special Expertise Index

Specialty & Special Expertise Index

Spec	Name	St	Pg	Spec	Name	St	Pg	Spec	Name	St	Pg
NS	Frempong-Boadu, A	NY	227	NS	Stieg, P	NY	230	N	Geller, E	NJ	749
NS	Fried, A	NJ	711	NS	Sundaresan, N	NY	230	N	Gendelman, S	NY	233
NS	Friedlander, M	NJ	879	NS	Tabar, V	NY	230	N	Gerber, O	NY	596
NS	Gamache, F	NY	227	NS	Vingan, R	NJ	711	N	Gilson, N	NJ	820
NS	Ghatan, S	NY	227	NS	Weiner, H	NY	231	N	Gizzi, M	NJ	800
NS	Ghogawala, Z	CT	915	NS	Wisoff, J	NY	231	N	Golbe, L	NJ	800
NS	Golfinos, J	NY	228	NS	Woo, H	NY	595	N	Goldstein, J	CT	952
NS	Goodman, R	NY	228	NS	Zampella, E	NJ	837	N	Gordon, N	NY	535
NS	Gutin, P	NY	228	NS	Zimmerman, G	CT	915	N	Green, M	NY	233
NS	Hartl, R	NY	228	NS	Zonenshayn, M	NY	443	N	Greer, D	CT	952
NS	Heary, R	NJ	749					N	Grenell, S	NY	400
NS	Hirschfeld, A	NY	442		**Neurology**			N	Gross, E	NY	649
NS	Hodosh, R	NJ	879	N	Ahluwalia, B	NY	649	N	Gross, J	CT	916
NS	Holtzman, R	NY	534	N	Alweiss, G	NJ	711	N	Gruber, M	NY	233
NS	Hubschmann, O	NJ	749	N	Anselmi, G	NJ	769	N	Haimovic, I	NY	535
NS	Jafar, J	NY	228	N	Apatoff, B	NY	231	N	Hainline, B	NY	535
NS	Kaiser, M	NY	228	N	Appelbaum, J	NY	480	N	Halperin, J	NJ	879
NS	Kaplitt, M	NY	228	N	Azhar, S	NY	443	N	Harden, C	NY	535
NS	Knightly, J	NJ	837	N	Bansil, S	NJ	879	N	Herbert, J	NY	233
NS	Kornel, E	NY	649	N	Belok, L	NY	231	N	Herbstein, D	NY	233
NS	Langer, D	NY	534	N	Belsh, J	NJ	799	N	Herman, M	NJ	820
NS	LaSala, P	NY	399	N	Blady, D	NJ	749	N	Herskovitz, S	NY	400
NS	Lavyne, M	NY	228	N	Blanck, R	NY	535	N	Heublum, M	NY	234
NS	Lee, S	NJ	799	N	Bodis-Wollner, I	NY	443	N	Hiesiger, E	NY	234
NS	Lee, T	NY	649	N	Brannagan, T	NY	231	N	Holland, N	NJ	821
NS	Leon, S	NY	595	N	Bressman, S	NY	231	N	Horvath, S	NY	234
NS	Levine, M	NY	534	N	Britton, C	NY	231	N	Jordan, B	NY	650
NS	Lipow, K	CT	915	N	Bronster, D	NY	231	N	Jutkowitz, R	NY	496
NS	McCormick, P	NY	229	N	Buckner, C	NY	443	N	Kaiser, P	NJ	780
NS	McKhann, G	NY	229	N	Butler, J	CT	915	N	Kanner, R	NY	535
NS	McLaughlin, M	NJ	780	N	Cafferty, M	NY	232	N	Katz, A	CT	953
NS	Mintz, A	CT	915	N	Casson, I	NY	480	N	Kaufman, D	NY	400
NS	Mittler, M	NY	534	N	Charles, J	NJ	769	N	Kay, A	NY	443
NS	Moore, F	NJ	711	N	Charney, J	NY	232	N	Keilson, M	NY	444
NS	Murali, R	NY	649	N	Chodosh, E	NJ	852	N	Kelemen, J	NY	535
NS	Nosko, M	NJ	799	N	Cohen, D	NY	595	N	Kessler, J	NY	536
NS	Onesti, S	NY	534	N	Cohen, J	NY	400	N	Klein, P	NJ	711
NS	Oppenheim, J	NY	576	N	Coll, R	NY	232	N	Knep, S	NJ	852
NS	Patel, A	NY	229	N	Cook, S	NJ	749	N	Kolodny, E	NY	234
NS	Perin, N	NY	229	N	Coyle, P	NY	596	N	Koppel, B	NY	234
NS	Piepmeier, J	CT	952	N	Crystal, H	NY	443	N	Kososky, C	NJ	780
NS	Post, K	NY	229	N	Cuzzone, L	CT	916	N	Kranzler, L	NY	650
NS	Przybylski, G	NJ	799	N	Daras, M	NY	232	N	Kula, R	NY	536
NS	Quest, D	NY	229	N	DeAngelis, L	NY	232	N	Kuzniecky, R	NY	234
NS	Rekate, H	NY	534	N	Devinsky, O	NY	232	N	Laban-Grant, O	NY	650
NS	Riina, H	NY	229	N	Dickoff, D	NY	649	N	Labar, D	NY	234
NS	Rosenblum, B	NJ	820	N	Drexler, E	NY	443	N	Lange, D	NY	234
NS	Rosner, S	NY	649	N	Duckrow, R	CT	952	N	Latov, N	NY	235
NS	Roth, P	NJ	711	N	Duncan, D	NY	649	N	Lazar, M	NJ	800
NS	Schulder, M	NY	534	N	Effron, C	NJ	711	N	Lepore, F	NJ	800
NS	Schwartz, A	NY	443	N	Engel, M	NY	232	N	Levin, K	NJ	711
NS	Schwartz, T	NY	229	N	Ettinger, A	NY	535	N	Levine, D	NY	235
NS	Sen, C	NY	230	N	Fahn, S	NY	232	N	Levine, S	NY	444
NS	Shahid, S	CT	915	N	Feinberg, T	NY	232	N	Levy, L	NY	536
NS	Shear, P	CT	915	N	Fellus, J	NJ	769	N	Libman, R	NY	536
NS	Simon, S	CT	915	N	Fink, M	NY	233	N	Lin, M	NY	235
NS	Sisti, M	NY	230	N	Foo, S	NY	233	N	Lipton, R	NY	400
NS	Snow, R	NY	230	N	Forster, G	NY	233	N	Litchman, C	CT	916
NS	Solomon, R	NY	230	N	Freddo, L	NY	400	N	Louis, E	NY	235
NS	Souweidane, M	NY	230	N	French, J	NY	233	N	Lublin, F	NY	235
NS	Spencer, D	CT	952	N	Friedlander, D	NJ	863	N	Luciano, D	NY	235
NS	Spitzer, D	NY	576	N	Gainey, P	NJ	820	N	Maccabee, P	NY	444
NS	Steinberger, A	NJ	711					N	Maniscalco, A	NY	444

Specialty & Special Expertise Index

Specialty & Special Expertise Index

Spec	Name	St	Pg
ObG	Leong, M	NY	538
ObG	Levine, R	NY	245
ObG	Levy, J	NY	401
ObG	Lind, L	NY	246
ObG	Luciani, R	NJ	750
ObG	Lustig, I	NY	246
ObG	Lynch, V	CT	953
ObG	Mack, L	NY	538
ObG	Maher, J	NY	446
ObG	Maloney, R	NY	652
ObG	Mann, C	NY	597
ObG	Margulis, E	NJ	880
ObG	Martens, M	NJ	821
ObG	Masson, L	NJ	769
ObG	Matalon, M	NY	597
ObG	McGovern, C	NY	652
ObG	Meacham, K	NY	652
ObG	Melnick, H	NY	246
ObG	Mendelowitz, L	NY	652
ObG	Meyer, M	NJ	713
ObG	Michel, K	NY	246
ObG	Mieszerski, L	NY	652
ObG	Minkoff, H	NY	446
ObG	Mohr, R	NJ	838
ObG	Nelson, W	NY	653
ObG	Nimaroff, M	NY	538
ObG	Olanescu, A	NY	481
ObG	Ordorica, S	NY	246
ObG	Ott, A	NY	597
ObG	Phillips, R	NY	246
ObG	Ponterio, J	NY	496
ObG	Quartell, A	NJ	750
ObG	Rathauser, R	NJ	801
ObG	Regard, M	NY	653
ObG	Reilly, J	NY	497
ObG	Reilly, K	NY	401
ObG	Reizis, I	NY	446
ObG	Rezvani, F	NJ	713
ObG	Rodke, G	NY	246
ObG	Rubenstein, A	NJ	714
ObG	Sadarangani, B	NY	246
ObG	Sailon, P	NY	246
ObG	San Roman, G	NY	597
ObG	Sanderson, R	NJ	863
ObG	Sassoon, R	NY	247
ObG	Schechter, M	CT	918
ObG	Scher, J	NY	247
ObG	Schwartz, J	NY	247
ObG	Segarra, P	NY	597
ObG	Seigel, M	NJ	821
ObG	Smilen, S	NY	247
ObG	Snyder, J	NY	247
ObG	Soffer, J	NJ	880
ObG	Steer, R	NJ	838
ObG	Sullum, S	NY	247
ObG	Szeto, M	CT	918
ObG	Toles, A	NY	538
ObG	Ugol, J	CT	918
ObG	Ullman, J	NY	653
ObG	Uy, V	NJ	769
ObG	Vasudeva, K	NY	538
ObG	Veloso, M	NY	538
ObG	Violi, C	CT	918

Spec	Name	St	Pg
ObG	Wallis, J	NJ	838
ObG	Waterstone, M	NY	247
ObG	Weinstein, D	CT	918
ObG	Wysoki, R	NY	653
ObG	Yale, S	NY	247
ObG	Yarberry-Allen, P	NY	247
ObG	Young, B	NY	248
ObG	Young, C	NY	401

Occupational Dermatology

Spec	Name	St	Pg
D	Cohen, D	NY	153
D	Cohen, S	NY	387

Occupational Disease & Injury

Spec	Name	St	Pg
OM	Mendelsohn, S	NY	538

Occupational Lung Disease

Spec	Name	St	Pg
OM	Kipen, H	NJ	802
Pul	Maxfield, R	NY	337
Pul	Redlich, C	CT	959

Occupational Medicine

Spec	Name	St	Pg
FMed	Levites, K	NY	590
IM	Altholz, J	NY	639
IM	Pappas, S	NY	642
IM	Schneider, S	NY	205
IM	Zarowitz, W	NY	643
OM	Gochfeld, M	NJ	801
OM	Kipen, H	NJ	802
OM	Landrigan, P	NY	248
OM	Mendelsohn, S	NY	538

Ocular Ultrasound

Spec	Name	St	Pg
Oph	Fisher, Y	NY	252

Oculoplastic & Orbital Surgery

Spec	Name	St	Pg
Oph	Elahi, E	NY	251
Oph	Leib, M	NY	255
Oph	Turbin, R	NJ	752
PlS	Spinelli, H	NY	319

Oculoplastic Surgery

Spec	Name	St	Pg
Oph	Della Rocca, R	NY	251
Oph	Di Leo, F	NY	598
Oph	Gordon, J	NY	654
Oph	Grasso, C	NY	481
Oph	Kazim, M	NY	254
Oph	Lauer, S	NY	255
Oph	Lisman, R	NY	255
Oph	Maher, E	NY	256
Oph	Milite, J	NJ	802
Oph	Moskowitz, B	NY	257
Oph	Pizzarello, L	NY	598
Oph	Relland, M	NY	258
Oph	Rodgers, I	NY	259
Oph	Schlessinger, D	NY	541
Oph	Schwarcz, R	NY	260
Oph	Stabile, J	NJ	715

Ophthalmic Pathology

Spec	Name	St	Pg
Oph	Friedman, A	NY	252
Oph	Rosenbaum, P	NY	402

Ophthalmic Plastic Surgery

Spec	Name	St	Pg
Oph	Angrist, R	NJ	863
Oph	Chern, R	NY	250
Oph	Garber, P	NY	539
Oph	Lauer, S	NY	255
Oph	Reich, R	NY	448

Ophthalmology

Spec	Name	St	Pg
Oph	Abramson, D	NY	248
Oph	Accardi, F	NY	248
Oph	Ackerman, J	NY	446
Oph	Aharon, R	NY	481
Oph	Altman, B	CT	919
Oph	Angioletti, L	NY	248
Oph	Angrist, R	NJ	863
Oph	Aries, P	NY	597
Oph	Asbell, P	NY	248
Oph	Auran, J	NY	248
Oph	Bansal, R	NY	653
Oph	Barile, G	NY	249
Oph	Barker, B	NY	249
Oph	Benedetto, D	NJ	770
Oph	Berke, S	NY	539
Oph	Berman, D	NY	446
Oph	Bhagat, N	NJ	751
Oph	Biser, S	NY	653
Oph	Blondo, D	NJ	802
Oph	Boniuk, V	NY	539
Oph	Braunstein, R	NY	249
Oph	Brecher, R	NY	447
Oph	Brown, A	NJ	714
Oph	Brown, C	NJ	714
Oph	Brustein, H	NY	653
Oph	Burke, P	NJ	714
Oph	Buxton, D	NY	249
Oph	Campolattaro, B	NY	249
Oph	Cangemi, F	NJ	751
Oph	Caputo, A	NJ	751
Oph	Casper, D	NY	249
Oph	Chaiken, B	NY	249
Oph	Chang, S	NY	249
Oph	Charles, N	NY	250
Oph	Chen, L	NJ	838
Oph	Chern, R	NY	250
Oph	Chess, J	NY	402
Oph	Chin, P	NJ	714
Oph	Cohen, B	NY	250
Oph	Cohen, L	NY	250
Oph	Coleman, D	NY	250
Oph	Confino, J	NJ	880
Oph	Constad, W	NJ	770
Oph	Cossari, A	NY	597
Oph	Cykiert, R	NY	250
Oph	D'Amico, D	NY	250
Oph	D'Aversa, G	NY	539
Oph	Davidson, L	NJ	751
Oph	Dayan, A	NY	250

Specialty & Special Expertise Index

Castle Connolly *Top Doctors: New York Metro Area* 16th Edition

Specialty & Special Expertise Index

Specialty & Special Expertise Index

Spec	Name	St	Pg
Oto	Frank, D	NY	543
Oto	Fried, M	NY	404
Oto	Garay, K	NJ	770
Oto	Gargano, R	NY	599
Oto	Genden, E	NY	280
Oto	Godin, D	NY	280
Oto	Gold, S	NY	280
Oto	Goldstein, S	NY	404
Oto	Gordon, M	NY	543
Oto	Gordon, N	CT	925
Oto	Green, R	NY	280
Oto	Grosso, J	NY	544
Oto	Guida, R	NY	280
Oto	Hammerschlag, P	NY	280
Oto	Hanson, M	NY	451
Oto	Har-El, G	NY	280
Oto	Henick, D	NJ	717
Oto	Ho, B	NJ	717
Oto	Hoffman, R	NY	280
Oto	Huo, J	NY	482
Oto	Jacobs, J	NY	281
Oto	Jacono, A	NY	544
Oto	Jahn, A	NY	281
Oto	Josephson, J	NY	281
Oto	Kacker, A	NY	281
Oto	Kase, S	NY	659
Oto	Kates, M	NY	659
Oto	Katz, H	NJ	717
Oto	Kay, S	NJ	803
Oto	Klarsfeld, J	CT	925
Oto	Klenoff, B	CT	925
Oto	Kohan, D	NY	281
Oto	Komisar, A	NY	280
Oto	Koufman, J	NY	281
Oto	Kraus, D	NY	281
Oto	Krespi, Y	NY	282
Oto	Krevitt, L	NY	282
Oto	Kuhel, W	NY	282
Oto	Kuriloff, D	NY	282
Oto	Kveton, J	CT	954
Oto	Kwartler, J	NJ	881
Oto	La Bagnara, J	NJ	853
Oto	La Marca, C	NY	482
Oto	Lachman, R	NJ	840
Oto	Lagmay, V	NY	451
Oto	Lalwani, A	NY	282
Oto	Lane, E	CT	925
Oto	Lawson, W	NY	282
Oto	Lazar, A	NJ	864
Oto	Lebovics, R	NY	282
Oto	Levin, R	CT	925
Oto	Levine, S	CT	925
Oto	Li, R	NJ	803
Oto	Lim, J	NY	282
Oto	Linstrom, C	NY	283
Oto	Lipinsky, E	NY	600
Oto	Litman, R	NY	600
Oto	Low, R	NJ	717
Oto	Markowitz, A	NY	283
Oto	Marotta, J	NY	600
Oto	Mattel, S	NJ	853
Oto	Mattucci, K	NY	544
Oto	Mazzara, C	NJ	803
Oto	Meiteles, L	NY	659
Oto	Michaelides, E	CT	955
Oto	Milgrim, L	NJ	717
Oto	Miller, A	NJ	803
Oto	Miller, P	NY	283
Oto	Moisa, I	NY	544
Oto	Morrow, T	NJ	753
Oto	Myssiorek, D	NY	283
Oto	Nass, R	NY	283
Oto	Parisier, S	NY	283
Oto	Perlman, P	NY	544
Oto	Persky, M	NY	283
Oto	Pincus, R	NY	283
Oto	Pollack, S	NY	284
Oto	Portnoy, W	NY	284
Oto	Rizk, S	NY	284
Oto	Roland, J	NY	284
Oto	Romo, T	NY	284
Oto	Rosen, A	NJ	717
Oto	Rosenbaum, J	NJ	804
Oto	Rosenberg, D	NY	284
Oto	Rosner, L	NY	544
Oto	Rossos, A	NJ	822
Oto	Rothstein, S	NY	284
Oto	Ryback, H	NY	659
Oto	Sacks, S	NY	284
Oto	Salzer, S	CT	925
Oto	Sasaki, C	CT	955
Oto	Scaccia, F	NJ	822
Oto	Schaefer, S	NY	285
Oto	Schantz, S	NY	285
Oto	Scharf, R	NJ	882
Oto	Scherl, M	NJ	717
Oto	Schley, W	NY	285
Oto	Schneider, K	NY	285
Oto	Sclafani, A	NY	285
Oto	Scott, J	NY	659
Oto	Selesnick, S	NY	285
Oto	Setzen, M	NY	544
Oto	Shah, D	NJ	822
Oto	Shapiro, B	NY	659
Oto	Shemen, L	NY	285
Oto	Shikowitz, M	NY	544
Oto	Shugar, J	NY	285
Oto	Singh, B	NY	286
Oto	Sinnreich, A	NY	498
Oto	Slavit, D	NY	286
Oto	Smith, R	NY	404
Oto	Snyder, G	NY	482
Oto	Soletic, R	NY	545
Oto	Sperling, N	NY	451
Oto	Stewart, M	NY	286
Oto	Stidham, K	NY	659
Oto	Storper, I	NY	286
Oto	Strome, M	NY	286
Oto	Sulica, R	NY	286
Oto	Surow, J	NJ	717
Oto	Tawfik, B	NY	545
Oto	Taylor, H	NJ	840
Oto	Tobias, G	NJ	717
Oto	Turk, J	NY	286
Oto	Urken, M	NY	286
Oto	Vambutas, A	NY	545
Oto	Vastola, A	NY	451
Oto	Vining, E	CT	955
Oto	Volpi, D	NY	287
Oto	Waner, M	NY	287
Oto	Wong, R	NY	287
Oto	Woo, P	NY	287
Oto	Yankelowitz, S	NY	404
Oto	Young, N	CT	955
Oto	Youngerman, J	NY	545
Oto	Zahtz, G	NY	545
Oto	Zalvan, C	NY	659
Oto	Zbar, L	NJ	753
Oto	Zelman, W	NY	545
Oto	Zimbler, M	NY	287

Otology

Spec	Name	St	Pg
Oto	Grosso, J	NY	544
Oto	Hanson, M	NY	451
Oto	Kay, S	NJ	803
Oto	Litman, R	NY	600
Oto	Mattucci, K	NY	544

Otology & Neuro-Otology

Spec	Name	St	Pg
Oto	Jahn, A	NY	281
Oto	Meiteles, L	NY	659

Otoplasty

Spec	Name	St	Pg
Oto	Shikowitz, M	NY	544

Otosclerosis

Spec	Name	St	Pg
Oto	Gordon, M	NY	543
Oto	Selesnick, S	NY	285
Oto	Sperling, N	NY	451

Ovarian Cancer

Spec	Name	St	Pg
GO	Abu-Rustum, N	NY	184
GO	Barakat, R	NY	184
GO	Brown, C	NY	184
GO	Caputo, T	NY	184
GO	Carlson, J	NJ	795
GO	Chi, D	NY	184
GO	Chuang, L	NY	637
GO	Curtin, J	NY	184
GO	Denehy, T	NJ	744
GO	Economos, K	NY	434
GO	Goldberg, G	NY	394
GO	Goldberg, M	NJ	795
GO	Herzog, T	NY	185
GO	Holcomb, K	NY	185
GO	Koulos, J	NY	185
GO	Lovecchio, J	NY	524
GO	Maiman, M	NY	494
GO	Menzin, A	NY	524
GO	Rodriguez, L	NJ	795
GO	Rutherford, T	CT	947
GO	Santin, A	CT	947
GO	Schwartz, P	CT	947
GO	Smith, H	NY	394
GO	Wallach, R	NY	185

Specialty & Special Expertise Index

Specialty & Special Expertise Index

Specialty & Special Expertise Index

Specialty & Special Expertise Index

Specialty & Special Expertise Index

Spec	Name	St	Pg	Spec	Name	St	Pg	Spec	Name	St	Pg
Ped	Esteban-Cruciani, N	NY	408	Ped	McAbee, G	NJ	807	Ped	Sugarman, L	NJ	723
Ped	Fernandes, D	NY	456	Ped	McCarton, C	NY	306	Ped	Traister, M	NY	308
Ped	Ferrier, G	NY	305	Ped	McHugh, M	NY	306	Ped	Versfelt, M	NY	667
Ped	Festa, R	NY	602	Ped	McMahon, D	NY	603	Ped	Visconti, E	NY	499
Ped	Freedman, R	CT	927	Ped	Mehta, U	NJ	883	Ped	Wager, M	NY	667
Ped	Freilich, S	NY	305	Ped	Meisler, S	NY	666	Ped	Weinberger, S	NY	308
Ped	Friedman, E	NY	552	Ped	Milanaik, R	NY	553	Ped	Weiner, R	NY	410
Ped	Galinkin, L	NY	552	Ped	Mini, K	CT	928	Ped	Weiss, C	NJ	723
Ped	Gately, A	NY	456	Ped	Mongillo, N	CT	928	Ped	Weissbrot, J	NY	667
Ped	Gerberg, L	NY	552	Ped	Monti, L	NY	306	Ped	Wisotsky, D	NJ	723
Ped	Glaser, A	NY	456	Ped	Morelli, A	CT	928	Ped	Wu, J	NY	457
Ped	Goldstein, J	NY	305	Ped	Morgan, J	CT	958	Ped	Yalamanchi, K	NJ	807
Ped	Goldstein, S	NY	482	Ped	Murphy, R	NY	306	Ped	Yorke, E	NJ	865
Ped	Gotfried, F	NJ	841	Ped	Murphy, R	NJ	823	Ped	Zimmerman, S	NY	308
Ped	Gould, E	NY	552	Ped	Namerow, D	NJ	722	Ped	Zoltan, I	NY	410
Ped	Green, A	NY	552	Ped	Nerwen, C	NY	553				
Ped	Grijnsztein, J	NY	552	Ped	Newman-Cedar, M	NY	306	**Pelvic & Acetabular Fractures**			
Ped	Gruenwald, L	NJ	757	Ped	O'Brien, D	NJ	722	OrS	Helfet, D	NY	269
Ped	Gruskay, J	CT	957	Ped	Oeffinger, K	NY	307				
Ped	Haber, P	NY	409	Ped	Oghia, H	NY	456	**Pelvic & Perineal Surgery**			
Ped	Hages, H	NJ	722	Ped	Oko, P	NJ	770	CRS	Fleischer, M	NY	427
Ped	Handler, R	NJ	841	Ped	Oppedisano, C	NY	409	CRS	Rezac, C	NJ	791
Ped	Hankin, D	NY	553	Ped	Palsky, G	NJ	783				
Ped	Harlow, P	NJ	722	Ped	Panza, R	NJ	883	**Pelvic Congestion Syndrome**			
Ped	Hartz, C	NY	666	Ped	Panzner, E	NJ	883	VIR	White, R	CT	964
Ped	Hedrick, D	CT	927	Ped	Parles, J	NY	603				
Ped	Hes, D	NY	305	Ped	Poon, E	NY	307	**Pelvic Imaging**			
Ped	Hirschman, A	NY	409	Ped	Popper, L	NY	307	DR	McCarthy, S	CT	945
Ped	Hyatt, A	NJ	722	Ped	Preis, O	NY	456	DR	Newhouse, J	NY	163
Ped	Igel, G	NY	409	Ped	Prezioso, P	NY	307				
Ped	Inamdar, S	NY	305	Ped	Prince, A	NY	307	**Pelvic Organ Prolapse Repair**			
Ped	Jackson, R	NY	456	Ped	Proskin, W	NY	666	CRS	Fleischer, M	NY	427
Ped	Juan, P	CT	927	Ped	Puder, D	NY	578	ObG	Brodman, M	NY	242
Ped	Kahn, M	NY	305	Ped	Quinn, J	NY	603	ObG	Goldstein, M	NY	244
Ped	Kaminer, R	NY	409	Ped	Rabinowicz, M	NY	553	ObG	Guess, M	CT	953
Ped	Kanter, A	NJ	722	Ped	Raucher, H	NY	307	ObG	Hines, B	CT	918
Ped	Kaplan, M	NY	602	Ped	Raymond, G	NJ	783	ObG	Olanescu, A	NY	481
Ped	Katz, A	NJ	865	Ped	Resmovits, M	NY	553	ObG	Segarra, P	NY	597
Ped	Katzenstein, M	NY	409	Ped	Richel, P	NY	666	ObG	Smilen, S	NY	247
Ped	Keith, M	NY	305	Ped	Rigtrup, E	NJ	757	ObG	Violi, C	CT	918
Ped	Klenk, R	CT	927	Ped	Robert, M	CT	958				
Ped	Klos, A	NJ	770	Ped	Romanowitz, H	CT	928	**Pelvic Reconstruction**			
Ped	Kolker, H	NY	603	Ped	Rosello, L	NY	307	GO	Smith, H	NY	394
Ped	Kolsky, N	NJ	722	Ped	Rosenbaum, M	NY	307	GO	Taylor, R	NJ	744
Ped	Korval, A	CT	927	Ped	Rosenfeld, S	NY	307	ObG	Evanko, J	NY	243
Ped	Kotin, N	NY	305	Ped	Sacker, I	NY	308	ObG	Leong, M	NY	538
Ped	Kurfist, L	NY	603	Ped	Sanford, M	NY	308	ObG	Lind, L	NY	246
Ped	Kushner, S	NJ	722	Ped	Saraiya, N	NJ	883	ObG	Mendelowitz, L	NY	652
Ped	Larson, S	NY	306	Ped	Schechter, M	NY	409	ObG	Quartell, A	NJ	750
Ped	Lazarus, G	NY	306	Ped	Schiz, S	CT	928				
Ped	Leavens-Maurer, J	NY	553	Ped	Schuss, S	NJ	723	**Pelvic Surgery**			
Ped	Levine, D	CT	928	Ped	Scofield, L	NJ	854	GO	Chambers, J	NY	433
Ped	Levitt, M	NY	666	Ped	Sergiou, H	NY	456	ObG	Ascher-Walsh, C	NY	242
Ped	Levitzky, S	NY	306	Ped	Shaywitz, S	CT	958	ObG	Bachmann, G	NJ	801
Ped	Levy, M	NY	553	Ped	Short, J	NY	499	ObG	Besser, G	CT	917
Ped	London, R	NY	666	Ped	Siegal, E	NY	578	ObG	Cooperman, A	NJ	750
Ped	Lubell, H	NY	666	Ped	Skripkus, A	NJ	770	ObG	Young, C	NY	401
Ped	Magner, J	CT	928	Ped	Softness, B	NY	308				
Ped	Manners, R	NY	603	Ped	Sosulski, R	NY	603				
Ped	Marcus, R	NJ	757	Ped	Stein, B	NY	308				
Ped	Marino, R	NY	553	Ped	Stein, R	NY	410				
Ped	Marks, L	CT	928	Ped	Strassberg, B	NY	410				
Ped	Mayers, M	NY	409	Ped	Suda, A	NJ	841				

Specialty & Special Expertise Index

Specialty & Special Expertise Index

Polycystic Ovarian Syndrome

Spec	Name	St	Pg
EDM	Albin, J	NY	629
EDM	Daud-Ahmad, S	NJ	699
EDM	Gelato, M	NY	589
RE	Brenner, S	NY	561
RE	Chang, P	NY	342
RE	Klein, J	NY	674
RE	Lydic, M	NY	606
RE	Schmidt-Sarosi, C	NY	345
RE	Tortoriello, D	NY	345

Polycythemia Rubra Vera

Spec	Name	St	Pg
Hem	Fruchtman, S	NY	189

Polymyalgia Rheumatica

Spec	Name	St	Pg
Rhu	Belilos, E	NY	562
Rhu	Lesser, R	NY	462
Rhu	Magid, S	NY	348
Rhu	Stern, R	NY	350

Polymyositis

Spec	Name	St	Pg
Rhu	Bernstein, L	NY	462
Rhu	Hutchinson, G	CT	961

Polypharmacology (Excess Medications)

Spec	Name	St	Pg
Ger	Sherman, F	NY	183

Porphyria

Spec	Name	St	Pg
CG	Desnick, R	NY	149

Portal Hypertension

Spec	Name	St	Pg
S	Emre, S	CT	961

Post Polio Syndrome/Rehabilitation

Spec	Name	St	Pg
PMR	Bach, J	NJ	758
PMR	Moldover, J	NY	310
PMR	Zimmerman, J	NJ	723

Post Traumatic Stress Disorder

Spec	Name	St	Pg
ChAP	Fornari, V	NY	473
Psyc	Caracci, G	NJ	759
Psyc	Levin, A	NY	670
Psyc	Markowitz, J	NY	327
Psyc	Schroeder, K	NY	579

Power Doppler Imaging

Spec	Name	St	Pg
DR	Adler, R	NY	160

Precancerous Lesions

Spec	Name	St	Pg
Oto	Boyle, J	NY	278

Preconception Planning

Spec	Name	St	Pg
ObG	Brightman, R	NY	242

Spec	Name	St	Pg
ObG	Brustman, L	NY	242

Pregnancy & Hematologic Abnormalities

Spec	Name	St	Pg
MF	Berkowitz, R	NY	209

Pregnancy After Age 35

Spec	Name	St	Pg
MF	Hutson, J	NY	209
ObG	Burns, L	NJ	852
ObG	Friedman, L	NY	244

Pregnancy Loss

Spec	Name	St	Pg
MF	Benito, C	NJ	836
MF	Meirowitz, N	NY	530
MF	Roshan, D	NY	210

Pregnancy Loss-Recurrent

Spec	Name	St	Pg
RE	Bronson, R	NY	606
RE	Keltz, M	NY	343
RE	Lydic, M	NY	606

Pregnancy-High Risk

Spec	Name	St	Pg
MF	Alvarez, M	NJ	706
MF	Berck, D	NY	643
MF	Bobby, P	CT	911
MF	Bond, A	CT	911
MF	Bush, J	NY	439
MF	Chandra, P	NY	439
MF	Chazotte, C	NY	397
MF	Copel, J	CT	949
MF	D'Alton, M	NY	209
MF	Devine, P	NY	644
MF	Eddleman, K	NY	209
MF	Fleischer, A	NY	529
MF	Genc, M	NY	209
MF	Gimovsky, M	NJ	747
MF	Gonzalez, D	NJ	819
MF	Grunebaum, A	NY	209
MF	Henderson, C	NY	397
MF	Inglis, S	NY	478
MF	Kalish, R	NY	209
MF	Klein, V	NY	530
MF	Lescale, K	NY	644
MF	Magriples, U	CT	949
MF	Meirowitz, N	NY	530
MF	Mootabar, H	NY	644
MF	Paidas, M	CT	949
MF	Patrick, S	NY	210
MF	Principe, D	NJ	707
MF	Rebarber, A	NY	210
MF	Rochelson, B	NY	530
MF	Roshan, D	NY	210
MF	Saltzman, D	NY	210
MF	Shevell, T	CT	912
MF	Stiller, R	CT	912
MF	Sullivan, C	NJ	851
MF	Warren, W	NJ	747
ObG	Apuzzio, J	NJ	750
ObG	Armbruster, R	NY	651

Spec	Name	St	Pg
ObG	Benedict, L	NY	537
ObG	Blair, E	CT	917
ObG	Brightman, R	NY	242
ObG	Buterman, I	NY	243
ObG	Coven, R	NJ	713
ObG	Cuteri, J	CT	917
ObG	Dor, N	NY	446
ObG	Florio, P	NY	652
ObG	Friedman, A	NJ	780
ObG	Gubernick, M	NY	244
ObG	Haratz-Rubinstein, N	NY	446
ObG	Iammatteo, M	NJ	838
ObG	Kessler, A	NY	245
ObG	Kim, J	NY	245
ObG	Lederman, S	NY	446
ObG	Luciani, R	NJ	750
ObG	Mack, L	NY	538
ObG	Meacham, K	NY	652
ObG	Mendelowitz, L	NY	652
ObG	Mieszerski, L	NY	652
ObG	Ordorica, S	NY	246
ObG	Rezvani, F	NJ	713
ObG	Sassoon, R	NY	247
ObG	Scher, J	NY	247
ObG	Steer, R	NJ	838
ObG	Szeto, M	CT	918
ObG	Toles, A	NY	538
ObG	Vasudeva, K	NY	538
ObG	Violi, C	CT	918
ObG	Weinstein, D	CT	918

Pregnancy-High Risk, Consultation

Spec	Name	St	Pg
ObG	Minkoff, H	NY	446

Pregnancy-Teenage

Spec	Name	St	Pg
MF	Chandra, P	NY	439

Preimplantation Genetic Diagnosis

Spec	Name	St	Pg
RE	Grazi, R	NY	461
RE	Grifo, J	NY	343

Premature Labor

Spec	Name	St	Pg
MF	Benito, C	NJ	836
MF	Chandra, P	NY	439
MF	Devine, P	NY	644
MF	Patrick, S	NY	210
ObG	Baker, D	NY	596

Prematurity/Low Birth Weight Infants

Spec	Name	St	Pg
NP	Boxer, H	NY	532
NP	Campbell, D	NY	398
NP	Golombek, S	NY	647
NP	Gudavalli, M	NY	440
NP	Hand, I	NY	479
NP	Hiatt, I	NJ	798
NP	Holzman, I	NY	222

Spec	Name	St	Pg
NP	La Gamma, E	NY	647
NP	Manginello, F	NJ	709
NP	Perlman, J	NY	223
NP	Shahrivar, F	NY	223
NP	Sun, S	NJ	748
ObG	Brustman, L	NY	242
Ped	Preis, O	NY	456
Ped	Weinberger, S	NY	308

Prenatal Diagnosis

Spec	Name	St	Pg
CG	Anyane-Yeboa, K	NY	148
CG	Gilbert, F	NY	427
CG	Hyman, D	NY	586
CG	Mahoney, M	CT	944
CG	Shapiro, L	NY	625
CG	Sklower Brooks, S	NJ	791
MF	Benito, C	NJ	836
MF	Bobby, P	CT	911
MF	Bond, A	CT	911
MF	Copel, J	CT	949
MF	D'Alton, M	NY	209
MF	Devine, P	NY	644
MF	Frieden, F	NJ	707
MF	Inglis, S	NY	478
MF	Laifer, S	CT	911
MF	Lescale, K	NY	644
MF	Meirowitz, N	NY	530
MF	Rochelson, B	NY	530
MF	Saltzman, D	NY	210
MF	Shevell, T	CT	912
MF	Smith, L	NJ	747
MF	Stiller, R	CT	912
ObG	Apuzzio, J	NJ	750
ObG	Lederman, S	NY	446

Prenatal Ultrasound

Spec	Name	St	Pg
MF	Frieden, F	NJ	707
MF	Stone, J	NY	210

Preventive Cardiology

Spec	Name	St	Pg
AM	Jacobson, M	NY	506
Cv	Andersen, H	NY	134
Cv	Berdoff, R	NY	134
Cv	Blum, M	NJ	831
Cv	Blumenthal, D	NY	135
Cv	Brown, D	NY	584
Cv	Chesner, M	NY	509
Cv	Eisenberg, S	NJ	692
Cv	Elkind, B	NJ	767
Cv	Epstein, S	NY	136
Cv	Fass, A	NY	619
Cv	Friedman, S	NY	136
Cv	Frishman, W	NY	620
Cv	Fuchs, R	NY	136
Cv	Fuster, V	NY	137
Cv	Gabelman, G	NY	620
Cv	Gardin, J	NJ	692
Cv	Gelbfish, J	NY	424
Cv	Gelles, J	NY	424
Cv	Gleckel, L	NY	510
Cv	Goldberg, N	NY	137
Cv	Goldberg, S	NY	510
Cv	Goodman, D	NY	137
Cv	Horowitz, S	CT	897
Cv	Inra, L	NY	138
Cv	Kay, R	NY	620
Cv	Keltz, T	NY	621
Cv	Landzberg, J	NJ	693
Cv	Lewis, B	NY	139
Cv	Mahalingam, B	NJ	775
Cv	Masri, B	NY	139
Cv	Matos, M	NY	621
Cv	Mercando, A	NY	622
Cv	Mintz, G	NY	511
Cv	Myerson, M	NY	140
Cv	Nash, I	NY	512
Cv	Neeson, F	CT	898
Cv	O'Brien, F	NY	140
Cv	Paiusco, A	NY	425
Cv	Phillips, M	NY	385
Cv	Porder, J	NY	141
Cv	Radwaner, B	NY	141
Cv	Raska, K	NJ	832
Cv	Reichstein, R	NY	141
Cv	Saroff, A	NJ	739
Cv	Schiffer, M	NY	142
Cv	Seinfeld, D	NY	142
Cv	Siegel, S	NY	143
Cv	Slama, R	NJ	873
Cv	Southren, D	NY	573
Cv	Spadaro, L	NY	513
Cv	Stein, R	NY	143
Cv	Unger, A	NY	144
Cv	Wein, P	NY	426
Cv	Weintraub, H	NY	144
Cv	Weisenseel, A	NY	144
Cv	Weiss, E	NJ	849
Cv	Winter, S	NY	492
Cv	Zimmerman, F	NY	623
FMed	Rednor, J	NJ	776
IC	Abittan, M	NY	529
IC	Innerfield, M	NY	575
IM	Blumberg, J	CT	908
IM	Case, D	NY	198
IM	Lipton, M	NY	203
IM	Sherman, I	NY	205
IM	Underberg, J	NY	206
IM	Warshafsky, S	NY	643
PCd	Langsner, A	NY	755

Preventive Medicine

Spec	Name	St	Pg
Cv	Porder, J	NY	141
FMed	Acosta, R	CT	902
FMed	Aponte, A	NY	589
FMed	Coloka-Kump, R	NY	390
FMed	Edelstein, M	NY	520
FMed	Filiberto, C	CT	903
FMed	Fisher, E	NY	475
FMed	Gottesfeld, P	NY	631
FMed	Greenblatt, L	NY	590
FMed	Istrico, R	NY	475
FMed	Lyon, V	NY	170
FMed	Morrow, R	NY	390
FMed	Moskowitz, G	NY	430
FMed	Sadovsky, R	NY	430
FMed	Sutton, I	NY	632
FMed	Vincent, M	NY	430
Ger	Callahan, E	NY	181
Ger	Ehrlich, A	NY	393
Ger	Feher, L	NY	182
Ger	Fogel, J	NY	182
Ger	Korc, B	NY	182
Ger	Paris, B	NY	433
IM	Ascheim, R	NY	198
IM	Baskin, D	NY	198
IM	Beyda, A	NY	477
IM	Bush, M	NY	198
IM	Cacciola, T	NJ	705
IM	Charap, P	NY	199
IM	Cohen, R	NY	199
IM	De Cosimo, D	NJ	746
IM	Dreyer, N	CT	908
IM	Ehrlich, M	NY	200
IM	Ellman, M	CT	949
IM	Etingin, O	NY	200
IM	Federman, A	NY	200
IM	Feltheimer, S	NY	200
IM	Fisher, L	NY	200
IM	Friedling, S	NY	593
IM	Friedman, J	NY	201
IM	Fukilman, O	NY	477
IM	Gelberg, B	NY	527
IM	Glassman, C	NY	574
IM	Glowacki, J	NJ	819
IM	Goldstein, P	NY	201
IM	Gorski, L	NY	527
IM	Greaney, E	NY	201
IM	Handelsman, R	NY	575
IM	Hauptman, A	NY	201
IM	Herzog, D	NY	640
IM	Kapoor, S	NY	641
IM	Karmen, C	NY	641
IM	Lamm, S	NY	203
IM	Leahy, M	NY	575
IM	Lewin, M	NY	203
IM	Lewin, N	NY	203
IM	Lodge, H	NY	204
IM	Logan, B	NY	204
IM	Molloy, E	CT	909
IM	Murray, S	NJ	778
IM	Olin, C	CT	909
IM	Pappas, S	NY	642
IM	Postley, J	NY	205
IM	Primas, R	NY	205
IM	Rakowitz, F	NY	528
IM	Rommer, J	NJ	747
IM	Rosch, E	NY	642
IM	Sander, N	NY	396
IM	Scaduto, P	NJ	835
IM	Silverman, D	NY	205
IM	Simon, T	NY	438
IM	Slogoff, F	CT	910
IM	Solomon, G	NY	206
IM	Spano, F	CT	910
IM	Teffera, F	NY	397
IM	Warshafsky, S	NY	643

Specialty & Special Expertise Index

Spec	Name	St	Pg
U	Boczko, S	NY	368
U	Breslin, D	NY	679
U	Fine, E	NY	369
U	Flanagan, M	CT	963
U	Giella, J	NY	580
U	Gribetz, M	NY	369
U	Harris, S	NY	567
U	Irwin, M	NY	466
U	Kaminetsky, J	NY	370
U	Katz, H	NJ	772
U	Katz, J	NJ	763
U	Lessing, J	NY	502
U	Lieberman, E	NY	568
U	Litvin, Y	NJ	826
U	Loo, M	NY	371
U	Lowe, F	NY	371
U	Margolis, E	NJ	732
U	Meisenberg, G	NY	466
U	Owens, G	NY	680
U	Peng, B	NY	372
U	Provet, J	NY	372
U	Raboy, A	NY	502
U	Romas, N	NY	372
U	Rosenthal, S	NY	466
U	Rotolo, J	NY	827
U	Sadeghi-Nejad, H	NJ	732
U	Schrager, A	NY	680
U	Strauss, B	NJ	764
U	Sunshine, R	NY	568
U	Tarasuk, A	NY	487
U	Trauzzi, S	NY	680
U	Williams, J	NY	374
U	Ziegelbaum, M	NY	569

Prostate Surgery

Spec	Name	St	Pg
U	Hajjar, J	NJ	732
U	Putignano, J	NY	680
U	Te, A	NY	374

PRP (Regenokine)

Spec	Name	St	Pg
PM	Schottenstein, D	NY	289

Pseudomotor Cerebri

Spec	Name	St	Pg
N	Lepore, F	NJ	800

Pseudotumor Cerebri

Spec	Name	St	Pg
Oph	Lesser, R	CT	953

Pseudoxanthoma Elasticum

Spec	Name	St	Pg
D	Lebwohl, M	NY	156
Oph	Fuchs, W	NY	253

Psoriasis

Spec	Name	St	Pg
D	Almeida, L	NJ	832
D	Bagel, J	NJ	775
D	Belsito, D	NY	152
D	Bickers, D	NY	152
D	Buchness, M	NY	152
D	Cohen, S	NY	387
D	Corey, T	NJ	696
D	Deitz, M	NY	428
D	Falcon, R	NY	515
D	Fox, A	NJ	860
D	Fried, S	NJ	696
D	Grossman, K	NJ	816
D	Grossman, M	NY	626
D	Hatcher, V	NY	155
D	Hisler, B	NY	516
D	Katz, S	NY	155
D	Lebwohl, M	NY	156
D	Lukash, B	NY	627
D	McCormack, P	NY	492
D	Notaro, A	NY	587
D	Possick, P	NJ	697
D	Savin, R	CT	945
D	Shupack, J	NY	159
D	Skrokov, R	NY	588
D	Soter, N	NY	159
D	Sturza, J	NY	628
D	Waldorf, D	NY	573
D	Walther, R	NY	159

Psoriasis/Eczema

Spec	Name	St	Pg
D	Danziger, S	NY	428
D	Evans, L	NY	626
D	Orlow, S	NY	157

Psoriatic Arthritis

Spec	Name	St	Pg
Rhu	Adlersberg, J	NY	346
Rhu	Barone, R	NY	674
Rhu	Berger, J	NY	674
Rhu	Danehower, R	CT	934
Rhu	Goodman, S	NY	347
Rhu	Greenwald, R	NY	562
Rhu	Lee, S	NY	348
Rhu	Marchetta, P	NY	348
Rhu	Mitnick, H	NY	349
Rhu	Nascimento, J	CT	934
Rhu	Schwartzfarb, L	NY	350
Rhu	Solomon, G	NY	350
Rhu	Wasser, K	NJ	825
Rhu	Yee, A	NY	351
Rhu	Yegudin-Ash, J	NY	675

Psychiatry

Spec	Name	St	Pg
Psyc	Addonizio, G	NY	669
Psyc	Adler, L	NY	321
Psyc	Almeleh, J	NY	321
Psyc	Alper, K	NY	321
Psyc	Appelbaum, P	NY	321
Psyc	Arkow, S	NY	321
Psyc	Aronoff, M	NY	321
Psyc	Aronson, T	NY	604
Psyc	Asnis, G	NY	411
Psyc	Attia, E	NY	322
Psyc	Badikian, A	NY	669
Psyc	Bailine, S	NY	557
Psyc	Barbuto, J	NY	322
Psyc	Basch, S	NY	322
Psyc	Bauman, J	NY	669
Psyc	Behr, R	NY	557
Psyc	Benjamin, J	NY	557
Psyc	Berkowitz, H	NY	457
Psyc	Berman, S	NY	557
Psyc	Bhatt, A	NY	557
Psyc	Bialer, P	NY	322
Psyc	Bogen, S	NY	669
Psyc	Bone, S	NY	322
Psyc	Borbely, A	NY	322
Psyc	Breitbart, W	NY	322
Psyc	Brenner, R	NY	482
Psyc	Brodie, J	NY	322
Psyc	Bronheim, H	NY	323
Psyc	Brown, R	NY	323
Psyc	Budman, C	NY	557
Psyc	Bukberg, J	NY	323
Psyc	Cabaniss, D	NY	323
Psyc	Caligor, E	NY	323
Psyc	Caracci, G	NJ	759
Psyc	Cherry, S	NY	323
Psyc	Chertoff, H	NJ	724
Psyc	Chung, H	NY	323
Psyc	Cohen, A	NY	323
Psyc	Coplan, J	NY	457
Psyc	Crasta, J	NY	557
Psyc	Devlin, M	NY	323
Psyc	Di Buono, M	NY	500
Psyc	Donnellan, J	NJ	866
Psyc	Douglas, C	NY	324
Psyc	Dulit, R	NY	669
Psyc	Eitan, N	NY	458
Psyc	Faber, M	NJ	759
Psyc	Fallon, B	NY	324
Psyc	Farkas, E	NJ	725
Psyc	Ferran, E	NY	324
Psyc	Finkel, J	NY	324
Psyc	First, M	NY	324
Psyc	Fox, H	NY	324
Psyc	Friedman, R	NY	324
Psyc	Fyer, A	NY	324
Psyc	Fyer, M	NY	324
Psyc	Gabel, R	NY	669
Psyc	Gelfand, J	NY	411
Psyc	Gewolb, E	NJ	771
Psyc	Goff, D	NY	325
Psyc	Goldberg, J	NY	458
Psyc	Goldenberg, D	NY	325
Psyc	Goldman, N	NY	325
Psyc	Goldstein, S	NY	325
Psyc	Gorman, L	NY	325
Psyc	Gupta, A	NY	557
Psyc	Gurevich, M	NY	558
Psyc	Gurland, F	NJ	725
Psyc	Harlam, D	NY	670
Psyc	Hart, C	CT	930
Psyc	Heiman, P	NY	411
Psyc	Heisman, A	NY	458
Psyc	Heller, S	NY	325
Psyc	Hindin, L	NJ	854
Psyc	Hoffman, R	NY	325
Psyc	Hollander, E	NY	325
Psyc	Idupuganti, S	NY	458
Psyc	Jacoby, J	NJ	771

Specialty & Special Expertise Index

Spec	Name	St	Pg
Psychiatry in Terminal Illness			
Psyc	Klagsbrun, S	NY	670
Psychiatry of Prostate Cancer			
Psyc	Roth, A	NY	330
Psychoanalysis			
ChAP	Fox, S	NY	145
ChAP	Hyler, I	NY	623
ChAP	Madigan, J	CT	943
Psyc	Basch, S	NY	322
Psyc	Bone, S	NY	322
Psyc	Bukberg, J	NY	323
Psyc	Cabaniss, D	NY	323
Psyc	Caligor, E	NY	323
Psyc	Cherry, S	NY	323
Psyc	Chertoff, H	NJ	724
Psyc	Goldenberg, D	NY	325
Psyc	Kalinich, L	NY	326
Psyc	Levitan, S	NY	327
Psyc	Lew, A	NY	670
Psyc	Michels, R	NY	328
Psyc	Olds, D	NY	329
Psyc	Rees, E	NY	329
Psyc	Samberg, E	NY	331
Psyc	Sawyer, D	NY	331
Psyc	Scharf, R	NY	331
Psyc	Shaw, R	NY	331
Psyc	Stone, M	NY	332
Psyc	Strain, J	NY	332
Psyc	Welsh, H	NY	334
Psychodynamic Psychotherapy			
Psyc	Berman, S	NY	557
Psyc	Cabaniss, D	NY	323
Psyc	Winters, R	NY	334
Psychoneuroimmunology			
Psyc	Schleifer, S	NJ	759
Psychopharmacology			
ChAP	Boorady, R	NY	145
ChAP	Coffey, B	NY	145
ChAP	Cohen, L	NY	623
ChAP	Koplewicz, H	NY	146
ChAP	Kron, L	NY	146
ChAP	Leventhal, B	NY	146
ChAP	Lewis, O	NY	146
ChAP	Newcorn, J	NY	146
ChAP	Perry, R	NY	146
ChAP	Rubinstein, B	NY	623
ChAP	Seaver, R	NY	623
ChAP	Silva, R	NY	624
ChAP	Slater, J	NY	624
ChAP	Williams, D	NY	513
Onc	Budman, D	NY	530
Psyc	Addonizio, G	NY	669
Psyc	Adler, L	NY	321
Psyc	Alper, K	NY	321

Spec	Name	St	Pg
Psyc	Arkow, S	NY	321
Psyc	Asnis, G	NY	411
Psyc	Bailine, S	NY	557
Psyc	Basch, S	NY	322
Psyc	Berman, S	NY	557
Psyc	Bhatt, A	NY	557
Psyc	Brodie, J	NY	322
Psyc	Brown, R	NY	323
Psyc	Caracci, G	NJ	759
Psyc	First, M	NY	324
Psyc	Fox, H	NY	324
Psyc	Friedman, R	NY	324
Psyc	Gabel, R	NY	669
Psyc	Goff, D	NY	325
Psyc	Goldstein, S	NY	325
Psyc	Gorman, L	NY	325
Psyc	Harlam, D	NY	670
Psyc	Hoffman, J	NY	325
Psyc	Jacoby, J	NJ	771
Psyc	Kahn, D	NY	325
Psyc	Kahn, J	NY	670
Psyc	Kaplan, G	NJ	884
Psyc	Katus, E	NY	558
Psyc	Kocsis, J	NY	326
Psyc	Leifer, M	NJ	784
Psyc	Levin, A	NY	670
Psyc	Levitan, S	NY	327
Psyc	Levy, M	NY	578
Psyc	Lindenmayer, J	NY	327
Psyc	Lipton, B	NY	327
Psyc	Markowitz, J	NY	327
Psyc	McMullen, R	NY	328
Psyc	Mendelowitz, A	NY	483
Psyc	Menza, M	NJ	808
Psyc	Meyers, B	NY	670
Psyc	Miller, D	NJ	884
Psyc	Milone, R	NY	670
Psyc	Mueller, F	CT	930
Psyc	Muskin, P	NY	328
Psyc	Nininger, J	NY	328
Psyc	Nucci, A	NJ	759
Psyc	Opler, L	NY	670
Psyc	Papp, L	NY	329
Psyc	Perry, B	NY	671
Psyc	Preven, D	NY	329
Psyc	Richardson, W	NJ	884
Psyc	Rosen, A	NY	330
Psyc	Rosen, B	NY	604
Psyc	Rubinstein, M	NY	330
Psyc	Scharf, R	NY	331
Psyc	Seaman, C	NY	331
Psyc	Shapiro, B	CT	931
Psyc	Shinbach, K	NY	332
Psyc	Siever, L	NY	332
Psyc	Silver, J	NY	332
Psyc	Sullivan, A	NY	483
Psyc	Sussman, N	NY	333
Psyc	Tardiff, K	NY	333
Psyc	Villafranca, M	NJ	885
Psyc	Wager, S	NY	333
Psyc	Wallack, J	NY	334
Psyc	Winters, R	NY	334

Spec	Name	St	Pg
Psychopharmacology-Consultation			
Psyc	McGrath, P	NY	328
Psychosomatic Disorders			
AM	Marks, A	NY	130
ChAP	Williams, D	NY	513
FMed	Lansing, M	NJ	776
Psyc	Coplan, J	NY	457
Psyc	Fallon, B	NY	324
Psyc	Gelfand, J	NY	411
Psyc	Gupta, A	NY	557
Psyc	Kalash, G	NY	483
Psyc	Lipton, B	NY	327
Psyc	Muhlbauer, H	NY	328
Psychotherapy			
ChAP	Hyler, I	NY	623
ChAP	Kron, L	NY	146
ChAP	Lewis, O	NY	146
ChAP	Madigan, J	CT	943
ChAP	Rosenfeld, A	CT	899
Psyc	Addonizio, G	NY	669
Psyc	Arkow, S	NY	321
Psyc	Bone, S	NY	322
Psyc	Bukberg, J	NY	323
Psyc	Caracci, G	NJ	759
Psyc	Cherry, S	NY	323
Psyc	Cohen, A	NY	323
Psyc	First, M	NY	324
Psyc	Fox, H	NY	324
Psyc	Gabel, R	NY	669
Psyc	Hart, S	CT	930
Psyc	Kahn, D	NY	325
Psyc	Kahn, J	NY	670
Psyc	Kalinich, L	NY	326
Psyc	Karasu, T	NY	326
Psyc	Katus, E	NY	558
Psyc	Levitan, S	NY	327
Psyc	Lew, A	NY	670
Psyc	Lipton, B	NY	327
Psyc	Meyers, B	NY	670
Psyc	Nininger, J	NY	328
Psyc	Olds, D	NY	329
Psyc	Opler, L	NY	670
Psyc	Preven, D	NY	329
Psyc	Rees, E	NY	329
Psyc	Sadock, V	NY	331
Psyc	Scharf, R	NY	331
Psyc	Seaman, C	NY	331
Psyc	Shaw, R	NY	331
Psyc	Sullivan, A	NY	483
Psyc	Swiller, H	NY	333
Psyc	Tamerin, J	CT	931
Psyc	Tardiff, K	NY	333
Psyc	Tolchin, J	NY	333
Psyc	Welsh, H	NY	334
Psyc	Zornitzer, M	NJ	759
Psychotherapy &			

Specialty & Special Expertise Index

Spec	Name	St	Pg
Pul	Thurm, C	NY	484
Pul	Trow, T	CT	959
Pul	Turetsky, A	CT	932
Pul	Villamena, P	NY	340
Pul	Volcovici, G	NY	673
Pul	Walser, L	NY	605
Pul	Weinberg, H	NY	673
Pul	Winter, S	CT	932
Pul	Wohlberg, G	NY	606
Pul	Wyner, P	NY	560
Pul	Yip, C	NY	340
Pul	Zupnick, H	NY	560

Pulmonary Disease/Immunocompromised

Spec	Name	St	Pg
Pul	Stover-Pepe, D	NY	339

Pulmonary Embolism

Spec	Name	St	Pg
DR	Ginsberg, M	NY	162
DR	Naidich, D	NY	163
Pul	Arcasoy, S	NY	335

Pulmonary Fibrosis

Spec	Name	St	Pg
Pul	Adams, F	NY	335
Pul	Bernardini, D	NY	605
Pul	DiCosmo, B	NY	672
Pul	Hammer, A	NY	459
Pul	Lederer, D	NY	337
Pul	McCalley, S	CT	932
Pul	Padilla, M	NY	338
Pul	Polkow, M	NJ	726
Pul	Posner, D	NY	338
Pul	Riley, D	NJ	809
Pul	Sussman, R	NJ	885
Pul	Thurm, C	NY	484

Pulmonary Hypertension

Spec	Name	St	Pg
Cv	Dresdale, R	NY	509
Cv	Horn, E	NY	138
Cv	Klapholz, M	NJ	739
Cv	Lachmann, J	NY	511
Cv	Pinney, S	NY	140
Cv	Poon, M	NY	585
Cv	Zucker, M	NJ	740
Pul	Demetis, S	NY	459
Pul	Glaser, M	NY	605
Pul	Krieger, A	NY	337
Pul	Padilla, M	NY	338
Pul	Shah, S	NJ	760
Pul	Steiger, D	NY	339
Pul	Steinberg, H	NY	560
Pul	Trow, T	CT	959

Pulmonary Infections

Spec	Name	St	Pg
Pul	Stover-Pepe, D	NY	339

Pulmonary Pathology

Spec	Name	St	Pg
Path	Klimstra, D	NY	290
Path	Travis, W	NY	291

Pulmonary Rehabilitation

Spec	Name	St	Pg
Pul	Novitch, R	NY	673
Pul	Raskin, J	NY	339
Pul	Rosen, M	NY	560
Pul	Sachs, P	CT	932
Pul	Silverman, J	NY	484

Pulmonary Vascular Disease

Spec	Name	St	Pg
Pul	Trow, T	CT	959

Pyschopharmacology

Spec	Name	St	Pg
Psyc	Zornitzer, M	NJ	759

R

Radiation Oncology

Spec	Name	St	Pg
RadRO	Adams, M	NY	500
RadRO	Ashamalla, H	NY	460
RadRO	Baumann, J	NJ	809
RadRO	Bodner, W	NY	413
RadRO	Bosworth, J	NY	560
RadRO	Braver, J	NJ	866
RadRO	Chadha, M	NY	340
RadRO	Chao, K	NY	340
RadRO	Cole, R	NJ	855
RadRO	Cooper, J	NY	461
RadRO	Dalton, J	NY	484
RadRO	Diamond, E	NY	560
RadRO	Donahue, B	NY	461
RadRO	Dowling, S	CT	932
RadRO	Dubin, D	NJ	727
RadRO	Ennis, R	NY	340
RadRO	Fang, D	CT	932
RadRO	Fass, D	NY	674
RadRO	Formenti, S	NY	340
RadRO	Gejerman, G	NJ	727
RadRO	Gewanter, R	NY	560
RadRO	Gliedman, P	NY	461
RadRO	Goodman, R	NJ	771
RadRO	Haas, A	NJ	809
RadRO	Haas, J	NY	561
RadRO	Haffty, B	NJ	810
RadRO	Harrison, L	NY	341
RadRO	Hayes, M	NY	341
RadRO	Higgins, S	CT	960
RadRO	Ingenito, A	NJ	727
RadRO	Isaacson, S	NY	341
RadRO	Kalnicki, S	NY	413
RadRO	Katz, A	NY	484
RadRO	Knisely, J	NY	561
RadRO	Lee, N	NY	341
RadRO	Lipsztein, R	NY	484
RadRO	Macher, M	NJ	810
RadRO	Marin, L	NY	561
RadRO	Masino, F	CT	933
RadRO	McCormick, B	NY	341
RadRO	McKenna, M	NJ	784

Spec	Name	St	Pg
RadRO	Moorthy, C	NY	674
RadRO	Mullen, E	NY	561
RadRO	Ng, J	NY	341
RadRO	Nori, D	NY	341
RadRO	Parashar, B	NY	341
RadRO	Park, T	NY	606
RadRO	Pathare, P	CT	933
RadRO	Peschel, R	CT	960
RadRO	Pollack, J	NY	561
RadRO	Potters, L	NY	561
RadRO	Roberts, K	CT	960
RadRO	Rosenbaum, A	NY	342
RadRO	Rotman, M	NY	461
RadRO	Schiff, P	NY	342
RadRO	Schwartz, L	NJ	885
RadRO	Sherr, D	NY	342
RadRO	Soffen, E	NJ	784
RadRO	Spera, J	CT	933
RadRO	Stock, R	NY	342
RadRO	Tinger, A	NY	674
RadRO	Varsos, G	NY	485
RadRO	Vialotti, C	NJ	727
RadRO	Wagman, R	NJ	760
RadRO	Weidhaas, J	CT	960
RadRO	Wilson, L	CT	960
RadRO	Wong, J	NY	843
RadRO	Yahalom, J	NY	342
RadRO	Zelefsky, M	NY	342

Radiation Therapy-Intraoperative

Spec	Name	St	Pg
RadRO	Harrison, L	NY	341

Radiofrequency Ablation

Spec	Name	St	Pg
CE	Costeas, C	NJ	738
CE	Iwai, S	NY	583
CE	Rubin, D	NY	618
CE	Sauberman, R	NJ	739

Radiofrequency Tumor Ablation

Spec	Name	St	Pg
VIR	Brown, K	NY	375
VIR	Solomon, S	NY	376

Radioimmunotherapy of Cancer

Spec	Name	St	Pg
NuM	Carrasquillo, J	NY	241
NuM	Fawwaz, R	NY	241
NuM	Pandit-Taskar, N	NY	241

Rare Skin Disorders

Spec	Name	St	Pg
D	Grossman, M	NY	626
D	Schwartz, R	NJ	741
D	Shupack, J	NY	159

Raynaud's Disease

Spec	Name	St	Pg
D	Franks, A	NY	154
Rhu	Schwartzman, S	NY	350

Specialty & Special Expertise Index

Spec	Name	St	Pg
RE	Taylor, H	CT	960
RE	Tortoriello, D	NY	345
RE	Treiser, S	NJ	866
RE	Warren, M	NY	345
RE	Weiss, G	NJ	728
RE	Witt, B	CT	933

Reproductive Genetics

Spec	Name	St	Pg
MF	Eddleman, K	NY	209
MF	MacMillan, W	NJ	797
ObG	Evans, M	NY	243

Reproductive Immunology

Spec	Name	St	Pg
RE	Bronson, R	NY	606

Reproductive Surgery

Spec	Name	St	Pg
RE	Davis, O	NY	343
RE	Kenigsberg, D	NY	606
RE	Noyes, N	NY	344
RE	Richlin, S	CT	933
RE	Sandler, B	NY	344

Respiratory Distress Syndrome

Spec	Name	St	Pg
CCM	Benjamin, E	NY	151
CCM	Cornell, J	NJ	696
NP	Hand, I	NY	479
NP	Siracuse, J	NY	440
NP	Sun, S	NJ	748
Pul	Multz, A	NY	559

Respiratory Failure

Spec	Name	St	Pg
CCM	Nierman, D	NY	473
NP	Hiatt, I	NJ	798
PCCM	Conway, E	NY	294
PCCM	Goltzman, C	NY	661
PCCM	Greenwald, B	NY	294
PCCM	Singer, L	NY	405
PCCM	Ushay, H	NY	405
Pul	Marino, W	NY	413
Pul	Niederman, M	NY	559
Pul	Thomashow, B	NY	340
Pul	Winter, S	CT	932

Retina/Vitreous Consultation

Spec	Name	St	Pg
Oph	Barile, G	NY	249
Oph	Fisher, Y	NY	252

Retina/Vitreous Surgery

Spec	Name	St	Pg
Oph	Chang, S	NY	249
Oph	Chess, J	NY	402
Oph	Cohen, B	NY	250
Oph	Coleman, D	NY	250
Oph	Dayan, A	NY	250
Oph	Douros, S	NY	447
Oph	Elbaba, F	NY	598
Oph	Fastenberg, D	NY	539
Oph	Friedman, R	NY	252
Oph	Gentile, R	NY	253

Spec	Name	St	Pg
Oph	Lee, C	NY	255
Oph	Muldoon, T	NY	257
Oph	Rosenthal, J	NY	259
Oph	Sachs, R	NJ	839
Oph	Weseley, P	NY	262
Oph	Yannuzzi, L	NY	262

Retinal Detachment

Spec	Name	St	Pg
Oph	Berman, D	NY	446
Oph	Bhagat, N	NJ	751
Oph	Cangemi, F	NJ	751
Oph	D'Amico, D	NY	250
Oph	Dayan, A	NY	250
Oph	Schiff, W	NY	259
Oph	Schubert, H	NY	259
Oph	Shabto, U	NY	260
Oph	Svitra, P	NY	541
Oph	Wong, R	NY	262
Oph	Zarbin, M	NJ	752

Retinal Disorders

Spec	Name	St	Pg
Oph	Angioletti, L	NY	248
Oph	Barile, G	NY	249
Oph	Chang, S	NY	249
Oph	D'Amico, D	NY	250
Oph	Eichler, J	NJ	751
Oph	Engel, H	NY	251
Oph	Ferrone, P	NY	539
Oph	Friedman, A	NY	252
Oph	Fromer, M	NY	252
Oph	Fuchs, W	NY	253
Oph	Gentile, R	NY	253
Oph	Odel, J	NY	258
Oph	Paccione, J	NY	258
Oph	Reppucci, V	CT	920
Oph	Sachs, R	NJ	839
Oph	Saffra, N	NY	448
Oph	Schubert, H	NY	259
Oph	Slakter, J	NY	260
Oph	Spaide, R	NY	261
Oph	Stein, A	NY	449
Oph	Svitra, P	NY	541
Oph	Tom, D	CT	953
Oph	Topilow, H	NJ	715
Oph	Unterricht, S	NY	449
Oph	Walsh, J	NY	261
Oph	Weber, P	NY	599
Oph	Weber, R	CT	921
Oph	Weiss, M	NY	262

Retinal Dosorders

Spec	Name	St	Pg
Oph	Dayan, A	NY	250

Retinitis Pigmentosa

Spec	Name	St	Pg
Oph	MacKay, C	NY	255
Oph	Solomon, S	NY	655

Retinoblastoma

Spec	Name	St	Pg
Oph	Abramson, D	NY	248

Spec	Name	St	Pg
Oph	Finger, P	NY	252
PHO	Dunkel, I	NY	297

Retinopathy of Prematurity

Spec	Name	St	Pg
Oph	Cangemi, F	NJ	751
Oph	Horowitz, M	NY	654
Oph	Most, R	NY	655
Oph	Shabto, U	NY	260
Oph	Topilow, H	NJ	715

Retroperitoneal Fibrosis

Spec	Name	St	Pg
Rhu	Solitar, B	NY	350
U	Stifelman, M	NY	374

Rett Syndrome

Spec	Name	St	Pg
PEn	Agarwal, C	NY	406

Rhabdomyosarcoma

Spec	Name	St	Pg
PHO	Wexler, L	NY	299

Rheumatic Fever

Spec	Name	St	Pg
Rhu	Gibofsky, A	NY	347

Rheumatic Heart Disease

Spec	Name	St	Pg
PCd	Cooper, R	NY	546

Rheumatoid Arthritis

Spec	Name	St	Pg
HS	Miller-Breslow, A	NJ	703
IM	Kazdin, H	NY	437
IM	Miguel, E	NJ	705
PRhu	Lehman, T	NY	302
Rhu	Adlersberg, J	NY	346
Rhu	Agus, B	NY	346
Rhu	Barone, R	NY	674
Rhu	Belilos, E	NY	562
Rhu	Belmont, H	NY	346
Rhu	Berger, J	NY	674
Rhu	Bernstein, L	NY	462
Rhu	Bienenstock, H	NY	462
Rhu	Blau, S	NY	562
Rhu	Blume, R	NY	346
Rhu	Brodman, R	NJ	885
Rhu	Burns, M	NY	675
Rhu	Cannarozzi, N	NJ	761
Rhu	Carsons, S	NY	562
Rhu	Crane, R	NY	346
Rhu	Danehower, R	CT	934
Rhu	Faller, J	NY	347
Rhu	Fields, T	NY	347
Rhu	Fischer, H	NY	347
Rhu	Fomberstein, B	NY	413
Rhu	Furie, R	NY	562
Rhu	Garner, B	NY	462
Rhu	Gibofsky, A	NY	347
Rhu	Goldberg, M	NJ	855
Rhu	Goldstein, M	NY	501
Rhu	Gonter, N	NJ	728
Rhu	Goodman, S	NY	347

Specialty & Special Expertise Index

S

Specialty & Special Expertise Index

Spec	Name	St	Pg
Sexual Addiction			
Psyc	First, M	NY	324

Spec	Name	St	Pg
Sexual Behavior-Compulsive			
Psyc	Krueger, R	NY	327

Sexual Development Problems			
ChAP	Rosenfeld, A	CT	899
PEn	Castro-Magana, M	NY	548

Sexual Differentiation Disorders			
PEn	Saenger, P	NY	661
PEn	Wilson, T	NY	601

Sexual Dysfunction			
AdP	Rosenberg, K	NY	129
FMed	Levy, A	NY	170
IM	Lamm, S	NY	203
ObG	Bachmann, G	NJ	801
ObG	Berman, A	NY	242
ObG	Coady, D	NY	243
Psyc	Sadock, V	NY	331
Psyc	Schore, A	NY	331
Psyc	Snyder, S	NY	332
U	Glassman, C	NY	679
U	Gribetz, M	NY	369
U	Kaminetsky, J	NY	370
U	Klein, G	NY	370
U	Lehrhoff, B	NJ	887
U	Seidman, B	NJ	887
U	Shulman, Y	NJ	772
U	Strauss, B	NJ	764
U	Werner, M	NY	680

Sexually Transmitted Diseases			
Inf	Augenbraun, M	NY	435
Inf	Johnson, D	NY	526
Inf	Lerner, C	NY	195
Inf	Robbins, N	NY	395
Inf	Scheer, M	NY	526
Inf	Smith, S	NJ	746
ObG	Baker, D	NY	596
ObG	Donovan, L	CT	918
PInf	Neu, N	NY	300

Short Bowel Syndrome			
PGe	Thompson, J	NY	406

Short Stature in Children			
PEn	Agdere, L	NY	452
PEn	Saenger, P	NY	661

Shoulder & Elbow Surgery			
OrS	Mendoza, F	NY	272
SM	Levine, W	NY	352

Spec	Name	St	Pg
Shoulder & Knee Injuries			
OrS	Maddalo, A	NY	657
SM	Gross, M	NJ	729
SM	Savatsky, G	NJ	729

Shoulder & Knee Reconstruction			
OrS	Splain, S	NY	450

Shoulder & Knee Surgery			
OrS	Brittis, D	CT	921
OrS	Garfinkel, M	NJ	802
OrS	Gladstone, J	NY	267
OrS	Nicholas, S	NY	272
OrS	Schob, C	NJ	753
OrS	Shebairo, R	NY	543
SM	Nisonson, B	NY	352

Shoulder Arthroscopic Surgery			
HS	Barron, O	NY	186
OrS	Bade, H	NJ	822
OrS	Cahill, J	NJ	715
OrS	Craig, E	NY	265
OrS	Fealy, S	NY	266
OrS	Flatow, E	NY	267
OrS	Hannafin, J	NY	268
OrS	Kraushaar, B	NY	577
OrS	Pollock, R	NJ	716
OrS	Rubin, C	NY	577
OrS	Ticker, J	NY	543
SM	Williams, R	NY	352

Shoulder Injuries			
OrS	Altman, W	NJ	715
OrS	Austin, K	NY	577
OrS	Drillings, G	NJ	852
OrS	Flatow, E	NY	267
OrS	Pollock, R	NJ	716
PMR	Malanga, G	NJ	883
SM	Gehrmann, R	NJ	761
SM	Halpern, B	NY	351
SM	Krinick, R	NY	351

Shoulder Instability			
SM	Cavaliere, G	NY	675
SM	Sclafani, M	NJ	825

Shoulder Reconstruction			
HS	Barron, O	NY	186
OrS	Barmakian, J	NJ	880
OrS	Decter, E	NJ	752
OrS	Gallick, G	NJ	881

Shoulder Replacement			
OrS	Craig, E	NY	265
OrS	Dines, D	NY	542
OrS	Fealy, S	NY	266
OrS	Flatow, E	NY	267
OrS	Mc Inerney, V	NJ	853

Spec	Name	St	Pg
OrS	Plancher, K	NY	273
OrS	Warren, R	NY	276

Shoulder Surgery			
HS	Choueka, J	NY	434
HS	Lisser, S	NJ	818
HS	Magill, R	NY	637
HS	Yang, S	NY	188
OrS	Abrams, J	NJ	781
OrS	Berman, M	NJ	715
OrS	Bigliani, L	NY	263
OrS	Bosco, J	NY	264
OrS	Compito, C	NY	265
OrS	Cunningham, J	CT	922
OrS	Cuomo, F	NY	265
OrS	D'Agostino, R	NY	542
OrS	Dines, D	NY	542
OrS	Doidge, R	NJ	716
OrS	Glashow, J	NY	267
OrS	Henshaw, D	CT	922
OrS	Jokl, P	CT	954
OrS	Karas, E	NY	657
OrS	Khabie, V	NY	657
OrS	Levitz, C	NY	542
OrS	Levy, H	NY	270
OrS	Lubliner, J	NY	271
OrS	Marx, R	NY	271
OrS	McCann, P	NY	271
OrS	McIlveen, S	NJ	716
OrS	Miller, S	CT	923
OrS	Montgomery, K	NJ	839
OrS	Morgan, D	NY	450
OrS	Plancher, K	NY	273
OrS	Rozbruch, J	NY	274
OrS	Schwartz, E	NY	481
OrS	Sethi, P	CT	924
OrS	Tabershaw, R	NY	599
OrS	Ticker, J	NY	543
OrS	Turtel, A	NY	276
OrS	Warren, R	NY	276
OrS	Weinstein, R	NY	658
OrS	Wickiewicz, T	NY	277
OrS	Zambetti, G	NY	277
OrS	Zuckerman, J	NY	278
SM	Altchek, D	NY	351
SM	Levy, A	NJ	761

Shoulder Tumors			
OrS	Wittig, J	NY	277

Sickle Cell Disease			
Hem	Billett, H	NY	395
Ped	Saraiya, N	NJ	883
PHO	Dasgupta, I	NY	406
PHO	Diamond, S	NJ	719
PHO	Drachtman, R	NJ	806
PHO	Flug, F	NJ	719
PHO	Guarini, L	NY	453
PHO	Kamalakar, P	NJ	756
PHO	Kulpa, J	NY	454
PHO	Miller, S	NY	454

Specialty & Special Expertise Index

Spec	Name	St	Pg
D	Lederman, J	NY	492
D	Leffell, D	CT	945
D	Levy, R	NY	627
D	Lombardo, P	NY	156
D	Lukash, B	NY	627
D	Machler, B	NJ	741
D	Mackler, K	NY	627
D	Maiocco, K	CT	900
D	Marghoob, A	NY	587
D	Mayer, F	CT	900
D	McCormack, P	NY	492
D	Morman, M	NJ	697
D	Moynihan, G	NY	587
D	Myskowski, P	NY	156
D	Naidorf, E	CT	900
D	Notaro, A	NY	587
D	Orbuch, P	NY	157
D	Oshman, R	CT	900
D	Ostad, A	NY	157
D	Pereira, F	NY	474
D	Podwal, M	NY	157
D	Possick, P	NJ	697
D	Prioleau, P	NY	157
D	Pruzan-Clain, D	CT	900
D	Prystowsky, J	NY	157
D	Ramsay, D	NY	157
D	Ratner, D	NY	158
D	Rigel, D	NY	158
D	Rosen, D	NY	387
D	Roth, J	NY	158
D	Safai, B	NY	158
D	Sarnoff, D	NY	516
D	Schliftman, A	NY	628
D	Schwartz, R	NJ	741
D	Sibrack, L	CT	900
D	Siegel, D	NY	588
D	Silverman, M	NY	516
D	Simon, S	NY	428
D	Skrokov, R	NY	588
D	Spinowitz, A	NY	516
D	Stillman, M	NY	628
D	Sweeney, E	NJ	697
D	Tanenbaum, D	NY	159
D	Tesser, M	NY	159
D	Treiber, R	NY	628
D	Waldorf, D	NY	573
D	Waldorf, H	NY	573
D	Walther, R	NY	159
D	Weinberger, G	NJ	874
D	Wong, A	NY	588
D	Wrone, D	NJ	792
D	Zirvi, M	NJ	874
D	Zweibel, S	NY	628
Onc	Pavlick, A	NY	218
Onc	Pfister, D	NY	218
Oto	Carniol, P	NJ	881
PlS	Granick, M	NJ	759
PlS	Groeger, W	NY	555
PlS	Karp, N	NY	316
PlS	Lesesne, C	NY	316
PlS	Roth, D	NY	669
RadRO	Cooper, J	NY	461
RadRO	Lee, N	NY	341

Spec	Name	St	Pg
S	Goydos, J	NJ	810

Skin Cancer & Moles

Spec	Name	St	Pg
D	Danziger, S	NY	428
D	Evans, L	NY	626
D	Katz, S	NY	155

Skin Cancer-Head & Neck

Spec	Name	St	Pg
Onc	Posner, M	NY	219

Skin Diseases

Spec	Name	St	Pg
D	Bagel, J	NJ	775
D	Brademas, M	NY	152
FMed	Moynihan, B	NY	520
FMed	Sutton, I	NY	632
FMed	Ziering, T	NJ	861
IM	Bernard, R	NY	593
IM	Fazio, N	NY	640

Skin Diseases in Transplants/Cancer

Spec	Name	St	Pg
D	Grossman, M	NY	626

Skin Diseases-Immunologic

Spec	Name	St	Pg
D	Liteplo, R	NY	387

Skin Infections

Spec	Name	St	Pg
D	Buchness, M	NY	152
D	Rudikoff, D	NY	387

Skin Laser Surgery

Spec	Name	St	Pg
D	Amin, S	NY	151
D	Avram, M	NY	152
D	Bank, D	NY	625
D	Basuk, P	NY	587
D	Biro, D	NY	427
D	Brancaccio, R	NY	428
D	Brauner, G	NJ	696
D	Bruckstein, R	NY	515
D	Clark, S	NY	153
D	De Pietro, W	NY	515
D	Downie, J	NJ	741
D	Geronemus, R	NY	154
D	Green, M	NY	154
D	Greenberg, R	NY	154
D	Grossman, M	NY	155
D	Hochman, H	NY	155
D	Leffell, D	CT	945
D	Levine, L	NY	516
D	Levy, R	NY	627
D	Lipper, G	CT	900
D	McCormack, P	NY	492
D	Milgraum, S	NJ	792
D	Oestreicher, M	CT	900
D	Ostad, A	NY	157
D	Polis, L	NY	157
D	Rapaport, J	NJ	697
D	Safai, B	NY	158

Spec	Name	St	Pg
D	Sarnoff, D	NY	516
D	Schliftman, A	NY	628
D	Schultz, N	NY	158
D	Shelton, R	NY	158
D	Siegel, E	NJ	742
D	Silverman, M	NY	516
D	Waldorf, H	NY	573
D	Wattenberg, D	NY	160
D	Wechsler, A	NY	160
D	Weiss, D	NJ	697
D	Wrone, D	NJ	792
D	Zweibel, S	NY	628
Oto	Brunner, E	NJ	782
Oto	Guida, R	NY	280
PlS	Gotkin, R	NY	555

Skin Tumors

Spec	Name	St	Pg
D	Feldman, P	NY	428
D	Savin, R	CT	945

Skin/Soft Tissue Infections

Spec	Name	St	Pg
Inf	Aufiero, P	NJ	777
Inf	Brause, B	NY	193
Inf	Helfgott, D	NY	194
Inf	Scheer, M	NY	526
Inf	Smith, P	NY	197
Inf	Soroko, T	NJ	746

Skull Base Surgery

Spec	Name	St	Pg
NS	Abrahams, J	NY	648
NS	Bruce, J	NY	227
NS	Chen, C	NY	227
NS	Davis, R	NY	595
NS	Eisenberg, M	NY	533
NS	Golfinos, J	NY	228
NS	Murali, R	NY	649
NS	Schulder, M	NY	534
NS	Stieg, P	NY	230
Oto	Close, L	NY	279
Oto	Frank, D	NY	543
Oto	Lalwani, A	NY	282
Oto	Meiteles, L	NY	659
Oto	Storper, I	NY	286

Skull Base Tumors

Spec	Name	St	Pg
NS	Bilsky, M	NY	226
NS	Chen, C	NY	227
NS	Jafar, J	NY	228
NS	Sen, C	NY	230
Oto	Costantino, P	NY	279
Oto	Har-El, G	NY	280
Oto	Kraus, D	NY	281
Oto	Persky, M	NY	283
Oto	Vining, E	CT	955
S	Shah, J	NY	360

Sleep & Snoring Disorders

Spec	Name	St	Pg
Oto	Youngerman, J	NY	545
Pul	Kupfer, Y	NY	459

Specialty & Special Expertise Index

Specialty & Special Expertise Index

Specialty & Special Expertise Index

Spec	Name	St	Pg
Thromboembolic Disorders			
Pul	Steiger, D	NY	339
Thrombolytic Therapy			
VIR	Aruny, J	CT	964
Thrombotic Disorders			
Hem	Ansell, J	NY	189
Hem	Billett, H	NY	395
Hem	Kempin, S	NY	190
Hem	Soff, G	NY	192
MF	Roshan, D	NY	210
Thymoma			
Onc	Aisner, J	NJ	797
Onc	Kris, M	NY	216
Onc	Rizvi, N	NY	219
T&CS	Camunas, J	NY	362
T&CS	Sanchez, J	CT	963
Thyroid & Parathyroid Cancer & Surgery			
Oto	Caruana, S	NY	278
Oto	Genden, E	NY	280
Oto	Urken, M	NY	286
Thyroid & Parathyroid Imaging			
NuM	Scharf, S	NY	242
Thyroid & Parathyroid Surgery			
Oto	Aferzon, M	CT	924
Oto	Drake, W	NJ	881
Oto	Frank, D	NY	543
Oto	Har-El, G	NY	280
Oto	Ho, B	NJ	717
Oto	Klarsfeld, J	CT	925
Oto	Komisar, A	NY	281
Oto	Kraus, D	NY	281
Oto	Krevitt, L	NY	282
Oto	La Bagnara, J	NJ	853
Oto	Lagmay, V	NY	451
Oto	Myssiorek, D	NY	283
Oto	Rosenbaum, J	NJ	804
Oto	Sacks, S	NY	284
Oto	Salzer, S	CT	925
Oto	Shah, D	NJ	822
Oto	Smith, R	NY	404
S	Auguste, L	NY	563
S	Chabot, J	NY	354
S	Heller, K	NY	356
S	Lee, J	NY	357
S	Rajdeo, H	NY	677
S	Rosenberg, V	NY	359
S	Schell, H	NJ	785
S	Shapiro, R	NY	360
Thyroid Cancer			
EDM	Davies, T	NY	167

Spec	Name	St	Pg
EDM	Hochstein, M	NJ	699
EDM	Mechanick, J	NY	168
EDM	Tuttle, R	NY	169
NuM	Goldfarb, C	NY	241
NuM	Goldsmith, S	NY	241
NuM	Pandit-Taskar, N	NY	241
NuM	Santos, E	NY	241
Onc	Pfister, D	NY	218
Oto	Boyle, J	NY	278
Oto	Branovan, D	NY	278
Oto	Brauer, R	CT	925
Oto	Kuhel, W	NY	282
Oto	Persky, M	NY	283
Oto	Salzer, S	CT	925
Oto	Schantz, S	NY	285
Oto	Shemen, L	NY	285
Oto	Singh, B	NY	286
Oto	Wong, R	NY	287
Path	Sanchez, M	NJ	718
S	Alfonso, A	NY	463
S	Roses, D	NY	359
S	Shah, J	NY	360
S	Sosa, J	CT	962
S	Sultan, R	NY	772
S	Udelsman, R	CT	962
Thyroid Disorders			
EDM	Agrin, R	NJ	793
EDM	Albin, J	NY	629
EDM	Arden-Cordone, M	CT	901
EDM	Balkin, M	NY	588
EDM	Baranetsky, N	NJ	742
EDM	Bergman, D	NY	165
EDM	Berkowitz, R	NJ	850
EDM	Bhatt, A	NY	518
EDM	Bitton, R	NY	518
EDM	Bleich, D	NJ	742
EDM	Bloomgarden, D	NY	630
EDM	Blum, C	NY	166
EDM	Blum, D	NY	630
EDM	Brand, H	NY	589
EDM	Brickman, A	NY	429
EDM	Brillon, D	NY	166
EDM	Bucholtz, H	NJ	793
EDM	Cam, J	NJ	767
EDM	Carlson, H	NY	589
EDM	Cobin, R	NJ	699
EDM	Cohen, C	NY	389
EDM	Cohen, N	NY	493
EDM	Das, S	NY	493
EDM	Friedman, S	NY	518
EDM	Fuhrman, R	NJ	874
EDM	Gelato, M	NY	589
EDM	Gewirtz, G	NJ	742
EDM	Giegerich, E	NY	429
EDM	Gioia, L	NY	589
EDM	Goldberg-Berman, J	CT	902
EDM	Goldenberg, A	NY	589
EDM	Goldman, J	NY	429
EDM	Goldman, M	NJ	699
EDM	Gordon, J	NY	518
EDM	Grajower, M	NY	389

Spec	Name	St	Pg
EDM	Greene, L	NY	167
EDM	Greenfield, M	NY	519
EDM	Guoth, M	CT	902
EDM	Guzman, R	NY	389
EDM	Hellerman, J	NY	630
EDM	Hochstein, M	NJ	699
EDM	Hoffman, R	NY	493
EDM	Hupart, K	NY	519
EDM	Jacobs, T	NY	167
EDM	Kantor, A	NY	630
EDM	Klyde, B	NY	167
EDM	Leibowitz, J	NY	630
EDM	Lomasky, S	NY	519
EDM	Maman, A	NJ	793
EDM	Margulies, P	NY	519
EDM	McConnell, R	NY	168
EDM	Mechanick, J	NY	168
EDM	Nassberg, B	NJ	817
EDM	Peck, V	NY	168
EDM	Poretsky, L	NY	168
EDM	Rennert, N	CT	902
EDM	Resta, C	NY	429
EDM	Rosenbaum, R	NJ	874
EDM	Rosenthal, R	NY	519
EDM	Rosman, L	NY	474
EDM	Rothman, J	NY	493
EDM	Selinger, S	NJ	874
EDM	Seltzer, T	NY	168
EDM	Seplowitz, A	NY	168
EDM	Shapiro, L	NY	519
EDM	Sherry, S	NJ	743
EDM	Silverberg, A	NY	429
EDM	Silverman, M	NJ	875
EDM	Spiler, I	NJ	793
EDM	Surks, M	NY	389
EDM	Tibaldi, J	NY	475
EDM	Tohme, J	NJ	699
EDM	Warman, J	NY	430
EDM	Wehmann, R	NJ	700
EDM	Weitzman, S	NY	589
EDM	Wexler, C	NY	589
EDM	Wiesen, M	NJ	700
EDM	Young, I	NY	169
EDM	Zonszein, J	NY	390
EDM	Zweig, S	NY	169
FMed	Sadovsky, R	NY	430
IM	Fiedler, R	NY	200
IM	Joy, M	NY	437
IM	Kennedy, J	NY	202
NuM	Goldfarb, C	NY	241
NuM	Strashun, A	NY	445
Oto	Tawfik, B	NY	545
Ped	Siegal, E	NY	578
PEn	Agdere, L	NY	452
PEn	Avruskin, T	NY	452
PEn	Carey, D	NY	547
PEn	Carpenter, T	CT	956
PEn	Chin, D	NJ	840
PEn	Frank, G	NY	548
PEn	Franklin, B	NY	294
PEn	Kohn, B	NY	295
PEn	Meyers-Seifer, C	NJ	823
PEn	Noto, R	NY	661

Specialty & Special Expertise Index

Specialty & Special Expertise Index

Spec	Name	St	Pg
DR	Goodman, K	NY	517
DR	Lerman, J	NY	429

Urology

Spec	Name	St	Pg
U	Andriani, R	CT	936
U	Armenakas, N	NY	367
U	Ashley, R	NY	567
U	Axelrod, S	NY	678
U	Bar-Chama, N	NY	367
U	Barone, J	NJ	867
U	Basralian, K	NJ	731
U	Beccia, D	NY	609
U	Benson, M	NY	367
U	Berdini, J	NJ	731
U	Berman, S	NY	367
U	Birkhoff, J	NY	368
U	Birns, D	NY	368
U	Blair, B	NY	678
U	Blaivas, J	NY	368
U	Bochner, B	NY	368
U	Boczko, J	NY	679
U	Boczko, S	NY	368
U	Boorjian, P	NJ	763
U	Breslin, D	NY	679
U	Brodherson, M	NY	368
U	Bruno, A	NY	567
U	Catanese, A	NJ	867
U	Chaikin, D	NJ	845
U	Choudhury, M	NY	679
U	Chun, T	NJ	731
U	Ciccone, P	NJ	763
U	Colberg, J	CT	963
U	Colton, M	NJ	845
U	Connor, J	NJ	845
U	D'Esposito, R	NY	567
U	DelPizzo, J	NY	368
U	Dillon, R	NY	368
U	Dodds, P	CT	937
U	Droller, M	NY	368
U	Eastham, J	NY	369
U	Ebani, J	NJ	826
U	Edelman, R	NY	567
U	Eshghi, A	NY	679
U	Esposito, M	NJ	732
U	Farrell, R	NY	486
U	Fine, E	NY	369
U	Fisch, H	NY	369
U	Flanagan, M	CT	963
U	Fleisher, M	NJ	811
U	Foster, H	CT	963
U	Fracchia, J	NY	369
U	Frey, H	NJ	732
U	Friedman, S	NY	465
U	Geltzeiler, J	NJ	826
U	Gershbaum, M	NY	567
U	Ghavamian, R	NY	416
U	Giella, J	NY	580
U	Girardi, S	NY	567
U	Glassberg, K	NY	369
U	Glassman, C	NY	679
U	Goldstein, M	NY	369
U	Grasso, M	NY	369
U	Grebler, A	NJ	826
U	Gribetz, M	NY	369
U	Grunberger, I	NY	465
U	Gupta, M	NY	370
U	Hajjar, J	NJ	732
U	Hall, S	NY	370
U	Hanna, M	NY	567
U	Harris, S	NY	567
U	Hennessy, W	CT	937
U	Hensle, T	NJ	370
U	Herr, H	NY	370
U	Horowitz, M	NY	465
U	Housman, A	NY	679
U	Irwin, M	NY	466
U	Jordan, M	NJ	763
U	Kaminetsky, J	NY	370
U	Kaplan, S	NY	370
U	Katz, A	NY	567
U	Katz, H	NJ	772
U	Katz, J	NJ	763
U	Katz, S	NJ	732
U	Kavoussi, L	NY	568
U	Kirschenbaum, A	NY	370
U	Klein, G	NY	370
U	Lanteri, V	NJ	732
U	Layne, J	NY	568
U	Lehrhoff, B	NJ	887
U	Lepor, H	NY	370
U	Lerner, S	NY	679
U	Lessing, J	NY	502
U	Levine, S	NJ	856
U	Lieberman, E	NY	568
U	Lindsay, G	NY	466
U	Linsenmeyer, T	NJ	764
U	Litvin, Y	NJ	826
U	Lizza, E	NY	371
U	Loo, M	NY	371
U	Lowe, F	NY	371
U	Margolis, E	NJ	732
U	Marks, J	NY	371
U	Matthews, G	NY	679
U	McGovern, T	NY	371
U	McKiernan, J	NY	371
U	Meisenberg, G	NY	466
U	Mellinger, B	NY	568
U	Mills, C	NY	609
U	Moldwin, R	NY	568
U	Muldoon, L	CT	937
U	Mulhall, J	NY	371
U	Munver, R	NJ	732
U	Nagler, H	NY	371
U	Nitti, V	NY	372
U	Owens, G	NY	680
U	Palese, M	NY	372
U	Passarelli, M	CT	963
U	Paul, E	NY	568
U	Peng, B	NY	372
U	Poppas, D	NY	372
U	Provet, J	NY	372
U	Putignano, J	NY	680
U	Raboy, A	NY	502
U	Ranta, J	CT	937
U	Reckler, J	NY	372
U	Reda, E	NY	680
U	Richards, S	NJ	811
U	Richstone, L	NY	568
U	Riechers, R	NY	680
U	Ring, K	NJ	887
U	Roberts, L	NY	680
U	Romas, N	NY	372
U	Rose, J	NJ	827
U	Rosenberg, G	NJ	732
U	Rosenthal, S	NY	466
U	Rossman, B	NJ	786
U	Rotolo, J	NJ	827
U	Russo, P	NY	372
U	Saada, S	NY	466
U	Sadeghi-Nejad, H	NJ	732
U	Samadi, D	NY	373
U	Sandhaus, J	NY	487
U	Savatta, D	NJ	764
U	Savino, M	NY	502
U	Sawczuk, I	NJ	733
U	Scardino, P	NY	373
U	Scherr, D	NY	373
U	Schiff, H	NY	373
U	Schlegel, P	NY	373
U	Schlussel, R	NY	373
U	Schrager, A	NY	680
U	Seidman, B	NJ	887
U	Shabsigh, R	NY	466
U	Shapiro, E	NY	373
U	Sheinfeld, J	NY	373
U	Shepard, B	NY	568
U	Shield, D	CT	937
U	Shulman, Y	NJ	772
U	Siegel, J	NY	680
U	Silva, J	NY	374
U	Silver, D	NY	466
U	Singh, D	CT	963
U	Sogani, P	NY	374
U	Solomon, M	NJ	811
U	Steigman, E	NJ	772
U	Stein, M	NY	416
U	Stifelman, M	NY	374
U	Stock, J	NJ	764
U	Stone, C	NJ	845
U	Strauss, B	NJ	764
U	Sunshine, R	NY	568
U	Taneja, S	NY	374
U	Tarasuk, A	NY	487
U	Te, A	NY	374
U	Tennenbaum, S	NJ	733
U	Tewari, A	NY	374
U	Tillem, S	NY	487
U	Trauzzi, S	NY	680
U	Vapnek, J	NY	374
U	Vasselli, A	NJ	786
U	Vates, T	NY	812
U	Viner, N	CT	937
U	Vitenson, J	NJ	733
U	Vukasin, A	NJ	786
U	Wainstein, S	NY	466
U	Wasnick, R	NY	609
U	Wasserman, G	NJ	733
U	Waxberg, J	CT	937

Specialty & Special Expertise Index

Specialty & Special Expertise Index

Alphabetical Listing of Doctors

Name	Specialty	Pg
A		
Aaronson, Beth (CT)	PMR	928
Abelow, Arthur (NY)	Ge	391
Abemayor, Elie (NY)	Ge	632
Abenavoli, Tancredi (NY)	IM	639
Aberg, Judith (NY)	Inf	193
Abittan, Meyer (NY)	IC	529
Ablaza, Valerie (NJ)	PlS	758
Abott, Michael (NY)	Pul	458
Abrahams, John (NY)	NS	648
Abramowitz, Avram (NY)	Onc	479
Abrams, Jeffrey (NJ)	OrS	781
Abrams, Martin (CT)	Onc	912
Abramson, David (NY)	Oph	248
Abramson, Sara (NY)	DR	160
Abright, A Reese (NY)	ChAP	144
Abrol, Sunil (NY)	T&CS	465
Abu-Rustum, Nadeem (NY)	GO	184
Abularrage, Joseph (NY)	Ped	482
Accacha, Siham (NY)	PEn	547
Accardi, Frank (NY)	Oph	248
Accurso, Charles (NJ)	Ge	861
Acker, Peter (NY)	Ped	665
Ackerman, Jacob (NY)	Oph	446
Ackert, John (NY)	Ge	170
Acosta, Rodrigo (CT)	FMed	902
Acquista, Angelo (NY)	Pul	334
Adams, David (NY)	T&CS	361
Adams, Francis (NY)	Pul	335
Adams, Marc (NY)	RadRO	500
Addonizio, Gerard (NY)	Psyc	669
Addonizio, Linda (NY)	PCd	292
Addrizzo-Harris, Doreen (NY)	Pul	335
Adelman, Mark (NY)	VascS	376
Adelman, Ronald (NY)	Ger	181
Adelsberg, Bernard (CT)	A&I	942
Ades, Joseph (NY)	IM	639
Adesman, Andrew (NY)	Ped	552
Adibi, Baback (NJ)	Cv	692
Adler, Edward (NY)	OrS	263
Adler, Harry (NY)	S	462
Adler, Howard (NY)	Ge	170
Adler, Jack (NY)	Pul	335
Adler, Kenneth (NJ)	Onc	836
Adler, Lenard (NY)	Psyc	321
Adler, Ronald (NY)	DR	160
Adler, Stephen (NY)	Nep	647
Adler-Klein, Debra (CT)	Inf	907

Name	Specialty	Pg
Adlersberg, Jay (NY)	Rhu	346
Aferzon, Mark (CT)	Oto	924
Afridi, Shariq (NJ)	Ge	776
Agarwal, Chhavi (NY)	PEn	406
Agarwal, Kishan (NJ)	PCd	804
Agarwal, Nanakram (NY)	S	414
Agdere, Levon (NY)	PEn	452
Aghajanian, Carol (NY)	Onc	210
Agin, Carole (NY)	PM	545
Agress, Harry (NJ)	NuM	712
Agri, Robyn (NJ)	PMR	783
Agrin, Richard (NJ)	EDM	793
Aguila, Helen (NJ)	PPul	756
Agus, Bertrand (NY)	Rhu	346
Aharon, Raphael (NY)	Oph	481
Ahlborn, Thomas (NJ)	S	729
Ahluwalia, Brij M Singh (NY)	N	649
Ahmad, Christopher (NY)	OrS	263
Ahmed, Tauseef (NY)	Onc	644
Ahn, Christina (NY)	PlS	312
Ahn, Jung (NY)	PMR	308
Aisenberg, James (NY)	Ge	170
Aisenberg, Javier (NJ)	PEn	719
Aisner, Joseph (NJ)	Onc	797
Ajl, Stephen (NY)	Ped	456
Akhund, Birjis (NY)	Onc	594
Akinboboye, Olakunle (NY)	Cv	472
Albin, Joan (NY)	EDM	629
Albom, Michael (NY)	D	151
Alderman, Elizabeth (NY)	AM	383
Aldrich, Thomas (NY)	Pul	412
Aledo, Alexander (NY)	PHO	297
Aledort, Louis (NY)	Hem	188
Alexander, Frederick (NJ)	PS	721
Alexiades, Michael (NY)	OrS	263
Alfonso, Antonio (NY)	S	463
Ali, Yousaf (NY)	Rhu	346
Alizadeh, Kaveh (NY)	PlS	554
Allegra, Donald (NJ)	Inf	835
Allen, Jeffrey (NY)	ChiN	147
Allen, Steven (NY)	Hem	525
Allendorf, Dennis (NY)	Ped	304
Almeida, Laila (NJ)	D	832
Almeleh, Jack (NY)	Psyc	321
Almeyda, Elizabeth (NY)	PlS	312
Aloia, John (NY)	EDM	518
Alper, Kenneth (NY)	Psyc	321
Alpert, Barbara (NY)	IM	639

Alphabetical Listing of Doctors

Name	Specialty	Pg	Name	Specialty	Pg
Altbaum, Robert (CT)	IM	908	Antony, Michael (NY)	Ge	391
Altchek, David (NY)	SM	351	Anyane-Yeboa, Kwame (NY)	CG	148
Alterman, Lloyd (NJ)	IM	877	Apatoff, Brian (NY)	N	231
Altholz, Jeffrey (NY)	IM	639	Aponte, Alex (NY)	FMed	589
Altman, Bruce (CT)	Oph	919	Apostolides, Paul (CT)	NS	914
Altman, Robin (NY)	Ped	665	Appel, David (NY)	Pul	412
Altman, Wayne (NJ)	OrS	715	Appel, Gerald (NY)	Nep	223
Altmann, Dory (NJ)	IC	797	Appelbaum, Jeffrey (NY)	N	480
Altmann, Karen (NY)	PCd	292	Appelbaum, Paul (NY)	Psyc	321
Altorki, Nasser (NY)	T&CS	362	Applebaum, Eric (NJ)	A&I	831
Altschul, Larry (NY)	Cv	584	April, Max (NY)	PO	301
Alvarez, Manuel (NJ)	MF	706	Aprile, Georgette (NY)	D	515
Alweiss, Gary (NJ)	N	711	Apuzzio, Joseph (NJ)	ObG	750
Ames, Richard (NY)	Nep	223	Apuzzo, Thomas (NY)	FMed	631
Amin, Hossam (NY)	Pul	458	Aranoff, Shera (NY)	D	151
Amin, Mahendra (NY)	IM	477	Arbour, Robert (NJ)	S	826
Amin, Milan (NY)	Oto	278	Arcasoy, Selim (NY)	Pul	335
Amin, Nikhil (NY)	PPul	663	Arcati, Anthony (NY)	FMed	520
Amin, Ravindra (NY)	GerPsy	433	Arcati, Robert (NY)	FMed	520
Amin, Snehal (NY)	D	151	Arden, Martha (NY)	AM	506
Amis, E Stephen (NY)	DR	387	Arden-Cordone, Mary (CT)	EDM	901
Amler, David (NY)	Ped	665	Arena, Francis (NY)	Onc	530
Ammazzalorso, Michael (NY)	IM	526	Arens, Raanan (NY)	PPul	407
Amodio, John (NY)	DR	428	Argenziano, Michael (NY)	T&CS	362
Amorosi, Edward (NY)	Hem	189	Aries, Philip (NY)	Oph	597
Amoruso, Robert (NJ)	Pul	854	Ariyan, Stephan (CT)	PlS	958
Amory, Spencer (NY)	S	353	Ark, Jon (NJ)	HS	777
Andaz, Shahriyour (NY)	T&CS	565	Arkow, Stan (NY)	Psyc	321
Andersen, Holly (NY)	Cv	134	Armbruster, Robert (NY)	ObG	651
Anderson, Patrick (NJ)	GO	744	Armenakas, Noel (NY)	U	367
Anderson, Richard (NY)	NS	226	Armento, Michael (NJ)	PMR	883
Andiman, Warren (CT)	PInf	956	Arnell, Tracey (NY)	CRS	149
Andrade, Joseph (NY)	Ped	408	Arno, Louis (NJ)	Pul	866
Andrei, Valeriu (NJ)	S	761	Arnold, Thomas (NY)	VascS	609
Andrews, Alan (NJ)	D	696	Arnon, Rica (NY)	PCd	292
Andriani, Rudy (CT)	U	936	Arnstein, Ellis (NY)	Ped	408
Andriola, Mary (NY)	ChiN	586	Aronne, Louis (NY)	IM	197
Anene, Okechukwu (NJ)	PCCM	805	Aronoff, Michael (NY)	Psyc	321
Angeli, Stephen (NJ)	IC	706	Aronson, Thomas (NY)	Psyc	604
Angioletti, Louis (NY)	Oph	248	Arpadi, Stephen (NY)	Ped	304
Angoff, Ronald (CT)	Ped	957	Arpino, Muthu (NJ)	Ger	744
Angrist, Richard (NJ)	Oph	863	Aruny, John (CT)	VIR	964
Anhalt, Henry (NJ)	PEn	882	Arvanitis, Michael (NJ)	CRS	816
Annabi, Iyad (NY)	FMed	631	Asarian, Armand (NY)	CRS	427
Ansell, Jack (NY)	Hem	189	Asbell, Penny (NY)	Oph	248
Anselmi, Gregory (NJ)	N	769	Ascheim, Robert (NY)	IM	198
Antaya, Richard (CT)	D	944	Ascher, Enrico (NY)	VascS	467
Anto, Maliakal (NY)	Cv	508	Ascher-Walsh, Charles (NY)	ObG	242
Anton, John (NY)	PlS	603	Ascherman, Jeffrey (NY)	PlS	312
Antonelle, Robert (NY)	Ge	632	Ashamalla, Hani (NY)	RadRO	460
Antonescu, Cristina (NY)	Path	289	Ashikari, Andrew (NY)	S	676

Alphabetical Listing of Doctors

Name	Specialty	Pg	Name	Specialty	Pg
Barley, Christopher (NY)	IM	198	Bellucci, Alessandro (NY)	Nep	532
Barmakian, Joseph (NJ)	OrS	880	Belmont, H Michael (NY)	Rhu	346
Barnard, Nicola (NJ)	Path	804	Belok, Lennart (NY)	N	231
Barone, Clement (NY)	DR	161	Belsh, Jerry (NJ)	N	799
Barone, Joseph (NJ)	U	867	Belsito, Donald (NY)	D	152
Barone, Richard (NY)	Rhu	674	Ben-Menachem, Tamir (NJ)	Ge	875
Barrett, Leonard (NY)	T&CS	565	Ben-Zvi, Jeffrey (NY)	Ge	171
Barrison, Adam (NJ)	Ge	875	Benchimol, Corinne (NY)	PNep	300
Barron, O Alton (NY)	HS	186	Bendo, John (NY)	OrS	263
Bartell, Abraham (NY)	ChAP	144	Benedetto, Dominick (NJ)	Oph	770
Bartlett, Jacqueline (NJ)	ChAP	740	Benedict, Leonard (NY)	ObG	537
Bartolomeo, Robert (NY)	Ge	520	Benedicto, Milagros (NY)	ObG	480
Barzegar, Hooshang (NY)	ObG	445	Benevenia, Joseph (NJ)	OrS	752
Basch, Samuel (NY)	Psyc	322	Beniaminovitz, Ainat (NY)	Cv	573
Bashevkin, Michael (NY)	Onc	439	Benisovich, Vladimir (NY)	Onc	479
Baskin, David (NY)	IM	198	Benito, Carlos (NJ)	MF	836
Baskin, Martin (NY)	Pul	335	Benjamin, Ernest (NY)	CCM	151
Baskind, Lawrence (NY)	Ped	665	Benjamin, John (NY)	Psyc	557
Basner, Robert (NY)	Pul	335	Benkov, Keith (NY)	PGe	296
Basralian, Kevin (NJ)	U	731	Bennett, Harvey (NJ)	ChiN	832
Bassett, Clifford (NY)	A&I	130	Benoff, Brian (NJ)	Pul	725
Bastawros, Mary (NY)	Ped	499	Benson, Mitchell (NY)	U	367
Basuk, Pamela (NY)	D	587	Bent, John (NY)	PO	407
Basuk, Paul (NY)	Ge	170	Benton, Marc (NJ)	Pul	843
Bateman, David (NY)	NP	222	Benvenisty, Alan (NY)	VascS	376
Bauer, Bertha (NY)	Rhu	346	Benzil, Deborah (NY)	NS	648
Bauman, Jonathan (NY)	Psyc	669	Beran, Nancy (NY)	IM	639
Bauman, Phillip (NY)	OrS	263	Beran, Samuel (NY)	PIS	667
Baumann, John (NJ)	RadRO	809	Berbari, Nicholas (NY)	IM	527
Baumgaertner, Michael (CT)	OrS	954	Berberian, Wayne (NJ)	OrS	752
Baydin, Jeffrey (NJ)	OrS	839	Berck, David (NY)	MF	643
Bazzy-Asaad, Alia (CT)	PPul	957	Berdini, Jeffrey (NJ)	U	731
Beauregard, Lou-Anne (NJ)	Cv	815	Berdoff, Russell (NY)	Cv	134
Beccia, David (NY)	U	609	Berenstein, Alejandro (NY)	NRad	239
Becker, Alfred (NY)	Rhu	579	Berezin, Marc (NY)	SM	579
Becker, David (NY)	D	152	Berezin, Stuart (NY)	PGe	662
Becker, Ina (NY)	ChAP	144	Berger, Bernard (NY)	D	587
Bederson, Joshua (NY)	NS	226	Berger, Jack (NY)	Rhu	674
Bednarek, Karl (NY)	Ge	171	Berger, Jeffrey (NY)	Ger	523
Behm, Dutsi (NY)	IM	436	Berger, Judith (NY)	Inf	395
Behr, Raymond (NY)	Psyc	557	Berger, Marvin (NY)	Cv	134
Beim, Robert (NJ)	ObG	880	Bergh, Paul (NJ)	RE	843
Belamarich, Peter (NY)	Ped	408	Bergman, Donald (NY)	EDM	165
Beldner, Steven (NY)	HS	186	Bergman, Kerry (NJ)	PS	882
Belenkov, Elliot (NY)	Onc	211	Bergmann, Steven (NY)	Cv	135
Belilos, Elise (NY)	Rhu	562	Bergtraum, Marcia (NY)	ChiN	514
Bell, Jonathan (CT)	A&I	895	Berke, Andrew (NY)	IC	529
Bell, Kevin (NJ)	IM	862	Berke, Stanley (NY)	Oph	539
Bellemare, Sarah (NY)	S	414	Berkey, Peter (NY)	Inf	638
Bello, Jacqueline (NY)	NRad	401	Berkowitz, Howard (NY)	Psyc	457
Bello, Mary (NJ)	FMed	700	Berkowitz, Leonard (NY)	Inf	435

Name	Specialty	Pg	Name	Specialty	Pg
Berkowitz, Norman (NY)	Ped	665	Bhattacharyya, Nishith (NJ)	PS	854
Berkowitz, Rhonda (NY)	D	625	Bia, Margaret (CT)	Nep	951
Berkowitz, Richard (NY)	MF	209	Biagiotti, Wendy (NY)	FMed	390
Berkowitz, Richard (NJ)	EDM	850	Bialer, Martin (NY)	CG	514
Berkwits, Kieve (CT)	PCd	926	Bialer, Philip (NY)	Psyc	322
Berman, Alvin (NY)	ObG	242	Biancaniello, Thomas (NY)	PCd	601
Berman, Daniel (NY)	IM	396	Bianchi, Mark (CT)	Oto	924
Berman, David (NY)	Oph	446	Bickers, David (NY)	D	152
Berman, Edward (CT)	IM	908	Bielory, Leonard (NJ)	A&I	872
Berman, Ellin (NY)	Onc	211	Bienenstock, Harry (NY)	Rhu	462
Berman, Mark (NJ)	OrS	715	Bierman, Fredrick (NY)	PCd	660
Berman, Russell (NY)	S	353	Bigliani, Louis (NY)	OrS	263
Berman, Sandra (NY)	IM	436	Bikoff, David (NJ)	PlS	724
Berman, Sheldon (NY)	Psyc	557	Bilezikian, John (NY)	EDM	166
Berman, Steven (NY)	U	367	Bilfinger, Thomas (NY)	T&CS	608
Bernard, Robert (NY)	IM	593	Billett, Henny (NY)	Hem	395
Bernard, Robert (NY)	PlS	667	Bilsky, Mark (NY)	NS	226
Bernardini, Dennis (NY)	Pul	605	Bindelglass, David (CT)	OrS	921
Bernardo, Salvatore (NJ)	FMed	817	Binder, Ralph (NY)	Pul	671
Bernhardt, Bernard (NY)	Onc	644	Binns, Joseph (NJ)	Ge	817
Bernik, Stephanie (NY)	S	353	Birch, Thomas (NJ)	Inf	704
Bernik, Thomas (NY)	VascS	377	Bird, Hector (NY)	ChAP	145
Bernstein, Brett (NY)	Ge	171	Birkhoff, John (NY)	U	368
Bernstein, Chaim (NY)	Pul	459	Birnbaum, Audrey (NY)	PGe	662
Bernstein, Charles (NY)	D	492	Birns, Douglas (NY)	U	368
Bernstein, David (NY)	Ge	521	Biro, David (NY)	D	427
Bernstein, Harvey (NY)	Ped	602	Bisaga, Adam (NY)	AdP	617
Bernstein, Larry (NY)	A&I	383	Bisberg, Dorothy (NJ)	PPul	756
Bernstein, Lawrence (NY)	Rhu	462	Biser, Seth (NY)	Oph	653
Bernstein, Michael (NY)	S	463	Bitan, Fabien (NY)	OrS	264
Bernstein, Robert (NY)	D	152	Bitton, Rachelle (NY)	EDM	518
Bernstein, William (NY)	Ped	578	Biviano, Angelo (NY)	CE	132
Berry, Richard (NY)	D	427	Biviano, Bernard (NY)	S	485
Berson, Barry (NY)	DR	161	Bivona, James (CT)	IM	908
Berson, Diane (NY)	D	152	Black, Henry (NY)	Nep	224
Besser, Gary (CT)	ObG	917	Blackwood, M Michele (NJ)	S	761
Besser, Louis (NY)	Cv	491	Blady, David (NJ)	N	749
Besser, Walter (NY)	OrS	481	Blair, Bryan (NY)	U	678
Bessey, Palmer (NY)	S	353	Blair, Emily (CT)	ObG	917
Bessler, Marc (NY)	S	353	Blair, Lester (NY)	Pul	336
Bethel, Colin (NJ)	PS	757	Blaivas, Jerry (NY)	U	368
Better, Donna (NY)	PCd	546	Blake, James (NY)	Cv	135
Bevelaqua, Frederick (NY)	Pul	335	Blanck, Richard (NY)	N	535
Beyda, Allan (NY)	IM	477	Blanco, Jody (NY)	ObG	242
Beyda, Bernadette (NY)	D	474	Blank, Ellen (NJ)	D	767
Beyerl, Brian (NJ)	NS	837	Blau, Sheldon (NY)	Rhu	562
Bhagat, Neelakshi (NJ)	Oph	751	Blaufox, Andrew (NY)	PCd	546
Bhansali, Rohan (NY)	Cv	508	Blei, Francine (NY)	PHO	297
Bharathan, Thayyullathil (NY)	IM	436	Bleiberg, Melvyn (NY)	Cv	618
Bhatt, Anjani (NY)	EDM	518	Bleich, David (NJ)	EDM	742
Bhatt, Ashok (NY)	Psyc	557	Bleicher, Robert (NJ)	Ge	850

Alphabetical Listing of Doctors

Name	Specialty	Pg	Name	Specialty	Pg
Bleiweiss, Ira (NY)	Path	290	Boone, Peter (CT)	OrS	921
Blick, Michael (NJ)	Cv	831	Boorady, Roy (NY)	ChAP	145
Blitzer, Andrew (NY)	Oto	278	Boorjian, Peter (NJ)	U	763
Blondo, Dennis (NJ)	Oph	802	Borah, Gregory (NJ)	PlS	807
Blood, David (NJ)	Cv	692	Borao, Frank (NJ)	S	826
Bloom, Norman (NY)	S	354	Borbely, Antal (NY)	Psyc	322
Bloom, Patricia (NY)	Ger	181	Borcich, Anthony (NY)	Ge	171
Bloomfield, Diane (NY)	Ped	408	Borek, Mark (NY)	Cv	584
Bloomgarden, David (NY)	EDM	630	Borer, Jeffrey (NY)	Cv	423
Bloomgarden, Zachary (NY)	EDM	166	Borg, Morton (NY)	PCd	292
Blum, Alan (NY)	Pul	558	Borgen, Patrick (NY)	S	463
Blum, Conrad (NY)	EDM	166	Borkowsky, William (NY)	PInf	299
Blum, Daniel (NY)	IM	477	Borriello, Raffaele (NY)	S	463
Blum, David (NY)	EDM	630	Boruchoff, Susan (NJ)	Inf	796
Blum, Jay (NJ)	A&I	789	Boscamp, Jeffrey (NJ)	PInf	719
Blum, Mark (NJ)	Cv	831	Bosco, Joseph (NY)	OrS	264
Blum, Ronald (NY)	Onc	211	Bosl, George (NY)	Onc	211
Blumberg, Joel (CT)	IM	908	Boss, William (NJ)	PlS	724
Blume, Ralph (NY)	Rhu	346	Bosso, John (NY)	A&I	573
Blumenfeld, Jon (NY)	Nep	224	Bostrom, Mathias (NY)	OrS	264
Blumenthal, David (NY)	Cv	135	Bosworth, Jay (NY)	RadRO	560
Blumstein, Meyer (NY)	Ge	521	Botwin, Clifford (NJ)	OrS	881
Boachie-Adjei, Oheneba (NY)	OrS	264	Botwinick, Nelson (NY)	HS	186
Bobby, Paul (CT)	MF	911	Bourla, Steven (NY)	Nep	533
Bobroff, Lewis (NY)	DR	574	Boxer, Harriet (NY)	NP	532
Bochner, Bernard (NY)	U	368	Boxer, Mitchell (NY)	A&I	506
Bochner, Ronnie (NJ)	ObG	801	Boxer, William (NY)	IM	198
Bockman, Richard (NY)	EDM	166	Boyd, D Barry (CT)	Hem	906
Boczko, Judd (NY)	U	679	Boyer, Joseph (NY)	PPul	663
Boczko, Stanley (NY)	U	368	Boyle, Jay (NY)	Oto	278
Bodenstein, Lawrence (NY)	PS	303	Brademas, Mary Ellen (NY)	D	152
Bodis-Wollner, Ivan (NY)	N	443	Bradley, Thomas (NY)	Onc	530
Bodner, William (NY)	RadRO	413	Brady, Mary (NY)	S	354
Bogen, Steven (NY)	Psyc	669	Bram, Harris (NJ)	PM	823
Bogin, Marc (NY)	Cv	491	Brancaccio, Ronald (NY)	D	428
Boim, Marilynn (NJ)	Ped	783	Brancaccio, William (NY)	DR	588
Bolognia, Jean (CT)	D	944	Brand, Howard (NY)	EDM	589
Bomback, David (CT)	OrS	921	Brandeis, Steven (NY)	CRS	149
Bomback, Fredric (NY)	Ped	665	Brandt, Fredric (NY)	D	152
Bonagura, Vincent (NY)	PA&I	546	Brandt, Lawrence (NY)	Ge	391
Bonaventura, Lisa (NJ)	IM	862	Brannagan, Thomas (NY)	N	231
Bond, Annette (CT)	MF	911	Branovan, Daniel (NY)	Oto	278
Bondi, Elliott (NY)	Pul	459	Brauer, Richard (CT)	Oto	925
Bone, Stanley (NY)	Psyc	322	Brauner, Gary (NJ)	D	696
Bonheim, Nelson (CT)	Ge	903	Braunstein, Richard (NY)	Oph	249
Bonilla, Mary Ann (NJ)	PHO	853	Brauntuch, Glenn (NJ)	Pul	726
Boniuk, Vivien (NY)	Oph	539	Brause, Barry (NY)	Inf	193
Boockvar, John (NY)	NS	226	Braver, Joel (NJ)	RadRO	866
Bookner, Scott (NY)	Ped	665	Brecher, Rubin (NY)	Oph	447
Boolbol, Robert (CT)	PM	926	Breda, Stephen (CT)	Oto	925
Boolbol, Susan (NY)	S	354	Breen, William (NY)	Cv	508

Alphabetical Listing of Doctors

Name	Specialty	Pg	Name	Specialty	Pg
Burton, Daniel (NY)	A&I	131	Cannarozzi, Nicholas (NJ)	Rhu	761
Busch-Devereaux, Erna (NY)	S	607	Canny, Christopher (CT)	Ped	957
Bush, Jacqueline (NY)	MF	439	Cantor, Michael (NY)	Ge	171
Bush, Michael (NY)	IM	198	Capasse, Jeanne (CT)	S	934
Busillo, Christopher (NY)	Inf	193	Caplivski, Daniel (NY)	Inf	193
Bussel, James (NY)	PHO	297	Capobianco, Luigi (NY)	FMed	520
Buterman, Irving (NY)	ObG	243	Capozzi, James (NY)	OrS	542
Butler, David (NJ)	ObG	713	Cappucci, Roger (NY)	Cv	618
Butler, James (CT)	N	915	Caputo, Anthony (NJ)	Oph	751
Butler, Mark (NJ)	OrS	864	Caputo, Thomas (NY)	GO	184
Butt, Ahmar (NY)	IM	436	Caracci, Giovanni (NJ)	Psyc	759
Buxton, Douglas (NY)	Oph	249	Cardiello, Gary (NJ)	IM	768
Buyon, Jill (NY)	Rhu	346	Cardoso, Erico (NY)	NS	442
Buzzeo, Louis (NY)	Nep	647	Carew, John (NY)	Oto	278
Byfield, Floyd (NY)	Ge	632	Carey, Dennis (NY)	PEn	547
Byk, Cheryl (NJ)	DR	742	Carlin, Elizabeth (NJ)	NP	709
Byrd, Lawrence (NJ)	Nep	748	Carlson, Gabrielle (NY)	ChAP	585
			Carlson, Harold (NY)	EDM	589
			Carlson, John (NJ)	GO	795
			Carlson, Michelle (NY)	HS	186
			Carney, Alexander (NJ)	Rhu	785
C			Carniol, Paul (NJ)	Oto	881
Cabaniss, Deborah (NY)	Psyc	323	Caron, Philip (NY)	Onc	644
Cabin, Henry (CT)	Cv	942	Carosella, Christine (NY)	IM	639
Caccavale, Robert (NJ)	T&CS	867	Carpenter, Duncan (NJ)	NS	710
Caccese, William (NY)	Ge	521	Carpenter, Thomas (CT)	PEn	956
Cacciola, Thomas (NJ)	IM	705	Carr-Locke, David (NY)	Ge	171
Cafferty, Maureen (NY)	N	232	Carrasquillo, Jorge (NY)	NuM	241
Cahan, Anthony (NY)	S	676	Carroccio, Alfio (NY)	VascS	377
Cahill, James (NJ)	OrS	715	Carroll, William (NY)	PHO	297
Cahill, John (NY)	PrM	320	Carson, Jeffrey (NJ)	IM	796
Cahill, Kevin (NY)	PrM	321	Carsons, Steven (NY)	Rhu	562
Cahill, Linda (NY)	Ped	408	Carter, Mitchel (NJ)	S	844
Cairo, Mitchell (NY)	PHO	662	Caruana, Salvatore (NY)	Oto	278
Calem-Grunat, Jaclyn (NJ)	DR	698	Carucci, John (NY)	D	153
Calhoun, Sean (NJ)	VIR	845	Caruso, Rocco (NY)	Onc	594
Caligiuri, Daniel (NY)	HS	434	Casale, Linda (CT)	Cv	896
Caligor, Eve (NY)	Psyc	323	Casden, Andrew (NY)	OrS	265
Callahan, Eileen (NY)	Ger	181	Case, David (NY)	IM	198
Callahan, Lisa (NY)	SM	351	Casino, Joseph (NY)	Pul	672
Calman, Neil (NY)	FMed	169	Casper, Daniel (NY)	Oph	249
Cam, Jenny Rose (NJ)	EDM	767	Casper, Theodore (NY)	Pul	412
Camacho, Fernando (NY)	Onc	397	Cassell, Lauren (NY)	S	354
Camacho, Margarita (NJ)	T&CS	763	Cassidy, Brian (NJ)	IM	796
Camel, Mark (CT)	NS	914	Casson, Ira (NY)	N	480
Cammisa, Frank (NY)	OrS	264	Castellano, Bartolomeo (NY)	Oto	498
Campbell, Deborah (NY)	NP	398	Castellano, Michael (NY)	Pul	500
Campolattaro, Brian (NY)	Oph	249	Castro-Magana, Mariano (NY)	PEn	548
Camunas, Jorge (NY)	T&CS	362	Castro-Malaspina, Hugo (NY)	Hem	189
Cancellieri, Russell (NY)	A&I	583	Catalano, Louis (NY)	HS	186
Cangemi, Francis (NJ)	Oph	751	Catanese, Anthony (NJ)	U	867

Alphabetical Listing of Doctors

Name	Specialty	Pg	Name	Specialty	Pg
Chronakos, John (CT)	Pul	931	Cohen, Michael (NY)	Cv	135
Chuang, Linus (NY)	GO	637	Cohen, Michel (NY)	Ped	304
Chun, Audrey (NY)	Ger	182	Cohen, Neil (CT)	Hem	906
Chun, Thomas (NJ)	U	731	Cohen, Neil (NY)	EDM	493
Chung, Henry (NY)	Psyc	323	Cohen, Richard (NY)	IM	199
Chung, Wendy (NY)	CG	149	Cohen, Robert (NY)	IM	199
Chung-Loy, Harold (NJ)	S	810	Cohen, Seth (NY)	Ge	172
Ciaburri, Daniel (NY)	T&CS	362	Cohen, Seymour (NY)	Onc	212
Ciccone, Patrick (NJ)	U	763	Cohen, Steven (CT)	DR	901
Cicogna, Cristina (NJ)	Inf	704	Cohen, Steven (NY)	D	387
Cioroiu, Michael (NY)	S	354	Cohn, Symra (NY)	IM	199
Cipriani, Ralph (CT)	Inf	907	Cohn, William (NY)	Ge	590
Cirello, Richard (NJ)	FMed	743	Coit, Daniel (NY)	S	354
Citron, Marc (NY)	Onc	531	Colaco, Rodolfo (NJ)	S	886
Clain, Michael (CT)	OrS	922	Colangelo, Daniel (NY)	IM	639
Claps, Richard (NJ)	DR	833	Colberg, John (CT)	U	963
Clark, Richard (NY)	D	587	Cole, Jeffrey (NJ)	PMR	758
Clark, Sheryl (NY)	D	153	Cole, Randolph (NJ)	Pul	726
Cleary, Joseph (NY)	S	676	Cole, Robert (NJ)	RadRO	855
Cleman, Michael (CT)	Cv	942	Cole, William (NY)	Cv	135
Cleri, Dennis (NJ)	Inf	777	Coleman, D Jackson (NY)	Oph	250
Close, Lanny (NY)	Oto	279	Coleman, Morton (NY)	Onc	212
Coady, Deborah (NY)	ObG	243	Colen, Helen (NY)	PlS	313
Coady, Michael (CT)	T&CS	936	Colenda, Maryann (NJ)	PA&I	718
Cobelli, Neil (NY)	OrS	403	Coll, Raymond (NY)	N	232
Cobin, Rhoda (NJ)	EDM	699	Collins, Eric (NY)	AdP	129
Coco, Maria (NY)	Nep	398	Collum, Robert (NJ)	IM	835
Coffey, Barbara (NY)	ChAP	145	Coloka-Kump, Rodika (NY)	FMed	390
Cofsky, Richard (NY)	Inf	435	Colon, Francisco (NJ)	PlS	842
Cohen, Alice (NJ)	Hem	745	Colton, Marc (NJ)	U	845
Cohen, Arnold (NY)	Psyc	323	Colyer-Aversa, Lori (NJ)	Ped	757
Cohen, Barry (NY)	IM	436	Compito, Catherine (NY)	OrS	265
Cohen, Barry (NJ)	Nep	779	Compito, Gerard (NJ)	DR	792
Cohen, Ben (NY)	Oph	250	Comrie, Millicent (NY)	ObG	445
Cohen, Bradley (NY)	S	607	Condemi, Giuseppe (NJ)	Onc	707
Cohen, Burton (NY)	DR	161	Condo, Dominick (NJ)	IM	768
Cohen, Carl (NY)	GerPsy	433	Confino, Joel (NJ)	Oph	880
Cohen, Charmian (NY)	EDM	389	Connery, Cliff (NY)	T&CS	363
Cohen, Daniel (NY)	Rhu	562	Connolly, Adrian (NJ)	D	741
Cohen, Daniel (NY)	N	595	Connolly, Mark (NJ)	T&CS	856
Cohen, David (NY)	Nep	224	Connor, Bradley (NY)	Ge	172
Cohen, David (NY)	D	153	Connor, John (NJ)	U	845
Cohen, Howard (NY)	Cv	135	Connor, Thomas (NJ)	PCd	754
Cohen, Joel (NY)	N	400	Connors, Richard (CT)	D	899
Cohen, Jonathan (NY)	Ge	172	Conroy, Daniel (NJ)	Cv	692
Cohen, Lawrence (NY)	Ge	172	Constad, William (NJ)	Oph	770
Cohen, Lee (NY)	ChAP	623	Constantiner, Arturo (NY)	IM	199
Cohen, Leeber (NY)	Oph	250	Constantinides, Minas (NY)	Oto	279
Cohen, Marc (NJ)	IC	747	Conte, Charles (NY)	S	564
Cohen, Martin (NY)	CE	618	Conway, Edward (NY)	PCCM	294
Cohen, Michael (NY)	Pul	558	Cook, Perry (NY)	Hem	189

Alphabetical Listing of Doctors

Alphabetical Listing of Doctors

Name	Specialty	Pg	Name	Specialty	Pg
Duncan, David (NY)	N	649	Eisenberg, Sheldon (NJ)	Cv	692
Dunkel, Ira (NY)	PHO	297	Eisenstat, Steven (NJ)	FMed	875
Dunston-Boone, Gina (CT)	MF	911	Eisenstat, Theodore (NJ)	CRS	791
Durante, Anthony (NY)	Oto	543	Eitan, Noam (NY)	Psyc	458
Dutcher, Janice (NY)	Onc	212	El-Sadr, Wafaa (NY)	Inf	193
Duva, Joseph (NY)	Ge	590	El-Tamer, Mahmoud (NY)	S	355
Dweck, Monica (NY)	Oph	447	Elahi, Ebrahim (NY)	Oph	251
Dworkin, Brad (NY)	Ge	633	Elamir, Mazhar (NJ)	Pul	771
Dworkin, Gregory (CT)	PPul	926	Elbaba, Fadi (NY)	Oph	598
Dwyer, James (NJ)	OrS	864	Eleff, Michael (NJ)	Onc	797
			Elefteriades, John (CT)	T&CS	962
			Elias, Steven (NJ)	VascS	733

E

Name	Specialty	Pg	Name	Specialty	Pg
			Elkind, Barry (NJ)	Cv	767
			Elkowitz, Marc (NY)	PlS	555
Eastham, James (NY)	U	369	Elliott, Andrew (NY)	OrS	266
Easton, Lon (NY)	Ped	666	Ellis, Earl (NY)	IM	436
Ebani, Jack (NJ)	U	826	Ellman, Matthew (CT)	IM	949
Economos, Katherine (NY)	GO	434	Ellozy, Sharif (NY)	VascS	377
Eddleman, Keith (NY)	MF	209	Elmann, Elie (NJ)	T&CS	731
Edelman, Bruce (NJ)	Oto	803	Emami, Arash (NJ)	OrS	853
Edelman, Robert (NY)	U	567	Emond, Jean (NY)	S	355
Edelson, Charles (NY)	OrS	656	Emre, Sukru (CT)	S	961
Edelson, Richard (CT)	D	944	Ende, Leigh (NJ)	HS	834
Edelstein, Barbara (NY)	DR	161	Eng, Margaret (NJ)	Inf	818
Edelstein, David (NY)	Oto	279	Engel, Harry (NY)	Oph	251
Edelstein, Gary (NY)	Ped	305	Engel, J Mark (NJ)	Oph	802
Edelstein, Martin (NY)	FMed	520	Engel, Lenore (NY)	ChAP	426
Eden, Edward (NY)	Pul	336	Engel, Mark (NJ)	Oph	821
Edis, Gloria (NY)	Ped	666	Engel, Murray (NY)	N	232
Edwards, Bruce (NY)	A&I	507	Engelhardt, Martin (NY)	IM	640
Edye, Michael (NY)	S	354	Engler, Mitchell (NJ)	Pul	726
Effron, Charles (NJ)	N	711	Englert, Christopher (NJ)	ObG	713
Efthimiou, Petros (NY)	Rhu	413	Ennis, David (NY)	IM	640
Eggers, Howard (NY)	Oph	251	Ennis, Francis (CT)	OrS	922
Egol, Kenneth (NY)	OrS	266	Ennis, Ronald (NY)	RadRO	340
Ehrenkranz, Richard (CT)	NP	951	Epstein, Lawrence (NY)	PM	287
Ehrlich, Amy (NY)	Ger	393	Epstein, Nancy (NY)	NS	534
Ehrlich, Conrad (CT)	DR	901	Epstein, Robert (NJ)	DR	792
Ehrlich, James (NY)	Ge	633	Epstein, Stanley (NY)	Cv	136
Ehrlich, Martin (NY)	IM	200	Erber, William (NY)	Ge	431
Ehrlich, Paul (NY)	PA&I	292	Ernst, Jerome (NY)	IM	396
Eichenbaum, Joseph (NY)	Oph	251	Errico, Thomas (NY)	OrS	266
Eichenfield, Andrew (NY)	PRhu	302	Escher, Jeffrey (NY)	Ger	636
Eichler, Joel (NJ)	Oph	751	Esformes, Ira (NJ)	OrS	716
Eichman, Gerard (NJ)	Cv	692	Eshghi, A Majid (NY)	U	679
Eilbott, David (CT)	IM	948	Eskreis, David (NY)	Ge	521
Eilen, Bonnie (NY)	ObG	651	Esposito, Donna (NY)	Oph	251
Einstein, Mark (NY)	GO	394	Esposito, Michael (NJ)	U	732
Eisenberg, Mark (NY)	NS	533	Esposito, Rick (NY)	T&CS	565
Eisenberg, Richard (NJ)	D	874	Esposito, Stephen (NY)	Ge	475
			Estabrook, Alison (NY)	S	355

Name	Specialty	Pg
Esteban-Cruciani, Nora (NY)	Ped	408
Etingin, Orli (NY)	IM	200
Ettinger, Alan (NY)	N	535
Evanko, John (NY)	ObG	243
Evans, Lydia (NY)	D	626
Evans, Mark (NY)	ObG	243
Evans, Steven (NY)	CE	133
Ezratty, Ari (NY)	Cv	509

F

Name	Specialty	Pg
Faber, Mark (NJ)	Psyc	759
Fagin, James (NY)	PA&I	546
Fahey, Thomas (NY)	S	355
Fahn, Stanley (NY)	N	232
Fahoum, Bashar (NY)	S	463
Fakharzadeh, Frederick (NJ)	HS	703
Falco, Thomas (NY)	Cv	584
Falcon, Ronald (NY)	D	515
Falk, Theodore (NJ)	A&I	691
Falkoff, Alan (CT)	FMed	903
Faller, Jason (NY)	Rhu	347
Fallon, Brian (NY)	Psyc	324
Fang, Bruno (NJ)	Onc	798
Fang, Deborah (CT)	RadRO	932
Fantasia, Michele (NJ)	PMR	807
Fantini, Gary (NY)	VascS	377
Farber, Bruce (NY)	Inf	526
Farber, Charles (NY)	Ge	521
Farber, Charles (NJ)	Onc	836
Faries, Peter (NY)	VascS	377
Farkas, Edward (NJ)	Psyc	725
Farkas, John (NJ)	Ge	850
Farrell, Matthew (CT)	FMed	903
Farrell, Robert (NY)	U	486
Farrer, William (NJ)	Inf	876
Fass, Arthur (NY)	Cv	619
Fass, Daniel (NY)	RadRO	674
Fastenberg, David (NY)	Oph	539
Fateh, Majid (NY)	RE	343
Faust, Glenn (NY)	VascS	569
Faust, Michael (NY)	Ge	172
Faust, Michael (NJ)	ObG	713
Fawwaz, Rashid (NY)	NuM	241
Fazio, Nelson (NY)	IM	640
Fazio, Richard (NY)	Ge	493
Fealy, Stephen (NY)	OrS	266
Federbush, Richard (NY)	IM	527
Federman, Alex (NY)	IM	200

Name	Specialty	Pg
Fefferman, Nancy (NY)	DR	161
Feghali, Joseph (NY)	Oto	404
Feher, Laszlo (NY)	Ger	182
Feigenbaum, Howard (NJ)	S	855
Fein, Alan (NY)	Pul	558
Fein, Deborah (NJ)	Nep	709
Fein, Frederick (NY)	Cv	509
Feinberg, Joseph (NY)	PMR	309
Feinberg, Joseph (NY)	PlS	555
Feinberg, Todd (NY)	N	232
Feinstein, Neil (NY)	Oph	447
Feintzeig, Irwin (CT)	Nep	914
Feit, Alan (NY)	Cv	423
Feit, David (NJ)	Ge	875
Feld, Michael (NY)	Cv	619
Felderman, Lenora (NY)	D	153
Feldman, B Robert (NY)	A&I	131
Feldman, David (NJ)	SM	844
Feldman, David (NY)	OrS	266
Feldman, Eric (NY)	Onc	212
Feldman, Jeffrey (NJ)	IM	877
Feldman, Philip (NY)	D	428
Feldman, Sheldon (NY)	S	355
Feldman, Stuart (NY)	Onc	644
Feldstein, Neil (NY)	NS	227
Fellus, Jonathan (NJ)	N	769
Felsenstein, Jerome (NY)	D	626
Feltheimer, Seth (NY)	IM	200
Fennell, Gail (CT)	IM	908
Fennoy, Ilene (NY)	PEn	294
Fenster, Mitchell (NY)	IM	640
Ferges, Mitchell (NJ)	Ge	861
Fernandes, David (NY)	Ped	456
Fernandes, John (NJ)	PCd	754
Fernandez, Harold (NY)	T&CS	565
Fernandez, Jacinto (NJ)	ObG	713
Fernbach, Barry (NJ)	Hem	704
Ferran, Elena Nascimbeni (NY)	Ge	173
Ferran, Ernesto (NY)	Psyc	324
Ferrante, Maurice (NJ)	IM	862
Ferrick, Kevin (NY)	CE	384
Ferrier, Genevieve (NY)	Ped	305
Ferrone, Philip (NY)	Oph	539
Ferrucci, Leonard (CT)	ObG	918
Ferrucci, Vito (CT)	ObG	918
Festa, Robert (NY)	Ped	602
Feteiha, Muhammad (NJ)	S	886
Feuer, Martin (NY)	IM	200
Fey, Christopher (CT)	DR	901
Fialk, Mark (NY)	Onc	645
Fiedler, Robert (NY)	IM	200

Alphabetical Listing of Doctors

Name	Specialty	Pg	Name	Specialty	Pg
Fiel, Stanley (NJ)	Pul	843	Fitzgerald, Denis (NJ)	Onc	819
Field, Barry (NY)	Ge	633	FitzGibbons, James (CT)	OrS	922
Field, Steven (NY)	Ge	173	Flamm, Eugene (NY)	NS	399
Fielding, George (NY)	S	355	Flanagan, Michael (CT)	U	963
Fields, Suzanne (NY)	Ger	591	Flanagan, Steven (NY)	PMR	309
Fields, Theodore (NY)	Rhu	347	Flatow, Evan (NY)	OrS	267
Fiest, Thomas (NJ)	Ge	817	Fleischer, Adiel (NY)	MF	529
Figgie, Mark (NY)	OrS	266	Fleischer, Lee (NY)	S	579
Filiberto, Cosmo (CT)	FMed	903	Fleischer, Marian (NY)	CRS	427
Filippone, Mark (NJ)	PMR	771	Fleischman, Jay (NY)	Oph	653
Filsoufi, Farzan (NY)	T&CS	363	Fleischman, Jean (NY)	Pul	484
Fine, Emily (CT)	ObG	953	Fleisher, Michael (NJ)	U	811
Fine, Eugene (NY)	U	369	Fleming, Gregory (NJ)	Oto	840
Fine, Jonathan (CT)	Pul	931	Flis, Raymond (NJ)	Nep	820
Fine, Paul (NJ)	Nep	837	Flood, Mary (NY)	Inf	193
Fine, Robert (NY)	Onc	213	Florakis, George (NY)	Oph	252
Fine, Stanley (NY)	A&I	472	Flores, Raja (NY)	T&CS	363
Finegold, Jonathan (NY)	Ge	633	Florio, Philip (NY)	ObG	652
Finger, Paul (NY)	Oph	252	Flug, Frances (NJ)	PHO	719
Fink, Matthew (NY)	N	233	Flynn, Maryirene (NY)	OrS	497
Finkel, Jay (NY)	Psyc	324	Flynn, Patrick (NY)	PCd	293
Finkelstein, Martin (NY)	Ger	182	Fochios, Steven (NY)	Ge	173
Finkelstein, Warren (NJ)	Ge	743	Fogel, Joyce (NY)	Ger	182
Finlay, Alexis (CT)	Oph	919	Fogel, Mitchell (CT)	Nep	914
Fiore, Amory (CT)	NS	915	Fogler, Richard (NY)	S	463
Fiore, John (NY)	Onc	594	Fojas, Antonio (NY)	IM	396
Fiorella, David (NY)	NRad	596	Foley, Carmel (NY)	ChAP	513
Fiorentino, Thomas (NY)	IM	640	Folman, Robert (CT)	Onc	912
First, Michael (NY)	Psyc	324	Fomberstein, Barry (NY)	Rhu	413
Fisch, Arthur (NJ)	Cv	832	Fonacier, Luz (NY)	A&I	507
Fisch, Harry (NY)	U	369	Fong, Raymond (NY)	Oph	252
Fischbach, Neal (CT)	Onc	912	Fong, Yuman (NY)	S	355
Fischer, Harry (NY)	Rhu	347	Fontana, Gregory (NY)	T&CS	363
Fish, Bernard (NY)	PCd	660	Foo, Sun-Hoo (NY)	N	233
Fishbach, Mitchell (NY)	Cv	619	Foong, Anthony (NY)	Ge	173
Fishbane-Mayer, Jill (NY)	ObG	243	Ford, Robert (NJ)	DR	792
Fisher, George (NY)	FMed	475	Forlenza, Thomas (NY)	Onc	495
Fisher, Laura (NY)	IM	200	Forley, Bryan (NY)	PlS	314
Fisher, Lawrence (CT)	Cv	897	Forman, Mark (NJ)	T&CS	763
Fisher, Margaret (NJ)	PInf	823	Forman, Scott (NY)	Oph	654
Fisher, Martin (NY)	AM	506	Formenti, Silvia (NY)	RadRO	340
Fisher, Rosemarie (CT)	Ge	946	Formica, Richard (CT)	Nep	951
Fisher, Yale (NY)	Oph	252	Fornari, Victor (NY)	ChAP	473
Fishkin, Michael (NY)	FMed	590	Fornier, Monica (NY)	Onc	213
Fishman, Allen (NY)	Oph	481	Forster, George (NY)	N	233
Fishman, David (NY)	GO	185	Forte, Francis (NJ)	Onc	707
Fishman, Donald (NY)	Pul	336	Fortunato, Franklin (NJ)	IM	746
Fishman, Eric (NY)	VascS	681	Foss, Francine (CT)	Onc	950
Fishman, Miriam (NJ)	D	696	Fost, Arthur (NJ)	PA&I	754
Fishman, Robert (CT)	IC	910	Foster, Craig (NY)	PlS	314
Fiske, Steven (NJ)	Ge	743	Foster, Harris (CT)	U	963

Alphabetical Listing of Doctors

Name	Specialty	Pg	Name	Specialty	Pg
Fou, Adora (NY)	S	676	Friedman, Alan (CT)	PCd	955
Fox, Alissa (NJ)	D	860	Friedman, Alan (NJ)	ObG	780
Fox, Herbert (NY)	Psyc	324	Friedman, Alan (NY)	Oph	252
Fox, James (NJ)	A&I	859	Friedman, David (NJ)	PS	721
Fox, John (NY)	IC	207	Friedman, David (NY)	PlS	314
Fox, Joyce (NY)	CG	514	Friedman, Deborah (NY)	PCd	660
Fox, Mark (NY)	Oto	658	Friedman, Eugene (NY)	Ped	552
Fox, Martin (NY)	Oph	252	Friedman, Howard (NY)	Cv	136
Fox, Sarah (NY)	ChAP	145	Friedman, Jeffrey (NY)	IM	201
Fracchia, John (NY)	U	369	Friedman, Lloyd (CT)	Pul	959
Frager, Joseph (NY)	Ge	391	Friedman, Lynn (NY)	ObG	244
Fragner, Paul (NY)	HS	637	Friedman, Richard (NY)	Psyc	324
Fragomen, Austin (NY)	OrS	267	Friedman, Ricky (NY)	ObG	244
Frances, Richard (NY)	AdP	129	Friedman, Robert (NY)	Oph	252
Francfort, John (NY)	S	607	Friedman, Sanford (NY)	Cv	136
Francis, Kathleen (NJ)	PMR	758	Friedman, Seth (NY)	EDM	518
Franck, Jeanne (NY)	D	516	Friedman, Stanley (NY)	DR	388
Frank, Douglas (NY)	Oto	543	Friedman, Steven (NY)	U	465
Frank, Graeme (NY)	PEn	548	Friedrich, Ivan (NJ)	Ge	701
Frank, Martin (NJ)	Hem	835	Frieri, Marianne (NY)	A&I	507
Frank, Michael (NY)	Ge	173	Frimer, Richard (NY)	Pul	672
Frank, Richard (CT)	Onc	912	Friscia, Philip (NY)	Onc	495
Franklin, Bonita (NY)	PEn	294	Frishman, William (NY)	Cv	620
Franks, Andrew (NY)	D	154	Frisoli, Anthony (NJ)	FMed	861
Franzetti, Carl (NY)	FMed	390	Frohman, Larry (NJ)	Oph	751
Freddo, Lorenza (NY)	N	400	From, Stuart (NJ)	A&I	691
Freed, Lisa (CT)	Cv	942	Fromer, Mark (NY)	Oph	252
Freedman, Gordon (NY)	PM	287	Frost, James (NJ)	S	886
Freedman, Jeffrey (NY)	Oph	447	Fruchtman, Steven (NY)	Hem	189
Freedman, Richard (CT)	Ped	927	Fuchs, Richard (NY)	Cv	136
Freeman, Leonard (NY)	NuM	401	Fuchs, Wayne (NY)	Oph	253
Freilich, Stephanie (NY)	Ped	305	Fuhrman, Robert (NJ)	EDM	874
Freiman, Hal (NY)	Ge	173	Fukilman, Oscar (NY)	IM	477
Frempong-Boadu, Anthony (NY)	NS	227	Fuks, Joachim (NY)	Onc	397
French, Jacqueline (NY)	N	233	Fulop, Robert (NY)	IM	494
Frenkel, Renata (NY)	A&I	131	Funt, David (NY)	PlS	555
Freund, Robert (NY)	PlS	314	Furie, Richard (NY)	Rhu	562
Frey, Howard (NJ)	U	732	Fuster, Valentin (NY)	Cv	137
Fried, Arno (NJ)	NS	711	Fyer, Abby (NY)	Psyc	324
Fried, Harry (NJ)	Ge	701	Fyer, Minna (NY)	Psyc	324
Fried, Karen (NY)	DR	161			
Fried, Kenneth (NJ)	S	729			
Fried, Marvin (NY)	Oto	404			
Fried, Richard (NY)	IM	200	# G		
Fried, Sharon (NJ)	D	696	Gabbay, Vilma (NY)	ChAP	145
Frieden, Faith (NJ)	MF	707	Gabel, Richard (NY)	Psyc	669
Friedlaender, Gary (CT)	OrS	954	Gabelman, Gary (NY)	Cv	620
Friedlander, Charles (NY)	Ge	173	Gabrilove, Janice (NY)	Onc	213
Friedlander, Devin (NJ)	N	863	Gaffney, Joseph (NJ)	PCd	804
Friedlander, Marvin (NJ)	NS	879	Gagliardi, Anthony (NJ)	Pul	760
Friedling, Steven (NY)	IM	593			

Alphabetical Listing of Doctors

Name	Specialty	Pg	Name	Specialty	Pg
Gaglio, Paul (NY)	Ge	391	Gejerman, Glen (NJ)	RadRO	727
Gagne, Paul (CT)	VascS	938	Gekowski, Kathleen (NJ)	Inf	777
Gainey, Patrick (NJ)	N	820	Gelato, Marie (NY)	EDM	589
Gajdos, Robert (NJ)	IM	851	Gelb, Bruce (NY)	PCd	293
Galanter, I Marc (NY)	AdP	129	Gelbard, Sandra (NY)	IM	201
Galinkin, Lawrence (NY)	Ped	552	Gelberg, Burt (NY)	IM	527
Gallagher, Mary (NY)	PEn	295	Gelbfish, Joseph (NY)	Cv	424
Gallagher, Pamela (NY)	PlS	555	Gelfand, Janice (NY)	Psyc	411
Galland, Leo (NY)	IM	201	Geller, David (NY)	OrS	403
Galler, Marilyn (NY)	Nep	480	Geller, Eric (NJ)	N	749
Gallick, Gregory (NJ)	OrS	881	Geller, Mark (NY)	DR	574
Gallin, Pamela (NY)	Oph	253	Geller, Peter (NY)	S	355
Galloway, Aubrey (NY)	T&CS	364	Gelles, Jeremiah (NY)	Cv	424
Gallucci, John (NJ)	PS	807	Gelmann, Edward (NY)	Onc	213
Gamache, Francis (NY)	NS	227	Geltzeiler, Jules (NJ)	U	826
Gambarin, Boris (NY)	IM	437	Genato, Romulo (NY)	S	463
Gammon, G Davis (CT)	ChAP	943	Genc, Mehmet (NY)	MF	209
Gamss, Jeffrey (NY)	Ge	431	Gendelman, Seymour (NY)	N	233
Ganchi, Parham (NJ)	PlS	854	Genden, Eric (NY)	Oto	280
Gandhi, Lajpat (NY)	ChAP	586	Gendler, Ellen (NY)	D	154
Gandhi, Rajinder (NJ)	PS	721	Gendler, Seth (NY)	Ge	633
Gannon, Christopher (NJ)	S	785	Genieser, Nancy (NY)	DR	161
Garan, Hasan (NY)	CE	133	Genn, David (NY)	Ge	633
Garay, Kenneth (NJ)	Oto	770	Gennace, Ronald (NJ)	OrS	716
Garay, Stuart (NY)	Pul	336	Gentile, Ronald (NY)	Oph	253
Garber, Perry (NY)	Oph	539	Gentilesco, Michael (NY)	ObG	596
Garcia, Mario (NY)	Cv	384	George, Liziamma (NY)	Pul	459
Gardenswartz, Mark (NY)	Nep	224	Geraci-Ciardullo, Kira (NY)	A&I	617
Gardin, Julius (NJ)	Cv	692	Geraghty, Michael (NY)	Onc	440
Gardner, James (NJ)	PlS	884	Gerard, Perry (NY)	NuM	651
Gardner, Peter (CT)	Ge	903	Gerber, Oded (NY)	N	596
Gardner, Sharon (NY)	PHO	298	Gerberg, Lynda (NY)	Ped	552
Garfinkel, Matthew (NJ)	OrS	802	Gerbino-Rosen, Ginny (NY)	ChAP	386
Gargano, Robert (NY)	Oto	599	Gerdes, Hans (NY)	Ge	173
Gargiulo, Juan (NY)	PM	600	Gerhard, Harvey (NJ)	Pul	866
Garner, Bruce (NY)	Rhu	462	German, Harold (NY)	IM	593
Garner, Steven (NY)	DR	428	Geronemus, Roy (NY)	D	154
Garrick, Renee (NY)	Nep	648	Gershbaum, Meyer (NY)	U	567
Garvey, Michael (NY)	Nep	224	Gerson, Charles (NY)	Ge	174
Garvey, Richard (CT)	S	935	Gesner, Matthew (NY)	PInf	454
Garvin, James (NY)	PHO	298	Getrajdman, George (NY)	VIR	375
Garzon, Maria (NY)	D	154	Gettenberg, Gary (NY)	Ge	431
Gass, Alan (NY)	Cv	620	Geuder, James (NJ)	VascS	733
Gately, Adrian (NY)	Ped	456	Gewanter, Richard (NY)	RadRO	560
Gayle, Lloyd (NY)	PlS	314	Gewirtz, George (NJ)	EDM	742
Gaynor, Mitchell (NY)	Onc	213	Gewirtz, Harold (CT)	PlS	929
Gazzara, Paul (NY)	IM	494	Gewirtz, Joan (CT)	Oph	919
Gecelter, Gary (NY)	S	564	Gewitz, Michael (NY)	PCd	660
Geders, Jane (NY)	Ge	633	Gewolb, Eric (NJ)	Psyc	771
Geer-Yan, Lisa (CT)	ObG	918	Gharibo, Christopher (NY)	PM	288
Gehrmann, Robin (NJ)	SM	761	Ghatan, Saadi (NY)	NS	227

Alphabetical Listing of Doctors

Name	Specialty	Pg	Name	Specialty	Pg
Goldfarb, C Richard (NY)	NuM	241	Goodman, Michael (NY)	IM	527
Goldfarb, Joel (NJ)	Ge	701	Goodman, Robert (NY)	NS	228
Goldfarb, Michael (NJ)	S	826	Goodman, Robert (NJ)	RadRO	771
Goldfischer, Mindy (NJ)	DR	698	Goodman, Susan (NY)	Rhu	347
Goldin, Daniel (NY)	IM	201	Goodstein, Carolyn (NJ)	A&I	691
Goldin, Howard (NY)	Ge	174	Goodwin, Charles (NY)	OrS	267
Goldman, Gary (NY)	ObG	244	Gordon, James (NY)	Oph	654
Goldman, Ira (NY)	Ge	522	Gordon, Jeffrey (NY)	EDM	518
Goldman, Jack (NY)	IM	640	Gordon, Marc (NY)	N	535
Goldman, Joel (NY)	EDM	429	Gordon, Mark (NY)	S	677
Goldman, Kenneth (NJ)	VascS	812	Gordon, Marsha (NY)	D	154
Goldman, Martin (NY)	Cv	137	Gordon, Michael (NY)	Oto	543
Goldman, Michael (NJ)	EDM	699	Gordon, Neil (CT)	Oto	925
Goldman, Neil (NY)	Psyc	325	Gordon, Richard (NJ)	Rhu	785
Goldman, Neil (NY)	A&I	617	Gordon, Richard (NY)	Pul	559
Goldschmidt, Howard (NJ)	Cv	693	Gorecki, Piotr (NY)	S	464
Goldsmith, Ari (NY)	PO	455	Gorenstein, Lyall (NY)	T&CS	364
Goldsmith, Stanley (NY)	NuM	241	Gorevic, Peter (NY)	Rhu	347
Goldstein, Carl (NJ)	Nep	878	Gorfine, Stephen (NY)	CRS	149
Goldstein, Daniel (NY)	T&CS	415	Gorkin, Janet (NY)	Nep	399
Goldstein, Jeffrey (NY)	OrS	267	Gorlick, Richard (NY)	PHO	406
Goldstein, Jonathan (NJ)	Cv	739	Gorman, Lauren (NY)	Psyc	325
Goldstein, Jonathan (CT)	N	952	Gorman, Robert (NJ)	FMed	743
Goldstein, Judith (NY)	Ped	305	Gorski, Lydia (NY)	IM	527
Goldstein, Marc (NY)	U	369	Gotfried, Fern (NJ)	Ped	841
Goldstein, Mark (NY)	Rhu	501	Gotkin, Robert (NY)	PlS	555
Goldstein, Martin (NY)	ObG	244	Gotlin, Robert (NY)	PMR	309
Goldstein, Michael (NY)	Oph	253	Gottesfeld, Peter (NY)	FMed	631
Goldstein, Paul (NY)	IM	201	Gottlieb, Beth (NY)	PRhu	551
Goldstein, Robert (NY)	PlS	410	Gotto, Antonio (NY)	Cv	137
Goldstein, Stanley (NY)	A&I	507	Gottridge, Joanne (NY)	IM	527
Goldstein, Steven (NY)	Oto	404	Gouge, Thomas (NY)	S	356
Goldstein, Steven (NJ)	ObG	821	Gould, Eric (NY)	Ped	552
Goldstein, Steven (NY)	Ped	482	Gould, Perry (NY)	Ge	522
Goldstein, Steven (NY)	ObG	244	Gould, Richard (NY)	Ge	634
Goldstein, Susanna (NY)	Psyc	325	Goy, Andre (NJ)	Onc	707
Goldweit, Richard (NJ)	Cv	693	Goyal, Arun (NY)	VascS	681
Golfinos, John (NY)	NS	228	Goydos, James (NJ)	S	810
Golombek, Sergio (NY)	NP	647	Grabowski, Wayne (NJ)	Oph	802
Goltzman, Carey (NY)	PCCM	661	Grace, William (NY)	Onc	213
Gomes, J Anthony (NY)	CE	133	Graff, Michael (NJ)	NP	820
Gomez, Henry (NY)	Cv	510	Graham, Alan (NJ)	VascS	812
Gomez, William (NJ)	OrS	782	Grajower, Martin (NY)	EDM	389
Gomolin, Irving (NY)	Ger	523	Granatir, Charles (NJ)	OrS	770
Gonter, Neil (NJ)	Rhu	728	Granet, Kenneth (NJ)	IM	819
Gonzalez, David (NJ)	MF	819	Granick, Mark (NJ)	PlS	759
Goodgold, Abraham (NJ)	IM	877	Grano, Vanessa (NY)	ObG	652
Goodman, Alan (NJ)	A&I	872	Grant, Linda (CT)	PMR	928
Goodman, Dennis (NY)	Cv	137	Grant, Robert (NY)	PlS	315
Goodman, Kenneth (NY)	DR	517	Grasso, Cono (NY)	Oph	481
Goodman, Mark (NY)	Cv	510	Grasso, Michael (NY)	U	369

Name	Specialty	Pg	Name	Specialty	Pg
Grasso, Michael (NJ)	Nep	749	Grelsamer, Ronald (NY)	OrS	268
Graver, L Michael (NY)	T&CS	486	Grendell, James (NY)	Ge	522
Gray, William (NY)	IC	207	Grenell, Steven (NY)	N	400
Grayson, Douglas (NY)	Oph	253	Grenis, Michael (NJ)	OrS	782
Grazi, Richard (NY)	RE	461	Gress, Frank (NY)	Ge	431
Greaney, Edward (NY)	IM	201	Gretz, Herbert (NY)	GO	637
Grebler, Arnold (NJ)	U	826	Gribbin, Dorota (NJ)	PMR	783
Greeley, Norman (NY)	A&I	422	Gribbon, John (NJ)	IM	747
Green, Abraham (NY)	Ped	552	Gribetz, Michael (NY)	U	369
Green, Jeffrey (CT)	Cv	897	Grieco, Michael (NY)	S	564
Green, Mark (NY)	N	233	Grifo, James (NY)	RE	343
Green, Michele (NY)	D	154	Grijnsztein, Jacob (NY)	Ped	552
Green, Peter (NY)	Ge	174	Grizzanti, Joseph (NJ)	Pul	855
Green, Richard (NY)	VascS	377	Grodberg, Michele (NJ)	D	697
Green, Robert (NY)	Oto	280	Grodman, Richard (NY)	Cv	491
Green, Stephen (NY)	Cv	510	Groeger, William (NY)	PlS	555
Green, Steven (NY)	OrS	267	Groff, Walter (NJ)	CRS	873
Green, Stuart (NY)	Rhu	462	Grosman, Irwin (NY)	Ge	431
Greenbaum, Allen (NY)	Oph	654	Gross, Dennis (NY)	D	155
Greenberg, Harly (NY)	Pul	559	Gross, Elliott (NY)	N	649
Greenberg, Howard (NY)	Onc	479	Gross, Gary (NJ)	A&I	815
Greenberg, Mark (NY)	Cv	384	Gross, Harvey (NJ)	FMed	700
Greenberg, Martin (NJ)	Pul	760	Gross, Ian (CT)	NP	951
Greenberg, Robert (NY)	D	154	Gross, Jay (NY)	CE	384
Greenberg, Robert (NY)	GerPsy	433	Gross, Jeffrey (CT)	N	916
Greenberg, Ronald (NY)	Ge	522	Gross, Jeffrey (NY)	IM	640
Greenberg, Rosalie (NJ)	ChAP	873	Gross, Joshua (NJ)	DR	698
Greenberg, Steven (NY)	Oph	654	Gross, Michael (NJ)	SM	729
Greenberg, Steven (NY)	Cv	510	Grossbard, Michael (NY)	Onc	214
Greenberg, Susan (NJ)	Onc	819	Grossi, Eugene (NY)	T&CS	364
Greenblatt, Louis (NY)	FMed	590	Grossi, Robert (NY)	VascS	378
Greene, Jeffrey (NY)	Inf	194	Grossman, Bernard (NJ)	Onc	778
Greene, Loren (NY)	EDM	167	Grossman, Edward (CT)	Ge	904
Greenfield, Martin (NY)	EDM	519	Grossman, Elliot (NJ)	ChiN	832
Greengart, Alvin (NY)	Cv	424	Grossman, Kenneth (NJ)	D	816
Greenman, James (NJ)	Inf	877	Grossman, Marc (NY)	D	626
Greenspan, Alan (NY)	D	154	Grossman, Melanie (NY)	D	155
Greenstein, Bruce (NY)	PlS	411	Grossman, Robert (NJ)	OrS	822
Greenstein, Stuart (NY)	S	414	Grossman, Susan (NY)	Nep	496
Greenwald, Blaine (NY)	GerPsy	476	Grosso, John (NY)	Oto	544
Greenwald, Brian (NY)	PMR	309	Grosso, Sue Jane (NJ)	DR	874
Greenwald, Bruce (NY)	PCCM	294	Grubb, William (NJ)	PM	804
Greenwald, David (NY)	Ge	391	Gruber, Michael (NY)	N	233
Greenwald, Joshua (NY)	PlS	668	Grubman, Samuel (NY)	A&I	131
Greenwald, Marc (NY)	CRS	514	Gruenstein, Steven (NY)	Hem	190
Greenwald, Robert (NY)	Rhu	562	Gruenwald, Laurence (NJ)	Ped	757
Greer, David (CT)	N	952	Grunberger, Ivan (NY)	U	465
Greer, Jeannete (NJ)	DR	860	Grunebaum, Amos (NY)	MF	209
Greif, Richard (NY)	Cv	620	Grunfeld, Lawrence (NY)	RE	343
Greisberg, Justin (NY)	OrS	268	Grunzweig, Milton (NY)	IM	437
Greisman, Stewart (NY)	Rhu	347	Gruskay, Jeffrey (CT)	Ped	957

Alphabetical Listing of Doctors

Name	Specialty	Pg	Name	Specialty	Pg
Gruss, Claudia (CT)	Ge	904	Hahn, John (NJ)	Ge	768
Gruss, Leslie (NY)	ObG	244	Haig, Scott (NY)	OrS	656
Guarini, Ludovico (NY)	PHO	453	Haight, David (NY)	Oph	253
Guarracini, Mary (NY)	PMR	578	Haimovic, Itzhak (NY)	N	535
Gubernick, Martin (NY)	ObG	244	Haines, Kathleen (NJ)	PRhu	721
Gudavalli, Madhu (NY)	NP	440	Hainline, Brian (NY)	N	535
Guerin, Bonni (NJ)	Onc	878	Hajjar, John (NJ)	U	732
Guess, Marsha (CT)	ObG	953	Halaas, Jeffrey (NY)	Onc	645
Guida, Louis (NY)	A&I	583	Halata, Michael (NY)	PGe	662
Guida, Robert (NY)	Oto	280	Hale, Elizabeth (NY)	D	155
Guillem, Jose (NY)	CRS	150	Hale, William (CT)	Ge	904
Guillen, Gregorio (NJ)	IM	797	Hall, Lisabeth (NY)	Oph	254
Guillory, Samuel (NY)	Oph	253	Hall, Simon (NY)	U	370
Gulati, Subhash (NY)	Onc	214	Hallal, Edward (NY)	IM	593
Gulrajani, Ramesh (NY)	Pul	459	Halperin, Ira (NY)	Hem	190
Guma, Michael (NJ)	Rhu	728	Halperin, John (NJ)	N	879
Gumbs, Andrew (NJ)	S	886	Halperin, Jonathan (NY)	Cv	137
Gumprecht, Jeffrey (NY)	Inf	194	Halpern, Allan (NY)	D	155
Gundy, Edward (NY)	OrS	656	Halpern, Brian (NY)	SM	351
Guoth, Maria (CT)	EDM	902	Halpern, Neil (NY)	CCM	151
Gupta, Adarsh (NY)	Psyc	557	Halpern, Steven (NJ)	PHO	719
Gupta, Jagdish (NY)	Ge	431	Hamburger, Max (NY)	Rhu	606
Gupta, Mantu (NY)	U	370	Hamet, Marc (NY)	VIR	681
Gupta, Prem (NY)	Cv	424	Hametz, Irwin (NJ)	D	816
Gupta, Sanjeev (NY)	Ge	391	Hamilton, Audrey (NJ)	Onc	862
Gurevich, Michael (NY)	Psyc	558	Hamilton, William (NY)	OrS	268
Gurland, Frances (NJ)	Psyc	725	Hammel, Jay (NY)	DR	517
Gurland, Mark (NJ)	HS	703	Hammer, Arthur (NY)	Pul	459
Gurubhagavatula, Sarada (NJ)	Onc	836	Hammer, Glenn (NY)	Inf	194
Gusmorino, Paul (NY)	PM	288	Hammer, Scott (NY)	Inf	194
Gutin, Philip (NY)	NS	228	Hammerman, Hillel (NY)	Ge	174
Gutowski, W Thomas (NJ)	OrS	782	Hammers, Lynwood (CT)	DR	945
Gutwein, Isadore (NY)	Ge	392	Hammerschlag, Paul (NY)	Oto	280
Guzik, Howard (NY)	Ger	523	Hamner, Daniel (NY)	SM	351
Guzman, Rodolfo (NY)	EDM	389	Hand, Ivan (NY)	NP	479
			Handelsman, Dan (NY)	PEn	661
			Handelsman, Richard (NY)	IM	575
			Handler, Robert (NJ)	Ped	841
			Hankin, Dorie (NY)	Ped	553

H

Name	Specialty	Pg	Name	Specialty	Pg
Haas, Alexander (NJ)	RadRO	809	Hanley, Gerard (NY)	Cv	424
Haas, Jonathan (NY)	RadRO	561	Hanna, Moneer (NY)	U	567
Haas, Steven (NY)	OrS	268	Hannafin, Jo (NY)	OrS	268
Haber, Gregory (NY)	Ge	174	Hanson, Matthew (NY)	Oto	451
Haber, Patricia (NY)	Ped	409	Har-El, Gady (NY)	Oto	280
Haber, Stuart (NY)	IM	201	Haramati, Linda (NY)	DR	388
Haddad, Joseph (NY)	PO	301	Haramati, Nogah (NY)	DR	388
Haffty, Bruce (NJ)	RadRO	810	Harangozo, Andrea (NJ)	Pul	809
Haft, Jacob (NJ)	Cv	693	Harary, Albert (NY)	Ge	174
Hagaman, John (NJ)	Cv	775	Haratz-Rubinstein, Natan (NY)	ObG	446
Hages, Harry (NJ)	Ped	722	Harden, Cynthia (NY)	N	535
			Harish, Ziv (NJ)	A&I	691

Name	Specialty	Pg	Name	Specialty	Pg
Harlam, Dean (NY)	Psyc	670	Helbraun, Mark (NJ)	CRS	695
Harlow, Paul (NJ)	Ped	722	Heldman, Jay (NJ)	D	697
Harman, John (NJ)	IM	778	Helfet, David (NY)	OrS	269
Harmon, Gregory (NY)	Oph	254	Helfgott, David (NY)	Inf	194
Harooni, Robert (NY)	Ge	476	Hellenbrand, William (CT)	PCd	956
Harpaz, Noam (NY)	Path	290	Heller, Debra (NJ)	Path	754
Harper, Harry (NJ)	Onc	707	Heller, Keith (NY)	S	356
Harrington, Elizabeth (NY)	VascS	378	Heller, Paul (NJ)	GO	834
Harrington, Martin (NY)	VascS	378	Heller, Stanley (NY)	Psyc	325
Harris, Dena (NY)	ObG	244	Hellerman, James (NY)	EDM	630
Harris, Leon (NY)	Pul	579	Hemmers, Philip (CT)	A&I	895
Harris, Loren (NY)	T&CS	465	Hen, Jacob (CT)	PPul	927
Harris, Michael (NJ)	PHO	719	Henderson, Cassandra (NY)	MF	397
Harris, Steven (NY)	U	567	Hendricks, Judith (NY)	IM	494
Harrison, Aaron (NY)	Ge	591	Henick, David (NJ)	Oto	717
Harrison, Louis (NY)	RadRO	341	Hennessy, William (CT)	U	937
Hart, Catherine (NY)	IM	201	Henschke, Claudia (NY)	DR	162
Hart, Sidney (CT)	Psyc	930	Henshaw, D Ross (CT)	OrS	922
Hartl, Roger (NY)	NS	228	Hensle, Terry (NJ)	U	370
Hartman, Alan (NY)	T&CS	566	Herbert, Joseph (NY)	N	233
Hartman, Barry (NY)	Inf	194	Herbin, Joseph (CT)	Inf	907
Hartz, Cindi (NY)	Ped	666	Herbst, Roy (CT)	Onc	950
Hartzband, Mark (NJ)	OrS	716	Herbstein, Diego (NY)	N	233
Harwin, Steven F (NY)	OrS	268	Herbstman, Robert (NJ)	PlS	808
Haselkorn, Joan (NY)	ObG	537	Herman, David (NJ)	Inf	862
Hashim, Sabet (CT)	T&CS	963	Herman, Martin (NJ)	N	820
Hassoun, Hani (NY)	Onc	214	Herman, Zeva (NY)	DR	162
Hatcher, Virgil (NY)	D	155	Hermele, Herbert (CT)	OrS	922
Hatsis, Alexander (NY)	Oph	540	Herold, Betsy (NY)	PInf	407
Hauptman, Allen (NY)	IM	201	Herr, Harry (NY)	U	370
Hausman, Michael (NY)	OrS	268	Herron, Daniel (NY)	S	356
Havens, Jennifer (NY)	ChAP	145	Hersh, Peter (NJ)	Oph	714
Hayes, Leslie (NY)	AM	422	Hershlag, Avner (NY)	RE	562
Hayes, Mary (NY)	RadRO	341	Hershman, Dawn (NY)	Onc	214
Hayworth, Robin (NY)	Oph	402	Hershman, Elliott (NY)	SM	351
Hayworth, Scott (NY)	ObG	652	Hershman, Ronnie (NY)	Cv	511
Healey, John (NY)	OrS	269	Herskovitz, Steven (NY)	N	400
Heary, Robert (NJ)	NS	749	Hertan, Hilary (NY)	Ge	392
Hecht, Alan (NY)	Cv	138	Hertz, Marc (NY)	DR	628
Hecht, Andrew (NY)	OrS	269	Hertzig, Margaret (NY)	ChAP	145
Hedrick, David (CT)	Ped	927	Herzlinger, Robert (CT)	NP	913
Heerdt, Alexandra (NY)	S	356	Herzog, David (NY)	IM	640
Hefter, Harold (NY)	D	516	Herzog, Thomas (NY)	GO	185
Heftler, Jeffrey (CT)	PMR	929	Hes, Dyan (NY)	Ped	305
Heier, Stephen (NY)	Ge	634	Hetzler, Peter (NJ)	PlS	824
Heim, John (NJ)	T&CS	811	Heublum, Michael (NY)	N	234
Heiman, Mark (CT)	Cv	897	Hiatt, I Mark (NJ)	NP	798
Heiman, Peter (NY)	Psyc	411	Hibbard, Claire (NY)	DR	628
Heinemann, Murk (NY)	Oph	254	Hicks, Patricia (NJ)	PA&I	718
Heisman, Alexander (NY)	Psyc	458	Hidalgo, David (NY)	PlS	315
Heitner, John (NY)	Cv	424	Hiesiger, Emile (NY)	N	234

Alphabetical Listing of Doctors

Name	Specialty	Pg	Name	Specialty	Pg
Higgins, Susan (CT)	RadRO	960	Hollister, Dickerman (CT)	Onc	913
Higgins, William (NY)	IM	640	Holtzman, Robert (NY)	NS	534
Hindenburg, Alexander (NY)	Onc	531	Holzer, Barry (NY)	ChAP	426
Hindin, Lee (NJ)	Psyc	854	Holzman, Ian (NY)	NP	222
Hindman, Steven (CT)	OrS	923	Hong, Andrew (NY)	PS	551
Hines, Brian (CT)	ObG	918	Hong, Joon Ho (NY)	S	464
Hines, William (CT)	Nep	914	Honig, Stephen (NY)	Rhu	348
Hiotis, Spiros (NY)	S	356	Hopkins, Arthur (NY)	IM	641
Hirsch, Andrew (NJ)	A&I	815	Horbar, Gary (NY)	IM	202
Hirsch, Bruce (NY)	Inf	526	Horn, Evelyn (NY)	Cv	138
Hirsch, Glenn (NY)	ChAP	146	Horner, Neil (NJ)	NRad	880
Hirsch, Lissa (NY)	ObG	244	Hornyak, Stephen (NY)	S	501
Hirschfeld, Alan (NY)	NS	442	Horovitz, Len (NY)	IM	202
Hirschman, Alan (NY)	Ped	409	Horowitz, Harold (NY)	Inf	194
Hirschman, Richard (NY)	Onc	214	Horowitz, Marc (NY)	Oph	654
Hirshaut, Yashar (NY)	Onc	214	Horowitz, Mark (NY)	U	465
Hirt, Paula (NY)	ObG	596	Horowitz, Mark (NY)	Rhu	348
Hisler, Barbara (NY)	D	516	Horowitz, Steven (CT)	Cv	897
Hjemdahl-Monsen, Craig (NY)	IC	643	Horvath, Susanna (NY)	N	234
Ho, Bryan (NY)	Oto	717	Horwitz, Steven (NY)	Onc	215
Ho, Sammy (NY)	Ge	392	Hotchkiss, Edward (NY)	IM	527
Hochman, Herbert (NY)	D	155	Hotchkiss, Robert (NY)	OrS	269
Hochstein, Martin (NJ)	EDM	699	Housman, Arno (NY)	U	679
Hochster, Howard (CT)	Onc	950	Howanitz, Nancy (NY)	D	626
Hockstein, Steven (NY)	ObG	245	Howes, Christopher (CT)	IC	911
Hoda, Syed (NY)	Path	290	Hricak, Hedvig (NY)	DR	162
Hodes, David (NY)	Pul	579	Hsu, Daphne (NY)	PCd	404
Hodes, Steven (NJ)	Ge	794	Hsueh, John Tzu-Lang (NY)	Cv	472
Hodges, David (NJ)	Cv	693	Hsuih, Terence (NY)	IM	437
Hodges, Laura (CT)	VIR	937	Hubbard, Christopher (NY)	OrS	269
Hodosh, Richard (NJ)	NS	879	Hubschmann, Otakar (NJ)	NS	749
Hoffman, Darryl (NY)	T&CS	364	Hudis, Clifford (NY)	Onc	215
Hoffman, Eileen (NY)	IM	202	Hughes, Peter (CT)	OrS	923
Hoffman, Janet (NY)	DR	517	Huh, Julie (NY)	D	587
Hoffman, Joel (NY)	Psyc	325	Hunt, William (CT)	Nep	914
Hoffman, Lloyd (NY)	PlS	315	Hunter, John (NY)	PlS	315
Hoffman, Michael (NY)	Rhu	563	Huo, Jerry (NY)	Oto	482
Hoffman, Pamela (CT)	IM	909	Hupart, Kenneth (NY)	EDM	519
Hoffman, Richard (NY)	EDM	493	Huprikar, Shirish (NY)	Inf	195
Hoffman, Robert (NY)	PrM	321	Huribal, Marsel (CT)	VascS	938
Hoffman, Ronald (NY)	Oto	280	Hurst, Lawrence (NY)	HS	591
Holcomb, Kevin (NY)	GO	185	Hurst, Wendy (NJ)	ObG	713
Holcombe, Randall (NY)	Onc	214	Hurwitz, Diana (NY)	D	626
Holder, Jonathan (NY)	OrS	657	Huston, Jan (NJ)	S	762
Holland, Claudia (NY)	ObG	245	Hutchinson, Gordon (CT)	Rhu	961
Holland, Elbridge (NJ)	FMed	833	Hutson, J Milton (NY)	MF	209
Holland, James (NY)	Onc	215	Hwang, Cheng-hong (NJ)	Pul	885
Holland, Neil (NJ)	N	821	Hyans, Peter (NJ)	PlS	884
Hollander, Eric (NY)	Psyc	325	Hyatt, Alexander (NJ)	Ped	722
Hollander, Gerald (NY)	Cv	424	Hyde, Phyllis (NY)	Hem	434
Holliday, Roy (NY)	DR	162	Hyler, Irene (NY)	ChAP	623

Name	Specialty	Pg
Hyman, David (NY)	CG	586
Hyman, George (NY)	Oph	447
Hyman, Jeffrey (NY)	IM	437
Hyman, Joshua (NY)	OrS	269
Hymes, Kenneth (NY)	Hem	190

I

Name	Specialty	Pg
Iammatteo, Matthew (NJ)	ObG	838
Ibelli, Vincent (NY)	FMed	574
Idupuganti, Sudharam (NY)	Psyc	458
Igel, Gerard (NY)	Ped	409
Ilowite, Norman (NY)	PRhu	407
Ilson, David (NY)	Onc	215
Imber, Gerald (NY)	PlS	315
Inabnet, William (NY)	S	356
Inamdar, Sarla (NY)	Ped	305
Ingenito, Anthony (NJ)	RadRO	727
Inglis, Steven (NY)	MF	478
Ingrassia, Joseph (NY)	FMed	574
Innerfield, Michael (NY)	IC	575
Inra, Lawrence (NY)	Cv	138
Inzucchi, Silvio (CT)	EDM	945
Irwin, Mark (NY)	U	466
Isaacs, Ellen (NY)	IM	641
Isaacson, Steven (NY)	RadRO	341
Isola, Luis (NY)	Hem	190
Isom, O Wayne (NY)	T&CS	364
Israel, Alan (NJ)	Hem	704
Israel, Jessica (NJ)	Ger	818
Israel, Shara (CT)	IM	909
Israeli, Ron (NY)	PlS	556
Issenberg, Henry (NY)	PCd	661
Istrico, Richard (NY)	FMed	475
Iswara, Kadirawelpillai (NY)	Ge	431
Itzkowitz, Steven (NY)	Ge	174
Iwai, Sei (NY)	CE	583

J

Name	Specialty	Pg
Jabs, Douglas (NY)	Oph	254
Jackson, Rosemary (NY)	Ped	456
Jacob, Brian (NY)	S	356
Jacob, Jessica (NY)	ObG	537
Jacobowitz, Glenn (NY)	VascS	378
Jacobowitz, Marilyn (NY)	Pul	672
Jacobs, Elliot (NY)	PlS	315
Jacobs, Jonathan (NY)	Inf	195

Name	Specialty	Pg
Jacobs, Joseph (NY)	Oto	281
Jacobs, Laurie (NY)	Ger	393
Jacobs, Michael (NY)	D	155
Jacobs, Morton (NY)	DR	162
Jacobs, Thomas (NY)	EDM	167
Jacobson, Ira (NY)	Ge	175
Jacobson, Marc (NY)	AM	506
Jacobson, Ronald (NY)	ChiN	624
Jacoby, Jacob (NJ)	Psyc	771
Jacono, Andrew (NY)	Oto	544
Jacowitz, Joel (NJ)	Cv	693
Jadonath, Ram (NY)	CE	508
Jafar, Jafar (NY)	NS	228
Jaffe, Alan (NY)	Ge	634
Jaffe, Fredrick (NY)	OrS	269
Jaffe, Herbert (NY)	Oph	447
Jaffin, Barry (NY)	Ge	175
Jagannath, Sundar (NY)	Onc	215
Jahn, Anthony (NY)	Oto	281
Jahre, Caren (NY)	NRad	240
Jaile-Marti, Jesus (NY)	NP	647
Jain, Subhash (NY)	PM	288
Jakubowski, Ann (NY)	Onc	215
Jamidar, Priya (CT)	Ge	946
Jarnagin, William (NY)	S	356
Jarowski, Charles (NY)	Onc	215
Jarrett, Mark (NY)	Rhu	501
Jauhar, Rajiv (NY)	Cv	511
Javit, Daniel J (NY)	VIR	375
Jawetz, Harold (NJ)	IM	851
Jayaram, Nadubeethi (NY)	OrS	497
Jelin, Abraham (NY)	PGe	453
Jelveh, Mansoor (NY)	Cv	511
Jennis, Andrew (NJ)	Onc	708
Jeremias, Allen (NY)	Cv	584
Johns, William (CT)	NuM	917
Johnson, Albert (NJ)	OrS	864
Johnson, Diane (NY)	Inf	526
Johnson, Robert (NJ)	AM	738
Johnson, Valerie (NY)	PNep	300
Jokl, Peter (CT)	OrS	954
Jones, Frank (NJ)	Psyc	808
Jones, Jacqueline (NY)	PO	301
Jones, Stephen (CT)	Ger	905
Jonna, Siva (NJ)	PCCM	805
Jordan, Barry (NY)	N	650
Jordan, Lawrence (NJ)	S	811
Jordan, Mark (NJ)	U	763
Joseph, John (NY)	IM	478
Joseph, Patricia (NY)	S	580
Josephson, Jordan (NY)	Oto	281

Alphabetical Listing of Doctors

Name	Specialty	Pg	Name	Specialty	Pg
Josephson, Lynn (NY)	S	677	Kaplan, Barry (NY)	Cv	511
Joy, Mark (NY)	IM	437	Kaplan, Gabriel (NJ)	Psyc	884
Juan, Paul (CT)	Ped	927	Kaplan, Jeffrey (CT)	Oph	919
Julie, Edward (NJ)	Cv	849	Kaplan, Jonathan (NY)	EDM	519
Jurcic, Joseph (NY)	Onc	215	Kaplan, Kenneth (NY)	Cv	620
Jutkowitz, Robert (NY)	N	496	Kaplan, Martin (NY)	Ped	602
			Kaplan, Matthew (NY)	PNep	454
			Kaplan, Rana (NY)	Pul	336
			Kaplan, Ronald (NY)	PM	288
K			Kaplan, Sherri (NY)	D	626
			Kaplan, Steven (NY)	U	370
Kabis, Suzanne (NJ)	Nep	863	Kaplitt, Michael (NY)	NS	228
Kacker, Ashutosh (NY)	Oto	281	Kaplovitz, Harry (NY)	PCd	452
Kadan-Lottick, Nina (CT)	PHO	956	Kapoor, Satish (NY)	IM	641
Kaell, Alan (NY)	Rhu	607	Kaporis, Athena (NY)	D	626
Kafantaris, Vivian (NY)	ChAP	473	Kappel, Bruce (NY)	Onc	531
Kagan, Peter (NJ)	S	729	Kapur, Sandip (NY)	S	356
Kahaleh, Michel (NY)	Ge	175	Karamitsos, Harry (NY)	ObG	245
Kahn, David (NY)	Psyc	325	Karanfilian, Richard (NY)	VascS	681
Kahn, Jeffrey (NY)	Psyc	670	Karas, Evan (NY)	OrS	657
Kahn, Leonard (NY)	Path	546	Karasu, Sylvia (NY)	Psyc	326
Kahn, Max (NY)	Ped	305	Karasu, T Byram (NY)	Psyc	326
Kahn, Oren (NY)	Ge	634	Karatoprak, Ohan (NJ)	FMed	700
Kairam, Indira (NY)	Ge	175	Karetzky, Monroe (NY)	Pul	412
Kaiser, Michael (NY)	NS	228	Karmen, Carol (NY)	IM	641
Kaiser, Paul (NJ)	N	780	Karp, Adam (NY)	Ger	182
Kaiser, Stephen (NY)	IM	437	Karp, George (NJ)	Hem	795
Kalash, Glenn (NY)	Psyc	483	Karp, Nolan (NY)	PlS	316
Kalchthaler, Thomas (NY)	Ger	636	Karpeh, Martin (NY)	S	357
Kaleya, Ronald (NY)	S	464	Karpinski, Richard (NY)	PlS	316
Kalikow, Kevin (NY)	ChAP	623	Karwowski, John (NY)	VascS	378
Kalinich, Lila (NY)	Psyc	326	Kasabian, Armen (NY)	PlS	556
Kalischer, Alan (NJ)	Cv	872	Kase, Steven (NY)	Oto	659
Kalish, Robin (NY)	MF	209	Kaskel, Frederick (NY)	PNep	407
Kalman, Arlene (CT)	Psyc	930	Kasper, William (NY)	Oph	540
Kalman, Jill (NY)	Cv	138	Kass, Lewis (NY)	PPul	664
Kalnicki, Shalom (NY)	RadRO	413	Kassapidis, Sotirios (NY)	Pul	484
Kamalakar, Peri (NJ)	PHO	756	Kassotis, John (NY)	CE	423
Kamen, Mazen (NY)	Cv	138	Kates, Matthew (NY)	Oto	659
Kaminer, Ruth (NY)	Ped	409	Kato, Tomoaki (NY)	S	357
Kaminetsky, Jed (NY)	U	370	Kattan, Meyer (NY)	PPul	302
Kaminsky, Donald (NY)	IM	202	Katus, Eli (NY)	Psyc	558
Kamler, Kenneth (NY)	HS	524	Katz, Aaron (NY)	U	567
Kanengiser, Steven (NJ)	PPul	720	Katz, Alan (NY)	RadRO	484
Kang, Harriet (NY)	ChiN	624	Katz, Amiram (CT)	N	953
Kang, Pritpal (NY)	Cv	424	Katz, Andrea (NJ)	Ped	865
Kanner, Ronald (NY)	N	535	Katz, Bruce (NY)	D	155
Kanter, Alan (NJ)	Ped	722	Katz, Edward (NY)	Cv	138
Kantor, Alan (NY)	EDM	630	Katz, Harry (NJ)	Oto	717
Kantrowitz, Niki (NY)	Cv	425	Katz, Henry (NY)	Ge	634
Kapel, Robert (CT)	Ge	904	Katz, Herbert (NJ)	U	772

Name	Specialty	Pg	Name	Specialty	Pg
Katz, Jack (NY)	Psyc	558	Kemeny, M Margaret (NY)	S	485
Katz, Jeffrey (NJ)	U	763	Kemeny, Nancy (NY)	Onc	216
Katz, Seymour (NY)	Ge	522	Kempin, Sanford (NY)	Hem	190
Katz, Steven (NJ)	U	732	Kenan, Samuel (NY)	OrS	542
Katz, Stuart (NY)	Cv	138	Kenet, Barney (NY)	D	156
Katz, Susan (NY)	D	155	Kenigsberg, Daniel (NY)	RE	606
Katzenelenbogen, Moshe (NY)	IM	437	Kenler, Andrew (CT)	S	935
Katzenstein, Martin (NY)	Ped	409	Kennedy, Gary (NY)	GerPsy	394
Kaufman, Alan (NY)	A&I	383	Kennedy, James (NY)	IM	202
Kaufman, Andrew (NJ)	PM	753	Kennedy, Timothy (NY)	S	414
Kaufman, David (NY)	N	400	Kennish, Arthur (NY)	IM	202
Kaufman, David (NY)	IM	202	Kenny, Raymond (NJ)	Ge	743
Kaufman, David (NY)	ChiN	147	Kent, Jennifer (NY)	IM	202
Kaufman, David (NY)	Cv	384	Kent, Joan (NY)	ObG	245
Kaufman, Matthew (NJ)	PlS	808	Kernan, Nancy (NY)	PHO	298
Kaufman, Richard (CT)	A&I	942	Kernan, Walter (CT)	IM	949
Kaufmann, Charles (NY)	Psyc	326	Kerner, Michael (NJ)	Ge	876
Kaul, Ashutosh (NY)	S	677	Kerr, Leslie (NY)	Rhu	348
Kaushik, Raj (NJ)	T&CS	856	Kerstein, Joshua (NY)	Cv	425
Kauvar, Arielle (NY)	D	156	Kesarwala, Hemant (NJ)	A&I	789
Kavanagh, Brian (CT)	OrS	923	Kesh, Sandra (NY)	Inf	638
Kavey, Neil (NY)	Psyc	326	Kessler, Alan (NY)	ObG	245
Kavookjian, Haik (CT)	HS	906	Kessler, Bradley (NY)	PGe	601
Kavoussi, Louis (NY)	U	568	Kessler, Edmund (NY)	PS	456
Kay, Arthur (NY)	N	443	Kessler, Jeffrey (NY)	N	536
Kay, Richard (NY)	Cv	620	Kessler, Leonard (NY)	Onc	531
Kay, Scott (NJ)	Oto	803	Kessler, Martin (NY)	PlS	556
Kazam, Ezra (NJ)	Oph	838	Kessler, William (NJ)	Hem	876
Kazdin, Hal (NY)	IM	437	Khabie, Victor (NY)	OrS	657
Kazim, Michael (NY)	Oph	254	Khaghan, Neda (CT)	Ge	904
Kazlow, Philip (NY)	PGe	296	Khalife, Michael (NY)	S	564
Kearney, Thomas (NJ)	S	811	Khan, Arfa (NY)	DR	517
Keefe, David (NY)	RE	343	Khandji, Alexander (NY)	NRad	240
Keilson, Marshall (NY)	N	444	Khilnani, Neil (NY)	VIR	375
Keiser, Harold (NY)	Rhu	413	Khimani, Karim (NJ)	Ger	876
Keith, Marie (NY)	Ped	305	Khouri, Philippe (NJ)	Psyc	784
Kelemen, John (NY)	N	535	Khoury, F Frederic (NY)	PlS	668
Keller, Adina (NY)	ObG	652	Khoury, Paul (NY)	DR	628
Keller, Alex (NY)	PlS	556	Khulpateea, Neekianund (NY)	GO	434
Keller, Andrew (CT)	Cv	897	Kierce, Roger (NJ)	ObG	852
Keller, Irwin (NJ)	NRad	800	Kiernan, Howard (NY)	OrS	270
Keller, Jeffrey (NY)	PO	663	Kim, Heakyung (NY)	PMR	310
Keller, Peter (NY)	Cv	385	Kim, Joyce (NY)	ObG	245
Keller, Steven (NY)	T&CS	415	Kim, Michelle (NY)	Ge	175
Kelly, Anna (NY)	NRad	240	Kim, Tae (NY)	PlS	668
Kelly, Bryan (NY)	OrS	270	Kim-Schluger, Hyung (NY)	Ge	175
Kelly, Michael (NJ)	OrS	716	Kimball, Annetta (NY)	Ge	175
Kelly, Stephen (NY)	Oph	254	Kimmelstiel, Fred (NY)	S	357
Kelsen, David (NY)	Onc	216	Kimura, Yukiko (NJ)	PRhu	721
Keltz, Martin (NY)	RE	343	King, Michael (CT)	DR	901
Keltz, Theodore (NY)	Cv	621	King, William (NY)	HS	187

Alphabetical Listing of Doctors

Name	Specialty	Pg	Name	Specialty	Pg
Kinkhabwala, Milan (NY)	S	414	Kobren, Steven (NY)	Cv	511
Kipen, Howard (NJ)	OM	802	Kocher, Jeffrey (NJ)	Inf	705
Kirschenbaum, Alexander (NY)	U	370	Kocsis, James (NY)	Psyc	326
Kirshblum, Steven (NJ)	PMR	758	Kodali, Susheel (NY)	IC	207
Kirshy, David (NY)	DR	588	Koenig, Eli (NY)	NP	440
Kirtane, Sanjay (NY)	Cv	472	Koenigsberg, Mordecai (NY)	DR	388
Kizelshteyn, Grigory (NY)	PM	660	Kofinas, George (NY)	RE	461
Klafter, Robert (NY)	Onc	216	Kohan, Darius (NY)	Oto	281
Klagsbrun, Samuel (NY)	Psyc	670	Kohn, Brenda (NY)	PEn	295
Klapholz, Ari (NY)	Pul	337	Kolenik, Steven (CT)	D	900
Klapholz, Marc (NJ)	Cv	739	Kolitz, Jonathan (NY)	Hem	525
Klapper, Daniel (NY)	Oph	254	Kolker, Adam (NY)	PlS	316
Klapper, Philip (NY)	Pul	412	Kolker, Harvey (NY)	Ped	603
Klar, Tobi (NY)	D	627	Kolodny, Edwin (NY)	N	234
Klares, Scott (NY)	Pul	672	Kolodny, Erwin (NY)	Pul	337
Klarsfeld, Jay (CT)	Oto	925	Kolsky, Neil (NJ)	Ped	722
Klausner, Stanley (NY)	S	608	Komisar, Arnold (NY)	Oto	281
Kleber, Herbert (NY)	AdP	129	Koniaris, Soula (NJ)	PGe	805
Klecz, Robert (NJ)	PMR	841	Konka, Sudarsanam (NY)	Cv	425
Kleeman, Harris (NY)	Cv	425	Kopec, Anna (NJ)	D	767
Klein, George (NY)	U	370	Kopelman, Rima (NJ)	Rhu	728
Klein, Jeffrey (NY)	RE	674	Kopf, Gary (CT)	T&CS	963
Klein, Natalie (NY)	Inf	526	Koplewicz, Harold (NY)	ChAP	146
Klein, Neil (CT)	IM	909	Koplin, Richard (NY)	Oph	254
Klein, Noah (NY)	Oph	254	Koppel, Barbara (NY)	N	234
Klein, Norman (NY)	A&I	422	Korc, Beatriz (NY)	Ger	182
Klein, Patricia (NJ)	N	711	Koreen, Amy (NY)	Psyc	604
Klein, Robert (NJ)	A&I	849	Korenstein, Deborah (NY)	IM	202
Klein, Victor (NY)	MF	530	Kornel, Ezriel (NY)	NS	649
Klein, Walter (NJ)	Ge	701	Korsten, Mark (NY)	Ge	392
Kleinberg, David (NY)	EDM	167	Korval, Arnold (CT)	Ped	927
Kleiner, Morton (NY)	Nep	496	Kosinski, Edward (CT)	Cv	897
Kleinman, Andrew (NY)	PlS	668	Kosofsky, Barry (NY)	ChiN	148
Kleinman, Paul (NY)	OrS	403	Kososky, Charles (NJ)	N	780
Klenk, Rosemary (CT)	Ped	927	Koss, Jerome (NY)	Cv	511
Klenoff, Bruce (CT)	Oto	925	Kostis, John (NJ)	Cv	789
Kliger, Alan (CT)	Nep	951	Kotin, Neal (NY)	Ped	305
Kligfield, Paul (NY)	Cv	138	Kotler, Donald (NY)	Ge	176
Kligler, Benjamin (NY)	FMed	169	Kotler, Lisa (NJ)	ChAP	695
Klimstra, David (NY)	Path	290	Kottler, William (NJ)	PPul	757
Kline, Gary (NJ)	T&CS	566	Kottmeier, Stephen (NY)	SM	607
Kline, Mitchell (NY)	D	156	Koufman, Jamie (NY)	Oto	281
Klos, Andrzej (NJ)	Ped	770	Koulos, John (NY)	GO	185
Kloss, Robert (CT)	Onc	913	Kowallis, George (NY)	Psyc	326
Klyde, Barry (NY)	EDM	167	Kozel, Joseph (NJ)	IM	768
Klimstra, David (NY)					
Knackmuhs, Gary (NJ)	Inf	704	Kozicky, Orest (NY)	Ge	634
Knapp, Albert (NY)	Ge	175	Kozin, Arthur (NY)	Nep	576
Knep, Stanley (NJ)	N	852	Kozlowski, Jeffrey (NJ)	Nep	710
Knightly, John (NJ)	NS	837	Kozuch, Peter (NY)	Onc	216
Knisely, Jonathan (NY)	RadRO	561	Krakovitz, Evan (NY)	CRS	625
Knopp, Edmond (NY)	NRad	240	Kramer, David (CT)	OrS	923

Castle Connolly *Top Doctors: New York Metro Area* 16th Edition

Alphabetical Listing of Doctors

Name	Specialty	Pg	Name	Specialty	Pg
Landau, Alan (CT)	Ge	904	Lebofsky, Martin (NY)	IM	641
Landau, Leon (NY)	Hem	395	Lebovics, Edward (NY)	Ge	635
Landau, Steven (NY)	Ge	634	Lebovics, Robert (NY)	Oto	282
Landers, David (NJ)	Cv	693	Lebowicz, Joseph (NY)	Onc	440
Landesman, Sheldon (NY)	Inf	435	Lebowitz, Mark (NY)	Oph	448
Landis, Gregg (NY)	VascS	487	Lebwohl, Mark (NY)	D	156
Landrigan, Philip (NY)	OM	248	Lebwohl, Oscar (NY)	Ge	176
Landzberg, Joel (NJ)	Cv	693	Lechner, Michael (NY)	IM	641
Lane, Edward (CT)	Oto	925	Leckman, James (CT)	ChAP	943
Lane, Joseph (NY)	OrS	270	Lederer, David (NY)	Pul	337
Lane, Lewis (NY)	HS	524	Lederman, Jeffrey (NY)	Inf	638
Lanfranchi, Angela (NJ)	S	867	Lederman, Josiane (NY)	D	492
Lang, Paul (NY)	A&I	507	Lederman, Martin (NY)	Oph	654
Lang, Samuel (NY)	T&CS	486	Lederman, Sanford (NY)	ObG	446
Lange, Dale (NY)	N	234	Lee, Alexander (NY)	PMR	310
Langer, David (NY)	NS	534	Lee, April (NY)	AM	491
Langer, Paul (NJ)	Oph	751	Lee, Carol (NY)	Oph	255
Langsner, Alan (NY)	PCd	755	Lee, Douglas (NY)	ObG	597
Lanman, Geraldine (NY)	Ger	523	Lee, Francis (NY)	OrS	270
Lannin, Donald (CT)	S	962	Lee, Haesoon (NY)	PPul	455
Lans, David (NY)	Rhu	675	Lee, Huey-Jen (NJ)	DR	742
Lansing, Martha (NJ)	FMed	776	Lee, James (NY)	S	357
Lansman, Steven (NY)	T&CS	678	Lee, Kwang (NY)	Psyc	604
Lanteri, Vincent (NJ)	U	732	Lee, Leonard (NJ)	T&CS	811
Lara, Jonathan (NJ)	Path	754	Lee, Marjorie (NY)	Pul	337
Larsen, John (NY)	PInf	299	Lee, Nancy (NY)	RadRO	341
Larson, Signe (NY)	Ped	306	Lee, Paul (NY)	T&CS	486
LaSala, Patrick (NY)	NS	399	Lee, Roberta (NY)	IM	203
Latov, Norman (NY)	N	235	Lee, Ronald (CT)	DR	901
Lau, Har Chi (NY)	S	677	Lee, S Howard (NJ)	NRad	863
Lauer, Simeon (NY)	Oph	255	Lee, Sang (NY)	CRS	150
Lauricella, Joseph (NJ)	IM	705	Lee, Sicy (NY)	Rhu	348
Lavyne, Michael (NY)	NS	228	Lee, Steve (NY)	HS	187
Lawson, William (NY)	Oto	282	Lee, Sun (NJ)	NS	799
Lax, James (NY)	Ge	176	Lee, Thomas (NY)	PS	602
Layne, Jeffrey (NY)	U	568	Lee, Thomas (NY)	NS	649
Lazar, Amy (NJ)	Oto	864	Leeds, Gary (NY)	FMed	169
Lazar, Eliot (NY)	Cv	139	Leeman, Benjamin (NY)	Pul	559
Lazar, Mark (NJ)	N	800	Leffell, David (CT)	D	945
Lazar, Robert (NY)	Ge	591	Lefkovitz, Zvi (NY)	DR	629
Lazarus, George (NY)	Ped	306	Lefkowitz, Mathew (NY)	PM	451
Lazarus, Herbert (NY)	PRhu	302	Legato, Marianne (NY)	IM	203
Lazarus, Laura (CT)	S	935	Lehach, Joan (NY)	A&I	383
Lazzaro, Douglas (NY)	Oph	448	Lehman, Thomas (NY)	PRhu	302
Lazzaro, Richard (NY)	T&CS	365	Lehrhoff, Bernard (NJ)	U	887
Le Benger, Kerry (NJ)	A&I	872	Lehrman, Gary (NY)	Pul	672
Leach, Thomas (NJ)	PlS	783	Lehrman, Stuart (NY)	Pul	673
Leahy, Mary (NY)	IM	575	Leib, Martin (NY)	Oph	255
Leavens-Maurer, Jill (NY)	Ped	553	Leibner, Donald (NJ)	A&I	789
Leb, Alvin (NY)	Ge	432	Leiboff, Arnold (NY)	CRS	586
Lebinger, Martin (NY)	Psyc	411	Leibowitz, Evan (NJ)	Rhu	728

Name	Specialty	Pg	Name	Specialty	Pg
Leibowitz, Jonas (NY)	EDM	630	Levine, David (NY)	N	235
Leichter, Donald (NJ)	PCd	882	Levine, David (NY)	OrS	270
Leifer, Bennett (NJ)	Ger	702	Levine, Dorothy (CT)	Ped	928
Leifer, Marvin (NJ)	Psyc	784	Levine, Evan (NY)	Cv	621
Leipsner, George (NJ)	FMed	700	Levine, Jeremiah (NY)	PGe	548
Leipzig, Rosanne (NY)	Ger	183	Levine, Joseph (NY)	CE	508
Leipziger, Lyle (NY)	PlS	556	Levine, Joshua (NY)	PlS	316
Leiter, Gila (NY)	ObG	245	Levine, Laurie (NY)	D	516
Leitner, Stuart (NJ)	Onc	748	Levine, Martin (NJ)	FMed	767
Lemercier, Maud (NY)	S	677	Levine, Mitchell (NY)	NS	534
Lenci, Margaret (NY)	Rhu	675	Levine, Randy (NY)	Hem	190
Lense, Lloyd (NY)	Cv	585	Levine, Richard (NY)	ObG	245
Lenzo, Salvatore (NY)	HS	187	Levine, Selwyn (NJ)	Pul	726
Leon, Martin (NY)	IC	207	Levine, Seth (NJ)	U	856
Leon, Steven (NY)	NS	595	Levine, Steven (CT)	Oto	925
Leonard, Daniel (NY)	Cv	621	Levine, Steven (NY)	N	444
Leonard, John (NY)	Hem	190	Levine, William (NY)	SM	352
Leong, Mary (NY)	ObG	538	Levitan, Stephan (NY)	Psyc	327
Leong, Pauline (NY)	IM	527	Levites, Kenneth (NY)	FMed	590
Lepor, Herbert (NY)	U	370	Levitt, Miriam (NY)	Ped	666
Lepore, Frederick (NJ)	N	800	Levitz, Craig (NY)	OrS	542
Lerma, Pauline (NJ)	Onc	779	Levitzky, Susan (NY)	Ped	306
Lerman, Bruce (NY)	CE	133	Levy, Adam (NY)	PHO	406
Lerman, Jay (NY)	D	627	Levy, Albert (NY)	FMed	170
Lerman, Jay (NY)	DR	429	Levy, Andrew (NJ)	SM	761
Lerner, Chester (NY)	Inf	195	Levy, Howard (NY)	OrS	270
Lerner, Elliot (NJ)	NRad	712	Levy, I Martin (NY)	OrS	403
Lerner, Seth (NY)	U	679	Levy, Joseph (NY)	PGe	296
Lerner, William (NJ)	Hem	818	Levy, Judith (NY)	ObG	401
Lescale, Keith (NY)	MF	644	Levy, Lauren (NJ)	DR	698
Lesesne, Carroll (NY)	PlS	316	Levy, Lewis (NY)	N	536
Leslie, Denise (NY)	DR	629	Levy, Michael (NY)	Psyc	578
Lesorgen, Philip (NJ)	RE	727	Levy, Miriam (NY)	DR	162
Lesser, Robert (NY)	Rhu	462	Levy, Morton (NY)	Ped	553
Lesser, Robert (CT)	Oph	953	Levy, Ross (NY)	D	627
Lessing, Jeffrey (NY)	U	502	Levy, Susan (CT)	ChiN	943
Lester, Mitchell (CT)	A&I	895	Lew, Arthur (NY)	Psyc	670
Lester, Thomas (NY)	Hem	637	Lewin, Margaret (NY)	IM	203
Lettera, James (CT)	T&CS	936	Lewin, Neal (NY)	IM	203
Levchuck, Sean (NY)	PCd	547	Lewin, Sharon (NY)	IM	203
Leventhal, Bennett (NY)	ChAP	146	Lewis, Benjamin (NY)	Cv	139
Levey, Robert (NY)	IM	437	Lewis, Blair (NY)	Ge	176
Levin, Alexander (NJ)	PM	804	Lewis, Dorothy (CT)	Psyc	959
Levin, Andrew (NY)	Psyc	670	Lewis, Owen (NY)	ChAP	146
Levin, David (NJ)	Nep	710	Lewis, Ronald (NY)	OrS	599
Levin, Frances (NY)	AdP	129	Lewis, Theophilus (NY)	S	464
Levin, Kenneth (NJ)	N	711	Lewko, Michael (NJ)	Rhu	855
Levin, Richard (CT)	Oto	925	Li, Ronald (NJ)	Oto	803
Levin, Sheryl (NY)	PMR	410	Liang, Vera (NY)	Psyc	604
Levin Carmine, Linda (NY)	AM	506	Libby, Daniel (NY)	Pul	337
Levine, Alice (NY)	EDM	167	Libman, Richard (NY)	N	536

Alphabetical Listing of Doctors

Name	Specialty	Pg	Name	Specialty	Pg
Libutti, Steven (NY)	S	414	Litchman, Mark (CT)	A&I	895
Licata, Joseph (NJ)	S	730	Liteplo, Ronald (NY)	D	387
Licciardi, Frederick (NY)	RE	344	Litman, Nathan (NY)	PInf	407
Licht, Arnold (NY)	Psyc	458	Litman, Richard (NY)	Oto	600
Lichtbroun, Alan (NJ)	Rhu	810	Litman, Steven (NY)	PM	600
Lichter, Stephen (NY)	Onc	440	Littlejohn, Charles (CT)	CRS	899
Lichtstein, Elliott (NJ)	Cv	694	Lituchy, Andrew (NY)	IC	529
Lieb, Mark (NY)	Cv	621	Litvin, Y Samuel (NJ)	U	826
Lieberman, David (NY)	Oph	448	Liu, David (NY)	Nep	225
Lieberman, Elliott (NY)	U	568	Liu, DeLong (NY)	Onc	645
Lieberman, Kenneth (NJ)	PNep	720	Liu, George (NY)	IM	204
Lieberman, Michael (NY)	S	357	Liva, Douglas (NJ)	Oph	714
Liebling, Anne (CT)	Rhu	961	Lizza, Eli (NY)	U	371
Liebling, Melissa (NJ)	DR	698	Lo, K M Steve (CT)	Onc	913
Liebling, Ralph (NY)	PlS	411	Lo Galbo, Peter (NY)	A&I	573
Liebmann, Jeffrey (NY)	Oph	255	Lodge, Henry (NY)	IM	204
Liftin, Alan (NJ)	D	741	Logan, Bruce (NY)	IM	204
Lightdale, Charles (NY)	Ge	177	Loganathan, Raghunandan (NY)	Pul	412
Ligresti, Louise (NJ)	Onc	708	Lois, William (NY)	S	464
Liguori, Michael (NY)	IM	203	Lomasky, Steven (NY)	EDM	519
Lim, Jessica (NY)	Oto	282	Lombardi, Joseph (NJ)	OrS	803
Lin, Michael (NY)	N	235	Lombardo, Gerard (NY)	Pul	460
Lind, Lawrence (NY)	ObG	246	Lombardo, James (NY)	Oph	448
Lindenmayer, Jean-Pierre (NY)	Psyc	327	Lombardo, Peter (NY)	D	156
Lindner, Paul (CT)	A&I	895	Lomonaco, Salvatore (NY)	ChAP	386
Lindsay, Gaius (NY)	U	466	Lonberg, Mathew (NY)	Onc	575
Link, Richard (CT)	Ge	904	London, Ronald (NY)	Ped	666
Linsenmeyer, Todd (NJ)	U	764	Longo, Walter (CT)	CRS	944
Linstrom, Christopher (NY)	Oto	283	Lonner, Baron (NY)	OrS	270
Lipetz, Jason (NY)	PMR	554	Loo, Marcus (NY)	U	371
Lipinsky, Edward (NY)	Oto	600	Lookstein, Robert (NY)	VIR	375
Lipner, Henry (NY)	Nep	441	Lopez, Clark (NY)	FMed	430
Lipow, Kenneth (CT)	NS	915	Lopez, Ralph (NY)	AM	130
Lipper, Graeme (CT)	D	900	Lorber, Daniel (NY)	EDM	474
Lippman, Alan (NJ)	Onc	748	Lorefice, Laurence (CT)	Psyc	930
Lippman, Jay (NY)	Oph	654	Loren, Gary (NJ)	PM	782
Lipsitz, Evan (NY)	VascS	416	Loria, Jeffrey (NY)	Ge	177
Lipson, David (NJ)	PlS	724	Lorich, Dean (NY)	OrS	270
Lipstein-Kresch, Esther (NY)	Rhu	563	LoRusso, Diane (NY)	DR	629
Lipsztein, Roberto (NY)	RadRO	484	Loughlin, Gerald (NY)	PPul	302
Lipton, Brian (NY)	Psyc	327	Louie, Eddie (NY)	Inf	195
Lipton, Jeffrey (NY)	PHO	549	Louis, Elan (NY)	N	235
Lipton, Mark (NY)	IM	203	Loulmet, Didier (NY)	T&CS	365
Lipton, Richard (NY)	N	400	Love, Barry (NY)	PCd	293
Lis, Eric (NY)	NRad	240	Lovecchio, John (NY)	GO	524
Lisman, Richard (NY)	Oph	255	LoVerme, Paul (NJ)	PlS	759
Liss, Donald (NJ)	PMR	723	Low, Ronald (NJ)	Oto	717
Liss, Howard (NJ)	PMR	723	Lowe, Franklin (NY)	U	371
Liss, Mark (NY)	Ge	635	Lowell, Barry (NJ)	Cv	832
Lisser, Steven (NJ)	HS	818	Lowenthal, Dennis (NJ)	Onc	878
Litchman, Charisse (CT)	N	916	Lowenthal, Diana (NY)	PPul	664

Name	Specialty	Pg
Lowy, Joseph (NY)	Pul	337
Lozner, Jerrold (NJ)	S	886
Lu, Bing (NY)	IM	437
Lu, Gabriel (NY)	PM	660
Lu, Stanley (NJ)	NRad	821
Lubat, Edward (NJ)	DR	698
Lubell, Harry (NY)	Ped	666
Lubitz, Arthur (NY)	A&I	132
Lublin, Fred (NY)	N	235
Lubliner, Jerry (NY)	OrS	271
Lucak, Susan (NY)	Ge	177
Lucariello, Richard (NY)	Cv	385
Luchs, Jonathan (NY)	DR	517
Luciani, Richard (NJ)	ObG	750
Luciano, Daniel (NY)	N	235
Ludwig, Shelly (NJ)	Ge	817
Lukash, Barbara (NY)	D	627
Lukash, Frederick (NY)	PlS	556
Luks, Howard (NY)	SM	676
Lundberg, Walter (CT)	Onc	950
Lundy, Edward (NY)	T&CS	580
Lunt, John (CT)	HS	906
Lusman, Paul (NY)	A&I	583
Lustbader, Ian (NY)	Ge	177
Lustig, Ilana (NY)	ObG	246
Lutwick, Larry (NY)	Inf	435
Lutz, Christopher (NY)	PMR	310
Lutz, Gregory (NY)	PMR	310
Lutzker, Letty (NJ)	NuM	750
Lux, Michael (NJ)	IC	877
Lyden, John (NY)	OrS	271
Lydic, Michael (NY)	RE	606
Lyman, Neil (NJ)	Nep	837
Lynch, Michael (CT)	OrS	923
Lynch, Thomas (CT)	Onc	951
Lynch, Vincent (CT)	ObG	953
Lynn, Robert (NY)	Nep	399
Lyon, Valerie (NY)	FMed	170

M

Name	Specialty	Pg
Ma, Dong (NY)	PMR	310
Macaulay, William (NY)	OrS	271
Maccabee, Paul (NY)	N	444
Maccia, Clement (NJ)	A&I	872
Macher, Mark (NJ)	RadRO	810
Machler, Brian (NJ)	D	741
Macina, Lucy (NY)	Ger	523
Mack, Laurence (NY)	ObG	538

Name	Specialty	Pg
MacKay, Cynthia (NY)	Oph	255
Mackessy, Richard (NJ)	OrS	881
Mackler, Karen (NY)	D	627
Mackool, Richard (NY)	Oph	481
Maclaren, Noel (NY)	PEn	295
MacMillan, William (NJ)	MF	797
Maddalo, Anthony (NY)	OrS	657
Madigan, Janet (CT)	ChAP	943
Magid, Steven (NY)	Rhu	348
Magill, Richard (NY)	HS	637
Maglaras, Nicholas (NJ)	IM	877
Magner, Joan (CT)	Ped	928
Magramm, Irene (NY)	Oph	256
Magriples, Urania (CT)	MF	949
Magro, Cynthia (NY)	Path	290
Magun, Arthur (NY)	Ge	177
Mahal, Pradeep (NJ)	Ge	876
Mahalingam, Banu (NJ)	Cv	775
Maharam, Lewis (NY)	SM	352
Maher, Elizabeth (NY)	Oph	256
Maher, John (NY)	ObG	446
Maheshwari, Vivek (NJ)	S	762
Mahoney, Maurice (CT)	CG	944
Maier, Herbert (NJ)	D	850
Mailloux, Lionel (NY)	Nep	533
Maiman, Mitchell (NY)	GO	494
Maiocco, Kenneth (CT)	D	900
Maizel, Barry (NY)	Ge	432
Maki, Robert (NY)	Onc	216
Malach, Barbara (NY)	IM	495
Malamud, Stephen (NY)	Onc	217
Malanga, Gerard (NJ)	PMR	883
Malaspina, Dolores (NY)	Psyc	327
Maldonado, Thomas (NY)	VascS	378
Malik, Asim (NY)	IM	438
Malik, Rubina (NY)	Ger	393
Malik, Sajid (NY)	Oph	540
Malits, Bella (NY)	PM	660
Mallozzi, Angelo (CT)	FMed	903
Maloney, Patrick (NY)	A&I	617
Maloney, Romelle (NY)	ObG	652
Malovany, Robert (NJ)	Pul	726
Malpeso, James (NY)	IC	495
Maman, Arie (NJ)	EDM	793
Manasseh, Donna-Marie (NY)	S	464
Mancini, Donna (NY)	Cv	139
Mandava, Suresh (CT)	Oph	919
Mandel, Eric (NY)	Oph	256
Mandel, Marc (NJ)	S	887
Mandel, Michael (NY)	Pul	673
Mandelbaum, Sidney (NY)	Oph	256

Alphabetical Listing of Doctors

Name	Specialty	Pg	Name	Specialty	Pg
Manevitz, Alan (NY)	Psyc	327	Marks, Andrea (NY)	AM	130
Manginello, Frank (NJ)	NP	709	Marks, David (NJ)	N	750
Mani, John (NY)	OrS	449	Marks, Jon (NY)	U	371
Mani, Susan (CT)	Cv	897	Marks, Laura (CT)	Ped	928
Maniatis, Theodore (NY)	Pul	500	Marks, Michael (CT)	OrS	923
Maniscalco, Anthony (NY)	N	444	Marks, Peter (CT)	Hem	948
Manjoney, Delia (CT)	Oph	919	Marks, Stephen (NY)	N	650
Mankes, Seth (NY)	DR	588	Marmur, Ellen (NY)	D	156
Mann, Charles (NY)	ObG	597	Marotta, James (NY)	Oto	600
Mann, J John (NY)	Psyc	327	Marron-Corwin, Mary (NY)	NP	223
Mann, Ronald (NY)	OrS	657	Marsan, Ben (CT)	VascS	938
Mann, Samuel (NY)	IM	204	Marsh, Franklin (NY)	Ge	178
Manners, Richard (NY)	Ped	603	Marsh, James (CT)	OrS	954
Manning, Eric (NJ)	Nep	820	Marshalko, Stephen (CT)	Cv	898
Manno, Joseph (NJ)	VascS	734	Marshall, Ian (NJ)	PEn	805
Mansour, E Hani (NJ)	S	762	Martens, Mark (NJ)	ObG	821
Mansouri, Hormoz (NY)	S	564	Martimucci, William (NY)	Ger	636
Marchetta, Paula (NY)	Rhu	348	Martin, Christopher (NY)	Ge	635
Marcus, Judith (NY)	PHO	298	Martin, Jeffrey (NY)	Oph	598
Marcus, Michael (NY)	PPul	455	Martins, Publius (NY)	Pul	500
Marcus, Norman (NY)	PM	288	Marush, Arthur (NY)	IM	438
Marcus, Ralph (NJ)	Rhu	728	Marx, Robert (NY)	OrS	271
Marcus, Richard (NJ)	Ped	757	Mascarenhas, Bento (NY)	Rhu	675
Marcus, Stuart (CT)	S	935	Masci, Joseph (NY)	Inf	477
Marder, Karen (NY)	N	235	Masciello, Michael (NY)	Cv	585
Marghoob, Ashfaq (NY)	D	587	Maselli, Frank (NY)	FMed	390
Margolis, Eric (NJ)	U	732	Masino, Frank (CT)	RadRO	933
Margulies, Paul (NY)	EDM	519	Maslak, Peter (NY)	Hem	191
Margulis, Elynne (NJ)	ObG	880	Masri, Bassem (NY)	Cv	139
Margulis, Stephen (NJ)	Ge	701	Masson, Lalitha (NJ)	ObG	769
Margulis, Steven (NY)	IM	641	Masterson, Raymond (NJ)	IM	819
Marin, Deborah (NY)	Psyc	327	Matalon, Martin (NY)	ObG	597
Marin, Geobel (NJ)	Ge	776	Matalon, Robert (NY)	Nep	225
Marin, Lorraine (NY)	RadRO	561	Matarasso, Alan (NY)	PlS	316
Marin, Michael (NY)	VascS	378	Matczuk, Agnieszka (CT)	A&I	895
Marino, A Michael (CT)	Pul	932	Matera, Cristina (NY)	RE	344
Marino, John (NY)	Onc	531	Math, Kevin (NY)	DR	162
Marino, Ronald (NY)	Ped	553	Mathias, Stephen (CT)	Oph	920
Marino, William (NY)	Pul	413	Matilsky, Michael (NY)	Cv	585
Marion, James (NY)	Ge	177	Matos, Jeffrey (NY)	CE	133
Marion, Robert (NY)	CG	386	Matos, Marshall (NY)	Cv	621
Markell, Mariana (NY)	Nep	441	Matossian, Cynthia (NJ)	Oph	781
Markenson, Joseph (NY)	Rhu	348	Matta, Raymond (NY)	Cv	139
Markovics, Sharon (NY)	A&I	507	Mattana, Joseph (NY)	Nep	533
Markowitz, Arlene (NY)	Oto	283	Mattel, Stephen (NJ)	Oto	853
Markowitz, Arnold (NY)	Ge	177	Mattes, Leonard (NY)	Cv	139
Markowitz, David (NY)	Ge	177	Matthews, Gerald (NY)	U	679
Markowitz, James (NY)	PGe	548	Mattison, Timothy (NY)	D	627
Markowitz, John (NY)	Psyc	327	Mattoo, Nirmal (NY)	Nep	480
Markowitz, Steven (NY)	CE	133	Mattucci, Kenneth (NY)	Oto	544
Marks, Alan (NY)	Oph	540	Mauer, Kenneth (CT)	Ge	904

Alphabetical Listing of Doctors

Name	Specialty	Pg	Name	Specialty	Pg
Mauri, Thomas (NY)	OrS	542	McKenna, Michael (NJ)	RadRO	784
Mauskop, Alexander (NY)	N	235	McKhann, Guy (NY)	NS	229
Maxfield, Roger (NY)	Pul	337	McKiernan, James (NY)	U	371
May, Louis (NY)	Ge	574	McKinley, Matthew (NY)	Ge	522
Mayer, Daniel (NY)	A&I	583	McKinsey, James (NY)	VascS	378
Mayer, Fern (CT)	D	900	McLaughlin, Mark (NJ)	NS	780
Mayer, Ira (NY)	Ge	432	McLeod, Gavin (CT)	Inf	907
Mayer, Lloyd (NY)	Ge	178	McMahon, Donna-Marie (NY)	Ped	603
Mayer, Stephan (NY)	N	236	McManus, Edward (NJ)	Inf	835
Mayers, Marguerite (NY)	Ped	409	McManus, Susan (NJ)	S	867
Mayers, Martin (NY)	Oph	402	McMeeking, Alexander (NY)	Inf	195
Mayeux, Richard (NY)	N	236	McMullen, Robert (NY)	Psyc	328
Maytal, Joseph (NY)	ChiN	514	McNamara, Joseph (CT)	PHO	956
Mazur, Eric (CT)	Hem	907	McPherson, Craig (CT)	CE	896
Mazza, David (NY)	A&I	132	McVeigh, Anne Marie (NY)	Oph	256
Mazzara, Carl (NJ)	Oto	803	McWhorter, Philip (CT)	S	935
Mc Inerney, Vincent (NJ)	OrS	853	Meacham, Kevin (NY)	ObG	652
McAbee, Gary (NJ)	Ped	807	Mears, John Gregory (NY)	Hem	191
McAllister, Peter (CT)	N	916	Mechanic, Laura (NY)	A&I	617
McAnally, James (NJ)	Nep	878	Mechanick, Jeffrey (NY)	EDM	168
McBride, Whitney (NY)	PS	664	Medici, Mark (NY)	OrS	577
McCain, Donald (NJ)	S	730	Medina, Emma (NY)	Cv	621
McCalley, Stuart (CT)	Pul	932	Medow, Norman (NY)	Oph	402
McCance, Sean (NY)	OrS	271	Meed, Steven (NY)	Rhu	348
McCann, Peter (NY)	OrS	271	Meere, Patrick (NY)	OrS	271
McCarthy, Joseph (NY)	PlS	316	Megibow, Alec (NY)	DR	163
McCarthy, Paul (CT)	PRhu	957	Mehrara, Babak (NY)	PlS	316
McCarthy, Shirley (CT)	DR	945	Mehrotra, Bhoomi (NY)	Onc	531
McCarton, Cecelia (NY)	Ped	306	Mehta, Davendra (NY)	CE	134
McClane, Steven (CT)	CRS	899	Mehta, Rajeev (NJ)	NP	798
McClelland, Shearwood (NY)	OrS	271	Mehta, Rekha (NY)	Ge	392
McClennan, Bruce (CT)	DR	945	Mehta, Uday (NJ)	Ped	883
McClung, John (NY)	Cv	621	Meighan, Dennis (CT)	Ge	904
McConnell, Robert (NY)	EDM	168	Meirowitz, Natalie (NY)	MF	530
McCormack, Patricia (NY)	D	492	Meirowitz, Robert (NJ)	Ge	776
McCormick, Beryl (NY)	RadRO	341	Meisenberg, Gene (NY)	U	466
McCormick, Paul (NY)	NS	229	Meisler, Susan (NY)	Ped	666
McDermott, John (NY)	Oph	256	Meiteles, Lawrence (NY)	Oto	659
McFarlane-Ferreira, Yvonne (NY)	PGe	453	Meixler, Steven (NY)	Pul	673
McGinn, Joseph (NY)	T&CS	501	Meizlish, Jay (CT)	Cv	898
McGinniss, George (CT)	OrS	923	Melamed, Jonathan (NY)	Path	290
McGovern, Catherine (NY)	ObG	652	Melillo, Nicholas (NJ)	Pul	809
McGovern, Margaret (NY)	CG	586	Meller, Jose (NY)	Cv	140
McGovern, Patrick (NJ)	S	772	Mellinger, Brett (NY)	U	568
McGovern, Peter (NJ)	RE	727	Mellman, Lisa (NY)	Psyc	328
McGovern, Thomas (NY)	U	371	Melman, Martin (NY)	IM	641
McGowan, Joseph (NY)	Inf	526	Melnick, Hugh (NY)	ObG	246
McGrath, Patrick (NY)	Psyc	328	Melone, Charles (NY)	HS	187
McHugh, Margaret (NY)	Ped	306	Melton, R Christine (NY)	Oph	256
McIlveen, Stephen (NJ)	OrS	716	Melville, Gordon (NJ)	DR	860
McKee, Heather (NY)	Oph	654	Menchell, David (NY)	A&I	472

Alphabetical Listing of Doctors

Name	Specialty	Pg	Name	Specialty	Pg
Mendelowitz, Alan (NY)	Psyc	483	Mickley, Diane (CT)	IM	909
Mendelowitz, Lawrence (NY)	ObG	652	Mickley, Steven (CT)	IM	909
Mendelsohn, Michael (NY)	PO	550	Middlesworth, William (NY)	PS	303
Mendelsohn, Sara (NY)	OM	538	Middleton, John (NJ)	Inf	796
Mendelson, Joel (NJ)	A&I	872	Mieszerski, Laura (NY)	ObG	652
Mendes, Donna (NY)	VascS	379	Mignone, Biagio (NY)	Oph	655
Mendes, John (NJ)	OrS	752	Miguel, Eduardo (NJ)	IM	705
Mendoza, Ernesto (NY)	S	485	Mikkilineni, Sushmita (NJ)	PPul	757
Mendoza, Francis (NY)	OrS	272	Milanaik, Ruth (NY)	Ped	553
Mendoza, Glenn (NY)	NP	575	Milano, Andrew (NY)	Ge	178
Menegus, Mark (NY)	Cv	385	Mildvan, Donna (NY)	Inf	195
Menezes, Placido (NY)	OrS	450	Miles, Daniel (NY)	ChiN	148
Menitove, Stephen (NY)	Pul	579	Milgraum, Sandy (NJ)	D	792
Ment, Laura (CT)	ChiN	943	Milgrim, Laurence (NJ)	Oto	717
Menza, Matthew (NJ)	Psyc	808	Milite, James (NJ)	Oph	802
Menzin, Andrew (NY)	GO	524	Miller, Aaron (NY)	N	236
Merav, Avraham (NY)	T&CS	678	Miller, Andrew (NJ)	Oto	803
Mercando, Anthony (NY)	Cv	622	Miller, Daniel (NY)	FMed	631
Meredith, Gary (NY)	Rhu	563	Miller, David (NJ)	Psyc	884
Merer, David (NY)	PO	663	Miller, David (NY)	Cv	140
Merhige, Kenneth (NY)	Oph	256	Miller, Dennis (NY)	Inf	195
Merker, Edward (NY)	FMed	631	Miller, Jane (NJ)	RE	727
Mermelstein, Erwin (NJ)	Cv	790	Miller, Jeffrey (NJ)	HS	834
Mermelstein, Harold (NY)	D	627	Miller, Kenneth (CT)	Rhu	934
Mermelstein, Steve (NY)	Pul	559	Miller, Kenneth (NJ)	IC	747
Merola, Andrew (NY)	OrS	450	Miller, Kevin (CT)	S	935
Merriam, John (NY)	Oph	256	Miller, Philip (NY)	Oto	283
Messana, Ida (NY)	IM	478	Miller, Rachel (NY)	Pul	338
Messerli, Franz (NY)	Cv	140	Miller, Richard (NJ)	Pul	760
Messina, John (NJ)	PCd	718	Miller, Scott (NY)	PHO	454
Messinger, David (NY)	IC	643	Miller, Seth (CT)	OrS	923
Metz, John (NJ)	FMed	793	Miller, Seth (NY)	Ge	522
Metzger, Scott (NJ)	PM	823	Miller, Theodore (NY)	DR	163
Metzl, Jordan (NY)	SM	352	Miller-Breslow, Anne (NJ)	HS	703
Meyer, Monica (NJ)	ObG	713	Mills, Carl (NY)	U	609
Meyer, Richard (NY)	Hem	191	Mills, Christopher (NY)	S	357
Meyers, Barnett (NY)	Psyc	670	Mills, Nancy (NY)	Onc	645
Meyers, Paul (NY)	PHO	299	Milman, Perry (NY)	Ge	522
Meyers, Philip (NY)	NRad	240	Milone, Richard (NY)	Psyc	670
Meyers-Seifer, Cynthia (NJ)	PEn	823	Milsom, Jeffrey (NY)	CRS	150
Miarrostami, Rameen (NY)	Pul	460	Milstein, David (NY)	NuM	401
Mich, Robert (NJ)	IC	878	Min, Albert (NY)	Ge	178
Michaelides, Elias (CT)	Oto	955	Mindel, Joel (NY)	Oph	257
Michaelson, Richard (NJ)	Onc	748	Miner, Charles (CT)	IM	909
Michaelson, Stephen (CT)	Cv	898	Mini, Katherine (CT)	Ped	928
Michel, Ketly (NY)	ObG	246	Minikes, Neil (NJ)	A&I	691
Michelassi, Fabrizio (NY)	S	357	Minkoff, Howard (NY)	ObG	446
Michelis, Mary Ann (NJ)	A&I	691	Minkowitz, Susan (NY)	IM	204
Michelis, Michael (NY)	Nep	225	Mintz, Abraham (CT)	NS	915
Michels, Robert (NY)	Psyc	328	Mintz, Guy (NY)	Cv	511
Michler, Robert (NY)	T&CS	415	Mirra, Suzanne (NY)	Path	452

Name	Specialty	Pg	Name	Specialty	Pg
Miskovitz, Paul (NY)	Ge	178	Morrissey, Nicholas (NY)	VascS	379
Mitchell, John (NY)	Oph	257	Morrow, Jon (CT)	Path	955
Mitnick, Hal (NY)	Rhu	349	Morrow, Monica (NY)	S	358
Mitnick, Julie (NY)	DR	163	Morrow, Robert (NY)	FMed	390
Mitsumoto, Hiroshi (NY)	N	236	Morrow, Todd (NJ)	Oto	753
Mittler, Mark (NY)	NS	534	Mosca, Ralph (NY)	T&CS	365
Mittman, Neal (NY)	Nep	441	Moses, Jeffrey (NY)	IC	208
Moazed, Kambiz (NY)	Oph	257	Moseson, Michael (NY)	CRS	515
Mogan, Glen (NJ)	Ge	744	Moshe, Solomon (NY)	ChiN	386
Mogil, Laurey (NY)	Oph	448	Moskovich, Ronald (NY)	OrS	272
Mohr, JP (NY)	N	236	Moskovits, Norbert (NY)	Cv	425
Mohr, Robert (NJ)	ObG	838	Moskovits, Tibor (NY)	Hem	191
Moisa, Idel (NY)	Oto	544	Moskowitz, Bruce (NY)	Oph	257
Mojtabai, Shaparak (NY)	IM	396	Moskowitz, Craig (NY)	Onc	217
Moldover, Jonathan (NY)	PMR	310	Moskowitz, George (NY)	FMed	430
Moldwin, Robert (NY)	U	568	Moskowitz, Richard (NJ)	CRS	832
Molinelli, Bruce (CT)	S	935	Most, Richard (NY)	Oph	655
Mollin, Joel (NY)	DR	474	Motiwala, Rajeev (NY)	N	236
Molloy, Edward (CT)	IM	909	Motzer, Robert (NY)	Onc	217
Molnar, Thomas (NY)	FMed	475	Moulton, Thomas (NY)	PHO	406
Molofsky, Walter (NY)	ChiN	148	Moussa, Ghias (NJ)	Cv	767
Monasebian, Douglas (NY)	PlS	317	Moynihan, Brian (NY)	FMed	520
Mondrow, Daniel (NJ)	Cv	790	Moynihan, Gavan (NY)	D	587
Mongillo, Nicholas (CT)	Ped	928	Muchnick, Richard (NY)	Oph	257
Monrad, E Scott (NY)	Cv	385	Mueller, F Carl (CT)	Psyc	930
Montero, Carlos (NY)	OrS	542	Mueller, Richard (NY)	Cv	140
Montgomery, Kenneth (NJ)	OrS	839	Muggia, Franco (NY)	Onc	217
Monti, Louis (NY)	Ped	306	Muhlbauer, Helen (NY)	Psyc	328
Moore, Anne (NY)	Onc	217	Mukherjee, Tanmoy (NY)	RE	344
Moore, Frank (NJ)	NS	711	Muldoon, Lawrence (CT)	U	937
Moore, Joanne (NY)	Psyc	328	Muldoon, Thomas (NY)	Oph	257
Moorjani, Harish (NY)	Inf	638	Mulford, Gregory (NJ)	PMR	841
Moorthy, Chitti (NY)	RadRO	674	Mulgaonkar, Shamkant (NJ)	Nep	749
Mootabar, Hamid (NY)	MF	644	Mulhall, John (NY)	U	371
Moqtaderi, Farideh (NY)	PM	288	Mullen, David (CT)	DR	901
Moraille, Pascale (NJ)	Psyc	771	Mullen, Edward (NY)	RadRO	561
Moreau, Donna (NY)	ChAP	146	Mullen, Michael (NY)	Inf	195
Morehouse, Helen (NY)	DR	388	Multz, Alan (NY)	Pul	559
Morelli, Alan (CT)	Ped	928	Mulvehill, Joseph (NY)	IM	204
Morello, Robert (NY)	Oph	655	Mulvey, Lauri (NJ)	Oph	781
Moreta, Henry (NY)	N	596	Munver, Ravi (NJ)	U	732
Morgan, Charles (CT)	Psyc	930	Muraca, Glenn (NY)	FMed	475
Morgan, Daniel (NY)	OrS	450	Murali, Raj (NY)	NS	649
Morgan, James (CT)	Ped	958	Murphy, Ramon (NY)	Ped	306
Moriarty, Daniel (NJ)	Onc	878	Murphy, Robert (NJ)	Ped	823
Morman, Manuel (NJ)	D	697	Murphy, Robyn (NJ)	DR	833
Morris, Elizabeth (NY)	DR	163	Murray, Henry (NY)	Inf	196
Morris, James (NY)	N	650	Murray, Simon (NJ)	IM	778
Morris, Robert (NY)	Oph	598	Muskin, Philip (NY)	Psyc	328
Morrison, R Sean (NY)	Ger	183	Musto, Anthony (CT)	Oph	920
Morrison, Susan (NJ)	PA&I	754	Mutterperl, Mitchell (NJ)	IM	768

Alphabetical Listing of Doctors

Name	Specialty	Pg	Name	Specialty	Pg
Myerson, Merle (NY)	Cv	140	Neistadt, L Daniel (NY)	DR	163
Myskowski, Patricia (NY)	D	156	Nelson, Alan (CT)	Ge	905
Myssiorek, David (NY)	Oto	283	Nelson, David (NY)	Oph	540
			Nelson, Deena (NY)	IM	204
			Nelson, John (NY)	Hem	638
			Nelson, John (NY)	OrS	657
N			Nelson, Judith (NY)	Pul	338
			Nelson, William (NY)	ObG	653
Nachajon, Roberto (NJ)	PPul	854	Neophytides, Andreas (NY)	N	236
Nachman, Sharon (NY)	PInf	602	Nepola, Neil (NY)	FMed	493
Nadelman, Robert (NY)	Inf	638	Nerwen, Clifford (NY)	Ped	553
Nadzam, Geoffrey (CT)	S	962	Neschis, Ronald (NY)	Psyc	670
Nagler, Harris (NY)	U	371	Neu, Natalie (NY)	PInf	300
Nagler, Jerry (NY)	Ge	178	Neuberg, Gerald (NY)	Cv	385
Nahass, Ronald (NJ)	Inf	862	Neuwirth, Michael (NY)	OrS	272
Nahm, Frederick (CT)	N	916	Nevin, Marie (NJ)	EDM	833
Naidich, David (NY)	DR	163	New, Maria (NY)	PEn	295
Naidorf, Ellen (CT)	D	900	Newburger, Amy (NY)	D	627
Najarian, James (NJ)	Nep	837	Newcorn, Jeffrey (NY)	ChAP	146
Najjar, Sessine (NJ)	Inf	850	Newhouse, Jeffrey (NY)	DR	163
Najjar, Souhel (NY)	N	496	Newman, Elliot (NY)	S	358
Naka, Yoshifumi (NY)	T&CS	365	Newman, Fredric (CT)	PlS	929
Nalbandian, Matthew (NY)	VascS	379	Newman, Lawrence (NY)	N	237
Namerow, David (NJ)	Ped	722	Newman, Leonard (NY)	PGe	662
Nanus, David (NY)	Onc	217	Newman, Scott (NY)	PlS	668
Napolitano, Joseph (NJ)	Oph	802	Newman, Stephen (NY)	N	536
Narins, Rhoda (NY)	D	627	Newman-Cedar, Meryl (NY)	Ped	306
Narula, Amarjot (NJ)	Psyc	725	Newmark, Ian (NY)	Pul	559
Narula, Pramod (NY)	PPul	455	Newton, Michael (NY)	Oph	257
Narwal, Shivinder (NY)	PGe	453	Ng, John (NY)	RadRO	341
Nascimento, Joao (CT)	Rhu	934	Ngai, Pakkay (NJ)	PPul	720
Nash, Bernard (NY)	Inf	592	Ngeow, Jeffrey (NY)	PM	288
Nash, Ira (NY)	Cv	512	Nguyen, Khanh (NY)	T&CS	365
Nash, Thomas (NY)	Pul	338	Nicholas, Stephen (NY)	OrS	272
Nass, Jack (NY)	Psyc	604	Nickerson, Katherine (NY)	Rhu	349
Nass, Richard (NY)	Oto	283	Nicosia, Thomas (NY)	Cv	512
Nass, Ruth (NY)	ChiN	148	Niederman, Michael (NY)	Pul	559
Nassberg, Barton (NJ)	EDM	817	Nierman, David (NY)	CCM	473
Natale, Benjamin (NJ)	Oph	880	Nightingale, Jeffrey (NY)	Oph	257
Nath, Sunil (NY)	Pul	484	Nikias, George (NJ)	Ge	701
Nattis, Richard (NY)	Oph	598	Nimaroff, Michael (NY)	ObG	538
Nauheim, Richard (NY)	Oph	540	Nini, Kevin (NJ)	PlS	808
Navot, Daniel (NJ)	RE	728	Nininger, James (NY)	Psyc	328
Neal, Wendy (NJ)	AM	738	Nisonson, Barton (NY)	SM	352
Nealon, Nancy (NY)	N	236	Nissenblatt, Michael (NJ)	Onc	798
Neelakantappa, Kotresha (NY)	Nep	441	Nitti, Victor (NY)	U	372
Neely, Michael (NY)	PMR	310	Nitzberg, Richard (NJ)	S	887
Neeson, Francis (CT)	Cv	898	Nizin, Joel (NJ)	CRS	695
Neibart, Eric (NY)	Inf	196	Nori, Dattatreyudu (NY)	RadRO	341
Neibart, Richard (NJ)	T&CS	826	Norton, Larry (NY)	Onc	217
Neiman, Deborah (NJ)	IM	862	Nosher, John (NJ)	VIR	812

Name	Specialty	Pg
Nosko, Michael (NJ)	NS	799
Notar-Francesco, Vincent (NY)	Ge	432
Notaro, Antoinette (NY)	D	587
Noto, Richard (NY)	PEn	661
Notterman, Robyn (NJ)	D	775
Nouri, Shahin (NY)	N	444
Novack, Stuart (CT)	Rhu	934
Novick, Brian (NY)	A&I	507
Novick, Mark (NY)	DR	163
Novitch, Richard (NY)	Pul	673
Nowak, Eugene (NY)	S	358
Noy, Ron (NY)	SM	352
Noyes, Nicole (NY)	RE	344
Nucci, Annamaria (NJ)	Psyc	759
Nucci-Sack, Anne (NY)	AM	130
Nunes, Edward (NY)	Psyc	328
Nussbaum, Michel (NY)	Ge	476

O

Name	Specialty	Pg
O'Brien, Daryl (NJ)	Ped	722
O'Brien, Francis (NY)	Cv	140
O'Connell, Joseph (CT)	PlS	929
O'Connor, Brian (NJ)	PCd	755
O'Connor, Owen (NY)	Onc	217
O'Connor, Patrick (CT)	IM	949
O'Donnell, Timothy (NJ)	Pul	843
O'Hea, Brian (NY)	S	608
O'Leary, Patrick (NY)	OrS	272
O'Malley, Grace (NY)	Oph	598
O'Malley, Martin (NY)	OrS	272
O'Reilly, Eileen (NY)	Onc	218
O'Reilly, Richard (NY)	PHO	299
O'Shaughnessy, Althea (NJ)	RE	785
Ober, David (NY)	N	576
Oberfield, Richard (NY)	Psyc	329
Oberfield, Sharon (NY)	PEn	295
Obstbaum, Stephen (NY)	Oph	258
Odaimi, Marcel (NY)	Onc	495
Odel, Jeffrey (NY)	Oph	258
Oeffinger, Kevin (NY)	Ped	307
Oestreicher, Mark (CT)	D	900
Offit, Kenneth (NY)	Onc	218
Oghia, Hady (NY)	Ped	456
Oh, William (NY)	Onc	218
Oh, Youn (NJ)	N	800
Oh, Young (NY)	OrS	657
Oko, Piotr (NJ)	Ped	770
Olanescu, Andrea (NY)	ObG	481

Name	Specialty	Pg
Olanow, C Warren (NY)	N	237
Olarte, Marcelo (NY)	N	237
Olds, David (NY)	Psyc	329
Oleske, James (NJ)	PInf	756
Olichney, John (NY)	IM	204
Olin, Craig (CT)	IM	909
Oliver, Gregory (NJ)	CRS	791
Olsewski, John (NY)	OrS	403
Olson, Robert (NJ)	PlS	865
Onesti, Stephen (NY)	NS	534
Ong, Lawrence (NY)	IC	594
Opler, Lewis (NY)	Psyc	670
Oppedisano, Carlyn (NY)	Ped	409
Oppenheim, Jeffrey (NY)	NS	576
Oppenheimer, John (NY)	IM	593
Oratz, Ruth (NY)	Onc	218
Orazi, Attilio (NY)	Path	290
Orbuch, Philip (NY)	D	157
Ordorica, Steven (NY)	ObG	246
Orentreich, David (NY)	D	157
Oribe, Emilio (NY)	N	480
Orlow, Seth (NY)	D	157
Ornstein, Matthew (NY)	Rhu	349
Orsher, Stuart (NY)	IM	204
Orsini, William (NJ)	D	816
Ortiz, Orlando (NY)	NRad	537
Osborne, Michael (NY)	S	358
Osei-Tutu, John (NY)	Psyc	411
Oshman, Robin (CT)	D	900
Osleeb, Craig (NY)	A&I	617
Osnoss, Kenneth (CT)	IM	909
Ossias, A Lawrence (NY)	Hem	191
Ostad, Ariel (NY)	D	157
Oster, Martin (NY)	Onc	218
Ostrer, Harry (NY)	CG	387
Ostriker, Glenn (CT)	Oph	920
Ostrow, Stanley (NY)	Onc	594
Ott, Allen (NY)	ObG	597
Ottaviano, Lawrence (NY)	Ge	178
Owens, George (NY)	U	680
Oz, Mehmet (NY)	T&CS	365
Ozkaynak, Mehmet Fevzi (NY)	PHO	662

P

Name	Specialty	Pg
Paccione, Jeffrey (NY)	Oph	258
Pace, Benjamin (NY)	S	486
Pachter, H Leon (NY)	S	358
Pacia, Steven (NY)	N	237

Alphabetical Listing of Doctors

Name	Specialty	Pg	Name	Specialty	Pg
Packer, Samuel (NY)	Oph	540	Patel, Aman (NY)	NS	229
Padgett, Douglas (NY)	OrS	272	Patel, Amit (NJ)	VascS	845
Padilla, Maria (NY)	Pul	338	Patel, Jitendra (NY)	Rhu	462
Paget, Stephen (NY)	Rhu	349	Pathare, Pradip (CT)	RadRO	933
Pahuja, Murlidhar (NY)	S	501	Patrick, Sharon (NY)	MF	210
Paidas, Michael (CT)	MF	949	Patrizio, Pasquale (CT)	RE	960
Paiusco, A Dino (NY)	Cv	425	Patterson, Francis (NJ)	OrS	753
Pak, Jayoung (NJ)	ChiN	740	Pattner, Austin (NJ)	Nep	710
Palaia, David (NY)	PlS	668	Paty, Philip (NY)	S	358
Palatt, Terry (NY)	T&CS	608	Paul, Edward (NY)	AdP	129
Palese, Michael (NY)	U	372	Paul, Elliot (NY)	U	568
Palestro, Christopher (NY)	NuM	537	Paul, Matthew (CT)	Oph	920
Palsky, Glenn (NJ)	Ped	783	Pavlakis, Steven (NY)	ChiN	426
Paltzik, Robert (NY)	D	516	Pavlick, Anna (NY)	Onc	218
Pandit-Taskar, Neeta (NY)	NuM	241	Pavlov, Helene (NY)	DR	164
Panella, Vincent (NJ)	Ge	701	Pawel, Michael (NY)	Psyc	329
Panicek, David (NY)	DR	163	Pearl, Michael (NY)	GO	591
Pannone, John (NY)	Nep	441	Pearlstein, Eric (NY)	Oph	448
Panza, Robert (NJ)	Ped	883	Pechman, Karen (NY)	PMR	667
Panzner, Elizabeth (NJ)	Ped	883	Peck, Valerie (NY)	EDM	168
Papadakos, Stylianos (NY)	IC	478	Pecker, Mark (NY)	IM	205
Papish, Steven (NJ)	Onc	836	Pecora, Andrew (NJ)	Onc	708
Papp, Laszlo (NY)	Psyc	329	Pedinoff, Andrew (NJ)	A&I	859
Pappas, Steven (NY)	IM	642	Pedley, Timothy (NY)	N	237
Pappas, Thomas (NY)	Cv	512	Pegler, Cynthia (NY)	AM	130
Pappert, Amy (NJ)	D	860	Pelavin, Martin (NJ)	IM	705
Parashar, Bhupesh (NY)	RadRO	341	Pellicci, Paul (NY)	OrS	273
Parekh, Aruna (NY)	NP	595	Pellicone, John (NY)	Pul	579
Parikh, Manish (NY)	IC	208	Peng, Benjamin (NY)	U	372
Paris, Barbara (NY)	Ger	433	Penzer, Jason (NY)	CRS	150
Parisier, Simon (NY)	Oto	283	Pepe, John (NY)	Nep	496
Park, Bernard (NJ)	T&CS	731	Pereira, Frederick (NY)	D	474
Park, Kenneth (NJ)	PM	718	Pereira, Stephen (NJ)	S	730
Park, Tae (NY)	RadRO	606	Perelstein, Eduardo (NY)	PNep	300
Parker, Robert (NY)	PHO	601	Perez-Soler, Roman (NY)	Onc	398
Parks, Michael (NY)	OrS	272	Perin, Noel (NY)	NS	229
Parles, James (NY)	Ped	603	Perin, Patrick (NJ)	A&I	691
Parnell, Vincent (NY)	PS	551	Perl, Harold (NJ)	NP	709
Parnes, Eliezer (NY)	Nep	442	Perlman, Barry (NY)	Psyc	671
Parness, Ira (NY)	PCd	293	Perlman, David (NY)	Inf	196
Parrish, Edward (NY)	Rhu	349	Perlman, Donald (NJ)	A&I	738
Pascal, Mark (NJ)	Onc	708	Perlman, Jeffrey (NY)	NP	223
Pasik, Deborah (NJ)	Rhu	843	Perlman, Philip (NY)	Oto	544
Pasmantier, Mark (NY)	Onc	218	Perron, Reed (NJ)	N	712
Pasquale, Jack (NY)	IM	478	Perrotti, John (NY)	PlS	317
Pass, Harvey (NY)	T&CS	365	Perry, Arthur (NJ)	PlS	865
Pass, Helen (CT)	S	935	Perry, Bradford (NY)	Psyc	671
Pass, Robert (NY)	PCd	405	Perry, Henry (NY)	Oph	540
Passarelli, Marianne (CT)	U	963	Perry, Richard (NY)	ChAP	146
Passaretti, David (CT)	PlS	930	Perry-Bottinger, Lynne (NY)	Cv	622
Passeri, Daniel (CT)	S	935	Persing, John (CT)	PlS	958

Name	Specialty	Pg	Name	Specialty	Pg
Persky, Mark (NY)	Oto	283	Politsky, Jeffrey (NJ)	N	879
Pesce, Joseph (CT)	D	900	Polkow, Melvin (NJ)	Pul	726
Peschel, Richard (CT)	RadRO	960	Pollack, Brian (CT)	Cv	898
Peterson, Stephen (NY)	IM	642	Pollack, Geoffrey (NY)	Oto	284
Petito, Frank (NY)	N	237	Pollack, Jed (NY)	RadRO	561
Petrone, Sylvia (NJ)	S	762	Pollack, Shoshannah (NJ)	D	850
Petrossian, George (NY)	IC	529	Pollak, Harvey (NY)	IM	528
Petrylak, Daniel (CT)	Onc	951	Pollina, Robert (NY)	VascS	609
Pettei, Michael (NY)	PGe	549	Pollock, Alan (NY)	Inf	196
Pfaff, H Charles (NY)	DR	164	Pollock, Jeffrey (NJ)	N	879
Pfeffer, Cynthia (NY)	Psyc	329	Pollock, Roger (NJ)	OrS	716
Pfister, David (NY)	Onc	218	Pollowitz, James (NY)	A&I	618
Philipp, Claire (NJ)	Hem	795	Polsky, Bruce (NY)	Inf	196
Phillips, Elizabeth (NY)	Onc	645	Pomerantz, Daniel (NY)	IM	642
Phillips, Howard (NY)	Oph	655	Pomeroy, John (NY)	ChAP	586
Phillips, Malcolm (NY)	Cv	385	Pomp, Alfons (NY)	S	358
Phillips, Robin (NY)	ObG	246	Ponamgi, Suri (NJ)	PlS	724
Pianka, George (NY)	OrS	657	Poneros, John (NY)	Ge	179
Picciano, Anne (NJ)	FMed	793	Ponterio, Jane (NY)	ObG	496
Piccione, Paul (NY)	Ge	432	Poole, John (NJ)	S	730
Piccirilli, Dora (NY)	FMed	631	Poon, Eric (NY)	Ped	307
Pici, Ralph (NY)	PMR	667	Poon, Michael (NY)	Cv	585
Picone, Frank (NJ)	A&I	815	Poplausky, Maurice (NY)	DR	629
Pidoriano, Arthur (NY)	OrS	658	Poppas, Dix (NY)	U	372
Pieczara, Beata (NJ)	Onc	708	Popper, Laura (NY)	Ped	307
Piepmeier, Joseph (CT)	NS	952	Porder, Joseph (NY)	Cv	141
Pile-Spellman, John (NY)	NRad	537	Poretsky, Leonid (NY)	EDM	168
Pincus, Emile (NJ)	ChAP	695	Porges, Andrew (NY)	Rhu	563
Pincus, Robert (NY)	Oto	283	Port, Abraham (NY)	DR	517
Pines, Jeffrey (NY)	Psyc	329	Port, Elisa (NY)	S	358
Pinke, James (CT)	Oph	920	Port, Jeffrey (NY)	T&CS	366
Pinke, Robert (NJ)	Oph	839	Portenoy, Russell (NY)	Hospice &	
Pinney, Sean (NY)	Cv	140	Palliative Med	193	
Pinsky, Steven (NY)	PM	545	Portlock, Carol (NY)	Onc	219
Pinto, Marguerite (CT)	Path	926	Portnoy, William (NY)	Oto	284
Piskun, Andrew (NJ)	OrS	803	Porwancher, Richard (NJ)	Inf	777
Pitchumoni, Capecomorin (NJ)	Ge	794	Posner, David (NY)	Pul	338
Pitman, Gerald (NY)	PlS	317	Posner, Jerome (NY)	N	237
Piwoz, Julia (NJ)	PInf	720	Posner, Marshall (NY)	Onc	219
Pizzarello, Louis (NY)	Oph	598	Possick, Paul (NJ)	D	697
Pizzurro, Joseph (NJ)	OrS	716	Post, Kalmon (NY)	NS	229
Plancher, Kevin (NY)	OrS	273	Post, Martin (NY)	Cv	141
Plestis, Konstadinos (NY)	T&CS	366	Postley, John (NY)	IM	205
Plumser, Allan (NJ)	Ge	794	Potter, Hollis (NY)	DR	164
Pochapin, Mark (NY)	Ge	178	Potter, William (CT)	Oph	920
Podell, Richard (NJ)	FMed	875	Potters, Louis (NY)	RadRO	561
Podwal, Mark (NY)	D	157	Powell, Jeffrey (NY)	EDM	630
Polatsch, Daniel (NY)	HS	187	Poynor, Elizabeth (NY)	GO	185
Polifroni, Nicholas (CT)	OrS	923	Prabhu, H Sudhakar (NY)	Cv	425
Polin, Richard (NY)	NP	223	Prager, Kenneth (NY)	Pul	338
Polis, Laurie (NY)	D	157	Prakash, Anaka (NJ)	Ge	768

Alphabetical Listing of Doctors

Name	Specialty	Pg
Preis, Oded (NY)	Ped	456
Preminger, Mark (NJ)	CE	692
Press, Robert (NY)	Inf	196
Presti, Salvatore (NY)	PCd	452
Pretto, Zorayda (NY)	EDM	630
Preven, David (NY)	Psyc	329
Prezant, David (NY)	Pul	413
Prezioso, Paula (NY)	Ped	307
Price, Andrew (NY)	OrS	273
Price, Gary (CT)	PlS	958
Price, Thomas (NY)	Cv	622
Primas, Ronald (NY)	IM	205
Prince, Alice (NY)	Ped	307
Prince, Andrew (NY)	Oph	258
Prince, Martin (NY)	DR	164
Principe, David (NJ)	MF	707
Prioleau, Philip (NY)	D	157
Procaccino, John (NY)	CRS	515
Proctor, Deborah (CT)	Ge	946
Proskin, Wendy (NY)	Ped	666
Provenzano, Anthony (NY)	Onc	645
Provet, John (NY)	U	372
Pruzan-Clain, Debra (CT)	D	900
Pruzansky, Mark (NY)	HS	187
Prystowsky, Janet (NY)	D	157
Prywes, Arnold (NY)	Oph	540
Przybylski, Gregory (NJ)	NS	799
Puccio, Carmelo (NY)	Onc	646
Pucillo, Anthony (NY)	Cv	622
Puder, Douglas (NY)	Ped	578
Pujol-Morato, Fernando (NY)	Inf	435
Pumill, Rick (NJ)	Cv	694
Purtill, William (NY)	VascS	569
Putignano, Joseph (NY)	U	680
Putman, Donald (NJ)	PCd	755
Putterman, Eric (NY)	SM	607
Pyo, Daniel (NJ)	PlS	842

Q

Name	Specialty	Pg
Qadir, Shuja (NY)	Cv	472
Quaegebeur, Jan (NY)	PS	303
Quagliarello, John (NY)	RE	344
Quagliarello, Vincent (CT)	Inf	948
Quartell, Anthony (NJ)	ObG	750
Quest, Donald (NY)	NS	229
Quinn, Joseph (NY)	Ped	603
Quittell, Lynne (NY)	PPul	664

R

Name	Specialty	Pg
Raab, Edward (NY)	Oph	258
Rabin, Aaron (NJ)	N	712
Rabinowicz, Morris (NY)	Ped	553
Rabinowitz, Simon (NY)	PGe	453
Rabinowitz, Stephen (CT)	Oph	920
Raboy, Adley (NY)	U	502
Rackoff, Paula (NY)	Rhu	349
Radin, Alan (CT)	IM	909
Radin, Allen (NY)	Rhu	349
Radwaner, Bradley (NY)	Cv	141
Raffalli, John (NY)	Inf	638
Rafizadeh, Farhad (NJ)	PlS	842
Ragnarsson, Kristjan (NY)	PMR	311
Ragno, Philip (NY)	Cv	512
Rago, Thomas (CT)	HS	906
Ragone, Philip (NY)	N	536
Ragukonis, Thomas (NJ)	PM	718
Rahaman, Jamal (NY)	GO	185
Rahmin, Michael (NJ)	Ge	702
Rai, Kanti (NY)	Hem	525
Rajdeo, Heena (NY)	S	677
Rajpal, Sanjeev (NY)	S	464
Rakos, Gerald (CT)	NP	913
Rakow, Joel (NJ)	DR	698
Rakowitz, Frederic (NY)	IM	528
Rakowski, Thomas (NJ)	Onc	708
Ralabate, James (CT)	IM	910
Raman, Bharathi (NY)	Ger	183
Ramaswamy, Prema (NY)	PCd	452
Rambler, Louis (NJ)	DR	698
Ramgopal, Mekala (NY)	Ge	476
Ramirez, Mark (NY)	Onc	398
Ramsay, David (NY)	D	157
Rand, James (NY)	Ge	476
Randolph, Audrey (NY)	PMR	667
Rangraj, Madhu (NY)	S	677
Raniolo, Robert (NY)	S	677
Ransom, Mark (NJ)	RE	855
Ranta, Jeffrey (CT)	U	937
Rao, Yalamanchi (NY)	A&I	422
Rao, Yalamanchili (NY)	A&I	491
Raoof, Suhail (NY)	Pul	460
Rapaport, Jeffrey (NJ)	D	697
Rapaport, Robert (NY)	PEn	295
Raphael, Bruce (NY)	Hem	191
Rapoport, David (NY)	Pul	338
Rapoport, Samuel (NY)	N	237
Raptis, George (NY)	Onc	219
Rashba, Eric (NY)	CE	583

Name	Specialty	Pg	Name	Specialty	Pg
Rashbaum, Ira (NY)	PMR	311	Remy, Prospere (NY)	Ge	392
Raska, Karel (NJ)	Cv	832	Ren-Fielding, Christine (NY)	S	359
Raskin, Elsa (CT)	PlS	930	Rennert, Nancy (CT)	EDM	902
Raskin, Jonathan (NY)	Pul	339	Rentrop, K Peter (NY)	Cv	141
Raskin, Keith (NY)	HS	187	Repice, Michael (NY)	Rhu	607
Rastegar, Asghar (CT)	Nep	952	Reppucci, Vincent (CT)	Oph	920
Rathauser, Robert (NJ)	ObG	801	Resmovits, Marvin (NY)	Ped	553
Ratner, Desiree (NY)	D	158	Resor, Louise (CT)	N	916
Ratner, Lloyd (NY)	S	358	Respler, Don (NJ)	PO	720
Ratner, Lynn (NY)	Onc	219	Resta, Christine (NY)	EDM	429
Raucher, Harold (NY)	Ped	307	Restifo, Richard (CT)	PlS	958
Rawlins, Bernard (NY)	OrS	273	Rettig, Michael (NY)	HS	188
Ray, Audell (NY)	Oph	655	Reuter, Victor (NY)	Path	291
Raymond, Gerald (NJ)	Ped	783	Rezac, Craig (NJ)	CRS	791
Raza, Azra (NY)	Onc	219	Rezvani, Fred (NJ)	ObG	713
Razaboni, Rosa (NY)	PlS	317	Rho, Dae (NY)	PMR	311
Rebarber, Andrei (NY)	MF	210	Rice, Stephen (NJ)	SM	825
Recht, Michael (NY)	DR	164	Rich, Daniel (NY)	OrS	543
Rechter, Lesley (NY)	FMed	520	Rich, Glenn (CT)	EDM	902
Reckler, Jon (NY)	U	372	Richards, Steven (NJ)	U	811
Reda, Dominick (NY)	Nep	648	Richardson, William (NJ)	Psyc	884
Reda, Edward (NY)	U	680	Richel, Peter (NY)	Ped	666
Reddy, Mallikarjuna (NY)	FMed	475	Richheimer, Michael (NY)	A&I	422
Reding, Michael (NY)	N	650	Richlin, Spencer (CT)	RE	933
Redlich, Carrie (CT)	Pul	959	Richman, Daniel (NY)	PM	289
Redner, Arlene (NY)	PHO	549	Richstone, Lee (NY)	U	568
Rednor, Jeffrey (NJ)	FMed	776	Richter, Edwin (CT)	PMR	929
Reed, William (NY)	S	565	Ricketti, Anthony (NJ)	A&I	775
Reede, Deborah (NY)	DR	429	Ridge, Gerald (NY)	IM	642
Rees, Ellen (NY)	Psyc	329	Rie, Jonathan (NY)	Nep	648
Regard, Monique (NY)	ObG	653	Rieber, Jonathan (NY)	Ge	179
Reich, Raymond (NY)	Oph	448	Riechers, Roger (NY)	U	680
Reich, Steven (NJ)	OrS	803	Rieder, Jessica (NY)	AM	383
Reicher, Oscar (NJ)	OrS	853	Rieger, Mark (NJ)	OrS	839
Reichstein, Robert (NY)	Cv	141	Rifkin, Matthew (NY)	DR	164
Reid, Malcolm (NY)	PMR	311	Rigel, Darrell (NY)	D	158
Reiffel, Robert (NY)	PlS	668	Rigolosi, Robert (NJ)	Nep	710
Reilly, James (NY)	ObG	497	Rigtrup, Edward (NJ)	Ped	757
Reilly, John (NY)	OrS	498	Riina, Howard (NY)	NS	229
Reilly, Kevin (NY)	ObG	401	Riles, Thomas (NY)	VascS	379
Reilly, Thomas (NY)	IM	478	Riley, David (NJ)	Pul	809
Reiner, Dan (NY)	S	565	Ring, Kenneth (NJ)	U	887
Reiner, Mark (NY)	S	359	Ritch, Robert (NY)	Oph	258
Reinitz, Elizabeth (NY)	Rhu	675	Ritterband, David (NY)	Oph	258
Reisberg, Barry (NY)	GerPsy	183	Rivera, Yadyra (NJ)	Onc	708
Reisner, Michelle (NJ)	Ger	768	Riviello, James (NY)	ChiN	148
Reison, Dennis (NJ)	Cv	694	Rizk, Samieh (NY)	Oto	284
Reizis, Igal (NY)	ObG	446	Rizvi, Hasan (NY)	Onc	594
Rekate, Harold (NY)	NS	534	Rizvi, Naiyer (NY)	Onc	219
Relkin, Norman (NY)	N	237	Robbins, Kim (CT)	Oph	920
Relland, Maureen (NY)	Oph	258	Robbins, Michael (NY)	Cv	472

Alphabetical Listing of Doctors

Name	Specialty	Pg	Name	Specialty	Pg
Robbins, Noah (NY)	Inf	395	Rose, Michael (NJ)	PlS	824
Robert, Marie (CT)	Ped	958	Rosell, Frank (NY)	T&CS	501
Roberti, M Isabel (NJ)	PNep	756	Rosello, Lori (NY)	Ped	307
Roberts, J Kirk (NY)	N	238	Roseman, Bruce (NY)	ChiN	624
Roberts, Kenneth (CT)	RadRO	960	Rosemarin, Jack (NY)	Ge	635
Roberts, Larry (NY)	U	680	Rosen, Allen (NJ)	PlS	759
Roberts, Matthew (NY)	OrS	273	Rosen, Arie (NJ)	Oto	717
Robilotti, James (NY)	Ge	179	Rosen, Arnold (NY)	Psyc	330
Robinson, Michael (NY)	PMR	578	Rosen, Bruce (NY)	Psyc	604
Robinson, Newell (NY)	T&CS	566	Rosen, Douglas (NY)	D	387
Roboz, Gail (NY)	Onc	219	Rosen, Evelyn (NY)	GerPsy	433
Robson, Mark (NY)	Onc	219	Rosen, Jeffrey (NY)	SM	485
Rochelson, Burton (NY)	MF	530	Rosen, Mark (NY)	Pul	560
Rochester, Carolyn (CT)	Pul	959	Rosen, Michael (NY)	Nep	648
Rochford, Joseph (NJ)	Psyc	866	Rosen, Nedra (NY)	IM	205
Rockman, Caron (NY)	VascS	379	Rosen, Norman (NY)	Onc	646
Rodeo, Scott (NY)	SM	352	Rosen, Robert (NY)	VIR	376
Rodgers, I Rand (NY)	Oph	259	Rosen, Tove (NY)	NP	223
Rodino, William (NY)	VascS	502	Rosenbaum, Alfred (NY)	RadRO	342
Rodke, Gae (NY)	ObG	246	Rosenbaum, Daniel (NY)	N	444
Rodriguez, Lorna (NJ)	GO	795	Rosenbaum, Jeffrey (NJ)	Oto	804
Rodriguez-Sains, Rene (NY)	Oph	259	Rosenbaum, Marlon (NY)	Cv	141
Roelke, Marc (NJ)	CE	739	Rosenbaum, Michael (NY)	Ped	307
Rogal, Gary (NJ)	Cv	739	Rosenbaum, Pearl (NY)	Oph	402
Rogers, David (NY)	VIR	487	Rosenbaum, Robert (NJ)	EDM	874
Roland, J Thomas (NY)	Oto	284	Rosenberg, Craig (NY)	PMR	603
Roland, Robert (NJ)	Inf	877	Rosenberg, David (NY)	Oto	284
Rolandelli, Rolando (NJ)	S	844	Rosenberg, Gene (NJ)	U	732
Romagnoli, Mario (NY)	Inf	196	Rosenberg, Kenneth (NY)	AdP	129
Romanelli, John (NY)	Oph	598	Rosenberg, Michael (NJ)	N	800
Romanello, Paul (NY)	Cv	141	Rosenberg, Michael (NY)	PlS	668
Romano, Alicia (NY)	PEn	661	Rosenberg, Vladimiro (NY)	S	359
Romano, Angela (NY)	PCd	547	Rosenberg, Zehava (NY)	DR	164
Romano, John (NY)	D	158	Rosenblatt, Ruth (NY)	DR	164
Romano, Rosario (NY)	IM	593	Rosenblatt, William (NY)	PlS	317
Romanowitz, Harry (CT)	Ped	928	Rosenblum, Bruce (NJ)	NS	820
Romas, Nicholas (NY)	U	372	Rosenblum, Marc (NY)	Path	291
Romero, Carlos (NY)	S	565	Rosenfeld, Alvin (CT)	ChAP	899
Romeu, Jose (NY)	Ge	179	Rosenfeld, David (NJ)	Psyc	725
Romita, Mauro (NY)	PlS	317	Rosenfeld, David (NY)	RE	562
Rommer, James (NJ)	IM	747	Rosenfeld, David (NJ)	DR	792
Romo, Thomas (NY)	Oto	284	Rosenfeld, Richard (NY)	PO	455
Roohi, Fereydoon (NY)	N	444	Rosenfeld, Stanley (NY)	DR	165
Roose, Steven (NY)	Psyc	330	Rosenfeld, Suzanne (NY)	Ped	307
Root, Barry (NY)	PMR	554	Rosenfeld, Walter (NJ)	AM	831
Rosa, Joseph (CT)	EDM	902	Rosengart, Todd (NY)	T&CS	608
Rosch, Elliott (NY)	IM	642	Rosenkilde, Carl (NY)	N	650
Rose, Donald (NY)	OrS	273	Rosenstein, Elliot (NJ)	Rhu	886
Rose, Elliott (NY)	PlS	317	Rosenstein, Roger (NJ)	HS	703
Rose, Howard (NY)	OrS	273	Rosenstock, Arthur (CT)	PlS	930
Rose, John (NJ)	U	827	Rosenstreich, David (NY)	A&I	383

Name	Specialty	Pg	Name	Specialty	Pg
Rosenthal, David (NY)	EDM	519	Rubenstein, Jack (NY)	IM	528
Rosenthal, Jeanne (NY)	Oph	259	Rubin, Cheryl (NY)	OrS	577
Rosenthal, Jesse (NY)	Psyc	330	Rubin, David (NY)	CE	618
Rosenthal, Kenneth (NY)	Oph	541	Rubin, James (NY)	A&I	132
Rosenthal, Richard (NY)	Psyc	330	Rubin, Kenneth (NJ)	Psyc	825
Rosenthal, Sheldon (NY)	U	466	Rubin, Kenneth (NJ)	Ge	702
Rosenwaks, Zev (NY)	RE	344	Rubin, Laurence (NY)	Oph	541
Rosenwasser, Melvin (NY)	HS	188	Rubin, Lorry (NY)	PInf	550
Roses, Daniel (NY)	S	359	Rubin, Marc (NJ)	Ge	777
Rosh, Joel (NJ)	PGe	841	Rubin, Moshe (NY)	Ge	179
Roshan, Daniel (NY)	MF	210	Rubin, Steven (NY)	Oph	541
Rosman, Lawrence (NY)	EDM	474	Rubino, Francesco (NY)	S	359
Rosner, Bruce (NJ)	Ge	777	Rubinoff, Mitchell (NJ)	Ge	702
Rosner, Louis (NY)	Oto	544	Rubinstein, Arye (NY)	A&I	384
Rosner, Richard (NY)	Psyc	330	Rubinstein, Boris (NY)	ChAP	623
Rosner, Saran (NY)	NS	649	Rubinstein, Mort (NY)	Psyc	330
Ross, Howard (NJ)	CRS	816	Rucker, Steve (NY)	IM	528
Ross, Marc (NY)	PMR	457	Ruddy, Michael (NJ)	Nep	779
Ross, Steven (NY)	Psyc	330	Ruderman, Marvin (NJ)	N	750
Rossakis, Constantine (NJ)	Cv	694	Rudick, A Joseph (NY)	Oph	259
Rossi, Dennis (NY)	DR	517	Rudikoff, Donald (NY)	D	387
Rossman, Barry (NJ)	U	786	Rudin, Eric (NY)	EDM	631
Rossos, Apostolos (NJ)	Oto	822	Rudman, Michael (NJ)	PM	865
Roston, Alfred (NY)	Ge	635	Rudolph, Daniel (CT)	Pul	932
Roth, Alan (NY)	FMed	475	Rudolph, Steven (NY)	N	444
Roth, Andrew (NY)	Psyc	330	Rudy, Bret (NY)	AM	130
Roth, Douglas (NY)	PIS	669	Ruggiero, Joseph (NY)	Onc	220
Roth, Jeffrey (NY)	D	158	Rundback, John (NJ)	VIR	733
Roth, Joseph (NJ)	Ge	702	Ruoff, Michael (NY)	Ge	179
Roth, Neil (NY)	SM	352	Rusch, Valerie (NY)	T&CS	366
Roth, Patrick (NJ)	NS	711	Rush, Thomas (NY)	Inf	638
Roth, Philip (NY)	NP	496	Rusk, Alice (CT)	N	916
Roth, Richard (NY)	Cv	573	Russakoff, L Mark (NY)	Psyc	671
Rothberg, Charles (NY)	Oph	598	Russell, Robin (NY)	Ger	393
Rothberg, Robert (NJ)	CRS	741	Russo, John (NJ)	IM	747
Rothman, Howard (NJ)	Cv	694	Russo, Paul (NY)	U	372
Rothman, Jeffrey (NY)	EDM	493	Rutherford, Thomas (CT)	GO	947
Rothschild, Michael (NY)	PO	301	Rutkovsky, Edward (NY)	Cv	512
Rothstein, Stephen (NY)	Oto	284	Rutkovsky, Lisa (NY)	PCd	482
Rotman, Marvin (NY)	RadRO	461	Ruzal-Shapiro, Carrie (NY)	DR	165
Rotolo, James (NJ)	U	827	Ryback, Hyman (NY)	Oto	659
Roubin, Gary (NY)	IC	208	Rydzinski, Mayer (NY)	Cv	473
Rowley, Scott (NJ)	Hem	704			
Roychowdhury, Sudipta (NJ)	NRad	801			
Roye, David (NY)	OrS	274	**S**		
Rozanski, Alan (NY)	Cv	141			
Rozanski, Reuben (NJ)	D	741	Saada, Simon (NY)	U	466
Rozbruch, Jacob (NY)	OrS	274	Saal, Stuart (NY)	Nep	225
Rozbruch, S Robert (NY)	OrS	274	Sabatino, Dominick (NY)	PHO	549
Rozenblit, Alla (NY)	DR	388	Sabbath, Kert (CT)	Hem	948
Rubenstein, Andrew (NJ)	ObG	714			

Alphabetical Listing of Doctors

Name	Specialty	Pg	Name	Specialty	Pg
Sabbatini, Paul (NY)	Onc	220	Salifu, Moro (NY)	Nep	442
Saberski, Lloyd (CT)	PM	955	Salik, Erez (CT)	DR	901
Sabetta, James (CT)	Inf	907	Salik, James (NY)	Ge	179
Sabharwal, Sanjeev (NJ)	OrS	753	Salimi, Mostafa (NJ)	Cv	849
Sable, Robert (NY)	Ge	392	Salky, Barry (NY)	S	359
Sabnani, Indu (NJ)	Hem	745	Salmon, Jane (NY)	Rhu	349
Saboeiro, Gregory (NY)	VIR	376	Salsitz, Edwin (NY)	IM	205
Sabry, M Zakir (NY)	PlS	317	Saltz, Leonard (NY)	Onc	220
Sacchi, Terrence (NY)	IC	439	Saltzman, Daniel (NY)	MF	210
Sacco, Margaret (NJ)	S	844	Saltzman, Martin (NY)	Nep	648
Sachar, David (NY)	Ge	179	Saltzman, Simone (NY)	Inf	395
Sachs, Jonathan (NJ)	Ge	777	Saltzman-Gabelman, Lori (NY)	IM	642
Sachs, Paul (CT)	Pul	932	Salvati, Eduardo (NY)	OrS	274
Sachs, R Gregory (NJ)	Cv	873	Salwitz, James (NJ)	Onc	798
Sachs, Ronald (NJ)	Oph	839	Salz, Alan (NJ)	Oph	864
Sachs, Stephen (NJ)	N	879	Salzer, Richard (NJ)	OrS	716
Sacker, Ira (NY)	Ped	308	Salzer, Stephen (CT)	Oto	925
Sacks, Michael (NY)	Psyc	330	Salzman, Jacqueline (NY)	Oph	655
Sacks, Steven (NY)	Oto	284	Samach, Michael (NJ)	Ge	834
Sacks-Berg, Anne (NY)	Inf	592	Samadi, David (NY)	U	373
Sadan, Sara (NY)	Onc	646	Samadi, Sharyar (NJ)	PO	720
Sadanandan, Swayam (NY)	PHO	454	Samberg, Eslee (NY)	Psyc	331
Sadarangani, Balvinder (NY)	ObG	246	Sami, Sherif (NY)	Psyc	558
Sadeghi, Hooshang (NJ)	N	769	Sampson, Hugh (NY)	PA&I	292
Sadeghi, Hossein (CT)	PPul	927	Samra, Said (NJ)	PlS	824
Sadeghi-Nejad, Hossein (NJ)	U	732	Samson, C Michael (NY)	Oph	259
Sadiq, Saud (NY)	N	238	Samuels, Jonathan (NY)	Rhu	349
Sadock, Virginia (NY)	Psyc	331	Samuels, Steven (NY)	Inf	592
Sadovsky, Richard (NY)	FMed	430	Samuels, Steven (NJ)	Psyc	725
Saenger, Paul (NY)	PEn	661	San Filippo, J Anthony (NY)	S	677
Safai, Bijan (NY)	D	158	San Roman, Gerardo (NY)	ObG	597
Safdieh, Joseph (NY)	N	238	Sanchez, Juan (CT)	T&CS	963
Saffra, Norman (NY)	Oph	448	Sanchez, Miguel (NJ)	Path	718
Safirstein, Benjamin (NJ)	Pul	760	Sanchez-Catanese, Betty (NJ)	IM	862
Safran, Steven (NJ)	Oph	781	Sander, Norbert (NY)	IM	396
Sage, Jacob (NJ)	N	800	Sanders, Abraham (NY)	Pul	339
Sagorin, Charles (NJ)	Onc	748	Sanders, Linda (NJ)	DR	742
Sagy, Mayer (NY)	PCCM	294	Sanderson, Rhonda (NJ)	ObG	863
Saha, Chanchal (NY)	T&CS	566	Sandhaus, Jeffrey (NY)	U	487
Sahar, David (NY)	Cv	385	Sandhu, Harvinder (NY)	OrS	274
Sailon, Peter (NY)	ObG	246	Sandler, Benjamin (NY)	RE	344
Saiman, Lisa (NY)	PInf	300	Sandoval, Claudio (NY)	PHO	662
Saland, Jeffrey (NY)	PNep	300	Sands, Andrew (NY)	OrS	274
Salas, Max (NJ)	PEn	805	Sanford, Marie (NY)	Ped	308
Salazer, Thomas (NJ)	Nep	710	Sanger, Joseph (NY)	NuM	241
Saleh, Anthony (NY)	Pul	460	Santamaria, Jaime (NJ)	Oph	802
Salem, Noel (NJ)	Rhu	728	Santilli, John (CT)	A&I	896
Salem, Ronald (CT)	S	962	Santin, Alessandro (CT)	GO	947
Salerno, William (NJ)	Cv	694	Santos, Elmer (NY)	NuM	241
Sales, Clifford (NJ)	VascS	887	Saponara, Eduardo (NY)	Onc	646
Salgado, Miran (NY)	N	445	Sara, Gabriel (NY)	Onc	220

Alphabetical Listing of Doctors

Name	Specialty	Pg	Name	Specialty	Pg
Saraiya, Narendra (NJ)	Ped	883	Scher, Howard (NY)	Onc	220
Sarnelle, James (CT)	S	936	Scher, Jonathan (NY)	ObG	247
Sarnoff, Deborah (NY)	D	516	Scherl, Ellen (NY)	Ge	180
Saroff, Alan (NJ)	Cv	739	Scherl, Michael (NJ)	Oto	717
Sarokhan, Alan (NJ)	OrS	881	Scherl, Sharon (NJ)	D	697
Sas, Norman (NY)	S	415	Scherr, Douglas (NY)	U	373
Sasaki, Clarence (CT)	Oto	955	Schiano, Thomas (NY)	Ge	180
Sasso, Louis (NY)	Pul	500	Schick, David (NY)	Cv	386
Sassoon, Robert (NY)	ObG	247	Schiff, Carl (NY)	Rhu	462
Satnick, Steven (NY)	A&I	583	Schiff, Howard (NY)	U	373
Sauberman, Roy (NJ)	CE	739	Schiff, Peter (NY)	RadRO	342
Sauer, Mark (NY)	RE	344	Schiff, Russell (NY)	PCd	547
Saul, Zane (CT)	Inf	907	Schiff, William (NY)	Oph	259
Saulino, Patrick (NJ)	Cv	860	Schiffer, Mark (NY)	Cv	142
Saunders, Craig (NJ)	T&CS	763	Schiller, Alan (NY)	Path	291
Saunders-Pullman, Rachel (NY)	N	238	Schiller, Myles (NY)	PCd	405
Savage, David (NY)	Hem	191	Schiller, Robert (NY)	FMed	170
Savatsky, Gary (NJ)	SM	729	Schiowitz, Emanuel (NY)	FMed	430
Savatta, Domenico (NJ)	U	764	Schiz, Steven (CT)	Ped	928
Savin, Ronald (CT)	D	945	Schlam, Everett (NJ)	FMed	743
Savino, Michael (NY)	U	502	Schlegel, Peter (NY)	U	373
Savino, Robert (CT)	EDM	902	Schleider, Michael (NJ)	Onc	709
Sawczuk, Ihor (NJ)	U	733	Schleifer, Steven (NJ)	Psyc	759
Sawyer, David (NY)	Psyc	331	Schleiter, Gary (CT)	Inf	908
Scaccia, Frank (NJ)	Oto	822	Schlesinger, Iris (NY)	OrS	658
Scaduto, Philip (NJ)	IM	835	Schlessinger, David (NY)	Oph	541
Scardino, Peter (NY)	U	373	Schley, W Shain (NY)	Oto	285
Scarpa, Nicholas (NJ)	Rhu	772	Schliftman, Alan (NY)	D	628
Schachne, Jeffrey (NY)	D	628	Schluger, Neil (NY)	Pul	339
Schaebler, David (NJ)	Onc	779	Schlussel, Richard (NY)	U	373
Schaefer, Steven (NY)	Oto	285	Schmerin, Michael (NY)	Ge	180
Schaeffer, Janis (NY)	PPul	550	Schmidt, Hans (NJ)	S	730
Schaeffer, Mark (NJ)	IM	778	Schmidt-Sarosi, Cecilia (NY)	RE	345
Schaer, Teresa (NJ)	IM	797	Schmierer, Jeffrey (CT)	Cv	898
Schanler, Richard (NY)	NP	532	Schnabel, Freya (NY)	S	359
Schantz, Stimson (NY)	Oto	285	Schneck, Gideon (NY)	Oph	599
Schanzer, Bernard (NJ)	N	879	Schneebaum, Cary (NY)	Ge	180
Scharf, Richard (NJ)	Oto	882	Schneider, Arlene (NY)	A&I	422
Scharf, Robert (NY)	Psyc	331	Schneider, Darren (NY)	VascS	379
Scharf, Stephen (NY)	NuM	242	Schneider, Kenneth (NY)	Oto	285
Schattman, Glenn (NY)	RE	345	Schneider, Lewis (NY)	Ge	180
Schaul, Neil (NY)	N	536	Schneider, Marcie (CT)	AM	895
Schechter, Justin (CT)	Psyc	930	Schneider, Robert (NY)	Onc	646
Schechter, Michael (CT)	ObG	918	Schneider, Samuel (NJ)	Psyc	784
Schechter, Miriam (NY)	Ped	409	Schneider, Stephen (NJ)	EDM	793
Scheer, Max (NY)	Inf	526	Schneider, Steven (NY)	IM	205
Schefer, Alan (NY)	HS	637	Schob, Clifford (NJ)	OrS	753
Schein, Jonah (NY)	Psyc	331	Schoen, Robert (CT)	Rhu	961
Scheinberg, David (NY)	Onc	220	Schoeneman, Morris (NY)	PNep	455
Schell, Harold (NJ)	S	785	Schoenfeld, Mark (CT)	CE	942
Scher, David (NY)	OrS	274	Schonfeld, Steven (NJ)	NRad	801

Alphabetical Listing of Doctors

Name	Specialty	Pg	Name	Specialty	Pg
Schor, Joshua (NY)	Ger	636	Schweitzer, Philip (NY)	Ge	392
Schore, Arthur (NY)	Psyc	331	Schwinn, Hans (NY)	FMed	590
Schottenstein, Douglas (NY)	PM	289	Scibetta, Maria (NJ)	IM	706
Schrager, Alan (NY)	U	680	Scigliano, Eileen (NY)	Hem	191
Schreiber, Carl (NY)	Cv	512	Sciortino, Patrick (NY)	Oph	448
Schreiber, Klaus (NY)	ChAP	623	Sclafani, Anthony (NY)	Oto	285
Schreiber, Michael (NY)	Pul	673	Sclafani, Lisa (NY)	S	608
Schroeder, Karl (NY)	Psyc	579	Sclafani, Michael (NJ)	SM	825
Schubach, Scott (NY)	T&CS	566	Sclafani, Salvatore (NY)	VIR	466
Schubert, Hermann (NY)	Oph	259	Scofield, Lisa (NJ)	Ped	854
Schubert, Romaine (NY)	ChiN	426	Scoppetuolo, Michael (NJ)	Onc	748
Schulder, Michael (NY)	NS	534	Scott, David (NY)	Nep	480
Schulhafer, Edwin (NJ)	A&I	859	Scott, John (NY)	Oto	659
Schulman, Ira (NY)	Cv	142	Scott, Richard (NJ)	RE	866
Schulman, Matthew (NY)	PlS	318	Scott, Susan (NY)	PlS	318
Schulman, Norman (NY)	PlS	318	Scott, W Norman (NY)	OrS	275
Schulman, Philip (NY)	Hem	592	Scriven, Richard (NY)	PS	602
Schulster, Rita (NY)	Pul	560	Scuderi, Giles (NY)	OrS	275
Schultz, Neal (NY)	D	158	Scully, Brian (NY)	Inf	196
Schulze, Paul (NY)	Cv	142	Seaman, Cheryl (NY)	Psyc	331
Schuss, Steven (NJ)	Ped	723	Seashore, Margretta (CT)	CG	944
Schuster, Edward (CT)	Cv	898	Seaver, Robert (NY)	ChAP	623
Schuster, Joseph (NJ)	IM	706	Seebacher, J Robert (NY)	OrS	658
Schuster, Michael (NY)	Hem	592	Seedor, John (NY)	Oph	260
Schwab, Frank (NY)	OrS	275	Seelagy, Marc (NJ)	Pul	784
Schwarcz, Robert (NY)	Oph	260	Segal-Maurer, Sorana (NY)	Inf	477
Schwartz, Allan (NY)	Cv	142	Segarra, Pedro (NY)	ObG	597
Schwartz, Amit (NY)	NS	443	Seidenberg, Roy (NY)	D	158
Schwartz, Bruce (NY)	Psyc	411	Seidenstein, Michael (NJ)	OrS	753
Schwartz, Charles (NY)	Cv	491	Seidman, Barry (NJ)	U	887
Schwartz, Evan (NY)	OrS	481	Seidman, Mitchell (NY)	Oph	449
Schwartz, Gary (NY)	Ge	523	Seifer, David (NY)	RE	461
Schwartz, Jeffrey (NY)	OrS	275	Seigel, Mark (NJ)	ObG	821
Schwartz, Joel (NY)	NRad	577	Seinfeld, David (NY)	Cv	142
Schwartz, Joseph (NJ)	EDM	699	Seinfeld, Fredric (NJ)	T&CS	785
Schwartz, Judith (NY)	ObG	247	Seiter, Karen (NY)	Onc	646
Schwartz, Kenneth (NY)	VascS	681	Sekiguchi, Raymond (CT)	FMed	903
Schwartz, Lawrence (NY)	DR	165	Selesnick, Samuel (NY)	Oto	285
Schwartz, Louis (NJ)	RadRO	885	Seliger, Glenn (NY)	N	577
Schwartz, Michael (NY)	Psyc	605	Selinger, Sharon (NJ)	EDM	874
Schwartz, Myron (NY)	S	359	Selman, Jay (NY)	N	650
Schwartz, Paula (NY)	Onc	531	Seltzer, Terry (NY)	EDM	168
Schwartz, Peter (CT)	GO	947	Selwyn, Peter (NY)	IM	396
Schwartz, Robert (NJ)	D	741	Selzer, Jeffrey (NY)	Psyc	483
Schwartz, Theodore (NY)	NS	229	Seminara, Donna (NY)	Ger	494
Schwartz, William (NY)	Cv	142	Sen, Chandranath (NY)	NS	230
Schwartzberg, Mori (NJ)	Rhu	825	Sena, Kanaga (CT)	N	916
Schwartzfarb, Lanny (NY)	Rhu	350	Sender, Joel (NY)	Pul	413
Schwartzman, Alexander (NY)	S	464	Sensakovic, John (NJ)	Inf	796
Schwartzman, Sergio (NY)	Rhu	350	Sepkowitz, Douglas (NY)	Inf	436
Schwarz, Steven (NY)	PGe	453	Sepkowitz, Kent (NY)	Inf	197

Name	Specialty	Pg	Name	Specialty	Pg
Seplowitz, Alan (NY)	EDM	168	Shaywitz, Sally (CT)	Ped	958
Serby, Michael (NY)	GerPsy	183	Shear, Perry (CT)	NS	915
Sergiou, Harry (NY)	Ped	456	Shebairo, Raymond (NY)	OrS	543
Serle, Janet (NY)	Oph	260	Sheikh, Shahid (NY)	Cv	622
Serur, Eli (NY)	GO	434	Shein, Leon (NY)	Nep	442
Sethi, Paul (CT)	OrS	924	Sheinart, Kara (NY)	N	238
Sett, Suvro (NY)	T&CS	678	Sheinfeld, Joel (NY)	U	373
Setton, Avi (NY)	NRad	537	Shell, Roger (NJ)	Cv	790
Setzen, Michael (NY)	Oto	544	Shelmet, John (NJ)	EDM	776
Sgaglione, Nicholas (NY)	OrS	543	Shelton, Ronald (NY)	D	158
Sgouros, Anthony (NY)	Ge	635	Shemen, Larry (NY)	Oto	285
Shabsigh, Ridwan (NY)	U	466	Shenoy, Rajesh (NY)	PCd	405
Shabto, Uri (NY)	Oph	260	Shepard, Barry (NY)	U	568
Shack, Robert (NJ)	S	762	Shepherd, Gillian (NY)	A&I	132
Shah, Darsit (NJ)	Oto	822	Sher, Ellen (NJ)	A&I	815
Shah, Jatin (NY)	S	360	Sheridan, Bernadette (NY)	FMed	430
Shah, Paresh (NY)	S	360	Sheris, Steven (NJ)	Cv	873
Shah, Pritesh (NJ)	Psyc	725	Sherling, Bruce (NY)	Pul	673
Shah, Smita (NJ)	Pul	760	Sherman, Frederic (NY)	IM	438
Shahid, Syed (CT)	NS	915	Sherman, Fredrick (NY)	Ger	183
Shahrivar, Farrokh (NY)	NP	223	Sherman, Howard (NY)	Ge	393
Shamamian, Peter (NY)	S	415	Sherman, Iris (NY)	IM	205
Shamoon, Fayez (NJ)	Cv	739	Sherman, John (NY)	PlS	318
Shamoon, Harry (NY)	EDM	389	Sherman, Mark (NY)	OrS	498
Shampain, Lawrence (NJ)	ChAP	790	Sherman, Raymond (NY)	Nep	225
Shams, Joseph (NY)	VIR	376	Sherman, Richard (NJ)	Nep	799
Shanahan, Andrew (NJ)	IC	778	Sherman, Scott (NY)	DR	517
Shane, Elizabeth (NY)	EDM	168	Sherman, Spencer (NY)	Oph	260
Shani, Jacob (NY)	IC	439	Sherman, Steven (NY)	Oph	449
Shapir, Yehuda (NY)	PCd	547	Sherman, Warren (NY)	Cv	142
Shapiro, Barry (NY)	Oto	659	Sherman, William (NY)	Onc	220
Shapiro, Bruce (CT)	Psyc	931	Sherr, David (NY)	RadRO	342
Shapiro, Ellen (NY)	U	373	Sherry, Stephen (NJ)	EDM	743
Shapiro, Eugene (CT)	PInf	957	Sheth, Parag (NY)	PMR	311
Shapiro, Kenneth (NY)	Nep	576	Shevell, Tracy (CT)	MF	912
Shapiro, Lawrence (NY)	EDM	519	Shield, Dennis (CT)	U	937
Shapiro, Lawrence (NY)	CG	625	Shifrin, Seth (NY)	SM	676
Shapiro, Marc (NY)	S	608	Shike, Moshe (NY)	Ge	432
Shapiro, Michael (NJ)	S	730	Shikowitz, Mark (NY)	Oto	544
Shapiro, Neil (NY)	Ge	635	Shim-Chang, Helen (NY)	D	158
Shapiro, Peter (NY)	Psyc	331	Shimony, Rony (NY)	Cv	142
Shapiro, Richard (NY)	S	360	Shinbach, Kent (NY)	Psyc	332
Shapiro, Warren (NY)	Nep	442	Shindler, Daniel (NJ)	Cv	790
Sharma, Samin (NY)	IC	208	Shinnar, Shlomo (NY)	ChiN	386
Sharon, David (NJ)	Onc	819	Shlofmitz, Richard (NY)	Cv	512
Sharon, Ezra (NY)	Rhu	485	Short, Joan (NY)	Ped	499
Sharpe, Arleen (NY)	FMed	631	Shugar, Joel (NY)	Oto	285
Shatkin, Jess (NY)	ChAP	147	Shulman, Julius (NY)	Oph	260
Shaw, Ronda (NY)	Psyc	331	Shulman, Melanie (NY)	N	238
Shayani, Steven (NY)	Cv	512	Shulman, Yale (NJ)	U	772
Shaywitz, Bennett (CT)	ChiN	943	Shum, Kee (NY)	Onc	479

Alphabetical Listing of Doctors

Name	Specialty	Pg	Name	Specialty	Pg
Shumko, John (NJ)	PMR	758	Simon, Clifford (NJ)	Pul	726
Shupack, Jerome (NY)	D	159	Simon, Jonathan (NJ)	Rhu	761
Shypula, Gregory (NJ)	Onc	798	Simon, Lawrence (NY)	S	580
Sibony, Patrick (NY)	Oph	599	Simon, Lloyd (NY)	IM	594
Sibrack, Laurence (CT)	D	900	Simon, Scott (CT)	NS	915
Sicherer, Scott (NY)	PA&I	292	Simon, Sheldon (NY)	OrS	275
Sicklick, Marc (NY)	A&I	507	Simon, Steven (NY)	D	428
Siderides, Elizabeth (CT)	Oph	920	Simon, Todd (NY)	IM	438
Sidoti, Paul (NY)	Oph	260	Simonson, Barry (NY)	OrS	543
Siegal, Elliot (NY)	Ped	578	Simotas, Alexander (NY)	PMR	311
Siegal, Michael (NY)	Cv	143	Simpson, David (NY)	N	238
Siegel, Beth (NY)	S	486	Simpson, Roger (NY)	PlS	556
Siegel, Daniel (NY)	D	588	Singer, Lewis (NY)	PCCM	405
Siegel, Eric (NJ)	D	742	Singer, Samuel (NY)	S	360
Siegel, Judy (NY)	U	680	Singh, Anup (NJ)	PNep	806
Siegel, Kenneth (CT)	N	916	Singh, Avtar (NY)	N	650
Siegel, Marc (NY)	IM	205	Singh, Bhuvanesh (NY)	Oto	286
Siegel, Randall (NJ)	VIR	812	Singh, Dinesh (CT)	U	963
Siegel, Robert (NY)	CCM	387	Singhal, Pravin (NY)	Nep	533
Siegel, Stephen (NY)	Cv	143	Sink, Ernest (NY)	OrS	275
Siegler, Eugenia (NY)	Ger	183	Sinnreich, Abraham (NY)	Oto	498
Siepser, Stuart (NJ)	Cv	849	Sipzner, Robert (NJ)	Nep	749
Sierocki, John (NJ)	Onc	779	Siracuse, Jeffrey (NY)	NP	440
Siever, Larry (NY)	Psyc	332	Siris, Ethel (NY)	EDM	169
Silberman, Deborah (NY)	Oph	449	Siris, Samuel (NY)	Psyc	483
Silberman, Mark Illan (NY)	PlS	556	Siskind, Steven (NY)	Cv	473
Silbert, Glenn (NJ)	Oph	715	Sisti, Michael (NY)	NS	230
Silbert, Paul (NJ)	N	821	Sivak, Mark (NY)	N	238
Silich, Robert (NY)	PlS	318	Sivitz, Jennifer (NJ)	PEn	755
Silva, Jose (NY)	U	374	Sklar, Charles (NY)	PEn	295
Silva, Raul (NY)	ChAP	624	Sklar, Jeffrey (NY)	D	516
Silva, Waldemar (NJ)	IM	835	Sklarek, Howard (NY)	Pul	605
Silver, Bennett (NJ)	Psyc	884	Sklarin, Nancy (NY)	Onc	221
Silver, David (NY)	U	466	Sklaroff, Herschel (NY)	Cv	143
Silver, Jonathan (NY)	Psyc	332	Sklower, Jay (NJ)	FMed	767
Silver, Lester (NY)	PlS	318	Sklower Brooks, Susan (NJ)	CG	791
Silver, Michael (NY)	Cv	622	Skluth, Myra (CT)	IM	910
Silverberg, Arnold (NY)	EDM	429	Skolnick, Lawrence (NJ)	NP	836
Silverberg, Nanette (NY)	D	159	Skolnik, Richard (NY)	PlS	318
Silverberg, Shonni (NY)	EDM	168	Skopicki, Hal (NY)	Cv	585
Silverman, Amy (NY)	ChAP	624	Skripkus, Aldona (NJ)	Ped	770
Silverman, Bernard (NY)	A&I	422	Skrokov, Robert (NY)	D	588
Silverman, Cary (NJ)	Oph	839	Skupski, Daniel (NY)	MF	478
Silverman, David (NY)	IM	205	Skuza, Kathryn (NJ)	PEn	805
Silverman, Joel (NY)	Pul	484	Slakter, Jason (NY)	Oph	260
Silverman, Lewis (NY)	Onc	221	Slama, Robert (NJ)	Cv	873
Silverman, Mark (NY)	D	516	Slamovits, Thomas (NY)	Oph	402
Silverman, Mitchell (NJ)	EDM	875	Slankard, Marjorie (NY)	A&I	132
Silverman, Rubin (NY)	Cv	386	Slater, Gary (NY)	S	360
Simberkoff, Michael (NY)	Inf	197	Slater, James (NY)	IC	208
Simmons, Rache (NY)	S	360	Slater, Jonathan (NY)	ChAP	624

Alphabetical Listing of Doctors

Alphabetical Listing of Doctors

Name	Specialty	Pg	Name	Specialty	Pg
Spector, Jason (NY)	PlS	318	Steele, Andrew (NY)	NP	532
Speiser, Phyllis (NY)	PEn	548	Steele, Mark (NY)	Oph	261
Spencer, Dennis (CT)	NS	952	Steer, Robert (NJ)	ObG	838
Spencer, Elizabeth Kay (NY)	ChAP	147	Steiger, David (NY)	Pul	339
Spera, John (CT)	RadRO	933	Steigman, Elliot (NJ)	U	772
Sperling, Neil (NY)	Oto	451	Stein, Adam (NY)	PMR	554
Spero, Charles (NY)	OrS	450	Stein, Alan (NY)	Inf	436
Spero, Marc (NY)	IM	206	Stein, Arnold (NY)	Oph	449
Speyer, James (NY)	Onc	221	Stein, Barry (NY)	Ped	308
Spicehandler, Debra (NY)	Inf	638	Stein, Daniel (NY)	RE	345
Spiegel, Michael (CT)	Rhu	934	Stein, David (NY)	Ge	393
Spielberg, Alan (NY)	Ge	591	Stein, Elliott (NJ)	Cv	873
Spielman, Joel (NJ)	OrS	839	Stein, Jeffrey (NY)	Ge	180
Spielvogel, David (NY)	T&CS	678	Stein, Jeffrey (NY)	VascS	379
Spiera, Harry (NY)	Rhu	350	Stein, Joel (NY)	PMR	311
Spiera, Robert (NY)	Rhu	350	Stein, Lawrence (NJ)	Ge	834
Spigland, Nitsana (NY)	PS	303	Stein, Mark (NY)	U	416
Spiler, Ira (NJ)	EDM	793	Stein, Mitchell (NY)	Oph	655
Spindola-Franco, Hugo (NY)	DR	388	Stein, Perry (NY)	PMR	457
Spinelli, Henry (NY)	PlS	319	Stein, Richard (NY)	Cv	143
Spinowitz, Alan (NY)	D	516	Stein, Ruth (NY)	Ped	410
Spinowitz, Bruce (NY)	Nep	480	Stein, Sidney (NY)	Pul	339
Spira, Robert (NJ)	Ge	744	Stein, Stefan (NY)	Psyc	332
Spitalewitz, Samuel (NY)	Nep	442	Steinberg, Charles (NY)	IM	206
Spitz, Henry (NY)	Psyc	332	Steinberg, Harry (NY)	Pul	560
Spitzer, Daniel (NY)	NS	576	Steinberg, L Gary (NY)	PCd	294
Spivack, Julie (CT)	Ge	905	Steinberger, Alfred (NJ)	NS	711
Spivak, Jeffrey (NY)	OrS	275	Steiner, Henry (NY)	S	464
Spivak, William (NY)	PGe	297	Steingart, Richard (NY)	Cv	143
Splain, Shepard (NY)	OrS	450	Steinhagen, Randolph (NY)	CRS	150
Spotnitz, Henry (NY)	T&CS	366	Steinherz, Laurel (NY)	PCd	294
Spriggs, David (NY)	Onc	221	Steinherz, Peter (NY)	PHO	299
Sproviero, Joseph (CT)	A&I	896	Stelzer, Paul (NY)	T&CS	366
Squitieri, Rafael (CT)	T&CS	936	Stern, Harvey (NY)	DR	389
Staats, Peter (NJ)	PM	823	Stern, Leonard (NY)	Nep	225
Stabile, John (NJ)	Oph	715	Stern, Richard (NY)	Rhu	350
Staeger-Hirsch, Christine (NY)	DR	629	Sternschein, Michael (NJ)	PlS	724
Staffenberg, David (NY)	PlS	319	Stewart, Allan (NY)	T&CS	366
Stafford, John (NY)	NP	647	Stewart, Michael (NY)	Oto	286
Stahl, Richard (CT)	PlS	958	Stidham, Katrina (NY)	Oto	659
Stam, Lawrence (NY)	Nep	442	Stieg, Philip (NY)	NS	230
Stanford, Paulette (NJ)	AM	738	Stifelman, Michael (NY)	U	374
Stangel, John (NY)	RE	674	Stiller, Robert (CT)	MF	912
Starc, Thomas (NY)	PCd	293	Stillman, Michael (NY)	D	628
Starke, Charles (NY)	IM	642	Stilwell, Anne (NY)	PM	498
Starker, Isaac (NJ)	PlS	842	Stock, Jeffrey (NJ)	U	764
Starker, Paul (NJ)	S	887	Stock, Richard (NY)	RadRO	342
Starkman, Harold (NJ)	PEn	840	Stone, Chester (NJ)	U	845
Starpoli, Anthony (NY)	Ge	180	Stone, Gregg (NY)	IC	208
Starr, Michael (NY)	Oph	261	Stone, Joanne (NY)	MF	210
Staszewski, Harry (NY)	Hem	525	Stone, Michael (NY)	Psyc	332

Alphabetical Listing of Doctors

Name	Specialty	Pg	Name	Specialty	Pg
Tamborlane, William (CT)	PEn	956	Teusink, J Paul (NY)	Psyc	333
Tamerin, John (CT)	Psyc	931	Tewari, Ashutosh (NY)	U	374
Tan, Mark (NY)	Rhu	607	Theofanidis, Stylianos (CT)	NP	913
Tan, Virak (NJ)	HS	745	Thomas, Byron (CT)	IM	910
Tancredi, Laurence (NY)	Psyc	333	Thomas, David (NY)	PMR	312
Taneja, Samir (NY)	U	374	Thomas, Gary (NY)	PM	289
Tanenbaum, Diane (NY)	D	159	Thomas, Mark (NY)	PMR	410
Tang, David (NY)	IM	642	Thomashow, Byron (NY)	Pul	340
Tank, Lisa (NJ)	Ger	703	Thompson, John (NY)	PGe	406
Tanoue, Lynn (CT)	Pul	959	Thomsen, Stephen (NJ)	Nep	769
Tanowitz, Herbert (NY)	Inf	395	Thomson, J Grant (CT)	HS	948
Tanzer, Floyd (NJ)	D	850	Thorne, Charles (NY)	PlS	319
Tap, William (NY)	Onc	222	Thornton, Scott (CT)	CRS	899
Tarasuk, Albert (NY)	U	487	Thurm, Craig (NY)	Pul	484
Tardiff, Kenneth (NY)	Psyc	333	Tibaldi, Joseph (NY)	EDM	475
Tartaglia, Joseph (NY)	Cv	622	Ticker, Jonathan (NY)	OrS	543
Tartell, Jay (NY)	DR	474	Tierney, Peter (NJ)	FMed	794
Tartini, Albert (NJ)	Nep	710	Tiger, Louis (NY)	Rhu	563
Tartter, Paul (NY)	S	360	Tillem, Steven (NY)	U	487
Tassiopoulos, Apostolos (NY)	VascS	609	Timpone, Leonard (NY)	IM	528
Taub, Peter (NY)	PlS	319	Tindel, Nathaniel (NY)	OrS	276
Taubin, Howard (CT)	Ge	905	Tinetti, Mary (CT)	Ger	947
Taubman, Lowell (NY)	IM	528	Ting, Andrew (NY)	PPul	302
Tavill, Michael (NJ)	PO	823	Ting, Jess (NY)	PlS	320
Tawfik, Bernard (NY)	Oto	545	Tinger, Alfred (NY)	RadRO	674
Tay, Steven (NY)	IM	206	Tiszenkel, Howard (NY)	CRS	473
Taylor, Howard (NJ)	Oto	840	Tittle, Shawn (CT)	T&CS	936
Taylor, Hugh (CT)	RE	960	Tiwari, Ram (NY)	Oph	402
Taylor, James (NY)	T&CS	609	Tobias, Daniel (NJ)	GO	834
Taylor, Noel (NY)	Psyc	333	Tobias, Geoffrey (NJ)	Oto	717
Taylor, Robert (NJ)	GO	744	Tobias, Hillel (NY)	Ge	180
Te, Alexis (NY)	U	374	Todd, George (NY)	VascS	380
Teffera, Fassil (NY)	IM	397	Tohme, Jack (NJ)	EDM	699
Teichholz, Louis (NJ)	Cv	694	Tolan, Robert (NJ)	PInf	806
Tello, Celso (NY)	Oph	261	Tolchin, Joan (NY)	Psyc	333
Telzak, Edward (NY)	Inf	396	Toles, Allen (NY)	ObG	538
Tempera, Patrick (NJ)	Ge	876	Tolston, Evelyn (NY)	A&I	132
Temple, Larissa (NY)	CRS	150	Tolunsky, Eugene (NY)	N	651
Tenenbaum, Joseph (NY)	Cv	143	Tom, David (CT)	Oph	953
Tenet, William (NY)	Cv	513	Tom, Jack (NY)	D	588
Tennenbaum, Steven (NJ)	U	733	Tomao, Frank (NY)	Onc	531
Tenner, Michael (NY)	NRad	651	Toomey, Kathleen (NJ)	Hem	861
Teodorescu, Victoria (NY)	VascS	379	Topilow, Arthur (NJ)	Hem	818
Teperman, Lewis (NY)	S	360	Topilow, Harvey (NJ)	Oph	715
Tepler, Melvin (NY)	OrS	450	Toppmeyer, Deborah (NJ)	Onc	798
Teplitz, Glenn (NY)	HS	525	Torman, Julie (NY)	Ge	636
Tepper, Howard (NJ)	PlS	884	Tornos, Carmen (NY)	Path	600
Terjanian, Terenig (NY)	Onc	495	Torrado-Jule, Carmen (NY)	PEn	498
Tesser, Mark (NY)	D	159	Torre, Arthur (NJ)	PA&I	754
Tessler, Sidney (NY)	Pul	460	Tortolani, Anthony (NY)	T&CS	465
Testa, Francine (CT)	ChiN	943	Tortoriello, Drew (NY)	RE	345

Name	Specialty	Pg	Name	Specialty	Pg
Tostanoski, Jean (NY)	Oph	656	Ullman, Joel (NY)	ObG	653
Toth, Patrick (NJ)	DR	699	Ullman, Thomas (NY)	Ge	181
Touliopoulos, Steven (NY)	OrS	482	Underberg, James (NY)	IM	206
Tousimis, Eleni (NY)	S	361	Underberg-Davis, Sharon (NJ)	DR	792
Tozzi, Robert (NJ)	PCd	719	Unger, Allen (NY)	Cv	144
Trachtman, Howard (NY)	PNep	300	Unger, Walter (NY)	D	159
Traeger, Eveline (NJ)	ChiN	873	Unis, George (NY)	OrS	276
Traister, Michael (NY)	Ped	308	Unterricht, Sam (NY)	Oph	449
Tranbaugh, Robert (NY)	T&CS	367	Upadhyay, Yogendra (NY)	Psyc	605
Traquina, Diana (NJ)	PO	806	Urban, William (NY)	OrS	450
Traube, Charles (NY)	Cv	425	Urbanek, Richard (NY)	D	492
Traube, Morris (NY)	Ge	181	Urken, Mark (NY)	Oto	286
Trauzzi, Stephen (NY)	U	680	Ushay, H Michael (NY)	PCCM	405
Travis, William (NY)	Path	291	Uy, Vena (NJ)	ObG	769
Treiber, Ruth (NY)	D	628			
Treiser, Susan (NJ)	RE	866			
Tria, Alfred (NJ)	OrS	864			
Trow, Terence (CT)	Pul	959	**V**		
Troy, Allen (CT)	OrS	924			
Troy, Kevin (NY)	Hem	192	Vad, Vijay (NY)	PMR	312
Tsai, James (CT)	Oph	954	Vahdat, Linda (NY)	Onc	222
Tuchman, Alan (NY)	N	239	Vaidya, Sudhir (NY)	FMed	632
Tuckman, David (NY)	HS	525	Vaillancourt, Philippe (NY)	PM	600
Tuerk-Mendelsohn, Lois (NY)	A&I	618	Valda, Victor (NJ)	PS	721
Tugal, Oya (NY)	PHO	663	Valenza, Joseph (NJ)	PMR	842
Tuhrim, Stanley (NY)	N	239	Valinoti, Anne Marie (NJ)	IM	706
Tuohy, Edward (CT)	Cv	898	Vallarino, Ramon (NY)	PMR	457
Turbin, Roger (NJ)	Oph	752	Vallone, Ambrose (NY)	PCd	547
Turcios, Nelson (NJ)	PPul	865	Vambutas, Andrea (NY)	Oto	545
Turecki, Stanley (NY)	ChAP	147	van Dyck, Christopher (CT)	GerPsy	947
Turetsky, Arthur (CT)	Pul	932	Van Engel, Daniel (NJ)	N	712
Turitto, Gioia (NY)	CE	423	Van Slooten, David (NJ)	N	712
Turk, Jon (NY)	Oto	286	Van Zee, Kimberly (NY)	S	361
Turner, Ira (NY)	N	536	Vapnek, Jonathan (NY)	U	374
Turro, James (NY)	IM	642	Vargas-Rodriguez, Ileana (NY)	PEn	296
Turtel, Andrew (NY)	OrS	276	Varriale, Philip (NY)	Cv	144
Turtel, Lawrence (NJ)	Oph	822	Varsos, George (NY)	RadRO	485
Turtel, Penny (NJ)	Ge	817	Vas, George (NY)	N	445
Tuttle, R Michael (NY)	EDM	169	Vasselli, Anthony (NJ)	U	786
Tyberg, Theodore (NY)	Cv	143	Vastola, A Paul (NY)	Oto	451
Tyshkov, Michael (NJ)	PGe	882	Vasudeva, Kusum (NY)	ObG	538
			Vaswani, Ashok (NY)	EDM	519
			Vates, Thomas (NJ)	U	812
			Vaughan, Margaret (NY)	Ger	637
U			Vazzana, Thomas (NY)	Cv	492
			Vega, Aida (NY)	IM	206
Uday, Kalpana (NY)	Nep	399	Velcek, Francisca (NY)	PS	304
Udell, Ira (NY)	Oph	541	Veloso, Manuel (NY)	ObG	538
Udelsman, Robert (CT)	S	962	Verga, Michele (NY)	PlS	320
Ugol, Jay (CT)	ObG	918	Verma, Rajiv (NJ)	PCd	755
Uhm, Kyudong (NJ)	Onc	851	Versfelt, Mary (NY)	Ped	667

Alphabetical Listing of Doctors

Name	Specialty	Pg	Name	Specialty	Pg
Vesole, David (NJ)	Hem	704	Wainstein, Sasha (NY)	U	466
Vester, John (NJ)	N	780	Waintraub, Stanley (NJ)	Onc	709
Vialotti, Charles (NJ)	RadRO	727	Walczyk, John (NY)	D	517
Vicencio, Alfin (NY)	PPul	551	Waldman, Seth (NY)	PM	289
Vickery, Carlin (NY)	PlS	320	Waldorf, Donald (NY)	D	573
Vieira, Jeffrey (NY)	IM	438	Waldorf, Heidi (NY)	D	573
Vietorisz, Esteban (CT)	Oph	921	Walfish, Jacob (NY)	IM	438
Vigorita, Vincent (NY)	Path	452	Walker, Audrey (NY)	ChAP	624
Villafranca, Manuel (NJ)	Psyc	885	Walker, Yvette (NY)	IM	397
Villamena, Patricia (NY)	Pul	340	Walkup, John (NY)	ChAP	147
Villongco, Raymond (NJ)	Ger	703	Wallach, Frances (NY)	Inf	197
Vincent, Miriam (NY)	FMed	430	Wallach, Robert (NY)	GO	185
Vinciguerra, Vincent (NY)	Onc	532	Wallack, Joel (NY)	Psyc	334
Vine, Anthony (NY)	S	361	Wallack, Marc (NY)	S	361
Vine, John (NJ)	D	775	Wallis, Joseph (NJ)	ObG	838
Viner, Nicholas (CT)	U	937	Walser, Lawrence (NY)	Pul	605
Vingan, Roy (NJ)	NS	711	Walsh, B Timothy (NY)	Psyc	334
Vining, Eugenia (CT)	Oto	955	Walsh, Christina (NJ)	Onc	819
Vintzileos, Anthony (NY)	MF	530	Walsh, Christine (NY)	PCd	405
Violi, Caterina (CT)	ObG	918	Walsh, Francis (CT)	IM	910
Visconti, Ernest (NY)	Ped	499	Walsh, Joseph (NY)	Oph	261
Viswanathan, Kusum (NY)	PHO	454	Walsh, Peter (NY)	ChAP	147
Viswanathan, Ramaswamy (NY)	Psyc	458	Walsh, Raymond (NY)	OrS	450
Vitale, Gerard (NY)	S	565	Walther, Robert (NY)	D	159
Vitale, Michael (NY)	OrS	276	Waner, Milton (NY)	Oto	287
Vitenson, Jack (NJ)	U	733	Wang, Beverly (NY)	Path	291
Vitting, Kevin (NJ)	Nep	851	Wang, Frederick (NY)	Oph	261
Vivek, Seeth (NY)	Psyc	483	Wang, John (NY)	Nep	225
Voellmicke, Kurt (NY)	OrS	658	Wang, Timothy (NY)	Ge	181
Vogel, James (NY)	Hem	192	Wangenheim, Paul (NJ)	Cv	740
Vogel, Louis (NY)	D	159	Wapner, Ronald (NY)	MF	210
Vogel, Mitchell (NJ)	Oph	852	Ward, Barbara (CT)	S	936
Vogelman, Arthur (NY)	Ge	476	Ward, Robert (NY)	PO	301
Vogiatzi, Maria (NY)	PEn	296	Wardlaw, Sharon (NY)	EDM	169
Vogl, Steven (NY)	Onc	398	Warman, Jacob (NY)	EDM	430
Volcovici, Guido (NY)	Pul	673	Warner, Robert (NY)	D	160
Volpe, Anthony (NJ)	IM	706	Warren, Floyd (NY)	Oph	261
Volpi, David (NY)	Oto	287	Warren, Michelle (NY)	RE	345
Vukasin, Alexander (NJ)	U	786	Warren, Ronald (NJ)	IM	778
			Warren, Russell (NY)	OrS	276
			Warren, Wendy (NJ)	MF	747
			Warshafsky, Stephen (NY)	IM	643
W			Warshofsky, Mark (CT)	IC	911
			Wasnick, Robert (NY)	U	609
Wachtel, Alan (NY)	Psyc	333	Wasser, Kenneth (NJ)	Rhu	825
Wager, Marc (NY)	Ped	667	Wasserheit, Carolyn (NY)	Onc	646
Wager, Steven (NY)	Psyc	333	Wasserman, Barry (NJ)	Oph	781
Wagle, Sharad (NJ)	Psyc	725	Wasserman, Eric (CT)	Oph	921
Wagman, Raquel (NJ)	RadRO	760	Wasserman, Gary (NJ)	U	733
Wagner, John (NY)	Nep	533	Wasserman, Hal (CT)	IC	911
Wagner, Rudolph (NJ)	Oph	752	Wasserman, Kenneth (NJ)	IM	706

Name	Specialty	Pg	Name	Specialty	Pg
Waters, Cheryl (NY)	N	239	Weinstein, Larry (NJ)	PlS	842
Waters, Paul (CT)	T&CS	936	Weinstein, Mark (NY)	IM	528
Waterstone, Melissa (NY)	ObG	247	Weinstein, Melvin (NJ)	Inf	796
Wattenberg, Debra (NY)	D	160	Weinstein, Paul (CT)	Onc	913
Wax, Michael (NJ)	Onc	878	Weinstein, Richard (NY)	OrS	658
Waxberg, Jonathan (CT)	U	937	Weinstein, Samuel (NY)	T&CS	416
Waxenbaum, Steven (NJ)	CRS	695	Weinstein, Toba (NY)	PGe	549
Waye, Jerome (NY)	Ge	181	Weinstock, Gary (NY)	A&I	508
Wayne, Peter (NY)	Ge	636	Weintraub, Howard (NY)	Cv	144
Waynik, Mark (CT)	Psyc	931	Weintraub, Joshua (NY)	VIR	376
Weber, Pamela (NY)	Oph	599	Weintraub, Michael (NY)	N	651
Weber, Richard (CT)	Oph	921	Weisbrot, Deborah (NY)	ChAP	586
Wechsler, Amy (NY)	D	160	Weiselberg, Lora (NY)	Onc	532
Weck, Steven (NY)	DR	518	Weisenseel, Arthur (NY)	Cv	144
Wedderburn, Raymond (NY)	S	361	Weiser, Kenneth (NY)	EDM	631
Weg, Arnold (NY)	Ge	476	Weiser, Martin (NY)	CRS	151
Weg, Ira (NY)	Cv	513	Weiser, Robert (NY)	VascS	467
Wehmann, Robert (NJ)	EDM	700	Weiser, Todd (NY)	T&CS	678
Wei, Fong (NJ)	Nep	779	Weisholtz, Steven (NJ)	Inf	705
Weidhaas, Joanne (CT)	RadRO	960	Weiss, Carol (NY)	AdP	130
Weiland, Andrew (NY)	HS	188	Weiss, Christopher (NJ)	Ped	723
Weill, Terry (NY)	Psyc	334	Weiss, Darryl (NJ)	D	697
Wein, Paul (NY)	Cv	426	Weiss, E Michael (NJ)	Cv	849
Weinberg, Gerard (NY)	PS	408	Weiss, Gabriella (NJ)	Inf	850
Weinberg, Harlan (NY)	Pul	673	Weiss, Gerson (NJ)	RE	728
Weinberg, Harold (NY)	N	239	Weiss, Jonathan (NY)	DR	629
Weinberg, Jeffrey (NY)	PMR	499	Weiss, Louis (NY)	Inf	396
Weinberg, Jerry (NY)	U	680	Weiss, Lynne (NJ)	PNep	806
Weinberg, Marc (NY)	Cv	585	Weiss, Melvin (NY)	IC	643
Weinberg, Martin (NJ)	Oph	715	Weiss, Michael (NY)	Oph	262
Weinberger, George (NJ)	D	874	Weiss, Paul (NY)	PlS	320
Weinberger, Jesse (NY)	N	239	Weiss, Rita (NY)	Onc	532
Weinberger, Judah (NY)	IC	208	Weiss, Robert (NY)	Ge	181
Weinberger, Michael (NY)	PM	289	Weiss, Robert (NJ)	U	812
Weinberger, Sylvain (NY)	Ped	308	Weiss, Robert (NY)	PNep	663
Weinblatt, Mark (NY)	PHO	549	Weiss, Robert (CT)	U	964
Weine, Gary (NJ)	IM	836	Weiss, Steven (NJ)	A&I	738
Weiner, Howard (NY)	NS	231	Weissbrot, Jay (NY)	Ped	667
Weiner, Kevin (NY)	PMR	499	Weissman, Gary (NY)	Ge	523
Weiner, Lon (NY)	OrS	276	Weissman, Ronald (NY)	Cv	622
Weiner, Michael (NY)	PHO	299	Weisstuch, Joseph (NY)	Nep	225
Weiner, Richard (NY)	Ped	410	Weitzman, Steven (NY)	EDM	589
Weinerman, Stuart (NY)	EDM	520	Weizman, Howard (NJ)	Nep	710
Weinfeld, Steven (NY)	OrS	277	Wells, Scott (NY)	PlS	320
Weingarten, Jacqueline (NY)	PCCM	405	Welsh, Howard (NY)	Psyc	334
Weingarten, Phyllis (NY)	Oph	577	Welshinger, Marie (NY)	GO	477
Weinreb, Jeffrey (CT)	DR	945	Wenig, Bruce (NY)	Path	291
Weinstein, David (CT)	ObG	918	Werner, Michael (NY)	U	680
Weinstein, Jay (NY)	IM	528	Wert, Sanford (NY)	OrS	451
Weinstein, Joseph (NY)	Oph	541	Wertheim, David (NY)	A&I	508
Weinstein, Joshua (NY)	Rhu	414	Wertheim, Iris (CT)	GO	905

Alphabetical Listing of Doctors

Name	Specialty	Pg	Name	Specialty	Pg
Wertkin, Martin (NY)	S	677	Wishner, Jerald (NY)	CRS	625
Weseley, Peter (NY)	Oph	262	Wisnicki, H Jay (NY)	Oph	262
Westrich, Geoffrey (NY)	OrS	277	Wisoff, Jeffrey (NY)	NS	231
Wetzler, Graciela (NY)	PGe	453	Wisotsky, David (NJ)	Ped	723
Wexler, Craig (NY)	EDM	589	Witt, Barry (CT)	RE	933
Wexler, Leonard (NY)	PHO	299	Witt, Marvin (NY)	IM	206
Wexler, Patricia (NY)	D	160	Witte, Arnold (NJ)	N	780
Wey, Philip (NJ)	PlS	808	Wittig, James (NY)	OrS	277
Whang, William (NY)	CE	134	Wiznia, Andrew (NY)	PA&I	404
Whelan, Richard (NY)	CRS	151	Wohlberg, Gary (NY)	Pul	606
Whelan, Thomas (CT)	Ge	905	Wolchok, Jedd (NY)	Onc	222
White, Robert (CT)	VIR	964	Wolf, David (NY)	Ge	636
White, Ronald (NJ)	CRS	695	Wolf, David (NY)	Hem	192
Whitley-Williams, Patricia (NJ)	PInf	806	Wolf, Ellen (NY)	DR	389
Whitman, Eric (NJ)	S	844	Wolf, Kenneth (NY)	Oph	402
Whitman, Hendricks (NY)	Rhu	351	Wolf, Steven (NY)	ChiN	148
Whitmore, Wayne (NY)	Oph	262	Wolf-Klein, Gisele (NY)	Ger	524
Wickiewicz, Thomas (NY)	OrS	277	Wolfe, Lawrence (NY)	PHO	549
Wickremesinghe, Prasanna (NY)	Ge	494	Wolfe, Mary (NY)	IM	643
Widmann, Mark (NJ)	T&CS	845	Wolfe, Scott (NY)	HS	188
Widmann, Roger (NY)	OrS	277	Wolff, Edward (NY)	IM	528
Wiesen, Mark (NJ)	EDM	700	Wolff, Steven (NY)	DR	165
Wilbur, Sabrina (NY)	CE	423	Wolfson, Robert (NY)	IM	643
Wilchinsky, Mark (CT)	OrS	924	Wolk, Michael (NY)	Cv	144
Wild, David (NJ)	Cv	695	Wollack, Jan (NJ)	ChiN	790
Williams, Daniel (NY)	ChAP	513	Wolodiger, Fred (NJ)	VascS	734
Williams, Gail (NY)	Nep	226	Wong, Anthony (NY)	D	588
Williams, Jill (NJ)	AdP	789	Wong, James (NJ)	RadRO	843
Williams, John (NY)	U	374	Wong, Michael (NJ)	Oph	781
Williams, Marcus (NJ)	Cv	695	Wong, Raymond (NY)	Oph	262
Williams, Mathew (NY)	T&CS	367	Wong, Richard (NJ)	Oph	781
Williams, Riley (NY)	SM	352	Wong, Richard (NY)	Oto	287
Willner, Joseph (NJ)	N	712	Woo, Henry (NY)	NS	595
Wilner, Philip (NY)	Psyc	334	Woo, Peak (NY)	Oto	287
Wilson, Arnold (NY)	OrS	403	Wormser, Gary (NY)	Inf	639
Wilson, Lynn (CT)	RadRO	960	Worth, David (NJ)	Rhu	886
Wilson, Thomas (NY)	PEn	601	Wright, Albert (NY)	S	464
Winant, John (NY)	A&I	775	Wrone, David (NJ)	D	792
Winchester, James (NY)	Nep	226	Wu, Chia (NJ)	Cv	740
Windsor, Russell (NY)	OrS	277	Wu, Hen-Vai (NJ)	Onc	863
Winslow, Robert (CT)	CE	896	Wu, Jason (NY)	Ped	457
Winston, Jonathan (NY)	Nep	226	Wyner, Perry (NY)	Pul	560
Winter, Robin (NJ)	FMed	794	Wysoki, Randee (NY)	ObG	653
Winter, Stephen (CT)	Pul	932	Wysolmerski, John (CT)	EDM	946
Winter, Steven (NY)	Cv	492	Wyszynski, Bernard (NY)	Psyc	412
Winterkorn, Jacqueline (NY)	Oph	481			
Winters, Richard (NY)	Psyc	334			
Winters, Stephen (NJ)	CE	831			
Wirz, Diane (CT)	N	917	**Y**		
Wisch, Nathaniel (NY)	Hem	192	Yablon, Steven (NY)	Nep	576
Wiseman, Paul (NY)	IM	206			

Alphabetical Listing of Doctors

Name	Specialty	Pg	Name	Specialty	Pg
Yaffe, Bruce (NY)	IM	207	Zakashansky, Konstantin (NY)	GO	186
Yagoda, Arnold (NY)	Oph	262	Zalkowitz, Alan (NJ)	Rhu	729
Yahalom, Joachim (NY)	RadRO	342	Zaloom, Robert (NY)	Cv	426
Yalamanchi, Krishan (NJ)	Ped	807	Zalvan, Craig (NY)	Oto	659
Yale, Suzanne (NY)	ObG	247	Zambetti, George (NY)	OrS	277
Yamane, Michael (NJ)	IM	778	Zampella, Edward (NJ)	NS	837
Yancovitz, Stanley (NY)	Inf	197	Zapolanski, Alex (NJ)	T&CS	731
Yang, Hee (NJ)	S	730	Zarbin, Marco (NJ)	Oph	752
Yang, Roger (NJ)	DR	860	Zaremski, Benjamin (NY)	IM	207
Yang, S Steven (NY)	HS	188	Zarich, Stuart (CT)	Cv	899
Yankelevitz, David (NY)	DR	165	Zarnegar, Rasa (NY)	S	361
Yankelowitz, Stanley (NY)	Oto	404	Zarowitz, William (NY)	IM	643
Yannuzzi, Lawrence (NY)	Oph	262	Zauber, N Peter (NJ)	Hem	745
Yarberry-Allen, Patricia (NY)	ObG	247	Zbar, Lloyd (NJ)	Oto	753
Yasgur, David (NY)	OrS	658	Zeale, Peter (NY)	IM	207
Yee, Arthur (CT)	Inf	908	Zeitels, Jerrold (NJ)	PlS	884
Yee, Arthur (NY)	Rhu	351	Zeitlin, Alan (NY)	S	486
Yegudin-Ash, Julia (NY)	Rhu	675	Zeldis, Steven (NY)	Cv	513
Yeh, Timothy (NJ)	PCCM	755	Zelefsky, Michael (NY)	RadRO	342
Yellin, Joseph (NY)	N	445	Zelenetz, Andrew (NY)	Onc	222
Yi, Peter (NJ)	Onc	779	Zelicof, Steven (NY)	OrS	658
Yiengpruksawan, Anusak (NJ)	S	730	Zelkowitz, Richard (CT)	Onc	913
Yip, Chun (NY)	Pul	340	Zellner, James (NY)	Oph	449
Yoo, Jinil (NY)	Nep	399	Zelman, Warren (NY)	Oto	545
Yoon, Sydney (NY)	DR	518	Zeltsman, Vadim (NY)	T&CS	566
Yorke, Eric (NJ)	Ped	865	Zerykier, Abraham (NY)	Oph	497
Youner, Craig (NY)	DR	474	Zevon, Scott (NY)	PlS	320
Young, Bruce (NY)	ObG	248	Zide, Barry (NY)	PlS	320
Young, Constance (NY)	ObG	401	Ziegelbaum, Michael (NY)	U	569
Young, George (NY)	U	375	Ziemba, David (NY)	IM	438
Young, Iven (NY)	EDM	169	Ziering, Thomas (NJ)	FMed	861
Young, Joshua (NY)	Oph	262	Zimbalist, Eliot (NY)	Ge	432
Young, Nwanmegha (CT)	Oto	955	Zimberg, Sheldon (NY)	Psyc	334
Young, Stuart (NY)	A&I	132	Zimbler, Marc (NY)	Oto	287
Youngerman, Jay (NY)	Oto	545	Zimmerman, Franklin (NY)	Cv	623
Youssef-Bessler, Manal (NJ)	Inf	746	Zimmerman, Gary (CT)	NS	915
Yudin, Howard (NY)	FMed	632	Zimmerman, Jerald (NJ)	PMR	723
Yung, Elizabeth (NY)	NuM	537	Zimmerman, Marc (NY)	Onc	575
Yurt, Roger (NY)	S	361	Zimmerman, Sol (NY)	Ped	308
			Zingale, Robert (NY)	S	608
			Zingler, Barry (NJ)	Ge	702
			Zinkin, Lewis (NJ)	CRS	791
			Zinkin, Noah (NY)	Ge	591

Z

Name	Specialty	Pg	Name	Specialty	Pg
Zaccaria, Alan (NJ)	PlS	824	Zirvi, Monib (NJ)	D	874
Zager, Robert (NJ)	Hem	745	Zisfein, Jerome (NY)	IC	529
Zagzag, David (NY)	Path	291	Zitsman, Jeffrey (NY)	PS	665
Zahtz, Gerald (NY)	Oto	545	Zolkind, Neil (NY)	Psyc	671
Zaidi, Syed (NJ)	Psyc	725	Zolkowski-Wynne, Joanna (CT)	AM	895
Zaidman, Gerald (NY)	Oph	656	Zoltan, Irving (NY)	Ped	410
Zairis, Ignatios (NJ)	T&CS	731	Zonenshayn, Martin (NY)	NS	443
			Zonszein, Joel (NY)	EDM	390

Alphabetical Listing of Doctors

Acknowledgments

The publishers would like to thank the entire staff for their many hours and days of intense and precise work on this guide in order to further its goal of assisting consumers in making the best healthcare choices.

Castle Connolly Executive Management:

Chairman — John K. Castle

President & CEO — John J. Connolly, Ed.D.

Vice President,
Chief Medical & Research Officer — Jean Morgan, M.D.

Vice President,
Chief Strategy & Operations Officer — William Liss-Levinson, Ph.D.

Vice President, Advertising — Mark McGinty

Senior Research & Healthcare Associate — Maryann Hynd, RN

Research Coordinators

Terysia Browne — Najette Miller

Tayler Chapman, DO — Yuliya Nagdimova

Neil Cohen — Zachary Preneta

Catherine Hoffman-Freiria — Mariadiep Vu

Book Layout, Database Management — Russell Hodgson

Office Manager — Marcie Samartino

Manager, Client Relations — Hilary Knerr

Manager, Client Relations & Communications — Nicki Hughes

Account Specialist — Adam Akmal-Gonzalez

Project Manager — John Santa

We also would like to extend our gratitude to the American Board of Medical Specialties (ABMS) for allowing us to use excerpts, especially the descriptions of medical specialties and subspecialties, from the text of their publication "Which Medical Specialist for You?"

Other Publications from Castle Connolly Medical Ltd.:
America's Top Doctors® for Cancer; Top Doctors: Chicago Metro Area; Top Doctors Southern California; Top Doctors Washington-Baltimore; Cancer Made Easier: New York—Metro Area, Eldercare and others...

Order online at http://www.castleconnolly.com/books

Healthcare Solutions

Castle Connolly's Healthcare Solutions is designed to help your employees and their loved ones navigate through the healthcare system with less stress, faster service and better outcomes. It is a high touch service with a hands-on health advocate to serve as a guide and dedicated healthcare champion 24 hours a day, 7 days a week, 365 days a year. Why have your most valued employees, your most critical asset, spend their time -- and possibly company time –coping with difficult and complex medical issues they may know little about, when Castle Connolly's Healthcare Solutions professionals can resolve them quickly and expertly. With one phone call, your employees will gain priority access to a global network of best-in-class medical professionals, Castle Connolly Top Doctors™, and higher quality patient resources. Our professional staff coordinates the entire process to provide consistency and support during their time of need.

Services include, but are not limited to, the following:

» Identifying top physicians and hospitals (nationally)

» Identifying reputable non-physician providers, such as Dieticians, Physical and Occupational Therapists, etc.

» Facilitating second opinions

» Defining complex medical terminology and situations

» Providing a list of tailored questions to discuss with your medical team

» Conducting medical research on your health condition

» Navigating the healthcare system

» Assisting with medical record retrieval and/or arranging a medical record review

» Identifying and assisting with eldercare issues

» Coordinating a hospital transfer

» Arranging medical transport or evacuation for travelers

» Coordinating with the employers' other vendors for continuity of care

Healthcare Solutions can be made available to your organization as a specific number of cases during the course of the year with the option to obtain more, or as a yearly retainer. Organizations may opt to make this service available for all of their employees, or to select groups such as high level executives or partners.

For further information on Healthcare Solutions, Corporate Membership, New Movers, and Doctor-Patient Advisor Program, please contact:

William Liss-Levinson, PhD.
VP, Chief Strategy & Operations Officer
212.367.8400, ext. 114
bliss-levinson@castleconnolly.com

Corporate Membership for Corporations & Organizations

This service enables an employer to assist employees in identifying Top Doctors to care for themselves and their families. It is a low-cost, non-intrusive service that will result in better care and, ultimately, lower healthcare costs. For as low as a few dollars per year, employees can have complete access to the Castle Connolly website and database of Top Doctors who were nominated by their peers and screened by the Castle Connolly physician-led research team.

Instead of simply choosing a doctor's name from the phone book or a plan directory, the employee can compare physician names to the Castle Connolly database of 30,000 plus Top Doctors and select from among the best doctors in the country. This will result in overall better care, lower costs and improved morale. Once an employee logs on to the Castle Connolly database, valuable background information is available on every Top Doctor such as: medical school, board certifications, fellowships, hospital affiliations, residencies and much more, to allow them to make the best informed decision they can make when selecting a doctor.

Top Doctors can have an enormous impact. For patients and their families, the value of receiving first-class medical care is great but unquantifiable – it is measured in quality and even length of life. Employers, however, can see the results in their bottom line. Faulty diagnoses and improper treatment take a toll in productivity and ripple out into higher workplace costs. No company should have to "make do" for weeks or months without a key employee or executive, when a Top Doctor may have solved the patient's problem quickly and efficiently. The effort to identify the best doctors from ordinary ones is justified by the money saved on incorrect treatments, unnecessary surgery and days lost from work.

The Corporate Membership is suited for employers of varying sizes and can also be of great value to professional, social, civic, fraternal and religious associations. Castle Connolly may also be able to adapt and tailor the presentation of the database to meet the specific corporate client's needs.

William Liss-Levinson, PhD.
VP, Chief Strategy & Operations Officer
212.367.8400, ext. 114
bliss-levinson@castleconnolly.com

New Movers Program

The Castle Connolly New Movers Program is designed to alleviate that concern, or even fear, as well as the time-consuming struggle to identify the right – and best – doctors and hospitals in one's new community or region. The service can be provided on a family basis (those living in the household) or for a single client. The service includes identifying primary care physicians, including Pediatricians, OB/GYN's, Internists and Family Practitioners as well as other specialists that may be needed: for example, Ophthalmologists, Allergists, Endocrinologists, Surgeons or others as required.

Perhaps nothing is more challenging to a family that has relocated to a new community than finding appropriate healthcare resources, especially physicians. While they can turn to recommendations from new neighbors and friends, or select names from the phone book or a plan directory, that is hardly adequate, especially if there are special healthcare needs in the family.

A Castle Connolly Health Advisor will identify two or three recommendations for up to six different medical specialties. If, for some reason the client wishes to change doctors within two months, Castle Connolly will identify new physicians in the same specialty. After the selection process occurs, the Health Advisor will make an introductory phone call to the physician's office. This typically facilitates faster appointments.

William Liss-Levinson, PhD.
VP, Chief Strategy & Operations Officer
212.367.8400, ext. 114
bliss-levinson@castleconnolly.com

Strategic Relationships

Castle Connolly Medical Ltd. has a number of strategic relationships that may be of interest to consumers and physicians.

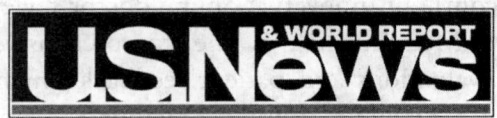

U.S. News & World Report and Castle Connolly created a strategic collaboration that will bring the Castle Connolly Top Doctors® database to online visitors to the U.S. News website. The online database went live on www.usnews.com in July 2011 and links with the U.S. News database of Best Hospitals. Consumers will be able to search the full database of Top Doctors across the nation, including all specialties and subspecialties. The detailed physician profiles, including designation of doctors affiliated with Castle Connolly's Partnership for Excellence hospital program, will be drawn from Castle Connolly's growing database of more than 32,000 physicians currently accessible online at www.castleconnolly.com.

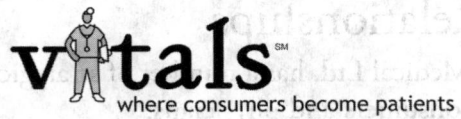

Vitals (www.vitals.com), an innovative online doctor review and comparison service from MDx Medical Inc., is the comprehensive source for vital information, peer evaluations and patient feedback on more than 700,000 doctors nationwide. Drawing upon prestigious information repositories, cutting-edge search and comparison technologies, and a robust patient feedback mechanism, Vitals has organized key information to help patients make an informed choice in their search for the right doctor. Castle Connolly and Vitals have a branding relationship in which those physicians who are Castle Connolly Top Doctors™ and appear on Vitals web sites have an icon indicating their status and recognition as a Castle Connolly Top Doctor.

In 2012, Castle Connolly will begin displaying insurance plans that are accepted by all physicians listed as Castle Connolly Top Doctors. An appointment scheduling feature will also appear on our site for those physicians who wish to participate in this feature. Additional information can be found at www.vitals.com.

Q sharecare

Sharecare is an interactive, social Q&A platform designed to greatly simplify the search for quality healthcare information and help consumers live their healthiest life. Sharecare has enlisted the nation's leading health experts, care providers, organizations, and brands to join the health and wellness conversation and empowering users with high-quality, relevant answers to their health questions from multiple expert perspectives and with interactive health and wellness tools to take action on what they've learned.

The website was launched in 2010 by Jeff Arnold, founder of WebMD, and Emmy—award winning host, Dr. Mehmet Oz, in partnership with Harpo Studios, Sony Pictures Television and Discovery Communications.

Castle Connolly teamed up with Sharecare in 2011. Dr. John Connolly, President and CEO of CCML, is one of the featured experts on Sharecare for healthcare choice questions. Find out more at www.sharecare.com

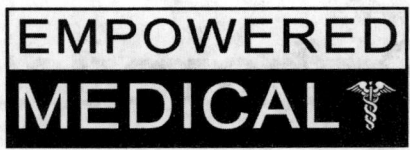

Empowered Doctor is a media, news and marketing service. Empowered Doctor produces syndicated consumer health reports. Its video and text news stories appear on major media websites, including CBS. Empowered Doctor also provides marketing services to hospitals, clinics and individual physicians by generating visibility in online search and social media. Empowered Doctor's clients benefit from the company's efficient methodologies for generating new patient referrals.

For more information call 888-333-1027 or visit www.empowereddoctor.com

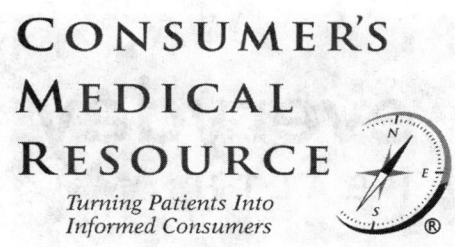

CONSUMER'S MEDICAL RESOURCE

Turning Patients Into Informed Consumers

Consumer's Medical Resource was started in 1996 to offer high-quality, high-impact employee benefit programs to help employees and their dependents, and has been a pioneer in Medical Decision Support® services. CMR addresses all medical conditions at any point within the continuum of care, by providing personalized, evidence-based medical research, information, access to genuine, in-person second opinions and support services to employees who face serious, complicated, and chronic illness, or would like to become well-informed healthcare consumers.

Leveraging a state-of-the-art integrated model of web, phone, and print-based services, CMR enables employees to fully understand and evaluate their options so they can make the most informed medical decisions possible with their doctors. The company is privately held and currently provides services to more than 600,000 Americans, achieving extremely high levels of user and customer satisfaction, improved clinical quality outcomes, and generated excellent ROI.

Castle Connolly and CMR are working together to provide Castle Connolly's various corporate services to CMR client companies and their employees.

For more information, please visit: http://www.consumersmedical.com.

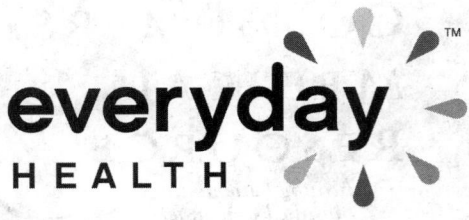

Everyday Health, Inc. comprises some of the nation's leading online health information resources. With over 25 comprehensive health websites including www.EverydayHealth.com, www.Carepages.com, PDRHealth.com and www.WhatToExpect.com, information and knowledge is accessible on a wide range of health topics such as lifestyle offerings in pregnancy, diet and fitness to in-depth medical content for condition prevention and management.

In addition to their commitment to provide consumers with health solutions that span the health spectrum, they also provide a wide range of content and advertising-based services to healthcare entities including hospitals, physicians and other healthcare professionals. Castle Connolly has formed a strategic relationship with Everyday Health to offer one of these services in particular; Reputation Management Solutions.

More than 150 million people search listings and online healthcare directories each month making it imperative for physicians and hospitals to consistently update and manage their information on local directories, reviews sites and social networks. Understandably, this is, at times, an unfeasible commitment. Everyday Health's Reputation Management Solutions provides online visibility information which shows exactly where listings appear on the web, information across hundreds of directory sites, identifying and tips on how to respond to negative reviews and much more.

For more information, please contact our Manager of Client Relations at (212) 367-8400 Ext. 135.

grandparents.com®
it's great to be grand.

Grandparents.com is dedicated to enhancing the lives of America's 70 million grandparents by fostering family connections, via child- and grandparent-friendly activities, travel ideas, compelling lifestyle features, expert advice, gift ideas, recipes, and more. Visitors have access to a range of tools, including groups, discussions, a homepage blog, photo sharing, and a Facebook page and Twitter feeds. Through the Grandparents.com Grand Deals page members can receive discounts and incentives they can use every day, in categories like gifts, clothes, and vitamins, plus exclusive opportunities to save on hotels, cruises, auto rentals, theme park trips, theatrical productions, and insurance. Grandparents can share their membership benefits with four extended family and household members. In 2010, Grandparents.com was ranked as the No. 3 website for seniors, boomers, and grandparents, following the U.S. Government and AARP. Castle Connolly provides access to its Top Doctors' database, its Doctor-Patient Advisor and New Movers programs for Grandparents.com members.

DrScore.com
PATIENTS SPEAK, DOCTORS LISTEN

Founded by Steven Feldman, M.D., DrScore.com is an interactive online survey site where patients can rate their physicians, as well as find a physician based on their service level preference.

The mission of DrScore.com is to improve medical care by giving patients a forum for rating their physician and by giving doctors an affordable, objective, non-intrusive means of documenting the quality of care that they provide. Visitors on Castle Connolly's website who are searching for "top doctors" have the option to also rate these and other physicians they have been to as patients, as well as to see if these physicians have been rated previously by other consumers on DrScore.com. Visitors to DrScore.com will be able to see if their doctors and/or other doctors are Castle Connolly "top doctors."

For more information, visit www.drscore.com.

The Good Works Health government-approved platform - www.goodworkshealth.com - offers physicians the opportunity to direct donations, based on the fair market value of their time, to charities of their choice in exchange for participation in educational programs.

Participating physicians can choose from more than a million approved charities to designate as the recipients of these donations. Good Works Health's unique platform reaches a growing community of medical professionals in many specialties that are motivated by the opportunity to do good works. Castle Connolly actively works with Good Works Health to promote these opportunities to its Castle Connolly Top Doctors®

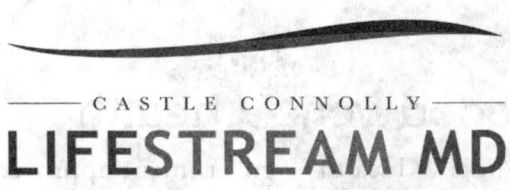

Castle Connolly Medical Ltd. has a strategic relationship with Castle Connolly LifeStream MD to provide a unique health advisory service designed for families and executives, especially those who travel regularly or may have more than one residence.

Each client is assigned a Castle Connolly LifeStream MD physician who is available to them by phone 24/7/365. A client call from anywhere in the world is answered promptly and the client is connected with their Castle Connolly LifeStream MD physician advisor.

The Castle Connolly LifeStream MD physician acts as a health manager assisting in navigation of an increasingly complex health care environment. The Castle Connolly LifeStream MD physician does not replace the member's primary physician or specialists, but provides additional independent counsel and services that provide security to our members either at home or while traveling.

In the United States, the Castle Connolly LifeStream MD physician will use the Castle Connolly database of Top Doctors to assure that the client is cared for in the best medical facilities by the top doctors. Assistance in securing timely appointments with specialists and records transfers is facilitated as needed. Outside of the United States, Castle Connolly LifeStream MD has an affiliation with International SOS, the world's largest and leading provider of travel medical assistance to assure the LifeStream MD member is cared for by the best doctors and hospitals available in that region or, if necessary, is transported to a place where that care is available.

National Physician of the Year Awards

Castle Connolly Medical Ltd. proudly hosted its seventh annual *National Physician of the Year Awards* on March 26, 2012 at The Pierre Hotel in New York City. It was a spectacular evening which allowed us to recognize both the outstanding honorees and the excellence of the many thousands of physicians throughout the nation.

The Genesis of the National Physician of the Year Award.

Each year we receive thousands of nominations from physicians and the medical leadership of major medical centers, specialty hospitals, teaching hospitals and regional and community medical centers across the United States as an integral part of our research, screening and selection process to identify *America's Top Doctors®*. The selected physicians, while spread across all fifty states and involved in more than 70 medical specialties and subspecialties, all share one distinguishing professional attribute: an unwavering dedication to their patients and to medicine as a whole. Each and every one of these outstanding medical professionals is a symbol of the clinical excellence that characterizes American medicine. In honor of these exemplary physicians, Castle Connolly Medical Ltd. has created the *National Physician of the Year Awards* to recognize the thousands of excellent, dedicated physicians across the United States. Our Medical Advisory Board selected the honorees from the hundreds nominated in a special nomination process conducted months before the event.

The honorees, Drs. Richard Edelson, Susan Mackinnon, and John M. Morton, are superb examples of excellence in clinical medical practice. In addition to these awards for Clinical Excellence, Castle Connolly Medical Ltd. honored Drs. Robert L. Brent and John G. Clarkson for their lifetime achievement in medicine. Ms. Marlo Thomas is a tireless fundraiser for St. Jude Children's Research Hospital and an exemplary recipient for the seventh National Health Leadership Award.

Each honoree received a beautiful and distinctive porcelain figurine created by the Boehm Porcelain Company exclusively for the National Physician of the Year Awards. The award features a golden caduceus, the symbol of the medical community, surrounded by a golden laurel wreath. Laurel wreaths were used by the ancients to crown and honor their leaders.

The caduceus and laurel rest upon a column accented by the signature Castle Connolly logo. By combining the caduceus and the laurel wreaths, the award embodies the excellence in medical achievement that the National Physician of the Year Awards celebrates each year.

2012 National Physician of the Year Awards Honorees

"Top Doctors Make a Difference™"

For Clinical Excellence

Richard Edelson, M.D.
Aaron B. and Marguerite Lerner Professor
Chairman of the Department of Dermatology
Yale School of Medicine.

Susan Mackinnon, M.D.
Chief of Plastic and Reconstructive Surgery
Washington University School of Medicine

John M. Morton, M.D., M.P.H., F.A.C.S.
Associate Professor of Surgery
Stanford University
Chief of Minimally Invasive Surgery,
Director of Bariatric Surgery and Surgical Quality

For Lifetime Achievement

Robert L. Brent, M.D., Ph.D., D.Sc.
Distinguished Professor of Pediatrics, Radiology and Pathology
Louis and Bess Stein Professor of Pediatrics at the Jefferson Medical College
and the Nemours/Alfred I. DuPont Hospital for Children

John G. Clarkson, M.D.
Dean Emeritus and Professor of Ophthalmology
Anne Bates Leach Eye Hospital/Bascom Palmer Eye Institute
Department of Ophthalmology
Miller School of Medicine at the University of Miami

National Health Leadership

Marlo Thomas
National Outreach Director
St. Jude Children's Research Hospital

2011 National Physician of the Year Awards Honorees

"Doctors Make a Difference"

For Clinical Excellence

Armando E. Giuliano, M.D., FACS, FRCSED
Chief of Science and Medicine
John Wayne Cancer Institute at Saint John's Health Center,
Santa Monica, CA

O. Wayne Isom, M.D.
Chairman of the Dept. of Cardiothoracic Surgery
New York Presbyterian-Weill Cornell Medical College

David W. Kennedy, M.D.
Otorhinolaryngology Professor at the
University of Pennsylvania

For Lifetime Achievement

George P. Canellos, M.D.
Served as Founding Chief of Medical Oncology at
Dana-Farber Cancer Institute;

Matthew D. Davis, M.D.
University of Wisconsin Medical Center
Chair, UW Opthalmology

National Health Leadership

Evelyn H. Lauder
Chairman of The Breast Cancer Research Foundation®

Previous National Physician of the Year Award Honorees

2010

Clinical Excellence
John B. Buse, M.D., Ph.D.
Director of the Diabetes Care Center, Professor, Chief of the Division of
Endocrinology and Executive Associate Dean for Clinical Research,
University of North Carolina School of Medicine, Chapel Hill

Larry Norton, M.D.
Deputy Physician-in-Chief, Memorial Hospital, Memorial Sloan-Kettering
Cancer Center, for Breast Cancer Programs
Medical Director of the MSKCC's Breast and Imaging Center, Evelyn H.
Lauder Breast Center

Ching-Hon Pui, M.D.
Department Chair of Oncology, St. Jude Children's Research Hospital
Medical Director of the St. Jude International Outreach China Program,
holder of the Fahad Nassar Al-Rashid Chair of Leukemia Research

Lifetime Achievement
Basil I Hirschowitz, M.D.
Director, Gastroenterology Division, The University of Alabama
Receipient of the Kettering Medal from the General Motors Cancer
Foundation; Friedenwald Medal of the AGA; the Schindler Medal and the
Crystal Award for lifetime contributions to Endoscopy by the ASGE;
honorary doctorate of Gothenburg University; honorary fellow of the Royal
Society of Medicine

Leonard Apt, M.D.
Professor of Ophthalmology Emeritus; Director Emeritus and Founder of
the Division of Pediatric Opthalmology and Strabismus, and Co-Director of
UCLA's Center for Child Blindness

National Health Leadership
Alexandra Reeve Givens and Matthew Reeve
Trustees, The Christopher & Dana Reeve Foundation

2009

Clinical Excellence
Carol R. Bradford, M.D.,
Professor and Chair
Department of Otolaryngology
University of Michigan Medical System

Diane E. Meier, M.D.,
Director, Center to Advance Palliative Care
Mount Sinai School of Medicine

Judd W. Moul, M.D.,
Chief of Urology
Duke University Medical Center

Lifetime Achievement
Emil J. Freireich, M.D., D. Sc. (Hon.),
Ruth Harriet Ainsworth Chair, Distinguished Teaching Professor
Director, Special Medical Education Programs
Director, Adult Leukemia Research Program
The University of Texas M.D. Anderson Cancer Center

Thomas E. Starzl, M.D., Ph.D.
Professor of Surgery, Emeritus
Distinguished Service Professor
University of Pittsburgh Medical Center

National Health Leadership
Page Morton Black
Chairman of the Board, Parkinson's Disease Foundation

****

2008

Clinical Excellence
Robert W. Carlson, M.D.
Medical Oncology
Stanford University Medical Center

Stanley Chang, M.D.
Ophthalmology
New York-Presbyterian Hospital

L. Dade Lunsford, M.D.
Neurological Surgery
University of Pittsburgh Medical Center

Lifetime Achievement
Jacqueline A. Noonan, M.D.
Pediatric Cardiology
University of Kentucky Medical Center

Robert W. Schrier, M.D.
Nephrology
University of Colorado Health Sciences Center

National Health Leadership
Suzanne and Robert Wright
Vice-Chair of the Board, General Electric Company
Co-founders of Autism Speaks™

****

2007

Clinical Excellence
Delos M. Cosgrove, M.D.
Chairman, Board of Governors
CEO and President
The Cleveland Clinic

Joseph G. McCarthy, M.D.
Lawrence D. Bell Professor of Plastic Surgery
Director, The Institute of Reconstructive Plastic Surgery
NYU Medical Center

Patrick C. Walsh, M.D.
University Distinguished Service Professor and Director of Urology
The James Buchanan Brady Urological Institute
The Johns Hopkins Hospital

Lifetime Achievement
Maria Delivoria-Papadopoulos, M.D.
Director, The Neonatal Intensive Care Unit
St. Christopher's Hospital for Children;
Professor of Pediatrics, Physiology and Obstetrics/Gynecology
Drexel University College of Medicine

National Health Leadership
The Honorable Nancy G. Brinker
Founder of Susan G. Komen for the Cure
Former U.S. Ambassador to Hungary

****

2006

Clinical Excellence
Bart Barlogie, M.D., Ph.D.
Director, Myeloma Institute for Research Therapy
University of Arkansas for Medical Services

Marilyn J. Bull, M.D.
Morris Green Professor of Pediatrics
Riley Hospital for Children

Michael J. Zinner, M.D.
Moseley Professor of Surgery
Harvard Medical School
Surgeon-in-Chief, Brigham & Women's Hospital

Lifetime Achievement
Michael E. DeBakey, M.D.
Chancellor Emeritus, Baylor College of Medicine

National Health Leadership
Princess Yasmin Aga Khan
Honorary Vice Chair
Alzheimer's Association

Castle Connolly and Social Media

Castle Connolly maintains Facebook, Twitter, LinkedIn and Sharecare accounts in an effort to keep consumers informed of the latest news not only regarding Castle Connolly Medical Ltd., its Top Doctors and Top Hospitals, but also reports on various health observances and events. A live Twitter feed can also be found on the homepage of www.castleconnolly.com.

Consumers who use our print guides, online database or refer to our regional magazine features can find up-to-date information about Castle Connolly, healthcare and medical news by logging onto these social networking sites:

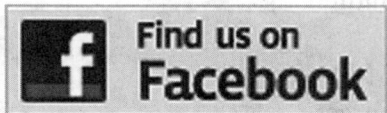

www.facebook.com/TopDoctors

Blog - Ask America's Top Doctors™
www.castleconnolly.com/blog

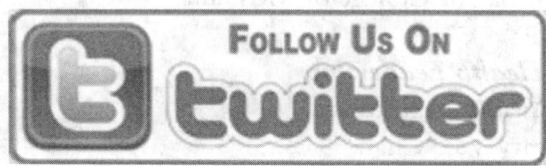

www.twitter.com/CastleConnolly

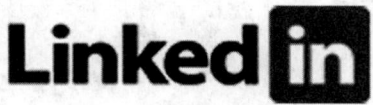

http://linkd.in/mP4Lmb (case sensitive)

Do you have a story about a Castle Connolly Top Doctor or Top Hospital that you want to share? If so, please email a link to the article to:

Nicki Hughes
Director of Client Relations & Research Operations
nhughes@castleconnolly.com

Castle Connolly has developed a website and online database – www.AmericasTopCosmeticDoctors.com – to enable consumers to search and identify top cosmetic specialists who have been nominated by their peers through an extensive selection process involving tens of thousands of American physicians. Nominated physicians' medical education, training, hospital appointments, disciplinary histories - and much more - are screened and reviewed by our physician-led research team. Those selected as top doctors may appear in a number of Castle Connolly guides/online databases, including www.AmericasTopCosmeticDoctors.com.

These doctors are specially trained in cosmetic procedures and spend the majority of their time in their medical practice doing cosmetic work. The Top Cosmetic Doctors whose profiles are included on this site are in one of only six medical specialties: Dermatology, Facial Plastic Surgery, Ophthalmology, Otolaryngology, Plastic Surgery or Surgery. The website also includes valuable information on how to select the right cosmetic doctor for you, as well as detailed information about some of the most common procedures.

For more information visit: www.AmericasTopCosmeticDoctors.com

Doctor-Patient Advisor for Individual Consumers

Doctor-Patient Advisor is a Castle Connolly Medical Ltd. service providing one-on-one consultations with a physician or nurse practitioner to individuals who have serious or complex medical problems or to anyone who feels he/she needs assistance finding the right physician for any purpose. Each client will receive personalized assistance in identifying the appropriate specialists for his/her condition, utilizing the Castle Connolly Medical Ltd. database of physicians and hospitals, as well as individual searches, to locate the best resources to meet the client's needs.

Fee: $375. For further information call (212) 367-8400 x 116.

Premium Membership to www.CastleConnolly.com

Reap the benefits of membership with Castle Connolly. Gain access to ALL online top doctor listings and get discounts on book purchases from our extensive catalog.

• Search among more than 30,000 Castle Connolly Top Doctor listings
• Search among select hospitals and centers of excellence
• Receive a 30% discount on all book purchases

Membership Levels:
• One year - $24.95
• Two years - $34.95

For more information visit: www.CastleConnolly.com/membership

Other Products From Castle Connolly

Castle Connolly Guides

Titles Include:

- *America's Top Doctors®*
- *America's Top Doctors® for Cancer*

And Many More

To order other Castle Connolly guides at a 15% discount please visit
http://www.CastleConnolly.com/books
When ordering use discount code: **NY16DOM**

Castle Connolly's Top Doctors Available Online

- Free Access to 20 -25% of Castle Connolly's Top Doctors
- Purchase Access to the entire database of more than 34,000 doctor profiles

http://www.castleconnolly.com/membership

Customer Feedback

We appreciate your comments regarding our guides. Please email us at
info@castleconnolly.com

Tepler

Swistel
Vapnek
Rosch
Milsom
Tahey

The Best in American Medicine
www.CastleConnolly.com